Resources for Instructor Success—

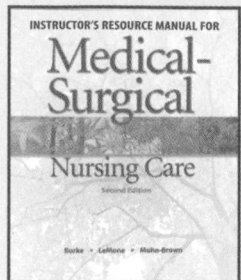

Instructor's Resource Manual
ISBN 0-13-188463-8
This manual contains a wealth of material to help faculty plan and manage their LPN/LVN nursing courses. It includes detailed learning outcomes, lecture outlines, teaching suggestions for the classroom and clinical settings, and more for each chapter. It also guides faculty how to assign and use the text-specific Companion Website, www.prenhall.com/burke and the Student CD-ROM that accompany the textbook. This supplement is available to faculty free upon adoption of the textbook.

Instructor's Resource CD-ROM
ISBN: 0-13-226999-6
This comprehensive resource CD-ROM provides Lecture Notes, Animations, and Illustrations integrated in PowerPoint presentations for use in the classroom. It also contains an electronic test bank and additional resources. The supplement is available to faculty free upon adoption of the textbook.

Companion Website Syllabus Manager
www.prenhall.com/burke
Faculty adopting this textbook have free access to the online Syllabus Manager feature of the Companion Website, www.prenhall.com/burke. Syllabus Manager offers a whole host of features that facilitate the students' use of the Companion Website, and allows faculty to post syllabi and course information online for their students. For more information or a demonstration of Syllabus Manager, please contact a Prentice Hall Sales Representative.

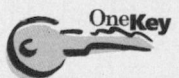 ## Online Course Management
OneKey is an integrated online resource that brings a wide array of supplemental resources together in one convenient place for both students and faculty. OneKey features everything you and your students need for out-of-class work, conveniently organized to match your syllabus. OneKey is an online course management solution that features interactive modules, text and image PowerPoints, animations, videos, case studies, and more. OneKey also provides course management tools so faculty can customize course content, build online tests, create assignments, enter grades, post announcements, communicate with students, and much more. Testing materials, gradebooks, and other instructor resources are available in a separate section that can be accessed by instructors only. OneKey content is available in three different platforms. A nationally hosted version is available in the reliable, easy-to-use CourseCompass platform. The same content is also available for download to locally hosted versions of BlackBoard and WebCT. Please contact your Prentice Hall Sales Representative for a demonstration or go online to **http://myphlip.pearsoncmg.com/OneKey/index.html.**

OneKey is all you need.
Convenience. Simplicity. Success.

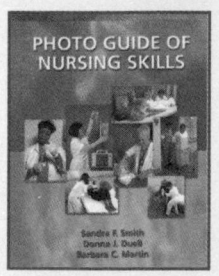

Photo Guide of Nursing Skills
Provides a full-color atlas of all basic and intermediate skills and its unique, easy-to-use format presents each procedure in logical steps—complete with appropriate illustrations, descriptions, and rationales. A critical thinking section focuses on unexpected outcomes.
ISBN: 0-8385-8174-9
Smith, Duell & Martin

ticin
skill
each

Basic
Inter
Phys
Mate
ISBN
Pedi

Critical Care Nursing Skills ISBN: 0-13-119264-7

Brief Table of Contents

Medical-Surgical

Nursing Care

Second Edition

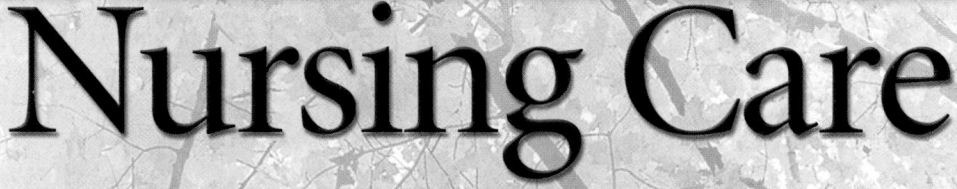

Karen M. Burke, RN, MS
Educational Consultant
Oregon State Board of Nursing
Portland, Oregon

Priscilla LeMone, RN, DSN, FAAN
Associate Professor Emerita
Sinclair School of Nursing
University of Missouri-Columbia
Columbia, Missouri

Elaine L. Mohn-Brown, RN, EdD
Faculty, ADN Nursing Program
Chemeketa Community College
Salem, Oregon

With new mental health unit by:
Linda Eby, RN, MN
Instructor of Nursing
Portland Community College
Portland, Oregon

PEARSON

Prentice
Hall

Upper Saddle River, New Jersey 07458

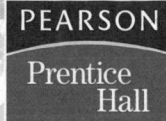

Library of Congress Cataloging-in-Publication Data

Burke, Karen M.
  Medical-surgical nursing care/Karen M. Burke, Priscilla LeMone,
Elaine L. Mohn-Brown; with new mental health unit by Linda Eby.
—2nd ed.
    p. ; cm.
  Includes bibliographical references and index.
  ISBN 0-13-171472-4
  1. Surgical nursing.   2. Nursing.   I. LeMone, Priscilla.   II. Mohn-Brown,
Elaine.   III. Title.
  [DNLM: 1. Nursing Care   methods.   2. Nursing Process
WY 150 B959m 2006]
RT41.B89 2006
617'.0231—dc22
                                                    2006010702

Publisher: Julie Levin Alexander
Publisher's Assistant: Regina Bruno
Editor-in-Chief: Maura Connor
Senior Acquisitions Editor: Kelly Trakalo
Senior Managing Editor: Marilyn Meserve
Associate Editor: Michael Giacobbe
Development Editor: Patricia Gillivan
Editorial Assistant: Emily Adler
Director of Marketing: Karen Allman
Senior Marketing Manager: Francisco Del Castillo
Marketing Coordinator: Michael Sirinides
Marketing Assistant: Patricia Linard
Director of Production and Manufacturing: Bruce Johnson
Managing Production Editor: Patrick Walsh
Production Liaison: Julie Li
Production Editor: Penny Walker, Techbooks
Media Product Manager: John Jordan
Manager of Media Production: Amy Peltier
New Media Project Manager: Tina Rudowski
Manufacturing Manager: Ilene Sanford
Manufacturing Buyer: Pat Brown
Senior Design Coordinator: Mary Siener
Interior Designer: Eva Ruutopold
Cover Designer: Mary Siener
Cover Images: (background) Perry Mastrovito/Jupiter Images (band) Getty
Images; Steve Satushek/Getty Images; Peter Haigh/Getty Images;
Morey Milbradt/Getty Images
Author Photographs: Karen Burke: Lamping Photography; Priscilla
LeMone: MU Sinclair School of Nursing; Elaine Mohn-Brown: Yeung &
Leix LLC.
Composition: Techbooks
Printing and Binding: Quebecor World
Cover Printer: Phoenix Color

Notice: Care has been taken to confirm the accuracy of information presented in this book. The authors, editors, and the publisher, however, cannot accept any responsibility for errors or omissions or for consequences from application of the information in this book and make no warranty, express or implied, with respect to its contents.

The authors and publisher have exerted every effort to ensure that drug selections and dosages set forth in this text are in accord with current recommendations and practice at time of publication. However, in view of ongoing research, changes in government regulations, and the constant flow of information relating to drug therapy and drug reactions, the reader is urged to check the package inserts of all drugs for any change in indications of dosage and for added warnings and precautions. This is particularly important when the recommended agent is a new and/or infrequently employed drug.

Pearson Education LTD.
Pearson Education Australia PTY, Limited
Pearson Education Singapore, Pte. Ltd
Pearson Education North Asia Ltd
Pearson Education Canada, Ltd.
Pearson Educación de Mexico, S.A. de C.V.
Pearson Education—Japan
Pearson Education Malaysia, Pte. Ltd
Pearson Education, Upper Saddle River

PEARSON
Prentice Hall

10 9 8 7 6 5 4 3 2 1
ISBN 0-13-171472-4

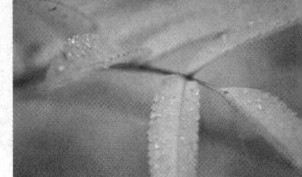

Student Success is built-in from the start...

Practical and vocational nurses from around the country told us that they needed two things to succeed as students in order to achieve their LPN/LVN licenses. First, they needed books that explain what the LPN/LVN needs to know and do. Second, they needed a variety of excellent review materials to reinforce their learning. ***Medical Surgical Nursing Care, 2e*** contains power-packed, built-in support to ensure your success throughout your LPN/LVN education.

As you start each chapter—

Brief Outlines preview what the chapter will cover for quick access and review.

Learning Outcomes identify what you can expect to learn from each chapter and help you focus your reading.

MediaLinks call your attention to the additional learning tools that are available on the CD-ROM and Companion Website that accompany your textbook, including:

Student CD-ROM
- Learning Outcomes
- Audio Glossary—key terms, definitions, and pronunciations
- NCLEX-PN® Review Questions— unique to this CD-ROM
- Animations & Videos—difficult concepts brought to life
- Procedure Checklists—for clinical reference
- Vocabulary Games

Companion Website
- Learning Outcomes
- Audio Glossary
- NCLEX-PN® Review Questions— unique to this website
- Case Studies—scenarios and questions
- Challenge Your Knowledge—visual critical thinking questions
- Matching Questions
- WebLinks—content-related hyperlinks
- ToolBox—handy reference materials
- Procedure Checklists

Chapter 22

The Respiratory System and Assessment

BRIEF Outline

Structure and Function of the Upper Respiratory System
The Nose and Sinuses
The Pharynx
The Larynx

Structure and Function of the Lower Respiratory System
The Lungs
Bronchi and Alveoli
Pulmonary Circulation
The Pleura
Rib Cage and Intercostal Muscles
Mechanics of Respiration
Factors Affecting Respiration

Respiratory Changes Associated with Aging

Assessment
Subjective Data
Physical Examination
Diagnostic Tests

LEARNING Outcomes

On completion of this chapter, you will be able to:
- Describe the structure and functions of the respiratory tract.
- Explain the mechanics of respiration.
- Describe assessment and data collection for respiratory function.
- Provide appropriate nursing care and teaching for clients undergoing diagnostic tests and procedures related to the respiratory system.

MediaLink

www.prenhall.com/burke
Use the address above to access the free, inter- active Companion Website created for this text- book. Get hints, instant feedback, and textbook references to chapter-related NCLEX-style questions. Link to other interesting sites.

Audio Glossary:
Use the Companion Website, or the CD-ROM disk enclosed with your textbook, to hear the pronunciation of key terms in this chapter.

Schiz...

Schizoph phrenia Affected ization; a to self an

Appro have sch proxima men, peo socioeco the late cence is set of sch

Video:Schizophrenia

MediaLink

MediaLink Tabs prompt you to explore videos, animations, and activities on the CD-ROM and Companion Website.

Makes need-to-know information easy to find and use...

Medical Surgical Nursing Care contains a large variety of color-coded boxes and tables providing important information for you to remember.

BOX 26-7   POPULATION FOCUS

Heart Disease in Women and Older Adults

Heart disease—myocardial infarction in particular—is the leading cause of death for women and older adults. In fact, more women than men die of heart disease every year. Women with symptoms of an acute myocardial infarction are likely to delay seeking treatment for several hours—an average of an hour longer than men. After an MI, the death rate for women is three times that of men, both in the hospital and within the first year.

Women and older adults are more likely than men to have a "silent" or unrecognized heart attack. Many women having an AMI experience epigastric pain and nausea, causing them to believe their pain is due to heartburn. Chest pain in women often occurs during mental stress or while resting. Shortness of breath is common, as is fatigue and weakness of the shoulders and upper arms.

Older people may seek treatment for vague complaints of difficulty breathing, confusion, fainting, dizziness, abdominal pain, or cough. Many older adults who experience AMI do not complain of chest pain. When these clients seek care with vague symptoms and a history of cardiovascular problems, an AMI should be suspected.

When teaching women and older adults about heart disease, emphasize the importance of seeking immediate medical care for manifestations of AMI. With prompt treatment, survival in both groups is improved.

Client Teaching, Population Focus and additional boxes help you prepare for your role as educators in health care settings.

BOX 32-3   CLIENT TEACHING

Pelvic Floor (Kegel) Exercises

■ Identify the pelvic muscles by:
   a. Attempting to stop the flow of urine during voiding and holding for a few seconds.
   b. Tightening the muscles of the vagina around a gloved finger or tampon.
   c. Tightening the muscles around the anus as though trying to avoid passing flatus.
■ Perform exercises: Tighten pelvic muscles, hold for 10 seconds, and relax for 10 to 15 seconds. Continue the sequence (tighten, hold, relax) for 10 repetitions.
■ Keep abdominal muscles and breathing relaxed while performing exercises.
■ Initially, exercises should be performed twice per day, working up to four times a day.
■ Exercise at a specific time each day or in conjunction with another daily activity (such as bathing or watching the news). Establish a routine, because these exercises should be continued for life.

BOX 26-5   ASSESSMENT

Assessing Clients with Angina Pectoris

SUBJECTIVE DATA

■ Pain: location, character (heavy, burning, tight, squeezing), intensity, radiation; timing (relationship to activity, meals, or other factors), duration; aggravating and relieving factors; associated manifestations
■ History of angina or other heart disease, previous or current treatment measures
■ Risk factors: family history of CHD; history of hypertension, diabetes, high blood cholesterol levels; smoking and alcohol intake, use of other recreational drugs; perceived stress levels and techniques used to manage stress; for women, age of menopause, use of hormone replacement therapy or oral contraceptives

OBJECTIVE DATA

■ Frequency and duration of angina; effectiveness of relief measures (oxygen, NTG, rest)
■ Vital signs and ECG tracing during anginal episode
■ Laboratory data: cardiac enzyme levels, serum cholesterol and glucose; hemoglobin and hematocrit (particularly following PCR or surgery).

Assessment boxes summarize data collected during assessment, common risk factors, and manifestations you might observe.

BOX 26-3   NURSING CARE CHECKLIST

Coronary Angiography and Percutaneous Transluminal Coronary Angioplasty

Before the Procedure

☑ Assess knowledge and understanding of the procedure. Reinforce teaching and provide additional information as needed.
☑ Provide routine preoperative care as ordered (see Chapter 9). ⚭
☑ Administer ordered cardiac medications with a small sip of water prior to the procedure unless contraindicated.
☑ Document and report any allergies to iodine, radiographic dyes, or seafood.
☑ Record height, weight, and vital signs. Record equality and amplitude of peripheral pulses; mark their locations.
☑ Explain that client will remain awake during the procedure, which lasts 1 to 2 hours. Sedation may be given, and a local anesthetic will be used where the catheter is inserted. A sensation of warmth (a "hot flash") and a metallic taste may be experienced as the dye is injected. A rapid pulse or a few "skipped beats" also are common during the procedure.

After the Procedure

☑ Provide routine postoperative care (see Chapter 9). ⚭
☑ Monitor vital signs, distal pulses, color, movement, sensation, temperature, and capillary refill of affected extremity as ordered, usually every 15 minutes for the first hour, every 30 minutes the next hour, hourly for 8 hours, and then every 4 hours.
☑ Monitor cardiac rhythm continuously. Report dysrhythmias, ECG changes, or chest pain to the charge nurse or physician.
☑ Maintain bed rest with the affected extremity extended and the head of the bed elevated no more than 30 degrees.
☑ Keep a pressure dressing in place over arterial access sites. Place a 5-lb. sandbag over the access site for 6 hours or as ordered. Check frequently for bleeding (if the access site is in the groin, check for bleeding under the buttocks).
☑ Unless contraindicated, encourage liberal fluid consumption.
☑ Administer medications as ordered.
☑ Monitor intake, output, and laboratory values. Report abnormal values to the physician.

Nursing Care Checklists provide handy summaries of important nursing interventions.

---

clinical ALERT

The cough reflex does not work if the person is unconscious.

Clinical Alerts call your attention to clinical roles and responsibilities for heightened awareness, monitoring, and/or reporting.

Learn to prioritize nursing actions and deliver safe, effective nursing care...

Nursing Care is presented in the five-step nursing process format, emphasizing the scope of practice for the LPN/LVN.

NURSING CARE

The priority for nursing care for the client with hemophilia is protection from injury and minimizing the risk for bleeding. Assessment of the client is similar to that for a client with leukemia.

Risk for Injury

- Monitor for signs of bleeding, including hematomas, ecchymoses, purpura, and obvious oozing or bleeding. *Careful assessment is necessary to identify hidden or occult bleeding.*
- Notify the charge nurse or physician at the first sign of bleeding. *Prompt intervention decreases the risk of hemorrhage.*
- If bleeding occurs, apply gentle pressure until bleeding ~~stops; apply ice or apply a~~ topical agent to stop bleed~~ing~~ ~~es reduce bleeding until definitive~~

NURSING PROCESS CARE PLAN
Client with Bladder Cancer

Ben Hussain is a 61-year-old man who became alarmed when his urine became bright red. Even though he had no other symptoms, he called his doctor. Urinalysis and cytology showed gross hematuria and abnormal cells. A cystoscopy and biopsy confirmed an invasive bladder tumor. He is admitted to the hospital for a radical cystectomy and ileal diversion.

Assessment. Mr. Hussain's admission history indicates that he has lost 10 to 15 pounds during the last few months. He has smoked two to three packs of cigarettes per day for 40 years, but he cut back to a pack a day about a year ago. Mr. Hussain says he is "a little nervous about surgery and what they're going to find." Ms. Mills, the admitting nurse, notes that he fidgets and talks rapidly throughout their interview. He is concerned about how he will handle the pain after surgery, because he has never been hospitalized before his cystoscopy. Physical assessment findings include BP 154/86; P 84; R 18; T 98.2°F (36.7°C) PO. He has scattered crackles throughout his lung fields. Mr. Hussain's urine is clear and bright pink. The remainder of his assessment is essentially normal.

Nursing Process Care Plans illustrate nursing care in a "real-life" scenario.

Documenting. Documentation includes the location, appearance, and size of lesions as well as the presence of nits. Record measures to protect the skin and client teaching including medications and ways to prevent transmission of infection or infestation.

Documenting gives you focus on what to include in your documentation as part of the nursing care process

---

Critical Thinking in the Nursing Process

1. How does cigarette smoking contribute to the increased risk of urinary tract tumors?
2. The first time Mr. Hussain changes his urostomy appliance, he experiences a leak. What hints can you give Mr. Hussain to prevent leaks from occurring?
3. How would you respond if Mr. Hussain said "I'm not only giving up on cigarettes, I'm also giving up on sex from here on"?

Critical Thinking questions allow you to apply your new knowledge to a specific client.

Priorities in Nursing Care. In the acute phase of psychosis, treatment should focus on the client's basic needs. Safety, nutrition, and rest are the priorities. Acute symptom management is also important.

Priority nursing diagnoses that often apply to clients with schizophrenia include Risk for Violence, Self-Directed or Other-Directed, Disturbed Thought Processes, Ineffective Coping, Impaired Social Interaction.

Priorities in Nursing Care focus your thinking on key assessments and interventions.

CONTINUING CARE

Planning and teaching for home care are important nursing responsibilities when caring for the client with a skin infection or infestation. Specific teaching for each type of illness follows.

Continuing Care focuses on your role preparing clients and families to achieve or maintain health after discharge.

BOX 22-2   PROCEDURE CHECKLIST

Obtaining a Throat Swab

- ☑ Obtain a sterile cotton swab or throat swab kit.
- ☑ Identify the client, explain the procedure, and provide for privacy.
- ☑ Place the client in a sitting position if possible.
- ☑ Use Standard Precautions.
- ☑ Ask the client to open the mouth, extend the tongue, and say "ah."
- ☑ Quickly swab the tonsils, reddened areas of the oropharynx, and any exudate.
- ☑ Insert the swab into the specimen container. Avoid contaminating the outside of the container or the swab.
- ☑ Label the container.
- ☑ Send the specimen and requisition to the laboratory.

SAMPLE DOCUMENTATION

10/27/06 Oropharynx red, patches of white exudate noted on tonsils and oropharynx. Throat swab (oropharynx, tonsils, and exudate) obtained and sent to lab for culture.
_____ J. Doene, LPN.

Note: Refer to a nursing fundamentals or skills text for more detailed instruction. Check state guidelines and facility policy before performing any procedure.

Procedure Checklists give you step-by-step instructions and rationales for nursing actions. Special icons in the procedures reinforce essential preliminary steps in client care. "Live" **documentation** at the end of each procedure demonstrates samples of good record-keeping.

Comprehensive reviews at the end of the chapter...

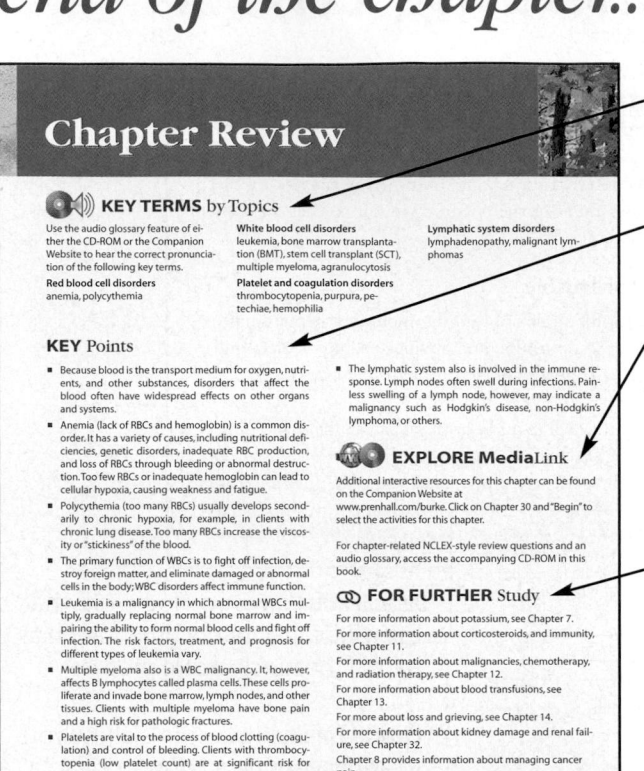

Chapter Review

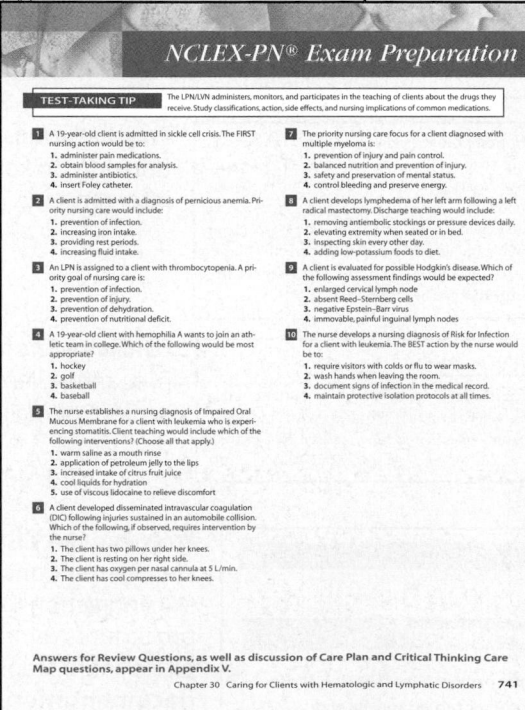

NCLEX-PN® Exam Preparation

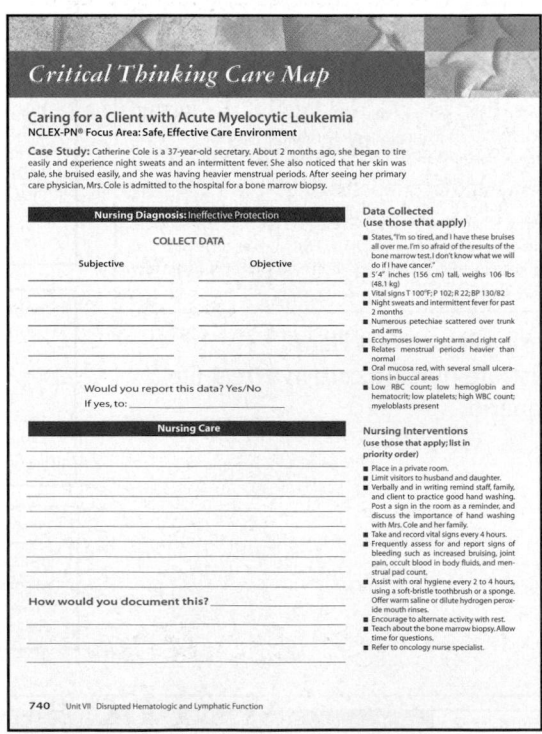

Critical Thinking Care Map

Key Terms by Topic link important new vocabulary to its content area in the chapter.

Key Points summarize need-to-know concepts from the chapter.

EXPLORE MediaLink encourages you to use the Student CD-ROM and Companion Website for a multi-modal review, regardless of your learning style.

For Further Study shows where related content areas are cross-referenced throughout the book.

NCLEX-PN® Exam Preparation includes:

- A Test-taking Tip with a focused study hint
- Bonus NCLEX-PN® style questions to review and practice taking tests with traditional and alternative question formats. Answers are found in Appendix V.

Critical Thinking Care Maps prepare you for success on NCLEX-PN®, in clinical, and on-the-job with a comprehensive review, including:

- NCLEX-PN® Focus Area
- Case Study
- Nursing Diagnosis
- Data Collection
- Reporting
- Nursing Care
- Documentation

Prepare for your career as an LPN/LVN...

After each unit in this book, use the **Thinking Strategically About** pages as an opportunity to reflect on the topics you have just read in the context of important themes across the LPN/LVN curriculum. Short scenarios and project ideas call for critical thinking about the unit's content from a variety of angles and enables you to progress through your education from a more integrated perspective.

Critical Thinking questions highlight specific challenges you will face as a new nurse and strive to provide the best possible care.

Coordination of Interdisciplinary Care challenges you to think about different health care settings and to envision the many health care workers who may participate in a client's care.

Management of Care questions highlight specific nursing interventions to take in different situations and the implications of care.

Communication and **Client Teaching** focus on communication and educational strategies to take with the patient and the family.

Time Management and **Priorities in Nursing Care** help you prioritize assessment and care.

Documenting and Reporting helps you practice what and how to document and report your findings.

Cultural Care Strategies build your confidence by providing information and scenarios to familiarize you with cultural patterns and differences.

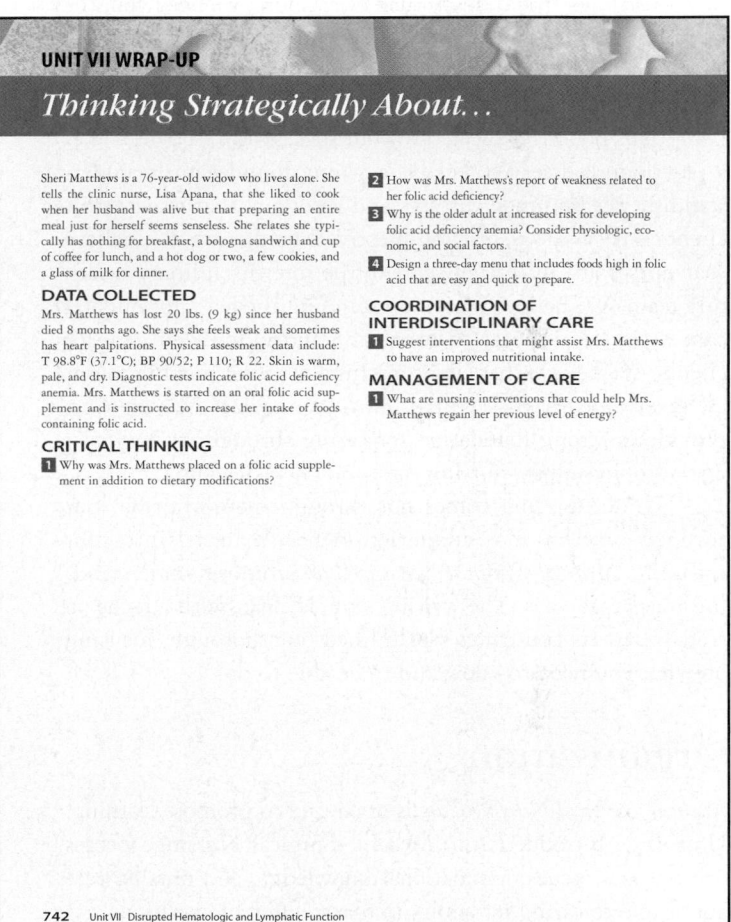

Medical-Surgical Nursing Care will be a key resource as you progress through your nursing courses and become a nurse.

The nature of nursing—grow with it!

Preface

The need for nurses is greater than ever before. There are no short-term solutions to this problem: as currently practicing nurses age and retire, so does the population as a whole, further increasing the need for health care services. Today, more than ever before, we need you, the nursing student, to succeed in your studies. Today, more than ever before, we need you, the nursing student, to enter the nursing profession. Today, more than ever before, we need you, the nursing student, to see nursing as a career, not just a job.

This book is dedicated to your success as a student and as a practicing nurse. We believe a strong foundation in understanding the common diseases and disorders that affect adult clients is necessary to provide effective nursing care. We believe that nurses are an integral part of the interdisciplinary health care team. We believe that understanding the basis for nursing care activities is vital to providing individualized care for clients. We believe that client teaching is a vital nursing role at all levels and in all settings. *Medical–Surgical Nursing Care* provides a strong foundation for caring through its emphasis on pathophysiology, nursing care, and client teaching.

Understanding comes not through memorization, but through practice and integration of new material into your thinking. *Medical–Surgical Nursing Care* promotes understanding in several ways. The writing style is clear, with a focus on readability. Its content is streamlined but thorough, focusing on what you need to know and to be able to do.

Organization

Medical–Surgical Nursing Care is organized to promote learning. Unit One, Introduction to Medical–Surgical Nursing, focuses on concepts, issues, foundational knowledge, and nursing care applicable to caring for adults in many different situations and settings. Unit I includes two chapters new to this edition: The Older Adult in Health and Illness and Essential Nursing Pharmacology. Unit II focuses on conditions that affect many people with a variety of underlying disorders. Units III through XII focus on diseases and disorders affecting adults. These disorders are organized by affected body systems (for example, common skin problems, gastrointestinal disorders, cardiac disorders). This edition includes an entirely new section (Unit XIII) that focuses on adult clients with mental health problems.

Each body system focus unit begins with a chapter that reviews the structure and function of the system, nursing assessment of that system, and commonly ordered diagnostic tests specifically related to that system with their nursing implications. Examples of nursing assessment documentation are included. These chapters provide a foundation for studying and learning about the disorders presented in subsequent chapters of the unit.

Each chapter begins with a **Brief Outline** of major topics included in that chapter. **Learning Outcomes** help focus and define your learning as you read and study the material.

Disorders affecting the body system are presented in a consistent format: the disorder is defined; its **pathophysiology**, signs and symptoms, and complications are explained; and **Interdisciplinary Care** (including diagnostic tests, medications, surgery, and other treatments) for the disorder is outlined. **Nursing Care** related to the disorder is presented in a nursing process format. When a disorder is major, very complex, or very common, major steps of the **Nursing Process** are provided. When it is not, the text provides an abbreviated, more focused discussion, similar to the focused assessment nurses perform. Because teaching and continuing care is a vital nursing consideration, discussion of each disorder concludes with **Continuing Care** and teaching for the client and family.

Nursing Process Care Plans following many major disorders bring the disorders to life. Clients rarely arrive in a health care setting as a pure medical diagnosis. As humans, clients bring all their roles and responsibilities as individuals, spouses, parents, children, workers, students, friends, and volunteers. They arrive as unique individuals influenced by their ethnicity, culture, and background. They arrive with psychosocial issues such as fear, guilt, or difficulty meeting financial responsibilities. They often arrive with other diseases and disorders complicating the current problem. The care plans in this text emphasize the holistic aspects of nursing care.

Critical Thinking Questions conclude each care plan. These questions allow you to practice your newfound learning and to expand your thinking beyond the immediate focus of the disease or disorder presented. Additional **Critical Thinking Self-Check Questions** are provided on the CD-ROM throughout nursing care chapters. They provide more case scenarios for you to use to test your knowledge and thinking skills. These self-check questions focus on the nursing roles of collecting assessment data and implementing nursing care. Each case is matched with hints to guide your critical thinking. They will help you learn to individualize your nursing care.

Each chapter concludes with features to reinforce and enhance your learning. **Key Terms by Topics** list the bold-faced key terms in the text by the topic under which they were defined. **Key Points** provide a summary of chapter content with reminders that you can use throughout your nursing career. **For Further Study** is a handy listing of cross-references within the chapter and the topics to which they apply. An interactive **Critical Thinking Care Map** at the conclusion of each disorders chapter provides a brief case study, assessment data, and a nursing diagnosis for a specific client. We then ask you, the student, to sort and prioritize the data and sample interventions, evaluate the results, and chart your findings.

Finally, **NCLEX-PN® Review Questions** and a **Test-Taking Tip** help you review the chapter material and practice your test-taking skills.

Finally, each unit concludes with a **Unit Wrap-Up** that encourages you to apply and integrate the knowledge you have gained.

Features

Throughout each chapter, you will find consistent features to facilitate and reinforce your learning.

- To avoid interrupting your reading by reaching for your medical dictionary, **Key Terms** are presented in boldface type. They are defined in the text and the glossary at the end of the book. Other important or unfamiliar terms are italicized and defined in the text.

- **Clinical Alerts** within the text emphasize information critical to providing effective, safe clinical nursing care.

- **Cultural Care Strategies,** including nursing implications and self-reflection questions, prepare students to deliver culturally sensitive adult nursing care.

- **Boxes** are color-coded by content for ease in identifying specific issues. (Examples of this are shown in the walk-through on page IV–V.)

- **Nursing Care Checklists** quickly summarize nursing care activities for particular procedures or surgeries.

- **Priorities in Nursing Care** emphasize the particular responsibilities and roles of the LPN and LVN as they provide nursing care.

- **Procedure Checklists** review key steps in performing previously learned nursing care procedures and provide Sample Documentation.

- **Pharmacology tables** highlight nursing implications and client teaching for drugs used to treat particular disorders.

- **Chapter and Unit reviews** allow for self-evaluation.

- **Bibliography** listings support further research.

- **MediaLinks** are provided for students who wish to investigate a topic further. Tabs in page margins identify added resources available in our electronic supplements or on the World Wide Web.

Acknowledgments

A project such as *Medical–Surgical Nursing Care* would not come into being without the contributions of many people.

First of all, we thank you, our students, past, present, and future, from whom we learn so much. It is your quest for learning and your enthusiasm for the profession you have chosen that stimulates us, invigorates us, and always keeps us honest and humble. You are the future of our profession.

Many nursing professionals provided invaluable expertise and input into this book. Our contributors provided their knowledge, skills, and time to this project, writing selected chapters and features of this book. Reviewers provide quality assurance for the book. They validate content, attend to details, and challenge our ways of thinking and expressing ourselves. Contributors and reviewers for *Medical–Surgical Nursing Care* are listed with their current affiliations following this preface.

A project such as this one requires the support, skills, and expertise of many people. We especially want to thank Julie Alexander, our publisher, for having the vision to create a line of books specifically for you, the practical/vocational nursing student. We also owe a debt of gratitude to Maura Connor, Editor-in-Chief for nursing, who provided unflagging support as *Medical–Surgical Nursing Care* grew from an idea into the book you are holding.

Throughout its initial development, champions of this project were Barbara Krawiec, the editor, and Rachel Bedard, the development editor. We thank Barbara for her vision and support of this book. She researched and developed the features and created a design to promote your interest and learning. We thank Rachel for forever encouraging us to stay with the vision: What do you, the student, need to know and be able to do?

Special thanks are also due to many others. Pat Gillivan, development editor for the second edition, kept us on track and attended to the details and consistency. Marilyn Meserve, managing editor, guided important aspects of the editorial process from behind the scenes. Michael Giacobbe, assistant editor, coordinated the supplements. Emily Adler, editorial assistant, attended to many details throughout this project (most of which happen without our knowledge or attention). Julie Li, production editor, moved parts in all directions, problem-solved and monitored quality. Patrick Walsh, managing production editor, and Ilene Sanford and Pat Brown, manufacturing managers, guided the scheduling, production, and manufacturing process. Lorretta Palagi did a superb copyediting job. Penny Walker and the capable staff of Techbooks transformed the manuscript to printed page. Cheryl Asherman, art director, and Mary Siener created a visually clear and inviting format. Bridget McDermott, research analyst, brought to life the voices of educators and students. John Jordan, Amy Peltier, and Tina Rudowski made all the media components happen. Harper Coles, marketing manager, Michael Sirinides, and Pat Linard enthusiastically worked to convey the features and benefits of these materials. To all of you we are most grateful!

About the Authors

Karen M. Burke, RN, MS

Karen M. Burke is the Education Consultant for the Oregon State Board of Nursing. She obtained her initial nursing education at Emanuel Hospital School of Nursing in Portland, Oregon, later completing baccalaureate studies at Oregon Health & Sciences University, and a master's degree at University of Portland. Ms. Burke has extensive clinical nursing experience in acute care and community-based settings, as well as more than 20 years of experience as a nurse educator and program administrator.

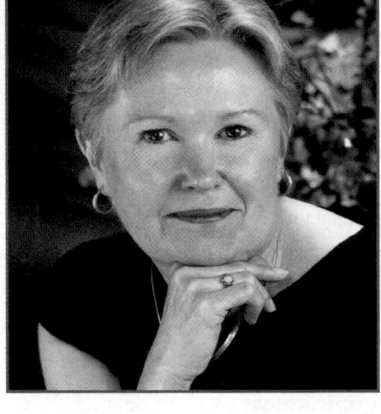

As a nurse educator, Ms. Burke is known as a leader and an innovator. She led the faculty of an associate degree nursing program in developing an online program to deliver nursing education to a distant rural community. Ms. Burke is actively involved in nursing education in Oregon, participating in the development of an educational consortium of a public university and local community colleges to deliver a common baccalaureate degree nursing curriculum around the state. She also is actively involved in the Oregon Nursing Leadership Council Education Committee, helping identify strategies to recruit and retain nursing faculty, develop innovative clinical models, and provide policy guidelines for use by all nursing education programs in the state. In addition, Ms. Burke is working with nursing leaders and educators to identify and develop strategic plans to more effectively educate and use practical nurses (LPNs) in Oregon. As education consultant to the Board, she works directly with new and existing practical and registered nursing programs to promote and maintain current and high-quality nursing education for the citizens of Oregon.

Ms. Burke strongly values the nursing profession and believes in the importance of a strong education in the art and science of nursing for all students entering the profession. She believes that her diverse experience as a nursing student, clinical nurse, and nurse educator and administrator has prepared her well to relate to nursing students in diverse educational settings.

Ms. Burke and her husband Steve love to garden, travel, and spend time with their extended family. Ms. Burke also enjoys a passion for quilting, accumulating and gradually completing multiple UFOs (unfinished objects).

Priscilla LeMone, RN, DSN, FAAN

Priscilla LeMone has spent most of her career as a nurse educator, teaching medical–surgical nursing and pathophysiology at all levels from diploma to doctoral students. She has a diploma in nursing from Deaconess College of Nursing (St. Louis, Missouri), baccalaureate and master's degrees from Southeast Missouri State University, and a doctorate in nursing from the University of Alabama-Birmingham. Dr. LeMone has retired from the Sinclair School of Nursing, University of Missouri-Columbia as Associate Professor Emerita.

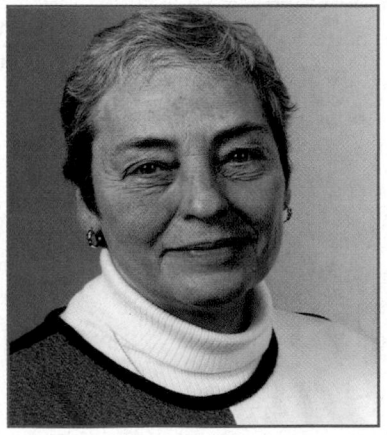

Dr. LeMone has received numerous awards for scholarship and teaching during her over 30 years as a nurse educator. She is most honored for receiving the Kemper Fellowship for Teaching Excellence from the University of Missouri-Columbia and the Unique Contribution Award from the North American Nursing Diagnosis Association, and for being selected as a Fellow in the American Academy of Nursing.

She believes that her education gave her solid and everlasting roots in nursing. Her work with students has given her the wings that allow her love of nursing and teaching to continue through the years.

Elaine L. Mohn-Brown, RN, EdD

Elaine L. Mohn-Brown received her Diploma in Nursing from Akron General Medical Center School of Nursing in Akron, Ohio. She has baccalaureate and master's degrees in nursing and health education from Metropolitan State College and University of Northern Colorado, and an EdD in higher education administration from Brigham Young University. She has worked in critical care units in Ohio and Colorado.

Her first teaching position was as a practical nursing instructor at Larimer County Vocational-Technical Center in Colorado. For the past 26 years, she has been on the faculty of the ADN Program at Chemeketa Community College in Salem, Oregon. Through thought-provoking classroom presentations and hands-on acute care

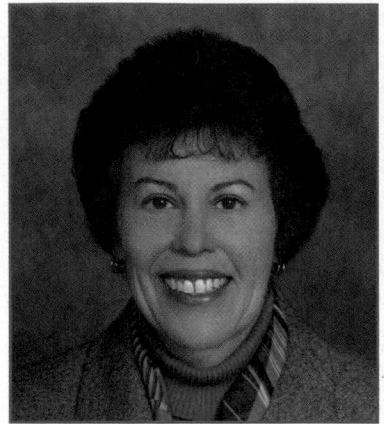

medical–surgical experiences, she has encouraged students to question and understand the rationale for their nursing care. She has implemented an extensive orientation program for novice nursing faculty at Chemeketa Community College and in 2005 developed *Clinical Teaching in Oregon,* a DVD to educate new clinical nursing faculty.

Dr. Mohn-Brown serves as a member of the Editorial Advisory Board for *Nurse Educator* and is a program evaluator for the Northwest Commission on Colleges and Universities. She has published nationally and conducts workshops at the national level. Her love of nursing and teaching has taken her to numerous international and national conferences.

When not working, she and her husband, Gene, spend time travelling and she enjoys flower gardening.

Linda Eby, RN, MN

Linda Eby received her baccalaureate and master's degrees in nursing from Oregon Health and Sciences University. She has 31 years of experience in nursing. Her nursing practice has been in critical care, home health/hospice, and psychiatric mental health nursing. As a Clinical Nurse Specialist in clinical genetics, she coordinated the Prenatal Genetics Clinic at OHSU. She has conducted workshops on teaching diverse students of nursing. As secretary of the American Federation of Teachers-Oregon, she serves as an advocate for the rights of education employees and students.

Ms. Eby has been teaching nursing at the community college level for 20 years. Her current teaching areas are nursing fundamentals, diabetes care, transcultural nursing, and psychiatric mental health nursing. She is the coordinator of a Nursing Student Success Program, which serves students who speak English as a non-native language, immigrant students, and other nontraditional students.

Ms. Eby loves and respects the profession of nursing even more now than she did 31 years ago. Fortunately, she has two wonderful daughters and two good dogs to provide balance in her life.

Contributor Team

Textbook Contributors

Mei R. Fu, PhD, RN
Chapter 12 Caring for Clients with Cancer
Medical–Surgical Nursing Clinical Specialist
Assistant Professor, Course Coordinator
Fundamentals of Nursing
College of Nursing, New York University
New York, NY

Karla Jones, RN, MS
Unit Wrap-Ups
Faculty
Department of Nursing
Treasure Valley Community College
Ontario, OR

Claudia Stoffel, MSN, RN
Caring for Clients Having Surgery
Instructor
Paducah Community College
Paducah, KY

Ruth Davidhizar, RN, DNS, CS, FAAN
Cultural Care Strategies
Professor and Dean of Nursing
Bethel College
Mishwaka, IN

Joyce Newman Giger, EdD, RN, CS, FAAN
Cultural Care Strategies
Professor, Graduate Studies, School of Nursing
University of Alabama at Birmingham
Birmingham, AL

Supplements

Student CD-ROM

Doris A. Clark, RN, BC, BSN
Instructor
Prince George's Community College
Largo, MD

Tammy Owen, MSN, RN
Instructor of Nursing
West Kentucky Community and Technical College
Paducah, KY

Companion Website (www.prenhall.com/burke)

Melissa Black RN, MSN, FNP
Nursing Instructor
Greenville Technical College
Greenville, SC

Traudel B. Cline, RN, MSN
Professor of Nursing
Milwaukee Area Technical College
Milwaukee, WI

Cheryl DeGraw, RN, MSN, CRNP
Faculty/Course Coordinator
Florence-Darlington Technical College
Florence, SC

Betty Kehl Richardson, RN, PhD, BC, LMFT, LPC
Professor Emeritus
Austin Community College
Austin, TX

Workbook

Melissa Black, RN, MSN, FNP
Nursing Instructor
Greenville Technical College
Greenville, SC

Instructor's Resource Manual

Diane M. Bligh, RN, MSN, CNS
Associate Professor, Nursing
Front Range Community College
Westminster, CO

Jo Anne Carrick, RN, MSN
Instructor
Penn State University
Sharon, PA

Cheryl DeGraw, RN, MSN, CRNP
Faculty/Course Coordinator
Florence-Darlington Technical College
Florence, SC

Margaret M. Gingrich, RN, MSN
Professor
Harrisburg Area Community College
Harrisburg, PA

Dawna Martich, RN, MSN
Manager, Training
American Healthways
Pittsburgh, PA

Linda Roy, RN, MSN, CRNP
Assistant Professor of Nursing
Montgomery County Community College
Blue Bell, PA

Reviewer Panel

Janice Ankenmann, RN, MSN, CCRN, FNP
Coordinator, LVN Program
Napa Valley College
Napa, CA

Rebecca Cappo, RN, BSN, MSN
Instructor, Allied Health Careers
Lenape Technical School
Ford City, PA

Janice Chapman, RN, BSN, MSN
Practical Nursing Instructor
Reid State Technical College
Atmore, AL

Traudel B. Cline, RN, MSN
Professor of Nursing
Milwaukee Area Technical College
Milwaukee, WI

Connie J. Frisch, RN, MA
PN Instructor
Central Lakes College
Brainerd, MN

Anita A. W. Garman, RN, MSN
Instructor
Emanuel/Modesto Junior College
Turlock, CA

Pamela Gwin, RNC
Director, Vocational Nursing Program
Brazosport College
Lake Jackson, TX

Julie Hansen, RN, BSN, MA
LPN Program Instructor
Southeastern Technical Institute
Sioux Falls, SD

Patti Kercher, RN, BSN
Practical Nurse Faculty
Montana State University Great Falls College of Technology
Great Falls, MT

Barbara Lee-Learned, MSN, RN
Nursing Faculty
Technical College of the Low Country
Beaufort, SC

Shirley Loffquist, RN, BSN
Practical Nursing Instructor
Central Lakes College
Brainerd, MN

Mary Marquardt, RN, BA
Practical Nursing Instructor
Central Lakes College
Brainerd, MN

Jennifer Ponto, RN, BSN
Faculty
South Plains College
Levelland, TX

LuAnn J. Reicks, RNC, BS, MSN
Instructor, PN Coordinator
Iowa Central Community College
Fort Dodge, IA

Esther Salinas, RN, MSN, MS ED
Associate Professor
Del Mar College
Corpus Christi, TX

Pat Schrull, MSN, MBA, M.Ed., RN
Professor
Lorain County Community College
Elyria, OH

Lyndi C. Shadbolt, MS, BSN
Associate Professor, VN Program Coordinator
Amarillo College
Amarillo, TX

Nancy Smith, BSN, MSN
Education Specialist
St. Joseph's Hospital of Atlanta
Atlanta, GA

Nancy Turner, RN, C, MSN
Associate Professor of Nursing
West Kentucky Community and Technical College
Paducah, KY

Ann Wood, RN, BSN
Nursing Faculty
Surry Community College
Dobson, NC

Contents

Introduction to Medical–Surgical Nursing

UNIT I

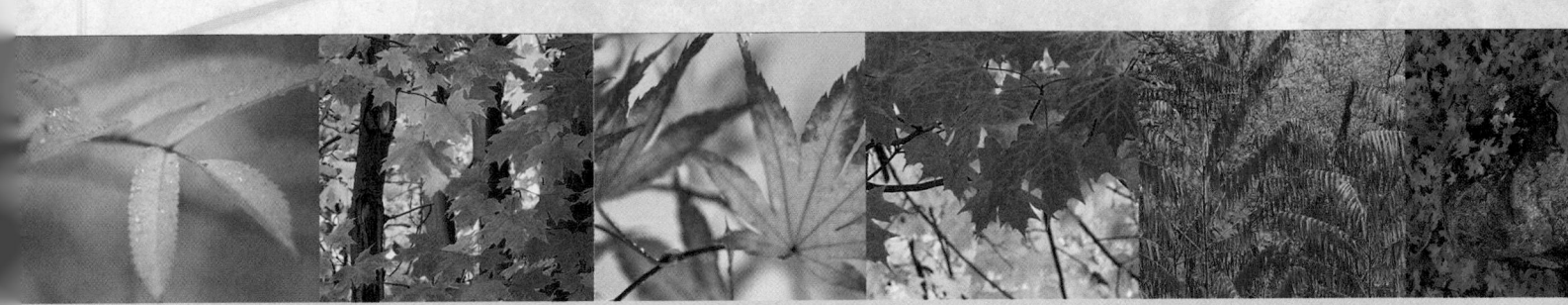

The Medical–Surgical Nurse

BRIEF Outline

LEARNING Outcomes

After completing this chapter, you will be able to:

- Describe the licensed practical/vocational nurse's role as caregiver, manager of care, advocate, and teacher.
- Discuss the steps of the nursing process: assessment, diagnosis, planning, implementation, and evaluation.
- Define critical thinking and explain how it contributes to nursing care.
- Explain how critical thinking and the nursing process are used to determine priorities of nursing care activities to promote, maintain, or restore health.
- Describe the importance of codes for nursing and nursing standards in medical–surgical nursing care.
- Discuss examples of legal and ethical dilemmas in client care.

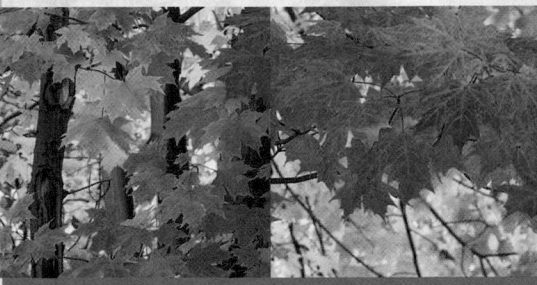

MediaLink

www.prenhall.com/burke
Use the address above to access the free, interactive Companion Website created for this textbook. Get hints, instant feedback, and textbook references to chapter-related NCLEX-style questions. Link to other interesting sites.

Audio Glossary:
Use the Companion Website, or the CD-ROM disk enclosed with your textbook, to hear the pronunciation of key terms in this chapter.

Medical–surgical nursing is the health care and illness care of adults. It is based on knowledge from the arts and sciences and is shaped by knowledge from nursing. The focus of medical–surgical nursing is the adult client's response to actual or potential disruptions in health. The adult requiring health care services is the *client*.

Medical–surgical nurses must address many issues simultaneously. The human responses for which nurses plan and implement care do not just result from changes in the structure and function of body systems. They also result from related and inseparable changes in the client's social, cultural, economic, and personal life. Beyond this, medical–surgical nurses provide care for people across the major part of the life span, ranging from their late teens to early 100s. The variety of individual health care needs and the wide range of clients' ages make medical–surgical nursing an ever-changing and challenging field.

This chapter serves as a broad overview of medical–surgical nursing practice. Topics include the roles of the licensed practical/vocational nurse (LPN/LVN), cultural sensitivity in nursing care, the steps of the nursing process, critical thinking, guidelines for practice, and legal and ethical dilemmas that may arise when providing care.

Roles of the LPN/LVN in Medical–Surgical Nursing Care

Health care today is a vast and complex system. It reflects changes in society, changes in the populations that require nursing care, and an emphasis on health promotion as well as illness care. The roles of the medical–surgical nurse have broadened in response to these changes. Medical–surgical nurses are not only caregivers but also managers of care, advocates, and teachers. The nurse assumes these roles to promote and maintain health, to prevent illness, and to help clients cope with disability or death in any setting.

THE NURSE AS CAREGIVER

Nurses have always been **caregivers** (people who provide personal, individual assistance), but the activities carried out within the caregiver role have changed tremendously. From 1900 to the 1960s, the nurse was almost always female; the primary definition of her caregiver role was to give personal care to the client and to carry out physicians' orders. The caregiver role for the nurse today is both independent and collaborative. Registered nurses (RNs) may independently make assessments, plan, and implement client care based on nursing knowledge and skills (Figure 1-1 ■). LPN/LVNs, in conjunction with RNs, carry out the same activities. All licensed nurses also *collaborate* (work cooperatively) with other members of the interdisciplinary health care team to implement and evaluate care.

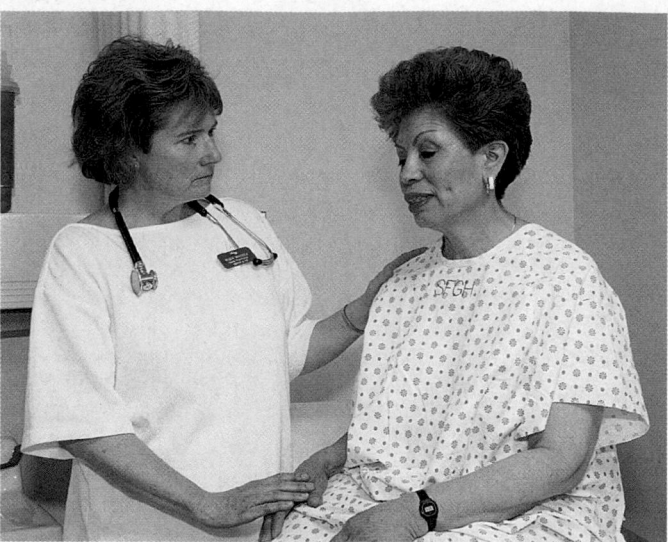

Figure 1-1. ■ In the role of caregiver, the nurse provides comprehensive, individualized care to the adult client. (Photographer: Richard Tauber.)

As a caregiver, the nurse practices both the science and the art of nursing. Using the nursing process as the framework for care, the nurse provides **interventions** (purposeful actions) to meet the physical, psychosocial, spiritual, environmental, and cultural needs of clients and families. Cultural awareness has become an increasingly important area in recent years. Box 1-1 ■ discusses culturally sensitive care in nursing.

The science (the knowledge) of nursing is translated into the art of nursing through caring. *Caring* is the means by which the nurse is connected with and concerned for the client. The nurse as caregiver is knowledgeable, skilled, understanding, and caring.

Nurses have always identified problems in client care and developed interventions to meet specific needs. Until recently, though, these activities were not conducted scientifically or communicated to other nurses through nursing literature. To develop the science of nursing, nursing knowledge must be established through clinical research and then published, so that the findings based on clinical evidence can be used by all nurses to improve client care. The nurse's role as a caregiver is increasingly based on evidence-based practice.

THE NURSE AS MANAGER OF CARE

All nurses must learn to coordinate care and to be leaders. Their jobs may require them to manage time, resources, the environment in which they provide care, and other people (such as support staff). Nurses develop the skills to direct, delegate, and coordinate activities and to evaluate the quality of care provided. In the role of leader and manager, the nurse takes responsibility for the quality of client care through a process called quality assurance. **Quality assurance** includes the quality control activities of evaluating, monitoring, or

BOX 1-1

CULTURALLY SENSITIVE NURSING

Culture is a set of socially inherited characteristics of a human group. People learn beliefs, practices, habits, likes, dislikes, customs, and rituals from their families and pass them on to their children. A person's *ethnic identity* includes belonging to a social group within a culture and a social system, and sharing a common religion, language, ancestry, and physical characteristics. (For example, a person's ethnic identity may be Irish Catholic; the person's culture might be American.) Culture gives shape and personal meaning to health or illness events. It also affects how the client relates to others within the health care environment.

The health care system serves clients who are culturally diverse in country of origin, health beliefs, sexual orientation, race, socioeconomic level, and age. However, nursing has been slow to address the need for culturally sensitive care. This is partly because the health care system is itself a culture, and still is primarily made up of white middle-class people. Prejudice and *ethnocentrism* (people's belief that their own cultural group's beliefs and values are the only acceptable ones) have often created barriers to culturally sensitive care.

Culturally sensitive care is important for nurses for the following reasons:

- The demographic and ethnic composition of the world, and the United States in particular, has changed markedly, but ethnic groups are not well represented among health care professionals.
- There is a growing awareness and acceptance of diversity and an increased willingness to maintain and support ethnic and cultural heritage.
- People of color and immigrants face limited access to health care.
- Nurses make up the largest force in health care delivery and therefore have tremendous potential to push for fairness and accessibility.
- Consumers are becoming increasingly aware of what constitutes competent and sensitive health care.

People of every culture have the right to have their cultural values known, respected, and addressed appropriately in nursing and other health care services. To provide nursing care that is culturally aware, nurses must develop a sensitivity to personal fundamental values about health and illness. They must accept the existence of differing values. They must be respectful of, interested in, and understanding of other cultures without being judgmental.

regulating the standard of services provided to the consumer. Clients are assured of quality care through professional and technical licensure of individual care providers; through accreditation of hospitals (e.g., by the Joint Commission on Accreditation of Healthcare Organizations, or JCAHO); through licensure of hospitals, pharmacies, and nursing homes; and through certification in specialty areas.

Quality assurance methods are used to evaluate the care of individual clients against established standards of care. In this process, documentation is reviewed, client surveys are conducted, nurses are interviewed, and nurse or client performance is directly observed. This information is then used to identify differences between actual practice and established standards and to develop a plan of action to resolve the differences. Later, the actions are assessed to determine whether they were effective in improving practice.

THE NURSE AS ADVOCATE

The client who enters the health care system is often unprepared to make independent decisions. The nurse as **advocate** (defined as one who speaks for another) actively promotes the client's rights to make decisions and choices. The nurse speaks for the client when necessary, mediates between the client and other persons, and protects the patient's right to self-determination (even when the nurse disagrees with the client's decision). As a client advocate, the nurse:

- Communicates with other health care team members.
- Provides client and family teaching.
- Assists and supports client decision making.
- Makes referrals.
- Identifies community and personal resources.

THE NURSE AS TEACHER

The teaching role of the nurse is important for many reasons. First, there is a greater emphasis on health promotion and illness prevention. Second, hospital stays are becoming shorter, so the client and family must provide continuing care at home. Third, the number of chronically ill in our society is rising as the overall population ages. All of these factors make the nurse's role as a teacher increasingly important.

The framework for the role of teacher is the teaching–learning process. Within this framework, the LPN/LVN, in conjunction with the RN, assesses learning needs, plans and implements teaching to meet those needs, and evaluates the effectiveness of the teaching. The nurse must have good interpersonal skills and be familiar with adult learning principles (Figure 1-2 ■).

Teaching is a major part of helping clients and their families know how to provide care at home. Because client and family education is such an important aspect of medical–surgical nursing care, we include information about what to teach for continuing care throughout this textbook.

Framework for Practice: The Nursing Process

The **nursing process** is the series of activities nurses perform as they provide care to clients. The nursing process is a model of care that differentiates nursing from other helping

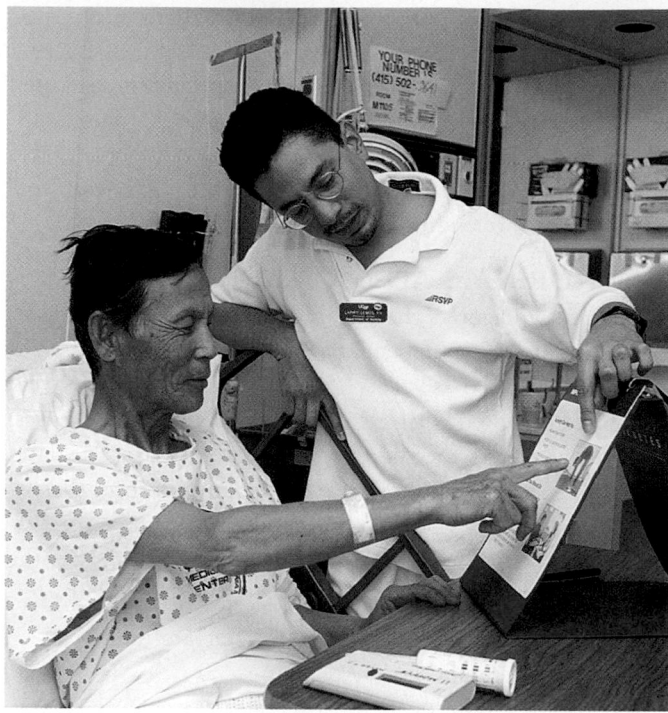

Figure 1-2. ■ The nurse's role as teacher is an essential component of care. As part of the discharge planning process, this nurse is providing teaching for self-care at home. (Photographer: Alain McLaughlin.)

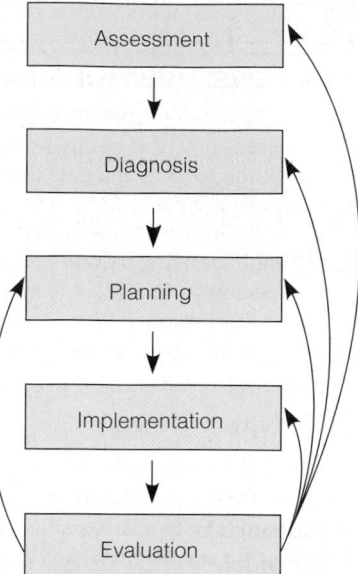

Figure 1-3. ■ Steps of the nursing process. Notice that the steps are interrelated and interdependent. For example, evaluation of the client might reveal the need for further assessment, additional nursing diagnoses, and/or a revision of the plan of care.

professions. It can be used in any setting in which the nurse provides care, from promoting wellness to coping with disability or death. Regardless of the situation, the nursing process includes activities that are specific, individualized, and concerned with the whole person—physical, emotional, and spiritual.

STEPS OF THE NURSING PROCESS

The nursing process has five interdependent steps: assessment, diagnosis, planning, implementation, and evaluation. They are most often used in a cyclic manner (Figure 1-3 ■).

The steps have been legitimized by the American Nurses Association's standards of practice and by state nursing practice acts. Licensing examinations, including the NCLEX-PN®, base their structure on this model of nursing care. Licensed practical/vocational nurses use all the steps of the nursing process except making a nursing diagnosis. However, they do provide information that supports a nursing diagnosis, and are often involved in identifying specific health problems of individual clients. A discussion of that step is included here so that you might see the entire process. Care plans that illustrate the nursing process are included throughout this textbook.

Assessment

Assessment, the first step of the nursing process, begins when the client first encounters the health care system and continues as long as the client requires care. During assessment, the nurse collects *data* (pieces of information) about the client's health status; these data are communicated either verbally or in written form. Accurate assessments are the basis for making accurate nursing diagnoses, for planning and implementing individualized care, and for evaluating the care that is given. (See guidelines for collecting assessment data in Chapter 5, ⟨⟨⟩⟩ and the assessment chapters that begin each disorders unit.)

Nurses assess clients in two ways:

1. The *initial assessment* includes a thorough history and physical assessment. It provides comprehensive data about health responses. It identifies factors that contribute to these responses in a specific individual. It begins the mutual process of establishing goals and outcomes of care with the client. An initial assessment is most often done when a client enters a health care setting, such as a physician's office or the hospital.

2. *Focused assessments* are continuous assessments that occur whenever the nurse interacts with the client (for example, at the beginning of each shift in the hospital). They enable the nurse to evaluate nursing actions and to determine whether interventions should continue or change to meet outcomes. They provide structure for documenting nursing care. They allow the nurse to identify responses to a disease process or treatment that was not present during the initial assessment, or to monitor the status of an actual or potential problem that was previously identified (Alfaro, 2005).

To make accurate assessments, nurses must have the competencies that are based on knowledge and skills. They must be able to assess the physical and mental status of the client and to use effective communication techniques. Nurses must be knowledgeable in anatomy, physiology, pathophysiology, and pharmacology. Finally, nurses must have a solid foundation of nursing knowledge and skills to provide safe and competent care.

Diagnosis

The American Nurses Association (ANA) has defined nursing as the "diagnosis and treatment of human responses to actual or potential health problems" (1980, p. 9). The registered nurse identifies these human responses in a **nursing diagnosis**, defined by NANDA International (formerly the North American Nursing Diagnosis Association) as "a clinical judgment about individual, family, or community responses to actual or potential health problems/life processes. Nursing diagnoses provide the basis for selection of nursing interventions to achieve outcomes for which the nurse is accountable" (NANDA, 2003, p. 263). Although no one list of nursing diagnoses is universally accepted, the work of NANDA is widely used. In 1988, the ANA accepted the NANDA system as the official system of diagnosis for the United States. Nursing diagnoses within the NANDA system are used in this book.

Nursing diagnoses identify two types of human responses: *actual* human responses and *potential* human responses. Nurses develop and implement a plan of care for actual responses; they also plan interventions to support health and prevent illness for potential human responses. Examples of nursing diagnoses are found throughout this textbook. (See also Appendix II, NANDA-Approved Nursing Diagnoses 2005–2006.)

Making a nursing diagnosis is a complex process that always involves uncertainty. Therefore, the nurse uses diagnostic reasoning to choose nursing diagnoses that best define the individual's health problems. Critical thinking, described in the next section, is used to make decisions about which label (or diagnosis) best describes the patterns of data, and to plan, develop, and evaluate nursing interventions. Many different frameworks exist for identifying patterns of human behavior. Some commonly used methods are basic human needs and body systems.

A diagnosis is written in two parts joined by the phrase *related to.* The first part of the statement is the human response that has been identified from the analysis of data. It identifies what needs to change in a specific client as a result of nursing interventions, and it also identifies the client outcomes that measure the change. The part of the statement that follows the *related to* phrase identifies the physical, psychosocial, cultural, spiritual, or environmental factors that cause or contribute to the response.

The PES method of writing a nursing diagnosis is frequently used in nursing practice (Gordon, 1994). Diagnoses written according to this method consist of three components:

1. The problem (P), which is the NANDA label
2. The etiology (E) of the problem, which names the related factors and is indicated by the phrase *related to*
3. The signs and symptoms (S), which are the defining characteristics and are indicated by the phrase *as manifested by.*

The following are examples of nursing diagnoses that are written using the PES method:

- *Anxiety* related to hospitalization as manifested by statements of nervousness and by crying
- *Bowel Incontinence* related to loss of sphincter control as manifested by involuntary passage of stool
- *Fatigue* related to the side effects of chemotherapy as manifested by the inability to carry out normal daily routines and statements of overwhelming exhaustion.

Planning

During the **planning** step, the nurse develops a list of nursing interventions (activities) and client **outcomes** (achievable goals) to promote healthy responses and prevent, reverse, or decrease unhealthy responses. Outcomes, which are mutually established by the client and nurse together, identify what the client will be able to do as a result of the nursing interventions. Both outcomes and nursing interventions are documented in a written plan of care that directs nursing activities, nursing documentation, and appropriate evaluation (Alfaro, 2005).

Nurses plan interventions for two types of client problems: those that require nursing management (stated as nursing diagnoses) and those that require collaborative management (collaborative or clinical problems). In *nursing management,* the nurse is guided by the diagnosis, initiates selected interventions, and is accountable for achieving outcomes. In *collaborative management* (pathophysiologic, treatment-related, personal, environmental, and maturational situations), nurses monitor for onset or changes in status, and both physician-initiated and nurse-initiated interventions are used to minimize complications.

EXPECTED OUTCOMES. Expected outcomes for nursing interventions are client centered, time specific, and measurable (e.g., "The client will demonstrate the ability to self-administer insulin injections by discharge"). Outcomes are classified into three domains: cognitive ("knowing"), affective ("feeling"), and psychomotor ("doing"). The nurse considers all three domains to ensure achievement of the desired therapeutic outcomes.

In contrast, expected outcomes for collaborative problems are goals for the nurse, usually written as statements that begin, for example, with "to detect and report early signs and symptoms of potential complications of . . ." and "to implement preventive and corrective nursing interventions ordered by . . ." (Alfaro, 2005). In many instances, these goals are not written down as part of the plan of care. Nursing interventions for collaborative problems may be ordered by the physician or by institutional policy, procedures, protocols, or standards.

The nursing plan consists of specific, individualized interventions. If, for example, the nurse identifies that a client is at risk for Deficient Fluid Volume, it is not enough for the nurse simply to encourage the client to drink more fluids. Together, the nurse and client must identify liquids the client prefers, times that will be best for drinking them, and the amount of fluid (in ounces or milliliters). The nurse must document this information on the written care plan. Only then does care truly become a part of the plan of care.

Implementation

The **implementation** step is the "doing" phase of the nursing process, during which the nurse carries out planned activities (interventions). Ongoing assessment of the client before, during, and after the intervention is essential. Although a plan may be appropriate, there are many variables that may make a change of plan necessary. For example, the nurse is not able to force fluids if the client is nauseated or vomiting.

When implementing the planned interventions, the nurse follows several important principles:

1. Set daily priorities, based on initial and focused assessments and on the client's condition, as reported during the change of shift report or as documented in the client's chart. Critical assessments take first priority. These include the status of invasive lines and fluids infusing or changes in health status during the preceding shift.
2. Be aware of how nursing interventions interrelate. For example, while giving a bath, the nurse can also assess physical and psychologic status, use therapeutic communication, teach the client, do range-of-motion exercises, and provide skin care.
3. Determine the most appropriate level of interventions for each client, based on health status and illness treatment. This may include any or all of the following:
   a. Directly perform the activity for the client.
   b. Assist the client to perform the activity.
   c. Supervise the client/family while they are performing the activity.
   d. Teach the client/family about health care.
   e. Monitor the client at risk for potential complications or problems.
4. Use available resources to provide interventions that are realistic and practical. This depends on the equipment

available, financial status of the client, and resources (including staff, agency, family, and community resources).
5. Document nursing interventions. This is the final part of implementation, and *it is a legal requirement.* There are many different ways of documenting care. Traditional narrative source-oriented and problem-oriented charting methods are often used. Other methods are focused charting, charting by exception, and electronic documentation.

Evaluation

The **evaluation** step of the nursing process allows the nurse to determine whether the plan was effective and to continue, revise, or terminate the plan. Evaluation is based on the expected outcomes that were established during the planning step. Although evaluation is listed as the last part of the nursing process, it actually takes place continuously throughout client care.

To evaluate a plan, the nurse collects data from the client, reviews the chart, and observes the client. The nurse then compares the status of the client with the expected outcomes. If the outcomes have been accomplished, the nurse may continue or terminate the plan. If the outcomes have not been accomplished, the nurse must continue to collect data and evaluate interventions.

BENEFITS OF THE NURSING PROCESS

The nursing process benefits all those involved in the health care setting. It helps nurses identify their special areas of practice. The nursing process provides a common reference system and common terminology to serve as a base for improving clinical practice. It also provides a framework for evaluating quality of care.

The nursing process benefits clients. The nursing process creates a structure for planned, individualized interventions. It involves the client in all steps of the process. It ensures continuity of care through the written care plan. The nursing process also benefits the health care setting through better resource utilization, increased client satisfaction, and improved documentation of care. As the 21st century progresses, increased research and theory development will continue to refine the nursing process.

THE NURSING PROCESS IN THE CLINICAL SETTING

With experience, the nursing process becomes an integral part of providing care and the nurse does not consciously stop and consider each step. For example, when caring for a client who is hemorrhaging, the nurse uses all five steps simultaneously to meet critical, life-threatening needs. In contrast, when considering the long-term needs of a client with a chronic illness or disability, the nurse makes in-depth assessments, determines goals jointly with the client, and documents care through a written plan that is revised as necessary by all nurses providing care.

Critical Thinking

Critical thinking is, most basically, thinking about your thinking. It is self-directed thinking that is focused on what to believe or do in a specific situation. It involves both attitudes and skills. Critical thinking occurs when the nurse uses knowledge to consider a client care situation and uses judgments and decisions about what to do in that situation. As you practice critical thinking, you must consider:

- The purpose of the thinking (e.g., is it to collect more data or is it to report your data to someone else?)
- How much knowledge you have
- What prejudices may influence your thinking (e.g., believing that all poor people are dirty or all old people are incapable of learning how to care for themselves) or whether you let your emotions affect your decision
- What information you need from others, such as your instructor, skilled clinical nurses, a textbook or a journal article, or the policies of the health care setting
- The ability to identify other possible options, evaluate the alternatives, and reach a conclusion.

It takes practice to integrate critical thinking into your attitudes and skills. Critical thinking exercises, titled *Critical Thinking Care Maps,* are included throughout this book to provide that practice. This chapter provides a sample Critical Thinking Care Map, plus suggestions for critical thinking and completing the exercise. In Appendix V, care map answers are provided to assist you in developing your critical thinking skills.

ATTITUDES AND MENTAL HABITS NECESSARY FOR CRITICAL THINKING

Thinking critically involves more than just cognitive (knowledge) skills. It is strongly influenced by the attitudes and mental habits one has. To think critically, you must focus your attention on your attitudes and how they affect your thinking. These attitudes and mental habits are:

- Being able to *think independently* so that you make decisions based on sound thinking and judgment. This means, for example, you are not influenced by negative comments from other health care providers about a client.
- Being willing to listen to and be fair in your evaluation of others' ideas and beliefs by having *intellectual courage.* This involves listening carefully to other ideas and thoughts and making a decision based on what you learn instead of how you feel.
- Having *intellectual empathy* by being able to put yourself in the place of another to understand that other person

better. For example, if you put yourself in the place of the person with severe pain, you are better able to understand why he or she is so upset when pain medications are late.

- Being fair minded and considering all viewpoints before making a decision through an *intellectual sense of justice* and being *intellectually humble.* This means you consider the viewpoints of others that may be different from yours before reaching a conclusion. You also realize that you are constantly learning from others. You are not afraid to say, "I don't know the answer to that question, but I will find out and let you know."
- Being *disciplined* so that you do not stop at easy answers, but continue to consider alternatives.
- Being *creative* and *confident in self.* Nurses often need to consider different ways of providing care and constantly look for better, more cost-effective methods. Confidence in one's decisions is gained through critical thinking.

CRITICAL THINKING SKILLS

Critical thinking skills are the mental abilities that are used for self-directed thinking. The major critical thinking skills are:

- *Divergent thinking*—when you collect data from a client, being able to sort out the relevant data from the data that are not relevant and explore possibilities to draw a conclusion. Abnormal data (such as a high body temperature or a rapid pulse) are usually considered relevant, and normal data are helpful but may not change the care you provide.
- *Reasoning*—having the ability to discriminate between facts and guesses. By using known facts, problems are solved and decisions are made in a systematic, logical way. For example, when you take a pulse you must know the facts of normal pulse rate for a person of this age, types of medications the client is taking that may alter the pulse rate, and the emotional and physical state of the client. Based on these facts, you are able to decide if the pulse rate is normal or abnormal.
- *Clarifying*—defining terms and noting similarities and differences. For example, when caring for a client with chronic pain, you must know the definition of chronic pain, and also know the similarities and differences between acute pain and chronic pain.
- *Reflection*—taking time to think about something. Reflection cannot take place in an emergency situation. However, as you reflect on your experiences in nursing, many of those experiences may in turn become alternatives when caring for a different client.

Critical thinking is an expected ability of all nurses. Using critical thinking to provide care that is structured by the nursing process allows the nurse to provide safe, effective, and individualized care.

This line provides an appropriate nursing diagnosis.

Sample Critical Thinking Care Map

This line provides the appropriate NCLEX-PN® focus area.

Caring for a Client with Impaired Mobility
NCLEX-PN Focus Area: Physiological Integrity: Reduction of risk potential

Case Study: Mrs. Jones is an 89-year-old woman who has been living in a long-term facility for the past 6 months. She has arthritis in her hips and knees and uses a walker to ambulate. Mrs. Jones has some impairment in hearing and often forgets to put on her glasses before getting out of bed. She takes a "water pill" and a "heart pill" for her congestive heart failure. You enter her room at 0730 to begin her morning care.

This information is provided to give you basic information about the client.

Risk for Falls

COLLECT DATA

Subjective	O	bjective
_____		_____
_____		_____
_____		_____
_____		_____
_____		_____
_____		_____

Would you report this data? Yes/No
If yes, to: _____

Nursing Care

_____
_____
_____
_____
_____
_____
_____
_____

How would you document this? _____
_____
_____

Data Collected
(use those that apply)

- States "I feel so dizzy today"
- BP 92/60
- P 56
- Uses walker to ambulate
- Skin is dry with little turgor
- Output 1100-0700 was 500 mL
- Urine light yellow
- States "I am nauseated"
- Vomits 75 mL of dark green–colored material
- Is not oriented to time or place, knows her name
- Has hearing and visual deficits
- Knee joints are swollen
- Refused to eat breakfast
- Takes digitalis and Lasix each morning at 0900

Nursing Interventions
(use those that apply)

- Place the bed in lowest position.
- Monitor for increased confusion.
- Inform Mrs. Jones of place and time as needed.
- Ask Mrs. Jones to ask for help when getting up.
- Ask Mrs. Jones to ask for help when ambulating.
- If symptoms persist, put Mrs. Jones on bed rest.
- Monitor vital signs and dizziness every 2 hours.
- Assist with sitting in chair and using walker.
- Record urine output every 2 hours.
- Do not give medications today.
- Ensure call bell is in reach.
- Force fluids.
- Provide midmorning snack to replace breakfast.

Carefully consider the data. What statements and data collected would increase Mrs. Jones's risk for falling? What data are subjective and what data are objective? What data are not relevant?

Subjective data: "I feel so dizzy."

Objective data: BP 92/60, P 56, not oriented to time and place, uses walker to ambulate, has hearing and visual deficits.

Irrelevant data: Dry skin with little turgor, urine color and output, "I am nauseated," vomits 75 mL, knee joints swollen, refuses breakfast, takes medications each morning.

Think about the data you have collected. Are any of the data abnormal? Do they increase the risk for falls? Are they important in preventing Mrs. Jones from falling? **Yes, report the data to the nurse in charge of the unit.**

This question allows you to practice your documentation. It is not necessary to document all the data or interventions for this exercise. For example, the assessment documentation might be:

730 States "I am dizzy" BP 92/60, P 56. Is not oriented to time and place, is oriented to person.
Mr. James, nurse manager notified.

J. Gomez, LVN

Consider the risk factors for falling identified in the data that were collected. Review the effect of dizziness, confusion, and hypotension on the ability to safely get out of bed and ambulate. Review the policy on fall-prevention programs in your health care clinical setting or in a current journal article. Make a decision about which interventions are relevant and which are not relevant.

Relevant interventions: Place bed in lowest position, monitor for increased confusion, inform client of place and time, ask client to ask for help when getting up and ambulating, put client on bed rest if symptoms persist, monitor vital signs and dizziness, assist with sitting in chair and using walker, ensure call bell is within reach.

Irrelevant interventions: Record urine output every 2 hours, do not give medications, force fluids, provide midmorning snack.

Note:

This sample is provided for the beginning student in medical–surgical nursing. As you learn more about pathophysiology, medications, and nursing care you will find there are more alternatives for consideration in this sample. For example, the medications Mrs. Jones is taking may cause dehydration and loss of potassium. These conditions may cause nausea, vomiting, and confusion. In turn, there would be an increased risk for falls. These data should be reported to the nurse in charge, who would report the data to the physician. The physician may order the medications to be held. The nurse would not omit the medications without a physician's order.

Guidelines for Nursing Practice

Nursing codes of ethics and standards guide nursing practice and protect the public. These guidelines are especially important because nurses encounter legal and ethical problems almost daily.

CODES FOR NURSES

An established code of ethics is one means that is used to define a profession. **Ethics** are principles of conduct. Ethical behavior is concerned with moral duty, values, obligations, and the distinction between right and wrong. Nursing codes of ethics provide a frame of reference for "professionally valued and ideal nursing behaviors that are congruent with the principles expressed in the Code for Nurses" (Ketefian, 1987, p. 13). Not only do they state ideal behaviors when making moral and ethical decisions; they also help define the roles of nurses.

The ANA Code for Nurses states principles of ethical concern. First published in 1950, the code was most recently revised in 2001. It guides the behavior of nurses and also defines nursing for the general public. Examples of the ANA code for nurses include these:

- The nurse's primary commitment is to the patient, whether an individual, family, group, or community.
- The nurse promotes, advocates for, and strives to protect the health, safety, and rights of the patient.
- The nurse owes the same duties to self as to others, including the responsibility to preserve integrity and safety, to maintain competence, and to continue personal and professional growth.

The National Association for Practical Nurse Education and Service (NAPNES) developed the code of ethics for licensed practical/vocational nurses that is outlined in Box 1-2 ■.

STANDARDS OF NURSING PRACTICE

A **standard** is a statement or criterion that can be used by a profession and by the general public to measure quality of practice. Established standards make each individual nurse accountable for practice. This means that each nurse who provides care has the responsibility or obligation to account for his or her own behaviors within that role. Professional nursing organizations develop and implement standards of practice to identify clearly the nurse's responsibilities to society.

The standards for NAPNES (2004) set a foundation for providing safe and competent nursing practice, guided by a commitment to ethical/legal principles (Box 1-3 ■). The ANA standards of clinical nursing practice (2004) outline standards for care (based on the nursing process) and professional performance, including quality of care, education, ethics, collaboration, and use of resources.

BOX 1-2

THE LICENSED PRACTICAL/VOCATIONAL NURSE CODE OF ETHICS
The Licensed Practical/Vocational Nurse shall:

1. Consider as a basic obligation the conservation of life and the prevention of disease.
2. Promote and protect the physical, mental, emotional and spiritual health of the patient and his/her family.
3. Fulfill all duties faithfully and efficiently.
4. Function within established legal guidelines.
5. Accept personal responsibility (for his/her acts) and seek to merit the respect and confidence of all members of the health team.
6. Hold in confidence all matters coming to his/her knowledge, in the practice of his/her profession, and in no way and at no time violate this confidence.
7. Give conscientious service and charge just renumeration.
8. Learn and respect the religious and cultural beliefs of his/her patient and of all people.
9. Meet his/her obligation to the patient by keeping abreast of current trends in health care through reading and continuing education.
10. As a citizen of the United States of America, uphold the laws of the land and seek to promote legislation that will meet the health needs of its people.

Source: National Association for Practical Nursing Education and Service, Inc. (2004). *Code of ethics.* Silver Springs, MD: Author.

Legal and Ethical Dilemmas in Nursing

A **dilemma** is a choice between two unpleasant alternatives. Nurses providing medical–surgical nursing care face dilemmas almost daily. Some common ones are discussed here briefly.

CLIENT RIGHTS

The client's right to refuse treatment (including surgery, medication, medical therapy, and food/fluids) at the end of life is sometimes a difficult area. As client advocate, the nurse must first establish that the client is mentally competent. The nurse then carefully explains the situation, the alternatives, and the potential harm from refusing treatment. Legally, the client must establish an *advance directive* on admission to a health care agency, stating the client's choice about preserving or prolonging life. (An advance directive, or *living will,* is a document in which a client formally states preferences for health care in the event that he or she later becomes mentally incapacitated. The client also names a person who has *durable power of attorney* to serve as a substitute decision maker to implement the client's stated preferences.) Documented advance directives become a part of the client's hospital record and are honored even if the client

---

BOX 1-3

NAPNES STANDARDS FOR NURSING PRACTICE OF LPN/LVN

1. The LPN/LVN provides individual and family-centered nursing care by:
   a. Utilizing appropriate knowledge, skills, and abilities
   b. Utilizing principles of the nursing process in meeting specific client needs in diversified health care settings
   c. Maintaining appropriate written documentation and utilizing effective communication skills with clients, family, significant others, and members of the health care team
   d. Executing principles of crisis intervention to maintain safety
   e. Providing appropriate education to clients, family, and significant others to promote health, facilitate rehabilitation, and maintain wellness
   f. Serving as a client advocate to protect client rights
   g. Serving as a client advocate to protect client rights
2. The LPN/LVN fulfills the professional responsibilities of the practical/vocational nurse by:
   a. Applying the ethical principles underlying the professions
   b. Following legal requirements
   c. Following the policies and procedures of the employing facility
   d. Cooperating and collaborating with all members of the health care team to meet the needs of family-centered nursing care
   e. Assuming accountability for his or her nursing actions
   f. Seeking educational opportunities to improve knowledge and skills
   g. Building skills to assure and increase postlicensure competence

Source: National Association for Practical Nurse Education and Service. (2004). *NAPNES standards of practice for licensed practical/vocational nurses.* Silver Spring, MD: Author.

---

becomes incompetent during the period of treatment. However, several states assert that artificial feeding cannot be rejected under living will statutes. The nurse must take responsibility for remaining informed about current laws in this area of practice.

Nurses respect the right to confidentiality of client information obtained from interviews or from the client's record. Most state nursing practice acts legally require nurses to uphold this right. However, the right to privacy and confidentiality becomes a dilemma when the nurse does not have access to information concerning the presence of acquired immune deficiency syndrome (AIDS) or human immunodeficiency virus (HIV) in clients under their care. Most states currently mandate that HIV test results can be given to another person only if the client provides written consent for the release of that information. Many health care providers believe that this law violates their own right to personal safety and so are actively working to change the law.

ISSUES OF DYING AND DEATH

Questions about who lives, who dies, and who decides often arise in the health care setting. These issues have become increasingly pressing as advances in technology extend the lives of people with chronic debilitating illness and major trauma. These changes have changed our ideas about living and dying. They have raised ethical conflicts about quality of life and death with dignity versus technologic methods of preserving life in any form. (See Chapter 14 ⚭ for further information about end-of-life care.)

CARING FOR THE CLIENT WITH AIDS

Despite great progress in controlling the course of the disease, the number of cases of HIV and AIDS continues to increase, and there is still no cure. AIDS occurs in heterosexual and homosexual men and women of all ages and at all socioeconomic levels. The disease inspires great fear and inflicts great physical, emotional, financial, and social havoc.

For nurses, AIDS poses a moral and ethical dilemma because of possible infection with the virus. According to the ANA, the nurse has a moral obligation to provide care for the client with AIDS unless the risk exceeds the responsibility. Most health care agencies have a written policy requiring nurses to provide care to clients with AIDS, except in certain circumstances, such as when a nurse is pregnant.

Note: The bibliography listings for this and all chapters have been compiled at the back of the book.

Chapter Review

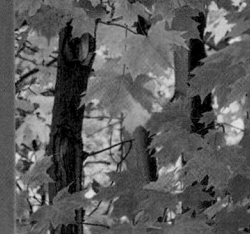

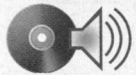 **KEY TERMS** by Topics

Use the audio glossary feature of either the CD-ROM or the Companion Website to hear the pronunciation of the following key terms.

Medical–surgical nurse
medical–surgical nursing

Roles of the nurse
caregivers, interventions, quality assurance, advocate

Framework for practice
nursing process, assessment, nursing diagnosis, planning, outcomes, implementation, evaluation

Critical thinking
critical thinking

Guidelines for nursing practice
ethics, standard

Legal and ethical dilemmas
dilemma

KEY Points

- Medical–surgical nurses promote health and provide care during illness or injury to adult clients. The roles of the medical–surgical nurse include caregiver, manager of care, client advocate, and teacher.

- The nursing process is a model of care that differentiates nursing from other health care providers. The five interdependent and cyclic steps of the nursing process are assessment, diagnosis, planning, implementation, and evaluation.

- Critical thinking is self-directed thinking that is focused on what to believe or do in a specific situation. It involves both attitudes and skills. Critical thinking and the nursing process are essential in nursing practice.

- Nursing codes of ethics (principles of conduct) and standards guide nursing practice and protect the public.

- Nurses often face dilemmas—a choice between two unpleasant alternatives—in clinical practice. Some dilemmas arise in the areas of client rights, issues of death and dying, and caring for clients with AIDS.

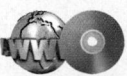 **EXPLORE Media**Link

Additional interactive resources for this chapter can be found on the Companion Website at www.prenhall.com/burke. Click on Chapter 1 and "Begin" to select the activities for this chapter.

For chapter-related NCLEX-style questions and an audio glossary, access the accompanying CD-ROM in this book.

FOR FURTHER Study

For more guidelines for collecting assessment data, see Chapter 5.

For NANDA diagnoses, see Appendix II.

For further information about end-of-life care, see Chapter 14.

NCLEX-PN® Exam Preparation

1 The nurse independently plans and implements client care based on:

  A. the physician's orders.
  B. the findings of other members of the health care team.
  C. nursing knowledge and skills.
  D. the wishes of the family.

2 The role of the nurse that is most evident when the nurse is protecting the client's rights is:

  A. caregiver.
  B. advocate.
  C. educator.
  D. manager.

3 The nurse is responsible for the *quality* of client care through a process called:

  A. quality assurance.
  B. delegation.
  C. nursing diagnosis.
  D. implementation.

4 The step of the nursing process in which the nurse collects data from clients is called:

  A. evaluation.
  B. diagnosis.
  C. implementation.
  D. assessment.

5 The step of the nursing process that is complex, involves uncertainty, and requires the nurse to use reasoning and critical thinking is:

  A. diagnosis.
  B. evaluation.
  C. assessment.
  D. planning.

6 Planned nursing interventions must be:

  A. determined by the nurse alone.
  B. specific and individualized.
  C. initiated by the physician.
  D. based on medical problems.

7 The nurse's role during the implementation phase of the nursing process is to:

  A. carry out planned activities.
  B. establish outcome criteria.
  C. identify client problems.
  D. evaluate the care given.

8 The final component of implementation that the nurse is legally required to complete is:

  A. setting priorities.
  B. assessing the client's condition.
  C. documenting interventions.
  D. teaching the client.

9 The public is protected and nursing practice is guided by:

  A. the nursing process.
  B. physicians' oversight.
  C. standardized procedures.
  D. standards and codes of ethics.

10 According to the ANA, the nurse has a moral obligation to provide care for the client with AIDS:

  A. when the client agrees to HIV testing.
  B. unless the risk exceeds the responsibility.
  C. only if a release of information is obtained.
  D. in all situations.

Answers for Review Questions appear in Appendix V.

Chapter 2

The Adult Client in Health and Illness

BRIEF Outline

LEARNING Outcomes

After completing this chapter, you will be able to:

- Compare and contrast the physical status, risks for alterations in health, and health behaviors of the young adult and the middle adult.
- Describe the functions and developmental stages and tasks of the family.
- Define health, the health–illness continuum, and the concept of high-level wellness.
- Explain factors affecting health status, health promotion, and health maintenance.
- Compare and contrast disease and illness.
- Describe the sequence of acute illness behaviors.
- Discuss chronic illness, including characteristics, needs of clients who are chronically ill, and the effects of chronic illness on the family.

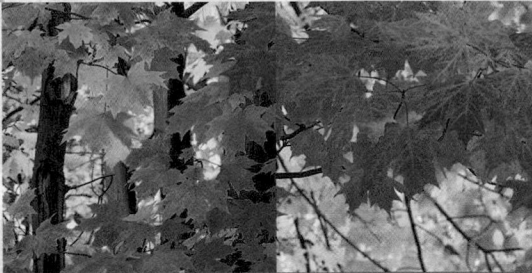

MediaLink

www.prenhall.com/burke
Use the address above to access the free, interactive Companion Website created for this textbook. Get hints, instant feedback, and textbook references to chapter-related NCLEX-style questions. Link to other interesting sites.

Audio Glossary:
Use the Companion Website, or the CD-ROM disk enclosed with your textbook, to hear the pronunciation of key terms in this chapter.

Gordon Hight, a 21-year-old college student, is admitted to the emergency room with multiple injuries and head trauma following a motorcycle crash. Mary Green, a 38-year-old homemaker, arrives at same-day surgery for biopsy of a tumor in her left breast. Sam Rosengarten, a 55-year-old attorney, is in the intensive care unit for treatment of a myocardial infarction. Margarite Schlefer, age 82, is receiving home health care following a fall that fractured her right hip. These examples demonstrate the striking variety among adult clients and the settings for their care—the focus of medical–surgical nursing.

Although growth and development are continuous processes throughout life, the adult years commonly are divided into three stages: the young adult (age 18 to 40), the middle adult (age 40 to 65), and the older adult (over age 65). With aging, specific changes occur in intellectual, psychosocial, and spiritual development, as well as in physical structures and functions. This chapter discusses the young and middle adult; Chapter 3 ⚭ provides information about the older adult.

Developmental Tasks of the Young and Middle Adult

The developmental tasks of adults, as described by Havighurst (1972), are divided into the young, middle, and adult years. From ages 18 to 35, young adults select and learn to live with a mate, have and raise children, have a job, manage a home, and take on civic responsibility. From ages 36 to 60, middle adults establish and maintain an economic standard of living, help adolescent children learn to become responsible adults, develop leisure activities, accept and adjust to the physical changes of middle age, and adjust to aging parents.

THE YOUNG ADULT

From age 18 to 25, the healthy young adult is at the peak of physical development. All body systems function at maximum efficiency. Then, during the 30s, some normal physiologic changes begin to occur. (A comparison of physical status for young adults during their 20s and 30s is shown in Table 2-1 ■.)

The nurse promotes health in the young adult by teaching the behaviors listed in Box 2-1 ■. Information about health for the young adult is primarily provided in community settings.

The young adult is at risk for **alterations in health** (a change from the normal health state) from accidents, sexually transmitted infections (STIs), substance abuse, and physical or psychosocial stressors. These risk factors may be interrelated.

Accidents are the leading cause of injury and death in people between ages 15 and 24 (Centers for Disease Control and Prevention [CDC], 2003). Most injuries and fatalities occur as

TABLE 2-1

Physical Status and Changes in the Young Adult Years

ASSESSMENT	STATUS DURING THE 20s	STATUS DURING THE 30s
Skin	Smooth, even temperature	Wrinkles begin to appear
Hair	Slightly oily, shiny Balding may begin	Graying may begin Balding may begin
Vision	Snellen 20/20	Some loss of visual acuity and accommodation
Musculoskeletal	Strong, coordinated	Some loss of strength and muscle mass
Cardiovascular	Maximum cardiac output 60–90 beats/min Mean BP: 120/80	Slight decline in cardiac output 60–90 beats/min Mean BP: 120/80
Respiratory	Rate: 12–20 Full vital capacity	Rate: 12–20 Decline in vital capacity

the result of motor vehicle crashes, but injuries and death also result from drowning, fire, use of firearms, occupational accidents, and exposure to environmental hazards. Accidental injury or death is often associated with the use of alcohol or other chemical substances or with psychologic stress.

Sexually transmitted infections include genital herpes, chlamydia, gonorrhea, syphilis, and acquired immune deficiency syndrome (AIDS). The young adult who is sexually active with a variety of partners and who does not use condoms is at greatest risk for development of these diseases.

Substance abuse is a major cause for concern in the young adult population. Although alcohol abuse occurs at all ages, it is greater in the 20s than during any other decade of the life span. Alcohol contributes to motor vehicle crashes and physical violence, and it is damaging to the developing fetus in pregnant women. It can also cause liver disease and nutritional deficits. Other substances that are commonly abused include nicotine, marijuana, amphetamines, cocaine, and crack. Cocaine and crack can cause death from cardiovascular effects and can lead to addiction and health problems in the baby born to an addicted mother. Smoking increases the risk of respiratory and cardiovascular diseases.

The young adult is subjected to a wide variety of physical and psychosocial stressors. Physical stressors that increase the risk of illness include environmental pollutants and work-related risks (e.g., electrical hazards, mechanical injuries, or exposure to toxins or infectious agents). Other

BOX 2-1

HEALTHY BEHAVIORS IN THE YOUNG ADULT
- Eat a variety of nutrient-dense foods and beverages within and among the basic food groups while choosing foods that limit the intake of saturated and trans fats, cholesterol, added sugars, salt, and alcohol.
- Choose a diet low in fat (30% or less of total calories), saturated fat (less than 10% of calories), and cholesterol (less than 300 mg daily). Choose foods high in fiber, low in sodium, and high in potassium.
- People with dark skin and those with little sunlight exposure should consume extra vitamin D from fortified foods or supplements.
- For females, maintain iron and adequate folate (a B vitamin) daily in the diet.
- Black individuals, who have an increased risk of hypertension, should aim to consume no more than 1,500 mg of sodium per day.
- Engage in at least 30 minutes of moderate-intensity physical activity, above usual activity, at work or home on most days of the week to help prevent chronic illnesses.
- Achieve physical fitness by including cardiovascular conditioning, stretching exercises for flexibility, and resistance exercises or calisthenics for muscle strength and endurance.
- Have regular physical examinations, including assessment every 3 years for cancer of the thyroid, ovaries, lymph nodes, and skin.
- Have a vision examination every 2 to 4 years.
- Practice good oral hygiene with teeth brushing and flossing, and have an annual dental checkup.
- For females, practice monthly breast self-examination and have a clinical breast examination every 3 years.
- For females, screening for cervical cancer (Pap test) should begin about 3 years after a woman begins having vaginal intercourse, but no later than 21 years. Screening should be done every year with regular Pap tests or every 2 years using liquid-based tests. At about age 30, women who have had three normal test results in a row may be screened every 2 to 3 years. Alternately, cervical cancer screening with HPV DNA testing and conventional or liquid-based cytology could be performed every 3 years (or more frequently, if risk factors such as a weakened immune system or an HIV infection are present). Women who are at high risk for hereditary nonpolyposis colon cancer should be offered a screening for endometrial cancer with endometrial biopsy beginning at age 35.
- For males, practice monthly testicular self-examination.
- Use sunscreen and avoid sunburn.

physical stressors include exposure to the sun, ingestion of chemical substances (e.g., caffeine, alcohol, nicotine), and pregnancy.

Many different and individualized psychosocial stressors may affect the young adult. Choices must be made about education, occupation, relationships, independence, and lifestyle. The young adult without an adequate education or job skills may face unemployment, poverty, homelessness,

and limited access to health care. Also, divorces in the United States are increasing. Three out of every five marriages end in divorce, and this number is even higher among young adults. Divorce often results in loneliness, feelings of failure, financial difficulties, domestic violence, and child abuse. The inability of the young adult to cope with these stressors may result in suicide, which ranks next to accidents as a major cause of death in this age group. Although difficult to prove, it is believed that some accidental deaths, especially when associated with substance abuse, are actually suicides.

THE MIDDLE ADULT

The middle adult, age 40 to 65, has physical status and function similar to that of adults in their 20s and 30s. However, many changes take place between ages 40 and 65 (Table 2-2 ■). The middle adult is at risk for alterations in

TABLE 2-2
Physical Changes in the Middle Adult Years

ASSESSMENT	CHANGES
Skin	Decreased turgor, moisture, and subcutaneous fat result in wrinkles. Fat is deposited in the abdominal and hip areas.
Hair	Loss of melanin in hair shaft causes graying. Hairline recedes in males.
Sensory	Visual acuity for near vision decreases (presbyopia) during the 40s. Auditory acuity for high-frequency sounds decreases (presbycusis); more common in men. Sense of taste diminishes.
Musculoskeletal	Skeletal muscle mass decreases by about age 60. Thinning of intervertebral disks results in loss of height (about 1 inch [2.5 cm]). Postmenopausal women may have loss of calcium and develop osteoporosis.
Cardiovascular	Blood vessels lose elasticity. Systolic blood pressure may increase.
Respiratory	Loss of vital capacity (about 1 L from age 20 to 60) occurs.
Gastrointestinal	Large intestine gradually loses muscle tone; constipation may result. Gastric secretions are decreased.
Genitourinary	Hormonal changes occur: menopause, women (↓ estrogen); andropause, men (↓ testosterone).
Endocrine	Gradual decrease in glucose tolerance occurs.

BOX 2-2

HEALTHY BEHAVIORS IN THE MIDDLE ADULT

- Eat a variety of nutrient-dense foods and beverages within and among the basic food groups while choosing foods that limit the intake of saturated and trans fats, cholesterol, added sugars, salt, and alcohol.
- Choose a diet low in fat (30% or less of total calories), saturated fat (less than 10% of calories), and cholesterol (less than 300 mg daily). Choose foods high in fiber, low in sodium, and high in potassium.
- People with dark skin and those with little sunlight exposure should consume extra vitamin D from fortified foods or supplements.
- Individuals with hypertension and blacks should consume no more than 1,500 mg of sodium each day.
- If weight loss is needed, aim for a slow, steady loss by decreasing caloric intake while maintaining an adequate nutrient intake and increasing physical activity.
- Include exercise as part of any weight-reduction program.
- Engage in at least 30 minutes of moderate-intensity physical activity, above usual activity, at work or home on most days of the week to help prevent chronic illnesses.
- Achieve physical fitness by including cardiovascular conditioning, stretching exercises for flexibility, and resistance exercises or calisthenics for muscle strength and endurance.
- Increase calcium intake (in perimenopausal women) to 800 mg daily.
- Consume high-fiber foods.
- Have an annual vision examination.
- Practice good oral hygiene with teeth brushing and flossing, and have a dental checkup one to two times a year.
- Have a physical examination annually, including assessment for cancer of the thyroid, testes, prostate, mouth, ovaries, skin, colon, and lymph nodes.
- For females, have a mammogram every year from age 40 on. Do a breast self-examination every month and have a breast examination annually.
- For females, have a Pap test as recommended for the young adult (see Box 2-1). Women who have had a total hysterectomy (with removal of the uterus and cervix) may choose to stop having Pap tests unless the surgery was done to treat cervical precancer or cancer. Women who are at high risk for hereditary nonpolyposis colon cancer should be offered a screening for endometrial cancer with endometrial biopsy beginning at age 35.
- For males, a prostate-specific antigen (PSA) blood test and a digital rectal examination (DRE) should be offered annually beginning at age 50. Men at high risk for prostate cancer (African American men and those who have a family history of father or brothers diagnosed with prostate cancer at an early age) should begin testing at age 45.
- Beginning at age 50, have one of the following to screen for colon cancer: yearly fecal occult blood test (FOBT) or fecal immunochemical test (FIT); flexible sigmoidoscopy every 5 years; yearly FOBT or FIT plus flexible sigmoidscopy every 5 years; double-contrast barium enema every 5 years; or colonoscopy every 10 years. Individuals who have an increased risk of colon cancer because of previous colon cancer, a personal history of chronic inflammatory bowel disease, a family history of colon cancer, or who have had adenomatous polyps should have screening more often.
- Use sunscreen and avoid sunburn.

health from obesity, cardiovascular disease, cancer, substance abuse, and psychosocial stressors. These factors may be interrelated.

The nurse promotes health in the middle adult by teaching the behaviors listed in Box 2-2 ■. Information about health for the middle adult may be provided in a variety of community settings, including outpatient clinics, occupational health clinics, and health care provider offices.

The middle adult often has a problem maintaining a healthy weight. Weight gain in middle adulthood is usually the result of continuing to consume the same number of calories while physical activity and basal metabolic rate decrease. Obesity affects all the major organ systems of the body, increasing the risk of atherosclerosis, hypertension, elevated cholesterol and triglyceride levels, and diabetes. Obesity is also associated with heart disease, osteoarthritis, and gallbladder disease.

The major cardiovascular risk factors, especially for coronary artery disease, include age, male gender, cigarette smoking, hypertension, elevated blood cholesterol levels, and

diabetes. Other contributing factors include obesity, stress, and lack of exercise. The middle adult is at risk for disorders of peripheral vascular, cerebrovascular, and cardiovascular disease.

Cancer is the third leading cause of death in adults between ages 25 and 64 in the United States, with one-third of cases occurring between ages 35 and 64. Cancers of the breast, colon, lung, and reproductive system are common in the middle years. The middle adult is at risk for cancer from environmental toxins as a result of increased length of exposure, and is also at risk from alcohol and nicotine use.

Although the middle adult may abuse a variety of substances, the most commonly abused are alcohol, nicotine, and prescription drugs. Excess alcohol use in the middle adult contributes to an increased risk of liver cancer, cirrhosis, pancreatitis, hyperlipidemia, and anemia. Alcoholism also increases the risk of accidental injury or death and disrupts careers and relationships. Cigarette smoking increases the risk of cancer, of chronic obstructive pulmonary disorders, and of cardiovascular disorders of the larynx, lung, mouth, pharynx, bladder, pancreas, esophagus, and kidney. The most commonly abused class of prescription drugs is tranquilizers.

The middle adult years are ones of change and transition, frequently resulting in stress. Both men and women must adapt to changes in physical appearance and function and accept their own mortality. Children may leave home or, as is becoming more common, choose to remain at home. Parents are aging, with illness and death probable. The middle adult thus becomes what has been called "the sandwich generation," caught between the need to care for both children and aging parents. Both men and women may make career changes, and approaching retirement becomes a reality. Divorce in the middle years is a major emotional, social, and financial stressor.

The Family of the Adult Client

Although some clients are totally alone in the world, most have one or more people who are significant in their lives. These significant others may be related or bonded to the client by birth, adoption, marriage, or friendship. Although not always meeting traditional definitions, people (or even pets) significant to the client are the client's family. The nurse includes the family as an integral component of care in all health care settings.

FAMILY DEFINITIONS AND FUNCTIONS

What is a family? The definition of a family changes as society changes. According to one definition, a **family** is a unit of people related by marriage, birth, or adoption (Duvall, 1977). An expanded definition states that a family is two or more people who are emotionally involved with each other and live close to each other. In a global society, it may not be possible for family members to live nearby, but they do remain emotionally involved.

Although every family is unique, all families have certain structural and functional features in common. *Family structure* (family roles and relationships) and *family function* (interactions among family members and with the community) provide support, guidance, and stability. The family carries out the tasks that are necessary for its survival and continuity:

- Providing shelter, food, clothing, and health care
- Sharing money, time, and space according to each member's needs
- Determining the roles and responsibilities of each member for the support, management, and care of the home and other family members
- Ensuring the socialization of members by raising them to take on increasingly responsible roles in the family and in society
- Establishing socially acceptable ways to interact with others through communication and the expression of feelings in areas such as love, anger, and sexuality

- Rearing and releasing children appropriately
- Relating to the community (neighborhood, school, church, work) and establishing rules for relatives, guests, and friends
- Maintaining morale and motivation, rewarding achievement, dealing with personal and family crises, setting attainable goals, and developing family loyalties and values.

DEVELOPMENTAL STAGES AND TASKS OF THE FAMILY

The family, just like the individual, has developmental stages and tasks. Each stage brings change and requires adaptation. Each new stage also brings family-related risk factors for alterations in health. The nurse must consider both the needs of the client at a specific developmental stage and the needs of the client within a family with specific developmental tasks:

1. *A couple.* Two people, living together with or without being married, are in a period of establishing themselves as a couple. Their tasks are to adjust to living together as a couple, establish a mutually satisfying relationship, relate to kin, and decide whether or not to have children.
2. *The family with infants and preschoolers.* The young family must adjust to being more than a couple. Family members must now support the needs and economic costs of more than two members. They must develop an attachment between parents and children, cope with lack of energy and privacy, and carry out activities that promote growth and development of the children.
3. *Family with school-age children.* The family with school-age children must adjust to the expanded world of children in school, encourage educational achievement, and promote joint decision making between children and parents.
4. *Family with adolescents and young adults.* The developmental tasks of this family unit focus on transition. Parents must provide a supportive home base and maintain open communications. They must balance freedom with responsibility and encourage adult children to become independent.
5. *Family with middle adults.* When the parents are middle aged and children are no longer at home, the parents' tasks are to maintain ties with older and younger generations, to plan for retirement, to reestablish their relationship, and (if necessary) to acquire the role of grandparents.
6. *Family with older adults.* The older adult family must adjust to retirement and aging. If a spouse dies, the surviving spouse must cope with the loss, adjust to living alone, or close the family home.

Health in the Adult Client

The World Health Organization (WHO) defines **health** as "a state of complete physical, mental, and social well-being, and not merely the absence of disease or infirmity" (WHO, 1974, p. 1). This definition is used as the classic definition of health. Even so, it does not take into account the many different levels of health a person may experience, or the fact that a person may be clinically described as ill and still define himself or herself as well. These additional factors, which greatly influence nursing care, include the health–illness continuum and high-level wellness.

THE HEALTH–ILLNESS CONTINUUM AND HIGH-LEVEL WELLNESS

The **health–illness continuum** represents health as a dynamic process, with high-level wellness at one extreme of the continuum and death at the opposite extreme (Figure 2-1 ■). Individuals place themselves at different locations on the continuum at specific points in time.

Dunn (1959) expanded the concept of a continuum of health and illness in his description of high-level wellness. Dunn described wellness as an active process influenced by the environment. He distinguished good health from wellness. Good health can be passive, a state of freedom from illness in which the individual is at peace with the environment. **High-level wellness,** on the other hand, is a way of functioning to reach one's maximum potential at a particular point in time (Dunn, 1959, p. 4).

A person's self-concept, environment, culture, and spiritual values all influence wellness. Care based on a framework of wellness encourages active involvement by both the nurse and the client to promote, maintain, or restore health. It also supports the philosophy of *holistic health care,* in which all aspects of a person (physical, psychosocial, cultural, spiritual, and intellectual) are considered as essential components of individualized care.

FACTORS AFFECTING HEALTH

Many different factors affect a person's health or level of wellness. These factors often interact to promote health or to become risk factors for alterations in health. Major factors affecting health follow.

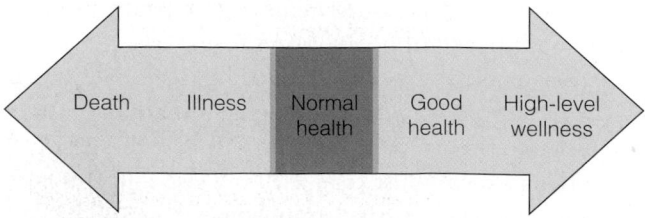

Figure 2-1. ■ The health–illness continuum

Genetic Makeup

Each person's genetic makeup influences health status throughout life. Genetic makeup affects personality, temperament, body structure, intellectual potential, and susceptibility to disruptions in health. Chronic illnesses associated with genetic makeup include sickle-cell disease, hemophilia, diabetes mellitus, and cancer.

Cognitive Abilities and Educational Level

Cognitive abilities are determined prior to adulthood. The level of cognitive development (education) affects whether people view themselves as healthy or ill and may also affect health practices. Cognitive abilities may be lessened by injuries to the brain and illnesses affecting the brain. Educational level affects the ability to understand and follow health guidelines. For example, if a person cannot read, written information about healthy behaviors and health resources is worthless.

Race, Ethnicity, and Cultural Background

Certain diseases occur at a higher rate in some races and ethnic groups than in others. For example, in the United States, hypertension is more common in African Americans, tuberculosis and diabetes mellitus are among the leading causes of illness in Native Americans, and eye disorders are more prevalent in Chinese Americans. A person's ethnic and cultural background also influences health values and behaviors, lifestyle, and illness behaviors. Every culture defines health and illness in a unique way. In addition, each culture has its own health beliefs and illness treatment practices.

Age, Gender, and Developmental Level

Age, gender, and developmental level are factors in health and illness. Cardiovascular disorders are uncommon in young adults, but their incidence increases after the age of 40. Heart attacks are more common in men than women until women are past menopause. Some diseases occur only in one gender or the other, for example, prostate cancer in men and cervical cancer in women.

Lifestyle and Environment

The components of a person's lifestyle that affect health status include patterns of eating, use of chemical substances (alcohol, nicotine, caffeine, legal and illegal drugs), exercise and rest patterns, and coping methods. Examples of altered responses are the relationship of obesity to hypertension, cigarette smoking to chronic obstructive pulmonary disease, a sedentary lifestyle to heart disease, and a high-stress career to alcoholism.

The environment has a major influence on health. Occupational exposure to toxic substances (such as asbestos and coal dust) increases the risk of pulmonary disorders. Air, water, and food pollution increase the risk of respiratory disorders, infectious diseases, and cancer. Seasonal temperature variations can result in hypothermia or hyperthermia, especially in the older adult.

Socioeconomic Background

Both lifestyle and environmental influences are affected by one's income level. The culture of poverty, which crosses all racial and ethnic boundaries, negatively influences health status. Living at or below the poverty level often results in crowded, unsanitary living conditions or homelessness. Housing is often overcrowded, lacks adequate heating or cooling, and is infested with insects and rats. Crowded living conditions increase the risk of transferring communicable diseases. Other problems include lack of infant and child care, lack of medical care for injuries or illness, inadequate nutrition, use of addictive substances, and violence.

Geographic Area

The geographic area in which one lives influences health status. Illnesses like malaria are more common in tropical areas of North America. Multiple sclerosis occurs with greater frequency in the northern United States and Canada. There are more cases of skin cancers in people living in sunny, hot areas, and more sinus infections among people living in areas with high humidity.

HEALTH PROMOTION AND MAINTENANCE

For many years, nursing care focused on the acutely ill client in the hospital setting. With changes in society and in health care, this emphasis is shifting toward prevention and community-based care. The focus of this book is not community health nursing. However, teaching health maintenance and providing activities and teaching for continuing care as a client moves among health care settings are two essential aspects of medical–surgical nursing.

Certain practices are known to promote health and wellness:

- Eating three balanced meals a day and including foods based on government recommendations (U.S. Department of Health and Human Services, 2005)
- Eating moderately to maintain a healthy weight
- Exercising 30 to 60 minutes a day
- Sleeping 7 to 8 hours each day
- Limiting alcohol consumption to a moderate amount
- Eliminating smoking
- Keeping sun exposure to a minimum by using sunscreen.

The nurse promotes health by teaching the activities that maintain wellness, by providing information about the characteristics and consequences of diseases when risk factors have been identified, and by supplying specific information about decreasing risk factors, such as recommended immunizations (see Table 2-3 ■). The nurse also promotes health by following healthy practices and serving as a role model.

TABLE 2-3

Routine Immunizations for Adults

VACCINE	INDICATIONS	DO NOT GIVE TO:
Measles-mumps-rubella	Anyone born after 1956 and never infected, or those likely to be exposed, such as those entering college or the military	Pregnant women, immunocompromised people, or anyone with a history of anaphylactic reaction to egg protein or neomycin
Tetanus and diphtheria toxoids	Anyone who has never been vaccinated should have the primary series, followed by booster every 10 years	None identified
Hepatitis B	Anyone likely to have repeated exposure (such as health care providers or sex partners of a known carrier) or who has had exposure (such as a needle-stick injury to a health care worker)	People with a history of anaphylactic reaction to common baker's yeast
Influenza A	Anyone at high risk for complications, health care providers, and those wanting immunity	Those with a high fever, or a history of anaphylactic reaction to egg protein
Pneumococcal pneumonia	Anyone at high risk for pneumonococcal disease and those over 65 years of age	Pregnant women
Varicella	Anyone never infected, especially health care providers and child care workers	Pregnant women, immunocompromised people, those who have received an immune globulin or a blood transfusion within 5 months, or those with a history of anaphylactic reactions to neomycin or gelatin

Illness in the Adult Client

The terms *disease* and *illness* are often used with the same meaning, but in fact they are different. In general, nursing is concerned with illness and medicine is concerned with disease.

DISEASE

Disease (literal meaning, "without ease") is a medical term describing disruptions in structure and function of the body or mind. Diseases may have mechanical causes, biologic causes, or normative causes. *Mechanical causes* of disease damage the structure of the body; they are the result of trauma or extremes of temperature. *Biologic causes* of disease affect body function; they are the result of genetic defects, aging, infestation and infection, changes in the immune system, and alterations in normal organ secretions. *Normative causes* are psychological but involve a mind–body interaction, so physical manifestations occur in response to the emotional disturbance (e.g., nausea).

The 10 leading causes of death in the United States are heart disease, cancer, stroke, chronic lower respiratory disease, unintentional injuries, diabetes, pneumonia/influenza, Alzheimer's disease, kidney disease, and systemic infection (septicemia). The cause of many diseases is still unknown. The following are generally accepted as common causes of disease:

- Genetic defects
- Developmental defects resulting from exposure to viruses, chemicals, or drugs that affect the developing fetus
- Biologic agents or toxins (including viruses, bacteria, and fungi)
- Physical agents, such as temperature extremes, radiation, and electricity
- Chemical agents, such as alcohol, drugs, strong acids or bases, and heavy metals
- Generalized response of tissues to injury or irritation
- Alterations in the production of antibodies, resulting in allergies or hypersensitivities
- Faulty metabolic processes (e.g., a production of hormones or enzymes above or below normal)
- Continued, unabated stress.

In all types of disease, disruptions in structure or function cause **manifestations** (signs and symptoms) that prompt a person to seek treatment. Although both subjective symptoms (such as pain, nausea, and anxiety) and objective signs commonly appear with disease, objective signs often predominate. Examples of objective signs include bleeding, vomiting, diarrhea, limitation of movement, swelling, visual disturbances, or changes in elimination. However, pain (a subjective symptom) is often the main reason a person seeks health care. (Disease classifications are provided in Table 2-4 ■.)

ILLNESS

Illness is the response a person has to a disease. This response is highly individualized, because the person responds not only to his or her own perceptions of the disease but also to the perceptions of others. Illness integrates pathophysiologic

TABLE 2-4	
Disease Classification Definitions	
CLASSIFICATION	**DEFINITION**
Acute	A disease that has a rapid onset, lasts a relatively short period of time, and is self-limiting
Chronic	A disease that has one or more of these characteristics: (1) is permanent, (2) leaves permanent disability, (3) causes nonreversible pathophysiology, (4) requires special training of the client for rehabilitation, (5) requires a long period of care
Communicable	A disease that can spread from one person to another
Congenital	A disease or disorder that exists at or before birth
Degenerative	A disease that results from deterioration or impairment of organs or tissues
Functional	A disease that affects function or performance but does not have manifestations of organic illness
Malignant	A disease that tends to become worse and cause death
Psychosomatic	A psychologic disease that is manifested by physiologic symptoms
Idiopathic	A disease that has an unknown cause
Iatrogenic	A disease that is caused by medical therapy

alterations; psychologic effects of those alterations; effects on roles, relationships, and values; and cultural and spiritual beliefs. A person may have a disease and not categorize himself or herself as ill, or may validate feelings of illness through the comments of others ("You don't look as though you feel well today").

Acute Illness

An **acute illness** occurs rapidly, lasts for a relatively short period of time, and is self-limiting. The condition responds to self-treatment or to medical–surgical intervention. Clients with uncomplicated acute illnesses usually have full recovery and return to normal pre-illness functioning.

The experience of being acutely ill is described as a sequence of behaviors for coping with the alterations in health and function caused by disease. Illness behaviors are highly individual, but the general stages were described by Suchman (1972):

1. In the first stage of an acute illness, a person experiences one or more manifestations that signal a change in normal health. The most significant of these is pain. Others are bleeding, difficulty breathing, swelling, or fever. When manifestations are mild or are familiar (such as symptoms of the common cold or influenza), the person usually uses over-the-counter medications or a traditional remedy for self-treatment. If the symptoms are relieved, no further action is taken. However, if the symptoms are severe or become worse, the person moves to the next stage.

2. In the second stage, the person assumes the sick role, accepting the symptoms as proof that an illness is present. The person usually discusses the symptoms with others and seeks support in deciding whether to get professional treatment or to stay home from school or work. People are self-preoccupied at this stage, focusing on alterations in function that result from the illness. If the illness is resolved, the person confirms health status with others and resumes normal activities. However, if manifestations remain or increase and others agree that no improvement has occurred, the person moves to the next stage.

3. The third stage is seeking medical care. In our society, a physician most often provides validation of illness. People who believe themselves to be ill (and who are encouraged by others to contact a health care provider) make the medical contact for diagnosis, prognosis, and treatment of the illness. If the medical diagnosis is of an illness, the person moves to the next stage. If the medical diagnosis does not support illness, the client may return to normal functioning or may seek a second opinion from a different health care provider.

4. The stage of assuming a dependent role begins when a person accepts the diagnosis and planned treatment of the illness. As the severity of the illness increases, so does the dependent role. During this stage, the person may enter the hospital for treatment and care. The person's responses to care depend on many different variables: the severity of the illness, the degree of anxiety or fear about the outcome, the loss of roles, the support systems available, individualized reactions to stress, and previous experiences with illness care.

5. The final stage of an acute illness is recovery and rehabilitation. The person now gives up the dependent role and resumes normal roles and responsibilities. As a result of education during treatment and care, the person may be at a higher level of wellness after recovery is complete. There is no set timetable for recovery from an illness; each person responds differently. Both the severity of the illness and the method of treatment affect the length of time required, as does the person's compliance with treatment plans and motivation to return to normal health.

Institutional health care focuses on the acute care needs of the ill client. Recovery begins in the hospital and is completed at home. This focus makes client education and continuity of care a major goal for nursing. It has also contributed to a shift in care settings. Increasing numbers of nurses now provide care in community settings and the home.

Chronic Illness

The term chronic illness describes many different lifelong pathologic and psychologic alterations in health. Chronic illness is the leading health problem in the world today, and it is estimated that the number of persons with chronic illnesses will triple by the year 2040. Current trends affecting an increased incidence of chronic illnesses include diseases of aging, diseases of lifestyle and behavior, the AIDS epidemic, and environmental factors.

The National Commission on Chronic Illness states that a **chronic illness** is any impairment or deviation from normal functioning that has one or more of the following characteristics:

- It is permanent.
- It leaves permanent disability.
- It is caused by nonreversible pathologic alterations.
- It requires special teaching of the client for rehabilitation.
- It may require a long period of care.

Chronic illness is also characterized by impaired function in more than one body system. Responses to the impaired function may occur in sensory perception, self-care abilities, mobility, cognition, and social skills. The demands on the individual and family as a result of these responses often last across the life span.

The intensity of a chronic illness and its related symptoms ranges from mild to severe, and the illness is usually characterized by periods of remission and exacerbation. During periods of **remission,** the person does not experience symptoms, even though the disease is still clinically present. During periods of **exacerbation,** the symptoms reappear. These periods of change do not appear in all chronic diseases.

Each person with a chronic illness has a unique set of responses and needs. The response of the person to the illness is influenced by many different factors:

- The point in the life cycle at which the onset of the illness occurs
- The type and degree of limitations caused by the illness
- The visibility of impairment or disfigurement
- The stigma attached to the impairment or disfigurement
- The pathophysiology causing the illness
- The relationship between the impairment and functioning in social roles
- Pain and fear

These factors are highly complex. They are interrelated within each person, resulting in individualized illness behaviors and needs. Because there are so many different chronic diseases and because the experience of each person with the illness is a mix of individualized responses, it is difficult to generalize about needs. However, almost all people with a chronic illness will need to do the following:

- Live as normally as possible, despite the symptoms and treatment that make them feel alienated, lonely, and different from others without the illness.
- Learn to adapt activities of daily living and self-care activities.
- Grieve over the loss of physical abilities, income, status, roles, and dignity.
- Learn to live with chronic pain.

- Follow a medical treatment plan.
- Maintain a positive self-concept and sense of hope.
- Maintain a feeling of being in control.
- Confront the possibility of death at an earlier age.

Some people with chronic illness successfully meet health-related needs; others do not. Research indicates that adaptation is influenced by variables such as anger, depression, denial, self-concept, locus of control, hardiness, and disability. Nursing interventions for the person with a chronic illness focus on education to promote independent functioning, reduce health care costs, and improve well-being and quality of life.

The client with a chronic illness may be hospitalized for diagnosis and treatment of acute exacerbations, but the care of the client is primarily provided at home by family members (such as a spouse). Chronic illness in a family member is a major stressor that may cause changes in family structure and function, as well as changes in performing family developmental tasks.

Many different factors affect family responses to chronic illness. Family responses in turn affect the client's response to and perception of the illness. Factors influencing response to chronic illness include personal, social, and economic resources; the nature and course of the disease; and demands of the illness as perceived by family members.

Client and family considerations for continuing care are integrated throughout this book. Chronically ill clients and families should be given information about helpful literature, self-help or support groups, and interactions with others with the same illness. Information provided by the nurse must be tailored to specific, current needs.

Note: The bibliography listings for this and all chapters have been compiled at the back of the book.

Chapter Review

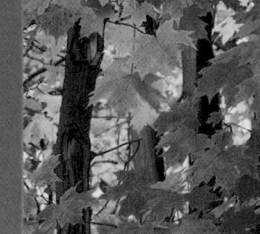

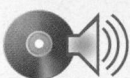 **KEY TERMS** by Topics

Use the audio glossary feature of either the CD-ROM or the Companion Website to hear the correct pronunciation of the following key terms.

Adult client
alterations in health

Family of the adult client
family

Health in the adult client
health, health–illness continuum, high-level wellness

Illness in the adult client
disease, manifestations, illness, acute illness, chronic illness, remission, exacerbation

KEY Points

- The young adult is at the peak of physical development. Risks for alterations in health include accidents, sexually transmitted infections, substance abuse, and physical or psychosocial stressors.

- The middle adult, although physically similar to the young adult, does have age-related changes. Risks for alterations in health include obesity, cardiovascular disease, cancer, substance abuse, and psychosocial stressors.

- All families have structure (family roles and relationships) and function (interactions with other family members and the community). The nurse must consider the needs of the client and the needs of the client's family when providing care.

- Health and illness are affected by many different factors. Nursing interventions to promote health are essential, no matter the degree of illness or the setting in which care is provided.

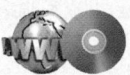 **EXPLORE MediaLink**

Additional interactive resources for this chapter can be found on the Companion Website at www.prenhall.com/burke. Click on Chapter 2 and "Begin" to select the activities for this chapter.

For chapter-related NCLEX-style questions and an audio glossary, access the accompanying CD-ROM in this book.

FOR FURTHER Study

Chapter 3 provides information about older adults. For more about nursing care for clients with substance abuse problems, see Chapter 52.

For more about teaching healthy food choices, see Figure 19-2, the Pyramid. USDA Food Guide

Critical Thinking Care Map

Caring for a Client with Early-Onset Diabetes

NCLEX-PN® Focus Area: Psychosocial Adaptation

Case Study: Alexis Burd has had the chronic illness diabetes mellitus (requiring daily insulin injections) since she was 4 years old. She is now 36 years old, is married, and has two teenage children. While you are weighing Alexis during her regular appointment at the diabetes clinic, she begins to cry and says, "I think this disease controls me more than I control it."

Nursing Diagnosis: Powerlessness

COLLECT DATA

Subjective	Objective
_____	_____
_____	_____
_____	_____
_____	_____
_____	_____
_____	_____
_____	_____

Would you report this data? Yes/No

If yes, to: _____

Nursing Care

_____
_____
_____
_____
_____
_____
_____
_____
_____
_____
_____

How would you document this? _____
_____
_____
_____

Data Collected
(use those that apply)

- Height: 5'3''
- Weight: 156 lbs
- Blood pressure: 126/64
- Fasting blood glucose: 180 (normal 110–130)
- States "I'm not a good mother anymore."
- States "I have done everything I was told to do."
- States "I think I will just stop taking my insulin."

Nursing Interventions
(use those that apply; list in priority order)

- Discuss weight-reduction diet.
- Discuss exercise plan.
- Listen carefully to Alexis's concerns.
- State "Tell me more about how you think diabetes controls you."
- Suggest that Alexis join a diabetes support group.
- Ask Alexis to keep a daily diary of self-management activities.

NCLEX-PN® Exam Preparation

TEST-TAKING TIP Do not read into the questions. When answering a question, remember that the only client you are considering is the one in the question.

1 The young adult is at risk for alterations in health from:

A. accidents, STIs, and substance abuse.
B. obesity, cardiovascular disease, and cancer.
C. chronic illness, stroke, and substance abuse.
D. injuries, pharmacologic therapy, and obesity.

2 What factor often causes the middle adult to gain weight?

A. maintaining calorie intake without increased physical activity
B. physical and psychosocial stressors
C. chronic illness such as arthritis and hypertension
D. normal physiologic changes of aging

3 In comparison to young adults, health promotion behaviors in middle adults include:

A. men no longer needing to do a testicular self-exam.
B. women having a mammogram at age 40.
C. having a vision examination every 4 years.
D. carrying out regular exercise that is strenuous.

4 Significant others related or bonded to the client by birth, adoption, marriage, or friendship are the client's family, and the nurse should:

A. ask them to step out when giving nursing care.
B. expect them to assist with care of the client.
C. speak with them regarding confidential client matters.
D. include them as an integral component of health care.

5 An active process that maximizes the potential capability of a person within the environment where he or she is functioning is known as:

A. health.
B. wellness.
C. continuum.
D. integration.

6 What factors affect a client's ability to understand health teaching?

A. race and ethnicity
B. cognitive abilities and educational level
C. lifestyle and environment
D. socioeconomic background and geographic area

7 The nurse, by following healthy practices, serves as a role model, which is one way to:

A. provide continuity of care.
B. provide acute care.
C. promote health.
D. identify risk factors.

8 The response a person has to disease is called:

A. illness.
B. biologic.
C. normative.
D. developmental.

9 What category of illness occurs rapidly, lasts for a short period, and is self-limiting?

A. remission
B. chronic
C. exacerbation
D. acute

10 Nearly all people with a chronic illness need:

A. to live as normally as possible.
B. to live in a health care facility.
C. to be assisted with activities of daily living.
D. large doses of pain relief medication.

Answers for Review Questions, as well as discussion of Critical Thinking Care Map questions, appear in Appendix V.

RECOGNIZING BIOLOGICAL VARIATIONS AMONG CULTURES

Mrs. Jamie Jean Johnson is a 38-year-old African American woman who is married and the mother of two daughters and one son, ages 16, 14, and 8, respectively. Mrs. Johnson was diagnosed at age 6 with sickle-cell anemia. For the last 5 years, she has remained largely asymptomatic. However, one evening she begins to complain of unbearable pain and is admitted to the hospital in sickle-cell crisis. When she arrives at the hospital, the nurse working in the emergency room takes a history and physical. She notes that Mrs. Johnson's admitting complaints include severe joint pains in both the upper and lower extremities, a temperature of 101.8°F, and shortness of breath. On physical examination, the nurse notes that Mrs. Johnson has coarse rales in the base of both lungs, and that her lips are cyanotic and dry. Her nail beds are also cyanotic, and capillary refill is slow. Initial laboratory examination reveals a hemoglobin of 8 g/dL. The nursing history reveals that Mrs. Johnson has also had problems drinking milk and eating certain dairy products for most of her adult life. In addition, she has begun to eat a great amount of ice. Mrs. Johnson tells the nurse that she craves ice and that it seems to satisfy her and is filling.

During the past three decades, a body of scientific knowledge about biological cultural differences has become evident. In fact, over this same time period, mushrooming literature about biocultural differences has resulted in a field of study known as biocultural ecology. Scientific facts about biological variations can aid the nurse in giving culturally appropriate health care.

Biological Variables Examples

Body weight

- African American men average 166.1 lb, and white men average 170.6 lb.
- African American women average 149.6 lb, and white women average 137.0 lb.
- African American women from 35 to 65 years of age are an average of 20 lb heavier than white women.
- Mexican Americans, on average, weigh more than whites due to truncal fat.
- Socioeconomic status is a predictor of obesity.
- *Nurses' note: Standardized height/weight charts may be inappropriate, because they are based on standard white measurements.*

Skin color

- With darker skin, it is more difficult to assess changes. Baseline skin color can be established using daylight or a 60-watt bulb. Examine least pigmented areas: palms, soles, abdomen, volar surfaces of forearms, buttocks. Also assess nail beds, conjunctiva, and mouth. Oral hyperpigmentation occurs in 50% to 90% of African Americans and in 10% to 50% of whites. The lips of some blacks have a natural bluish hue.

Other visible physical characteristics

- Mongolian spots are more common in African Americans, Asian Americans, Native Americans, and Mexican Americans.
- Keloids are more common in African Americans.

Enzyme and genetic variations

- Many diseases have a genetic linkage. Trauma does not.

Drug interactions and metabolism

- Isoniazid—Up to 60% of whites inactivate this drug slowly and are at risk for peripheral neuropathy. Also, 40% of African Americans, 10% to 40% of Native Americans and Eskimos, and 10% to 15% of Orientals inactivate this drug slowly.
- Primaquine—One hundred million people worldwide (about 35% of African Americans) lack enzyme to digest primaquine and so cannot use it for treatment of malaria.

Disease incidence

- Tuberculosis—Some Native American groups have an incidence 7 to 15 times higher than non–Native Americans. African Americans have an incidence 3 times higher than white Americans.

- Diabetes has a high incidence among Seminoles, Pimas, and Papagos but is rare among Alaskan Eskimos. Diabetes is the seventh leading cause of death in U.S. whites, blacks, Chinese, and Filipinos; it is the fourth leading cause among Native Americans.

Hypertension

- Among African Americans, hypertension has an earlier onset, is more severe, and has a higher mortality than among whites; 35% of African Americans over 40 years of age are hypertensive.
- Prevalence increases with age and is higher in less educated individuals. In young adulthood and early middle age, men are more affected than women; after middle age, the reverse is true.
- *Nurses' note*: *Alertness to risk factors can allow early detection, medical maintenance, and reduced mortality.*

Sickle-cell anemia

- This is a common genetic disorder that affects more than 70,000 Americans. African Americans are the primary group affected, although it also occurs in people from Asia Minor, India, the Mediterranean region, and Caribbean areas.
- *Nurses' note*: *Early recognition and treatment of crisis symptoms are essential.*

(The astute nurse should recognize from the presenting symptoms in the case scenario that Mrs. Johnson is in sickle-cell crisis and needs immediate hospitalization.) Pain control is a crucial concern.

AIDS

- Incidence among African Americans and Hispanics is increasing. African Americans constitute one-eighth of all Americans, but one-fourth of Americans with AIDS. Hispanic Americans constitute one-twelfth of all Americans, but one-seventh of Americans with AIDS.

Lactose intolerance

- Intolerance affects 66% of Mexican Americans and 90% of African Americans, Orientals, and Ashkenazic Jews.
- Most affected clients only need to restrict, not eliminate, lactose-containing foods. Nutritional supplements are not usually needed; pregnant or lactating women may be the exception.

Pica

- Consumption of nonfood items may have originated among undernourished populations. Examples are eating dirt, clay, or ice.

Nursing Implications

- Be aware that people differ in their susceptibility to disease because of biological variations. Data relative to all the significant variables of a racial group are essential for complete assessment.
- Remember that a relationship exists between race and body weight, skin color, other visible physical characteristics, enzymatic and genetic variations, and risk for certain diseases.
- Many diseases, with the exception of trauma, can be linked to a genetic influence. Many common diseases like diabetes or heart disease have both a genetic and an environmental cause. People of certain races may be more susceptible to some diseases or conditions.

Self-Reflection Questions

1. What is your understanding of the role that biological variations play in susceptibility to disease by race?
2. Have you been educated in a system that does not acknowledge biological variation among racial groups?
3. How can you render culturally competent care to persons of different racial, ethnic, or cultural groups without overgeneralizing or stereotyping?

Chapter 3

The Older Adult Client in Health and Illness

LEARNING Outcomes

After completing this chapter, you will be able to:

- Describe what is meant by the term *old*, including who is considered an *older adult*.
- Discuss selected theories of aging, including those involving genetics, immunity, free radicals, and apoptosis.
- Define ageism, incorporating common myths of older adults.
- Compare and contrast cognitive, psychosocial, moral, and spiritual development of the older adult to that of the young and middle adult.
- Explain age-related physical and psychosocial changes common to older adults.
- Describe common threats to the health of the older adult, including chronic illness, accidental injuries, medication management, and dementia and confusion.
- Incorporate actions to promote health and quality of life into nursing care of the older adult.

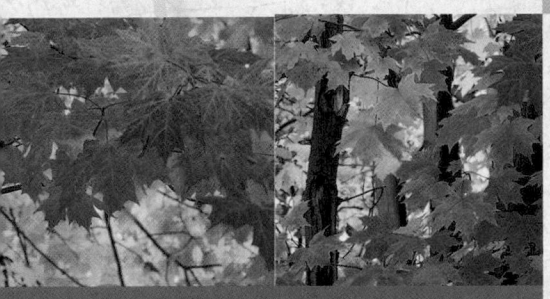

MediaLink

www.prenhall.com/burke
Use the address above to access the free, interactive Companion Website created for this textbook. Get hints, instant feedback, and textbook references to chapter-related NCLEX-style questions. Link to other interesting sites.

Audio Glossary:
Use the Companion Website, or the CD-ROM disk enclosed with your textbook, to hear the pronunciation of key terms in this chapter.

Growing older is not always easy, but it happens to everyone who lives long enough. As one ages, physical and psychosocial processes are altered, developmental tasks continue to influence choices and behaviors, and changes may occur in living arrangements, employment, and income. Added to those areas of adjustment are the very real possibility of loss of a spouse and significant others, changes in role and status, and disruptions in health.

The older adult population (those age 65 years and older) is increasing more rapidly than any other age group. In the last century, the number of adults in the United States living to age 65 or older more than tripled. That percentage is projected to be slightly more than 20% by the year 2030, with the largest increase occurring in adults over the age of 75 (Figure 3-1 ■). At that time the life expectancy is projected to be 78.5 years. Currently, the life expectancy in North America is 77.7 years, with the white population living about 5 years longer than African Americans (Medical News Today, 2005).

The increase in the number of older adults has important implications for nursing. The aging of America will result in a huge demand for health care and social services. Clients needing health care in all settings will be older. They will require nursing interventions and teaching designed specifically to meet their needs. Although **gerontologic nursing** (care of the older adult) is a nursing specialty area, it is also an integral component of medical–surgical nursing (Figure 3-2 ■).

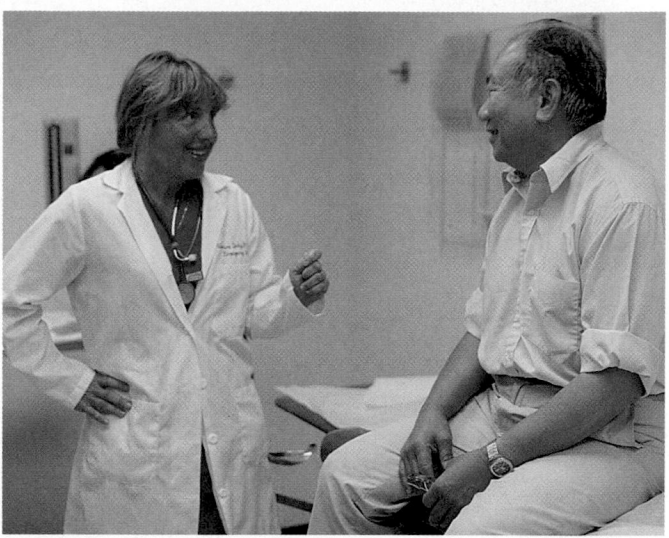

Figure 3-2. ■ The older population is increasing more rapidly than any other age group, making gerontologic nursing a major part of medical–surgical nursing. (Photographer: Richard Tauber.)

What Is Old?

Aging is defined in a number of ways. To some, aging is seen as a universal process beginning at birth. To others, aging is viewed as being "old" or reaching "older adulthood," with people defining *aging* in terms of personal meaning and experience. Based on the 1935 Social Security Act, reaching the age of 65 years has been established as the criterion for

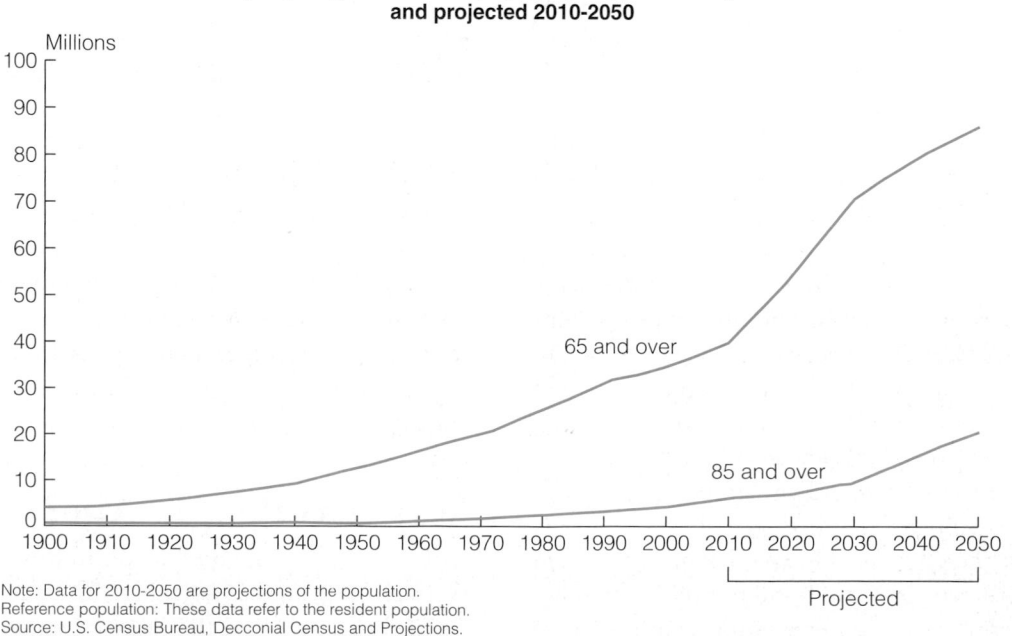

Number of people age 65 and over, by age group, selected years 1900-2000 and projected 2010-2050

Note: Data for 2010-2050 are projections of the population.
Reference population: These data refer to the resident population.
Source: U.S. Census Bureau, Decconial Census and Projections.

Figure 3-1. ■ Number of people age 65 and over, by age group, for selected years 1900–2000 and projected 2010–2050. (*Source:* Federal Interagency Forum on Aging-Related Statistics. [2004]. *Older Americans 2004: Key Indicators of Well-Being.*)

TABLE 3-1

Age and Socioeconomic Characteristics of Older Adults

CHARACTERISTIC	INFORMATION
Average life expectancy remaining on reaching one's 65th birthday	Men: 16.4 years Women: 19.4 years
Number of older adults	Men: 14.8 million Women: 20.8 million
Married	Men: 73% Women: 41%
Older women	50% of those over age 75 live alone About 50% over age 65 are widows
Live alone	31% of those who are noninstitutionalized live alone
Caring for grandchildren	400,000 grandparents age 65 or over have the primary responsibility for their grandchildren who live with them
Median income per year	Men: $19,436 Women: $11,406
Sources of income	Social Security: 91% Assets: 58% Pensions: 40% Earnings: 22%
Living below the poverty line	3.6 million
Completed high school education	70%

Source: Department of Health & Human Services, Administration on Aging. (2003). *Statistics—A Profile of Older Americans: 2003—the Older Population.*

retirement and eligibility for economic and health care benefits. However, most experts in gerontology agree that there is no one age that defines a person as "old" (Miller, 2004).

The older adult period begins at age 65, but it can be further divided into three periods: the "young-old" (age 65 to 74), the "middle-old" (age 75 to 84), and the "old-old" (age 85 and over). The rapid increase projected in the aging population by the 2030s is largely the result of the "baby boom," which refers to the increased number of people born in the post–World War II period from 1946 to 1964. To illustrate the effect on the population, people born from 1946 to 1950 resulted in a 55% increase in the number of 50- to 54-year-olds in the 2000 census. By 2030, those people will be part of the middle-old age group (U.S. Census Bureau, 2001).

In addition to the effect of the baby boom, the United States has experienced growth in migration from other countries. As a result, minority older adults comprise more than 16% of all older Americans, and their numbers are expected to increase even more dramatically than the older white population. For example, the population of white older adults is projected to increase by 81%, whereas minority older adults will increase as follows: African Americans, 128%; Asian Americans, 301%; Hispanic Americans, 322%; and American Indian and Alaska Native, 193% (Agency on Aging, 2001). These numbers have major implications for nurses in providing culturally competent care to an older population.

In addition to characteristics unique to age, the older population also has socioeconomic characteristics that differ from those of younger adults, as well as gender and racial group differences. Age and socioeconomic characteristics are outlined in Table 3-1 ■.

Why Do People Age?

Although there is no one answer to this question, different theories (best guesses by experts in an area) have been developed to try to find the cause of aging. It is known that aging is a complex process with great individual variation. The major theories of aging are categorized as biologic and senescence.

Biologic aging theories examine the basic aging processes that affect all living organisms and try to explain age-related changes. There are many different theories; selected ones include the following:

- Genetic theories emphasize the role of genes in aging. A major idea in this theory is that of a predetermined life span; for example, in humans, about 110 years. Proponents of this theory believe that normal human cells divide 50 times in 110 years and are genetically programmed to begin to deteriorate and stop dividing after that time.
- Immunity theories are based on the knowledge that components of the immune system are affected by aging. Because of this effect, called *immunosenescence,* a person has fewer defenses against foreign organisms with aging. Therefore, the older adult is more susceptible to chronic illnesses such as cancer, arthritis, cardiovascular disease, and Alzheimer's disease.
- The free-radical theory (free radicals are very unstable and reactive molecules, formed during metabolism and in response to environmental pollutants) in which free radicals interact with and damage cellular components, such as lipids and proteins. Antioxidants are among the major protective mechanisms of the body; however, these may become less effective with aging.
- Apoptosis theory is concerned with the mechanisms of cell death (in this case, not the same as necrosis) that maintain normal cell structure and numbers in tissues. Apoptosis is a normal process that occurs throughout life, regulated by opposing genes. With aging, the process becomes imbalanced or ineffective, and the disability and degeneration common to increasing age are seen.

Longevity and **senescence** (aging) theories focus on why people live as long as they do. Studies have found that the factors that influence a long and healthy life include genetic factors, physical environment, physical activity throughout life, consumption of moderate amounts of alcohol, sexual activity persisting into advanced years, dietary factors, and social environment. Other theories have been developed to explain the relationships between aging and health behaviors, and to design interventions to delay the onset of senescence (aging) and chronic illness.

Ageism and Common Stereotypes about Older Adults

Ageism is a form of prejudice (like racism) in which older adults are stereotyped by characteristics found only in a small number of their age group. Basic to the prejudice of ageism is the belief that all older people are different and will remain different; as a result, they do not experience the same needs, desires, and concerns. In an industrial society that values productivity, retired people may be considered to have "outlived their usefulness." In addition, younger generations often lose ties with the older generation because of increased mobility of the family, so many young adults lack experiences with older relatives.

Older adults may be incorrectly pictured as being rigid and narrow minded, unable to learn, unreliable because of memory problems, too old to enjoy sexual pleasure, or childlike and dependent. Many older adults dread growing older, because they believe others will see them as poor, lonely, in frail health, and housed in a nursing home during their final years. These characteristics and descriptions are not true of most older adults. Myths about older adults, compared to the realities of aging, are outlined in Table 3-2 ■. Health care workers may have negative perceptions of older adults, and need to understand that most older adults are healthy and want to maintain their level of health and function as long as possible.

Most older people are satisfied with their lives, enjoying retirement and the time to do more of the things they have not had time to do before. The majority have adequate incomes, live in their own homes, maintain close ties with their families, and maintain an interest in community activities.

TABLE 3-2	
Common Myths about Older Adults	
MYTH	REALITY
Families do not care for older members.	Their families provide 80% of the care of older adults.
Most older adults live in nursing homes.	Only about 5% of older adults live in nursing homes.
Most older adults are sick.	Almost half of all older adults rate their health as good or excellent.
Older adults are incapable of learning new knowledge and skills.	Although the speed that new information is processed becomes slower with age, older adults are capable of learning new things.
Older adults are not interested in sex.	Although sexual activity may be less frequent, the ability to perform and enjoy sexual activity lasts well into the 90s in healthy older adults.
All older adults have problems with constipation and incontinence.	Constipation results from inactivity and diet, not aging. Incontinence is not a part of aging and requires medical attention.

Developmental Aspects of Aging

Although older adults do not continue to grow and develop physically, they do develop in other areas of life and have well-defined stages and tasks.

COGNITIVE DEVELOPMENT

Cognition is a term used to mean the ability to perceive and understand one's world. Cognitive function does not normally change with aging. Intelligence continues to develop and increase well into the 60s, and learning continues throughout life. Older adults do often take longer to process information and to respond, especially in new environments. Nurses should allow extra time when teaching older adults, and should slow the pace of care for those who are ill. Mild short-term memory loss is often experienced, but is managed with lists and calendars. Long-term memory usually remains intact. Dementing diseases do occur and cause cognitive impairment, as discussed later in the chapter.

PSYCHOSOCIAL DEVELOPMENT

Although a person's self-concept and sense of identity remain relatively stable throughout the life span, the way in which the older adult feels about self is often the result of the type of person he or she was before reaching later years. For example, the person who successfully met challenges and made adjustments will be more likely to consider himself or herself healthy and remain socially active. On the other hand, a person who has had difficulty coping with life may find retirement, loss of a spouse, or an illness to be devastating. An early psychosocial theory, called *disengagement theory,* proposed that as people age they become more introspective and focused on self, withdrawing from usual roles and interactions with others. This has been proven untrue; rather as societal interactions decrease (e.g., as a result of retirement), older adults increase their close relationships with family and friends.

Erikson (1963) identified ego integrity versus despair and disgust as the last stage of human development. During this stage, which begins at about 60 years of age, adults begin to reflect on their lives. If they are satisfied, they accept the past as a part of the present along with acceptance of physiologic decline without fear of death. In the process, older adults like to tell stories of their past in what is called *life review* or **reminiscence.** This allows the older adult to relive and restructure life experiences and is part of achieving ego integrity. The same process can be used therapeutically to facilitate coping with change, such as treatment for an illness or moving to a residential care facility. Examples of activities to facilitate reminiscence are listed in Box 3-1 ■.

Havighurst (1972) believed the major tasks of old age centered on maintaining social contacts and relationships, with successful aging depending on one's ability to adapt

---

BOX 3-1

EXAMPLES OF ACTIVITIES TO ENCOURAGE REMINISCENCE
- Choose a comfortable place to sit and talk.
- Use open-ended questions to encourage the person to talk about both negative and positive life events.
- Encourage the person to write about his or her life and share it with family and friends.
- Tape record the person telling the stories, and play this oral history back as appropriate.
- Ask the person to write about significant events on or near the year they occurred (forming a time line of their life).
- Ask family members to bring in pictures or scrapbooks that depict events in the person's life.
- Encourage the person to develop a family tree. Many sources are now available on the Internet about genealogy.

---

to age-related roles. He described the developmental tasks for later maturity as adjusting to decreasing physical strength and health, adjusting to retirement and reduced income, adjusting to death of a spouse, establishing an affiliation with one's age group, adjusting and adapting social roles in a flexible way, and establishing a satisfactory physical living arrangement.

MORAL AND SPIRITUAL DEVELOPMENT

According to Kohlberg (1969), older adults have completed the stages of moral development, and are at the conventional level, following society's rules and meeting the expectations of others. Spiritually, most older adults integrate faith and truth to see the reality of their own beliefs, trusting in a greater power and believing in the future. By integrating the past and future into the present, the older adult facilitates acceptance of where one is in life without regretting past mistakes or fearing the future in a process of self-transcendence (Reed, 1996). With aging, spirituality and transcendence are sources of strength when faced with inevitable changes and loss. Many older adults openly express their spiritual beliefs with pictures, bibles, and religious items such as rosaries or crucifixes. It is very important for health care providers to respect the older adult's views and take proper care of these items if the older adult is not able to do so.

Experiencing and Adapting to Change

The older adult is a member of a unique population in the world today. Older adults have lived the longest and experienced the most change, both in themselves and in the society in which they live. Adaptation is necessary with advancing age because of limitations involving one's spouse, loss of health, or changing economic ability and living arrangement. Numerous role changes are necessary, and lost roles must be replaced with those that are satisfying to the person. Depending on the ability to adapt to change, older adults may live out their remaining years happy and at peace or be in a state of conflict and confusion.

AGE-RELATED PHYSICAL CHANGES

As we age, the number of cells of the body is gradually reduced. Lean body mass decreases, but fat tissue increases until one is in the 60s. Bone mass and intracellular fluids tend to decrease. As a result, older adults are at increased risk for bone fractures from falls and trauma, and from dehydration in response to illness or environmental heat.

Many physical changes are obvious, including hair graying and loss, wrinkled skin, baggy eyelids, facial hair in women,

and a reduction in height by about 2 inches by age 80 years. These changes are gradual over time and are highly individualized. Some people look old at 50, whereas others still retain a youthful appearance when they are 70. Other age-related changes affect specific body systems, as summarized in Table 3-3 ■. More detailed information is provided in each assessment chapter of this book, and nursing actions specific to age-related physical changes are integrated throughout the text.

Most older adults adjust their lifestyle over time to accommodate age-related changes. Although continued physical activity and exercise are important, regular periods of rest are also needed. With decreasing body reserves, the older adult is at increased risk for both acute and chronic illnesses. As a result,

TABLE 3-3

Age-Related Physical Changes in the Older Adult

ASSESSMENT	CHANGES
Skin	■ Decreased turgor and sebaceous gland activity result in dry, wrinkled skin. ■ Melanocytes cluster, causing "age spots" or "liver spots."
Hair and nails	■ Scalp, axillary, and pubic hair thins; nose and ear hair thickens. ■ Women may develop facial hair. ■ Nails grow more slowly; may become thick and brittle.
Sensory	■ Visual field narrows, and depth perception is distorted. ■ Pupils are smaller, reducing night vision. ■ Lenses yellow and become opaque, resulting in distortion of green, blue, and violet tones and increased sensitivity to glare. ■ Production of tears decreases. ■ Sense of smell decreases. ■ Age-related hearing loss progresses, involving middle- and low-frequency sounds. ■ Threshold for pain and touch increases. ■ Alterations in proprioception (sense of physical position) may occur.
Musculoskeletal	■ Loss of overall mass, strength, and movement of muscles occurs; tremors may occur. ■ Loss of bone structure and deterioration of cartilage in joints result in increased risk of fractures and in limitation of range of motion.
Cardiovascular	■ Systolic blood pressure rises. ■ Cardiac output decreases. ■ Peripheral resistance increases, and capillary walls thicken.
Respiratory	■ Continued loss of vital capacity occurs as the lungs become less elastic and more rigid. ■ Anteroposterior chest diameter increases. ■ Although blood carbon dioxide levels remain relatively constant, blood oxygen levels decrease by 10% to 15%.
Gastrointestinal	■ Production of saliva decreases, and a decrease in the number of taste buds decreases accurate receptors for salt and sweet. ■ Gag reflex is decreased, and stomach motility and emptying are reduced. ■ Both large and small intestines have some atrophy, with decreased peristalsis. ■ The liver decreases in weight and storage capacity; gallstones increase; pancreatic enzymes decrease.

(continued)

TABLE 3-3

Age-Related Physical Changes in the Older Adult (continued)

ASSESSMENT	CHANGES
Genitourinary	■ Kidneys lose mass, and the glomerular filtration rate is reduced (by nearly 50% from young adulthood to old age). ■ Bladder capacity decreases, and the micturition reflex is delayed. Urinary retention is more common. ■ Men may have an enlarged prostate gland. ■ Reproductive changes in men include decreased testosterone and sperm count; smaller testes; increased time to achieve an erection and penis is less firm when erect. ■ Reproductive changes in women include decreased estrogen, vaginal lubrication, and breast tissue; atrophy of the vagina, uterus, ovaries, and urethra; and increased alkalinity of vaginal secretions.
Endocrine	■ Pituitary gland loses weight and vascularity. ■ Thyroid gland becomes more fibrous, and plasma T_3 decreases. ■ Pancreas releases insulin more slowly; increased blood glucose levels are common. ■ Adrenal glands produce less cortisol.

diet modifications and prescribed medications may be necessary, as well as learning to live with some pain from common chronic illnesses such as arthritis. The older adult is at greater risk for injuries from accidents and falls, and may need to curtail driving or use some type of assistive device to remain mobile. All of these factors cause some loss of independence.

AGE-RELATED PSYCHOSOCIAL CHANGES

Psychosocial changes for the older adult include the illness or death of a spouse, decreased or limited income, retirement, isolation from friends and family because of distance, lack of transportation, or relocation to a long-term health care facility. A further change may be role loss or reversal, for example, when the wife becomes the caretaker of her chronically ill husband.

Widowhood

Life changes immeasurably when a spouse dies, even though it is a common event. Suddenly the remaining spouse is faced with not only adjusting to the loss of the loved person, but also to living alone. **Widowhood** (loss of a spouse) affects more women than men, both because women live longer and because most older men are married. Many older women find that income from the husband's pension or retirement is discontinued or reduced, necessitating living on a sharply reduced income. Sexual desires are unfulfilled and the number of single friends is limited. However, after the initial grief diminishes, most widows adjust well.

Retirement

The loss of one's role as a worker through retirement is a major adjustment for aging adults. When one's work is the primary interest and focus of life, activities, and social contacts, separation from employment leaves a large void. In addition, income may be significantly reduced, despite pensions and

Social Security benefits, with retirement income often being half of the income earned when employed. However, many retirees take advantage of more free time to become more active in volunteer activities, to join senior citizen groups for socialization, and to do things they enjoy but have not previously had time to do (Figure 3-3 ■).

Living Arrangements

Although almost all older adults would prefer to live in their own homes, and many do, it is not always possible. The ability to function safely and independently at home alone depends on one's functional health, transportation, income, and family or support systems. Many older adults, even though in poor health, can continue living at home with some assistance from home health services, home delivered meals, and senior

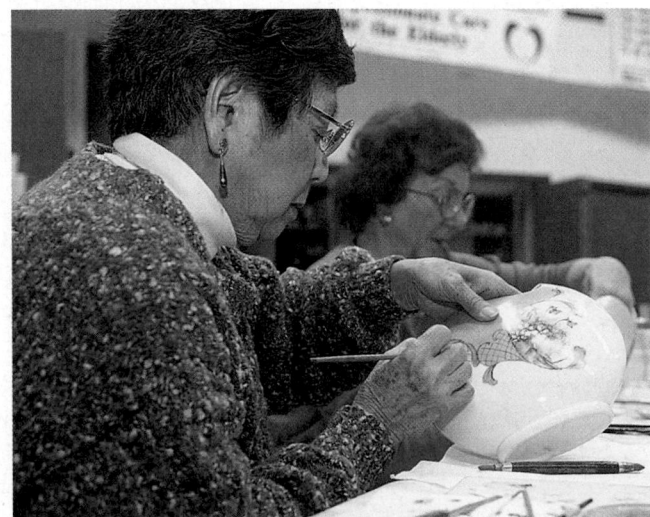

Figure 3-3. ■ Many older adults find creative outlets during retirement. (Photographer: Elena Dorfman.)

transportation. Assisted-living housing for older adults is becoming more common, providing housekeeping, meals, and health care services. Some areas now provide "aging-in-place" models, where people are provided the care needed as they advance in age. There are many different types of housing options for older adults; a selected few are described as follows:

- Home modification, such as replacing door knobs with handles, replacing faucet handles with levers, and installing grab bars in bathrooms, may allow older adults to remain in their own home.
- Senior retirement communities offer rental apartments or houses for people who are mobile and can care for themselves. Meals may be available, housekeeping services may be provided (at additional cost), social and recreational activities are carried out, and transportation is provided.
- Residential care facilities provide services that include room, meals, personal care, and medical care.
- Long-term care facilities provide skilled nursing care, including meals, personal care, and medical care. Bedrooms and bathrooms may be shared.

Health of the Older Adult

The older adult is at risk for alterations in health from a variety of causes, including chronic illnesses, accidental injuries, medication management, and dementia. This section provides a broad overview of the health care problems and needs of the older adult; more specific information is found throughout the book.

CHRONIC ILLNESS

Approximately 40% of all older adults report having a limitation caused by a chronic illness, with more than 80% having at least one disability and 50% having at least two (Centers for Disease Control and Prevention [CDC], 2004). The most frequently occurring conditions in the older adult are arthritis, hypertension, hearing and vision impairments, cardiovascular diseases, cataracts, sinusitis, orthopedic disorders, diabetes, and Alzheimer's disease. These conditions can cause years of pain, disability, and loss of function and independence before resulting in death. The leading causes of death are heart disease, cancer, and stroke.

In the older adult, the accumulation of years of exposure to environmental hazards such as sun and noise may be manifested by skin cancer or impaired hearing. The older adult (especially the older male) may develop respiratory disorders, from years of smoking or from exposure to pollutants in the work environment. The older adult with limited income may live in substandard housing and may suffer heat- or cold-related illness and even death.

As described by the CDC (2004), new challenges have been created by the increase in life span and the increasing incidence of chronic illness in older adults. Currently, Medicare

spending has increased seven-fold compared to 20 years ago, and is expected to double again by 2010. By 2030, health care spending will increase by 25% simply because the population will be older. Nearly 79% of people who need long-term care live at home or in a community setting rather than an institution. As a result, 59% of the adult U.S. population either is or expects to be a family caregiver. The value of family caregivers, considered "free," is estimated to be $257 billion a year.

Some suggested areas for teaching older adults how to cope with chronic illness follow:

- Encourage them to assume responsibility for their own health care by getting as much information from as many sources as possible.
- Try to define what has been lost, so as to develop alternate ways to regain those lost functional abilities.
- Recognize that behavior that is appropriate for acute illness may not be adaptive when a person is chronically ill.
- Deal with emotional realities and go forward with life.
- Try to accept the way things are at this moment in time.
- Be positive.

ACCIDENTAL INJURIES

Injuries in the older adult cause many different problems: illness, financial burden, hospitalization, self-care deficits, loss of independence, and even death. The risk of injury is increased by normal physical changes that accompany aging, by changes in health, by environmental hazards, and by lack of support systems. The three major causes of injury in the older adult are falls, fires, and motor vehicle crashes. Of these causes, falls that result in hip fractures are the most significant in terms of long-term disability and death.

Older adults should practice the following to avoid injury:

- Have adequate lighting in all rooms of the house including stairs, basements, and bedrooms. Use nightlights in bedrooms, bathrooms, and halls.
- Avoid sitting or standing rapidly; if dizziness occurs, remain in one position until dizziness is gone.
- Have handrails installed by the toilet and in the shower or bathtub.
- Do not use throw rugs.
- Install smoke alarms.
- Never step into a tub or shower without checking the temperature of the water.
- Always wear corrective lenses and/or hearing aids when driving.
- Do not drive a car after taking medications that cause drowsiness or dizziness.

clinical ALERT

Elder abuse and neglect further increase the risk of injury or illness.

MEDICATION MANAGEMENT

The average older adult in the community has 11 prescriptions filled each year. Although older adults constitute 13% of the total population, they consume 34% of all prescriptions (CDC, 2004). Older adults also consume over-the-counter medications in addition to those prescribed. While these medications do make life more comfortable for the older adult, they carry a risk of adverse drug reactions and interactions as a result of drug–drug interactions and a decreased ability of the liver and kidneys to detoxify and excrete substances. Adverse effects such as dizziness, numbness, dehydration, anorexia, nausea, and diarrhea can have more serious consequences than in younger adults. These consequences include falls, depression, confusion, hallucinations, and malnutrition. Factors contributing to problems with medication management in this age group include decreased metabolism, nutritional problems, visual deficits, memory changes, cost, and noncompliance.

Nurses must have knowledge of medications, and how their effects may differ for older adults. For example, older adults should not take or be given barbiturates, such as pentobarbital (Nembutal), because they are highly addictive and increase the risk of drug–drug interactions, or the narcotic meperidine (Demerol), which can accumulate and cause seizures. Other drugs to avoid because of their toxic effects include the antidepressants amitriptyline (Elavil) and doxepin (Sinequan), the antihypertensive methyldopa (Aldomet), and gastrointestinal antispasmodics hyoscyamine (Anaspaz) and propantheline (Pro-Banthine). Both coumadin and digoxin are commonly prescribed for older adults and have a high risk of toxicity. Pharmacology is discussed in Chapter 6. ∞

BOX 3-2

HEALTHY BEHAVIORS IN THE OLDER ADULT

- Eat a variety of nutrient-dense foods and beverages within and among the basic food groups while choosing foods that limit the intake of saturated and trans fats, cholesterol, added sugars, salt, and alcohol.
- Choose a diet low in fat (30% or less of total calories), saturated fat (less than 10% of calories), and cholesterol (less than 300 mg daily). Choose foods high in fiber, low in sodium, and high in potassium.
- People with dark skin and those with little sunlight exposure should consume extra vitamin D from fortified foods or supplements.
- Individuals with hypertension and blacks should consume no more than 1,500 mg of sodium each day.
- Increase calcium intake to 1,200 mg daily.
- If weight loss is needed, aim for a slow, steady loss by decreasing caloric intake while maintaining an adequate nutrient intake and increasing physical activity.
- Make exercise a part of life, carrying out regular exercise that is moderately strenuous, is consistent, and avoids overexertion; exercise for 30 to 60 minutes every day, if possible.
- Have an annual vision examination, including a test for glaucoma. (Medicare covers a test for glaucoma every 12 months for people at high risk).
- Practice good oral hygiene with teeth brushing and flossing and have a dental checkup one to two times a year.
- Have a physical examination annually, including blood studies for glucose and cholesterol. (Medicare covers a one-time physical examination if conducted within the first 6 months of having Medicare Part B. Tests for diabetes are covered, with number of times per year depending on number of risk factors. Medicare covers costs for cholesterol, lipids, and triglyceride levels every 5 years.)
- For women, have a bone density examination. (Bone density examinations are covered by Medicare every 24 months [or more if medically necessary] for those at risk for osteoporosis.)
- For women, have a mammogram every year. Do a breast self-examination every month and have a breast examination annually. (Medicare covers mammograms once every 12 months for all women age 40 and older.)
- For women, have an annual pelvic examination and Pap test as recommended by their health care provider. Women who have had a total hysterectomy (with removal of the uterus and cervix) may choose to stop having Pap tests unless the surgery was done to treat cervical precancer or cancer. Women who are at high risk for hereditary nonpolyposis colon cancer should be offered a screening for endometrial cancer with endometrial biopsy beginning at age 35. (Medicare covers a pelvic examination and Pap test every 24 months for all women and once every 12 months for those at high risk.)
- For men, a prostate-specific antigen (PSA) blood test and a digital rectal examination (DRE) should be offered annually. Men at high risk (African American men and those who have a family history of father or brothers diagnosed with prostate cancer at an early age) should begin testing at age 45. (Medicare covers a DRE and PSA test once every 12 months for all men over age 50.)
- Have one of the following to screen for colon cancer: yearly fecal occult blood test (FOBT) or fecal immunochemical test (FIT); flexible sigmoidoscopy every 5 years; yearly FOBT or FIT plus flexible sigmoidoscopy every 5 years; double-contrast barium enema every 5 years; or colonoscopy every 10 years. Individuals who have an increased risk of colon cancer because of previous colon cancer, a personal history of chronic inflammatory bowel disease, a family history of colon cancer, or who have had adenomatous polyps should have screening more often. (Medicare pays for one or more of these depending on the test prescribed and the level of risk.)
- Use sunscreen and avoid sunburn.
- Obtain an annual influenza immunization and have the pneumonia vaccine at age 65. (Medicare pays for an annual influenza shot once a year in the fall or winter and covers the cost of the pneumoccal shot, which most people only need once.)

Note: Medicare pays costs of examinations only for people with Medicare coverage.

DEMENTIA AND CONFUSION

Although growing older is often associated with becoming demented, this is not true. **Dementia** is a term used to refer to different kinds of organic disorders that progressively affect cognitive function, and it is **not** a part of the normal aging process. Although there are various dementias, the one most devastating to the older population, as well as society as a whole, is Alzheimer's disease (AD). AD is the most common degenerative neurologic illness and the most common cause of cognitive impairment (Porth, 2005). Scientists do not know what causes AD, but they do know that age is the most important risk factor, with the number of people with AD doubling every 5 years after age 65. It is believed that as many as 4.5 million Americans have AD, with almost half of those 85 years and older having the disease (Alzheimer's Disease Education and Referral Center, 2004). The early symptoms of AD, such as loss of concentration and forgetfulness, are frequently missed because the same symptoms are common with aging. However, it is important to note that AD is not considered a normal part of aging. AD is discussed in detail in Chapter 39. ⚭

Sometimes, confusion and depression in an older adult are mistaken for true dementia. It is important to assess for other causes, including circulatory or metabolic problems, electrolyte imbalances, effects of medications, or nutritional deficiencies. An older adult may also become confused when too many changes or losses occur at one time or when he or she is moved to a different environment. A type of confusion called **sundowning syndrome** may also occur, in which the older adult becomes confused after dark.

Nursing Care to Promote Health

Older adults get the same benefits from health teaching that young adults and middle adults do. They should never be viewed as being "too old" to learn healthy living practices. However, nurses should adapt teaching methods to this age group, such as by using charts and literature with large print. Hospitals, long-term care facilities, retirement centers, outpatient clinics, senior citizen centers, and other community settings all provide health education for the older adult. The nurse promotes health in the older adult by encouraging the behaviors listed in Box 3-2 ■, and by providing nursing care as outlined in Table 3-4 ■.

It is important to remember that illness and loss of independence are not inevitable consequences of aging. The following actions, described by the CDC (2004) to improve older Americans' health and quality of life are:

■ **Healthy lifestyles:** People who are physically active, eat a healthy diet, do not use tobacco, and practice other healthy

---

TABLE 3-4

Nursing Care to Promote Health in Older Adults

FUNCTIONAL AREA	NURSING ACTIONS
Physiologic function	■ Establish a baseline, and monitor for changes on an ongoing basis. ■ Review beliefs about current health status and health problems. ■ Maintain a list and periodically review use of prescribed, over-the-counter, and herbal or supplemental medications. ■ Provide nursing care to maintain physical status, such as skin care and assisting with activities of daily living.
Psychosocial function	■ Discuss major stressors, such as illness, injury, hospitalization, or change in living arrangements. ■ Assess and encourage use of sources of support and strength, including family, friends, pets, community resources, and cultural and spiritual values and rituals. ■ Encourage independent decision making about care. ■ Encourage life review and reminiscence. ■ Encourage self-care. ■ Develop plans of care that are individualized to the client's background, interests, capabilities, values, culture, and lifestyle.
Cognitive function	■ Ensure eyeglasses and hearing devices are used; ensure lenses are clean and batteries are good. ■ Slow pace of activities. ■ Wait for responses during conversations. ■ Encourage interaction with other people.
Sleep and rest	■ Discourage excessive napping. ■ Assess and use information about normal bedtime, time for rising, and bedtime rituals. ■ Assess effects of pain, medications, and anxiety on sleep.

(continued)

TABLE 3-4

Nursing Care to Promote Health in Older Adults (continued)

FUNCTIONAL AREA	NURSING ACTIONS
Nutrition	■ Assess for lost or damaged teeth and state of dentures if present. ■ Assist with oral care as necessary. ■ Provide food the client is able to chew and swallow. ■ Assess height, weight, eating patterns, and food choices. ■ Suggest programs such as Meals-on-Wheels if appropriate.
Elimination	■ Assess frequency of urinary elimination, including problems with urinary incontinence. ■ Assess normal times for bowel movements. ■ Monitor frequency and consistency of bowel movements, and if a problem is present, consider effects of diet, activity, and medications. ■ Review diet for fiber and fluid intake.
Activity and exercise	■ Assess mobility; ensure assistive devices (such as a cane or walker) are available. ■ Consider effects of illness, surgery, medications, and changes in diet and fluid intake on strength and motor function. ■ Recommend moderate exercise 30 minutes each day.
Safety	■ Assess ability to swallow. ■ Review medications with the client, including type, dosage, and times of administration. ■ Ensure an environment that is free of clutter and well lit. Suggest removing throw rugs and using night-lights. ■ Discuss safety of neighborhood and community.
Sexuality	■ Assist as necessary with hygiene, hair care, clean clothing, makeup, and shaving. ■ Maintain a clean, odor-free environment. ■ Ask preferred name. ■ Respect belongings. ■ Discuss safer sex if appropriate. ■ Discuss vaginal lubricants with women; refer men for evaluation of erectile dysfunction if appropriate.

behaviors reduce their risk for chronic illnesses and have half the rate of disability as those who do not (Figure 3-4 ■).

■ **Early detection of diseases:** Screening to detect chronic diseases (with examinations such as mammograms and colonoscopies) when they are early in their course and most treatable can save many lives.

■ **Immunizations:** Immunizations for influenza and pneumonia reduce the risk of hospitalization and death. More than 40,000 people age 65 and older die each year of influenza and pneumonia.

■ **Injury prevention:** Falls are the most common cause of injuries to older adults. More than one-third of adults age 65 and older fall each year, and of that number, 20% to 30% have moderate to severe injury that reduces mobility and independence.

■ **Self-management techniques:** Programs to teach older Americans self-management techniques for illnesses such as diabetes and arthritis can reduce both the pain and the costs of chronic disease.

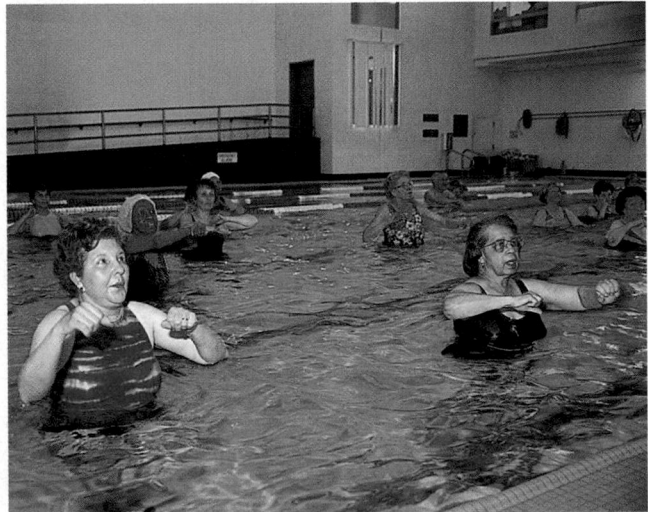

Figure 3-4. ■ A regular program of exercise is important for maintenance of joint mobility and muscle tone and can promote socialization. (Photographer: Elena Dorfman.)

Chapter Review

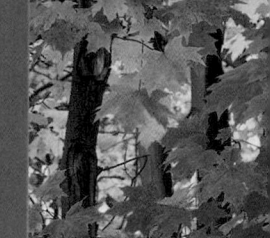

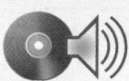 **KEY TERMS** by Topics

Use the audio glossary feature of either the CD-ROM or the Companion Website to hear the correct pronunciation of the following key terms.

Aging
gerontologic nursing, senescence, ageism

Developmental aspects
cognition
reminiscence
psychosocial changes
widowhood

Health of the older adult
dementia
sundowning syndrome

KEY Points

- Aging may be defined in many ways, including age in years as well as by personal definition. Older adulthood may be divided into three periods: "young-old" (ages 65 to 74), "middle-old" (ages 75 to 84), and "old-old" (ages 85 and over). The rapid increase in older adults in the United States is the result of the baby boom and increased growth of minority populations.

- The theories of why people age include genetics, immune factors, free radicals, and cell death (apoptosis). Scientists also study the factors that influence having a long and healthy life, which include genetic inheritance, physical environment, physical activity, and diet.

- Ageism is a form of prejudice in which older adults are stereotyped by characteristics found in only a small number of their age group. Most older adults are satisfied with their lives, have adequate income, live in their own homes, are close to family and friends, and take part in community activities.

- Older adults continue to have developmental tasks. Cognition does not normally change with age. As people age it is important for them to review their lives through reminiscence in order to achieve ego integrity. Most older adults are at the moral development stage of the conventional level, and find strength in spirituality and transcendence.

- Aging does bring physical changes as well as the strong probability of psychosocial changes involving widowhood, retirement, and living arrangements.

- The older adult is at risk for alterations in health from chronic illnesses, accidental injuries, medication management, and dementia.

- Nursing care to promote health in older adults includes teaching healthy behaviors and encouraging healthy lifestyles, preventive medicine (including screening examinations and immunizations), injury prevention, and self-management of illness.

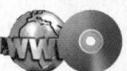 **EXPLORE MediaLink**

Additional interactive resources for this chapter can be found on the Companion Website at www.prenhall.com/burke. Click on Chapter 3 and "Begin" to select the activities for this chapter.

For chapter-related NCLEX-style questions and an audio glossary, access the accompanying CD-ROM in this book.

FOR FURTHER Study

Pharmacology is discussed in Chapter 6.

For information about loss and end-of-life care, see Chapter 14.

For more on Alzheimer's disease, see Chapter 39.

For NANDA diagnoses, see Appendix II.

NCLEX-PN® Exam Preparation

TEST-TAKING TIP Only change an answer for a multiple-choice question if you have misread or misinterpreted the question because your first answer is usually the correct one.

1 What is the major factor in the projected increase in the number of older adults during the next 30 years?

A. a significant decrease in chronic illness in older adults
B. decreased physical effects of longevity
C. increased number of people known as "baby boomers"
D. increased efforts to provide effective home care

2 The immunity theory of aging supports the idea of immunosenescence, meaning people have fewer defenses against foreign organisms with aging. What results from this?

A. increased risk of chronic illnesses
B. people living a predetermined life span
C. decreased tolerance of environmental pollutants
D. an imbalance in cell regeneration and cell death

3 A member of your health team says, "Oh, that old lady in Room 232 won't be able to learn how to take her own pulse." What is this an example of?

A. reality
B. ageism
C. critical thinking
D. nursing process

4 Which of the following statements is true of cognitive function in the older adult?

A. "The ability to learn new skills ends at about age 45."
B. "Dementia is inevitable as one reaches the 70s."
C. "Long-term memory loss interferes with learning."
D. "Cognitive function normally does not change."

5 You are caring for an older woman in a long-term care facility. She says, "When I was ten years old, my parents took me to the circus and I had such a good time." What does this statement facilitate?

A. problems with short-term memory
B. achievement of ego integrity
C. inability to cope with change
D. increasingly living in the past

6 What two terms might best describe the time following widowhood?

A. loss, loneliness
B. bitterness, sadness
C. peace, strength
D. friends, family

7 You are caring for an older man who has been hospitalized for treatment of pneumonia. He says, "I want to be able to live in my own home, but I don't know if I can." What topic would you discuss with him?

A. need for nursing home care
B. services of the local community center
C. educational opportunities at a local college
D. assistance from home health services

8 Which of the following chronic diseases is a leading cause of death in older adults?

A. pneumonia
B. influenza
C. stroke
D. arthritis

9 You are caring for an older adult who is caring for herself at home alone. What would you assess on a regular basis to facilitate safety?

A. her temperature, pulse, and respirations
B. prescribed and over-the-counter medications
C. amount of food in her refrigerator
D. condition of the windows in her house

10 Which of the following nursing actions will facilitate cognitive function in an older adult?

A. Give a complete bed bath.
B. Ensure the television is on.
C. Monitor ability to use walker or cane.
D. Ensure hearing aid battery strength.

Answers for Review Questions appear in Appendix V.

Settings of Care

BRIEF Outline

LEARNING Outcomes

After completing this chapter, you will be able to:

- Define community-based nursing care.
- Identify types of community-based health care services.
- Discuss the components of home health and the roles of the home health nurse.
- Describe nursing care guidelines and special considerations for home health care.
- Apply the nursing process to care of the client in the home.
- Describe the philosophy of and nursing care to facilitate rehabilitation.

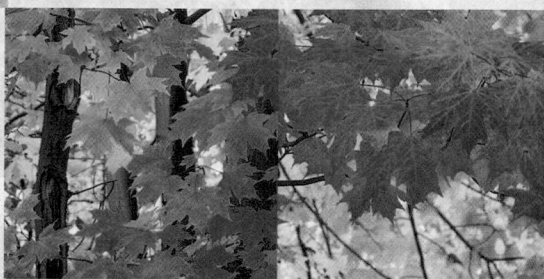

MediaLink

www.prenhall.com/burke

Use the address above to access the free, interactive Companion Website created for this textbook. Get hints, instant feedback, and textbook references to chapter-related NCLEX-Style questions. Link to other interesting sites.

Audio Glossary:

Use the Companion Website, or the CD-ROM disk enclosed with your textbook, to hear the pronunciation of key terms in this chapter.

As recently as two decades ago, clients went to the hospital for almost all health care services, including diagnostic tests and minor surgery. Now, hospitals have become primarily acute-care centers with services focused on high-technology care for severely ill or injured people or for people having major surgery. Even these clients rarely remain in the hospital for long periods of time. They are moved as rapidly as possible to less acute-care settings within the hospital and then to community-based care. Health care has changed from a pay-for-service inpatient method of delivery to a managed-care, community-based system. This shift in health care settings has changed the way nurses provide interventions to promote and restore health. Although many nurses are still employed in hospitals, nursing care is increasingly provided outside the hospital setting.

Community-Based Nursing Care

A community is many things. Encompassing a specific geographic area, a community may be a small neighborhood in a major urban city or a large area of rural residents. Communities have in common the characteristics of people, area, social interaction, and common ties. However, each community is unique. People who live in a community may share a culture, history, or heritage. Although a community is where people live, have homes, raise families, and carry on daily activities, people within a community often cross community boundaries to work or to seek health care.

In contrast to community health nursing, which focuses on the health of the community, **community-based nursing** focuses on culturally competent individual and family health care needs. Nurses practicing community-based care provide direct services to individuals to manage acute or chronic health problems and to promote self-care. Nursing care is based on a philosophy that directs nursing care for clients wherever they are, including where they live, work, play, worship, and go to school.

Nurses provide community-based care in many different settings. Depending on their level of education, they do activities that range from leading support groups in a hospital (for individuals and family members diagnosed with illnesses such as cancer or diabetes), to managing a free-standing clinic, to providing care in the client's home.

Types of Community-Based Health Care Services

Many different types of community-based health care services are available, including community-based health centers and clinics, day care programs, long-term care facilities,

---

BOX 4-1

COMMUNITY-BASED NURSING CARE SETTINGS

- Hospitals
  Inpatient care
  Outpatient (ambulatory) surgery
  Outpatient diagnostics and treatments
  Cardiac rehabilitation
  Support groups
  Education groups
- County health departments
- Senior centers
- Long-term care
- Parish nursing
- Adult day care centers
- Homeless shelters
- Mobile vans
- Mental health centers
- Schools
- Crisis intervention centers
- Ambulatory surgery centers
- Alcohol/drug rehabilitation
- Health care provider offices
- Health care clinics
- Free clinics
- Urgent care centers
- Rural health centers
- Home care
- Hospice care
- Industry
- Jails and prisons

---

parish nursing, and meals-on-wheels. Box 4-1 ■ illustrates the varied settings within the community in which a nurse may provide care.

COMMUNITY CENTERS AND CLINICS

Community centers and clinics may be directed by physicians, advanced practice nurses in collaboration with physicians, or advanced practice nurses who work independently (depending on state regulations). These health care settings may be located within a hospital, be part of a hospital but located in another area, or be independent of a hospital base. Health care centers and clinics provide a wide range of services and often meet the health needs of clients who are unable to get care elsewhere. This group includes the homeless, the poor, those with substance abuse problems, those with sexually transmitted infections, and the victims of violent or abusive behavior. Licensed practical/vocational nurses are often employed in community centers and clinics to carry out basic assessments (such as weights and vital signs), to assist the physician or advanced practice nurse with examinations, and to teach the client any needed self-care activities.

DAY CARE PROGRAMS

Day care programs, such as senior centers, are usually found in a location where people gather for social, nutritional, and recreational purposes. These programs vary from community to community. Meals may be provided at low cost. Adult day care also provides a great service for working families who are caregivers for family members with chronic illnesses who require supervision during the day.

LONG-TERM CARE FACILITIES

People who are mentally or physically unable to care for themselves independently may require health care and help with activities of daily living in a **long-term care** facility. The care may be a short stay for rehabilitation, or it may last for years. Many different types of long-term care facilities are available, including skilled care, intermediate and long-term care, transitional (from the acute care setting) care, assisted living facilities, nursing homes, retirement centers, and residential institutions for people of all ages who have disabilities.

The number of long-term care facilities has increased for several reasons. Care of clients at home after increasingly short hospital stays is often beyond the abilities of the client and family. Such clients are often transferred to a long-term facility for care until they can use home care. In addition, many older adults do not have any family available to provide care but can no longer safely care for themselves. More and more older adults are moving to retirement centers, where they remain independent as long as they can, and then have nursing care and other services (such as meals) readily available.

Nursing homes are long-term facilities that provide care primarily for older adults. The focus is on maintaining client function and independence. Concern for the clients' well-being, and increased knowledge of the importance of the environment, has resulted in more homelike surroundings that include plants, birds, and pets. Legislation to maintain standards of quality assurance in the nursing home industry was mandated by the 1987 Omnibus Budget Reconciliation Act (OBRA).

The roles of the nurse in long-term care include providing direct care, serving as a unit manager, and teaching and supervising other health care providers. Almost all long-term care facilities require that care given to residents be performed only by or under the direct supervision of a licensed nurse. The licensed practical/vocational nurse, directed by the registered nurse, provides direct care, administers medications, and supervises the care administered by nursing aides.

PARISH NURSING

Parish nursing and **block nursing** are nontraditional ways of providing health promotion and health restoration nursing interventions to specific groups of people. Both of these types of care are community based and meet the needs of people often underserved by the traditional health care system.

A nurse who practices parish nursing works with the pastor and staff of a faith community to promote health and healing through counseling, referrals, teaching, and assessment of health care needs. A parish nurse may be employed by a hospital and contracted by a church, employed directly by a church, or work as a volunteer with the congregation of a church. The parish nurse helps bridge gaps between members of the church and the health care system.

MEALS-ON-WHEELS

Many communities have a food service, usually called Meals-on-Wheels, for older people who do not have assistance in the home with food preparation. A hot, nutritionally balanced meal is delivered once a day, usually at noon. Volunteers often deliver the meals, providing not only nutrition but also a friendly, caring visit each day.

Home Health Care

Nursing care in the home differs in many ways from nursing care in a hospital setting. Nurses are invited into homes as guests; they cannot assume entry as they do in formal clinical settings. The environment belongs to the client, who retains control. Every nursing action must communicate respect for these boundaries. Nurses must establish trust and rapport quickly, because most home health nurses are with each client for only 1 hour a few times a week. Home care is the responsibility of a group of health care providers collaborating as a team, with a physician responsible for the orders for care, the registered nurse completing an initial assessment and developing the plan of care, the practical nurse providing nursing interventions and directing the care provided by nursing aides, and the nursing assistant providing physical care.

Home health care includes health and social services, provided to the chronically ill, disabled, or recovering person in his or her own home. Home care is also provided as a person nears the end of life, in a program called *hospice* (hospice care is discussed in Chapter 14). Home care is usually provided when a person needs help that cannot be provided by a family member or friend on an ongoing basis for a period of time. Among clients who benefit from home health care services are those who:

- Cannot live independently at home because of age, illness, or disability
- Have illnesses such as congestive heart failure, heart disease, kidney disease, respiratory diseases, diabetes mellitus, or muscle–nerve disorders

- Are terminally ill and want to die with comfort and dignity at home (see Chapter 14) ⚭
- Do not need inpatient hospital or nursing home care but require additional assistance
- Need short-term help at home because of outpatient surgery

Services provided within the home include professional nursing care, home health care assistance, physical therapy, speech therapy, occupational therapy, medical social worker services, and nutritional services. Clients receiving home health care services are under the care of a physician, with the focus of care being treatment or rehabilitation. Nursing care is provided by registered nurses or licensed practical/vocational nurses based on physician orders. These nurses give direct care, supervise other health care providers, coordinate client care with the physician, advocate for the client and family, and teach family members and friends how to care for the client.

HISTORY OF HOME CARE

The concept of nurses meeting health care needs in the home and community is not new. Although many sources say the birth of home care in the United States occurred when the Boston Dispensary's first home care program opened in 1796, it wasn't until visiting nursing associations were established in the late 1800s that care of the sick in their own homes took hold.

At that time, few hospitals were available to handle the health and illness problems of a nation experiencing both rapid growth in its cities and a large influx of immigrants. Illness and hygiene problems resulted from substandard living and working conditions. In response, several philanthropic individuals and organizations sponsored nurses to visit the sick poor in their homes.

The role of the nurse then, as today, was to advocate for the client, provide direct care, and educate the client. Both illness care and health promotion were the nurse's principal focus.

The passage of Medicare in 1965, Medicaid in 1970, the addition of hospice benefits in 1973, and the introduction of diagnosis-related groups in 1983 have dramatically affected home care. In 1965, Medicare legislation entitled the nation's elderly to home care services, primarily skilled nursing and other therapies of a curative or restorative nature. This same benefit was extended to certain younger Americans with disabilities in 1973. As a result, between 1967 and 1980, the number of Medicare-certified home health agencies nearly doubled.

This number doubled again when diagnosis-related groups were introduced. **Diagnosis-related groups (DRGs)** are categories for reimbursement of inpatient services. The DRG system pays a predetermined amount of money for the care of different persons with the same medical diagnosis. DRGs were introduced in an effort to control the rapidly increasing costs of health care. Prior to their introduction, Medicare reimbursed hospitals on a cost-plus basis, paying for the actual cost of caring for an individual plus other allowable expenses, such as depreciation of facilities and administrative costs.

Today, approximately 20,000 providers deliver home health care services to 7.6 million people who require care because of acute illness, chronic health conditions, permanent disability, or terminal illness (National Association for Home Care, 2004). This number is predicted to grow, making home health an exciting and challenging setting for nursing care.

HOME HEALTH AGENCIES

Home health agencies are either public or private organizations that provide skilled nursing and other therapeutic services in the client's home. All home health agencies must meet uniform standards for licensing, certification, and accreditation. Home health agencies include the following:

- *Official or public agencies.* These are agencies operated by state or local governments, financed primarily by tax funds. Most official agencies offer home care, health education, and disease-prevention programs in the community.
- *Voluntary or private not-for-profit agencies.* These agencies are supported by donations, endowments, charities such as the United Way, and third-party reimbursement. They are governed by members of a volunteer board of directors, which usually represent the community they serve.
- *Private, proprietary agencies.* Most of these agencies are for-profit organizations and are governed by either individual owners or national corporations. Although some of these agencies participate in third-party reimbursement, others rely on "private-pay" sources.
- *Institution-based agencies.* These agencies operate under a parent organization, such as a hospital. The home health agency is governed by the sponsoring organization, and the mission of both is similar. Often, most of the home health referrals come from the parent organization.

COMPONENTS OF HOME HEALTH CARE

This discussion provides basic information about the requirements and standards for home care nursing in general. Rules and regulations for home care and for nursing licensure mandate at what level of education the nurse must be to carry out activities. Nurses who practice home care do so within a system where clients, referrals and reimbursement sources interact.

Home Care Clients

The client in home health is both the person receiving care and the person's family. The client's family is not limited to persons related by birth, adoption, or marriage, but may be lovers, colleagues, other significant people, and even animals.

Even though home care is provided to clients of all ages, age and functional disability are the main predictors of need for home care services. A national survey by the Agency for Health Care Policy and Research found that (1) about half of all home care clients are over the age of 65, and (2) the number of home care services that are needed seems to increase with the client's age (National Association for Home Care, 2004).

Family dynamics are more visible in the home. As the nurse becomes a familiar presence and the family's behavior relaxes, the nurse can gain a clearer and more complete picture of family issues and relationships, lifestyle choices, and coping patterns.

"Families of one" are a worrisome reality for home health nurses. Today, more older adults are living alone. Some may have current or potential caregivers nearby; others have no one. These people often require considerable nursing support to remain strong, independent, and resourceful. Caring for "families of one" can take a toll on even the strongest home health nurse. Some nurses have reported calling between visits, keeping in touch after discharge, and driving by on days off because they have such difficulty "letting go" of their concerns about these clients.

Finally, caregiver burden is not easily hidden in the home. Millions of Americans are taking care of relatives and friends with disabilities, and many of the caregivers are themselves older adults. Health care planners picture the home as a place where all kinds of medical services can occur, but they may give little thought to how people manage. Few ever ask whether families can cope with the level of care they are expected to assume. Caregiving is now recognized as a complex activity that requires adjustment in family living patterns, relationships, and finances. For some families, the crisis of caregiving is short lived, but for others it lasts for years. As a result, caregivers are at great risk for both physical and emotional illness. The success of home care heavily depends on the supports in place, so it is crucial to address the needs of the support network.

Referrals for Home Care

A referral source is a person who recommends home health services and supplies the agency with details about the client's needs. A referral source can be a physician, nurse, social worker, therapist, or discharge planner. Families sometimes generate their own referrals, either by approaching one of the sources already mentioned or by calling a home health agency directly. When the family seeks a referral and the agency feels that the client qualifies for services, the agency contacts the client's physician and requests a referral on the client's behalf.

The nurse considers making a referral to a home health agency, a hospice, or a community resource if the client has a need for formal follow-up beyond the present clinical setting. Hospital discharge planners, social workers, organizations for the aged, and local nonprofit agencies usually have a good command of the services and support groups available in their communities.

The nurse must talk to clients and their caregivers about their concerns related to home management. It is quite common for family members to disagree about whether additional help is necessary. Steps the nurse can take include leading an informal family meeting in which everyone shares concerns and asking about the family's insurance coverage for home health care. Suggesting services when families have no funds to pay for them only adds to the problem. For clients with limited means, the nurse can identify staff who are knowledgeable about funding and consult with them. It is always important for the nurse to avoid making assumptions. Intelligent, well-educated, and financially secure clients can be just as overwhelmed by illness as the less educated and the poor. Everyone is a referral candidate.

If the family feels that no help is necessary and the nurse feels otherwise, the nurse may suggest an evaluation visit, explaining that the situation may look different once the client is home. If family members continue to refuse, the nurse lets them know that the door is never closed and gives them contacts in the community to call independently if their needs change.

Once a referral is made and an initial set of physician orders is obtained, a nursing assessment visit is scheduled to identify the client's needs. If the input of another provider, such as a physical therapist, is necessary to complete the initial assessment, the nurse arranges for this visit. Data may be collected and the treatment plan formulated through collaboration of the LPN/LVN and RN. Home care cannot begin without a physician's order and cannot proceed without a physician-approved treatment plan.

At the nursing assessment visit, the nurse identifies client needs and begins to formulate the plan of care. Box 4-2 ■ lists Medicare's required data for the nursing plan of care. The plan of care is sent back to the physician for review and approval. The physician's signature on the plan of care authorizes the home health agency's providers to continue with services and also serves as a contract indicating agreement to participate in the care of the client on an ongoing basis.

BOX 4-2

MEDICARE'S REQUIRED DATA FOR THE PLAN OF CARE

1. All pertinent diagnoses
2. A notation of the beneficiary's mental status
3. Types of services, supplies, and equipment ordered
4. Frequency of visits to be made
5. Client's prognosis
6. Client's rehabilitation potential
7. Client's functional limitations
8. Activities permitted
9. Client's nutritional requirements
10. Client's medications and treatments
11. Safety measures to protect against injuries
12. Discharge plans
13. Any other items the home health agency or physician wishes to include

Source: Medicare Health Insurance Manual-11, Section 204.2.

Reimbursement Sources for Home Care

A reimbursement source is a party that pays for home health services. Medicare is home care's largest single reimbursement source. Other reimbursement sources include Medicaid, public funding, private insurance, public donation, and self-pay.

The treatment (or care) plan formulated by the home health agency providers and authorized by the physician is used by the reimbursement source. Only interventions identified on the treatment plan are paid for. The reimbursement source evaluates each treatment plan to determine whether the goals and plans set forth by the professional providers match the needs assessed. Periodically, the reimbursement source may ask for the home health provider's notes to substantiate what is being done in the home. Therefore, accurate documentation is critical.

Medicare's regulations for reimbursement are the model for many other third-party payers. Medicare has specifically defined what skilled services will be reimbursed in home health. Medicare does not reimburse visits made to support general health maintenance, health promotion, or clients' emotional or socioeconomic needs. There are very specific criteria that both client and nurse must meet in order to secure Medicare reimbursement. The client must meet all of the following criteria:

- The client must be in need of "reasonable and necessary" home care with a "skilled need."
- The client must be essentially homebound.
- The client must have a plan of care that meets the necessary Medicare criteria.
- The client must require interventions on an intermittent basis only.

Medicare will reimburse only when the skilled provider performs at least one of the following tasks:

- Teaching about a new or acute situation
- Assessing an acute process or a change in the client's condition
- Performing a skilled procedure or a hands-on service requiring the skill, knowledge, ability, and judgment of a licensed nurse.

ROLES OF THE HOME HEALTH NURSE

The roles of the home health nurse are similar to those of nurses in any setting: provider of care, educator, and advocate (discussed in Chapter 1). ◐◑

Provider of Care

Home health nurses usually are not involved in providing personal care for clients (bathing, changing linens, etc.). Routine personal care usually is provided by the family or by a home health aide arranged for by the nurse. However, if a personal care need arises during the course of the skilled visit (e.g., if a client has an incontinent episode), the nurse typically either bathes and changes the client or assists the caregiver to do so before moving on to the skilled activities planned for the visit.

The nurse uses the nursing process to assess, diagnose, plan and implement care, and evaluate client needs. During the course of this process, home health nurses frequently perform specific procedures and treatments, such as physical assessments, care of intravenous lines, ostomy care, wound care, and pain management. The assessments and interventions for each home visit are documented. In addition, Medicare requires completion of an assessment form called the outcome and assessment information set (OASIS). This form represents core items of a comprehensive assessment and plan of care for the adult home care client and is the basis for measuring patient outcomes.

Teacher

Clients need help understanding their situations, making health care decisions, and changing health behaviors. It is unrealistic to believe that clients can be taught everything they need to know during a short hospital stay. The nurse should recommend a home health referral for anyone who needs follow-up teaching.

When preparing clients for discharge, the nurse focuses on safety and survival first. Even if health education is to continue with home care, a day or two may elapse before the nurse arrives. The nurse must not discharge clients without giving them the right information and supplies to get them through the first few days at home.

Clients must have complete information about their medications. They must be given a list of manifestations of

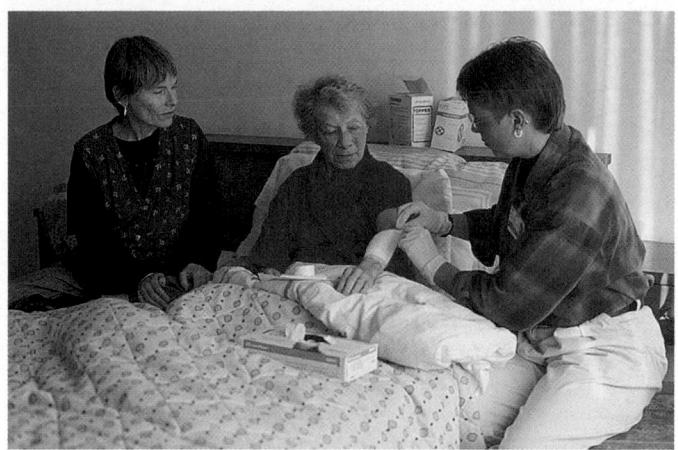

Figure 4-1. ■ The home health nurse often provides client education. This nurse is teaching the client and family member how to apply dressings. (Photographer: Richard Tauber.)

complications they should report to their doctor. Finally, they must be able to manage any necessary treatments at least minimally. This means not only performing procedures safely but also knowing how to obtain necessary supplies in the community.

Most of the home health nurse's time is spent teaching about illness care and disease prevention (Figure 4-1 ■). Often, the greatest educational challenge is to motivate the client. Even the most dedicated nurses can have trouble discovering what will make the client want to learn and how to focus the client on what is most important. Despite the work involved, the nurse's reward is knowing that clients have learned to manage independently. Because the nurse's role as educator is increasingly important, continuing care is included in the discussion of every major disorder in this text.

Advocate

As client advocate, the nurse explores, informs, supports, and affirms the choices of clients. As a protector of client rights, the nurse discusses advance medical directives, living wills, durable power of attorney for health care, and the home health agency's bill of rights. Box 4-3 ■ provides an example of a home health agency's bill of rights.

During the course of care, clients may need help negotiating the complex medical system (especially in regard to medical insurance), accessing community resources, recognizing and coping with required changes in lifestyle, and making informed decisions. When the family's desires differ from those of the client, advocacy can be a challenge. It is impossible for the nurse to please everyone. If a conflict arises, the nurse must remain the primary client's advocate, regardless of any negative response from the family.

GUIDELINES FOR HOME HEALTH NURSING CARE

ANA Standards

Home health nurses are responsible for adhering to the same codes and standards that guide all other nurses. These codes and standards (see Chapter 1) ⚭ guide nursing practice and protect the public. The American Nurses Association (ANA) has established *ANA Standards for Home Health Nursing Practice* and *ANA Standards of Community Health Nursing* as a basis for the practice of nursing in the home. The standards reflect the current state of knowledge in the field of home and community health nursing and should be the criteria for evaluating quality care.

National Association for Home Care Bill of Rights

Another source of guidance regarding home care is the National Association for Home Care (NAHC) bill of rights. The Home Care Bill of Rights grew out of a comprehensive code of ethics the NAHC adopted in 1982. In 1987, Congress made it a requirement for all home health agencies to use this bill of rights. Although home health agencies may make additions to the NAHC's original bill of rights, they are required by law to review it with all home health clients on the initial visit.

Ethical and Legal Guidelines

The legal issues in home health center on privacy and confidentiality, client access to health information, freedom from unreasonable restraint, witnessing of documents, informed consent, and negligence or malpractice. Nurses can best avoid lawsuits by familiarizing themselves with the standards of practice, providing care that is consistent with standards and with their agency's policies, and documenting all care fully and accurately according to agency guidelines.

SPECIAL CONSIDERATIONS IN HOME HEALTH CARE

Safety and infection control in the home are priority concerns for the home health nurse. Other considerations are outlined in Table 4-1 ■.

Safety

Safety assessment in the home is a nursing responsibility and a legal requirement. Nurses cannot close their eyes to an unsafe environment. On the first and later visits, the nurse must alert the family to unsafe and hazardous conditions, suggest remedies, and document the family's response to the nurse's suggestions. In particular, nurses must remain alert to the following conditions:

■ How clients handle stairs
■ How they manage their own care if they are alone

BOX 4-3

A HOME HEALTH AGENCY'S BILL OF RIGHTS

The agency acknowledges the client's rights and encourages the client and family to participate in their plan of care through informed decision making. In accordance with this belief, each client/family member will receive, prior to admission, the following bill of rights and responsibilities.

1. The client and the client's property will be treated with respect by the program's staff.
2. The client will receive care without regard to race, color, creed, age, sex, religion, national origin, or mental or physical handicap.
3. The client has the right to be free from mental and physical abuse.
4. The client's medical record and related information are maintained in a confidential manner by the program.
5. The client will receive a written statement of the program's objectives, scope of services, and grievance process prior to admission.
6. The client, family, or guardian has the right to file a complaint regarding the services provided by the program without fear of disruption of service, coercion, or discrimination.
7. The client will be advised of the following in advance of service:
   a. Description of services and proposed visit frequency.
   b. Overview of the anticipated plan of care and its likely outcome.
   c. Options that may be available.
8. The client/family is encouraged to participate in the plan of care. The client will receive the necessary information concerning the client's condition and will be encouraged to participate in changes that may arise in care.
9. The program shall provide for the right of the client to refuse any portion of planned treatment to the extent permitted by law without relinquishing other portions of the treatment plan, except where medical contraindications exist. The client will be informed of the expected consequences of such action.
10. The client has a right to continuity of care:
    a. Services provided within a reasonable time frame.
    b. A program that is capable of providing the level of care required by the client.
    c. Timely referral to alternative services, as needed.
    d. Information regarding impending discharge, continuing care requirements, and other services, as needed.
11. The client will be informed of the extent to which payment will be expected for items or services to be furnished to clients by Medicare, Medicaid, and any other program that is funded partially or fully with federal funds. On admission, the client will be informed orally and in writing of any charges for items and services that the program expects will not be covered on admission. The client will be informed of any change in this amount as soon as possible, but no later than within 25 days after the program is made aware of the change.
12. On request, the client may obtain
    a. An itemized bill.
    b. The program's policy for uncompensated care.
    c. The program's policy for disclosure of the medical record.
    d. Identity of health care providers with which the program has contractual agreements, insofar as the client's care is concerned.
    e. The name of the responsible person supervising the client's care and how to contact this person during regular business hours.
13. The client has the right to obtain medical equipment and other health-related items from the company of the client's choice and assumes financial responsibility for such. The program's staff will assist in obtaining supplies and physician approvals as needed.
14. The client/family is responsible for
    a. Giving the program accurate, necessary information.
    b. Being available and cooperative during scheduled visits.
    c. Assisting, as much as possible, in the plan of care.
    d. Alerting the staff to any problems as soon as possible.

Source: Adapted from the Patient Bill of Rights and Responsibilities, Bon Secours Home Health and Hospice. Baltimore, MD.

- The presence of a smoke detector in the home (the fire department will often install one free if notified)
- The presence of bathroom safety equipment
- Electrical hazards
- Slippery throw rugs, clutter, or furniture arrangements that may cause a fall
- Expired medications
- Inappropriate clothing or shoes
- Cooking or smoking habits that may start a fire
- An inadequate food supply
- Poorly functioning utilities
- Signs of abusive behavior
- Safe handling of medical gases, such as oxygen.

Obviously, nurses cannot go into homes and change the family's living space and lifestyle, but they can register their concern and reactions if the situation could lead to an injury or if they suspect abuse or neglect. Within the home and community setting, ignoring an unsafe environment is considered nursing negligence. Documentation should address what information the nurse has covered, the family's response to the teaching, and assessment of their ongoing practice of safety precautions.

Infection Control

Infection control in the home centers on protecting clients, caregivers, and the community from the spread of disease. Within the home, nurses may encounter clients with infectious or communicable diseases, clients who are immunocompromised, or clients with multiple access devices, drainage tubes, or draining wounds. The home presents a challenging

TABLE 4-1	
Suggestions for Effective Home Health Care	
WHAT IS IMPORTANT?	**WHAT TO DO**
Making the first contact with the client	■ Suggest someone else be with the client during the first home visit, just to "help them listen." ■ Stress important information and repeat it on following visits. ■ Speak slowly and directly to the client. ■ Allow client and family members time to process the information.
Establishing trust and rapport	■ Find common ground; establish that the nurse is a guest in the client's home. ■ Offer suggestions that include the client's right to say "no." ■ Maintain a respectful distance from the client. ■ Notice and respect family values and customs. ■ Listen carefully to stories.
Assessing the overall home environment	■ Note sights, sounds, and smells. ■ Note dress, tone of voice, and body language. ■ Note visiting patterns of family members and significant others. ■ Note the appearance of the living space, yard, sidewalk, and neighborhood.
Promoting client's ability to learn	■ Teach information needed for safety until the next home visit. ■ Set priorities by a need-to-know, want-to-know, ought-to-know basis. ■ Teach while providing care whenever possible.
Paying attention to the needs of the client	■ Limit distractions as much as possible, but ask before turning off music or television. ■ Be honest about allergies to pets or difficulty hearing because of noise.
Being flexible	■ Enter the home with a plan, but be prepared to modify it. ■ Set goals *with* the client, not *for* the client.

environment for infection control. Nurses must teach the importance of effective hand washing, the use of gloves, the disposal of wastes and soiled dressings, the handling of linens, and the practice of standard precautions.

NURSING PROCESS IN HOME HEALTH CARE

The nursing process is the same for home care as for any other setting. Differences lie in assessing how the home's unique environment affects the need or problem and in using outcome criteria and mutual participation to plan goals and interventions.

Assessing

Assessment begins when the nurse calls the client to arrange a visit. That telephone call can yield much information. How alert, oriented, and stressed does the client (or family) seem to be? Does the client know the reason for the home health referral? How open to intervention do the client and family seem to be? Have they encountered any difficulties since discharge from the prior setting? Are there any supplies they need on the first visit? Because most agencies require submission of a plan of care within 48 hours of the first home visit, careful and complete data collection is essential. Nurses also collect information on an ongoing basis.

The nurse must collect the information requested on the tools and forms contained in the agency's admission packet. Many packets include a physical and psychosocial database; an OASIS assessment form; a medication sheet; forms for pain assessment, spiritual assessment, financial assessment; and a family roster. Through interviewing, direct observation, and physical assessment, the nurse gains as clear and accurate a picture of the client as possible.

Diagnosing

After the initial assessment is completed, the actual or potential client problems are identified. The label of the problem (the nursing diagnosis) varies from agency to agency. No matter which method is used, meaningful statements describing the client's issues must be part of the home health record. These statements, based on data collection, are used to organize care and to justify reimbursement. Although it is the RN (not the LPN or LVN) who makes the nursing diagnosis, LPNs and LVNs contribute greatly to this process.

Planning

Planning includes setting priorities, establishing goals, and deciding on interventions to meet the needs of the client. The greatest level of success occurs when clients feel ownership of the plan. For this reason, planned interventions and expected outcomes should be client centered, realistic, achievable, and mutually agreed on. Goals and expected outcomes should be documented clearly in timed, measurable, and observable terms. These measures help clients and care providers focus their work together and evaluate the effectiveness of care. The expected outcomes are a way for the reimbursement source to judge the appropriateness of the plan of care.

Implementing

The home health nurse implements the plan of care that was mutually developed with the client. Some interventions may be carried out by another agency provider, by a paraprofessional brought in by the nurse case manager, or by the client.

Evaluating

Evaluation involves (1) comparing the plan of care with the goals that are achieved from visit to visit, and (2) reviewing the client's progress toward goals in order to determine the client's eligibility for discharge. Because reimbursement sources require that all skilled services be justified, many home health agency charts include space to evaluate the client's response to interventions and to document a plan of care for the next scheduled visit.

Rehabilitation

Rehabilitation is the process of learning to live to one's maximum potential with a chronic impairment and the resulting functional disability. Rehabilitation nursing is based on a philosophy that each person has a unique set of strengths and abilities that can enable him or her to live with dignity, self-worth, and independence. This philosophy applies to clients with both acute and chronic illnesses. Many rehabilitative services are provided in community-based settings.

The terms *impairment, disability,* and *handicap* are often used as synonyms, but they have different meanings. An **impairment** is a disturbance in structure or function resulting from physiologic or psychologic abnormalities. A **disability** is the degree of observable and measurable impairment. A **handicap** is the total adjustment to disability that limits functioning at a normal level. For example, following a motorcycle crash, Kim Rushin had damage to her left leg that resulted in an impairment in the ability to flex her knee. This resulted in a 50% disability of that leg and caused a handicap because Kim was a school bus driver and could no longer operate the bus safely. See the Critical Thinking Care Map on health promotion for Kim at the end of this chapter.

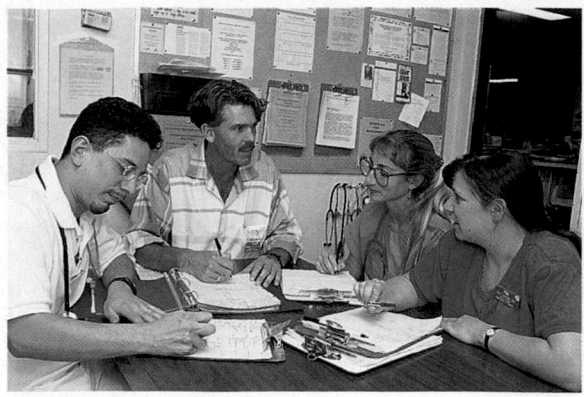

Figure 4-2. ■ The rehabilitation team discusses the client's plan of care. (Photographer: Alain McLaughlin.)

INTERDISCIPLINARY CARE

Rehabilitation promotes reintegration into the client's family and community through a team approach. The plan of care includes many different aspects of the client's life: physical function, mental health, interpersonal relationships, social interactions, and vocational status. This comprehensive consideration of the client requires the expertise of a team of health care providers. The rehabilitation team usually meets weekly to discuss the achievement of client goals (Figure 4-2 ■). As a part of this comprehensive plan of care, the following points are included:

■ Assessing the level of function
■ Developing an individualized and holistic plan of care, with ongoing evaluation of outcomes
■ Including the family in the plan of care
■ Implementing discharge planning to ensure a smooth transition to home.

NURSING CARE IN REHABILITATION

The nurse provides care for the chronically ill client of all ages and with many types of disability. The 20-year-old man with quadriplegia from a spinal cord injury has needs that are different from those of the 75-year-old woman who has had a stroke and is unable to move her left arm or speak. However, the plan of care developed for each of these clients considers common factors in assessing and planning individualized interventions.

Assessment of the client's needs begins with the first contact and continues throughout care. Assessment includes functional level and self-care abilities, educational needs, psychosocial needs, and the home environment. It is critical to determine the client's and family's priorities before establishing any plan of care. Questions for assessment include the following:

■ What is the client's present level of physical function (mobility, self-care, communication, skin integrity, bowel and bladder function)?

- What are the client and family short-term and long-term goals?
- Are those goals realistic and attainable?
- What concerns are verbalized by the client and family (financial, work, housing, school, transportation, sexual activities, social activities, relationships)?
- What stage of grief and loss is present (denial, anger, bargaining, acceptance)?
- To what home environment will the client be going?
- What resources are available to assist reintegration (personal, support, community, federal)?

Nursing interventions to assist rehabilitation are revised to meet client and family needs as the client progresses toward reintegration. In the acute-care stage, the nurse focuses on interventions that will prevent complications. As recovery progresses, the nurse develops and implements individualized teaching plans for the client and family. General areas of interventions include the following:

- Preventing infection
- Maintaining correct body alignment, position, and range of motion
- Preventing skin breakdown
- Providing adequate nutrition and fluids
- Providing care as necessary and appropriate, with the goal of achieving a level of independence that is realistic for the client
- Referrals to community agencies (nursing care, special equipment or supplies, support groups, counseling, physical therapy, occupational therapy, respiratory therapy, vocational guidance, house cleaning, meals).

To ensure continuity of care during rehabilitation, the home health nurse is often involved in the plan of care during the acute-care stage. Continued education and support of the client and family are essential. The achievement of self-care and mobility does not guarantee that the client can function independently in all areas.

Note: The bibliography listings for this and all chapters have been compiled at the back of the book.

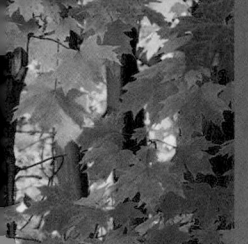

Chapter Review

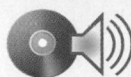 **KEY TERMS** by Topics

Use the audio glossary feature of either the CD-ROM or the Companion Website to hear the correct pronunciation of the following key terms.

Community-based nursing care
community-based nursing

Types of community-based health care services
long-term care, parish nursing, block nursing

Home health care
home health care, diagnosis-related groups (DRGs)

Rehabilitation
rehabilitation, impairment, disability, handicap

KEY Points

- Community-based nursing care focuses on individual and family health care needs, with nurses providing care in a variety of community settings, including community centers and clinics, day care programs, churches, long-term care facilities, and homes.

- Long-term care facilities provide health care and activities of daily living for people who are mentally or physically unable to care for themselves.

- Home health agencies are organizations that provide skilled nursing and other therapeutic services in the client's home. Nurses make the initial visit and collect data to develop a plan of care. The plan of care is implemented and evaluated within the special characteristics of the home as a nursing care setting.

- Rehabilitation nursing care is often provided in community-based settings. The goal of rehabilitation nurses is to assist clients to again become a part of their family and community.

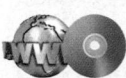 **EXPLORE Media**Link

Additional interactive resources for this chapter can be found on the Companion Website at www.prenhall.com/burke. Click on Chapter 4 and "Begin" to select the activities for this chapter.

For chapter-related NCLEX-style questions and an audio glossary, access the accompanying CD-ROM in this book.

FOR FURTHER Study

For more information about nursing roles and nursing codes and standards, see Chapter 1.

For further information about caring for clients who are terminally ill and want to die with comfort and dignity at home, see Chapter 14.

Critical Thinking Care Map

Caring for a Client with a Handicap
NCLEX-PN® Focus Area: Coping and Adaptation

Case Study: After seriously damaging her left leg in a motorcycle crash 6 months ago, Kim Rushin is no longer able to drive a school bus safely. As part of the rehabilitation team that is caring for Kim, what data would you collect and what interventions would you suggest?

Nursing Diagnosis: Deficient Knowledge: Overcoming Handicap from Knee Injury

COLLECT DATA

Subjective	Objective
_____	_____
_____	_____
_____	_____
_____	_____
_____	_____
_____	_____

Would you report this data? Yes/No

If yes, to: _____

Nursing Care

_____
_____
_____
_____
_____
_____
_____
_____
_____
_____
_____
_____

How would you document this? _____
_____
_____
_____

Data Collected
(use those that apply)

- Age 28
- Unmarried
- Height 5′6″
- Weight 140 lbs
- BP 120/72
- Unable to bend left leg more than 15 degrees
- States "I can't keep my present job."
- States "I don't know where to go for help."

Nursing Interventions
(use those that apply; list in priority order)

- Teach crutch-walking techniques.
- Perform passive range-of-motion exercises on Kim's left leg.
- Suggest career counseling.
- Ask Kim if she has ever considered other types of employment.
- Recommend that Kim join Weight Watchers or similar group.
- Refer Kim to vocational rehabilitation services.
- Suggest that Kim take more time to adjust.

NCLEX-PN® Exam Preparation

1   Nursing care provided directly to clients wherever they are, including where they live, work, play, worship, and go to school, is known as:

   A. home health nursing.
   B. community health nursing.
   C. community-based nursing.
   D. parish nursing.

2   Community-based health care services may include:

   A. obstetrical services.
   B. day care centers.
   C. emergency departments.
   D. surgery units.

3   When the family's desires differ from those of the client, the home care nurse must:

   A. remain the primary client's advocate.
   B. try to please everyone.
   C. avoid negative responses from the family.
   D. call the physician to resolve the conflict.

4   In order for home care to receive Medicare reimbursement, certain criteria must be met. Which of the following are necessary? (Choose all that apply.)

   A. The client must need help with cooking and cleaning.
   B. The client must have a "skilled need."
   C. The client must have an income below poverty level.
   D. The client must be essentially homebound.
   E. The client must have a plan of care.

5   Clients cannot realistically be taught everything they need to know during today's shortened hospital stays. Therefore, a client needing follow-up teaching should:

   A. have a home health referral.
   B. have more frequent physician appointments.
   C. have the option to increase his or her hospital stay.
   D. rely on family for continued care.

6   In the home, one nursing responsibility and legal requirement is:

   A. identifying caregiver burden.
   B. respecting client boundaries.
   C. completing a safety assessment.
   D. honoring family customs.

7   Nursing interventions for unsafe and hazardous conditions in the home would include:

   A. changing the unsafe home environment regardless of client wishes.
   B. ignoring the unsafe environment, allowing the client freedom to choose his or her own lifestyle.
   C. threatening to discontinue home care if the environment is not made safe.
   D. alerting the client/family, suggesting remedies, and documenting the response.

8   The process of learning to live to one's maximum potential with a chronic impairment/functional disability is:

   A. long-term care.
   B. rehabilitation.
   C. reintegration.
   D. infection control.

9   Rehabilitation includes many different aspects of the client's life such as physical, mental, social, and vocational status. This comprehensive consideration of the client requires:

   A. an interdisciplinary approach to care.
   B. primarily nursing care.
   C. focusing on the physical disability.
   D. short-term care.

10   Before establishing any plan of care in rehabilitation, it is important to:

   A. guarantee the client independence in all areas of functioning.
   B. determine the priorities of needs from the client's and family's perspective.
   C. establish a rapport with the family.
   D. complete all physical exercises.

Answers for Review Questions, as well as discussion of Critical Thinking Care Map questions, appear in Appendix V.

Chapter 5

Guidelines for Client Assessment

BRIEF Outline

Purposes of a Client Assessment
Types of Assessment
Obtaining a Health History
Methods of Physical Examination
   Inspection
   Palpation
   Percussion
   Auscultation
The Physical Examination
   General Survey
   Skin, Hair, and Nails
   Head and Neck
   Thorax and Abdomen
   Extremities
   Mental Status
Documentation

LEARNING Outcomes

After completing this chapter, you will be able to:

- Discuss the purposes of a client assessment.
- Describe the types of client assessment.
- Compare sources and accuracy of assessment data.
- Describe components of the health history.
- Demonstrate the methods of physical examination.
- Prepare a client for a physical examination.
- Describe the body systems and characteristics assessed in a physical examination.
- Document a health assessment.

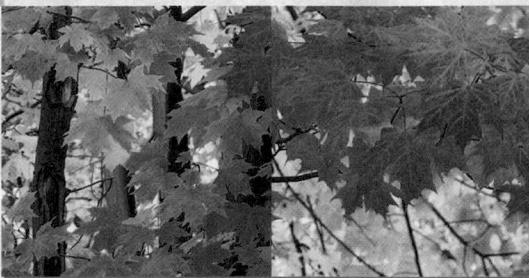

MediaLink

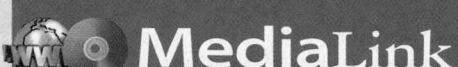

www.prenhall.com/burke
Use the address above to access the free, interactive Companion Website created for this textbook. Get hints, instant feedback, and textbook references to chapter-related NCLEX-style questions. Link to other interesting sites.

Audio Glossary:
Use the Companion Website, or the CD-ROM disk enclosed with your textbook, to hear the pronunciation of key terms in this chapter.

One of the most important aspects of nursing care is assessment. **Assessment** is the process of collecting data (pieces of information) that provides information about the client's individualized health care needs. It is the first step in the nursing process, providing the base for the planning, implementation, and evaluation of client care. Assessment by nurses is mandated by nursing standards, nurse practice acts, accrediting bodies, and institutional policies. Depending on state nurse practice acts and agency or institutional protocol, licensed practical/vocational nurses may do most components of the physical assessment, or they may only do selected parts that are within the scope of their defined practice. This chapter provides information about all components of a physical assessment to serve as a knowledge base.

Purposes of a Client Assessment

The purposes of a client assessment are to:

- Collect objective data about the client. **Objective data** (also called *signs*) are observable or measurable pieces of information. Objective data can be seen, heard, touched, or smelled. Examples of objective data are the color of urine, vital signs, moisture on skin, and breath odor. Laboratory results are also objective data.
- Collect subjective data from the client. **Subjective data** (also called *symptoms*) are experiences only the client can describe. Examples of subjective data are nausea, pain, and itching.
- Collect information about the client's family, community, culture, ethnicity, and religion.
- Identify past and present client behaviors that support health or increase the risk of illness.
- Identify data that suggest risk for or actual health problems. (The RN will label these problems as *nursing diagnoses*.)

This chapter provides guidelines for conducting the two components of a health assessment: a health history and physical examination. Information about health assessments is included in the first chapter of each unit that discusses a disrupted body system function. The term **manifestations** is used throughout this book to refer to objective and subjective data that are associated with specific illnesses. It is important to remember that documenting (recording) the client assessment is as important as conducting it.

Types of Assessment

The type of assessment varies depending on the setting, the situation, and the needs of the client. The types of assessment are an initial comprehensive assessment, an ongoing partial assessment, and a focused assessment.

COMPREHENSIVE ASSESSMENT

When a client first enters a health care setting, a comprehensive assessment of the client's health history and physical status is conducted. This provides a baseline for comparing later assessments. The comprehensive assessment may be the responsibility of one health care professional or of different members of the health care team. For example, when a client enters the hospital setting for inpatient care and receives a comprehensive assessment, a nurse may collect data about the client's health history, the physician may perform a complete physical examination, and a nursing technician may take vital signs and weight. In a community or home setting, the nurse usually collects all of the assessment data.

PARTIAL ASSESSMENT

An ongoing partial assessment is one that is conducted on a regular basis throughout the client's care. It usually reviews any problems that have been identified to determine if changes have occurred or if new problems are present. A partial assessment is conducted in any type of setting, although the timing may differ. In the hospital, the nurse conducts a partial assessment at the beginning of each shift. In the home, a partial assessment is conducted at each visit (which may vary from daily to once a week).

FOCUSED ASSESSMENT

A focused assessment (through both a focused interview and a focused physical examination) is one that is conducted to assess a specific client problem. For example, assessment for a client who has abdominal pain includes assessing body temperature; frequency of bowel movements; pain with urination; any associated trauma; menstrual history (for women); and the location, duration, and type of pain experienced. It does not include assessment of musculoskeletal function or visual acuity. A focused assessment is also a part of other nursing responsibilities, such as when the nurse takes an apical pulse before administering a drug that affects the heart rate. An *emergency assessment* is a special type of focused assessment. It is a very rapid assessment to determine life-threatening situations. The practice of assessing the ABCs (Airway, Breathing, Circulation) before beginning cardiopulmonary resuscitation is an example of an emergency assessment.

Sources and Accuracy of Assessment Data

Data may be collected from primary or secondary sources. The client is the best source of data and is the primary source. However, if the client is very young, very ill, unconscious, or confused, data may be collected from secondary sources. Secondary sources include the client's family or friends, the client records (such as medical records and laboratory data), and other health care professionals.

Data that are collected must be accurate and factual. General guidelines for ensuring this include the following:

- Compare subjective and objective data. If the client says "I feel like I have a fever," compare the statement to an actual measurement of body temperature.
- Consider factors that may interfere with accurate measurements. The client who has just walked up three flights of stairs may have an increased pulse rate that is unrelated to a disease process.
- Clarify statements made by the client. If the client says, "I have this terrible pain in my stomach," ask the client to point to the area of pain (which may be abdominal rather than gastric).
- Double-check data that are very high or low, such as a pulse of 120 or a blood pressure of 60/20.
- Do not jump to conclusions. The older adult client's dry skin with decreased turgor may be a result of aging; it may not mean the client is dehydrated.

Obtaining a Health History

The health history is a collection of subjective and objective data that provide an overall picture of the client's health status (Table 5-1 ■). The data are collected through an interview with the client. Many health care institutions and agencies have specific forms with standardized questions to use in conducting the health history. Although these may vary, most contain the data listed in Table 5-1.

During the health history, principles of therapeutic communication help you collect accurate data. Most importantly, use words the client can understand, and listen carefully. Sit in a relaxed posture and maintain eye contact. This open body language tells the client that you are interested in what is being said. Barriers to collecting accurate data include offering advice, acting disgusted or defensive, disagreeing, offering false assurance, and jumping to conclusions.

Open-ended questions ("Tell me about what brought you to the clinic today") give the client the chance to provide more information than closed-ended questions ("Did you come here today because of your back pain?"). Avoid

TABLE 5-1

Information Included in a Health History

COMPONENT	INFORMATION
Biographical data	Name, address, age, gender, marital status, occupation, religious preference, health care financing, usual source of medical care (primary health care provider)
Reason for health care visit (chief complaint)	Documented in client's own words
History of present illness	When symptoms began Whether onset was sudden or gradual Exact location of the problem Character of the problem (such as type of discharge or intensity of pain) Other associated symptoms Type of self-treatment
Past medical history	Childhood illnesses Childhood immunizations Allergies Accidents and injuries Hospitalizations All current prescribed and over-the-counter medications
Family history of health and illness	Ages of brothers/sisters, parents, grandparents Health status of living relatives and cause of death if no longer living
Lifestyle	Amount, frequency, and use of tobacco, alcohol, and street drugs Type and amount of foods eaten each day Sleep patterns Any difficulty with activities of daily living Type and amount of exercise Education and occupation Support systems (family, friends, community) Expectations of treatment and care

"why" questions ("Why didn't you come last week when you first noticed this problem?"). "Why" questions often make the client feel threatened or foolish. Closed-ended questions are appropriate in emergency situations, when specific information must be collected quickly.

It is very important to be sensitive to cultural differences between yourself and the client. Cultural differences influence how both verbal and nonverbal communications are interpreted. Culture and ethnicity, as well as the family in which one grew up and the community in which one lives, also influence health beliefs, health behaviors, and health treatments.

If the client does not speak the same language as the nurse, a translator is necessary to assist with the interview. The room should be arranged so the client can see both the nurse and the translator at the same time. Look at the client, not the translator, and ask questions one at a time in clear, concise terms.

Methods of Physical Examination

Physical examination is a skill that takes practice. The four basic methods of physical examination are inspection, palpation, percussion, and auscultation. The methods of physical examination used depend on the nurse's level of education, knowledge, and skill acquired through clinical practice, and on institutional or agency policy. The four basic methods of physical examination are introduced next.

INSPECTION

Inspection is the method of observing the client in a careful and deliberate manner, using the senses of seeing, smelling, and hearing to observe abnormal findings. Some body systems are inspected with special equipment; for example, an otoscope is used to inspect the ear canal and tympanic membrane. Inspection is the first method used in an assessment of the whole body or of each body system. The guidelines for inspection are:

- The room temperature should be comfortable. If the room is too hot or too cold, it may alter the appearance of the client's skin and change his or her behavior.
- Use good lighting. Dim light can obscure abnormalities, and fluorescent lights can change the perception of skin color.
- Look before touching.
- Completely expose the body part being inspected.
- Compare symmetric (matching) parts (e.g., eyes, ears, arms, legs).
- Inspect for these characteristics: color, size, symmetry, patterns, location, consistency of tissue, movement, behavior, odors, sounds.

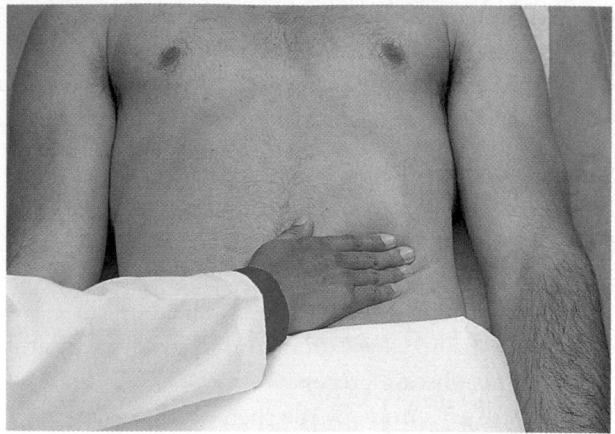

Figure 5-1. ■ The position of the hand for light palpation. (Photographer: Richard Tauber.)

PALPATION

Palpation is the method of using the hands to touch and feel. Light and moderate palpation are used most often by nurses. Light palpation is performed by placing your hand lightly on the surface to palpate for pulses, tenderness, skin texture, skin temperature, and skin moisture (Figure 5-1 ■). To perform moderate palpation, the hand is placed on the skin surface and the surface is depressed 1 to 2 cm (1/2 to 3/4 inch). A circular motion is used to feel for the size, shape, or mobility of underlying structures such as masses or body organs (Table 5-2 ■). A distended urinary bladder may be assessed with moderate palpation. The guidelines for palpation are:

- Make sure hands are clean and warm and fingernails are short.
- Follow Standard Precautions as appropriate.
- Use the pads of the fingers to palpate pulses, texture, size, shape, and crepitus (air in subcutaneous tissue).
- Assess for the characteristics listed in Table 5-2.

TABLE 5-2

Characteristics Assessed by Palpation

CHARACTERISTIC	DESCRIPTORS
Consistency	Soft, hard, filled with fluid
Mobility	Movable, fixed
Moisture	Wet, dry
Pulse strength	Strong, weak, full, bounding, thready
Shape	Regular, irregular
Size	Small, medium, large
Temperature	Warm, cold
Texture	Rough, smooth

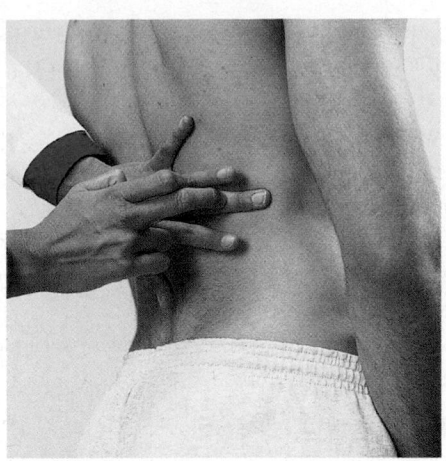

Figure 5-2. ■ Indirect percussion. Use the finger of one hand to tap the finger of the other. (Photographer: Richard Tauber.)

PERCUSSION

Percussion is the method of tapping the body to produce sound waves. The sounds produced are used to assess underlying structures. Although percussion can be used to assess the density of tissue and the size and shape of organs, it is used most often to assess abdominal structures. Tympany is a characteristic loud, drumlike sound heard over an organ that is filled with air, such as the intestines. In actual practice, nurses do not often use percussion.

The guidelines for percussion are:

- Make sure hands are clean and warm and fingernails are short.
- Follow Standard Precautions as appropriate.
- To use direct percussion, use one or more fingertips to tap over the area being assessed.
- To use indirect percussion (Figure 5-2 ■):
  - Place the middle finger of your nondominant hand over the area to be percussed.
  - Use the pad of the middle finger of your dominant hand to strike the area between the knuckle and the fingernail of the hand over the body part.
  - Deliver two quick taps by flexing your wrist and listen to the tone.

AUSCULTATION

Auscultation is the method that uses a stethoscope to listen for body sounds, including those of the heart, blood moving through a blood vessel, bowel, and lungs. Sounds are described in a variety of ways, depending on the body part being assessed. Sounds are generally classified according to intensity (loud/soft), pitch (high/low), duration, and quality (crackles, wheezes, etc.). Auscultation is also used to assess the apical pulse.

General guidelines for auscultation are:

- Make sure hands are clean and warm and fingernails are short.
- Follow Standard Precautions as appropriate.
- Make the environment as quiet as possible.
- Auscultate over bare skin.
- Press the diaphragm of the stethoscope firmly on the body part being assessed to listen to normal heart sounds, breath sounds, and bowel sounds (all of which are high pitched).
- Hold the bell of the stethoscope lightly on the body part being assessed to listen to low-pitched sounds, such as abnormal heart sounds and vascular sounds.

Preparation for a Physical Examination

Before beginning the examination, the nurse should ensure that the room temperature is comfortable, that the area is quiet, and that adequate lighting is available. All equipment that will be used should be clean and in good working order. The nurse should wash his or her hands before and after the assessment. Gloves should be worn and Standard Precautions followed if either the nurse or the client has an open cut or abrasion, if the client has drainage from a cut or wound, if body fluids or excretions are being collected, and for any examination of the mucous membranes, genitalia, or rectum. If there is any possibility of being splashed with fluids or secretions, the nurse should wear a mask and protective eye goggles.

The purpose and techniques of the physical examination should be explained to the client to decrease anxiety and feelings of embarrassment. Although the examination is not painful, it may be difficult for some clients to sit or lie in a position necessary for a specific assessment, especially if the client is in pain or is older. The length of the examination should be adjusted to the physical condition and age of each client. The nurse should be aware of normal changes in structure and function that occur with aging because they can affect client tolerance and the data that are collected. Normal age-related changes in the older adult are outlined in Box 5-1 ■, and are further described in each assessment chapter.

If at all possible, the nurse should conduct the physical examination in a private location at a time agreeable to the client. For a complete physical examination, the nurse should (if needed) assist the client in removing clothing and putting on a gown. The client should empty the bladder before the examination to facilitate abdominal assessment. A drape should be placed over the client so that only the body part being assessed is exposed. The nurse should also determine if any positions are contraindicated during the examination.

MediaLink Video: Prepping the Exam Room

BOX 5-1	FOCUS ON OLDER ADULTS

Age-Related Assessment Findings in the Older Adult

Skin, Hair, and Nails
- Dry and wrinkled skin
- Thin scalp and body hair (men may be bald)
- Facial hair in women
- Loss of hair pigment
- Areas of pigmentation and moles
- Thickened and yellowed nails

Eyes and Ears
- Cataracts (opacity of the lens)
- Decreased visual acuity (*presbyopia*)
- Decreased hearing acuity (*presbycusis*)

Mouth
- Loss of teeth
- Presence of dentures

Heart and Lungs
- Increased respiratory rate
- Increased blood pressure
- Increased, but weaker, heart rate

Abdomen
- Decreased frequency of bowel sounds
- More frequent voiding, including at night

Extremities
- Blood vessels more prominent and less straight
- Peripheral pulses sometimes more difficult to palpate
- Decreased muscle mass and strength
- Decreased range of motion
- Stooped posture

Mental Status
- Slower response to questions
- Occasional confusion in unfamiliar surroundings

The Physical Examination

A comprehensive physical examination (Table 5-3 ■) can be conducted in a system-by-system or head-to-toe sequence. Some parts of the examination, such as a rectal examination, male and female genitalia with a pelvic examination, internal eye examination, and external ear canal examination are most often conducted by an advanced practice nurse or physician and are not included here. The following discussion of a basic physical examination provides structure for a head-to-toe assessment.

GENERAL SURVEY

The general survey provides the nurse with information about the client's overall appearance and behavior, as well as vital signs and height and weight. Data for the general survey are collected from the first meeting with the client and continue through the physical examination or during nursing care. The following information is assessed:

- Facial expressions, mood, speech patterns
- Hygiene, grooming, odors
- Posture, physical deformities, ability to move and walk
- Manifestations of illness, such as difficulty breathing, pain, swelling
- Vital signs (temperature, pulse, respirations, blood pressure)
- Height and weight

SKIN, HAIR, AND NAILS

The skin, hair, and nails make up the integumentary system and often provide a general indication of the client's overall health. These structures are assessed by inspection and palpation in conjunction with other body parts during a head-to-toe physical examination.

The skin varies in color from pale white to dark brown, depending on race and individual characteristics. It is normally warm, smooth, dry, and intact. Various diseases and injuries or environmental exposure may change the color, moisture, or continuity of the client's skin (see Chapters 45 and 46). ⬤ Changes in color are more difficult to assess in dark-skinned people (such as Native Americans, African Americans, Hispanics, those of Mediterranean descent, and Caucasians who are deeply suntanned). Abnormal assessments are described below:

- *Cyanosis.* Cyanosis is a blue or gray discoloration of the skin that is the result of a decreased level of oxygen in the blood. Cyanosis in people with dark skin is often seen as a dullness in color.
- *Pallor.* Pallor, or paleness of the skin, is most often the result of a loss of blood. Pallor may be assessed over the entire body, or only in the lips, nail beds, and conjunctiva (white area) of the eyes. People with dark skin often are ashen gray or appear slightly yellowish.
- *Jaundice.* Jaundice is a yellow color of the skin and mucous membranes. It is caused by liver or gallbladder disease, or by an excessive breakdown of red blood cells. Jaundice is usually seen first in the eyes, and then in the skin and mucous membranes. Darker skin does not show jaundice, but it can be seen in the eyes, oral mucous membranes, and palms and soles.
- *Erythema.* Erythema is redness of the skin. It may appear during a fever, in response to inflammation or allergy, or from a sunburn.
- *Ecchymosis.* Ecchymosis is a purple discoloration resulting from a collection of blood in the subcutaneous tissues. *Petechiae* are small red spots caused by capillary bleeding. The location and size of the discolorations should be documented.

TABLE 5-3

Guidelines for a Physical Examination

COMPONENT	METHODS AND AREAS OF ASSESSMENT
General survey	Inspection, Auscultation ■ General appearance, posture, gait, thought process, speech patterns ■ Vital signs ■ Height and weight
Integument	Inspection, Palpation ■ Skin: Color, moisture, temperature, turgor, lesions (color, size, shape) ■ Hair: Distribution, texture, infection, infestation ■ Nails: Shape, angle at nail bed, color, texture
Eyes	Inspection, Palpation ■ Eyebrows: Hair distribution, alignment, movement ■ Eyelashes: Distribution, direction of curl ■ Eyelids: Skin texture, symmetrical closure, ability to blink ■ Conjunctiva: Color, texture, lesions ■ Lacrimal glands: Pain, infection, edema, tearing ■ Cornea: Transparency, reflex ■ Pupils: Color, shape, symmetrical size, reaction to light, accommodation, convergence ■ Extraocular muscles: Coordination ■ Visual acuity: Near and distance vision
Ears	Inspection, Palpation ■ Auricles: Color, symmetrical size, position, texture, pain ■ External ear: Cerumen (wax), infection, blood ■ Hearing acuity: Voice tones, watch tick
Nose/Sinuses	Inspection, Palpation ■ External nose: Shape, size, color, discharge, pain ■ Nasal cavities: Patency, mucosa, discharge, lesions, location of septum ■ Sinuses: Pain
Mouth/Oropharynx	Inspection, Palpation ■ Lips/buccal mucosa: Symmetrical, color, moisture, lesions ■ Teeth/gums: Number of teeth; dental care, caries; gum color, adherence of gums to teeth ■ Tongue: Position, color, texture, movement, moisture, swelling, ulceration, masses, lesions ■ Palate/uvula: Color, shape, bony growth, lesions; position of uvula ■ Oropharynx/tonsils: Color, size, discharge
Neck	Inspection, Palpation, Auscultation ■ Neck muscles: Movement, range of motion, pain, swelling, masses ■ Lymph nodes: Size, pain ■ Carotid arteries, thyroid: Presence of *bruits* (soft rushing sound heard through bell of stethoscope)
Breasts/Axilla	Inspection, Palpation ■ Breasts: Size, shape, symmetrical, color, swelling, pain, masses, lesions ■ Areola: Size, shape, symmetrical, color, masses, lesions ■ Nipples: Size, shape, position, color, discharge, lesions, masses, retraction ■ Axillary lymph nodes: Size, pain, nodules
Thorax/Lungs	Inspection, Palpation, Auscultation ■ Thorax: Shape, symmetrical, spinal curves, skin lesions, pain, masses, expansion ■ Lungs: Breath sounds, respiratory patterns
Cardiovascular	Inspection, Palpation, Auscultation ■ Precordium: Location of point of maximum impulse, pulsations ■ Heart: Heart sounds, rate and rhythm of contractions ■ Peripheral pulses: Strength, symmetrical, volume

(continued)

TABLE 5-3	
Guidelines for a Physical Examination (continued)	
COMPONENT	METHODS AND AREAS OF ASSESSMENT
	Peripheral veins: Visibility, symmetrical, pain Circulation: Skin color, temperature, skin changes, nail changes, lesions, edema, capillary refill
Abdomen	Inspection, Auscultation, Percussion, Palpation Skin: Lesions, color Abdomen: Contour, distention, movements Bowel sounds: Audible, timing Bladder: Size, pain
Musculoskeletal	Inspection, Palpation Muscles: Symmetrical, size, tone, movement, contractures, pain, masses Bones: Symmetrical, alignment, pain Spine: Curves
Neurologic	Inspection, Palpation, Percussion Motor function/balance: Gait, ability to stand on one foot and walk heel to toe Fine motor movement: Ability to repeatedly touch nose with hand, pat knees with palms and backs of hands, run down opposite shin Sensory/light touch: Ability to distinguish between sharp and dull touch Cranial nerves: Ability to smell, see, clench teeth, move eyes, have facial expressions, hear, taste, feel touch, swallow, shrug shoulders against resistance, protrude tongue Reflexes: Type of response (using percussion hammer)

■ *Lesions.* Lesions are alterations in the surface of the skin. *Wounds* may be the result of an injury or a surgical incision. A *scar* is a healed wound. Other types of lesions are bites, scratches, blisters, warts, moles, acne, burns, and rashes. When assessing lesions, document the size, shape, location, drainage, odors, and associated pain.

■ *Turgor.* This term refers to the fullness or elasticity of the skin. With normal turgor, skin can be pinched up in a fold, and when released it immediately returns to its previous shape. *Dehydration* decreases the skin's turgor, so

that skin folds remain elevated (like a tent) or return to shape very slowly. *Edema,* or excess fluid in tissues, is manifested by swelling covered by tight, shiny skin. Edema may be caused by trauma, heart disease, peripheral vascular disease, kidney disease, or overhydration. Edema is often measured by palpating with the fingers; if the skin remains indented, the term *pitting edema* is used. The scale used to describe pitting edema is 0 + none, 1+ = trace (2 mm), 2+ = moderate (4 mm), 3+ = deep (6 mm), and 4+ = very deep (8 mm) (Figure 5-3 ■).

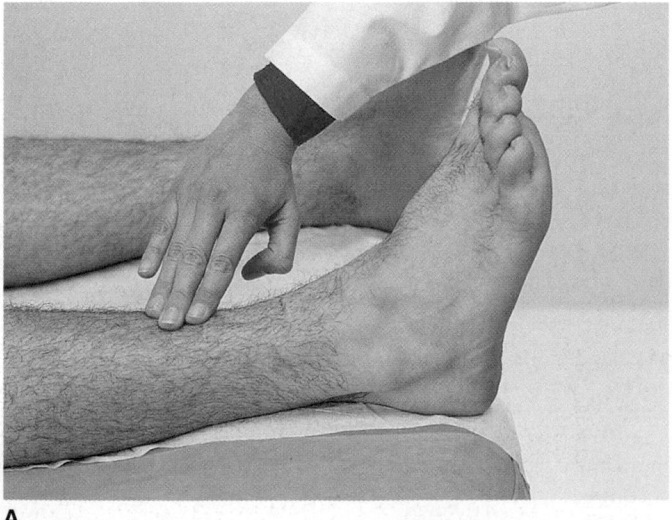

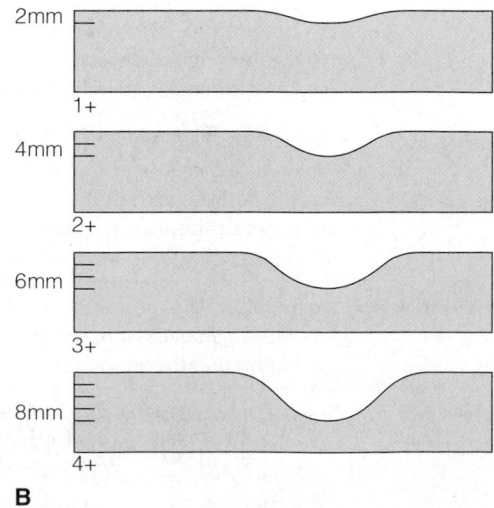

A   **B**

Figure 5-3. ■ Assessing edema. (**A**) Palpating for edema over the tibia. (Photographer: Richard Tauber.) (**B**) Four-point scale for grading edema.

The nails are inspected for shape, color, and consistency. The hair is inspected for color, texture, and distribution. *Alopecia* (loss of hair on the head or all of the body) may result from hereditary factors (specific to the hair on the head in men), infection, inadequate nutrition, or treatment of cancer with chemotherapy or radiation therapy. *Hirsutism* (excessive hair) is often caused by hormone disorders.

HEAD AND NECK

A basic physical examination of the head and neck includes assessing the skull, face, eyes, ears, nose and sinuses, mouth, and lymph nodes. These structures are assessed by inspection and palpation. More advanced physical assessment techniques, not discussed here, use the ophthalmoscope to examine the internal eye and the otoscope to examine the tympanic membrane and internal nasal structures.

Skull and Face

The skull and face are inspected for shape and proportion and should be symmetrical. If the skull appears abnormally large, its circumference should be measured with a tape measure. The face is inspected for color, symmetry, and distribution of hair. The facial muscles and nerves are assessed by asking the client to raise the eyebrows, puff out the cheeks, smile, and show the teeth. Abnormal findings that should be documented are edema around the eyes *(periorbital edema),* inability to move a part of the face, and any abnormal movements such as tremors or tics.

Eyes

The external structures of the eyes (including the eyebrows, eyelids, eyelashes, and lacrimal glands) are inspected. The eyes and eyebrows should be in alignment, the eyelashes should curl outward, and the eyelids should cover the eyes equally. The lacrimal gland is palpated for tenderness. The conjunctiva should be white. The pupils are normally black and round. When a client has a cataract, the pupil appears white or cloudy. Other abnormal findings are dilation *(mydriasis)* or constriction *(miosis)* of one or both pupils (see Figure 5-4 ◾). The pupils are also assessed for reaction to light, accommodation, and convergence. The procedures for these assessments are outlined in Box 5-2 ◾.

Visual acuity is often measured with a Snellen's chart (Figure 5-5 ◾) and can be done with or without corrective lenses (eyeglasses or contact lenses). The client is placed 20 feet from the chart and asked to cover one eye. The client is

BOX 5-2	ASSESSMENT

Assessing the pupils

REACTION TO LIGHT

- Ask the client to look straight ahead.
- Using a penlight, bring the light from the side of the client's face and briefly shine the light on one pupil. Observe the response of the pupil (it should normally constrict).
- Repeat the procedure with the other eye.

ACCOMMODATION

- Hold your finger about 10 to 15 cm (4 to 6 inches) from the bridge of the client's nose.
- Ask the client to look at your finger, then at a distant object, and then back at your finger. Observe the response of the pupils. They should normally constrict when looking at your finger (a near object) and dilate when looking at the distant object.

CONVERGENCE

- Move your finger toward the client's nose from a distance of about 15 cm (6 inches) and observe the eyes. Normally, the pupils move toward the nose, assuming a cross-eyed appearance (convergence).

asked to read the smallest possible line of letters with the uncovered eye. This procedure is repeated with the other eye. Each line on the chart has a fraction on the side, with the top number always being 20 (the distance at which a person with normal vision can read the line of letters). The bottom number indicates the vision of the person being tested and larger numbers represent poorer vision. Visual acuity is documented as the smallest line of letters that can

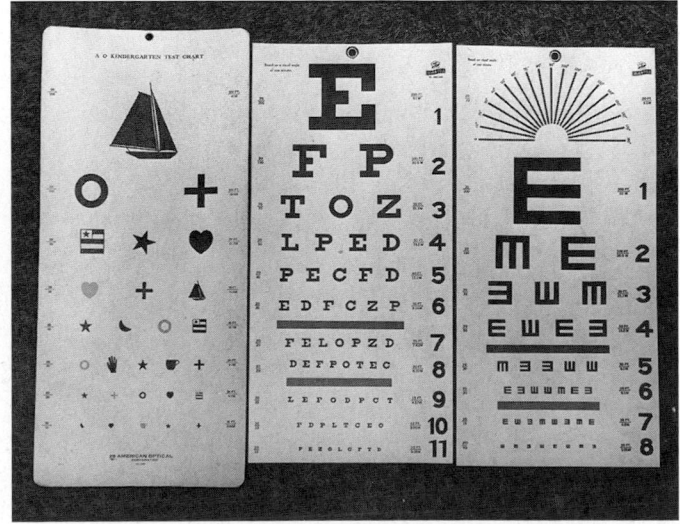

Figure 5-5. ◾ Types of eye charts: the preschool children's chart (left), Snellen's standard chart (center), and the Snellen E chart for clients who are unable to read (right).

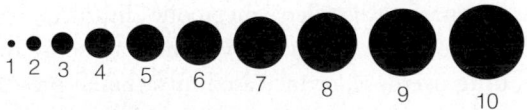

Figure 5-4. ◾ Size of pupil in millimeters.

be read with only two errors. For example, normal vision is 20/20, whereas a person with visual problems may have a visual acuity of 20/100. The visual acuity for each eye is documented, and use of corrective lenses is noted. (See Chapter 40 ⬮⬯ for disorders of the ear and eye.)

Ears

Inspect the external ears for location, symmetry, lesions, redness, and drainage. Gently palpate the external ears for tenderness and swelling. An estimate of hearing may be made by asking the client to cover one ear as you whisper a word while standing about 1 to 2 feet away out of the client's line of vision (to prevent lip-reading). Repeat with the other ear.

Nose and Sinuses

To test the patency of the client's nostrils, have the client occlude one side at a time and then inhale and exhale. A penlight can be used to assess the mucous membranes in the lower nasal passages. Abnormal findings include swelling, bleeding, discharge, and a crooked (deviated) septum. The sinuses are assessed by gentle palpation over the frontal and maxillary sinuses, noting any tenderness or pain.

Mouth

Ask the client to open the mouth widely. Inspect the lips, the oral mucous membranes, the tongue, the teeth, and the gums. The lips, mucous membranes, gums, and tongue should be pink, smooth, and moist. The teeth should be in good repair. There should be no bad odors. Abnormal findings are swelling, redness, pallor, drainage, lesions, or poor dental hygiene.

Lymph Nodes

Palpate the lymph nodes of the head and neck (Figure 5-6 ⬛). The lymph nodes normally are not palpable. If they are palpable, assess for size, location, consistency, and tenderness.

THORAX

Assessment of the thorax in a head-to-toe examination includes the chest and back, the lungs, the heart, and the breasts. The assessment techniques most often used are inspection and auscultation, with palpation also used to assess the breasts and lymph nodes in the axilla.

Chest and Back

The color, size, shape, muscles, and breathing movements of the chest and back are inspected. The color should be the same as the face and neck. Bilateral sides of the chest and back should be symmetrical, with equal expansion and relaxation during respirations. The thorax should have a greater transverse (side-to-side) diameter than anteroposterior (front-to-back) diameter. The reverse (referred to as a *barrel chest*) is seen in clients with chronic obstructive pulmonary diseases. The scapulae should be

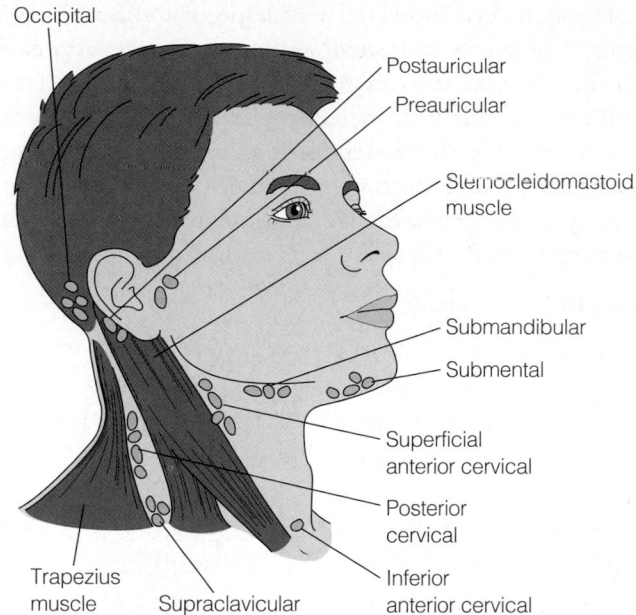

Figure 5-6. ⬛ Lymph nodes of the head and neck.

equal in height, and the spine should be aligned midline with normal curves (concave cervical and convex thoracic). Abnormal findings of the thoracic spine include *kyphosis* (increased thoracic curve) and *scoliosis* (lateral deviation). In clients with respiratory difficulty, the intercostal and upper thoracic muscles may *retract* (pull in) on inhalation.

Lungs

The lungs are assessed by inspection of the external thorax and by auscultation with a stethoscope. Inspection can be used to determine respiratory rate, depth, and rhythm. The rate is normally 12 to 20 regular breaths per minute (known as *eupnea*) in the adult. Respiratory rates may increase to more than 24 breaths per minute (*tachypnea*) in response to exercise, to fever, and to illnesses that cause an increase in the amount of carbon dioxide or a decrease of oxygen in the blood. Respiratory rates may decrease to less than 10 breaths per minute (*bradypnea*) in a client with an increase in intracranial pressure or in response to certain narcotic drugs.

The normal depth and rhythm of respirations is about equal during inspiration and expiration, but may abnormally be very deep or shallow. A client may also have increased respiratory rate and depth (*hyperventilation*) or decreased respiratory rate and depth (*hypoventilation*) in response to factors such as respiratory disorders, metabolic disorders, fear, and drug overdose. *Cheyne–Stokes respirations,* a response to organ failure, drug overdose, or increased intracranial pressure, are manifested by regular periods of alternating deep and rapid respirations followed by apnea. Other abnormal respiratory findings are *dyspnea* (difficulty breathing), *orthopnea* (breathing more easily in an upright position), and *apnea* (periods in which there is no breathing).

Auscultation is used to assess normal and abnormal (or *adventitious*) breath sounds. To auscultate the chest, the client should be in a sitting position. Warm the stethoscope diaphragm before placing it on the client's chest and ask the client to breathe slowly and deeply through the mouth. A regular pattern of auscultation should be used, beginning above the clavicle or scapula and moving the diaphragm down at regular intervals to the bottom of the ribs. Compare and document sounds for both the right and left lungs.

There are several different types of abnormal breath sounds. Noisy respirations are often labeled *stertorous.* *Crackles,* heard most often during inspiration, are crackling sounds made as air moves through secretions in the airways. *Wheezes* are high-pitched continuous sounds heard on both inspiration and expiration. Wheezes are heard when secretions, swelling, or tumors narrow the small airways. A grating sound indicates a *pleural friction rub,* resulting from an inflamed pleura rubbing against the chest wall.

While assessing the lungs, it is important to note if the client has a cough, and to ask if and when sputum is coughed up. If the cough is productive of sputum, note the color, amount, and consistency. Depending on the cause, sputum may be clear, yellow, green, or blood tinged and may be thin or thick. Additional documentation is necessary if the client is receiving oxygen. Record how it is administered (i.e., by mask or nasal cannula) and at what rate (in liters per minute). (See also Chapters 23 and 24. ⚭)

Heart

The heart is assessed by auscultation for heart sounds to take an apical pulse. The equipment used is a stethoscope with a diaphragm. The diaphragm should be warmed before placement on the client's chest, and the room should be quiet so sounds can be heard without difficulty. The nurse assesses the rate and rhythm of the heart and the normal heart sounds. Assessing abnormal heart sounds is an advanced assessment technique.

The apical impulse is used as a landmark for taking an apical pulse. This landmark is located at the fourth or fifth left intercostal space in the midclavicular line (Figure 5-7 ■). It may often be palpated as a slight tap against the fingers. The apical pulse is the most accurate pulse measurement. It should be taken if there is any question about the peripheral pulse or if the client is taking a medication that affects heart rate. The apical pulse is taken for 1 full minute; the normal rate for adults ranges from 60 to 100 beats per minute.

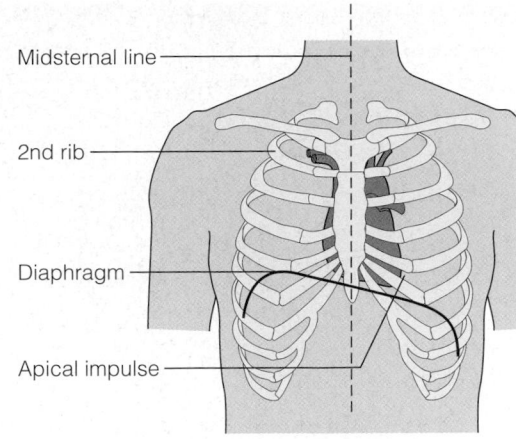

Figure 5-7. ■ Location of the apical impulse.

The first heart sound heard (S$_1$) is the "lub" of "lub-dub." This is a low-pitched sound that occurs as the mitral and tricuspid valves close. The second heart sound (S$_2$) is the "dub" of "lub-dub." This sound is not as low pitched and is shorter than the first heart sound. It occurs as the aortic and pulmonic valves close. Both sounds normally occur within 1 second or less, and are counted together to determine the heart rate.

clinical ALERT

Remember to count only once for each two sounds that are heard, and to count for 1 full minute when taking an apical pulse. It is helpful always to begin counting when the second hand of your watch is on 12 (to avoid forgetting when you began counting).

While assessing the heart rate, it is important to note whether the rhythm is regular or irregular, and whether the sounds are strong or weak. An irregular pattern of heartbeats is called a *dysrhythmia* (see Chapter 27). ⚭ The client should also be asked about any other symptoms that might indicate heart disease, such as swelling of the feet, pain in the chest, difficulty breathing, fatigue, and dizziness. During an assessment for a client who complains of chest pain, also assess skin color for cyanosis or pallor; pulse, blood pressure, and respirations; location, duration, and intensity of the pain; and any other accompanying manifestations such as nausea or loss of consciousness.

Breasts and Axillary Lymph Nodes

The breasts of both men and women are assessed by inspection and palpation. The breasts are inspected for size, symmetry, skin condition, nipple condition, and discharge. Normally, the color is the same as that of the chest, the breasts are bilaterally symmetrical (although slight variations are normal), the areola and nipples are bilaterally

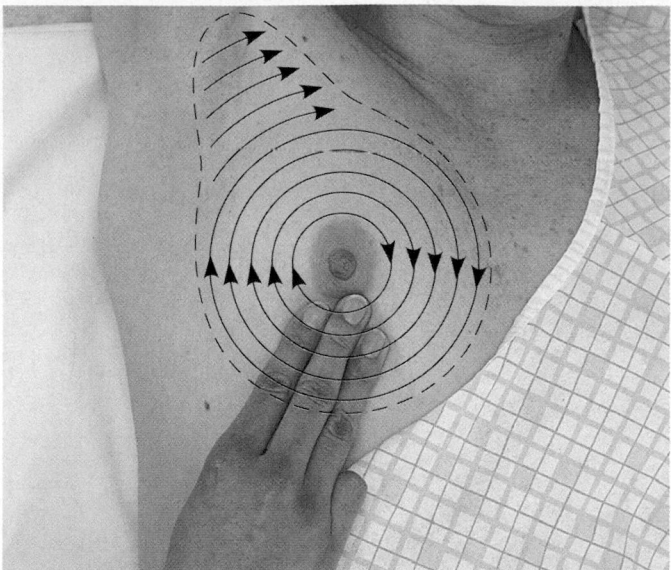

Figure 5-8. ■ Possible pattern for palpation of the breast. (Photographer: Richard Tauber.)

equal in size and color, and there is no sign of skin dimpling or redness, or discharge from the nipples.

The breasts are gently palpated by using the pads of the first three fingers to compress the breast tissue against the chest wall (Figure 5-8 ■). Breast tissue normally is firm with a granular consistency. Assess for tenderness or pain, abnormal consistency, or the presence of a mass. If the breasts feel nodular, ask the woman about a diagnosis of fibrocystic breast disease as well as the time of her last period (if she is still menstruating). While palpating the breasts, also palpate well into the axilla for the presence of pain and enlarged lymph nodes. If present, document size and consistency. Any abnormal findings are documented by quadrant (upper inner, upper outer, lower inner, lower outer). Ask women about a history of breast cancer, self-breast examinations, and mammograms (if age appropriate). (See Chapter 35. ⊙⊙)

ABDOMEN

Abdominal assessment includes inspecting the exterior abdomen, auscultating bowel sounds to determine intestinal function, and palpating the urinary bladder when a client has not been voiding. Because palpation may alter bowel sounds, the sequence of examination is inspection, auscultation, and palpation. Percussion and moderate to deep palpation of the abdomen are more advanced assessments and are not discussed here. Before beginning an abdominal assessment, be sure your hands are warm. For documentation purposes, mentally divide the abdomen into four quadrants (right upper, right lower, left upper, left lower) and know the underlying organs of each quadrant (Figure 5-9 ■).

Exterior Abdomen

The abdomen is normally slightly rounded, with the umbilicus midline. Fine white or silver-colored lines (*striae*) may be visible; they result from skin being stretched by weight gain or pregnancy. There should be no visible masses. If the abdomen is distended, ask questions about any changes in usual patterns of bowel movements and urination.

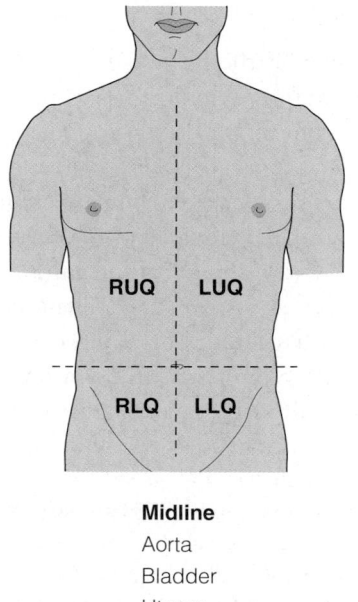

Midline
Aorta
Bladder
Uterus

◯ = Umbilicus

Right Upper Quadrant (RUQ)
Liver and gallbladder
Pylorus
Duodenum
Head of pancreas
Right adrenal gland
Portion of right kidney
Hepatic flexure of colon
Portions of ascending and transverse colon

Left Upper Quadrant (LUQ)
Left lobe of liver
Spleen
Stomach
Body of pancreas
Left adrenal gland
Portion of left kidney
Splenic flexure of colon
Portions of transverse and descending colon

Right Lower Quadrant (RLQ)
Lower pole of right kidney
Cecum and appendix
Portion of ascending colon
Bladder (if distended)
Right ovary and salpinx
Right spermatic cord
Right ureter

Left Lower Quadrant (LLQ)
Lower pole of left kidney
Sigmoid colon
Portion of descending colon
Bladder (if distended)
Left ovary and salpinx
Uterus (if enlarged)
Left spermatic cord
Left ureter

Figure 5-9. ■ The four quadrants of the abdomen, with anatomic location of organs within each quadrant.

Bowel Sounds

Bowel sounds are auscultated to assess intestinal function. Warm the diaphragm of the stethoscope and gently place it on the abdominal skin, listening in all four quadrants. Bowel sounds are clicks and gurgles made as intestinal contents move through bowel and should always be present. They normally occur every 5 to 20 seconds. Bowel sounds that occur less often are referred to as *hypoactive,* and those that occur more often are referred to as *hyperactive.* Hypoactive or absent bowel sounds may result from abdominal surgery, paralysis of the intestinal wall *(paralytic ileus),* or advanced intestinal obstruction. Hyperactive bowel sounds are heard during diarrhea and in the early stage of intestinal obstruction (see Chapter 20). ⚭

Urinary Bladder

The urinary bladder, if distended with urine, may be gently palpated in the midline of the abdomen above the symphysis pubis. If a client has not voided for 8 to 10 hours, or if the voidings are frequent and in small amounts, palpating a distended urinary bladder is essential to identify the need for further interventions to empty the bladder (see Chapter 32). ⚭

EXTREMITIES

The extremities are assessed for color, temperature, lesions, condition of hair and nails, peripheral circulation, and muscle strength. Skin color and temperature should be similar to that of the face. Hair distribution is normally symmetrical on arms and legs, and nails should be intact. Clients with peripheral vascular disease often have abnormal assessments, including decreased or absent pulses; cool, pale, shiny skin; absence of hair; and thickened nails (see Chapter 28). ⚭

Peripheral Circulation

Peripheral pulses are assessed by noting the rate, rhythm, and strength of the pulse at various locations, including the temporal, carotid, brachial, radial, femoral, popliteal, posterior tibial, and dorsalis pedis arteries (Figure 5-10 ■). The pulse is taken by gently compressing the artery against an underlying bone with the tips of the middle three fingers. During a physical examination, or if abnormalities are assessed, bilateral pulses should be palpated and compared (although both carotid arteries should never be palpated at the same time). If peripheral pulses are abnormal or cannot be palpated, a Doppler ultrasound can be used to determine the rate.

The normal pulse rate in an adult is from 60 to 100 beats per minute. A rapid heart rate (ranging from 100 to 180 beats per minute) is labeled *tachycardia.* Tachycardia can be caused by many different factors, including pain, anxiety, fever, and heart disease. A slow heart rate (less than 60 beats per minute) is labeled *bradycardia.* Bradycardia can be caused by medications, increasing age, or disorders of the

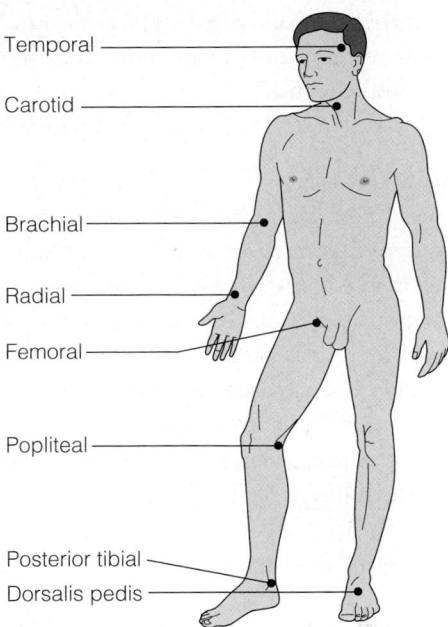

Figure 5-10. ■ Body sites at which peripheral pulses are most easily palpated.

cardiac conduction system. The rhythm of the heartbeat (the pattern of pulsations and pauses) should be regular. An abnormal rhythm should be reported. The *amplitude* is normally strong. The amplitude can be documented as:

- 0 or absent—no pulsation is felt
- 1+ or thready—pulsations are not easily palpated and disappear with slight pressure
- 2+ or weak—although stronger than a thready pulse, disappears with light pressure
- 3+ or normal—pulsations are palpated easily and only disappear with moderate pressure
- 4+ or bounding—pulsations are strong and do not disappear with moderate pressure.

If the radial pulse is irregular, an apical–radial pulse may be taken. This procedure requires two nurses who simultaneously count the apical pulse and the radial pulse for 1 minute. A difference in the rate is called a *pulse deficit,* and is caused by heartbeats that are weak or are not all reaching the peripheral arteries.

Capillary refill also provides information about peripheral circulation. To assess capillary refill, the nurse squeezes the client's fingernail or toenail until it turns white, then releases the pressure and observes the time for normal color to return. The return is normally immediate.

Musculoskeletal

Musculoskeletal function is initially assessed by observing the client's posture, ability to move, walk, and carry out activities of daily living. Range of motion of joints may be observed during the physical examination. Muscle strength is often assessed through hand grips and feet pushes. The nurse asks the client to grasp the nurse's index and middle finger and squeeze, and to push the soles of the feet against the nurse's hands. Muscle strength should be bilaterally equal.

MENTAL STATUS

Mental status is most often assessed by determining the client's level of awareness (*orientation*) and degree of wakefulness or ability to be aroused (*level of consciousness*). These are not the same conditions; a client may be conscious but disoriented.

The client's level of awareness is assessed by orientation to time, place, and person. When awareness is lost, the usual sequence of loss is time orientation, followed by place orientation, and then person orientation. It is important to remember that pain, trauma, illness, and a change in surroundings may make it difficult for clients to know the exact day and date. The following questions can be used to assess orientation:

- *Time*—What is the date today? What day of the week is today? What was our last holiday?
- *Place*—Where are you now? What state do we live in?
- *Person*—What is your name? How old are you?

Level of consciousness can be assessed and labeled as follows:

- *Awake and alert.* Client is fully awake, responds to verbal requests, and is oriented to time, place, and person.
- *Lethargic.* Client appears drowsy or asleep but can be awakened by calling his or her name and gently shaking.
- *Stuporous.* Client is deeply asleep most of the time and can be awakened only by shouting and shaking, responds to painful stimuli by making purposeful movements, and verbally responds but may make inappropriate responses.
- *Comatose.* Client cannot be aroused, even with painful stimuli; some reflexes (such as the gag reflex) may still be present.

Documentation

Data from the initial comprehensive assessment provide a foundation for the development and application of the nursing process. Documentation of ongoing focused assessments identifies improvement or worsening of identified health problems, provides information to help diagnose new problems, and serves as a means of communication among all members of the health care team. In addition, documentation of assessments provides the base for evaluation of health care outcomes, provides evidence to support health care cost reimbursements, and is legal evidence of the health status of the client at that point in time.

Each institution or agency has its own requirements for the timing and method of documentation. The types seen most often are the traditional narrative form, the checklist or standardized form (ranging from an initial admission record to a flow sheet for vital signs), and the nursing minimum data set (used in long-term care facilities). Increasingly, documentation is entered into a computer, where it becomes part of a database that is shared within and between health care settings. With this method, for example, a nurse caring for a client in the home would have access to previous assessment data and would not have to repeat the entire procedure, nor would the client have to repeat all the information.

To document factually and accurately, follow these principles:

- *Document as soon as possible.* It is difficult to remember information accurately for long periods of time.
- *Document legibly or make computer entries accurately.* Errors in documentation must legally be corrected in the format approved by the health care institution or agency. Check the policy of your institution.
- *Organize the data in a logical way.* The health history is generally documented before the physical examination. If the health care setting uses a specific framework for organizing the data, data are documented within this framework. When documenting the health history, present health problems are described beginning with onset of the problem.
- *Avoid inferences and judgments.* An inference is a statement about something unknown based on observation. For example, the nurse should not write "Obesity and body odor indicate little knowledge of nutrition and hygiene" or "Requests pain medication although obviously is not in pain."
- *Record findings rather than methods of assessment.* A detailed description of the method of assessment is unnecessary. For example, when recording a blood pressure, the nurse writes "BP 120/70," not "The diaphragm of the stethoscope was placed over the brachial artery and the sounds were auscultated."
- *Write concisely, using approved abbreviations and grammar.* It is not necessary to use entire sentences or to begin the narrative with the words "the client." Group phrases, such as "Bowel sounds heard in all four quadrants," rather than "The client has bowel sounds in the right upper and lower quadrants and left upper and lower quadrants." Use only those abbreviations approved by policy in the setting. Avoid jargon and slang words unless they are direct quotes.
- *Do not use the word "normal" for normal findings.* It is better to write what was assessed, such as "Breath sounds clear in both lower lungs," rather than "Breath sounds normal."
- If the agency uses documents called "charting by exception," document only abnormal findings.

Note: The bibliography listings for this and all chapters have been compiled at the back of the book.

Chapter Review

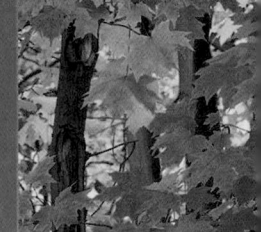

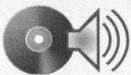 **KEY TERMS** by Topics

Use the audio glossary feature of either the CD-ROM or the Companion Website to hear the correct pronunciation of the following key terms.

Guidelines for client assessment

assessment

Purposes of a client assessment

objective data, subjective data, manifestations

Methods of physical examination

inspection, palpation, percussion, auscultation

KEY Points

- Assessment is the process of collecting data that provides information about the client's individualized health care needs. Nurses collect this data through the client assessment, comprised of a health history and a physical examination.

- The primary source of data is the client.

- The health history, collected through an interview of the client, provides subjective data.

- The four methods of physical examination are inspection, palpation, percussion, and auscultation. The skills of physical examination take practice.

- A comprehensive physical examination is conducted in a head-to-toe sequence. If a focused or emergency assessment is being conducted, the nurse assesses only the specific client problem.

- Documenting assessments factually and accurately provides the base for evaluation of health care outcomes, provides evidence to support health care cost reimbursements, and is legal evidence of the health status of the client at that point in time.

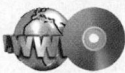 **EXPLORE MediaLink**

Additional interactive resources for this chapter can be found on the Companion Website at www.prenhall.com/burke. Click on Chapter 5 and "Begin" to select the activities for this chapter.

For chapter-related NCLEX-style review questions and an audio glossary, access the accompanying CD-ROM in this book.

FOR FURTHER Study

For more information about intestinal disorders, see Chapter 20.

For more information about respiratory disorders, see Chapters 23 and 24.

For more information about dysrhythmias, see Chapter 27.

For more information about assessing peripheral circulatory disorders, see Chapter 28.

For more information about urinary disorders, see Chapter 32.

For more information about female reproductive and breast disorders, see Chapter 35.

For more information about ear and eye disorders, see Chapter 40.

For more information about skin disorders, see Chapters 45 and 46.

Critical Thinking Care Map

Caring for a Client with Risk for Excess Fluid Volume

NCLEX-PN® Focus Area: Coordinated Care

Case Study: Cath Cole, age 62, has a long history of congestive heart failure. She lives in a small apartment with her cat, Tom. She states, "You know, I have had many problems with water in my lungs and my legs swell something awful." Cath is supposed to take her "heart pill" and "water pill" every day, but she ran out of money and couldn't buy any this month. Although a low-sodium diet has been prescribed, Cath eats anything she wants.

Nursing Diagnosis: Risk for Excess Fluid Volume

COLLECT DATA

Subjective	Objective
_____	_____
_____	_____
_____	_____
_____	_____
_____	_____
_____	_____
_____	_____

Would you report this data? Yes/No

If yes, to: _____

Nursing Care

_____

_____

_____

_____

_____

_____

_____

_____

_____

How would you document this? _____

_____

_____

Data Collected
(use those that apply)

- Height: 5'5"
- Weight: 125 lbs
- Blood pressure: 180/96
- Pupils cloudy, conjunctiva red
- States she has chronic infection in her sinuses
- Kyphosis present
- R = 30, crackles and wheezes present
- Apical pulse = 108, irregular
- Bowel sounds present in all four quadrants
- 4+ edema from toes to knees in both legs
- Has not taken medications for more than a week
- Does not follow prescribed diet

Nursing Interventions
(use those that apply; list
in priority order)

- State "Why didn't you ask for help with your medicines?"
- Ask Cath if she would consider being seen by a social worker.
- Monitor vital signs on a regular basis.
- State "You need to follow your diet."
- Monitor breath sounds, apical pulse, and peripheral pulses.
- Measure circumference of lower legs.

NCLEX-PN® Exam Preparation

1 When the nurse collects a urine specimen and notes the color of the urine, this assessment data is referred to as:

A. comprehensive.
B. objective.
C. subjective.
D. secondary.

2 A focused assessment for a client complaining of abdominal pain would include assessing the client's:

A. legs.
B. vision.
C. bowel movements.
D. blood pressure.

3 It is preferable to collect assessment data from secondary sources instead of directly from the client when the:

A. client is irritable or agitated.
B. client is very young, unconscious, or confused.
C. client's family prefers to speak for him or her.
D. client's medical records are available.

4 The health history data are collected through an interview with the client. Questions that give the client a chance to provide more information are called:

A. yes or no.
B. why.
C. closed ended.
D. open ended.

5 A basic method of physical examination that uses the hands to touch and feel is called:

A. inspection.
B. auscultation.
C. palpation.
D. percussion.

6 The first thing that the nurse should do in preparing for a physical examination is:

A. wash his or her hands.
B. don gloves and mask.
C. set up the equipment.
D. position the client.

7 Two nurses are checking a client's pulse for a pulse deficit. The nurse taking the apical pulse counts the pulse as 100. The nurse taking the radial pulse counts the pulse as 85. What is the pulse deficit? _____

8 Mrs. Haynes developed a bowel obstruction following abdominal surgery 3 days ago. To monitor peristalsis, the nurse would:

A. inspect the abdomen.
B. auscultate the abdomen.
C. percuss the abdomen.
D. palpate the abdomen.

9 Mr. Scott has a history of alcohol abuse and has developed cirrhosis of the liver. The nurse might expect to observe what change in skin color?

A. mottling
B. erythema
C. jaundice
D. cyanosis

10 Documenting the client assessment is as important as the actual assessment. Identify the documentation that is most correctly stated.

A. Breath sounds normal.
B. The client had bowel sounds in the right upper and lower quadrants and the left upper and lower quadrants.
C. BP 120/70.
D. Client obese, indicating lack of knowledge about nutrition.

Answers for Review Questions, as well as discussion of Critical Thinking Care Map questions, appear in Appendix V.

CULTURAL CARE STRATEGIES

APPRECIATING VARIATIONS IN FACIAL EXPRESSION WHEN RELATING TO THE CLIENT FROM ANOTHER CULTURE

The home health care supervisor received an angry call from Mrs. Espanito, a Mexican American woman who had been the recipient of a home health care visit that day by a nurse. Mrs. Espanito explained that her infant was crying and feverish today, and it was undoubtedly because the nurse had complimented the baby but had not touched the infant during the compliment. Mrs. Espanito felt the nurse had given the infant the evil eye. Mrs. Espanito explained that in Mexican culture, babies are considered very weak and susceptible to the power of an envious glance. A simple compliment without touching a child can bring on the evil eye. While touching a child during a compliment can neutralize the power of the evil eye, no touch had occurred, and therefore she felt her child had become sick from the glance of the nurse.

Throughout the world, facial expression and eye contact are considered an important part of the communication message (Giger & Davidhizar, 1999). From birth, individuals learn how to communicate nonverbally and how to interpret different facial expressions and eye behaviors. Because nursing occurs in an interpersonal arena, nurses need to be aware of facial expression and eye behavior and the meaning that different cultures may associate with facial expressions.

Facial Expression

Facial expression is commonly used as a guide to a person's feelings. A constant stare with immobile facial muscles is generally an indication of coldness. However, it can also be an indication of shock, guardedness, or fear. In an individual with schizophrenia or Parkinson's disease it may be a symptom of the disease process. Facial expression is usually only one part of the total verbal and nonverbal communication that an individual provides. It is important to use facial expression in conjunction with other information to draw conclusions about another's feelings.

The meanings of facial expression vary among persons from different cultures. For example, Italian, Jewish, African American, and Hispanic persons tend to smile readily and use many facial expressions, gestures, and words to communicate feelings. Persons in other cultures (including the Irish, the English, and northern Europeans) tend to use less facial expression and to be less responsive. Facial expression can also convey the opposite meaning from the one that is felt; for example, Oriental people may conceal negative emotions with a smile (Sue & Sue, 1990).

Eye Behavior

Eye contact is a valuable source of information. Typically, individuals look at each other for 3 to 10 seconds in a glance. For many people, longer contact arouses anxiety (Argyle & Dean, 1965). Most Caucasians value eye contact. They may equate avoidance of eye contact with rudeness, disrespect, or lack of attention. Fleeting eye contact may suggest insecurity, shyness, anxiety, or, in some cases, rejection. Embarrassment, guilt, fear, or anger may be interpreted from eye contact.

Because eye contact is learned in a family and cultural context, patterns of eye behavior can sometimes be related to cultural groups. For example, most Mexican American and African American people are comfortable with eye contact (Giger & Davidhizar, 1999). Oriental people and some Native Americans tend to have difficulty with eye contact; they may relate eye contact to impoliteness and an invasion of privacy. Some Filipinos may interpret eye contact that is diverted as a sign of a witch. Some cultures may associate eye contact with the "evil eye" (Henderson & Primeaux, 1981).

Nursing Implications

■ *Assess facial expression for possible cultural significance.* Most individuals use facial expression to reveal feelings. However, since facial expression is learned in a cultural context, the nurse should use an understanding of the individual's culture when interpreting the meaning of a facial expression.

■ *Assess eye behavior for possible cultural significance.* Since individuals are unique, nurses should interpret eye behavior in the context of other available interpersonal information. Since eye behavior is learned in a cultural context, the cultural significance of eye behavior should also be considered.

■ *Be aware that your health care team members may use culturally oriented communication behaviors that make others uncomfortable.* When the communication of a coworker makes you uncomfortable, it is important to assess whether the communication difference is related to cultural behavior.

Self-Reflection Questions

1. What facial and eye behavior do you use in communicating with others?

2. What eye behavior of others makes you uncomfortable?

3. What facial and eye behavior in clients or staff would you interpret as negative or hostile?

Chapter 6

Essential Nursing Pharmacology

BRIEF Outline

Drug Sources and Names
Drug Legislation and Resources
Pharmacokinetics
  Absorption
  Distribution
  Metabolism (Biotransformation)
  Excretion
  Pharmacokinetics in Older Adults
Pharmacodynamics
  Drug Effectiveness
  Dose–Response Relationship
  Variables in Drug Response
  Drug Interaction
  Adverse Drug Reactions

LEARNING Outcomes

After completing this chapter, you will be able to:

- Explain the four types of names given to each drug.
- Identify laws that govern the prescription, storage, and administration of drugs.
- Describe the processes of pharmacokinetics: absorption, distribution, metabolism, and excretion.
- Identify how pharmacodynamics affect drug action.
- Explain the six rights of medication administration and the importance of each right.
- Apply the nursing process to administering medications.

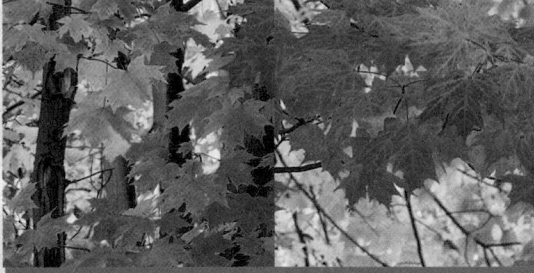

MediaLink

www.prenhall.com/burke
Use the address above to access the free, interactive Companion Website created for this textbook. Get hints, instant feedback, and textbook references to chapter-related NCLEX-style questions. Link to other interesting sites.

Audio Glossary:
Use the Companion Website, or the CD-ROM disk enclosed with your textbook, to hear the pronunciation of key terms in this chapter.

The study of drugs and their uses in the body is called **pharmacology.** Drugs can be used to prevent disease, aid in the diagnosis and treatment of disease, and restore or maintain body system function. For many disease conditions, drug therapy is the only treatment available to control or cure the disease. In other disease processes, the goal may be relief of symptoms in order to increase the client's quality of life.

The nurse is responsible for understanding how medications affect clients as well as the legal implications for administering medications. This chapter focuses on drug standards and legislation, pharmacokinetics, and pharmacodynamics. The nurse's role in applying the nursing process during medication administration is also presented.

Drug Sources and Names

Drugs are made from natural resources including plants, animal tissue, and minerals. Some drugs are produced synthetically in the laboratory, while others are developed through genetic engineering. Synthetic drugs have the advantage of being made in large quantities, possibly reducing the cost when compared to that of natural drugs. Genetic engineering uses recombinant DNA techniques to put together DNA material from different organisms to form new drugs. An example of a product of this process is Humalin® insulin, which is used to manage diabetes mellitus.

All drugs have four names: chemical, generic, trade, and official. The *chemical name* describes the chemical compounds and molecular structure of the drug. Chemical names are long and seldom used; for example, acetylsalicylic acid. For this reason, drugs are given a shorter name called a nonproprietary or *generic name.* The nonproprietary name is approved by the United States Adopted Names (USAN) Council. Thus, acetylsalicylic acid is known by its generic name, aspirin. The *trade name,* sometimes called a brand name, identifies drugs sold by a specific manufacturer. The symbols ® or ™ (trademark) after the drug signify that the trade name is registered. A common trade name for aspirin is Bufferin®. The *official name* is usually the trade name. Official names are listed in the *United States Pharmacopeia–National Formulary (USP-NF).*

Laws regulate generic and nongeneric drugs with respect to the amount and purity of each drug. Only a small amount of active ingredient is in every tablet, leaving the rest of the tablet to be filled with nonmedicinal substances. Although a generic drug is therapeutically equal to its trade name drug, some clients may not receive the same therapeutic effect. It is unclear why a few clients may not receive the same effect. In many states, the law requires pharmacists to fill prescriptions with the generic form. However, a prescriber can direct the pharmacist to fill a prescription with a specific trade name drug. Some prescription drug plans have a higher copay amount when generic drugs are not prescribed. Clients may request the generic form in order to decrease their copay amount. Note also that a prescription may not be listed on an insurance company's formulary, resulting in additional costs to the client.

Nurses must be familiar with both the generic and trade name for a drug in order to prevent potential errors. Physicians are encouraged to write prescriptions by using both names. To recognize the difference between generic and trade names, the generic is listed first in small letters with the trade name capitalized and placed in parentheses after it, for example, digoxin (Lanoxin).

Drug Legislation and Resources

Several drug laws are important in nursing practice. In 1906, the Pure Food and Drug Act was passed to protect the public by restricting the manufacture and sale of drugs. This act was replaced in 1938 by the Food, Drug, and Cosmetic Act, which added new regulations regarding labeling and packaging of drugs as well as requiring drug companies to perform toxicity tests on lab animals. Under the U.S. Department of Health and Human Services, the Food and Drug Administration (FDA) enforces this legislation.

The Controlled Substances Act of 1970 identifies and regulates the manufacture and sale of narcotics and dangerous drugs. Under this law, five schedules (Table 6-1 ■) of drugs

TABLE 6-1		
Schedule for Controlled Substances		
SCHEDULE	**DEFINITION**	**EXAMPLES**
Schedule I	■ Drugs with high abuse potential and no accepted medical use	■ Heroin, peyote
Schedule II	■ Drugs with high abuse potential and accepted medical use	■ Opioid analgesics (morphine, codeine, meperidine); cocaine; amphetamines
Schedule III	■ Drugs with moderate abuse potential and accepted medical use	■ Drugs containing an opioid plus a non-narcotic (Vicodin, Lortab)
Schedule IV	■ Drugs with low abuse potential and accepted medical use	■ Benzodiazepines (diazepam [Valium], chloral hydrate, phenobarbital)
Schedule V	■ Drugs with limited abuse potential and accepted medical use	■ Narcotics used in small amounts for antitussive and antidiarrheal purposes

based on abuse potential and medical effectiveness have been developed. For instance, Schedule I drugs (e.g., heroin, peyote) have the highest abuse potential without any proven medical use in the United States. This act is administered by the Drug Enforcement Administration (DEA), under the Department of Justice. Anyone who possesses a controlled substance without a prescription is subject to fines, imprisonment, or both. In addition, special DEA duplicate prescription pads must be used when a prescriber prescribes certain controlled substances.

All health care facilities are required to have narcotic control systems in place. Policies must be in place regarding use, drug wastage, and documentation. Narcotics are always locked up and only authorized persons have access to the keys.

Nurses require reliable and up-to-date drug information to give medications safely and accurately. Given that numerous new drugs and medicinal agents are approved and marketed each year, textbooks quickly become outdated. In the acute-care setting, the *Hospital Formulary* may be the most readily available and accurate source of drug information. *Facts and Comparisons* is a loose-leaf notebook that contains drug information that is updated monthly. The *Physicians' Desk Reference* (PDR) is the most widely used drug reference in the United States. Package inserts that accompany drugs are another resource to check. The following Internet sites also provide drug information: Food and Drug Administration (www.fda.gov) and RxMed (www.rxmed.com).

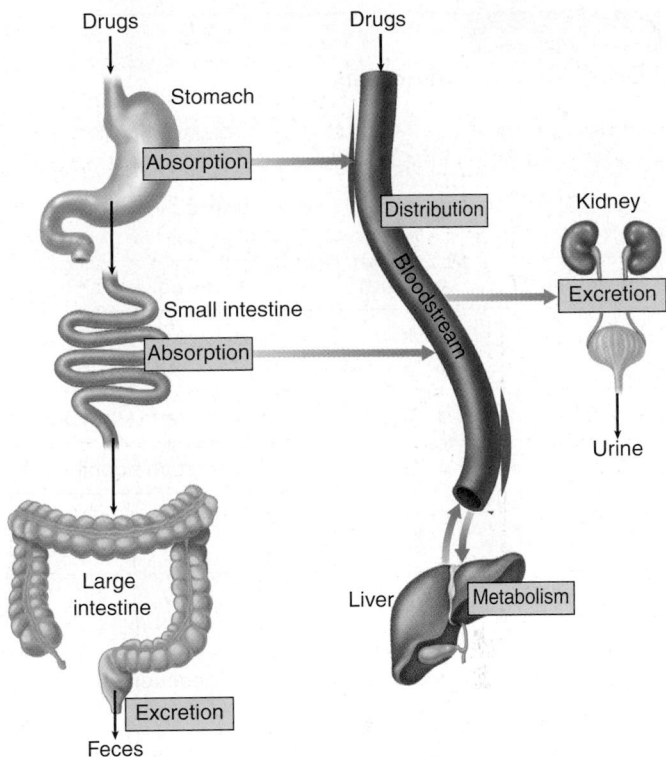

Figure 6-1. ■ The four processes of drug movement (pharmacokinetics): absorption, distribution, metabolism, and excretion. (From *Core Concepts in Pharmacology*, by N. Holland & M. P. Adams, 2003, Upper Saddle River, NJ. Reprinted with permission.)

Pharmacokinetics

Pharmacokinetics is the study of how drugs are processed by the body. It describes the steps that occur from the time a client is administered a drug until it is eliminated from the body. Specific processes that make up pharmacokinetics include absorption, distribution, metabolism (or biotransformation), and excretion (Figure 6-1 ■).

ABSORPTION

Absorption is the first step in the passage of a drug through the body. The absorption process occurs from the time a drug enters the body until it enters the body fluids that carry the drug to its site(s) of action. A drug's absorption rate is important in identifying how soon the drug becomes available to exert its action. If the drug is not absorbed properly, it may not reach its targeted organs or tissues.

Oral preparations are swallowed and dissolved by gastric juices before they reach the small intestine. They must pass through the GI lining and blood vessels before they gain access to the blood. *Sublingual* (under the tongue) or *buccal* (placed in the inner lining of the cheeks) drugs enter the bloodstream through the lining of the mouth. Topical ointments enter through the skin, and rectal suppositories are absorbed through the mucous membranes into the blood.

Transdermal (applied to the skin) patches absorb drugs slowly into the body and usually have a longer duration of action.

Parenteral (injectable) drugs, such as *subcutaneous* (below the skin) and *intramuscular* (into a muscle) drugs, are absorbed faster than oral drugs. Drugs given via the *intradermal* route (injection into dermis) are also absorbed faster than oral drugs and are used to test for diseases (e.g., tuberculosis) and allergies. Intravenous drugs have the fastest absorption rate because they are delivered directly into the bloodstream. Other medication routes include ear, eye, nose, and inhalation. Common routes and drug examples are listed in Table 6-2 ■.

DISTRIBUTION

After a drug is absorbed, it is distributed to various organs and tissues. Several factors affecting drug distribution include blood flow, plasma protein binding, and the blood–brain barrier. Within minutes after absorption into the bloodstream, a drug is delivered to those organs (heart, liver, kidney, and brain) with the largest blood supply. When blood supply from the heart is reduced, adequate tissue levels of a drug are difficult to attain. Drug delivery to other internal organs, muscle, skin, and fat is slower and may take from minutes to hours.

TABLE 6-2

Drug Absorption Routes

ADMINISTRATION ROUTE	ABSORPTION SITE	COMMON MEDICATION EXAMPLE
Oral (PO)	■ Stomach/intestine	■ Antibiotics
Sublingual (SL)	■ Mouth	■ Nitroglycerin
Topical	■ Skin	■ Hydrocortisone ointment
Vaginal	■ Vagina	■ Nystatin (antifungal)
Rectal	■ Rectum	■ Acetaminophen
Intradermal	■ Just under the skin	■ TB testing
Subcutaneous (SC)	■ Subcutaneous tissue	■ Insulin
Intramuscular (IM)	■ Muscle	■ Meperidine
Intravenous (IV)	■ Blood	■ Antibiotics

Following absorption in the bloodstream, most drugs bind with the plasma proteins, especially albumin, which transports the drug to its site of action. However, because the albumin molecule is too large to pass through the capillary wall, the drug must be released from the albumin to be available to the tissues. Thus, drugs bound to albumin have slower absorption, resulting in a longer duration of action. For example, warfarin (Coumadin), an anticoagulant, lasts longer and can accumulate, increasing the client's risk for bleeding.

Drug distribution to the brain is limited because of the blood–brain barrier. (See Chapter 38 ⟳ for further information on the blood–brain barrier). The blood–brain barrier protects the central nervous system against severe toxic drug effects by preventing access to the cerebrospinal fluid. However, some drugs such as anesthetics can cross into the brain.

METABOLISM (BIOTRANSFORMATION)

Drug metabolism refers to the process by which the body changes a drug from its original chemical structure into a form that can be readily eliminated or excreted. This is also called **biotransformation.** The metabolism of most drugs takes place in the liver. Microsomal enzymes (drug-metabolizing enzymes) in the liver break down the drug and also detoxify any potentially harmful substances to the body. Liver diseases such as hepatitis and cirrhosis inhibit enzyme action, which results in excess drug accumulation in the body.

Oral drugs, absorbed from the gastrointestinal tract, move from the intestine into the liver before passing into the systemic circulation. This means that for drugs metabolized

extensively in the liver, only a portion of the drug dose will ever reach its action site. This is referred to as a *first-pass effect* (Figure 6-2 ■). In order for a client to receive a therapeutic effect, the oral dose is often much greater than a parenteral dose (e.g., an IM or IV dose), which bypasses the liver.

EXCRETION

The common pathways of drug excretion are the kidneys, lungs, and the large intestine (in feces). The kidney is the most important organ of drug excretion. Drugs are eliminated either unchanged or as metabolites in urine. Kidney damage may impair excretion, lead to drug accumulation, and increase the potential for severe adverse reactions. The respiratory system is only involved with excretion when a drug changes into a gaseous form, as do, for example, anesthetics. Biliary excretion involves the drug being taken up by the liver, released into the bile, and eliminated in the feces. Drugs excreted by this process remain in the body longer than those excreted by other means.

PHARMACOKINETICS IN OLDER ADULTS

Older adults, aged 65 or older, often have at least one chronic health problem for which they take medications.

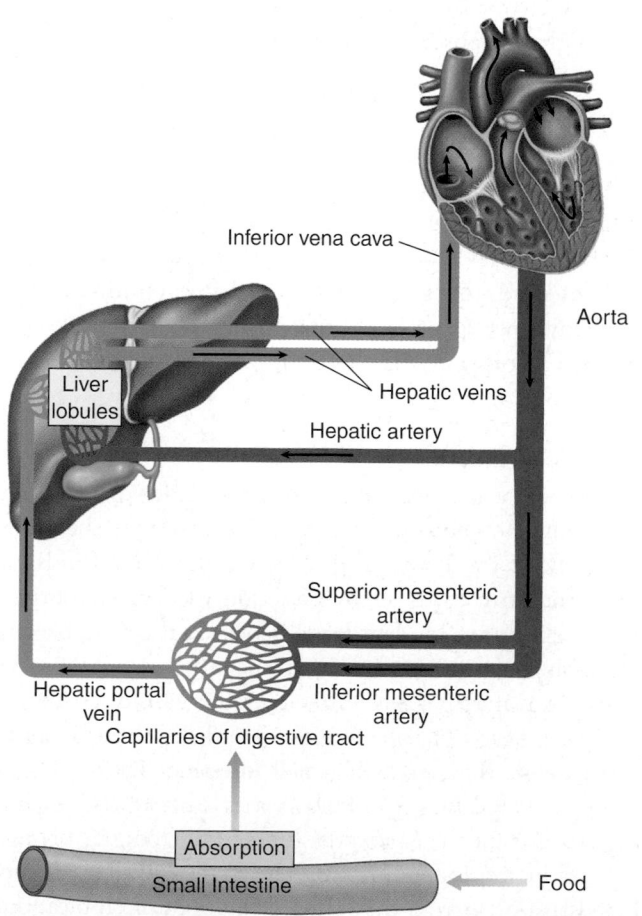

Figure 6-2. ■ First-pass effect. (From: *Core Concepts in Pharmacology,* by N. Holland & M. P. Adams, 2003, Upper Saddle River, NJ. Reprinted with permission.)

Labels in figure: Inferior vena cava; Aorta; Liver lobules; Hepatic veins; Hepatic artery; Superior mesenteric artery; Hepatic portal vein; Inferior mesenteric artery; Capillaries of digestive tract; Absorption; Small Intestine; Food

MediaLink ● **Drug Metabolization**

Pharmacokinetic Changes in Older Adults

Absorption
- Decreased gastric emptying time
- Decreased gastric pH

Distribution
- Decreased lean body weight
- Increased body fat
- Decreased serum albumin levels

Metabolism
- Reduced liver blood flow
- Decreased metabolism of drugs

Excretion
- Reduced kidney blood flow
- Decreased glomerular filtration rate

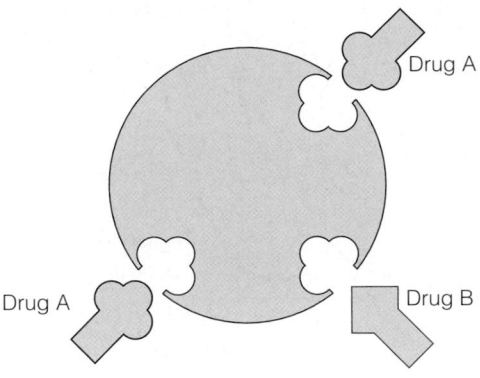

Figure 6-3. ■ Receptor site action: Drug A fits into the receptor site like a key into a lock to initiate a drug reaction. Drug B does not fit into this receptor site; therefore, no drug action occurs at this site.

Many take at least four or more prescription drugs daily as well as about 40% of the over-the-counter (OTC) drugs sold. Physiologic changes occur in the older adult, that affect the normal pharmacokinetic processes (Box 6-1 ■). The practice of *polypharmacy* (use of many prescribed and OTC drugs at the same time) along with the pharmacokinetic changes often leads to drug toxicity in the older adult. Some studies indicate that 15% to 20% of hospitalizations of older adults are related to adverse medication reactions.

clinical ALERT

Changes in mental status may mistakenly be associated with aging rather than the use of multiple drugs.

Pharmacodynamics

Pharmacodynamics is the study of how drugs produce their effects in the body to result in a pharmacologic response. Drug action begins after a drug attaches itself to a specific area on the cell, called a *receptor site* (Figure 6-3 ■). By binding to the receptor, a drug can either initiate or block a cell response. Drugs that combine with a specific receptor to cause a pharmacologic response are called **agonists.** For example, morphine is an agonist, binding to receptors in the central nervous system (CNS) to decrease pain. **Antagonists** are drugs that prevent a receptor response or block a normal cellular response. Naloxone (Narcan) blocks the depression of the CNS caused by narcotic agonists such as morphine. Antihistamines block the normal release of histamine to stop allergy symptoms.

Drugs can have a *local* or *systemic* effect depending on the location and action on the cell receptors. Examples of drugs with a local effect include eye, ear, and nose drops, lozenges, skin ointments, and suppositories. Systemic drugs, such as narcotics for pain relief, must travel through the bloodstream to affect cells or tissues.

DRUG EFFECTIVENESS

The effectiveness of a drug depends on its action and dose. Each drug has an onset, peak, and duration of action. *Onset of action* is the time it takes for a drug to reach an effective blood level and to initiate a body response. The onset can be slow, intermediate, or rapid depending on the route of administration and pharmacokinetic principles. *Peak action* occurs when the drug achieves its highest blood concentration. The length of time that a drug has a pharmacologic effect is called its *duration of action*.

The length of time that a drug remains effective depends on its half-life. **Half-life** is the amount of time needed for elimination processes to decrease the original blood concentration by 50% (one-half). For example, if a 650-mg dose of a drug with a half-life of 3 hours is administered, it takes 3 hours for 325 mg (50%) of the drug to be eliminated. However, the half-life increases in clients with liver or kidney disease because of impaired metabolism or impaired elimination of the drug.

A drug's therapeutic effect depends on maintaining a constant serum level of drug. Drugs that are eliminated rapidly from the body need more frequent dosing throughout the day. Most drugs require several doses or several days to achieve their desired drug effect. In certain clinical situations, it may be necessary to reach therapeutic drug levels rapidly. In these cases, a **loading dose** (an initial higher-than-normal dose of drug) is given, usually intravenously, to quickly produce the desired result. Following the loading dose, smaller *maintenance* doses are given to maintain the drug level within a therapeutic range. A common example of this practice is the administration of digoxin (Lanoxin) to a client in acute heart failure. (See Chapter 26 ⊘ for more information on heart failure.)

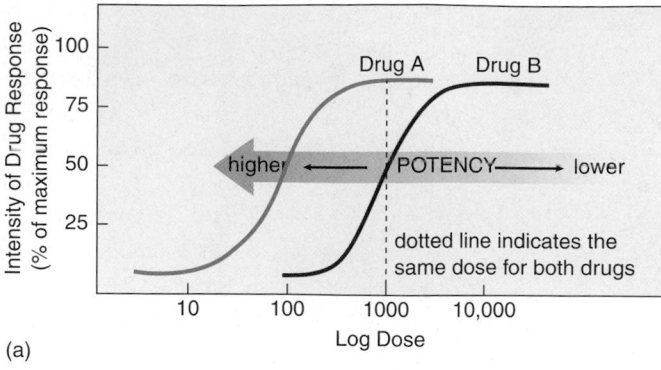

(a)

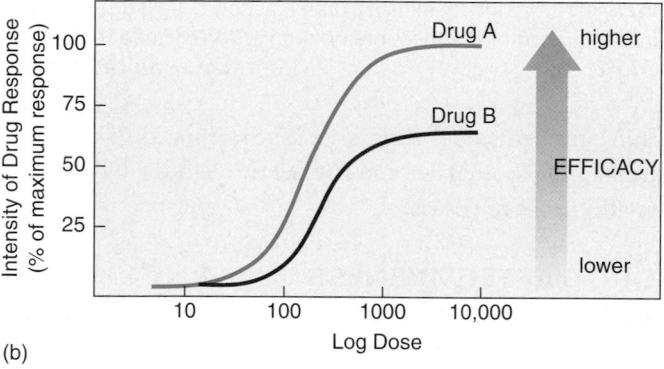

(b)

Figure 6-4. ■ Potency and efficacy. (**A**) Drug A has a higher potency than drug B. (**B**) Drug B has a higher efficacy than drug B. (From *Core Concepts in Pharmacology*, by N. Holland & M. P. Adams, 2003, Upper Saddle River, NJ. Reprinted with permission.)

DOSE–RESPONSE RELATIONSHIP

The response to any drug depends on the amount of drug given. As the dose increases, so does the response until a maximum response is attained. Potency and efficacy are two factors used to determine dose responsiveness. *Potency* is the relationship between the dose of the drug and the intensity of its effect. A more potent drug will achieve effects similar to another drug. However, the more potent drug can be administered in a smaller dose. For example, 10 mg of morphine equals 1 mg of hydromorphone (Dilaudid). It is clear that hydromorphone is more potent, however, the doses are equally effective. A dose–response curve is used to plot the potency of drugs (Figure 6-4A ■).

Efficacy refers to a drug's maximum effect. The efficacy of a drug is seen on the dose–response curve when it reaches a plateau (Figure 6-4B). For example, acetaminophen effectively controls mild to moderate pain; meperidine (Demerol) effectively controls all levels of pain. This makes meperidine a more effective pain reliever than acetaminophen. Once a drug is at its plateau, a further increase in dose will not increase its effectiveness.

Some drugs have a **ceiling effect,** which means that there is a dose limit to produce a specific effect. For instance, acetaminophen (Tylenol) has a ceiling effect of 4,000 mg per day. Doses exceeding the ceiling effect usually cause undesirable results, such as liver toxicity with acetaminophen.

VARIABLES IN DRUG RESPONSE

Drug response varies in each client even when the same dose and dosage regimen are followed. Factors that contribute to this variation include age, body weight, genetics, ethnicity, disease conditions, and emotional state.

Age

Infants, children, and older adults are more sensitive to drug actions than middle-aged adults. The very young have an immature liver and kidneys, which slow drug metabolism and excretion. Altered pharmacokinetics in older adults increases and prolongs the effects of drugs.

Body Weight

Dosage is often prescribed in relation to a client's weight. Clients who are underweight or overweight may require different doses. The usual adult dose of a drug is based on individuals between 18 and 65 years old and weighing 150 pounds (70 kg). Some drug doses are calculated on body weight (milligrams per kilograms), such as drugs given to pediatric clients.

Genetics

Drugs are expected to have predictable results. However, in some clients given the same drug in the same dose, the results vary. Some may not achieve the therapeutic effect, while others experience adverse effects. Some people lack certain drug-metabolizing enzymes as a result of their genetic makeup. When an enzyme is missing, drug metabolism slows, increasing the risk for prolonged drug effects and possible serious consequences. Other clients do not lack enzymes but rather have an increased metabolic rate. They may need higher doses or more frequent drug administration to overcome the rapid metabolism of the drug.

Ethnicity

Ethnicity also plays a role in drug response. For example, in African Americans some antihypertensive drugs are less effective than in Caucasians. Asian clients may need lower doses of the antianxiety drug alprazolam (Xanax) and the antipsychotic agent haloperidol (Haldol).

Disease Conditions

Liver disease alters metabolism, while kidney disease decreases excretion. Cardiac conditions, such as heart failure, reduce the heart's pumping ability, decreasing all pharmacokinetic processes. Inflammatory bowel disorders (Crohn's disease, ulcerative colitis) can either increase or decrease absorption. Hyperthyroidism and fever increase metabolism, causing a shorter duration and faster elimination. Hypothyroidism slows a person's metabolic rate, which prolongs drug action. Malnutrition lowers the concentration of albumin, which is necessary for plasma protein binding.

Emotional State

Clients' expectations about their drug therapy may affect the outcome. Usually individuals with a positive attitude respond better to drug therapy. In contrast, clients who are depressed may not respond as well. Expectations and attitudes also influence whether individuals will follow their drug regimen.

DRUG INTERACTIONS

Drug interaction refers to the effects that occur when the actions of one drug are affected by another drug. The most common types of interactions are called additive, synergism, and potentiation. An **additive** effect develops when two drugs with similar actions are taken. Additive effects increase the sum of the effects of the two drugs. Combining aspirin with codeine increases pain relief and usually lowers the dose of each drug, resulting in fewer toxic effects. However, a dangerous situation occurs when alcohol is consumed with sedative drugs, because the combination increases their sedative effect.

When two drugs given together cause a greater response than each drug given separately, it is called **synergism.** A client may receive two different drugs for hypertension, lowering blood pressure in two different ways. The combined effect of these two drugs more effectively lowers the blood pressure than either one by itself.

Potentiation is when the action of one drug increases the effect of the second drug. Clients who take anticoagulants are advised against taking aspirin because the two drugs together increase the risk for bleeding.

Other drug interactions develop during the pharmacokinetic process. For instance, antacids decrease absorption of drugs in the gastrointestinal tract. This action affects such drugs as digoxin (cardiac drug), isoniazid (antitubercular drug), and tetracycline (antibiotic). Another interaction occurs in smokers. Nicotine increases the action of the drug-metabolizing enzymes, causing rapid metabolism of medications. Drug dosages in smokers would have to be increased to obtain therapeutic results similar to those for nonsmokers.

Drug incompatibilities can occur while preparing or administering intramuscular or intravenous medications. A drug *incompatibility* is defined as a chemical or physical reaction between two drugs. This reaction can either inactivate one of the drugs or cause a precipitate (discoloration or particles) to form. For example, Lantus insulin (antidiabetic) forms a precipitate when mixed with regular insulin.

clinical ALERT

Before combining or administering two drugs together, consult with a pharmacist or a drug compatibility chart.

Food–Drug Interactions

Food can increase, decrease, or delay drug absorption. Diets high in vitamin K (dark-green leafy vegetables) reduce the absorption of warfarin (anticoagulant). The calcium in milk and milk products binds with tetracycline (antibiotic), reducing its absorption. A high carbohydrate diet increases absorption of levodopa (antiparkinsonian drug). However, protein delays the absorption of levodopa and theophylline (bronchodilator). Grapefruit juice can increase the metabolism of numerous drugs, especially calcium channel blockers, caffeine, and cholesterol-lowering drugs.

A more toxic reaction develops when foods with tyramine (aged cheeses, aged beer, Chianti wine, and yogurt) are consumed while taking monoamine oxidase (MAO) inhibitors. Combining tyramine food with the MAO inhibitor could cause a hypertensive crisis or stroke.

clinical ALERT

Before administering oral medications, determine whether they should be given before, with, or after meals.

Over-the-Counter Drugs

Over-the-counter (OTC) drugs can be purchased without a prescription. About 60% of all medications are classified as OTCs. The FDA is responsible for maintaining the safety of this drug class. Common OTCs include analgesics for pain, antacids, antihistamines, cough and cold medications, eyedrops, hemorrhoid products, herbal supplements, laxatives, sleep aids, vitamin supplements, and weight loss aids. Some OTCs such as ibuprofen were once prescription drugs.

OTCs allow the consumer to treat minor illnesses. Usually they are an effective, inexpensive way to manage common health problems for a short period of time. However, OTCs are not without potential problems. Clients may delay seeking medical care, resulting in serious or life-threatening consequences. Drug interactions can occur with prescription drugs or other OTCs. Individuals with liver and kidney disease should avoid OTCs unless recommended by their health care provider.

Herbal Therapy

The practice of using herbal therapy has existed for thousands of years. Many cultures believe that herbs can prevent or cure health problems. For the past two decades there has been increased interest in products without preservatives or additives, resulting in greater use of herbal therapy and other nontraditional remedies. This led the National Institutes of Health to establish the National Center for Complementary and Alternative Medicine (NCCAM). NCCAM has developed five categories of complementary and alternative therapies.

BOX 6-2	COMPLEMENTARY THERAPIES

Common Herbal Therapies

- Aloe
- Black cohosh
- Chamomile
- Echinacea
- Feverfew
- Garlic
- Gingko
- Ginseng
- Goldenseal
- Saw palmetto
- St. John's wort
- Valerian

In the early 1990s the FDA threatened to ban all herbal remedies. Based on public outcry, Congress passed the Dietary Supplement Health and Education Act of 1994. It reclassified herbal remedies as dietary supplements. However, the safety and effectiveness of herbal therapies are not regulated. In addition, manufacturing regulations are not standardized. Allergic, adverse, and toxic reactions can develop from herbal remedies just like with OTC and prescription drugs.

Herbal therapy comes in a variety of forms, including dried or fresh herbs, teas, ointments, oils, syrups, and tinctures. The most common herbal remedies are listed in Box 6-2 ■. Their uses can be found throughout this textbook as they relate to specific disease conditions.

Clients should be taught to avoid taking herbal remedies if pregnant or nursing. They should not be given to infants or children. All clients are advised to contact their health care provider before substituting an herb for a prescription drug. Herbal remedies should be considered medicines and, therefore, used cautiously.

clinical ALERT

Caution clients to read the drug label for contraindications and adverse reactions before taking any OTC or herbal remedy.

ADVERSE DRUG REACTIONS

The desired action of all drugs is achievement of a *therapeutic effect*. However, drugs are not without the potential to cause harm. Adverse drug reactions (ADRs) can develop that range from mild to severe—even death. The most frequent adverse drug reactions include side effects, allergies, idiosyncratic effects, and toxic effects.

Side effects are anticipated effects from a therapeutic drug dose. Most often they are mild. For example, opioid analgesics may cause nausea and constipation, whereas antihistamines are known to cause drowsiness and dry mouth. Gastric irritation is a common side effect following the administration of corticosteroids and aspirin. Side effects can develop within a few hours of starting a new drug or can be delayed for weeks.

Drug *allergy* occurs when an individual becomes sensitized to a specific drug, producing antibodies against the drug (antigen). Subsequent administration of the drug leads to an antigen–antibody reaction. Reaction between the antibody and antigen causes damage to body tissues. The injured cells release histamine that generates the characteristic symptoms of an allergy. These include hives, rashes, itching, and nasal secretion. Severe allergic reactions, called *anaphylaxis,* begin within minutes of exposure. They produce hypotension, tachycardia, and bronchoconstriction; without immediate treatment death may result. (See Chapter 13 🔗 for further information about anaphylaxis and anaphylactic shock.)

clinical ALERT

Always check a client's allergy status before administering any drug.

When a very small percentage of the population develops an unusual or unexpected response, the reaction is termed an *idiosyncratic effect*. The response may be opposite the desired effect, such as agitation from a sedative drug. Often idiosyncrasy is triggered by a genetic difference not found in most individuals.

Toxic effects denote harmful, undesired effects (e.g., persistent vomiting) or the possibility of organ damage. Most drugs are capable of producing toxic effects when administered in high doses. For example, clients taking excessive amounts of opioid narcotics are at risk for severe respiratory depression and possibly death. Toxicity can also develop when serum drug levels exceed the therapeutic range. Drugs with a narrow therapeutic range, such as digitalis, aminoglycoside antibiotics, and anticonvulsants, are monitored through serum blood levels to prevent toxic effects.

Because most drugs are metabolized in the liver and excreted in the kidneys, these organs can suffer potential damage. Liver damage (*hepatotoxicity*) results from an overdose of acetaminophen. Aminoglycosides can damage the kidneys (*nephrotoxicity*) as well as the eighth cranial nerve, causing *ototoxicity*.

Other organs most often affected include the blood, GI, skin, and lungs. Bone marrow suppression (anemia, thrombocytopenia, and leukopenia) results from chemotherapy agents. Gastrointestinal toxicity includes GI ulceration, bleeding, or pseudomembranous colitis (a severe form of colitis). Severe skin reactions such as exfoliative dermatitis and Stevens–Johnson syndrome can develop. Some antibiotics and chemotherapy drugs may cause drug-induced asthma or pneumonitis.

Drugs that cause birth defects are known to have a *teratogenic effect*. They must be avoided in pregnant women. Other drugs with a *carcinogenic effect* may promote the growth of cancerous tumors.

NURSING CARE

The nursing care process is a systematic process for providing care to clients. The five-step process of assessing, diagnosing, planning, implementing, and evaluating when correctly applied to drug therapy can reduce the potential for errors. The nursing care process also promotes the sound decision making that is necessary for safe drug administration.

ASSESSING

Assessment begins by collecting data on the client's medication history. When first meeting the client, assess weight, age, health status, and any disease conditions. The nurse conducts a nonjudgmental interview about medication use and any factors that could affect the client's compliance with a medication schedule (Box 6-3 ■). When information cannot be obtained from the client, contact family members and check the chart for the client's history. The client's level of education and understanding is included during assessment.

A physical examination is performed to determine whether the client has physical or mental problems that could affect his or her ability to take any medication. The nurse assesses for hearing and visual deficits, swallowing ability, and manual dexterity. Clients with mental disorders may have difficulty remembering or understanding how to take their medications. Those with reading deficits may be unable to follow the directions on a drug label. The nurse should review pertinent laboratory test values such as liver and kidney function studies, WBC count, hemoglobin, hematocrit, electrolytes, and albumin levels.

DIAGNOSING AND PLANNING

Diagnosing focuses on identifying the client's actual and potential health problems based on the assessment data. The LPN contributes to the development of the nursing diagnosis. Several nursing diagnoses can be selected for clients receiving drug therapy. The following are examples of appropriate nursing diagnoses:

- Deficient Knowledge
- Ineffective Health Maintenance
- Noncompliance
- Risk for Injury related to side effects

During the planning step, the nurse reviews the drug's purpose, recommended dose, potential side effects, and therapeutic effects. The nurse plans when medications are scheduled according to the physician's orders. Factors to consider include drug–food or drug–drug interactions and frequency of dosing. In addition, the nurse plans client teaching about taking medications at home.

IMPLEMENTING

This step involves the actual nursing interventions used to administer drug therapy. Before giving any medication, an authorized health care provider must either write or verbally state an order. All medication orders must include the following information:

- Client's name
- Date and time order was written
- Drug with dose, route, and frequency
- Any special instruction for administration
- Physician's or health care provider's signature

clinical ALERT

Never implement an order that is incomplete, unclear, or written illegibly.

Different types of drug orders are used to direct when the nurse should administer drugs. *Routine orders* are applied until a discontinuation order is written. Some agencies have an automatic stop date, which encourages the physician to reevaluate the client's condition and either reorder, change, or stop the drug. A *standing order* is used for a specific condition in which a drug is to be given. For example, "Give acetaminophen (Tylenol) 650 mg suppository for temperature above 101.6°F." *Stat orders* are to be done immediately, and *prn orders* are to be implemented when the client needs them.

BOX 6-3

MEDICATION HISTORY

- Use of prescription and OTC drugs, and herbal remedies
- Purpose and response to current drugs
- Types of allergies—drugs, food, animal dust, plants
- Allergic reactions, side or toxic effects to current or past drugs
- Use of alcohol, nicotine, caffeine, contraceptives, or street drugs
- Presence of liver, kidney, GI, or heart diseases
- Attitude about taking medications
- Compliance with drug therapy
- Financial resources
- Access to family, friends, or neighbors
- Dietary habits and cultural influences

The nurse is responsible for carrying out an order as it is written. The nurse cannot change an order without clarifying it with the health care provider who wrote the order. It is the nurse's duty to clarify any unclear orders.

To administer drugs safely, the nurse is expected to follow the "Six Rights" so that the potential for errors is reduced:

- Right drug
- Right client
- Right time
- Right route
- Right dose
- Right documentation.

Right Drug. Before administering any medication, always compare the drug label to the medication administration record (MAR) three times: (1) Compare the drug before taking it from the shelf or drawer. (2) Compare on removing the ordered amount of drug from the container. (3) Compare again before returning the container to the shelf or drawer, or with unit-dose packaging, as the drug is placed into the client's hand.

clinical ALERT

Never administer medications that someone else has prepared.

Right Client. Check the client's name against an identifying wristband (in the hospital setting) and the MAR. When the wristband is unclear or missing, ask the client for identifying data such as first, middle, and last name.

Right Time. Check the time for giving the drug with the MAR. Follow the routine times according to the facility's policies. Failure to administer drugs at the correct times is a medication error.

Right Route. Check the physician's order and the MAR to verify the correct route for administering the drug. Be aware of changes in the client's health that could alter the route; for instance, a client who is vomiting probably cannot take oral medications. The physician must be notified to change the route. Before crushing any medications, check with the pharmacist.

Right Dose. Be sure the dose matches the amount stated on the MAR and falls within the usual dose range for the drug. The *unit-dose system* (individually packaged drugs) has helped to reduce medication errors. If dose calculations are necessary, have another licensed health care worker check them.

Right Documentation. Chart medications immediately after giving them, including drug, dose, route, date and time, and nurse's initials. Record and report immediately any

unusual client reaction to a medication or inability or refusal to take the prescribed drug.

clinical ALERT

Never chart a medication before giving it because it increases the risk of missing a dose.

Medication Errors

Medication errors occur in all health care facilities. The National Coordinating Council for Medication Error Reporting and Prevention (NCC MERP) defines a medication error as "any preventable event that may cause or lead to inappropriate medication use or patient harm while the medication is in the control of the healthcare professional, patient, or consumer." Although nurses are the primary individuals administering medications, errors can occur at any point in the process. The most common types of errors causing client death include the wrong dose, wrong drug, and wrong route.

Any medication error must be reported immediately to the nurse in charge. The next steps are to assess the client followed by notification of the client's physician. Many health care facilities require the physician to make a follow-up visit to see the client. The nurse who made the error is expected to complete an incident report. This is an objective, factual account of how the error occurred so that future errors can be prevented.

clinical ALERT

Failure to report an error violates the standard of professional care.

In addition to always following the Six Rights of medication administration, nurses can implement other strategies to prevent errors. For instance, an unfamiliar abbreviation, unusual drug name or dose, confusing drug name, or ambiguous drug orders should signal a need for follow-up. While transcribing medication orders to the MAR, use only acceptable abbreviations and symbols as developed by Joint Commission on Accreditation of Healthcare Organizations (JCAHO).

While the nurse prepares the client's medications, it is essential to think about why each drug is prescribed. The nurse should ask the following questions: "Does the drug make sense for the client's diagnosis? Has the client achieved the desired therapeutic effect?"

During drug preparation, several principles should be followed. It is unacceptable to use the dropper of one medication to administer another drug. When the pharmacy has dispensed multiple tablets, ampules, or vials to provide a single dose, the nurse should question the dose. If a dose seems unusually small or large, ask the pharmacist or physician for a clarification. As a final safety check, the MAR is taken into the client's room and the drug is compared to the MAR before administering it to the client.

Clients can also assist in preventing errors. When a client questions the color of a tablet or capsule, the number of pills, or an injection instead of a pill, recheck the MAR and physician orders. If a client reports an allergy to a medication, do not give it, and verify the order with the client's physician.

The overall goal of medication administration is client safety. To accomplish this goal, everyone involved in writing medication prescriptions, dispensing, and administering must make a conscious effort to prevent medication errors.

EVALUATING

The success of the nursing interventions is measured by evaluating the client's outcomes. The client should exhibit manifestations that the medication is effective. For exam-ple, pain should decrease following analgesic therapy. The nurse determines if the client has developed side effects or any drug interactions. Evaluate the success of the teaching session with the client.

CONTINUING CARE

Another important aspect of medication administration is client teaching. The client should know the following information: name, dose, route, and purpose of the drug, special storage or preparation directions, and any expected or unusual side effects. Clients must also understand the need for follow-up tests or evaluation related to their drug therapy. To ensure accurate drug information is provided, give the client approved, preprinted drug information sheets. Following client teaching, the information presented is documented in the chart.

Note: The bibliography listings for this and all chapters have been compiled at the back of the book.

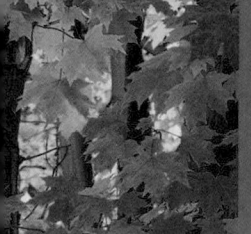

Chapter Review

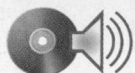 **KEY TERMS** by Topics

Use the audio glossary feature of either the CD-ROM or the Companion Website to hear the correct pronunciation of the following key terms.

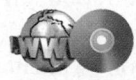 **Essential nursing pharmacology**
pharmacology

Pharmacokinetics
pharmacokinetics, biotransformation

Pharmacodynamics
pharmacodynamics, agonist, antagonist, half-life, loading dose, ceiling effect, additive, synergism, potentiation

KEY Points

- Medications are substances that alter body function to prevent or treat disease, aid in diagnosis, and restore or maintain function.

- The processes of absorption, distribution, metabolism, and excretion make up the pharmacokinetic action of a drug.

- Adverse drug reactions range from expected side effects to toxic effects. The most common toxic effects include liver and kidney damage.

- Safe medication administration means implementing the "Six Rights" in order to prevent a medication error.

- Preventing medication errors requires everyone to make a commitment to client safety.

EXPLORE MediaLink

Additional interactive resources for this chapter can be found on the Companion Website at www.prenhall.com/burke. Click on Chapter 6 and "Begin" to select the activities for this chapter.

For chapter-related NCLEX-style questions and an audio glossary, access the accompanying CD-ROM in this book.

FOR FURTHER Study

Further information about anaphylaxis and anaphylactic shock is given in Chapter 13.

See Chapter 26 for more information on heart failure.

Chapter 38 provides further information on the blood–brain barrier.

NCLEX-PN® Exam Preparation

1 Decreased serum albumin levels in the older adult would affect which part of the pharmacokinetic process?

A. excretion
B. metabolism
C. distribution
D. absorption

2 The nurse receives the following order: Lasix 40 PO BID. Dr. Lowe. What action should the nurse take?

A. Call the physician for a complete dosage.
B. Give the medication as ordered.
C. Wait until the physician calls the unit.
D. Call the physician for a time to start the drug.

3 Which of the following drug examples indicates a synergistic drug response?

A. aspirin and an anticoagulant drug
B. two different antihypertensive drugs
C. nicotine and an anticonvulsant drug
D. alcohol and a sedative drug

4 To prevent a medication error, the nurse should:

A. check illegible handwriting with another nurse.
B. accept atypical drug names as a new medication.
C. use the dropper of one medication to administer another.
D. question the use of multiple tablets to provide a single dose.

5 In which of the following clients is an adverse drug reaction most likely to occur?

A. a four-year-old with croup
B. a 35-year-old with pneumonia
C. a 50-year-old with kidney disease
D. a 60-year-old with osteoarthritis

6 List the order of drug absorption from the most rapid route to the least rapid route.

A. subcutaneous (SC)
B. oral (PO)
C. transdermal
D. intravenous (IV)
E. sublingual
F. intramuscular (IM)

7 The physician prescribes Vicodin for a patient experiencing pain. Under what category of controlled substances is this drug found?

A. Schedule V
B. Schedule IV
C. Schedule III
D. Schedule II

8 What is the most important factor in administering medications to a 1-year-old infant?

A. weight of the child
B. age of the child
C. ethnicity of the child
D. sex of the child

9 When digoxin (Lanoxin) is started, a larger than normal dose may be given. This is called a:

A. scheduled dose.
B. maintenance dose.
C. therapeutic dose.
D. loading dose.

10 The nurse is reviewing information on a medication in a drug handbook and notices that the drug is teratogenic. Which of the following clients should not receive this medication?

A. clients with renal failure
B. pregnant clients
C. children under 10 years old
D. clients older than 65 years

Answers for Review Questions appear in Appendix V.

Thinking Strategically About...

You are a newly graduated LPN assigned to a medical–surgical unit. You have been assigned to three clients.

Mr. Ramos is a 58-year-old male who was admitted for a prostatectomy (TURP) this morning. He is predominantly Spanish speaking, though he knows a few words of English and understands a little if he is spoken to slowly. He has returned from surgery. Initially he was sedated but he is becoming more alert. He appears agitated and is yelling loudly at his roommate, who puts on his call light to summon the nurse. The roommate states, "Mr. Ramos is trying to climb out of bed and he is frightening me."

Mr. Drew is a 53-year-old male who was admitted directly from his physician's office with chest pain. His BP is 168/90 with tachycardia (heart rate 102). He is diaphoretic and is complaining of nausea.

Mr. Melezack is a 64-year-old male who had a colon resection 3 days ago. His NG tube has been clamped and he has been started on clear liquids. It was reported that he tolerated them well. The doctor has ordered that the tube can be removed if there is no nausea or vomiting.

TIME MANAGEMENT

You have received report. Using your knowledge of three clients' diagnoses and present needs, prioritize your care for the shift.

CRITICAL THINKING

Mr. Ramos is frightening his roommate and trying to climb out of bed. He has an IV line and a three-way catheter that is draining dark red urine with clots. Outline the steps you would take to protect Mr. Ramos from himself and to relieve the concerns of the roommate.

CLIENT TEACHING

Mr. Drew's lab work has come back. You observe that his CPK values are within normal limits and that his chest pain is relieved with sublingual nitroglycerin spray. He will be discharged in the morning and you are to begin his discharge planning. In your teaching plan, state what activities would decrease the chance of recurrent angina and the risk factors that need to be controlled to decrease heart disease.

DOCUMENTING AND REPORTING

The client care assistant reports to you that Mr. Melezack is complaining of abdominal pain. He has vomited and asks to see you right away. After you go to his room to assess his present status, you will need to document and report your finding to the appropriate individuals. Write a medical record entry, using the Focus Charting method. State what information needs to be reported and to whom.

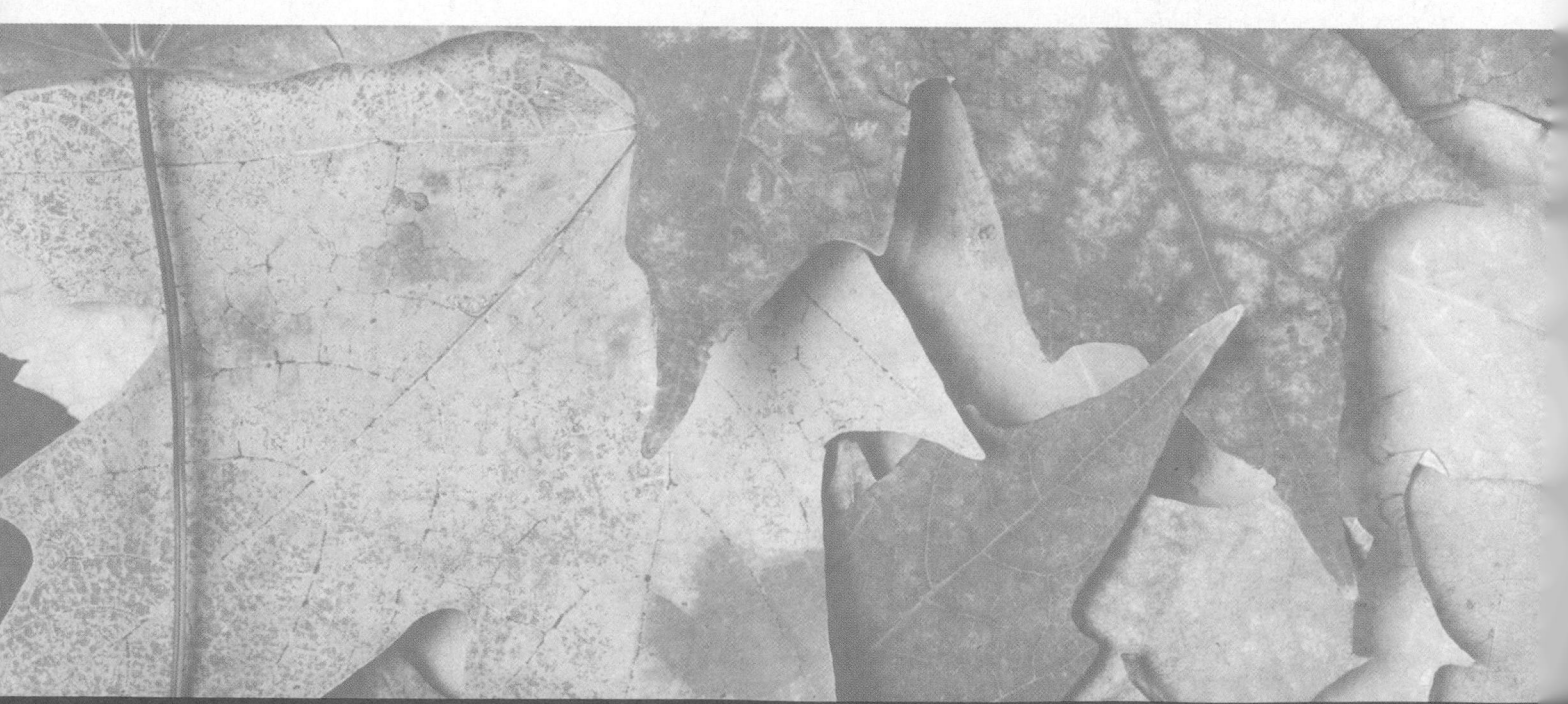

Foundations of Medical–Surgical Nursing

UNIT II

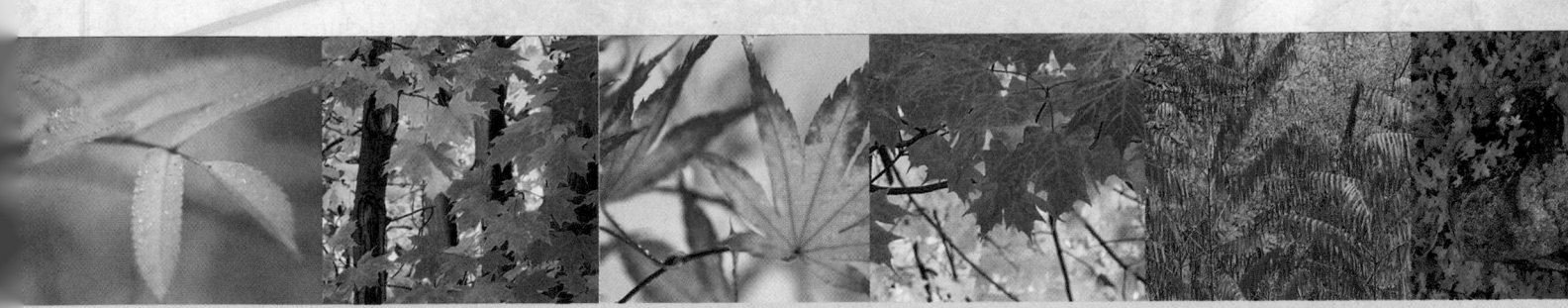

Chapter 7

Caring for Clients with Altered Fluid, Electrolyte, or Acid–Base Balance

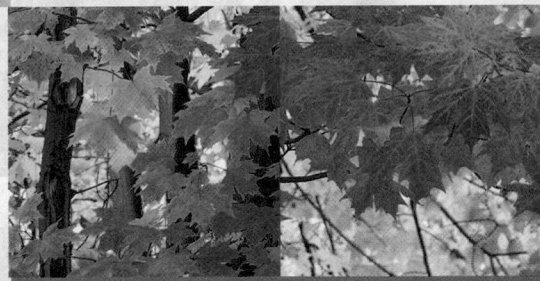

BRIEF Outline

Fluid and Electrolyte Balance

Structure and Function

Fluid Volume Deficit

Fluid Volume Excess

Sodium Imbalance

Potassium Imbalance

Calcium Imbalance

Magnesium Imbalance

Phosphorus Imbalance

Acid–Base Disorders

Acid–Base Regulation

Types of Acid–Base Imbalances

LEARNING Outcomes

After completing this chapter, you will be able to:

- Identify the functions and regulatory mechanisms that maintain water, electrolyte, and acid–base balance in the body.

- Compare and contrast the causes and effects of fluid volume, electrolyte, and acid–base imbalances.

- Identify tests used to diagnose and monitor treatment of fluid, electrolyte, and acid–base disorders.

- Recognize normal and abnormal values of electrolytes in the blood.

- Use arterial blood gas results to identify the type of acid–base imbalance present in a client.

- Provide appropriate nursing care and teaching for clients with fluid, electrolyte, or acid–base disorders.

MediaLink

www.prenhall.com/burke

Use the address above to access the free, interactive Companion Website created for this textbook. Get hints, instant feedback, and textbook references to chapter-related NCLEX-style questions. Link to other interesting sites.

Audio Glossary:

Use the Companion Website, or the CD-ROM disk enclosed with your textbook, to hear the pronunciation of key terms in this chapter.

Normal life processes depend on a relatively stable state within the body. **Homeostasis** is the body's tendency to maintain a state of physiologic balance in constantly changing conditions. For the body to function and survive, the volume, electrolyte composition, and pH of body fluids all must remain within a relatively narrow and constant range. Disorders in fluid volumes, electrolyte concentrations, and hydrogen ion concentration (pH) often occur in response to illness and trauma. Nursing care related to homeostasis focuses on assessing for imbalances and their manifestations, and intervening to prevent or correct imbalances.

FLUID AND ELECTROLYTE BALANCE

Structure and Function

BODY FLUID COMPOSITION

Water is the primary component of body fluids. Water has a number of vital functions in the body:

- It transports nutrients and oxygen to the cells, and waste products such as carbon dioxide away from the cells.
- It provides a medium for metabolic reactions within cells.
- It insulates and helps regulate and maintain body temperature.
- It provides form for body structure and acts as a shock absorber.
- It acts as a lubricant.

About 60% of total body weight is water, but this amount varies with age, gender, and body fat. In people over age 65, body water may decrease to 45% to 50% of total body weight. The proportion of water to total body weight is smaller in an obese person, because fat cells contain comparatively little water. Adult females have a higher percentage of body fat and a lower percentage of body water than males.

To maintain normal fluid balance, water intake and output should be approximately equal. The average daily fluid intake and output usually is about 2,500 mL. Water enters the body through ingested fluids and foods. It also is produced by the cells during metabolism. Water is lost in urine, feces, and sweat, and when we exhale air from the lungs.

Besides water, body fluids contain solutes such as oxygen, dissolved nutrients, waste products of metabolism such as carbon dioxide, and electrolytes.

Electrolytes are substances that *dissociate* (separate) in solution to form *ions* (charged particles). *Cations* are positively charged electrolytes; *anions* are negatively charged electrolytes. Electrolytes have many functions:

- They help regulate water and acid–base balance.
- They contribute to enzyme reactions.
- They are essential to neuromuscular activity.

The concentration of most electrolytes in body fluids is measured in milliequivalents per liter of water (mEq/L). A *milliequivalent* is a measure of the combining power of the ion. For example, 100 mEq of sodium (Na^+) can combine with 100 mEq of chloride (Cl^-) to form sodium chloride (NaCl), or table salt. Some electrolytes (e.g., calcium) may be measured by weight, in milligrams per deciliter of water (mg/dL). Table 7-1 ■ lists normal laboratory values for electrolytes.

BODY FLUID DISTRIBUTION

Body fluid is classified by its location. **Intracellular fluid (ICF)** is within the cells; it accounts for about 40% of total body weight (Figure 7-1 ■). ICF contains solutes such as electrolytes, glucose, and oxygen. ICF is essential for normal cell function.

Extracellular fluid (ECF) is outside of cells; it accounts for about 20% of total body weight. ECF is found in three compartments:

- *Interstitial fluid* is in the spaces between most of the cells of the body (about 15% of total body weight).
- *Intravascular fluid* or *plasma* is in the arteries, veins, and capillaries (about 5% of total body weight).
- *Transcellular fluid* includes cerebrospinal fluid, urine, digestive secretions, perspiration, and small amounts of fluid found within organs and joints (<1% of total body weight).

TABLE 7-1

Normal Laboratory Values for Electrolytes, Osmolality, and Urine Specific Gravity

ELECTROLYTES	
Sodium (Na)	135–145 mEq/L
Potassium (K^+)	3.5–5.0 mEq/L
Calcium (Ca^{2+})	8.5–10 mg/dL
Magnesium (Mg^{2+})	1.3–2.1 mEq/L or 1.6–2.6 mg/dL
Chloride (Cl^-)	98–106 mEq/L
Bicarbonate (HCO_3^-)	22–26 mEq/L
Phosphate/phosphorus (PO_4^{2-})	2.5–4.5 mg/dL
Serum osmolality	275–295 mOsm/kg
Urine specific gravity	1.010–1.035 mEq/L

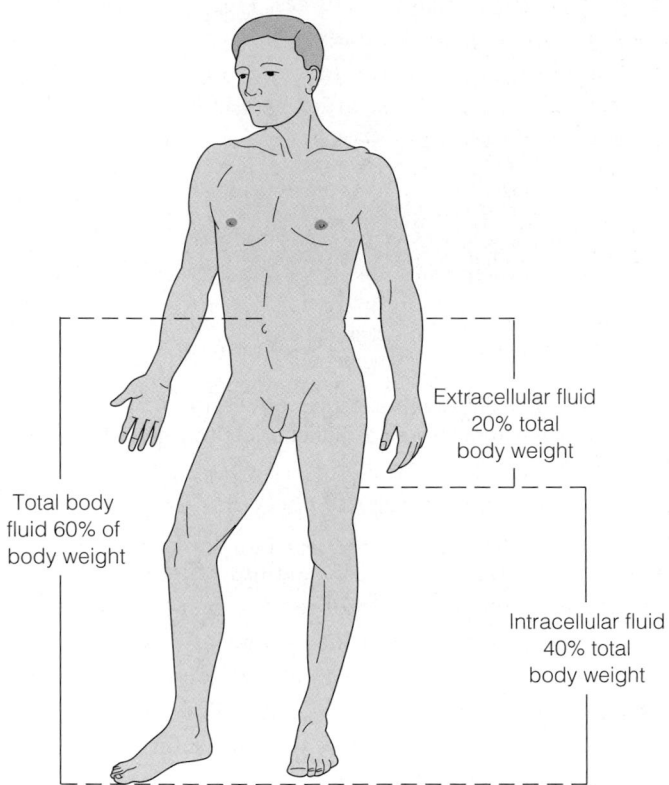

Figure 7-1. ■ A comparison of the major fluid compartments of the body.

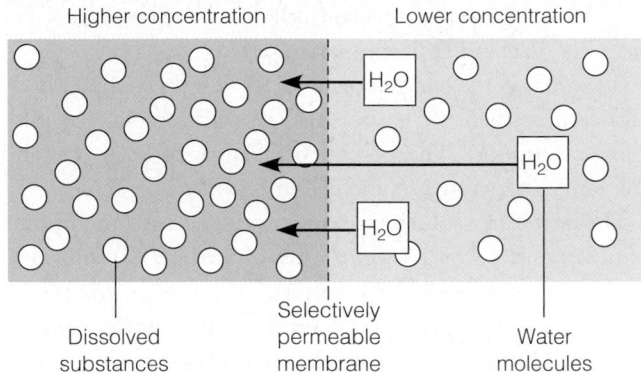

Figure 7-3. ■ Osmosis. Water moves across a selectively permeable membrane from an area of low solute concentration to an area of high solute concentration.

ECF transports oxygen and nutrients to cells, and waste products away from the cells. For example, plasma transports oxygen from the lungs and glucose from the gastrointestinal tract to the tissues. Waste products of metabolism such as carbon dioxide are carried away from the tissues to the lungs and the kidneys for elimination.

Electrolytes are found in both fluid compartments, but the electrolyte composition of ICF and ECF differs (Figure 7-2 ■). Sodium (Na^+), chloride (Cl^-), and bicarbonate (HCO_3^-) are the principal extracellular electrolytes. The principal intracellular electrolytes are potassium (K^+), magnesium (Mg^{2+}), and phosphate (PO_4^{2-}).

BODY FLUID MOVEMENT

Membranes such as the cell membrane and capillary walls separate the body fluid compartments. These membranes are *selectively permeable;* that is, they allow water and some solutes (e.g., oxygen, carbon dioxide, electrolytes, and glucose) to cross, but block proteins and other large molecules. Water and solutes move across these membranes by the processes of osmosis, diffusion, filtration, and active transport.

Osmosis

In the process of **osmosis,** water moves across a membrane from an area of lower solute concentration to an area of higher solute concentration (Figure 7-3 ■). Osmosis continues until the solute concentration on both sides of the membrane is equal. For example, if a selectively permeable membrane separates pure water from a salt solution, water moves into the

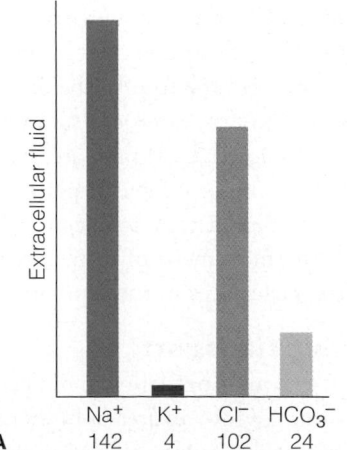

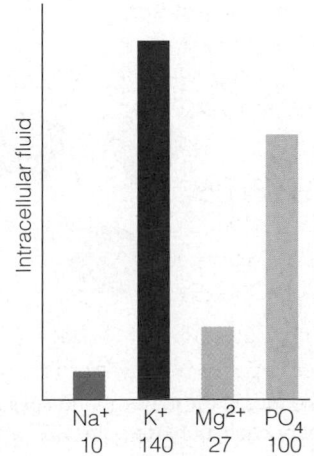

Figure 7-2. ■ The principal electrolytes (in milliequivalents) of (**A**) extracellular fluid and (**B**) intracellular fluid.

salt solution. Osmosis is responsible for water movement between the ICF and ECF compartments.

Osmolality is the concentration of all solutes within a body fluid compartment. It is measured in milliosmoles per kilogram (mOsm/kg). The normal osmolality of both ICF and ECF ranges between 275 and 295 mOsm/kg (see Table 7-1).

The power of a solution to draw water across a membrane is known as the *osmotic pressure* of the solution. All solutes in a solution contribute to its osmotic pressure. In the blood, plasma proteins, especially albumin, exert osmotic pressure, helping to hold water within the blood vessels.

Tonicity refers to the effect of the osmotic pressure of a solution on cells within that solution. *Isotonic* solutions (such as normal saline, 0.9% sodium chloride solution) have the same concentration of solutes as plasma. Cells placed in an isotonic solution do not gain or lose water (Figure 7-4 ■).

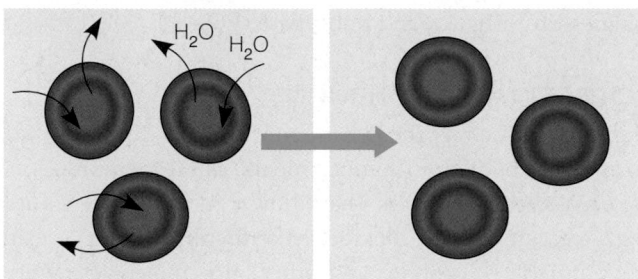

A Isotonic solution

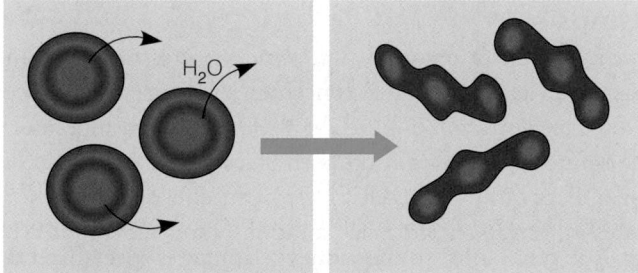

B Hypertonic solution

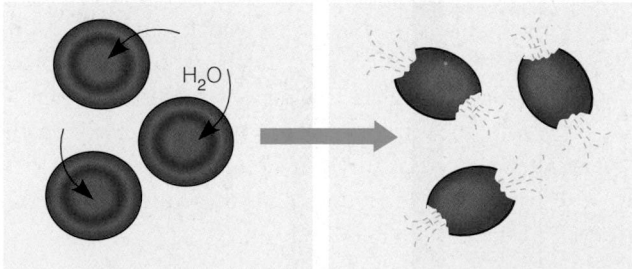

C Hypotonic solution

Figure 7-4. ■ The effect of changes in the concentration of solutions on red blood cells. (**A**) Cells neither gain nor lose water, size, or shape in isotonic solutions. (**B**) Cells lose water and shrink in hypertonic solutions. (**C**) Cells absorb water, swell, and burst in hypotonic solutions.

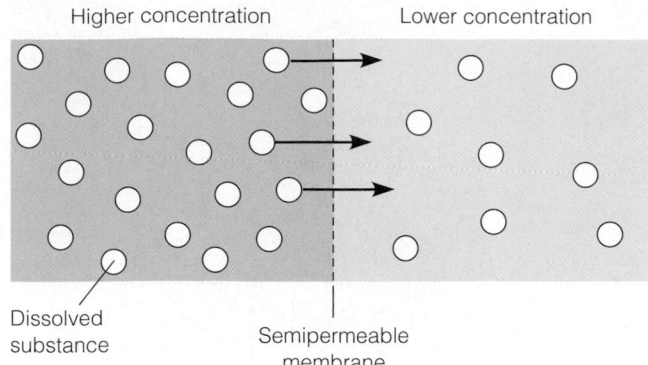

Figure 7-5. ■ In diffusion, molecules move across a semipermeable membrane from an area of higher solute concentration to an area of lower concentration.

Hypertonic solutions (e.g., 3% sodium chloride solution) have a greater concentration of solutes than plasma. A cell placed in a hypertonic solution shrinks as water is drawn out of it into the solution. *Hypotonic* solutions (such as 0.45% sodium chloride) have a lower solute concentration than plasma. A cell placed in a hypotonic solution swells as water moves into it. The cell may burst.

Diffusion

Diffusion is the process in which solutes move from an area of high solute concentration to an area of low concentration to become evenly distributed (Figure 7-5 ■). There are two types of diffusion. *Simple diffusion* occurs by the random movement of solutes. Solutes such as oxygen and carbon dioxide move from plasma to the interstitial space and into cells by simple diffusion. Large water-soluble molecules such as glucose move into cells by a process of *facilitated diffusion*. Proteins within the cell membrane act as carriers to help large molecules cross the membrane.

Filtration

Filtration is the process in which water and solutes move across capillary membranes driven by fluid pressure. Fluid (or *hydrostatic*) pressure is created by the pumping action of the heart and by gravity. At the arterial end of capillaries, this pressure pushes water and solutes into the interstitial space, an area of lower fluid pressure. At the venous end of the capillary, the osmotic force of plasma proteins draws fluid back into the capillary. A balance of filtration and osmosis regulates the movement of water between the intravascular and interstitial spaces in the capillary beds of the body.

Active Transport

Active transport allows molecules to move across cell membranes into an area of higher solute concentration. This movement requires cellular energy (adenosine triphosphate or ATP) and a carrier mechanism. The sodium–potassium

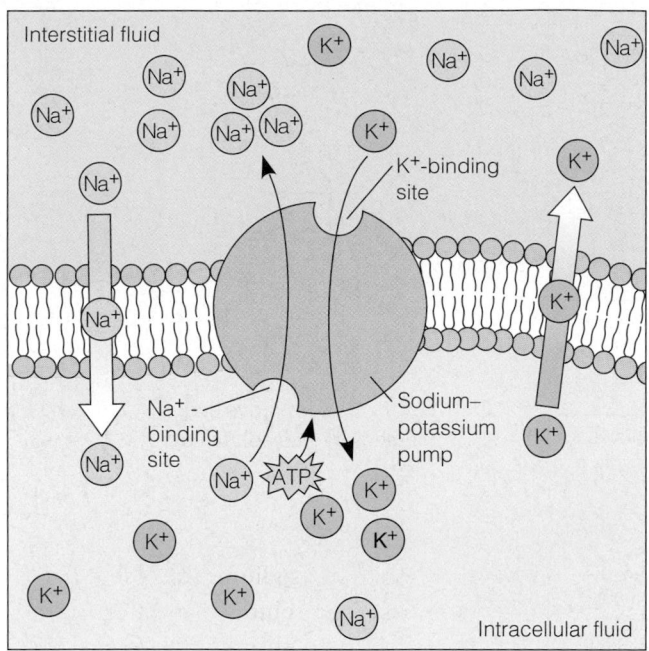

Figure 7-6. ■ The sodium–potassium pump. Active transport moves sodium and potassium ions across cell membranes against their concentration gradients.

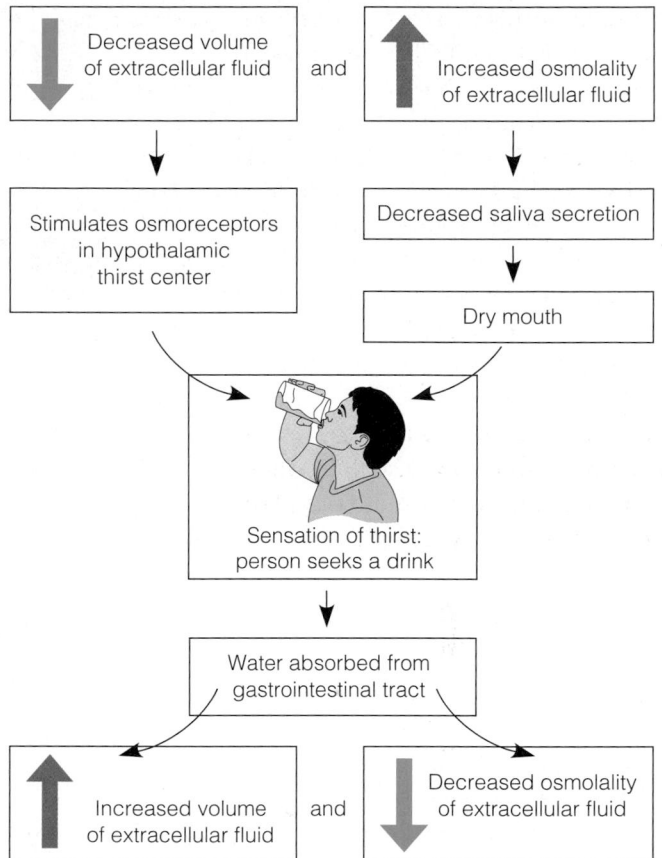

Figure 7-7. ■ Factors stimulating water intake through the thirst mechanism.

pump is an important example of active transport (Figure 7-6 ■). High concentrations of potassium within cells are maintained because cells actively move potassium from interstitial fluid (where the potassium concentration is about 5 mEq/L) into intracellular fluid (K^+ concentration about 150 mEq/L). Sodium is "pumped" from ICF into ECF.

BODY FLUID REGULATION

Homeostasis depends on a number of mechanisms and processes that regulate the balance between fluid intake, output, and distribution. These regulatory mechanisms include thirst, the kidneys, the renin–angiotensin–aldosterone mechanism, antidiuretic hormone, and atrial natriuretic factor.

Thirst

Thirst is the primary regulator of water intake. It plays an important role in maintaining fluid balance and preventing dehydration. The thirst center in the brain is stimulated when the blood volume drops because of water losses or when the solute content (osmolality) of body fluids increases (Figure 7-7 ■). The thirst mechanism declines with age, so older adults are more vulnerable to dehydration. Clients with impaired consciousness or who are unable to respond to thirst also are at risk.

Kidneys

The kidneys are primarily responsible for regulating fluid volume and electrolyte balance in the body. In adults, about 170 liters of plasma are filtered by the kidneys every day. About 99% of this filtrate is reabsorbed, and only about

1,500 mL of urine are produced. By selectively reabsorbing water and electrolytes, the kidneys maintain the volume and osmolality of body fluids.

Renin–Angiotensin–Aldosterone System

The *renin–angiotensin–aldosterone system* helps maintain intravascular fluid balance and blood pressure (Figure 7-8 ■). A fall in blood flow to the kidneys stimulates specialized receptors in the kidney to produce renin (an enzyme). Renin converts angiotensinogen (a plasma protein) in the blood into angiotensin I. In the lungs, angiotensin I is converted to angiotensin II by angiotensin-converting enzyme (ACE). Angiotensin II constricts blood vessels, which raises blood pressure. It also stimulates thirst, releases aldosterone (a hormone) from the adrenal cortex, and acts directly on the kidneys, causing them to retain sodium and water. Aldosterone also promotes sodium and water retention by the kidneys, restoring blood volume.

Antidiuretic Hormone

Antidiuretic hormone (ADH) regulates water excretion from the kidneys. Receptors in the hypothalamus detect changes in osmolality and blood volume, stimulating ADH production and release as needed. When ADH is present, more

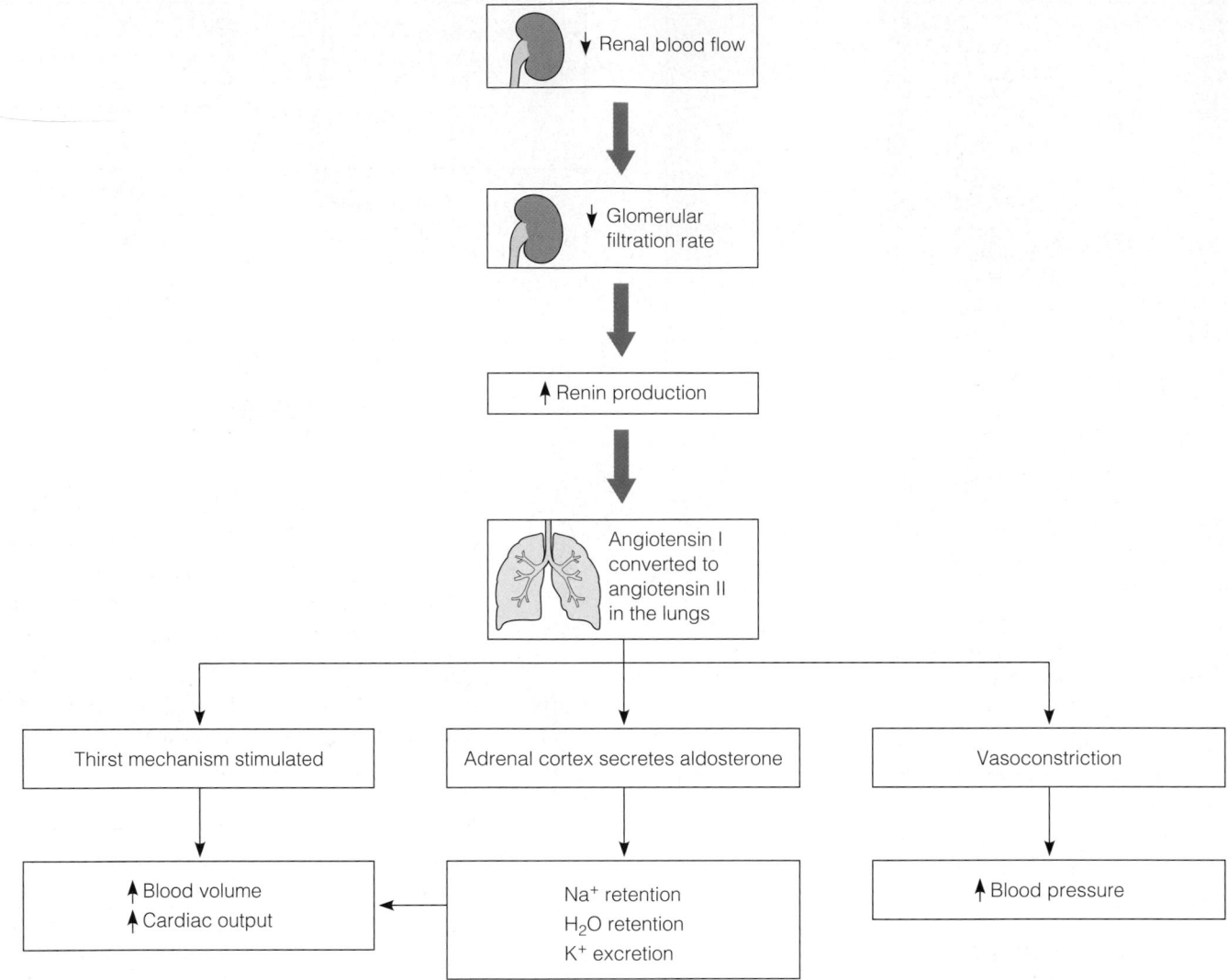

Figure 7-8. ■ The renin–angiotensin–aldosterone system.

water is reabsorbed in the kidney. Urine output falls, blood volume is restored, and serum osmolality drops as the water dilutes body fluids (Figure 7-9 ■).

Disorders of ADH production affect urine output. In *diabetes insipidus,* ADH is not produced. The lack of ADH impairs water reabsorption in the kidney, resulting in copious, very dilute urine output. The thirst mechanism is stimulated and the client drinks additional fluids, maintaining high urine output. In the *syndrome of inappropriate ADH secretion (SIADH),* excess ADH is released. More water is reabsorbed, fluid volume increases, and urine output is scant and concentrated. (See Chapter 16 ⊙⊙ for more information about diabetes insipidus and SIADH.)

Atrial Natriuretic Peptide

Atrial natriuretic peptide (ANP) is a hormone released by cells in the atria of the heart in response to stretching from fluid overload. ANP inhibits renin secretion and blocks the se-

cretion and effects of aldosterone. In doing so, it promotes sodium and water loss, and causes blood vessels to dilate.

Fluid Volume Deficit

Fluid volume deficit (FVD) may be due to excessive fluid losses, insufficient fluid intake, or both. The most common causes are vomiting, diarrhea, or gastrointestinal suctioning. Other common causes are listed in Table 7-2 ■. Inadequate fluid intake may result from decreased thirst sensation, limited access to fluids, difficulty swallowing, or lack of awareness of the need to replace fluids. Older adults are at particular risk for fluid volume deficits (Box 7-1 ■).

PATHOPHYSIOLOGY AND MANIFESTATIONS

Fluid volume deficit is characterized by a decrease in extracellular fluids. Usually, both water and electrolytes are lost from the body. Initial manifestations are related to *hypovolemia,* or

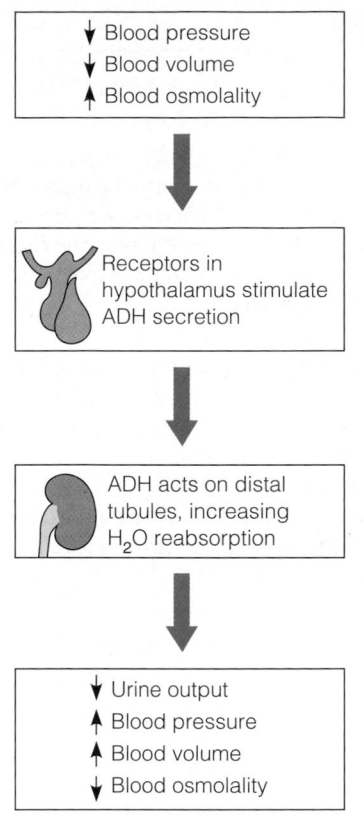

Figure 7-9. ■ The effect of antidiuretic hormone (ADH) release.

decreased circulating blood volume. Manifestations of FVD are related to the cause and severity of the imbalance. With rapid fluid losses, manifestations may be seen within minutes or hours. With gradual losses, interstitial fluid shifts into the vascular space to maintain blood volume. A significant amount of ECF may be lost by the time symptoms develop (see Table 7-2). In many cases, the extent of fluid loss can be estimated by the amount of total body weight lost:

- Mild FVD—2% to 4% weight loss

TABLE 7-2		
Fluid Imbalances		
	FLUID VOLUME DEFICIT	**FLUID VOLUME EXCESS**
Causes	GI fluid losses Excess urine output: diuretics, diabetes Hemorrhage Sweating Fever Draining wounds, burns Fluid shifts (third-spacing) Inadequate fluid intake	Renal failure Heart failure Cirrhosis of the liver Medications Excess fluid intake Excess sodium intake
Manifestations	Fatigue, altered mentation Postural hypotension Tachycardia Weak, thready peripheral pulses Weight loss Flat neck veins, ↓ CVP Dry skin, poor turgor Decreased urine output, concentrated urine	Hypertension Tachycardia Full, bounding peripheral pulses ↑ Respiratory rate Moist crackles, wheezes Weight gain Distended neck veins, ↑ CVP Dependent edema
Lab Values	↑ Serum osmolality ↑ Hematocrit ↑ Urine-specific gravity	↓ Serum osmolality ↓ Hematocrit ↓ Urine specific gravity

- Moderate FVD—5% to 7% loss
- Severe FVD—8% or greater loss

Third-Spacing

Third-spacing is a shift of fluid from the vascular space into an area where it is not available for physiologic processes (e.g., the bowel or the peritoneal cavity). Fluid may also become trapped within soft tissues following trauma or burns. Fluid loss due to third-spacing can be difficult to detect, because the weight may remain stable, and intake and output records may not show the loss.

INTERDISCIPLINARY CARE

In addition to the history and physical examination, laboratory tests and invasive monitoring help determine and monitor fluid status.

Diagnostic Tests

- *Serum electrolytes* may show increased sodium levels if the fluid loss is primarily water. If both water and sodium have been lost, the sodium level may be normal or low. Serum potassium levels often are low.
- *Serum osmolality* is high when primarily water has been lost; if both water and sodium are lost, it may be normal.
- The *hematocrit* may be elevated due to loss of intravascular fluid volume and concentration of the blood cells.
- *Urine specific gravity* and *osmolality* are high due to increased concentration of the urine as the kidneys attempt to conserve water.
- The *central venous pressure (CVP)* (pressure in the right atrium or vena cava) may be measured to help determine fluid status. The normal CVP (measured by manometer) ranges from 2 to 8 cm water. A low CVP indicates inadequate fluid volume; a high CVP occurs in fluid overload, heart failure, and some lung disorders. The procedure for measuring CVP using a manometer is outlined in Box 7-2 ■. Hemodynamic monitoring equipment generally is used to measure CVP. Clients requiring hemodynamic monitoring usually are placed in intensive or coronary care units. See Chapter 27 ⬀ for more information about hemodynamic monitoring.

Fluid Management

Depending on the severity of the deficit, fluids and electrolytes may be replaced orally, *enterally* (into the gastrointestinal tract), or intravenously. Whenever possible, oral or enteral (nasogastric or gastrostomy tube) fluid replacement is preferred. The client is encouraged to drink increased amounts of fluid. Whenever possible, fluids that also contain electrolytes (e.g., commercial products such as sports drinks or Pedialyte) are preferred for fluid replacement to avoid potential electrolyte imbalances resulting from pure water intake.

BOX 7-2

MEASURING CENTRAL VENOUS PRESSURE WITH A MANOMETER

Central venous pressure is used to evaluate fluid volume status. The CVP catheter is inserted into the right atrium or vena cava through a large vein. Nursing responsibilities related to CVP include explaining the procedure to the client and family and monitoring the pressure at regular intervals. The steps in measuring CVP are as follows:

1. Explain what is being done.
2. Mark the level of the right atrium on the lateral chest wall. This is usually at the fourth intercostal space, midaxillary line. This mark is the reference point for all measurements.
3. Place the client in the same position for each reading, usually supine with the head of the bed flat.
4. Use a carpenter's level to make sure the 0 on the manometer is level with the mark on the client's chest for each measurement (see figure).

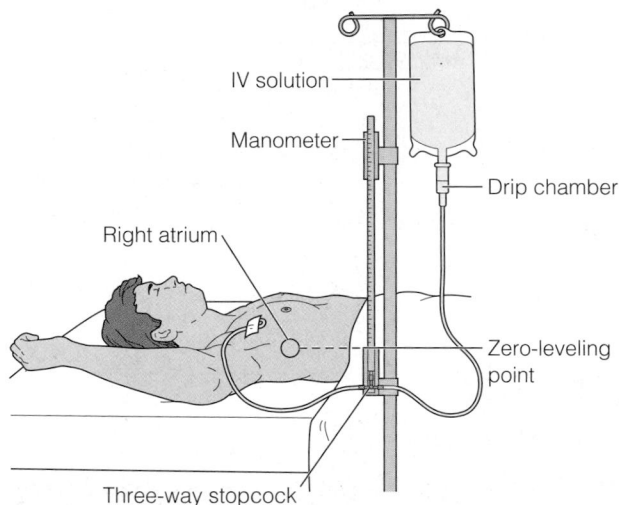

5. Remove any air bubbles in the line.
6. Turn the stopcock to allow fluid to flow into the manometer, filling it a few centimeters above the expected reading. Then turn the stopcock to open the line between the manometer and the client. The fluid level will fall and then reach a point at which it fluctuates with the client's breathing. This point is recorded as the CVP.
7. After the measurement is taken, turn the stopcock so that the fluid again flows from the fluid source to the client.
8. Document the reading on the vital sign or CVP flow sheet.

Intravenous Therapy

In acute situations, intravenous fluids are necessary. Intravenous (IV) delivery effectively supplies fluids directly into the blood, and can be used to replace electrolytes as well. While IV fluids generally require a physician's order, the nurse is responsible for initiating, monitoring, and maintaining parenteral fluid replacement. A fluid challenge may be ordered to evaluate

BOX 7-3	NURSING CARE CHECKLIST

Intravenous Infusion

☑ Identify the type, amount, and duration of the infusion from the physician's order.

☑ Calculate the appropriate flow rate or infusion pump settings based on the order and type of infusion set used.

- To determine the amount to infuse each hour, divide the total amount of fluid to be infused by the number of hours over which the infusion is to be run.

- To determine the amount to infuse per minute, divide the total amount to be infused by the number of minutes over which the infusion is to be run (e.g., an 8-hour infusion runs over 480 minutes).

- To determine the number of drops per minute, use the following formula:

$$\frac{\text{Amount to be infused} \times \text{drop factor of infusion set}}{\text{Total time of infusion in minutes}}$$

  For example

$$\frac{1000 \text{ mL} \times 10 \text{ drops/mL}}{480 \text{ minutes}} = 21 \text{ drops/min}$$

☑ Verify that the correct solution is being infused. If the solution in incorrect, slow the rate of flow to a minimum to maintain the patency of the catheter and change the solution to the correct one. Document and report the error per agency protocol.

☑ Observe the rate of flow every hour. Regularly compare the rate of flow with the infusion schedule. Slow an infusion that is too fast; report an infusion that is running too slow. It may be unsafe to increase the rate of flow to "catch up" with the infusion schedule. Notify the physician or follow agency protocol for adjusting the rate.

☑ Check the patency and integrity of the system:

- Check solution container position; increase its height as needed to maintain gravity flow.

- Check fluid level in the drip chamber; if less than half full, squeeze the chamber to add fluid. If too full, invert the solution container and squeeze the chamber to empty fluid.

- Inspect tubing for kinks or obstructions. Position tubing to avoid tension on the intravenous catheter, dangling below the insertion site, and occlusion by the client's weight.

- Check for catheter patency: Lower the solution container below the infusion site, and observe for blood return. Lack of blood return may indicate partial occlusion or catheter dislodgement from the vein.

- If the tip of the catheter is against the vein wall or a valve, reposition it slightly, using care to avoid contamination or dislodging of the catheter.

- Check for leaks in the system. Tighten connections. If unable to repair a leak or if the connection has become contaminated, replace the infusion set. Estimate the amount of fluid lost if significant.

☑ Inspect the insertion site for infiltration, inflammation, or bleeding.

- *Infiltration*, fluid flow into interstitial tissues caused by dislodging the catheter from the vein, is manifested by local swelling, coolness, pallor, and discomfort at the IV site. If present, stop the infusion and remove the catheter. Restart the infusion at another site. Apply a warm compress to the site to promote reabsorption of the fluid.

- *Phlebitis*, inflammation of a vein, results from injury to the vein due to mechanical trauma or chemical irritation. It is characterized by redness, warmth, and swelling at the insertion site and burning pain along the vein. If detected, discontinue the infusion and apply a warm compress to the site.

- Oozing or bleeding into the surrounding tissues can occur while the infusion is in place, but usually occurs after the needle has been removed. Apply a sterile pressure dressing and inspect frequently for continued bleeding.

☑ Instruct the client to avoid stress or tension on the tubing or infusion site, and to notify the nurse if the solution container is nearly empty, the flow rate changes, there is blood in the tubing, or the infusion site is painful or swollen.

☑ Document the solution infusion, its flow rate, assessment data, and any measures taken to correct problems.

fluid status when a fluid volume deficit is suspected. Box 7-3 ■ outlines nursing care for the client receiving IV fluids.

The fluid administered depends on the type and rapidity of the fluid loss. Isotonic electrolyte solutions (0.9% NaCl or Ringer's solution) are used to expand blood volume or to replace abnormal losses (e.g., loss of gastric fluid via nasogastric suction). Five percent dextrose in water (D_5W) is used to treat total body water deficits. Hypotonic saline solution (0.45% NaCl) or mixed solutions are used as maintenance solutions to provide electrolytes and water. (See Table 7-3 ■.)

Intravenous solutions usually are supplied in plastic bags of various sizes from 50 to 1,000 mL. Glass containers may be used for solutions or medications that are incompatible with plastic. Glass containers require an air vent to allow air to enter the bottle as the fluid flows into the client. Plastic bags collapse as the fluid flows out, making an air vent unnecessary. IV fluids must be sterile and free from contamination. Before administering, inspect the container and solution for evidence of tampering, clarity, and expiration date. Do not administer any solution that is questionable or

TABLE 7-3

Commonly Administered Intravenous Fluids

FLUID	TONICITY	USES
0.9% NaCl (Normal saline)	Isotonic	Restore intravascular volume Replace extracellular fluid Replace sodium losses
0.45% NaCl (½ normal saline)	Hypotonic	Replace water losses Maintain sodium and chloride levels
3% NaCl	Hypertonic	Correct sodium depletion
5% dextrose in water (D_5W)	Isotonic	Replace water losses Correct hypernatremia (excess sodium)
10% dextrose in water ($D_{10}W$)	Hypertonic	Replace water losses Provide calories (340 kcal/L)
20% dextrose in water ($D_{20}W$)	Hypertonic	Promote diuresis Provide calories (680 kcal/L)
50% dextrose in water ($D_{50}W$)	Hypertonic	Treat severe hypoglycemia Provide calories (1,700 kcal/L)
5% dextrose in 0.45% NaCl (D_5 ½ NS)	Isotonic	Maintain fluid level Replace water losses Maintain sodium and chloride levels
Ringer's solution (balanced electrolyte solution)	Isotonic	Replace fluid losses Maintain intravascular volume
Lactated Ringer's solution (electrolyte solution with buffer)	Isotonic	Replace fluid losses Prevent acidosis

may have been contaminated. IV bottles or bags are changed before they are completely empty to prevent air from entering the IV line. All IV bags are changed at least every 24 hours, regardless of how much solution remains, to reduce the risk of bacterial growth.

IV poles are used to hang the solution container. They may be free standing, attached to the bed, or hanging from the ceiling. The pole height is adjustable to promote gravity flow of the IV solution.

An infusion set is used to connect the solution container to the IV catheter or needle. This equipment varies by manufacturer, so the nurse must become familiar with that used by the agency. Infusion sets usually include an insertion spike, a drip chamber, a roller valve or screw clamp, tubing with secondary ports, and a protective cap over the needle adapter (Figure 7-10 ■). The sterile insertion spike is inserted into the solution container. The drip chamber allows the nurse to observe the amount of fluid being administered. Administration sets commonly deliver 10 to 20 drops/mL of solution. This information is found on the package. When smaller amounts of solution are given (e.g., less than 50 mL per hour), a microdrip set that delivers

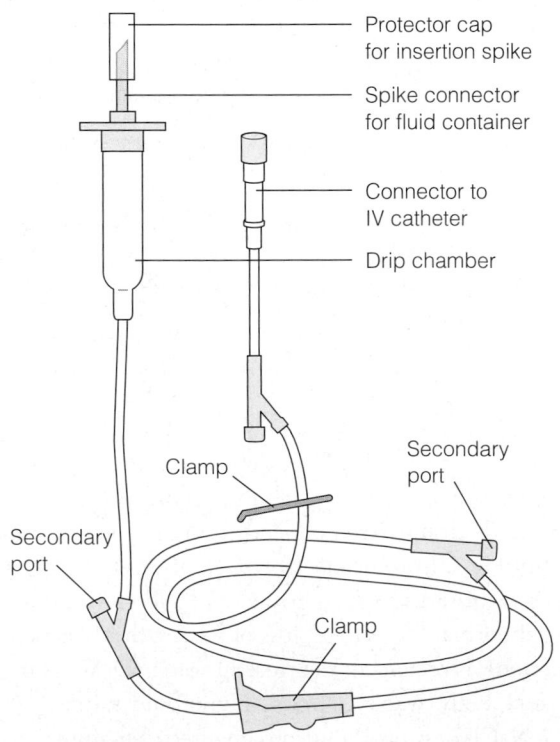

Figure 7-10. ■ A standard IV administration set.

60 drops/mL of solution is used. The rate of flow is controlled by a roller valve or screw clamp, which compresses the lumen of the tubing. A protective cap over the needle adapter maintains sterility of the end of the tubing until it is attached to the IV needle, catheter, or venous access device. A special infusion set may be required when an infusion pump or controller is used. IV tubing and the site dressing is changed every 24 to 72 hours. Box 7-4 ■ outlines the process for changing an IV solution container, tubing, and the IV site dressing.

Infusion pumps or devices control the rate of an infusion. They also have alarms that are triggered by air in the tubing or low solution levels in the IV bag. Infusion pumps reduce the risk of administering fluids too rapidly or too slowly. It is vital to use an infusion pump when medications such as heparin are added to the IV solution. Infusion control devices vary by manufacturer; the nurse must become familiar with the devices used within each agency.

Catheters and needles are used to administer IV infusions. Over-the-needle catheters are commonly used. The

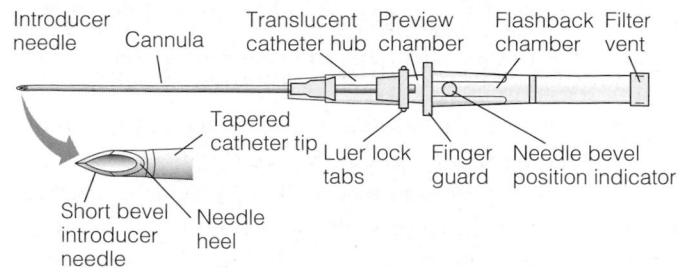

Figure 7-11. ■ An over-the-needle IV catheter.

plastic catheter fits over a needle used to pierce the skin and vein wall (Figure 7-11 ■). Once in the vein, the needle is withdrawn, leaving the catheter in place. IV catheters promote comfort, allow more mobility, and are less likely to become dislodged from the vein, allowing fluid to flow into interstitial spaces *(infiltrate)*. Butterfly, or wing-tipped, needles with plastic flaps attached to the shaft may be used, particularly for very small veins. The flaps are used to direct the needle during insertion. Once in place, the flaps are flattened against the skin and secured with tape.

BOX 7-4	PROCEDURE CHECKLIST

Changing an Intravenous Bag, Tubing, and Site Dressing

Before the Procedure

☑ Verify the order or agency protocol for bag, tubing, and dressing changes.

☑ Gather equipment: IV container with correct type and amount of solution, fluid administration set, timing label, appropriate antiseptic for cleansing site, transparent dressing, tape.

During the Procedure

☑ Use Standard Precautions throughout the procedure.

☑ Verify the physician's order for solution type, added medications, and infusion rate.

☑ Select the appropriate solution (generally supplied by the pharmacy); verify that it is the correct solution (and medication, if appropriate) and amount for the client.

☑ Calculate the drip rate.

☑ Mark the timing strip with start time, appropriate amount to be delivered per hour, and end time; apply the strip to the container, taking care to avoid covering the label.

☑ Open the infusion set (see Figure 7-10). Maintaining sterility of the spike and IV solution, insert the spike into the solution container.

☑ Prime the tubing, keeping the IV catheter connection sterile. Close the drip regulator.

☑ Identify the client and explain the procedure.

☑ Assess the IV site for infiltration, bleeding, phlebitis; appearance of the dressing; date and time of previous dressing change.

☑ Prepare dressing supplies. Prepare transparent dressing for application, tear two or more strips of tape for securing tubing, open antiseptic swabs.

☑ Place a towel or clean absorbent pad under the extremity to prevent soiling bed linens. Be sure the IV and tubing, and all dressing supplies are within easy reach.

☑ Remove soiled dressing and tape to expose catheter connection.

☑ Clamp the tubing on the existing infusion, and carefully loosen the tubing from the IV catheter or needle, securing the catheter with the nondominant hand.

☑ Remove the used IV tubing and securely attach the new tubing to the IV catheter or needle; open the regulator clamp to restart the infusion.

☑ Continuing to hold the IV catheter or needle, clean the IV site, following agency protocol.

☑ Apply transparant dressing to IV insertion site. Secure tubing with tape to prevent inadvertent tension on the catheter or needle with movement.

☑ Label the dressing, with the date and time of the dressing change and your initials.

☑ Regulate the IV flow rate as ordered.

Note: Refer to a nursing fundamentals or skills text for more detailed instruction. Check state guidelines and facility policy before performing any procedure.

The type of IV access device and insertion site depend on a number of factors: client age and condition of veins, duration of the infusion, and type of solution to be infused. For adults, veins in the hand and arm (the metacarpal, basilic, and cephalic veins) are commonly used (Figure 7-12 ■). The radius and ulna splint the veins of the arm, reducing catheter movement during activities such as eating. Larger veins are used when solutions are to be rapidly infused and for solutions that may irritate vein walls. Although the veins in the antecubital space can be easily accessed for venipuncture, they are usually reserved for blood draws, IV medications, and insertion of a peripherally inserted central catheter (PICC) line. Insertion of an IV catheter and initiation of an infusion are outlined in Box 7-5 ■.

When the duration of IV therapy will be extended or the site used to administer medications that irritate vein walls, a

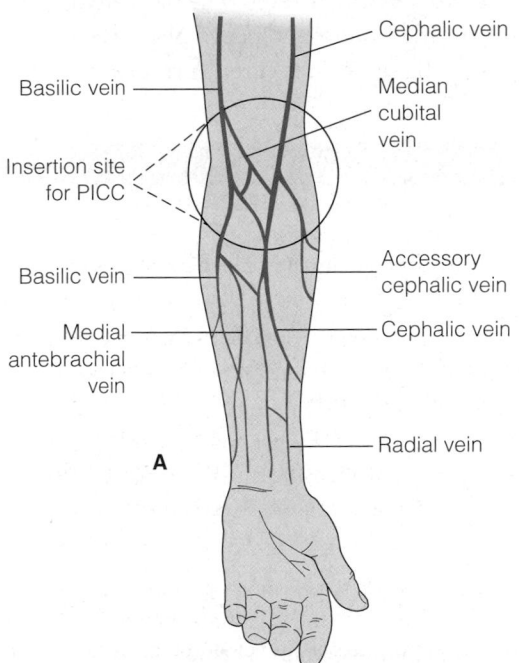

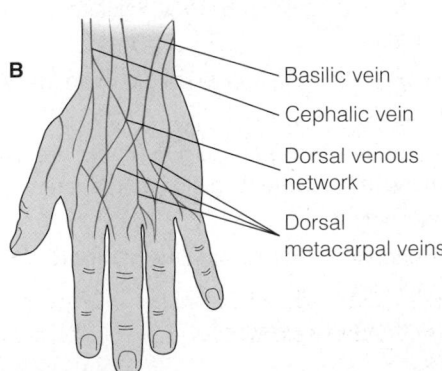

Figure 7-12. ■ Commonly used venipuncture sites of the (**A**) arm and (**B**) hand. Figure A also shows the site used for a peripherally inserted central catheter (PICC).

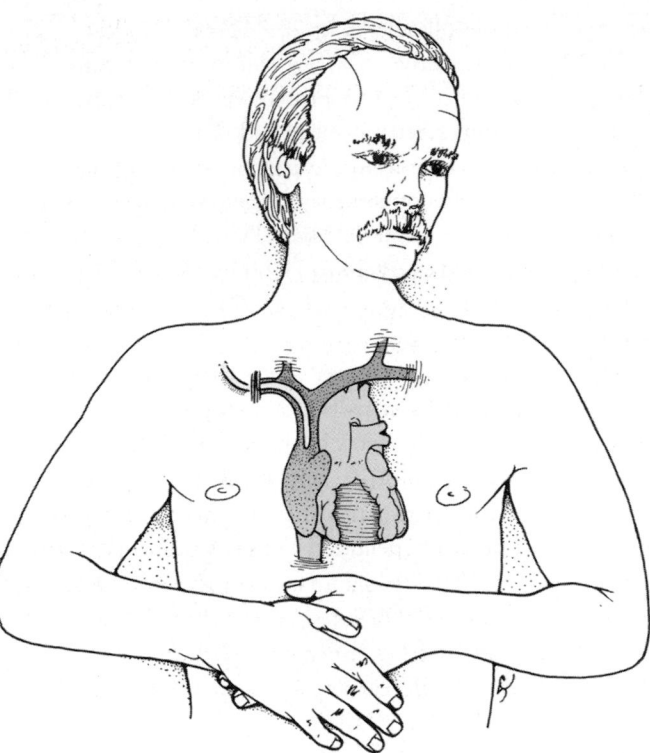

Figure 7-13. ■ A central venous catheter inserted via the right subclavian vein.

central venous catheter or an implantable IV access device or port may be used. Central venous catheters usually are inserted into the subclavian or jugular vein, with the distal tip of the catheter in the superior vena cava, just above the right atrium (Figure 7-13 ■). Implantable ports, tunneled catheters (e.g., Hickman catheters), and PICC lines often are used for long-term intravenous access, for example, when a client is receiving chemotherapy. Because these devices remain in place for long periods of time, there is a risk of infection and occlusion.

NURSING CARE

ASSESSING

Nursing assessment of the client with an actual or potential fluid volume deficit is outlined in Box 7-6 ■. Throughout the assessment, the nurse is alert for manifestations of fluid volume deficit (Table 7-2).

clinical ALERT

Assess skin turgor over the sternum in older adults. Loss of subcutaneous tissue in aging makes the skin of the arms a less reliable indicator of fluid status.

BOX 7-5	PROCEDURE CHECKLIST

Initiating an Intravenous Infusion

Before the Procedure

☑ Verify the order, including the solution to be used, any medications to be added, and the time and the rate of the infusion.

☑ Obtain the ordered solution from the pharmacy.

☑ Gather equipment: Infusion set, IV pole, infusion controller if appropriate, intravenous catheter or needle, clean gloves, IV insertion set (tourniquet, cleansing pads and/or solutions, sterile gauze, occlusive dressing, tape), clean protective absorbent pad.

☑ Prepare the infusion: Apply a medication label to the container as appropriate (if not applied by the pharmacy), and a timing strip or label per agency procedure. Using sterile technique, attach the tubing to the solution container, and fill the drip chamber and tubing with solution. Close the drip regulator. Maintain sterility of all connections.

☑ Identify the client, provide for privacy, and explain the procedure. Allow time for questions.

During the Procedure

☑ Use Standard Precautions throughout the procedure.

☑ Select the insertion site. If possible use the nondominant arm, selecting a vein that is relatively straight (see Figure 7-12). Choose a site that allows normal arm movement to the extent possible and where the tip of the catheter will not be at a joint.

☑ Place a clean protective pad or towel under the arm to protect linens or furniture.

☑ If necessary, apply heat to the extremity (using a heating pad or hot, damp towel) for 10 to 15 minutes to promote blood flow and venous distention.

☑ Cleanse the site according to agency protocol. Use a circular motion, starting at the insertion site and working outward for several inches. Allow site to dry. Do not touch the site once it has been cleansed.

☑ Prepare IV catheter/needle, dressing, and tape while site dries.

☑ Apply tourniquet firmly approximately 12 cm (5 in.) or more above (proximal to) the site (see accompanying figure). Apply

the tourniquet tight enough to occlude venous return, but loose enough to allow arterial flow (check pulse distal to the tourniquet). Ask the client to open and close the fist to distend the vein; if necessary, tap or flick the vein above or below the cleansed site to promote distention.

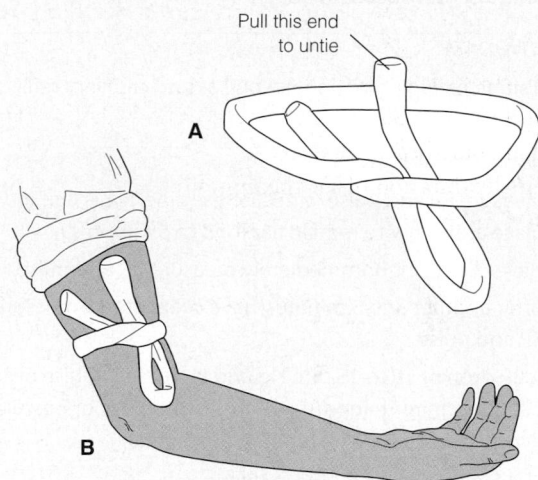

☑ Using the nondominant hand, pull the skin taut below the insertion site. Holding the catheter and/or needle at a 10- to 15-degree angle and the bevel up, pierce the skin and vein wall in a smooth, controlled motion. Once blood appears, reduce the angle and advance the catheter and/or needle into the vein, using appropriate technique for the device.

☑ Release the tourniquet. Holding the catheter/needle in place, remove the sterile cap from the IV tubing; remove the needle from an over-the-needle catheter, and attach the tubing to the catheter.

☑ Open the drip regulator and adjust to maintain flow.

☑ Apply dressing to site per agency protocol. Secure IV tubing to prevent tension on the IV catheter or on connections. Label the dressing with the time, date, type of infusion device or catheter, and your initials.

☑ Adjust flow rate to maintain ordered rate of infusion.

Note: Refer to a nursing fundamentals or skills text for more detailed instruction. Check state guidelines and facility policy before performing any procedure.

DIAGNOSING, PLANNING, AND IMPLEMENTING

Priorities in Nursing Care. Restoring blood and fluid volume is the priority of care for the client with fluid volume deficit. Low blood volume, usually due to a total body fluid

volume deficit, increases the client's risk for injury due to falls, impaired mental status, and kidney failure.

Deficient Fluid Volume

■ Monitor intake and output (I&O). Report a urine output of less than 30 mL/hr to the charge nurse or primary care

BOX 7-6	ASSESSMENT

Assessing for Fluid Volume Deficit

SUBJECTIVE DATA
- Complaints of weakness, thirst
- Recent weight loss
- Risk factors: strenuous exercise (particularly in warm weather); acute illness (e.g., fever, nausea, vomiting, diarrhea); chronic diseases such as diabetes

OBJECTIVE DATA
- Vital signs, including peripheral pulses and capillary refill
- Weight
- Orthostatic vital signs:
  - Measure BP and pulse with client supine; leave cuff in place and allow to remain flat for 3 to 5 minutes.
  - Have client sit up; immediately measure BP and pulse.
  - After another 3 to 5 minutes, have client stand; measure BP and pulse.
  - A BP drop of 10 to 15 mm Hg and increase in pulse of 10 beats per minute (bpm) indicates orthostatic or postural hypotension (an indicator of hypovolemia).
- Mental status, level of consciousness
- Color and moisture of skin and mucous membranes; skin temperature
- Observe jugular veins
- Assess skin turgor: Gently pinch up a fold of skin on the forearm or over the sternum. Turgor is good if the skin returns immediately to previous shape; poor when it remains tented
- Auscultate breath and bowel sounds
- Laboratory results: hematocrit, serum osmolality

provider. *Urine output of less than 30 mL/hr indicates poor kidney perfusion and a risk for renal failure.*
- Measure urine specific gravity. *Urine specific gravity is normally 1.010 to 1.035. A reading higher than 1.025 may indicate fluid volume deficit.*
- Assess vital signs, CVP, and peripheral pulses every 4 hours. *Hypotension, tachycardia, and weak peripheral pulses indicate hypovolemia. CVP is used to evaluate fluid replacement.*
- Weigh daily with standard conditions (same time of day, approximately the same clothing, balanced scale). *Rapid weight changes often reflect changes in fluid balance. Research studies have shown weight to be a more accurate indicator of overall fluid volume status than I&O records.*
- If a fluid challenge is ordered, assess vital signs, urine output, breath sounds, and mental status prior to fluid administration, and every 10 to 15 minutes during the challenge. *A large amount of fluid may be given very*

rapidly in a fluid challenge. Clients with impaired cardiac or renal status may develop signs of a fluid overload during the challenge.*
- Provide oral fluids as ordered. Identify the client's beverage preferences; monitor fluid intake. *Oral fluids are used to replace lost fluids and relieve thirst.*
- Administer intravenous fluids as ordered. *Clients with severe fluid volume deficit or who are unable to tolerate oral fluids may require intravenous fluid replacement to restore blood volume.*
- Assess laboratory values: electrolytes, serum osmolality, and hematocrit. *Electrolyte levels, serum osmolality, and hematocrit may fall with rehydration. Continue to assess these values to ensure they remain within normal limits.*

Risk for Injury

- Institute safety precautions, including keeping the bed in a low position, using side rails, and raising the client slowly from the supine to sitting or sitting to standing position. *The client with orthostatic hypotension is at risk for dizziness, fainting, or falling with rapid position changes.*
- Teach client to get up slowly, sitting on the side of the bed for several minutes before standing. *These measures reduce orthostatic hypotension and the client's risk for injury.*

EVALUATING

Collect data related to fluid volume status (such as stable vital signs and weight) and safety to evaluate the effectiveness of nursing measures for the client with a fluid volume deficit.

Documentation. Document continuing assessment data, as well as the effectiveness of interventions. Note the client's ability and willingness to take oral fluids, as well as the amount of fluids consumed. Monitor for and document possible adverse effects of treatment, such as shortness of breath or abnormal breath sounds.

CONTINUING CARE

Assess the client's resources for home care and for preventing future problems with fluid losses (Box 7-7 ■). Provide verbal and written instructions:

- Instruct about recommended fluid intake.
- Avoid overexposure to heat and exercise (adjust activity level and fluid intake in hot weather).
- If vomiting, take small frequent amounts of ice chips or clear liquids (weak tea, flat cola, or ginger ale).
- Be aware that coffee, tea, alcohol, and large amounts of sugar increase urine output and can cause fluid loss.
- Replace fluids lost through diarrhea with fruit juices or bouillon rather than large amounts of tap water.
- Monitor weight, reporting changes of more than 3 to 5 pounds in a week to primary care provider.

Assessing for Discharge Fluid Volume Imbalance

- Ability to perform activities of daily living (ADLs), access fluids
- Knowledge:
  - Risks for fluid deficit (e.g., vomiting, diarrhea, strenuous exercise during hot weather, diuretic therapy, chronic diseases such as diabetes mellitus); preventive measures; early manifestations
  - Risks for fluid excess (e.g., heart, kidney, or liver failure; medications); preventive measures; early manifestations; low-sodium diet, fluid restrictions
- Home environment: appropriate heating and cooling; access to clean water and other fluids; cooking facilities
- Availability and knowledge of caregivers to assist with ADLs, monitor fluid intake, and assist with fluid or dietary restrictions as ordered

Teach older adults and their caregivers to prevent fluid volume deficit. Suggest offering preferred fluids on a regular basis throughout the day and using alternative sources of liquid (such as gelatin, broth, or ice cream). Discuss the importance of providing additional water to clients who are receiving enteral nutrition via tube feedings.

Fluid Volume Excess

Fluid volume excess usually results from sodium and water retention. It is rarely a problem in healthy adults. However, older adults, people with chronic or debilitating illnesses, and clients receiving intravenous therapy are at risk.

PATHOPHYSIOLOGY

Fluid volume excess is caused by excess sodium in the body that leads to water retention. Conditions that can lead to sodium and water retention include heart failure, cirrhosis of the liver, kidney failure, and endocrine conditions that affect ADH and aldosterone release. Sodium and water are retained in approximately the same proportion as is present in ECF.

MANIFESTATIONS AND COMPLICATIONS

Excess fluid tends to remain within the extracellular space, leading to the primary manifestations of **hypervolemia** (excess intravascular fluid) and interstitial **edema** (excess fluid in body tissues). Manifestations related to hypervolemia include tachycardia and bounding peripheral pulses, increased respiratory rate with crackles on auscultation, distended neck veins, and an increased CVP. The blood pressure often is elevated. Interstitial edema causes weight gain and edema of dependent tissues (the lower extremities in ambulatory clients and the back and sacrum in bedridden clients). When fluid volume excess is associated with kidney disease, edema

may be generalized, affecting tissues around the eyes and the upper extremities as well. Causes and manifestations of fluid volume excess are listed in Table 7-2.

Heart failure not only is a potential cause of fluid volume excess, it may be a complication of the problem. The heart may be unable to handle the workload caused by excess fluid, leading to failure. See Chapter 27 ∞ for more information about heart failure.

INTERDISCIPLINARY CARE
Diagnostic Tests

Diagnostic tests to determine the severity and possible causes of fluid volume excess may include the following:

- *Serum electrolytes* and *serum osmolality* often remain within normal limits in fluid volume excess.
- *Hemoglobin* and *hematocrit* levels may be reduced due to dilution of the blood by excess fluid.
- *Liver* and *kidney function tests* (see Chapters 18 and 31) ∞ may be done to help determine the cause of fluid volume excess.

Diet and Fluid Management

Because sodium retention is a primary cause of fluid volume excess, a sodium-restricted diet often is prescribed. People require about 500 mg of sodium per day, but Americans typically consume about 4 to 5 grams daily, mostly from salt, processed foods, and foods themselves. A mild sodium restriction can be achieved by reducing the amount of salt in recipes by half, by not using the salt shaker at the table, and by avoiding foods that contain high levels of sodium either naturally or because of processing (Box 7-8 ■). In moderate and severely sodium-restricted diets, salt and all foods containing significant amounts of sodium are avoided altogether.

FOODS HIGH IN SODIUM

High in Added Sodium

- *Processed meat and fish*—bacon, sausage, smoked fish, luncheon meat and other cold cuts
- *Selected dairy products*—buttermilk, cottage cheese, cheeses, ice cream
- *Processed grains*—graham crackers, most dry cereals
- *Canned goods*—meats, vegetables, soups
- *Snack foods*—salted popcorn, nuts, potato chips/pretzels, gelatin desserts
- *Condiments and food additives*—barbecue sauce, saccharin, catsup, pickles, chili sauce, soy sauce, meat tenderizers, salted margarine, Worcestershire sauce, salad dressings

Naturally High in Sodium

- Brains, kidney, oysters, shrimp, clams, crab, lobster
- Dried fruit
- Spinach, carrots

Fluid intake also may be restricted in clients who have fluid volume excess. The amount of fluid allowed per day is prescribed by the care provider. All fluid intake must be calculated, including fluid in meals and fluid used to administer medications orally or intravenously. Box 7-9 ■ ■ provides guidelines for clients on a fluid restriction.

Medications

Diuretics, which promote sodium and water excretion, may be prescribed. Three classes of diuretics are commonly used: loop diuretics, thiazide diuretics, and potassium-sparing diuretics (Table 7-4 ■).

NURSING CARE

ASSESSING

Preventing fluid volume excess and early identification of its manifestations are important nursing responsibilities. Assessment data to collect for clients at risk for or with fluid volume excess are listed in Box 7-10 ■.

BOX 7-9 | **NURSING CARE CHECKLIST**

Fluid Restriction Guidelines

☑ Subtract requisite fluids (e.g., ordered IV fluids, fluids in which IV medications are mixed) from total daily allowance.

☑ Divide remaining fluid allowance:
- Day shift: ½ of total
- Evening shift: ¼ to ⅓ of total
- Nights: Remainder.

☑ Explain the fluid restriction to the client and family members.

☑ Work with client to determine preferred fluids and intake pattern.

☑ Offer fluids in small glasses (allows perception of a full glass).

☑ Offer ice chips (which, when melted, are approximately half of the frozen volume).

☑ Provide frequent mouth care and opportunities to rinse mouth.

☑ Provide sugarless chewing gum (if allowed) to reduce thirst.

TABLE 7-4

Nursing Implications for Pharmacology: Fluid Volume Excess

DRUG GROUP/DRUGS	ACTION/USES	NURSING IMPLICATIONS (FOR ALL DRUG GROUPS)	CLIENT TEACHING (FOR ALL DRUG GROUPS)
Loop diuretics Furosemide (Lasix) Ethacrynic acid (Edecrin) Bumetanide (Bumex) Torsemide (Demadex)	Loop diuretics inhibit sodium and water reabsorption in the loop of Henle and increase potassium loss in the distal tubule. As a result, loop diuretics promote sodium, chloride, potassium, and water excretion.	Obtain baseline weight and vital signs. Monitor intake and output, weight, VS, skin turgor, and edema. Report manifestations of volume depletion: dizziness, orthostatic hypotension, tachycardia, muscle cramping. Loop and thiazide diuretics cause potassium wasting. Monitor serum electrolytes (especially potassium) and blood glucose. Notify physician of abnormal values. Notify the physician if the client is receiving a loop diuretic with another ototoxic drug such as an aminoglycoside antibiotic.	The drug will increase the amount and frequency of urination. Take the drugs in the morning and afternoon to avoid having to get up at night to urinate. Change position slowly to avoid dizziness. Report the following to your primary health care provider: flulike symptoms, weakness, dehydration, thirst, dizziness; trouble breathing; or swelling of face, hands, or feet. Weigh yourself at the same time every day, and report sudden gains or losses. Try to avoid using the salt shaker when eating. If the drug increases potassium loss, eat foods high in potassium, such as orange juice and bananas. Unless restricted, drink 6 to 8 glasses of water daily.
Thiazide diuretics Bendroflumethiazide (Naturetin) Chlorothiazide (Diuril) Chlorthalidone (Hygroton) Hydrochlorothiazide (HydroDIURIL) Metolazone (Diulo) Polythiazide (Renese) Others	Thiazide diuretics promote the excretion of sodium, chloride, potassium, and water by decreasing their reabsorption in the distal tubule.		
Potassium-sparing diuretics Spironolactone (Aldactone) Amiloride HCl (Midamor) Triamterene (Dyrenium)	Potassium-sparing diuretics promote excretion of sodium and water by inhibiting sodium–potassium exchange in the distal tubule.		

BOX 7-10	ASSESSMENT

Assessing for Fluid Volume Excess

SUBJECTIVE DATA

- Complaints of cough, shortness of breath, difficulty sleeping or breathing when lying down
- Recent changes in fluid intake, output, or weight
- Risk factors such as renal failure, heart failure, cirrhosis of the liver, or an endocrine disorder; medications such as corticosteroid drugs (e.g., prednisone), nonsteroidal anti-inflammatory drugs (NSAIDs)

OBJECTIVE DATA

- Vital signs, peripheral pulses, and weight
- Mental status, level of consciousness
- Presence of peripheral or facial edema; color and moisture of skin and mucous membranes
- Observe for distended jugular or distal veins
- Auscultate breath sounds for crackles, wheezes; heart sounds for S_3 (heard immediately after S_2) and/or S_4 (heard immediately before S_1)

DIAGNOSING, PLANNING, AND IMPLEMENTING

Priorities in Nursing Care. Excess fluid volume and hypervolemia can have serious consequences for clients, particularly the elderly. The heart may not be able to adapt to increased blood volume, leading to heart failure. Congestion of the pulmonary vascular system can impair gas exchange, affecting tissue oxygenation. For this reason, the excess fluid volume is the priority nursing care focus.

Excess Fluid Volume

Monitoring clients with fluid volume excess is important, and is particularly critical in older clients because of age-related changes in cardiac and renal function.

- Monitor daily weights and intake and output. Report weight or fluid gain to the charge nurse or physician. *Daily weights are one of the most important gauges of fluid balance. Two kilograms (approximately 5 pounds) of weight gain is equivalent to 2 liters of fluid gain.*
- Monitor edema, particularly in the lower extremities and the sacral and periorbital areas. *Localized edema tends to occur in dependent tissues such as the lower extremities of ambulatory clients and the sacrum in bedridden clients. Periorbital edema indicates generalized edema.*
- If fluid restriction is prescribed, carefully monitor fluid intake. Instruct the client and significant others about the restriction and how to accurately measure fluid intake. *All sources of fluid intake, including ice chips, should be strictly monitored to avoid excess fluid.*

- Provide oral hygiene as needed. *Oral hygiene contributes to client comfort and keeps mucous membranes intact; it also helps relieve thirst if fluids are restricted.*
- Encourage the client to rest frequently in bed or a recliner with the feet elevated. *Bed rest promotes excretion of excess fluid by promoting its reabsorption into blood vessels and excretion by the kidneys.*
- Place in semi-Fowler's or Fowler's position if dyspnea is present. *Semi-Fowler's position improves lung expansion and promotes fluid excretion.*

Risk for Impaired Skin Integrity

Edema, which results from excess fluid in the interstitial spaces, decreases the delivery of nutrients to tissues and increases their susceptibility to injury.

- Reposition at least every 2 hours. *Frequent change of position minimizes tissue pressure.*
- Assess vulnerable pressure areas—particularly tissues over bony prominences—with each position change, and provide skin care. *Edematous tissue over bony prominences is more prone to tissue breakdown.*
- Minimize tissue pressure by providing an alternating pressure mattress, foot cradles, and other devices. *An egg crate mattress distributes pressure over a wider area of the body surface and reduces pressure over bony prominences. A foot cradle minimizes the pressure that bedding can exert on the feet and lower extremities.*

EVALUATING

To evaluate the effectiveness of nursing care for clients with fluid volume excess, collect assessment data, evaluating for changes in vital signs, weight, ease of breathing, and relief of edema. Assess skin integrity and the need for additional measures to protect skin and underlying tissues from injury.

Documentation. Document continuing assessment data and the client's response to treatment. Document teaching about fluid and sodium restrictions and the client's understanding of foods to eat and those to avoid.

CONTINUING CARE

Assess the client's and family's readiness and ability to provide home care after an episode of fluid volume excess (see Box 7-8). Focus on prevention in teaching. Emphasize the importance of taking medications as prescribed and avoiding foods that are high in sodium. Instructions for a low-sodium diet are found in Box 7-11 ■. Provide verbal and written instructions:

- Discuss amount and type of fluids allowed, including a specific plan if fluids are restricted.

BOX 7-11	CLIENT TEACHING

Teaching Clients About a Low-Sodium Diet

- The body needs less than 1 teaspoon (about 500 mg) of salt per day. About one-third of sodium intake comes from adding salt during cooking and at the table; one-fourth to one-third comes from processed foods; and the rest comes from food and fluids naturally high in sodium.
- In place of salt or salt substitutes, use herbs, spices, lemon juice, vinegar, and wine as flavoring when cooking. The taste for salt will eventually diminish.
- Use salt substitutes sparingly if at all; they often taste bitter instead of salty in large amounts, and contain significant amounts of potassium.
- Low-sodium salt substitutes may contain half the sodium of regular salt.
- Read labels. Salt, monosodium glutamate, baking soda, and baking powder contain significant amounts of sodium. Processed foods list the sodium content. Some nonprescription drugs (such as laxatives and antacids) contain high amounts of sodium.

- Describe ways to reduce sodium intake when buying and preparing foods.
- To reduce dependent edema, change positions often, elevate feet and legs when sitting, avoid crossing legs, and wear support hose and clothing that do not impair circulation.
- To reduce the risk of damage to edematous tissue, shop in the afternoon for shoes that do not require "breaking in," and avoid walking barefoot.
- Use more than one pillow or a recliner chair for sleeping if orthopnea is a problem.
- Weigh daily and report sudden increases of more than 2 pounds to your doctor.

NURSING PROCESS CARE PLAN
Client with Excess Fluid Volume

Dorothy Rainwater is a 45-year-old former high school principal who is hospitalized with acute renal failure. She is expected to recover from this acute illness, but she currently has very little urine output.

Assessment. Mike Penning, Ms. Rainwater's evening shift nurse, notes that her output for the previous 24 hours is 250 mL; this low output has been constant for the past 8 days. She has gained 1 lb (0.45 kg) in the past 24 hours. Ms. Rainwater is on a fluid restriction of 500 mL plus the amount of her output for the previous day.

Mr. Penning collects the following assessment data: T 98.6°F, BP 160/92, P 102, with obvious neck vein distention, R 28, with crackles and wheezes; head of bed elevated 30 degrees; periorbital and sacral edema noted, 3+ pitting edema in feet bilaterally; skin pale and shiny. Alert and oriented; responds appropriately to questions; states she is thirsty, slightly nauseated, and extremely tired.

Diagnosis. The current nursing diagnoses for Ms. Rainwater are as follows:

- *Excess Fluid Volume* related to acute renal failure
- *Risk for Impaired Skin Integrity* related to edema
- *Risk for Impaired Gas Exchange* related to pulmonary congestion
- *Activity Intolerance* related to fluid volume excess, fatigue, and weakness

Expected Outcomes. The expected outcomes specify that Ms. Rainwater will:

- Regain fluid balance, as evidenced by weight loss, decreasing edema, and normal vital signs.
- Experience decreased dyspnea.
- Maintain intact skin and mucous membranes.
- Increase activity levels as prescribed.

Planning and Implementation. The following nursing interventions are planned and implemented:

- Weigh q12hr at 0600 and 1800.
- Monitor vital signs and breath sounds q4hr.
- Intake and output q4hr.
- Restrict fluids as follows: 375 mL, 0700 to 1500; 275 mL, 1500 to 2300; 100 mL, 2300 to 0700. Prefers water or apple juice.
- Turn every 2 hours, following schedule posted at the head of bed. Inspect skin, and provide skin care when turned; avoid vigorous massage.
- Provide oral care every 2 to 4 hours; allow to brush own teeth (caution not to swallow water). Use moistened applicators as desired.
- Keep head of bed at 30 to 40 degrees; prefers two small soft pillows under her head.
- Up at bedside in recliner for 20 minutes b.i.d. Monitor carefully for fatigue and weakness as activity level increases.

Evaluation. At the end of the shift, Mr. Penning notes that Ms. Rainwater gained no weight, and her urinary output during his shift is 300 mL. Her vital signs remain unchanged, but her crackles and wheezes have decreased, and she states that she can breathe more easily. Her skin and mucous membranes are intact. She enjoyed sitting in the chair at her bedside and did not experience any shortness of breath.

Critical Thinking in the Nursing Process

1. Why are Ms. Rainwater's respiratory rate, blood pressure, and pulse elevated?
2. Explain how elevating the head of the bed 30 degrees makes breathing easier.
3. Outline a plan for teaching Ms. Rainwater about diuretics.
4. Suppose Ms. Rainwater says, "I would really like to have all my fluids at once instead of spreading them out." What would be your reply, and why?

Sodium Imbalance

Sodium (Na^+), the most plentiful electrolyte in ECF, has a normal serum range of 135 to 145 mEq/L. Sodium regulates ECF volume and distribution, and contributes to neuromuscular activity and acid–base balance. Because of the close relationship between sodium and water balance, disorders of fluid volume and sodium often occur together. Sodium imbalances affect the osmolality of ECF. When sodium levels are low (*hyponatremia*), water is drawn into the cells of the body, causing them to swell. In contrast, high sodium levels in ECF (*hypernatremia*) draw water out of body cells, causing them to shrink (see Figure 7-4).

Although the body requires only about 500 mg of sodium per day, many people consume more than 10 times that amount. Sodium excretion is controlled by the kidneys. The kidneys work together with the renin–angiotensin–aldosterone system and atrial natriuretic peptide to retain or excrete sodium. They usually maintain ECF sodium concentration within its usual range despite variations in daily intake.

HYPONATREMIA

Hyponatremia (serum sodium < 135 mEq/L) usually results from loss of sodium from the body. It may also be caused by water gains that dilute ECF. Hyponatremia affects the function of voluntary and involuntary muscles (such as the gastrointestinal tract). Brain cells swell, leading to neurologic manifestations such as headache and possible brain damage. The causes, manifestations, and laboratory values of hyponatremia are shown in Table 7-5 ■. Serum sodium levels of less than 110 to 120 mEq/L are considered critical, necessitating immediate intervention.

TABLE 7-5		
Sodium Imbalances		
	HYPONATREMIA	**HYPERNATREMIA**
Causes	Excess sodium loss through kidneys, skin, or GI tract (vomiting, diarrhea, gastric suctioning or irrigation, enemas with water) Excess sodium excretion due to diuretic medications, kidney or endocrine disorders Water gains related to kidney disease, heart failure, or cirrhosis of the liver Syndrome of inappropriate secretion of antidiuretic hormone (SIADH) Excessive hypotonic IV fluids	Altered thirst or inability to respond to thirst Hyperventilation Profuse sweating Diarrhea Diabetes insipidus Oral electrolyte solutions or hyperosmolar tube-feeding formulas Excess IV fluids such as normal saline, 3% or 5% sodium chloride, or sodium bicarbonate
Manifestations	Anorexia, nausea, vomiting, abdominal cramping, and diarrhea Headache Mental status changes Hyperreflexia, muscle twitching, and tremors Convulsions and coma	Thirst Restlessness, weakness Altered mental status, decreasing level of consciousness, seizures Muscle irritability Dry, sticky mucous membranes Postural hypotension Hot, dry skin, fever, and decreased sweating
Lab Values (normal 135–145 mEq/L or 135–145 mmol/L)	Serum sodium < 135 mEq/L Critical value < 110–120 mEq/L *Other lab values* Serum osmolality < 280 mOsm/kg	Serum sodium > 145 mEq/L Critical value > 160 mEq/L *Other lab values* Serum osmolality > 295 mOsm/kg

Interdisciplinary Care

Serum electrolytes and *serum osmolality* levels are drawn. Values for sodium and osmolality are low, reflecting an excess of water in relation to the amount of sodium in the body. A *24-hour urine specimen* may be ordered to evaluate sodium excretion and help identify the cause of hyponatremia. See Box 31-3 ⬛⬛ for nursing responsibilities in collecting a 24-hour urine specimen.

If hyponatremia is mild, increased intake of foods high in sodium may restore normal sodium balance (see Box 7-6). Oral fluids often are restricted. If the client is unable to eat or drink, or if hyponatremia is severe, sodium-containing intravenous fluids may be administered. Normal saline (0.9% NaCl) may be given, or a 3% or 5% NaCl solution may be used cautiously to replace sodium and draw fluid out of the intracellular fluid compartment. A loop diuretic such as furosemide (see Table 7-4) may be administered along with sodium replacements to remove excess water.

HYPERNATREMIA

Hypernatremia (serum sodium concentration > 145 mEq/L) almost never occurs in people with an intact thirst mechanism and access to water. Hypernatremia results either from a gain of sodium in excess of water or from a loss of water in excess of sodium. Because excess sodium causes ECF to become hyperosmolar, water moves out of cells, leading to cellular dehydration. Dehydration of brain cells causes neurologic manifestations such as confusion and a decreasing level of consciousness. Cellular dehydration also causes dry, sticky mucous membranes. Causes of excess water loss or excess sodium intake, as well as manifestations and laboratory values of hypernatremia, are summarized in Table 7-5. Serum sodium levels greater than 160 mEq/L are considered critical, requiring immediate intervention.

Interdisciplinary Care

Hypernatremia is treated by adding water (oral or hypotonic intravenous solutions such as D_5W or 0.45% NaCl) to correct any water deficit. Diuretics may also be given to increase sodium excretion, and a low-sodium diet may be prescribed. Hypernatremia is corrected slowly (over a 48-hour period) to avoid rebound cerebral edema as water shifts back into the dehydrated brain cells.

NURSING CARE

Nurses need to identify and monitor clients at risk for sodium imbalances. Hyponatremia is often associated with therapeutic measures such as IV fluid administra-

tion, gastrointestinal suction, or tap-water enemas. Diuretics such as furosemide and thiazide diuretics cause increased sodium excretion and contribute to a risk for hyponatremia.

Hypernatremia, on the other hand, usually is associated with an inability to access fluids or to respond to the thirst sensation. Clients who are elderly, debilitated, or confused are at highest risk for hypernatremia.

ASSESSING

Assessment of clients experiencing or at risk for sodium imbalance involves collection of subjective and objective data.

- *Subjective data:* current manifestations (such as nausea, vomiting, abdominal cramps, muscle weakness, headache) and their duration; precipitating factors such as heavy perspiration, vomiting, diarrhea, water deprivation; perception of thirst; current medications and any chronic diseases such as heart or kidney disease, cirrhosis of the liver, or diabetes insipidus (See Chapter 16 ⬛⬛ for more information about diabetes insipidus.)
- *Objective data:* mental status; vital signs including temperature and orthostatic vitals; peripheral pulses; manifestations of fluid volume excess or deficit
- *Laboratory values:* monitor serum sodium levels and serum osmolality, as well as levels of other serum electrolytes such as potassium

DIAGNOSING, PLANNING, AND IMPLEMENTING

Priorities in Nursing Care. Sodium levels in the body have a significant role in regulating water balance, therefore a risk for imbalanced fluid volume and its consequences are the highest priority nursing diagnoses.

Risk for Imbalanced Fluid Volume

- Monitor intake and output, and weigh daily. *Fluid excess or deficit may occur in clients with sodium disorders.*
- Maintain oral and intravenous fluid intake as prescribed. Monitor serum sodium levels and osmolality. Report rapid changes in serum sodium and osmolality. *Body water and sodium are replaced gradually to prevent cerebral edema or fluid volume excess.*
- In clients who are receiving normal saline or IV solutions with a higher sodium concentration, monitor for signs of hypervolemia (increased blood pressure and CVP, tachypnea, tachycardia, gallop rhythm, shortness of breath, crackles). *Hypertonic saline solutions may cause fluid retention and lead to heart failure, particularly in the elderly or people with preexisting heart problems.*

- Explain ordered fluid restrictions, how much fluid is allowed over 24 hours, and how to measure fluid volumes. *Fluid intake may be restricted in clients with a sodium imbalance; teaching increases understanding and compliance.*

Risk for Injury

- Assess muscle strength and tone by asking client to squeeze your fingers, to hold the arms flexed while you pull downward, and to push both feet against your hands. *Muscle weakness resulting from sodium imbalance increases the risk for falling.*
- Assess for mental status changes, such as lethargy, altered or decreased level of consciousness, confusion, and seizures. Monitor behavior, mental status, and orientation. *Baseline data and ongoing assessments are critical because changes in serum sodium and serum osmolality may affect neurologic status and safety.*
- Maintain a quiet environment, and institute seizure precautions as indicated: Keep the bed in its lowest position, side rails up and padded, and airway at the bedside. *A quiet environment reduces neurologic stimulation. Seizures often occur unexpectedly. Safety precautions reduce risk of injury from seizure.*

EVALUATING

To evaluate the effectiveness of nursing interventions for clients with sodium imbalances, collect data related to fluid balance, serum sodium level, and freedom from injury. Monitor laboratory values, reporting lack of response to treatment or overcorrection of the imbalance.

Documenting. Document continuing assessment data throughout treatment, including the client's mental status and any changes that occur. Document teaching provided to help prevent future episodes of sodium imbalance.

CONTINUING CARE

Athletes, people who do heavy labor in a hot environment, and older adults without access to air conditioning during hot weather are at risk for developing hyponatremia if they replace fluid losses with water. Teaching to prevent hyponatremia includes the following:

- Manifestations of mild hyponatremia, including nausea, cramps in the abdomen, and muscle weakness
- The importance of drinking liquids containing sodium and other electrolytes (such as Gatorade and other sports drinks) at frequent intervals when perspiring heavily, when environmental temperatures are high, or if experiencing prolonged watery diarrhea

- The importance of regular checkups to monitor electrolytes if taking a potent diuretic or on a low-sodium diet

People with impaired thirst or a condition that interferes with normal sodium balance require teaching to prevent hypernatremia. Emphasize the importance of adequate water intake and discuss ways to ensure that water needs are met. Teach clients and caregivers about a low-sodium diet if prescribed (see Box 7-9). When helping the client plan a low-sodium diet, include cultural foods and identify nondietary sources of sodium, such as softened water or over-the-counter medications.

Potassium Imbalance

Potassium (K^+), the primary intracellular cation, is vital for cell metabolism and for cardiac and neuromuscular function. The normal serum (ECF) potassium level is 3.5 to 5.0 mEq/L, while the potassium concentration of intracellular fluid is 140 to 150 mEq/L. The sodium–potassium pump sustains this significant difference in concentrations between ICF and ECF.

To maintain normal potassium levels in the body, potassium must be replaced every day. Virtually all foods contain potassium, although some foods and fluids are richer sources than others. The kidneys eliminate potassium very efficiently; even when potassium intake is stopped, the kidneys continue to excrete potassium. The hormone aldosterone contributes to potassium regulation by the kidneys. When aldosterone is present, more potassium is excreted; when it is absent, potassium is retained.

Potassium shifts into and out of the cells constantly. For example, it shifts into or out of the cells in response to changes in hydrogen ion concentration (pH, discussed later in this chapter), as the body strives to maintain a stable acid–base balance. This movement can significantly affect the serum potassium level.

HYPOKALEMIA

Hypokalemia (abnormally low serum potassium, <3.5 mEq/L) usually results from excess potassium loss. However, many hospitalized clients are at risk for hypokalemia because of inadequate intake. Clients who are NPO for extended periods, as well as clients with anorexia nervosa (see Chapter 19) ⊘ are at risk for inadequate intake of potassium.

Excess potassium may be lost through the kidneys or the gastrointestinal (GI) tract (Table 7-6 ■). Drugs such as diuretics, corticosteroids, and some antibiotics are a major cause of excess potassium loss from the kidneys. GI losses may be caused by severe vomiting, diarrhea, or excessive ileostomy drainage.

TABLE 7-6		
Potassium Imbalances		
	HYPOKALEMIA	**HYPERKALEMIA**
Causes	Excess GI losses: vomiting, diarrhea, ileostomy drainage	Renal failure
	Renal losses: diuretics, corticosteroids; hyperaldosteronism	Potassium-sparing diuretics
		Adrenal insufficiency
	Inadequate intake (NPO, anorexia nervosa)	Excess potassium intake (e.g., excess potassium replacement)
	K^+ shift into cells (alkalosis, tissue repair)	Administering aged blood
		K^+ shift out of cells (acidosis, tissue damage)
Manifestations	Dysrhythmias and ECG changes	Tall, peaked T waves, dysrhythmias, heart block, cardiac arrest
	Nausea and vomiting	
	Anorexia	Nausea, abdominal cramping, diarrhea
	Decreased bowel sounds or ileus	Muscle weakness, paresthesias, flaccid paralysis
	Muscle weakness or leg cramps	
Lab Values (normal 3.5–5.0 mEq/L or 3.5–5.0 mmol/L)	Serum potassium < 3.5 mEq/L	Serum potassium > 5.0 mEq/L
	Critical value < 2.5 mEq/L	Critical value > 6.5 mEq/L

A temporary shift of potassium into the intracellular space may occur because of alkalosis, rapid tissue repair (e.g., following a burn or trauma), or high blood insulin levels.

Hypokalemia affects the transmission of nerve impulses and the normal contractility of smooth, skeletal, and cardiac muscle. All clients with serum potassium values of 3.5 mEq/L or less should be closely monitored. Manifestations of hypokalemia generally are not seen until the serum K^+ level falls below 3.0 mEq/L. Values lower than 2.5 mEq/L are considered to be critical. Serious and potentially life-threatening cardiac dysrhythmias are a major concern, particularly in clients who are receiving digitalis to treat heart failure (see Chapter 27). ⚭ The manifestations of hypokalemia are summarized in Table 7-6.

Interdisciplinary Care

DIAGNOSTIC TESTS. *Serum potassium levels* are drawn. *Arterial blood gases (ABGs)* may be ordered to determine acid–base status, because hydrogen ion balance (pH) and serum potassium levels are linked. An *electrocardiogram (ECG)* is done to evaluate cardiac rhythm and assess for characteristic changes associated with hypokalemia.

POTASSIUM REPLACEMENT. Potassium replacement therapy (by mouth or intravenously) is implemented both to prevent and to treat hypokalemia. Commonly prescribed potassium supplements, their actions, and nursing implications are described in Table 7-7 ▪. Several days of therapy may be required to correct hypokalemia.

Increased intake of foods high in potassium may be recommended for clients at risk for hypokalemia, either to prevent its occurrence or to supplement pharmacologic therapy. Box 7-12 ▪ lists foods and fluids that are high in potassium.

HYPERKALEMIA

Hyperkalemia (abnormally high serum potassium > 5 mEq/L), results from inadequate potassium excretion, excessive potassium intake, or a shift of potassium from the ICF to the ECF. The major cause of hyperkalemia is impaired renal excretion (see Table 7-6). Excess potassium intake often occurs when people use potassium-based salt substitutes while taking potassium-sparing diuretics. Administration of aged blood can also lead to hyperkalemia, because the potassium concentration of blood increases during storage. Burns and crushing injuries release potassium

BOX 7-12	

FOODS HIGH IN POTASSIUM
- *Fruits*—apricots, avocados, bananas, cantaloupe, dates, oranges, raisins
- *Vegetables*—carrots, cauliflower, mushrooms, peas, potatoes, spinach, tomatoes
- *Meat and fish*
- *Milk and milk products*

TABLE 7-7			
Nursing Implications for Pharmacology: Hypokalemia			
DRUG GROUP/DRUGS	ACTION/USES	NURSING IMPLICATIONS	CLIENT TEACHING
Potassium Sources Potassium acetate (Tri-K) Potassium bicarbonate (K Care ET) Potassium citrate (K-Lyte) Potassium chloride (K-lease, Micro-K10, Apo-K) Potassium gluconate (Kaon Elixir, Royonate)	Potassium is used to prevent and treat hypokalemia. It is rapidly absorbed from the gastrointestinal tract. Potassium chloride is the agent of choice, because low chloride levels often accompany low potassium.	When giving oral potassium: 1. Dilute or dissolve effervescent, soluble, or liquid potassium in fruit or vegetable juice or cold water. 2. Chill to increase palatability. When giving parenteral potassium: 1. Administer slowly. 2. Never administer undiluted. 3. Assess injection site frequently for pain and inflammation. 4. Use an infusion control device. Monitor intake and output. Monitor serum potassium levels; do not administer if serum K^+ is > 5.0 mEq/L.	Take as prescribed; do not skip a dose or double your prescribed dose unless instructed to do so by your physician. Take potassium supplements with meals to reduce gastric irritation. Do not chew enteric-coated tablets or allow them to dissolve in the mouth; this may affect the potency and action of the medications. Do not use salt substitutes when taking potassium (most salt substitutes are potassium based). Do not take potassium supplements if you are also taking a potassium-sparing diuretic.

from cells into ECF. In acidosis, hydrogen ion moves into the cells and potassium shifts out into ECF as the body attempts to maintain a normal pH.

Hyperkalemia alters neuromuscular function. Its most harmful effects are on cardiac function, with a risk for dysrhythmias, heart block, and cardiac arrest. The strength of cardiac contractions decreases as the potassium level rises. It also affects skeletal and smooth muscle, causing weakness and GI symptoms. Levels higher than 6.5 mEq/L are considered critical, carrying a high risk for cardiac arrest.

clinical ALERT

Remember: Both *hypo*kalemia and *hyper*kalemia affect cardiac function and can result in serious, even fatal, dysrhythmias.

Interdisciplinary Care

Managing hyperkalemia focuses on returning the serum potassium level to normal by treating the underlying cause and avoiding additional potassium intake.

DIAGNOSTIC TESTS. *Serum electrolytes* are monitored, because low calcium and sodium levels may increase the effects of hyperkalemia. *ABGs* are measured to determine whether acidosis is present. *ECG monitoring* of heart rate and rhythm is performed to evaluate the effects of hyperkalemia on cardiac function.

MEDICATIONS. Mild hyperkalemia may be reversed by treating the cause (e.g., correcting acidosis) or by discontinuing drugs that caused it. Loop diuretics such as furosemide (Lasix) promote renal excretion of potassium. A cation exchange resin, sodium polystyrene sulfonate (Kayexalate), may be given orally or rectally (by enema) to remove excess potassium by exchanging sodium for potassium in the intestinal tract. In the client with renal failure, hemodialysis and peritoneal dialysis are used to manage hyperkalemia (see Chapter 32). ⌘

For moderate to severe hyperkalemia, intravenous insulin and glucose may be given to drive potassium into the cells. Intravenous sodium bicarbonate has a similar effect. Calcium gluconate may also be given to block the effects of hyperkalemia on the heart.

NURSING CARE

Nursing care focuses on early identification and reporting of abnormal serum potassium levels and monitoring cardiac status.

ASSESSING

- Subjective data: current manifestations (e.g., anorexia, nausea, vomiting, abdominal discomfort, muscle weakness, heart palpitations) and their duration; use of medications such as diuretics and the type of diuretic used (see Table 7-4), drugs associated with potassium loss (e.g., corticosteroids); use of salt substitutes; compliance with prescribed potassium supplements and dietary intake of foods and fluids.
- Objective data: mental status, vital signs including apical pulse and orthostatic vitals; abdominal distention and bowel sounds; muscle strength and tone
- Laboratory data: serum potassium level; as indicated, serum glucose and arterial blood gas results

DIAGNOSING, PLANNING, AND IMPLEMENTING

Priorities in Nursing Care. The client with a potassium imbalance is at risk for injury due to its potential effects on the heart, as well as muscle weakness resulting from the imbalance.

Risk for Injury

- Carefully monitor serum potassium levels in clients at risk for imbalances, and notify the charge nurse or physician of abnormal levels (<3.5 mEq/L or >5 mEq/L). *Early identification of a potassium imbalance allows prompt treatment and reduces the risk for injury from very high or very low potassium levels.*

clinical ALERT

Immediately report critical values (<2.5 mEq/L or >6.5 mEq/L). Critical values are associated with a high risk of cardiac dysrhythmias and cardiac arrest.

- Monitor for manifestations of potassium imbalance, such as muscle weakness, nausea and anorexia, abdominal cramping, or decreased bowel sounds. *Weakness and GI manifestations of potassium imbalance increase the risk for injury from falls or aspiration of vomitus.*
- Closely monitor clients receiving sodium bicarbonate or sodium polystyrene sulfonate (Kayexalate) for fluid volume excess. *Increased sodium levels can cause water retention.*
- Closely monitor the ECG of clients receiving calcium gluconate, particularly if the client also is on digitalis. *Digitalis toxicity may develop when calcium gluconate and digitalis are given concurrently.*

Decreased Cardiac Output

- Monitor vital signs, including apical pulse. Chart and report any irregularities. *Disruptions of heart rhythm are more easily detected by listening to the apical pulse than by palpating peripheral pulses.*
- Place on a cardiac monitor and observe for changes in heart rhythm or pattern (e.g., prolonged PR interval, ST segment and T-wave changes, and the presence of U waves). (See Chapter 26 ◯◯ for more explanation of ECG waveforms.) Notify the physician of changes. *A monitor allows early identification and intervention for life-threatening dysrhythmias.*
- Monitor clients taking digitalis for signs of digitalis toxicity (see Chapter 27). ◯◯ *Hypokalemia increases the risk for digitalis toxicity.*
- Monitor intravenous potassium infusions closely. Dilute intravenous potassium as recommended, and administer using an electronic infusion device. *Administering more than 40 mEq of potassium per hour is not safe.*
- Promote comfort by slowing the intravenous infusion rate or applying an ice pack to the IV site if necessary. *Potassium may cause local irritation to the vein wall.*

clinical ALERT

Do not administer undiluted potassium directly into the vein. Potassium usually is mixed to a concentration of 20 to 40 mEq/L of solution and should not exceed 60 mEq/L. The rate of infusion should not exceed 20 to 40 mEq of potassium per hour. Evaluate the serum potassium level during therapy. In clients requiring rapid potassium replacement, monitor the ECG. Too rapid administration of intravenous potassium may cause cardiac dysrhythmias and death.

EVALUATING

Collect data related to the client's serum potassium level, safety, and cardiovascular status to evaluate the effectiveness of nursing interventions for clients with potassium imbalances.

Documenting. Document continuing assessment data, including laboratory test results, and the client's compliance with and response to treatment. Document teaching provided, and the client's and family's understanding of instructions.

CONTINUING CARE

Discharge planning for clients with potassium imbalances focuses on teaching about prescribed medications (potassium supplements or diuretics), diet, and the importance of regular follow-up assessments. Include the family, a significant other, or a caregiver in teaching as indicated. Provide both written and verbal instructions. Provide a list of salt substitutes and foods high in potassium, with instructions for their use (see Box 7-10). Instruct clients taking supplemental forms of potassium and potassium-sparing diuretics to avoid salt substitutes that contain potassium. Instruct clients with chronic renal failure to avoid foods high in potassium. Discuss measures to make potassium supplements more palatable: Dilute liquid potassium supplements with water or juices, or mix with sherbet or gelatin. Emphasize the importance of regular laboratory tests as ordered by the physician. Teach the client taking digitalis to count the pulse before taking the medication. Report a rate of less than 60 to the primary health care provider.

NURSING PROCESS CARE PLAN
Client with Hypokalemia

Rose Ortiz is a 72-year-old woman who is being treated for mild heart failure with digoxin (Lanoxin) 0.125 mg, hydrochlorothiazide (Oretic) 75 mg orally (PO) daily, and a mildly sodium-restricted diet (2 g daily). For the last several weeks, Ms. Ortiz has been feeling weak and sometimes faint, light-headed, and dizzy. Her physician ordered serum electrolytes drawn, which showed a potassium level of 2.4 mEq/L. Potassium chloride solution (Kaochlor, 20 mEq/15 mL) PO twice daily is prescribed, and the clinic nurse does a nursing assessment prior to teaching Ms. Ortiz about her care.

Assessment. Ms. Ortiz has adhered to her sodium-restricted diet and has been taking her prescribed medications. She occasionally takes an additional "water pill" when her ankles swell. She says she is reluctant to take the potassium the doctor has ordered because her neighbor says it causes "heartburn." Physical assessment findings include T 98.4, P 70, R 20, and BP 138/84.

Diagnosis. The following nursing diagnosis is identified for Ms Ortiz:

- *Risk for Ineffective Health Maintenance* related to lack of knowledge of side effects of diuretic therapy and of foods high in potassium

Expected Outcomes. The expected outcomes specify that Ms. Ortiz will:

- Have a potassium level within normal limits (3.5 to 5.0 mEq/L).
- Verbalize understanding of the side effects of diuretic therapy.
- State measures to avoid gastrointestinal irritation when taking oral potassium.
- Identify potassium-rich foods.

Planning and Implementation. The following nursing interventions are planned and implemented:

- Discuss the side effects of diuretic therapy, and explain how taking additional diuretics may have contributed to her hypokalemia.
- Explain the need for the prescribed potassium and its role in reversing her muscle weakness.
- Instruct to take the potassium supplement after breakfast and supper, diluted in 4 oz of juice or water, and sipped slowly over a 5- to 10-minute period. Instruct her to call if gastric irritation occurs.
- Discuss dietary sources of potassium, and provide a list of potassium-rich foods (see Box 7-10).

Evaluation. On a follow-up visit 1 week later, Ms. Ortiz says that her symptoms have been resolved. She is taking her prescribed drugs as directed. She also reports that she has increased her intake of potassium-rich foods. Her potassium level is within normal limits.

Critical Thinking in the Nursing Process

1. What did Ms. Ortiz do that contributed to her hypokalemia?
2. What additional teaching at the time that digitalis and hydrochlorothiazide were prescribed might have prevented Ms. Ortiz from developing hypokalemia? How could the nurse reinforce this teaching?
3. Mrs. Ortiz states that she gets "terrible stomach cramps" from eating fresh fruits and vegetables. What suggestions could the nurse provide to increase her potassium intake?

Calcium Imbalance

Calcium (Ca^{2+}) is one of the most abundant ions in the body. Most of it is in the bones and teeth; a small amount is in the ECF. The normal adult total serum calcium concentration is 8.5 to 10.0 mg/dL. About half of extracellular calcium is ionized; the rest is bound to protein, phosphate, or other ions.

Ionized calcium is essential to a number of body processes. It affects neuromuscular irritability, nerve impulse transmission, muscle contraction and relaxation, blood clotting, and hormone secretion. It is vital in maintaining heart rhythm and contraction.

Three hormones interact to regulate serum calcium levels: parathyroid hormone (PTH), calcitriol (a metabolite of vitamin D), and calcitonin. When serum calcium levels fall, the parathyroid glands secrete PTH. PTH mobilizes calcium from the bones, increases calcium absorption in the intestines, and promotes calcium reabsorption by the kidneys (Figure 7-14 ■). Calcitriol assists these processes.

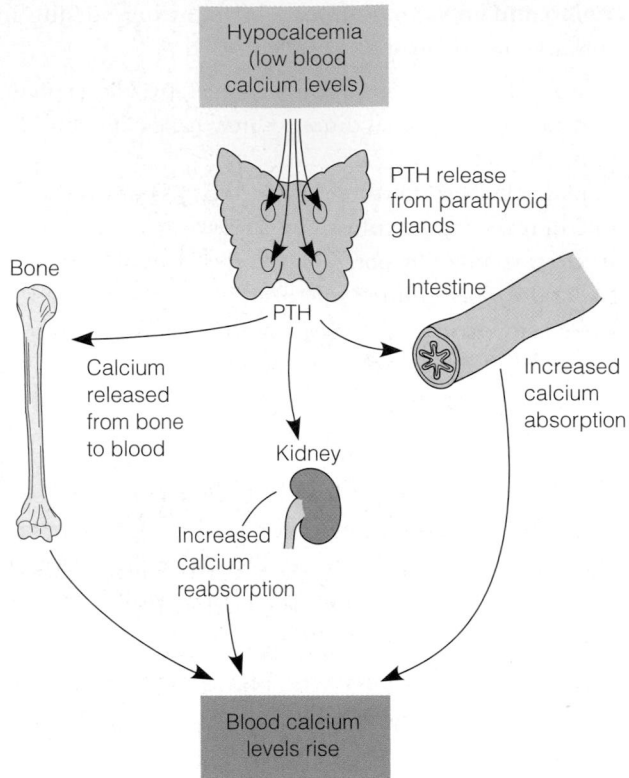

Figure 7-14. ■ Low serum calcium levels stimulate parathyroid hormone release, increasing serum calcium levels by triggering its release from bone, absorption in the intestine, and reabsorption in the kidneys.

Calcitonin is secreted by the thyroid gland in response to high serum calcium levels. Calcitonin has the opposite effect of PTH: It inhibits the movement of calcium out of bone, reduces intestinal absorption of calcium, and promotes urinary calcium excretion.

HYPOCALCEMIA

Hypocalcemia is a serum calcium of less than 8.5 mg/dL. People at risk for hypocalcemia include those who have had their parathyroid glands removed, older adults (especially women), and alcoholics. Older adults often consume less milk and milk products (good sources of calcium) and may have less exposure to the sun (a source of vitamin D). They may be less active, leading to loss of calcium from bones. They are more likely to be taking drugs that interfere with calcium absorption or promote calcium excretion (e.g., furosemide). Older women are at particular risk after menopause because of estrogen deficiency. Alcohol consumption reduces intestinal absorption of calcium and interferes with other processes that help maintain serum calcium levels.

Hypocalcemia can result from decreased total body calcium stores or low levels of calcium in ECF with normal amounts of calcium stored in bone. Many disorders can cause hypocalcemia (Table 7-8 ■). *Hypoparathyroidism,* usually due to surgical removal of the parathyroid glands, is the

most common cause. Hypoparathyroidism also may result from total thyroidectomy or radical neck surgery (see Chapter 16). ⬭ Hypocalcemia is common in clients with acute pancreatitis (see Chapter 21). ⬭ It often accompanies hypomagnesemia, common in malnourished alcoholics.

The manifestations of hypocalcemia are caused by insufficient ionized calcium in ECF. Calcium has a sedative effect on neuromuscular transmission. When calcium levels are low, neuromuscular excitability increases. **Tetany** (a group of symptoms caused by this increased excitability) is the most characteristic and serious consequence of hypocalcemia. Manifestations of tetany are *paresthesias* (numbness and tingling around the mouth and in the hands and feet) and muscle spasms. Chvostek's sign (facial muscle spasm when the facial nerve is tapped in front of the ear) and Trousseau's sign (carpal spasm that occurs when blood flow to the lower arm is restricted) also may be present (Figure 7-15 ■). Other manifestations are listed in Table 7-8. Critically low values, <6 mg/dL, may lead to respiratory or cardiac arrest or convulsions.

Interdisciplinary Care

DIAGNOSTIC TESTS. The *total serum calcium* will be less than 8.5 mg/dL, and ionized calcium (the active form) generally is about 50% of that. *Serum magnesium* is measured because hypocalcemia is often associated with hypomagnesemia. *Serum phosphate* is measured because there is a relationship between phosphorus and calcium levels (i.e., the serum level of one often rises as the other falls, and vice versa). *Parathyroid hormone (PTH)* is measured to identify hypoparathyroidism as a possible underlying cause. The *ECG* shows changes in the waveforms and dysrhythmias, such as bradycardia (slow heart rate) or ventricular tachycardia (a very rapid ventricular rate).

CALCIUM REPLACEMENT. Oral calcium preparations, increased dietary intake of calcium, and oral vitamin D are used to increase calcium levels in clients with chronic hypocalcemia. Vitamin D may be given as well to increase GI absorption of calcium.

In acute hypocalcemia, intravenous calcium (calcium chloride, calcium gluconate, or calcium gluceptate) is given to prevent or treat tetany. Calcium may be given by slow IV push or by infusion. It is given with caution to clients taking digitalis, because it increases the risk of digitalis toxicity. (See Table 7-9 ■.)

HYPERCALCEMIA

Hypercalcemia (serum calcium > 10.0 mg/dL) usually results from increased calcium release (*resorption*) from the bones. Increased calcium intake and decreased renal excretion of calcium are other causes.

TABLE 7-8

Calcium Imbalances

	HYPOCALCEMIA	HYPERCALCEMIA
Causes	Parathyroidectomy or neck surgery Acute pancreatitis Inadequate dietary intake Lack of sun exposure (vitamin D) Lack of weight-bearing exercise Drugs: loop diuretics, calcitonin, furosemide Hypomagnesemia (alcohol abuse, some chemotherapy)	Hyperparathyroidism Some cancers (lung, breast, multiple myeloma) Prolonged immobilization Paget's disease Excess milk or antacid intake Renal failure
Manifestations	Neuromuscular ■ Tetany: paresthesias, muscle spasms, laryngospasm, seizures ■ Positive Chvostek's sign ■ Positive Trousseau's sign Behavioral ■ Anxiety, confusion, psychoses Cardiovascular ■ ↓ Cardiac output ■ ↓ BP ■ Dysrhythmias Gastrointestinal ■ Abdominal cramping ■ Diarrhea	Neuromuscular ■ Muscle weakness ■ ↓ Deep tendon reflexes Behavioral ■ Confusion, impaired memory, bizarre behavior ■ Psychoses Cardiovascular ■ Dysrhythmias ■ ↑ BP Renal ■ ↑ Urine output Gastrointestinal ■ Constipation ■ Anorexia, nausea, vomiting
Lab values (normal 8.5–10.0 mg/dL or 2.12–2.57 mmol/L)	Serum calcium < 8.5 mg/dL Critical value < 6 mg/dL	Serum calcium > 10 mg/dL Critical value > 13 mg/dL

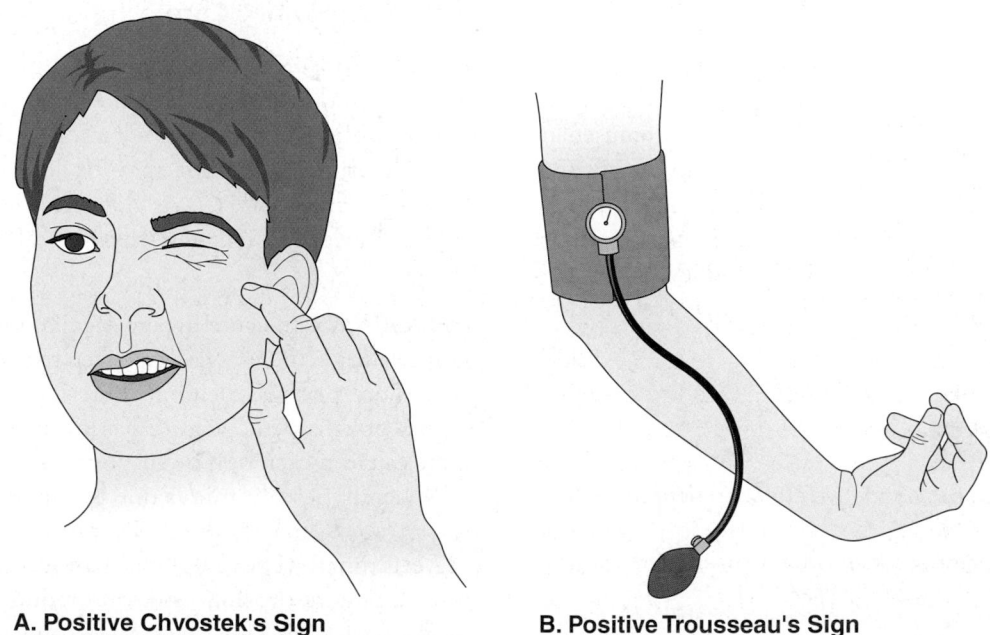

A. Positive Chvostek's Sign   **B. Positive Trousseau's Sign**

Figure 7-15. ■ (**A**) Positive Chvostek's sign and (**B**) positive Trousseau's sign.

TABLE 7-9

Nursing Implications for Pharmacology: Hypocalcemia

DRUG GROUP/DRUGS	ACTION/USES	NURSING IMPLICATIONS	CLIENT TEACHING (FOR ALL DRUG GROUPS)
Oral calcium Calcium carbonate (BioCal, Calsam, Caltrate, OsCal, Tums) Calcium gluconate Calcium lactate	Oral calcium preparations are used to increase calcium levels in the body.	Administer oral calcium 1–1.5 hours after meals. Calcium absorption is improved by concurrent administration of vitamin D.	A daily intake of 1,000–1,500 mg of calcium is recommended for adults. Older adults should consume 1,500 mg/day. Milk and milk products are a good source of calcium. If you have a tendency to form kidney stones, talk to your doctor before taking calcium supplements. Smoking and alcohol consumption interfere with calcium absorption. Regular physical exercise that involves weight bearing (walking, bicycling, weight training) helps maintain calcium stores in the bone and can help prevent osteoporosis.
Intravenous calcium Calcium gluconate Calcium chloride	Intravenous calcium is used to treat acute hypocalcemia. It also may be ordered postoperatively for clients who have had neck surgery such as parathyroidectomy, thyroidectomy, or radical neck surgery.	Administer into a central line or large peripheral vein. Dilute calcium solutions with normal saline or administer by infusion to reduce irritation of the vein. Monitor IV site closely; stop the infusion if infiltration occurs. Closely monitor ECG and serum calcium levels.	

Increased resorption of calcium from the bones may result from *hyperparathyroidism* and excess PTH secretion, prolonged immobilization, or certain malignancies (such as lung and breast cancers and multiple myeloma). Excess PTH also impairs renal excretion of calcium, as does kidney failure. Other causes of hypercalcemia are listed in Table 7-8.

The effects of hypercalcemia largely depend on the degree of serum calcium elevation and the length of time over which it develops. The primary effects are neuromuscular. Calcium has a sedative effect on neuromuscular transmission, which affects skeletal, smooth, and cardiac muscles. Excess calcium in cerebrospinal fluid affects behavior, and excess calcium in the urine can lead to kidney stones. Review Table 7-8 for the manifestations of hypercalcemia by body systems.

clinical ALERT

Remember, calcium has a sedative effect on neuromuscular transmission. Therefore:

Hypocalcemia → *Increased* neuromuscular excitability, muscle twitching, spasms, and possible tetany

Hypercalcemia → *Decreased* neuromuscular excitability, muscle weakness, and fatigue

Hypercalcemia can lead to complications such as peptic ulcer disease and pancreatitis. Critically high serum calcium levels, greater than 13 mg/dL, may cause complete heart block and cardiac arrest.

Interdisciplinary Care

DIAGNOSTIC TESTS. Hypercalcemia is diagnosed by measuring *serum calcium levels. Serum PTH* is measured to identify possible hyperparathyroidism. Levels are increased in hyperparathyroidism but may be low in other cases of hypercalcemia. An *ECG* is done to identify changes in impulse transmission and rhythm related to hypercalcemia.

MEDICATIONS. In acute hypercalcemia, intravenous normal saline solution (0.9% NaCl) is given to restore fluid volume and dilute plasma calcium. Diuretics such as furosemide (Lasix) or ethacrynic acid (Edecrin) may be given to promote calcium excretion by the kidneys.

When hypercalcemia is due to excess bone resorption, *biphosphonates* may be used. This group of drugs, including etidronate (Didronel) and pamidronate (Aredia), inhibit bone resorption and can reduce serum calcium levels with few side effects. Phosphates may be prescribed to inhibit bone resorption and reduce intestinal absorption of calcium. Other drugs used to treat hypercalcemia include calcitonin or intravenous plicamycin (Mithracin) to inhibit bone resorption, and glucocorticoids to decrease GI absorption of calcium and increase its excretion.

NURSING CARE

ASSESSING

Clients who have or are at risk for calcium imbalance are assessed for the following:

- Heart rate and rhythm
- Respiratory rate and effort; laryngeal *stridor* (a high-pitched, harsh sound heard during inspiration)
- Mental status and neuromuscular function
- Manifestations of tetany (tingling around mouth and fingers, muscle twitching or cramps, hyperactive reflexes)
- Serum calcium, magnesium, phosphate, and albumin levels

DIAGNOSING, PLANNING, AND IMPLEMENTING

Priorities in Nursing Care. The mental and neuromuscular effects of calcium imbalances place the client at significant risk for injury due to falls, airway impairment, dysrhythmias, or seizures.

Risk for Injury

- Institute safety precautions for clients who have mental changes resulting from hypercalcemia. *Changes in mental status may impair the client's judgment and ability to maintain his or her own safety.*

> ### clinical ALERT
>
> Frequently monitor airway and respiratory status. Report any changes, such as respiratory stridor or increased respiratory rate and effort. These may indicate laryngeal spasm, a respiratory emergency that requires immediate intervention to maintain adequate ventilation of the lungs.

- Monitor cardiovascular status, including heart rate and rhythm and blood pressure. *Calcium imbalances can affect heart contractility, leading to decreased cardiac output, dysrhythmias, and hypotension.*
- Place clients receiving intravenous calcium replacement on a cardiac monitor. *Clients receiving intravenous calcium may develop dysrhythmias.*

- Provide a quiet environment. Institute seizure precautions: Raise padded side rails and keep an airway at the bedside. *A quiet environment reduces central nervous system stimuli. The client with tetany is at risk for developing seizures.*
- If excess bone resorption has occurred, use caution when turning, transferring, or ambulating the client. *Bone may fracture more easily if excess calcium has been lost.*
- Ambulate clients as soon as allowed and encourage weight-bearing activity. *These measures help move calcium into bone, lowering serum calcium levels and reducing the risk of fracture.*
- Promote fluid intake to keep the client well hydrated and maintain dilute urine. Encourage fluids such as prune or cranberry juice. *The client is at risk for developing calcium renal stones. These juices help maintain acid urine, which inhibits calcium stone formation.*
- Keep emergency resuscitation equipment available. *Cardiac arrest may occur with extremely high serum calcium levels.*

EVALUATING

In addition to monitoring serum calcium levels, collect assessment data such as mental status, muscle strength, deep tendon reflexes, and cardiovascular status to evaluate the effectiveness of interventions for clients with calcium imbalances. Monitor laboratory results to evaluate the effectiveness of interdisciplinary interventions.

Documenting. Document continuing assessment data, as well as nursing and medical interventions implemented to restore calcium balance. Document the client's understanding of the condition, teaching provided, and compliance with treatment measures.

CONTINUING CARE

Assess risk factors for future episodes of calcium imbalance, such as poor dietary intake, cigarette smoking, alcohol consumption, lack of exposure to sunlight, and lack of weight-bearing exercise. Evaluate the client's knowledge and understanding of measures to prevent calcium imbalances. Discuss dietary sources of calcium and vitamin D; provide a list of foods that are high in calcium (Box 7-13 ■).

BOX 7-13

FOODS HIGH IN CALCIUM
- Milk and milk products
- Canned salmon and sardines
- Rhubarb
- Broccoli, collard greens, spinach
- Soy flour, tofu

Encourage taking prescribed oral calcium and vitamin D replacements as directed; caution to avoid excess doses of vitamin D supplements. Advise the client to increase fluid intake to at least 2,000 to 3,000 mL per day. Instruct clients who are at high risk for kidney stone formation to increase the intake of fluid and acid-ash foods (meats, fish, poultry, eggs, cranberries, plums, prunes). Discuss the relationship between weight-bearing activities and maintaining bone calcium. Help the client identify activities that fit with his or her lifestyle. Finally, instruct the client to increase dietary fiber and fluid to maintain normal bowel function and avoid constipation.

Magnesium Imbalance

About two-thirds of the magnesium (Mg^{2+}) in the body is in bones; one-third is within the cells; 1% is in ECF. The normal serum magnesium concentration is 1.3 to 2.1 mEq/L or 1.6 to 2.6 mg/dL. Magnesium is critical to intracellular metabolism. Extracellular magnesium affects neuromuscular irritability and contractility. Excess ECF magnesium depresses skeletal muscle contraction and central nervous system activity. A deficit causes increased irritability of the nervous system, cardiac dysrhythmias, and peripheral va-

sodilation. Serum magnesium values less than 1 mg/dL or higher than 4.7 mg/dL are considered to be critical.

Magnesium enters the body in the foods we eat. It is abundant in green vegetables, grains, nuts, meats, and seafood. The kidneys regulate extracellular magnesium levels by conserving or excreting it as needed.

HYPOMAGNESEMIA

Hypomagnesemia (serum magnesium < 1.3 mEq/L or 1.6 mg/dL) is usually due to a total body deficit of magnesium. In fact, body stores of magnesium may be depleted even when the serum magnesium level is within normal limits.

Chronic alcoholism is one of the most common causes of hypomagnesemia (Table 7-10 ■).

Hypomagnesemia has direct effects on body processes; it also affects potassium and calcium metabolism. Manifestations of hypomagnesemia usually do not occur until the serum level drops below 1 mEq/L. Neuromuscular excitability is increased in hypomagnesemia. Electrical conduction in the heart is affected, as is central nervous system function. The manifestations of hypomagnesemia are also listed in Table 7-10.

TABLE 7-10		
Magnesium Imbalances		
	HYPOMAGNESEMIA	**HYPERMAGNESEMIA**
Causes	Chronic alcoholism GI losses (intestinal suction, vomiting and diarrhea, ileostomy) Impaired intestinal absorption Increased renal excretion: drugs (loop diuretics, aminoglycoside antibiotics), kidney disease	Renal insufficiency or failure Excess intake of antacids, laxatives Excess magnesium administration
Manifestations	*(Generally seen with serum levels < 1 mEq/L)* Neuromuscular ■ Muscle weakness, tremors ■ Tetany ■ Positive Chvostek's and Trousseau's signs Gastrointestinal ■ Dysphagia Cardiovascular ■ Dysrhythmias ■ Peripheral vasodilation ■ ECG changes CNS ■ Seizures ■ Mental status changes	Neuromuscular ■ Muscle weakness ■ ↓ Deep tendon reflexes Gastrointestinal ■ Nausea and vomiting Cardiovascular ■ Vasodilation (facial flushing, sweating, feeling of warmth) ■ ↓ BP ■ Bradycardia ■ Cardiac arrest CNS ■ Lethargy, drowsiness ■ Respiratory depression, paralysis ■ Coma
Lab Values (normal 1.6–2.6 mg/dL or 0.6–1.0 mmol/L)	Serum magnesium < 1.6 mg/dL (0.6 mmol/L) Critical value < 1 mg/dL	Serum magnesium > 2.6 mg/dL (1.0 mmol/L) Critical value > 4.7 mg/dL

BOX 7-14

FOODS HIGH IN MAGNESIUM
- Green, leafy vegetables
- Legumes
- Whole grains
- Bananas, oranges, grapefruit
- Dairy products
- Meat
- Seafood

HYPERMAGNESEMIA

Hypermagnesemia (serum magnesium level > 2.1 mEq/L or 2.6 mg/dL) is often caused by renal insufficiency or failure. It also may develop in clients who take excess amounts of magnesium-containing antacids or laxatives, and when magnesium solutions are given to treat complications of pregnancy.

Elevated serum magnesium levels interfere with neuromuscular transmission and depress the central nervous system. Hypermagnesemia also affects the cardiovascular system and respiratory function. With mild hypermagnesemia, nausea and vomiting, hypotension, facial flushing, sweating, and a feeling of warmth occur. Table 7-10 summarizes the manifestations of hypermagnesemia.

Interdisciplinary Care

Prevention is important for both hypomagnesemia and hypermagnesemia. Identifying clients at risk and treatments that increase the risk of altered serum magnesium levels can prevent adverse effects.

In clients who are able to eat, a mild deficiency may be corrected by increasing the intake of magnesium-rich foods (Box 7-14 ■), or by using oral magnesium supplements (for example, magnesium-containing antacids). The use of these supplements is limited by their tendency to cause diarrhea.

Magnesium also can be given intravenously or by deep intramuscular injection. Serum magnesium levels and deep tendon reflexes are monitored frequently during treatment. Depressed deep tendon reflexes indicate high serum magnesium levels and a need to stop treatment.

Hypermagnesemia is treated by withholding all medications and solutions that contain magnesium. In clients with renal failure, excess magnesium is removed by hemodialysis or peritoneal dialysis (see Chapter 32). ⚭ With extremely high magnesium levels, intravenous calcium is given to counteract the cardiac effects of magnesium. Some clients may require mechanical ventilation to maintain respirations.

NURSING CARE

Nursing interventions for clients with magnesium imbalances focus on carefully monitoring individuals at risk, assessing signs and symptoms, implementing safety measures, teaching the client and family, and administering prescribed medications.

Assess clients at risk for magnesium imbalances for:
- Serum magnesium levels and other electrolytes, particularly potassium, calcium, and phosphate
- Manifestations of neuromuscular excitability, such as muscle twitching, tremors, grimaces, paresthesias, leg cramps, and hyperactive reflexes
- Changes in GI function, such as nausea, vomiting, anorexia, diarrhea, and abdominal distention
- Changes in cardiovascular function, such as hypotension, dysrhythmias, and changes in cardiac conduction. In clients receiving digitalis, monitor for digitalis toxicity.

Closely monitor serum magnesium levels and deep tendon reflexes in clients receiving intravenous magnesium solutions. Refer to the section on calcium imbalances for measures to reduce the risk of injury related to increased neuromuscular excitability.

CONTINUING CARE

Teach clients about foods that are high in magnesium (see Box 7-12) and provide information about magnesium supplements. Teach clients who have high magnesium levels to avoid magnesium-containing medications, including antacids, mineral supplements, cathartics, and enemas. Provide a list of magnesium-containing medications. Refer clients for whom alcohol abuse is a problem to a treatment program. Discuss support systems for alcoholics such as Alcoholics Anonymous, Al-Anon, and/or Al-a-Teen.

Phosphorus Imbalance

The normal serum phosphorus level in adults is 2.5 to 4.5 mg/dL. Phosphorus is found in all body tissues, but most of it is combined with calcium in bones and teeth. Phosphorus is the primary anion in ICF. Within cells, phosphorus is important for energy (ATP) production, metabolism, and red blood cell function. Although a very small portion of phosphorus (1%) is in ECF, it is essential for normal neuromuscular activity. Phosphate, the ionized form of phosphorus, is responsible for its physiologic effects. Phosphate is abundant in many foods, including meat, fish, poultry, eggs, milk products, and legumes. The kidneys regulate serum phosphorus levels, excreting excess phosphorus or retaining it if phosphate intake is low. An inverse relationship exists between phosphorus and calcium levels: When one increases, the other decreases. Thus, regulatory mechanisms that maintain calcium levels in the body also affect phosphorus levels.

TABLE 7-11

Phosphorus Imbalances

	HYPOPHOSPHATEMIA	HYPERPHOSPHATEMIA
Causes	■ Decreased GI absorption or increased renal excretion ■ Shift from ECF into cells ■ Alcoholism Iatrogenic causes ■ IV glucose administration ■ Total parenteral nutrition without phosphorus ■ Aluminum- or magnesium-based antacids ■ Insulin administration ■ Diuretic therapy	Acute or chronic renal failure Impaired excretion Increased phosphate intake or absorption Shift into ECF from: ■ Chemotherapy ■ Muscle tissue trauma ■ Sepsis ■ Severe hypothermia ■ Heat stroke
Manifestations	Neurologic ■ Irritability, confusion ■ Paresthesias ■ Ataxia, lack of coordination ■ Seizures, coma Hematologic ■ Tissue hypoxia ■ Hemolytic anemia ■ ↓ WBC function, ↑ risk of infection Muscle ■ Muscle pain, weakness ■ Respiratory failure Cardiac ■ Chest pain ■ ↓ Cardiac output ■ Dysrhythmias	Circumoral and peripheral paresthesias Muscle spasms Tetany Soft tissue calcification
Lab Values (normal 2.5–4.5 mg/dL or 0.8–1.45 mmol/L)	Serum phosphorus < 2.5 mg/dL Critical value < 1 mg/dL	Serum phosphate > 4.5 mg/dL

Hypophosphatemia (serum phosphorus < 2.5 mg/dL) may indicate a phosphorus deficit, or it may occur when phosphate shifts out of ECF into the cells. Decreased absorption of phosphate from the GI tract or increased excretion of phosphate by the kidneys can lead to a deficit of phosphorus. Iatrogenic (treatment-related) causes of hypophosphatemia are common (Table 7-11 ■). Alcoholism can cause severe hypophosphatemia.

The manifestations of hypophosphatemia (see Table 7-11) are caused by a lack of intracellular phosphate. Cellular energy resources for vital processes are depleted. The ability of red blood cells to transport oxygen is affected, resulting in tissue hypoxia.

Hyperphosphatemia (serum phosphate > 4.5 mg/dL) usually results from acute or chronic renal failure and impaired phosphorus excretion. It may be caused by increased phosphate intake or absorption. Phosphate is released into ECF when cells are damaged or destroyed (see Table 7-11).

When serum phosphate levels are high, the excess phosphate combines with calcium. The primary manifestations of hyperphosphatemia (Table 7-11) relate to the resulting hypocalcemia rather than to high phosphate levels themselves.

INTERDISCIPLINARY CARE

Management of phosphate imbalances focuses on preventing an imbalance in clients at risk and treating any underlying disorder causing phosphate imbalance.

For mild hypophosphatemia improved nutrition may be enough. Unless contraindicated, milk may be recommended because it supplies phosphate, calcium, and potassium. Oral phosphorus supplements may be prescribed, but common adverse effects (nausea and diarrhea) may limit their effectiveness. For severe hypophosphatemia, intravenous phosphate solutions may be ordered.

For hyperphosphatemia, agents such as aluminum hydroxide (Amphogel) that bind with phosphate may be used to lower serum phosphate levels. Dialysis may be used to remove excess phosphate. In clients with adequate renal function, intravenous normal saline may promote phosphate excretion. In severe hyperphosphatemia, glucose and insulin may be given to drive phosphate into the cells, lowering the serum phosphate level.

NURSING CARE

Identifying clients at risk for phosphate imbalances is an important nursing responsibility. Monitor serum phosphorus levels closely in malnourished clients, alcoholics, clients with renal failure, and clients being treated for diabetic ketoacidosis. Assess for and report manifestations of phosphate imbalance (paresthesias, muscle weakness and pain, or changes in mental status). Protect clients with severe hypophosphatemia from infection. Administer intravenous phosphate solutions carefully, observing for signs of hyperphosphatemia or other electrolyte imbalances (particularly potassium and calcium).

Teach at-risk clients and their families how to prevent and recognize manifestations of phosphate imbalance. Discuss the effects of phosphorus-binding antacids and phosphate-containing laxatives and enemas. Provide information about appropriate alternatives to these products and directions for their use. Teach clients that a well-balanced diet provides adequate phosphate. Milk and milk products, meats, and legumes (such as dried beans) are particularly rich in phosphate. Stress the importance of good nutrition, particularly with clients for whom alcohol is a problem. Provide information about alcohol treatment programs such as Alcoholics Anonymous. Instruct clients to mix powdered oral phosphorus supplements with very cold water or juice to make them more palatable.

ACID–BASE DISORDERS

For optimal cell function, the concentration of hydrogen ions (H^+) in body fluids must remain relatively constant. Hydrogen ions determine the relative acidity of body fluids. Acids release hydrogen ions in solution; bases (or alkalis) accept hydrogen ions in solution. The hydrogen ion concentration of a solution is measured as its **pH,** from 0 to 14, with 7 being neutral. The relationship between hydrogen ion concentration and pH is inverse; that is, as hydrogen ion concentration increases, the pH falls, and the solution becomes more acidic. As hydrogen ion concentration falls, the pH rises, and the solution becomes more alkaline or basic. The normal pH of body fluids is slightly basic, ranging from 7.35 to 7.45.

Acid–Base Regulation

Acids are continually produced by metabolic processes in the body. These acids may be either volatile or nonvolatile acids. *Volatile acids* can be eliminated from the body as a gas. Carbonic acid (H_2CO_3) is the only volatile acid produced in the body. It dissociates into carbon dioxide (CO_2) and water (H_2O). The carbon dioxide is eliminated from the body through the lungs. All other acids produced in the body (e.g., lactic acid, hydrochloric acid, phosphoric acid, and sulfuric acid) are *nonvolatile acids.* These must be metabolized or excreted from the body in fluid. Most acids and bases in the body are weak (close to a pH of 7).

Three systems work together in the body to maintain a normal pH despite continuous acid production: buffers, the respiratory system, and the renal system.

BUFFER SYSTEMS
Buffers prevent major changes in pH by attaching to or releasing hydrogen ion. When body fluid becomes excessively acid, buffers bind with hydrogen ions to minimize the change in pH. If body fluids become too basic or alkaline, buffers release hydrogen ion, restoring the pH. Although buffers act within a fraction of a second, their capacity to maintain pH is limited. The major buffer systems of the body are the bicarbonate–carbonic acid buffer system, phosphate buffer system, and protein buffers.

Bicarbonate is a weak base; when an acid is added to the system, it combines with bicarbonate, and the pH changes only slightly. Carbonic acid is a weak acid produced when carbon dioxide dissolves in water. If a base is added to the system, it combines with carbonic acid, and the pH remains within the normal range. The normal serum bicarbonate level is 24 mEq/L, and that of carbonic acid is 1.2 mEq/L. Thus, the ratio of bicarbonate to carbonic acid is 20:1. As long as this ratio is maintained, the pH remains within the 7.35 to 7.45 range (Figure 7-16 ■). When a strong acid is added to ECF, bicarbonate is depleted, changing the 20:1 ratio. The pH then drops below 7.35. If a strong base is added, carbonic acid is

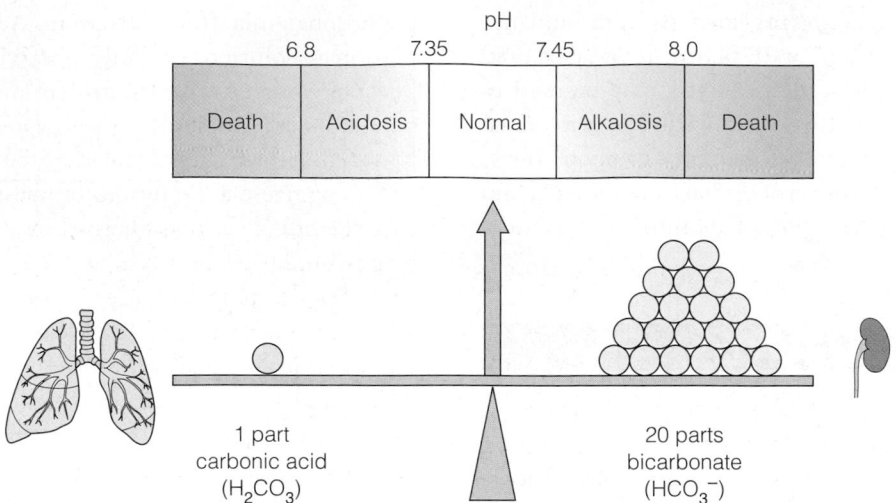

Figure 7-16. ■ As long as the ratio of bicarbonate to carbonic acid is 20:1, the pH remains within the normal range of 7.35 to 7.45.

depleted, the 20:1 ratio is altered, and the pH rises above 7.45.

Inorganic phosphates and plasma proteins serve a lesser role as buffers in ECF, although they are important intracellular buffers. Within red blood cells, hemoglobin also acts as a buffer.

RESPIRATORY SYSTEM

The respiratory system (including the respiratory center of the brain) regulates carbonic acid in the body by eliminating or retaining carbon dioxide. Carbon dioxide is a potential acid; when combined with water, it forms carbonic acid. Acute increases in either carbon dioxide or hydrogen ions in the blood stimulate the respiratory center in the brain to increase the rate and depth of respirations. This eliminates carbon dioxide from the body; carbonic acid levels fall, bringing the pH to a more normal range. This compensation for increased hydrogen ion concentration occurs within minutes. It becomes less effective over time, however. Clients with chronic lung disease may have consistently high carbon dioxide levels in their blood.

Alkalosis, by contrast, depresses the respiratory center. The rate and depth of respirations decrease, and carbon dioxide is retained. The retained carbon dioxide then combines with water to restore carbonic acid levels and bring the pH back within the normal range.

RENAL SYSTEM

The renal system responds more slowly to changes in pH (hours to days). It is responsible for the long-term regulation of acid–base balance in the body. The kidneys regulate bicarbonate levels in ECF and can either excrete or retain hydrogen ion as needed. When excess hydrogen ions are present and the pH falls, the kidneys excrete hydrogen ions and retain bicarbonate. When bicarbonate levels are high, the kid-

neys retain hydrogen ion and excrete bicarbonate to restore acid–base balance.

Types of Acid–Base Imbalances

Acid–base imbalances fall into two major categories: *acidosis* and *alkalosis.* **Acidosis** occurs when the hydrogen ion concentration increases above normal and the pH falls below 7.35. **Alkalosis** occurs when the hydrogen ion concentration decreases below normal and the pH rises above 7.45. Acid–base imbalances are further classified as *metabolic* or *respiratory* disorders. In *metabolic disorders,* the primary change is in bicarbonate concentration. In *metabolic acidosis,* the amount of bicarbonate is decreased in relation to the amount of acid in the body (Figure 7-17A ■). *Metabolic alkalosis,* by contrast, occurs when there is an excess of bicarbonate (Figure 7-17B). In *respiratory disorders,* the primary change is in the concentration of carbonic acid. *Respiratory acidosis* occurs when carbon dioxide is retained, increasing the amount of carbonic acid in the body (Figure 7-18A ■). When too much carbon dioxide is "blown off," carbonic acid levels fall, and *respiratory alkalosis* develops (Figure 7-18B).

Acid–base disorders are further defined as primary (simple) and mixed. *Primary (simple) disorders* usually are due to one cause. For example, respiratory failure often causes respiratory acidosis; renal failure usually causes metabolic acidosis. With primary disorders, the amount of change in pH may be minimized by *compensatory* responses by the acid–base regulatory system. The kidneys compensate for simple respiratory imbalances by altering bicarbonate production and hydrogen ion excretion; the lungs compensate for simple metabolic imbalances by changing the rate and depth of respirations. *Mixed disorders* occur when both metabolic and respiratory imbalances are present. For

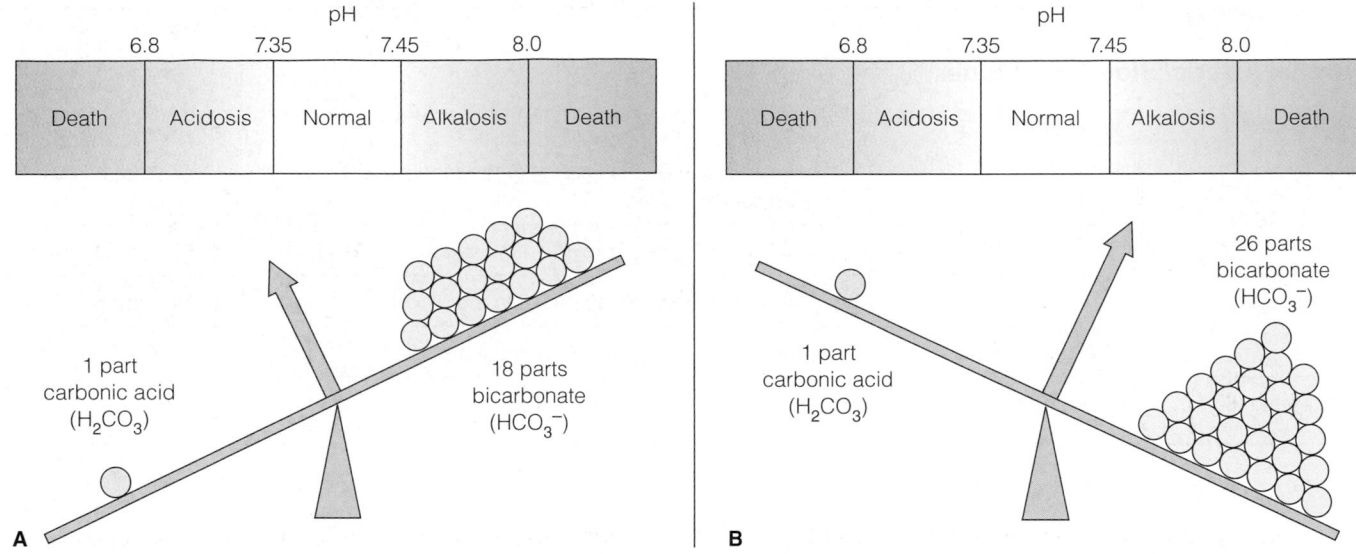

Figure 7-17. ■ Metabolic acid–base imbalances. (**A**) Metabolic acidosis. (**B**) Metabolic alkalosis.

example, a client in cardiac arrest develops a mixed respiratory and metabolic acidosis due to respiratory arrest and hypoxia of body tissues that affects normal cell metabolism.

ASSESSMENT OF ACID–BASE BALANCE

Acid–base balance is evaluated by measuring *arterial blood gases (ABGs)*. The elements measured are the $PaCO_2$, the PaO_2, bicarbonate, and pH. Normal ABG values are listed in Table 7-12 ■. Arterial blood is used because it reflects acid–base balance throughout the entire body and allows evaluation of oxygenation.

clinical ALERT

In contrast to veins, arteries are high-pressure vessels. ABGs are drawn by a registered nurse, respiratory therapist, or laboratory technician who has had specialized training. After the sample has been drawn, apply firm pressure to the puncture site for at least 5 minutes to prevent bleeding into the surrounding tissues.

The $PaCO_2$ measures the amount of dissolved carbon dioxide in the blood. The $PaCO_2$ is regulated by the lungs.

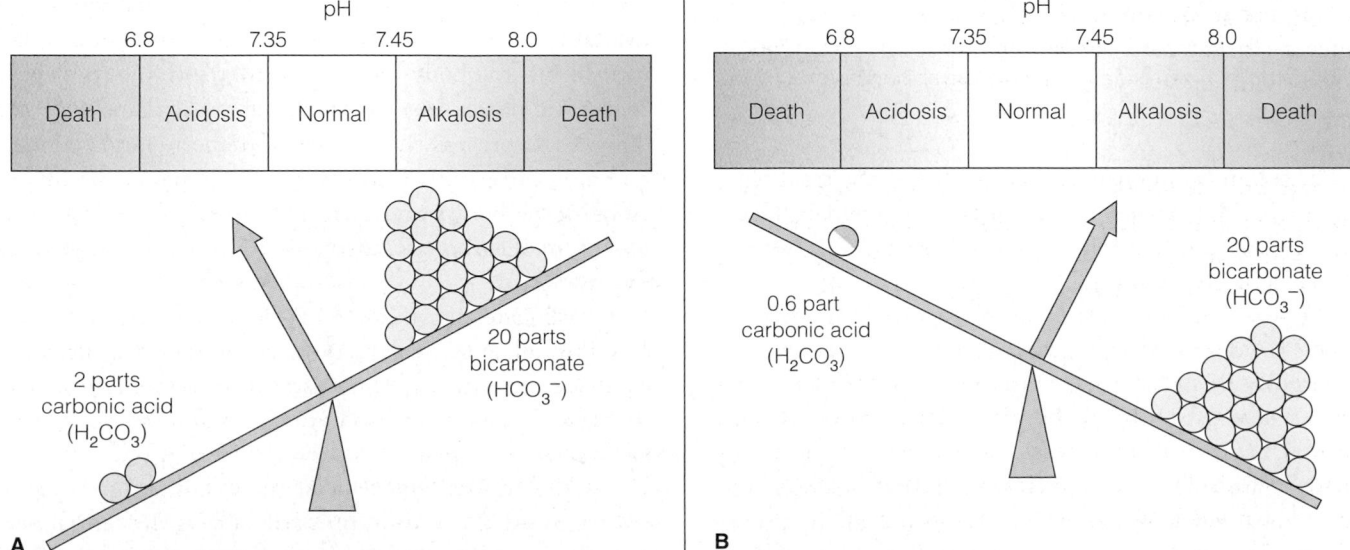

Figure 7-18. ■ Respiratory acid–base imbalances. (**A**) Respiratory acidosis. (**B**) Respiratory alkalosis.

TABLE 7-12			
Normal Arterial Blood Gas Values			
COMPONENT	NORMAL VALUE	SIGNIFICANCE	CRITICAL VALUES
pH	7.35–7.45	Relative acidity or alkalinity of the blood; hydrogen ion concentration	<7.20 or >7.60
Paco$_2$	35–45 mm Hg (Torr)	Amount of carbon dioxide dissolved in the blood	<20 or >70 mm Hg
Pao$_2$	80–100 mm Hg (Torr)	Amount of oxygen dissolved in the blood	<40 mm Hg
HCO$_3^-$	22–26 mEq/L	Bicarbonate concentration in the blood	
Base excess (BE)	−3.0–+3.0	Buffering capacity of the blood	

The normal value is 35 to 45 mm Hg. A Paco$_2$ of less than 35 mm Hg is known as *hypocapnia;* a Paco$_2$ greater than 45 mm Hg is *hypercapnia.*

The *Pao$_2$* measures the amount of oxygen dissolved in the plasma. Only about 3% of oxygen in the blood is in solution; most oxygen is carried by hemoglobin. However, it is the dissolved oxygen that is available to the cells for metabolism. As dissolved oxygen diffuses out of plasma into the tissues, more is released from hemoglobin. The normal value for Pao$_2$ is 80 to 100 mm Hg. A Pao$_2$ of less than 80 mm Hg indicates **hypoxemia.** The Pao$_2$ level is valuable for evaluating respiratory function but is not used as a primary measurement in determining acid–base status.

clinical ALERT

The abbreviations Paco$_2$ and Pao$_2$ often are used interchangeably with Pco$_2$ and Po$_2$. The "P" stands for partial pressure: the pressure exerted by the gas dissolved in the blood. The "a" indicates that the sample is arterial blood. Because these measurements rarely are done on venous blood, the "a" often is deleted from the abbreviation.

The serum bicarbonate (HCO$_3^-$) reflects the renal regulation of acid–base balance. It often is referred to as the *metabolic component* of arterial blood gases. The normal HCO$_3^-$ is 22 to 26 mEq/L.

The *base excess (BE)* also may be reported on ABGs. It reflects the degree of acid–base imbalance; it represents the amount of acid or base that must be added to a blood sample to achieve a pH of 7.4. The normal base excess is −3.0 to +3.0.

ABGs are analyzed to identify acid–base disorders and their probable cause, determine the extent of the imbalance, and monitor treatment. When analyzing ABG results, it is important to use a systematic approach (see Box

7-15 ■). First, evaluate each individual measurement, then look at the interrelationships to determine the client's acid–base status.

Metabolic Acidosis

Metabolic acidosis may be caused by excess acid or inadequate bicarbonate in the body. It is characterized by a low pH (<7.35) and a low bicarbonate level (<22 mEq/L). When metabolic acidosis develops, the respiratory system attempts to return the pH to normal by increasing the rate and depth of respirations. Carbon dioxide elimination increases, and the Paco$_2$ falls (<35 mm Hg).

PATHOPHYSIOLOGY AND MANIFESTATIONS

Metabolic acidosis rarely is a primary disorder; it usually develops during the course of another disease (Table 7-13 ■). Insufficient oxygen to support cell metabolism leads to the production of lactic acid. When inadequate glucose is available for cell metabolism (due to starvation or a lack of insulin), the body breaks down fatty tissue to meet its metabolic needs. In this process, fatty acids are released. This is the process that occurs in diabetic ketoacidosis, a common cause of metabolic acidosis. Renal failure, which impairs the body's ability to excrete excess hydrogen ion and form bicarbonate, also is a common cause of metabolic acidosis.

Bicarbonate-rich fluid from the small intestine can be lost through intestinal suction, severe diarrhea, ileostomy drainage, or fistulas. Administering excess chloride solutions (e.g., NaCl or ammonium chloride) can lead to metabolic acidosis as well.

In all acid–base imbalances, the manifestations may be subtle. Metabolic acidosis primarily affects the central nervous system, GI tract, and cardiovascular function. Deep, rapid respirations (Kussmaul's respirations or hyperventila-

---

BOX 7-15   NURSING CARE CHECKLIST

Interpreting Arterial Blood Gases

1. Look at the pH.
   - ☑ pH < 7.35 = acidosis
   - ☑ pH > 7.45 = alkalosis
2. Look at the $Paco_2$.
   - ☑ $Paco_2$ < 35 mm Hg = hypocapnia; more carbon dioxide is being exhaled than normal.
   - ☑ $Paco_2$ > 45 mm Hg = hypercapnia; carbon dioxide is being retained.
3. Evaluate the pH–$Paco_2$ relationship for a possible respiratory problem.
   - ☑ If the pH is < 7.35 (acidosis) and the $Paco_2$ is > 45 mm Hg (hypercapnia), retained carbon dioxide is causing *respiratory acidosis.*
   - ☑ If the pH is > 7.45 (alkalosis) and the $Paco_2$ is < 35 mm Hg (hypocapnia), low carbon dioxide levels are causing *respiratory alkalosis.*
4. Look at the bicarbonate.
   - ☑ If the HCO_3^- is < 22 mEq/L, bicarbonate levels are lower than normal.
   - ☑ If the HCO_3^- is > 26 mEq/L, bicarbonate levels are higher than normal.

5. Evaluate the pH, HCO_3^-, and base excess (BE) for a possible metabolic problem.
   - ☑ If the pH is < 7.35 (acidosis), the HCO_3^- is < 22 mEq/L, and the BE is < −3 mEq/L, low bicarbonate levels are causing *metabolic acidosis.*
   - ☑ If the pH is > 7.45 (alkalosis), the HCO_3^- is > 26 mEq/L, and the BE is > +3 mEq/L, high bicarbonate levels are causing *metabolic alkalosis.*
6. Look for compensation.
   - ■ *Renal compensation:*
     - ☑ In respiratory acidosis (pH < 7.35, $Paco_2$ > 45 mm Hg), the kidneys retain HCO_3^- to buffer the excess acid, so the HCO_3^- is > 26 mEq/L.
     - ☑ In respiratory alkalosis (pH > 7.45, $Paco_2$ < 35 mm Hg), the kidneys excrete HCO_3^- to minimize the alkalosis, so the HCO_3^- is < 22 mEq/L.
   - ■ *Respiratory compensation:*
     - ☑ In metabolic acidosis (pH < 7.35, HCO_3^- < 22 mEq/L), the rate and depth of respirations increase, increasing carbon dioxide elimination, so the $Paco_2$ is < 35 mm Hg.
     - ☑ In metabolic alkalosis (pH > 7.45, HCO_3^- > 26 mEq/L), respirations slow, and carbon dioxide is retained, so the $Paco_2$ is > 45 mm Hg.

---

tion) are characteristic of metabolic acidosis, as the body tries to eliminate excess acid by "blowing off" carbon dioxide. See Table 7-13 for the manifestations of metabolic acidosis.

INTERDISCIPLINARY CARE

The focus of treatment for acute metabolic acidosis is the underlying cause. (See Chapter 17 ↺ for treatment of diabetic ketoacidosis and Chapter 32 ↺ for treatment of renal failure.)

In addition to ABGs, *serum electrolytes* are measured. The serum potassium is usually greater than 5 mEq/L as potassium ions shift out of cells in exchange for hydrogen ions. Serum potassium levels are measured throughout treatment for metabolic acidosis because hypokalemia can develop as the acidosis is corrected. An *ECG* is done to evaluate the effects of metabolic acidosis on cardiac function.

Bicarbonate may be given to correct the acid–base imbalance, particularly when the pH is less than 7.2. Overtreatment is avoided, because it may lead to metabolic alkalosis, hypokalemia, dysrhythmias, and possible tetany. Other basic solutions that may be given to correct metabolic acidosis include lactate, acetate, or citrate solutions.

clinical ALERT

Closely monitor serum potassium levels during treatment of metabolic acidosis. As the acidosis is corrected, potassium shifts into the cells. This can lead to hypokalemia and cardiac dysrhythmias.

NURSING CARE

ASSESSING

Collect subjective assessment data, including symptoms of anorexia, nausea, abdominal discomfort, fatigue, or lethargy. Ask about precipitating factors such as diarrhea, aspirin ingestion, chronic diseases such as diabetes or renal failure, and current medications.

Obtain objective data including mental status and level of consciousness; vital signs including respiratory rate and depth; apical and peripheral pulses; skin color and temperature; and urine output.

TABLE 7-13			
Causes and Manifestations of Primary Acid–Base Imbalances			
IMBALANCE	**LAB VALUES**	**COMMON CAUSES**	**MANIFESTATIONS**
Metabolic acidosis	pH < 7.35 HCO_3^- < 22 mEq/L Compensation: $Paco_2$ < 35 mm Hg Serum K^+ usually > 5 mEq/L	Increased acid production ■ Lactic acidosis ■ Ketoacidosis (diabetes mellitus, starvation, or alcoholism) ■ Salicylate toxicity Decreased acid excretion ■ Renal failure Increased bicarbonate loss ■ Diarrhea, ileostomy drainage, intestinal fistula Increased chloride ■ Renal tubular acidosis	CNS ■ Headache ■ Confusion ■ Decreased level of consciousness GI ■ Anorexia ■ Nausea and vomiting Cardiovascular ■ Vasodilation; warm, flushed skin ■ Decreased cardiac output Respiratory (compensatory) ■ Increased rate and depth (hyperventilation)
Metabolic alkalosis	pH > 7.45 HCO_3^- > 26 mEq/L Compensation: $Paco_2$ > 45 mm Hg Serum potassium often < 3.5 mEq/L	Increased acid loss or excretion ■ Vomiting, gastric suction ■ Hypokalemia Increased bicarbonate ■ Alkali ingestion (bicarbonate of soda) ■ Excess bicarbonate administration	■ Dizziness ■ Paresthesias (around mouth and fingers and toes) ■ Carpopedal spasm (+ Trousseau's sign) ■ Hyperactive DTRs (deep tendon reflexes) ■ Depressed respirations (compensatory)
Respiratory acidosis	pH < 7.35 $Paco_2$ > 45 mm Hg Compensation: HCO_3^- > 26 mEq/L	Acute respiratory acidosis ■ Acute respiratory conditions ■ Narcotic overdose ■ Chest trauma ■ Respiratory arrest Chronic respiratory acidosis ■ Chronic respiratory conditions ■ Multiple sclerosis, other neuromuscular diseases ■ Stroke	Acute respiratory acidosis ■ Feeling of fullness in head ■ Mental cloudiness, decreasing level of consciousness ■ Dizziness, muscle twitching, seizures ■ Warm, flushed skin ■ Cardiac dysrhythmias Chronic respiratory acidosis ■ Dull headache ■ Weakness
Respiratory alkalosis	pH > 7.45 $Paco_2$ < 35 mm Hg Compensation: HCO_3^- < 22 mEq/L	■ Anxiety-induced hyperventilation ■ Fever ■ Early salicylate intoxication ■ Hyperventilation with mechanical ventilator	↓ Cerebral blood flow ■ Light-headedness ■ Inability to concentrate ↓ Calcium ionization ■ Paresthesias around mouth and distal extremities Hyperventilation syndrome ■ Palpitations, shortness of breath, chest tightness ■ Tremulousness, sweating, dry mouth ■ Feeling of panic ■ Loss of consciousness, seizures

Monitor laboratory results, including ABGs and serum electrolytes. Report changes that are not within expected ranges for treatment.

DIAGNOSING, PLANNING, AND IMPLEMENTING

Priorities in Nursing Care. An acid environment affects cell function. This is most apparent in the effects of acidosis on heart and neurologic function. These effects direct nursing care priorities.

Decreased Cardiac Output

Metabolic acidosis decreases the strength of heart contractions, slows the heart rate, and increases the risk of dysrhythmias.

■ Monitor vital signs, peripheral pulses, and capillary refill. *Hypotension, diminished pulse strength, and slowed capillary refill may indicate decreased cardiac output.*

- Monitor ECG pattern for dysrhythmias. Notify the physician of changes. *Dysrhythmias further decrease cardiac output, which may worsen acidosis.*
- Monitor laboratory values, including arterial blood gases, serum electrolytes, serum creatinine, and blood urea nitrogen (BUN). *Frequent monitoring of laboratory values helps evaluate treatment effectiveness and identify potential problems.*

Risk for Injury

- Monitor mental status, level of consciousness, and muscle strength. *As the pH falls, mental function declines, causing confusion and a decreasing level of consciousness. This increases the risk for injury.*
- Institute safety precautions as necessary: Keep the bed in its lowest position with side rails up. *These measures help protect the client from injury resulting from confusion or disorientation.*
- Keep clocks, calendars, and familiar objects at the bedside. Orient to time, place, and circumstances as needed. Allow significant others to remain with the client as much as possible. *An unfamiliar environment and altered thought processes can further increase the risk for injury. Significant others provide a sense of security and reduce anxiety.*

Risk for Excess Fluid Volume

Administering bicarbonate to correct acidosis increases the risk for hypernatremia and fluid volume excess.

- Obtain daily weights. *Daily weights are an accurate indicator of fluid balance.*
- Monitor intake and output. Obtain hourly urine outputs as indicated, reporting an output of less than 30 mL/hr. *Heart failure and inadequate renal perfusion may lead to decreased urine output.*
- Monitor respiratory status and CVP. *Increasing dyspnea, adventitious lung sounds, and high CVP readings indicate excess fluid volume. Report to the care provider.*
- Assess for edema in dependent tissues and periorbital areas. *Dependent or generalized edema may indicate excess fluid volume.*

Nursing care also includes measures to treat the underlying disorder, such as diabetic ketoacidosis. Refer to the chapters on diabetes (Chapter 17) ∞ and renal failure (Chapter 32) ∞ for specific interventions.

EVALUATING

To evaluate the effectiveness of nursing care, monitor the client's cardiac output, safety, and fluid balance, as well as laboratory results for ABGs and serum electrolytes.

Documenting. Document the care and interventions provided, and the client's response (e.g., improved mental functioning, fewer cardiac dysrhythmias) to interventions.

Document continuing assessments, including assessments of fluid balance.

CONTINUING CARE

Discharge planning focuses on the underlying cause of the metabolic acidosis. Teach the client who has developed ketoacidosis as a result of diabetes mellitus, starvation, or alcoholism about diet and medications. Refer for treatment of alcoholism and to a support group such as Alcoholics Anonymous. Discuss the importance of day-to-day management of renal failure (e.g., diet and dialysis) to prevent future problems with metabolic acidosis. With clients who developed acidosis as a result of diarrhea or ileostomy drainage, provide information about strategies to prevent or treat diarrhea, and when to call their primary care provider.

Metabolic Alkalosis

Metabolic alkalosis may be caused by loss of acid or excess bicarbonate in the body. It is characterized by a high pH (>7.45) and a high bicarbonate level (>26 mEq/L). When metabolic alkalosis develops, the respiratory system attempts to return the pH to normal by slowing the respiratory rate. Carbon dioxide is retained, and the $PaCO_2$ increases (>45 mm Hg).

PATHOPHYSIOLOGY AND MANIFESTATIONS

Vomiting or gastric suction often leads to loss of hydrogen ions from the body. Gastric secretions are highly acidic (pH 1–3). Hypokalemia also reduces hydrogen ion concentration, as the kidneys excrete hydrogen ion in exchange for potassium. In addition, when potassium shifts out of the cells to maintain potassium levels in ECF, hydrogen ion shifts into the cells.

Excess bicarbonate usually results from ingestion of antacids that contain bicarbonate (such as soda bicarbonate or Alka-Seltzer) or overzealous administration of bicarbonate to treat metabolic acidosis. Review Table 7-13 for common causes of metabolic alkalosis.

Alkalosis affects calcium ionization in ECF. Because of this, the manifestations of both metabolic and respiratory alkalosis are similar to those of hypocalcemia. As the respiratory system compensates for metabolic alkalosis, respirations are depressed (see Table 7-13).

INTERDISCIPLINARY CARE

Treatment of metabolic alkalosis focuses on diagnosing and correcting the underlying cause. Serum electrolytes are monitored; hypokalemia (<3.5 mEq/L) and hypochloremia (<95 mEq/L) are often present. The potassium level is closely monitored during treatment, because correcting the alkalosis may affect serum potassium.

Treatment includes restoring normal fluid volume and administering potassium chloride and sodium chloride solutions. Chloride is necessary for the kidneys to excrete excess bicarbonate. Potassium helps restore intra- and extracellular potassium levels, allowing the kidneys to more effectively retain hydrogen ion. Sodium chloride is given to treat accompanying fluid volume deficits. When the pH is critically high (>7.6), an acidifying solution such as dilute hydrochloric acid or ammonium chloride may be given.

NURSING CARE

ASSESSING

Obtain the following assessment data related to metabolic alkalosis:

- Current symptoms, such as numbness and tingling, muscle spasms, or dizziness; any precipitating factors such as bicarbonate ingestion or vomiting, current medications
- Objective data: vital signs including apical pulse, rate and depth of respirations; muscle strength; and deep tendon reflexes
- Laboratory data: ABGs, serum electrolytes

DIAGNOSING, PLANNING, AND IMPLEMENTING

Priorities in Nursing Care. A high pH (alkalosis) inhibits the respiratory center of the brain, slowing respirations as the body attempts to retain carbonic acid to balance the excess of bicarbonate. This places the client at risk for impaired gas exchange, the priority for nursing care.

RISK FOR IMPAIRED GAS EXCHANGE

- Monitor respiratory rate, depth, and effort. Monitor oxygen saturation continuously; report an oxygen saturation level of less than 95% (or as ordered). *Depressed respirations can lead to hypoxemia and impaired tissue oxgenation. An oxygen saturation of less than 90% indicates significant problems.*
- Monitor mental status and level of consciousness (LOC). Report decreasing LOC or behavior changes such as restlessness, agitation, or confusion. *Changes in mental status or behavior may be early signs of hypoxia.*
- Place in semi-Fowler's or Fowler's position as tolerated. *Elevating the head of the bed improves ventilation and gas exchange.*
- Schedule nursing care activities to allow rest periods. *The hypoxemic client has limited energy reserves, requiring frequent rest and limited activities.*

- Administer oxygen as ordered or necessary to maintain oxygen saturation levels. *Supplemental oxygen can help maintain blood and tissue oxygenation despite depressed respirations.*

Deficient Fluid Volume

Clients with metabolic alkalosis often have an accompanying fluid volume deficit.

- Assess intake and output; monitor hourly if indicated. *Urine output of less than 30 mL/hr indicates inadequate renal perfusion and an increased risk for acute renal failure and inadequate tissue perfusion.*
- Monitor vital signs, CVP, and peripheral pulses at least every 4 hours. *Hypotension, tachycardia, low CVP, and weak, easily obliterated peripheral pulses indicate hypovolemia.*
- Weigh daily. *Rapid weight changes accurately reflect fluid balance.*
- Administer intravenous fluids as ordered using an infusion pump. Monitor for dyspnea, tachypnea, tachycardia, increased CVP, jugular vein distention, and edema. *Rapid fluid replacement may lead to hypervolemia.*
- Monitor serum electrolytes, osmolality, and ABG values. *Rehydration and administration of potassium chloride will affect both acid–base and fluid and electrolyte balance. Careful monitoring is important to identify changes.*

EVALUATING

Collect data related to the client's respiratory status, tissue oxygenation, and fluid balance to evaluate the effectiveness of nursing interventions for clients with metabolic alkalosis.

Documenting. Document nursing and interdisciplinary care provided, continuing assessment data, and the client's and family's understanding of the condition and its causes.

CONTINUING CARE

Planning and teaching for home care of the client who has experienced metabolic alkalosis focus on the underlying cause of the imbalance. Teach clients how to prevent and manage problems such as acute gastroenteritis that can lead to excessive vomiting (see Chapter 19). ∞ Discuss the importance of adequate potassium in the diet, foods high in potassium (see Box 7-10), and potassium supplements with clients for whom hypokalemia contributed to metabolic alkalosis. Teach clients to avoid using bicarbonate-based antacids, and suggest alternatives.

Respiratory Acidosis

Respiratory acidosis is caused by an excess of dissolved carbon dioxide, or carbonic acid. It is characterized by a pH of less than 7.35 and a $PaCO_2$ greater than 44 mm Hg. Respiratory acidosis may be either acute or chronic in nature.

In chronic respiratory acidosis, the bicarbonate is higher than 26 mEq/L as the kidneys compensate by retaining bicarbonate.

PATHOPHYSIOLOGY AND MANIFESTATIONS

Both acute and chronic respiratory acidosis are caused by alveolar hypoventilation leading to carbon dioxide retention. Hypoxemia (low oxygen in the arterial blood) frequently accompanies respiratory acidosis.

Acute respiratory acidosis occurs due to an acute failure of ventilation. Chest trauma, aspiration of a foreign body, acute pneumonia, and overdoses of narcotic or sedative medications can lead to acute respiratory acidosis. In acute respiratory acidosis, the $PaCO_2$ rises rapidly and the pH falls markedly. The serum bicarbonate initially is unchanged because the compensatory response of the kidneys occurs over hours to days.

Chronic respiratory acidosis is associated with chronic respiratory or neuromuscular conditions such as chronic obstructive pulmonary disease (COPD), asthma, cystic fibrosis, or multiple sclerosis. These conditions affect alveolar ventilation because of airway obstruction, structural changes in the lung, or limited chest wall expansion. Most clients with chronic respiratory acidosis have chronic obstructive pulmonary disease with chronic bronchitis and emphysema (see Table 7-13). In chronic respiratory acidosis, the $PaCO_2$ increases over time and remains elevated. The kidneys retain bicarbonate, increasing bicarbonate levels, and the pH often remains close to the normal range.

The manifestations of acute and chronic respiratory acidosis differ. An acute rise in $PaCO_2$ causes manifestations of hypercapnia (elevated serum carbon dioxide levels). Carbon dioxide dilates cerebral blood vessels, causing a feeling of fullness in the head and mental cloudiness. Rapid and dramatic changes in ABGs can lead to unconsciousness and cardiac arrest.

Clients with chronic respiratory acidosis may have few symptoms because carbon dioxide levels rise gradually, allowing compensatory changes to occur. See Table 7-13 for other manifestations of acute and chronic respiratory acidosis.

clinical ALERT

In clients with chronically high blood levels of carbon dioxide, hypoxemia becomes the primary stimulus to breathe. Administering oxygen at a high flow rate may suppress respirations and lead to acute respiratory failure.

INTERDISCIPLINARY CARE

Clients with acute respiratory failure usually require treatment in the emergency department or intensive care unit to restore adequate ventilation and gas exchange. Hypoxemia often accompanies acute respiratory acidosis, so oxygen is administered as well. Supplemental oxygen is used with caution for clients with chronic respiratory acidosis.

Bronchodilator drugs may be given to open the airways. Antibiotics may be ordered to treat respiratory infections. If excess narcotics or anesthetic has caused acute respiratory acidosis, drugs to reverse their effects may be given. Pulmonary hygiene measures, such as breathing treatments or percussion and drainage, may be used to clear airways and support ventilation. Adequate hydration is important to promote removal of respiratory secretions. Intubation and mechanical ventilation may be necessary for some clients in respiratory acidosis. (See Chapter 24 ⬭ for more information about mechanical ventilation and its nursing implications.)

NURSING CARE

ASSESSING

Assessment data related to respiratory acidosis includes the following:

- *Subjective data:* current symptoms such as headache, difficulty thinking, blurred vision; any precipitating factors such as drug use or infection; chronic diseases such as cystic fibrosis or COPD; current medications
- *Objective data:* mental status and level of consciousness vital signs; skin color and temperature; rate and depth of respirations, lung sounds
- *Laboratory data:* ABGs, serum electrolytes.

DIAGNOSING, PLANNING, AND IMPLEMENTING

Priorities in Nursing Care. Ineffective gas exchange in the lungs is the primary cause of respiratory acidosis, and the focus of nursing care. When gas exchange is impaired, oxygen saturation levels fall and tissues receive inadequate oxygen to meet metabolic needs.

Impaired Gas Exchange

- Frequently assess respiratory status (rate, depth, effort, and oxygen saturation levels) and LOC. *Decreasing respiratory rate, effort, oxygen saturation level, and LOC may indicate worsening of the client's condition.*
- Promptly report ABG results to the physician and respiratory therapist. *Rapid changes in carbon dioxide or oxygen levels may indicate a need to modify the treatment plan.*
- Place in semi-Fowler's to Fowler's position as tolerated. *Elevating the head of the bed promotes lung expansion and gas exchange.*

- Administer oxygen as ordered. Carefully monitor response. Reduce the oxygen flow rate or percentage and immediately report decreased level of consciousness. *Supplemental oxygen can suppress the respiratory drive in clients with chronic respiratory acidosis.*

Ineffective Airway Clearance

In some instances, for example, a client with acute asthma or chronic bronchitis, obstruction of the airways impairs the flow of gases to and from the alveoli, affecting gas exchange.

- Frequently auscultate breath sounds. *Increasing adventitious sounds or decreasing breath sounds (faint or absent) may indicate worsening airway clearance due to obstruction or fatigue.*
- Encourage the client with chronic respiratory acidosis to use pursed-lip breathing. *Pursed-lip breathing helps maintain open airways throughout exhalation, promoting carbon dioxide elimination.*
- Frequently reposition and encourage client to get out of bed as tolerated. *Movement and ambulation promote airway clearance and lung expansion.*
- Encourage fluid intake of up to 3,000 mL per day as tolerated or allowed. *Fluids help liquefy secretions and hydrate respiratory mucous membranes, promoting airway clearance.*
- Administer medications such as inhaled bronchodilators as ordered. *Inhaled bronchodilators help relieve bronchial spasm, dilating airways.*
- Provide percussion, vibration, and postural drainage as ordered. *Pulmonary hygiene measures such as these help loosen respiratory secretions so they can be coughed out of airways.*

EVALUATING

Collect data such as ABG results, oxygen saturation levels, mental status, skin color, lung sounds, activity tolerance, and ease of respirations to evaluate the effectiveness of nursing interventions for the client with respiratory acidosis.

Documenting. Document continuing assessment data, as well as the client's response to interventions. Document care and teaching provided, as well as the client's and family's understanding of the disorder and measures to prevent future episodes of respiratory acidosis.

CONTINUING CARE

Planning and teaching for discharge focus on the problem that caused the client to develop respiratory acidosis. Clients with acute respiratory acidosis resulting from acute pneumonia or chest trauma may need only teaching to prevent future problems. If acute respiratory acidosis was secondary to a narcotic overdose, determine if the drug was prescribed or an illicit street drug. Provide teaching to the client who requires narcotic medication on a continuing basis. Refer the client using illicit drugs to a substance abuse

counselor, treatment center, or Narcotics Anonymous as appropriate.

For clients with chronic lung disease, discuss ways to avoid future episodes of acute respiratory failure. Encourage the client to be immunized against pneumococcal pneumonia and influenza. Discuss ways to avoid acute respiratory infections and measures to take when respiratory status is further compromised.

Respiratory Alkalosis

Respiratory alkalosis is always caused by hyperventilation leading to a carbon dioxide deficit. It is characterized by a pH greater than 7.45 and a $PaCO_2$ of less than 35 mm Hg.

PATHOPHYSIOLOGY AND MANIFESTATIONS

In acute respiratory alkalosis, the pH rises rapidly as the $PaCO_2$ falls. The bicarbonate level remains within normal limits because the kidneys require time to increase bicarbonate elimination. Anxiety-induced hyperventilation is the most common cause of acute respiratory alkalosis. Other causes are listed in Table 7-13. Low carbon dioxide levels cause cerebral blood vessels to constrict, reducing blood flow. The manifestations of respiratory alkalosis relate to this cerebral vasoconstriction and decreased calcium ionization (which also occurs in metabolic alkalosis). Table 7-13 lists the manifestations of respiratory alkalosis.

INTERDISCIPLINARY CARE

Anxiety-induced respiratory alkalosis is treated by instructing the client to breathe slowly into a paper bag or rebreather mask. This allows the client to rebreathe exhaled carbon dioxide, which increases $PaCO_2$ levels and reduces the pH. A sedative or antianxiety agent may be given. In other cases, such as salicylate intoxication or excessive ventilation by a mechanical ventilator, treatment is aimed at the underlying cause of the hyperventilation.

NURSING CARE

Priorities in Nursing Care. The priority of care for the client with respiratory alkalosis is restoring an effective breathing pattern to prevent excess loss of carbon dioxide.

Ineffective Breathing Pattern

- Assess respiratory rate, depth, and ease. Monitor vital signs (including temperature) and skin color. *Assessment data can help identify the underlying cause, such as a fever or hypoxia.*
- Obtain subjective assessment data such as circumstances leading up to the current situation, current health and recent illnesses or medication use, as well as current

manifestations. *Subjective data provide cues to the cause and circumstances of hyperventilation.*

- Reassure the client that he or she is not having a heart attack and that symptoms will resolve when breathing returns to normal. *Manifestations of hyperventilation and respiratory alkalosis such as dyspnea, chest tightness or pain, and palpitations can mimic those of a heart attack.*

- Instruct client to maintain eye contact and breathe with you to slow the respiratory rate. *These measures help make the client aware of respirations and provide a sense of support and control.*

- Have the client breathe into a paper bag. *This allows the client to rebreathe exhaled carbon dioxide, increasing the $PaCO_2$ and decreasing the pH.*

- Protect from injury. *If hyperventilation continues, the client may lose consciousness, causing respirations and acid–base balance to return to normal.*

- Refer clients with repeated episodes of hyperventilation or a chronic anxiety disorder for counseling. *Counseling can help the client develop strategies for dealing with anxiety.*

CONTINUING CARE

Planning and teaching for home care are directed toward the underlying cause of hyperventilation. If anxiety precipitated the episode, discuss anxiety-management strategies. Refer the client and family to a counselor if appropriate. Teach how to identify a hyperventilation reaction and breathe into a paper bag to manage it at home.

Note: The bibliography listings for this and all chapters have been compiled at the back of the book.

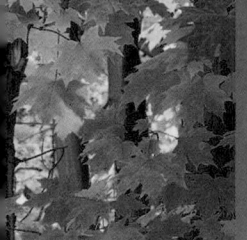

Chapter Review

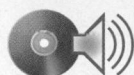 **KEY TERMS** by Topics

Use the audio glossary feature of either the CD-ROM or the Companion Website to hear the correct pronunciation of the following key terms.

Physiologic balance

homeostasis

Structure and Function

electrolytes, intracellular fluid (ICF), extracellular fluid (ECF), osmosis, diffusion, filtration, active transport

Fluid volume excess

hypervolemia, edema

Potassium imbalance

hypokalemia, hyperkalemia

Calcium imbalance

tetany

Acid–base disorders

pH, buffers, acidosis, alkalosis, metabolic acidosis, metabolic alkalosis, respiratory acidosis, respiratory alkalosis, hypoxemia

KEY Points

- The volume and composition of body fluid is normally maintained by a balance of fluid and electrolyte intake; elimination of water, electrolytes, and acids by the kidneys; and hormonal influences. Change in any of these factors can lead to a fluid, electrolyte, or acid–base imbalance that affects health.

- Fluid, electrolyte, and acid–base imbalances can affect all body systems, especially the cardiovascular system, the central nervous system, and the transmission of nerve impulses.

- Fluid and sodium imbalances commonly are related; both affect serum osmolality.

- Both hypokalemia and hyperkalemia affect cardiac conduction and function. Carefully monitor cardiac rhythm and status in clients with very low or very high potassium levels.

- Calcium imbalances primarily affect neuromuscular transmission: Too little calcium causes increased neuromuscular irritability; too much calcium depresses neuromuscular transmission. Magnesium imbalances have a similar effect.

- Acid–base imbalances may be caused by either metabolic or respiratory problems.

- Buffers, lungs, and kidneys work together to maintain acid–base balance in the body. Buffers respond to changes almost immediately; the lungs respond within minutes; the kidneys, however, require hours to days to restore normal acid–base balance.

- The lungs compensate for metabolic acid–base imbalances by excreting or retaining carbon dioxide. This is accomplished by increasing or decreasing the rate and depth of respirations.

- The kidneys compensate for respiratory acid–base imbalances by producing and retaining or excreting bicarbonate, and by retaining or excreting hydrogen ions.

- Careful monitoring of respiratory and cardiovascular status, mental status, neuromuscular function, and laboratory values is an important nursing responsibility for all clients with fluid, electrolyte, or acid–base imbalances.

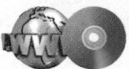 **EXPLORE Media**Link

Additional interactive resources for this chapter can be found on the Companion Website at www.prenhall.com/burke. Click on Chapter 7 and "Begin" to select the activities for this chapter.

For chapter-related NCLEX-sytle questions and an audio glossary, access the accompanying CD-ROM in this book.

FOR FURTHER Study

See Chapter 16 for more information about diabetes insipidus and SIADH.

For more information on diabetic ketoacidosis, see Chapter 17.

See Chapter 18 for more information about liver function tests.

Anorexia nervosa and GI disorders are discussed in Chapter 19.

For more on clients with acute pancreatitis, see Chapter 21.

For more about mechanical ventilation, see Chapter 24.

For more about ECG waveforms and cardiac disorders, see Chapters 26 and 27.

For more on water reabsorption, urine concentration, and renal function tests see Chapter 31.

See Box 31-3 for nursing responsibilities in collecting a 24-hour urine specimen.

For more information on clients with renal failure, see Chapter 32.

Caring for a Client with Acute Respiratory Acidosis

NCLEX-PN® Focus Area: Physiologic Adaptation

Case Study: Marlene Hitz, age 76, is eating lunch with her friends when she suddenly begins to choke and is unable to breathe. After several minutes of trying, an attendant at the senior center successfully dislodges some meat caught in Ms. Hitz's throat using the Heimlich maneuver. Ms. Hitz is taken by ambulance to the emergency department for follow-up.

Nursing Diagnosis: Impaired Gas Exchange

COLLECT DATA

Subjective	Objective
_____	_____
_____	_____
_____	_____
_____	_____
_____	_____
_____	_____
_____	_____

Would you report this data? Yes/No

If yes, to: _____

Nursing Care

_____

_____

_____

_____

_____

_____

_____

_____

How would you document this? _____

_____

_____

_____

Data Collected
(use those that apply)

- T 98.2°F, P 102, R 36 and shallow, BP 146/92
- Skin warm and dry
- Alert but not oriented to time or place
- Responds slowly to questions
- Restless
- Oxygen at 4 L/min per nasal cannula
- D_5 ½ NS running intravenously at 50 mL/hr
- Chest x-ray normal
- ABGs: pH 7.38 (normal 7.35 to 7.45), Pa_{CO_2} 48 mm Hg (normal 35 to 45 mm Hg), Pa_{O_2} 92 mm Hg (normal 80 to 100 mm Hg), HCO_3^- 24 mEq/dL (normal 22 to 26 mEq/L)

Nursing Interventions
(use those that apply; list in priority order)

- Monitor ABGs, to be redrawn in 2 hours.
- Monitor respiratory status and vital signs every 15 minutes for the first hour, then hourly.
- Assess mental status, LOC, and color of skin, nail beds, and oral mucous membranes hourly.
- Maintain a calm, quiet environment.
- Reorient to setting and explain all activities.
- Keep side rails in place, and place call bell within reach.

NCLEX-PN® Exam Preparation

1 Which of these clients would most likely develop dehydration after surgery?

   A. 24-year-old male diagnosed with an inguinal hernia
   B. 70-year-old female with ovarian cancer
   C. 65-year-old male with prostate cancer
   D. 19-year-old female with a badly fractured leg

2 A client has been diagnosed with deficient antidiuretic hormone (ADH). Which assessment finding should the nurse anticipate?

   A. increased serum osmolality
   B. dilute urine
   C. decreased thirst
   D. normal blood pressure

3 The nurse assessing a client in the emergency department notes dry, sticky mucous membranes; weak peripheral pulses; and tachycardia. The primary nursing diagnosis should be:

   A. Deficient Fluid Volume.
   B. Impaired Skin Integrity.
   C. Risk for Injury.
   D. Decreased Cardiac Output.

4 A client admitted to the medical floor has muscle spasms and a positive Chvostek's sign. In obtaining the history, the nurse notes that the client had a thyroidectomy 6 weeks ago. Based on this finding, the nurse anticipates that the physician will order a lab test for:

   A. sodium.
   B. potassium.
   C. magnesium.
   D. calcium.

5 A client presents with muscle weakness, tremors, and confusion. Laboratory testing reveals a serum magnesium level of 0.9 mg/dL. The nurse recalls that a common cause of hypomagnesemia is

   A. kidney failure.
   B. excessive antacid use.
   C. chronic alcoholism.
   D. lack of sun exposure.

6 A client is hyperventilating due to anxiety. Which of the following lab values indicates an altered acid–base balance?

   A. pH 7.51
   B. $Paco_2$ 38 mm Hg
   C. HCO_3^- 22 mEq/L
   D. Pao_2 95 mm Hg

7 The nurse knows that a client's low bicarbonate level may be caused by:

   A. gastrointestinal suction.
   B. constipation.
   C. use of baking soda for indigestion.
   D. alcohol abuse.

8 A client with hyperkalemia is admitted to the medical floor. Which of the following complications of this electrolyte imbalance does the nurse monitor most closely for?

   A. paralytic ileus
   B. cardiac dysrhythmias
   C. fluid retention and edema
   D. kidney stones

9 The nurse administered the prescribed dose of furosemide (Lasix). To evaluate the effectiveness of the drug, the nurse should assess:

   A. weight.
   B. apical pulse.
   C. breath sounds.
   D. fluid intake PO.

10 The nurse is caring for a client being treated for diabetic ketoacidosis (metabolic acidosis). Which laboratory value should the nurse monitor closely as the acidosis is corrected?

   A. hemoglobin and hematocrit
   B. serum potassium
   C. urine specific gravity
   D. serum magnesium

Answers for Review Questions, as well as discussion of Care Plan and Critical Thinking Care Map questions, appear in Appendix V.

Chapter 8

Caring for Clients in Pain

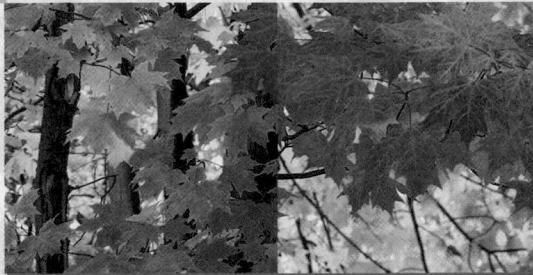

BRIEF Outline

Physiology of Pain
Types of Pain
Factors Affecting Client Response to Pain
Interdisciplinary Care

LEARNING Outcomes

After completing this chapter, you will be able to:

- Define pain.
- Describe the steps of pain conduction: transduction, transmission, perception, and modulation.
- Identify the characteristics of acute and chronic pain.
- Differentiate characteristics of the four types of acute pain.
- Identify factors that may affect a client's response to pain.
- Describe pain rating scales and their use in assessing pain.
- Explain the nurse's role in administering medications to reduce or relieve pain.
- Describe nonpharmacologic interventions clients may use in reducing or relieving pain.
- Identify several myths and misconceptions about pain and pain management.
- Use the nursing process in care of clients experiencing pain.

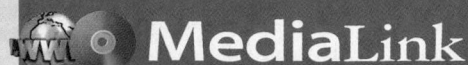

MediaLink

www.prenhall.com/burke
Use the address above to access the free, interactive Companion Website created for this textbook. Get hints, instant feedback, and textbook references to chapter-related NCLEX-style questions. Link to other interesting sites.

Audio Glossary:
Use the Companion Website, or the CD-ROM disk enclosed with your textbook, to hear the pronunciation of key terms in this chapter.

There are many accepted definitions of pain. McCaffery and Beebe (1989, p. 7) define **pain** as "whatever the person experiencing it says it is, and existing whenever the person says it does." This definition recognizes that the client is the only person who can accurately describe his or her own pain. If the client says he or she has pain, the client is in pain. All pain should be considered real. It is a well-known fact that pain can negatively affect the whole body. This definition considers the person as its main focus and should guide nursing assessment and care.

Pain is a subjective response to physical and psychologic stressors. All people feel pain at some point during their lives. Although pain is unwelcome, it often serves as a warning of potentially health-threatening conditions. Each pain event is a unique, personal experience. It can be affected by biologic, psychologic, cognitive, social, cultural, and spiritual factors. Pain is the most common reason for seeking health care.

Because it is subjective, pain presents a real challenge to nurses. Usually nurses assess clear objective manifestations of a disorder, such as skin color or decreased pulse. In assessing pain, however, the nurse must rely on the client's description and nonverbal cues to indicate the type, location, duration, and intensity of pain.

Unfortunately, pain management can be inadequate in all types of health care settings. Several factors influence how pain is perceived and managed. Often, physicians and nurses do not understand the newer concepts about pain management. The public and health care professionals fear addiction. The nurse's own bias can positively or negatively affect how a client's pain is managed. Because pain is subjective, the nurse may judge whether the client is actually experiencing pain. This is not the nurse's role. Nurses have an obligation to react positively to the client's report of pain and a responsibility to minimize or eliminate pain.

In 1997, the American Pain Society designated pain assessment as the "fifth vital sign." Because vital signs are routinely monitored, it was felt that by including pain, more client problems would be addressed. Health care facilities and nursing organizations are adopting and implementing this proposal.

National and state regulating agencies recognize the importance of assessing and treating pain. Standards for pain management have been developed by the Agency for Health Care Policy and Research, and the Joint Commission for the Accreditation of Healthcare Organizations (JCAHO). Nurses working in JCAHO-accredited facilities are expected to comply with these standards. These standards focus on the client's right to appropriate pain assessment and intervention and the health care professional's responsibility to treat pain.

TABLE 8-1 **Pain Stimuli**	
CAUSATIVE FACTOR	**EXAMPLE**
Inflammation	Sore throat
Impaired blood flow	Angina
Invasive tumor	Colon cancer
Obstruction	Kidney stone
Spasm	Colon cramping
Stretching or straining	Sprained ankle
Fractures	Fractured hip

Physiology of Pain

The ability of the body to produce pain depends on **nociceptors.** Nociceptors are nerve endings in the skin, viscera, blood vessels, muscle, and joints that are activated when *noxious* (unpleasant) stimuli are applied. Various noxious stimuli start the pain process (Table 8-1 ■). Once tissue damage occurs from the noxious stimuli, inflammation begins. Inflammation causes the release of bradykinin and prostaglandins, which also activate the nociceptors. So pain impulses are initiated both by direct tissue damage and by the release of internal chemicals. The intensity and duration of the stimuli determine the sensation. Long-lasting, intense stimulation produces greater pain than does brief, mild stimulation.

PAIN CONDUCTION

The conduction of pain impulses involves four steps: transduction, transmission, perception, and modulation (Figure 8-1 ■).

TRANSDUCTION. Transduction is the change of a noxious stimulus into an electrical action potential stimulus that sends impulses throughout the central nervous system. Pain is transmitted through large afferent A-delta and small C nerve fibers to the spinal cord. A-delta fibers are *myelinated* (covered with an insulating sheath). They transmit impulses rapidly and produce the sharp, well-defined pain sensations usually associated with acute pain. C fibers are not myelinated and transmit pain impulses more slowly. C-fiber pain is diffuse, usually chronic, and described as dull, burning, or aching.

Both A-delta and C fibers are involved in most injuries. For example, if a person bangs an elbow, A-delta fibers transmit this pain stimulus within 0.1 second. The person feels this pain as a sharp, localized, smarting sensation. One or more seconds after the blow, the person experiences a duller, aching, diffuse sensation of pain impulses carried by the C fibers.

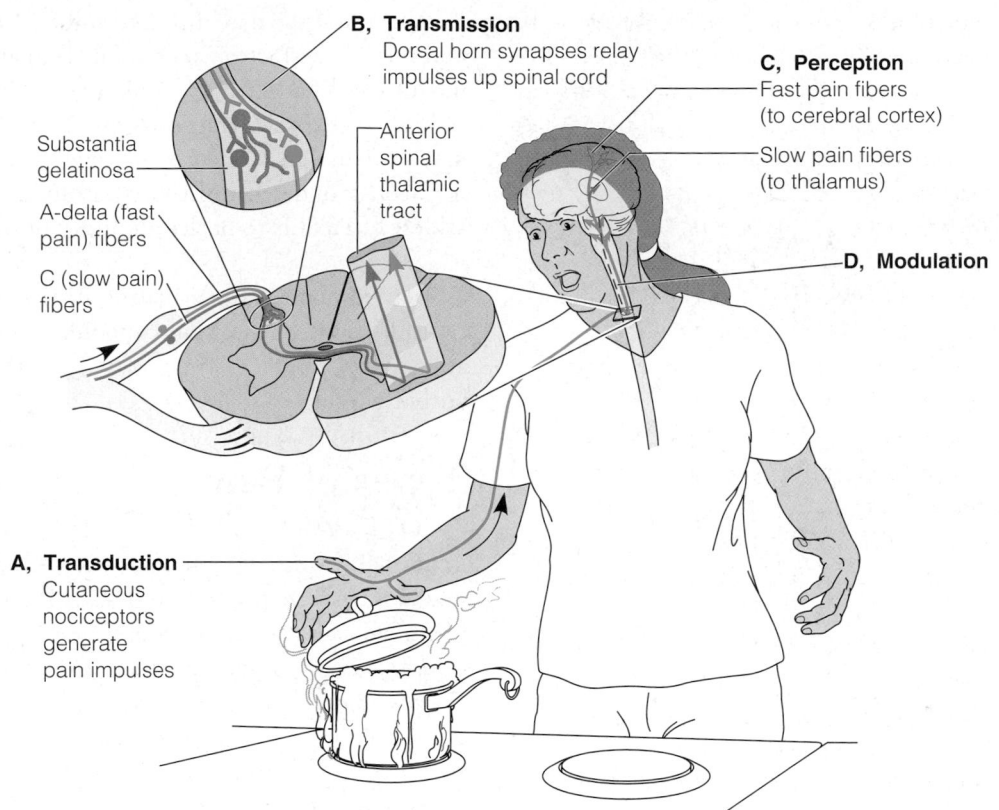

B, Transmission
Dorsal horn synapses relay impulses up spinal cord

C, Perception
Fast pain fibers (to cerebral cortex)
Slow pain fibers (to thalamus)

Substantia gelatinosa

A-delta (fast pain) fibers

C (slow pain) fibers

Anterior spinal thalamic tract

D, Modulation

A, Transduction
Cutaneous nociceptors generate pain impulses

Figure 8-1. ■ Pain conduction. (**A**) **Transduction:** Cutaneous nociceptors send impulses to spinal cord. (**B**) **Transmission:** Impulses synapse in the substantia gelatinosa. (**C**) **Perception:** Pain impulses processed in the thalamus and cerebral cortex. (**D**) **Modulation:** Along efferent fibers from cerebral cortex to substantia gelatinosa, pain may be inhibited or modulated.

TRANSMISSION. Transmission, the second step, involves sending the impulses from the *afferent* (sensory nerve that transmits impulses toward the CNS) neurons to the dorsal horn in the spinal cord, where they *synapse* (transmit an impulse) in the substantia gelatinosa. Substance-P helps send the impulse across the synapse. From here the impulses travel to the spinothalamic tracts and ascend to the thalamus and cerebral cortex.

PERCEPTION. Perception is the processing of pain impulses in the thalamus and cerebral cortex. During this step, pain impulses are perceived and interpreted. The client experiences pain when the sensation reaches a conscious level.

Pain threshold and pain tolerance are part of the perception step. **Pain threshold** is the point at which each person recognizes pain. Newer research suggests that pain intensity and duration vary among people. If a client reports more pain than is expected, the nurse should investigate further.

Pain tolerance is the amount and duration of pain a person can stand before seeking relief. Again, pain tolerance varies. Sometimes mild pain can be tolerated longer than severe, intense pain. Each person's tolerance is not to be judged as acceptable or unacceptable by health care providers. Instead, it should be accepted as a basis for pain management.

MODULATION. Modulation is the last step of pain conduction, in which the body attempts to decrease the perception of pain. Descending pathways of efferent fibers run from the cerebral cortex to the substantia gelatinosa in the dorsal horn. Along these fibers, pain may be inhibited or modulated. The body's naturally occurring **endorphins** (endogenous morphines) are released in response to afferent noxious stimuli or from efferent impulses. Endorphins bind with opiate receptors on the neurons and inhibit the release of substance-P. This process stops the pain impulse transmission (Figure 8-2 ■).

GATE-CONTROL THEORY OF PAIN

In 1965, Melzack and Wall developed the *gate-control theory* of pain. This theory states that when pain impulses travel from the skin to the substantia gelatinosa in the dorsal horn of the spinal cord, the substantia gelatinosa can either open or close the "gate" to transmit pain impulses to the brain.

Whether the gate is opened or closed in the substantia gelatinosa depends on the amount of stimulation the large and small nerve fibers receive. If more small-diameter C fibers are stimulated, the gate is open, and pain impulses travel uninhibited to the brain. In contrast, if more

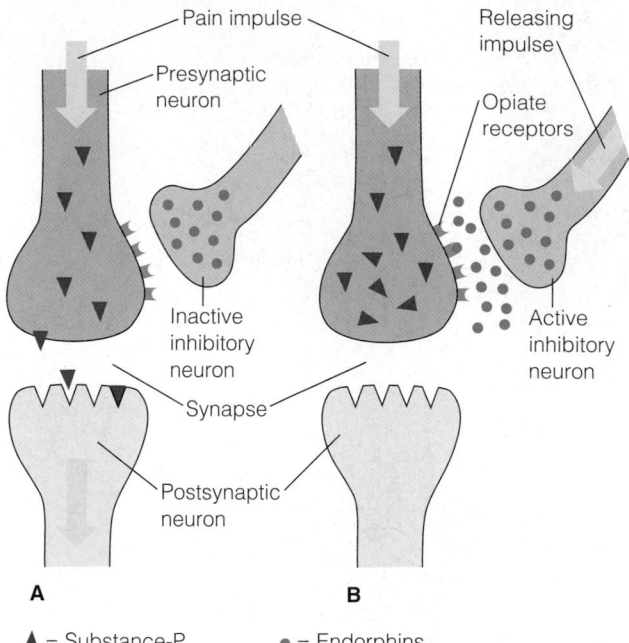

▲ = Substance-P   ● = Endorphins

Figure 8-2. ■ **(A)** Substance-P transmits pain impulse across synapse between presynaptic neuron and postsynaptic neuron. **(B)** During modulation, endorphins are released from inhibitory neuron, which prevents the release of substance-P, and pain impulse is inhibited.

large-diameter A-delta fibers are stimulated, the gate is closed and pain is inhibited (Figure 8-3 ■).

Stimulation of the A-beta or touch fibers closes the gate and "turns away" pain impulses. Massaging a stubbed toe activates A-beta fibers, so it reduces intensity and duration of the pain.

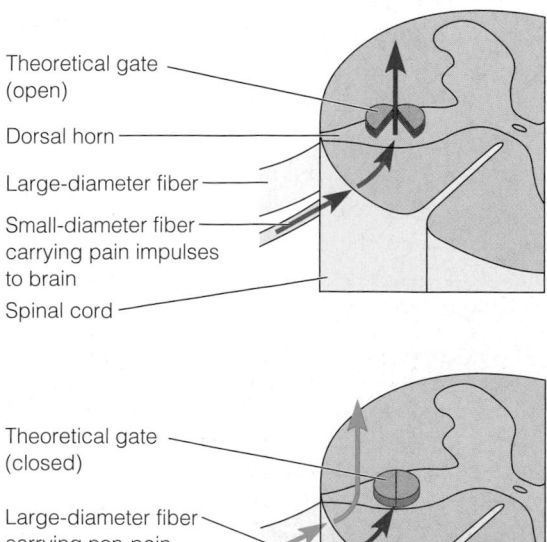

Figure 8-3. ■ Diagram of gate-control theory. When small-diameter C fibers are stimulated, the gate is open and pain is transmitted. When large-diameter A-delta fibers are stimulated, the gate is closed and pain transmission is stopped.

Pain impulses may also be inhibited in the brainstem. Opioids or distraction techniques signal receptors in the medulla, which in turn stimulate nerve fibers in the spinal cord to block pain transmission. This regulation process may explain why a client who experiences severe pain may not feel it under certain circumstances. For example, an athlete often fails to notice an injury until the competition is over.

New research is investigating further the complex relationship between pain and modulation. Possible genetic and sensory influences may play a greater role than previously thought.

Types of Pain

ACUTE PAIN

Acute pain is usually temporary, has a sudden onset, and is localized. It normally lasts for less than 6 months and has an identified cause. Acute pain is caused by tissue injury from trauma, surgery, or inflammation. Examples of acute pain include sprains, toothache, needle sticks, and muscle spasms. Acute pain may warn of actual or potential injury to tissues. Pain can initiate the fight-or-flight response. Physical responses to pain include tachycardia, rapid and shallow respirations, increased blood pressure, dilated pupils, sweating, and pallor. The person with acute pain may be anxious and fearful. Acute pain is classified into four major types:

1. *Cutaneous pain* arises from the skin or superficial tissues. This type of pain is described as sharp, cutting, burning, and well localized. When blood vessels are involved, individuals may describe the pain as throbbing.
2. *Deep somatic pain* results from injury to deep body structures such as muscles, bones, ligaments, tendons, and joints. It is characterized as dull and diffuse.
3. *Visceral pain* comes from the body organs lined with viscera. Visceral pain is deep, dull, and poorly localized and is associated with nausea and vomiting, hypotension, and weakness. It may be referred to another area of the body.
4. **Referred pain** starts in one site but is perceived in another area, distant from the site of the stimuli (Figure 8-4 ■).

CHRONIC PAIN

Chronic pain is prolonged pain, usually lasting longer than 6 months. There may not be an identifiable cause, and often it is unresponsive to conventional medical treatment. Chronic pain is more complex than acute pain. Clients with chronic pain are often depressed, withdrawn, immobile, irritable, or controlling. They may experience social withdrawal, fatigue, and reduced activity level. The autonomic nervous system is unaffected because the body adapts to the constant presence of pain.

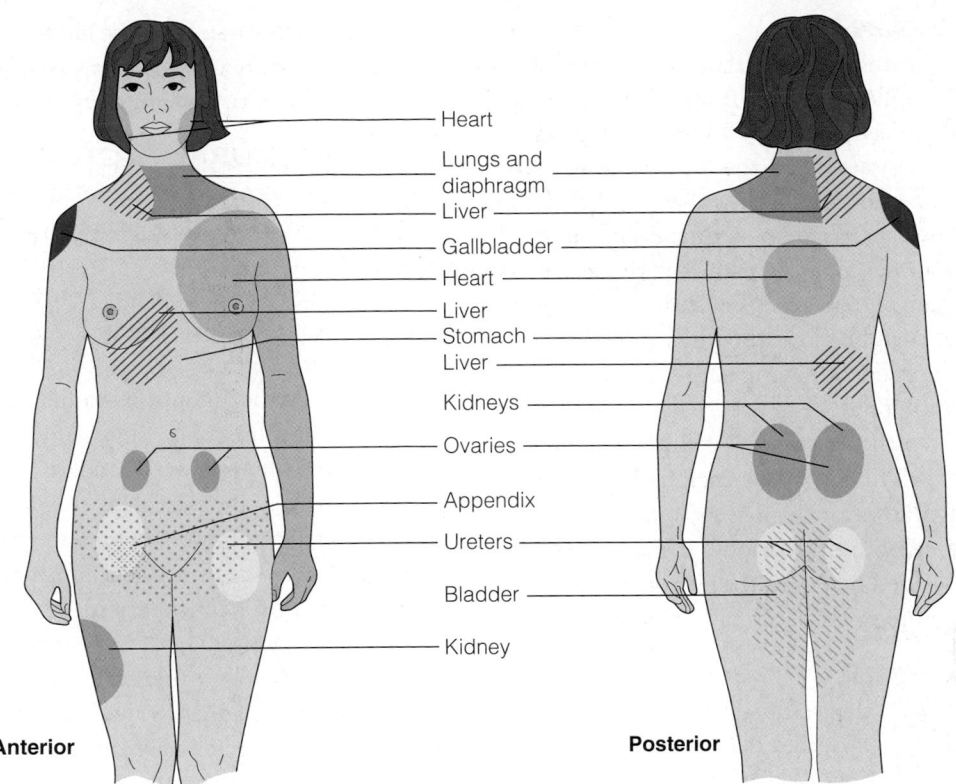

Heart
Lungs and diaphragm
Liver
Gallbladder
Heart
Liver
Stomach
Liver
Kidneys
Ovaries
Appendix
Ureters
Bladder
Kidney

Anterior

Posterior

Figure 8-4. ■ Referred pain begins in one site but is felt in another area. For example, pain from an inflamed gallbladder may be felt in the shoulder, or angina from ischemia of the heart muscle may be felt in the left arm or jaw.

Chronic pain may be nonmalignant pain or malignant pain. *Chronic nonmalignant pain* is "pain that has lasted 6 months or longer, is on-going, is not due to life-threatening causes, has not responded to currently available treatments, and may continue for the remainder of the patient's life" (McCaffery & Pasero, 1999, p. 471). Examples of this category include low back pain, arthritis, chronic abdominal pain (Crohn's disease), migraine headache, peripheral neuropathy, and neuralgia.

Chronic malignant pain or *cancer pain* is due to cancer. Cancer pain can result from the disease itself (tumor pressing on nerves or other structures, stretching of viscera, or metastasis to the bones). It may be associated with chemotherapy and radiation therapy. Cancer pain requires multiple pharmacologic and nonpharmacologic approaches, as discussed later. (A comparison of the characteristics of acute and chronic pain is found in Table 8-2 ■.)

TABLE 8-2
Comparison of Acute and Chronic Pain

ACUTE PAIN	CHRONIC PAIN
Pain lasts less than 6 months. Results from specific tissue injury (e.g., surgery, trauma). Pain is localized. Resolves when specific injury heals.	Pain lasts more than 6 months. Chronic malignant from cancer; chronic nonmalignant (e.g., low back pain, headache). Pain areas are hard to identify. May have no foreseeable end except for death.
Autonomic Responses Blood pressure, pulse, and respiration are increased. Pupils are dilated. Skin is diaphoretic, pale, cool.	**Autonomic Responses** Vital signs are normal. Pupils are normal. Skin is dry, warm, normal color.
Psychologic Responses Anxious, facial grimacing, guarding, crying.	**Psychologic Responses** Sense of depression, hopelessness, frustration. Decreased sleep and appetite.

NEUROPATHIC PAIN

Neuropathic pain is pain caused by damage to the central nervous system or peripheral nerves. Brain tumors, stroke, or trauma can result in central nerve injury, causing burning or tingling pain sensations in the affected area. **Allodynia** (pain that results from a stimulus that usually would not cause pain) is a unique feature of neuropathic pain. The other common type of neuropathic pain is peripheral neuropathy, a complication of diabetes. (See Chapter 17 ⬤⬤ for further discussion of peripheral neuropathy.)

Phantom limb pain occurs following surgical or traumatic amputation of a limb. The client experiences pain in the missing body part even though there is complete awareness that the limb is gone. This pain may include itching, tingling, or pressure sensations, or it may be more severe, including burning or stabbing sensations. It may be due to stimulation of the severed nerves at the site of the amputation. Treatment is complex and often unsuccessful.

PSYCHOGENIC PAIN

Psychogenic pain is pain that results from emotional rather than physical causes. Typically, the client has had a long history of severe pain complaints that are real. If psychogenic pain persists, it may lead to physiologic changes, such as muscle tension, which may produce further pain. This condition may result from interpersonal conflicts or a desire to avoid a stressful or traumatic situation. Depression is often present.

Factors Affecting Client Response to Pain

Just as individual pain thresholds differ, so do responses to pain. A person's response is shaped by age, sociocultural factors, emotional state, past experiences with pain, the meaning of pain, and the client's knowledge base. Pain tolerance may be decreased by repeated episodes of pain, fatigue, anger, anxiety, and sleep deprivation. On the other hand, it may be increased by medications, alcohol, warmth, distraction, and spiritual practices.

AGE

In the past it was assumed that as people age, pain perception decreases. There is no scientific evidence to prove that age reduces pain perception or sensitivity to pain. What is true is that older adults often have at least one chronic disease condition associated with pain. Chronic diseases that are more common in the elderly include arthritis, low back pain, and diabetic neuropathy. Elders tend to underreport pain. They may believe that pain is a part of growing older or that it is unacceptable to show pain. They might fear drug addiction. They may ignore pain or self-medicate with over-the-counter medications. If they do report pain, health care providers often discount it. All of these factors increase the older adult's risk of injury or serious illness.

SOCIOCULTURAL FACTORS

Family and culture strongly influence a person's response to pain. From childhood, people learn from their families what behavior is expected when they experience pain. Expected behaviors range from being stoic to feeling comfortable requesting pain medication. Pain behaviors are the way a client expresses his or her pain. They should not be used to judge the amount of pain an individual client has. Despite many misconceptions, men and women respond similarly to pain. Cultural standards play a powerful role in how much pain an individual should tolerate, what types of pain to report and to whom, and what kind of treatment to seek. In some cultures, one family member or the entire extended family may expect to be involved in pain management decisions.

The nurse's sociocultural values and beliefs also influence pain treatment. If these values and beliefs differ from the client's, the nurse may have difficulty accepting the client's pain behaviors. It is important for the nurse to understand how ethnicity and culture affect pain expression and management, and to respect cultural differences.

EMOTIONAL STATUS

Pain perception can be affected by the client's emotional status. Different emotional factors affect how a person handles pain. Clients experiencing acute pain usually have some degree of anxiety. The anxious client can develop tense muscles that can add to the pain. This is why relaxation and guided imagery are helpful in relieving or decreasing pain. The presence or absence of support people can influence how a client perceives pain.

PAST EXPERIENCES WITH PAIN

Previous experiences with pain influence how the person reacts to a current pain episode. If the person's childhood experiences with pain were positive, then the adult usually will have a healthy attitude toward pain. If, however, the person's experiences were unfavorable, then future responses to pain will be negative.

Nurses play an important role in how clients view their pain. When the nurse is helpful and caring, the client is less anxious about future pain. However, when the client has unrelieved pain or a nonsupportive nurse, the client fears how future pain will be managed. The client's anxiety, in turn, increases pain.

MEANING OF PAIN

The meaning associated with the pain affects the pain experience. For example, the pain of labor to deliver a baby is experienced differently from the pain following removal of a major organ for cancer. Individuals usually associate pain with the potential for disability, loss of role, and death. For this reason, it is important for clients to understand the *etiology* (source) and *prognosis* (predicted outcome) of their pain.

The client who perceives advantages from the sick role may be motivated to maintain pain. These advantages, called *secondary gain,* may include support from others and avoidance of disagreeable work or stressful social obligations. Such clients may require assistance not only to treat the pain but also to learn new ways for handling personal stresses.

KNOWLEDGE DEFICIT

Misunderstanding the source, outcome, and meaning of pain can negatively affect the pain experience. If the client understands pain, it is easier for the nurse to teach the client about pain and pain management strategies. It is important for the nurse to assess the client's readiness to learn, use teaching methods appropriate for the client and family, and evaluate the level of learning. Teaching content should include the pain process and the plan of care. The nurse should encourage clients to describe what pain relief measures work best for them. Also, clients should learn how to let family know about their pain and how they can help promote effective pain management.

Interdisciplinary Care

Effective pain relief involves collaboration among a variety of health care professionals. Pain clinics are independent centers, run by a team of health care professionals who use a variety of approaches to manage chronic pain. These therapies may include medications, herbs, biofeedback, hypnosis, acupuncture, and massage. Hospice provides care and support for terminally ill clients and their families.

MEDICATIONS

Medication is the most common approach to pain management. These drugs include nonopioids, opioids, and adjuvant analgesics. The nurse is responsible for assessing the side effects of the medications, evaluating the medication's effectiveness, and providing client teaching. The nurse's role in pain relief also includes being a client advocate as well as a direct caregiver.

Types of Medications

Analgesics are pharmacologic agents used to relieve or reduce pain. The pharmacologic agents most commonly ordered to provide *analgesia* (pain relief) are the nonopioids, opioids, and adjuvant analgesics.

NONOPIOIDS. Nonopioids are drugs used for pain that are not derived from opium. They include acetaminophen (Tylenol) and nonsteroidal anti-inflammatory drugs (NSAIDs). Acetaminophen reduces pain and fever but does not have an anti-inflammatory effect. It does not produce adverse effects on the kidney, gastric lining, or platelets.

NSAIDs act on the peripheral nervous system. They reduce pain by interfering with prostaglandin synthesis. Examples are aspirin, ibuprofen, and ketorolac. NSAIDs are the treatment of choice for mild pain and continue to be effective when combined with narcotics for moderate to severe pain. However, they have an *analgesic ceiling.* This means that increasing the dose beyond a certain dosage will not increase its pain relief effect. NSAIDs can cause gastric ulcers and increase bleeding. (Nursing implications and client teaching guidelines for acetaminophen and NSAIDs are found in Table 8-3 ■.)

OPIOIDS. Opioids are derivatives of the opium plant. They produce analgesia by binding to opioid receptors in the central nervous system, especially the brain and spinal cord. Opioids are subdivided into two groups: opioid agonists (e.g., morphine, meperidine, and codeine) and opioid agonist–antagonists (e.g., buprenorphine and nalbuphine). Both opioid categories are given for moderate to severe pain. Nursing responsibilities and client teaching recommendations for opioids are found in Table 8-3.

ADJUVANT ANALGESICS. Adjuvant analgesics are drugs with other specific uses that can provide analgesia in clients with chronic nonmalignant and cancer pain. They include anticonvulsants, antidepressants, systemic anesthetics, corticosteroids, and psychostimulants. Anticonvulsants include such drugs as carbamazepine (Tegretol), clonazepam (Klonopin), and phenytoin (Dilantin). Antidepressants include amitriptyline (Elavil) and doxepin (Sinequan). An example of a systemic anesthetic is bupivacaine (Marcaine). Corticosteroids include dexamethasone (Decadron) and methylprednisolone (Solu-Medrol). The psychostimulant methylphenidate (Ritalin) is also useful.

Anticonvulsants are used for diabetic neuropathy and neuralgia. *Antidepressants* promote normal sleeping patterns in clients with chronic pain. They are useful in treating neuropathic pain. *Systemic anesthetics* can be injected into nerves for a nerve block or given via the intraspinal route for cancer pain. Metastatic bone cancer pain may be relieved by using *corticosteroids. Psychostimulants* decrease sedation from opioids without decreasing pain relief in persons with cancer.

Routes of Administration

The route of administration affects the amount of medication needed to relieve pain. For example, oral doses of some narcotics may need to be five times greater than parenteral doses to achieve the same amount of pain relief. Of course, different

MediaLink · Naproxen

TABLE 8-3

Nursing Implications for Pharmacology: Acetaminophen, NSAIDs, Opioids

CLASS/DRUGS	PURPOSE	NURSING RESPONSIBILITIES	CLIENT TEACHING
Acetaminophen (Tylenol)	It is given to decrease pain and fever but not inflammation.	Give with a full glass of water.	Take with a full glass of water.
NSAIDs ■ Aspirin ■ Ibuprofen (Motrin) ■ Piroxicam (Feldene) ■ Ketorolac (Toradol) ■ Naproxen (Naprosyn)	NSAIDs are given for mild to moderate pain; provide antipyretic and anti-inflammatory effects.	Give with meals or a full glass of water. Do not give aspirin with other NSAIDs. Monitor for signs of GI bleeding. If given for fever, monitor client's temperature.	Take with meals or a full glass of water. Do not take more than the recommended amount. Do not take aspirin or alcohol with other NSAIDs. Monitor for GI bleeding (e.g., black stools).
Opioid Agonists ■ Codeine ■ Fentanyl ■ Hydrocodone ■ Hydromorphone (Dilaudid) ■ Meperidine (Demerol) ■ Morphine sulfate ■ Oxymorphone (Numorphan) ■ Propoxyphene (Darvocet) **Opioid Agonist–Antagonists** ■ Buprenorphine (Buprenex) ■ Nalbuphine (Nubain)	Opioids are used to manage moderate to severe pain. They bind to opiate receptors in the brain to alter the perception of pain. They are addictive, causing psychologic and physical dependence.	Record the appropriate information in the narcotic inventory sheet. Follow institution policy for wasting any narcotic. Monitor for side effects of sedation, respiratory depression, urinary retention, constipation, nausea, and vomiting. Keep naloxone available to treat respiratory depression.	Opioids used to treat severe pain are unlikely to cause addiction. Do not drink alcohol. Do not take over-the-counter drugs without MD approval. Increase fluids and fiber to prevent constipation. The drugs often cause dizziness, drowsiness, and impaired thinking; use caution when driving or making decisions. Do not increase dosage or take extra doses without discussing with MD.

narcotics have different recommended dosages. Consulting an equianalgesic dosage chart helps to ensure that **equianalgesic doses** of different narcotics given by different routes will have the same analgesic effect (Table 8-4 ■).

ORAL. The oral (PO) route is usually the simplest to administer for the client and the nurse, although special nursing care may be required when the client has difficulty swallowing or is confused. The nurse must know whether medications are given with food or can be chewed. In addition, the nurse is responsible for making sure that the medication is actually swallowed.

RECTAL. The rectal route is useful for clients who cannot swallow. Morphine, hydromorphone, and oxymorphone are available in this form. To be effective, any rectal medication must be placed above the rectal sphincter. The rectal route is effective and simple, but the client may not accept it.

TRANSDERMAL. The transdermal ("patch") form of medication is simple and painless and delivers a continuous level of medication (Figure 8-5 ■). Transdermal medications are expensive but easy to store and apply. The only opioid available

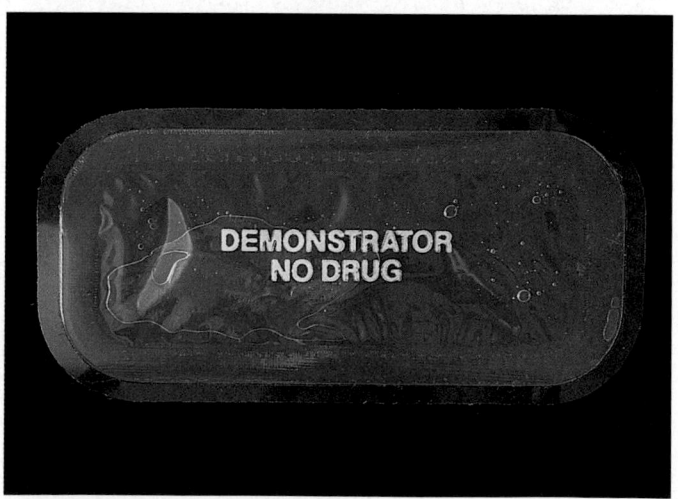

Figure 8-5. ■ Transdermal patch. To apply the patch, clip any hair from the upper body, clean the site with clear water, and dry it. Apply immediately after opening the package by placing it in the palm and pressing firmly onto the prepared site for 30 seconds. Be sure that contact is complete around the edges. A patch lasts for 72 hours, and the next patch is applied on a different site.

TABLE 8-4

Equianalgesic Dosage Chart

ANALGESIC	DOSAGE (MG)	DURATION (HOURS)	NURSING CONSIDERATIONS
Opioid Agonists			
Morphine sulfate	10 IM 30 PO	4–5 IM 4–5 PO	**MS 10 mg IM is the analgesic dose to which all other IM and PO doses in this table are considered equianalgesic.**
Codeine	130 IM 200 PO	4 IM 4 PO	Often given together with aspirin or acetaminophen for mild to moderate pain.
Hydrocodone	30 PO	4–6	Combined with acetaminophen (Vicodin) for mild to moderate pain.
Hydromorphone (Dilaudid)	1.5 IM 7.5 PO	4 IM 4 PO	More potent than morphine for severe pain; monitor client closely during first doses.
Meperidine (Demerol)	75 IM 300 PO	3 IM 2–4 PO	Produces a metabolite, normeperidine, causing CNS irritability and tremors. Occurs with chronic or high-dose therapy. PO dose of 300 mg is the equianalgesic dose but *not* recommended.
Oxycodone	20 PO	3–4	Combined with acetaminophen (Tylox, Percocet) for mild to moderate pain.
Oxymorphone (Numorphan)	1–1.5 IM	3–6	Used for moderate to severe pain.
Propoxyphene (Darvon)	500 PO	4–6	Give only recommended dose of 65–130 mg PO for short-term mild pain. 500 mg is the equianalgesic dose but **never** give 500 mg due to risk of toxicity.
Opioid Agonist–Antagonists			
Buprenorphine (Buprenex)	0.3 IM	6	Used for moderate to severe pain.
Butorphanol (Stadol)	2 IM	3–4	Given preop and postop for moderate to severe pain.
Nalbuphine (Nubain)	10 IM	3–6	Given preop and postop for moderate to severe pain.
Pentazocine (Talwin)	60 IM 180 PO	3–4 IM 3–4 PO	May be used for moderate to severe pain but has limited use due to short half-life.

Sources: LeMone, P., & Burke, K. M. (2004). *Medical-surgical nursing.* Upper Saddle River, NJ: Prentice Hall Health; McCaffery, M., & Pasero, C. (1999). *Pain: Clinical manual.* St. Louis, MO: Mosby; and Abrams, A. C. (2004). *Clinical drug therapy* (7th ed.) Philadelphia: Lippincott.

for the transdermal route is fentanyl (Duragesic). The fentanyl patch is used to treat moderate to severe cancer pain. If breakthrough pain occurs, short-acting medications are added.

Topical analgesic agents such as capsaicin (Zostrix) are used to relieve pain related to arthritis, diabetic neuropathy, and neuralgia from herpes zoster infection. Capsaicin is derived from cayenne peppers and acts by depleting substance-P in the nerve endings.

INTRAMUSCULAR. Although the intramuscular (IM) route is still used for pain management, it has limited usefulness. It has several problems, including uneven absorption from the muscle, pain during administration, and with chronic use can cause abscesses. It is, however, useful for clients who need acute pain relief when nausea and gastric distress prevent oral administration (e.g., the client with a migraine headache accompanied by nausea).

INTRAVENOUS. The intravenous (IV) route provides the most rapid onset, usually ranging from 1 to 15 minutes. Medication can be given by drip, bolus, or **patient-controlled analgesia (PCA),** a pump with a handheld button that allows clients to manage their own pain (Figure 8-6 ■). The medication dose and interval between doses are programmed into the PCA pump so that the client does not receive an overdose. The PCA pump allows clients to feel somewhat in control of their pain relief. The commonly ordered drugs include morphine, hydromorphone, fentanyl, and meperidine.

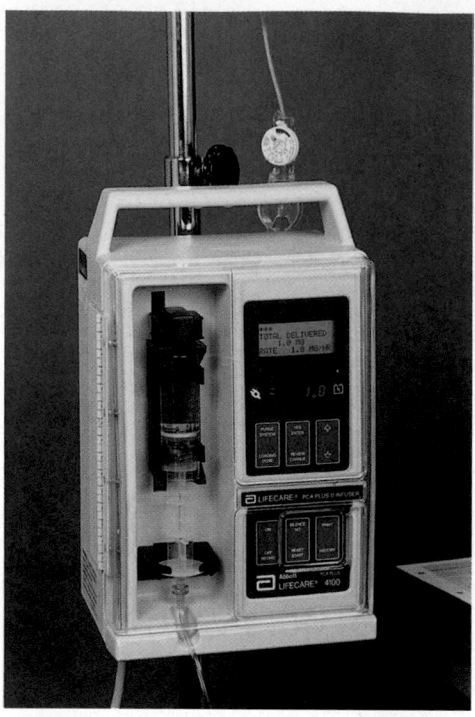

Figure 8-6. ■ PCA unit allows the client to self-manage severe pain. It can be mounted on an intravenous pole.

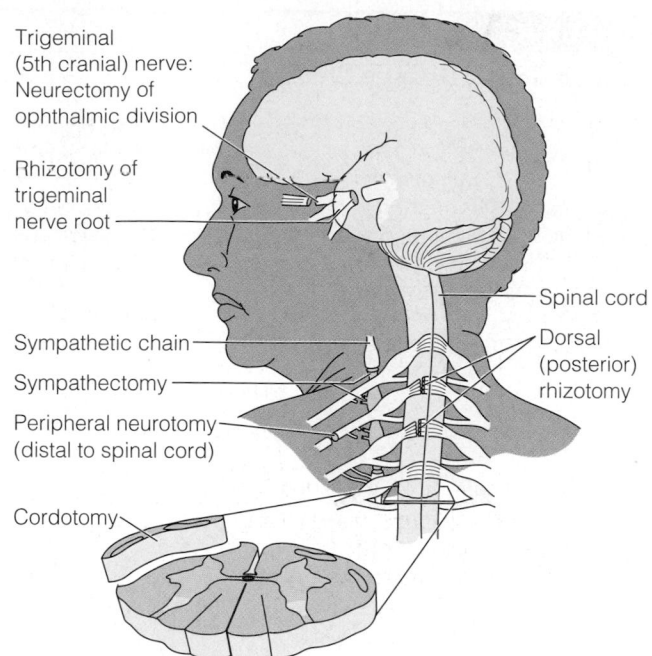

Trigeminal
(5th cranial) nerve:
Neurectomy of
ophthalmic division

Rhizotomy of
trigeminal
nerve root

Spinal cord

Sympathetic chain

Dorsal
(posterior)
rhizotomy

Sympathectomy

Peripheral neurotomy
(distal to spinal cord)

Cordotomy

Figure 8-7. ■ Surgical procedures are used to treat severe pain that does not respond to other types of management. They include cordotomy, neurectomy, sympathectomy, and rhizotomy.

SUBCUTANEOUS. The subcutaneous continuous infusion (SCCI) route is used as an alternative for chronic cancer pain management. A subcutaneous needle, placed in the upper arm or thigh, is connected to a continuous infusion of medication. This route is painful and often disliked by clients.

INTRASPINAL. The intraspinal route delivers drugs directly into the spinal column and then to the brain. This method is invasive and requires experienced nursing care. Box 8-1 ■ provides nursing implications for clients receiving intraspinal analgesia.

NERVE BLOCKS. In a nerve block, local anesthetics are injected into or near a nerve to reduce unrelenting pain. Sometimes this procedure is used to locate the source of pain before permanent blocking is done. Permanent nerve blocking is done with a neurolytic agent that destroys the nerve. Neurolytic blocks are reserved for terminally ill clients because of the risks of weakness, paralysis, and bowel and bladder dysfunction. Temporary nerve blocks may give the client enough relief to feel hopeful that pain relief is possible.

SURGERY

As a pain-relief measure, surgery is performed only after all other methods have failed. Clients need to understand thoroughly the implications of surgery for pain relief. The common surgical procedures (Figure 8-7 ■) are as follows:

CORDOTOMY. A *cordotomy* is an incision into the anterolateral tracts of the spinal cord to interrupt the transmission of pain. It is difficult to isolate the nerves responsible for upper body pain, so this surgery is most often performed for pain in the abdominal region and legs, including severe pain from terminal cancer.

NEURECTOMY. A *neurectomy* is the removal of a nerve. It is sometimes used for pain relief. A peripheral neurectomy is the severing of a nerve at any point distal to the spinal cord.

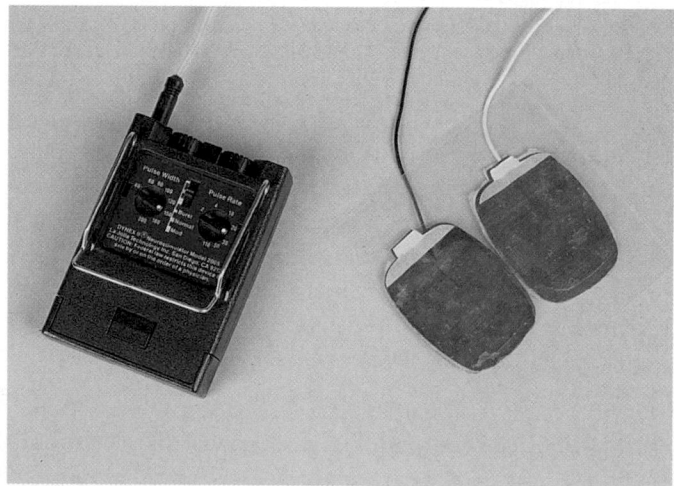

Figure 8-8. ■ TENS unit. Electrodes that deliver low-voltage electrical stimuli are placed directly on the client over painful areas. (Courtesy of Rehabilicare, Inc., Tampa, FL.)

BOX 8-1

NURSING CARE OF THE CLIENT RECEIVING INTRASPINAL ANALGESIA

Intraspinal analgesia is used to manage chronic, cancer, and severe postoperative pain. The intraspinal route may be either intrathecal (into the subarachnoid space) or epidural (into the epidural space). Opioids such as morphine and fentanyl and local anesthetics like bupivacaine (Marcaine) are given. Opioids act on the opiate receptors in the central nervous system; anesthetics block conduction of pain impulses. This method provides complete pain relief but produces side effects. The opioids may cause pruritus (itching), urinary retention, nausea, sedation, and respiratory depression. Local anesthetics can cause motor and sensory deficits.

Procedure

The physician places a catheter into the epidural space, attaches a tube to an infusion pump, and starts the medication infusion. A portable or implantable pump may deliver a narcotic infusion that lasts for a few days.

Nursing Care

- Monitor pulse, blood pressure, respirations, and pulse oximetry every 15 minutes for the first 2 to 3 hours and then every hour for the first 24 hours.
- Have naloxone, a narcotic antagonist, at bedside to reverse respiratory depression.
- Monitor for effectiveness of pain relief.
- Monitor intake and output.
- Monitor for motor and sensory deficits.

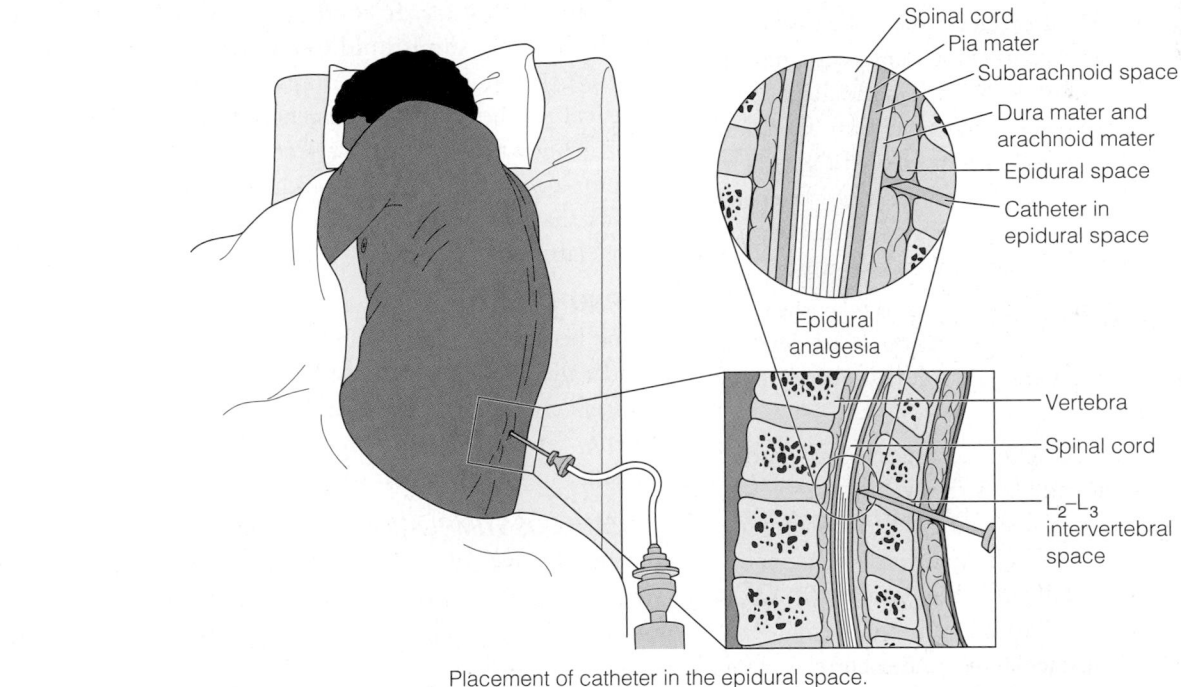

Placement of catheter in the epidural space.

SYMPATHECTOMY. Because sympathetic nerves produce and transmit the pain sensation, a *sympathectomy* may reduce pain by destroying the involved sympathetic nerve with an injection or incision. Usually, nerves in the lumbar or cervical region are considered for this procedure.

RHIZOTOMY. Rhizotomy is severing of the dorsal spinal roots to relieve the pain of cancer of the head, neck, or lungs. This is done by surgically cutting the nerve fibers, injecting a chemical such as alcohol or phenol into the subarachnoid space, or using a radio-frequency current to selectively destroy pain fibers.

TRANSCUTANEOUS ELECTRICAL NERVE STIMULATION (TENS)

A transcutaneous electrical nerve stimulation (TENS) unit is a low-voltage transmitter connected by wires to electrodes that are placed on the client (Figure 8-8 ■). The client experiences a vibrating sensation at the electrodes, which decreases pain. Clients can adjust the voltage to achieve maximum pain relief. The advantages of TENS units are avoidance of drug side effects and client control. Disadvantages are its cost and the need for training.

A TENS unit is most commonly used to relieve chronic benign pain and acute postoperative pain. The nurse or physical therapist explains the manufacturer's directions, where to place the electrodes, and the importance of placing the electrodes on clean, unbroken skin. The client is taught how to assess the skin daily for signs of irritation.

COMPLEMENTARY THERAPY

Nonpharmacologic interventions are often used together with analgesics to treat pain. They may be used for all types of pain, but their success is highly individual. Nonpharmacologic methods include acupuncture, biofeedback, relaxation, distraction, hypnotism, and cutaneous stimulation.

ACUPUNCTURE. Acupuncture is an ancient Chinese system of pain relief that involves inserting needles into specific points on the body. It is believed that acupuncture enhances energy flow (Qi) along pathways called meridians, which restores the body's healing mechanisms. Only care providers with special training can use this method. Acupuncture and acupressure are fairly well-accepted therapies for pain.

BIOFEEDBACK. Biofeedback uses electronic instruments to measure brain waves, muscle contraction, and skin temperature, and then "feeds" this information back to the client. Electrodes are placed on the client's skin and an amplification unit transforms data into visual cues, such as colored lights. The client learns to recognize stress-related responses and to replace them with relaxation responses. The goal is for the client to initiate those actions that cause relaxation independently.

RELAXATION. Relaxation involves learning to relax the body and mind. The primary goal of relaxation is to decrease muscle tension and anxiety. Some examples of relaxation activities are as follows:

- *Diaphragmatic breathing.* The client assumes a comfortable position in a quiet room and keeps the eyelids closed. The client inhales and exhales slowly, using the diaphragm to help extend the breath. (The technique for diaphragmatic breathing is described and illustrated in Chapter 9.) 🔗
- *Progressive muscle relaxation.* The client is taught to tighten one group of muscles slowly and then relax them

completely. The client should repeat the sequence for all parts of the body. Audiotapes may guide the client through this process.
- *Guided imagery.* To distract clients from their pain and produce relaxation, clients use their imagination to create a scene that is pleasurable and relaxing. The nurse assists the client through the steps of imagery. Clients should understand that several sessions may be necessary before they experience some pain relief.
- *Meditation.* The client empties the mind of all sensory data and may concentrate on a single object, word, or idea. This activity can produce a deeply relaxed state. A variety of exercises can induce the meditative state, and all are relatively easy to learn. Many books and tapes on meditation are available commercially.

DISTRACTION. Distraction focuses the client's attention away from the pain and onto something that the client finds more pleasant. It is often used in labor and is best used when the pain is mild to moderate. Examples of distracting activities are listening to music, tapping out a musical rhythm with the fingers or foot, and humor. Humor is known to be highly effective in pain relief. Laughing for 20 minutes or more produces an increase in endorphins that may continue pain relief even after the client stops laughing.

HYPNOTISM. Hypnosis is a trance-like state in which the mind becomes extremely suggestible. For this technique to work, the client must be fully relaxed and believe in the concept. It usually requires a skilled practitioner, but some clients can hypnotize themselves. Hypnosis has been successful in modifying pain.

CUTANEOUS STIMULATION. Cutaneous stimulation seems to be an effective pain reliever because it closes the "gate" in the substantia gelatinosa. Cutaneous stimulation may be accomplished by massage and the application of heat and cold (Table 8-5 ■).

TABLE 8-5			
Methods of Cutaneous Stimulation			
METHOD	TECHNIQUE	USES	NURSING IMPLICATIONS
Massage	The nurse performs massage to back, shoulders, or feet.	May be soothing and relaxing to decrease pain.	Ask the client about accepting a massage.
Heat	Nurse applies a hot-water bottle, heating pad, or hot moist towels to client's body. A hot shower or bath may also be effective.	May reduce muscle spasms and pain. Works best for localized pain.	Protect the client from burns. Heat should be applied for about 20–30 minutes.
Cold	Nurse applies waterproof bags filled with ice, gel packs, or cool damp towels to the client's body.	May reduce muscle spasm and arthritic joint pain. Usually more effective than heat for pain relief.	Monitor for excessive redness or blisters. Cold should be applied for about 20–30 minutes.

NURSING CARE

Nursing care of the client in pain presents more of a challenge than other illnesses or injuries. Whether pain is acute or chronic, the goal of nursing care is to assist the client to achieve optimal control of the pain. To accomplish pain control, the nurse uses a combination of medications and nonpharmacologic pain-relief strategies.

ASSESSING

The first step in relieving the client's pain is to conduct an accurate, unbiased, and thorough assessment of the client's pain. A comprehensive pain assessment ensures adequate and appropriate interventions. The nurse should assess the client's perceptions, physiologic responses, and behavioral responses.

Client Perceptions

Because pain is subjective, the client's perceptions provide the most reliable indicator about the type and degree of pain. The McGill Pain Questionnaire is one tool for assessing the client's pain (Figure 8-9 ■). A thorough pain assessment will ensure a complete database for pain management (Box 8-2 ■).

Pain intensity is assessed by using a pain rating scale (several scales are illustrated in Figure 8-10 ■). For clients who do not understand English or numerals, a scale using colors may be helpful. Another resource is the "Wong–Baker Faces Pain Rating Scale," which ranges from a happy face to one with a huge frown.

The nurse must thoroughly explain the purpose of the pain rating scale. When a word descriptor scale is used, verify that the client can read and understand the language

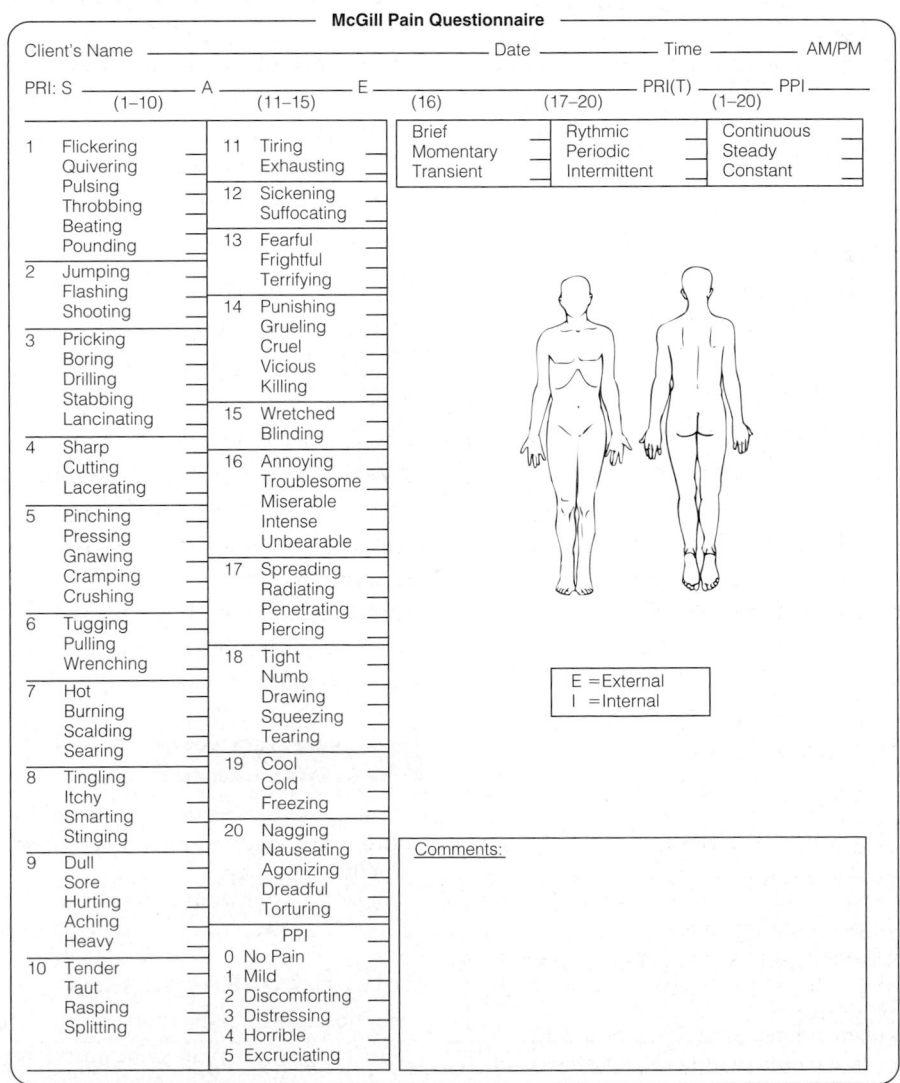

Figure 8-9. ■ The McGill Pain Questionnaire.
(© Ronald Melzack, 1970.)

BOX 8-2 | **ASSESSMENT**

Assessing For Pain

SUBJECTIVE DATA
Location

- Where does it hurt?
- Does the pain radiate?
- Is the pain superficial or deep?

Onset, Pattern, Duration, Quality

- When did the pain start?
- Did it begin gradually or suddenly?
- Is it constant or intermittent?
- Does it occur in cycles (e.g., same time each day)?
- How often does it appear?
- How long does the pain last?
- Is the pain throbbing, dull, aching, sharp, stabbing, prickling, burning?

Precipitating, Aggravating, and Relieving Factors

- What seems to trigger the pain?
- What seems to make the pain worse (e.g., movement, position changes, coughing, straining, or eating)?
- What seems to make the pain better (e.g., rest, sleep, food, pain medications, standing, or sitting)?

Intensity

- How strong is the pain? (Have client rate the pain using a rating scale.)

Other Problems

- Does the pain cause nausea, vomiting, anorexia, or insomnia?
- Does pain interfere with activities at home, work, or social interactions?
- Are there other diseases or conditions (e.g., arthritis)?

Methods of Pain Relief

- What has helped control pain in the past?
- What has not worked to relieve the pain?

OBJECTIVE DATA

- Vital signs: blood pressure, pulse, respirations.
- Assess skin moisture and color; pupils for dilation.
- Observe appearance for signs of grimacing, clenching jaws or fist, guarding, drawing up into fetal position, lying rigidly, restlessness.
- Observe behavioral responses: moaning, sighing, crying, becomes quiet, withdraws from others, appears frightened, has sad facial expression.
- Gently palpate painful area; identify possible trigger points.

---

being used. If a numerical scale is used, be sure the client can count to 10. It is often helpful to use the client's own words when describing the pain. The client should understand that

reporting pain is important for recovery, not just for achieving temporary comfort.

Physiologic Responses

Physiologic changes result from stimulation of the sympathetic nervous system. Objective manifestations include muscle tension; tachycardia; rapid, shallow respirations; increased blood pressure; dilated pupils; sweating; and pallor. They usually occur in the presence of acute pain. However, absence of physiologic signs does not mean absence of pain. In clients with prolonged pain, the body adapts to the pain stimulus and there may not be physiologic changes. The client with chronic pain may have an unexpressive, tired facial appearance.

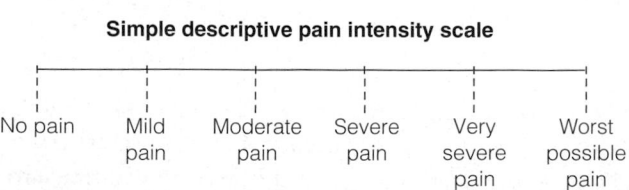

Figure 8-10. ■ Examples of commonly used pain scales. Other examples include pictures of faces (from happy and relaxed to sad and frowning), or colors from bright red (terrible pain) to light blue (no pain).

> **clinical ALERT**
>
> Assess clients for pain every time you check blood pressure, pulse, respirations, and temperature because pain is the fifth vital sign.

Behavioral Responses

Behavioral responses to pain may or may not match the client's report of pain. The nurse must accept the client's pain rating regardless of the client's behaviors. For example, one client may rate pain at an 8 on a 0-to-10 scale while

BOX 8-3

MISCONCEPTIONS ABOUT PAIN MANAGEMENT

MISCONCEPTION	CORRECTION
People who frequently ask for opioid pain medications are addicted.	Research shows that addiction from opioids is rare. If the client is asking for pain medication, pain relief is probably inadequate.
It is best to wait until a client has pain before giving medication.	Anticipating pain and offering pain relief ahead of time can significantly lessen the pain.
Postoperative pain is best treated with intramuscular injections.	The most commonly ordered postoperative pain medication is meperidine (Demerol) IM. This is a poor choice because it is short acting, can irritate tissues, and produces normeperidine, a CNS stimulant.
It is dangerous to give an opioid and a nonsteroidal anti-inflammatory drug (NSAID) at the same time.	These medications do not need to be given at different times. The opioid acts on the CNS; the NSAID acts on the peripheral nervous system. By combining them, the client receives better pain management.
Opioid medication is too risky to be used in chronic pain.	Other methods should be tried first; if they prove ineffective, opioids should be added.

Sources: Data adapted from McCaffery, M., & Pasero, C. (1999). *Pain: Clinical manual*. St. Louis, MO: Mosby; and LeMone, P., & Burke, K. M. (2004). *Medical-surgical nursing* (3rd ed.). Upper Saddle River, NJ: Prentice Hall Health.

laughing or walking down the hall; another may deny pain completely while tachycardic, hypertensive, and grimacing. Discrepancies between the client's report of pain and behavioral responses may result from cultural factors, coping skills, fear, denial, or the use of relaxation or distraction techniques.

Clients often deny pain for a variety of reasons. They may fear injections. Fears of developing addiction or physical dependence may exist. Sometimes clients believe they will be labeled as an addict if they ask for analgesics. **Addiction** is a condition of seeking drugs habitually (other than for a medical purpose) and of not being able to give them up without adverse effects. **Physical dependence** occurs when the body adapts to chemical substances over an extended period of time; abrupt cessation of the substance causes withdrawal symptoms (see Chapter 52).

Sometimes there is a misinterpretation of terms. The client may think that aching, soreness, or discomfort does not qualify as pain. Also, clients may think that health care providers know when they are experiencing pain. Some clients may deny pain as an attempt to deny that anything is wrong with them. Other clients believe that "as-needed" medications are given only if their pain rating is high.

The nurse should not assume that a sleeping client is without pain. Pain is physically exhausting. Unrelieved pain leaves clients fatigued. Sometimes clients sleep out of fatigue rather than because they are pain free.

DIAGNOSING, PLANNING, AND IMPLEMENTING

Numerous misconceptions about pain and its management exist among clients and health care professionals. Before appropriate nursing care can be delivered, the nurse must explore these misconceptions and understand the facts. Box 8-3 ■ lists a few common misconceptions and their corrections.

Managing pain in the older adult requires special considerations. Box 8-4 ■ lists guidelines and rationale for managing pain in the elderly.

Acute Pain

■ Believe the client is experiencing pain. *By believing the client, the nurse reduces anxiety, which may lessen pain.*

clinical ALERT

Do not assume the older client or cognitively impaired client cannot identify the intensity of pain.

■ Discuss with the client his or her desired level of pain relief and any fears about proposed interventions. *Understanding the client's goals and fears will help the nurse determine suitable pain relief methods.*

■ Individualize the choice of medication, route, dose, and interval between doses. *Because each client absorbs, metabolizes, and excretes medications differently, the nurse carefully*

BOX 8-4	FOCUS ON OLDER ADULTS

Pain Management Guidelines for the Older Adult

GUIDELINE	RATIONALE
■ Reduce initial opioid dose by 25%, then carefully titrate dose based on client response.	■ Drug absorption, distribution, metabolism, and excretion decrease with age; therefore, monitor dosages carefully.
■ Avoid giving benzodiazepines such as diazepam (Valium) or lorazepam (Ativan).	■ They cause delirium, increasing the risk for injury.
■ Use all NSAIDs with caution and monitor for side effects.	■ The elderly are four times more likely to develop peptic ulcers.
■ Closely monitor long-term use of acetaminophen.	■ Acetaminophen can accumulate and cause liver toxicity.
■ Choose NSAIDs like ibuprofen (Motrin) and naproxen (Naprosyn).	■ They have shorter half-lives, so they will not accumulate and cause toxicity.
■ Avoid using meperidine, and propoxyphene (Darvon).	■ They produce toxic metabolites with long half-lives, leading to more adverse effects.
■ Choose morphine or hydromorphone for severe pain.	■ They have short half-lives and less chance for toxicity.
■ Monitor closely for sedation and respiratory depression with opioid use.	■ Decreased renal and liver clearance rates increase potential opioid side effects.
■ Avoid the IM route.	■ It is painful, absorption is unreliable, and there is less muscle mass in the elderly.
■ Assess frequently for signs of constipation.	■ Elderly are prone to constipation before adding opioids, which also cause constipation.

selects an analgesic based on the client's needs. When frequent injections are needed, consider the intravenous route.

■ Adjust the analgesic regimen by using a flow sheet (Figure 8-11 ■). The dose can be adjusted within prescribed limits according to the client's response. Adjustments should be considered:

■ When the client feels most of his or her pain an hour after administration (dose too low).

■ When dose causes significant side effects such as respiratory depression (dose too high).

■ When most of the pain returns before the next scheduled dose (interval too long). The pain flow sheet records the effectiveness of each pain intervention. It is the nurse's role to inform the physician if the prescribed medication, route, dose, and interval do not meet the client's needs.

■ Use a preventive approach. Administer pain analgesics at regular, scheduled intervals around the clock (ATC) when the client's pain is expected for at least 12 of the next 24 hours. PRN (as-needed) administration is appropriate for unpredictable pain. It should be administered before pain becomes severe and before painful procedures such as a dressing change or physical activities. Preventive approaches allow clients to know that their pain needs will be met. They help reduce anxiety about the return of pain and may result in decreased doses, fewer side effects, and less time in pain. Physical activity may increase, so problems caused by immobility can be avoided.

■ Use a balanced analgesia approach by administering nonopioids and opioids when ordered. Nonopioids act on the peripheral nervous system; opioids act on the central nervous system. Combining these medications improves pain relief and lowers the incidence of side effects.

■ Demonstrate use of self-administered PCA. PCA allows clients more control over their pain relief.

■ Use nonpharmacologic measures (e.g., relaxation, distraction, heat, or cold) as appropriate. Nondrug measures by the nurse or client's family can provide pain relief with minimal risk to the client. They should not be substituted for medications but rather combined with them.

■ Provide comfort measures, such as changing positions, back massage, oral care, skin care, and changing bed linens. Basic comfort measures promote physical and emotional well-being.

■ Avoid actions that increase pain, for example, jarring the bed or moving the client too quickly out of bed. By avoiding actions that increase pain, the nurse shows a caring attitude.

■ Teach the client to request pain medication before the pain becomes severe. This strategy prevents the client from experiencing highs and lows of pain relief.

■ Use an equianalgesic dosage chart when changing doses or medications. If the client is receiving inadequate pain relief or is being switched from a parenteral to an oral route, an equianalgesic dosage chart helps the client maintain adequate pain relief.

■ Monitor effectiveness of pain relief measures at least every 2 hours and ATC. Planned assessments prevent inconsistent pain relief for the client.

PAIN FLOWSHEET

Client: Mrs. J   **Age:** 55   **Physician:** Dr. Masson   **Date:** 4/12/06
Diagnosis: 4/12/06 Abdominal hysterectomy
Pain rating scale: 0 to 10 (0 = no pain, 10 = worst pain)
Analgasic ordered: Morphine 6-12 mg. IM q 4 hours

Date and Time	Pain rating	Analgesic	Vital signs R, P, BP	Level of arousal	Other: Nausea and vomiting, bowel function	Initials
4/12/06 14:00	10	MS 10 mg. IM	24, 90, 138/88	Awake, "I have sharp pain in my stomach. It really hurts to move."	Denies nausea and vomiting. No bowel tones since returning from surgery at 1300.	KC
14:30	8		22			KC
15:00	4		20	"The pain is much less than before."		KC
16:30	4		18	"Pain is about the same."		EB
17:45	7		20	"The pain is coming back."	No nausea or vomiting.	EB
18:10	8	MS 10 mg. IM	20, 88, 130/82	"The pain isn't quite as bad as before, but it still hurts a lot."		EB
18:30	8		20	"Pain is a little less."		EB

Figure 8-11. ■ A flow sheet for nursing documentation of pain management.

Chronic Pain

Chronic nonmalignant pain can occur throughout the body. This type of pain may accompany chronic diseases or occur as the result of an injury (e.g., low back pain). Because chronic pain is prolonged, different interventions are used by the nurse.

- Discuss client's expectations about pain relief and management. *The nurse and the client need to understand whether the pain can be resolved or significantly lessened.*
- Teach the client and family about the nature of chronic pain and various pain relief methods. *Inclusion of the family enables them to support the client better.*
- Administer nonopioids, adjuvant, and opioid pain medications as ordered and needed. *The type of chronic pain determines the combination of analgesics needed by the client.*
- When opioid analgesics are ordered, use the oral route. *Chronic pain is usually long term, so the parenteral route is unacceptable.*
- Encourage the client to use noninvasive methods of pain management, such as relaxation, distraction, and cuta-

neous stimulation. *These techniques are useful in managing chronic pain.*
- Promote rest and proper nutrition. *Chronic pain is physically exhausting.*
- Consult with health care team about referral to multidisciplinary pain management facility. *Clients with unresolved pain problems may need more advanced pain management techniques or referral to a pain clinic.*

Cancer Pain

Clients with cancer usually do not develop pain until the later stages of the disease. Their pain may be acute or chronic. Cancer-related pain requires many different approaches. (Chapter 12 ∞ discusses care of the client with cancer.)

- Discuss goals of care with the client. *These goals may include the amount of pain the client will tolerate in order to participate in activities of daily living. The nurse needs to understand these goals and help the client meet them.*

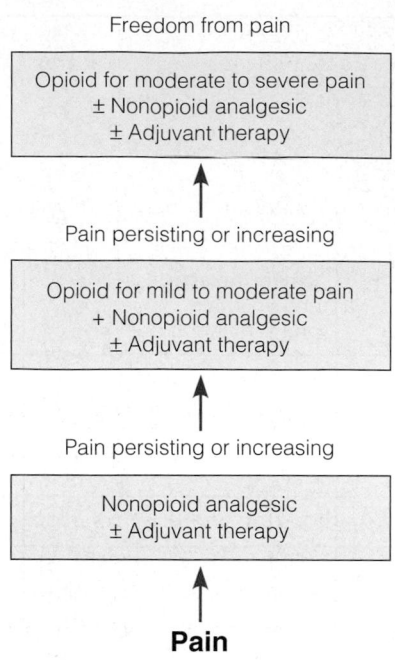

Freedom from pain

Opioid for moderate to severe pain
± Nonopioid analgesic
± Adjuvant therapy

↑

Pain persisting or increasing

Opioid for mild to moderate pain
+ Nonopioid analgesic
± Adjuvant therapy

↑

Pain persisting or increasing

Nonopioid analgesic
± Adjuvant therapy

↑

Pain

Figure 8-12. ■ The WHO three-step analgesic ladder.
(Courtesy of World Health Organization.)

- Encourage client and family to express concerns about opioid use. *Fears of addiction may prevent the client from obtaining adequate pain relief.*
- Administer a combination of nonopioid, opioid, and adjuvant analgesics according to the World Health Organization (WHO) analgesic ladder (Figure 8-12 ■). *The three steps of the analgesic ladder are used progressively until the cancer pain is relieved or at least reduced to an acceptable level.*
- Give analgesics ATC. *Clients with cancer pain usually have persistent pain. Consistent administration should prevent peaks and valleys of pain relief.*
- Have analgesics available for breakthrough pain. *As cancer progresses, clients will experience breakthrough pain. They need fast-acting analgesics to control it.*
- Give analgesics orally. *The oral route is safe and easy to administer. When clients cannot take their medications orally, the transdermal, rectal, intravenous, and intraspinal routes should be used.*

clinical ALERT

For clients with cancer, who need frequent analgesic doses, avoid the IM route because it is painful.

- Teach the patient about **opioid tolerance**—the loss of opioid effectiveness with chronic use. For the client to receive the same amount of pain relief, increased doses are required. *Clients need to understand why they need increased doses.*
- Aggressively treat adverse effects of analgesics (see following nursing diagnosis). *Sedation, respiratory depression, nausea, and constipation are the common adverse effects of opioids.*

- Add noninvasive pain management strategies. *Noninvasive strategies are helpful in managing cancer pain.*
- Refer to support groups and pastoral counseling. *Clients and families need emotional and spiritual resources.*

Risk for Injury: Side Effects of Opioid Analgesics

The four main side effects of opioid therapy are sedation, respiratory depression, constipation, and nausea. Usually, side effects develop at the beginning of narcotic therapy. Only sedation and respiratory depression may subside with long-term use.

- *Sedation* often occurs at the start of opioid therapy or when the dose is increased. This results from opioids acting on the central nervous system. Assess the client's sedation level every 1 to 2 hours for the first 8 to 12 hours. *Sedation precedes respiratory depression. Monitor the client frequently during initial opioid therapy or increased dosage changes.*
- If pain relief is adequate and sedation is clinically significant, consult with physician about reducing the dose. *The goal is to decrease sedation, yet maintain pain relief.*
- Add a mild stimulant such as caffeine during the day. *Mild stimulants may offset the opioid sedative effects.*
- All opioid analgesics are capable of causing *respiratory depression.* Most of the time the altered respiratory function is not life threatening or clinically significant. Monitor sedation and respiratory rate and depth every 1 to 2 hours during the first 24 hours the client receives opioids. *Clients are at risk for respiratory depression when they start on opioids.*

clinical ALERT

Respiratory depression is clinically significant when there is a decrease in rate and depth of respirations from the client's baseline.

- Encourage deep breathing and use of incentive spirometry. *These measures help counteract respiratory depression.*
- If the client is unresponsive to physical stimulation, has shallow respirations, and respiratory rate of less than 8 breaths per minute with pinpoint pupils, naloxone (Narcan) may be required. *Naloxone, an opioid antagonist, reverses the effects of opioids.*
- *Constipation* is the most common side effect of opioids. They decrease gastric emptying and peristalsis, which increases the client's risk for developing constipation. Auscultate abdomen for presence of bowel tones. *Reduced bowel tones mean decreased peristalsis.*
- Encourage at least eight glasses of water per day. *Increased fluid intake promotes moist, soft stool.*

- Encourage a diet high in bulk and fiber such as beans, carrots, bran cereals and breads, and prunes. *This type of diet improves stool consistency and promotes passage through the colon.*
- Promote activity and exercise as tolerated. *Increased movement stimulates peristalsis.*
- Give a stool softener or stimulant during the opioid therapy. *An aggressive bowel regimen is needed to prevent and treat opioid-induced constipation.*
- Monitor client's bowel pattern carefully. *Monitoring is essential to prevent further complications of constipation.*
- *Nausea* may occur during the beginning of opioid therapy but usually decreases with longer use. It is caused by stimulation of a trigger zone in the brain and slowed gastric motility. Give an antiemetic such as ondansetron (Zofran) or prochlorperazine (Compazine). *These medications decrease nausea.*
- Provide frequent oral care. *Oral care helps to decrease bad tastes in the mouth.*
- Provide a clean-smelling environment. *Reducing unpleasant odors decreases the potential for nausea.*
- Have patient try to eat dry toast or crackers. *Dry foods tend to decrease nausea.*
- If nausea continues from opioid use, add a nonopioid or adjuvant medication before reducing opioid dose. *To maintain client's pain relief yet decrease nausea, add other pain medications.*
- For chronic nausea with advanced cancer, give metoclopramide (Reglan). *This medication increases gastric motility.*

EVALUATING

Evaluation focuses on determining the effectiveness of pain management strategies. The nurse collects data on the client's report of pain relief, physical responses, and emotional behaviors.

The nurse documents subjective and objective assessment findings related to the client's pain. Document the client's pain relief in response to pain medications and non-pharmacologic measures. Be sure to include effectiveness of interventions for managing opioid side effects. Record client teaching about pain medications and noninvasive pain management strategies.

CONTINUING CARE

Clients can learn to manage most types of pain at home. The nurse should explain about expected pain, when it will happen, what it feels like, and what to do to help oneself during the event. Education should decrease anxiety about the unknown and provide the client with a means of controlling the pain.

All instructions should be in writing so that the client can take them home. The following teaching points should be included for the client and family:

- Specific drugs, including the frequency, potential side effects, possible drug interactions, and any special precautions such as taking with food or avoiding alcohol
- How to administer the drugs (if given by any route other than oral)
- Importance of taking pain medications before the pain becomes severe
- How to manage opioid side effects (e.g., constipation)
- How to keep a diary or log about pain, including what makes it better or worse
- Explain about addiction and drug tolerance
- Importance of scheduling periods of rest and sleep
- Contact person with phone number if pain becomes worse
- Reminder to store narcotics away from small children or grandchildren

The client and family may need additional information about pain clinics or support groups in the community. Also, they may need help with finding resources for finances, care, and hospice.

NURSING PROCESS CARE PLAN
Client with Pain

Susan Akers, 37 years old, is being seen at an outpatient clinic for a 3-year history of neck and shoulder pain. She believes the pain is caused by lifting heavy objects at work, but she says now household chores make it worse. She misses work about three times a month from her pain. About twice a month the pain becomes so intense that she needs meperidine (Demerol) injections at the local emergency department. She takes Darvocet-N 100 and Valium usually two to three times a day without complete relief.

Assessment. Ms. Akers rates her pain during an acute episode as a 7 on a 0-to-10 scale. When she raises her arms above shoulder level, it causes sharp pain.

Diagnosis. The main nursing diagnosis for Ms. Akers is "Chronic pain related to muscle inflammation."

Expected Outcomes. The expected outcomes for the plan of care are that Ms. Akers will:

- After 5 days on regularly scheduled analgesics report a decrease in pain from 7 to 3–4 on a 0–10 scale.
- Modify activities at work and at home, especially when pain is intense.

Planning and Implementation. The following interventions are implemented for Ms. Akers:

- Consult with a physician for new opioid and nonopioid analgesic prescription.
- Teach Ms. Akers about her medications, as well as the side effects and how to treat them.
- Teach Ms. Akers relaxation and distraction techniques.
- Discuss with Ms. Akers and her children ways for dividing the household tasks between everyone.

Evaluation. A week later Ms. Akers reports that the pain medications have decreased her pain to a 2–3 on a 0–10 scale. She says she has been reassigned to a position that requires no lifting and that her children are helping with the household tasks.

Critical Thinking in the Nursing Process

1. Ms. Akers asks you how often she should take her pain medications. You tell her to (a) take them on a regular basis or (b) wait until she experiences pain. Which action would you choose, and why?
2. If Ms. Akers experienced acute pain, what assessment findings would the nurse expect to see?
3. What suggestions should the nurse give to Ms. Akers for treating constipation?

Note: The bibliography listings for this and all chapters have been compiled at the back of the book.

Chapter Review

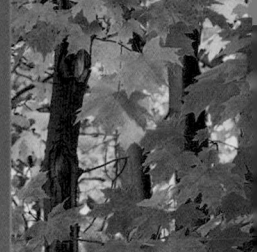

 **KEY TERMS** by Topics

Use the audio glossary feature of either the CD-ROM or the Companion Website to hear the correct pronunciation of the following key terms.

Client in pain

pain

Physiology of pain

nociceptors, pain threshold, pain tolerance, endorphins

Types of pain

acute pain, referred pain, chronic pain, neuropathic pain, allodynia, psychogenic pain

Interdisciplinary care

analgesics, nonopioids, opioids, equianalgesic dose, patient-controlled analgesia (PCA)

Nursing care

addiction, physical dependence, opioid tolerance

KEY Points

- Pain affects an individual both physically and emotionally.

- Pain is transmitted through the four steps of transduction, transmission, perception, and modulation.

- Acute pain is usually a short-term event while chronic pain is prolonged.

- Pain management includes medications such as nonopioids, opioids, and adjuvant analgesics and nonpharmacologic therapies including relaxation, distraction, massage, and TENS.

- Nonopioids are used to manage mild to moderate pain; opioids are given for moderate to severe pain; and adjuvant analgesics are used in chronic pain.

- Clients receiving opioids must be monitored for side effects of sedation, respiratory depression, nausea, and constipation.

- The nurse assumes an important role in assessing the client's pain and working collaboratively with the physician to implement appropriate pain-reducing methods.

- All pain relief measures must incorporate an individualized and preventive approach.

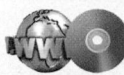 **EXPLORE Media**Link

Additional interactive resources for this chapter can be found on the Companion Website at www.prenhall.com/burke. Click on Chapter 8 and "Begin" to select the activities for this chapter.

For chapter-related NCLEX-style review questions and an audio glossary, access the accompanying CD-ROM in this book.

FOR FURTHER Study

The technique for diaphragmatic breathing is described and illustrated in Chapter 9.

For in-depth discussion about care of the client with cancer, see Chapter 12.

For further discussion of peripheral neuropathy, see Chapter 17.

For more on drug dependency, see Chapter 52.

Critical Thinking Care Map

Caring for a Client with Pain
NCLEX-PN® Focus Area: Physiologic Adaptation

Case Study: Mrs. Bruski, 98 years old, has returned to her room following a colon resection. Four hours later the nurse enters Mrs. Bruski's room and finds her lying on her side with her eyes closed. When the nurse asks about her pain, she says, "It hurts right here," as she points to her lower abdomen. She describes the pain as dull and rates it at a 7 on a 0–10 scale. She complains of feeling thirsty and cold. She says, "I just wish I could sleep. I feel so tired."

Nursing Diagnosis: Acute Pain

COLLECT DATA

Subjective	Objective
_____	_____
_____	_____
_____	_____
_____	_____
_____	_____
_____	_____
_____	_____

Would you report this data? Yes/No
If yes, to: _____

Nursing Care

_____
_____
_____
_____
_____
_____
_____
_____
_____
_____
_____
_____

How would you document this? _____
_____
_____
_____

Data Collected
(use those that apply)

- Says she feels cold
- Pulse 100
- Dull pain in lower abdomen
- Temperature 99°F
- "It hurts right here."
- Blood pressure 150/92
- Rates pain at a 7
- Lying on her side with eyes closed
- Complains of being thirsty
- "I'm tired. I wish I could sleep."

Nursing Interventions
(use those that apply; list in priority order)

- Teach Mrs. Bruski to use the incentive spirometer.
- Give acetaminophen (Tylenol) 650 mg PO q 4 hours PRN.
- Offer a back massage at HS.
- Give morphine sulfate 8 mg IM q 4 hours prn.
- Listen attentively to Mrs. Bruski.
- Teach Mrs. Bruski a relaxation technique.

Knowledge of medications and medication administration is a frequently tested subject on NCLEX. The nurse should also monitor the effects of medication on the client, including therapeutic and adverse reactions. Responses to NCLEX questions should focus on physiologic status. Pain is often considered psychologic, but this should not be considered the primary answer.

1 Client reports a history of constant low back pain for the past 7 months. In planning care for client, the nurse recognizes this type of pain as:

A. acute pain.
B. chronic pain.
C. cutaneous pain.
D. neuropathic pain.

2 A client complains of pain in her abdomen radiating to the left shoulder. The nurse explains this type of pain is:

A. visceral.
B. deep somatic.
C. referred.
D. cutaneous.

3 Client has pain related to a brain tumor that required multiple pharmacologic approaches. This pain is classified as:

A. acute pain.
B. neuropathic pain.
C. referred pain.
D. chronic malignant pain.

4 Client has a below-the-knee amputation of her right leg. She reports pain in her right foot and requests pain medication. The appropriate nursing intervention is to:

A. report the symptoms to the charge nurse.
B. remind the client that her foot has been amputated.
C. administer pain medication.
D. offer a back rub.

5 Client has a history of gastric ulcer. The nurse recognizes this client should avoid which of the following analgesics?

A. ibuprofen (Motrin)
B. acetaminophen (Tylenol)
C. meperidine (Demerol)
D. codeine sulfate (Codeine)

6 Client complains of pain in his surgical incision. To assess the severity of his pain, which of the following would be most effective?

A. Observe his facial expressions.
B. Assess his vital signs.
C. Ask if the pain is mild, moderate, or severe.
D. Ask the client to describe the pain using a scale of 0–10.

7 Client, age 75, complains of arthritic pain in her left hip. Which of the following analgesics will provide the least risk of accumulation and toxicity for this client?

A. meperidine (Demerol)
B. ibuprofen (Motrin)
C. acetaminophen (Tylenol)
D. propoxyphene (Darvon)

8 Client receives morphine sulfate 10 mg intravenously for severe abdominal pain. Thirty minutes later client is unresponsive to physical stimulation. His breathing is shallow with respiratory rate of 8. Which of the following medications should the nurse expect to be administered?

A. lorazepam (Ativan)
B. diazepam (Valium)
C. naloxone (Narcan)
D. ketorolac (Toradol)

9 A client is prescribed naproxen (Naprosyn) 500 mg for treatment of osteoarthritis. Teaching for home care should include:

A. discontinuing the medication when the pain is relieved.
B. limiting alcohol intake to three servings/day.
C. taking with meals to decrease gastric irritation.
D. combining with aspirin to enhance analgesic effect.

10 Client, age 67, is receiving codeine 60 mg PO every 3 to 4 hours prn for pain. A priority nursing implication is to:

A. assess bowel sounds every 4 hours.
B. limit fluids to 1,000 mL/day.
C. assess respiratory rate every 4 hours.
D. monitor for evidence of gastrointestinal bleeding.

Answers for Review Questions, as well as discussion of Care Plan and Critical Thinking Care Map questions, appear in Appendix V.

RESPONDING TO PAIN AS A CROSS-CULTURAL VARIABLE

Mr. Chu, a 48-year-old Chinese client, refused pain medication following surgery. When asked by the nurse about whether he needed pain medication, he said his discomfort was bearable and he could survive without any medication. Later, the nurse noticed he was restless and perspiring. Again, the nurse offered pain medication. Again, he refused, saying her responsibilities were far more important than his discomfort and he did not want to impose. The nurse knew that many Chinese are taught self-restraint and that some Chinese view the needs of the group as more important than individual needs. She also knew that some Chinese individuals have been taught it is polite to say no the first time an offer is extended. The nurse said, "Mr. Chu, it will help you recover sooner if you are able to relax. I have time to get it for you and would like to do that. If I bring you some medication, will you take it?" Mr. Chu smiled, look relieved, and said, "Yes, you are very kind."

Pain is a universal experience of human existence, but it is not a concrete entity. McCaffery and Thorpe (1988) stated: "Pain is whatever the experiencing person says it is, existing whenever the experiencing person says it does." Today, this phrase is often quoted when holistic pain management is discussed.

Holistic pain management involves consideration of the physical, emotional, social, and spiritual components of pain. It also includes consideration of the client in the context of family, culture, past experiences, and the meaning of the event being experienced (Davidhizar, Shearer, & Giger, 1997). Culture shapes beliefs and behaviors related to pain and influences the way pain is expressed.

Affective Response to Pain

Cultural responses to pain have been divided into two categories: stoic and emotive. Stoic clients are those who tend to "grin and bear it." Emotive people are more likely to verbalize their feelings of pain. A child raised in a Jewish home may react to a physical injury stoically, saying, "It does not hurt much," while a child raised in a Hispanic home may react to the same injury very demonstratively.

Communication of Pain

Words used to describe symptoms differ among cultures. A nurse may understand what is said by a client from the same cultural background, but have less understanding of a client from another culture who uses different terms, is less fluent in English, or speaks another language.

Nonverbal communication also differs among cultures. A client may feel that he or she is communicating the level of pain nonverbally and does not need to describe it. However, the nurse may not recognize culturally unique communications of pain (Giger & Davidhizar, 1999).

Biological Variations and Cultural Reaction to Pain

People within cultural groups may differ biologically in their reaction to pain and to pain medication. For example, when white clients and Chinese clients were compared for reactions to morphine, white clients reported less pain but greater incidence of drug-induced gastrointestinal effects (Levy, 1993).

Nursing Implications

- *Assess individuals in pain from a holistic and cultural perspective.* A "meaning-centered" approach must be used when assessing the client in pain. This approach includes an assessment not only of what the client is saying verbally and nonverbally, but also of personal meanings that pain may have for that person.

- *Avoid reacting judgmentally to the client who is demonstrative about pain.* When a client's reaction to pain appears excessive, the nurse should appreciate that the behavior may be customary in the client's culture and that any other behavior would be considered abnormal. The nurse should react with sensitivity and provide emotional support.

- *Provide appropriate care to promote health in a client who may have a stoic reaction to pain.* When the client is stoic, the nurse may need to be more directive in controlling pain. The nurse should assess for physiological symptoms of pain and tell the client why intervention will help recovery.

- *Recognize differences in responses to pain among health team members.* If team members are stoic themselves, they may be less responsive to complaints of pain by clients.

Self-Reflection Questions

1. What is your attitude toward pain— your own and others'?

2. How do you think your family has shaped your attitude toward pain?

3. How do you react when you are around people who have different reactions to pain than yours?

Chapter 9

Caring for Clients Having Surgery

BRIEF Outline

Types and Settings for Surgery
Informed Consent
Phases of the Surgical Experience
Preoperative Care
   Physiology Review
Intraoperative Phase
Postoperative Phase
   Postanesthesia Recovery
   Wound Healing
   Common Postoperative Complications
Ambulatory Surgery

LEARNING Outcomes

After completing this chapter, you will be able to:

- Describe the classifications of surgical procedures.
- Identify laboratory and diagnostic tests used in the perioperative period.
- Describe nursing implications for medications prescribed for the surgical client.
- Discuss appropriate nursing care for the client in the preoperative, intraoperative, and postoperative phases of surgery.
- Identify variations in perioperative care for the older adult.
- Describe principles of pain management for postoperative pain control.
- Compare and contrast outpatient and inpatient surgery.
- Use the nursing process to provide care for the client undergoing surgery.

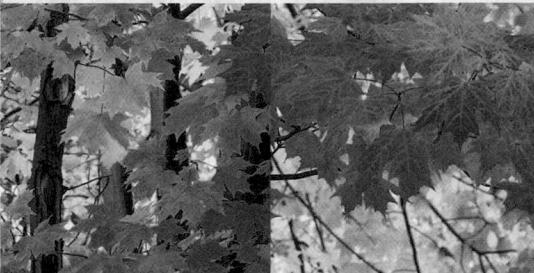

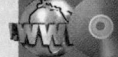 **MediaLink**

www.prenhall.com/burke
Use the address above to access the free, interactive Companion Website created for this textbook. Get hints, instant feedback, and textbook references to chapter-related NCLEX-style questions. Link to other interesting sites.

Audio Glossary:
Use the Companion Website, or the CD-ROM disk enclosed with your textbook, to hear the pronunciation of key terms in this chapter.

Surgery is an invasive medical procedure used to diagnose, treat, or cure illness, injury, or deformity. Although surgery is a medical treatment, the nurse assumes an active role in caring for the client before, during, and after surgery. The licensed practical/vocational nurse (LPN/LVN) collaborates with members of the health care team to prepare the client prior to surgery, prevent complications, and promote optimal recovery following surgery.

Perioperative nursing care requires knowledge and understanding of:

- Surgical anatomy
- Anticipated functional disruptions related to the surgery
- Potential consequences of disrupted function
- Risk factors and potential complications of the surgery
- The emotional and psychosocial effects of the surgery on the client and family.

Types and Settings for Surgery

Surgical procedures can be classified according to purpose, risk, and urgency (Table 9-1 ■). Based on this information, nursing care can be individualized to meet client needs well.

The client may have either inpatient surgery or ambulatory surgery. **Inpatient surgery** requires admission to a hospital before the procedure and inpatient nursing care following the procedure. Inpatient surgery may be a planned event or an unanticipated emergency situation. Although the length of stay for surgical clients has declined during the past two decades, many major procedures still require inpatient stays of 3 to 4 days or more following surgery.

Ambulatory surgery (or *outpatient surgery*) is defined as a surgical procedure performed on a client who does not require inpatient care. The procedure may be performed under local or general anesthesia, but the client is able to return home without assistance following treatment. Special considerations related to ambulatory care are discussed at the end of the chapter.

Ambulatory or outpatient surgery may be performed in a physician's office, free-standing ambulatory surgery center, or in the operating suites and facilities of a hospital, depending on the complexity of the procedure, the anesthesia required, and the surgeon's preference.

Informed Consent

Informed consent is a legal document required for certain diagnostic procedures or therapeutic measures, including surgery. This legal document protects the client, nurse, physician, and health care facility. Informed consent includes the following information:

- The need for the procedure in relation to the diagnosis
- A description and purpose of the proposed procedure
- Possible benefits and potential risks
- Likelihood of a successful outcome
- Alternative treatments or procedures available
- Anticipated risks should the procedure not be performed
- Physician's advice as to what is needed
- Right to refuse treatment or withdraw consent.

The surgeon who performs the procedure is responsible for obtaining the client's informed consent. The surgeon should

---

TABLE 9-1

Classification of Surgical Procedures

	CLASSIFICATION	FUNCTION	EXAMPLE
Purpose	Diagnostic	Determine or confirm a diagnosis	Breast biopsy
	Ablative	Remove diseased organ or extremity	Appendectomy, amputation
	Constructive	Build tissue/organs that are absent	Repair of cleft palate (congenital anomalies)
	Reconstructive	Rebuild tissue/organ that has been damaged	Skin graft after a burn, total joint replacement
	Palliative	Alleviate symptoms of a disease (not curative)	Bowel resection in client with terminal cancer
	Transplant	Replace organs/tissue to restore function	Heart, lung, liver, kidney transplant
Risk	Minor	Minimal physical assault with minimal risk	Removal of skin lesions, dilation and curettage (D&C), cataract extraction
	Major	Extensive physical assault and/or serious risk	Transplant, total joint replacement, cholecystectomy, colostomy, nephrectomy
Urgency	Elective	Suggested though no foreseen ill effects if postponed	Cosmetic surgery, cataract surgery, bunionectomy
	Urgent	Necessary to be performed within 1 to 2 days	Heart bypass surgery, amputation resulting from gangrene, fractured hip
	Emergency	Performed immediately	Obstetric emergencies, bowel obstruction, ruptured aneurysm, life-threatening trauma

discuss the preceding information with the client and family in language they can understand. Ideally, the nurse should be present during this time. Later, the nurse can discuss and clarify as needed what was presented. If the client's questions or concerns were not answered, or if the nurse questions the client's understanding, the nurse should contact the surgeon. The surgeon is responsible for supplying further information before the client signs the informed consent form. After a thorough discussion of the informed consent, the nurse may witness the client's signature on the form (Figure 9-1 ■). The nurse also signs the form, indicating that the correct person signed the form and that the client was alert and aware of what was being signed.

Hospital policies specify criteria and procedures for obtaining surgical consent. These policies identify who can sign the consent, circumstances in which the consent may be signed by someone other than the client, and the procedure to follow if a signature cannot be obtained. Most states require clients ages 18 and over to sign their own consent, and a parent or legal guardian to sign for clients under age 18. Married minors may sign their own consent for surgery, regardless of age. **Emancipated minors** (individuals under age 18 who are responsible for their own welfare and live independently from their parents) also sign their own consent. The signature of a legal guardian is required for adults who are mentally challenged or who have been determined by the courts to be incompetent to make their own medical decisions. In life-threatening situations when surgery is required but the client is unable to sign the consent, every effort is made to contact *next of kin* (as specified by facility policy) for consent. If next of kin cannot be located and continued delay would be life threatening, a court order may be obtained, or the surgeon may assume responsibility for proceeding without consent. The nurse carefully documents the steps taken to obtain consent and the circumstances dictating the need for surgery.

When obtaining informed consent from older adults, allow adequate time for the client to process information, ask questions, and make decisions with the assistance of professionals and family members. The input of adult children and other family members is almost always represented in the older adult's decision to proceed with surgery. The nurse works closely with both the client and family members to provide teaching and emotional support.

clinical ALERT

Follow facility policy related to signing of informed consent. Spouses, children, and significant others cannot sign the informed consent instead of the capable, adult surgical client.

Phases of the Surgical Experience

Perioperative nursing care incorporates the three phases of the surgical experience: preoperative, intraoperative, and postoperative. The **preoperative phase** begins when the decision for surgery is made and ends when the client is transferred to the operating room. The **intraoperative phase** begins with the client's entry into the operating room and ends with admittance to the postanesthesia care unit (PACU, or recovery room). The **postoperative phase** begins with the client's admittance to the postanesthesia recovery area and ends with the client's complete recovery from the surgical intervention.

Preoperative Care

The focus of the preoperative phase of the surgical experience is on:

- Obtaining informed consent for surgery
- Identifying client risk factors and needs prior to and during surgery
- Physical and psychologic preparation of the client
- Educating the client and family about the surgery, expected outcomes, and the recovery process.

PHYSIOLOGY REVIEW

Surgery is a physical stressor that evokes the general stress response. An understanding of the stress response and its effect on the client is vital when providing care for the client undergoing surgery. Three major organ systems are involved in the stress response: the nervous system, endocrine system, and immune system.

The sympathetic nervous system is activated and norepinephrine is released from sympathetic nerve endings. Norepinephrine, together with epinephrine from the adrenal glands, increases the heart rate, and improves cardiac output and blood flow to skeletal muscles. Gastrointestinal tract motility and secretions decrease in response to these substances. Cortisol (from the adrenal cortex), together with other hormones such as glucagon and growth hormone, helps maintain blood glucose levels, providing fuel to the cells. However, cortisol also suppresses the immune response and healing processes.

Surgery also presents significant psychosocial stress for the client and family. Anxiety is a common psychologic response to impending surgery. The level of anxiety the client and family experiences is unique and depends on the significance of the procedure to the individuals. For example, a client scheduled to have a biopsy to rule out cancer may be more anxious than a client undergoing gallbladder removal. The level of anxiety affects the

M.R. # _____

SAINT FRANCIS MEDICAL CENTER

Informed Consent to Operation, Administration of Anesthetics, and to the Rendering of Other Medical Services

1. I do hereby authorize and direct _____ M.D./D.O/D.D.S., my physician, and/or such associates or assistants of his choice, to perform operation or procedure:

   _____

   _____

   upon _____ (patient's name). I understand that the above named physician and his associates or assistants are employed by me and will be occupied solely with performing such operation or procedure.

2. The nature of the operation or procedure has been explained to me by my physician or his/her physician associate and no warranty or guarantee has been made as to result or cure. I have been advised that additional surgical and/or medical procedures treatment services, medications, or interventions may be deemed necessary during the course of the operation or procedure consented hereto, and I fully consent to such additional procedures and treatment which, in the opinion of my physician, are deemed necessary or desirable for the well being.

   My physician or his/her physician associate has explained the following to me to my satisfaction:

   - The potential risk, benefits, and side effects/complications.
   - Reasonable alternatives and relevant risks, benefits and side effects related to alternative including possible results of not receiving care, treatment and services.
   - Potential problems related to recuperation.
   - Likelihood of achieving care, treatment and service goals.
   - If indicated, any limitations on the confidentiality of information learned from or about myself.

3. I hereby authorize and direct the above named physician and/or his associates or assistants or those working under his direction to provide for _____ (patient's name) such additional services as he or they may deem reasonable and necessary, including, but not limited to, the administration and maintenance of anesthesia, blood or blood derivatives, and the performance of services involving pathology and radiology and I hereby consent thereto. The possible risks and complications of blood transfusions and the administration of anesthetics have also been explained to me.

4. I understand also that the persons in attendance at such operation or procedure for the purpose of administering anesthesia, and the radiologists in attendance at such operation or procedure for the purpose of performing radiological (x-ray)/the pathologist in attendance at such operation or procedures for the purpose of performing pathology service are not the agents, servants or employees of Saint Francis Medical Center nor of any physician, but are independent health care providers who are employed by me in the same way that my surgeon and physician are employed by me.

5. **Sedation/Analgesia**: I consent to the administration of medication as appropriate during the procedure. My physician and/or his/her physician associate has explained the risks, benefits, side effects/complications (which may include allergic reation to medications or reactions effecting respiratory or cardiac status) and alternatives of Sedation/Analgesia. In the event of an emergency or additional procedures becomes necessary, I consent to the administration of anesthetics as may be necessary or advisable by the physician responsible for this service.

6. I hereby authorize the Medical Center pathologist or personnel to use their discretion in the disposal of any severed tissue or member.

7. I hereby grant permission for Saint Francis Medical Center to obtain clinical photographs for educational purposes or for my patient record as deemed necessary by my physician.

8. **The exception to this consent:** (If none, write "none.") _____

   _____ and I assume full responsibility for these exceptions.

_____ _____
PATIENT'S SIGNATURE DATE WITNESS SIGNATURE DATE

If the patient is a minor or incompetent or is unable to sign, the following must be completed:

I hereby certify that I am the (relationship) _____ of the above named patient who

is unable to sign because _____ ,

and I am fully authorized to give the consent herein granted. _____

  SIGNATURE DATE

_____ _____
WITNESS SIGNATURE DATE WITNESS SIGNATURE DATE

665-004 (1427) BS / Rev. 7/04

Figure 9-1. ■ Informed consent to operation, administration of anesthetics, and the rendering of other medical services. (Courtesy of St. Francis Medical Center, Cape Girardeau, MO.)

client's ability to learn new information and understand instructions, as well as physical responses to anesthetics and perceived postoperative pain.

Surgical Risk Assessment

Assessment of the client's overall health status and specific risk factors for surgery is vital during the preoperative phase. This information is used by the surgeon in deciding on the type and extent of the procedure to be performed, by the anesthesiologist/nurse anesthetist in determining the safest anesthetic for use, and the nurse in planning care during all phases of the surgical experience. Table 9-2 ■ identifies selected surgical risk factors and their nursing implications.

INTERDISCIPLINARY CARE

Diagnostic Tests

Laboratory and diagnostic tests are obtained prior to surgery to provide baseline data and to detect problems that may place the client at risk during and after surgery. These studies are performed within a week prior to elective

TABLE 9-2

Nursing Implications for Surgical Risk Factors

FACTOR	ASSOCIATED RISK	NURSING IMPLICATIONS
Advanced age	Age-related changes affect physiologic, cognitive, and psychosocial responses to surgery; increase risk for adverse responses to anesthesia and postoperative medications; impair immune defenses and delay wound healing.	Closely monitor vital signs, response to anesthesia and medications, level of consciousness and orientation, renal status, and wound healing. Promptly report signs of infection (temperature may remain within normal range).
Obesity	Increased risk for delayed wound healing, wound dehiscence, infection, pneumonia, atelectasis, thrombophlebitis, dysrhythmias, and heart failure.	Promote weight reduction if time permits. Monitor closely for wound, pulmonary, and cardiovascular complications postoperatively. Encourage coughing, turning, and diaphragmatic breathing exercises and early ambulation.
Malnutrition	Increased risk for adverse outcomes of surgery (shock, organ system failure). Increased risk for impaired wound healing, infection and sepsis.	Minimize duration of fasting or diet restriction associated with surgery. With the physician and dietitian, promote a well-balanced, high-calorie, high-protein diet. Weigh daily. Monitor wound healing and for signs of infection. Monitor WBC, hemoglobin, hematocrit, and serum albumin.
Dehydration/electrolyte imbalance	Increased risk for cardiovascular instability, dysrhythmias, and heart failure. Increased risk for acute renal failure, paralytic ileus, impaired wound healing, pressure ulcers, and venous thrombosis.	Administer intravenous fluids as ordered. Monitor vital signs, intake and output. Monitor for signs of electrolyte imbalance. Monitor serum electrolytes, osmolality, and hematocrit. Restore oral intake as soon as possible. Ensure safety when ambulating.
Cardiovascular disorders	Increased risk of cardiovascular instability, shock, hypotension, venous thrombosis, pulmonary embolism, stroke, and fluid volume overload.	Monitor vital signs, including apical pulse rate, regularity, and rhythm, respiratory rate and ease, and general condition. Assess skin color. Assess for chest pain, lung congestion, and peripheral edema. Provide early postoperative ambulation.
Respiratory disorders	Increased risk for respiratory complications such as bronchitis, atelectasis, and pneumonia. Respiratory depression from general anesthesia and acid–base imbalance may also occur.	Closely monitor respirations, pulse, and breath sounds. Encourage coughing, turning, deep-breathing exercises, use of incentive spirometer, and early ambulation.

(continued)

TABLE 9-2

Nursing Implications for Surgical Risk Factors (continued)

FACTOR	ASSOCIATED RISK	NURSING IMPLICATIONS
Diabetes mellitus	Increased risk for cardiovascular disease, delayed wound healing, and wound infection; unstable blood glucose levels during and after surgery.	Monitor blood glucose and electrolyte levels. Assess for signs of hypoglycemia and hyperglycemia.
Renal and liver dysfunction	Poor tolerance of general anesthesia; increased risk for fluid and electrolyte imbalances, decreased metabolism and excretion of drugs.	Monitor fluid status. Monitor response to drugs. Monitor intake and output. Monitor laboratory values for renal and liver function (BUN, creatinine, bilirubin, liver enzymes).
Alcoholism	Often associated with malnourished status; may require more anesthesia; at risk for hemorrhage and delayed wound healing.	Monitor for signs of delirium tremens. Monitor diet. Assess for evidence of bleeding. Monitor serum electrolytes, hemoglobin, and hematocrit.
Smoking	Increased risk for respiratory complications such as pneumonia, atelectasis, and bronchitis because of increased mucous secretions and a decreased ability to expel them.	Encourage to quit smoking. Monitor for respiratory complications. Encourage coughing and breathing exercises. Promote early ambulation.
Medications	Interaction between anesthetics and some medications increases risk for respiratory complications, bleeding, hypotension, and circulatory collapse.	Inform anesthesiologist and surgeon of all prescribed and over-the-counter medications.
Anticoagulants	Increased risk for intraoperative and postoperative bleeding.	Monitor for bleeding. Assess PT/PTT values, hemoglobin, and hematocrit.
Diuretics	Increased risk for fluid and electrolyte imbalances, cardiovascular instability. Some affect blood glucose levels.	Monitor intake and output and serum electrolytes. Assess cardiovascular and respiratory status. Monitor blood glucose.
Antihypertensives/antidepressants	Increase the hypotensive effects of anesthesia.	Closely monitor blood pressure.

surgery, and immediately prior to surgery in emergency situations. The information is used to help guide the choice of anesthetic, prepare for anticipated complications or problems during surgery, and help determine postoperative care.

The most common preoperative laboratory and diagnostic tests performed are *complete blood count* (CBC), *serum electrolytes* (Na^+, K^+, Cl^-), *coagulation studies* (prothrombin time [PT], partial thromboplastin time [PTT]), *urinalysis, chest x-ray,* and *electrocardiogram* (ECG) (Table 9-3 ■). The urinalysis is obtained to evaluate renal function and to rule out urinary tract infection and pregnancy. Additional laboratory tests are performed as needed. For example, if the client has a history of diabetes mellitus, blood glucose levels are monitored before, during, and after surgery.

The chest x-ray provides baseline information about the size, shape, and condition of the heart and lungs. Pulmonary complications, such as chronic lung disease or pneumonia, may require postponement of surgery for further evaluation or treatment.

The ECG is ordered for clients who are undergoing general anesthesia, are over age 40, or have a history of cardiovascular disease. The ECG is used to evaluate the cardiac status of the client and identify new or preexisting cardiac conditions. The client's surgery may be postponed or canceled if a life-threatening heart condition is discovered.

clinical ALERT

Monitor
Monitor laboratory test values and results of diagnostic tests for the preoperative patient.

Report
Report abnormal values to the charge nurse or physician.

TABLE 9-3

Laboratory Tests for Perioperative Assessment

TEST	NORMAL VALUE	SIGNIFICANCE OF INCREASED VALUES	SIGNIFICANCE OF DECREASED VALUES	NURSING IMPLICATIONS
Hemoglobin (Hgb)	12–16 g Females 14–18 g Males	Dehydration, excessive plasma loss	Fluid overload, excessive blood loss, anemia	Monitor intake and output, vital signs, assess for bleeding.
Hematocrit (Hct)	37–47% Females 40–54% Males	Polycythemia		
White blood cell count (WBC)	5–10 mm^3	Infection/inflammation process	Immune deficiencies	Monitor for signs of inflammation and infection.
Platelet count	200,000–300,000	Malignancies	Clotting disorders, chemotherapy	Assess for signs of bleeding at incision site and drainage tubes. Assess for hematoma.
Potassium (K$^+$)	3.5–5.0 mEq/L	Renal failure, dehydration, cell damage	Diuretics, malnutrition	Monitor cardiac and GI status; monitor intake and output.
Chloride (Cl$^-$)	98–106 mEq/L	Dehydration, renal dysfunction	Side effects of diuretics, vomiting, NG suctioning	Monitor lab values; monitor intake and output.
Sodium (Na$^+$)	135–145 mEq/L	Kidney dysfunction, IV fluids containing sodium chloride	Side effects of diuretics, vomiting, NG suctioning	Monitor lab values; monitor intake and output, and mental status.
Prothrombin time (protime, or PT) and partial thromboplastin time (PTT)	10–13 sec 22–32 sec	Clotting disorders, anticoagulant therapy, side effects of other drugs affecting clotting time	Increased risk for venous thrombosis (DVT)	Monitor lab values. Assess for bleeding from incision, urine, and hematoma formation. Encourage leg exercises, ambulation.
Urinalysis	Glucose negative Protein negative WBC negative RBC negative Bacteria negative Ketones negative	May indicate urinary tract infection, impaired kidney function, malnutrition, or diabetes mellitus.		Monitor and report abnormal values.

Medications

The surgical client may be given preoperative medications 45 to 60 minutes before the scheduled surgery, although frequently no drugs are administered until the client is in the surgical suite. Preoperative drugs may be ordered to sedate the client, reduce anxiety, enhance the actions of anesthetics, induce amnesia to minimize unpleasant surgical memories, increase comfort during preoperative procedures, reduce gastric acidity and volume, increase gastric emptying, decrease nausea and vomiting, and reduce the incidence of aspiration by drying oral and respiratory secretions. Table 9-4 ■ outlines commonly prescribed preoperative medications. The nurse is responsible for administering these drugs prior to surgery.

Physical Preparation

Physical preparation of the client for surgery may include the following:

- *Marking the operative site* is done while the client is awake and before any sedation is given. The site is clearly and unambiguously (e.g., do not use an X as it could be interpreted to mean "not this one") identified with an indelible marker that will remain visible after the skin preparation. When a stoma is to be created during surgery, an enterostomal therapist works with the client and surgeon to identify and mark the appropriate stoma location. Whenever a specific side of the body, extremity, or digit (e.g., finger or toe) is involved, marking the operative site is vital.

Diazepam

MediaLink

TABLE 9-4

Preoperative Medications and Nursing Implications

DRUG GROUP/NAME	DOSE AND ROUTE	ACTION/USES	NURSING IMPLICATIONS
Benzodiazepines			
■ Midazolam (Versed)	3–5 mg IM, IV	Decrease anxiety and produce sedation	Monitor for respiratory depression, hypotension, drowsiness, and lack of coordination.
■ Diazepam (Valium)	5–20 mg PO	Induce amnesia	
■ Lorazepam (Ativan)	1–4 mg IM, IV	May induce substantial amnesia	
Opioid Analgesics			
■ Morphine	5–15 mg IM, IV	Decrease anxiety, provide analgesia, allow reduced anesthetic dose	Monitor for respiratory depression, nausea, vomiting, orthostatic hypotension, and pruritus.
■ Meperidine (Demerol)	50–150 mg IM, IV		
H₂ Receptor Antagonists			
■ Cimetidine (Tagamet)	300 mg IV, IM, PO	Reduce gastric acid volume and concentration	Monitor for confusion and dizziness in older adults.
■ Famotidine (Pepcid)	20 mg IV		
■ Ranitidine (Zantac)	50 mg IV, IM, PO		
Antiemetics			
■ Metoclopramide (Reglan)	10 mg IV	Enhance gastric emptying	Monitor for sedation and extrapyramidal reaction (involuntary movement, muscle tone changes, and abnormal posture).
■ Droperidol (Inapsine)	2.5–10 mg IM	Tranquilizer	
Anticholinergics			
■ Atropine sulfate	0.4–0.6 mg IM, IV	Reduce oral and respiratory secretions to decrease risk of aspiration; decrease risk of vomiting and laryngospasm	Monitor for confusion, restlessness, and tachycardia. Prepare client to expect a dry mouth.
■ Glycopyrrolate (Robinul)	0.1–0.3 mg IM, IV		

■ *Skin preparation* is performed to reduce the number of bacteria on the skin in the surgical area. These procedures are often performed in the surgical suite immediately prior to the procedure. The areas to be prepped are determined by the type and location of surgery to be performed. Client allergies to iodine, seafood (which may indicate an iodine allergy), or other topical agents are determined before skin preparation, because many antiseptic soaps and solutions contain iodine or other allergenic substances.

■ Any moles, warts, rashes, or lesions within the surgical site are noted and documented.

■ The area to be prepared is cleansed by having the client shower and shampoo or by washing the surgical site before transferring the client to the surgical suite. The choice of cleansing agent may be determined by agency policy or the surgeon.

■ Hair may be removed from the surgical site, using clippers, depilatory, or razor. Because inappropriate hair removal techniques can damage the skin and increase the risk for infection, hair removal should be done by trained and skilled personnel and as close to the time of surgery as possible. Clippers are the safest for removing hair. Depilatories may cause skin reactions, and razors can disrupt skin integrity. If a razor is to be used, wet the hair, skin, and razor with soapy water prior to shaving to reduce skin trauma.

■ *An indwelling (Foley) catheter* may be inserted to reduce the risk of injury to the bladder during abdominal surgery. It also provides a means to assess urinary output accurately during extensive surgery.

■ *Bowel preparation* may be necessary to prevent introduction of bacteria into the peritoneum during surgery on the bowel. This may include administration of enemas or medications (e.g., GoLYTELY) to evacuate the bowel prior to surgery. Bowel prep may be initiated by the client prior to admission to the hospital or by the nurse for inpatients. Oral antibiotics also may be ordered to reduce resident bacteria in the bowel. The nurse should explain the procedures thoroughly to the patient and document evaluation of patient understanding. See Table 20-4 for nursing responsibilities related to medications used for bowel preparation.

■ *Withholding of food and fluids* may be part of preparation for surgery. Clients are instructed to withhold all food and fluids for a specific period of time prior to surgery. Current evidence supports continuing intake of clear liquids up until about 2 hours before surgery, and fasting for the remaining time. The surgeon and the anesthesiologist determine the exact amount of time the patient should be NPO. Fasting reduces the risk of aspiration of stomach contents during surgery, especially if the patient receives general anesthesia. The nurse should explain the importance of following these instructions. Clients with a history of chronic medical problems such as diabetes mellitus, hypertension, or heart disease often are allowed to take their medications prior to surgery. The nurse must verify this with the physician and instruct the client to take the medications with a minimal amount of water.

NURSING CARE

The LPN/LVN plans and implements care with the registered nurse to meet the needs of the client. In many facilities, the LPN/LVN obtains focused assessment data and may perform presurgical procedures such as starting an IV, inserting a Foley catheter, and preparing the surgical area. Refer to the agency's position description and the state nurse practice act to determine the role of the practical nurse in applying the nursing process for a client undergoing surgery.

ASSESSING

Thorough assessment by the nurse is critical for the preoperative client. The practical/vocational nurse contributes to the assessment by collecting focused assessment data to identify physiologic and psychologic alterations that require nursing and/or medical intervention.

- *Subjective data:* reason for surgery, current complaints or symptoms, reaction or feelings about proposed surgery;

completion of prescribed preoperative preparation (e.g., bowel preparation, shower, last food and fluid intake); current health status; chronic diseases or conditions, current medications; allergies to medications, topical agents, other substances (e.g., latex, iodine, seafood); smoking history, alcohol intake, use of recreational or street drugs; previous surgeries and their outcomes, any problems experienced during or following previous surgeries

- *Objective data:* apparent general health, mobility, mental status and level of consciousness, ability to communicate; vital signs including apical and peripheral pulses, respiratory rate and depth, and temperature; weight; lung sounds; abdominal assessment including bowel sounds, distention, tenderness to palpation; urine color and clarity.

DIAGNOSING, PLANNING, AND IMPLEMENTING

The nurse identifies problems, plans care, and develops nursing interventions to meet client needs and prevent complications during the perioperative period.

Priorities in Nursing Care. Assuring that the client is appropriately informed, managing possible anxiety, and ensuring complete assessment and adequate physical preparation of the client prior to surgery are the priorities of nursing care in the preoperative phase. A nursing care checklist for the day of surgery is provided in Box 9-1 ■.

Deficient Knowledge

- Assess client's current level of knowledge. *This allows the nurse to prioritize teaching, provide new information, and*

BOX 9-1	NURSING CARE CHECKLIST

Day of Surgery

- ☑ Verify that the informed consent form has been signed prior to administering preoperative medications.

- ☑ Ensure that identification, blood, and allergy bands are correct, legible, and secure.

- ☑ Assist with bathing, grooming, and changing into operating room gown as needed.

- ☑ Ensure that the client takes nothing by mouth (NPO) for the prescribed period. Notify the anesthesiologist if fasting orders have not been followed.

- ☑ Reinforce and clarify teaching.

- ☑ Remove nail polish and makeup to facilitate circulatory assessment during and after surgery.

- ☑ Remove hair pins and jewelry. A ring may be protected and secured with tape to the finger if the patient is unable or unwilling to remove it.

- ☑ Clearly mark operative site if not already completed or if instructed to do so.

- ☑ Complete skin or bowel preparation as ordered.

- ☑ Insert an indwelling catheter, intravenous line, or nasogastric tube as ordered.

- ☑ Remove dentures, artificial eye, and corrective lenses, and store them in a safe place.

- ☑ Leave a hearing aid in place if the client cannot hear without it, and notify the operating room nurse.

- ☑ Verify documentation of height and weight in the chart (for dosage of anesthesia).

- ☑ Verify presence of ordered laboratory and diagnostic test reports in the chart.

- ☑ Instruct to empty the bladder immediately before the preoperative medication is administered (unless an indwelling catheter is in place).

(continued)

BOX 9-1	NURSING CARE CHECKLIST (continued)

☑ Administer preoperative medication as scheduled (see Table 9-4).

☑ Ensure safety following medication administration by placing the client on bed rest with the side rails up and the call light within reach.

☑ Obtain and record vital signs.

☑ Provide ongoing supportive care to the client and family.

☑ Complete the preoperative surgical checklist. Document all preoperative care in the appropriate location, such as the pre-operative surgical checklist, the medication record, and the nurses' notes.

☑ Verify the client's identity and surgical site with the surgical personnel.

☑ Assist with transferring the client from the bed to the gurney.

☑ Prepare room for postoperative care, including making the surgical bed and ensuring that anticipated supplies and equipment are in the room.

BOX 9-2	CLIENT TEACHING

Preoperative Exercises

Diaphragmatic Breathing Exercise

Diaphragmatic (abdominal) breathing exercises help to prevent pulmonary complications. Risk factors for atelectasis or pneumonia include general anesthesia, abdominal or thoracic surgery, prolonged immobility, history of smoking, chronic lung disease, obesity, and advanced age.

1. Explain to the client that the diaphragm is a muscle that makes up the floor of the thoracic cavity and assists in breathing. When the client breathes in deeply, the diaphragm flattens, promoting lung expansion, ventilation, and blood oxygenation. When the client exhales, the diaphragm contracts inward and upward and helps to expel air.
2. Place the client in Fowler's position.

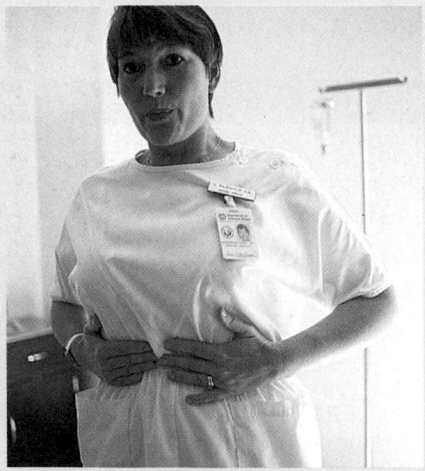

Demonstrating diaphragmatic breathing exercise.
(Photographer: Elena Dorfman.)

3. Ask the client to place hands lightly on the abdomen (see figure).
4. Instruct to breathe in deeply through the nose, allowing the chest and abdomen to expand.
5. Have the client hold the breath for a count of 5.
6. Instruct to exhale completely through pursed (puckered) lips, allowing the chest and abdomen to deflate.

7. Have the client repeat the exercise five times consecutively. Encourage to perform diaphragmatic breathing exercises every 1 to 2 waking hours if possible.

Coughing Exercise

Coughing exercises are also taught to reduce the risk for pulmonary complications. The purpose of coughing is to loosen, mobilize, and remove pulmonary secretions. *Splinting* (holding something firm over) the incision decreases the discomfort associated with coughing.

1. Assist the client in following steps 1 through 4 for diaphragmatic breathing.
2. Instruct to splint the incision with interlocked hands or a pillow (see figure).

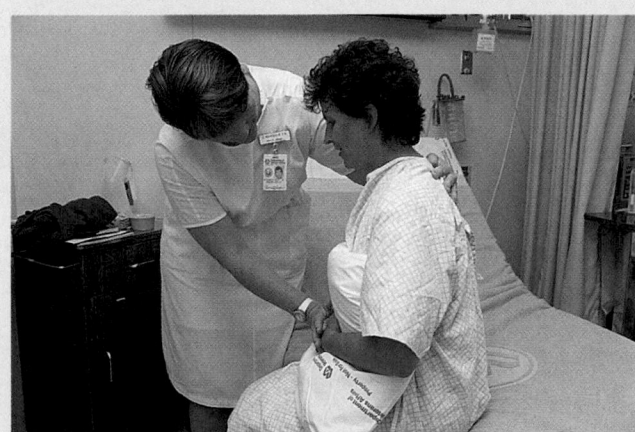

Splinting abdomen while coughing. (Photographer: Elena Dorfman.)

3. Tell the client to take three deep breaths and then cough contracting abdominal muscles.
4. Instruct to repeat the exercise five times consecutively every 2 hours while awake, taking short rest periods between coughs, if necessary.

Leg, Ankle, and Foot Exercises

Leg exercises are taught to reduce the risk for developing deep venous thrombosis (blood clot formation and inflammation in a deep vein). Risk factors for venous thrombosis include

reinforce prior knowledge about the surgical procedure and post-operative course of treatment.

■ Assist the client to obtain information about expectations during the intraoperative and postoperative phase. Refer to the physician for detailed information about the surgical procedure. *The surgeon provides information so the client can make an informed decision about care.*

■ Teach postoperative breathing exercises, turning, coughing, deep breathing, and leg exercises. (See Box 9-2 ■) *This knowledge helps prevent postoperative complications.*

■ Collaborate with physician concerning postoperative pain control. Discuss pain management with the client. *This assures the client that pain will be managed and makes the client an integral member of the pain management process.*

Anxiety

The nurse's ability to listen actively to both verbal and non-verbal messages is essential to establishing a trusting relationship with the client and family. Therapeutic communication can help the client and family identify fears

---

decreased mobility preoperatively or postoperatively; a history of peripheral circulation disorders; and cardiovascular, pelvic, or lower extremity surgeries.

As the leg muscles contract and relax, blood is pumped back to the heart, promoting cardiac output and reducing venous stasis. Besides promoting venous blood return from the extremities, leg exercises also maintain muscle tone and range of motion, which facilitates early ambulation.

Teach the client to perform the following exercises while lying in bed (see drawings):

b. With feet together, point toes toward the head and then to the foot of the bed. Repeat this pumping action 10 times, and then relax.

Encourage to perform leg, ankle, and foot exercises every 1 to 2 hours while awake, depending on the client's needs and ambulatory status, the physician's preference, and institutional protocol.

Turning in Bed

Clients may need to be taught to turn in bed. This normally simple task may be very difficult after surgery, particularly ab-

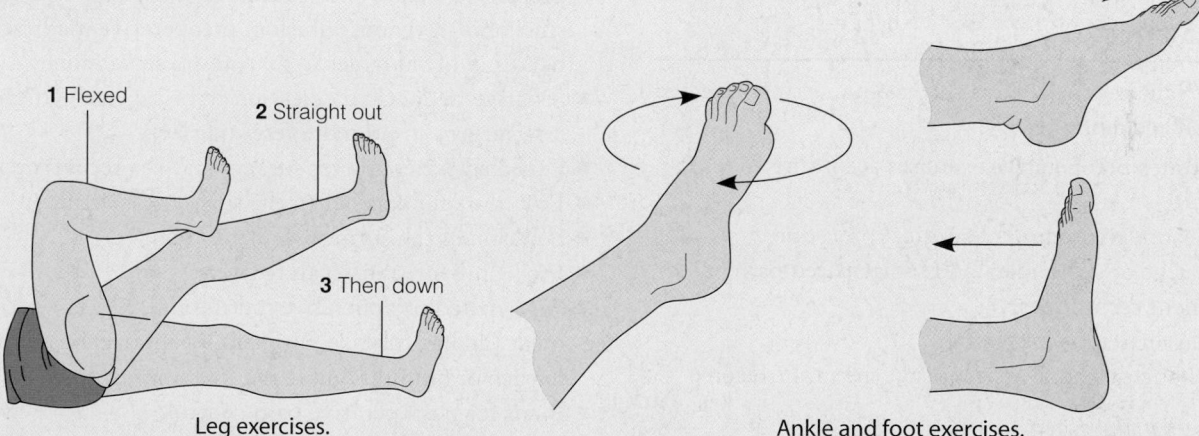

Leg exercises.

Ankle and foot exercises.

1. *Muscle pumping exercise:* Contract and relax calf and thigh muscles at least 10 times in a row.
2. *Leg exercises:*
   a. Bend the knee and raise it toward the chest.
   b. Straighten out leg and hold for a few seconds before lowering the leg back to the bed.
   c. Repeat exercise five times with one leg, then do them with the other leg.
3. *Ankle and foot exercises:*
   a. Rotate both ankles by making complete circles, first to the right and then to the left. Repeat five times and then relax.

dominal surgery. The client may need to splint the incision with the hand and a small pillow or blanket. Analgesics can be given to ease postoperative discomfort involved with turning. Encourage the client to turn every 2 hours while awake.

1. Instruct to grasp the side rail toward the direction to be turned, to rest the opposite foot on the mattress, and to bend the knee.
2. Instruct to roll over in one smooth motion by pulling on the side rail while pushing off with the bent knee.
3. Pillows may need to be positioned behind the back to help the client maintain a side-lying position. The older client may also need padding over pressure points between the knees and ankles to prevent decubitus ulcer formation.

and concerns. The nurse plans nursing interventions and supportive care to reduce the client's anxiety level and assist the client to cope successfully with the stressors encountered during the perioperative period.

- Assess specific source(s) of anxiety. *Common fears include loss of control, pain, death, disfigurement, disability, and disturbing diagnosis and prognosis. The unfamiliar environment increases anxiety. Assessment provides the basis for planning specific nursing interventions.*
- Answer all questions thoroughly and honestly. Refer to appropriate resources as needed. *Honesty establishes trust and helps relieve anxiety.*
- Allow expression of fears. Use active listening. *Listening helps the client identify fears and clarify concerns.*
- Refer to clergy or spiritual support of client's choice. *Spiritual support provides comfort to most clients.*

Disturbed Sleep Pattern

- Assess usual sleep pattern. *This identifies alterations in pattern. Anxiety prior to surgery often results in sleep disturbance.*
- Provide environment with minimal stimuli prior to surgery. *A relaxing environment encourages sleep.*
- Collaborate with physician to obtain sleep medication. *Adequate rest reduces the risk of complications and contributes to more effective induction of anesthesia.*

EVALUATING

The nurse evaluates the client's success in meeting expected outcomes. The client:

- Demonstrates preoperative exercises according to teaching plan.
- Verbalizes understanding of surgical procedure.
- States that he or she understands anticipated pain management techniques.
- States that anxiety is decreased.
- Sleeps 8 hours without interruption the night before surgery.

Documenting. Document the client's and family's understanding of and emotional response to the planned procedure. Fully document all assessment data and preoperative preparation performed, including skin marking and preparation, bowel preparation and results, medications administered, and other procedures.

Preoperative Teaching

Client teaching is an essential nursing responsibility in the preoperative period. Client education combined with emotional support has positive physical and psychologic effects. Surgical clients receiving client education and/or supportive interventions have less pain and anxiety, experience fewer complications, are discharged sooner, are more satisfied with their care, and return to normal activities sooner than clients who are not adequately prepared. These positive outcomes

may be attributed in part to the perceived sense of control the client gains through the nurse's teaching.

Nurses develop and implement the preoperative teaching plan. Teaching should begin as soon as the client is aware of the upcoming surgery. Most teaching is carried out prior to surgery, because postsurgical pain and the effects of anesthesia can significantly diminish the ability to learn.

The amount of information desired varies from client to client. The nurse must assess the client's need for and readiness to accept information. The teaching is determined partly by the particular surgical procedure being performed. Client teaching that helps to reduce postsurgical risk for most patients is included in Box 9-2.

Besides teaching measures to decrease the risk of complications, the nurse provides other preoperative information to prepare the client and family for surgery:

- Laboratory and diagnostic tests to be performed, including reason for the tests and preparations
- Any prescribed preparation, such as shower with antibacterial soap, bowel preparation
- Time family should arrive if surgery is scheduled in early morning
- Preparations for the day of surgery: nothing by mouth (NPO) as instructed prior to a morning surgery, skin preparation, indwelling catheter or bladder elimination, start of intravenous infusion, preoperative medication, handling of valuables (e.g., rings, watch, money)
- Sedative/hypnotic medication to be taken the night before surgery to promote rest and sleep
- Expected timetable for surgery and the recovery room
- Procedure for transfer to the surgery department
- Location of the surgical waiting room
- Procedure for transfer to recovery room
- Anticipated postoperative routine and devices or equipment (drains, tubes, equipment for intravenous infusions, oxygen or humidifying mask, dressings, splints, casts)
- Plans for postoperative pain control.

NURSING PROCESS CARE PLAN
Preoperative Care for Client Having Inpatient Surgery

Martha Overbeck is a 74-year-old widow of German descent who lives alone in a senior citizens' housing complex. She is active in the housing complex's activities, as well as in the Lutheran church. She is in good health and is independent; however, she has become progressively less active as a result of arthritic pain and stiffness. Mrs. Overbeck has degenerative joint changes that have particularly affected her right hip. On the recommendation of her physician and following a discussion with her friends, Mrs. Overbeck has been admitted to the hospital for an elective right total hip replacement. Her surgery has been scheduled for 8:00 A.M. the following day.

Mrs. Eva Jackson, a close friend and neighbor, accompanies Mrs. Overbeck to the hospital. Mrs. Overbeck explains that her friend will help in her home and assist her with the wound care and prescribed exercises.

Assessment. Gloria Nobis, LVN, completes the admission assessment for Mrs. Overbeck. Mrs. Overbeck appears to be an alert, oriented, healthy 74-year-old client. She is 30 pounds over her ideal weight. Mrs. Overbeck states she has pain and some stiffness in her weight-bearing joints, particularly her right hip. Enteric-coated aspirin 650 mg four times daily is the only medication she has been taking. Preadmission laboratory tests are normal except for a slightly elevated clotting time (which suggests an increased risk for bleeding). The x-ray film of her right hip reveals degenerative joint changes indicative of osteoarthritis.

Mrs. Overbeck confides that although she has faith that her surgery will be successful, she feels uneasy. She cannot identify exactly why she is apprehensive. She states she has had a number of restless nights since her decision to have surgery. She has never had major surgery and is not familiar with the hospital routine.

Diagnosis. The following nursing diagnoses are identified for Mrs. Overbeck and are included in her preoperative plan of care:

- *Anxiety* related to unfamiliar environment (hospital) and upcoming surgery
- *Deficient Knowledge* related to lack of information about the perioperative surgical experience
- *Disturbed Sleep Pattern* related to environmental changes (hospitalization) and anxiety response

Expected Outcomes. The expected outcomes established in the plan of care specify that Mrs. Overbeck will:

- Describe an increase in psychologic and physiologic comfort.
- Verbalize an understanding of perioperative events to occur.
- Demonstrate turning, coughing, deep-breathing exercise, and leg exercises.
- Report sleeping soundly from 10:00 P.M. to 7:00 A.M.

Planning and Implementation. Ms. Nobis plans and implements the following interventions to assist Mrs. Overbeck in the preoperative surgical phase:

- Establish a therapeutic relationship with Mrs. Overbeck and her friend.
- Provide reassurance and comfort by acknowledging concerns and conveying understanding.
- Familiarize Mrs. Overbeck with hospital routines.
- Initiate perioperative teaching to include:
  - Preparation for surgery
  - A visit from the operating room nurse and anesthesiologist

- Coughing, turning, and deep-breathing exercises
- Leg exercises
- Written materials describing total hip replacements.
- Help Mrs. Overbeck identify factors that interfere with her ability to sleep.
- Decrease noise, lighting, and disturbances between 10:00 P.M. and 7:00 A.M.
- Encourage the use of prescribed hypnotic/sedative medications to assist in sleep prior to surgery.

Evaluation. By the end of the shift, Ms. Nobis assesses that Mrs. Overbeck's anxiety has diminished. Mrs. Overbeck confirms that she feels more comfortable about the upcoming surgery. She is able to describe the preoperative preparations that will occur the following morning, events that are most likely to occur in surgery and the recovery room, and routine postoperative nursing care following her total hip replacement. She states that she will take the hypnotic/sedative prescribed to help her sleep. She asks Ms. Nobis to convey to the evening and night nurses that she would like to have her door closed and lights off except for the one in the bathroom.

Critical Thinking in the Nursing Process

1. What teaching would you implement with Mrs. Overbeck and her friend to prepare them for the first 72 hours of postoperative recovery?
2. What consultations may be appropriate for you to make to other health care providers to assist Mrs. Overbeck before and after surgery?
3. Develop a care plan for Mrs. Overbeck for the nursing diagnosis "Deficient Knowledge related to lack of information about preoperative care."

Intraoperative Phase

The intraoperative phase begins when the client is admitted to the operating room and ends when the client is admitted to the PACU. The duration of this phase of the perioperative experience depends on the type and extent of the surgery being performed, as well as any problems or complications that develop during surgery.

On entry into the surgical suite, the *Universal Protocol* for preventing surgery on the wrong person, the wrong site, or performing the wrong procedure is followed. A "time-out" is taken immediately before starting the procedure to conduct a final verification of the correct client, procedure, and site. This is a process of active communication among surgical team members. The surgery itself does not begin until all questions or concerns are resolved (JCAHO, 2003).

INTERDISCIPLINARY CARE

The Surgical Team

The surgeon, surgical assistant(s), anesthesiologist and/or certified registered nurse anesthetist (CRNA), circulating nurse, scrub nurse, and certified surgical technologist (CST) constitute the surgical team. Because the intraoperative environment is so complex, members must function as a coordinated unit. The surgeon and anesthesiologist maintain primary roles in managing the client physiologically; nurses are responsible for maintaining the safety of the client and the environment, monitoring client status, and providing psychologic support.

The *surgeon* is the physician performing the procedure and the head of the surgical team. All medical actions and judgments are the surgeon's responsibility.

The *surgical assistant* works closely with the surgeon in performing the operation. The number of assistants varies according to the complexity of the procedure. The assistant may be another physician, a nurse, a physician's assistant, or other trained personnel. The LPN/LVN may assume this role with specialized training. The assistant performs such duties as exposing the operative site, retracting nearby tissue, sponging or suctioning the wound, tying off bleeding vessels, and suturing or assisting with suturing of the surgical wound.

The *anesthesiologist* (a physician) or *certified registered nurse anesthetist (CRNA)* (an advanced practice nurse) administers anesthesia and assumes responsibility for the client's general well-being during surgery. The anesthesiologist or CRNA evaluates the client preoperatively, administers medications, transfuses blood or blood products, infuses intravenous fluids, continuously monitors physiologic status, alerts the surgeon to developing problems and treats problems as they arise, and supervises the client's recovery in the PACU.

The *circulating nurse* is a registered nurse who coordinates and manages a wide range of activities before, during, and after the surgical procedure. The circulating nurse oversees the physical aspects of the operating room and its equipment. The circulating nurse assists with transferring and positioning the client, preparing the surgical site, ensuring that no break in aseptic technique occurs, and counting all sponges and instruments. The circulating nurse assists other team members and documents intraoperative nursing activities, medications, blood administration, placement of drains and catheters, and length of the procedure. The circulating nurse is at all times an advocate for the safety and well-being of the client.

The *scrub nurse* (or *certified surgical technologist*) handles sutures, instruments, and other equipment immediately adjacent to the sterile field (Figure 9-2 ■). This role requires technical skills, manual dexterity, and in-depth knowledge of the anatomic and mechanical aspects of a particular surgery. LPNs/LVNs often assume the role of scrub nurse, acquiring skills through facility training programs or a formal surgical technology program.

Medications

Anesthesia is the use of chemical substances to produce loss of sensation, reflex loss, or muscle relaxation during a surgical procedure, with or without the loss of consciousness.

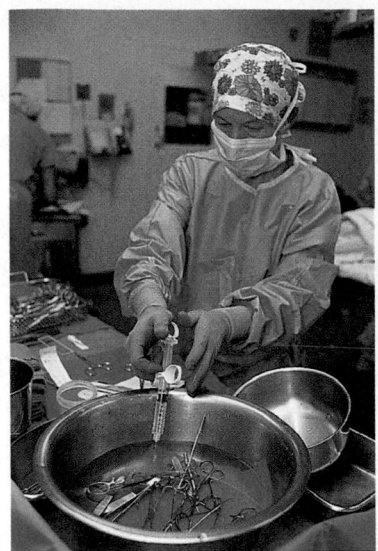

Figure 9-2. ■ A scrub nurse in the operating room. (Photographer: Alain McLaughlin.)

Factors that influence the type of anesthesia used include the surgery to be performed and the client's medical and surgical history, age and health status, and preferences.

GENERAL ANESTHESIA. *General anesthesia* is administered by inhalation or the intravenous route. It produces central nervous system depression resulting in loss of consciousness and amnesia. The client perceives no pain, skeletal muscles relax, and reflexes diminish. Advantages of general anesthesia include rapid excretion of the anesthetic agent and prompt reversal of its effects when desired. Additionally, general anesthesia can be used with all age groups and most surgical procedures.

Its disadvantages include risks associated with circulatory and respiratory depression. Clients with serious respiratory or circulatory diseases, such as emphysema or heart failure, are at greater risk for these complications.

The phases of general anesthesia are as follows:

1. The *induction phase* begins when the anesthetic agent is administered and ends when the client is ready for the surgical procedure to begin. During this phase, airway patency is achieved with endotracheal intubation. The client is positioned and the skin is prepared during this phase.

2. The *maintenance phase* begins with surgical incision and continues until the procedure nears completion. The anesthesiologist maintains the proper depth of anesthesia while constantly monitoring such parameters as heart rate, blood pressure, respiratory rate, temperature, and oxygen and carbon dioxide levels.

3. The *emergence phase* begins as the client "emerges" from the anesthetic agents and continues until the client is ready to leave the operating room. The endotracheal tube is removed (*extubation*) once the client has reestablished voluntary breathing. Airway patency is critical

during this period, because extubation may cause bronchospasm or laryngospasm.

REGIONAL ANESTHESIA. In *regional anesthesia,* medication is instilled around the peripheral nerves to block transmission of nerve impulses in a particular area. Regional anesthesia produces analgesia, relaxation, and reduced reflexes. The client is awake and conscious during the surgical procedure but does not perceive pain. Regional anesthesia has several subclassifications:

- *Surface or topical.* Anesthesia is applied to the skin or mucous membranes to block nerve impulses at that site. Wounds of the skin or burns are anesthetized using a cocaine solution, lidocaine (Xylocaine), or benzocaine.
- *Local nerve infiltration.* Lidocaine or tetracaine is injected around a local nerve to depress nerve sensation over a limited area of the body. This technique may be used when a skin or muscle biopsy is obtained or when a small wound is sutured.
- *Nerve blocks.* An anesthetic agent is injected at the nerve trunk to produce a lack of sensation over a specific body area, like the hand.
- *Epidural blocks.* Local anesthetic agents are injected into the epidural space, outside the dura mater of the spinal cord. This may be used for surgeries of the abdomen and lower extremities.
- *Spinal anesthesia.* A local anesthetic is injected into the subarachnoid space. Surgeries of the lower abdomen, perineum, and lower extremities are likely to use this type of regional anesthesia. Leakage of cerebrospinal fluid (CSF) from the needle insertion site may reduce CSF pressure and cause postoperative headaches. Bed rest, maintaining hydration, and applying pressure to the infusion site combat this common side effect.

CONSCIOUS SEDATION. **Conscious sedation** is a type of anesthesia that provides analgesia and amnesia but allows the client to remain conscious. An increasing number of surgical and diagnostic procedures are performed using conscious sedation. A combination of opioids and sedative intravenous medications produces the pharmacologic effects. Opioids include morphine sulfate, meperidine hydrochloride (Demerol), and fentanyl (Sublimaze). Sedatives include diazepam (Valium) and midazolam (Versed). During conscious sedation, the client can independently maintain an open airway and respond to verbal and physical stimulation.

Common adverse effects include venous thrombosis, phlebitis, local irritation, confusion, drowsiness, hypotension, and apnea. Naloxone hydrochloride (Narcan) and flumazenil (Romazicon) are used as needed to reverse conscious sedation. The client must be monitored before, during, and after the procedure when using conscious sedation. In most facilities, the RN is responsible for administering the medication and assessing and monitoring the client during the procedure. The

LPN/LVN may be responsible for preparing the client for the procedure and monitoring the client after the procedure.

Infection Control

Surgery disrupts a major defense system, the skin. In addition, hormones released during the general stress response suppress the immune system. As a result, procedures used to prevent contamination of the surgical site are vital to prevent infection. *Surgical asepsis* is followed to prevent introduction of all microbes that can cause disease into the surgical wound.

SURGICAL ATTIRE. Strict dress codes in the surgical department facilitate infection control, reduce cross-contamination between the surgery department and other hospital units, and promote the health and safety of clients and personnel. All personnel in the surgical department wear surgical attire to minimize bacterial shedding and reduce wound contamination.

The surgical department is divided into three zones:

1. Unrestricted zones permit access by persons in hospital uniforms or street clothes, and allow limited access for communicating with operating room personnel.
2. Semirestricted zones require scrub attire, including a scrub suit, shoe covers, and a cap or hood (Figure 9-3A ■). Hallways, work areas, and storage areas are semirestricted.
3. Restricted zones, within operating rooms, require personnel to wear masks, sterile gowns, and gloves in addition to appropriate scrub attire (see Figure 9-3B). The entire surgical attire is changed between procedures and whenever soiled or wet.

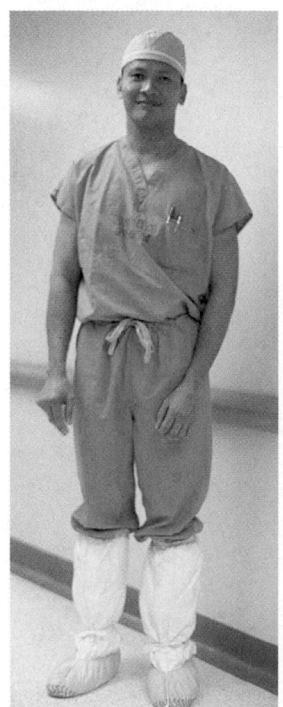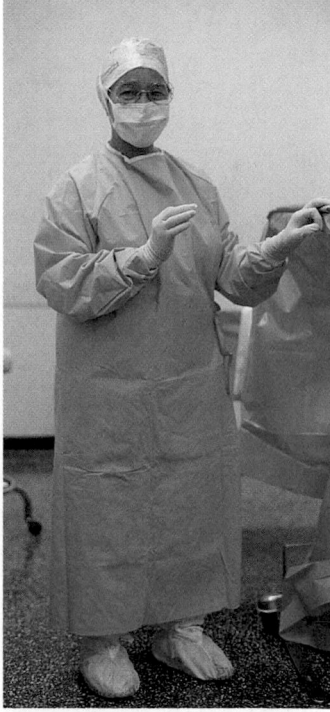

Figure 9-3. ■ **(A)** Surgical attire. **(B)** Sterile surgical attire. (Photographer: Richard Tauber.)

THE SURGICAL SCRUB. The surgical scrub, using a sponge or brush and antimicrobial soap, is required for all personnel who participate directly in the procedure. Skin cannot be sterilized, but it is considered "surgically clean" following the scrub. The purposes of the surgical scrub are to:

- Remove dirt, skin oils, and transient microorganisms from hands and forearms.
- Increase client safety by reducing microorganisms on surgical personnel.

- Leave an antimicrobial residue on the skin to inhibit growth of microbes for several hours.

Following the 5- to 10-minute surgical scrub, hands and arms are dried with sterile towels.

SITE PREPARATION. The client's skin is cleansed in the surgical department to decrease microorganisms on the skin and reduce the possibility of wound infection (Figure 9-4 ■). The surgeon also may order hair removed from the proposed incision area. Generally, the area from which hair is removed

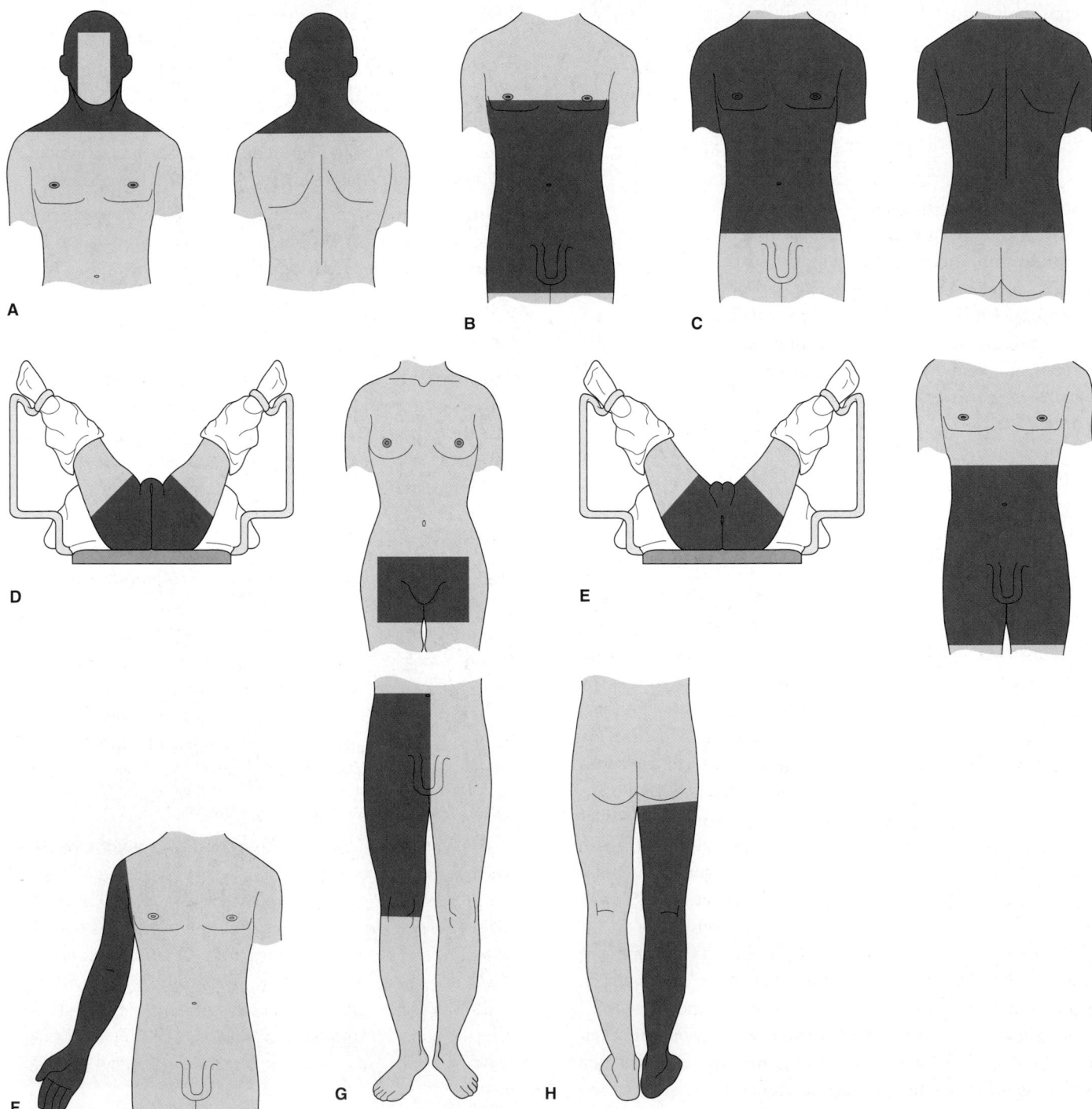

Figure 9-4. ■ Surgical areas to be scrubbed. (**A**) Head surgery. (**B**) Abdominal surgery. (**C**) Thoracoabdominal surgery. (**D**) Gynecologic surgery. (**E**) Genitourinary surgery. (**F**) Forearm, elbow, or hand surgery. (**G**) Hip surgery. (**H**) Lower leg or foot surgery.

Older Adult Undergoing Surgery

Because of *cardiovascular and tissue changes* associated with aging, surgeries lasting longer than 2 hours place the older adult at increased risk for complications. The older adult is more prone to hypotension, hypothermia, and hypoxemia resulting from anesthesia and the cool temperature in the operating room.

Intraoperative *positioning* of arthritic joints can result in postoperative joint pain that is unrelated to the surgical procedure. The older client is at increased risk for skin breakdown and delayed wound healing because of decreased subcutaneous fat tissue and reduced peripheral circulation. Elderly clients undergoing lengthy surgeries have increased risk of this complication.

Some older adults have *hearing or visual impairments*. Sensory impairments, coupled with an unfamiliar environment, can make the operating room a frightening, disorienting place. By effectively communicating with the client, the nurse can provide support and reassurance to minimize these factors.

is slightly wider than the planned incision in case the incision must be extended. Disposable, sterile supplies are used, in accordance with aseptic techniques. Hospital policy and surgeon preference should be followed.

Positioning

The client is positioned on the operating table for exposure of the operative site and access for administration of anesthesia (Table 9-5 ■). Careful positioning is crucial to prevent injury to the client. Pressure, rubbing, or shearing forces can damage the tissue over bony prominences. If normal joint range of motion is exceeded, muscle and joint injuries can occur. Improper positioning also can lead to sensory and motor dysfunction and nerve damage. Pressure on peripheral blood vessels can decrease venous return to the heart and negatively affect the blood pressure. Oxygenation of the blood can be decreased if lung expansion is impaired.

The anesthetized client cannot respond to discomfort. It is the surgical team's responsibility to position the client for the best surgical advantage and for safety and comfort. The circulating nurse follows agency policy, the surgeon's preference, and the client's history to ensure optimal positioning, and continuously assesses the client. Box 9-3 ■ lists special considerations for the older adult undergoing surgery.

NURSING CARE

Nurses assume many roles in caring for the client during the intraoperative phase. The nurse's focus, however, is on maintaining client safety. In addition to contributing to client assessment, the circulating nurse is responsible for monitoring surgical asepsis, counting sponges and instruments to ensure none are left in the surgical wound, and monitoring traffic flow within the room.

ASSESSING

The nurse verifies identity, the type and site of surgery, and previously obtained assessment data on receiving the client in the surgical suite. During the procedure, the nurse collaborates with the anesthesiologist or CRNA to collect and relate objective assessment data such as vital signs and peripheral pulses to the surgical team.

clinical ALERT

Carefully identify the client on admission to the operating room. Ensure that the surgical consent form accurately describes the scheduled procedure. Immediately inform all surgical personnel of any discrepancies.

DIAGNOSING, PLANNING, AND IMPLEMENTING

Priorities in Nursing Care. Maintaining the client's physiologic and psychologic safety is the priority of nursing care during the intraoperative period.

Risk for Perioperative Positioning Injury

- Assess for potential risk factors, including history of arthritis or other musculoskeletal disorders and lack of optimal tissue integrity due to aging or nutritional status. *Information provides a basis for planning and may direct modification of planned positioning.*
- Notify the surgeon if the planned position must be adjusted. *This ensures client safety yet provides the means to accomplish the surgical procedure.*
- Use safety belts to secure client to stretcher and operating room table, ensuring that distal circulation is unimpaired. *Belts reduce risk of falls when client's awareness is decreased.*
- Provide padding to bony prominences on clients at risk for tissue breakdown due to prolonged pressure. *Padding prevents excessive pressure on body parts.*

Risk for Infection

- Assess sterility of all instruments and supplies used in the operating room. *Surgical asepsis decreases risk of introducing pathogens during the surgical procedure.*
- Report results of lab studies that may indicate systemic infection or altered immune status. *Client may require prophylactic antibiotics.*
- Follow instructions related to surgical shaves and skin prep. *Preparation reduces bacteria at surgical site, but, if done improperly, may damage the skin, increasing the risk for infection.*
- Inform any member of the surgical team if breaks or potential breaks in technique are observed (e.g., tears in sterile gloves, contamination of equipment or surgical

TABLE 9-5

Common Surgical Positions

POSITION AND USE	POSSIBLE ADVERSE EFFECTS AND NURSING INTERVENTIONS
(a) The *dorsal recumbent* or *supine position* is used for abdominal surgeries, some thoracic surgeries, and some surgeries on the extremities. 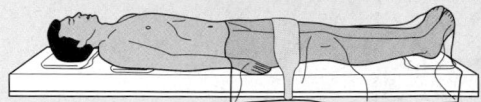	This position may cause excessive pressure on posterior bony prominences, such as the back of the head, scapulae, sacrum, and heels. Pad these areas with soft materials. To avoid compression of blood vessels and sluggish circulation, ensure that the knees are not flexed. Use trochanter rolls or other padding to avoid internal or external rotation of the hips and shoulders.
(b) The *semi-sitting position* is used for surgeries on the thyroid and neck areas. 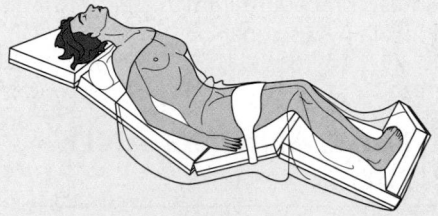	This position can lead to postural hypotension and venous pooling in the legs. It may promote skin breakdown on the buttocks. Sciatic nerve injury is possible. Assess for hypotension. Ensure that knees are not sharply flexed. Use soft padding to prevent nerve compression.
(c) The *prone position* may be used for spinal fusion and removal of hemorrhoids. 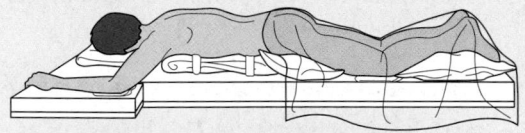	This position causes pressure on the face, knees, thighs, anterior ankles, and toes. Pad bony prominences, and support the feet under the ankles. To promote optimum respiratory function, raise the client's chest and abdomen and support with padding. Corneal abrasion could occur if the eyes are not closed or are insufficiently padded.
(d) The *lateral chest position* is used for some thoracic surgeries as well as hip replacements. 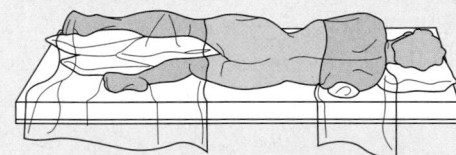	This may cause excessive pressure on the bony prominences on the side on which the client is positioned. Ensure adequate padding and support, especially on the downside arm. The weight of the upper leg may cause peroneal nerve injury on the downside leg. Both legs must therefore be padded.
(e) The *lithotomy position* is used for gynecologic, perineal, or rectal surgeries. 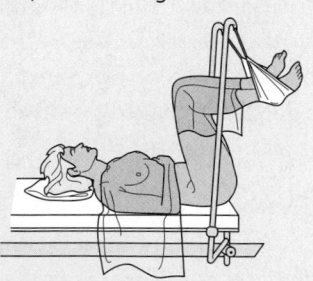	This position causes an 18% decrease (from a standing position) in vital capacity of the lungs. Monitor respirations, and assess for hypoxia and dyspnea. The lithotomy position can lead to joint damage, peroneal nerve damage, and damage to peripheral blood vessels. To avoid injury, ensure adequate padding, and manipulate both legs into the stirrups simultaneously.
(f) The *jackknife position* is used for proctologic surgeries, such as removal of hemorrhoids, and for some spinal surgeries. 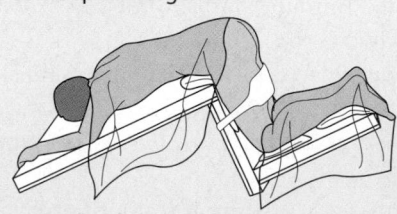	This position causes a 12% decrease (from a standing position) in vital capacity of the lungs. Monitor respirations, and assess for hypoxia and dyspnea. In this position, the greatest pressure is felt at the bends in the table. Therefore, the client is supported with pads at the groin and knees, as well as at the ankles. Padding of the chest and knees helps prevent skin breakdown. Padding and proper positioning help prevent pressure on the ear, the neck, and the nerves of the upper arm.

instruments). *The circulating nurse is responsible for ensuring strict aseptic technique is followed in the operating room.*

Risk for Imbalanced Body Temperature

Surgical clients are at risk for injury due to the cool environment of the operating room. Hyperthermia may occur from the effects of anesthesia, administration of cool intravenous fluids, or medications used during the intraoperative phase.

■ Assess temperature prior to induction of anesthesia. *This provides baseline data.*

■ Assess environmental temperature and client response. *Temperature can be modified to maintain client's body temperature.*

■ Note changes in temperature, and intervene as soon as possible (e.g., provide cooling or warming blanket). *Prompt response reduces risk for injury.*

Risk for Aspiration

■ Assess fasting status. *Data provide a basis for decision making about postponing or canceling surgery. A nasogastric tube may be inserted.*

■ Report consumption of food or fluids during the prescribed fasting period to the surgeon and anesthesiologist. *Surgery may be delayed or canceled.*

■ Insert nasogastric tube if ordered. *Clients requiring emergency surgery may have eaten. Anesthetic agents may also contribute to aspiration risk. Removal of stomach contents reduces risk of aspiration.*

EVALUATING

The nurse evaluates whether or not expected outcomes are met. Validation includes:

■ Client is free from injury during the intraoperative period.

■ Client's body temperature remains within normal limits during the intraoperative period.

■ No evidence of breaks in aseptic technique during the intraoperative period.

Documenting. Document assessment data, care provided, sponge and instrument counts, and any adverse events that occur during surgery using the appropriate forms.

Postoperative Phase

The postoperative phase of the surgical experience begins in the postanesthesia recovery unit (PACU) and ends when wound healing and functional recovery are complete.

POSTANESTHESIA RECOVERY

Postanesthesia recovery begins when the client is transferred from the operating room to the PACU. During this critical period, vital signs and the surgical site are carefully moni-

tored to determine the response to the surgical procedure, and to detect significant changes. Hydration status is carefully assessed and maintained to prevent cardiovascular and renal complications. Assessing mental status and level of consciousness are ongoing nursing responsibilities in the PACU. Pain level is assessed and managed through careful analgesic administration to promote comfort. The client may require repeated orientation to time, place, and person. Emotional support is essential during this vulnerable period.

WOUND HEALING

Healing varies, depending on factors such as age, nutritional status, general health, and the type and location of the wound.

Some tissues heal by cell regeneration; in others, connective scar tissue fills the wound to restore structural integrity of the surgical site. Wounds heal by primary, secondary, or tertiary intention (Figure 9-5 ■):

1. Healing by **primary intention** occurs when the wound is uncomplicated and clean and has sustained little

Primary intention

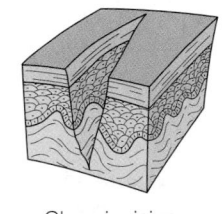 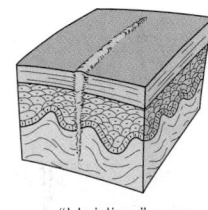

Clean incision   Early suture   "Hairline" scar

Secondary intention

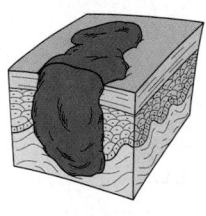 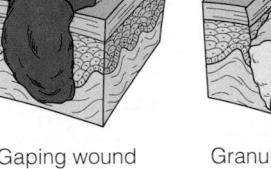 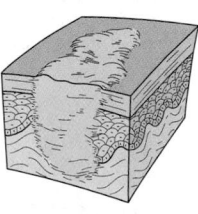

Gaping wound   Granulation tissue   Large scar
with blood clot   fills in wound

Tertiary intention

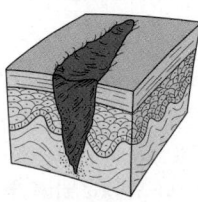 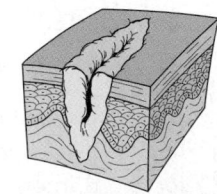 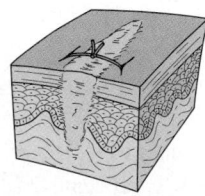

Contaminated wound   Granulation tissue   Closure with
                                               wide scar

Figure 9-5. ■ Wound healing by primary, secondary, and tertiary intention.

tissue loss. The edges of the incision are well *approximated* (have come together well) with sutures or staples. This type of incision heals quickly with very little scarring.

2. Healing by **secondary intention** occurs when the wound is large, gaping, and irregular. Tissue loss prevents approximation of wound edges, so the wound fills by granulation. This type of wound takes longer to heal, is more prone to infection, and develops more scar tissue.

3. Healing by **tertiary intention** occurs when substantial time passes before a wound is sutured. Infection is more likely. Wound edges are not approximated, so tissue is replaced by granulation. Closure of the wound may result in a wide scar.

Wound healing occurs in three phases: the inflammatory phase, the proliferative phase, and the remodeling phase.

The *inflammatory phase* begins with the surgical incision. Physiologic mechanisms to maintain hemostasis and promote blood clotting are activated. (See Chapter 29 ⬥ for more information about clotting processes.) Blood vessels initially constrict, then dilate and become more permeable to bring plasma and blood cells to the site. Phagocytic WBCs remove invading organisms and debris from the area. These cells also release growth factors to stimulate tissue repair.

The *proliferative phase* begins within 2 to 3 days after surgery. Fibroblasts (connective tissue cells that synthesize collagen, growth factors, and other wound healing elements) and vascular endothelial cells proliferate to form granulation tissue. This tissue initially is fragile and bleeds easily. Epithelial cells proliferate at the wound edges to form a new surface.

Sutures or staples are removed during this phase of wound healing. Wound strength is only about 10% of normal tissue strength at the time of their removal, but increases significantly during the next 4 weeks (Porth, 2005). Sutures or staples may be removed over a period of several days, with initial removal of every third suture/staple, then half of the remaining sutures/staples, and finally all remaining. Strips of tape or Steri-Strips may be used to maintain approximation of wound edges that are not fully healed.

During the *remodeling phase,* scar tissue is remodeled by a process of collagen synthesis and breakdown to increase its strength. This phase begins about 3 weeks after surgery and can continue for 6 or more months.

Wound Drainage

Wound drainage (*exudate*) results from the inflammatory process that occurs in the first two stages of wound healing. (See Chapter 10 ⬥ for more information about the inflammatory process.) The drainage is composed of escaped fluid and cells from the rich blood supply that surrounds the wound. Drainage is described as serous, sanguineous, or purulent:

- *Serous drainage* contains mostly the clear portion of the blood (serum). The drainage appears clear or slightly yellow and is thin in consistency.
- *Sanguineous drainage* contains a combination of serum and red blood cells and has a thick, reddish appearance. This is the most common drainage from an uncomplicated surgical wound.
- *Purulent drainage* is composed of white blood cells, tissue debris, and bacteria. Purulent drainage results from infection. Its consistency is greater than serous or sanguineous drainage, and the color varies by infecting organism. It may have an unpleasant odor. Purulent drainage should be reported to the surgeon.

Box 9-4 ■ describes and illustrates wound drainage devices that decrease pressure in the wound area by removing excess fluid.

COMMON POSTOPERATIVE COMPLICATIONS

A number of factors place the client at risk for postoperative complications. Nursing care before, during, and after surgery is aimed at preventing and/or minimizing the effects of these complications.

Cardiovascular Complications

HEMORRHAGE. **Hemorrhage** is excessive loss of blood. A *concealed* hemorrhage occurs internally from a bleeding vessel that is unsutured or that has been eroded by a drainage tube. An *obvious* hemorrhage occurs externally from a dislodged or ill-formed clot at the wound. Hemorrhage also may result from clotting abnormalities due to a coagulation disorder or medications.

A *venous* hemorrhage oozes out quickly and is dark red. An *arterial* hemorrhage is bright red blood that flows freely. Either type of hemorrhage will cause hypovolemic shock if enough blood is lost from the circulation.

Assessment findings depend on the amount and rate of blood loss. Restlessness and anxiety are observed in the early stage of hemorrhage. The heart rate is increased, but the blood pressure may remain normal. Frank bleeding may be obvious or may only be noted by turning or repositioning the client if blood pools under the back or buttocks. Manifestations of hypovolemic shock may be noted (see Box 13-3 ⬥).

SHOCK. **Shock** is a life-threatening postoperative complication that results from insufficient blood flow to vital organs. *Hypovolemic shock,* the most common type in the postoperative client, results from decreased circulating fluid volume from blood loss, severe vomiting, or prolonged diarrhea. The greater the loss of fluid volume, the more severe the symptoms.

DEEP VENOUS THROMBOSIS (DVT). *DVT* is the formation of a *thrombus* (blood clot) that develops in deep veins,

BOX 9-4

WOUND DRAINAGE DEVICES

A Penrose **drain** (see figure A below), used for passive wound drainage, promotes healing from the inside to the outside. The use of a drain decreases the risk of abscess formation. The safety pin in the Penrose drain prevents the exposed end from slipping down into the wound.

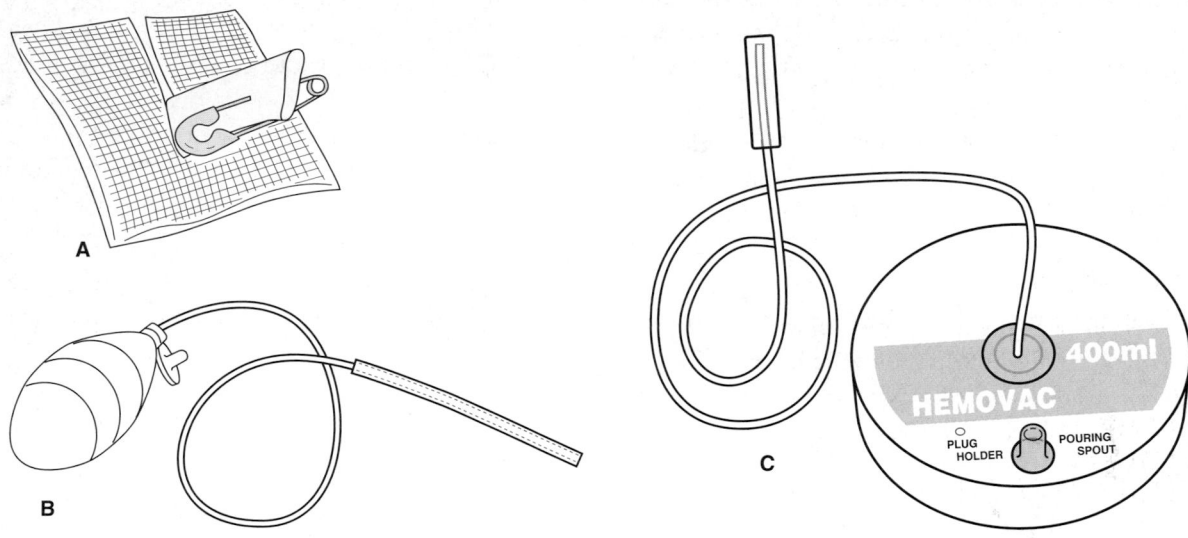

Wound care focuses on cleaning around the drain with a prescribed solution, such as sterile normal saline, and replacing the precut gauze dressing as necessary to keep the surrounding skin dry and to encourage further drainage. An absorbent dressing is placed over the drain and gauze (not shown).

Wound **suction** devices promote drainage of fluid from the wound, decreasing pressure on healing tissues and reducing abscess formation. Shown are the Jackson Pratt (figure B) and Hemovac (figure C) wound suction devices.

The frequency with which the device is emptied depends on the time elapsed since surgery, type of surgery, amount of drainage, and agency policy. For example, immediately after surgery the nurse may empty the device every 15 to 60 minutes. As drainage decreases, the device is emptied every 2 to 4 hours (per policy). Amount, color, consistency, and odor of drainage are documented.

Drains and suction devices usually are removed on the second to fourth day after surgery. Removal causes minor discomfort. Following removal, the drain site is cleaned, and a sterile dressing is applied.

usually of the lower extremities or pelvis. It may result from a combination of factors, including trauma during surgery, pressure applied under the knees, and sluggish blood flow during and after surgery. Risk factors for DVT include:

- Orthopedic surgery to lower extremities; urologic, gynecologic, or obstetric surgeries; or neurosurgery
- Varicose veins
- History of thrombophlebitis or pulmonary emboli
- Age over 40
- Obesity
- Infection
- Malignancy

Common assessment findings of DVT reveal pain or cramping in the involved calf or thigh. Redness, edema, and warmth of the entire extremity may be present. DVT also may be asymptomatic. A positive *Homans' sign* (pain in the calf on dorsiflexion of the affected foot; see Box 28-14 🔗) may be noted.

PULMONARY EMBOLISM. A *pulmonary embolism* is a blood clot or other substance that lodges in a pulmonary artery. It commonly occurs as a consequence of DVT, when a portion of the thrombus dislodges and travels to the lung. Other risk factors for pulmonary emboli include fat emboli (which may complicate large bone fracture or orthopedic surgeries) and amniotic fluid emboli, an obstetric complication.

Signs and symptoms of a pulmonary embolism include mild to moderate dyspnea, chest pain, diaphoresis, anxiety, restlessness, rapid respirations and pulse, dysrhythmias, cough, and cyanosis. Sudden death can occur if a major pulmonary artery is completely blocked.

Respiratory Complications

Common postoperative respiratory complications include pneumonia and atelectasis.

PNEUMONIA. *Pneumonia* (inflammation of lung tissue) is caused either by infection or by inflammation due to a foreign substance in the lung. Retained pulmonary secretions due to an ineffective cough and decreased mobility are the most common risk factor in surgical clients. Other risk factors include aspiration of oral or gastric secretions and an impaired cough reflex due to endotracheal intubation or anesthetic drugs.

Manifestations of pneumonia include (see also Table 24-1 ⊙⊙):

- Moderate to high fever
- Rapid pulse and respirations
- Chills (may be present initially)
- Productive cough (depending on the type of pneumonia)
- Dyspnea
- Chest pain
- Crackles and wheezes.

Treating the infection, supporting respiratory efforts, promoting lung expansion, and preventing the organisms' spread are the goals in caring for the client with pneumonia.

ATELECTASIS. Atelectasis is incomplete expansion or collapse of lung tissue. It results in inadequate ventilation and retained pulmonary secretions. Assessment findings commonly observed include dyspnea, diminished breath sounds over the affected area, anxiety, restlessness, crackles, and cyanosis. Promoting lung expansion and systemic tissue oxygenation is a goal in the care of the client with atelectasis (see also Chapter 24 ⊙⊙).

Elimination Complications

Common postoperative complications associated with elimination include urinary retention (see Chapter 32 ⊙⊙) and altered bowel elimination (see Chapter 20 ⊙⊙). Urinary retention may occur due to postoperative positioning, the effects of anesthesia and narcotics, inactivity, altered fluid balance, anxiety, or surgical manipulation in the pelvic area.

Bowel elimination frequently is altered after abdominal or pelvic surgery. Return to normal gastrointestinal function may be delayed by general anesthesia, narcotic analgesia, decreased mobility, or altered fluid and food intake during the perioperative period. It is important to frequently assess bowel sounds and abdominal distention, and to ambulate the client as early as possible to encourage normal gastrointestinal function.

Wound Complications

INFECTION. Despite all the measures designed to prevent contamination of the surgical wound, infection is a common complication. Other common assessment findings of an infected wound include redness, warmth, and edema around the edges of the incision. The client may have a fever, chills, and increased respiratory and pulse rates.

DEHISCENCE. Dehiscence is separation of the incision (Figure 9-6A ■). When dehiscence occurs, the wound

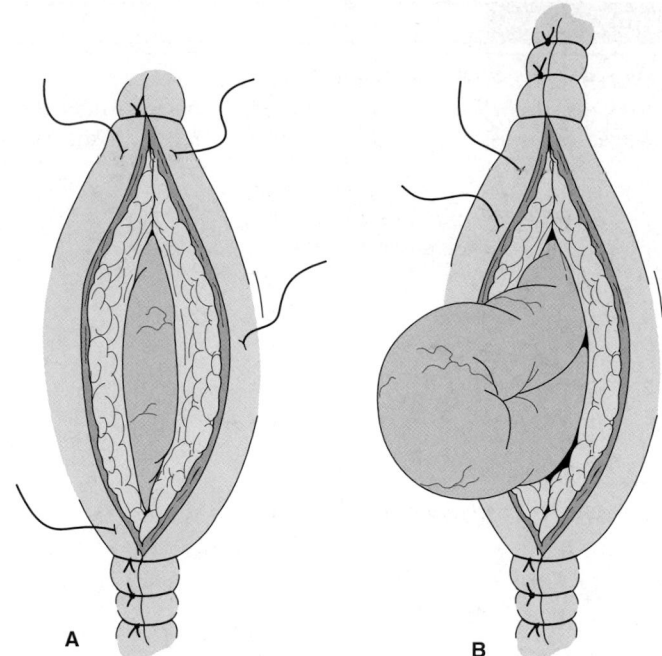

Figure 9-6. ■ Wound complications. (**A**) Dehiscence. (**B**) Evisceration.

should be covered immediately with a sterile dressing moistened with normal saline and the surgeon notified. Treatment depends on the extent of wound disruption. If the dehiscence is extensive, the client returns to surgery for wound closure.

EVISCERATION. Evisceration is the protrusion of body organs from a wound dehiscence (see Figure 9-6B). Like dehiscence, this serious complication may occur immediately following surgery, after forceful straining (coughing, sneezing, or vomiting), or may result from delayed wound healing. Protruding organs are covered with moist sterile dressings or towels and the surgeon is notified. Emergency surgery is necessary to repair evisceration.

Special Considerations for Older Adults

The older adult is at increased risk for postoperative complications because of physiologic, cognitive, and psychosocial changes associated with aging. The nursing care plan is modified to account for these normal changes and provide for safe, supportive care. Sensory deprivation is responsible for much of the confusion experienced by the older adult. Eyeglasses and hearing aids should be returned to the client as soon as possible after surgery. Early ambulation is vital to prevent complications associated with immobility (pneumonia, skin and tissue breakdown). The older adult's nutritional status often is compromised prior to surgery; prompt reinstitution of feeding is vital to promote wound healing, immune function, and recovery.

INTERDISCIPLINARY CARE

Diagnostic Tests

Diagnostic tests commonly ordered during the postoperative period include:

- *Hemoglobin* and *hematocrit* to monitor for undetected bleeding
- *Serum osmolarity* and *electrolytes* to evaluate fluid volume status and electrolyte balance
- *Blood glucose levels,* particularly in diabetic clients, to monitor the effects of stress and blood glucose management
- *Therapeutic drug levels* if antibiotic therapy is ordered
- *Chest x-ray* if manifestations of pneumonia, atelectasis, or heart failure develop
- *Oxygen saturation levels* are monitored continuously in the initial postoperative period to ensure adequate tissue oxygenation.

Medications

Management of acute postoperative pain is of primary concern to the client, surgeon, and nurse. Established, severe pain is more difficult to treat than pain that is at its onset. Initially, postoperative analgesics are administered at regular intervals or via a patient-controlled analgesia (PCA) device to maintain a therapeutic blood level. As-needed (prn) administration allows blood levels to fall below the therapeutic range; delays in medication administration further increase pain intensity and make its management more difficult. (Chapter 8 discusses care of the client in acute pain.)

Nonsteroidal anti-inflammatory drugs (NSAIDs) (e.g., ibuprofen, ketorolac tromethamine [Toradol]) are administered to treat mild to moderate postoperative pain and as adjuncts to opioid analgesics. They should be given soon after surgery (orally, parenterally, or rectally) along with opioids unless contraindicated. NSAIDs allow for lower dosages of opioid analgesics and, therefore, fewer side effects. Certain NSAIDs, such as ketorolac, when given in higher doses after surgery, may only be administered safely for 2 to 3 days before the dosage must be reduced. NSAIDs can be given safely to older clients, but the nurse should observe closely for side effects, especially gastric, hepatic, and renal toxicity.

Opioid analgesics, such as morphine and its derivatives, are the foundation for managing moderate to severe postoperative pain. Opioid dosage requirements vary greatly from one client to another, so the dosage must be individually tailored.

Contrary to the belief of many health care providers, physical dependence and tolerance to opioid analgesics are uncommon in short-term postoperative use. Also, when opioid analgesics are used to treat acute pain, they rarely lead to psychologic dependence and addiction.

Older clients tend to experience a higher peak effect and longer duration of pain control with opioids, therefore, the older client should be monitored closely for signs of respiratory depression.

Fluid and Nutrition Management

Fluids commonly are administered intravenously until the client is fully awake and bowel sounds are present. Balanced electrolyte solutions are commonly used to prevent electrolyte imbalance related to fasting. Potassium chloride may be added to the intravenous solution if nasogastric suction is in place or fasting will be prolonged. (See Chapter 7 ⬭ for more information about intravenous fluid management.)

Oral fluids and feeding are resumed as soon as possible, based on the type of surgery performed, the client's mental status, and resumption of peristalsis. Recent studies have shown a significant risk for protein-calorie malnutrition (PCM) in the postoperative client when fasting is necessary for 12 or more hours. PCM slows wound healing and impairs immune defenses, increasing the risk for postoperative complications. Total parenteral nutrition may be required for clients who are unable to resume oral intake for several days or more. See Chapter 19 ⬭ for more information about PCM, total parenteral nutrition, and the nurse's role in caring for clients with nutritional disorders.

Other Therapies

Oxygen may be administered in the initial postoperative period to support tissue oxygenation and healing. Use of the incentive spirometer often is prescribed hourly (during waking hours) for the first 24 hours, then at least every 2 hours until discharge. The incentive spirometer promotes deep breathing and lung expansion, helping prevent pneumonia and atelectasis.

NURSING CARE

Nursing care of the postoperative client focuses on preventing and monitoring for wound complications, as well as complications involving other organ systems. Once stable and awake, the client is transferred from the PACU to the care unit. The PACU nurse communicates information about client's condition and postoperative orders to the unit nurse.

ASSESSING

After major surgery, the client is assessed every 15 minutes during the first hour and, if stable, every 30 minutes for the next 2 hours, and then every hour during the subsequent 4 hours. Then assessments are carried out every 4 hours, unless the client's condition changes or protocol dictates a more frequent schedule

- *Subjective data:* pain (location, intensity, duration, character), effect of analgesia; presence of nausea or other noxious sensations; ability to deep breathe, use incentive spirometer, move in bed or from bed to chair; other concerns.
- *Objective data:* level of consciousness, mental status; skin color, temperature, moisture; vital signs including temperature and oxygen saturation; breath sounds and depth; bowel sounds, abdominal distention, tenderness; operative site, including condition of wound and dressings, surrounding tissues, presence of drainage, evidence of active bleeding (may require checking under the back or buttocks); peripheral vascular assessment as indicated, including pulse strength and equality, capillary refill, color and temperature, presence of edema, movement and sensation
- *Laboratory results:* hemoglobin and hematocrit; serum glucose, electrolytes, and osmolality; any abnormal values or significant changes from preoperative or expected results.

DIAGNOSING, PLANNING, AND IMPLEMENTING

After the initial assessment and ensuring the client's safety (lowering the bed, raising the side rails, and placing the call light within reach), the nurse reviews the postoperative orders. Specific orders to be noted include: activity level, diet, medications for pain and nausea, antibiotics (if ordered), continuation of preoperative medications, frequency of vital sign assessments, administration of intravenous fluids, and laboratory tests. In most institutions, preoperative orders must be specifically reordered following surgery because the client's condition is assumed to have changed. If a previously ordered drug for a chronic condition (such as a cardiac drug or insulin) is not included in the postoperative orders, it is the nurse's responsibility to contact the physician to ensure that discontinuation of the drug was intended, not unintentional.

Priorities in Nursing Care. Nursing care priorities during the postoperative phase are pain management, prevention of postoperative complications, and teaching the client and family about post-discharge care.

Acute Pain

Pain is expected after surgery. Pain management involves the interdisciplinary care team, including the client, physician, and nurse. Managing acute postoperative pain is an important nursing role and responsibility. The client should be made aware of how much pain to anticipate, the importance of relieving postoperative pain to recovery, and methods available to relieve pain (see Chapter 8). ⚭ After discussing options with the client, health care providers must respect the client's personal preferences.

- Assess level of pain at least hourly during the initial postoperative period, then at least every 4 hours or whenever vital signs are obtained. Have patient describe pain on a scale of 0 to 10 (where 0 is no pain and 10 is the worst pain). *Controlling postoperative pain not only promotes comfort but also facilitates coughing, turning, deep-breathing exercises, early ambulation, and healing. Rating the pain provides a more objective description and helps the nurse to choose pain medication appropriate to severity of the pain.*
- Identify location and source of pain. *Assessment data are used to plan interventions. Identifying the location of the pain is important to distinguish between expected pain related to the surgery and pain associated with potential complications such as pneumonia or angina.*
- Administer pain medication as prescribed. *Medication provides comfort and allows the client to rest. Regular analgesic administration maintains a therapeutic blood level for more effective pain relief.*
- Initiate nonpharmacologic approaches to pain management such as relaxation, distraction, and imagery techniques. *These techniques complement pain medication.*
- Evaluate effectiveness of pain medication within 30 to 45 minutes of administration. *Effectiveness may indicate a need for change of dosage or medication.*
- Document administration of pain medication. Communicate to all members of the health care team. *Documentation and communication ensure continuity of care.*

Risk for Injury (Hemorrhage)

- Apply one or more sterile gauze pads and a snug pressure dressing to the area. If external bleeding is severe, apply mechanical pressure with gloved hands. *Pressure assists the coagulation process. Increased pressure may be necessary to achieve coagulation.*
- Notify physician of excessive bleeding or a fall in hemoglobin or hematocrit levels. *Medical intervention is needed to correct the complication.*
- Monitor vital signs, level of consciousness, skin color and temperature frequently. *Data are used to assess physiologic response to the event.*

clinical ALERT

Promptly report vital signs outside the client's normal or expected range. Tachycardia may be an early sign of internal hemorrhage.

- Establish or maintain intravenous access. *Rapid infusion of fluids may be necessary to maintain or replace fluid volume.*
- Monitor urine output. Report output less than 30 mL per hour to the charge nurse or physician. *Low urine output may be an early sign of decreased cardiac output due to blood loss.*
- Prepare client and family for emergency surgery. *Surgery may be necessary to locate and repair the source of bleeding.*

Ineffective Tissue Perfusion

Deep venous thrombosis in the postoperative client usually results from venous stasis related to immobility. Nursing care focuses on preventing this potentially life-threatening complication.

- Assess peripheral pulses, color and temperature of extremities, and Homans' sign at least every 4 hours. Report changes or abnormal findings to the physician. *This provides early detection of signs of DVT.*
- Encourage postoperative leg exercises at least every 2 hours. Encourage early ambulation. *Exercise prevents venous stasis, and enhances venous return.*
- Administer anticoagulants as prescribed. *Anticoagulants prevent platelet aggregation and decrease the risk of clot formation.*
- Monitor laboratory values for clotting times. *This information is used to determine dosage of anticoagulant medications.*
- Apply thigh-high antiemboli stockings or pneumatic compression devices as ordered. *Antiembolism stockings and pneumatic compression devices promote venous return.*

Impaired Gas Exchange (Pulmonary Embolus)

- Frequently assess and record general condition and vital signs. *Frequent assessment allows early detection of manifestations of pulmonary embolism or other respiratory complications.*
- Immediately notify the charge nurse and physician if manifestations of impaired gas exchange or pulmonary embolism develop. *Stabilizing respiratory and cardiovascular functioning is vital to protect physiologic function. Intensive care and monitoring are critical.*
- Maintain bed rest, with the head of the bed elevated. *This position facilitates breathing and promotes gas exchange.*
- Provide oxygen as ordered and monitor oxygen saturation. *This supports respiratory status and detects a deteriorating condition early.*
- Administer prescribed intravenous fluids. *Circulating volume must be maintained.*
- Administer prescribed anticoagulants. *This prevents development of additional clots.*

Ineffective Breathing Pattern

- Assess vital signs, breath sounds, and general condition. *Clients who are chronically ill or malnourished, who have a history of chronic lung disease, and the elderly are at increased risk for these complications. Data allow early detection and evaluation of treatment.*
- Elevate the head of the bed. *This facilitates lung expansion.*
- Encourage the client to turn, cough, and perform deep-breathing exercises at least every 2 hours. *This mobilizes secretions and supports airway clearance.*
- Assist with and encourage incentive spirometry and nebulizer treatments as ordered. *These expand alveoli and facilitate airway clearance.*

- Ambulate as condition permits and as prescribed. *Ambulation reduces the risk of complications related to immobility.*
- Maintain fluid intake to at least 2,000 mL/day if condition permits. *Fluid liquefies secretions for easier clearance.*

Risk for Infection (Surgical Incision)

- Assess vital signs, including temperature. *Elevated pulse, respirations, or temperature may indicate infection.*
- Assess the incision (approximation of the edges, sutures, staples, or drains) and surrounding tissue. *Integrity of the incision site reduces risk factors. Redness, warmth, or edema of the incision or surrounding tissue may indicate infection.*
- Evaluate wound discharge (color, odor, and amount). *Purulent sound drainage may indicate the presence of wound infection.*
- Maintain medical asepsis (use good handwashing technique) and standard precautions. Use aseptic technique during dressing changes and handling of tubes and drains. *Asepsis reduces risk of introducing microorganisms into surgical wounds.*
- Maintain hydration and nutritional status. *Nutrition facilitates healing.*

Risk for Urinary Retention

- Assess for bladder distention if the client has not voided within 7 to 8 hours after surgery or if the client is urinating small amounts frequently. *Early detection of urinary retention provides information for intervention.*
- Increase daily oral fluid intake to 2,500 to 3,000 mL as condition permits. *This facilitates renal function.*
- Insert a straight or indwelling catheter if ordered. *Emptying the bladder provides comfort.*
- Assist patient to void by:
  - Assisting and providing privacy when the client uses a bedpan.
  - Helping the client to use the bedside commode or to walk to the bathroom.
  - Assisting male clients to stand to void.

These measures help promote normal urinary elimination.

Risk for Constipation

- Auscultate bowel sounds every 4 hours while client is awake. Assess the abdomen for distention. Determine whether the client is passing flatus. Monitor for passage of stool, including amount and consistency. *A distended abdomen with absent bowel sounds may indicate paralytic ileus. These measures evaluate presence or absence of peristalsis.*
- Encourage early ambulation within prescribed limits. *Mobility stimulates peristalsis.*
- Facilitate a daily fluid intake of 2,500 to 3,000 mL unless contraindicated. *Fluids provide moisture and facilitate passage of stool.*

- Provide privacy when the client is using the bedpan, bedside commode, or bathroom. *Privacy provides relaxation and facilitates bowel elimination.*

EVALUATING

Careful evaluation of the postoperative client's progress is essential to prevent development of complications and prompt intervention should they occur. Expected outcomes include:

- Client is free of wound or systemic infection.
- Remains free of manifestations of venous thrombosis.
- Oxygen saturation remains at least 90%.
- Client voids within 6 hours of return from surgery and at least 1,000 mL in 24 hours.
- Breath sounds remain clear.
- Client performs incentive spirometry exercises at least every 4 hours.
- Bowel sounds are active in all four quadrants within 24 hours of abdominal surgery.

Documenting. Document initial postoperative and continuing assessments, including any abnormal or unexpected data. When the physician or charge nurse is notified of abnormal or unexpected data, document notification and the care provider's response. Document pain level with vital signs, noting the effectiveness of analgesia and other pain relief measures. Note appearance of the surgical wound, including presence of any bleeding or drainage on the dressing or within the wound. Document intake and output, including intravenous fluids, oral intake, urinary output, drainage from wound suction devices, and any emesis or abnormal fluid losses. Note ability and willingness to ambulate and assume self-care activities. Document all teaching and the client's and family's understanding and ability to demonstrate care.

CONTINUING CARE

Because the postoperative phase does not end until recovery is complete, the nurse's role is vital as the client nears discharge. To prepare the client to recuperate at home, provide information and support as needed for self-care. Written guidelines, directions, and information should accompany all aspects of teaching, especially when teaching involves a large amount of unfamiliar detail. The nurse must be organized in order to educate the client and family during the brief hospital stay. The most common teaching needs are as follows:

- *Wound care.* Demonstrate and explain the procedure, then ask the client and family to participate in care. Have the client or caregiver demonstrate the procedure in return. Ideally, teaching is carried out over several days, evaluated, and reinforced.
- *Manifestations of a wound infection.* Teach the client what is normal and what should be reported to the physician.

- *How and when to take a temperature.*
- *Limitations or restrictions on activities* (lifting, driving, bathing, sexual activity, return to work or school, and other physical activities).
- *Control of pain.* If analgesics are prescribed, discuss the dosage, frequency, purpose, common side effects, and symptoms to report to the physician. Reinforce the use of relaxation, distraction, imagery, or other pain-control techniques that the client has found useful in controlling postoperative pain.

Ambulatory Surgery

Ambulatory (also called *outpatient* or *same-day*) *surgery* is performed on a nonhospitalized client under local or general anesthesia or conscious sedation. Many surgical procedures are performed in an ambulatory care setting. The client may be discharged immediately after the procedure, or remain for a short period of postoperative recovery and observation. Surgeries such as cataract removal with or without lens implant, hernia repair, tubal ligation, vasectomy, dilation and curettage (D&C), and biopsy are routinely performed on an outpatient basis. More complicated procedures such as laparoscopic gallbladder removal and simple mastectomy may also be performed on an outpatient basis. The client's responses following surgery drive the decision for discharge or admission to a short-stay unit (less than 24 hours) or an inpatient facility for further observation.

Ambulatory surgery has advantages and disadvantages. The client recovers more quickly in the home and is less likely to be exposed to pathogens that could lead to a wound infection. Disadvantages include limited time and opportunity for assessment of client needs and teaching for home care. The increased number and complexity of procedures and client acuity present a challenge to the perioperative nurse.

Many similarities exist in nursing care of the inpatient and ambulatory surgical client. Physical care is provided in much the same manner in the preoperative, intraoperative, and postoperative phases of surgery. Postanesthesia care focuses on restoring hemodynamic status and recovery from anesthesia. The client returns from the PACU to the ambulatory surgery unit for monitoring and teaching for discharge.

The major differences are in the extent of teaching and emotional support that must be provided. The ambulatory surgical client must cope with additional stress produced by the need to learn a great deal of information in a short span of time. The nurse teaches self-care to the client and family in both the preoperative and postoperative periods. Clients with complicated health problems or who are undergoing complex surgical procedures require more extensive teaching and emotional support. Figure 9-7 ■ shows a standard outpatient care plan form.

OUTPATIENT CARE PLAN

Outpatient Surgery Center
Directions: Each unit, please check "Yes" or "No" and initial appropriate space in column on right.

Client's Name _____ Date _____

NURSING DIAGNOSES	CLIENT OUTCOME STANDARDS	Goal Met	OPTI	PREOP	OR	PACU	OBS
I. A. Anxiety related to knowledge deficit regarding surgical procedure. B. Fear related to risk of death, alteration of body image, or change in lifestyle. C. Impaired verbal communication related to anxiety. D. Impaired verbal communication related to preoperative medication/sedation. E. Impaired verbal communication related to language barrier. F. Ineffective individual or family coping related to perceived threat of surgery or surgical outcome. G. Noncompliance related to sensory alteration, fear, anxiety. H. Sensory–perceptual alteration related to inadequate tissue perfusion, or preexisting deficits.	**I.** The client demonstrates knowledge of the physiologic and psychological responses to surgical intervention. Comments _____	Yes No					
II. A. Potential for infection related to: Type of operative procedure Wound classification Tissues transected Length of procedure Preexisting disease process Obesity Length of preoperative hospitalization Implants Presence/insertion of invasive/indwelling lines	**II.** The client is free from infection. Comments _____	Yes No					
III. A. Potential for impaired skin integrity related to: Positioning Preexisting disease process Pooling of prep solutions under client Improper placement of electrical dispersive pad Impaired circulation Poor tissue perfusion Allergic reactions to chemical agents	**III.** The client's skin integrity is maintained. Comments _____	Yes No					
IV. A. Potential for injury related to: Electrical hazards Positioning Retained foreign objects External constriction of peripheral circulation Chemical agents (ETO or Glutaraldehyde residuals, irritants, allergans) B. Impaired gas exchange related to: Positioning Inadequate airway Obesity C. Impaired physical mobility related to positioning.	**IV.** The client is free from injury related to positioning; extraneous objects; or chemical, physical, and electrical hazards. Comments _____	Yes No					
V. A. Potential for fluid and electrolyte imbalance related to: Type of surgical procedure Excessive blood loss Shock, trauma	**V.** The client's fluid and electrolyte balance is maintained. Comments _____	Yes No					
VI. A. Potential for altered or ineffective participation in rehabilitation related to: Ineffective coping mechanisms Anxiety due to surgical outcomes Lack of resources for self-care after discharge	**VI.** The client participates in the rehabilitation process. Comments _____	Yes No					

Figure 9-7. ■ Outpatient care plan form. (Courtesy of Southwest Texas Methodist Hospital.)

Following ambulatory surgery, the client is discharged when the institution's criteria are met. Discharge criteria may include:

- Vital signs stable.
- Able to stand and walk without dizziness or nausea.
- Pain controlled or alleviated.
- Able to urinate.

- Oriented or returned to preoperative mental status.
- Client and family/caregiver demonstrate understanding of postoperative instructions.

Note: The bibliography listings for this and all chapters have been compiled at the back of the book.

Chapter Review

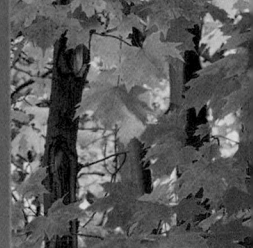

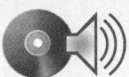 **KEY TERMS** by Topics

Use the audio glossary feature of either the CD-ROM or the Companion Website to hear the correct pronunciation of the following key terms.

Types and settings for surgery
inpatient surgery, ambulatory surgery

Informed consent
informed consent, emancipated minors

Phases of the surgical experience
preoperative phase, intraoperative phase, postoperative phase

Intraoperative phase
anesthesia, conscious sedation

Postoperative Phase
primary intention, secondary intention, tertiary intention, hemorrhage, shock, dehiscence, evisceration

KEY Points

- Perioperative nursing includes care of the client through three phases: preoperative, intraoperative, postoperative.
- Care of the surgical client should focus on psychologic as well as physiologic risk factors.
- Thorough nursing assessment is key to identifying potential risk factors that may lead to perioperative complications.
- Nursing interventions are developed to prevent development of perioperative complications.
- Control of postoperative pain is a major concern of the surgical client.
- Patient education is a critical tool to prepare the client for the perioperative experience. Inclusion of family members and caregivers is essential for success of the nursing plan of care.
- Major postoperative complications include respiratory and cardiovascular disorders, infection, hemorrhage, and elimination disorders.
- Collaboration of all members of the health care team is essential to achieve an optimal outcome for the surgical client.

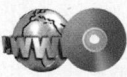 **Explore MediaLink**

Additional interactive resources for this chapter can be found on the Companion Website at www.prenhall.com/burke. Click on Chapter 9 and "Begin" to select the activities for this chapter.

For chapter-related NCLEX-style review questions and an audio glossary, access the accompanying CD-ROM in this book.

FOR FURTHER Study

See Chapter 7 for more information about fluid management.

For more information about assessing and managing pain in clients, see Chapter 8.

Chapter 10 covers inflammation and infections.

Shock is discussed in detail in Chapter 13.

See Chapter 19 for more information about nutritional disorders.

For further study about nursing care of constipation and bowel preparation for surgery, see Chapter 20.

For more about promoting lung expansion and systemic oxygenation, see Chapter 24.

For assessment of Homans' sign, see Box 28-15.

For more information about clotting processes, see Chapter 29.

For more information about urinary retention, see Chapter 32.

Critical Thinking Care Map

Caring for a Client after Surgery
NCLEX-PN® Focus Area: Safety and Infection Control

Case Study: Mrs. Wilson, age 80, is 3 days post total hip replacement of her right hip. Daniel Moore, LPN, is assigned to her care. Mr. Moore performs a complete head-to-toe assessment and determines that Mrs. Wilson is alert and oriented. Her skin is warm and moist. Mrs. Wilson states she has slight discomfort with incisional pain of 3 on a scale of 0-to-10. She complains of feeling alternately warm and chilled. Vital signs are T 101°F, P 100, R 24, BP 134/82. She is on a soft diet and states she is "drinking lots of fluids." An intravenous solution of dextrose and water is infusing at 100 mL/hr per infusion pump. No redness or edema is noted at the infusion site. Mrs. Wilson is receiving ciprofloxacin hydrochloride (Cipro) PO every 8 hours. She has a gauze dressing to the right hip incision. The dressing is intact with a 3-cm area of light brown drainage. Mr. Moore removes the dressing and notes the incision is red and edematous with a 2-cm opening. Steri-Strips are in place, and a Jackson Pratt drain is in place. Mr. Moore empties 25 mL of dark red drainage from the device. Mrs. Wilson has a Foley catheter in place with 250 mL of clear, light amber urine in the bag.

When assessing Mrs. Wilson's lower extremities, Mr. Moore finds her feet pink and warm with rapid capillary refill. Dorsalis pedis and posterior tibial pulses are strong and equal bilaterally. Mr. Moore notes slight pitting edema in the right foot and ankle. Sensation and ability to move both extremities are noted. Review of lab work reveals Hgb 11.3 g, Hct 38.4%, WBC 13,000 mm^3.

Nursing Diagnosis: Risk for Infection

COLLECT DATA

Subjective	Objective
_____	_____
_____	_____
_____	_____
_____	_____

Would you report this data? Yes/No

If yes, to: _____

Nursing Care

_____
_____
_____
_____
_____
_____

How would you document this? _____
_____
_____

Data Collected
(use those that apply)

- Alert and oriented
- Incisional pain
- T 101°F, P 100
- Jackson Pratt drain in place
- WBC 13,000 mm^3
- IV infusing at 100 mL/hr
- Pedal pulses strong
- Light brown drainage on dressing
- Foley has 250 mL clear, light amber urine
- Incision red, edematous, 2-cm opening
- Complains of feeling warm and has chills
- Cipro 250 mg q 8 hr
- States she is "drinking lots of fluids"

Nursing Interventions
(use those that apply; list in priority order)

- Empty Jackson Pratt drain q 4 hr.
- Monitor vital signs, especially temperature and pulse, q 4 hr. Report temperature above 100°F to charge nurse.
- Assess pedal pulses q 8 hr.
- Provide extra blankets for warmth.
- Change dressing, using aseptic technique, twice per day.
- Assess wound status with each dressing change.
- Tylenol 325 mg PO q 4 hr for temperature above 100°F.
- Cleanse wound with normal saline qd, per physician's order.
- Monitor urinary output.
- Maintain fluid intake at least 2,000 mL/day.
- Administer pain medications as needed.
- Administer antibiotics as ordered.
- Collect sample of wound drainage, send to lab for culture and sensitivity.

NCLEX-PN® Exam Preparation

1 A client is scheduled for a thyroidectomy. Which of the following would be an appropriate preoperative nursing diagnosis?

A. *Infection, Risk for* (surgical wound)
B. *Aspiration, Risk for*
C. *Deficient Knowledge* (surgical procedure)
D. *Urinary Retention*

2 A man is admitted to the ambulatory surgery unit in preparation for a hernia repair. Which of the following lab results noted by the nurse may require medical intervention?

A. hemoglobin 13.4, hematocrit 44
B. potassium 2.8
C. platelets 280,000
D. blood urea nitrogen (BUN) 10

3 A client asks the nurse to explain possible complications she might experience as a result of her total abdominal hysterectomy. The most appropriate response by the nurse would be:

A. "I will contact your physician to discuss this with you."
B. "Let's not worry about complications. You will be just fine."
C. "Why are you worried about complications?"
D. "There are many potential complications. Let's discuss them."

4 A client is 5 hours postoperative. He has an IV infusing at 125 mL/hr. He has not voided and complains of pain in his lower abdomen. All of the following are appropriate nursing actions. Place them in the order in which the nurse would perform them.

A. Assist Mr. Harris to stand to void.
B. Assess the bladder for distention.
C. Notify the physician of inability to void.
D. Prepare to perform a straight catheterization.
E. Run water in the sink.

5 A client has been taught coughing exercises prior to surgery. Which one of the following actions indicates a need for further teaching?

A. He splints his incision with a pillow.
B. He takes a deep breath through his nose prior to coughing.
C. He positions himself supine and flat in bed.
D. He coughs forcefully after the deep breath.

6 The client's surgical incision is healing by primary intention. Which assessment finding should the nurse expect?

A. Wound edges are approximated.
B. Wound exudate is present.

C. The wound is large, gaping, and irregular.
D. Granulation tissue is evident.

7 A teenage girl, age 16, and her husband, age 23, present to the outpatient center to complete her preoperative procedures. The appropriate procedure for completion of the surgical consent would be to:

A. have the husband sign the consent for the wife.
B. have the girl sign the consent.
C. have the husband co-sign the consent.
D. contact the girl's parents to sign the consent.

8 The nurse assesses a postoperative client on return to the nursing unit. The following data are collected:

    1:15 P.M.: T 99°F, P 92, R 20, BP 120/80, alert, oriented
    1:30 P.M.: T 98°F, P 100, R 24, BP 116/68, sleeping
    1:45 P.M.: T 98°F, P 116, R 28, BP 100/54, restless
    2:00 P.M.: T 97°F, P 130, R 32, BP 90/50, restless, drowsy

The appropriate INITIAL nursing action would be to:

A. assess the surgical dressing.
B. notify the physician.
C. position the client flat with the feet elevated 8 to 12 inches.
D. increase the IV infusion rate.

9 A client had a right total hip replacement 3 days ago. The LPN/LVN assesses a positive Homans' sign in the left leg. The MOST important action by the nurse at this time would be to:

A. document the findings.
B. notify the physician.
C. place the client on complete bed rest.
D. assess the extremity for signs of thrombus formation.

10 A client asks if she should take her medications for hypertension and diabetes the morning of surgery. The MOST appropriate response by the nurse would be:

A. "No, the anesthesiologist will monitor your blood pressure and blood glucose."
B. "NPO means nothing by mouth."
C. "Yes, take them with no more than a glass of water."
D. "I will clarify this with your physician."

Answers for Review Questions, as well as discussion of Care Plan and Critical Thinking Care Map questions, appear in Appendix V.

Chapter 10

Caring for Clients with Inflammation and Infection

BRIEF Outline

Inflammation
Pathophysiology
Interdisciplinary Care

Infection
Pathophysiology
Interdisciplinary Care

LEARNING Outcomes

After completing this chapter, you will be able to:

- Explain the steps of the inflammatory process.
- State the five cardinal manifestations of acute inflammation.
- State the purpose of diagnostic tests used to identify inflammation and infection.
- Describe the chain of infection.
- Identify common nosocomial infections.
- Explain age-related changes in older adults that increase their risk for infection.
- Identify the common antimicrobial medications, nursing implications, and client teaching guidelines.
- Describe the guidelines for Standard and Transmission-based Precautions.
- Use the nursing process to collect data, establish outcomes, provide individualized care, and evaluate responses for clients with inflammation and infections.

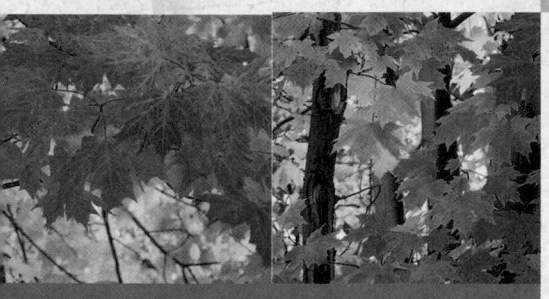

MediaLink

www.prenhall.com/burke
Use the address above to access the free, interactive Companion Website created for this textbook. Get hints, instant feedback, and textbook references to chapter-related NCLEX-style questions. Link to other interesting sites.

Audio Glossary:
Use the Companion Website, or the CD-ROM disk enclosed with your textbook, to hear the pronunciation of key terms in this chapter.

Inflammation

Inflammation is a "nonspecific" response to an injury, meaning the same sequence of events occurs regardless of the cause. Inflammation brings fluid, dissolved substances, and blood cells into the interstitial tissues where an injury has occurred. Its purpose is to destroy the harmful agent, limit spread to other tissues, and begin the healing process. Inflammation develops as soon as one or more harmful invaders injure the body's cells.

PATHOPHYSIOLOGY

Normally, the skin and mucous membranes act as the body's first line of defense, preventing an invasion by external organisms. Mucous membranes lining the inner surfaces of the body trap microorganisms and other foreign substances. These are removed by other protective mechanisms such as ciliary movement in the respiratory tract or the washing action of tears and urine. Many body fluids contain bactericidal substances that provide barrier protection. These include acid in the gastric fluid and lysosomes in tears, nasal secretions, and saliva.

External or internal agents can destroy the body's defense mechanisms and trigger the inflammatory process. Inflammation can be caused by the following factors:

■ Mechanical injuries, such as cuts or surgical incisions
■ Physical damage, such as burns
■ Chemical injury from toxins or poisons
■ Microorganisms, such as bacteria, viruses, or fungi
■ Extremes of heat or cold
■ Immunologic responses, such as hypersensitivity reactions
■ Ischemic damage or trauma, such as a stroke or myocardial infarction

The inflammatory response involves three steps:

1. *Vascular response.* Initially, the blood vessels around the injured area constrict briefly. Then they dilate as chemical mediators, such as histamine, bradykinin, and prostaglandins, are released. Blood flow to the injured area increases, causing redness and warmth. It also raises local hydrostatic pressure (pressure within the capillary), which causes capillaries to leak fluid into surrounding tissues. The result is edema at the injury site and dilution of the organisms or toxins in the area. The chemical mediators and edema are responsible for pain and impaired function.

2. *Cellular response.* As blood flow increases to the injured tissues, white blood cells (WBCs) move into the area. *Neutrophils,* the first white blood cells to respond, usually arrive within 90 minutes. They move from inside the capillary to the injured tissue by a process known as **diapedesis** (Figure 10-1 ■).

Neutrophils and **macrophages** (large white blood cells that develop from monocytes) ingest harmful bacteria and dead tissue cells in a process called **phagocytosis**

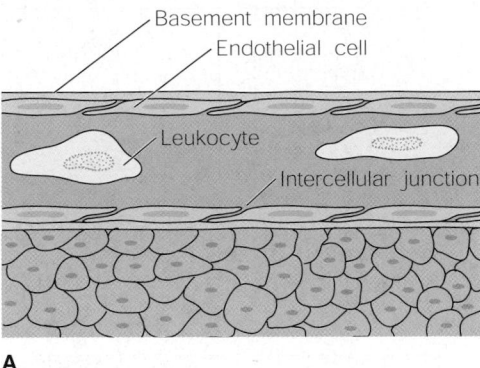

A

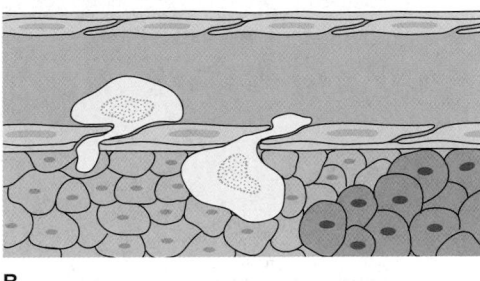

B

Figure 10-1. ■ **(A)** Leukocytes in the circulation. **(B)** Diapedesis, the process of leukocytes moving from inside the capillary to injured tissue.

(see Figure 10-2 ■). Once neutrophils have ingested their full capacity of bacteria, they die. The accumulation of dead neutrophils, dead bacteria, and tissue debris forms *pus.* Bacteria such as staphylococci, streptococci, and neisseriae often cause purulent drainage.

3. *Healing and tissue repair.* After neutrophils die, macrophages clean up the site for healing. In minor injuries, the inflammatory process and healing restore normal structure and function. If the injury is more extensive, new cells are produced to replace the functional tissue. Most cells can regenerate or reproduce (except for nerve, skeletal muscle, and cardiac muscle cells). When regeneration is impossible, collagen scar tissue replaces the destroyed tissue through a process known as *repair.* Scar tissue, which is composed of a different cell type from the original cell, fills in the empty space left by the injury. It often has less strength than the original tissue, and so is more vulnerable to future injury. (See Chapter 9 ⬭ for more on the healing process.) Box 10-1 ■ discusses age-related changes related to inflammation in the older adult.

Acute Inflammation

Inflammation may be either acute or chronic. *Acute inflammation* is a short-term reaction of the body to any tissue damage. It is immediate and usually lasts less than 1 to 2 weeks. Once the harmful agent is removed, the inflammation subsides. Healing and tissue repair occur, and the

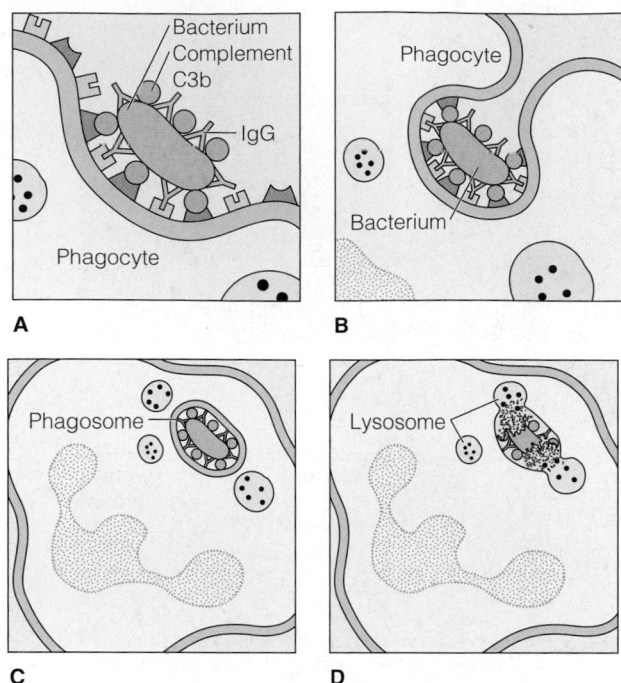

Figure 10-2. ■ The process of phagocytosis. **(A)** Opsonization coats the surface of the bacterium with IgG (an antibody) and complement. **(B)** The bacterium is bound to and engulfed by the phagocyte. **(C)** The phagosome is ingested into the cytoplasm of the phagocyte. **(D)** Lysosomes fuse with the phagosome, releasing digestive enzymes and destroying the antigen.

body returns to normal or near-normal function. Acute inflammation produces local and systemic manifestations.

LOCAL MANIFESTATIONS. Local manifestations develop at and around the site of injury. The degree of functional loss depends on the location and extent of the injury. Increased tissue damage results in more swelling, pain, and functional impairment. The amount of prostaglandin release determines whether pain is immediate or delayed.

Sometimes the inflammatory process does not end immediately with healing and tissue repair. **Cellulitis** develops when inflammation spreads to the surrounding connective tissues. In other circumstances, pus develops and accumulates in pockets called **abscesses.** Abscesses are the body's way of walling off the infection. Abscesses may need to be artificially drained with a procedure called **incision and drainage** (I&D). Inflammation may also cause the formation of a **fistula** (an abnormal tubelike passage from one body cavity to another cavity). More extensive treatment is necessary to manage a fistula.

Clients with diabetes mellitus are at an increased risk for poor wound healing and cellulitis. High blood glucose levels seem to alter phagocytic function and to damage the capillaries. Both these changes impair wound healing. Once a wound heals, it loses some of its original strength, so the diabetic client has a higher incidence of leg and foot ulcers.

SYSTEMIC MANIFESTATIONS. One systemic response to inflammation is enlargement of the lymph nodes (**lymphadenitis**). This process occurs when bacteria, phagocytes, and destroyed lymph tissue accumulate in the affected lymph node. Enlarged lymph nodes are palpable in the groin, axillae, and neck (Figure 10-3 ■). Loss of appetite and fatigue develop as the body tries to conserve energy during the inflammatory process. **Leukocytosis** (increased WBC production) supports inflammation and phagocytosis.

Another systemic manifestation is fever. Fever inhibits the growth of many microorganisms and may increase tissue repair. Macrophages release chemicals called **endogenous pyrogens** that act on the temperature control center in the hypothalamus to elevate the temperature set point. As the temperature rises, the client complains of being cold and shivers because the blood vessels constrict to conserve heat. Once the new set point is reached, the body attempts to cool itself by vasodilation and sweating. Fever should end when the microorganism is destroyed or antibiotics or antipyretics are given. Clients who are immunosuppressed may not experience a fever. Local and systemic manifestations of inflammation are summarized in Box 10-2 ■.

clinical ALERT

In 25% of the elderly, fever is low grade or absent. Older clients may have a serious infection with a 98.6°F temperature. The best indicator of a serious infection is delirium or a change in mental function.

BOX 10-1	FOCUS ON OLDER ADULTS

Inflammatory Changes in the Older Adult

In the older adult, the skin becomes thinner, drier, and more fragile, increasing the potential for injury. The combination of decreased blood flow from atherosclerosis and fewer macrophages results in slower wound healing. The phagocytic activity of the neutrophils lessens with age and impairs local resistance to infection. Older adults also take more medications that interfere with inflammation and healing. The cardinal signs of inflammation—redness, heat, and swelling—tend to be diminished or absent in older adults.

BOX 10-2	

MANIFESTATIONS OF INFLAMMATION

Local Manifestations	Systemic Manifestations
■ Redness	■ Fever
■ Warmth	■ Tachycardia
■ Edema	■ Increased respiratory rate
■ Pain	■ Loss of appetite
■ Loss of function	■ Fatigue
	■ Enlarged lymph nodes
	■ WBC count >10,000/mm³

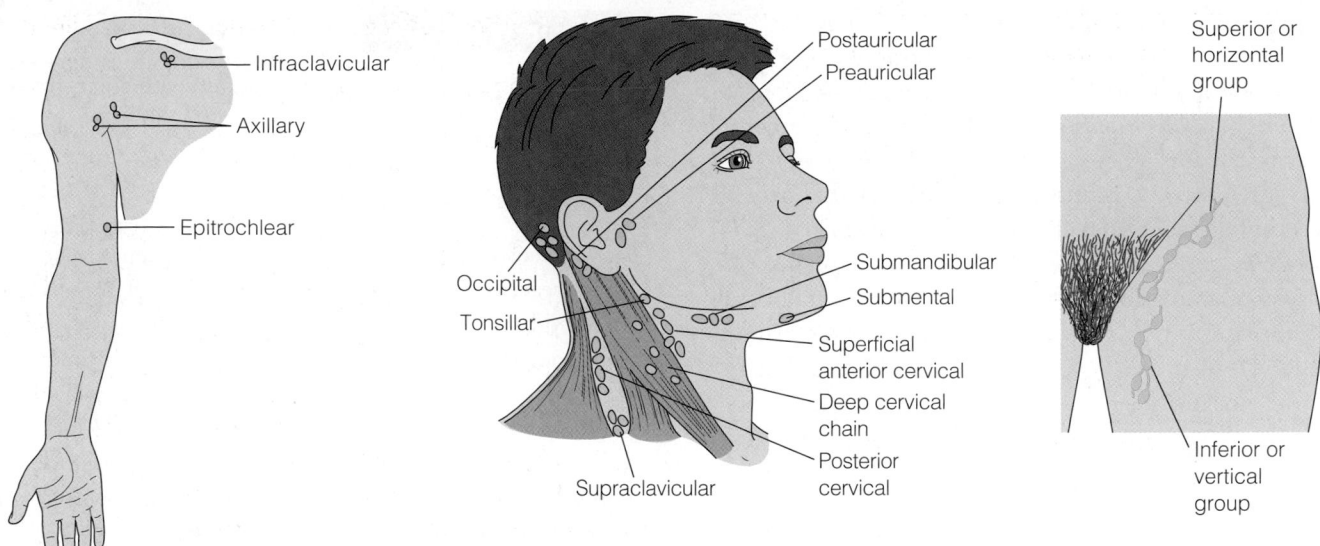

Figure 10-3. ■ Lymph nodes that may be assessed by palpation.

Chronic Inflammation

Chronic inflammation is slower in onset and lasts weeks to months or years. It may develop when the acute inflammatory process has been ineffective in removing the offending agent. For example, in tuberculosis, the mycobacteria resist phagocytosis. *Mycobacterium tuberculosis* can survive for many years and emerge only when the client's immune system is compromised. Chronic inflammation may also develop from constant irritation by chemicals or physical irritants such as talc, asbestos, or silica.

INTERDISCIPLINARY CARE

Management of the client with an inflammation focuses on promoting healing. Care is generally supportive, allowing the client's own physiologic processes to remove foreign matter and damaged cells. The client is encouraged to rest and drink more fluids. A well-balanced diet with vitamin supplements also promotes healing. The client may receive anti-inflammatory medications and antibiotics.

Diagnostic Tests

Diagnostic tests can identify the source and extent of inflammation. The following diagnostic tests may be ordered:

■ *WBC count with differential* provides information about five leukocytes: neutrophils, eosinophils, basophils, monocytes, and lymphocytes. It measures the percentage of the total WBC made up by each type of leukocyte and provides clues about the type of inflammation (Table 10-1 ■).

TABLE 10-1		
White Blood Cell Count and Differential		
CELL TYPE AND NORMAL VALUE	**INCREASED**	**DECREASED**
Total WBCs: 4,500–10,000 per mm³	*Leukocytosis:* Acute infection, tissue necrosis, trauma, stress	*Leukopenia:* Anemia, viral infections, autoimmune diseases
Neutrophils: 55–70%	*Neutrophilia:* Acute infection, inflammatory diseases, myelocytic leukemia	*Neutropenia:* Viral diseases, aplastic anemia
Eosinophils: 1–3%	*Eosinophilia:* Allergies, parasitic diseases, autoimmune disorders	*Eosinopenia:* Stress, Cushing's syndrome
Basophils: 0.5–1%	*Basophilia:* Inflammation, leukemia	*Basopenia:* Acute stress, hypersensitivity reactions
Monocytes: 2–6%	*Monocytosis:* Viral diseases, parasitic diseases	*Monocytopenia:* Bone marrow depression, corticosteroids
Lymphocytes: 25–35%	*Lymphocytosis:* Lymphocytic leukemia, viral infections, chronic bacterial infection	*Lymphocytopenia:* Cancer, leukemia, Cushing's syndrome, renal failure

Source: Data compiled from Pagana, T. J., & Pagana, K. D. (2003). *Mosby's diagnostic and laboratory test references* (6th ed.). St. Louis, MO: Mosby.

With inflammation, leukocytosis (a WBC count of $>10,000/mm^3$) typically occurs. **Leukopenia** (a WBC count of $<4,500\ mm^3$) may indicate a viral infection.

- *Erythrocyte sedimentation rate* (ESR or sed rate) is a nonspecific test that can detect generalized inflammation. Normal levels are <20 mm/hr; significant increases may be seen in both acute and chronic inflammation.
- *C-reactive protein* (CRP) test can identify the presence of active inflammation and tissue necrosis but cannot specify the site. It may show inflammation quicker than the ESR.
- *Cultures* of the blood and other body fluids are also ordered to determine whether infection is the cause of inflammation.

Medications

The medications prescribed to relieve the effects of inflammation include antibiotics, acetaminophen, anti-inflammatory agents, and corticosteroids.

Antibiotics are used to treat infection and prevent infection from interfering with the healing process. If an infection is present, a culture and sensitivity test is done to determine the most effective antibiotic. Anti-infective therapy is discussed in greater depth later in the chapter under infectious diseases.

Acetaminophen (Tylenol) does not have an anti-inflammatory effect. It is used by clients to reduce the pain associated with inflammation. Acetaminophen does have an antipyretic effect. It decreases fever by acting directly on the hypothalamic heat-regulating center.

Although inflammation is a beneficial process to prepare injured tissue for healing, it can have harmful effects. When inflammation presents a danger to the client, anti-inflammatory medications are prescribed. Anti-inflammatory medications fall into four broad groups: salicylates; other non-steroidal anti-inflammatory drugs (NSAIDs), COX-2 inhibitors, and corticosteroids.

Aspirin (acetylsalicylic acid, or ASA) and NSAIDs have a similar action. They produce anti-inflammatory, antipyretic, and analgesic effects. Clients receive varying degrees of relief with aspirin and different NSAIDs. Sometimes several different drugs are tried before the client reports any relief. All of these medications can produce gastrointestinal (GI) irritation and the possibility of bleeding. Indomethacin is the most toxic NSAID; it should be limited to short-term therapy (see Table 10-2 ■).

Cyclooxygenase-2 (COX-2) inhibitors are used to manage pain and inflammation without producing the GI irritation or bleeding associated with aspirin and NSAIDs. They act by blocking the production of prostaglandins.

clinical ALERT

Aspirin should not be given to children with chickenpox or influenza, because it can cause Reye's syndrome, which is acute encephalopathy.

Corticosteroid therapy is prescribed for acute hypersensitivity reactions, such as poison oak, or for inflammation unrelieved by aspirin or NSAIDs. Corticosteroids are also used to manage chronic inflammatory diseases such as arthritis, but they do not cure disease. Steroid medications cause adverse reactions. They suppress the immune and inflammatory responses as well as delay healing; therefore, they should be used cautiously. Remember the following principles when administering corticosteroids:

- Use the smallest effective dose.
- An alternate-day dose schedule may decrease suppression of adrenal gland activity.
- Never stop steroid therapy abruptly. Taper the dose gradually so that adrenal gland function can return to normal.
- Harmful side effects increase with higher doses and prolonged therapy.

The nursing implications of caring for a client receiving corticosteroid medications are presented in Chapter 16 (see Table 16-3 ⬤).

Wound Care

Minor wounds may require no more then gentle cleansing with soap and water. If wounds are more extensive, wound care may involve irrigations and debridement of necrotic tissue. To prevent additional wound damage, the nurse cleanses the site with sterile normal saline or commercially prepared nontoxic wound cleansers such as Comfeel (Coloplast Corporation) or ClinisWound (Sage Laboratories). Hydrogen peroxide, povidone–iodine (Betadine), and sodium hypochlorite (Dakin's solution) have a drying effect on the tissue. They can also inhibit the healing process. They should be used as a last resort. Because granulation tissue in a healing wound is fragile and bleeds easily, wound care must be performed gently. (See wound care in Chapter 9 ⬤.)

Fluid and Diet Treatment

Inflammation and wound healing require adequate nutrition, blood supply, and oxygenation. *Malnutrition* makes the phagocytes ineffective so that there is a delayed inflammatory response. The macrophages cannot prepare the wound site for healing. If an infection develops, it interferes with effective wound healing. *Inadequate circulation* cannot deliver sufficient oxygen and nutrients or remove waste products. Without normal circulation the injury site cannot heal properly.

TABLE 10-2

Nursing Implications for Pharmacology: Anti-Inflammatory Drugs

DRUG GROUP/DRUGS	PURPOSE	NURSING RESPONSIBILITIES	CLIENT TEACHING
Salicylates ■ Aspirin (acetylsalicylic acid)	Aspirin is a nonsteroidal anti-inflammatory drug with analgesic, antipyretic, and antiplatelet effects.	Do not give to clients with peptic ulcers, with gastritis, or taking anticoagulants. Give with food or milk to prevent gastric irritation. Notify the physician for signs of black or bloody stools, coffee-ground emesis, or tinnitus.	Take with food or milk to avoid gastric irritation. Report any dark stools, unusual bleeding, bruising, blurred vision, or ringing in the ears. Do not use with other drugs containing aspirin. Discard tablets with vinegar-like odor.
Nonsteroidal Anti-Inflammatory Drugs (NSAIDs) ■ Fenoprofen calcium (Nalfon) ■ Ibuprofen (Motrin, Advil) ■ Indomethacin (Indocin) ■ Ketorolac (Toradol) ■ Naproxen (Anaprox, Naprosyn) ■ Piroxicam (Feldene) ■ Ketoprofen (Orudis)	NSAIDs are used to reduce pain and inflammation.	Give cautiously to patients with bleeding disorders, peptic ulcers or gastritis, and renal disease. Give with food or milk to decrease gastric irritation. Monitor for heartburn, gastrointestinal bleeding, a change in urination, or bloody urine.	Take with food or milk as ordered. Report changes in vision or hearing; a change in urination or bloody urine; coffee-ground emesis or blood in the stool. *Avoid the use of alcohol while taking NSAIDs.*
Cyclooxygenase-2 Inhibitors ■ Celecoxib (Celebrex) ■ Valdecoxib (Bextra)	COX-2 inhibitors are used to decrease pain and inflammation but with reduced GI side effects or bleeding.	Do not give to clients with sulfa allergy. Monitor for GI bleeding with long-term use.	Take with full glass of water. Notify doctor before taking with warfarin (Coumadin) or aspirin.

The client with an inflammation or wound requires a well-balanced diet to promote healing. When clients develop protein deficiency, their risk for poor wound healing and infection increases. Inflammation produces **catabolism,** a condition in which body tissues are broken down. During healing, the desired result is tissue building (**anabolism**). Diets low in calories and essential nutrients lead to catabolism and impaired healing.

Encourage the client to eat a diet high in carbohydrates, protein, and vitamins. Carbohydrates are important to meet energy demands and to support leukocyte function. Protein is necessary for tissue healing and the production of antibodies and WBCs. Some vitamins and minerals are also important. Vitamin A fosters capillary formation and tissue growth. B-complex vitamins promote wound healing. Vitamin C is necessary for collagen synthesis. Vitamin K is essential for blood clotting. Minerals, especially zinc, are important for tissue growth, skin integrity, and immune function.

Complementary Therapy

Aloe gel from the aloe vera plant is applied topically to treat minor skin irritations such as sunburns. Topical camphor is used to provide pain relief from cold sores and warts. To reduce the inflammation of bruises and strains, comfrey may be used topically.

NURSING CARE

Priorities in Nursing Care. The nursing care needs of the client with an inflammatory process are related to the manifestations of inflammation and altered tissue integrity. Priority nursing diagnoses include Pain, Impaired Tissue Integrity, and Risk for Infection.

ASSESSING

The nurse must collect assessment data to help determine the extent to which the inflammatory process is interfering

BOX 10-3	ASSESSMENT

Assessing Clients with Inflammation

SUBJECTIVE DATA

- Present health status:
  - General health and nutritional status.
  - Describe any injuries.
  - Describe any redness, warmth, swelling, or pain.
  - Is drainage associated with current injury or previous procedure? Is drainage clear or purulent?
  - Changes in appetite or energy level.
- Past medical history:
  - Any frequent infections?
  - Use of anti-inflammatory medications, corticosteroids, or antibiotics.

OBJECTIVE DATA

- Vital signs: blood pressure, pulse, respirations, temperature.
- Height and weight.
- Observe client for fatigue and listlessness.
- Assess ability to move injured area and amount of pain.
- Assess circulation to affected area.
- Inspect skin and surrounding area of injury for redness and warmth, purulent drainage, odor, and poor healing.
- Measure size (depth and width) of wounds.
- Palpate the skin for the presence of edema.
- Palpate for enlarged lymph nodes.
- Monitor and report abnormal results of WBC count with differential, ESR, CRP.

with the client's life. Data can also identify risk factors for complications and can determine the type of medical intervention (Box 10-3 ■).

DIAGNOSING, PLANNING, AND IMPLEMENTING

When caring for a client with inflammation, it is important for the nurse to monitor for increased temperature, pulse, and respiratory rate. It is essential to observe the color, consistency, and odor of any wound drainage, and to report any abnormal findings.

Acute Pain

Along with redness, warmth, swelling, and impaired function, pain is one of the cardinal manifestations of inflammation. Depending on the cause, affected area, and degree of inflammation, pain may be acute and immobilizing or chronic.

- Give anti-inflammatory medications as prescribed. *These medications can lessen the pain resulting from inflammation.*
- Give mild analgesic medications as prescribed. *Although most analgesics do not reduce inflammation, they may decrease pain perception.*
- Remind the client that rest is important for acutely inflamed tissue. *Strenuous activity or exercising an inflamed body part may increase discomfort and cause tissue damage.*
- Apply cold or heat therapy as ordered. Remove ice pack or heating pad after 10 minutes and check the client's skin. (For cold, note bluish color or a feeling of numbness; for heat, observe for redness.) *For an acute injury, cold reduces swelling and relieves pain. After the initial stage, heat increases blood flow to the affected tissue and promotes absorption of edema. It is important to monitor the client's skin for untoward effects and to prevent injury to the skin.*

clinical ALERT

Use heat or cold application cautiously in older adults who have fragile skin and are at risk for tissue injury.

- Elevate the inflamed area if possible. *Elevation promotes venous return and reduces swelling.*

Impaired Tissue Integrity

Both an injury and the inflammatory response to it can lead to impaired skin integrity. The nurse must prevent any additional skin problems.

- Provide protective devices, such as an eye patch, over the injured area. *Protective devices aid in comfort and healing.*
- Clean inflamed tissue gently; use water or normal saline only. *Soap and harsh cleansing agents can cause drying and further tissue damage.*
- Encourage the client to balance rest with active and passive exercises. *Rest decreases metabolic demands and promotes cell growth. Activity promotes circulation.*
- Encourage the client to eat a well-balanced diet with adequate carbohydrates, protein, vitamins, and minerals. If the client is NPO or unable to eat an adequate diet, suggest parenteral nutrition, between-meal supplements, or multivitamin supplements. *A well-balanced diet promotes immune function and healing.*

Risk for Infection

The inflammatory response is meant to protect the client against microorganisms. However, when intact skin is broken (as in a healing wound), the risk for infection increases.

- Monitor the client's temperature, pulse, and respirations at least every 4 hours. *Increased vital signs usually indicate inflammation. A temperature of 101°F (38.3°C) or above indicates infection.*
- Culture purulent or odorous wound drainage. *Wound culture is used to determine the infectious organism and appropriate antibiotic therapy.*
- Provide fluid intake of 2,500 mL per day unless otherwise contraindicated. *Adequate hydration helps maintain blood flow and nutrient supply to the tissues. Fluids may be limited for the client with heart failure.*
- Use proper hand washing techniques (including at least 15 seconds of friction). *Hand washing is the fundamental tool for preventing the spread of infection to a susceptible person.*
- Wear sterile gloves when providing wound care. *Sterile gloves prevent further wound contamination and the spread of infection to other clients.*

EVALUATING

To evaluate the effectiveness of care for a client with acute inflammation, collect data about the presence of redness, heat, swelling, loss of function, and swelling. For the client with systemic inflammation, note vital signs, appetite, energy level, and lymph nodes.

The nurse should document the client's vital signs, type and location of pain, and the color, consistency, and odor of any wound drainage. In addition, describe the client's response to any heat or cold therapy ordered. Document teaching related to prescribed medications, fluid intake, well-balanced diet, and wound care at home.

CONTINUING CARE

Client and family teaching should focus on understanding the inflammatory process, its cause, and its management. When planning for home care, assess the client's ability to perform self-care at home. Remind the client to avoid other members of the household with infections. Teaching is also important to prevent actions that could lead to infection.

Provide the client with the following verbal and written instructions:

- Increase fluid intake to 2,500 mL (approximately 2½ quarts) per day, unless contraindicated.
- Eat a well-balanced diet that is high in carbohydrates, protein, vitamins, and minerals.
- Use good hand washing techniques (wash for at least 15 seconds with friction) when caring for wounds and after using the bathroom.

- Elevate the inflamed area to reduce swelling and pain.
- Apply heat or cold for no longer than 20 minutes at a time to reduce the risk of tissue damage from burns or frostbite.
- Take all medications as prescribed. Review the use, expected effects, and side effects of anti-inflammatory medications. Notify the physician if adverse effects occur.
- Rest acutely inflamed tissue. Do not engage in strenuous activity until the inflammation has subsided.

Infection

Microorganisms invade humans in order to grow and reproduce. Contact between humans and microorganisms is often beneficial to both. For example, the normal flora of the skin, mucous membranes, and gastrointestinal tract play an important part in the body's defense system. However, all microorganisms are capable of producing **infection** (growth and invasion of microorganisms that leads to disease), especially when an individual is in poor health.

Infectious diseases have existed throughout history. Modern medicine, antibiotic therapy, immunizations, and public health measures that protect food and water supplies have significantly reduced the prevalence of infectious diseases in many parts of the world. Although smallpox has been eliminated, malaria, typhoid, and tuberculosis are still common in many developing nations. In spite of vaccines and anti-infective drugs, new strains of bacteria for sexually transmitted infections (STIs), tuberculosis, and antibiotic-resistant strains of *Staphylococcus* and *Streptococcus* have emerged. Tuberculosis remains on the rise in the United States because organisms are resistant to antitubercular medications. New strains of human immunodeficiency virus (HIV) and newer diseases such as Lyme disease and *Hantavirus* pulmonary syndrome challenge modern medicine to find new treatments. Even diseases that once were unrelated to microorganisms now have an infectious disease connection; for example, *Helicobacter pylori* seems to be the underlying cause of chronic gastritis.

To a certain extent, modern medicine has contributed to the development of microorganisms. For example, invasive procedures that use metal and plastic prosthetic devices provide potential sites for infection. **Immunosuppression** (inability of the immune system to provide adequate immunity) is part of the medical consequence for organ recipients. Clients who receive immunosuppressive therapy following organ transplant or chemotherapy are, therefore, more susceptible to infection.

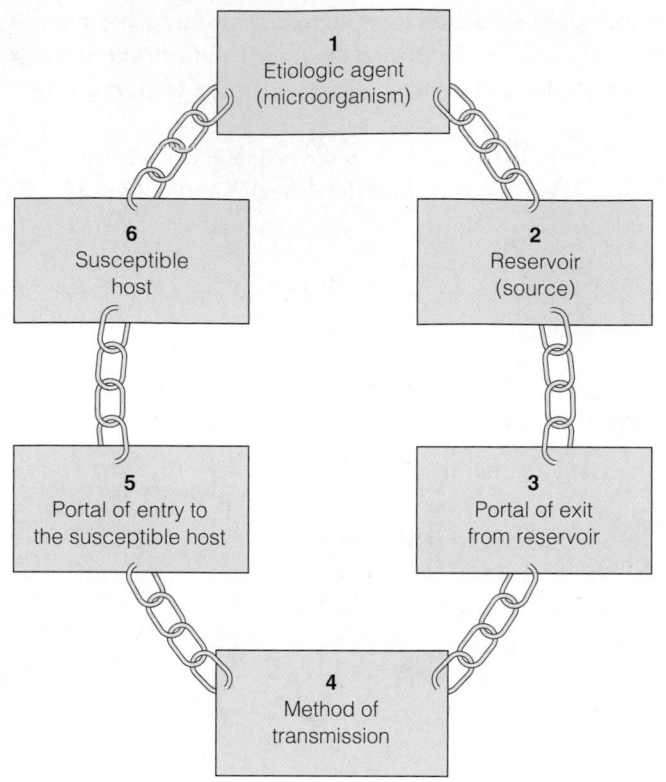

Figure 10-4. ■ The chain of infection.

PATHOPHYSIOLOGY

Chain of Infection

For an individual to develop an infection, the **chain of infection** must be in place. Key elements of the chain include (1) a microorganism, (2) a reservoir, (3) a portal of exit from the reservoir, (4) a mode of transmission from the reservoir to the host, and (5) an entry point into a (6) susceptible host (Figure 10-4 ■). Each element is presented in more detail in the following discussion.

MICROORGANISMS. **Pathogens** are microorganisms that are capable of causing disease. Common pathogens include bacteria, mycoplasma, rickettsiae, chlamydia, viruses, fungi, protozoans, helminths, and arthropods (Box 10-4 ■). Each organism causes a different reaction in the host.

For microorganisms to result in disease, several factors are required, including virulence and invasiveness. **Virulence** is the power of a microorganism to cause infection. It is affected by the number of organisms, the host's health, and whether toxins are produced. For example, measles has a low virulence, but rabies has a high virulence. An organism's ability to invade and multiply in a host determines its **invasiveness.** Microorganisms that produce enzymes or toxins are better able to resist the host's defenses and can easily

---

BOX 10-4

PATHOGENIC ORGANISMS

Bacteria
Bacteria are single-celled organisms. They have different shapes: round *(cocci),* rod shaped *(bacilli),* or spiral *(spirochete).* Bacteria can adapt to different environments: *Aerobes* require oxygen for survival; *anaerobes* survive without oxygen. In the laboratory, they are classified by staining properties: *gram-positive* bacteria stain purple and *gram-negative* bacteria stain red. Common bacterial infections include *Streptococcus pneumoniae, Staphylococcus aureus,* and *Escherichia coli.*

Mycoplasma
Although similar to bacteria, mycoplasma are smaller. They are more resistant to antibiotics such as penicillins and cephalosporins.

Rickettsiae and Chlamydia
Rickettsiae and chlamydia have some features similar to bacteria and viruses. Rickettsiae infect the cells of arthropods (e.g., fleas, ticks, and lice) without causing disease. When they are transmitted from these vectors to humans, they cause diseases such as typhus. Chlamydia are transmitted by direct contact and can cause sexually transmitted infections.

Viruses
Viruses are the smallest pathogens. They are incapable of reproducing outside of a living cell. They use the host's metabolic and reproductive materials to multiply. Viruses consist of a protein shell

around a DNA or RNA core. Some viruses are short lived, such as rhinovirus (the common cold). Latent viruses remain dormant in the host until they are reactivated, for example, herpes zoster (shingles) and fever blisters (cold sores). Human immunodeficiency virus (HIV) is classed as a retrovirus. Oncogenic viruses may be able to transform normal cells into cancer cells.

Fungi
Fungi are prevalent throughout the world, but few are capable of causing disease in humans. They grow in two forms: yeasts and molds. Fungal infections can be mild, affecting the skin and subcutaneous tissue. Some fungi, such as *Pneumocystis carinii,* can cause life-threatening opportunistic infections in the immunocompromised host.

Protozoans, Helminths, and Arthropods
Protozoans, helminths, and arthropods are considered parasites. Protozoans are single-celled organisms transmitted from host to host, indirectly through contaminated water, or by an arthropod vector. Helminths are wormlike parasites (e.g., roundworms, tapeworms, and flukes). They are transmitted via eggs or larvae that usually are excreted by humans in urine or feces. They enter other humans through food contaminated by urine or feces or through broken skin. Arthropod parasites, such as scabies (mites), lice, and fleas, typically infest external body surfaces, causing localized tissue damage and inflammation. Transmission is by direct contact with the arthropod or its eggs.

Sources: Data adapted from Porth, C. M. (2005). *Pathophysiology: Concepts of altered health states* (7th ed.). Philadelphia: Lippincott Williams & Wilkins.

TABLE 10-3

Common Infectious Diseases and the Causative Organism

DISEASE	CAUSATIVE ORGANISM
Chickenpox	Varicella zoster
Gonorrhea	*Neisseria gonorrhoeae*
Foodborne hepatitis	Hepatitis A virus
Bloodborne hepatitis	Hepatitis B, C, or D
Herpes simplex	Human herpesvirus 1 and 2
Impetigo	*Staphylococcus aureus*
Influenza	Influenza virus A, B, or C
Lyme disease	*Borrelia burgdorferi*
Meningitis	*Haemophilus influenzae*
Meningococcal meningitis	*Neisseria meningitidis*
Pneumococcal pneumoniae	*Streptococcus pneumoniae*
Rabies	Rabies virus
Respiratory syncytial disease	Respiratory syncytial virus
Ringworm	*Microsporum* species
Rubella	Rubella virus
Streptococcal pharyngitis	*Streptococcus pyogenes*, Group A
Syphilis	*Treponema pallidum*
Tetanus	*Clostridium tetani*
Tuberculosis	*Mycobacterium tuberculosis*

invade the body. For example, *Staphylococcus aureus* releases an enzyme that increases its resistance to certain antibiotics.

Bacteria may release **exotoxins** (from *Staphylococcus, Streptococcus,* or tetanus bacteria) or **endotoxins** (from gram-negative bacteria). Also, diseases such as botulism and cholera release deadly bacterial exotoxins. Gram-negative organisms that produce endotoxins can cause septic shock. (Common infections and their causative organisms are noted in Table 10-3 ■.)

RESERVOIR AND PORTAL OF EXIT. The reservoir is where the pathogen lives and multiplies. Humans, animals, insects, and nonliving or inanimate objects such as equipment, needles, and utensils act as reservoirs. Infectious diseases are usually transmitted from human sources who have the clinical disease. People who have the disease but do not show any clinical manifestations are called **carriers.** For an infection to escape its reservoir, it must have a portal of exit.

Pathogens exit humans through respiratory secretions, gastrointestinal and genitourinary body fluids, skin or mucous membrane lesions, or the blood.

MODE OF TRANSMISSION. Pathogens move from their reservoir to a susceptible host by several routes: direct or indirect contact, droplet or airborne transmission, or a vector. *Direct contact* includes person-to-person spread or contact with infected body fluids or contaminated food or water. *Indirect contact* occurs when the infectious agent is carried on inanimate objects, such as dirty eating utensils.

Droplet transmission involves large, moist droplets released during sneezing, talking, and coughing. Contaminated droplets can be sprayed to another person within a 2- to 3-foot radius. In *airborne transmission,* small respiratory particles are carried by air currents and then inhaled by the host. For example, tuberculosis is spread by airborne transmission. *Vectors* are insects and animals (such as flies, mosquitoes, or rodents) that act as intermediate hosts between the source and host.

Pathogenic organisms must be able to survive their transport from the reservoir to a host. Over time, they have developed mechanisms to resist drying and unfavorable temperatures (e.g., tetanus bacteria produce spores).

PORTAL OF ENTRY. An organism needs a portal of entry to gain access into the host. Portals of entry include eyes; mouth; respiratory, gastrointestinal, and genitourinary tracts; broken skin; and blood.

HOST. The susceptible host is the final link in the chain of infection. The concepts of normal flora, colonization, infection, and disease are important to how bacteria can affect a host. Normal flora (resident bacteria) work in harmony with the host and provide a benefit such as the normal flora in the intestinal tract. **Colonization** occurs when pathogenic microorganisms live in the host but do not cause injury or initiate the inflammatory response. For example, *Staphylococcus aureus* may colonize on the skin. Infection indicates that pathogenic bacteria have triggered the inflammatory process, such as when *S. aureus* enters a surgical wound, causing redness, heat, and pain. **Infectious disease** is the illness that results from an infection.

Whether an infection develops depends on microbe virulence and host resistance. The following factors help the host resist infection:

- Physical barriers, such as the skin and mucous membranes
- Hostile environment created by acid stomach secretions, urine, and vaginal secretions
- Antimicrobial factors in saliva, tears, and prostatic fluid
- Coughing, sneezing, and the cilia in the respiratory tract
- Neutrophils and macrophages.

When host resistance is compromised, the host becomes *susceptible* to infection. Invasive procedures (urinary catheters, chest tubes, IV lines) penetrate the body's physical barriers. The very young and very old may have underdeveloped or failing immune systems. Clients who are malnourished, have AIDS, or have cancer and are being treated with chemotherapy or radiation therapy have increased susceptibility. Susceptibility is lowered when a person receives an immunization or has previously developed the disease.

Stages of the Infectious Process

Infectious disease usually follows a predictable course through five stages as it develops in the host:

1. The *initial stage* is the incubation period. The pathogen actively reproduces but does not cause symptoms. Some diseases have short incubation periods (such as food poisoning due to *Salmonella*). On the other hand, HIV infection has an incubation period of months to years.

2. In the *prodromal stage,* symptoms begin to appear, although they are often vague and nonspecific. The client will report general malaise, fever, muscle aches and pains, headache, and fatigue.

3. During the *acute stage,* the pathogen continues reproducing and disperses rapidly. Manifestations become obvious and reflect the specific organism and site. Usually, the client develops a fever, chills, tachycardia, and tachypnea. Infections of an internal organ cause an inflammatory response. The client may have tenderness over the site or show signs of altered function, such as hematuria in kidney infections. If the infectious process continues over an extended period, clients show signs of increased catabolism and malnutrition. They lose weight and their muscles become weak. Sometimes products of the immune process, formed in other sites than the primary infection, cause an inflammatory reaction. For example, a sore throat caused by a streptococcal infection may result in glomerulonephritis.

4. In the *convalescent stage,* the infection is contained and the pathogen is continually destroyed. At this point, affected tissues are repaired and symptoms disappear.

5. During the last stage, *resolution,* the infection is totally eliminated from the body without residual manifestations. Clients with chronic infections never reach the convalescent and resolution stages.

Complications

Complications may be associated with the type of infecting organism and its virulence. They also may be related to the physical condition of the host. As discussed earlier, if the host is immunosuppressed, the body's normal defenses are missing. Immunosuppression causes not only poor wound healing but also slower disease resolution.

Microorganisms such as bacteria, fungi, and viruses can enter the bloodstream causing *bacteremia, fungemia,* or *viremia.* If gram-negative organisms release their toxins into the bloodstream, the client develops *septicemia* (infection in the blood). Septicemia in an immunosuppressed host can lead to septic shock. Septic shock is a systemic inflammatory response to infection resulting in inadequate blood flow to the internal organs; unless treated aggressively, it can lead to widespread cell and tissue injury, organ failure, and death. (See in-depth discussion in Chapter 13 ⚭.)

***NOSOCOMIAL INFECTIONS.* Nosocomial infections** are infections acquired in a health care setting, such as a hospital or long-term care facility. More than 2 million clients a year develop a nosocomial infection while hospitalized. Hospital-acquired infections increase the client's hospital stay and are costly in terms of diagnosis and treatment. The frequency of nosocomial infections varies according to the type of clients, the severity of illness, and the number of health care workers within each facility.

Numerous factors can affect whether the hospitalized client develops a nosocomial infection (Box 10-5 ■). In addition, clients in the hospital are exposed to numerous health care personnel who may transmit microorganisms between clients. Often, visitors carry infectious diseases that they unknowingly transmit to ill clients. Even such items as thermometers, blood pressure cuffs, and wheelchairs can carry nosocomial organisms. Some of the pathogens that typically cause nosocomial infections include *Escherichia coli, Staphylococcus aureus,* Group A streptococci, and *Enterococcus.* Urinary tract infections are the number-one infection, usually due to urinary catheterization and urologic procedures. Postoperative infections may result from wound contamination during surgery, for example, when *E. coli,* normally found in the colon, is accidentally transferred to another site via contaminated instruments. Other common infection sites are the respiratory tract and the bloodstream.

BOX 10-5

RISK FACTORS FOR NOSOCOMIAL INFECTIONS

- Chronic diseases (e.g., renal disease, lung disease, cancer, AIDS, diabetes, peripheral vascular disease, pressure ulcers, dermatitis)
- Morbid obesity
- Long-term use of corticosteroids, chemotherapy, radiation therapy
- History of frequent antibiotic use
- Major surgery such as heart, lung, or intra-abdominal surgeries, or organ transplant
- Invasive procedures (e.g., urinary catheter, peripheral and central IV lines, respiratory care procedures, percutaneous endoscopic gastrostomy [PEG] feeding tube, dialysis)
- Prosthetic devices: vascular grafts, heart valves, orthopedic joints
- Infections in other sites
- Burns
- Length of hospital stay
- Very young and very old age

The nurse assumes a key role in recognizing clients who are at risk for nosocomial infections. It is the nurse's responsibility to use consistently the principles of medical and surgical asepsis and assist other health care personnel to follow these principles when caring for clients. When necessary, limit visitors to prevent overcrowding in the client's room.

Another factor contributing to the rise in nosocomial infections is long-term or inappropriate use of antibiotics. Every time an antibiotic is given, a few hardy bacteria survive. When these bacteria reproduce, they pass along their antibiotic resistance. If a client does not complete the course of antibiotic therapy, an entire generation of resistant bacteria can survive to reproduce. Then, when a new infection occurs, the client may need a stronger antibiotic. This process, if repeated frequently enough, can establish a pattern of *antibiotic resistance*. The most common antibiotic-resistant microorganisms include methicillin-resistant *Staphylococcus aureus* (MRSA), vancomycin-resistant *Enterococcus* (VRE), and

penicillin-resistant *Streptococcus pneumococci* (PRSP). MRSA, VRE, PRSP, and *Clostridium difficile*–associated diarrhea (CDAD, another nosocomial infection) are discussed in the following subsections.

Methicillin-Resistant *Staphylococcus aureus* (MRSA). Staphylococci normally live in the mucous membranes of the respiratory tract and on the skin. MRSA is a type of staphylococcal infection that survives the antibiotic methicillin. It exists not only in hospitals but also in the community. The general population and health care workers can be silent carriers, because the colonized bacteria grow in the anterior part of the nose.

In health care facilities, MRSA is transmitted on the hands of health care workers. After exposure, it can live on a person's hands for more than 3 hours. Clients with MRSA infections may be isolated using Contact Precautions (see Table 10-4 ■ for further guidelines). When providing direct care, gowns

---

TABLE 10-4

Transmission-Based Precautions

CATEGORY	INFECTIOUS DISEASES	PURPOSE	PRECAUTIONS
Airborne Precautions	Pulmonary tuberculosis, varicella (chickenpox), measles	Reduce transmission of airborne droplets or dust particles containing the infectious agent.	Private room with private bathroom. Use negative pressure (pulls air from hall inward when someone enters the room); otherwise, keep door closed. Particulate air filter for TB cases. Place mask on client if transport needed.
Droplet Precautions	Meningitis, pneumonia, influenza, mumps, pertussis, diphtheria, adenovirus	Reduce transmission of large droplets generated during coughing, sneezing, talking, or procedures such as suctioning. Can infect others if droplets land on conjunctivae, nasal mucosa, or mouth.	Private room with bathroom facilities. Wear mask when working within 3 feet of client. Place mask on client if transport is required.
Contact Precautions	Acute diarrhea including VRE, CDAD; MRSA; herpes and varicella; respiratory syncytial virus (RSV); skin, wound, or urinary tract infection with multidrug-resistant organisms; *Staphylococcus aureus* infections; hepatitis A in incontinent clients	Reduce transmission by direct skin-to-skin contact or indirect contact with a contaminated object. Direct contact may occur between clients or during direct care activities such as bathing or turning clients.	Private room with bathroom facilities. Don gloves when entering room and remove before leaving room. Change gloves after contact with infective material. Wear gown and gloves when giving direct care or touching contaminated surfaces. Leave blood pressure cuff, stethoscope, and thermometer in room. Wash hands immediately after removing gloves.

and gloves must be worn. Serious MRSA infections are treated with intravenous vancomycin. However, vancomycin may be losing its effectiveness. Recent cases of *vancomycin intermediate Staphylococcus aureus (VISA)* and *vancomycin-resistant Staphylococcus aureus (VRSA)* have occurred in the United States. They were successfully treated with other antibiotics, but the medical community fears that new, totally antibiotic-resistant microorganisms will emerge.

Vancomycin-Resistant *Enterococcus* (VRE). Enterococci are primarily found in the GI and female genital tracts as part of the normal flora. VRE, the second most common nosocomial infection, developed in the past 10 years from overuse of different antibiotics. VRE is spread by direct contact from client to client or health care worker to client. The bacteria can live on equipment or environmental surfaces such as over-bed tables. Clients and health care workers can carry the colonized bacteria into a health care facility.

Once VRE is confirmed, the client is isolated using Contact Precautions (see Table 10-4). These include wearing gloves and gowns when providing direct care and dedicating essential equipment (a thermometer, blood pressure cuff, and stethoscope) to the affected client.

Penicillin-Resistant *Streptococcus pneumoniae* (PRSP). *Streptococcus pneumoniae* is the most common cause of community-acquired pneumonia (CAP). Now it has developed into a resistant form, penicillin-resistant *Streptococcus pneumoniae* (PRSP). Unlike MRSA and VRE, PRSP is transmitted by droplets from the respiratory tract and requires Transmission-based Droplet Precautions (see Table 10-4).

Clostridium difficile–Associated Diarrhea (CDAD). *Clostridium difficile* is an anaerobic gram-positive bacillus that produces two endotoxins that cause damage to the mucosal lining of the bowel. Because the organism forms spores, it can live for months on environmental sources. Antibiotic therapy reduces the bowel's normal flora, allowing the growth of *C. difficile.*

Manifestations may range from mild diarrhea to the life-threatening condition of pseudomembranous colitis. The client is placed in a private room with Contact Precautions (see Table 10-4). Again, gowns and gloves are worn when providing direct client care. Because CDAD is easily transmitted, equipment such as thermometer, stethoscope, and blood pressure cuff must be left in the client's room. Mild diarrhea is treated with fluid and electrolyte replacement and discontinuation of any antibiotic therapy. Clients with severe cases receive metronidazole (Flagyl) as well as fluids, electrolytes, and nutritional support.

COMMUNITY-ACQUIRED INFECTIONS. Community-acquired infections are usually referred to as *communicable diseases,* be-

cause they can be transmitted to other people. Smallpox, diphtheria, polio, mumps, measles, rubella, pertussis, and tetanus are long-standing communicable diseases. Other community-acquired infections include influenza, community-acquired pneumonia, MRSA, hepatitis A, and tuberculosis. Smallpox is the only communicable disease to have been completely eradicated. In the United States, most of these communicable diseases are under control through immunization programs. (See Chapter 11 for more information on immunizations.)

Communicable diseases are monitored from an international to a local level. The World Health Organization (WHO) focuses on controlling disease throughout the world. In Atlanta, Georgia, the Centers for Disease Control and Prevention (CDC) (a federal government agency) is responsible for monitoring, controlling, and preventing infectious diseases. It routinely publishes guidelines and recommendations to use in caring for clients with infections. State and local health departments work cooperatively with the CDC to manage diseases in their area. Physicians and health care facilities are expected to report any communicable disease to their local health department.

Emerging Infectious Diseases. Emerging infectious diseases are defined as diseases that have increased in the past 20 years or threaten to increase in the near future. Several factors contribute to this threat: worldwide food supply and distribution, international travel, increased crowding in cities, resistant microorganisms, and poor sanitation.

Public health officials remain concerned about multidrug-resistant tuberculosis (TB) and HIV. Other new emerging diseases include West Nile virus, severe acute respiratory syndrome (SARS), and monkeypox. Also, diarrheal diseases are increasing throughout the world and the United States. Infectious diarrhea results from organisms such as *E. coli, Salmonella, Shigella, Campylobacter,* and *Giardia,* which are transmitted by contaminated food or water.

WHO and CDC are responsible for protecting the public from infectious diseases. The role of the nurse is education and prevention of the spread of infectious diseases. Through the efforts of the health care community, the battle against these new infections may be won.

Biologic Threat Infections. Following the terrorist attacks on September 11, 2001, and the development of anthrax cases in the United States, the threat of the use of biologic weapons is increasing. The most likely pathogens to be used for this purpose include anthrax, smallpox, botulism, plague, and viral hemorrhagic fevers.

Anthrax is an acute bacterial infection caused by *Bacillus anthracis,* a gram-positive, spore-producing organism. It can be contracted by inhalation, ingestion, and skin contact. The spores cannot be destroyed by sunlight or temperature and remain viable for years.

Inhalation anthrax carries the highest mortality rate. At first, the client exhibits flulike symptoms that progress to respiratory failure and shock. Clients who ingest the spores develop fever, nausea, vomiting, abdominal pain, and bloody diarrhea. Skin contact produces an itching papule progressing to a painless fluid-filled vesicle. Those with positive anthrax exposure are treated prophylactically with oral ciprofloxacin (Cipro) or doxycycline (Doxycin).

In 1980, WHO certified that smallpox had been eradicated. Routine smallpox vaccination was discontinued in 1972, leaving people under the age of 30 at risk for the disease if it is used as a weapon. Even those who received smallpox vaccinations are no longer immune because antibody levels only last up to 30 years. Smallpox spreads by direct contact or by inhalation of respiratory droplets. Symptoms include a high fever, malaise, and headache followed by a vesicular/pustular rash, which appears simultaneously on the face and extremities. Anyone exposed to smallpox should be vaccinated and monitored closely.

Health care providers should be alert to unusual illness patterns that could indicate an infectious disease outbreak. Indicators of a biologic agent release include increased disease among people in the same geographic area (e.g., people who attended the same event); the disease is unusual for the clients' age, such as chickenpox in adults; and a client presents with symptoms of a rare disease. Any one of these factors should be reported to the public health authorities to identify the infectious disease source and to prevent further exposure.

INFECTIOUS PROCESS IN OLDER ADULTS. Infections are a leading cause of disease and death in older adults. Those older than 75 years of age have a higher rate of infections. The geriatric client is especially prone to several infectious diseases. Part of their increased risk is related to the physiologic changes of aging. (Common infections in older adults, as well as associated factors, are outlined in Table 10-5 ■.)

In addition to physiologic changes, the following factors can increase the risk for infectious disease:

- Decreased activity level related to musculoskeletal, neurologic, or balance problems
- Poor nutrition and an increased risk of dehydration
- Chronic diseases, such as diabetes mellitus, cardiac disease, and renal disease
- Chronic medication use
- Lack of recent influenza and pneumococcal vaccinations

- Altered mental status and dementias
- Hospitalization or residence in a long-term care facility.

Although the older adult is at increased risk for infection, he or she may not exhibit the classic manifestations of infection. Fever may be mild or absent. (It is not unusual for an older client's normal temperature to range from 96 to 98°F.) The white blood cell count may be only slightly elevated. Confusion is a frequent atypical sign of infection in older adults, along with restlessness, fatigue, and mild behavioral changes. Even older adults with sepsis may only appear slightly disoriented and tachypneic.

If an infection is suspected, the physician will order a chest x-ray, urinalysis and culture, and complete blood count. The nurse must complete a baseline assessment and be alert for subtle changes in the client's mental status or behavior. Other important data to collect include fluid and diet intake, urinary output, respiratory and cardiovascular assessment, and activity level. Early diagnosis and prompt treatment will improve outcomes for the older adult. Nursing implications for common infectious diseases in older adults are provided in Table 10-5.

INTERDISCIPLINARY CARE

Most clients with infectious diseases need little or no medical care. However, medical treatment can be lifesaving in an overwhelming infection or an immunocompromised host.

The client's history and manifestations can limit the number of possible infectious agents. Asking about recent activities may provide the necessary clues. For instance, family members who all came down with vomiting and diarrhea within 12 hours after a picnic probably do not have the flu.

Once the infecting agent and disease are identified, the type of therapy is selected for each client. Viral infections may need only supportive care, such as providing rest and fluids. Skin infections may respond to a topical agent. Severe systemic infections may require long-term intravenous antibiotic therapy.

Diagnostic Tests

Diagnostic tests assess the client's response to infection, identify the infecting organism, and monitor progress of the medical intervention. The following laboratory tests may be ordered:

- *WBC count* provides clues about the infecting organism and the body's immune response to it (see Table 10-1). The normal WBC count ranges from 4,500 to 10,000/mm^3.
- *WBC differential* is also ordered. During acute infections, more mature neutrophils are produced. If the infection is severe, the body may require more neutrophils than are

TABLE 10-5

Special Population: Common Infectious Diseases in Older Adults, Age-Related Changes, and Nursing Implications

DISEASE WITH CONTRIBUTING FACTORS	AGE-RELATED CHANGES	NURSING IMPLICATIONS
Urinary Tract Infections (UTIs) UTIs are a leading cause of bacteremia and sepsis. UTIs often result from poor hygiene, improper cleansing after bowel elimination, and the presence of a urinary catheter.	Loss of bladder tone, reduced bladder contractility, and decreased mucosal barrier lead to UTIs. Also, incomplete bladder emptying causes residual urine that provides a breeding ground for bacteria.	Monitor for manifestations of burning and urgency. Teach clients to clean properly after bowel elimination. Increase fluids to increase urinary output unless contraindicated by cardiac status. Provide cranberry juice to reduce UTI. Give antibiotics as ordered.
Pneumonia and Influenza Older adults are prone to community-acquired and nosocomial pneumonia. Influenza A and pneumococcal pneumonia can be deadly to those with chronic cardiac and respiratory diseases.	Decreased ciliary action, poor chest expansion, shallow breathing, and reduced cough inhibit removal of inhaled organisms. Impaired swallow reflex from CVA increases risk of aspiration pneumonia.	Monitor for manifestations of increased respiratory rate, listlessness, anorexia, and confusion. (Cough and pleuritic chest pain are often absent.) Recommend annual influenza vaccine and pneumococcal vaccine every 7 years. Give antibiotics as ordered.
Tuberculosis Increased incidence especially in long-term care facilities. Usually recurs from a previous infection.	Altered immune function with decreased phagocytosis reduces ability to ward off TB infection. See other respiratory changes above.	Monitor for weight loss, anorexia, and weakness. (Classic signs of night sweats and fever are absent.) Give anti-TB drugs and monitor closely for side effects.
Skin Infections Due to *S. aureus* and *Streptococcus* A and B; and fungal infections causing candidiasis.	Thinning of skin, loss of elasticity, and decreased sensation increase the skin's vulnerability and invasion of organisms.	Wash hands for 15 seconds with friction to reduce disease transmission. Give antibiotics or antifungals as ordered.
Herpes Zoster or Shingles Reactivation of a latent varicella (chickenpox) virus.	Altered immune system function reduces ability to prevent virus reactivation.	Give analgesics, steroids, antivirals, and topical ointments to alleviate symptoms.
Decubitus Ulcers Increased risk due to chronic diseases, reduced mobility, dehydration, and poor nutrition.	Thinning of skin, loss of elasticity, and decreased sensation reduce skin integrity.	Maintain skin integrity by turning, removing wet linens and clothing, using pressure mattresses, and gently massaging reddened skin areas. Perform wound care as indicated.

made. The bone marrow responds by releasing immature neutrophils called *bands*. This condition is termed *a shift to the left* (Figure 10-5 ■). Eventually the band cells mature and assist in fighting the infection.

■ *Cultures of the wound, blood, or other infected body fluids* may be obtained. Using sterile technique, a specimen is collected and immediately taken to the laboratory. There, it is placed in or on a special culture medium. The culture is placed in an incubator to encourage growth of the organism outside the body. Most cultures take 24 to 36 hours to grow. Then the culture is examined under the microscope to identify the offending microorganism.

■ *Sensitivity studies* determine which antibiotics are most effective against the identified pathogen. Often, several antibiotics are listed. The health care professional selects the appropriate drug based on host and pathogen factors. (See following Medications section for additional information.)

■ *Antibiotic peak and trough levels* monitor therapeutic blood levels of a prescribed medication, especially

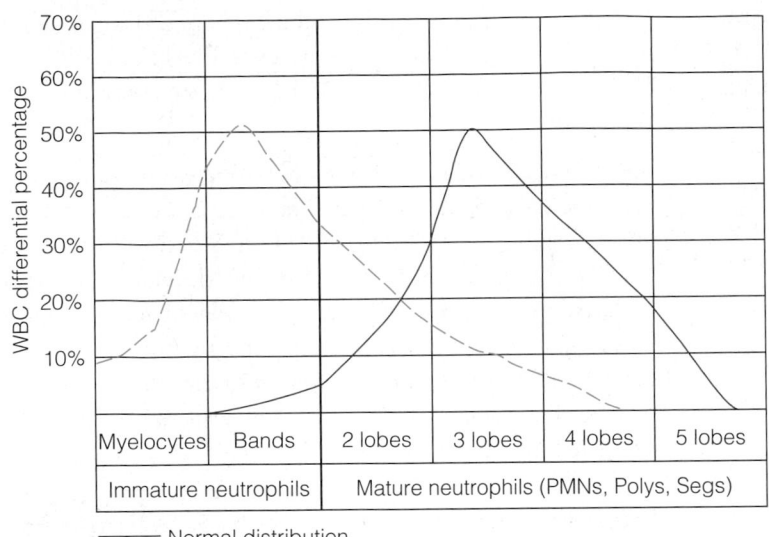

Type of WBC	Normal differential	Shift to left
Myelocytes	0%	Present
Band neutrophils (Bands)	3 to 5%	Increased
Mature neutrophils (Segs, Polys, PMNs)	55 to 70%	May be stable, increased, or decreased

Figure 10-5. ■ Neutrophils by stage of maturity and normal distribution in the blood versus shift to left caused by severe infection.

aminoglycosides. It is important to maintain drug levels within a *therapeutic range,* the amount of drug that will effectively destroy pathogens while producing few toxic effects. By measuring blood levels at the predicted *peak* (1 hour after IM injection and 30 minutes after IV infusion) and *trough* (lowest level, usually just before the next scheduled dose), the physician can determine whether the client is maintaining a level within the therapeutic range.

Other diagnostic tests may confirm an infectious diagnosis in a specific organ. Two of the common tests are:

- *Lumbar puncture,* done to obtain cerebrospinal fluid (CSF) for examination and culture if meningitis or encephalitis is suspected. (See Box 38-3 ⏺⏺ for nursing responsibilities related to lumbar puncture.)
- *Ultrasound examination,* used to detect abscesses or evaluate organ function. An echocardiogram assesses cardiac function and is ordered when pericarditis or endocarditis is suspected. Renal ultrasonography may reveal defects in the urinary tract that would predispose the client to infection.

Medications

Management of infectious diseases focuses on administering *antimicrobials* (drugs capable of killing or incapacitating pathogens). Antimicrobial therapy includes antibiotic, antifungal, antiviral, or antiparasitic drugs. Antibiotics are classified according to the way they interfere with bacterial growth. **Bacteriostatic** agents inhibit the growth of microorganisms. Tetracyclines, macrolides, and sulfonamides are bacteriostatic preparations. **Bactericidal** agents kill the microorganism and include penicillin, cephalosporin, and

aminoglycoside antibiotics. In addition, antibiotics have either a narrow spectrum or broad spectrum of action. **Narrow-spectrum antibiotics** act against a limited number of pathogens, whereas **broad-spectrum antibiotics** inhibit a wide variety of microbes.

Antimicrobials can be applied topically or administered by oral, intramuscular, intravenous, interperitoneal, or intrathecal routes. Oral and intravenous routes are most commonly used.

A culture and sensitivity test should be done before antimicrobial therapy is started. If antibiotics are started before the culture is collected, they could interfere with organism growth on the culture medium. When clients are scheduled for surgery or invasive procedures that could cause an infection, they are started on **prophylactic** (preventive) anti-infective therapy.

Selection of an appropriate antimicrobial is based on its effectiveness, level of toxicity, ease of administration, and cost effectiveness. The health care professional must also consider several factors about the client, such as:

- History of allergic reactions
- Client's age and childbearing status
- Client's present health status; presence of malnutrition, cancer, or AIDS
- Renal and hepatic function
- Site and extent of the infection
- History of chronic diseases and other drug therapy.

Many microorganisms can develop resistance to one or more antimicrobial agents. This means that the pathogen lives and grows in the presence of the antimicrobial. Resistance occurs because the pathogen develops a new form or **mutation,** allowing the organism to survive. Overuse of

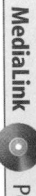

antibiotics and insufficient medication doses are the most frequent causes.

Several factors contribute to antimicrobial resistance. Clients may expect to receive antibiotics every time they are ill, no matter whether the organism is bacterial or viral. When antibiotics are given for viral infections, bacteria learn to thrive in an antibiotic environment. Also, the use of broad-spectrum rather than narrow-spectrum drugs can lead to multidrug-resistant strains of bacteria.

Finally, the way the client takes an antibiotic can contribute to drug resistance. When a client fails to take all of the prescribed doses, the pathogen is inadequately destroyed, and new microbe mutations can occur. The nurse must teach clients the importance of completing their drug prescriptions.

As with all drug therapy, antimicrobials can cause adverse reactions. Allergic responses, toxicity to the liver, kidneys, ears, and bone marrow, and superinfections may develop. A **superinfection** is a new infection that appears because the antibiotic has eliminated normal bacterial flora. For example, yeast infections called candidiasis (or *thrush*) will appear in the mouth or vaginal area.

ANTIBIOTIC DRUGS. Medications used to treat bacterial infections are generally known as **antibiotics.** They were first developed more than 50 years ago. New antibiotics are constantly being developed to overcome the multidrug-resistant bacteria. Antibiotics fall into different classes of drugs with related chemical structure and activity. Some are effective only against gram-positive bacteria; others are effective only against gram-negative organisms. Newer broad-spectrum antibiotics have activity against a wide variety of bacteria, including both gram-positive and gram-negative forms. (Antibiotic drugs, action, nursing implications, and client teaching for each class are summarized in Table 10-6 ■.)

ANTIFUNGAL AGENTS. Fungal infections can be superficial or systemic. Topical antifungal preparations are used to treat superficial infections such as candidiasis, tineas, and ringworm. One of the most frequently ordered drugs is nystatin (Mycostatin) for treating candidiasis. Vaginal preparations are available to treat vaginal yeast infections.

Amphotericin B (Fungizone) is a systemic antifungal agent for parenteral administration. It is used to treat severe, life-threatening fungal infections including histoplasmosis, coccidioidomycosis, and candidiasis. Fluconazole (Diflucan) is preferred over amphotericin B because it is less toxic and is available in oral and parenteral forms. (Nursing responsibilities are listed in Table 10-7 ■.)

ANTIVIRAL DRUGS. Viral infections can be as mild as the common cold, chronic like herpes infections, or life threatening like acquired immunodeficiency syndrome (AIDS). Antiviral therapy is relatively new and quite limited

because new viruses can reproduce before a drug is developed. The drugs in this class are expensive and fairly toxic to the client. Common antiviral agents are summarized in the Table 10-7.

ANTIPARASITIC AGENTS. Drugs used to treat parasitic infections are as varied as the organisms that cause them. Generally, these drugs are expensive and often toxic. Quinine was one of the first antiparasitic drugs developed to treat malaria. Quinine is very toxic, but newer forms such as chloroquine (Aralen), primaquine, and hydroxychloroquine (Plaquenil) are widely used as antimalarial drugs. Metronidazole (Flagyl) is used to treat protozoan infections and is discussed in Table 10-6.

Infection Prevention and Control Techniques

Prevention is the most important control measure for nosocomial infections and begins with health care workers. Health care personnel wear clean clothing and follow good hygiene practices. Most infectious organisms are spread by direct contact with health care workers. *Effective hand washing (at least 15 seconds, using friction and antimicrobial soap) is the single most important measure in infection control.* Although hand washing remains the key to infection control, the convenience of using antimicrobial foam or gel increases health care worker's compliance for hand cleansing. They also should keep immunizations current and should not care for clients when ill with an infectious disease or open skin lesions. The nurse also assumes an important role in determining when invasive procedures such as urinary catheterization are needed. Catheterization increases the incidence of urinary tract infection (UTI), so the nurse must decide whether another choice for managing incontinence might be workable.

Controlling the spread of infectious diseases in the hospital or long-term care setting is essential. Each health care facility follows infection control guidelines developed by the CDC. Each institution also develops its own specific policies for handling biologic waste disposal, housekeeping and sterilization procedures, and employee health standards. Other policies outline the frequency for changing urinary drainage bags or intravenous bags and tubing. For instance, intravenous bags are changed every 24 hours and tubing every 24 to 72 hours.

The Occupational Safety and Health Administration (OSHA) is responsible for reducing the risk of exposure to infectious diseases. It publishes mandatory guidelines about routine training to prevent bloodborne pathogens and TB. Institutions that do not follow OSHA standards face penalties and fines.

ISOLATION PRECAUTIONS. The CDC developed and implemented two tiers of isolation precautions to be used in health care facilities. These two tiers are Standard Precautions and

TABLE 10-6

Nursing Implications for Pharmacology: Antibiotic Therapy

CLASS/DRUGS	PURPOSE	NURSING RESPONSIBILITIES	CLIENT TEACHING
Penicillins *Natural* ■ Penicillin G ■ Penicillin V *Penicillinase-Resistant* ■ Cloxacillin (Tegopen) ■ Dicloxacillin (Dynapen) ■ Nafcillin (Unipen) ■ Oxacillin (Prostaphlin) *Ampicillins* ■ Amoxicillin (Amoxil) ■ Ampicillin (Polycillin) *Extended-Spectrum* ■ Carbenicillin (Geocillin) ■ Mezlocillin (Mezlin) ■ Piperacillin (Pipracil) ■ Ticarcillin (Ticar) *Penicillin/Beta-Lactamase Inhibitors* ■ Amoxicillin and clavulanate (Augmentin)	Penicillins are bactericidal and effective against streptococci, staphylococci, meningococci, and gonococci organisms. They are safe, effective, and have a low toxicity. Penicillin is ordered in units or milligrams. They are available in PO, IM, and IV forms.	Check for allergies before giving the first dose. Do not give to anyone with an allergy to penicillin or cephalosporins. Assess the client for an allergic response: rashes, hives, and itching. Notify the MD immediately. Monitor for anaphylaxis. In an outpatient setting, ask client to wait 30 minutes after an IM injection. Monitor for white patches in mouth or a vaginal discharge due to candidiasis. An antifungal drug may be needed while the antibiotic is continued.	Take as ordered to prevent developing resistant organisms. Shake suspensions well before pouring them. Take with a full glass of water 1 hour before or 2 hours after meals. If any signs of an allergic reaction occur, stop the drug and contact the physician. Notify the physician if white patches are noted on the oral mucosa or if vaginitis develops. Eat yogurt or buttermilk to prevent fungal infection but do not take these products within 1 hour of taking the drug.
Cephalosporins *First Generation* ■ Cefazolin (Ancef) ■ Cephalexin (Keflex) *Second Generation* ■ Cefaclor (Ceclor) ■ Cefoxitin (Mefoxin) ■ Cefuroxime (Zinacef) *Third Generation* ■ Cefoperazone (Cefobid) ■ Cefotaxime (Claforan) ■ Ceftazidime (Fortaz) ■ Ceftizoxime (Cefizox) ■ Ceftriaxone (Rocephin) *Fourth Generation* ■ Cefepime (Maxipime)	Cephalosporins are related structurally to the penicillins so there may be a cross-sensitivity between them. First generation act against gram-positive organisms; second and third generation are more effective against gram-negative organisms; fourth generation act against gram-positive and -negative organisms. They are used preoperatively and to treat skin, soft tissue, respiratory and urinary tract.	Check for allergic response to cephalosporins or penicillins. Give with food or milk to reduce GI upset. Give IM injections into large muscle site. Monitor IV site for phlebitis or local pain at IM site. Monitor for decreased output and elevated blood urea nitrogen (BUN) in older clients. Monitor for diarrhea; if blood or mucus appears, notify MD immediately.	Take all of the prescribed drug as ordered. Take with food or milk to reduce GI upset. Eat yogurt or drink buttermilk to prevent oral or vaginal infections. Notify MD if skin rashes, hives, vomiting, severe diarrhea, anal or vaginal itching, or mouth sores develop.
Aminoglycosides ■ Amikacin (Amikin) ■ Netilmicin (Netromycin) ■ Gentamicin (Garamycin) ■ Streptomycin ■ Kanamycin (Kantrex) ■ Tobramycin (Nebcin)	Aminoglycosides are used against serious gram-negative organisms; *Pseudomonas, E. coli, Klebsiella.* They are combined with other antibiotics to provide a greater effect.	Monitor for ototoxicity (ringing in the ears) and nephrotoxocity (decreased urine output, elevated BUN and serum creatinine). Monitor peak and trough levels. Increase fluid intake to 2,000–3,000 mL/day. Give IV drugs one hour apart from other IV antibiotics. Give IM deep into a large muscle.	If adverse effects occur, stop the drug and notify the MD. Monitor daily weights. A sudden weight gain may indicate adverse effects on the kidney.
Fluoroquinolones ■ Ciprofloxacin (Cipro) ■ Gatifloxacin (Tequin)	Fluoroquinolones act against gram-positive and gram-negative	Increase fluid intake to 2,000–3,000 mL/day.	Check label before taking with food.

(continued)

TABLE 10-6

Nursing Implications for Pharmacology: Antibiotic Therapy (continued)

CLASS/DRUGS	PURPOSE	NURSING RESPONSIBILITIES	CLIENT TEACHING
■ Levofloxacin (Levaquin)	organisms to treat respiratory, GI, GU, and soft tissue infections. They are given in PO and IV forms.	Monitor for decreased urine output.	Drink 6–8 glasses of water per day. Avoid exposure to sunlight; notify MD if skin rashes or redness occur.
Tetracyclines ■ Tetracycline (Achromycin) ■ Demeclocycline (Declomycin) ■ Doxycycline (Vibramycin)	Tetracyclines act against gram-positive and gram-negative bacteria to treat chlamydia, severe acne, and when the client is allergic to other antibiotics. Tetracyclines are not used during pregnancy or in children under 5 to prevent tooth discoloration.	Do not give with milk/milk products or antacids. Monitor for signs of nausea, vomiting, and diarrhea. Monitor for thrush, vaginal or anal itching. Report signs to the physician.	Do not take with milk/milk products or antacids. Take dose with a full glass of water. Avoid sun exposure and wear protective clothing to reduce risk of sunburn. Avoid exposing drug to light, extreme heat, and humidity.
Sulfonamides ■ Sulfamethiazole (Thiosulfil Forte) ■ Sulfamethoxazole (Gantanol) ■ Trimethoprim-sulfamethoxazole (Bactrim, Septra) ■ Sulfisoxazole (Gantrisin) ■ Mafenide (Sulfamylon)	Oral sulfonamides treat UTIs by bacteriostatic action. Trimethoprim-sulfamethoxazole is used for *Pneumocystis carinii* pneumonia (PCP). Sulfamylon is applied topically for burns.	Give with a full glass of water. Increase fluid intake to 2,000–3,000 mL/day. Monitor for skin rash, itching, easy bruising, or bleeding gums and notify MD. For burns, apply thin layer of sulfamylon with sterile gloves.	Take drug with full glass of water. Drink 2–3 quarts of fluids per day. Avoid sun exposure to reduce sunburn. Notify physician if skin rash, itching, hives, easy bruising, or bleeding gums develop.
Macrolides ■ Erythromycin (E-Mycin, Ilosone) ■ Azithromycin (Zithromax) ■ Clarithromycin (Biaxin)	Macrolides are used for gram-positive and gram-negative organisms causing skin/soft tissue and respiratory infections; for clients allergic to penicillin. Zithromax and Biaxin act longer and have fewer GI side effects.	Give with a full glass of water. Check whether to give with or without food. Monitor for nausea, vomiting, diarrhea, dark urine, jaundice. Use cautiously in pregnancy and those with liver disease.	Take with a full glass of water. Check label for taking with or without food. Notify physician if GI upset is severe or if dark urine or yellowish-tinge of eyes appear.
Miscellaneous Drugs ■ Metronidazole (Flagyl) ■ Vancomycin (Vancocin)	Flagyl is effective for protozoans causing amebiasis, giardiasis, and trichomoniasis. Flagyl is given prophylactically for anaerobic gram-negative bacteria before and after colon surgery. Vancocin is used for severe gram-positive infections such as MRSA.	*Flagyl:* Give with meals to decrease GI upset. Inform client that drug causes a metallic taste and urine turns dark. Increase fluid intake to 2,000–3,000 mL/day. Notify MD if dizziness, headache, tingling of extremities, or seizures occur. *Vancocin:* Give IV dose over 1 hour. Monitor closely for Red Man syndrome—severe rash, flushing, and hypotension. Monitor for ototoxicity and nephrotoxicity.	*Flagyl:* Take with meals to decrease GI upset. Drink 2–3 quarts of water daily. Avoid alcohol during therapy to prevent flushing, nausea, vomiting, and headache. Notify physician if dizziness, headache, tingling of extremities, or seizures occur. *Vancocin:* Report tinnitus, hearing loss, or decreased urine output immediately.

TABLE 10-7

Nursing Implications for Pharmacology: Antifungal and Antiviral Drugs

CLASS/DRUGS	PURPOSE	NURSING RESPONSIBILITIES	CLIENT TEACHING
Antifungal Drugs ■ Amphotericin B (Fungizone) ■ Clotrimazole (Lotrimin) ■ Fluconazole (Diflucan) ■ Ketoconazole (Nizoral) ■ Miconazole (Monistat) ■ Nystatin (Mycostatin)	Antifungals treat oral and vaginal candidiasis, ringworm histoplasmosis, and cryptococcosis. May be applied topically or given PO and IV.	Follow Standard Precautions when cleaning skin lesions and applying topical medications. Have client swish nystatin suspension in mouth for 2–3 minutes before swallowing. Premedicate with Tylenol and/or Demerol to prevent rigors with amphotericin B.	For topical agents, wash and dry the area before applying the medication. Swish nystatin suspension in mouth for 2–3 minutes before swallowing. Follow instructions for using vaginal preparations. Notify physician of unusual fatigue, decreased appetite, vomiting, dark urine, jaundice, or diarrhea.
Antiviral Drugs ■ Amantadine (Symmetrel) ■ Acyclovir (Zovirax) ■ Ganciclovir (Cytovene) ■ Ribavirin (Virazole) ■ Vidarabine (Vir-A) ■ Zidovudine (AZT, Retrovir)	Antivirals treat influenza A, herpesvirus, and opportunistic viral infections in AIDS. Specific antiretroviral drugs reduce viral loads in HIV. May be given PO, IV, or topical.	Apply topical agents with gloves. For IV acyclovir: increase fluid intake to 2,000–3,000 mL/day and monitor for fatigue, headache, and seizures. Monitor for signs of bone marrow suppression. See Chapter 11 for discussion of antiretroviral drugs. ⦾	Take drugs as prescribed. Cleanse area and apply topical ointment with gloves. Keep acyclovir in tight, light-resistant container. Report unusual fatigue, headache, and seizures. Discuss sexual abstinence during active herpes infection.

Transmission-based Precautions. To determine the need for isolation precautions, the nurse must consider the microorganism, the mode of transmission, and susceptibility of hospital staff and other clients. For example, clients with active tuberculosis are highly contagious and must be placed in Airborne Precautions.

Standard Precautions. **Standard Precautions** are guidelines to protect the health care worker as well as prevent transmission to other clients. These guidelines are used with all clients, whether they are known to have an infectious disease or not. All health care workers who have direct contact with clients or with their body fluids or have indirect contact, such as by emptying trash, changing linens, or cleaning the room must use Standard Precautions. Standard Precautions apply to (1) blood; (2) all body fluids, secretions, and excretions except sweat, regardless of whether they contain visible blood; (3) nonintact skin; and (4) mucous membranes.

Barrier protection prevents exposure of skin and mucous membranes to blood and body fluids. Barrier protection involves using gloves, gowns, masks, or goggles as appropriate. Standard Precautions are outlined in Box 10-6 ■.

Transmission-Based Precautions. Some infectious diseases require added techniques in addition to Standard Precautions. The three types of **Transmission-based Precautions** are Airborne Precautions, Droplet Precautions, and Contact Precautions. Transmission-based Precautions may

BOX 10-6

STANDARD PRECAUTION GUIDELINES

- Wash hands immediately after touching blood, body fluids, secretions and excretions, mucous membranes, nonintact skin, and contaminated items; between client contact; and after removing gloves.
- Wear clean, nonsterile gloves when touching blood, body fluids, secretions and excretions, mucous membranes, nonintact skin, and contaminated items.
- Change gloves between tasks on the same client.
- Wear mask, eye protection, face shield, gown, or plastic apron to avoid being splashed or sprayed with blood, body fluids, secretions, and excretions.
- Remove soiled protective clothing as soon as client care is completed.
- Do not recap or break needles; dispose of needles and other sharp objects in puncture-proof containers. Use one-handed "scoop" technique or a special needle-recapping device.
- Clean spills immediately with 1:10 bleach solution or facility-recommended germicide.
- Handle used client equipment and linen carefully to prevent self- and clothing contamination, and transfer of organisms to other clients. Place in leak-proof bags and follow institution's policies regarding double-bagging.
- Place the client who may contaminate the environment in a private room with a private bathroom.

Source: Adapted from CDC (2004). *Standard Precautions* (developed in 1996). Available at www.cdc.gov/ncidod/hip/ISOLAT/std_prec_excerpt.htm

be combined for diseases that have multiple routes of transmission. (Specific guidelines for Transmission-based Precautions were outlined earlier in Table 10-4.)

Complementary Therapies

Oral echinacea is taken to decrease inflammation and to prevent the common cold and influenza. It should be used for less than 8 weeks at a time. Anyone who is currently taking immunosuppressants (see Table 11-7 🔗) should not take echinacea because it stimulates immune function.

NURSING CARE

Priorities in Nursing Care. Nursing management of clients with an infection or infectious disease focuses on prevention, health promotion, and health maintenance. Prevention includes assessing the client's risk for infection, immune function, and the need for immunizations. Health promotion and maintenance activities include monitoring vital signs; administering prescribed antibiotics; using aseptic technique and infection control measures; and promoting rest, activity, and nutritional intake.

ASSESSING

Before implementing nursing care, the nurse must collect assessment data. These data can help determine the extent to which an infection or infectious disease is interfering with the client's life, can identify risk factors for complications, and can be used by the physician to determine the type of medical intervention needed (Box 10-7 ■). The nurse must also assess for risks of nosocomial infection from invasive procedures and therapies.

DIAGNOSING, PLANNING, AND IMPLEMENTING

Individuals with an acute infection or infectious disease may require hospitalization until the crisis is resolved. Those with chronic infections or side effects from the infectious disease process may need care in long-term care facilities or at home. Priority nursing diagnoses are Risk for Infection, Imbalanced Nutrition, and Ineffective Thermoregulation.

Risk for Infection

Clients may enter health care facilities with inadequate physical defenses, malnutrition, or chronic diseases. In addition, they may be exposed to drug-resistant microorganisms. It is vital that nurses in health care facilities follow all of the standards for infection prevention and control.

■ Admit clients with known or suspected infections to a private room. *This minimizes risk to other clients.*

BOX 10-7	ASSESSMENT

Assessing Clients with Infection

SUBJECTIVE DATA

■ Present health status:
  ■ General health and nutritional status.
  ■ Fever: How long has the fever existed? Has client had chills?
  ■ Describe cough and/or sputum.
  ■ Sore throat, congestion, runny or stuffy nose.
  ■ Anorexia, nausea, vomiting, abdominal pain, diarrhea.
  ■ Weakness, malaise, muscle aches, joint pains, headache.
  ■ Pain on urination, odor, urgency, frequency, flank pain.
  ■ Vaginal discharge—color, odor, itching.
  ■ Describe any rash.
  ■ Presence of animal or insect bite.
■ Past medical history:
  ■ Any infections or exposure to infectious person.
  ■ Treatment for tuberculosis or sexually transmitted disease.
  ■ Has the client been tested for HIV?
  ■ Use of antipyretics, antimicrobials.
  ■ Immunization history.
  ■ Any travel overseas?

OBJECTIVE DATA

■ Vital signs: blood pressure, pulse, respirations, temperature.
■ Height and weight.
■ Observe for fatigue, shortness of breath, and altered mental status.
■ Assess for dehydration: increased thirst, dry mucous membranes, decreased skin turgor.
■ Auscultate chest for crackles and wheezes.
■ Inspect sputum, stool, genitourinary excretions for amount, color, consistency, and odor.
■ Inspect throat for redness.
■ Palpate the skin for the presence of any rash.
■ Palpate for enlarged lymph nodes.
■ Monitor WBC and C&S report; report abnormal findings.

■ Wash hands thoroughly on entering and leaving the client's room. *Hand washing removes microorganisms from the skin and prevents transmission of infection to or from the client.*
■ Use Standard Precautions for all clients. *Standard Precautions significantly reduce the risk of disease transmission during client care.*
■ Use Transmission-based Precautions when appropriate. *Transmission-based Precautions reduce the spread of disease by airborne, droplet, or direct and indirect methods.*

- Explain to the client and family the reasons for isolation precautions. *Clients with isolation precautions may feel neglected or dirty. Explaining the reasons and procedures can enhance understanding and acceptance.*
- Place a mask on the client or cover all infectious lesions or wounds completely when transporting the client to other parts of the facility for diagnostic or treatment procedures. *These measures minimize air contamination and the risk to visitors and personnel.*
- Collect a culture and sensitivity (C&S) specimen as ordered. *C&S can identify infectious organisms and determine the most effective antibiotics.*

clinical ALERT

Collect the specimen before administering the first dose of antibiotics to ensure adequate organisms for culture.

- Administer prescribed antimicrobial agents. *Antimicrobial agents are given to destroy invading microorganisms.*
- Notify all personnel who have contact with the client about the diagnosis. *Personnel must take appropriate precautions, particularly for clients with diseases requiring category-specific isolation.*
- Ensure that visitors wear appropriate protective garments before they enter the client's room. *Protective wear reduces visitors' risk of infection.*
- Follow facility guidelines for disposal of contaminated tissues, dressings, or other material, and for removal of soiled linens and equipment from the client's room. *These measures prevent the transmission of pathogenic organisms.*

Imbalanced Nutrition

Fever, especially prolonged high fever, increases the body's metabolism. Inadequate nutrition may prolong the infectious process.

- Encourage a high-calorie, high-protein diet. *Increased calories and protein are needed to meet increased metabolic demands.*
- Provide liquid or soft, easily digested foods. *Difficult-to-digest foods increase heat production. If the client has a sore throat, liquids and soft food are easier to swallow.*
- Encourage client to choose appealing foods. *Clients with a systemic infection often lose their appetite. If they can choose foods they like, it may stimulate their appetite.*
- Minimize offensive odors from draining wounds. *Decreasing odors may increase the client's appetite.*

Ineffective Thermoregulation

Clients with an infectious disease usually develop a fever. Although fever serves a useful purpose, abnormally high fevers can put the client at risk for other complications.

- Monitor temperature, pulse, and respirations at regular intervals. *This helps to determine the fever pattern and effects on other body systems.*

clinical ALERT

Monitor temperature between 5 P.M. and 7 P.M. because the body's temperature cycle peaks during these hours.

- Increase oral fluid intake to 2,500 mL/day, as appropriate, for the client's cardiopulmonary status. *Fever can cause dehydration; increased fluid intake reduces this risk. Fluids are given cautiously to clients with cardiopulmonary disease to prevent fluid overload.*
- Administer IV fluid and electrolytes as ordered. *If fluid loss is severe, client will need IV electrolyte solutions.*
- Record intake and output at least every 8 hours. *Decreased urine output may indicate dehydration.*
- Give prescribed antipyretics as ordered for an elevated temperature. *Antipyretics lower the body's temperature; however, they decrease WBC activity, especially phagocytosis. Some microorganisms can be destroyed when the body reaches a certain temperature.*
- Provide tepid baths, place ice packs in the groin and axilla, or cover with a hypothermia blanket only if temperature is greater than 104°F. *These methods can reduce fever too rapidly, causing more shivering and increased temperature. Be sure to wrap ice bags in a towel to prevent tissue damage.*

clinical ALERT

Use ice packs, cool/tepid baths, or hypothermia blanket cautiously to prevent unnecessary shivering.

- Maintain bed rest. *Bed rest conserves energy and reduces metabolic demands.*
- When the client becomes diaphoretic, bathe and replace wet gowns and linen. *Personal hygiene promotes client comfort.*
- Monitor the client for decreased level of consciousness and seizures. *High fevers can cause dehydration, leading to an altered mental status and seizures.*

EVALUATING

Evaluate effectiveness of nursing care by collecting the following data: temperature remains normal for 24 hours, no signs of dehydration, clear breath sounds, and cultures negative for pathogens. Also, evaluate whether the client takes precautions to prevent spread of an infection and is completing any ordered antibiotics.

Documentation. Document assessment findings related to increased temperature and pulse and the presence of dehydration. Note whether the client can increase oral fluid intake and eat a high-calorie, high-protein diet.

CONTINUING CARE

Client and family teaching focuses on promoting client recovery, preventing spread of infection to others, and preventing potential complications. Instructions should include the following points:

- Wash hands after touching infected wounds or lesions, coughing, sneezing, blowing the nose, using the bathroom, before preparing food or eating, or before wound care.
- Take all prescribed antibiotics until the prescription is completed even after symptoms are relieved.
- Notify your health care provider if any of the following occurs:
  - No improvement in symptoms within 24 to 48 hours after antibiotic therapy is started, or recurring symptoms after antibiotic therapy is completed.
  - Itching, rash, difficulty breathing; signs of superinfection such as vaginitis, oral candidiasis, or diarrhea; persistent high fever, change in alertness, or activity.
  - Adverse reactions, such as gastrointestinal distress, that interfere with completion of the prescription.
- Do not share medication with family members or others.
- Wear Medic-Alert bracelet noting medication allergies.
- Increase fluid intake to at least 2.5 quarts per day and eat a well-balanced diet.
- Prevent the spread of infection to others by:
  - Avoiding crowds and contact with infectious persons
  - Using disposable tissues when coughing or sneezing
  - Practicing safe food handling practices
  - Not sharing personal hygiene items
  - Using safe sex practices
  - Keeping the home clean; disinfecting with 1:10 bleach solution for blood spills.
- Keep immunizations current. If they are not up to date, discuss where immunizations can be obtained.

NURSING PROCESS CARE PLAN
Client with MRSA Infection

Mr. Frank Kendall, 87 years old, is transferred from a nearby long-term care facility to the medical unit of the community hospital. Mr. Kendall has been in the long-term care facility for 6 months following a cerebrovascular accident (CVA). Two months ago he was in the hospital for urosepsis. He has been widowed for 9 months. One daughter lives 1,000 miles away and has visited him only once in the past 6 months.

The nurse from the long-term care facility reports that he is too weak to get out of bed by himself. He has a poor appetite and seems frail. About 1 month ago he developed a large decubitus ulcer on the sacral area that is not healing.

Assessment. On admission, vital signs are BP 150/84, P 92, R 24, T 100°F (37.7°C), weight 165 lbs, and height 5'10". He is listless, with decreased right arm and leg movement, thin extremities, and poor skin turgor. He answers the nurse's questions without looking at her. The decubitus ulcer on the sacral area measures 7 cm long, 4 cm wide, 1.5 cm deep, with yellowish-green drainage. The wound edges are red and tender. He grimaces as the nurse assesses the wound. An intravenous line is inserted and 5% dextrose/0.45 normal saline is started at 75 mL/hr. After 24 hours a preliminary culture report shows MRSA in the decubitus ulcer. The nurse implements Contact Precautions for Mr. Kendall.

Diagnosis. The following nursing diagnoses are developed for Mr. Kendall:

- *Imbalanced Nutrition: Less than Body Requirements* related to poor appetite
- *Impaired Skin Integrity* related to large decubitus ulcer
- *Acute Pain* related to decubitus ulcer
- *Hopelessness* related to recent widowhood and CVA

Expected Outcomes. The expected outcomes established in the plan of care specify that:

- Mr. Kendall will increase dietary intake.
- Wound will show signs of healing.
- Wound cultures will no longer show a MRSA infection.
- Mr. Kendall will report that pain is decreased.
- He will communicate feelings about his situation.

Planning and Implementation. Ms. Thompson, RN, implements the following interventions:

- Monitor daily weight, intake and output, and hydration status.
- Assess for risk of aspiration during eating and drinking.
- Identify foods Mr. Kendall likes and dislikes.
- Provide small, frequent, high-protein meals.
- Consult with a dietitian regarding supplemental foods such as Ensure.
- Monitor serum albumin levels.
- Assess skin every 8 hours; keep clean and dry.
- Turn at least every 2 hours; minimize time Mr. Kendall lies on his back; and prevent shearing.
- Consult with physician for an air/water mattress or specialized bed (e.g., Clinitron Bed).

- Follow Contact Precautions; meticulously wash hands before and after care.
- Premedicate before dressing changes or wound care.
- Use aseptic technique to provide wound care to decubitus ulcer.
- Administer antibiotics as ordered.
- Determine level of pain using a 0-to-10 pain scale.
- Administer pain medications prn.
- Encourage Mr. Kendall to discuss his feelings and concerns.
- Arrange for social services to talk to his daughter.

Evaluation. After a month in the hospital Mr. Kendall's wound culture is negative for MRSA. The wound is showing signs of healing. His daughter has visited him twice. He smiles occasionally and interacts with the staff more positively. Mr. Kendall's appetite has improved and he no longer needs supplemental feedings. He reports that his pain is tolerable. He understands that he has to return to the long-term care facility until his wound heals completely. His daughter plans to move him to her home sometime in the near future.

Critical Thinking in the Nursing Process

1. What type of isolation garments should the nurse wear while providing care to Mr. Kendall?
2. How did Mr. Kendall contract MRSA?
3. List three strategies to prevent the transmission of MRSA to other clients.

Note: The bibliography listings for this and all chapters have been compiled at the back of the book.

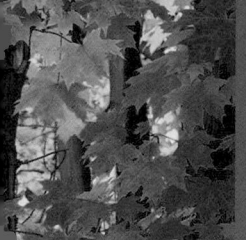

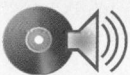 **KEY TERMS** by Topics

Use the audio glossary feature of either the CD-ROM or the Companion Website to hear the correct pronunciation of the following key terms.

Inflammation
inflammation, diapedesis, macrophages, phagocytosis

Acute inflammation
cellulitis, abscesses, incision and drainage, fistula, lymphadenitis,

leukocytosis, endogenous pyrogens, leukopenia

Chronic inflammation
catabolism, anabolism

Infection
infection, immunosuppression, chain of infection, pathogens, virulence, invasiveness, exotoxins, endotoxins, carriers, colonization, infectious disease, nosocomial infections

Collaborative care of infections
bacteriostatic, bactericidal, broad-spectrum antibiotics, narrow-spectrum antibiotics, prophylactic, mutation, superinfection, antibiotics

Infection control
Standard Precautions, Transmission-based Precautions

KEY Points

- The body is protected from microorganisms by the skin, physical barriers such as coughing, and chemical defenses.

- Cardinal manifestations of local inflammation are redness, warmth, pain, edema, and loss of function.

- The chain of infection includes a microorganism, a reservoir, a portal of exit from the reservoir, a mode of transmission from the reservoir, and an entry point into a susceptible host.

- Fever and WBC count greater than 10,000/mm^3 may indicate a generalized infection.

- Antibiotics, antiviral, antifungal, and antiparasitic medications are the common medications used to manage infections.

- Older adults are at greater risk for developing pneumonia, influenza, and urinary tract and skin infections than are younger adults.

- Hand washing is the most important measure in preventing nosocomial infections.

- Two tiers of isolation are (1) Standard Precautions and (2) Transmission-based Precautions.

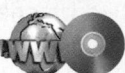 **EXPLORE MediaLink**

Additional interactive resources for this chapter can be found on the Companion Website at www.prenhall.com/burke. Click on Chapter 10 and "Begin" to select the activities for this chapter.

For chapter-related NCLEX-style review questions and an audio glossary, access the accompanying CD-ROM in this book.

FOR FURTHER Study

For more on the healing process and wound care, see Chapter 9.

For more information on immunizations and a discussion of retroviral drugs, see Chapter 11.

For in-depth discussion on septic shock, see Chapter 13.

For more on the client receiving corticosteroid medications, see Table 16-3.

Box 38-3 lists the nursing responsibilities related to the lumbar puncture procedure.

Critical Thinking Care Map

Caring for a Client Exposed to *Staphylococcus aureus*
NCLEX-PN® Focus Area: Reduction of Risk Potential

Case Study: Mr. Fields, age 76, was transferred from a long-term nursing care facility for a mild left-side stroke. He has an intravenous line and Foley catheter in place. Mr. Fields weighs 140 lbs and is 6' tall. He shares a hospital room with another client who is diagnosed with *Staphylococcus aureus* pneumonia. Mr. Fields' vital signs are BP 158/90, P 88, R 24, T 99°F.

Nursing Diagnosis: Risk for Infection

COLLECT DATA

Subjective	Objective
_____	_____
_____	_____
_____	_____
_____	_____
_____	_____
_____	_____

Would you report this data? Yes/No

If yes, to: _____

Nursing Care

_____
_____
_____
_____
_____
_____
_____
_____
_____
_____
_____

How would you document this? _____
_____
_____

Data Collected
(use those that apply)

- Roommate with *S. aureus* pneumonia
- Pale coloring
- Weight 140 lbs
- Urine output 200 mL for shift
- Temperature 99°F
- Dislikes being in the nursing home
- Pressure ulcer on right great toe
- History of Type 2 diabetes

Nursing Interventions
(use those that apply; list in priority order)

- Provide a diet high in protein.
- Place in protective isolation.
- Monitor vital signs every 4 hours.
- Monitor skin for further breakdown.
- Increase fluid intake as tolerated.
- Prevent food from pocketing on the right side of his mouth.

NCLEX-PN® Exam Preparation

1 A client, age 82, has been admitted to your surgical unit after 3 days in the intensive care unit following a colon resection. His vital signs are stable and his urinary bag contains 300 mL of clear yellow urine. Which of the following information is most important to determine if the client is at risk for developing a nosocomial infection?

A. Foley catheter insertion during surgery
B. use of an antibiotic for 1 week prior to surgery
C. weight of 150 lbs
D. poor venous circulation in the left leg

2 Your client is scheduled for a left knee replacement. Which of the following lab values must you report to the physician immediately?

A. WBC count of 7,000
B. WBC count of 3,500
C. WBC count of 15,000
D. WBC count of 4,500

3 Prior to the administration of aspirin to your client with rheumatoid arthritis, it is most important to assess:

A. the age of the client.
B. the client's use of alcohol.
C. the expiration date of the medication.
D. the client's allergy history.

4 A client has been taking penicillin G for a staph infection. Three days after beginning the drug, she returns to your clinic. She complains of vaginal itchiness and redness. You suspect that the client has developed vaginitis. Your response to the client should be:

A. "Oh, don't worry about that. It will go away after you finish the medication."
B. "I will let the doctor know right away."
C. "Its just vaginitis. We'll give you something for it."
D. "Okay. Are you having any other problems?"

5 You are planning discharge care for your client who has suffered numerous abrasions sustained in a motor vehicle accident. Which of the following should be included in the discharge instructions?

A. Discontinue the antibiotics once the redness has subsided.
B. A slight fever is common and should not be reported.
C. Drink at least 2 quarts of water per day.
D. Wash your hands carefully before changing the wound dressings.

6 Which medication treatment would the nurse anticipate for the client with a diagnosis of MRSA?

A. vancomycin (Vancocin)
B. erythromycin (E-Mycin)
C. fluconazole (Diflucan)
D. acyclovir (Zovirax)

7 A 70-year-old male client was admitted to the medical floor with a diagnosis of left periorbital cellulitis. Based on this diagnosis, which of the following interventions should the nurse include in the client's care plan in order to promote the healing process?

A. Administer IV antibiotics as ordered.
B. Maintain bed rest.
C. Medicate the client around the clock with IM morphine.
D. Monitor the WBC count.

8 Which of the following conditions indicate that an infection has become systemic?

A. A fistula forms.
B. Lymphadenitis is observed.
C. Abscesses form in the area of infection.
D. Cellulitis begins to develop.

9 Your AIDS client has been diagnosed with *Pneumocystis carinii* pneumonia. Your client asks you what type of "bug" causes this illness. You state that *Pneumocystis carinii* is a:

A. virus.
B. fungus.
C. bacteria.
D. protozoan.

10 An elderly woman was admitted on your shift with varicella. What type of isolation precautions should be used for this client?

A. Droplet Precautions
B. Contact Precautions
C. Airborne Precautions
D. Standard Precautions

Answers for Review Questions, as well as discussion of Care Plan and Critical Thinking Care Map questions, appear in Appendix V.

CONSIDERING CULTURAL VARIATIONS RELATED TO ENVIRONMENTAL CONTROL

Mrs. Jones, 43, a white woman from Appalachia, is admitted to a small Appalachian hospital in respiratory distress and reports she has had difficulty getting her breath for the past 3 days. She has a persistent cough, which she reports having had for 8 months. The nurse doing the admission notes that she is emaciated, has ashen color, tires easily, and has a productive cough. When the nurse asks why she has not sought treatment, she responds, "Sickness is God's will. Whatever will be will be. I have tried some herbal remedies but they have not done much good. It is my time to go. I guess I'm ready, although I wish I could stay and see my children get married."

The term *environmental control* refers to the ability of a person to plan activities that control nature. Environmental control also refers to people's perception that they can direct factors in the environment. Feelings of control are an important part of responding to illness and of taking actions to promote health. Thus, it is important to assess each client for beliefs related to locus of control.

Locus of Control

Individuals may be described as having internal or external locus of control (Rotter, 1966). An individual who feels that actions and outcomes are related to *internal control* feels some power over future behaviors and situations. Personal actions are considered to be important in influencing events.

The term *external control* describes the belief that events are unpredictable and are influenced by outside forces such as luck, change, or fate. Individuals who believe in external feelings of control believe that efforts and rewards are not related to each other. The locus-of-control construct can be applied to a variety of phenomena including the weather, preventive health, curative actions, and feelings of well-being (Giger

& Davidhizar, 1999). An individual who believes in internal locus of control is more likely to comply with treatment and to take preventive actions related to future health. On the other hand, an individual who believes that compliance with treatment and health are unrelated will have little motivation to develop behaviors that influence the future or enhance health.

The culturally competent nurse should be aware that people with an Appalachian, Hispanic, or Puerto Rican cultural orientation may have an external locus of control. Northern Europeans or African Americans may have either an internal or external locus of control (Kluckhohn & Strodtbeck, 1961). Many North Americans have a strong internal locus of control and believe they are in control of their own destiny. The beliefs of some Native Americans, Chinese Americans, and Japanese Americans do not include the locus-of-control construct, but focus on harmony with nature.

Folk or traditional medicine beliefs and practices may be part of a person's world view and belief about what will influence health. Folk medicine beliefs classify illness or diseases as natural or unnatural. Folk medicine differs from Western medicine in the way in which illness is explained and treated. Alternative and traditional therapies provide options for treatment other than relying on medication or surgery.

Nursing Implications

- *Assess the client for locus of control.* The nurse needs to appreciate that individuals differ, and that actions to seek health care or to promote health may depend on culturally based locus-of-control orientation.

- *Show respect for folklore and folklore practices.* The nurse should appreciate that persons from diverse cultural backgrounds may have deeply ingrained beliefs about how to attain and maintain health. These beliefs may be linked to the natural and supernatural worlds, may adversely affect the physician–client or nurse–client relationship, and may influence the individual's decision to follow or not to follow prescribed treatment recommendations.

- *Try to incorporate folklore practices with Western medicine.* Rather than disregarding folklore practices, it is important to incorporate beliefs of the client with practices of Western medicine. When folk beliefs of the client are respected and incorporated into the nurse's plan of care, the client may be more cooperative and have a better response to nursing interventions.

Self-Reflection Questions

1. What are your beliefs about internal or external locus of control?

2. Can you relate your beliefs to early parental teaching?

3. Do you have any folk beliefs that are outside the scope of Western medicine?

4. What folk beliefs have you encountered in your client interactions?

Chapter 11

Caring for Clients with Altered Immunity

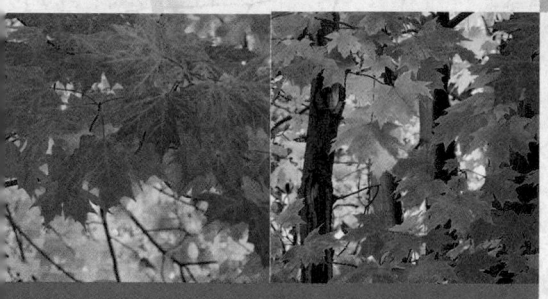

BRIEF Outline

Overview of the Immune System
Natural and Acquired Immunity
Altered Immune Responses
Autoimmune Disorders
Organ/Tissue Transplant
Impaired Immune Responses and the Client with HIV

LEARNING Outcomes

After completing this chapter, you will be able to:

- Describe the functions of the lymphoid organs and tissues.
- Compare natural and acquired immunity and active and passive immunity.
- List recommended immunizations for adult clients.
- Identify laboratory and diagnostic tests used to diagnose and monitor immune response.
- Describe the nursing implications for medications ordered for clients with altered immunity.
- Teach clients with altered immune responses and their families.
- Use the nursing process to collect data, establish outcomes, provide individualized care, and evaluate responses for the client experiencing altered immunity.
- Identify three ways to prevent the transmission of HIV infection.
- Identify laboratory tests used to diagnose HIV and to monitor HIV progression.
- Provide the nursing management of a client with AIDS, including medications and diet therapy.

The human body is constantly bombarded by foreign invaders such as bacteria, viruses, parasites, insect venoms, and transfusions. Because the body provides the perfect host environment, microbes try to break through the skin and mucous membrane barriers. The role of the immune system is either to keep out the foreign substances or, once they break through the defenses, to destroy them.

Sometimes the immune system malfunctions, causing allergies or autoimmune diseases such as rheumatoid arthritis. Diseases, such as human immunodeficiency virus (HIV) infection and multiple-drug-resistant tuberculosis, also affect the immune system.

Overview of the Immune System

The immune system is a complex network of cells and organs that protect the body against infection-causing microorganisms, foreign substances, and cancerous cells. Three defense mechanisms provide this protection. The first line of defense involves the skin, mucous membranes, and body secretions. If these defenses are penetrated, the body's inflammatory response is activated within seconds as the second line of defense. It is a nonspecific response in which white blood cells engulf and neutralize any harmful invaders. (See Chapter 10 ⊘⊘ for more information on inflammation.) A much slower response involves the third line of defense: immunity. The immune response provides specific immunity with T lymphocytes and B lymphocytes.

The immune system can recognize the body's own cells (self) and foreign cells (nonself). Normally, the body's immune defenses coexist peacefully with any cell marked as "self." When any nonself substance (**antigen**) invades the body, the immune system responds. Antigens can be bacteria, viruses, or tissues transplanted from another person. If the immune system perceives transplanted tissues or organs as nonself, they may be rejected. Sometimes, harmless substances such as dog hair or pollen set up an allergic response. This kind of antigen is called an **allergen.** In other circumstances, the immune system mistakes self for nonself and attacks it. The result is autoimmune diseases.

IMMUNE SYSTEM COMPONENTS

The immune system consists of cells and organs that produce the immune response. These components may be involved in the nonspecific inflammatory response, the specific immunologic response, or both.

Leukocytes

Leukocytes, or white blood cells (WBCs), are the primary cells involved in nonspecific and specific immune system responses. Leukocytes start as stem cells in the bone marrow. They are moved throughout the body by the circulatory system. This mobility allows them to detect, attack, and destroy any foreign invaders at the site of involvement.

The normal number of circulating leukocytes is 4,500 to 10,000 cells per cubic millimeter of blood as indicated on the WBC count. If an infection develops, additional WBCs are released from the bone marrow, leading to *leukocytosis* (increased WBC count). The WBC differential test identifies the percent of the total number of WBCs for each type of leukocyte.

From the original stem cells, leukocytes develop into three major groups of WBCs: granulocytes, monocytes, and lymphocytes (Table 11-1 ■). Granulocytes make up the greatest number of normal blood leukocytes. Monocytes are the largest leukocyte. Lymphocytes are subdivided into B-cell lymphocytes, T-cell lymphocytes, and natural killer (NK) cells (Figure 11-1 ■). T cells and B cells are the basis for the specific immune response and are discussed further in this chapter.

Natural killer (NK) cells survey the body for potential foreign invaders such as viruses and malignant cells. Unlike B and T cells, which attack only specific infected cells or malignant cells, natural killer cells can attack any target identified as foreign. They assume a key role in destroying early malignant cells. The functions of all leukocytes are closely interrelated.

Lymphoid Organs and Tissues

The organs and tissues of the immune system are found throughout the body. They are called lymphoid organs because they are home to the lymphocytes. The *lymphoid system* consists of the bone marrow, thymus, spleen, lymph nodes, and lymphoid tissue scattered in the connective tissues and mucosa (Figure 11-2 ■). The bone marrow and thymus are considered primary or central lymphoid organs. The spleen, lymph nodes, and other peripheral lymphoid tissue (e.g., the tonsils and appendix) are secondary lymphoid organs.

Bone marrow is the soft tissue in the hollow center of all bones. Red bone marrow produces blood cells from the stem cells. In adults, red marrow is located in the ends of the long bones, as well as in the pelvis, skull, sternum, ribs, and vertebrae. Yellow bone marrow is found in the other bones; it stores fat for an energy reserve.

The *thymus gland* is located in the neck area above the heart and behind the sternum. The gland is fully developed at puberty, and gradually decreases in size and function over a person's life span. Its main function is to mature lymphocytes into T cells.

The *spleen,* the largest lymphoid organ, is found in the upper left quadrant of the abdomen. The spleen has both white pulp and red pulp. White pulp contains macrophages, which destroy bacteria in the blood. Red pulp filters out damaged or aged RBCs and stores blood for future use. The spleen is not essential for life. If it is removed, the liver and the bone marrow assume its functions.

TABLE 11-1

Cells of the Immune System

TYPE OF LEUKOCYTE	FUNCTION
Granulocytes ■ Neutrophils ■ Eosinophils ■ Basophils	Involved in inflammatory response; make up 60–80% of normal blood leukocytes. First to appear after an injury; involved in phagocytosis. Involved in phagocytosis; protect against parasites; part of allergic response. Protect mucosal surfaces; secrete histamine during allergic reactions.
Monocytes	Involved in inflammatory response; mature into macrophages. Trap and phagocytize foreign substances and cellular debris.
Lymphocytes ■ T lymphocytes 　■ Helper T cells (T4) 　■ Suppressor T cells (T8) 　■ Cytotoxic T cells	Involved in specific immune response; make up 20–40% of circulating leukocytes. Provide cell-mediated immunity; mature in thymus gland. Turn on immune system function: 　Stimulate B cells to produce antibodies. 　Release lymphokines to destroy viral infections and cancer cells. 　Involved in hypersensitivity reactions and graft tissue rejection. Turn off immune system function. Kill tumor cells, viral-infected cells, and foreign tissue.
■ B lymphocytes 　■ Plasma cells 　■ Memory cells	Responsible for humoral immunity; mature in bone marrow. Produce antibodies (immunoglobulins). Produce specific antibody when reexposed to a specific antigen.
■ Natural killer cells	Kill virus-infected and tumor cells.

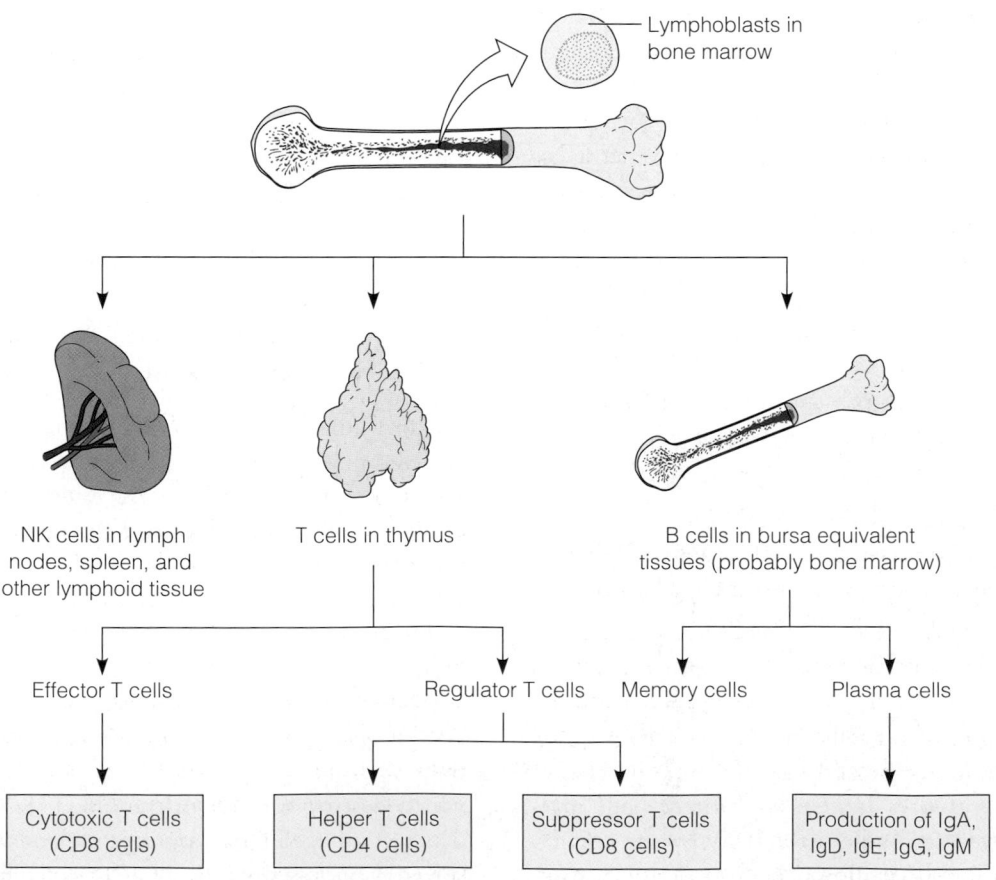

Figure 11-1. ■ The development and differentiation of lymphocytes from the lymphoid stem cell (lymphoblasts).

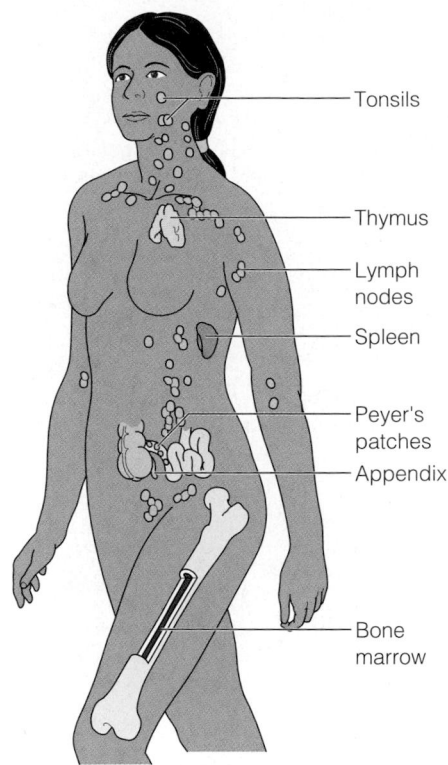

Figure 11-2. ■ The lymphoid system: the central organs of the thymus and bone marrow, and the peripheral organs, including the spleen, tonsils, lymph nodes, and Peyer's patches.

Labels: Tonsils, Thymus, Lymph nodes, Spleen, Peyer's patches, Appendix, Bone marrow

The *lymphatic system* includes the lymph nodes, lymphatic vessels, and lymph. *Lymph* is a clear, protein-containing fluid. *Lymphatic vessels* transport lymph to the lymph nodes. *Lymph nodes,* small bean-shaped encapsulated tissues, are distributed throughout the body (concentrated in the neck, axillae, abdomen, and groin). In the lymph nodes, T and B lymphocytes and macrophages filter out and destroy foreign products. The lymph nodes can become tender and palpable when a person develops a systemic infection. Clumps of specialized lymphoid tissue are also located in the tonsils, adenoids, appendix, and Peyer's patches in the intestines. They protect the body from inhaled foreign agents or ingested pathogens.

Recognition of Self

The effectiveness of the immune system depends on whether it can differentiate normal body tissue (self) from foreign tissue (nonself). Each body cell has cell surface markers that are unique to each person. These are known as *human leukocyte antigens (HLA).* A person's HLA characteristics are coded within a large cluster of genes known as the *major histocompatibility complex (MHC).* The possibility of two people having the same HLA is rare except in identical twins. Some siblings may have similar HLA. In organ transplants, matching the HLA as closely as possible tends to decrease rejection.

HUMORAL IMMUNITY AND CELL-MEDIATED IMMUNITY

When antigens enter the body, a specific immune response occurs. The immune system recognizes the particular antigens (viruses, bacteria, or transplanted tissue) and destroys them without harming itself. Unlike a localized inflammatory response, the immune response is systemic. The immune response also has memory. Repeated exposures to an antigen produce a more rapid response.

A person whose immune system identifies and effectively destroys antigens is said to be **immunocompetent.** When the immune response is altered, health problems such as hypersensitivity (allergy and autoimmune disorders) may occur. Immunodeficiency diseases or malignancies develop when the immune system is incompetent or cannot respond effectively.

Humoral Immunity

B-cell lymphocytes (B cells) are responsible for **humoral immunity.** When an antigen enters the body, T cells activate B cells, which differentiate into plasma cells and memory cells (Figure 11-3 ■). Plasma cells produce antibodies or **immunoglobulins** (Ig) that are released into the bloodstream.

An **antibody** is an immunoglobulin molecule that binds to and inactivates a specific antigen. Immunoglobulins make up the gamma globulin portion of the blood proteins. Antibodies fall into five classes of immunoglobulins: IgG, IgM, IgA, IgD, and IgE. Each has a slightly different structure and function (Table 11-2 ■).

Memory cells remember a prior exposure to a particular antigen even if they have been inactive for years. When exposed to the same antigen, they convert into plasma cells and inactivate the antigen. This rapid response means that either a person avoids the disease or the second infection is milder. Memory cells are responsible for acquired immunity against diseases such as measles or chickenpox.

Cell-Mediated Immunity

T-cell lymphocytes (T cells) are the foundation for **cell-mediated** (or cellular) **immunity** (Figure 11-4 ■). There are three types of T cells: (1) helper T cells, (2) suppressor T cells, and (3) cytotoxic T cells.

Helper T cells, also known as CD4+ cells, are responsible for switching on the immune system. They also recognize antigens such as a virus or transplanted tissue. **Suppressor T cells** (CD8 cells) limit the immune response so that the body does not destroy itself. These cells are important in preventing autoimmune disorders. **Cytotoxic T cells** can destroy cancer cells, cells of transplanted organs, and grafted tissues. They are vital in the control of viral and bacterial infections.

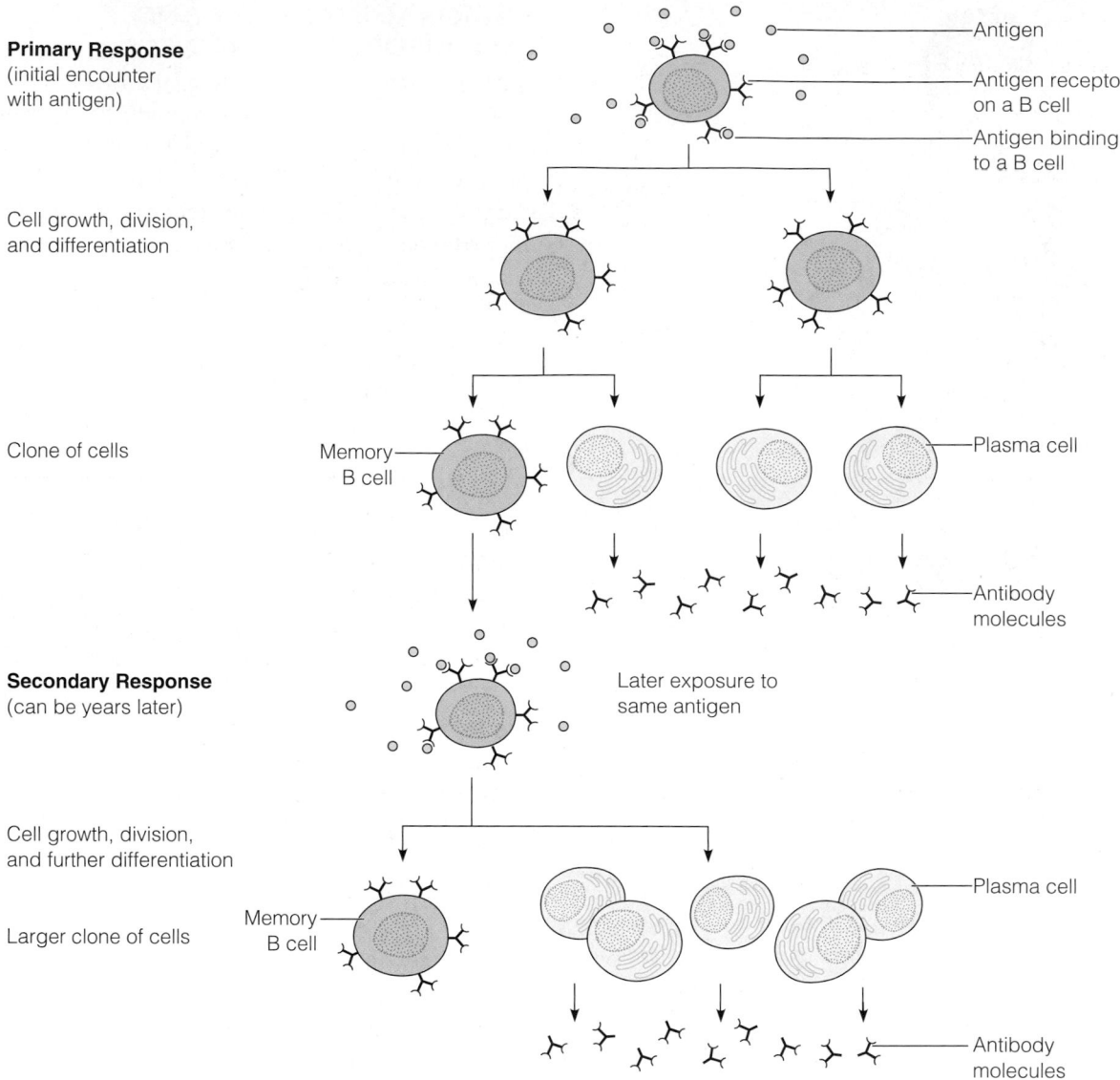

Figure 11-3. ■ Humoral immunity. *Primary response:* During first exposure to an antigen, B cells are stimulated to become plasma cells and produce antibodies or memory cells. *Secondary response:* With reexposure to the same antigen, the memory cells respond rapidly with antibody production.

IMMUNE FUNCTION IN THE OLDER ADULT

As immune function declines with aging, there is an increased susceptibility to infections and a diminished immune response. The thymus gland atrophies and, by age 60, it no longer is functional. Although the total number of T cells remains the same, T-cell function and reproduction decrease. T lymphocytes cannot eliminate foreign invaders as well as when the person was younger.

With these changes, cell-mediated immune function declines. Immune memory against such diseases as chickenpox and tuberculosis weakens. In the older person, reactivation of the chickenpox virus leads to herpes zoster (shingles). Immunoglobulins, especially IgG, decrease, followed by a reduced antibody response to influenza, tetanus, and pneumococcus immunizations.

There is also a rise in autoantibody production that may increase the potential for autoimmune diseases. Some autoimmune diseases (such as myasthenia gravis, rheumatoid arthritis, and multiple sclerosis) start in young adulthood or middle age and cause progressive damage.

External factors that may influence immune function include exposure to excessive ultraviolet radiation, environmental pollution, and poor nutrition. An older person's genetic background and history of chronic and past illness may also impair the immune system. Even with all of these influences, some older individuals have an immune system as effective as that of younger persons.

TABLE 11-2

Immunoglobulin Characteristics and Functions

CLASS	PERCENTAGE OF TOTAL	CHARACTERISTICS AND FUNCTION
IgG	75%	Found in intravascular and interstitial compartments. Most abundant Ig; also known as gamma globulin. Active against bacteria, bacterial toxins, and viruses. Crosses placenta providing immune protection to neonate.
IgA	10–15%	Found in saliva, sweat, tears, mucus, bile, colostrum, and vaginal secretions. Provides local protection to prevent entry of bacteria and viruses especially through the respiratory and gastrointestinal tracts.
IgM	5–10%	High concentrations in the blood; less in the lymph. First antibody formed and lasts about 1 week. Reacts effectively against bloodborne bacteria and viruses.
IgD	1%	Found on surface of B cells. Exact function unknown; may bind antigens to B-cell surface.
IgE	<1%	Found on mast cells and basophils. Stimulates release of chemical mediators such as histamine and bradykinin that cause allergic reactions and hypersensitivity responses such as anaphylaxis. Acts in preventing helminth (worm) infections.

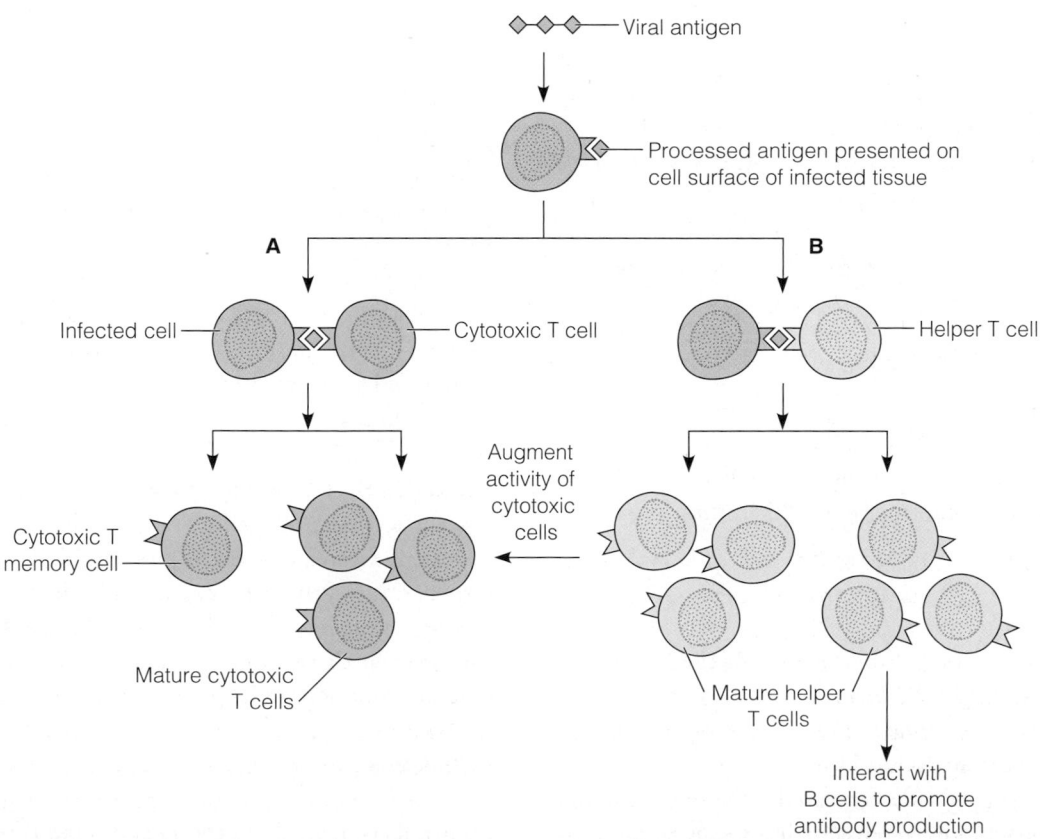

Figure 11-4. ■ Cellular immunity. (**A**) An infected cell with an antigen on its surface binds with a receptor site on a cytotoxic T or a helper T cell. The cytotoxic T cell produces memory cells or mature cytotoxic cells. (**B**) The helper T cell assists the cytotoxic activity of the cytotoxic cells and stimulates B cells to produce antibodies.

Natural and Acquired Immunity

There are three types of immunity: natural, active, and passive. Immunity results from activating humoral or cell-mediated responses. In the immunocompetent client, the immune response eliminates the antigen and either prevents the disease or promotes recovery.

PATHOPHYSIOLOGY

Natural immunity or innate immunity is a person's resistance to foreign substances, which occurs because of gender, race, heredity, age, or health status. Natural immunity does not produce an immune response. Individuals are naturally protected because of their physical and chemical barriers.

Active immunity can be *naturally acquired* by actually developing the disease or *artificially acquired* through an immunization. Either way, the body produces plasma and memory cells against specific antigens. Children may naturally acquire active immunity when exposed to mumps or measles. If reexposed later in life, the memory cells should protect them against these diseases. Active immunity can last from years to a lifetime, depending on the disease.

Immunization or vaccination against highly contagious diseases such as influenza provides artificially acquired active immunity. Immunizations require the body to actively initiate an immune response. This process can take days to weeks to complete. Vaccines do not produce disease but rather stimulate the B cells to remember a specific disease.

Passive immunity involves injecting serum with ready-made antibodies from other humans or animals. Once these antibodies are used up (a few weeks or months), their protection is lost. For example, human immune globulin or gamma globulin is given to clients when they are exposed to hepatitis A. This is known as *artificially acquired* passive immunity. *Naturally acquired* passive immunity occurs when neonates receive antibodies from their mothers via the placenta.

INTERDISCIPLINARY CARE

Interdisciplinary care focuses on assessing the client's immune status and promoting acquired immunity to prevent disease.

Diagnostic Tests

■ *Serum immunoglobulins* measure the level of IgA, IgD, IgE, IgG, and IgM (see Table 11-2). IgG levels are increased during acute infections. Decreased levels of IgG, IgA, and IgM are found in malignancies.

■ *Antibody titer testing* may determine whether a client has developed antibodies in response to an infection or immunization. Antibodies for hepatitis, rubella, and infectious mononucleosis can be identified. An elevated titer level indicates the presence of antibodies.

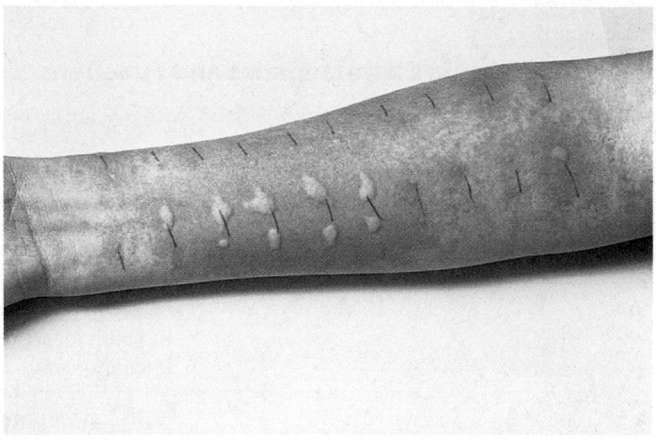

Figure 11-5. ■ Skin testing on the forearm showing induration (hardness) and erythema (redness) typical of a positive response to an antigen. (*Source:* Photo Researchers, Inc.)

■ *Skin testing* can detect impaired cell-mediated immunity. A known antigen such as streptokinase, tuberculin purified protein derivative (PPD), or *Candida albicans* is injected intradermally. The site is assessed in 24 to 48 hours for signs of *induration* (hardening of skin) and redness. An induration of 10 mm in diameter is a positive reaction (Figure 11-5 ■), indicating previous exposure and sensitization to the antigen. No reaction, or **anergy,** indicates depressed cell-mediated immunity.

Immunizations

Immunizations or **vaccines** are suspensions of live, *attenuated* (weakened), or killed microorganisms that promote active immunity against a specific organism. Special treatment makes them incapable of causing disease. Some vaccinations are combined to protect against several diseases. The most common combinations in the United States are MMR (measles-mumps-rubella) and DTP (diphtheria-tetanus-pertussis). (Recommended adult immunizations are found in Table 11-3 ■.)

Inactivated vaccines are made by killing the disease-producing microorganism with heat or chemicals. For example, each year a new influenza vaccine is made, containing the three strains of influenza most likely to occur in the upcoming winter. These vaccines stimulate a weaker immune response, so yearly influenza immunizations are required.

Live, attenuated vaccines (like the MMR) are made by growing the disease-producing organism under special laboratory conditions. The process causes the organisms to lose their virulence or disease-producing power.

Toxoids contain an inactivated toxin that is produced by a microbe. They are made harmless by exposing them to chemicals or heat. Diphtheria and tetanus toxoids are combined into a single immunization (Td for adults, DT for children). New vaccines (such as hepatitis B) are being developed by using recombinant genetic engineering. Some

TABLE 11-3

Recommended Immunizations for Adults

VACCINE	TYPE	DOSE	INDICATIONS	PRECAUTIONS AND NURSING IMPLICATIONS
Measles-mumps-rubella (MMR)	Live, attenuated virus	0.5 mL SC	One dose for those 19–49 years of age, if vaccination history unreliable. Two doses for those 19–49 years of age with occupational exposure.	Do not administer to pregnant females; pregnancy should be avoided for 4 weeks after vaccination. Do not give to immunosuppressed clients (AIDS, cancer); those with a history of anaphylaxis or allergy to eggs.
Tetanus and diphtheria toxoids (Td)	Attenuated toxoid	0.5 mL IM	If never immunized, give series of 3 injections. Give booster every 10 years, and after a contaminated wound.	Do not give in the first trimester of pregnancy or to a client with a history of anaphylactic reaction to horse serum.
Hepatitis B (recombinant) (Recombivax B)		1 mL IM (20 mcg/mL)	Series of 3 doses; initial and at 1 and 6 months.	Do not administer to clients allergic to yeast. Give in deltoid site only.
Influenza (Fluzone)	Inactivated virus	0.5 mL IM	Yearly for clients >50 years of age; in nursing homes; or with chronic pulmonary, renal, or cardiovascular diseases, or diabetes.	Do not give to clients with a history of anaphylactic reaction to eggs or to acutely ill clients.
FluMist	Live, attenuated virus	Intranasal	Yearly for those healthy clients 5–49 years of age.	Do not give to those taking salicylates or who are immunocompromised.
Pneumonococcal (Pneumovax-23)	Bacterial	0.5 mL IM	One dose for clients >65 years of age. First dose for age 2–64 with chronic diseases and a booster 5 years after first dose.	Do not give to those with a history of anaphylactic reactions.

Note: For pediatric clients, please consult a pediatric textbook for recommended immunizations.

vaccines are made from portions or subunits of the antigen; one such vaccine protects clients against pneumonia caused by *Streptococcus pneumoniae.*

Hepatitis B vaccine is recommended for everyone at high risk for exposure to blood or other body fluids. It is mandated by the Occupational Safety and Health Administration (OSHA) for all health care workers. Other high-risk populations include intravenous drug users, sexual partners of infected individuals, clients on hemodialysis, prison guards, and athletic coaches.

People traveling outside the United States and Canada should receive vaccines against diseases that are found in certain regions of the world. Additional vaccines might include cholera, yellow fever, and typhoid.

When a client has been exposed to a specific disease, immune globulins made from human or animal sources are given to provide passive immunity. Human sources carry less risk for an allergic reaction and are available for hepatitis A and B, tetanus, varicella, rabies, measles, rubella, and respiratory syncytial virus.

Animal immune serums are made by injecting an antitoxin into an animal, allowing antibodies to develop, then withdrawing blood and preparing a serum for human injection. Antitoxins are used against diphtheria, tetanus, rabies, and botulism. Antivenins, another form of passive immunization, are given after a client has been bitten by potentially lethal snakes or spiders.

A *sensitivity test* should be done before the first immunization to determine allergy to horse serum or eggs. The test dose is injected intradermally; if no hives appear after 20 minutes, the selected vaccine is given.

Immunization side effects can range from mild local reactions to **anaphylaxis** (an acute, immediate allergic reaction). Local reactions at the injection site include redness, swelling, tenderness, and muscle ache. Giving the vaccine in the dominant arm of the client reduces the local discomfort, because arm movement helps to increase absorption of the solution. Warm compresses may also be beneficial. Sometimes the client may experience systemic manifestations such as fever or malaise. Anaphylaxis is most likely with horse serum injections.

NURSING CARE

Nurses have an important role in preventing the spread of communicable diseases. This includes encouraging immunizations. Factors that may prevent active use of immunization programs are religious beliefs, poverty, and unfamiliarity with the health care system (e.g., among immigrants). Also, many people simply neglect routine immunization in adulthood. The result is increased risk for infectious disease among all people.

Before immunizations are given, the nurse should collect assessment data to determine whether immunization is appropriate (Box 11-1 ■).

Nursing care focuses on preventing injury from the vaccination and on providing client education.

Risk for Injury

- Check the expiration date and the manufacturer's instructions for administration guidelines, dosage, routes, sites, precautions, and contraindications. *Outdated vaccines may not provide protection against the specific disease. Some sites have better absorption than others.*

BOX 11-1	ASSESSMENT

Assessing Clients: Immune Status

SUBJECTIVE DATA
- Present health status:
  - General health status.
  - Exposure to any infections? Any fever or infections, especially upper respiratory?
  - Swollen glands in neck, axilla, or groin?
  - Pregnancy status?
  - Any immunosuppressive diseases (e.g., AIDS, cancer), chemotherapy, or radiation therapy?
  - Chronic pulmonary, cardiac, or renal disorders or diabetes?
- Past medical history:
  - History of infectious diseases.
  - Immunization history: For which diseases and dates of immunizations? Any adverse effects? Any foreign travel that required immunizations?
  - Allergy to horse serum or eggs?
  - Ever received tetanus toxoid for any wounds?

OBJECTIVE DATA
- Vital signs: blood pressure, pulse, respirations, temperature.
- Height and weight.
- Observe client for any signs of infection.
- Assess for any skin lesion, rashes, or impaired healing.
- Monitor and report antibody titer and skin testing results.

- Do not administer any immunization to a client with an upper respiratory infection or other infection. *Infections can increase the inflammatory reaction from an immunization.*
- Do not administer oral polio vaccines (OPV) or MMR to immunosuppressed clients or to clients who are in close household contact with an immunosuppressed person. *Live virus vaccines can cause disease in the immunosuppressed client or can transmit disease to close household contacts during the initial postvaccination period.*

clinical ALERT

Observe the client for 20 to 30 minutes following vaccination, because allergic reactions usually occur within this time frame.

- Keep epinephrine 1:1000 readily available when administering immunizations. *Epinephrine causes vasoconstriction and reduces laryngospasm; in acute anaphylaxis, it can be life-saving.*

CONTINUING CARE

Provide instructions in the following areas:

- Appropriate immunizations and recommended schedules for initial vaccination and boosters.
- How and where to obtain immunizations. County or public health departments may offer immunization clinics at a lower cost than private physicians or urgent care clinics.
- Possible side effects of the immunization, as well as the need to observe the client for up to 30 minutes following a vaccine for possible adverse reactions.
- Self-care measures for side effects such as warm compresses over the injection site and taking acetaminophen (Tylenol) for fever.
- The need to report immediately any adverse reactions such as fever, rash, itching, or shortness of breath.
- Importance of maintaining permanent immunization records.

Altered Immune Responses

HYPERSENSITIVITY REACTIONS

Normally, the immune system protects humans against foreign substances, but sometimes it overreacts. **Hypersensitivity** is an altered immune response to an antigen that results in harm to the client. Hypersensitivity responses include hay fever, blood transfusion reactions, and organ transplant rejections. The tissue response to a hypersensitivity reaction may be simply a runny nose or itchy eyes, or it may be life threatening, leading to blood cell hemolysis or anaphylaxis.

TABLE 11-4

Types of Hypersensitivity Reactions

TYPE	CAUSES	PATHOPHYSIOLOGY	EXAMPLES
I—Immediate hyper-sensitivity	Pollens, foods, insect bites, animal dander, and drugs	Allergen binds to IgE antibodies that are attached to mast cells in connective tissue, skin, and mucous membranes where they release histamine. Histamine constricts smooth muscle and causes peripheral vasodilation leading to watery, itchy eyes; runny nose; rash; hives; or anaphylaxis.	Allergic asthma, hay fever, insect sting reactions, food allergies, anaphylaxis
II—Cytotoxic hyper-sensitivity	Incompatible blood	IgG or IgM antibodies bind with an antigen such as ABO or Rh. This triggers an autoimmune destruction of the target cell, causing a systemic reaction.	Blood transfusion reactions, hemolytic disease of the newborn
III—Immune hyper-sensitivity	Horse antitoxin; extra-cellular bacteria, fungi, and viruses	IgG or IgM antibody–antigen complexes form in the circulation and begin the inflammatory process.	Serum sickness, systemic lupus erythematosus, rheumatoid arthritis
IV—Delayed hyper-sensitivity	Chemicals or plants; skin tests with fungi or my-cobacteria; foreign tissues	T lymphocytes interact with an antigen and activate the inflammatory response. Reactions may be delayed for 24–72 hours after exposure.	Contact dermatitis, tuberculin skin test; graft or tissue transplant reaction

There are four types of hypersensitivity reactions (Table 11-4 ■). Types I, II, and III have an immediate tissue response and are caused by the humoral system. Type IV has a delayed response and results from the cell-mediated system. (See Chapter 13 ◯◯ for substances that may cause anaphylaxis.)

LATEX ALLERGY

A unique hypersensitivity response is latex allergy. Once the natural rubber latex is removed from the tree, more than 200 chemicals may be added to prevent degradation. Latex allergy results from reaction to the chemicals or to the latex proteins. Latex proteins can enter the body through the skin and mucous membranes, by invasive lines and tubes, or by inhalation. Box 11-2 ■ lists common products of natural rubber latex.

Type I and type IV allergic reactions to latex may occur. Type I response, a reaction to the natural rubber proteins, may occur within minutes of exposure. Symptoms range from mild (hives, itching, and generalized edema) to severe (wheezing, dyspnea, feeling of faintness, laryngospasm, and cardiac arrest). Type IV response results from an allergic reaction to the processing chemicals. Manifestations develop from 1 to 48 hours later and include local redness and itching.

Prevention of adverse reactions is most important. Ask clients about their allergy history, including food allergies. There seems to be a cross-sensitivity between latex allergy and certain foods, such as avocados, bananas, kiwi, pineapples, and chestnuts. Instruct clients with known latex sensitivity to wear a Medic-Alert bracelet. Many hospitals have created latex-free carts that are used for clients with latex allergies.

Since 1998 all medical products must identify that they contain latex. The National Institute for Occupational

BOX 11-2

NATURAL RUBBER LATEX PRODUCTS
Home
- Balloons
- Condoms, diaphragms
- Band-Aids

Health Care Setting
- Ace bandages (brown)
- Jobst elastic stocking
- Bulb syringes
- Blood pressure cuffs and tubing
- Gloves
- Intravenous tubing
- Tourniquets
- Wound drains
- Rubber stoppers in medication vials
- Rubber dams used in dental work
- Stethoscopes
- Urinary catheters
- Mattress covers

TABLE 11-5

Nursing Implications for Pharmacology: Antihistamines

CLASS/DRUGS	PURPOSE	NURSING RESPONSIBILITIES	CLIENT TEACHING
Antihistamines ■ Diphenhydramine (Benadryl) ■ Chlorpheniramine (Chlor-Trimeton) ■ Hydroxyzine (Vistaril)	Antihistamines block H_1 histamine receptors to relieve allergic rhinitis and anaphylactic reactions such as urticaria and angioedema.	Give cautiously to older adults who are taking other medications. Monitor for side effects: excessive sedation, dizziness, palpitations, or urinary retention. Encourage a fluid intake of 2,500–3,000 mL/day unless contraindicated. Give Benadryl before blood transfusion or diagnostic tests that use contrast media as ordered.	Take only one antihistamine at a time. If drowsiness occurs, do not drive or operate machinery while taking this medication. Do not drink alcohol. Use hard candy, gum, ice chips, or mouth rinses to relieve dryness. Stop the drug and notify the physician if excessive sedation, dizziness, palpitations, or urinary retention occurs.

Safety and Health (NIOSH) recommends that health care workers with latex allergies use powder-free gloves with reduced protein content. When handling noninfectious material, they should wear non-latex gloves. Manufacturers are trying to develop latex-free alternatives that also provide safe barrier protection.

INTERDISCIPLINARY CARE

A key aspect of management is identifying allergens so that exposure is minimized. A complete history of all of the client's allergies is obtained, including medications, foods, animals, plants, and other materials. The type of hypersensitivity response is documented, as are onset, manifestations, and usual treatment. Several tests may be ordered:

■ A *radioallergosorbent test (RAST)* measures the amount of IgE to specific allergens. This test is very expensive and is time consuming, but poses no risk for an anaphylactic reaction.

■ *Skin tests* are used to identify specific allergens to which a person may be sensitive. Allergens used for testing are based on the client's history. Test solutions are injected intradermally or by a prick or patch on the back or arms.

■ The *prick test* may be done first to avoid a systemic reaction. A drop of allergenic solution is placed on the skin and the skin is punctured through the drop. A positive test yields a wheal and redness within 15 to 20 minutes.

■ An *intradermal test* involves a small amount of allergen being injected on the forearm or intrascapular area. Several allergens can be tested by allowing ½- or ¼-inch intervals between injections. A plain diluent is injected opposite the test site. A positive test yields a wheal and redness within 15 to 20 minutes (see Figure 11-5).

■ In a *patch test,* a 1-inch patch impregnated with the allergen is applied to the skin for 48 hours. Positive responses range from mild redness to severe redness, papules, or vesicles.

Medications

Treatment focuses on avoiding the offending allergen, but sometimes medications provide symptomatic relief. Antihistamines, nasal and oral decongestants, and corticosteroids are usually ordered. Epinephrine is given during an acute anaphylactic reaction (see Chapter 13).

Antihistamines are the major class of drugs for treating symptoms of hypersensitivity responses. (Nursing care for the client receiving antihistamines is outlined in Table 11-5 ■.)

Nasal decongestants such as oxymetazoline (Afrin) and oral decongestants such as pseudoephedrine (Sudafed) may relieve allergy symptoms. Overuse of Afrin may result in decreased effectiveness and rebound nasal congestion. Remind clients to see their health care provider if symptoms last longer than a week. Decongestants should be used for less than 5 days.

Glucocorticoids are used in systemic and topical hypersensitivity responses. They have an anti-inflammatory effect. Short-term corticosteroid therapy is used for severe asthma, allergic contact dermatitis, and some immune-complex disorders. Corticosteroids in topical forms or delivered by inhaler may be used for longer periods of time with few side effects.

Another option is **desensitization,** a form of immunotherapy that involves injecting small doses of the allergen weekly. Over time, antibodies develop to block the allergic IgE response. This process can take years to accomplish symptomatic relief.

NURSING CARE

Nursing care is directed toward prevention of adverse effects and providing prompt, effective treatment. Prior to administering any medication, ask the client's allergy history, including the allergic response and its treatment. If the client experienced rash, hives, or difficulty breathing, check with the physician before giving the drug.

clinical ALERT

When a client receives a new medication, observe closely. Even without any past allergic reaction, the client is still at risk for anaphylaxis.

A second exposure increases the risk for a reaction and increases the severity of the reaction. While the client is hospitalized, ask about allergies to latex, skin cleansers, and radiopaque dyes. When a suspected hypersensitivity reaction occurs, stop the intravenous medication or transfusion immediately.

With a type I hypersensitivity response, the first priority is managing the client's airway. The client with a type II hypersensitivity reaction may need aggressive treatment to control bleeding. A type III reaction is treated by removing the antigen and stopping the inflammatory response. Treatment of type IV reactions includes eliminating the antigen and giving anti-inflammatory drugs. Antihistamines may relieve the client's discomfort. (Chapter 13 ⚭ discusses management of anaphylaxis and transfusion reactions.)

CONTINUING CARE

Most hypersensitivity responses can be treated by the client or family with little or no medical intervention. Teaching should include the following points:

- Tell clients to inform health care personnel of all allergens.
- Encourage clients to wear a Medic-Alert bracelet or tag identifying allergies.
- Instruct the client and family members on how to give emergency injections of epinephrine.
- Teach clients to use prescribed and over-the-counter medications as recommended.
- For the client with contact dermatitis, discuss appropriate skin care.

Autoimmune Disorders

In **autoimmune disorders,** the immune system mistakes self for nonself, and the body reacts against its own cells. **Autoantibodies** (antibodies made against self-antigens) attack various body tissues, leading to tissue damage and chronic inflammation. Autoimmune disorders can affect any tissue, cell group, or organ. When the inflammatory process involves multiple organs, the client is said to have a systemic autoimmune disorder. Selected autoimmune disorders are listed in Box 11-3 ■.

BOX 11-3

AUTOIMMUNE DISORDERS

CELL OR ORGAN SPECIFIC	SYSTEMIC
Blood	Rheumatoid arthritis
Idiopathic thrombocytopenia purpura	Scleroderma
Endocrine System	Systemic lupus erythematosus
Graves' disease	
Thyrotoxicosis	
Type 1 diabetes mellitus	
Addison's disease	
Central Nervous System	
Multiple sclerosis	
Muscles	
Myasthenia gravis	
Gastrointestinal System	
Pernicious anemia	
Ulcerative colitis	

Certain families have a greater incidence of autoimmunity. Autoimmune disorders are more common in females and the elderly. Clients may develop more than one autoimmune disorder. The onset of an autoimmune disorder is frequently associated with a severe physical or psychological stressor.

PATHOPHYSIOLOGY

It is unclear exactly how autoimmune disorders develop. Several theories have been proposed:

- Trauma, drugs, radiation, and infections alter body tissues so that the body no longer recognizes itself, and autoantibodies are produced.
- Bacteria such as group A beta-hemolytic *Streptococcus* may cross-react with the heart muscle, causing heart damage.
- Viruses may alter tissues that are not usually antigenic. This may be the cause of multiple sclerosis and Type 1 diabetes mellitus.

Manifestations vary according to the tissues or organs affected. Most often, the client shows signs and symptoms of the inflammatory process (pain, fatigue, and fever). Autoimmune disorders are characterized by periods of acute flare-ups followed by no symptoms. As these diseases progress, remission periods become less frequent.

INTERDISCIPLINARY CARE

Diagnostic Tests

Diagnosis of an autoimmune disorder is usually based on the client's clinical manifestations. Serum assays are helpful to identify increased levels of antibodies. Other laboratory and diagnostic tests more specific to the suspected disorder are ordered. Symptoms can be managed, but a cure is unlikely.

- The *antinuclear antibody (ANA)* test is used to screen for systemic lupus erythematosus (SLE). *Lupus erythematosus (LE) cell prep* is also used to detect SLE and monitor its treatment. Like the ANA, the LE cell prep is nonspecific for SLE. Positive results may be seen in rheumatoid arthritis or drug-induced lupus from penicillin, tetracycline, Dilantin, and oral contraceptives.
- *Rheumatoid factor (RF)* is an immunoglobulin present in the serum of approximately 80% of clients with rheumatoid arthritis.

Medications

Treatment of autoimmune disorders focuses on relieving symptoms. Because there is chronic inflammation, anti-inflammatory medications such as aspirin, nonsteroidal anti-inflammatory drugs (NSAIDs), COX-2 inhibitors, and corticosteroids may be prescribed (see Chapters 10 and 16 ⚭).

Other slow-acting anti-inflammatory drugs may be added to the treatment plan. Disease-modifying antirheumatics are given to clients with rheumatoid arthritis. These drugs include gold salts, hydroxychloroquine (Plaquenil), and penicillamine. They are discussed further in Chapter 43. ⚭ Cytotoxic drugs may be used in combination with plasmapheresis in treating many autoimmune disorders.

NURSING CARE

Nursing care is individualized for the client with an autoimmune disorder. Clients are taught stress reduction techniques, good nutrition, and medication uses and side effects. Most clients can be managed in outpatient settings. Interventions for the following nursing diagnoses should be included in the nursing care plan:

- *Fatigue* related to inflammatory effects of autoimmune disorder
- *Acute* and *Chronic Pain* related to inflammation
- *Impaired Physical Mobility* related to pain and activity intolerance
- *Ineffective Coping* related to chronic disease process
- *Disturbed Body Image* related to joint deformity, rashes, and altered body function
- *Ineffective Protection* related to immune disorder

CONTINUING CARE

Because autoimmune disorders are chronic, the client and family need to understand their long-term effects. They must learn about medications and possible side effects.

During periods of remission, clients may not appear ill, and it may be difficult for the family to understand their needs. Often, these clients are at risk for unproven remedies and quackery. Nurses can provide psychologic support, listening, teaching, and referral to local support groups and state or national agencies.

Organ/Tissue Transplant

At one time, transplants were considered an experimental treatment option. Now they have become fairly common. Skin, cornea, bone, and heart valve transplants are done more frequently and require less extensive tissue matching. Kidney, heart, and liver transplants are no longer considered extraordinary procedures. However, these surgeries cannot be considered lightly. They cost from $40,000 to $250,000. (Medicare will cover the costs of kidney, liver, and heart transplants.) The client must also be able to afford the yearly cost of medications.

Organ and tissue transplants are used when clients with cancer need healthy cells; for example, those with leukemia may need stem cells. They are also used when an organ is about to fail or has irreversible disease, or when part of the body is destroyed as in transplant of skin to a burn victim.

Transplant success is closely tied to matching antibodies of the donor and the recipient. As discussed earlier, HLA antigens are unique to the individual. Although identical twins may have the same HLA type, the chance is reduced to one in four for siblings, and less than one in several thousand for unrelated individuals. Matching the HLA type of the donor decreases, but does not eliminate, the potential for transplant rejection.

PATHOPHYSIOLOGY

An **autograft** (a transplant of the client's own tissue) is the most successful type of tissue transplant. Skin grafts are the most common examples of autografts. Increasingly, **autologous** (self) bone marrow transplants and blood transfusions are being used to reduce the immune response. When the donor and recipient are identical twins, the term **isograft** is used. These grafts are usually successful, with only mild rejection episodes.

Most often, organ and tissue transplants are **allografts** (grafts between members of the same species). Because of the growing number of transplant candidates, allografts from living donors are needed to fill the shortage of organs. Living donors do not have to be blood relatives. Whole or partial organs are donated (one kidney, the lobe of the liver or lung, and part of the pancreas tail). Bone marrow transplant (BMT) is exclusively from a living donor.

Organs are obtained most often from cadavers. Donors must meet the criteria for brain death; be less than 70 years old; and be free from diabetes, hypertension, cancer, HIV, hepatitis B, and hepatitis C. The organ is removed immediately before or after cardiac arrest and is preserved until transplanted into the waiting recipient. Organ donation is coordinated by the United Network for Organ Donation, a federally funded organization (see also Chapter 13 ⬭).

A **xenograft** (transplant from an animal species to a human) is the least successful type of transplant and is seldom used. The one exception is the use of pig skin as a temporary covering for a massive burn.

Tissue typing determines the **histocompatibility** (histo = cell; the ability of cells and tissues to survive transplantation without rejection). Tissue typing identifies HLA type and blood types (ABO, Rh) of the donor and recipient, as well as any preformed antibodies to the donor's HLA antigens.

Transplant rejection is stimulated by humoral and cell-mediated immune responses. It typically begins 24 hours after the transplant, although it may develop immediately. Rejection episodes are characterized as follows (Table 11-6 ■):

1. *Hyperacute rejection:* The grafted organ initially appears pink and healthy, but then turns soft and white and is usually lost.
2. *Acute rejection:* The client shows signs of the inflammatory process. Manifestations are related to the specific organ, for example, elevated blood urea nitrogen (BUN) and creatinine; liver enzyme and bilirubin elevations; or elevated cardiac enzymes and signs of heart failure.
3. *Chronic rejection:* This results from antibodies and complement being deposited in the transplant vessel walls. Narrowing of the vessels causes decreased blood flow and ischemia. The organ eventually fails.

Graft-versus-host disease (GvHD) is a frequent complication of bone marrow transplant. When there is no close match between donor and recipient HLA antigen, immunocompetent cells in the grafted tissue attack other body tissues, especially the skin, liver, and intestine. Acute GvHD occurs within the first 100 days following a transplant. A maculopapular rash begins on the palms of the hands and soles of the feet. The rash may spread over the entire body, eventually causing the epidermis to shed. Intestinal symptoms are abdominal pain, nausea, and bloody diarrhea. Chronic GvHD has a poor prognosis.

INTERDISCIPLINARY CARE

Pre- and post-transplant care focuses on reducing the risk of tissue rejection. Laboratory tests are used to identify a suitable donor and to monitor the immune response to the transplant. Immunosuppressive medications are often the key to successful organ transplants.

Diagnostic Tests

Basic diagnostic tests are done prior to surgery (complete blood count [CBC] and differential, urinalysis, chemistry panel, coagulation studies, arterial blood gases, an electrocardiogram, and chest x-ray). Other laboratory studies are ordered specifically before organ or tissue transplantation:

- *Blood type* and *Rh factor* of both donor and recipient
- *Cross-matching* of the client's serum against the donor's lymphocytes to identify preformed antibodies
- HLA *histocompatibility testing* to identify donors with an HLA type close to that of the recipient
- *Mixed lymphocyte culture (MLC) assay tests* to determine histocompatibility between the donor and the recipient.

TABLE 11-6			
Transplant Rejection Episodes			
TYPE	CAUSE	PRESENTATION	TREATMENT
Hyperacute	Preexisting antibodies (usually associated with previous transplant) immediately react against the ABO and HLA antigens of the donor organ.	Occurs within minutes to hours or days of the transplant. Rapid deteriorization of organ function	Transplant cannot usually be saved. Prevent with cross-match and by using antimetabolite and anti-inflammatory drugs before surgery.
Acute	Antigens on the donor organ (usually from a cadaver) trigger the release of cytotoxic T cells that attack the foreign organ.	Occurs within 4 days to 4 months after the transplant. Signs of inflammation (fever, swelling, redness, and tenderness over graft site) and impaired organ function	Most common and treatable type of rejection. Increase immunosuppression using steroids, cyclosporines, monoclonal antibodies, or anti-lymphocyte globulins.
Chronic	Probably antibody-mediated response; may also involve inflammatory damage to the lining or vessel walls of the transplant.	Occurs 4 months to years after the transplant. Gradual deterioration of organ function	Changing to another immunosuppressive drug may help, but usually transplant is lost, requiring retransplant.

Various diagnostic tests may detect signs of transplant rejection. Ultrasonography or magnetic resonance imaging (MRI) of the transplanted organ can evaluate its size, perfusion, and function. Tissue biopsies of the transplanted organ can provide evidence of tissue rejection.

Medications

Preoperatively, antibiotic and antiviral drugs may be prescribed, such as trimethoprim-sulfamethoxazole (Septra, Bactrim), acyclovir (Zovirax), and ganciclovir (Cytovene).

Postoperatively, a combination of immunosuppressive drugs is given to prevent tissue rejection. Drug selection is based on the transplanted tissue or organ and the preference of the medical center.

Corticosteroids, prednisone (Deltasone), and methylprednisolone (Solu-Medrol) reduce the inflammatory response and decrease the production of T-helper cells and cytotoxic cells. Although beneficial, corticosteroids have numerous side effects: poor wound healing, fluid retention, hypertension, gastrointestinal (GI) distress, increased sodium and glucose levels, and muscle weakness. (Corticosteroids are discussed further in Chapter 16.)

Cytotoxic agents such as azathioprine (Imuran) and cyclosporine (Sandimmune) have been used as immunosuppressants since the 1970s. *Monoclonal antibodies* and *antilymphocyte globulins* are newer agents. (Nursing responsibilities and client teaching for immunosuppressive agents are outlined in Table 11-7 ■.)

TABLE 11-7

Nursing Implications for Pharmacology: Immunosuppressive Agents

CLASS/DRUGS	PURPOSE	NURSING RESPONSIBILITIES	CLIENT TEACHING
Cytotoxic Agents ■ Azathioprine (Imuran) ■ Cyclophosphamide (Cytoxan) ■ Cyclosporine (Sandimmune) ■ Methotrexate (Rheumatrex) ■ Mycophenolate (Cellcept) ■ Tacrolimus (Prograf)	Cytotoxic agents treat cancer and prevent tissue or organ rejection reactions.	Use meticulous hand washing to prevent infection. Notify the MD if WBCs fall below 4,000 or platelets below 75,000. Monitor BUN, creatinine, and liver enzymes. Increase fluids to maintain output. Monitor for bleeding gums, bruising, petechiae, or tarry stools. Monitor for oral candidiasis; client may need an antifungal drug.	Follow directions for taking the medications. Avoid large crowds and people with infections. Report signs of infection, any bleeding, reduced urine output, and jaundice. Do not take aspirin or ibuprofen. Use contraception to avoid pregnancy; drugs could harm the fetus. Wear protective clothing and use sunscreens. Wear Medic-Alert tag.
Monoclonal Antibody ■ Muromonab-CD3 or OKT3 (Orthoclone) ■ Basiliximab (Simulect) ■ Daclizumab (Zenapax)	A mouse is injected with an antigen that produces a specific monoclonal antibody. The antibody is harvested from the mouse and given by IV route to prevent organ transplant rejection.	Obtain chest x-ray before therapy starts. Premedicate the client as ordered to reduce potential side effects. Monitor closely for side effects of chills, fever, tremor, dyspnea, chest pain, or wheezing.	Discuss potential side effects and the need to report symptoms promptly. Explain that side effects may occur during the first two doses, requiring close observation at that time.
Antilymphocyte Globulins ■ Antilymphocyte globulin (ALG) ■ Antithymocyte globulin (ATG)	These drugs are given to horses or rabbits to produce antibodies. They are removed from the, animal, refined, and given IV to the client. They are used after an organ transplant to cause immunosuppression.	Before the initial dose, perform skin test to test for allergy to horse serum. Premedicate as ordered. Monitor for anaphylaxis during the infusion. Monitor client's WBC and platelet count daily.	Explain the need for special precautions and close monitoring during the IV infusion. Report any side effects to the nurse immediately.

NURSING CARE

The client who has undergone an organ or tissue transplant has immediate and long-term nursing care needs. Immediately after the transplant, the client is transferred to the critical care or transplant unit and is monitored closely. Both the physical and psychosocial needs of client and family must be considered.

Risk for Infection

- Monitor vital signs and temperature frequently. Assess for abnormal wound drainage, changes in body secretions, complaints of pain, or behavior changes. Culture abnormal wound drainage. *Incisions, invasive lines and tubes, nutritional deficits, immunosuppressive drugs, and chronic disease all increase the potential for infection. The client on immunosuppressive therapy is more susceptible to infection, but the usual signs and symptoms may be absent. To prevent life-threatening complications, assess the client constantly and start appropriate interventions immediately.*
- Ensure meticulous hand washing by all caregivers before providing direct care. *Hand washing provides first-line defense against infection and cross-contamination.*

clinical ALERT

Use strict aseptic technique in changing dressings and caring for invasive catheters such as intravenous lines and indwelling urinary catheters to reduce risk of transferring microorganisms to the client.

- Monitor CBC, especially WBC differential; report changes to the physician. *An elevated WBC count with a shift to the left may be an early indication of infection.* (See Chapter 10. ⬯)
- Initiate protective isolation precautions as indicated by facility policy and the client's immune status. Screen staff, family, and visitors for signs of infection. *These procedures further protect the severely immunocompromised client from infection.*
- Encourage deep breathing and coughing. *This mobilizes respiratory secretions and reduces the potential for atelectasis and pneumonia.*
- Provide adequate nutrition with supplementary feedings or parenteral nutrition if necessary. *Adequate nutrition is important for healing and immune system function.*
- Provide frequent mouth care. *Meticulous mouth care reduces oral microorganisms and helps maintain an intact mucous membrane lining.*
- Change intravenous bags and tubing at least every 24 hours, and change peripheral intravenous sites every 48 to 72 hours, unless contraindicated. Remove invasive

catheters and lines as soon as possible. *Changing lines and sites helps reduce bacterial contamination. Fewer invasive lines mean fewer sites for bacterial invasion.*
- Monitor for potential adverse effects of medication:
  - Bleeding due to thrombocytopenia
  - Fluid retention with edema and possible hypertension
  - Anorexia, nausea, vomiting, and abdominal pain
  - Decreased urine output from renal toxicity
  - Jaundice from hepatic toxicity
  - Bone or joint pain.

  Medications used to maintain immunosuppression and to preserve the allograft have many potential adverse effects that can alter normal protective and homeostatic mechanisms.

Risk for Impaired Tissue Integrity: Allograft

- Administer immunosuppressive therapy as ordered. *Agents that suppress the immune response reduce transplant rejection.*
- Assess the client for signs of graft rejection: tenderness, redness, and swelling over the site; sudden weight gain, edema, and hypertension; chills and fever; malaise; and an increased WBC count and sedimentation rate. Report any changes immediately. *The risk for transplant rejection is highest in the initial postoperative period, but it is never completely eliminated. The client with a bone marrow transplant has the additional risk of developing graft-versus-host disease. Early identification allows adjustment of medication regimens and may preserve the graft.*
- Monitor tests of organ function. Report changes to the physician. *A decline in function of the transplanted organ (e.g., a rising BUN and creatinine in the renal transplant client) may be an early indication of transplant rejection.*
- In the client who has had a bone marrow transplant, assess for and report signs of GvHD immediately. Look for maculopapular rash, erythema of the skin and possible desquamation, hair loss, abdominal cramping and diarrhea, jaundice with elevated bilirubin and liver enzymes (aspartate transaminase [AST], alanine transaminase [ALT]). *GvHD is a potentially lethal complication. It requires immediate intervention.*
- Stress to the client the importance of maintaining immunosuppressive therapy and of reporting signs of graft rejection promptly. *The risk for transplant rejection is never completely eliminated.*

Anxiety

- Assess the client's level of anxiety by noting restlessness, tension, apprehension, fear, facial expression, and poor eye contact. *Clients may have difficulty talking about their fears and anxieties about organ rejection. When the transplant comes from a living donor, clients may also worry about the condition of the donor. Nonverbal cues help to identify anxiety.*

- Use opening statements such as "Facing an organ transplant must be very stressful." Listen attentively. *Encouragement and active listening help identify issues that can lead to problem solving.*
- Stay with the client as much as possible. When leaving, tell the client when you will return. Also encourage family members to remain with the client as much as possible. *Time the nurse spends with the client promotes trust. The presence of family helps reduce anxiety.*
- Provide clear, concise information and directions. *Highly anxious clients have difficulty focusing and retaining information.*
- Encourage the use of coping behaviors that were useful in the past. If necessary, consult with a mental health specialist. Encourage client and family to meet other transplant recipients. *Past coping mechanisms may work again. A specialist can help the client deal with feelings. Hearing about the success and problems of others can reduce anxiety.*

CONTINUING CARE

Thorough client education is necessary before the client with a transplant is discharged. The client and family need to understand the long-term treatment regimen as well as any lifestyle changes.

Provide verbal and written instructions about the following points:

- Signs and symptoms of transplant rejection and the importance of notifying the physician should these occur
- How to monitor temperature, blood pressures, pulse, and weight
- The importance of following the prescribed medication regimen; understanding interactions with other medications and appropriate OTC drugs; and maintaining a medication record
- Side effects of immunosuppressive drug therapy. Include management techniques for minor side effects. Indicate which side effects should be reported to the physician
- The importance of avoiding exposure to infectious diseases, especially upper respiratory infection (URI), influenza, or pneumonia. Wearing a mask when going outside is helpful. Good hand washing technique is essential
- The importance of oral hygiene and regular visits to the dentist
- Dietary needs and expected changes associated with medications
- The importance of avoiding damage to the skin. Steroids increase the fragility of the skin. Any injury could allow microorganisms to enter

- Wearing a Medic-Alert bracelet or tag identifying the client as a transplant patient receiving immunosuppressive drug therapy
- The importance of follow-up visits to the physician or clinic.

Impaired Immune Responses and the Client with HIV

When function of either the B cells or T cells is impaired, the result is an immunodeficiency disorder. Immunodeficiency disorders can be inherited, acquired through infection, or produced unintentionally by immunosuppressive drugs.

Primary immunodeficiency is a rare congenital disorder that is usually found in infants and young children. In addition to a higher risk for infection, these children have more autoimmune diseases and cancer.

Secondary immunodeficiency is acquired and results in impaired immune function. One or more factors can cause immunodeficiency: stress, malnutrition, trauma, age, viral infections, cancer, or drugs. Infection with the human immunodeficiency virus (HIV) may lead to **acquired immunodeficiency syndrome (AIDS)**, the final, fatal stage of HIV infection and the most well-known secondary immunodeficiency.

AIDS was first identified in 1981 among homosexual males in Los Angeles and New York who had developed an unusual opportunistic infection. By 1982, the Centers for Disease Control (CDC) acknowledged the presence of a new infection involving immune system deficits and associated opportunistic disorders. In 1985 the **human immunodeficiency virus (HIV)** was isolated as the cause of AIDS.

By December 2003, the CDC estimated that 850,000 to 950,000 people were living with HIV infection, with a third of them unaware of their HIV status. An estimated 40,000 new HIV infections develop each year in the United States. AIDS is the fifth leading cause of death among adults ages 25 to 44; however, the death rate has been slowly decreasing since 1995.

Among men with new HIV infections, 60% were men who had sex with men (homosexuals, bisexuals, prisoners), 25% injected drugs, and 15% had heterosexual contact. Of the women, 75% were infected through heterosexual contact and the remainder through IV drug use. African American and Hispanic males make up 70% of AIDS cases; women of these ethnic groups represent 82% of cases in females. The number of AIDS cases in women increased from 7% in 1985 to 26% of newly reported cases in 2003 (National Institute of Allergy and Infectious Diseases [NIAID], 2004). Pediatric AIDS cases (children under 13) are also more prevalent in African American and Hispanic families.

By the end of 2003, approximately 35.7 million adults and 2.1 million children under the age of 15 were living with HIV/AIDS worldwide and in nearly every country (NIAID, 2004). The highest incidence is in sub-Saharan Africa and Southeast Asia, but it is increasing rapidly in eastern Europe and central Asia. In Africa, the life expectancy is decreasing due to the large number of HIV-infected people.

There are three main routes of transmission: (1) direct person to person through sexual contact; (2) direct injection with contaminated blood, blood products, or needles; and (3) mother to fetus. HIV is transmitted through blood, semen, vaginal secretions, the placenta, and breast milk. It can also be found in saliva, but no known cases have been transmitted by saliva.

Certain behaviors increase the risk for contracting HIV. The most common behavior is intercourse with an infected partner. Sexual relations by anal, oral, or vaginal routes without the use of a condom is the major risk factor. Sharing of needles and other drug paraphernalia is the second leading risk factor for IV drug users. Multiple sexual partners, heterosexual intercourse with an infected drug user, and exchanging sex for drugs or money are major risk factors for women. Hemophiliacs who received intravenous clotting factors and people infected through blood transfusion represent less than 2% of the cases.

Among the general population of the United States, HIV infection is very low. HIV is not transmitted by casual contact such as sneezing, coughing, handshaking, hugging, dry kissing, or sharing eating utensils or linens. There is no evidence that it can be transmitted by mosquitoes. Blood donation also poses no risk, because only new, sterile equipment is used.

A small but real occupational risk exists for health care workers. The main exposure routes are needle-stick injuries or nonintact skin and mucous membranes. A needle-stick injury poses a 0.3% risk of becoming HIV positive. Mucosal exposures, such as splashing in the eyes or mouth, pose a much smaller risk.

PATHOPHYSIOLOGY

HIV is a retrovirus, which means it reproduces in a "backward" manner. Instead of reproducing from deoxyribonucleic acid (DNA) to ribonucleic acid (RNA), it uses RNA to make DNA copies. After the virus enters the bloodstream, it attaches to CD4+ T4 helper lymphocytes. CD4 is a receptor antigen on the T4 helper surface.

Once inside the CD4+ cell, the virus sheds its protein coat and releases an enzyme called **reverse transcriptase** to convert the RNA to DNA (Figure 11-6 ■). Then the viral DNA inserts itself into the host cell DNA and duplicates during normal cell division. At this point, the virus may remain latent or produce new RNA with the assistance of an enzyme called *protease* to form very small virus particles (buds). These buds have the ability to move to other CD4+ cells where they disrupt and eventually destroy the host cell. Billions of HIV buds are produced and destroyed each day along with CD4+ cells. The loss of helper T cells leads to the immunodeficiencies seen with HIV infection. The infection eventually overwhelms the body's immune system (Figure 11-7 ■).

The virus may remain inactive in infected cells for years. During this stage, B-cell antibodies are produced in a process known as **seroconversion.** These antibodies can be detected 6 weeks to 6 months after the initial infection.

A diagnosis of HIV infection is based on the client's history and risk factors, physical examination, laboratory studies, and manifestations. HIV infection and AIDS in adolescents and adults are classified according to the CDC system. This system uses CD4+ T-cell counts and clinical manifestations to diagnose a client.

Manifestations

Clinical manifestations of HIV infection range from no symptoms (after the initial mononucleosis-like onset), to severe immunodeficiency with multiple opportunistic infections and cancers in the late stages (Box 11-4 ■).

Following the primary infection, clients enter a long-lasting asymptomatic period (about 10 years). The virus can be transmitted to others during this time. The next stage is acute infection, characterized by persistent generalized lymphadenopathy lasting 3 or more months. It is unclear exactly what causes a client to progress from HIV infection to AIDS. However, once clients are diagnosed with AIDS, they are at risk for developing multiple opportunistic infections and cancers. AIDS affects almost all organ systems. The client with AIDS has a poor prognosis, but newer treatments and medications enable clients to live longer.

Opportunistic Infections

Opportunistic infections are infections that develop in clients with compromised immunity. Clients with AIDS are more likely to develop opportunistic infections when their CD4+ count falls below 200. These infections mostly affect the respiratory, gastrointestinal, and neurologic systems.

RESPIRATORY SYSTEM

Pneumocystis carinii Pneumonia. ***Pneumocystis carinii* pneumonia (PCP)** (a fungus-like organism that rarely causes disease in clients with an intact immune system) is the most common opportunistic infection. However, early and aggressive treatment with HAART (highly active antiretroviral therapy) medications has reduced the

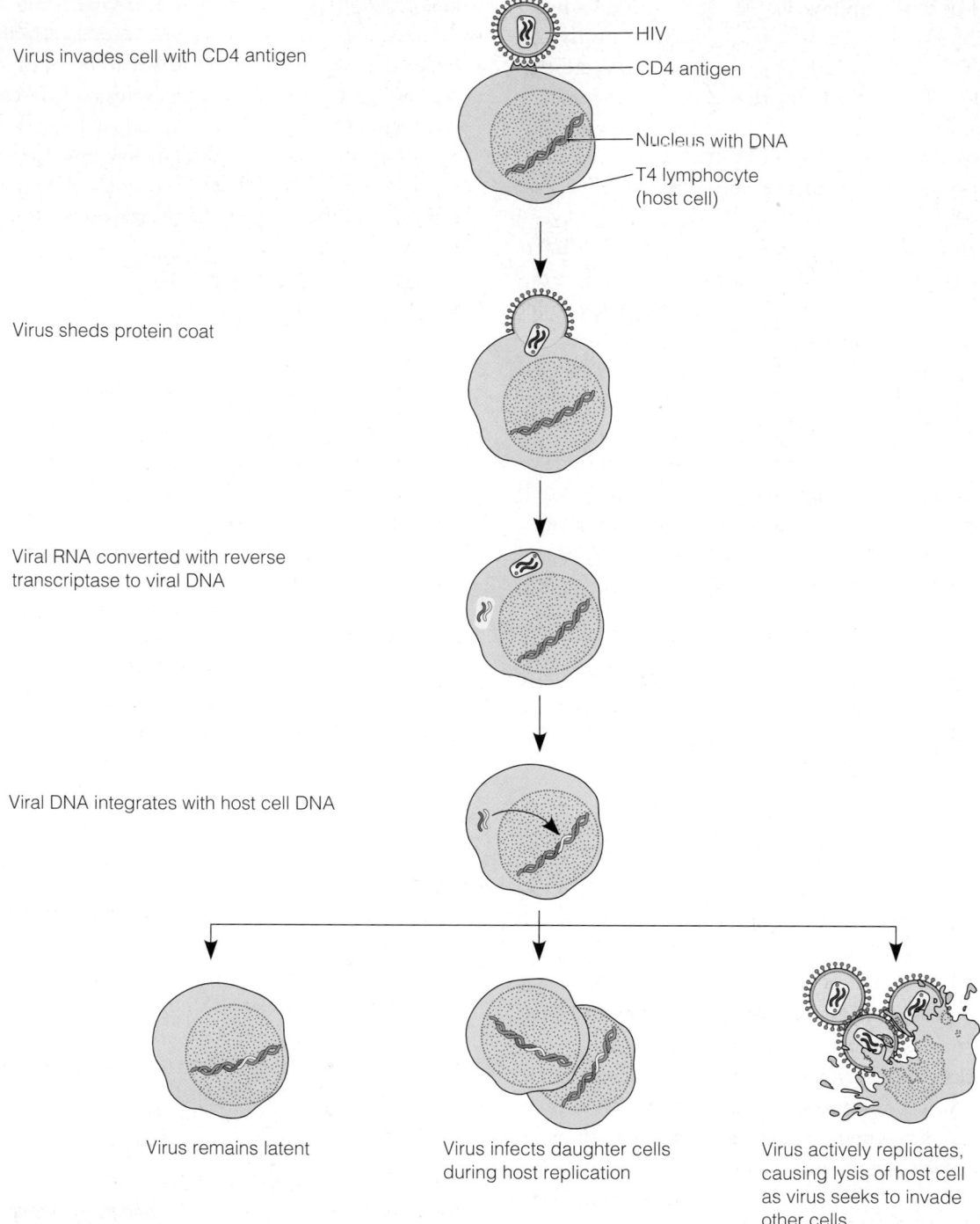

Virus invades cell with CD4 antigen

HIV

CD4 antigen

Nucleus with DNA

T4 lymphocyte
(host cell)

Virus sheds protein coat

Viral RNA converted with reverse
transcriptase to viral DNA

Viral DNA integrates with host cell DNA

Virus remains latent

Virus infects daughter cells
during host replication

Virus actively replicates,
causing lysis of host cell
as virus seeks to invade
other cells

Figure 11-6. ■ How HIV infects and destroys CD4 cells.

incidence. Without HAART and prophylactic treatment, the prognosis is poor.

PCP settles in the lungs and damages the lung alveoli. The client may experience fever, nonproductive cough, shortness of breath, dyspnea, tachypnea, crackles, decreased breath sounds, and cyanosis. Diagnosis is made by chest x-ray or bronchoscopy. A chest x-ray will show diffuse infiltrates. The bronchoscopy is used to obtain sputum for a culture.

Tuberculosis.   Tuberculosis (TB) is caused by *Mycobacterium tuberculosis*. It usually invades the lungs but can also be found in the bone marrow, kidneys, and central nervous system. Tuberculosis in AIDS clients is increasing as are multiple-drug-resistant strains. Co-infection with TB significantly decreases the client's survival time.

TB is diagnosed by the Mantoux test; however, clients with a CD4+ cell count below 200 may not react to it. A

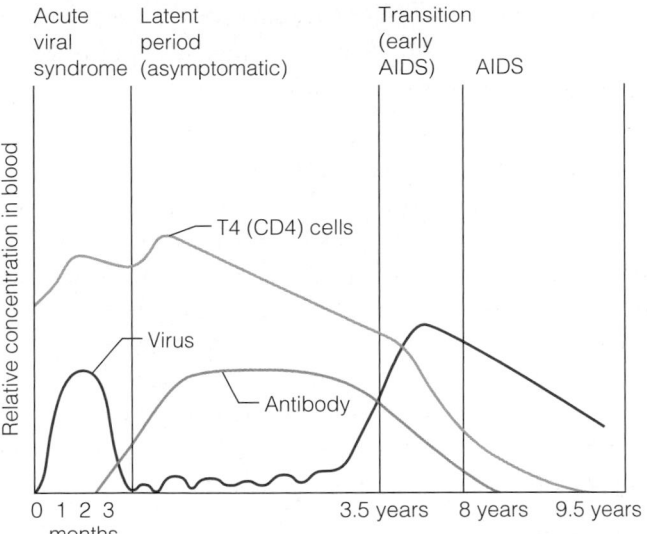

Figure 11-7. ■ The progression of HIV infection. The primary infection begins shortly after contracting the virus, corresponding with a rapid rise in viral levels. Antibodies are formed and remain throughout the infection. Late in the disease, viral activity increases destroying CD4 (T4) cells. Antibody levels gradually decrease as immune function is impaired.

follow-up chest x-ray provides a more accurate diagnosis. Persistent cough, night sweats, fever, fatigue, and weight loss are seen in clients with pulmonary tuberculosis.

***Mycobacterium avium* Complex (MAC).** MAC is caused by a bacterial organism found in the food, water, and soil. MAC affects nearly every organ and has a high mortality rate. The most common manifestations are a high fever, diarrhea, and weight loss.

GASTROINTESTINAL SYSTEM

Candidiasis. Oral candidiasis or *thrush* (a fungal infection caused by *Candida albicans*) occurs in most clients with AIDS. It is characterized by white patches in the mouth that may extend to the esophagus and stomach. Clients may complain of mouth soreness and an unpleasant taste. Esophagitis may lead to painful swallowing, an inability to eat, and malnutrition. In women, vaginal candidiasis is frequent and often recurs.

Cryptosporidiosis. The protozoan *Cryptosporidium* is normally found in birds, fish, reptiles, and humans. Transmission occurs from ingesting contaminated water or food or from human-to-human contact. The organism settles in the small intestine. AIDS clients experience large watery, nonbloody diarrhea that often causes dehydration, electrolyte imbalances, and malnutrition. Diagnosis is made by sending a stool sample for ova and parasites.

Wasting Syndrome. In the later stages of AIDS, most clients develop wasting syndrome. This is described as an

---

BOX 11-4

Manifestations of HIV Infection

1. **Primary Infection**
   - Fever
   - Sore throat
   - Arthralgias and myalgias
   - Headache
   - Rash
   - Nausea, vomiting, and abdominal cramping

2. **Asymptomatic Infection**
   - None; converts to seropositive status

3. **Acute Infection**
   - Persistent generalized lymphadenopathy
   - General malaise, fatigue
   - Low-grade fever
   - Night sweats
   - Involuntary weight loss
   - Diarrhea

4. **AIDS and Opportunistic Disorders**
   A. Respiratory
      - *Pneumocystis carinii* pneumonia
      - *Mycobacterium tuberculosis*
      - *Mycobacterium avium* complex
   B. Gastrointestinal
      - Candidiasis
      - Cryptosporidiosis
      - Wasting syndrome
   C. Neurologic
      - Cryptococcosis
      - Toxoplasmosis
   D. Other infections
      - Herpes simplex 1 and 2, herpes zoster
      - Cytomegalovirus (CMV)
      - Pelvic inflammatory disease
      - Human papillomavirus
   E. HIV encephalopathy
   F. Secondary cancers
      - Kaposi's sarcoma
      - Non-Hodgkin's lymphoma

---

unplanned weight loss of 10% along with chronic diarrhea or an unexplained fever. Fatigue, nausea, vomiting, and oral lesions lead to poor food intake, and chronic diarrhea results in malabsorption of nutrients. The client appears emaciated (Figure 11-8 ■).

NEUROLOGIC SYSTEM. **Toxoplasmosis** and **cryptococcosis** are parasitic infections with *Toxoplasma gondii* and *Cryptococcus neoformans*. Toxoplasmosis can cause encephalitis. Cryptococcosis settles in the lungs but can travel to the brain or meninges, causing meningitis. Symptoms for both conditions include headache, fever, stiff neck, altered mental status, and seizures.

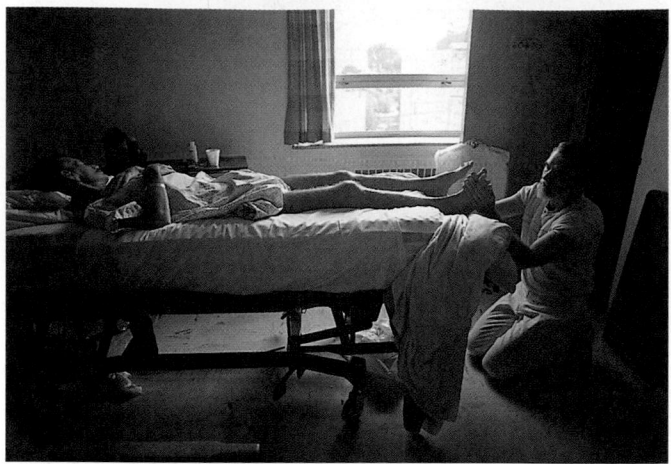

Figure 11-8. ■ Wasting syndrome in a client with AIDS. (Photographer: Alain McLaughlin.)

Other Infections

Herpes simplex 1 and 2 frequently develop in clients with AIDS. Type 1 infections involve the oral cavity, while type 2 infections develop in the genital and anal regions. Large groups of painful lesions form in the affected areas. When the lesions rupture, the virus is easily transmitted to other parts of the body and to caregivers.

Cytomegalovirus (CMV) is part of the herpesvirus family. It can affect the retina, the gastrointestinal tract, or lungs. CMV is the primary cause of blindness in AIDS clients.

Women with AIDS have a high incidence of pelvic inflammatory disease (PID). They seem to contract the **human papillomavirus**, which increases their risk for cervical cancer.

HIV Encephalopathy

HIV encephalopathy is caused by HIV acting directly on the brain. It results in progressive deterioration of cognitive, motor, and behavioral functioning. Typical manifestations include forgetfulness, difficulty concentrating, confusion, leg weakness, and clumsiness. Clients lose interest in personal hygiene, work, and social activities. In the later stages, the client may develop tremors, incontinence, and paraplegia.

Secondary Cancers

KAPOSI'S SARCOMA (KS). Kaposi's sarcoma is the most common cancer associated with HIV infection. Tumors develop in the lining of small blood vessels, causing reddish-purple lesions on the skin and mucous membranes. Initially, the lesions are painless but may become painful as the disease progresses. Tumors within body organs can disrupt function or cause bleeding. Diagnosis is made by tissue biopsy.

LYMPHOMAS. Lymphomas are malignancies of the lymphocytes, lymph nodes, the spleen, and bone marrow. AIDS clients develop either non-Hodgkin's lymphoma or primary lymphoma of the brain. Symptoms may be vague or reflect brain involvement, such as headache and changes in mental status.

INTERDISCIPLINARY CARE

New treatments are being investigated, but research has not yet found a cure for HIV infection and AIDS. Because an AIDS diagnosis eventually means death, preventive strategies are most important. Clients at risk for HIV infection need help in identifying their HIV status. Once a positive diagnosis is made, they should be taught how to maintain their health and prevent opportunistic infections. Health care workers and support persons play a key role in providing emotional and psychosocial support.

Prevention

Vaccines against HIV infection are being investigated but to date, none have been successfully developed. Education and counseling are the key elements for HIV prevention.

The nurse first focuses on sex education. All sexually active individuals need to know how HIV is spread. The only safe sex practices are (1) no sex, (2) long-term monogamous sexual relations between two uninfected people, and (3) mutual masturbation without direct contact. Clients who engage in sexual activity must understand and practice safer sex (Box 11-5 ■).

It is often difficult to find and educate injection drug users. People in this group should never share needles, syringes, or other drug paraphernalia. Needle-exchange programs provide a sterile needle and syringe in exchange for a used one. A fresh solution of household bleach and water in a 1:10 ratio is effective to clean injection paraphernalia when sterile supplies are unavailable. This population also should be taught safe sex practices. Most heterosexual HIV transmission occurs between injection drug users and their partners.

Screening of voluntary blood donors and donated blood supplies has reduced the risk of transmission by transfusion. However, it is possible for HIV to be transmitted during the time between contracting the virus and developing detectable antibodies (the *window period*). The window period usually lasts from 6 weeks to 6 months. For this reason, it is important for persons to donate their own blood prior to an anticipated surgery.

Health care workers can prevent most exposures to HIV by using Standard Precautions. With Standard Precautions, all body fluids are treated as if they are infectious, and barrier precautions are used to prevent skin, mucous membrane, or percutaneous exposure to them.

Any health care worker who is exposed to blood or receives a needle-stick injury should report it immediately to an employee health department. They should be tested at regular intervals for a year and receive appropriate counseling.

BOX 11-5

GUIDELINES FOR SAFER SEX

- Limit the number of sexual partners, preferably to one.
- Do not engage in unprotected sex, especially if HIV status of partner is unknown.
- When entering into a new monogamous relationship, both partners should undergo HIV testing initially. If both are negative, practice abstinence or safer sex for 6 months, followed by retesting.
- Use latex condoms for oral, vaginal, or anal intercourse; avoid natural or animal skin condoms, which allow HIV to pass through.
- Do not use an oil-based lubricant (e.g., petroleum jelly), which can damage the condom.
- Store condoms in cool, dry place and prevent damage to condom.
- Apply and remove condom properly; do not reuse condoms.
- Do not swallow urine or semen.
- Women should carry and use a female condom.
- Remember that oral contraceptives provide no protection against HIV.
- Engage in safer sexual practices that are less damaging to sensitive tissues (e.g., mutual masturbation, avoiding anal or oral sex).
- Do not use drugs or alcohol.
- Do not share needles, razors, toothbrushes, sexual toys, or other items that may be contaminated with blood or body fluids.
- If HIV positive:
  a. Do not engage in unprotected sexual activity.
  b. Inform all current and former sexual partners of HIV status.
  c. Inform all health care personnel—primary care providers, physicians, and dentists, in particular—of HIV status.
  d. Do not donate blood, plasma, blood products, sperm, organs, or tissue.
  e. If female, do not become pregnant.

The CDC recommends postexposure prophylaxis with azidothymidine (AZT) therapy after a needle-stick injury from an HIV-positive client. Treatment must be started *within 1 to 2 hours* after exposure and continued for 4 weeks. Research confirms that follow-up treatment with AZT can reduce the rate of infection.

Diagnostic Tests

- *Enzyme-linked immunosorbent assay (ELISA)* is the first screening test used to determine the presence of HIV antibodies (not presence of the virus itself). The client must give informed consent before the test is performed. An infected client may test negative during the window period. If the test is positive, a second test is done to confirm it. When the second test is positive, the Western blot assay is done.
- *Ora quick rapid HIV-1 antibody test* is a test to provide HIV results in 20 minutes by obtaining a blood sample from a finger stick. Positive results must be confirmed by the Western blot assay.
- *Western blot assay* is a reliable test that is used to confirm that the client is HIV seropositive.
- *HIV viral load tests* measure the amount of HIV viral activity. Viral loads are used to monitor disease progression and response to antiretroviral medications. Levels greater than 5,000 to 10,000 copies/mL indicate the need for treatment.
- *CD4+ cell count* is used to confirm progression from HIV infection to AIDS. The normal range for the CD4+ count is 800 to 1,200 mm^3. AIDS is defined not only by the presence of opportunistic infections but also by a CD4+ count of less than 200/mm^3 or a percentage of CD4 lymphocytes of less than 14%. CD4 counts are recommended every 3 to 6 months for all people with HIV disease.
- *CD4+ : CD8+ ratio* measures the ratio of helper T cells to suppressor T cells (normal 2:1). With decreased immune function, the ratio is reversed.
- *CBC* detects anemia, leukopenia, and thrombocytopenia, which are often present in HIV infection.

Tests may be ordered to diagnose secondary cancers and opportunistic infections. *Tuberculin skin testing* can identify tuberculosis infection. *Magnetic resonance imaging (MRI)* and a *computed tomography (CT) scan* of the brain can identify lymphomas and other opportunistic infections. *Cultures* of urine, blood, stool, spinal fluid, and sputum identify PCP, toxoplasmosis, cryptosporidiosis, and cryptococcosis.

Medications

Antiretroviral medications are given (1) to reduce the client's viral load, (2) to maintain CD4+ cell counts above 500, and (3) to treat opportunistic infections and malignancies. Four classes of antiretroviral drugs are used: nucleoside reverse transcriptase inhibitors (NRTIs), non-nucleoside reverse transcriptase inhibitors (NNRTIs), protease inhibitors, and fusion inhibitor. Highly active antiretroviral therapy (HAART), the standard for treating HIV infection, combines three or four of the antiretroviral drugs. (Each drug group, with nursing responsibilities, is discussed in Table 11-8 ■.)

Before clients begin the HAART protocol, they should understand the benefits and risks as well as the effects on their daily life. They will need to take multiple medications at specific times throughout the day, and the HAART drugs cost more than $20,000 per year. This does not include the cost of other medications to treat or prevent opportunistic infections or cancers. Antiretrovirals cause adverse reactions that affect quality of life. For these reasons, clients with HIV must be fully committed to the treatment plan and be partners in their care.

TABLE 11-8

Nursing Implications for Pharmacology: Clients Receiving Antiretroviral Agents

CLASS/DRUGS	PURPOSE	NURSING IMPLICATIONS	CLIENT TEACHING
Nucleoside Reverse Transcriptase Inhibitors (NRTIs)			
■ Zidovudine (AZT, Retrovir, ZDV) ■ Didanosine (ddI, Videx) ■ Zalcitabine (ddC, HIVID) ■ Stavudine (d4T, Zerit) ■ Lamivudine (3TC, Epivir) ■ Abacavir (ABC, Ziagen) ■ Zidovudine plus lamivudine (Combivir)	NRTIs inhibit action of reverse transcriptase to prevent HIV reproduction.	Give at the ordered times around the clock. If a dose is missed, call the MD. Assess for bone marrow suppression: anemia, leukopenia, granulocytopenia. Monitor the client's CBC. Give epoetin (Epogen) or filgrastim (Neupogen) to treat anemia and neutropenia. Monitor CD4+ counts and viral load for drug effectiveness.	Take drug at ordered times to maintain serum blood levels. Report all side effects. Have regular blood tests: viral load, CD4+ counts, CBC, kidney or liver to monitor for drug toxicity. Notify physician if any signs of infection occur: sore throat, fever, swollen lymph nodes.
Non-Nucleoside Reverse Transcriptase Inhibitors (NNRTIs)			
■ Nevirapine (Viramune) ■ Delavirdine (Rescriptor) ■ Efavirenz (Sustiva)	NNRTIs block HIV reproduction.	Give at the ordered times around the clock. Monitor for skin rash, nausea, and headache. Monitor CD4+ counts and viral load for drug effectiveness.	Take drug at ordered times to maintain serum blood levels. Report side effects. Have regular blood tests: viral load, CD4+ counts, liver to monitor for drug toxicity. Notify physician if any signs of infection occur: sore throat, fever, swollen lymph nodes.
Protease Inhibitors			
■ Indinavir (Crixivan) ■ Ritonavir (Norvir) ■ Nelfinavir (Viracept) ■ Saquinavir (Fortovase) ■ Amprenavir (Agenerase) ■ Lopinavir/Ritonavir (Kaletra)	Protease inhibitors block the production of the HIV protease enzyme, which is needed to make mature virions.	Give at the ordered times around the clock. Assess for GI upset: nausea, vomiting, diarrhea. Monitor liver studies for signs of toxicity and CD4+ counts and viral load for drug effectiveness.	Take drug at ordered times to maintain serum blood levels. Have regular blood tests: viral load, CD4+ counts, liver to monitor for drug toxicity. Notify physician if any signs of infection occur.
Fusion Inhibitor			
■ Enfuvirtide (Fuzeon)	Fusion inhibitor prevents virus from entering CD4+ cells.	Assess for skin reaction (slight redness, itching)	Notify physician if skin reaction worsens.

Treatment is started when the client (1) shows severe symptoms of HIV infection or is diagnosed with AIDS, (2) the viral load is greater than 55,000 copies, or (3) the CD4+ cell count is less than 350. Usually, the client is given two NRTIs and one protease inhibitor. Single drugs are avoided to prevent drug resistance.

If successful, the drug regimen should reduce the viral load to less than 50 copies in 2 to 8 weeks. However, not all clients experience the same results. Some clients cannot tolerate the multiple medications, side effects, or strict dosing schedule. Resulting feelings of despair, depression, and hopelessness may require antidepressants and counseling.

As mentioned earlier, the client may need medications for opportunistic infections and malignancies associated with HIV infection and AIDS. Many of these disorders cannot be eliminated, but pharmacologic agents attempt to control their devastating effects (Table 11-9 ■).

Many clients at some point need central venous access devices, such as a Groshong catheter, to draw blood and to give medications, transfusions, and parenteral nutrition.

TABLE 11-9

Pharmacologic Treatment of Opportunistic Infections and Malignancies

CONDITION	TREATMENT	POTENTIAL ADVERSE EFFECTS
Infections		
Pneumocystis carinii pneumonia	Trimethoprim-sulfamethoxazole (TMP-SMX, Bactrim) Pentamidine (Septra)	Nausea, anorexia, rashes, fever, hypotension, cough
Tuberculosis	Antitubercular drugs	See Chapter 24
Mycobacterium avium complex	Clarithromycin (Biaxin) Azithromycin (Zithromax) Ciprofloxacin (Cipro)	Diarrhea, hepatotoxicity Headache, nausea, vomiting Nausea, abdominal pain, rash
Candidiasis Oral thrush	Clotrimazole troches (Lotrimin) Nystatin suspension (Mycostatin)	Nausea Nausea, epigastric pain
Recurrent vaginitis	Ketoconazole (Nizoral)	Nausea, hepatotoxicity
Cryptococcosis	Fluconazole (Diflucan)	Jaundice, rash
Herpes simplex	Acyclovir (Zovirax)	Vomiting, diarrhea, headache
Malignancies		
Kaposi's sarcoma	Chemotherapy with (doxorubicin) bleomycin and vincristine Radiation therapy Alpha-interferon	Nausea, vomiting, bone marrow suppression, alopecia Same as for chemotherapy plus possible radiation burns Mental status changes, chills, fever
Lymphoma	Chemotherapy	Nausea, vomiting, bone marrow suppression, alopecia

(See Chapter 30 ⚭ for nursing care of the client with an intravenous access device.)

The following immunizations are recommended for all HIV-infected clients: pneumococcal, influenza, hepatitis B, and *Haemophilus influenzae b* vaccines. Persons with a positive PPD and negative chest x-ray film are given isoniazid (INH) for one year. When the client's CD4+ cell count falls to less than 200, prophylactic treatment for PCP is begun, usually with TMP-SMX.

Research has not found a successful vaccine, partly because new viral forms emerge constantly. Another roadblock is that so far animal testing has been unsuccessful, and the ethics of human testing has not been resolved. So, the best control method for HIV is prevention.

COMPLEMENTARY THERAPY

Complementary therapies are used primarily to manage client problems caused by opportunistic infections and cancers. For instance, ginger root may be given to reduce nausea and vomiting from cancer chemotherapy. Goldenseal seems to decrease fungal infections such as *Candida albicans* but high doses may cause nausea, vomiting, and diarrhea.

Several herbal supplements may decrease the effectiveness of antiretroviral drugs, mainly the non-nucleoside reverse transcriptase inhibitors and protease inhibitors. Clients with AIDS who are considering herbal therapy must consult their primary care provider before taking St. John's wort or garlic.

NURSING CARE

Priorities in Nursing Care. Because HIV and AIDS can affect all body systems, the client needs physical and psychosocial support. Initially, the nurse focuses on prevention, maintaining a healthy lifestyle, education, and coping with a terminal illness. If the client develops opportunistic infections and malignancies, direct care becomes more important. Nursing care for the AIDS client needs to address such issues as Infective Individual Coping, Risk for Infection, Imbalanced Nutrition: Less than Body Requirements, Impaired Skin Integrity, Fatigue, Ineffective Breathing Pattern and Disturbed Thought Processes.

Nurses are providing care for clients with HIV infection on medical–surgical, maternal–child, and pediatric units,

BOX 11-6	ASSESSMENT

Assessing Clients with HIV Infection and Aids

SUBJECTIVE DATA

- Present health status:
  - General health status.
  - Any difficulty swallowing, weight loss, anorexia, abdominal pain, or diarrhea?
  - Rashes or lesions on skin or in mouth.
  - Complaints of fatigue, weakness, difficult walking.
  - Insomnia or night sweats.
  - Headaches, confusion, forgetfulness, personality changes, visual changes.
  - Fever, nonproductive cough, shortness of breath, difficulty breathing.
  - Any swollen lumps in neck, axillae, or groin.
  - Drug or alcohol use.
- Past medical history:
  - Any screening tests for TB or HIV?
  - Sexual history (unprotected sex, multiple partners, anal intercourse).
  - History of tuberculosis, STDs, hepatitis, or other infectious diseases.
  - Use of any immunosuppressive drugs.

- Exposure to blood, blood products, or needles.
- Ever receive a blood transfusion?

OBJECTIVE DATA

- Vital signs: blood pressure, pulse, respirations, temperature.
- Height and weight.
- Observe for poor nutritional status: thinness, sunken eyes, muscle wasting.
- Carefully observe client for lethargy, depression, inability to concentrate, memory loss, tremors, slurred speech, aphasia. Manifestations may be due to toxoplasmosis or cryptococcosis.
- If possible, have client walk in the room; observe for ataxia and poor coordination.
- Inspect oropharynx with penlight and tongue depressor for gray-white patches *(Candida)*.
- Inspect skin for discolorations (KS).
- Inspect genital area for lesions or discharge from candidiasis or STIs.
- Palpate lymph nodes in neck, axillae, and groin for swelling or tenderness.
- Auscultate lungs for crackles and wheezing.
- Monitor and report results out of expected range for HIV viral load, CD4+ cell count, CD4+ : CD8+ ratio, and CBC.

as well as in hospices, clinics, and home settings. They must respect these clients' right to confidentiality. The nurse should never discuss a client's diagnosis except with the health care team.

ASSESSING

The nurse must collect a database before selecting the appropriate nursing interventions. The database can help determine the extent to which HIV infection and AIDS is affecting the client's life and can identify potential complications (Box 11-6 ■).

DIAGNOSING, PLANNING, AND IMPLEMENTING

Individuals with HIV may require acute and chronic care throughout their illness.

Ineffective Coping

- Assess the client's support network and coping skills. *Once clients learn of HIV seropositive status, they face an uncertain future and social stigma. They may feel guilty about their chosen lifestyle and the way the disease was contracted. As the disease progresses, social isolation and body image changes*

can tax their coping skills. The nurse helps clients identify available people and skills.

- Provide continuity of care. Spend time actively listening to the client. *This promotes trust and a caring atmosphere for the client to express feelings and work through issues related to HIV infection.*
- Support positive coping behaviors, client decisions, actions, and achievements. *As the client's self-esteem is enhanced, coping improves.*
- Promote and support the client's social network. *The client will need others in order to cope with the diagnosis and disease progression.*
- Provide referral to counselors, support groups, and agencies. Include addresses and phone numbers for local and national information resources and hot lines. Encourage the client, family, and significant others to participate in support groups. *Resource persons and groups can provide information and support. Support groups decrease the risk of social isolation and encourage clients to find ways to cope.*

Risk for Infection

- Wash hands before and after all care. Use Standard Precautions for all clients. Use aseptic technique when performing invasive procedures. *Hand washing and Standard Precautions reduce the risk of disease transmission. Asepsis prevents nosocomial infections in hospitals or long-term care facilities.*

- Monitor for signs of infection (e.g., chills, sweating; burning on urination; shortness of breath; redness, tenderness, or drainage from wounds). Monitor WBC count. *Remember, immunocompromised clients may not have a fever; the nurse must look for other signs of infection.*
- Culture lesions, blood, urine, and sputum as ordered. *Cultures may identify infections or determine the effectiveness of medications.*
- Clean client's nails frequently. *Fungal infections are common under the nails.*
- Administer antiretrovirals and other anti-infective drugs as ordered. *These medications help control the HIV infection and may prevent opportunistic infections.*

Imbalanced Nutrition: Less than Body Requirements

- Consult with dietitian to identify client's nutritional needs. *The dietitian can plan appropriate meals, supplements, and the need for parenteral nutrition.*
- Serve small portions of soft foods and avoid hot or spicy foods. Limit fluids before and with meals. *Small portions do not overwhelm the client. Soft foods are easily digested. Very hot or spicy foods can irritate the client's mouth when lesions are present. Excess fluids decrease appetite and food intake.*
- Provide a diet high in protein and kilocalories. *A high-protein, high-kilocalorie diet provides nutrients to meet the client's increased metabolic needs.*
- Assist the client with eating as needed. Encourage client to rest before meals. *Fatigue and weakness can prevent the client from eating an adequate diet.*
- Provide frequent oral hygiene. *Oral hygiene improves comfort and appetite and reduces the risk of mucosal lesions.*
- Provide supplementary vitamins and enteral feedings, such as Ensure. *This improves the client's nutritional status and caloric intake.*
- Give appetite stimulants such as megestrol (Megace) and dronabinol (Marinol) as ordered. *Both drugs may increase appetite and promote weight gain.*
- Offer topical anesthetics such as Xylocaine viscous to clients with mouth lesions. Give antiemetics prior to meals and antidiarrheals after stools as ordered. *A topical anesthetic may reduce pain and improve oral intake. Antiemetics reduce nausea and improve food intake. Antidiarrheals improve nutrient absorption*

clinical ALERT

Avoid high-fiber foods that can increase intestinal motility and diarrhea.

- Monitor weight and albumin levels. *These measures promote early intervention to prevent anemia and wasting syndrome. Albumin levels reflect the client's nutritional status.*

Impaired Skin Integrity

- Monitor lesions for signs of infection or impaired healing. *Maintaining skin integrity is important because of the progressive and debilitating nature of AIDS. Infection or poor tissue perfusion not only impairs healing but may lead to further skin breakdown.*
- Turn the client at least every 2 hours with a turn sheet. *Turning decreases stress over bony prominences, improves circulation, and promotes healing. A turn sheet prevents skin shearing.*
- Use pressure and egg crate mattresses, or sheepskin pads for elbows and heels. *These devices reduce pressure on skin.*
- Wash skin with mild, nondrying soaps and pat dry gently. *Clean, dry skin is a barrier to infection. Gentle drying prevents skin tears.*

clinical ALERT

Apply A&D ointment to reddened areas in the rectal area to prevent skin damage from diarrhea.

- If blisters are present, leave intact, and cover with a transparent film (e.g., Tegaderm). *Covering may prevent bacterial invasion and promote healing.*
- Trim fingernails regularly. Teach client to avoid scratching. If the client is confused, apply mitts or soft restraints to prevent scratching, and check circulation of hands and fingers frequently. *Scratching with long fingernails can damage skin, increasing risk of infection. Tight or restrictive restraints or mitts may decrease circulation.*
- Encourage ambulation. If the client is confined to bed, encourage active or passive range-of-motion exercises. *Activity increases circulation, decreases pressure and skin breakdown, and maintains muscle tone.*

Fatigue

- Balance activities with rest periods and assist with activities of daily living (ADLs) if necessary. *Fatigue may be related to low energy levels, medication side effects, or the emotional stress of the disease. Establishing realistic activity goals helps the client perform activities when energy levels are the highest, and gives the client a sense of accomplishment.*
- Provide supplemental oxygen as ordered. *Anemia and hypoxemia reduce oxygen to the cells, leading to fatigue.*
- Identify energy-saving techniques (e.g., sitting for a shower; using a cane, walker, or wheelchair). *Energy-saving techniques enable the client to do more activities throughout the day. Assistive devices help conserve energy.*

- Refer to physical or occupational therapist as needed. *Physical therapy and occupational therapy exercises can increase muscle strength and tone.*

Ineffective Breathing Patterns

- Promote coughing and deep breathing. Instruct client to use incentive spirometer. Suction airway as needed. *Thick secretions (as in PCP infection) reduce the flow of oxygen to the tissues. These interventions promote lung expansion and mobilize secretions.*
- Monitor oxygen levels with pulse oximetry. If less than 90%, give supplemental oxygen. *Oxygen levels should be above 90% to provide adequate oxygen to tissues and cells.*
- Increase fluid intake as tolerated. *Increased fluids will thin secretions and make them easier to expectorate.*
- Place client in semi- or high Fowler's position. *Elevating the head of the bed reduces abdominal pressure against the diaphragm and prevents aspiration.*
- Give anti-infective medications according to culture and sensitivity tests. *Anti-infective medications help control opportunistic infections.*

Disturbed Thought Processes

- Use simple, short sentences. Always call client by name. *Cognitive and neurologic functioning may be altered by brain malignancies and HIV infection of the central nervous system. These measures decrease confusion and help the client remain oriented.*
- Reorient to time and place frequently. Provide calendar, clock, radio, TV, and a room with a window. *Frequent reorientation may be necessary during acute periods of confusion.*
- Provide quiet room with minimal lights at night. *Excess noise and bright lights confuse the client between day and night.*
- Apply a bed alarm if client tends to get out of bed unassisted. Move the client closer to the nurses' station or place in a monitored room. *The client may experience confusion and impaired judgment. Bed alarms alert nursing staff to check on client's safety. Staff can monitor the client more easily if the room is close or is a monitored room.*
- Encourage family and significant others to socialize with the client. *Contacts with familiar persons can help maintain reality orientation.*
- Maintain safe environment by removing excess furniture, placing call bell within client's reach, and padding side rails as needed. *If motor coordination is altered, clients may injure themselves. These measures can decrease the risk for injury.*

Other Nursing Diagnoses

With a disease such as HIV infection, the list of possible nursing diagnoses is long. Some additional nursing diagnoses to consider are:

- *Powerlessness* related to terminal disease
- *Pain* related to Kaposi's sarcoma and peripheral neuropathy

- *Risk for Caregiver Role Strain* related to care needs of the client with HIV
- *Impaired Home Maintenance* related to fatigue and weakness
- *Ineffective Sexuality Patterns* related to HIV infection.

EVALUATING

Evaluate effectiveness of care by collecting data related to client's overall health, absence of opportunistic infections, laboratory values especially CD4+ cell count, and the ability to care for self at home.

Documenting. Documentation includes the client's vital signs and the presence of any manifestations, which indicate opportunistic infections or cancers. Record the client's response to antiretroviral therapy and other interventions for managing opportunistic infections. The nurse documents client teaching about medications, diet, infection prevention strategies, and safe sex guidelines.

CONTINUING CARE

Most clients with HIV infection and AIDS are cared for in the home. The client and significant others need thorough teaching. They should understand HIV infection and AIDS, disease transmission, and the stages of the disease including opportunistic infections. Provide the client and family with current factual information so they can plan their future. Discuss the myths, misperceptions, and prejudices that accompany this diagnosis.

Teach the client and family how to maintain optimal health. Discuss diet and nutritional intake, balancing rest and exercise, stress reduction, lifestyle changes, and safe sexual practices. Teach them that the client needs a diet high in protein and calories to meet increased metabolic needs and maintain weight. Activity and rest periods should be balanced to prevent unnecessary fatigue.

Provide instruction on hand washing techniques and disinfection procedures for the home. Teach them to clean bathrooms and kitchens daily with disinfectant. Emphasize that all blood spills should be cleaned up immediately by using a 1:10 dilution of bleach and water (½ cup bleach to 5 cups water).

Teach care providers to use gloves when handling the client's secretions or excretions, to wash hands before and after providing direct care, and to wash the client's laundry separately in hot water with 10% bleach. Teach that separate dishes, glassware, and utensils are not necessary, provided they are washed in hot, soapy water. Inform clients that they can assist with food preparation as long as they are feeling well.

Teach strategies to avoid opportunistic infections. Emphasize the importance of avoiding large crowds and people with infectious diseases. Inform clients of the risks of having birds and cats in the home (they can carry toxoplasmosis, cryptosporidiosis, and MAC). Advise clients to avoid changing cat litter boxes or bird cages. Teach the client to wash all raw fruits and vegetables before eating them; to cook all meat, fish, and eggs; and to avoid unpasteurized milk.

Encourage the client to stop smoking and to eliminate alcohol and recreational or illicit drugs because they may decrease health status. Provide contact with a social worker for referral to the appropriate clinic or agency.

Teach clients and families the signs and symptoms of opportunistic infections and malignancies. They must report a fever, sore throat, night sweats, cough, dyspnea, chest pain, swollen glands, diarrhea, headaches, and skin lesions. Discuss the need for regular follow-up with their health care provider and routine laboratory testing.

Teach the client and significant others about the use and adverse effects of prescribed medications. Provide guidelines for helping the client adapt to the fixed medication schedules. Be sure the client understands the importance of complying with the medication regimen.

If necessary, provide information about home health care, hospice, and respite care. Provide referrals to local care providers, home health services, support groups, and social agencies as needed. When the client's disease progresses to the advanced stage, give the caregiver instructions on intravenous nutrition and medication delivery systems.

NURSING PROCESS CARE PLAN
Client with HIV Infection

Sara Lu is a 26-year-old elementary schoolteacher who lives with her parents and two younger sisters. During her yearly physical exam, she complains of feeling fatigued, a persistent sore throat, intermittent bouts of diarrhea, and mild shortness of breath for about a month. Normally, she is very physically active. She is planning to be married in 6 months. Ms. Lu states that she has had unprotected sexual relations only with her fiancé. Seven years ago she had open heart surgery to repair a mitral valve defect. The physician orders a mononucleosis test, ELISA, Western blot test, CD4 T-cell count, and an erythrocyte sedimentation rate (ESR). She is to return to the office in a week.

Assessment. On Ms. Lu's follow-up visit, she tells Carole Kee, RN, that she still has flulike symptoms but has improved somewhat. She is less active than usual and is worried about her health. Her appetite is poor because of a sore mouth, and she has lost 10 lbs during the past month. She has noted white patches on her tongue and cheeks.

A chest x-ray is normal. The results of her laboratory tests are as follows:

- ELISA: positive for antibodies against HIV
- Western blot analysis: positive for antibodies against HIV
- ESR: increased
- CD4+ T-cell count: 599/mm^3 (normal range is 800 to 1,200).

Ms. Lu's physical examination reveals that she has enlarged lymph nodes in her neck, white patches on her oral mucosa, and is somewhat dehydrated. Vital signs are BP 100/70; R 20; P 90; T 99.9°F (37.7°C).

Ms. Lu is told the results of her laboratory tests and the medical diagnosis of HIV infection. Ms. Lu is distressed and wants to know how this happened, its meaning, whether she has infected her loved ones, and whether she will get better. She is admitted to the hospital for short-term care.

Diagnosis. The following nursing diagnoses are developed for Ms. Lu:

- *Imbalanced Nutrition: Less than Body Requirements* related to mouth soreness
- *Risk for Deficient Fluid Volume* related to decreased fluid intake and diarrhea
- *Risk for Infection* related to altered immunity
- *Anxiety* related to diagnosis and fear
- *Deficient Knowledge* about the HIV disease process

Expected Outcomes. The expected outcomes established in the plan of care specify that Ms. Lu will:

- Maintain adequate dietary intake.
- Return hydration status to normal.
- Remain free of infections and any complications.
- Discuss anxiety and fears.
- State ways to prevent HIV transmission to others, including safer sex practices.

Planning and Implementation. Ms. Kee plans the following interventions to be implemented:

- Monitor daily weight, intake and output, and hydration status.
- Suggest strategies for decreasing anorexia and nausea.
- Provide a consult with a dietitian.
- Provide oral care before and after meals.
- Monitor serum albumin levels.
- Assess bowel sounds and monitor elimination pattern.
- Administer antiemetic and antidiarrheal medications as ordered.
- Increase fluid to 2,500 mL daily.
- Use strict aseptic technique for all invasive procedures.
- Give antiretroviral and antibiotics as ordered.
- Encourage physical activity as possible.

- Encourage Ms. Lu to discuss her feelings and concerns.
- Avoid false reassurances.
- Suggest testing for her fiancé.
- Teach about HIV/AIDS, a nutritionally balanced diet, adequate fluid intake, avoiding people with infectious diseases, safe sex practices, and ways to prevent HIV transmission.

Evaluation. Ms. Lu is eager to learn about her illness. She also wants her fiancé and family to attend the teaching sessions with her. Ms. Lu is taking home an antifungal medication, diet plans, and a schedule for increased exercise. She will return in 1 month for a follow-up physical.

Critical Thinking in the Nursing Process

1. Are the laboratory results for Ms. Lu a true indication that she is HIV positive? What additional tests might be ordered?
2. What is the most likely source of Ms. Lu's infection?
3. Ms. Lu says that her fiancé would like to have a child. How will you counsel her regarding pregnancy and childbearing?

Note: The bibliography listings for this and all chapters have been compiled at the back of the book.

Chapter Review

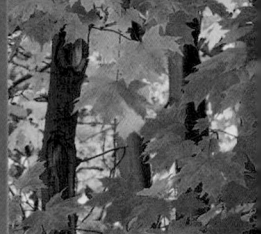

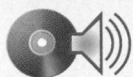 ## KEY TERMS by Topics

Use the audio glossary feature of either the CD-ROM or the Companion Website to hear the correct pronunciation of the following key terms.

Immune system
antigen, allergen, leukocytes, natural killer (NK) cells

Humoral and cell-mediated immunity
immunocompetent, B-cell lymphocytes (B cells), humoral immunity, immunoglobulins, antibody, memory cells, T-cell lymphocytes (T cells), cell-mediated immunity, helper T cells, suppressor T cells, cytotoxic T cells

Immunity
natural immunity, active immunity, passive immunity, anergy, immunizations, vaccines, toxoid, anaphylaxis, hypersensitivity, desensitization

Autoimmune disorders and transplants
autoimmune disorders, autoantibodies, autograft, autologous, isograft, allografts, xenograft, histocompatibility

Client with HIV
acquired immunodeficiency syndrome (AIDS), human immunodeficiency virus (HIV), reverse transcriptase, seroconversion, *Pneumocystis carinii* pneumonia (PCP), toxoplasmosis, cryptococcosis, herpes simplex 1 and 2, cytomegalovirus (CMV), human papillomavirus

KEY Points

- The immune system consists of leukocytes, lymphoid organs (bone marrow, thymus, spleen, lymph nodes), and peripheral lymph tissues such as the tonsils and appendix.

- Active immunity provides long-term immunity either by developing the disease or by an immunization. Passive immunity is short term and involves injecting serum with ready-made antibodies for other humans or animals.

- Hypersensitivity reactions range from mild such as hay fever to severe (e.g., blood transfusion reactions, anaphylaxis, and organ transplant rejections).

- Autoimmune disorders develop when the body fails to identify self from nonself (e.g., rheumatoid arthritis).

- The human immunodeficiency virus (HIV) is the cause of acquired immunodeficiency syndrome (AIDS).

- HIV attacks helper T4 lymphocytes, which decreases a person's ability to remain immunocompetent and increases the risk for developing opportunistic infections.

- The ELISA and Western blot tests detect antibodies to identify if a person is infected with HIV.

- The client with HIV is managed with a combination of antiretroviral medications, such as zidovudine (AZT).

- Health teaching focuses on safer sex practices, adverse drug reactions, nutrition, and ways to reduce opportunistic infection, to prevent transmission, and to maintain self-care.

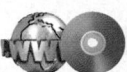 ## EXPLORE MediaLink

Additional interactive resources for this chapter can be found on the Companion Website at www.prenhall.com/burke. Click on Chapter 11 and "Begin" to select the activities for this chapter.

For chapter-related NCLEX-style review questions and an audio glossary, access the accompanying CD-ROM in this book.

FOR FURTHER Study

See Chapter 10 for more in-depth discussion of inflammation.

For discussion of elevated WBC count with a shift to the left, see Chapter 10 and Figure 10-5.

For pharmacologic treatment of autoimmune disorders, see Chapters 10 and 16.

For substances that may cause anaphylaxis and for management of anaphylactic reactions, see Chapter 13.

For more on organ donation, see Chapter 13.

For more on corticosteriods, see Chapter 16.

See Chapter 30 for nursing care of the client with an intravenous access device.

For pharmacologic treatment of clients with rheumatoid arthritis, see discussion in Chapter 43.

Critical Thinking Care Map

Caring for a Client with *Pneumocystis carinii* Pneumonia
NCLEX-PN® Focus Area: Physiologic Integrity

Case Study: A 42-year-old male client is admitted to the medical floor with *Pneumocystis carinii* pneumonia. Two years ago he was diagnosed with AIDS and has "felt good" until last week when he started to feel tired. His CD4+ T-cell count dropped from 500 to 400/mm³. The nurse notes a dry cough and hears crackles in the bases. He says, "I get really short of breath when I walk." He complains of being cold, yet the room temperature is normal.

Nursing Diagnosis: Ineffective Breathing Pattern

COLLECT DATA

Subjective

_____
_____
_____
_____
_____
_____

Objective

_____
_____
_____
_____
_____
_____

Would you report this data? Yes/No

If yes, to: _____

Nursing Care

_____
_____
_____
_____
_____
_____
_____
_____
_____
_____
_____

How would you document this? _____
_____
_____
_____

Data Collected
(use those that apply)

- States, "Short of breath when I walk."
- BP 140/84
- Crackles in the posterior bases
- T 100.8°F
- Complains of being cold
- Easily fatigued
- Purple spots on both arms
- 4-lb weight loss in last month
- Dry cough
- RR 28, shallow
- Pulse oximetry = 88%
- Night sweats
- CD4+ T-cell count = 400 mm³

Nursing Interventions
(use those that apply; list in priority order)

- Instruct in use of incentive spirometer.
- Provide quiet room with minimal lights.
- Collect sputum culture.
- Monitor oxygen levels with pulse oximetry.
- Encourage coughing and deep breathing.
- Provide frequent oral hygiene.
- Increase fluid intake as tolerated.
- Place in semi-Fowler's position.
- Monitor weight daily.
- Give nasal oxygen at 3 L/min.

NCLEX-PN® Exam Preparation

1 A client was given an immunization for influenza 10 minutes ago. Which of these statements, if made by the client, would indicate that the client has a correct understanding of the discharge instructions?

A. "I must be having a severe reaction; my arm is red."

B. "My ride is here. I have to leave now."

C. "I'll put a heating pad on my arm when I get home."

D. "I'll be back in two weeks to get my second shot."

2 A nursing assistant tells you that she is allergic to pineapples. Your best response should be:

A. "Make sure you don't eat foods with pineapple as an ingredient."

B. "I'm allergic to peanuts. What symptoms do you get?"

C. "You must have a type I hypersensitivity reaction."

D. "I will order you some latex-free gloves for your client care."

3 A client arrives in the clinic complaining of a swollen lip after being stung by a bee. The nurse's first priority would be to:

A. assess the respiratory status.

B. ask the client about prior episodes with insect bites.

C. administer epinephrine.

D. explain the allergic reaction pathophysiology.

4 The physician has ordered azathioprine (Imuran) for a post–kidney transplant recipient. Which of the following teaching instructions must be emphasized to the client?

A. Increase PO fluids to 2,000 mL/day.

B. Avoid large crowds.

C. Limit activity to walking.

D. Expect urine output to be normal.

5 When a client diagnosed with HIV says to the nurse, "I guess hugging my little girl is out of the question now," the best response by the nurse would be:

A. "HIV is not transmitted by casual kissing or hugging."

B. "I'm sorry, but you don't want to infect your child."

C. "Perhaps you can show your affection in other ways."

D. "You're right; you must not share your utensils either."

6 When assessing a client who has recently been diagnosed with HIV, the nurse should expect the client to have which of these symptoms?

A. diarrhea

B. *Pneumocystis carinii* pneumonia

C. sore throat

D. night sweats

7 Which of these safe sex guidelines should be included in teaching a client who is HIV positive?

A. Use oil-based lubricants.

B. Oral contraceptives are effective in preventing transmission.

C. Anal sex is acceptable if a condom is used.

D. Do not reuse condoms.

8 A client reports a persistent cough, night sweats, fever, fatigue, and weight loss. The Mantoux test is assessed at 10 mm. The most likely condition that the nurse expects is:

A. *Mycobacterium avium* complex.

B. tuberculosis.

C. candidiasis.

D. cryptosporidiosis.

9 When caring for a client with HIV encephalopathy, which of these nursing interventions should be given priority?

A. Obtain vital signs every 4 hours.

B. Assess the client's support system.

C. Serve small portions of soft foods.

D. Remove excess furniture from the room.

10 A client who is undergoing chemotherapy for Kaposi's sarcoma states, "I'm just too sick to eat." Which of these actions should the nurse take?

A. Remove the tray of food.

B. Administer nausea medication prior to meals.

C. Encourage fluids with meals.

D. Give appetite stimulants as ordered.

Answers for Review Questions, as well as discussion of Care Plan and Critical Thinking Care Map questions, appear in Appendix V.

Chapter 12

Caring for Clients with Cancer

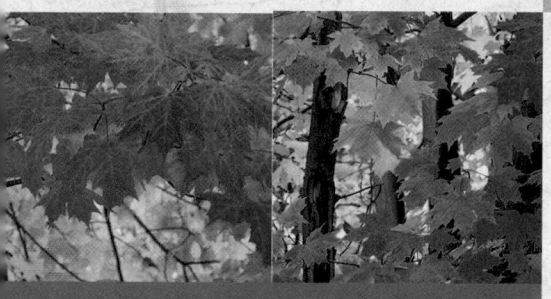

BRIEF Outline

Cancer, the Nurse, and the Health Care Team
Cancer Incidence and Trends
    Carcinogenesis
    Risk Factors
    Early Detection
Effects and Manifestations of Cancer
Nursing Interventions for Oncologic Emergencies
    Superior Vena Cava Syndrome
    Pericardial Effusion and Cardiac Tamponade
    Sepsis and Septic Shock
    Spinal Cord Compression
    Obstructive Uropathy
    Hypercalcemia
    Hyperuricemia
    Tumor Lysis Syndrome

LEARNING Outcomes

After completing this chapter, you will be able to:
- Define cancer and differentiate benign from malignant neoplasms.
- Discuss the pathophysiology of cancer and factors associated with carcinogenesis.
- Describe the effects of cancer on the body.
- Describe the laboratory and diagnostic tests used for cancer diagnosis.
- Discuss the use of surgery, radiation therapy, chemotherapy, and biotherapy in the treatment of cancer.
- Provide teaching for the client and family experiencing cancer.
- Use the nursing process as a framework for providing individualized care for the client with cancer.

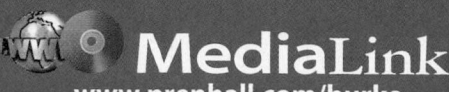

Cancer is a group of complex diseases characterized by uncontrolled growth of abnormal tumor cells. The manifestations of cancer vary depending on which body system is affected and what type of tumor cells are involved. People of any age, gender, ethnicity, or geographic region can be affected by this disease. Despite research that has shed more light on this life-threatening disease, the death rate from cancer remains at 41%. The fear caused by even a possible diagnosis of cancer is considerable. Cancer, "the big C," brings forth feelings of hopelessness and helplessness.

This chapter focuses on cancer as a disease and its treatment. It discusses nursing care appropriate for most clients with cancer. Discussions of cancers that affect specific body systems (e.g., laryngeal cancer, lung cancer) are found in corresponding chapters in the text.

Cancer, the Nurse, and the Health Care Team

Cancer develops when normal cells mutate into abnormal, deviant cells that grow uncontrollably and continue to reproduce within the body. Cancer is not one disease, but a constellation of many diseases. Because cancer can affect any body tissue and has many different manifestations, care of the client with cancer can be complex.

Cancer is a disruptive and life-threatening experience that affects all aspects of the clients and their significant others. Nursing interventions address the wholistic and chronic nature of this disease. Nursing care for clients with cancer occurs in a variety of community-based, ambulatory, and acute-care settings. Cancer is treated with a combination of therapies, many of which have devastating effects on the client and family. Finally, nurses are actively involved in cancer care through education, early detection of potentially malignant growths, rehabilitation and long-term follow-up of clients, and terminal care.

Oncology is the study of cancer; *oncologists* are physicians who specialize in caring for clients with cancer. Oncologists may be medical doctors, surgeons, radiologists, immunologists, or researchers. Often, the client with cancer has the benefit of an interdisciplinary team of physicians, registered nurses (RNs), licensed practical/vocational nurses (LPNs/LVNs), and other health care professionals working together to provide the most effective treatment and care.

Cancer Incidence and Trends

Approximately 1,372,910 new cancer cases were diagnosed in 2005 according to the American Cancer Society (ACS) (2005a). Cancer is a disease associated with aging: 76% of cancer diagnoses occur after age 55. In the United States, breast cancer is the most frequently diagnosed cancer in women (211,240 new cases in 2005), and prostate cancer is the most common cancer in men (232,090 new cases during 2005). Lung and bronchus cancer and colorectal cancer rank second and third in incidence in both men and women. Cancer affects different ethnic groups disproportionately. African American men have a significantly higher incidence of prostate cancer than white men, whereas melanoma mainly occurs in white Americans (ACS, 2005a).

Only heart disease has a higher mortality rate than cancer. Statistics show that 1 in every 4 deaths in the United States is caused by cancer (ACS, 2005a). In 2005, about 70,280 Americans died of cancer—more than 1,500 people per day. Lung cancer remains the leading cause of cancer deaths, accounting for approximately 29% of all cancer deaths (ACS, 2005a). Information about the most recent cancer cases and mortality rates are available on the World Wide Web at www.cancer.org.

With advances in cancer prevention, early detection, and treatment, the 5-year survival rate for individuals with cancer continues to improve in the United States. However, minority ethnic groups bear a disproportionate burden of cancer. African Americans have the highest mortality rate for all cancers among all ethnic groups (ACS, 2005b). Although breast cancer occurs more commonly in white women than in African American and Chinese American women, the survival rate is 89% for white women compared to only 75% for African Americans and 55% for Chinese American women (ACS, 2005b; Aziz & Rowland, 2002). Similar disparities are seen in survival rates for colorectal, prostate, and endometrial cancers in these ethnic groups. Lack of health insurance, lower incomes, unequal access to health care, knowledge deficit, cultural beliefs and attitudes, and language barriers have been identified as the influential factors contributing to this disparity (Aziz & Rowland, 2002; Facione, Giancarlo, & Chan, 2000; Haynes & Smedley, 1999; Wu & Yu, 2003).

PATHOPHYSIOLOGY

Mature normal cells of the body are uniform in size and have nuclei characteristic of the tissue to which the cells belong. Within the cell nucleus, chromosomes containing deoxyribonucleic acid (DNA) molecules carry the genetic information that controls protein synthesis. The genetic information coded in the DNA of every gene is translated into the protein structures that determine the type, maturity, and function of a cell. Any change or disruption in a gene can result in an inaccurate "blueprint" that can produce an abnormal cell, which may then become cancerous.

A **neoplasm** (*neo* = new; *plasm* = tissue) is a mass of abnormal cells that grows independently of its surrounding structures and has no physiologic purpose. It is often called a *tumor* (from the Latin word for "swelling"). Neoplasms grow at a rate unrelated to the needs of the body, do not benefit the host, and in some cases are actively harmful. Neoplasms typically are classified as benign or malignant, based on their potential to damage the body and on their growth characteristics.

Benign Neoplasms

Benign neoplasms are localized growths with well-defined borders; they are frequently encapsulated. Benign neoplasms tend to respond to the body's controls. They grow slowly and often remain stable in size. Because they are usually encapsulated, they often are easily removed and tend not to recur. However, they can be destructive if they crowd surrounding tissue and obstruct the function of organs. For example, a benign meningioma (from the meninges of the brain and spinal cord) can increase intracranial pressure and progressively impair the person's cerebral function. Unless the meningioma is successfully removed, rising intracranial pressure will eventually lead to coma and death.

Malignant Neoplasms

In contrast, **malignant** neoplasms grow aggressively and do not respond to the body's controls. They have an irregular shape and cut through surrounding tissues, causing bleeding, inflammation, and *necrosis* (tissue death) as they grow. When health care professionals use the term *cancer*, they are referring to a malignant neoplasm. Malignant neoplasms can recur after surgical removal of the primary and secondary tumors and after other treatments. (Table 12-1 ■ compares benign and malignant neoplasms.)

Malignant tumors compress, and cancer cells easily separate from the neoplasm, allowing them to move into surrounding body fluids and tissues. Malignant cells may break away from the primary tumor, traveling through the blood

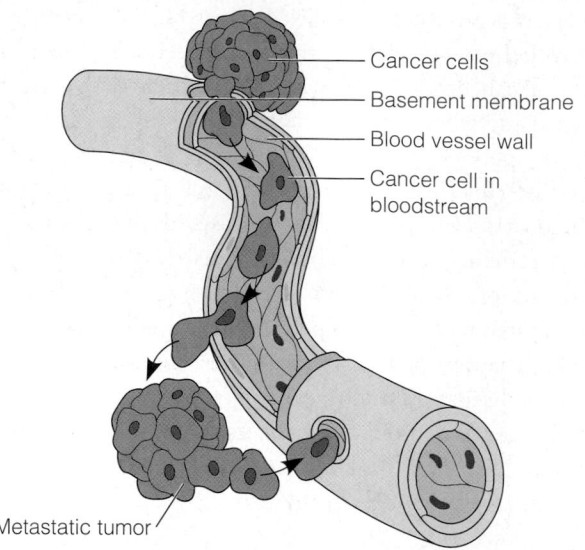

Figure 12-1. ■ Metastasis through the bloodstream. Cancer cells disrupt the basement membrane in the blood vessel and gain access into the circulation. Once in the blood, only about 1 cell in 1,000 escapes immune detection, but that can be enough. Undetected cells move out of the blood, entering new tissue. Once in the new site, the malignant cells multiply and establish a metastatic tumor.

Labels: Cancer cells; Basement membrane; Blood vessel wall; Cancer cell in bloodstream; Metastatic tumor

or lymph to invade other tissues of the body. The ability of cancer cells to invade adjacent tissues and travel to distant organs is considered their most dangerous characteristic. Both the secondary tumor they form and the process by which malignant neoplasms spread are called **metastasis.**

Metastasis can travel as an embolism in the blood or lymph or shed cells into body cavities. A blood or lymph-borne metastasis allows a new tumor to be established in a distant organ (Figure 12-1 ■). The malignant cells enter the circulation, survive in the blood, exit the circulation, and implant in a new tissue. About 60% of metastatic lesions occur in this manner. Malignant cells from a colon cancer may be seeded directly into the peritoneal cavity, establishing a new tumor in the mesenteric epithelium.

For metastasis to occur, the cancerous cells must avoid detection by the immune system. Thus, impairment or suppression of the immune system is a major factor in the establishment of metastatic lesions. The most common sites of metastasis are the lymph nodes, liver, lungs, bones, and brain (Table 12-2 ■).

It is estimated that 50% of all cancers have metastasized by the time the tumor is identified. This may account for the current 41% death rate and supports the need for client education to speed early diagnosis. The time it takes for metastasis to occur is extremely variable and often difficult to predict. Some cancers, such as basal cell carcinomas, do not metastasize. The aggressiveness and location of the tumor, as well as the tumor's ability to escape immune detection, determine whether and how rapidly metastasis takes place.

TABLE 12-1

Comparison of Benign and Malignant Neoplasms

BENIGN	MALIGNANT
Local	Invasive
Cohesive	Noncohesive
Well-defined borders	Does not stop at tissue border
Pushes other tissues out of the way	Invades and destroys surrounding tissues
Slow growth	Rapid growth
Encapsulated	Metastasizes to distant sites
Easily removed	Not always easy to remove
Does not recur	Can recur

TABLE 12-2

Various Cancers and Sites of Metastases

PRIMARY TUMOR	COMMON METASTATIC SITES
Bronchogenic (lung)	Spinal cord, brain, liver, bone
Breast	Regional lymph nodes, vertebrae, brain, liver
Colon	Liver, lung, brain, ovary
Prostate	Bladder, bone (especially vertebrae), liver
Malignant melanoma	Lung, liver, spleen, regional lymph nodes

CARCINOGENESIS

Cancer is primarily a disorder of gene expression, beginning with transformation of a single normally functioning cell into a cancer cell. Because cancer is not a single disease, it is likely that no single cause can be identified. It appears that most cancers result from the interaction of genetic and internal factors with environmental factors, or **carcinogens** (cancer-causing agents).

Carcinogens damage cellular DNA. It appears that damage to and mutation of multiple genes is necessary to transform a cell into a cancer cell. Six or more gene mutations may be necessary for a malignant tumor cell to develop. Carcinogenesis occurs in a process of steps, from *initiation* and proliferation of the mutant cell, *promotion* of abnormal cell growth, and *progression* of the abnormal, mutant cells to malignancy. As the malignancy continues to progress, its cells become increasingly abnormal, differing significantly from cells of the tissue in which the tumor arose. The period of time between the damage to the DNA and detection of a tumor may be as long as 10 to 20 years.

Specific genes control cell growth, replication, and replacement. Normally, damage to any of these genes is repaired by DNA repair genes. All cells in the body have **oncogenes** (genes capable of promoting uncontrolled cellular growth), which normally are repressed. Invading viruses or other carcinogens may "switch on" a cell's oncogenes or damage DNA repair genes. As a result, the rate of cell replication accelerates and normal inhibitory factors that prevent uncontrolled cell growth are suppressed. This allows the transformed cell to develop into a tumor that invades other body tissues.

Tumor suppressor genes (*antioncogenes*) inhibit tumor cell proliferation. When these genes are inactivated, tumor growth is unregulated. Mutations of certain tumor suppressor genes are linked to the leading causes of cancer deaths: lung, breast, and colon cancers. For a tumor to grow, it must be supplied with blood. The growth of new blood vessels (*angiogenesis*) within the tumor also is genetically controlled.

Some researchers suspect that cancerous cells form continuously within the body. The healthy immune system recognizes these cells as "foreign" and destroys them. A tumor takes hold and grows only when it escapes immune surveillance (e.g., people who are immunocompromised). For example, clients with acquired immune deficiency syndrome (AIDS), who have a decreased number of helper T lymphocytes, have a much higher than normal incidence of certain cancers.

Carcinogens

Viruses, drugs, hormones, and chemical and physical agents are known to cause cancer or have strong links to certain kinds of cancers. Certain *viruses* can cause cancer by modifying the genes of the cells they invade. Human immunodeficiency virus (HIV) infects helper T lymphocytes and monocytes, and impairs the person's protection against cancers such as lymphoma and Kaposi's sarcoma. Hepatitis B virus is believed to cause primary liver cancer. Papillomaviruses, which cause benign warts, are associated with malignant melanoma and cervical, penile, and laryngeal cancers. Vaccines to prevent and treat virus-induced cancers are under investigation.

Certain *drugs* and *hormones* are also related to the development of cancer. Chemotherapeutic drugs and recreational drugs (e.g., heroin) cause immune suppression. Hormones, such as estrogen, have been linked to cervical, endometrial, and breast cancers.

Many *chemicals* have been identified as carcinogens, including many occupational hazards encountered in the workplace. Environmental carcinogens include polycyclic hydrocarbons, found in soot; arsenic, found in pesticides; wood and leather dust; polymer esters, used in plastics and paints; carbon tetrachloride; and asbestos. Some foods also contain carcinogens added during preparation or preservation, such as nitrosamines and nitrosindoles found in pickled, salted foods. In some cases, food contaminants produce carcinogenic chemicals.

Excessive *exposure to radiation* causes increased rates of cancer. Both solar radiation from ultraviolet rays and ionizing radiation from industrial or medical sources are carcinogenic. Radon, a naturally formed radioactive gas found in the basements of many homes, is a known carcinogen. People who have lived in areas where nuclear weapons testing has been carried out or whose ground water has been polluted by nuclear wastes are also at increased risk for developing cancers.

Although everyone comes into contact with a vast number of carcinogens, not everyone develops cancer. Other factors, such as genetic predisposition, an impaired immune response, and repeated exposure to the carcinogen, are necessary for a cancer to develop.

RISK FACTORS

Risk factors make an individual or a population vulnerable to a specific disease or other unhealthy outcome. Some risk factors are controllable; others are not. Knowledge and assessment of risk factors are especially important in counseling clients and families regarding cancer prevention.

Noncontrollable Risk Factors

Noncontrollable risk factors include heredity, age, gender, and poverty. Inherited genetic defects have been identified in some types of cancer (breast, colorectal, lung, and prostate). For example, women who inherit a BRCA gene mutation have an 80% lifetime risk of developing breast cancer and a 10% to 60% lifetime risk of developing ovarian cancer (depending on which BRCA oncogene is inherited).

Age is a risk factor, with about 80% of all cancers occurring in people over age 55. One possible factor involved in this increased risk is that at least five cycles of genetic mutations seem to be necessary to cause permanent damage to afflicted cells. Evidence indicates that the immune response is altered with aging, and cells are damaged over time. Also, long-term exposure to carcinogenic agents is usually necessary for cancer to develop. Hormonal changes that occur with aging can be associated with cancer. Postmenopausal women receiving exogenous estrogen have an increased risk for breast and uterine cancers. Older men are at risk for prostate cancer, possibly due to breakdown of testosterone into carcinogenic forms. See Box 12-1 ■ for a discussion about cancer and older adults.

Gender is a risk factor for certain types of cancer. For example, thyroid cancer and breast cancer occur more commonly among females; bladder cancer and prostate cancer are seen more often among males.

Cancer statistics show that *poverty* is a risk factor for cancer. Inadequate access to health care, especially preventive counseling and screening for early detection, may be a major factor. Some factors that usually come under the category of lifestyle risks, such as diet and stress, may not be controllable in this population.

Controllable Risk Factors

Controllable or lifestyle risk factors include stress, diet, weight, occupation, infection, tobacco, drug and alcohol use, and sun exposure. Continuous unmanaged *stress* can keep certain hormones (e.g., epinephrine and cortisol) at high levels, leading to systemic "fatigue" and impaired immune surveillance. Emotional and physical isolation, unexpressed anger, depression, and hopelessness tend to suppress energizing chemicals in the body and depress immune responses.

Some *foods* such as nitrosamines and nitrosindoles are considered carcinogenic. Excessive frying or broiling of foods increases the risk for certain cancers (e.g., gastric). Other substances that are believed to increase cancer risk include sodium saccharine and red food dyes. *Obesity* has been linked to hormone-dependent cancers such as malignancies of the breast, bowel, ovary, endometrium, and prostate.

BOX 12-1	FOCUS ON OLDER ADULTS

Cancer and the Older Adult

Cancer is the second leading cause of death in people over age 65. The incidence of cancer increases with age, probably as a result of the accumulated exposure to carcinogens and age-related declines in the action of the immune system. Hormonal changes (estrogen, testosterone) may also predispose older adults to cancer. The most commonly seen cancers in older women are colorectal, breast, lung, pancreatic, and ovarian. In older men, lung, colorectal, prostate, pancreatic, and gastric cancers occur most frequently.

The importance of screening and early detection of cancer does not diminish with age. Unfortunately, older adults may be less likely to undergo cancer screening or seek treatment for cancer due to fear, depression, cognitive impairments, poor access to health care, or financial constraints. Some older adults (and health care providers) mistake cancer symptoms for normal age-related changes and do not seek appropriate health care. When they do seek treatment, chronic conditions may mask the usual symptoms associated with cancer.

Older adults are at greater risk for side effects associated with cancer treatment (especially chemotherapy) because of age-related physiologic changes and chronic conditions associated with aging. The incidence of toxic effects on the heart and central nervous system is increased. Fatigue, problems related to immobility and functional decline, and risk for infection also occur more frequently in older adults. The nurse needs to monitor the client closely and consider the effect of aging on responses to the disease and its treatment.

Teach the older client and family about the warning signs of cancer. Stress the importance of seeking health care if any of the warning signs develop. Encourage clients to schedule an annual physical examination. Teach women how to perform a breast self-exam (BSE) and emphasize the importance of continuing BSE and regular mammography after menopause. Teach men the early signs of prostate cancer, and encourage them to have an annual digital rectal exam.

Occupational risk factors include excessive exposure to solar rays (e.g., farmers, construction workers), chemicals such as benzenes, and particulate matter such as asbestos or coal dust. Health care workers (x-ray technicians, biomedical researchers) are exposed to ionizing radiation and carcinogenic substances. Although federal standards exist to protect workers from hazardous substances, employees may feel they lack the power to prevent violations or worry that reporting violations may cost them their job.

Specific *infections* increase the risk of cancer, but can be avoided through lifestyle modification. For example, genital herpes and papillomavirus-induced genital warts (linked to cancer) can often be prevented by following safer sex practices (e.g., monogamy, use of condoms). Hepatitis B, spread through blood and body fluids, is a significant risk factor for liver cancer.

CAUTION MODEL

1. Change in bowel or bladder function
2. A sore that does not heal
3. Unusual bleeding or discharge
4. Thickening or lump in breast or other parts of the body
5. Indigestion or difficulty swallowing
6. Obvious or recent change in a wart or mole
7. Nagging cough or hoarseness

Source: American Cancer Society.

Lung cancer is highly preventable because of the relationship of cigarette *smoking* and lung cancer. The larger the dose and the longer the use of tobacco, the higher the risk for developing cancer. The carcinogenic substances in tobacco are weak; therefore, stopping smoking can minimize or even reverse the damage. Research has shown a significantly lower lung cancer death risk for former smokers compared to current smokers. Smokers who quit before age 50 decrease their death risk by 50% in the next 15 years (ACS, 2005a). Tobacco is also related to cancers of the lip, mouth and pharynx, larynx, esophagus, stomach, colon, rectum, pancreas, cervix, bladder, liver, kidney, and myeloid leukemia. Long-term exposure to secondhand smoke increases the risk for lung or bladder cancers in nonsmokers.

Alcohol promotes cancer by enhancing the contact between carcinogens such as those in tobacco and the stem cells that line the oral cavity, larynx, and esophagus (Porth, 2005). People who both smoke and drink a considerable amount of alcohol daily have an increased risk for oral, esophageal, and laryngeal cancers. *Recreational drugs* suppress the immune system, and drug use often is associated with an unhealthy lifestyle that increases general cancer risk. Marijuana has been shown to cause chromosomal damage.

As the protective ozone layer thins, more of the sun's damaging *ultraviolet radiation* reaches the earth. Since the early 1970s, the incidence of melanoma has increased an average of 4% per year. Incidence rates are more than 10 times higher in whites than in blacks. Sun-related skin cancers are now considered to be a problem for all people, regardless of skin color, but people of Northern European extraction with very fair skin, blue or green eyes, and light-colored hair are most vulnerable. Elderly people with decreased pigment are also more at risk, even those with darker skin.

EARLY DETECTION

Early detection and treatment significantly influence the prognosis of people with cancer. Many people do not seek early diagnosis and treatment because of denial, fear and anxiety, stigma, or the absence of specific early signs.

Screening procedures (mammograms, occult blood stool tests, etc.) may be lifesaving.

The American Cancer Society promotes early cancer detection through promotion of cancer awareness and guidelines for screening procedures. Although no longer in use by the ACS, the CAUTION model (Box 12-2 ■) is helpful to promote awareness of common symptoms that may indicate cancer. For people without symptoms, the ACS recommends incorporating a cancer checkup into periodic health examinations. This general cancer checkup includes health counseling, teaching self-examination techniques when appropriate, and, depending on age and gender, examination for cancers of the thyroid, oral cavity, skin, lymph nodes, testes, and ovaries (ACS, 2005a). Box 12-3 ■ lists ACS recommendations for specific screening exams. Nurses should encourage all clients to schedule regular cancer checkups.

AMERICAN CANCER SOCIETY GUIDELINES FOR CANCER SCREENING

Breast

- Routine breast self-examination starting at age 20, prompt reporting of any change in breast tissue to health care provider
- Clinical breast examination every 3 years from age 20 to 39 and yearly thereafter
- Annual screening mammography starting at age 40; women at increased risk may have more frequent mammography or other tests such as breast ultrasound exams

Colon and Rectum

Beginning at age 50, a combination of the following exams:

- Annual fecal occult blood test or fecal immunochemical test
- Flexible sigmoidoscopy every 5 years
- Colonoscopy every 10 years.
- Double-contrast barium enema every 5 years

Cervix/Uterus

- Pelvic examination and Papanicolaou (Pap) test every 2 years for sexually active girls and any women over 18; less often for women with three consecutive negative results, more frequently if certain risk factors are present; women over age 70 who have had three or more consecutive normal Pap tests in previous 10 years may stop screening exams
- At age 35, women with risk for hereditary nonpolyposis colon cancer should be offered annual endometrial biopsy to screen for endometrial cancer

Prostate

Beginning at age 50; age 45 for African American men and those with a strong family history:

- Annual digital rectal exam
- Prostate-specific antigen (PSA) test

Source: American Cancer Society.

MediaLink

Video: Skin Cancer

Effects and Manifestations of Cancer

Although the manifestations and effects of cancer vary with the type and location of the tumor, certain effects are usually observed (Box 12-4 ■). For manifestations of specific cancers, see information about types of cancers in the chapters that follow.

Pain is ranked as one of the most serious concerns of clients, families, and oncology health care professionals. Cancer pain may be *acute,* with a well-defined pattern of onset, and related to the diagnosis or treatment. It may be *chronic,* lasting more than 6 months and frequently lacking the objective manifestations of acute pain. Chronic pain may alter personality, functional abilities, and lifestyle; it may disrupt compliance with treatment and quality of life.

Cancer pain often is due to direct tumor involvement (about 70% of pain experienced by people with cancer). The tumor may stretch pain-sensitive tissues or press directly on pain receptors. Metastases in other organs or in bone can activate pain and pressure receptors as well.

Emotional responses (e.g., fear) to the disease and treatment contribute to the pain experience, as does the fatigue associated with the disease and its treatment. For the dying client, pain may be intensified by feelings of hopelessness.

BOX 12-4

COMMON GENERAL MANIFESTATIONS OF CANCER

- Pain: acute and chronic
- Bone marrow suppression: anemia, leukopenia, thrombocytopenia
  - Fatigue, exercise intolerance
  - Increased incidence of infections
  - Bruising, petechiae, occult or obvious bleeding or hemorrhage
- Anorexia–cachexia syndrome: recent weight loss, poor appetite, early satiety
- Disrupted organ function:
  - Voice hoarseness (laryngeal cancer)
  - Cough, shortness of breath (lung or bronchus cancer)
  - Difficulty eating, swallowing (esophageal or gastric cancer)
  - Jaundice (liver cancer)
  - Constipation, changes in stool caliber (colorectal cancer)
  - Hematuria (bladder or kidney cancer)
  - Difficulty urinating (prostate cancer)
  - Abnormal uterine bleeding (cervical or endometrial cancer)
  - Personality, cognitive, mental status changes (brain tumor)
- Paraneoplastic syndromes: altered blood chemistries, manifestations of hormone or electrolyte imbalance

---

Disruption of function may result from obstruction or pressure (e.g., urine retention from prostatic tumors obstructing bladder neck or urethra) caused by the tumor. Resulting anoxia and necrosis affect the function of involved organs or tissues.

Bone marrow suppression is a common effect of cancer and its treatment, leading to anemia, leukopenia (decreased white blood cells), and thrombocytopenia (low platelet levels). Bone marrow function may be suppressed by the invasion of the marrow by malignant cells, poor nutrition, and treatments such as chemotherapy and radiation therapy. Acute or chronic bleeding may contribute to the anemia. Anemia, in turn, contributes to fatigue experienced by the client. Leukopenia can impair the ability to fight infections. The immune system commonly is suppressed in clients with cancer.

Infection is common due to impaired immune defenses and direct effects of the tumor. Tumors may involve two organs, such as the bowel and bladder, leading to urinary tract infection. They may become necrotic, leading to septicemia. Tumors that grow near the surface of the body can erode through to the surface, providing a site for the entry of microorganisms.

Hemorrhage may be caused by tumor erosion through blood vessels. Thrombocytopenia impairs blood clotting and contributes to the risk for serious bleeding. Hemorrhage can be serious enough to cause life-threatening hypovolemic shock.

The **anorexia–cachexia syndrome** is common in clients with cancer. The metabolic rate increases as cancer cells reproduce, and the cancer cells divert nutrients from normal cells. The tumor secretes substances that alter taste and smell and produce early satiety (a sensation of fullness). Pain, infection, and depression contribute to anorexia. Cancer cells support their growth processes by breaking down (*catabolizing*) body tissue and muscle proteins (Figure 12-2 ■). Unexplained rapid weight loss is often the symptom that brings the client to a health care provider.

Some cancers produce excessive amounts of hormones and other substances, leading to *paraneoplastic syndromes.* As a result, the client may develop symptoms of Cushing's syndrome (see Chapter 16 ⬤⬤) or fluid and electrolyte imbalances. Hypercalcemia is a common manifestation of paraneoplastic syndromes.

PSYCHOLOGIC RESPONSES

People exhibit a variety of psychologic and emotional responses to a diagnosis of cancer. Some see it as a death sentence; they experience overwhelming grief and may give up hope. Others feel guilt and consider cancer a punishment for past behaviors. Common emotions are grief, anger, powerlessness, fear, isolation, and concern about body image and sexual dysfunction.

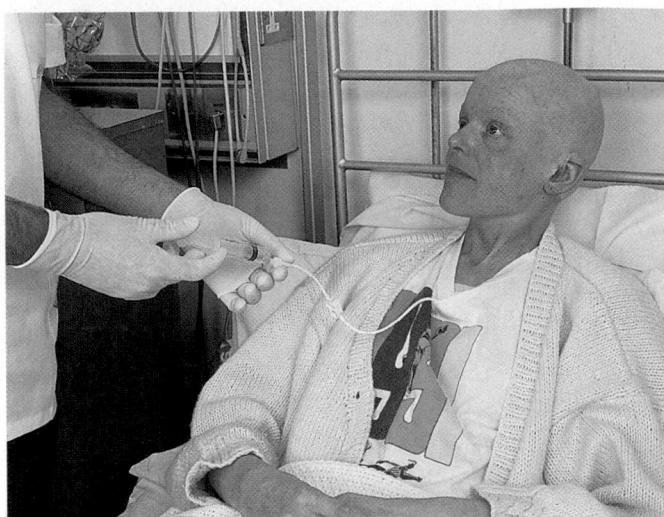

Figure 12-2. ■ Cachexic person with cancer. Cancer robs its host of nutrients and increases body catabolism of fat and muscle to meet its demands. Also note alopecia (hair loss) related to chemotherapy. (*Source: Simon Fraser/Photo Researchers, Inc.*)

INTERDISCIPLINARY CARE

The ACS identifies four major goals of interdisciplinary care for clients with cancer: (1) to eliminate the tumor or malignant cells (cure), (2) to prevent metastasis (control), (3) to reduce cellular growth and tumor burden, and (4) to promote functional abilities and provide pain relief to those whose disease does not respond to treatment (palliation). These goals may overlap. Cancer may be treated with surgery, radiotherapy, chemotherapy, and biotherapy. Often a combination of several treatment modes is used.

Diagnostic Tests

A number of laboratory and diagnostic tests are used to diagnose cancer and monitor progress and treatment.

TUMOR MARKERS. Tumor markers are substances or proteins produced or secreted by malignant cells that are found in the blood. Commonly used tumor markers include:

- Cell surface proteins (CA 125, CA 19-9, CA 50, others)
- Oncofetal antigens that normally are present during fetal development but normally found in only very small amounts in adults (α-fetoprotein [AFP], CEA, others)
- Cell enzymes such as prostate-specific antigen (PSA) and alkaline phosphatase
- Hormones such as ACTH, ADH, calcitonin, hCG, and prolactin
- Markers of tissue injury such as lactic dehydrogenase (LDH), uric acid
- Antibodies to specific cancer antigens (monoclonal antibodies).

High levels of a known tumor marker require follow-up diagnostic studies. The primary use of tumor markers, however, is to determine the client's response to therapy and to detect residual disease.

OTHER LABORATORY TESTS. Other laboratory tests such as the complete blood count (CBC) and studies of specific organ function (e.g., liver function tests, renal function tests, pancreatic enzyme levels, thyroid hormone levels) may be used to evaluate organ function and provide information about the effects of potential metastasis.

IMAGING STUDIES. X-ray imaging, computed tomography, ultrasonography, magnetic resonance imaging, radioisotope scans, and angiography can locate abnormal tissues or tumors.

- *X-ray imaging* is the least expensive and least invasive diagnostic procedure for screening. X-ray imaging cannot distinguish well between cysts and tumors, and cannot usually detect tumors smaller than 1 cm in size.
- *Computed tomography (CT) scans* reveal subtle differences in tissue densities and are much more accurate than X-ray studies. CT scans are useful in screening for renal cell, gastrointestinal tumor, and lymph node involvement. Contrast media may be used to enhance the image. Ask the client about possible allergies to iodine, seafood, or X-ray contrast prior to the exam.
- *Ultrasonography* uses reflected sound waves to examine body tissues and structures. Ultrasonography is noninvasive and requires no exposure to radiation. It is increasingly used to detect and monitor tumors in breast tissue, the prostate, and other organs.
- *Magnetic resonance imaging (MRI)* produces images from radio-frequency signals emitted by the body. Although expensive, it is preferred to diagnose head and neck tumors. Because a strong magnet is used, inquire about the presence of a pacemaker or joint prosthesis prior to the procedure. MRI procedures can produce a feeling of claustrophobia; preparation, support, and reassurance of the client are important.
- *Radioisotope (nuclear) scans* use a special scanner to detect specific radioisotopes administered orally or by injection. In most cases, no special radiation precautions are necessary.
- *Angiography* may be performed when the tumor's location cannot be identified precisely by other methods or the tumor must be visualized before surgery. Fluoroscopy or serial x-ray films trace the movement of radiopaque dye injected into a major blood vessel. Disrupted flow in the vessel indicates tumor location. The exam may also identify blood vessels that supply the tumor, allowing the surgeon to know where to ligate vessels safely. See Box 25-3 ⚭ for nursing care of the client undergoing angiography.

DIRECT VISUALIZATION. Direct visualization procedures using a rigid or flexible fiberoptic scope are invasive but allow inspection of organs and usually permit biopsy of suspicious lesions or masses. Commonly used visualization procedures include the following:

- *Sigmoidoscopy* (inspection of the sigmoid colon)
- *Colonoscopy* (inspection of the entire large bowel)
- *Cystoscopy* (inspection of the urethra and bladder)
- *Bronchoscopy* (inspection of the right and left bronchi)
- *Endoscopy* (inspection of the upper gastrointestinal tract)
- *Laryngoscopy* (inspection of the larynx)
- *Laparoscopy* (inspection of abdominal organs).

All require some client preparation (e.g., food restriction, bowel cleaning), cause some discomfort, and may require sedation or anesthesia. Some may be performed in the physician's office or specialty ambulatory clinic.

EXPLORATORY SURGERY. Exploratory surgery with biopsy also allows direct visualization of suspected malignancies. The client undergoes the usual preoperative preparation for the type of surgery anticipated (see Chapter 9 ⌼).When the tumor is exposed, a sample of tissue (biopsy) is sent to the pathology laboratory for a rapid "frozen-section" histologic examination. If the initial report is negative, the benign mass is usually removed to prevent further symptoms. If the report is positive for cancer, the tumor, often adjacent lymph nodes, and any other suspicious tissue are resected. These are sent to the pathology laboratory for further analysis. The client then receives the usual postoperative care.

CYTOLOGIC EXAMINATION. Tissue samples obtained through biopsy, shedded cells, or collection of secretions are microscopically examined. Cytologic examination can determine the tissue of origin, as well as the stage and grade of the tumor (see later section). Biopsy specimens are collected by exfoliation (a Papanicolaou smear or bronchial washings), aspiration of fluid (like pleural or cerebrospinal fluid), or needle aspiration (solid tumors of breast, lung, or prostate). Body secretions, such as sputum or urine, are also examined. Lymph nodes are biopsied to determine the presence of metastasis.

Psychologic Support during Diagnosis

Preparing for and awaiting the results of diagnostic tests can be stressful, creating extreme anxiety. In addition to coping with the possibility of a life-threatening or life-changing disease, clients often have to go through a series of uncomfortable, even painful, diagnostic procedures. They have important decisions to make that hang on the outcome of those tests. Many unspoken questions may exist:

- Do I have cancer?
- If so, what kind, and how serious?
- Has it spread?

- Will I survive?
- What kind of treatment is needed?
- How will this affect my lifestyle?
- How will this affect family members and friends?

Nurses can provide valuable help during this very difficult time of cancer diagnosis by keeping clients actively involved in managing their life and disease. The LPN can help clients by sitting down with them as soon as they enter the health care system and soliciting questions regarding what the client already knows about the oncoming diagnostic procedures. Initiating the interaction with objective questions and encouraging clients to share their knowledge and experience are effective strategies to facilitate their sense of control.

It is essential that clients understand required test preparation, especially when preparation is done at home. Clients also need to know what to expect during the test, such as nausea or flushing from radioactive dye. A phone call the evening before the procedure to verify the client's understanding and to answer questions can be very supportive.

As clients begin to feel more comfortable with the nurse, they may express concerns, fears, and other emotions. The nurse should avoid giving advice and false reassurance, but listen and be supportive, sharing appropriate information when needed. Being nonjudgmental and providing nonverbal support may facilitate more open communication with clients who are not ready to discuss concerns or those who appear angry. An atmosphere of calmness, warmth, caring, and respect can ease the tension and often unspoken terror of this initial period.

Support of and communication with the client's significant others is extremely important. Family members often try to be strong for the client but may have many fears and emotional concerns they do not feel comfortable expressing. The nurse needs to be available to the family without the client present to allow them to talk without feeling the need to edit for the client's benefit. This can help family members manage their own difficulties in coping with their loved one's potential cancer diagnosis.

Tumor Classification, Grading, and Staging

Malignant tumors are classified using a standardized system. This system consists of *tumor classification* (naming its origin), *tumor grading* (describing its aggressiveness), and *tumor staging* (describing its spread within or beyond the tissue of origin):

1. *Classification.* Tumors are classified and named by the tissue or cell of origin; adjectives are added to further specify the location. For example, an adenocarcinoma of the breast arises in glandular or ductal epithelial cells; osteogenic sarcoma is a bone tumor; and leukemias involve white blood cell precursors, e.g., myeloid

TABLE 12-3

TNM Staging Classification System

STAGE		MANIFESTATIONS
Tumor	T_0	No evidence of primary tumor
	T_{IS}	Tumor *in situ*
	T_1, T_2, T_3, T_4	Ascending degrees of tumor size and involvement
Nodes	N_0	No abnormal regional nodes
	N_{1a}, N_{2a}	Regional nodes—no metastasis
	N_{1b}, N_{2b}, N_{3b}	Regional lymph nodes—metastasis suspected
	N_x	Regional nodes cannot be assessed clinically
Metastasis	M_0	No evidence of distant metastasis
	M_1, M_2, M_3	Ascending degrees of metastatic involvement of the host including distant nodes

leukemia. Other tumors are named for the discoverer of that particular cancer, such as Burkitt's lymphoma or Hodgkin's lymphoma.

2. *Grading.* Tumor grading evaluates cell differentiation and estimates the rate of growth. Cells that are well differentiated (most closely resemble normal cells of the tissue) are the least malignant and earn a grade of 1. Grade 4 is reserved for the least differentiated (appear significantly different than normal cells) and most aggressively malignant cells. Grading criteria may vary with different locations and types of tumors.

3. *Staging.* Staging refers to the relative size of the tumor and extent of the disease. The TNM classification system is commonly used to stage tumors. T stands for the relative tumor size and invasiveness, N indicates the presence and extent of lymph node involvement, and M denotes distant metastases. Table 12-3 ■ outlines the TNM system. Although the TNM system is generalized for all solid tumors, it is frequently adapted for specific types of cancers.

Other systems use specific coding to differentiate types and locations of tumors. These provide a shorthand for staging and grading tumors and provide guidelines for treatment. For example, oncologists may use either an A-B-C-D staging and grading system or a modified TNM system for evaluating prostate cancer.

Surgery

Surgery is used to diagnose and stage more than 90% of all cancers and as a primary treatment for more than 60%. Whenever possible, the tumor is removed entirely. This sometimes requires creation of new structures to maintain body function. For example, if the sigmoid colon and rectum are removed, the remaining healthy segment of the bowel is brought out through a *stoma* (a created opening) in the abdominal wall, providing a permanent *colostomy* for bowel elimination. Surgery can also alter normal body function by destroying nerves and the lymph system; for example, prostate surgery may lead to incontinence and impotence, and lymph node dissection may lead to lymphedema (swelling) in the affected areas (Fu, 2004).

Not all cancer surgery is so radical. Surgery may remove the tumor and a nonessential portion of organ or tissue. An organ whose function can be replaced chemically, like the thyroid, may be removed. When one of a pair of organs is removed, the unaffected organ can take over (e.g., the lung or kidney).

If the tumor is *nonresectable* (cannot be removed) or has metastasized, surgery may be used as a palliative measure, to promote function of the involved organs, to relieve pain, or to reduce the bulk of the tumor so that other treatments are more effective. Surgery is often used in combination with radiation therapy, chemotherapy, or biologic therapies. Reconstructive surgery also may be part of the treatment plan (e.g., breast reconstruction following mastectomy). See Chapter 9 ∞ and discussion of specific cancers in the chapters that follow for nursing care of the client undergoing surgery to treat a malignancy.

Radiation Therapy

Radiation therapy is the treatment of choice for some tumors. Radiation causes lethal injury to DNA. It is used to kill the tumor, to reduce its size, to decrease pain, or to relieve obstruction, and when beginning metastases are suspected. *External radiation* places the source of radiation at a distance from the client and delivers a relatively uniform dose. *Brachytherapy* is internal; the radioactive material (*implant*) is placed directly into the tumor site, delivering a high dose to the tumor and a lower dose to the normal tissues around it. It requires special safety measures (Box 12-5 ■). A combination of these two therapies is often used.

In brachytherapy, the radiation source is sealed in tubes, containers, wires, seeds, capsules, or needles that are inserted into the affected tissue or body cavity. An implant may be temporary or permanent. Internal radiation may also be ingested or injected as a solution into the bloodstream or a body cavity or be introduced into the tumor through a catheter. The radioactive substance may transmit rays outside the body or be excreted in body fluids.

External radiation does not place family members at risk because the client does not emit radioactive particles. Implanted or ingested radiation, however, can be dangerous for those

---

BOX 12-5

CAREGIVER SAFETY: BRACHYTHERAPY

- Maintain the greatest possible distance from the source of radiation.
- Spend the minimum amount of time close to the radiation source.
- Shield yourself from the radiation with lead gloves and aprons whenever possible.
- If you are pregnant, do not provide care for the client receiving brachytherapy.
- If you work routinely near radiation, wear a monitoring device to measure whole-body exposure.
- Avoid direct exposure to radioisotope containers (do not touch the container).
- Keep clients with implanted radioisotopes in a private room with private bath and as far away from other hospitalized persons as possible.
- Use special care to dispose of body fluids of clients with unsealed implanted radioisotopes. Use specially marked containers for disposal.
- Handle bed linen and clothing with care and according to agency protocol.
- Use long-handled forceps to place any dislodged implants into a lead container.
- Consult with the radiation therapy department if there are questions or problems in caring for these clients.

---

living with, caring for, or treating the client. Box 12-6 ■ discusses nursing care for the client receiving radiation therapy.

Potential adverse effects of radiation therapy include skin damage (blanching, erythema, sloughing), ulcerations of mucous membranes, vulnerability to infection, bone marrow suppression, gastrointestinal effects (nausea, vomiting, diarrhea, bleeding), exudate in the lungs (called *radiation pneumonia*), and fistulas or necrosis of adjacent tissues.

Chemotherapy

Chemotherapy disrupts malignant and rapidly dividing cells by interrupting cell metabolism and replication. It reduces the cell's ability to synthesize needed enzymes and chemicals. Chemotherapy may work during specific phases of the cell cycle or through the entire cell cycle.

Chemotherapy can cure some cancers (leukemias, lymphomas, some solid tumors). It may be used to decrease tumor size, as an adjunct to surgery or radiation, or to prevent or treat suspected metastases. Chemotherapy is also used in conjunction with *biologic response modifiers (BRMs)* in some types of advanced cancers. BRMs modify the antitumor response of the body. All chemotherapy has adverse or toxic effects; the type and severity of these effects depend on the drugs and doses used.

Most chemotherapy regimens involve combinations of drugs given over varying periods of time. Treatment is given in cycles with rest periods in between. Treatment is continued until the disease enters remission or the particular protocol is abandoned (due to lack of improvement or toxic effects) and a new one is tried.

Several courses of chemotherapy are necessary because a fixed percentage of cells are killed with each course, reducing the tumor burden. The goal is to reduce the number of malignant cells until the body's immune system can finish the job. In general, this involves giving the maximum amount of chemotherapy the client can tolerate.

During chemotherapy, clients may experience psychologic and emotional distress. The need to plan activities around chemotherapy treatments and adverse effects can impair the ability to work, manage a household, function sexually, or participate in social and recreational activities. Weight loss and alopecia may prompt feelings of powerlessness and depression. The nurse can assist clients by carefully evaluating symptoms, providing specific interventions as indicated, and providing opportunities to express fears, concerns, and feelings. The nurse should encourage clients to participate in their care and facilitate their sense of control over their life as much as possible. Specific interventions are discussed later in the chapter under the appropriate nursing diagnoses.

COMMON ADVERSE AND TOXIC EFFECTS OF CHEMOTHERAPY.
Most drugs used for chemotherapy target cells at a certain point in the cell cycle. Cells that are rapidly dividing are the most vulnerable to damage by these drugs. Cells in certain body tissues such as the bone marrow, GI tract, hair follicles, and the testes have rapid growth cycles, making them vulnerable to the effects of chemotherapy.

Bone marrow suppression is common, resulting in reduced numbers of red blood cells (erythrocytes), white blood cells (leukocytes), and platelets (thrombocytes) As a result, clients often become anemic experiencing fatigue and exercise intolerance. Low white blood cell counts (leukopenia) increase the risk for infection and impair the client's ability to fight off infections that develop. Thrombocytopenia (low platelet counts) impairs clotting, and can result in serious bleeding or hemorrhage.

Colony-stimulating factors (CSFs), or hematopoietic growth factors, often are given to "rescue" the bone marrow following chemotherapy. CSFs regulate the growth and differentiation of blood cells, and are used to help reduce bone marrow suppression. Bone pain is a common side effect of therapy with these agents. Clients also may experience fevers, chills, anorexia, muscle aches, and lethargy.

Common toxic effects of chemotherapy on the GI tract include *stomatitis* (inflammation of the oral cavity), *nausea* and *vomiting,* and *diarrhea.* Stomatitis interferes with the ability to eat and drink, potentially leading to malnutrition. Nausea and vomiting can be severe, resulting from direct effects of the drug on vomiting centers. Administering an antiemetic drug prior to chemotherapy administration can reduce nausea and vomiting. Diarrhea, which can

BOX 12-6 NURSING CARE CHECKLIST

Clients Receiving Radiation Therapy

Nursing Responsibilities for Both External and Internal Radiation Therapy

☑ Working with the interdisciplinary team, carefully assess for, manage, and document any complications.

☑ Assist in documenting the results of the therapy; for example, clients receiving radiation for metastases to the spine will show improved neurologic functioning as tumor size diminishes.

☑ Provide emotional support, relief of discomfort, and opportunities to talk about fears and concerns. For some clients, radiation therapy is a last chance for cure or relief of physical discomfort.

☑ Document nursing care and the client's responses to radiation therapy.

☑ Document teaching, including evaluation and achievement of learning goals, and the need for further client and family instruction.

External Radiation

Prior to the start of treatments, the treatment area is specifically identified by the radiation oncologist and marked with colored semipermanent ink. Treatment is usually given 5 days per week for 15 to 30 minutes per day over 2 to 7 weeks.

Nursing Responsibilities

☑ Monitor for and document adverse effects: skin changes, such as blanching, erythema, desquamation (shedding of the epidermis), sloughing, or hemorrhage; ulcerations of mucous membranes; nausea and vomiting, diarrhea, or gastrointestinal bleeding.

☑ Assess respiratory function, including lung sounds. Document dyspnea, changes in respiratory pattern, or abnormal lung sounds.

☑ Identify and document medications the client is receiving during radiation therapy.

☑ Monitor white blood cell counts and platelet counts for significant decreases. Report changes to the charge nurse or physician.

Client and Family Teaching

☑ Wash the radiation site with plain water only, no soap; do not apply deodorant, lotions, medications, perfume, or powder to the site during treatment. Do not wash off the treatment marks.

☑ Do not rub, scratch, or scrub treated skin areas. If it is necessary to shave the treated area, use an electric razor.

☑ Apply neither heat nor cold to the treatment site.

☑ Inspect the skin for damage or changes, and report these as well as any mouth sores or pain, difficulty swallowing or breathing, or other problems to the radiologist or physician.

☑ Wear loose, soft clothing over the treated area.

☑ Protect skin from sun exposure during treatment and for at least 1 year after radiation therapy. Wear protective clothing and use sun-blocking agents with a sun protection factor (SPF) of at least 15.

☑ External radiation poses no risk for radiation exposure to other people, even with intimate physical contact.

☑ Be sure to get plenty of rest and eat a balanced diet.

Internal Radiation
Nursing Responsibilities

☑ Place the client in a private room.

☑ Limit family and caregiver visits to 10 to 30 minutes; have visitors sit at least 6 feet from the client.

☑ Monitor for and document adverse effects such as burning sensations, excessive perspiration, chills and fever, nausea and vomiting, or diarrhea.

☑ Assess for evidence of fistulas or necrosis of adjacent tissues (e.g., cloudy, malodorous urine), documenting and reporting manifestations to the charge nurse or physician.

Client and Family Teaching

☑ While a temporary implant is in place, stay in bed and rest quietly to avoid dislodging the implant unless otherwise instructed.

☑ During outpatient treatments, avoid close contact with others.

☑ Dispose of excretory materials in special containers or in a toilet not used by others as instructed by the radiologist.

☑ Carry out daily activities as able; get extra rest if fatigued.

☑ Eat a balanced diet; frequent, small meals often are better tolerated.

☑ Contact the nurse or physician for any concerns or questions after discharge.

---

lead to a fluid volume deficit, often can be managed by including constipating foods (e.g., cheese) and foods high in fiber in the diet.

Other important toxic effects of chemotherapy drugs include *reversible alopecia* (hair loss), *teratogenic* (defect-producing) *effects* on a developing fetus, *irreversible sterility* in males, *hyperuricemia* (high uric acid levels in the blood), and, in the long term, an increased risk for cancer (*carcinogenesis*) due to DNA damage by chemotherapy agents.

CHEMOTHERAPEUTIC DRUG CLASSES. The major classes of chemotherapeutic agents are alkylating agents, antimetabolites, cytotoxic antibiotics, plant derivatives, and hormones. Table 12-4 ■ gives the classifications of chemotherapeutic

TABLE 12-4			
Nursing Implications for Pharmacology: Chemotherapeutic Drugs			
DRUG CLASSIFICATIONS/ DRUGS	TARGET MALIGNANCIES	ADVERSE EFFECTS OR SIDE EFFECTS	NURSING IMPLICATIONS
Alkylating Agents Mechlorethamine (Mustargen)	Hodgkin's disease Lymphosarcoma Lung cancer Chronic leukemia	Nausea and vomiting Bone marrow depression Hyperuricemia	Maintain good hydration. Administer antiemetics prior to chemotherapy. Monitor CBC with differential, uric acid. Assess for infection, bleeding. Institute bleeding precautions as indicated.
Busulfan (Myleran)	Chronic myelogenous leukemia	Bone marrow depression Renal failure Pulmonary fibrosis	Monitor CBC, BUN, serum creatinine. Maintain adequate fluid intake. Assess for infection, bleeding. Assess lungs for coarse, loud crackles. Institute bleeding precautions as needed.
Cyclophosphamide (Cytoxan)	Lymphomas Multiple myeloma Leukemias Adenocarcinoma of lung and breast	Hemorrhagic cystitis Renal failure Alopecia Stomatitis Liver dysfunction	Encourage daily fluid intake of 2–3 L during treatment. Monitor WBCs, BUN, serum creatinine, liver enzymes. Teach ways to manage hair loss.
Antimetabolites Methotrexate	Acute lymphoblastic leukemia Osteosarcoma Gestational trophoblastic carcinoma	Oral and gastrointestinal ulcerations Anorexia and nausea Bone marrow depression	Monitor CBC with differential, BUN, uric acid, creatinine. Assess oral mucous membranes; treat ulcers prn. Assess for infection, bleeding. Institute bleeding precautions as needed.
5-Fluorouracil (5-FU)	Colon carcinoma Rectal carcinoma Breast carcinoma Gastric carcinoma Pancreatic cancer	Stomatitis Alopecia Nausea and vomiting Gastritis Enteritis Diarrhea Bone marrow depression	Monitor CBC with differential, BUN, uric acid. Administer antiemetics prn. Assess for infection, bleeding. Evaluate hydration and nutrition status. Teach oral care for stomatitis. Teach care for hair loss. Institute bleeding precautions as needed.
Antitumor Antibiotics Doxorubicin (Adriamycin)	Acute lymphoblastic leukemia (ALL) Acute myeloblastic leukemia Neuroblastoma Wilms' tumor Breast, ovarian, thyroid, lung cancer	Stomatitis Alopecia Nausea and vomiting Gastritis Enteritis Diarrhea Bone marrow depression Cardiac toxicity	Monitor ECG for dysrhythmias; assess for abnormal heart sounds, heart failure. Monitor CBC with differential, BUN, uric acid. Administer antiemetics prn. Assess for infection, bleeding. Evaluate hydration and nutrition.

TABLE 12-4

Nursing Implications for Pharmacology: Chemotherapeutic Drugs (continued)

DRUG CLASSIFICATIONS/ DRUGS	TARGET MALIGNANCIES	ADVERSE EFFECTS OR SIDE EFFECTS	NURSING IMPLICATIONS
		Changes in urine color (red or orange)	Teach oral care for stomatitis. Teach care for hair loss. Instituted bleeding precautions as needed.
Bleomycin (Blenoxane)	Squamous cell carcinoma Lymphosarcoma Reticulum cell sarcoma Testicular carcinoma Hodgkin's disease	Mucocutaneous ulcerations Alopecia Nausea and vomiting Chills and fever Pneumonitis and pulmonary fibrosis	Check for fever 3–6 hours after administration. Monitor chest x-ray reports. Assess respiratory status, and report coarse rales. Evaluate hydration and nutrition status. Teach oral care for stomatitis. Assess for infection. Teach care for hair loss.
Plant Alkaloids Vincristine (Oncovin)	Combination therapy for acute leukemia, Hodgkin's and non-Hodgkin's lymphomas, rhabdomyosarcoma, neuroblastoma, Wilms' tumor	Areflexia Muscle weakness Peripheral neuritis Constipation Paralytic ileus Mild bone marrow depression	Assess neuromuscular function. Monitor CBC with differential. Evaluate gastrointestinal function. Manage constipation.
Vinblastine (Velban)	Combination therapy for Hodgkin's disease, lymphocytic and histocytic lymphoma, Kaposi's sarcoma, advanced testicular carcinoma, unresponsive breast cancer	Areflexia Alopecia Nausea and vomiting Bone marrow depression	Assess neuromuscular function. Monitor CBC with differential. Administer antiemetics prn. Teach ways to manage hair loss. Assess for infection, bleeding.
Etoposide, also called VP-16 (VePesid)	Nonresponsive testicular tumors Small-cell lung cancer	Alopecia Hypotension with rapid infusion	Hydrate adequately before administration. Administer over 60 minutes. Monitor vital signs every 15 minutes during administration and every 2–4 hours thereafter. Teach ways to manage hair loss.
Prednisone	Combination therapy for many tumors Leukemia Lymphoma	Fluid retention Hypertension Steroid diabetes Emotional lability Silent bleeding ulcers Increased risk for infection	Monitor vital signs. Administer diuretics as ordered. Check blood glucose regularly. Evaluate mental status. Administer oral medications with food. Administer proton-pump inhibitors, H_2 blockers, and antacids as ordered.

(continued)

TABLE 12-4

Nursing Implications for Pharmacology: Chemotherapeutic Drugs (continued)

DRUG CLASSIFICATIONS/ DRUGS	TARGET MALIGNANCIES	ADVERSE EFFECTS OR SIDE EFFECTS	NURSING IMPLICATIONS
			Monitor WBC with differential. Monitor for signs of systemic infection.
Diethylstilbestrol (DES)	Advanced breast and prostrate cancers	Fluid retention Feminization Uterine bleeding	Monitor vital signs. Administer diuretics prn as ordered. Explain reason for feminization to men, bleeding to women. Monitor for excessive bleeding.
Tamoxifen (Nolvadex)	Breast cancer	Hot flashes Nausea and vomiting	Teach ways to manage hot flashes. Explain reason for hot flashes. Administer antiemetics as ordered.
Paclitaxel (Taxol)	Ovarian cancer, breast cancer, non–small-cell lung cancer, head and neck cancer	Hypersensitivity reactions including dyspnea, urticaria, flushing, and hypotension Cardiotoxicity Peripheral neuropathy Alopecia Mucositis Nausea and vomiting	Administer prophylactic histamine blockers. Monitor for dysrhythmias, chest pain, palpitations, and changes in hemodynamic status. Assess neuromuscular function. Teach care for hair loss. Teach oral care for stomatitis. Administer antiemetics prn.
Miscellaneous Drugs Cisplatin (CDDP) (Platinol)	Combination and single therapy for metastatic testicular and ovarian cancers, advanced bladder cancer, head and neck tumors, non–small-cell lung carcinoma, osteogenic sarcoma, neuroblastoma	Bone marrow depression Renal tubular damage Deafness	Monitor WBC with differential and platelets, BUN, creatinine, uric acid. Monitor for signs of infection, bleeding. Evaluate hearing; check for tinnitus. Ensure that client is well hydrated before administering. Encourage 2–3 L of fluid intake daily.

drugs, common examples, target malignancies, adverse effects and side effects, and nursing implications.

PREPARATION AND ADMINISTRATION. Chemotherapeutic drugs can be administered orally, intramuscularly, intravenously, intrathecally (into the subarachnoid space), or by direct injection into the tumor itself or the intraperitoneal or intrapleural body cavities. They are prepared and

administered under specific safety guidelines to protect the health care worker.

Vascular access devices (VADs) are commonly used to administer chemotherapy drugs, especially when several cycles of treatment over weeks or months are required. These devices allow the drug to be injected into a large central vein, reducing local irritating effects of the drug on vein walls and the risk of *extravasation* of the drug into subcutaneous tissue.

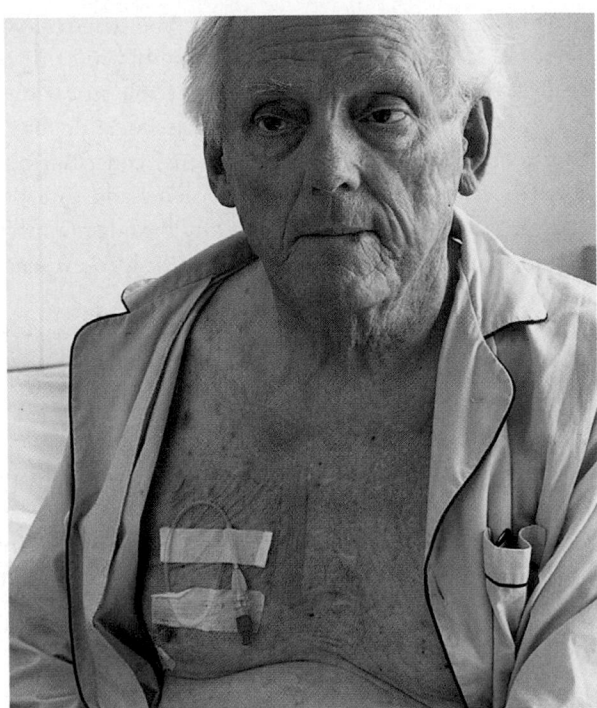

Figure 12-3. ■ A tunneled vascular access device (VAD) for long-term chemotherapy.

VADs are also used to administer parenteral nutrition, for pain management (see Chapter 8 ⊘), or for frequent blood draws to monitor blood counts. Types of VADs include peripherally inserted central catheters (PICC lines); tunneled catheters into a major vein, such as a Hickman or Groshong catheter (Figure 12-3 ■); and surgically implanted ports, such as Mediport.

Chemotherapy generally is administered by RNs who are trained and certified in chemotherapy administration. Practical nurses frequently are responsible for monitoring adverse effects during and after chemotherapy administration.

Biotherapy

Biotherapy is immunotherapy used to treat solid tumors, hematologic malignancies, and bone marrow transplants and as supportive therapy for myelosuppressive chemotherapy. Biotherapy includes injection of monoclonal antibodies, cytokines, hematopoietic growth factors, natural killer cells, and newer agents that specifically target abnormal DNA within malignant cells.

Biotherapy often is accompanied by serious adverse and toxic effects (Fu et al., 2002; Legha et al., 1998). Interleukin-2 can cause acute changes in renal, cardiac, liver, gastrointestinal, and mental functioning. Alpha-interferon causes mental slowing, confusion, and lethargy. When used in combination with 5-fluorouracil or interleukin-2, it may cause severe flulike symptoms, with chills and fever of 103 to 106°F (39.4 to 41.1°C), nausea, vomiting, diarrhea, anorexia, severe fatigue,

---

BOX 12-7	NURSING CARE CHECKLIST

Immunotherapy

Nursing Responsibilities

☑ Monitor for and document adverse effects: mental slowing, confusion, and lethargy; severe flulike symptoms (chills and fever, nausea, vomiting, diarrhea, anorexia, severe fatigue); stomatitis; acute hypertension.

☑ Monitor renal and liver function tests, cardiac enzyme levels (CK, cardiac troponins).

☑ Assess for the desired response to therapy (e.g., reduced effects of the tumor).

☑ Assess coping and teach new strategies as needed.

☑ Monitor and manage fatigue and depression.

☑ Encourage self-care and participation in decision making.

☑ Closely supervise clients with altered mental functioning.

☑ Teach medication administration (subcutaneous, ambulatory pumps), equipment care, and site or catheter care to the client and caregivers.

☑ Document assessments, nursing activities, and teaching, including ability to demonstrate medication administration and catheter care.

Client and Family Teaching

☑ Minimize fever and flulike symptoms: increase fluid intake, take analgesic and antipyretic medications, and maintain bed rest until symptoms abate.

☑ Notify care provider if unable to maintain fluid intake or manage symptoms.

---

and stomatitis. The toxic effects are probably exaggerations of the normal systemic effects that these substances cause when fighting infection. Nursing care of clients receiving immunotherapy is discussed in Box 12-7 ■.

Bone Marrow or Stem Cell Transplant

Bone marrow transplant (BMT) often is used with or following chemotherapy or radiation, particularly in treating hematologic cancers. In *allogeneic* BMT, the bone marrow of a healthy donor (often from a sibling with closely matched tissue) is infused into the client with the illness. In *autologous* BMT, the client's own bone marrow is aspirated during a period of disease remission, frozen and stored, and then infused if the disease recurs.

Allogeneic *stem cell transplant (SCT)*, an alternative to bone marrow transplant, results in replacement of the recipient's blood cell lines (WBCs, RBCs, and platelets) with cells derived from donor stem cells. Donor tissue must be closely matched with that of the recipient. Hematopoietic growth factors are administered to the donor for 4 to 5 days to increase the concentration of stem cells in peripheral blood, allowing it to be used instead of bone marrow. Stem cells also are prevalent in umbilical cord blood. This may be stored and used in some cases (Kasper et al., 2005).

Prior to BMT or SCT, high doses of chemotherapy and/or total body irradiation are used to destroy malignant cells in the bone marrow. The marrow or peripheral blood containing stem cells is then infused through a central venous line. Prior to and immediately following BMT or SCT, the client is critically ill and at significant risk for infection and bleeding due to depletion of WBCs and platelets.

GRAFT-VERSUS-HOST DISEASE. Allogeneic BMT or SCT may precipitate *graft-versus-host disease (GVHD),* which develops when immune cells of the donated bone marrow identify the recipient's body tissue as foreign. Consequently, T cells in the donated marrow attack the liver, skin, and gastrointestinal tract, causing skin rashes and sloughing, diarrhea, gastrointestinal bleeding, and liver damage. *Acute GVHD* develops within days of the transplant, whereas *chronic GVHD* develops later, 100 or more days after the transplant. GVHD is treated with antibiotics and steroids; immunosuppressive drugs also may be used if necessary.

Complementary Therapies

Although advances in cancer treatment have increased the 5-year survival rate, the uncertainty of cure and reoccurrence of cancer often impels some clients to look for complementary therapies. It is estimated that approximately 30% to 50% of patients with cancer may have used some kind of complementary therapies, which are increasingly accepted as appropriate adjuncts to traditional medical care. Common complementary therapies for cancer include botanical agents, nutritional supplements, dietary regimens, mind–body modalities, spiritual approaches, and miscellaneous therapies. Box 12-8 ■ provides information about commonly used complementary therapies.

Nurses need to understand common complementary therapies to provide safe, effective nursing care, because these therapies can affect the client's response to prescribed treatments. It is also important for nurses to provide truthful, nonjudgmental responses to questions or inquiries about complementary therapies from clients with cancer. Nurses should encourage clients to report the use of any complementary therapies to their primary care provider and oncologist to prevent harmful interactions of the therapies with their medical treatment plan.

NURSING CARE

Nursing care for the client with cancer occurs in a variety of settings, including acute and long-term care, ambulatory care, the home, and in hospice settings. The practical/vocational nurse is an integral member of the interdisciplinary health care team, and plays an important role in caring for clients with cancer. Practical nurses are responsible for conducting focused assessment of the client, contributing to the identification of nursing care problems and care planning, delivering direct care, providing and reinforcing client and family teaching, and contributing to evaluation of the effectiveness of care.

Nurses should educate all clients about cancer risk factors, as well as preventive strategies and lifestyle changes to reduce their risk. At the same time, nurses should reassure clients with cancer that they are not responsible for having acquired the disease. Once a cancer diagnosis is established, assist and support clients during their treatment, recovery, and rehabilitation. When cure is not possible, nurses provide comfort for the client and significant others during the dying process.

ASSESSING

Practical/vocational nurses collect focused assessment data to evaluate the responses of clients with cancer to the disease and its treatment. It is important to be alert for adverse effects of cancer treatments, manifestations of infection or bleeding, decreased blood cell counts, and psychosocial or spiritual distress.

Subjective Data

During a focused interview, the nurse collects significant data, including:

- History of the disease, including signs and symptoms that led the client to seek health care
- Current symptoms or problems related to the disease or treatment, such as pain, nausea, or depression
- Other current or chronic diseases, such as diabetes; current medications
- Any known allergies to drugs, foods, or other substances
- Understanding of the treatment plan
- Expectations of the treatment plan
- Functional limitations and effect of the disease or treatment on current lifestyle and family responsibilities/relationships
- Support systems or caretakers the client can rely on
- Coping strategies and how well they are working; effective coping strategies used in the past.

It is important to ask clients with cancer about the presence of an advance directive for treatment should the client be unable to express his or her preferences. As appropriate, inquire about end-of-life decisions, such as designated caregivers, knowledge of hospice care, presence of a will, and desires for a service and burial or cremation.

BOX 12-8

COMMON COMPLEMENTARY THERAPIES FOR CANCER

TYPES AND EXAMPLES	DESCRIPTIONS
Botanical agents: echinacea, Essiac, ginseng, green tea, pau d'arco, and Hoxsey	Herbs are believed to be the most "natural" and "safe" plants ingested; the safety of many botanical agents hasn't been proved, especially used in conjunction with medical treatment.
Nutritional supplements: vitamins, minerals, enzymes, amino acids, essential fatty acids, and proteins (such as shark cartilage)	Nutritional supplements are believed to promote health and to help cure cancer. The safety of compounds such as vitamins is established; however, in megadoses, many nutritional supplements can be toxic and may interact with therapeutic agents such as chemotherapy.
Dietary regimens: grape diet, carrot juice diet, garlic, onions, and liver	The ingestion of only natural substances is believed to purify the body and slow the growth of cancer. The effectiveness of these dietary regimens still needs to be established.
Mind–body modalities: relaxation, meditation, or imagery	The harmony of mind and body is believed to facilitate physiologic and psychologic healing. Recent research has shown that these modalities helped clients adjust to the experience of cancer.
Energy healing: therapeutic touch and healing touch	The human body is believed to be an energy field and cancer the result of a disturbed energy field. Energy therapies promote healing by treating the body's energy field. In therapeutic touch, the hands are passed over the body without touching it to restore energy imbalances and innate healing forces. Healing touch uses a series of energy healing techniques to restore the harmony and balance of the body. Clinical practice and research has shown positive effects of energy healing in a variety of clients.
Spiritual approaches: faith healing, prayer, prayer groups or chains	Faith in God or a higher power of the universe is believed to promote healing. Research has shown that faith in God or a higher power also helped people with cancer to adjust to the experience of cancer.
Miscellaneous therapies	Aromatherapy has been used to relieve nausea, vomiting, or retching and to decrease anxiety. Aromatherapy might not be appropriate for clients who are highly sensitive to strong fragrances. Music, art, and humor therapies have also been used to help reduce anxiety, express feelings of loss, and promote optimism.

Objective Data

A complete physical assessment is conducted to establish a baseline against which to evaluate later changes. It is especially important to document current general health status, current manifestations, nutritional status using anthropomorphic measurements, hydration, and laboratory results.

- General appearance: apparent state of health, alertness, interaction; voice quality and pattern of speaking; posture, muscle mass, weight for height; ability to move, sit easily; use of any assistive devices
- Vital signs including temperature; current weight; intake and output
- Skin and mucous membranes: color, moisture, temperature and condition; condition of hair and nails; skin turgor; presence of lesions, *petechiae* (small red spots that do not blanch with pressure), bruises, areas of inflammation (red, hot, tender)
- Cardiorespiratory: respiratory pattern and ease, lung sounds; heart rate, rhythm, and sounds; strength and equality of peripheral pulses; color and temperature of extremities, capillary refill; presence of edema
- Abdomen: shape, contour; bowel sounds; presence of tenderness to light palpation; visible or palpable swelling or masses
- Laboratory data: CBC including differential and platelet count; serum electrolytes, osmolality, albumin and total protein, BUN and creatinine, glucose, bilirubin, liver enzymes; urinalysis; specific tests for organ function or cancer markers

DIAGNOSING, PLANNING, AND IMPLEMENTING

Priorities in Nursing Care. The goals of nursing care for clients with cancer focus on providing support and managing specific physical and emotional responses to the disease and its treatment. Nursing care also focuses on promoting rehabilitation and function for survivors and helping others maintain their dignity and comfort in the dying process. Nursing care includes the whole family from the onset of diagnosis through treatment and the ultimate outcome. Only the most common diagnoses are discussed here.

Physiologic needs are the priority for nursing care; however, it is important to remember that clients with cancer and their families also have significant psychosocial and emotional needs.

Chronic Pain

- Frequently assess comfort and the effectiveness of current measures, using a standardized pain scale (see Chapter 8 ⏺). *Changes in tumor size with treatment or lack of response to treatment, as well as therapies to treat cancer can affect the amount and type of pain experienced by the client. Continuing assessment is necessary to ensure effective pain relief.*
- Provide relief that allows clients to function as they wish and, for terminally ill clients, to die relatively free of pain. *Providing pain relief at the level desired allows the client to maintain control and function at an optimal level.*
- Administer prescribed medications in combination and to the maximum prescribed dose as needed to maintain comfort and prevent breakthrough pain. *A combination of medications, including nonsteroidal anti-inflammatory drugs, over-the-counter analgesics, and mild (e.g., oxycodone) to potent (e.g., morphine, hydromorphone) narcotic analgesics may be required to manage the client's pain.*
- Continue to try combinations and increasing dosages or alternate drugs until maximal pain relief is achieved, balanced with client's need to function. *When narcotic doses are increased gradually, there is no limit to the amount the client can receive, as long as adverse reactions can be managed.*
- Administer medication on a regular schedule (e.g., every 2 to 4 hours) with additional medication to cover breakthrough pain. *A regular schedule of medication will provide the patient with greater pain relief.*
- Closely monitor the client receiving analgesia per patient-controlled analgesia (PCA), continuous drip, pump, or alternate mechanism for effective pain relief and manifestations of toxicity or overdose. *Although PCA and analgesic pumps are very safe and well controlled, frequent assessment of the drug effects on the client is necessary to ensure safe and effective care.*

Ineffective Protection

- Monitor vital signs including temperature. *Fever and sympathetic nervous system responses, such as increased pulse and respiration, are common early signs of infection.*

clinical ALERT

Severely immunosuppressed patients may have infection without fever.

- Monitor white blood cell counts frequently, especially when bone marrow suppression is a risk due to chemotherapy. *Early identification and reporting of decreasing WBC counts allow institution of infection precautions and corrective actions to restore immune status.*
- Teach the client and significant others to avoid crowds, small children, and people with infections when the WBC count is at *nadir* (lowest point) and to practice careful personal hygiene. *During periods of leukopenia, even minor infections can be very dangerous. The immunosuppressed client also is susceptible to infection from normal host organisms (opportunistic infections).*
- Protect skin and mucous membranes from injury. Teach good hygiene, use of moisturizing lotion to prevent dryness and cracking, frequent position changes for the bedfast client, and immediate attention to skin breaks or lesions. *Intact skin is the first line of defense against infection.*
- Encourage to consume a diet high in protein, minerals, and vitamins, especially vitamin C. *Improved nutrition decreases the risk of infection. Vitamin C has been shown to help prevent certain infections.*
- Monitor vital signs and assess for obvious or occult bleeding: excessive bruising; bleeding gums, oral mucous membranes; emesis, stool, and urine for visible or occult blood; vaginal bleeding; prolonged bleeding from puncture sites; neurologic or mental status changes; complaints of abdominal pain, diminished bowel sounds. *Early identification of bleeding helps prevent significant blood loss and potential shock.*
- Avoid invasive procedures such as rectal temperatures and suppositories, urinary catheterization, and parenteral injections if possible. Diagnostic procedures such as biopsy or lumbar puncture should not be done if the platelet count is less than 50,000. *Invasive procedures can cause tissue trauma and bleeding. Procedures that use large-bore needles should be delayed until the platelet count is increased.*
- Apply pressure to injection sites for 3 to 5 minutes, and to arterial punctures for 15 to 20 minutes. *Pressure prevents prolonged bleeding by prompting hemostasis and clot formation.*
- Instruct to avoid forcefully blowing or picking the nose, forceful coughing or sneezing, and straining to have a bowel movement. *These activities can damage mucous membranes, increasing the risk for bleeding.*

Risk for Injury

- Assess frequently for manifestations of obstruction or organ dysfunction (e.g., the brain, lungs, liver, or urinary system). *Early detection allows medical intervention before the problem becomes a crisis.*
- Teach the client and family to differentiate minor from serious problems. Box 12-9 ■ provides guidelines to identify problems that must be reported or that require emergency services. *Guidelines for when to call the doctor provide an anxiety-reducing safety net for the client and family and promote early detection of complications.*
- Monitor laboratory values; report abnormal findings or significant changes to physicians immediately. *If the cancer impairs organ function or creates ectopic sites of hormone production, laboratory values provide an early indication of this development and are reported so treatment can be instituted to restore homeostasis.*

Imbalanced Nutrition: Less than Body Requirements

- Assess current eating patterns, including likes and dislikes, and identify factors that impair food intake. *This permits an individualized plan based on the client's needs and preferences.*
- Evaluate degree of malnutrition using height–weight charts, skin fold measurements, body mass (see Chapter 19 ⚭), and laboratory values for total serum protein, serum albumin and globins, total lymphocyte count, serum transferrin, hemoglobin, and hematocrit. *These data provide an objective determination of nutritional status.*
- Teach ways of maintaining good nutrition by using the Food Guide Pyramid (see Figure 19-2 ⚭) and adapting to any medical restrictions and preferences. *Clients comply better with food plans that are tailored to their needs.*
- Manage problems that interfere with eating:
  - Encourage the client with food aversions to eat whatever is appealing. *It is better for the client to eat something to maintain calorie intake, even if it is not nutritionally balanced.*
  - Eat small, frequent meals. *These are more easily digested and absorbed and usually better tolerated by the client with anorexia.*
  - Encourage to try icy cold foods (such as ice cream) or more highly seasoned dishes if food has no taste. *Chemotherapy and radiation therapy may harm taste buds. Strong seasonings and coldness make food more enjoyable.*
  - Encourage cold, bland semisoft and liquid foods for the client with stomatitis. Have the client use an anesthetic mouthwash prior to eating. *These foods are less irritating to sensitive mucous membranes. Reducing*

BOX 12-9   CLIENT TEACHING

When to Call for Help

Instruct the client or family member to call when:

- Oral temperature greater than 101.5°F (38.6°C)
- Severe headache; significant increase in pain at usual site, especially if the pain is not relieved by the medication regimen; or severe pain at a new site
- Difficulty breathing
- New bleeding from any site, such as rectal or vaginal bleeding
- Confusion, irritability, or restlessness
- Withdrawal, greatly decreased activity level, or frequent crying
- Verbalizations of deep sadness or a desire to end life
- Changes in body functioning, such as inability to void or severe diarrhea or constipation
- Changes in eating patterns, such as refusal to eat, extreme hunger, or a significant increase in nausea and vomiting
- Appearance of edema in the extremities or significant increase in edema already present

Instruct to seek emergency care if the client:

- Is having significant difficulty breathing or if the lips or face has a bluish tinge
- Becomes unconscious or has a convulsion
- Exhibits unmanageable behavior, such as being physically abusive, hurting self, or engaging in uncontrollable activity

---

discomfort with a local anesthetic can make chewing and swallowing easier.

- Administer antiemetic medications. Encourage low-fat meals with dry foods such as crackers and toast; to avoid liquids with meals; and to sit upright for an hour after meals. Remove emesis basins and encourage oral hygiene before eating. *Dry, low-fat foods are more readily tolerated by the nauseated client. Removing odors and supplies associated with nausea and vomiting can reduce nausea.*
- Encourage use of nutritional supplements (Ensure, Isocal) and multivitamin and mineral tablets with meals. Suggest increasing calories by adding ice cream or frozen yogurt to the liquid supplement or commercial protein–carbohydrate powders to milk or fruit juice. *Food intake of most cancer clients is less than what is needed to maintain or gain weight. These supplements can add calories and nutrients in a manner often tolerated by the client.*
- Teach to keep a food diary to document daily intake. *When clients see how little is being consumed, they may eat more. A food diary also helps the nurse keep a calorie count and*

alerts the physician if more drastic nutritional measures, such as parenteral nutrition, need to be considered.

Impaired Tissue Integrity: Oral Mucous Membranes

- Carefully assess and evaluate for impaired tissue integrity: ulcerations on the tongue and oropharyngeal mucosa due to chemotherapy; herpes simplex type 1 lesions; a white, yellow, or tan coating with dry, red, fissured tissue underneath indicative of a fungal infection (*Candida*); red, swollen, gums that bleed with minimal or no trauma; or *xerostomia* (excessive dryness of the oral mucous membranes) due to chemotherapy or radiation. *Accurate assessment and documentation are vital for care planning by the interdisciplinary team.*

- Instruct to clean teeth gently in the morning, after meals, and at bedtime. Use a very soft toothbrush, and obtain a new toothbrush monthly. If gums are bleeding, clean teeth with toothpaste and a soft cloth over finger. Floss gently with waxed floss (unless contraindicated by risk for bleeding), and use a non-alcohol-based mouthwash after brushing. Dentures should be soaked nightly in hydrogen peroxide. *Disrupted mucous membranes allow normal oral bacteria into the systemic circulation, potentially leading to sepsis in the immunocompromised person. Reducing oral flora by frequent hygiene decreases the risk of infection.*

- Culture any oral lesions, and report the problem to physician. *Identifying the cause of the infection, whether viral, fungal, or bacterial, allows the physician to prescribe the appropriate treatment.*

- Advise the client with xerostomia to use lubricating and moisturizing agents, such as Gatorade, sugarless gum, and Blistex. Avoid putting sharp instruments or utensils in the mouth. Advise to have necessary dental work done by a dental oncologist. Chlorhexidine mouthwash (Peridex) may be used. *These measures protect gums from trauma and decrease risk of hemorrhage.*

- Administer medications as ordered: acyclovir (viral infections), systemic antibiotics (bacterial infections), Nystatin or clotrimazole solution or lozenges (fungal infections), viscous lidocaine or combination mouthwashes before meals and as needed. *These agents reduce pain and inflammation. Knowing the contents of each mouthwash can prevent hypersensitivity reactions (e.g., to lidocaine).*

Anxiety

Clients with cancer, especially those with poor coping skills, may exhibit overt signs of anxiety, such as trembling, irritability, increased blood pressure, pallor, or poor eye contact. The client may report insomnia and feelings of tension, or express concerns about perceived changes caused by the disease and fear of future events.

- Carefully assess the level of anxiety versus the real threats of the current situation. *A client in panic may need medical intervention with appropriate medications. Those with moderate or even severe anxiety often can be managed through listening, counseling, and teaching new skills.*

- Convey warmth and empathy, and listen nonjudgmentally. *A client who feels safe will more easily express feelings and thoughts, and may be more willing to try new behaviors as suggested.*

- Encourage the client to acknowledge and express feelings, no matter how inappropriate they may seem. *Acknowledging and expressing feelings help diminish anxiety and direct energy toward healing, as well as lay the groundwork for new coping behaviors.*

- Review past coping strategies and introduce new strategies as appropriate. Explain why inappropriate strategies (repressing anger, turning to alcohol) are not helpful. *The client will be more willing to build on strategies that worked in the past and may be more able to reject inappropriate strategies if shown why they did not work in past crises.*

- Identify community resources, such as crisis hot lines and support groups. *The client's support systems may be lacking or having their own difficulties dealing with the cancer diagnosis. Programs such as "I Can Cope," sponsored by the ACS, provide education, counseling, and support in a group setting with other cancer patients.*

- Provide specific information about the disease, treatment, and what may be expected, especially for those clients with obvious misinformation. Avoid advice and false reassurance. *Knowing what to expect gives the client a sense of control and the ability to make decisions. Discussions about symptom management as part of the treatment plan can significantly relieve anxiety.*

- Provide a safe, calm, and quiet environment for the client in panic. Stay with the client, and administer antianxiety medications as ordered. *Being present and displaying calmness and confidence can protect the client from injury and prevent further panic. If the panic does not subside, report to the physician for medication management.*

- Use crisis intervention strategies to promote growth in the client and significant others, regardless of the outcome of the disease. A referral to a mental health professional may be helpful. *With help, people can transform a major crisis from an experience of defeat and despair to one of personal and spiritual growth.*

Deficient Knowledge

The nurse plays an important role in preparing clients with cancer and their families for planned cancer treatment strategies such as surgery or chemotherapy.

- Before surgery, provide the opportunity to ask questions and to discuss concerns and fears. *In some cases, the client may want to discuss alternative treatment options that are available.*

- Explain the specific surgical procedure and any anticipated alterations to the client's body. *Some surgeries will require major lifestyle adjustments, such as a colostomy.*
- Prior to surgery, set up a conference for the client with the oncologist and surgeon. *This will provide an opportunity to clarify the planned surgery and follow-up treatment.*
- When a vascular access device (VAD) such as a Groshong or Hickman catheter is inserted, teach clients and family members to observe for redness, swelling, pain, or exudate at the insertion site; and swelling of the neck or skin near the VAD. Teach how to flush catheters and provide site care on a regular basis. *The risk of infection, catheter obstruction, and extravasation of fluid into surrounding tissue are the main problems associated with VADs.*
- Instruct the client and family members to assess and monitor for signs and symptoms of toxic side effects of chemotherapy. *This will alert the nurse to the onset of toxicity. Indicators of organ toxicities, such as nephrotoxicity or cardiac toxicity, must be reported immediately to the physician.*
- Teach clients undergoing chemotherapy to dispose of used equipment and excretions safely. *Excretion of chemotherapy is primarily through the urine.*

Disturbed Body Image

- Discuss the meaning of the loss or change for the client. *A seemingly trivial loss may have a big impact on the client's life. Likewise, a major loss may not be as important as the nurse imagines. The nurse must evaluate each situation in terms of the reactions of the specific client.*
- Observe and evaluate the client's interaction with significant others. *People may unintentionally reinforce negative feelings about body image or the client may perceive rejection where none exists.*
- If appropriate, allow the client to engage in denial, but do not participate in it. (If a client won't look at the wound, the nurse may say, "I am going to change the dressing to your breast incision now.") *Denial is a protective mechanism and should not be challenged, but it also should not be promoted. A matter-of-fact and empathetic attitude will help the client accept the change.*
- Encourage the client and significant others to express their feelings about the situation and to identify new coping strategies. Give matter-of-fact responses to questions and concerns, and enlist family and friends in reaffirming the client's worth. *A supportive, safe environment promotes acceptance and encourages new coping strategies. It also reaffirms that the client's worth is not lessened by physical changes.*
- Teach the client or significant others to participate in care of the affected body area. Support and validate their

efforts. *Active involvement in providing care empowers the client and significant others, promotes closeness, and reduces the risk of rejection. Positive reinforcement encourages these behaviors to continue.*

- Teach specific strategies for minimizing physical changes (skin care during radiation therapy, dressing to enhance appearance and disguise change in a body part). *Early intervention can limit negative effects and promote recovery. Involvement gives the client some control in a difficult situation.*
- Teach ways to reduce the *alopecia* (hair loss) from chemotherapy or radiation therapy and to enhance appearance until hair grows back:
  - Discuss the pattern and timing of hair loss. *This allows the client to plan for and cope with changes and incorporate coping strategies into daily activities.*
  - Encourage the client to wear cheerful head coverings, coordinated with usual clothing. *Attractive head coverings protect the head while allowing the client to feel attractive and well dressed.*
  - Advise that hair will grow back after chemotherapy, but that its color and texture may be different. Refer the client to a good wig shop before hair loss occurs. *Hair color and texture can be matched to minimize obvious changes in appearance. The client who knows what to expect may experience less anxiety and distress.*
  - Refer the client to support programs such as "Look Good . . . Feel Better," sponsored by the ACS and the Cosmetic, Toiletry, and Fragrance Association Foundation. *A support group can diminish feelings of isolation and provide practical tips for managing problems. For a list of community resources available to clients with cancer, refer to a local phone book.*

Anticipatory Grieving

- Use active listening, silence, and nonverbal support to provide an open environment to discuss feelings realistically and to express anger or other negative feelings. *This helps the client and family members express feelings and confront the possibility of the loss or death. Although 59% of people with cancer recover fully, facing death and making preparations can be a healthy response that allows the client and family to work through the dying process and achieve growth, or to cope with changes in body image and lifestyle (see Chapter 14 ⬯).*
- Answer questions about illness and prognosis honestly, always encouraging hope. *This allows realistic assessment of and planning for their situation. It also helps combat feelings of hopelessness and depression.*
- When cure is no longer an option and the disease is terminal, discuss hospice care with the client and family. *Hospice services provide support and comfort for the client and family, promoting their sense of control through the dying process.*

- Encourage the dying client to make funeral and burial plans ahead of time and to be sure the will is in order. Make sure the necessary phone numbers can be easily located. *This gives the client a sense of control and frees family members of these concerns when the client is most in need of their support.*
- Encourage the client to continue taking part in activities he or she enjoys, including keeping a job as long as possible. *The client keeps a sense of continuity of life even in the face of severe losses.*

EVALUATING

Evaluate the effectiveness of nursing care for the client with cancer through ongoing assessment and care planning. Measures that are ineffective, such as pain management, will need to be changed or modified and the effectiveness evaluated over time. The family or significant others can also provide data about the effectiveness of the plan of care.

Documenting. Cancer is a chronic condition, requiring lengthy treatment. Initial and ongoing documentation of assessment data, plans of care and interdisciplinary interventions, and the effectiveness of these interventions is vital. Carefully document any changes in assessment data and responses to those changes (such as modification of the treatment plan or nursing care plan). Document the client's and family's psychologic responses and coping strategies throughout the process. Document all teaching provided and the client's and family's apparent understanding and acceptance of information. Note when reinforcement of teaching is necessary.

CONTINUING CARE

Prevention. The ACS makes specific recommendations for cancer prevention, in addition to the screening measures discussed earlier in this chapter. Based on these recommendations, nurses should provide the following teaching:

- Avoid tobacco use, secondhand smoke, and excessive alcohol use.
- Eat a variety of healthy foods, primarily from plant sources (whole grains, fruits, and vegetables); limit consumption of red meats and processed meats.
- Maintain a healthy weight; if overweight or obese, lose weight.
- Consume ample amounts of antioxidant foods, such as those containing beta carotene (a vitamin A precursor), vitamins E and C, and omega-3 oils.
- Take certain medications and hormones, such as estrogen or tamoxifen, only under close medical supervision.
- Limit exposure to ionizing radiation (x-rays, radon) and ultraviolet (UV) radiation from the sun.

- Avoid exposure to known and potential carcinogenic chemicals such as benzene, asbestos, vinyl chloride, arsenic, and others. If employed in an industry where such chemicals are employed, use personal protective equipment and devices to limit exposure.
- Limit expose to viral diseases associated with certain cancers by using safer sex practices (see Chapter 36 ⬮⬮) and avoiding use of recreational and illicit drugs.
- Improve immunity by maintaining a healthy lifestyle and managing stress.

In addition, encourage people to report to the public health department any known leaking of chemicals or radioactive materials into the water or air. Also report any noted increase in the incidence of cancer, especially of one specific type, in the community.

Rehabilitation. Rehabilitation from cancer not only involves regaining strength and function, recovering from surgery or chemotherapy, and learning to live with an altered body part or appliance, but also recovery from associated psychologic and emotional turmoil.

Rehabilitation centers provide physical therapy, occupational therapy, speech therapy, job retraining, and an opportunity to rest before resuming life responsibilities. Many clients convalesce at home, with the support of nursing assessment and counseling, direct care, and teaching. Hygiene and home maintenance can be provided by a certified home health aide. Physical and occupational therapists provide muscle strengthening, mobility training (especially with prostheses), and home safety teaching.

Psychologic rehabilitation of cancer survivors addresses quality-of-life issues. Employment may be a problem, health insurance may be canceled, and life insurance may be difficult to get following a diagnosis of cancer. Relationships may have suffered from the strain the illness placed on significant others and the essential self-focusing required for recovery. In contrast, both the client and significant others may have undergone personal and spiritual growth leading to a new and enriching period of their lives.

Self-help groups are available in many communities to support people through the cancer experience. Clients and families need to be informed about the many resources that are available through community agencies as well as the survivor support groups.

Home Care. Teach the client and significant others or caregivers how to manage the client at home. In addition to teaching outlined in the nursing interventions section, discuss problems that may result from the type of cancer and the treatment received. Provide information on how to manage these problems and when to call the physician. Teach wound care to the client with an open wound or draining lesion, and provide a referral to a home health nurse to monitor progress. Explain special diets clearly, or refer the client to a dietitian before discharge. Carefully review home care instructions with the client and family, making sure they understand medications to be taken, any other treatments, and when to see the doctor for follow-up care. Provide or order equipment and supplies needed for home care, especially any special bed or equipment for mobility and safety in the home. For the client who needs complex care, such as parenteral nutrition, provide a referral to a home health nurse before discharge. Because the hospital stay is often short, make follow-up phone calls for several days after discharge, and provide a number to call for concerns and questions.

Hospice Care. Hospice care allows cancer clients with terminal disease to elect to die at home or in a home-like setting When a client and family choose hospice care, they are usually deciding against additional hospitalizations, except those required to manage reversible problems. Hospice clients also refuse resuscitation measures (see Chapter 14 ⏺). The multidisciplinary hospice team usually includes:

- A nurse case manager, who works directly with the client and family, and coordinates the activities of the other disciplines. The nurse (or another nurse familiar with the client) is usually on call 24 hours a day and makes home visits frequently. The nurse is often with the family when the client dies
- A physician who collaborates with the nurse case manager about medications and treatments and may make periodic home visits
- An anesthesiologist or pharmacist to manage pain control and watch for drug interactions
- An infusion therapist, who provides equipment, supplies, solutions, and expertise for intravenous medications or nutrition. This person is usually on call 24 hours a day to trouble-shoot equipment problems
- A social worker who helps identify resources and who assists with grief work, general support, and counseling as needed
- A physical therapist who teaches safe procedures for mobility and moving the client
- A home health aide who provides physical care and assists the family with household chores
- Volunteers who provide companionship for the client and respite to the family for short periods of time.

Many hospice services are connected with an inpatient respite care unit, where the client can receive 24-hour care for up to several weeks. This source provides the necessary care to the client if a family member becomes ill or needs to be relieved temporarily of the tremendous burden of caring for a dying loved one. Clients who do not have family available for support during the dying process may be admitted to a "hospice house," a home-like setting in which the client receives care and hospice support.

NURSING PROCESS CARE PLAN
Client with Cancer

James Casey is a 72-year-old man who has been under medical care for chronic obstructive pulmonary disease, post-myocardial infarction, and type 1 diabetes mellitus for over 15 years. He lost his wife due to lung cancer 5 years ago and still "misses her terribly." He reports smoking two packs of cigarettes a day for 52 years, one to two six-packs of beer a week, one "bourbon and water" a night, and "a lot of sugar-free junk food." He quit smoking 2 years ago, when he could no longer walk a block without considerable shortness of breath, and just quit drinking alcohol a few weeks ago at his physician's insistence. About a year ago, he had a basal-cell carcinoma removed from his right ear. Six months ago, he underwent two 6-week courses of chemotherapy for bladder cancer. The latest report indicates that the cancer has returned and no further chemotherapy would be useful. Surgery was considered but his other medical problems would compromise his chances of survival, so Mr. Casey decided to forgo further treatment and to be managed at home through hospice care. His daughter, Mary Walsh, and her family have moved in with him to provide care and support during his final months. The daughter says she is glad to be able to spend this time with her father. She has been informed of the physical and emotional stress this will entail.

Assessment. The hospice nurse, Ms. Jackson, completes a health history and physical examination during her first two home visits. She gathers this information over 2 days to conserve his strength and allow more time for him and his daughter to talk about their concerns.

During the assessment, Ms. Jackson notes that Mr. Casey is pale and thin, with a wasted appearance and a worried facial expression. His blood pressure is 90/50; apical pulse is 102 and regular; respiratory rate 24; breath sounds are clear but diminished in the bases; oral temperature is 96.8°F.

Last week a tunneled Groshong catheter as a VAD was placed in the right anterior chest. There is no drainage, redness, or swelling at the site.

Mr. Casey states that he spends most of his time either in bed or sitting up in a chair in his room. He says he has no energy and is unable to walk to the bathroom alone or take care of his own personal hygiene. He complains of severe back pain no longer adequately relieved by alternating Percodan and Vicodin every 2 to 4 hours. The nurse rates Mr.

Casey's functional level as capable of only limited self-care, confined to bed or chair 50% or more of waking hours. He tells the nurse that his daughter "is working day and night to help me and is looking awfully tired."

Ms. Walsh reports that Mr. Casey is eating very poorly: He has a small bowl of oatmeal for breakfast, soup and crackers for lunch, and only fruit juice for dinner. Mr. Casey says that he has no appetite and eats just to please his daughter. He does drink at least three to four glasses of water a day plus juice. His finger-stick blood sugars remain within normal range. His current weight is 120 pounds, down from 180 pounds a year ago. He has lost about 30 pounds over the last 2 months.

Laboratory values from his visit with the doctor show the following:

Total protein: 4.1 (normal range: 6.0 to 8.0 g/dL)
Albumin: 2.2 (normal range: 3.5 to 5.0 g/dL)
Hemoglobin: 10.2 (normal range: 13.5 to 18.0 g/dL)
Hematocrit: 30.5 (normal range: 40.0 to 54.0%)
Blood urea nitrogen (BUN): 30 (normal range: 5 to 25 mg/dL slightly higher in older people)
Creatinine: 2.2 (normal range: 0.5 to 1.5 mg/dL).

Diagnosis. The nursing diagnoses for Mr. Casey (and significant others) include the following:

- *Imbalanced Nutrition: Less than Body Requirements* related to anorexia and fatigue
- *Risk for Caregiver Role Strain* related to severity of her father's illness and lack of help from other family members
- *Chronic Pain* related to progression of disease process
- *Impaired Physical Mobility* related to pain, fatigue, and beginning neuromuscular impairment
- *Risk for Impaired Skin Integrity* related to impaired physical mobility and malnourished state

Expected Outcomes. The expected outcomes established in the plan of care specify that:

- Mr. Casey will increase his oral intake and show improvement in his serum protein values.
- His daughter will be able to maintain her supportive caretaking activities as long as Mr. Casey needs them.
- Mr. Casey will have minimal pain for the rest of his life.
- Mr. Casey will be able to continue his current activity level.
- Mr. Casey will have intact skin.

Planning and Implementation. The following interventions are planned and implemented during Mr. Casey's care:

- Ask Mr. Casey what his favorite foods are, and ask his daughter to offer him a small portion of one of these foods each day.
- Encourage Mr. Casey to drink up to four cans of Ensure Plus with Fiber a day, sipping them throughout the day.
- Talk with the physician about trying a medication to stimulate the appetite.
- Have a home health aide assist with personal care and some household tasks.
- Talk with Ms. Walsh about her adult children providing some assistance. Offer to talk with them if she is uncomfortable doing so.
- Request a volunteer to spend up to 4 hours a day, twice a week with Mr. Casey so that Ms. Walsh can attend to outside activities and chores.
- Talk with the physician, and work out a pain-control program using the VAD and a patient-controlled analgesia (PCA) infusion pump with a continuous morphine infusion.
- Call the infusion therapist to set up the equipment and supplies (including the medication) for the morphine infusion.
- Teach Mr. Casey and his daughter how to use the pump and about the side effects of the morphine infusion, including those requiring assistance.
- Leave detailed instructions regarding medication storage and care of the pump, along with the telephone number of the infusion therapist.
- Instruct Ms. Walsh to allow ample rest periods between each activity Mr. Casey must carry out, such as taking a shower or using the commode.
- Order a hospital bed, a special foam pad for Mr. Casey's bed and chair, and a bedside commode from the medical supply house.
- Instruct Ms. Walsh and the home health aide in proper skin care, and to report any beginning lesions immediately to the nurse.

Evaluation. Mr. Casey increased his oral intake a little and drank one or two cans of Ensure a day. His weight remained at about 120 pounds until his death 2 weeks later. Ms. Walsh was very grateful for the extra help from the home health aide and the volunteer, but could not bring herself to ask her son and daughter for help and did not want the nurse to do so. She did become more rested and reported that "we had some wonderful 3:00 A.M. talks when he couldn't sleep."

Mr. Casey was started on 20 mg of morphine per hour with boluses of 10 mg four times a day. This medication relieved his pain quite well; after 2 days he was alert enough most of the time to carry on a normal conversation and able to walk to the bathroom with help until 2 days before he died.

The hospital bed simplified Mr. Casey's care and made it much easier for him to rest comfortably and change position. His skin remained intact and in good condition. Mr. Casey died peacefully in his sleep, about 2 weeks after care was started.

Critical Thinking in the Nursing Process

1. What other tests could have been done to evaluate Mr. Casey's nutritional status?
2. Mr. Casey had severe back pain. What were the possible pathophysiologic reasons for his pain?
3. If Mr. Casey's daughter, Ms. Walsh, had a nursing diagnosis of Ineffective Individual Coping, what would you include in a teaching plan to help her learn new coping strategies?

Nursing Interventions for Oncologic Emergencies

Clients with cancer may experience a number of emergency situations associated with their disease or its treatment. These emergencies require astute observation, accurate judgment, and rapid action once the problem has been identified. In all cases, notifying the physician or emergency team immediately is the first step. A brief description of some of the more common oncologic emergencies with nursing interventions follows.

SUPERIOR VENA CAVA SYNDROME

The superior vena cava can be compressed by mediastinal tumors or adjacent thoracic tumors. The most common cause is lung cancer. Signs and symptoms may develop slowly. Facial and arm edema are early signs. As the problem progresses, pleural effusion and tracheal edema cause respiratory distress, dyspnea, cyanosis, and, eventually, altered consciousness and neurologic deficits. Nursing interventions include the following:

- Provide respiratory support with oxygen, and prepare for tracheostomy.
- Monitor vital signs.
- Administer corticosteroids (e.g., dexamethasone) as ordered to reduce edema.
- If the disorder is due to a clot, administer fibrinolytic or anticoagulant drugs as ordered.
- Provide a safe environment, including seizure precautions.

After the emergency is managed, the client often receives radiation or chemotherapy to reduce the tumor size.

PERICARDIAL EFFUSION AND CARDIAC TAMPONADE

Malignant *pericardial effusion* may develop secondary to lung or esophageal cancers or due to metastases. It can compress the heart, restrict heart movement, and result in a cardiac tamponade. The signs of cardiac tamponade are those of circulatory collapse or cardiogenic shock: hypotension, tachycardia, tachypnea, dyspnea, cyanosis, increased central venous pressure, anxiety, restlessness, and impaired consciousness.

Muffled heart sounds and weak or absent peripheral pulses during the inspiratory phase of breathing may be early manifestations of cardiac tamponade. Manifestations suggesting cardiac tamponade should immediately be reported to the physician. Nursing interventions include the following:

- Start oxygen and alert respiratory therapy for other respiratory support as needed.
- Monitor vital signs and prepare for hemodynamic monitoring.
- Bring crash cart to bedside.
- Set up for and assist physician with a pericardial tap (pericardiocentesis). (See Chapter 27. ⚭)
- Reassure the client.

SEPSIS AND SEPTIC SHOCK

Tumor necrosis in a client who is immunosuppressed and/or malnourished can result in sepsis. Bacteria enter the blood, grow rapidly, and produce septicemia. The sepsis, which is usually gram-negative, progresses to systemic shock and eventually results in multisystem failure (see Chapter 13 ⚭). Manifestations appear in two phases. The first phase is characterized by vasodilation and hypovolemia; high fever; peripheral edema; hypotension; tachycardia; tachypnea or Kussmaul's respirations; hot, flushed skin with creeping mottling beginning in the lower extremities; and anxiety or restlessness. Without treatment, the shock progresses to the second phase and more classic signs of shock: hypotension; rapid, thready pulse; respiratory distress; cyanosis; subnormal temperature; cold, clammy skin; decreased urinary output; and altered mentation. Identifying the problem while the client is still in the first phase is crucial to the client's survival. In addition to promptly notifying the physician, nursing interventions include:

- Monitor infusion of colloidal solutions (plasma volume expanders, such as albumin) and balanced salt solutions as ordered.
- Monitor hemodynamic values (arterial and venous pressure, pulmonary artery pressure, cardiac output) to evaluate the effects of rehydration and detect early signs of overload.
- Provide oxygen and other respiratory support as needed.
- Assist with obtaining cultures of wound drainage, urine and sputum, and blood cultures.
- Administer prescribed broad-spectrum antibiotics until the specific organism is identified.
- Provide a safe environment when mentation is altered; provide support and reassurance for the anxious client.

SPINAL CORD COMPRESSION

Spinal cord compression is usually associated with pressure from expanding tumors of the breast, lung, or prostate;

lymphoma; or metastatic disease. It can lead to irreversible paraplegia. Early symptoms include progressive back and leg pain, numbness, paresthesias, and coldness. Later, bowel and bladder dysfunction occur and, finally, neurologic dysfunction progressing to weakness and paralysis. Treatment often consists of radiation or surgical decompression, but early detection is essential. Nursing interventions include the following:

- Perform neurologic checks every shift for clients with advanced cancers of the breast, lung, prostate, or lymphoma.
- Thoroughly assess all complaints of back pain or sensory changes.
- Notify physician if spinal cord compression is suspected, and prepare for magnetic resonance imaging (MRI).
- Administer corticosteroids (e.g., dexamethasone) as ordered to reduce cord edema and protect function.

OBSTRUCTIVE UROPATHY

Clients with intra-abdominal, retroperitoneal, or pelvic malignancies (prostate, cervical, or bladder cancers) may experience obstruction of the bladder neck or the ureters. Bladder neck obstruction usually manifests as urinary retention, flank pain, hematuria, or persistent urinary tract infections; ureteral obstruction is often not evident until renal failure develops. Nursing interventions include the following:

- Investigate and report complaints of flank pain or urinary retention.
- Monitor serum BUN, creatinine, and potassium, reporting elevated levels.
- Send a specimen of any foul-smelling urine for culture.
- Report hematuria to the physician immediately.
- Catheterize the client with acute retention as ordered.

HYPERCALCEMIA

Hypercalcemia is associated with cancers of the breast, lung, esophagus, thyroid, head, and neck and with multiple myeloma. Bone metastases may also cause hypercalcemia. (Hypercalcemia is discussed in Chapter 7. ⚭) Clients often present with nonspecific symptoms (fatigue, anorexia, polyuria, constipation). Neurologic symptoms include muscle weakness, lethargy, and diminished reflexes. Without treatment, hypercalcemia progresses with alterations in mental status, psychotic behavior, cardiac dysrhythmias, seizures, coma, and death. Nursing interventions include the following:

- Monitor serum calcium, phosphate, alkaline phosphatase, electrolytes, BUN, and creatinine levels.
- Monitor pulse and cardiac rhythm.
- Administer intravenous solutions of normal saline as ordered to increase urinary calcium excretion.

- Administer corticosteroids and calcitonin as ordered.
- Maintain bed rest until calcium levels decrease.

HYPERURICEMIA

Hyperuricemia usually develops as a complication of rapid necrosis of tumor cells after vigorous chemotherapy for lymphomas and leukemias. Uric acid crystals are deposited in the urinary tract, causing renal failure and uremia. Symptoms of hyperuricemia include nausea, vomiting, lethargy, and oliguria. Nursing interventions focus on prevention and include the following:

- Increase intravenous hydration to ensure urinary output of approximately 3 L a day for 48 hours prior to chemotherapy.
- Administer allopurinol (antigout drug) per recommended dosage and schedule or teach the client the importance of taking the prescribed drug for 48 hours prior to chemotherapy.
- Administer daily sodium bicarbonate as ordered to alkalinize the urine and thereby prevent uric acid crystallization.
- Monitor serum uric acid levels and urine pH.
- If signs of uremia occur, insert a Foley catheter and monitor urinary output as well as serum BUN, creatinine, and potassium levels.

TUMOR LYSIS SYNDROME

Tumor lysis syndrome (TLS) is a life-threatening emergency most commonly seen in clients undergoing initial chemotherapy for hematologic cancers such as leukemias or lymphomas. TLS is characterized by metabolic abnormalities including hyperuricemia, hyperphosphatemia, hyperkalemia, hypocalcemia, and lactic acidosis (Cantril & Haylock, 2004; Holdsworth & Nguyen, 2003). These metabolic abnormalities increase the risk for cardiac dysfunction and renal failure. The syndrome develops when the body is unable to excrete the metabolic by-products and intracellular contents from a massive and rapid cell death, resulting in their accumulation in the bloodstream (Cairo & Bishop, 2004). Manifestations and potential consequences of TLS include nausea, vomiting, lethargy, edema, fluid overload, heart failure, cardiac dysrhythmias, seizures, muscle cramps, tetany, syncope and possible sudden death (Cairo & Bishop, 2004; Cantril & Haylock, 2004). Nursing interventions focus on prevention and management of TLS:

- Identify clients at risk, including people with high-grade lymphomas, acute leukemia, those with elevated serum uric acid, potassium, and phosphorus levels, and those with impaired renal function.
- Administer allopurinol as ordered prior to and during chemotherapy; stress to the client the importance of taking the drug as ordered.

- Promote adequate hydration to maintain a urinary output of at least 150 mL/hr.
- Administer sodium bicarbonate as ordered to alkalinize urine to promote uric acid excretion.
- Administer oral phosphate binder such as aluminium hydroxide as ordered to promote the excretion of phosphate through the bowel.

- As indicated, administer sodium polystyrene sulfonate (Kayexalate) to promote potassium excretion via the bowel.

Note: The bibliography listings for this and all chapters have been compiled at the back of the book.

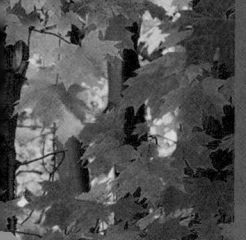

Chapter Review

 **KEY TERMS** by Topics

Use the audio glossary feature of either the CD-ROM or the Companion Website to hear the correct pronunciation of the following key terms.

Cancer
cancer, oncology, neoplasm, benign, malignant, metastasis, carcinogens

Theories of carcinogenesis
oncogenes

Effects of cancer
anorexia–cachexia syndrome

KEY Points

- Cancer can affect people of any age, gender, ethnicity, or geographic region.
- Many cancer risk factors are controllable; prevention is key.
- Clients with cancer need a great deal of emotional support because fear and anxiety are common responses to a diagnosis of cancer.
- Cancer treatment is aimed at cure, control, or palliation of symptoms.
- Cancer may be treated through surgery, radiotherapy, chemotherapy, and biotherapy.
- Early detection and treatment influence the prognosis of people with cancer most.
- All people should have regular cancer checkups.
- Cancer pain is the most feared symptom.

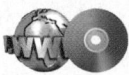 **EXPLORE MediaLink**

Additional interactive resources for this chapter can be found on the Companion Website at http://www.prenhall.com/burke. Click on Chapter 12 and "Begin" to select the activities for this chapter.

For chapter-related NCLEX-style review questions and an audio glossary, access the accompanying CD-ROM in this book.

FOR FURTHER Study

For more information on hypercalcemia, see Chapter 7.

For more information about caring for clients in pain, see Chapter 8.

For more information on preoperative preparation, see Chapter 9.

For more information on shock and multisystem failure, see Chapter 13.

For more on the death and dying issues and hospice care, see Chapter 14.

For more information about Cushing's syndrome and other endocrine disorders, see Chapter 16.

For more information about nutrition and the Food Guide Pyramid, see Figure 19-2.

Box 26-3 provides information about nursing care of the client undergoing angiography.

Pericardial taps are discussed on Chapter 27.

Chapter 36 discusses safer sex practices.

Caring for a Client Undergoing Chemotherapy for Cancer

NCLEX-PN® Focus Area: Physiologic Integrity: Reduction of Risk Potential

Case Study: Maria Hernandez, a 78-year-old Hispanic woman, was diagnosed with colon cancer and had a colon resection 6 months ago. When she comes in for chemotherapy, she reports that she has been progressively anorexic and nauseated since beginning chemotherapy of 5-fluorouracil (5-FU). She states "I just can't eat. My mouth is so sore and it hurts to swallow. I've lost so much weight."

Nursing Diagnosis: Imbalanced Nutrition: Less than Body Requirements

COLLECT DATA

Subjective

_____

_____

_____

_____

_____

_____

Objective

_____

_____

_____

_____

_____

_____

Would you report this data? Yes/No

If yes, to:_____

Nursing Care

_____

_____

_____

_____

_____

_____

_____

_____

_____

_____

_____

How would you document this? _____

_____

_____

_____

Data Collected
(use those that apply)

- Height: 5'4"
- Weight: 102 lbs.
- Pale skin with poor turgor
- Blood pressure: 134/76
- Apical pulse: 88, regular
- Lungs clear to auscultation
- Pale skin with poor turgor
- Hemoglobin: 13.4
- White blood count: 6,500
- Oral mucous membranes red and swollen
- Bowel sounds present in all four quadrants
- Hair dry and brittle
- Concentrated urine

Nursing Interventions
(use those that apply; list in priority order)

- Administer pain medications.
- Administer antiemetics.
- Assist Mrs. Hernandez with ambulation.
- Assess hemoglobin and hematocrit.
- Encourage fluid intake.
- Monitor vital signs every 4 hours.
- Suggest referral for counseling.
- Suggest eating soft bland foods at room temperature.
- Offer high-protein drinks.
- Instruct on using soft toothbrush or toothette for oral hygiene.
- Administer pain medications.

NCLEX-PN® Exam Preparation

1 A client with a history of lung cancer complains of nausea, anorexia, and upper right quadrant pain. The nurse suspects

A. an adverse effect of the prescribed chemotherapy.
B. metastasis of the tumor to the liver.
C. superior vena cava syndrome.
D. extension of the tumor to involve the diaphragm.

2 A client whose father was recently diagnosed with colon cancer asks the nurse what she can do to reduce her risk of developing the disease. The nurse responds that

A. because colorectal cancer risk is primarily genetically determined, she cannot change her risk.
B. the cause of most cancers, including colon cancer is unknown, so she should simply maintain a healthy lifestyle.
C. research has shown that a diet rich in whole grains, fruits, and vegetables with limited red meat consumption is associated with a lower risk for colon cancer.
D. it is vital that the client undergo annual colonoscopy for early detection of precancerous lesions or polyps in the bowel.

3 A client diagnosed with lung cancer reports he is having difficulty sleeping and often feels tense. The most appropriate initial nursing intervention would be to:

A. encourage expression of his or her feelings about the cancer diagnosis.
B. offer an antianxiety drug such as Ativan (lorazepam).
C. document the client's status in the medical record.
D. collaborate with the physician to obtain an order for sleep medication.

4 Following surgery to remove a colon tumor, a client refuses to care for his colostomy. Appropriate nursing intervention would be to:

A. teach a family member to perform colostomy care.
B. inform the client that he must learn to change the colostomy bag.
C. tell the client to turn his head away while colostomy care is performed.
D. refer the client for psychologic counseling.

5 A client anticipates alopecia as a result of chemotherapy. The nurse can best assist her to cope with this result by:

A. purchasing a wig for the client.
B. suggesting that the client ask her physician about a possible alternative drug regimen.
C. scheduling a consultation with a hairdresser when she loses her hair.
D. encouraging her to choose a wig or other head cover before losing her hair.

6 A client reports a 15-pound weight loss due to anorexia during a course of chemotherapy. The serum albumin level is 2.0. Appropriate nursing interventions include (select all that apply):

A. stress the importance of consuming foods with high nutritional value.
B. request double portion meals for the client.
C. assess food likes and dislikes and encourage small frequent meals.
D. encourage hot foods such as soup and broth to provide calories.
E. encourage use of nutritional supplements such as Ensure.

7 A client is receiving internal radiation to the cervix. The nurse discovers the implant in the client's bed. The appropriate action would be to:

A. remove the client from the room.
B. use long-handled forceps to place the implant in a lead container.
C. discard the implant in the trash receptacle.
D. flush the implant in the toilet.

8 A client is receiving external radiation for treatment of lung cancer. Client teaching for care of the skin in the marked area includes:

A. apply antibacterial ointment daily.
B. cleanse the skin with mild soap and water.
C. avoid rubbing or scratching treated skin areas.
D. avoid contact with others to eliminate radiation risk.

9 A client complains of nausea and vomiting following her daily chemotherapy treatment. The MOST appropriate nursing intervention would be to:

A. provide antiemetic medication 30 to 40 minutes prior to each treatment.
B. withhold food and fluids until after each treatment.
C. schedule chemotherapy for bedtime.
D. provide clear liquids until chemotherapy is finished.

10 A client experiences bone marrow depression as a result of chemotherapy. Which of the following would the nurse expect to find?

A. nausea and vomiting
B. alopecia
C. temperature 102°F
D. platelet count 200,000

Answers for Review Questions, as well as discussion of Care Plan and Critical Thinking Care Map questions, appear in Appendix V.

RESPONDING TO BELIEFS RELATED TO DEATH, DYING, AND GRIEF FROM A CULTURAL PERSPECTIVE

Mr. Fazil, 68, a Muslim from Afghanistan, is dying of pancreatic cancer. His brother remains constantly at the bedside where he recites verses from the Koran. When staff offer to sit with Mr. Fazil so the brother can go to the cafeteria, he refuses, saying his voice reciting the Koran must be the last words Mr. Fazil hears before he dies. The nurse offers to bring him some food and he accepts this offer, provided he is able to perform hand washing rites before eating. The brother requests that a private room be provided for other family members including the women of the family where they can meet and grieve together. The brother also requests that he be given all the information concerning Mr. Fazil's status so that he can give this information to the other family members. The women in the family are not permitted in Mr. Fazil's room.

One of the most challenging aspects of providing care for dying people and their families is rendering care that is relevant to cultural, racial, ethnic, and religious needs. There is no universally applicable view of grief. Rather, grief practices and responses to death and dying vary depending on cultural orientation. It is important to determine how the nurse can assist in bereavement and the dying process in a culturally competent manner.

Mourning practices and methods of communicating grief vary across and within cultural groups. For example, for some Chinese individuals, wailing is an essential part of proper mourning. Among African Americans, it has been said that wailing shows how much the family cared about the individual (Perry, 1993). Buddhists use chanting during the dying process. Chanting is thought to facilitate a calm and peaceful atmosphere for the caregivers, thus indirectly helping the dying person. Crying is the most common expression of grief among cultures. Crying serves to bind individuals who mourn together. In some cultures, grief is expressed through singing and dancing.

Mourning customs related to social organization are important. Individuals may wish to mourn in private, with family members, or with a community group. In some families, such as many Asian families, having the extended family present and involved in decision making is important. This can be problematic when the head of the family group is still resident in Asia. Talamanes, Lawler, and Espino (1995) note that involving Hispanic family members in decision making is important. Issues related to gender role must also be considered. For example, Hispanic, Amish, and Asian American families may have male-dominated decision making. In some cultures grief expression may be related to the social position, age, and sex of the deceased. In a country with high infant mortality, the death of an infant may not be considered as "important" as it is in Western culture. In Chinese society, husbands require "greater mourning" than wives. Rosenblatt et al. (1976) suggested that this might be a cross-cultural constant, since the average time of mourning by widows was found to be 304 days, and by widowers 215 days.

Many cultures are rich in rituals surrounding death. For instance, some Hindus perceive death as a passage from one existence to another. Thus, preparation of the body for cremation involves bathing the remains in a milk and yogurt solution, which symbolically cleanses the soul of the deceased. When a married Indian women dies, she traditionally is placed in a white wedding sari; a man is dressed in a plain off-white East Indian suit. Religious prayers and chanting are continuous before and after death to promote safe passage of the soul. Russian family members—after washing, dressing, and placing the body in the coffin—may keep vigil over the coffin for hours prior to the wake and funeral. They may place a black wreath on the door of the deceased person's home. If the individual is Catholic or Russian Orthodox, a priest uses holy oil to anoint the deceased person while making the sign of the cross and saying specific prayers. At the funeral, each member of the Russian Orthodox family may symbolically place a few grains of soil into the coffin.

Nursing Implications

- *Assess individuals for personal beliefs related to death and dying.* Nurses should appreciate that clients' practices related to grief, dying, and death may be significantly different from their own and may be related to cultural practices.
- *Assist the client and family to grieve and practice death rituals to meet individual needs.* By respecting personal beliefs, the nurse can facilitate grieving in a culturally appropriate manner.

Self-Reflection Questions

1. What beliefs related to grief, death, and dying do you have?

2. Are you flexible in allowing people from different cultures to practice their own traditions in relation to bereavement, the dying process, and death rituals?

3. What can you do to increase your knowledge of bereavement and death practices?

Chapter 13

Caring for Clients Experiencing Shock, Trauma, or Critical Illness

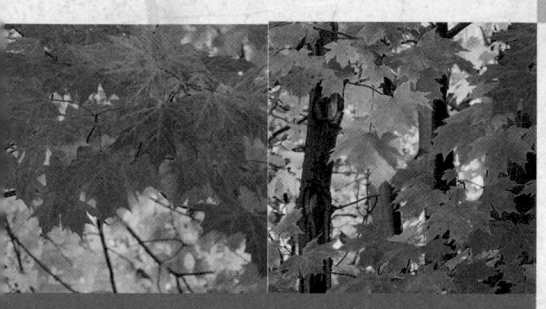

BRIEF Outline

The Client in Shock
Pathophysiology
Types of Shock
Complications of Shock

The Client Experiencing Trauma
Causes and Types of Trauma
Effects of Traumatic Injury
Environmental Injuries
Poisonings

The Client Experiencing a Critical Illness

LEARNING Outcomes

After completing this chapter, you will be able to:

- Identify the three stages of shock.
- Identify the common causes for each type of shock: hypovolemic, anaphylactic, cardiogenic, septic, and neurogenic.
- Describe the pathophysiology and manifestations of the five types of shock.
- Explain the nursing care of the client in shock.
- State the nursing implications for administering fluid replacement solutions.
- Identify common traumatic injuries.
- Describe emergency management of clients with traumatic injuries.
- Use the nursing process to collect data, establish outcomes, provide individualized care, and evaluate responses for the client experiencing shock or trauma.
- Describe the effects of a critical care unit on the client and family.
- Discuss the legal and ethical considerations of organ donation.

MediaLink

www.prenhall.com/burke
Use the address above to access the free, interactive Companion Website created for this textbook. Get hints, instant feedback, and textbook references to chapter-related NCLEX-style questions. Link to other interesting sites.

Audio Glossary:
Use the Companion Website, or the CD-ROM disk enclosed with your textbook, to hear the pronunciation of key terms in this chapter.

The Client in Shock

Shock is a life-threatening condition, characterized by inadequate blood flow to the tissues and cells. Shock is identified according to its underlying cause. Types of shock include the following:

- **Hypovolemic shock** (low-volume shock)—caused by lack of circulating blood volume, for example, rapid blood loss through hemorrhage.
- **Anaphylactic shock**—caused by immunologic reactions that trigger abnormal dilation of blood vessels, for example, an allergic drug reaction.
- **Cardiogenic shock**—caused by failure of the heart's pumping action, for example, myocardial infarction.
- **Septic shock**—caused by toxins produced from an overwhelming infection, for example, bacterial infection caused by *Pseudomonas*.
- **Neurogenic shock**—caused by changes in sympathetic tone of blood vessels, for example, spinal cord injury.

All types of shock progress through the same stages and exert similar effects on body systems.

PATHOPHYSIOLOGY

To maintain homeostasis, all cells require a consistent supply of oxygen and removal of metabolic wastes. The cardiovascular system regulates homeostasis through three basic factors: an adequate blood flow, a correctly functioning heart (pump), and normal blood vessel diameter to maintain tissue perfusion. When one or more of these factors are altered, normal cell function is disrupted. Consequently, tissue perfusion may be inadequate to sustain normal cellular metabolism. The result is the clinical syndrome known as shock. The manifestations of shock result from the body's attempt to maintain vital organ (heart and brain) function. When shock is prolonged or severe, hypoxia occurs and cells die. Unless shock is stopped, organs fail and death will result.

Stages of Shock

The three stages of shock are compensated, progressive, and irreversible. Box 13-1 ■ lists the fairly distinct manifestations of each stage. Early treatment focuses on preventing the client from reaching the irreversible stage.

COMPENSATED STAGE. The *compensated stage* of shock occurs when decreased blood volume significantly reduces the heart's cardiac output as seen in hypovolemic and cardiogenic shock. In anaphylactic, septic, and neurogenic shock, the blood vessels vasodilate. Vasodilatation causes blood to remain in the blood vessels instead of returning to the heart. As a result, blood pressure drops and normal tissue perfusion cannot be maintained. At this point, the body initiates several mechanisms to maintain blood pressure and preserve the vital organs:

1. Baroreceptors in the aortic arch sense the drop in blood pressure and stimulate the sympathetic nervous system (SNS), which releases epinephrine and norepinephrine. These "fight-or-flight" hormones constrict arterial blood vessels and increase the heart's rate and strength to contract. Arterial constriction causes the body to **shunt** (push) blood from the kidneys, skin, and gastrointestinal tract to the heart and brain. All of these effects increase venous return to the heart, increase cardiac output, and increase oxygen supply to the body's tissues.

2. As blood flow to the kidneys decreases, the **renin–angiotensin system** (a blood pressure regulation system, see also Chapters 7 and 31 ⚭) is activated. Renin stimulates the production of angiotensin II, a potent vasoconstrictor that raises blood pressure. Angiotensin II signals the adrenal cortex to release aldosterone. Aldosterone causes the kidneys to reabsorb water and sodium, which increases circulating blood volume and also the blood pressure.

MediaLink
Shock

BOX 13-1

MANIFESTATIONS FOUND IN EACH STAGE OF SHOCK

MANIFESTATION	COMPENSATED STAGE	PROGRESSIVE STAGE	IRREVERSIBLE STAGE
Level of consciousness	Oriented, can follow simple commands; restless	Confused; listless; decreased response to painful stimuli	Lethargy to coma; no reflex response
Speech	Clear	Slurred	Incoherent to absent
Blood pressure	Normal to slightly decreased	<90 mm Hg	Falling to unobtainable
Pulse rate	>100 beats/min	>150 beats/min, irregular	Slow and irregular
Peripheral pulses	Thready	Weak, thready	Absent
Respirations	>20/min	>30/min, shallow, possible crackles	Slow with Cheyne–Stokes respiration
Skin	Pale, cool, moist	Cold, clammy; possible cyanosis	Cold, cyanotic, mottled
Urinary output	<30 mL/hr	<20 mL/hr	Anuria
Bowel sounds	Decreased	Absent	Absent

3. Low blood volume stimulates the posterior pituitary gland to release antidiuretic hormone (ADH) or vasopressin. ADH increases water reabsorption and helps to increase blood pressure.

If effective treatment is provided during the compensated stage, the client should not experience any permanent damage. When the underlying cause cannot be reversed, shock advances to the progressive stage.

PROGRESSIVE STAGE. When the compensatory mechanisms fail, the *progressive stage* of shock occurs. Without adequate tissue perfusion, the body's organ functions deteriorate. Unless this stage of shock is treated rapidly, the client's prognosis is poor.

The progressive stage produces numerous effects on the body's organs (Figure 13-1 ■):

1. *Cardiovascular:* A decrease in cardiac output reduces blood flow to the coronary arteries. The heart muscle receives less oxygen. The imbalance between oxygen supply and demand results in muscle **ischemia** (reduced blood supply to an organ), dysrhythmias, and a myocardial infarction.

2. *Respiratory:* Decreased pulmonary blood flow alters the exchange of oxygen and carbon dioxide between the alveoli and capillaries. Oxygen levels decrease and carbon dioxide levels increase leading to respiratory acidosis (see Chapter 7 ⦾).

3. *Gastrointestinal (GI) and liver:* Blood shunted from the GI tract and liver to the heart and brain causes the GI organs to become ischemic. This results in ulceration of the gastric mucosa and the development of stress ulcers (see Chapter 19 ⦾). The lining of the small intestine sloughs off, allowing intestinal bacteria to enter the abdominal cavity and move into the circulation, which leads to sepsis. Impaired gastric and intestinal motility may cause paralytic ileus.

At first, the liver increases glucose production to compensate for the stress of shock. As shock progresses the liver fails, leading to hypoglycemia. The liver's *Kupffer cells* (phagocytes that destroy bacteria) cannot function, so bacteria multiply, causing an overwhelming bacterial infection.

4. *Neurologic:* Decreased blood flow to the brain alters mental status and orientation. The client's level of consciousness

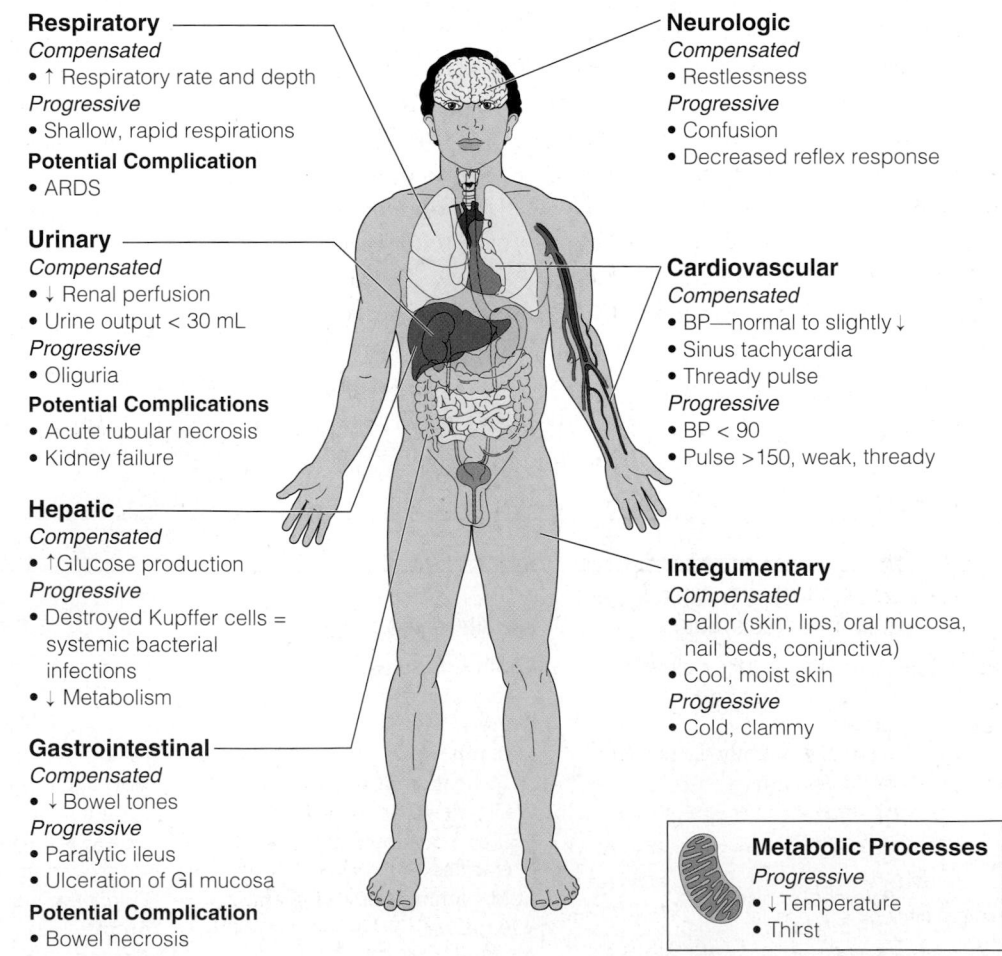

Respiratory
Compensated
• ↑ Respiratory rate and depth
Progressive
• Shallow, rapid respirations
Potential Complication
• ARDS

Urinary
Compensated
• ↓ Renal perfusion
• Urine output < 30 mL
Progressive
• Oliguria
Potential Complications
• Acute tubular necrosis
• Kidney failure

Hepatic
Compensated
• ↑Glucose production
Progressive
• Destroyed Kupffer cells = systemic bacterial infections
• ↓ Metabolism

Gastrointestinal
Compensated
• ↓ Bowel tones
Progressive
• Paralytic ileus
• Ulceration of GI mucosa
Potential Complication
• Bowel necrosis

Neurologic
Compensated
• Restlessness
Progressive
• Confusion
• Decreased reflex response

Cardiovascular
Compensated
• BP—normal to slightly ↓
• Sinus tachycardia
• Thready pulse
Progressive
• BP < 90
• Pulse >150, weak, thready

Integumentary
Compensated
• Pallor (skin, lips, oral mucosa, nail beds, conjunctiva)
• Cool, moist skin
Progressive
• Cold, clammy

Metabolic Processes
Progressive
• ↓Temperature
• Thirst

Figure 13-1. ■ Multisystem effects of shock.

deteriorates and may progress to coma. Cerebral edema and irreversible brain cell damage may occur.

5. *Renal:* Blood shunting to the heart and brain reduces flow through the kidneys. Urine output decreases, and the client develops *oliguria* (low urine output). Prolonged reduced renal blood flow leads to acute renal failure.

6. *Skin and temperature:* In most types of shock, blood vessels in the skin vasoconstrict, leading to skin color changes. Caucasian clients appear pale. Persons with darker skin (such as those of African, Hispanic, or Mediterranean descent) have pale lips, oral mucous membranes, nail beds, and conjunctiva. Activation of the sweat glands causes cool, moist skin that may become cold. As metabolism decreases, so does the body's temperature.

IRREVERSIBLE STAGE. If shock progresses to the irreversible stage, tissue and cellular death becomes so widespread that treatment cannot reverse the damage. **Multiple organ dysfunction syndrome (MODS)** is an irreversible complication of shock in which the body's systems fail and the client eventually dies.

Types of Shock

HYPOVOLEMIC SHOCK. Hypovolemic shock is the most common type. It is caused by a decrease in intravascular volume. Normally, about two-thirds of the body's fluids are found in the intracellular compartment and the remaining third is in the extracellular compartment. The extracellular compartment is divided into intravascular and interstitial fluids. To remain in balance, each compartment must maintain the correct amount of fluid (see Chapter 7). 🔗

The decrease in circulating volume may result from:

- Loss of blood volume (hemorrhage) due to trauma, surgery, GI bleeding, hemophilia
- Internal fluid shifts (third-spacing) as a result of cirrhosis with ascites, pleural effusion, pancreatitis, intestinal obstruction
- Loss of body fluids through persistent and severe vomiting, diarrhea, or continuous nasogastric suctioning; massive diuresis from diuretics or diabetes insipidus
- Loss of fluids through the skin as a result of profuse diaphoresis or burns.

The pathophysiology of hypovolemic shock as seen in Figure 13-2 ■ can occur alone or develop along with other types of shock. Manifestations reflect the stage of shock the client is experiencing (Box 13-2 ■). They depend on the client's age, general health, severity of injury or illness, length of time before treatment started, and the rate of volume loss. Hypovolemic shock caused by fluid losses or internal fluid shifts may have more subtle manifestations.

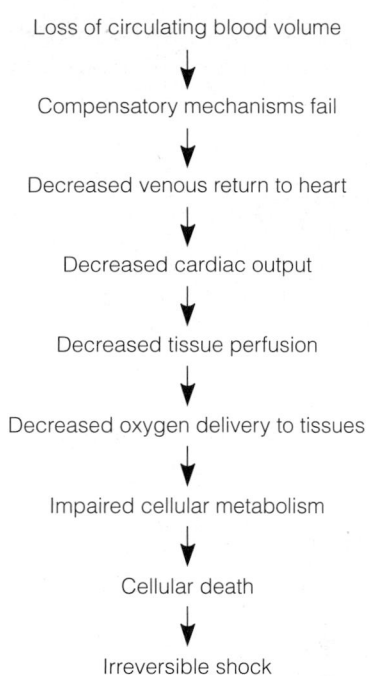

Loss of circulating blood volume

↓

Compensatory mechanisms fail

↓

Decreased venous return to heart

↓

Decreased cardiac output

↓

Decreased tissue perfusion

↓

Decreased oxygen delivery to tissues

↓

Impaired cellular metabolism

↓

Cellular death

↓

Irreversible shock

Figure 13-2. ■ The pathophysiology of hypovolemic shock.

ANAPHYLACTIC SHOCK. Anaphylaxis is caused by a severe allergic reaction and, when severe, can progress to anaphylactic shock. Almost any *antigen* (foreign substance) can trigger an anaphylactic response. Antigens can enter the body by injection, ingestion, or through the skin or respiratory tract. Some common causes of anaphylactic shock are:

- Foods, such as legumes (nuts, seeds), shellfish, egg whites, milk, chocolate, tomatoes, and strawberries
- Stings and bites of insects
- Snake venom
- Substances used to diagnose and treat disease, such as antibiotics, vaccines, local anesthetics, iodine dyes, blood, and narcotics
- Other substances such as latex, pollen, and molds or food additives.

When a person is first exposed to an antigen, the body produces antibodies against it. The initial antigen–antibody

---

BOX 13-2

INITIAL MANIFESTATIONS OF HYPOVOLEMIC SHOCK

- Restlessness and anxiety
- Decreased blood pressure
- Rapid, weak pulse
- Thirst
- Tachypnea, dyspnea
- Pale, cool, moist skin
- Decreased urine output
- Weakness

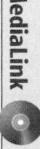

MediaLink

Hypovolemic Shock

response usually produces no harmful effects, but it sensitizes the person to the antigen. With each future exposure, the antigen reacts with the antibodies and anaphylaxis may occur.

clinical ALERT

Anaphylactic reactions are more severe when the antigen enters the body by the intravenous route or when a second exposure occurs.

An antigen–antibody reaction stimulates mast cells to release histamine and other chemical mediators into the circulation. These substances cause widespread vasodilation and make capillaries more permeable. The shift of fluids results in hypotension and **relative hypovolemia** (fluid shifts from vascular space into interstitial space, so that blood pools in the tissues). Blood volume is reduced, tissue perfusion is impaired, and cell metabolism is altered. Other effects include inflammation, bronchoconstriction, and cutaneous reactions. Manifestations of anaphylaxis may begin on immediate contact with the antigen. Anaphylactic shock, a severe form of anaphylaxis, is a life-threatening emergency and requires immediate intervention to prevent death within a matter of minutes. People with known allergies should wear a Medic-Alert bracelet. Health care providers should carefully assess and document allergies or previous drug reactions. A summary of the manifestations found in anaphylactic shock is listed in Box 13-3 ■.

CARDIOGENIC SHOCK. Cardiogenic shock occurs when the heart fails to act as an effective pump, so cardiac output and adequate tissue perfusion cannot be maintained. Myocardial infarction is the most common cause of cardiogenic shock. The amount of myocardial damage determines the severity and progression of shock. (Other cardiac disorders that can cause cardiogenic shock are discussed more thoroughly in Chapter 27. ◯◯)

BOX 13-3

MANIFESTATIONS OF ANAPHYLACTIC SHOCK

- **Skin:** Generalized itching, flushing, sensation of warmth, urticaria (hives), angioedema (edema of eyelids, lips, and tongue)
- **Neurologic:** Restlessness, apprehension, anxiety, decreased level of consciousness
- **Respiratory:** Difficulty breathing, wheezing, laryngospasm, stridor, rales
- **Cardiovascular:** Hypotension, tachycardia
- **Gastrointestinal:** Nausea, vomiting, diarrhea

BOX 13-4

MANIFESTATIONS OF CARDIOGENIC SHOCK

- Systolic pressure < 90 mm Hg
- Rapid, weak, thready pulse
- Distended neck veins
- Rapid, labored respirations; crackles
- Pale, cold, moist skin
- Restlessness, agitation, or disorientation
- Oliguria to anuria

In cardiogenic shock, the ventricles fail to pump blood into the circulatory system. This leads to a decreased **stroke volume** (the amount of blood ejected from the heart each minute). Excess blood is left in the ventricle with each beat. This blood backs up into the lungs, leading to pulmonary edema. When cardiac output drops, the client becomes hypotensive. A compensatory rise in heart rate increases myocardial oxygen consumption and decreases coronary perfusion. This burdens an already overworked myocardium, so eventually it fails. Common manifestations of cardiogenic shock are listed in Box 13-4 ■.

SEPTIC SHOCK. Septic shock usually results from an overwhelming gram-negative bacterial infection (i.e., *Pseudomonas, Escherichia coli, Klebsiella*), but also may follow gram-positive infections (e.g., *Staphylococcus* and *Streptococcus*). Common sources of these pathogens include the hospital environment and health care workers. The following risk factors increase the chance for developing septic shock:

- Extremes of age (<1 year, >65 years)
- Chronic debilitating diseases or conditions:
  - Cancer, AIDS, or malnutrition
  - Burns or decubitus ulcers
  - Diabetes mellitus
- Surgery, invasive lines or tubes (IV or central venous lines, urinary catheters, tracheostomy or endotracheal tube)
- Drug therapy (chemotherapy, corticosteroids, long-term antibiotic therapy).

Septic shock begins with **septicemia** (the presence of pathogens and their toxins in the blood). The invading bacteria multiply faster than the body can kill them. As bacteria are destroyed, endotoxins are released into the bloodstream. The endotoxins damage tissues and starve the cells of oxygen and nutrients. The damaged cells release histamine and other chemicals to dilate peripheral blood vessels and increase capillary permeability. As in anaphylactic shock, fluids shift from intravascular space to interstitial space, resulting in relative hypovolemia. *Microemboli* (tiny blood clots) form in the capillaries, causing further cell damage and death. Septic shock has an early phase and a late phase; manifestations

---

BOX 13-5

MANIFESTATIONS OF SEPTIC SHOCK

Early (Warm) Septic Shock

- Normal to decreased blood pressure
- Tachycardia
- Rapid respirations
- Warm, flushed, dry skin
- Alert, anxious
- Normal urine output
- Elevated body temperature

Late (Cold) Septic Shock

- Profound hypotension
- Rapid, thready pulse; arrhythmias
- Rapid, shallow respirations with crackles
- Cold, cyanotic extremities
- Confused to lethargic to comatose
- Oliguria to anuria
- Decreased body temperature

BOX 13-6

MANIFESTATIONS OF NEUROGENIC SHOCK

- Hypotension
- Bradycardia
- Warm, dry skin
- Anxiety, restlessness
- Decreased urine output
- Lowered body temperature

---

of each are summarized in Box 13-5 ■. Death may result from respiratory, cardiac, or renal failure.

Toxic shock syndrome (TSS) is caused by a toxin-producing form of *Staphylococcus aureus*. It usually affects menstruating women between 15 and 19 who use tampons. Toxins from the bacteria enter the bloodstream and circulate throughout the body, causing the septic shock process to begin. The client may have a high fever, vomiting, and diarrhea. The client's condition worsens and can be fatal without treatment.

NEUROGENIC SHOCK. Neurogenic shock results from an interruption in the sympathetic nervous system. The problem can result from damage to the vasomotor center in the medulla or from loss of impulse transmission (seen in a spinal cord injury above the T6 level). Other causes include head injury, spinal anesthesia, opiate drug overdose, and insulin reactions.

Without sympathetic nervous system impulses, the blood vessels dilate, leading to massive peripheral vasodilation. Blood pools in the venous and capillary beds, leading to inadequate tissue perfusion. Thermoregulation is impaired because the cutaneous blood vessels lose vasomotor tone. Without appropriate treatment, organ failure and death can occur. Manifestations of neurogenic shock are listed in Box 13-6 ■.

Complications of Shock

The two most common complications of shock are **acute respiratory distress syndrome (ARDS)** and **disseminated intravascular coagulation (DIC).** Both disorders usually develop once the client has entered the progressive stage of shock.

ARDS is characterized by acute respiratory failure due to damage to the alveoli. When alveolar capillaries become more permeable, fluid and proteins leak into the alveoli, causing a type of pulmonary edema. The client with ARDS may require mechanical ventilation. See Chapter 24 ⊙⊙ for more information about ARDS and mechanical ventilation.

DIC is an acute condition characterized by simultaneous bleeding and clotting throughout the body. Tissue damage triggers an abnormal activation of the body's clotting mechanisms. There is widespread, continuous clot formation, which consumes all of the clotting factors, resulting in generalized bleeding. Clots are deposited in the capillaries, reducing blood flow to the skin and causing *mottling* (discoloration). Initially, the client bleeds from puncture sites and incisions. Treatment is aimed at replacing the platelets and clotting factors while protecting the client from injury. See Chapter 30 ⊙⊙ for more information about DIC and its treatment.

INTERDISCIPLINARY CARE

Successful management of shock requires early recognition and treatment. The nurse is expected to identify early manifestations of shock. Once a diagnosis of shock is made, medical management focuses on treating the underlying cause, increasing oxygenation, and improving tissue perfusion. The common interventions include oxygen therapy, fluid and blood replacement, and pharmacologic therapy.

Diagnostic Tests

No single diagnostic test can determine shock. However, the following tests may be ordered to help identify the type of shock and to assess the client's physical status:

- Blood hemoglobin and hematocrit, to identify decreases associated with hypovolemic shock resulting from hemorrhage. Hemoglobin levels below 5 g/dL and hematocrit levels below 15% should be reported immediately to a physician.
- Arterial blood gases (ABGs), to measure oxygen and carbon dioxide levels and pH. As shock progresses, metabolic acidosis develops from anaerobic metabolism.
- Serum sodium and serum potassium levels; the first decreases and the second increases in the progressive stage.

BOX 13-7

PREHOSPITAL EMERGENCY CARE OF THE CLIENT EXPERIENCING HEMORRHAGE

1. Scan the area for potential hazards (e.g., fire).
2. Call for help.
3. Ensure adequate airway; assist with ventilation as needed.
4. Assess for cause of hemorrhage.
5. Control external bleeding by applying direct pressure to the local site. If an extremity is involved, elevate it to stop venous bleeding. When bleeding continues, apply pressure to an arterial pressure point.
6. Apply a tourniquet *only as a last resort*.
7. Assess for manifestations of shock, which may include:
   a. Decreased blood pressure
   b. Rapid, thready pulse
   c. Rapid, shallow respirations
   d. Cool, pale, moist skin
   e. Thirst
   f. Restlessness
   g. Changes in level of consciousness.
8. Keep the client's trunk and head flat and legs slightly elevated. (Use this position *only* when no head injury exists.)
9. Cover the client to maintain warmth.
10. Do not give the client anything by mouth.
11. Use touch and verbal communication to reduce apprehension and anxiety.

- Blood glucose levels; these increase in early shock but decrease as shock worsens.
- Blood urea nitrogen (BUN) and serum creatinine levels, to measure renal function. Decreased renal perfusion reduces renal function, so the BUN and creatinine levels increase.
- Blood cultures, to identify the causative organism in septic shock.
- White blood cell count (WBC) is elevated in the client with septic shock.
- Serum cardiac markers (creatine kinase, CK-MB, and troponins [a myocardial muscle protein]); these are elevated following a myocardial infarction and in cardiogenic shock.
- X-ray studies, computerized tomography (CT) scans, magnetic resonance imaging (MRI), and peritoneal lavage may determine the extent of injury or locate sites of internal hemorrhage.

Oxygen Therapy

To reverse shock, adequate oxygenation and tissue perfusion must be restored. The first step is to ensure that the client has a patent airway. If necessary, a nasal or oral airway may be inserted. When excess secretions obstruct the airway, the nurse must be prepared to suction the client.

All clients in shock should receive oxygen therapy. This may be given by a nonrebreather mask at 12 to 15 L/min to maintain the PaO_2 greater than 90 mm Hg. If the client develops respiratory distress, the nurse should anticipate endotracheal intubation and mechanical ventilation. (Care of the client requiring ventilatory assistance is discussed in Chapter 24. ●)

Discussion of specific measures used to treat the different types of shock follows.

Hypovolemic Shock

Hypovolemic shock resulting from trauma or hemorrhage requires immediate emergency care. This care begins as soon as medical rescuers arrive on the accident scene and continues through transport to the emergency department (ED). At the emergency scene, intravenous fluids are started and pneumatic antishock garments may be applied. Because shock can progress so rapidly, treatment needs to begin within the first hour following an injury if at all possible (the "golden hour" of trauma care). Failure to begin emergency treatment within the first hour increases the client's risk for death. Box 13-7 ■ summarizes the prehospital emergency care for a client in hypovolemic shock.

PNEUMATIC ANTISHOCK GARMENT. The **pneumatic antishock garment (PASG),** also called military antishock trousers (MAST), is applied following a traumatic injury (Figure 13-3 ■). The device is used to raise blood pressure and can be used to stabilize pelvic and femoral fractures. Only specially trained personnel can apply or remove PASGs.

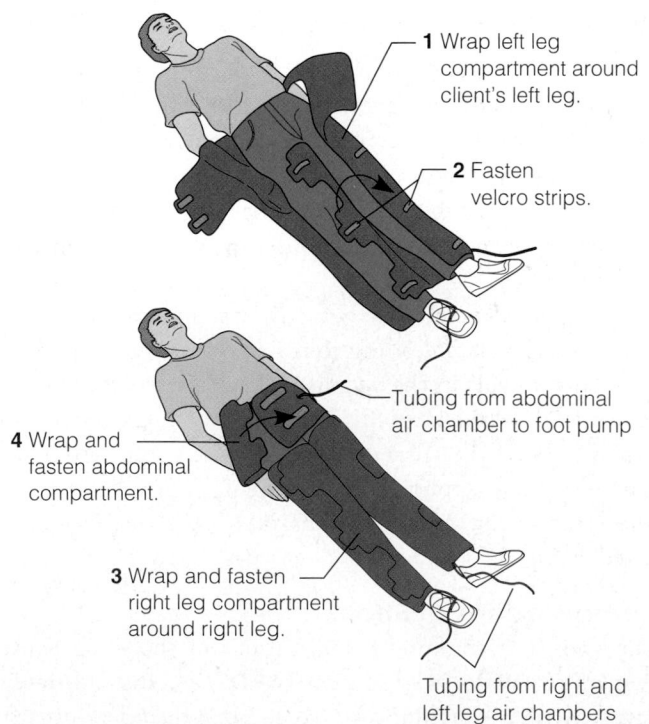

1 Wrap left leg compartment around client's left leg.

2 Fasten velcro strips.

Tubing from abdominal air chamber to foot pump

4 Wrap and fasten abdominal compartment.

3 Wrap and fasten right leg compartment around right leg.

Tubing from right and left leg air chambers

Figure 13-3. ■ Pneumatic antishock garments provide rapid, emergency treatment of shock.

FLUID REPLACEMENT. The main goal for clients with hypovolemic shock is to restore intravascular volume. Intravenous fluids are used alone or in combination with colloids, blood, or blood products. The type and amount of fluid chosen depends on the type of fluid lost. Usually, fluid replacements are given in a 3:1 ratio (300 mL fluid for every 100 mL of fluid loss).

Crystalloid solutions contain electrolytes dissolved in water. The most commonly ordered intravenous solutions are normal saline (0.9%) and lactated Ringer's. Both isotonic solutions increase volume in the intravascular and the interstitial spaces. These solutions are given during the emergency phase while the client's blood is being typed and cross-matched. See Chapter 7 ⚭ for more information about crystalloid solutions and intravenous therapy.

clinical ALERT

Large infusions of crystalloid solutions can lead to pulmonary edema. Monitor the client closely for signs of respiratory distress.

Colloid solutions contain proteins that increase osmotic pressure. (Osmotic pressure holds fluid within the vessels so that the plasma volume expands.) Colloid solutions include albumin, plasma protein fraction, dextran, and hetastarch. (Nursing implications for administering colloids are discussed in Table 13-1 ■.)

Blood and blood products used in treating hemorrhage are obtained from a donor and given as a *transfusion* (an infusion of blood or blood components) to the client (Table 13-2 ■). State and institutional policies vary about whether LPNs/

LVNs can administer transfusions. Nurses are responsible for knowing their scope of practice.

Each person has one of four blood types: A, B, AB, or O. Blood group antigens A and B form the basis for ABO blood categorization. The presence or absence of these inherited antigens determines one's blood type (type A has A antigen, type B has B antigen, and type AB has both). Persons with neither antigen have blood type O.

A protein on the red blood cell membrane determines the Rh of a person's blood. Rh-positive blood has the protein, Rh-negative blood does not (Table 13-3 ■).

Before a client can receive a blood transfusion, a blood **type and cross-match** (test to determine donor and recipient ABO types and Rh groups) must be done. Blood is also tested for hepatitis A, hepatitis B, and human immunodeficiency virus (HIV).

Despite rigorous type and cross-matching procedures, blood transfusion reactions may still occur. The most common is a febrile reaction, which typically begins during the first 15 minutes of the transfusion. In a *febrile reaction,* the client's antibodies react to the donor's white blood cells, causing fever and chills. (General guidelines for monitoring blood transfusions are found in Table 13-4 ■.)

When hemorrhage causes hypovolemic shock, the client may receive whole blood or red blood cells (RBCs). The goal is to increase the client's hematocrit and hemoglobin levels to near-normal values. Trauma victims may receive a type O blood transfusion while the type and cross-match is done.

Some emergency departments and trauma centers use autotransfusion for the client with multiple injuries and/or severe shock. **Autotransfusion** is the collection,

---

TABLE 13-1

Nursing Implications for Pharmacology: Colloid Solutions

DRUG GROUP/DRUGS	ACTION	NURSING IMPLICATIONS	CLIENT TEACHING
Colloid solutions (plasma expanders) ■ Albumin 5% or 25% (Albuminar, Buminate) ■ Plasma protein fraction (Plasmanate) ■ Dextran 40 or 70 (Gentran 40 or 70) ■ Hetastarch (Hespan)	■ Colloid solutions expand blood volume and are used to treat hypovolemic shock. ■ Albumin and plasma protein fraction come from healthy human donors. ■ Dextran and hetastarch are made synthetically.	■ Before infusion, take client's vital signs and assess lung and heart sounds. ■ Take vital signs according to institutional policy (usually every 15–60 minutes). ■ Monitor for manifestations of heart failure or pulmonary edema (dyspnea, cyanosis, cough, crackles, wheezes). If these appear, notify the physician immediately.	■ The solutions are helping to maintain blood volume. ■ Vital signs are taken frequently to ensure the client's safety.

TABLE 13-2

Blood and Blood Products

TYPE	COMPOSITION	USE
Whole blood	Contains RBCs, plasma, and clotting factors.	Replaces blood volume and increases oxygen carrying capacity in hemorrhage and shock.
Packed red cells	Contains some platelets; very little plasma.	Increases oxygen-carrying capacity of blood.
Platelets	Contains only platelets.	Controls bleeding in clients with platelet deficiencies.
Fresh frozen plasma	Contains all clotting factors except platelets.	Expands blood volume; can be administered to any blood group or type, because it contains no RBCs; takes 30–60 minutes to thaw.
Cryoprecipitate	Contains factor VIII, factor XIII, and fibrinogen.	Treats clients with clotting factor deficiencies.

Note: Each hospital has its own policy about blood transfusions. The nurse must learn and follow those policies.

filtration, and retransfusion of a client's own blood. Blood from the chest cavity is the typical source for an auto-transfusion.

Anaphylactic Shock

When an anaphylactic reaction develops, the client needs immediate intervention. First priorities are a patent airway and supplemental oxygen, followed by drug therapy. Epinephrine, given subcutaneously or intravenously, is the drug of choice to restore arterial blood pressure and promote bronchodilation. Antihistamines such as diphenhydramine (Benadryl) reverse the effects of histamine. Corticosteroids are given to prevent a delayed reaction to the antigen. If respiratory distress continues, aminophylline or nebulized albuterol (Proventil) is ordered to reverse bronchospasm. Once the client's condition is stable, the client must be monitored for reappearance of signs and symptoms of anaphylaxis. The effects of the causative antigen may last for hours.

TABLE 13-4

Nursing Implications for Pharmacology: Blood Transfusions

NURSING IMPLICATIONS	CLIENT TEACHING
■ Take and record baseline vital signs. ■ Stay with the client during the first 15 minutes of the transfusion. ■ Monitor for manifestations of a transfusion reaction. ■ Take and record vital signs according to institutional policy. ■ If a transfusion reaction occurs, take the following actions: a. Stop the transfusion immediately, and notify the nurse. Start normal saline slowly. b. Take vital signs and assess for manifestations. c. Follow institutional policy for saving the blood bag, returning it to the laboratory, and collecting urine and venous blood samples. d. Continue to monitor the client and provide prescribed interventions to treat the reaction according to physician orders.	Immediately report any warm feelings, chills, itching, feelings of weakness or fainting, or difficulty breathing.

TABLE 13-3

Blood Group and Rh Types and Compatibilities

BLOOD GROUP	COMPATIBLE DONOR BLOOD GROUPS
O	O
A	A, O
B	B, O
AB	A, B, AB, O
Rh	**Compatible Donor**
Rh positive	Rh pos, Rh neg
Rh negative	Rh neg

Note: Group O is often called the universal donor, and group AB is called the universal recipient. Do not infuse if types are not compatible according to the chart!

Cardiogenic Shock

Cardiogenic shock usually results from an acute myocardial infarction. Oxygen is given to prevent further heart muscle damage. Drug therapy and mechanical devices are prescribed to raise blood pressure and improve cardiac output. These clients are acutely ill and are best managed in a critical care unit. Several intravenous medications are used to treat cardiogenic shock. **Vasopressor drugs** such as dopamine (Intropin) and norepinephrine (Levophed) produce vasoconstriction, which raises the client's blood pressure. **Positive inotropic drugs,** Dobutamine (Dobutrex) and amrinone (Inocor), increase the force of myocardial contraction so that cardiac output increases. Nitroglycerin (Tridil) may be used to improve the pumping action of the heart. Diuretics and digoxin (Lanoxin) may be given if the client shows signs of heart failure. Antidysrhythmic drugs regulate the client's heart rhythm.

In addition to medications, two mechanical devices can also help improve blood circulation: the intra-aortic balloon pump (IABP) and the ventricular assist device (VAD). (See Chapter 26 ⚭ for further discussion.)

Septic Shock

One of the first steps in managing septic shock is to identify the causative organism. Using aseptic technique, specimens of blood, urine, wounds, and sputum are collected and sent for culture and sensitivity. Intravenous fluids are given to counteract the massive vasodilation caused by the release of bacterial endotoxins. Intravenous antibiotics, such as aminoglycosides and third-generation cephalosporins, are started immediately. Once the organism is positively identified, antibiotic therapy may be changed. If clients become unstable, they should be transferred to the critical care unit.

Neurogenic Shock

Treatment of neurogenic shock varies according to its cause. Intravenous fluids are ordered to reverse the peripheral vasodilation, so blood pressure and tissue perfusion are restored. If neurogenic shock is caused by severe pain, appropriate analgesics should be given. Clients receiving spinal anesthesia should have the head of the bed raised to prevent the anesthetic from moving up the spinal cord. (Management of clients with spinal cord injury is presented in Chapter 39. ⚭)

NURSING CARE

The nurse assumes an important role in preventing shock as well as potential complications.

ASSESSING

Assessment data collected by the nurse can determine the severity of the shock condition. The manifestations for each type of shock can be found in the previous discussion. Restlessness, tachycardia, and slight anxiety are common early symptoms with a fall in blood pressure occurring later. It is important to recognize and notify the physician at this early stage. Frequent assessment of the client in shock is done at least every hour. When the client's condition worsens, assessments may be as often as every 5 to 10 minutes.

DIAGNOSING, PLANNING, AND IMPLEMENTING

Priorities in Nursing Care. Nursing care for the client in shock focuses on monitoring overall tissue perfusion and on meeting the psychosocial needs of the client and family. Two major nursing diagnoses appropriate for the client with hypovolemic shock are Ineffective Tissue Perfusion and Anxiety. Ineffective tissue perfusion is the highest priority.

Ineffective Tissue Perfusion: Cardiopulmonary, Peripheral, Cerebral, Renal

- Monitor skin color, temperature, turgor, and moisture. *Decreased tissue perfusion is shown by pale, cool, moist skin. When hemoglobin levels drop, cyanosis may occur.*
- Monitor cardiopulmonary function every 15 to 30 minutes by assessing blood pressure, heart rate and rhythm, rate and depth of respirations, lung sounds, and peripheral pulses (include presence, equality, rate, rhythm, and quality). If unable to palpate pulses, use a Doppler ultrasound device. If a line is inserted, measure central venous pressure (CVP). *Vital signs help identify the stage of shock. As shock progresses, BP drops; the pulse becomes rapid, weak, and thready. Decreased lung perfusion causes crackles, wheezes, and dyspnea. Capillary refill is prolonged. Peripheral pulses (dorsalis pedis and posterior tibial) are weak or nonpalpable. CVP measures fluid status; low findings indicate decreased blood volume (normal = 5 to 15 cm).*
- Monitor oxygen saturation by attaching a pulse oximeter to the client. *Oxygen saturation should be maintained between 94% and 100% with oxygen therapy.*
- Assess for restlessness, confusion, mental status changes, and decreased level of consciousness. *These indicate decreased cerebral perfusion.*
- Monitor intake and urinary output per Foley catheter hourly, using a urometer. Measure daily weight and fluid loss such as emesis and gastric and chest tube drainage. Estimate fluid loss from profuse perspiration and wound drainage. *This evaluates fluid status and renal blood flow.*

clinical ALERT

Urinary output less than 30 mL/hr indicates reduced renal perfusion and an increased risk for acute renal failure.

- Monitor bowel sounds, abdominal distention, and abdominal pain. *Decreased gastrointestinal blood flow reduces bowel motility and peristalsis; paralytic ileus may result.*
- Assess for sudden sharp chest pain, dyspnea, cyanosis, anxiety, and restlessness. *Hemoconcentration and increased platelet aggregation may result in pulmonary emboli.*

clinical ALERT

Assess for irregular heart rate and chest pain because these indicate decreased coronary artery perfusion and increased risk for myocardial infarction.

- Monitor body temperature. *An elevated body temperature increases oxygen requirements.*
- Maintain client on bed rest, and provide a calm, quiet environment. Place the client in a modified Trendelenburg position as tolerated (Figure 13-4 ■). *Bed rest decreases the workload of the heart. The modified Trendelenburg position increases venous return to the heart. Do not use this position for clients in cardiogenic shock.*

Anxiety

Clients with hypovolemic shock may have experienced a traumatic injury that has required major surgery and a transfer to a critical care unit. Other types of shock also are associated with critical illness or injury, such as acute myocardial infarction, head injury, or spinal cord injury. Throughout these events, the client and family are frightened, anxious, and often emotionally isolated. While the nurse's first priority must be to provide emergency care, the psychosocial needs of the client and family also must be met.

- Acknowledge the client's anxiety and fear. *This helps validate the client's feelings.*
- Remain with and explain procedures to the client. Listen carefully to client. Speak slowly and calmly, using short sentences. Use touch to provide support. *These measures provide reassurance to the client and help reduce anxiety.*

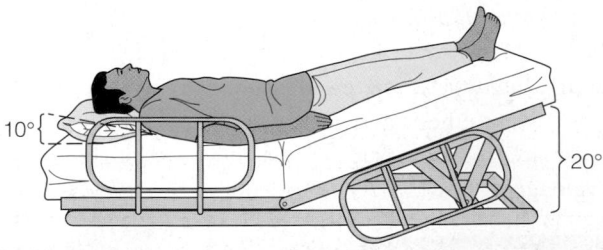

Figure 13-4. ■ Modified Trendelenburg position. Position the client with the lower extremities elevated approximately 20 degrees (knees straight), trunk horizontal, and the head elevated about 10 degrees.

- Provide comfort measures (e.g., calm, quiet environment, back rub). *Comfort measures can reduce the client's anxiety.*
- Provide time, space, and privacy for family members. *Allowing the family access to the client reduces anxiety and gives both the client and the family some feeling of control.*
- Provide anticipatory guidance to prepare for recovery or death. *If the prognosis is poor, this helps the family begin the grieving process.*
- Keep the client's family informed. *They need information on which to make their decisions.*

EVALUATING

Evaluate the effectiveness of care by noting whether the client's vital signs are stabilized. Also, the nurse notes the client's tissue perfusion: alert and oriented; warm, dry skin, urine output > 30 mL/hr, and palpable pedal pulses.

Documentation focuses on the client's vital signs, orientation level, skin temperature and presence of moisture, urine output, and quality of pedal pulses. Record the client's response to acute interventions such as oxygen therapy and fluid replacement.

CONTINUING CARE

Shock must be fully resolved before a client can be discharged. Although the client has survived the shock episode, recovery from the original medical problem may be delayed. Teach the family that a lengthy recovery often leads to depression and that the client will need a supportive and nurturing environment. Teach clients who have experienced an anaphylactic reaction how to prevent a future reaction. Emphasize the following key points before discharge:

- Avoid known allergens.
- Notify health care professionals of allergies.
- If allergic to insect stings, avoid wearing bright colors, perfumes, and scented hair sprays when outdoors.
- If allergic to foods, read package labels. When eating out, ask how meals are prepared and what ingredients are used.
- Wear a Medic-Alert bracelet or necklace.
- Advise client to carry an emergency kit for anaphylaxis.
- Review manifestations of anaphylaxis.
- Seek medical attention immediately when symptoms occur.

NURSING PROCESS CARE PLAN
Client with Septic Shock

Huang Mei Lan is a 43-year-old single woman who had surgery 4 days ago for recurrent breast cancer. She is underweight, weak, and depressed. Despite her multiple problems, she never complains or asks for pain medication. A central line and a urinary catheter are in place. On her fourth postoperative day, Mrs. Canote, her primary nurse, finds Ms. Huang huddled in the middle of the bed, shivering violently.

Assessment. T 104°F, P 110, R 30, and BP 96/66. Her skin is hot, dry, and flushed with poor turgor. She is alert and oriented, but is restless and appears anxious. She is nauseated and has diarrhea. Her WBC count is elevated. Blood, sputum, urine, and wound cultures are collected. She is diagnosed as having septic shock. Intravenous solutions of lactated Ringer's and of a broad-spectrum antibiotic are begun until the organism and its portal of entry are identified. Ms. Huang's condition worsens. Her blood pressure continues to drop, her skin becomes cool and cyanotic, and she has periods of disorientation. She is transferred to the critical care unit. As she is being prepared for the transfer she begins to cry and asks, "Am I going to die?"

Diagnosis. The following nursing diagnoses are established for Ms. Huang:

- *Deficient Fluid Volume* related to vomiting, diarrhea, high fever, and hypotension
- *Impaired Gas Exchange* related to rapid respirations
- *Ineffective Tissue Perfusion* related to hypotension and massive vasodilation
- *Anxiety* related to feelings that illness is worsening and is potentially life threatening

Expected Outcomes. The expected outcomes for the plan of care are that Ms. Huang will:

- Maintain adequate circulating blood volume.
- Regain and maintain arterial blood gas parameters within normal limits.
- Regain and maintain stable hemodynamic levels.
- State her feelings of fear and anxiety.

Planning and Implementation. The following nursing interventions are implemented for Ms. Huang. Assessments are done frequently to monitor her condition.

- Monitor mental status and level of consciousness.
- Monitor arterial blood pressure; rate, rhythm, and quality of pulses; central venous pressure; pulmonary artery pressure; and cardiac output.
- Assess color and character of skin.
- Monitor results of arterial blood gases, blood counts, clotting times, and platelet counts.
- Monitor respiratory rate, rhythm, and breath sounds.
- Monitor temperature every 2 hours.
- Monitor urinary output hourly, reporting any output of less than 30 mL/hr.
- Explain procedures and provide oral and skin care, turning, and positioning.

Evaluation. Despite intensive nursing and medical care, Ms. Huang's condition remains critical. The interventions are continued.

Critical Thinking in the Nursing Process

1. What stage of shock was Ms. Huang experiencing when Ms. Canote first entered her room? Provide supporting evidence.
2. Why was the lactated Ringer's solution started on Ms. Huang?
3. Why would the nursing diagnosis Impaired Skin Integrity be appropriate for Ms. Huang?

The Client Experiencing Trauma

Persons who need urgent medical care enter the medical system through the emergency department (ED). Severely injured clients may require transport to a regional trauma center. Treatment in the ED is provided by nurses and doctors with special training in emergency care. Emergency nurses take care of clients of all ages with a wide range of medical problems. This type of nursing requires a broad knowledge base, solid observation skills, and the ability to provide care in an unpredictable environment.

The goals of emergency care are to stabilize the critically ill, prevent deterioration of a client's condition, and promote optimal function. To accomplish these goals, clients must be prioritized when they enter the ED. **Triage** systems identify who will receive medical attention first. The most common triage categories are emergent, urgent, and nonurgent. During disasters such as earthquakes or tornadoes, a tag triage system is used. Clients are tagged as "red" *(emergent),* "yellow" *(urgent),* "green" *(nonurgent),* and "black" *(dead or expected to die).*

CAUSES AND TYPES OF TRAUMA

Trauma is defined as an injury caused by physical force (motor vehicle crashes, falls, drowning, gunshots, burns, stabbing, or other physical assaults). Trauma is the number one cause of death for persons under the age of 35 and is the fifth leading cause of death in the United States for all age groups. At highest risk are males between the ages of 15 and 24 years; geriatric clients are also at risk (Box 13-8 ■).

BOX 13-8	FOCUS ON OLDER ADULTS

Geriatric Risks for Trauma

The elderly are hospitalized for trauma twice as often as the general population. Falls commonly cause trauma in those over age 65. The fall may be caused by acute or chronic medical conditions, environmental factors, or simply the aging process. Persons over age 75 also experience a high fatality rate following a motor vehicle crash. Elderly pedestrians are at a higher risk for being struck by a motor vehicle, because they don't move as quickly when crossing the street or cannot see traffic lights well.

Traumatic injuries can result in temporary physical impairment, permanent disability, or death.

Traumatic injury occurs suddenly, leaving the client and family with little time to prepare for its consequences. Nurses serve as a vital communication link between the injured client and the family. They help the client and family cope with the client's current injury, as well as understand the potential long-term effects of this injury.

Minor or Major Trauma

Whether intentional or accidental, trauma causes injury to one or more body parts. *Minor trauma* involves a single body part or system and is usually treated in the ED. A fractured collarbone, a small second-degree burn, and a cut requiring stitches are all considered minor trauma. *Major* or *multiple trauma* involves serious single-system injury (such as traumatic amputation of a leg) or multiple-system injuries. Multiple trauma victims require immediate emergency care.

Blunt or Penetrating Trauma

Trauma also may be classified as blunt or penetrating. *Blunt trauma* does not cause a break in the skin. It can result in greater internal damage than appears on the surface. Common blunt forces are motor vehicle crashes, falls, assaults, and contact sports. *Penetrating trauma* results from foreign objects that pierce the body. The most common sources are knives, bullets, shotgun blast, or impaled, sharp objects. The penetrating object often damages the intestines, liver, spleen, and vascular system. Again, the external appearance of the wound does not determine the extent of internal damage.

EFFECTS OF TRAUMATIC INJURY

Traumatic injuries have serious consequences that must be identified and treated rapidly. Some common effects of traumatic injury are the following:

- *Airway obstruction* can be caused by blood, teeth, the tongue, or vomitus in a client's airway. Once the cervical spine is immobilized with a cervical collar, oxygen is given. The airway may be cleared by suctioning. Clients with severe airway obstruction may require intubation with an endotracheal tube (Figure 13-5 ■).
- *Pneumothorax* results from air in the pleural space causing partial or complete lung collapse. Blunt and penetrating injuries to the chest may be the cause. A *tension pneumothorax* develops when air continually enters the chest cavity but cannot exit. In the ED, a chest tube is inserted to reinflate the lung. See Chapter 24 🔗 for more information about pneumothorax.
- *Hemorrhage* in the trauma client may be external or internal (see prehospital care in Box 13-7 on page 290). When an artery is severed, the bleeding must be controlled

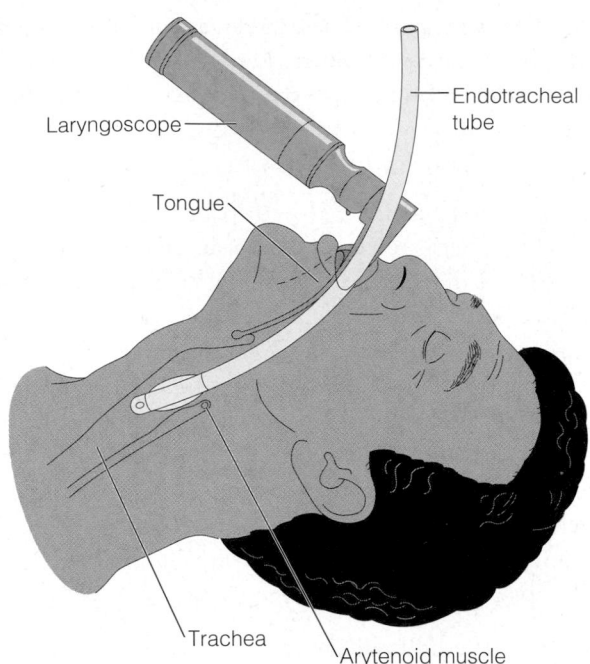

Figure 13-5. ■ Intubation with insertion of an endotracheal tube (ETT). When a client is experiencing respiratory distress, oxygen can be given into the external opening of the tube.

immediately (Figure 13-6 ■). Internal hemorrhage may lead to blood pooling in several body cavities. For example, chest trauma may cause bleeding into the pleural space. A pelvic fracture may lead to bleeding in the

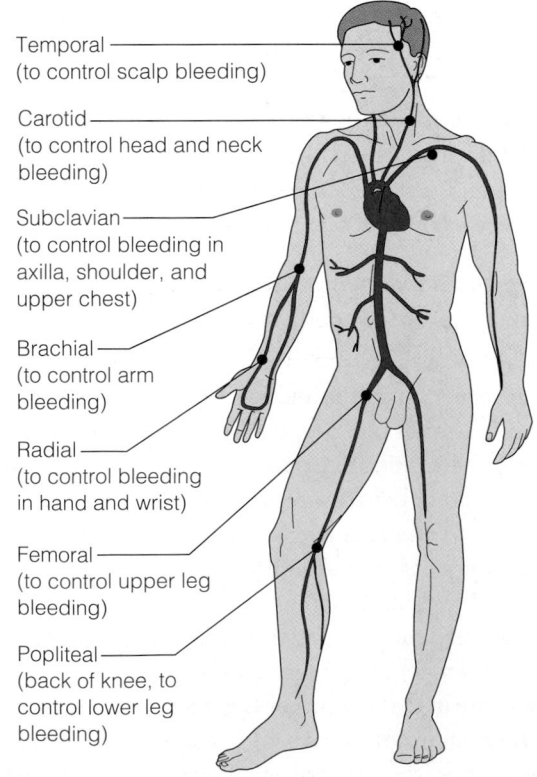

Figure 13-6. ■ The major pressure points used to control bleeding.

retroperitoneal region. The nurse must identify the cause, location, and extent of blood loss.

- *Hypovolemic shock* may be caused by hemorrhage from blunt or penetrating injuries, long-bone or pelvic fractures, major vessel injuries, traumatic amputation, or plasma loss from burns or crush injuries (see earlier discussion).
- *Neurologic injuries* most often include traumatic brain injury (TBI) with spinal cord injury occurring less frequently. Both injuries can have a permanent, devastating outcome. Most head and spinal cord injuries result from motor vehicle crashes; other causes include falls, sports injuries, and assault.
- *Gastrointestinal* and *genitourinary injuries* can be caused by blunt and penetrating injuries. Liver and spleen injuries are the main sources of life-threatening hemorrhage. Peritonitis can occur when damaged intestines leak bile and stool into the peritoneum. Motor vehicle crashes cause most of the renal injuries.

clinical ALERT

Never remove a penetrating object. Removal may cause internal injuries or possible nerve damage.

- *Musculoskeletal injuries* are frequently seen in the ED. Injury includes damage to bone, soft tissue, nerves, or blood vessels. Common manifestations of musculoskeletal injuries are swelling, bone protrusion, obvious deformity, abnormal motion, pain, and a pulseless extremity. See Chapter 42 ⟲⟳ for more information about musculoskeletal injury.
- *Integumentary injuries* are not usually as serious, except for burns (see Chapter 46 ⟲⟳). The nurse must assess both the skin and the underlying structures for any sign of injury. Injuries to the integument are often contaminated with dirt, debris, or foreign objects that increase the client's risk for infection. The four main skin injuries are contusions, abrasions, puncture wounds, and lacerations (Figure 13-7 ■).
- *Psychologic effects on the client* are a consequence of trauma. The client will feel anxious and insecure in the unfamiliar surroundings. It is important for the nurse to provide explanations about treatment procedures and reassure the client frequently.
- *Psychosocial effects on the family* are also a consequence of trauma. Death or serious injury may change family dynamics. The suddenness and seriousness of the event predispose families to psychologic crisis. Families may exhibit shock, fear, numbness, anxiety, guilt, hostility, or anger.

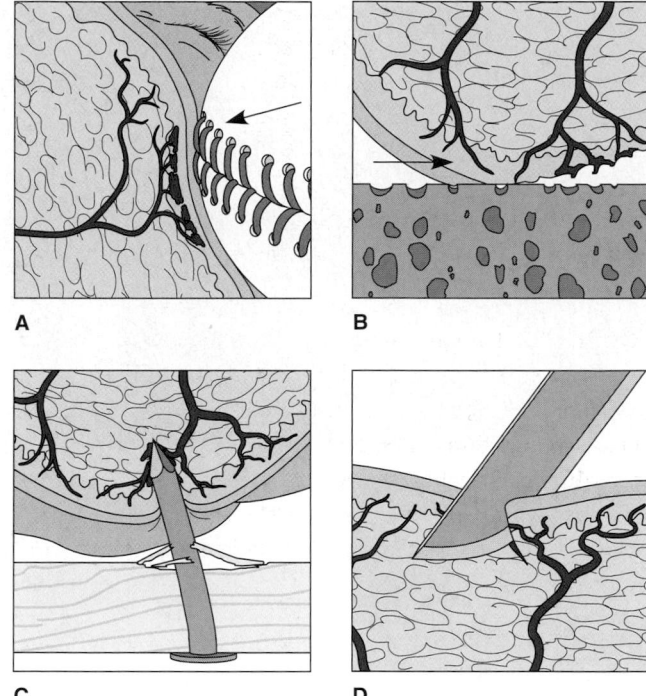

Figure 13-7. ■ (**A**) Contusions (bruises) do not cause a break in the skin. (**B**) Abrasions (scrapes) occur when a partial layer of skin is removed. (**C**) Puncture wounds occur when the integument is penetrated by a sharp or blunt object. (**D**) Lacerations are irregular tears in the skin.

INTERDISCIPLINARY CARE

The trauma client requires collaborative care at the accident scene before arriving in the ED (see Box 13-7, page 290). This type of care may be provided by emergency medical technicians (EMTs), paramedics, flight nurses, or physicians. Flight nurses are educated in trauma care and air transport techniques. They can perform advanced techniques such as intubation or chest tube insertion.

At the accident scene, life-threatening problems must be identified and treated immediately. Before other treatments are started, the client may require basic life support and advanced cardiac life support. The client's cervical spine is immobilized at once by placing the client on a spine board and applying a cervical collar (Figure 13-8 ■). If the client's airway is patent, high-flow oxygen is started. Direct pressure may be applied to control active external bleeding. One or two intravenous lines with IV fluids are started.

As soon as the client's condition is stabilized, the client is transported rapidly to the ED or trauma center. Ground ambulances and air ambulances (e.g., specially staffed and equipped helicopters or fixed-wing aircraft) are used. Once the trauma client arrives at the ED, team members provide medical and nursing care. These team members may include an ED physician, ED nurses, trauma surgeon, anesthesiologist, laboratory technicians, radiologist, and respiratory therapist.

MediaLink Video: Spinal Immobilization

MediaLink Video: Administration of Oxygen

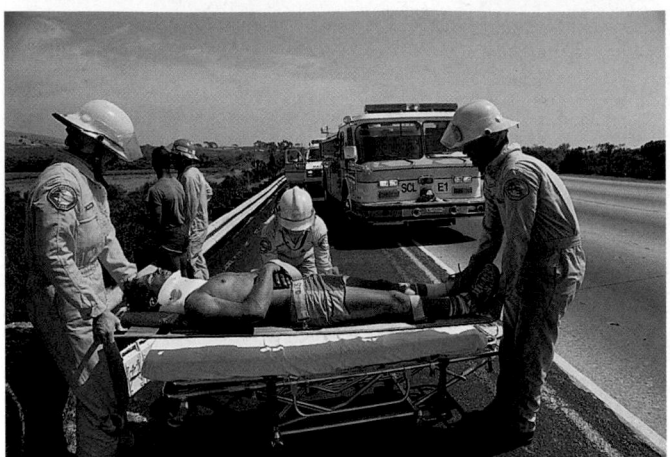

Figure 13-8. ■ Application of a cervical collar at an accident scene immobilizes the cervical spine and prevents further injury to the spinal cord. (*Source:* Spencer Grant/Photo Researchers, Inc.)

Diagnostic Tests

The type of diagnostic tests obtained depend on the client's injuries. Besides the tests used to rule out shock, the following tests may be ordered:

■ Blood alcohol levels measure the amount of alcohol in a client's blood (20% to 50% of people who are injured may be intoxicated).

■ Urine drug screen determines the presence of cocaine, heroin, or amphetamines.

■ Pregnancy test for any woman of childbearing age rules out the potential for pregnancy and fetal injury.

■ Diagnostic peritoneal lavage identifies the presence of blood in the peritoneal cavity, which may indicate abdominal injury.

■ Computerized tomography (CT) scan locates injuries to the brain, skull, spinal cord, chest, and abdomen.

■ Magnetic resonance imaging (MRI) identifies brain and spinal cord injuries.

Emergency Surgery

Surgery is indicated when the client remains in shock despite resuscitation and there is no obvious external sign of blood loss. Nurses prepare the client for emergency surgery by undressing the client and removing jewelry, dentures, or other loose objects. Place an identification bracelet on the client. Report the extent of the injury, allergies and past medical history (if obtainable), and completed nursing interventions to the operating room nurse.

It is important for the emergency or trauma nurse to speak with the family as soon as possible and keep them informed about what is happening to their family member. Unfortunately, family members or significant others may not have time to see their loved one before transfer to the operating room.

Forensic Considerations

Sometimes injuries involve criminal activity that requires legal investigation. The nurse's role is to identify, store, and properly transfer potential evidence for medical–legal investigations. All evidence must be marked and sealed in tamper-proof containers.

The nurse must not cut through any clothing containing potential evidence such as blood stains or bullet holes. Each clothing item is placed in an individual breathable container, such as a paper bag, and labeled appropriately. Bullets or knives are labeled with the identifying source and given to the proper authorities. Entrance and exit wounds must be recorded in the chart. Photographs may be needed of wounds and clothing.

The client's hands may yield important evidence, such as powder burns on the skin or tissue or hair samples beneath the fingernails. Paper bags should be placed over the client's hands if the presence of evidence is suspected.

NURSING CARE

Nursing care of the client who has suffered a serious injury starts with a primary assessment and includes collaborative interventions to manage any life-threatening injuries.

ASSESSING

In the emergency department, the nurse ensures that the cervical spine is immobilized and then performs a five-step primary assessment: airway, breathing, circulation, disability, and exposure. The ABCs are assessed and managed first. Then the nurse assesses for the degree of disability related to neurologic functioning. A baseline neurologic assessment should include the client's level of consciousness and pupillary reaction to light. In the exposure step, the nurse removes the client's clothes and examines all body surfaces for obvious injuries. The nurse also obtains a brief history, client allergies, and past medical history.

A Foley catheter is inserted to monitor urinary output. If there is a risk for aspiration, a nasogastric tube is placed. The client is attached to a cardiac monitor. At least two intravenous lines are used to give IV fluids, blood components, inotropic drugs, and vasopressors as needed, to treat hypovolemic shock. The emergency nurse monitors the client closely for shivering or chills. Warm blankets and warmed IV solutions are used to prevent hypothermia. If the client has penetrating wounds, a tetanus prophylaxis such as tetanus toxoid or human toxin–antitoxin may be given.

DIAGNOSING, PLANNING, AND IMPLEMENTING

Priorities in Nursing Care. The post-trauma client has many nursing care problems. Two of the most common are actual or potential problems with infection, and mobility.

Risk for Infection

Traumatic injuries often occur in a dirty environment. Projectiles entering the body carry dirt and debris into the wound. Open fractures provide an entry point for bacteria and dirt. Even after surgery, wounds can remain contaminated.

- Use strict aseptic technique when inserting catheters, suctioning, or changing dressings. *Trauma clients are at a greater risk for infection.*
- Monitor wounds for odor, redness, heat, swelling, purulent drainage, increased pain under casts, and increased drainage over the wound area. Be sure dressings do not restrict circulation. Avoid tape; instead, use mesh or stretch gauze to hold dressings in place. Prevent cross-contamination between wounds. *Because the skin is the first line of defense against infection, the nurse must monitor for signs of infection and prevent any new breaks in the skin.*
- Take vital signs and temperature every 2 to 4 hours. *An elevated body temperature and pulse are indicators of an infection.*
- Provide adequate fluids and nutrition. *Adequate fluids, calories, and protein are essential to wound healing.*
- Monitor for manifestations of sepsis. *Clients with traumatic injuries are at a high risk for developing sepsis.*

Impaired Physical Mobility

- Provide active or passive exercises to affected and unaffected extremities at least once every 8 hours. Do not perform exercises if active bleeding or edema is present. *Exercise improves muscle tone, maintains joint mobility, improves circulation, and prevents contractures. Immobility due to trauma increases the risk for complications of the skin, cardiovascular, gastrointestinal, respiratory, musculoskeletal, and renal systems.*
- Assist the client to turn, cough, and deep breathe at least every 2 hours. *Changing positions, coughing, and deep breathing reduce the risk of skin and respiratory complications.*
- When the client cannot be moved and positioned easily, consult with the physician regarding the use of a specialty bed such as the kinetic continuous rotation bed (Figure 13-9 ■). *Continuous motion helps prevent pneumonia, venous stasis, urinary stasis, and bone loss.*
- Monitor the lower extremities every 8 hours for deep venous thrombosis (DVT): heat, swelling, and pain. Measure the circumference of the thigh and calf each day. Remove antiemboli stockings for 1 hour during each shift and assess the skin for changes. *When injury occurs to the vein and blood flow becomes sluggish, a thrombus (clot) forms. DVT is a major risk for pulmonary embolism.*

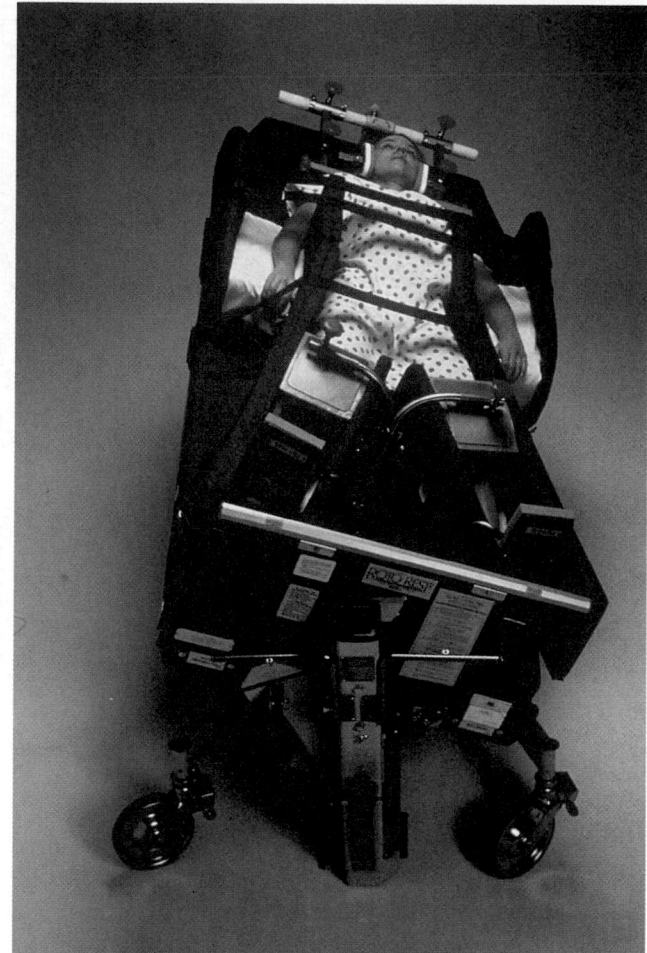

Figure 13-9. ■ A kinetic continuous rotation bed reduces complications of immobility for a client with multiple injuries. (KCI Roto Rest® Delta Kinetic Treatment Table Courtesy of Kinetic Concepts, Inc., San Antonio, TX.)

EVALUATING

Evaluate the effectiveness of nursing care by collecting data related to the absence of infection and complications from immobility. As the client recovers, evaluate the client's progress toward maximum wellness.

Because the trauma client is usually managed in the critical care unit, documentation is specific to the client's injuries. Once transferred to a medical–surgical unit, the nurse documents the client's progress toward recovery.

CONTINUING CARE

The nurse's main responsibility is to prepare the client and family for discharge and promote maximum wellness. Before discharge, determine potential home modifications. (For example, if the client's bedroom is on an upper floor, first-floor sleeping arrangements may be necessary until healing has occurred.) Review when and how to take the medications and their potential side effects. Provide

BOX 13-9

HOME SAFETY TIPS

- Be alert in order to avoid potentially harmful conditions or activities.
- Don't drink and drive or use any mechanical/electrical equipment.
- Wear a protective helmet when riding a bicycle, motorcycle, skateboard, or scooter.
- Follow equipment safety precautions when operating power tools.
- Wear safety belts and secure children in a child safety seat or safety belt.

Bathroom

- Use nonskid mats or strips in shower or tub.
- Install handrails in shower or tub and by the toilet as needed.
- Use night-light in bathroom.
- Use tub bench for unsteady persons.
- Set water heater below 115°F.

Kitchen

- Turn pot handles away from the edge of the stove.
- Keep flammable liquids, paper towels, and pot holders away from the burners.
- Keep a fire extinguisher near the stove.

Floors and Stairways

- Keep entryways, halls, and stairways well lit.
- Remove clutter and trailing cords from pathways inside and outside.
- Install handrails and antiskid strips on stairways.
- Secure or remove scatter rugs.
- Use nonskid shoes on waxed floors.

Other

- Use a stepladder to reach high objects.
- Use good lifting technique when lifting heavy objects.
- Install smoke alarms in the kitchen and on every floor.
- Keep firearms unloaded and locked in a secure place.

information as needed about special diets. Discuss the client's rehabilitation plan and identify transportation concerns. Emphasize the need for follow-up appointments with the physician. Discuss with the family emotional changes that the client may experience (e.g., insomnia, nightmares, and reliving the incident). If the family has lost a loved one, provide a referral for grief counseling.

Preventive Health Teaching. Injury is a major health problem in the United States. The nurse is in a unique position to provide preventive education, after assessing for individual risk factors (weakness, poor vision, and risky behaviors). Safety education should be taught in emergency departments, doctors' offices, clinics, schools, and health fairs.

Because many injuries occur at home, individuals should also know how to make their homes safer. Box 13-9 ■ lists common safety tips.

ENVIRONMENTAL INJURIES

A variety of medical emergencies can result from excessive exposure to heat or cold. This section presents prehospital and basic ED care for clients with environmental emergencies.

Hyperthermia (elevated core body temperature) occurs when the body is exposed to excessive heat. Normally, the body regulates its temperature through sweating and peripheral vasodilation. When the temperature and humidity exceed the body's regulatory mechanisms, heat exhaustion and heat stroke develop. *Heat exhaustion* results from increased sweating and electrolyte loss, which causes hypovolemia. It is characterized by profuse sweating, weakness, nausea, and cool skin. Individuals with heat exhaustion should be placed in a cool area and given oral fluids. Loosen clothing and apply cool, wet towels. Victims who are very young or elderly, or who do not improve within 30 minutes, should be taken to the nearest hospital.

Heat stroke involves a rapid rise in temperature, often above 106°F, because the body cannot cool itself. It is not common but is a medical emergency. Manifestations include altered mental status; hot, dry skin; hypotension; tachycardia; and tachypnea. Heat stroke victims must be cooled immediately. This is done by removing the client's clothes and placing cold packs to the groin, axillae, and back of the neck. The client can be misted with cool water but never immersed in icy water (shivering produces more heat). As soon as possible, the client is transported to an emergency department. If the temperature has not dropped to 102°F, a cooling blanket is used. The client is given 100% oxygen immediately to compensate for the increased metabolic rate. Monitor the client closely for acute renal failure and seizures.

Hypothermia (core body temperature is below 95°F) results from exposure to cold temperatures. Infants are at higher risk because they have less body fat. Older adults also have an increased risk. Mild hypothermia is characterized by shivering and slowed mental functioning. As the victim's temperature drops, muscle coordination is lost, heart, respiratory, and neurologic functions slow; eventually death results.

In cases of mild hypothermia, move the client to a warm place, remove wet clothing, and cover with warm blankets. Clients with moderate to severe hypothermia should be transported immediately to a nearby hospital. On arrival in the ED, the client is warmed slowly with blankets, radiant heat lamps, or an external warming blanket. Warmed intravenous solutions may be given, along with warmed peritoneal lavage. Respiratory therapy includes warmed, humidified oxygen. The client is monitored closely for signs of cardiac arrest.

POISONINGS

A *poison* is any chemical substance that damages body structures. Poisons enter the body through ingestion, inhalation, and skin contamination. Common ingested poisons include corrosives such as lye, toilet bowl cleaners, and bleach; plants; and drugs such as aspirin, antidepressants, and benzodiazepines. Most inhalation injuries occur in the home from carbon monoxide, natural gas, chlorine, and some pesticides. Skin contamination occurs from pesticides and industrial chemicals.

When poisoning is suspected, call the local poison control center immediately. They can provide guidelines for appropriate treatment. Some poisonings can be managed at home, but most require treatment in the ED. When the client arrives in the ED, the first priority is to assess the client's airway, breathing, and circulation, and then to identify the poison. The medical staff will recommend the appropriate antidote or an elimination method.

Ingested poisons may be treated by giving activated charcoal orally or through a gastric lavage; this binds to the poison for expulsion in the stool. Syrup of ipecac induces vomiting but its use has decreased during the past decade. It is contraindicated for corrosive poisons, which must be diluted with milk or water. Other elimination methods include gastric lavage, cathartics, whole-bowel irrigation, and hemodialysis. Clients who have inhaled poisonous substances need supplemental oxygen. Contaminated skin must be drenched immediately with running water and all clothes must be removed. Anyone assisting the client should wear protective clothing to prevent secondary exposure.

Poisonings can be prevented. Box 13-10 ■ summarizes prevention tips.

BOX 13-10

GUIDELINES TO PREVENT POISONING

- Use dangerous chemicals only in well-ventilated areas.
- Wear protective clothing such as gloves and goggles.
- Do not mix common household cleaning products.
- Keep all products in their original containers with the label attached.
- Use poison symbols to identify dangerous substances.
- Keep all poisons and medicines locked away.
- Identify poisonous plants and keep them away from children.
- Never call medicine "candy."
- Use childproof safety caps.
- Always take medications in a well-lit room to prevent an error.
- Post the local Poison Control Center telephone number by the phone.

The Client Experiencing a Critical Illness

Clients with shock or traumatic injuries are best treated in a critical care unit or *intensive care unit (ICU)*. These highly specialized units are designed to provide care to clients in the critical phase of an illness. ICU nurses and physicians have advanced knowledge in the latest medical and technological methods. The critical care nurse constantly monitors the acutely ill client for life-threatening situations and initiates nursing actions as needed. Because of the critical condition of these clients, the ICU nurse may care for only one or two clients.

PSYCHOSOCIAL EFFECTS

The critical care environment is overwhelming to clients. They are under artificial lighting and are attached to strange machines that make sounds. The environment and the constant nursing care often lead to sensory overload and sleep deprivation. Unfamiliar voices and the lack of personal touch from family members result in sensory deprivation and increase the client's stress level.

The nurse can reduce sensory overload by monitoring noise levels and limiting conversation directly to the client. Adding a calendar and clock to the client's room, or playing a favorite radio station or tape, may reorient the client. The client's psychologic well-being can be increased by encouraging the family to touch the client. Uninterrupted rest periods are beneficial, but rest must be balanced with the client's need for family and with the need for hourly monitoring.

ICU psychosis (acute confusion after 2 to 3 days in the ICU) develops rapidly and is generally reversible. Older adults are more prone to this condition. Common features include altered attention span, memory loss, confusion, and visual and auditory hallucinations. Sedatives or psychotropic drugs may be given, but often they can make the condition worse. ICU psychosis usually decreases once the client's sensory-perceptual problems and sleep deprivation are resolved, but it is distressing to the client and family.

Although a critical illness affects the client most, it also affects family roles and functions. The family fears death of a loved one. They are anxious about all of the equipment surrounding the client and the potential for pain. They worry about finances and permanent changes in family roles. The nurse can assist the family by giving them a short status report every time they visit. If possible, involve the family in the client's daily care. Each family member should be assessed for signs of exhaustion. When necessary, the nurse should consult a social worker and chaplain to help obtain resources for the family. When the family's needs can be met, they are able to provide greater support to the client.

ORGAN DONATION

Under the Uniform Anatomical Gift Act, consent for organ donation may be given not only by the donor but also by a spouse, adult child, parent, adult sibling, or guardian. Most states require health care providers to ask family members about organ donation. Nurses should know their hospital's organ and tissue donation policies. The following organs and tissues can be donated: kidneys, heart, lungs, pancreas, intestines, liver, cornea, bones, bone marrow, and skin.

Before donation is considered, the family is notified of the client's grave prognosis. They should be given the option of donating the client's organs but should realize that organ donation is an option, not an obligation. The family should be encouraged to ask questions and express their feelings in making this difficult decision. A grief counselor or clergy can provide emotional support to the family. Even if the client carries an organ donor card, many institutions will not remove any organs without a signature from a family member or other authorized person.

Before organs can be removed, the client must be declared brain dead. **Brain death criteria** are clinical signs used to determine whether a comatose client is brain dead (Box 13-11 ■). Once brain death has been confirmed, the

---

BOX 13-11

BRAIN DEATH CRITERIA

- Cause of coma accounts for loss of brain function
- Irreversible condition
- Unresponsive coma (absence of motor and reflex movements)
- No spontaneous respirations; $Paco_2$ greater than 60 mm Hg
- Absent brainstem functions (no pupillary, corneal, and gag reflexes)
- Isoelectric (flat) electroencephalogram (EEG)
- Persistence of these signs for 30 minutes to 1 hour

---

family must also agree with the diagnosis and be allowed time to prepare for the client's death as well as they can.

When the decision has been made to proceed with organ donation, the Organ Procurement Organization is notified (1-800-24-DONOR). Nurses should know the agency in their region that is responsible for organ procurement.

Note: The bibliography listings for this and all chapters have been compiled at the back of the book.

Chapter Review

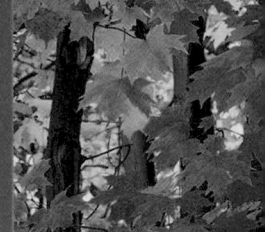

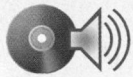 **KEY TERMS** by Topics

Use the audio glossary feature of either the CD-ROM or the Companion Website to hear the correct pronunciation of the following key terms.

Client in shock

shock, shunt, renin–angiotensin system, hypovolemic shock, anaphylactic shock, cardiogenic shock, septic shock, neurogenic shock, multiple organ dysfunction syndrome (MODS), ischemia, anaphylaxis, relative hypoxemia, stroke volume, septicemia, toxic shock syndrome (TSS), acute respiratory distress syndrome (ARDS), disseminated intravascular coagulation (DIC), pneumatic antishock garment (PASG), type and cross-match, autotransfusion, vasopressor drugs, positive inotropic drugs

Client experiencing trauma
triage, heat stroke

Client experiencing a critical illness
ICU psychosis, brain death criteria

KEY Points

- Shock is characterized by inadequate blood flow and oxygen to cells and tissues.

- Without immediate recognition and treatment, shock progresses through the compensated, progressive, and irreversible stages and can result in death.

- Nursing management of hypovolemic shock includes providing oxygen therapy, intravenous fluids, blood or blood products, cardiac support, and client support.

- Trauma is the leading cause of death in young people. It can be prevented by following common safety guidelines such as wearing a seat belt or helmet when riding a bicycle.

- Clients experiencing a traumatic accident, are assessed in the emergency department for airway, breathing, circulation, disability, and exposure.

- The critical care unit is overwhelming to clients and families. The nurse plays an important role in reducing the psychosocial effects while caring for the acutely ill client.

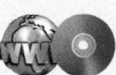 **EXPLORE Media**Link

Additional interactive resources for this chapter can be found on the Companion Website at http://www.prenhall.com/burke. Click on Chapter 13 and "Begin" to select the activities for this chapter.

For chapter-related NCLEX-style review questions and an audio glossary, access the accompanying CD-ROM in this book.

FOR FURTHER Study

For further information about regulatory systems and their effects on the kidneys, see also Chapters 7 and 31.

For further information about changes with respiratory acidosis, see the Respiratory Acidosis section in Chapter 7.

For further information about fluid compartments, crystalloid solutions, and IV therapy, see Chapter 7.

For more information about how stress ulcers develop, see Chapter 19.

For more information about pneumothorax, ARDS, and care of the client requiring ventilatory assistance, see Chapter 24.

For more information about the intra-aortic balloon pump (IABP) and the ventricular assist device (VAD), see Chapter 26.

For more information about cardiac disorders that can cause cardiogenic shock, see Chapter 27.

See Chapter 30 for more information about disseminated intravascular coagulation.

For more information about management of clients with spinal cord injury, see Chapter 39.

Chapter 42 provides more information about musculoskeletal injuries.

See Chapter 46 for more information about caring for clients with burns.

Caring for a Client at an Accident Scene

NCLEX-PN® Focus Area: Physiologic Integrity

Case Study: You are driving down a rural road and see a car swerve back and forth across the road. It hits a patch of ice and strikes a utility pole. There is no one else in sight and you stop. You find a young man alone in the car who says his name is Paul Thompson. He is not wearing a seat belt.

Nursing Diagnosis: Risk for Ineffective Tissue Perfusion

COLLECT DATA

Subjective	Objective

Would you report this data? Yes/No

If yes, to: _____

Nursing Care

_____
_____
_____
_____
_____
_____
_____
_____
_____
_____

How would you document this? _____
_____
_____
_____

Data Collected
(use those that apply)

- Scalp is bleeding
- Allergic to penicillin
- Skin slightly pale and dry
- Is awake
- Complains of being thirsty
- Left leg is twisted at an odd angle
- Shallow, slow respirations
- Does not drink alcohol
- Rapid radial pulse rate
- Says his dad will be really mad that he wrecked the car
- Denies any difficulty breathing
- Complains of left leg pain
- Wears glasses

Nursing Interventions
(use those that apply; list in priority order)

- Splint Paul's left leg.
- Ask how the accident happened.
- Give him a few sips of water.
- Cover scalp wound with a clean cloth.
- Cover client with a blanket.
- Keep head and neck in neutral position.
- Assist him out of the car.
- Call for help.
- Lay him on the ground and elevate his feet and legs.
- Look for hazards in the area.

NCLEX-PN® Exam Preparation

1 Your client has an order to receive 2 units of packed red blood cells (PRBCs) for postoperative bleeding. During the transfusion of the first unit, your client tells you that he is having chills. List the actions in the sequence in which the nurse should perform them.

A. Take the client's vital signs.
B. Notify your charge nurse.
C. Start a normal saline infusion.
D. Stop the infusion.
E. Send the blood bag to the laboratory.

2 A client was admitted to your unit at 6:00 A.M. following a motor vehicle accident. One of her diagnoses is hypovolemia due to blood loss. At 10:00 A.M. you observe that the client's Foley catheter bag has approximately 50 mL of dark, tea-colored urine. Which of the following actions would be the most appropriate at this time?

A. Ask the client if she feels light-headed.
B. Check the client's CBC results.
C. Assess the client's pain level.
D. Check the Foley catheter tubing for kinks.

3 A client is admitted to the intensive care unit following surgery for an abdominal aneurysm repair. Her vital signs are stable and her dressing is dry and intact. She is restless and repeatedly states that she might die. Which of the following nursing diagnoses would be the most appropriate to add to her care plan?

A. Infection, Risk for
B. Anxiety
C. Deficient Knowledge
D. Confusion, Acute

4 You are working in a community hospital ED. A 50-year-old man with a diagnosis of a first-degree burn to the left forearm is complaining that he has been waiting to be seen for 3 hours. Your best response would be:

A. "I know; this place has a history of long waiting times."
B. "There are other clients here that are a lot worse than you and they are not fussing."
C. "I understand your concerns. I will check to see how much longer it will be."
D. Just ignore the client and he will stop complaining.

5 A client broke her pelvis during a horse riding accident. Her son found her several hours after the accident had occurred. On arrival at the ED she was confused and her skin was cold and clammy. No bowel sounds were present. Her apical pulse was 180 with thready and weak radial pulses. In which stage of shock might the client's condition be categorized?

_____

6 A 65-year-old man on your unit is diagnosed with advanced cirrhosis of the liver. Vital signs: P 130, R 32, BP 110/60, T 100.4°F. The physician states that the client is in shock. Which of the following would most accurately describe this type of shock?

A. hypovolemic
B. anaphylactic
C. septic
D. cardiogenic

7 Which of the following statements by a client being treated for a severe reaction to a bee sting indicates that additional teaching might be needed?

A. "I'm going to order a Medic-Alert bracelet right away."
B. "My pharmacist can tell me which anti–bee sting medication will be best for me."
C. "I'll just stay away from bees and not worry about them."
D. "I'm going to tell my family what to do if I get stung again."

8 When assessing a client who has suffered a heat stroke, what clinical manifestation should the nurse expect to find?

A. cool skin
B. profuse sweating
C. nausea and vomiting
D. severely elevated temperature

9 When managing cardiogenic shock and heart failure, the nurse expects to administer several medications including a diuretic such as furosemide (Lasix). Which of the following findings indicate that the diuretic is effective?

A. The client's blood pressure increases.
B. There is a significant increase in urine output.
C. The client's level of consciousness improves dramatically.
D. The client's irregular heartbeat has stabilized.

10 Your elderly client has recovered from a traumatic injury to the right hip from a fall in his bathroom. He will be going home with a walker for ambulation. Which of the following is most important to discuss prior to the discharge?

A. transportation to his doctor's appointment
B. the client's ability to ambulate with his walker
C. social services consult for Meals-on-Wheels
D. home safety tips

Answers for Review Questions, as well as discussion of Care Plan and Critical Thinking Care Map questions, appear in Appendix V.

Chapter 14

Loss, Grief, and End-of-Life Care

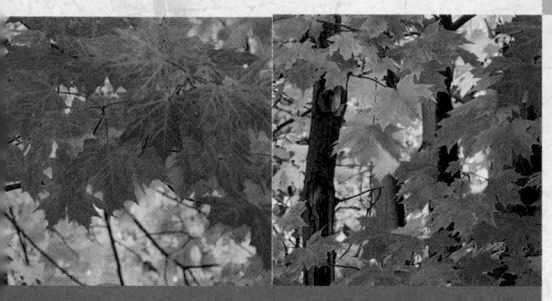

BRIEF Outline

Loss, Grief, and Death
Experiencing and Resolving Loss
Family and Other Support Systems
Spirituality
Rituals of Mourning
Nurses' Responses to Client's Loss

End-of-Life Care
Legal and Ethical Issues

Settings and Services for End-of-Life Care
Hospice
Palliative Care
Physiologic Changes in the Dying Client
Support for the Client and Family
Death
Interdisciplinary Care
Nursing Care

LEARNING Outcomes

After completing this chapter, you will be able to:

- Define loss, grief, and death.
- Explain the stages of loss, with commonly experienced emotional responses.
- Discuss factors that influence responses to loss and reflect on one's own responses to loss and death.
- Discuss legal and ethical issues of dying, including advance directives, living wills, do-not-resuscitate orders, and euthanasia.
- Assess physiologic changes in the dying client and signs of death.
- Use the nursing process to collect data and provide interventions for the client who is experiencing loss and is at the end of life.

Loss, Grief, and Death

Loss occurs when a valued object, person, body part, or situation that was formerly present is lost or changed and can no longer be seen, felt, heard, known, or experienced. A loss may be temporary or permanent, complete or partial, subjective, physical, or symbolic. Losses that occur in any phase of the life cycle may produce grief responses as intensely painful as those observed in the death experience. Only the person who experiences it can determine the meaning of the loss. The order of importance varies, but people most commonly fear the loss of those items listed in Box 14-1 ■.

The stress of loss may initiate physical or emotional changes in a person or family. To deal with the resulting changes, people must resolve their feelings about the loss, through a process called *grief work*. **Grief** is the emotional response to loss and its accompanying changes. *Grieving* may be thought of as the internal process the person uses to work through the response to loss. *Mourning* describes the actions or expressions of the bereaved (symbols, clothing, and ceremonies) that make up the outward signs of grief.

Death, the most critical loss of all, is defined in a variety of ways. A commonly used definition of death is an irreversible cessation of circulatory and respiratory functions or irreversible cessation of all functions of the entire brain, including the brainstem. Generally, the following characteristics must be present (in some cases for at least 24 hours) for death to be declared: a lack of responsiveness, a lack of movement or breathing, a lack of reflexes, and a flat encephalogram.

Although death is an inevitable part of life, it is often an immensely difficult loss both for the person who is dying and for his or her loved ones. Death may be accidental (such as from trauma or a drug overdose). It may be the end of a long and painful struggle with a terminal illness such as cancer, AIDS, or heart disease. It may also be purposeful, if a person commits suicide.

BOX 14-1

THE MOST COMMON FEARS OF LOSS

- Health
- Social status
- Possessions
- Lifestyle
- Sexual functioning
- Body part
- Death
- Marital relationship (i.e., through divorce)
- Reproductive functioning
- Stable relationships

EXPERIENCING AND RESOLVING LOSS

Medical–surgical nurses practicing in all types of settings care for clients who are experiencing loss and are in various stages of the grieving process. Grief is highly individual. The grief process may range from discomforting to debilitating; it may last a day or a lifetime, depending on what the loss means to the person experiencing it.

Kübler-Ross's (1969, 1978) research on death and dying provides one framework for understanding the stages of coping with an impending or actual loss. Kübler-Ross was careful to state that not all people dealing with a loss go through these stages or go through them in the sequence described. She identified stages of death and dying, but repeatedly stressed the danger of labeling a "stage" prematurely. She emphasized that her goal was to describe observations of how people come to terms with loss. She observed that some or all of the stages discussed next may occur during the grieving process and may reappear as the person experiences the loss.

Denial

A person may react with shock and disbelief after receiving word of an actual or potential loss. People may make such statements as "This can't be happening to me" or "This can't be true." This initial stage of denial serves as a buffer. During denial, the person or family mobilizes defenses to cope with the situation.

Anger

In the anger stage, the person resists the loss. The anger, described as "acting out," is often directed toward family and health care providers.

Bargaining

The bargaining stage serves as an attempt to delay the reality of the loss. The person makes a secret bargain with God, expressing a willingness to do anything to postpone the loss or change the prognosis. This is the individual's plea for an extension of life or the chance to "make everything right" with a dying family member or friend.

Depression

Upon realizing the full effect of the actual or perceived loss, the person enters a stage of depression and prepares for the impending loss by working through the struggle of separation. While grieving over "what cannot be," the person may either talk freely about the loss or withdraw from others.

Acceptance

Some people who are dying reach a stage of acceptance in which they may appear to have no emotions. The struggle is past, and the emotional pain is gone. If the person has experienced the loss of a loved one or other valued object, he or

TABLE 14-1
Development of the Concept of Death

AGE	BELIEFS/ATTITUDES ABOUT DEATH
3	Fears separation; lacks comprehension of permanent separation.
3–5	Believes death is like sleeping and is reversible. Expresses curiosity about what happens to the body.
6–10	Understands finality of death. Views own death as avoidable. Associates death with violence. Believes wishes can be responsible for death.
11–12	Reflects views of death expressed by parents. Expresses interest in afterlife as an understanding or mortality develops. Recognizes death as irreversible and inevitable.
13–21	Usually has a religious and philosophic view of death but seldom thinks about it. Views own death as distant or a challenge, acting out defiance through reckless behavior. Previously held developmental awareness of death may still be present.
22–45	Does not think about death unless confronted with it. Emotionally distances self from death. Attitude toward death influenced by religious and cultural beliefs.
46–65	Experiences the death of parents or friends. Accepts own mortality. Experiences waves of death anxiety. Puts life in order to prepare for death and decrease anxiety.
66 and older	Fears lingering, incapacitating illness. Views death as inevitable but from a philosophical viewpoint, that is, as freedom from pain and illness or as a spiritual reunion with deceased friends and loved ones.

MediaLink Video: Emotional, Social, & Spiritual Needs

she begins to come to terms with the loss and resumes activities with an air of hopefulness for the future.

Differences in a person's understanding of and reaction to loss are affected by the person's developmental stage. In general, as people age and experience life transitions, they are more able to understand and accept the losses associated with those transitions (Table 14-1 ■).

FAMILY AND OTHER SUPPORT SYSTEMS

Grieving is painful and lonely. Reactions to loss are affected by how much social support people feel they have. Lack of a support system has been identified as one factor that may delay grief work. Even if the client is reacting to the loss in an expected manner, feelings of isolation and withdrawal behaviors are often observed. Clients need encouragement to reestablish contact with significant others in their lives to allow them to share their grief. If the client is not making progress in grief work, the nurse may need to explain to the client the benefit of sharing his or her grief with significant others. Some losses may lead to social isolation, placing clients at high risk for dysfunctional grief reactions. For example, survivors of people with AIDS often report feeling excluded by the deceased person's family and by health care providers. Factors that can interfere with successful grieving include:

- Perceived inability to share the loss
- Lack of social recognition of the loss
- Ambivalent relationships prior to the loss
- Traumatic circumstances of the loss.

A well-functioning family usually rallies after the initial shock and disbelief, and the family members provide support for each other during all phases of the grieving process. After a loss, the well-functioning family is able to shift roles, levels of responsibility, and ways of communicating.

The nurse needs to be alert for the negative as well as positive effects the family may have on the grieving client. For example, the dying client may ask someone the family perceives as an outsider to be near, and the family may respond with anger to this "intrusion." Similarly, certain family members may have hurt feelings or be angry if the client is unresponsive to them. Well-meaning family members also may try to shield the client from the pain of grieving. Because no two people grieve alike, the nurse must assess the individual family members' reactions to the loss. The family and the client rarely experience anger, denial, and acceptance in unison. While one member is in denial, another may be angry because "not enough is being done."

SPIRITUALITY

Spirituality is at the core of human existence, integrating and transcending the physical, emotional, intellectual, and social dimensions (Reed, 1996). The principles, values, personal philosophy, and meaning of life may be called into question when the client responds to an actual or perceived loss. Because of a fear of intruding on personal beliefs and practices, the nurse often feels at a loss when implementing interventions that would help the client respond to a loss and meet spiritual needs.

TABLE 14-2

Cultural Aspects of Dying and Death

CULTURE/ETHNICITY	NURSING INTERVENTIONS
Native American	Some tribes prefer not to openly discuss terminal prognosis and DNR decisions, as negative thoughts may make inevitable loss occur sooner. Suggest a family meeting to discuss care and end-of-life issues. If the family feels comfortable, all members of the family and close friends may remain 24 hours a day (eating, joking, singing). Mourning is done in private, away from the dying person. After death, the family may hug, touch, sing, and stay close to the deceased.
Black/African American	Suggest that the family have a family meeting or talk with their minister or family elder. Client may decide to have older family member disclose a poor prognosis. Care for the dying family member is often done at home until death is imminent.
Chinese American	Ensure the head of the family is present when terminal illness is discussed. The client may not want to discuss approaching death. Special amulets or cloths may be brought from home. Family members may prefer to bathe the body after death.
Iranian	Information about a terminal illness should be presented by a trusted member of the health care team to the family, and never to the client when he or she is alone. Most Iranians believe in *tagdir* (will of God) in life and death as a predestined journey. When death occurs, notify the head of the family first. DNR decisions are often made by the family. The family may want to bathe the body.
Mexican American	Based on the belief that worry may make health worse, the family may want to protect the client from seriousness of illness. The information is often handled by an older daughter or son. Extended family members are obligated to pay respects to the sick and dying, although pregnant women do not care for dying persons or attend funerals. May prefer that the client die at home. Prayers, amulets, and rosary beads are used, and the priest should be notified. Death is seen as an important spiritual event. The family may bathe the body and spend time with the body.
Vietnamese	Consult head of family before telling client about a terminal illness. Entire family will make DNR decision, often with assistance from the priest or monk. Often prefer to die at home. Family should have extra time with the body, and may cry loudly and uncontrollably. Spiritual/religious rites are often conducted in the room.

Source: Adapted from Lipson, J. G., Dibble, S. L., & Minarik, P. A. (Eds.). (1996). *Culture & nursing care: A pocket guide.* San Francisco: UCSF Nursing Press.

Developing a trusting relationship with the client and family helps the nurse overcome discomfort in dealing with the spiritual aspects of care, even when the client and nurse have different views. For example, the nurse should be accepting and nonjudgmental if the client initially expresses a belief that the loss is punishment for some past misdeed or failure "to do right." Even spiritually healthy clients need time to challenge their beliefs and values before moving on to the next stage of grieving.

As the client becomes aware of the full effect of the loss, spiritual beliefs and rituals often provide comfort and help the client to find meaning in the loss. The nurse provides spiritual support by listening as the client analyzes beliefs and values, begins to put the loss in perspective, and expresses interest in getting on with life.

RITUALS OF MOURNING

The rituals of mourning are an important part of the work of mourning and grieving a loss. Culture is the primary factor that dictates the rituals of mourning (Table 14-2 ■). The funeral ceremony serves the needs of the bereaved as they gather to share their loss. Through the ceremony, people symbolically express triumph over death and deny the fear of death. Through rituals, the survivors publicly adapt to the loss. This adaptation does not decrease the suffering they will continue to feel, but it does move them toward reinvesting emotionally in the future.

NURSES' RESPONSES TO CLIENT'S LOSS

To give effective nursing care, nurses need to take time to analyze their own feelings and values related to loss and the expression of grief. The nurse's conscious or unconscious reactions to the client's responses to the loss will influence the outcome of interventions. When assessing the physical symptoms of grief, for example, the nurse may believe the client's behavior is exaggerated and out of proportion to the loss suffered. However, even a brief moment of self-reflection will help the nurse approach the interaction more objectively.

End-of-Life Care

Nurses care for dying clients in intensive care units, emergency rooms, hospital units, long-term care facilities, and the home. Regardless of the setting, the client's wishes about death should be respected.

End-of-life nursing care that ensures a peaceful death was mandated by the International Council of Nurses' (1997) and further supported by the American Association of Colleges of Nursing (AACN) (1999a). The principles of hospice care are basic to end-of-life care: that people live until the moment they die, that care until death may be offered by a variety of health care providers, and that such care is coordinated, sensitive to diversity, offered around the clock, and incorporates the physical, psychologic, social, and spiritual concerns of the patient and the patient's family. Listed here are selected competencies necessary for nurses to provide high-quality end-of-life care as defined by the AACN (1999a):

- Promote the provision of comfort care to the dying as an active, desirable, and important skill, and an integral component of nursing care.
- Communicate effectively and compassionately with the patient, family, and health care team members about end-of-life issues.
- Recognize one's own attitudes, feelings, values, and expectations about death and the individual, cultural, and spiritual diversity existing in those beliefs and customs.
- Demonstrate respect for the patient's views and wishes during end-of-life care.
- Use scientifically based standardized tools to assess symptoms (e.g., pain, dyspnea [breathlessness], constipation, anxiety, fatigue, nausea/vomiting, and altered cognition) experienced by patients at the end of life.
- Use data from symptom assessment to plan and intervene in symptom management using state-of-the-art traditional and complementary approaches.
- Assist the client, family, colleagues, and oneself to cope with suffering, grief, loss, and bereavement in end-of-life care.

LEGAL AND ETHICAL ISSUES

Issues such as those involved in advance directives and living wills, euthanasia, and quality of life are especially important to nurses in upholding the specific care requests of their clients.

Advance Directives

Advance directives are legal documents that allow a person to plan for health care and/or financial affairs in the event of incapacity. (Types of advance directives are defined in Box 14-2. ■) A **durable power of attorney for health care** (or *health care proxy*) is a legal document

---

BOX 14-2

TYPES OF ADVANCE DIRECTIVES

- **Living will:** A document that provides written directions about life-prolonging procedures; provides instructions when a person can no longer communicate in a life-threatening situation.
- **Health care surrogate:** An individual selected to make medical decisions when a person is no longer able to make them for him- or herself.
- **Durable power of attorney:** A document that can delegate the authority to make health, financial, and/or legal decisions on a person's behalf. It must be in writing and must state that the designated person is authorized to make health care decisions.

---

written by a competent (mentally healthy) adult that gives another competent adult the right to make health care decisions on his or her behalf if he or she cannot. The legal authority is limited to decisions about health care. A **living will** is a legal document that formally expresses a person's wishes regarding life-sustaining treatment in the event of terminal illness or permanent unconsciousness. It is not a type of durable power of attorney and usually does not designate a substitute decision maker. It is the responsibility of the nurse as client advocate to request and record the client's preference for care and include it in the plan of care. The nurse's documentation helps communicate these preferences to the other members of the health care team.

All facilities that receive Medicare and Medicaid funds are required to provide clients with written information and counseling about advance directives and the institution's policies governing them. The specific terms of this requirement are found in the Patient Self-Determination Act (PSDA). A copy of the signed advance directive must be kept in the client's medical record, but clients do not have to sign it in order to be treated. Nurses are the ones in close contact with clients, so they are often left with unresolved feelings about the moral, ethical, and legal aspects of their actions. Although advance directives do not ease the pain of seeing clients die, they do help nurses provide clients with the care the clients have chosen.

Do-Not-Resuscitate Orders

A **do-not-resuscitate (DNR) order** (or "no-code") is written by the physician for the client who is near death. This order is usually based on the wishes of the client and family that no cardiopulmonary resuscitation be performed for respiratory or cardiac arrest. A **comfort measures only order** indicates that no further life-sustaining interventions are necessary and that the goal of care is a comfortable, dignified death. Confusing or conflicting DNR orders create dilemmas, because nurses are involved in resuscitation and either begin CPR or ensure that unwanted attempts do not occur. The American Nurses Association (ANA) recommends that guidelines and policies be developed to help resolve conflicts between clients and their families, between clients and health care professionals, and among health care professionals.

Euthanasia

Euthanasia (from the Greek for painless, easy, gentle, or good death) is now commonly used to signify a killing that is prompted by some humanitarian motive. There are many arguments for and against euthanasia, and nurses have often found themselves at the center of the debate. As a result, nurses have pushed for the development of appropriate guidelines and procedures for DNR orders. When no such orders exist, the nurse faces a dilemma. Certainly, there are situations in which the nurse's role is clear. For example, it is considered malpractice to participate in "slow codes" (in which the nurse does not hurry to alert the emergency team when a terminally ill client without a DNR order stops breathing).

The natural death laws seek to preserve the notion of voluntary versus involuntary euthanasia. In voluntary euthanasia, the competent adult client and a physician, nurse, or adult friend or relative make the decision to terminate life. Involuntary euthanasia ("mercy killing") is performed without the client's consent. Because care settings offer many complex and technologic interventions, it is not likely that the ethical aspects of euthanasia will soon be resolved. However, advance directives do give clients a much more active role in decisions about their own care.

Settings and Services for End-of-Life Care

Settings and services for end-of-life care range from the critical care unit in a hospital to the client's own home. Because people are increasingly choosing to die at home, two models of care that focus on the dying client's quality of life—hospice and palliative care—are described in this section.

HOSPICE

Hospice is a model of care (rather than a place of care) for clients and their families when faced with a limited life expectancy. Hospice care is initiated for clients as they near the end of life; it emphasizes quality rather than quantity of life. The client and the family are included in the plan of care. Emotional, spiritual, and practical support is provided based on the wishes of the client and the needs of the family. Hospice regards dying as a normal part of life; it provides support for a dignified and peaceful death. It is palliative

(takes care of the comfort needs of the whole person) rather than curative.

PALLIATIVE CARE

Palliative care is focused on the relief of physical, mental, and spiritual distress for individuals who have an incurable illness. It primarily is planned and implemented to alleviate symptoms such as pain, nausea, dyspnea, confusion, anxiety, and wounds. The goal of palliative care is to improve the quality of life for the person.

Although palliative care may be provided by a single person, it usually involves the combined efforts of an interdisciplinary team, including physicians, nurses (registered nurses and licensed practical/vocational nurses), social workers, chaplains, home health aides, and volunteers. Care is provided in the client's home (or long-term care facility, senior living facility, hospice home, or hospital). The expected outcomes of care are directed by interventions to manage current manifestations of the illness and to prevent new manifestations from occurring.

PHYSIOLOGIC CHANGES IN THE DYING CLIENT

Death may occur rapidly or slowly. Physiologic changes are a part of the dying process. As death nears, these changes result in any or all of the manifestations listed in Box 14-3 ■.

- *Weakness and fatigue.* Weakness and fatigue cause discomfort, especially in joints, and contribute to an increased risk for pressure ulcers (see Chapter 45 ⬤).
- *Anorexia and decreased food intake.* Although anorexia and a decrease in food intake are normal in the dying client, the family often views this as "giving up." Anorexia may be a protective mechanism; the breakdown of body fats results in ketosis, which leads to a sense of well-being and helps decrease pain. Parenteral or enteral feedings do not improve symptoms or prolong life and may actually cause discomfort. As weakness and difficulty in swallowing

---

BOX 14-3

MANIFESTATIONS OF IMPENDING DEATH
- Difficulty talking or swallowing
- Nausea, flatus, abdominal distention
- Urinary and/or bowel incontinence, constipation
- Decreased sensation, taste, and smell
- Weak, slow, and/or irregular pulse
- Decreasing blood pressure
- Decreased, irregular, or Cheyne–Stokes respirations
- Changes in level of consciousness
- Restlessness, agitation
- Coolness, mottling, and cyanosis of the extremities

progress, the gag reflex is decreased and clients are at increased risk for aspiration if oral foods are given.

- *Fluid and electrolyte imbalances.* Decreased oral fluid intake is normal at the end of life and does not cause distress. Parenteral fluids are sometimes given to decrease delirium, but they may cause increased edema, breathlessness, cough, and respiratory secretions. If the client has edema or ascites (a collection of fluid in the abdominal cavity), excess body water is present, so dehydration is not a problem.
- *Hypotension and renal failure.* As cardiac output decreases, so does intravascular blood volume. As a result, renal perfusion decreases and the kidneys cease to function. Urinary output is scanty. The client will have tachycardia, hypotension, cool extremities, and cyanosis with skin mottling.
- *Neurologic dysfunction.* Neurologic dysfunction results from any or all of the following: decreased cerebral perfusion, hypoxemia, metabolic acidosis, sepsis, an accumulation of toxins from liver and renal failure, the effects of medications, and disease-related factors. These changes may result in a decreased level of consciousness or agitated delirium. Clients with terminal delirium may be confused, restless, or agitated. Moaning, groaning, and grimacing may accompany the agitation and are often misinterpreted as pain. Level of consciousness may decrease to the point where the client cannot be aroused. Although decreased consciousness and agitation are both normal states at the end of life, they are very distressing to the client's family. A client near death often has altered cerebral function, so the nurse must stand near the bedside and speak clearly.

clinical ALERT

Hearing is thought to be the last sense a dying client loses; the nurse should never whisper or engage in conversation with the family as if the client were not there.

- *Respiratory changes.* Respiratory changes are normal at this time. The client may have dyspnea, apnea (periods of not breathing), or Cheyne–Stokes respirations (see Chapter 24), ∞ and may use accessory muscles to breathe. Fluids accumulated in the lungs and oropharynx may lead to what is sometimes called "the death rattle." Oxygen may not relieve these manifestations.
- *Bowel and bladder incontinence.* Loss of sphincter control may lead to incontinence of feces, urine, or both.
- *Pain.* Pain is a common problem for clients at the end of life, and is what people often say they fear the most. It is

of utmost importance to keep the client comfortable through general comfort measures and by administering ordered medications for pain and anxiety.

clinical ALERT

At the end of life, there is no maximum allowable dose for opioids such as morphine sulfate; the dose should be increased to whatever is necessary to relieve pain. (See Chapter 8 ∞ for further information about pain medications.)

SUPPORT FOR THE CLIENT AND FAMILY

As the client's condition deteriorates, the nurse's knowledge of the client and family guides the care provided. It may be necessary to provide opportunities for clients to express personal preferences about where they want to die and about funeral and burial arrangements. If the family feels that this is morbid, the nurse explains that it helps clients to keep a sense of control as they approach death.

The client needs the opportunity to say goodbye to others. The nurse encourages and supports the client and family as they terminate relationships as a necessary part of the grief process. The nurse acknowledges that termination is painful and, if the client or family desires, stays with them during this time. Family members are often afraid to be present at the moment of death, yet dying alone is the greatest fear expressed by clients.

DEATH

The manifestations listed in Box 14-4 ∎ are seen after death occurs and are the basis for pronouncing death. They appear gradually and not in any special order. Pronouncement of death is legally required by a physician or other health care provider to confirm death. The time of death, with any related data, is documented in the client's chart.

The nurse may also fear being present at the moment of the client's death. In fact, Kübler-Ross (1969) noted that the nurse's fear of death frequently interferes with the ability to provide support for the dying client and family. Thoughts such as "Please, God, don't let him die on my

---

BOX 14-4

MANIFESTATIONS OF DEATH

- Absence of respirations, pulse, and heartbeat
- Fixed and dilated pupils; eyes may stay open
- Release of stool and urine
- Waxen color (pallor) as blood settles to dependent areas
- Drop in body temperature
- Lack of reflexes
- Flat encephalogram

shift" are common, and they express the nurse's emotional turmoil in dealing with the task. Nurses who have worked through their own feelings about death and dying are more at ease in assisting the dying client toward a peaceful death.

After the death, the family is encouraged to acknowledge the pain of loss. The nurse's presence and support as the bereaved express their sorrow, anger, or guilt can help them resolve their grief. It is important for the bereaved not to suppress the pain of grieving with drugs. By accepting variations in the expression of grief, the nurse supports the family's grief reactions and helps prevent dysfunctional grieving. Dysfunctional grieving is an extended and unsuccessful resolution of grief.

Resolution of grief begins with acceptance of the loss. The nurse can encourage this acceptance by maintaining open, honest dialogue and by providing the family with the opportunity to view, touch, hold, and kiss the person's body. As family members realize the finality of the death, they are often comforted by the presence of the nurse who cared for the client during the final days.

Postmortem Care

Normally, the nurse documents the time of death (required for the death certificate and all official records), notifies the physician, and assists the family (if needed) in choice of a funeral home. If the client dies at home, death must be pronounced before the body is removed. In some states and in some situations, nurses can pronounce death. For specifics, consult state practice acts, laws, and agency policy. All jewelry, except a wedding ring, is removed and given to the family. The body is kept in place until the family is ready and gives permission. If an autopsy is required or requested, the body must be left undisturbed (e.g., do not remove any tubes) for transportation to the medical examiner.

clinical ALERT

The bodies of deceased clients with known infections that require body and body fluid precautions or isolation (such as tuberculosis or AIDS) should be tagged accordingly. Soiled items should be disposed of appropriately, and nondisposable items should be cleaned.

Documentation of the death is completed by sending a completed death certificate to the funeral home (for a death in the home), or by completing the required paperwork and sending the body to the morgue or funeral home (for a death in the hospital or long-term care setting).

Nurses' Grief

The nurse who has developed a close relationship with the client who has died may experience strong feelings of grief.

Crying with families (at one time considered unprofessional) is now recognized as simply an expression of empathy and caring. Sharing grief with the family after the death of a loved one helps both the nurse and family to cope with their feelings about the loss. Taking time to grieve after the death of a client provides a release that can help prevent "blunting" of feelings, a problem often experienced by nurses who care for terminally ill clients.

Nurses working with critically or terminally ill clients should be aware that witnessing a client's death and the family's grief may reactivate feelings about some unresolved grief in their own lives. In these cases, nurses may need to reflect on their responses to their own losses. Also, nurses who work with dying clients need support from peers and other professionals to work through the often overwhelming feelings that result from dealing with death, grief, and loss (Figure 14-1 ■). A national education program, the End-of-Life Consortium (ELNEC) project, has been created to develop a core of expert academic and clinical staff educators who can better prepare nurses for end-of-life care (AACN, 2004).

INTERDISCIPLINARY CARE

Interventions for loss and grief may be planned and implemented by any or all members of the health care team. Nurses and social workers may provide interventions to help clients or families adapt to a loss. They may also make referrals to mental health professionals (grief counselors, social services), support groups, chaplains, or legal or financial assistance agencies.

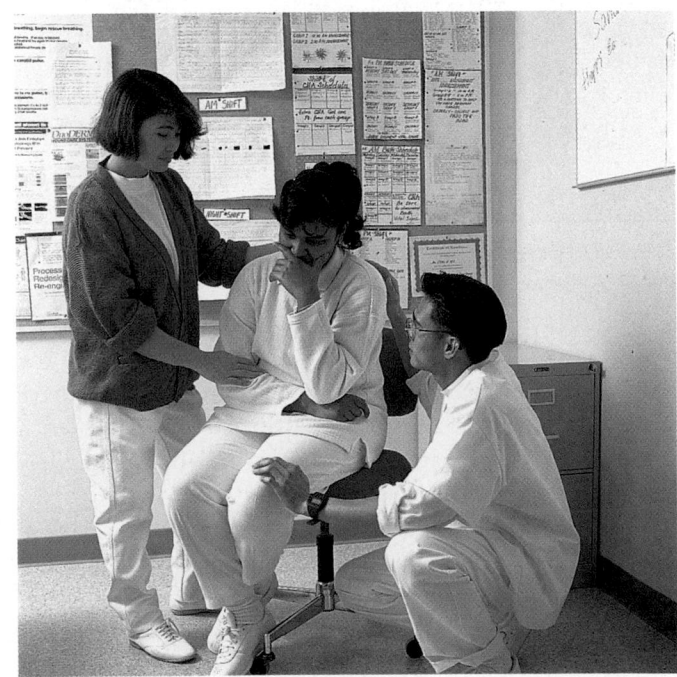

Figure 14-1. ■ Nurses who work with dying clients need support from their colleagues to work through their often overwhelming feelings of grief. (Photographer: Richard Tauber.)

BOX 14-5	NURSING CARE CHECKLIST

Providing Physical Comfort for the Client Nearing Death

- ☑ Maintain clean skin and bed linens.
- ☑ Use a draw sheet to turn the client as often as possible and as is comfortable for the client.
- ☑ Position the client to promote comfort and protect bony areas with padding. Reposition the client and raise the head of the bed if fluids accumulate in the upper airways and back of the throat.
- ☑ Use bed pads or insert a Foley catheter (if ordered) for urinary incontinence.
- ☑ Use gentle massage to improve circulation and shift edema.
- ☑ Provide small, frequent sips of fluids, ice chips, or Popsicles.
- ☑ Provide oral care, using a soft moist brush or glycerin swab.
- ☑ Clean secretions from the eyes and nose.
- ☑ Administer ordered pain medications as needed to maintain comfort.
- ☑ Administer oxygen as prescribed to relieve dyspnea.

NURSING CARE

Priorities in Nursing Care. Nursing care of clients and family members who are experiencing loss, grief, or death must be holistic; that is, it must consider physical, emotional, cultural, and spiritual needs. The nursing process is used to organize a plan of care to provide comfort and facilitate grief resolution. Comfort measures for the client nearing death are outlined in Box 14-5 ■.

ASSESSING

Before collecting data to plan and implement care for the client experiencing a loss, the nurse must consider the individual's response. Approaches for collecting data depend on the age of the client and the circumstances under which the nurse encounters the client. The nurse observes for changes in sensory processes and asks questions about the client's sleeping and eating patterns, activities of daily living, general health status, and pain.

Clients may experience one or more physical reactions as they become aware of a loss. Gastrointestinal symptoms occur frequently (indigestion, nausea or vomiting, anorexia, weight gain or loss, constipation, or diarrhea). The shock and disbelief that accompany a loss may cause shortness of breath, a choking sensation, hyperventilation, or loss of strength. Some clients also report insomnia, preoccupation with sleep, fatigue, and decreased or increased activity level.

Crying and sadness are normal during grieving. Crying may make the client feel exhausted and may interfere with carrying out daily activities. However, a person who is unable to cry may have difficulty completing the mourning process.

The nurse must assess the client's concerns about pain, especially if the client has cancer or another painful illness. Knowledge of pain theories and pain assessment can help the nurse assess the need for pain medication (see Chapter 8 ⚭).

It is important for the nurse to explore the client's spiritual beliefs and practices, because they greatly influence reactions to loss. The spiritually healthy client has inner resources that help him or her work through the grief process. Faith, prayer, trust in God or a superior being, perception of a purpose in life, or belief in immortality are examples of the inner resources that may sustain the client during an actual or perceived loss (Reed, 1996).

Clients often perceive a loss as punishment from God for wrongdoing or for failing to remain faithful to their religious practices. Clients may suddenly turn to religion to seek comfort or to cope with feelings of despair, helplessness, hopelessness, or guilt. They may utter anguished statements such as "Why, God?" or "Please help me, God." The nurse assesses and reports the client's verbalization of such feelings.

It is more important for the nurse to focus on the meaning of the loss to the client than to place the client in a stage or phase of grief. The caring and sensitivity of the nurse's questions will influence the amount of information the client will be willing to reveal. Asking such questions as "Why do you feel this way?" or "What does this loss mean to you?" is less helpful than making a statement such as "This must be difficult for you." This last sentence conveys the nurse's genuine interest in hearing how the client feels about the loss.

The nurse may not be able to collect much information during a brief initial contact. However, as trust is built, the client may reveal the meaning of the relationship and the circumstances surrounding the loss. By establishing trust during the first stages of the nurse–client relationship, the nurse will be better able to assess the effect of the loss. If the relationship was a significant one, the nurse will observe intense grief. The client may state, "I know I can't go on without him/her." The client may even feel anger at the person for having left, whether through death, divorce, or separation. The losses associated with changes in body image or work role may produce similar feelings.

DIAGNOSING, PLANNING, AND IMPLEMENTING

Anticipatory Grieving

Anticipatory grieving is a combination of intellectual and emotional responses and behaviors by which people adjust their self-concept in the face of a potential loss. Their response may be normal or problematic. Anticipatory grieving may be a response to one's own future death; to potential loss of body parts or functions; to potential loss of a significant person, animal, or possession; or to potential loss of a social role.

- Assess for factors that are causing or contributing to the grief. Ask about support systems, how many losses have occurred, relationship with the lost person, significance of the body part, and previous experiences with loss and grief. *Grief and mourning occur when a person experiences any type of loss.*
- Use open-ended questions to encourage the person to share concerns and the possible effect on the family unit. *Grief resolution cannot occur until the client acknowledges the loss.*
- Promote a trusting nurse–client relationship by:
  - Allowing enough time for communications
  - Speaking clearly, simply, and to the point
  - Listening
  - Being honest in responses to questions, and not giving unrealistic hope
  - Offering support
  - Demonstrating respect for the person's age, culture, religion, race, and values. *An effective nurse–client relationship begins with acceptance of the client's feelings, attitudes, and values related to the loss. If the client is ready to talk, then the nurse's listening and presence are the most appropriate interventions (Figure 14-2* ∎*).*

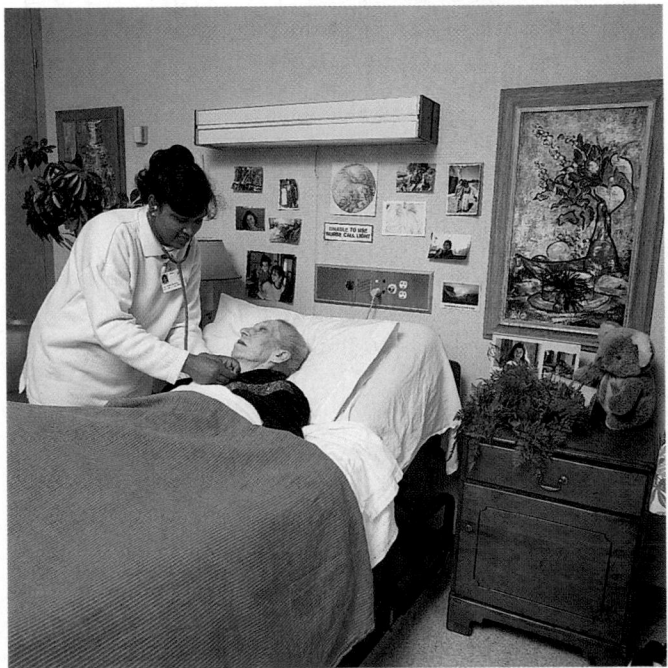

Figure 14-2. ∎ The nurse establishes a trusting nurse–client relationship through therapeutic communications and by demonstrating respect for the person's age, culture, religion, race, and values. (Photographer: Richard Tauber.)

- Ask about the client's strengths and weakness in coping with the anticipated loss. Current responses are influenced by past experiences with loss, illness, and death. *Socioeconomic and cultural backgrounds, as well as cultural and spiritual beliefs and values, affect a person's ability to adapt to loss.*
- Teach the client and family the stages of grief. *This helps them to be aware of their emotions in each stage, and reassures them that their reactions are normal.*
- Provide time for decision making. *In periods of stress, people may need extra time to make informed decisions.*
- Provide information about appropriate resources, including support from family, friends, and support groups, community resources, and legal/financial aides. *Support from others decreases feelings of loneliness and isolation and facilitates grief work.*

Death Anxiety

Death anxiety is worry or fear related to death or dying. It may be present in clients who have an acute life-threatening illness, who have a terminal illness, who have experienced the death of a family member or friend, or who have experienced multiple deaths in the same family.

- Explore the client's knowledge of the situation. For example, ask, "What has your doctor told you about your condition?" *This informs you about the client's knowledge base about the condition and about his or her ability to make informed decisions.*
- Ask the client to identify specific fears about death. *This provides data about any unrealistic expectations or misperceptions.*
- Determine the client's perceptions of strengths and weakness in coping with death. *Identifying past strengths can help the client cope with loss, illness, and death.*
- Ask the client to identify needed help. *This determines whether available resources are adequate.*
- Encourage independence and control in decisions about treatment and care. *This promotes self-esteem, decreases feelings of powerlessness, and allows the client to retain dignity in dying.*
- Facilitate client's access to culturally appropriate spiritual rituals and practices. *This provides spiritual comfort.*
- Explain advance directives and assist with them if necessary. *Advance directives help ensure that the client's wishes for end-of-life care are carried out.*
- Encourage life review and reminiscence. *Life review is self-affirming.*
- Encourage activities such as listening to music, aromatherapy, massage, or relaxation exercises. *These activities decrease anxiety.*

BOX 14-6	NURSING CARE CHECKLIST

End-of-Life Checklist

☑ Take time a day or so before appointments with your health care provider to think about the questions you need answered and concerns you want to discuss. It is often a good idea to keep a pad of paper and a pen handy so you can write down things as they come to you.

☑ Do not hesitate to have your doctor explain your diagnosis again if you didn't understand the explanation the first time, or if you missed some key points. The same goes for details about using medications and possible side effects.

☑ You may wish to have a friend or family member go with you to medical appointments.

☑ When you visit the doctor, take an up-to-date list of all medications (prescribed and over-the-counter) you are currently taking.

☑ If you have physical pain, tell your health care provider. You will probably be asked to rate your pain on a scale of 1 (no pain) to 10 (severe pain). Your rating helps determine what pain relief measures are appropriate.

☑ It is a good idea to ask your health care provider about hospice services well before you are likely to need them.

☑ Your family and close friends should be aware of your treatment preferences (such as the existance of a do-not-resuscitate order). You might consider documenting your wishes in a living will.

☑ Think about asking and appointing someone you trust to make your health care decisions, in case the moment comes when you can no longer make them yourself.

☑ If you are feeling depressed or anxious or need emotional support, consider talking to a pastor, chaplain, rabbi, or other trusted person in your faith community. If necessary, ask your health care provider to recommend someone to help you sort out your feelings.

☑ Avoid withdrawing from social activities. Keep communicating with your family, friends, and the people who help care for you. If you are open with them, you are more likely to get the care you need.

Source: Data from the United States Senate Special Committee on Aging. (2000). *End-of-life care checklist for seniors.* Available at www.advancedseniorsolutions.com/end_of_life_care%20v2.htm

■ Suggest keeping a journal or leaving a written legacy. *A written document provides continuing support to others after death.*

EVALUATING

Evaluate the effectiveness of nursing care for loss and grief by collecting data from statements by the client that support grief resolution, such as "I am beginning to accept the fact that my father is gone." The plan of care for the dying client is effective if the client has a comfortable and dignified death.

CONTINUING CARE

Nurses teach clients and families to carry out the physical skills that are necessary to the client's care. They also provide information on identifying signs of deterioration and obtaining additional sources of support (from hospice, home health care agencies, and public health departments). Encourage families to identify friends and other family members who can help out either routinely or occasionally. At discharge, provide the client or family with information for contacting the appropriate support groups. Box 14-6 ■ provides a checklist for older adults as they near end of life, but the information is useful for anyone. Box 14-7 ■ provides general guidelines for teaching clients and families about grief.

BOX 14-7	CLIENT TEACHING

Teaching for Clients Experiencing a Loss

■ Encourage both children and adults to discuss expected or impending loss and to express feelings.
■ Teach problem-solving skills.
  ■ Define what the possible changes and problems are related to the predicted loss.
  ■ Develop potential strategies for dealing with problems.
  ■ List pros and cons of each strategy.
  ■ Decide which strategies might be most useful to try first to solve potential problems associated with loss.
■ Identify persons who are at risk for potential dysfunctional grieving: those who present a brave, stoic front; clients with a history of multiple losses; socially isolated individuals; people who feel their social network is not supportive; and clients with a history of dealing ineffectively with loss.
■ Teach individuals and families how to support a person who is dealing with an impending loss:
  ■ Explain what to expect with a loss: sadness, fear, rejection, anger, guilt, and loneliness.
  ■ Teach signs of grief resolution:
    ■ No longer living in the past, becoming future oriented
    ■ Breaking ties with the lost object or person (Acute stages often shows signs of resolving in 6 to 12 months.)
    ■ The possibility of having painful "waves" of grief years after the loss, especially on the anniversary of the loss and in response to "triggers" such as pictures, events, songs, or memories
■ Identify community agencies that may be helpful to people responding to loss.

NURSING PROCESS CARE PLAN
Client Experiencing Loss

Pearl Rogers is a 79-year-old African American woman who is admitted to the Methodist Home Nursing Center. Mrs. Rogers lived with her husband of 58 years until his death 9 months ago. She had one son, who died in an auto accident 2 years ago, and she has one daughter who lives nearby. After her husband's death, Mrs. Rogers lived with her daughter until her admission to the nursing center. Mrs. Rogers has become increasingly agitated and helpless, complaining constantly of pain. Her daughter states that Mrs. Rogers is chronically constipated, has difficulty sleeping, and has stopped taking part in all social activities, including weekly church services. She cries frequently. Extensive medical testing prior to her admission to the nursing center revealed Mrs. Rogers has arthritis but no other pathologic disorder.

Assessment. When Mrs. Rogers arrives at the nursing center, she is admitted by Sandy Sutphin, LPN. Mrs. Rogers tells Ms. Sutphin, "I'm a sick woman, and no one will listen to me! I can't walk, I'm so weak. My head hurts, and I'm always sick at my stomach. I haven't had a bowel movement in a week, and I never sleep more than three hours a night." Ms. Sutphin completes data collection and works with her manager to develop a plan of care for Mrs. Rogers.

Diagnosis. The following nursing diagnoses are made for Mrs. Rogers:

- *Dysfunctional Grieving* related to stress of husband's death
- *Sleep Pattern Disturbed* related to grieving
- *Constipation* related to inactivity

Expected Outcomes. The expected outcomes established in the plan of care are that Mrs. Rogers will:

- Discuss her losses, use constructive coping mechanisms, and discuss positive and negative aspects of the loss.
- Fall asleep within 20 to 30 minutes after retiring and remain asleep for 7 to 8 hours.
- Have a bowel movement at least every other day.

Planning and Implementation. The following interventions are planned and implemented during care of Mrs. Rogers:

- Promote trust: Show empathy and caring, demonstrate respect for her culture and values, offer support and reassurance, be honest, engage in active listening.
- During one-to-one interactions, encourage Mrs. Rogers to recognize normal grieving behavior. Assist her in labeling her feelings: anger, fear, loneliness, guilt, and isolation.

- Explore previous losses and the ways in which the client has coped.
- Encourage Mrs. Rogers to express her feelings of anger. Do not become defensive, and explain to her family that anger helps her feel as though she has some control over her environment, even though she has no control over her loss.
- Encourage Mrs. Rogers to participate in her spiritual practices.
- Provide afternoon activities for Mrs. Rogers as indicated by the occupational therapist.
- Provide evening care: warm sponge bath; clean, warm bed; night-light; soft music for relaxation; closed door.
- Provide measures that assist in bowel function: Encourage exercise as tolerated, including walks and rocking in a rocking chair. Offer foods that stimulate bowel movements (such as fruits, vegetables, and high-fiber cereals). Increase fluid intake. Provide privacy: Close the door, ensuring that the emergency call bell is within reach, and do not interrupt. Assure Mrs. Rogers that a nurse will be there to help her clean herself if she needs one, and have toilet paper, soap, warm water, and a cloth available to promote her dignity.
- Administer a mild laxative and/or stool softener to Mrs. Rogers, if ordered and necessary, but discontinue as soon as possible.

Evaluation. After 4 weeks at the nursing center, Mrs. Rogers states, "I don't feel any better, but I know I have to accept my situation." Although Mrs. Rogers states that she doesn't feel better, she now walks the length of the hall several times a day, is sleeping better, and has regular bowel movements. Mrs. Rogers is also less withdrawn, has greatly reduced the time she spends crying, and has openly discussed her feelings related to her husband's death, including her anger at the loss of her son and her husband less than 2 years apart. She has attended chapel services on Sunday for the past 2 weeks. She plays cards with the other residents 2 or 3 afternoons a week.

Critical Thinking in the Nursing Process

1. How might the nursing staff involve Mrs. Rogers's daughter in developing and implementing her mother's plan of care?
2. Suppose Mrs. Rogers said that she did not want any help, that she just wanted to be left alone to die. How would you respond?
3. What factors in Mrs. Rogers's current life would support the nursing diagnosis of Social Isolation?

Note: The bibliography listings for this and all chapters have been compiled at the back of the book.

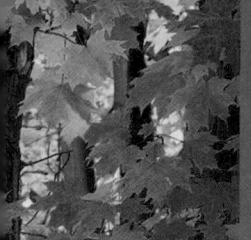

Chapter Review

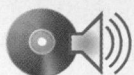 **KEY TERMS** by Topics

Use the audio glossary feature of either the CD-ROM or the Companion Website to hear the correct pronunciation of the following key terms.

Loss, grief, and death
loss, grief, death
End-of-life care
advance directives, durable power of

attorney for health care, living will, do-not-resuscitate (DNR) order, comfort measures only order, euthanasia, hospice, palliative care

KEY Points

- When a valued object, person, body part, or situation is lost or changed, the experience of loss occurs. Grief is the emotional response to loss. Grieving responses are individualized to each person, but commonly include the stages of denial, anger, bargaining, depression, and acceptance.

- Death is an immensely difficult loss for both the person who is dying and for his or her loved ones. Grief work is often facilitated by family, friends, and spiritual practices.

- The dying person may control his or her own care through advance directives, living wills, and a durable power of attorney for health care. The client and family may request that the physician write a do-not-resuscitate (DNR) order.

- As death nears, specific physiologic changes take place. These changes result in manifestations that indicate impending death. Death is pronounced when respiratory and circulatory functions stop or when all brain function ceases.

- Nursing care for clients who experience loss, grief, or death is implemented to meet the physical, emotional, and spiritual needs of the client and family. Nurses must also be aware of their own responses to these experiences to provide care more effectively.

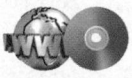 **EXPLORE Media**Link

Additional interactive resources for this chapter can be found on the Companion Website at www.prenhall.com/burke. Click on Chapter 14 and "Begin" to select the activities for this chapter.

For chapter-related NCLEX-style review questions and an audio glossary, access the accompanying CD-ROM in this book.

FOR FURTHER Study

For further information about fear of pain, see Chapter 8. Chapter 45 provides more information on pressure ulcers. For further information about respiratory changes, see Chapter 24.

Caring for a Client Experiencing a Loss

NCLEX-PN® Focus Area: Psychosocial Adaptation

Case Study: Tom Moore was involved in a serious automobile accident on his way to work and was pronounced dead on arrival at the emergency room. Tom and his wife, Sara, were married for more than 30 years. During that time, Sara did not work outside the home and Tom took care of all the finances. One year after Tom's death, Sara has her annual physical checkup.

Nursing Diagnosis: Dysfunctional Grieving

COLLECT DATA

Subjective

_____
_____
_____
_____
_____
_____

Objective

_____
_____
_____
_____
_____
_____

Would you report this data? Yes/No

If yes, to: _____

Nursing Care

_____
_____
_____
_____
_____
_____
_____
_____
_____
_____

How would you document this? _____
_____
_____

Data Collected
(use those that apply)

- Weight loss of 25 lbs
- B/P 110/70
- States, "I can't stand being alone."
- States, "I am still angry at Tom for dying."
- Difficulty sleeping
- States, "My knees sometimes feel like sandpaper inside."
- Unable to continue normal routines
- Has joined a grief support group at her church

Nursing Interventions
(use those that apply; list in priority order)

- Discuss time needed to resolve a loss.
- Explain grief reactions.
- Ignore statements and conduct basic physical assessment.
- Encourage expression of feelings.
- State, "I can't talk about that right now—I'm too busy."
- State, "This must have been very difficult for you."
- State, "I know it's hard, but you will be okay."

NCLEX-PN® Exam Preparation

1 The grief process may range from discomforting to debilitating, and it may last a day or a lifetime, depending on:

A. whether the loss is temporary or permanent.
B. what the loss means to the person experiencing it.
C. the religion of the person experiencing the loss.
D. the educational level of the person experiencing the loss.

2 A client has been diagnosed with terminal cancer and is reacting with hostility and abruptness to her family and the hospital staff. She tells them to leave her alone. The client is most likely in the stage of:

A. denial.
B. anger.
C. bargaining.
D. acceptance.

3 Factors that affect an individual's reaction to loss include:

A. age and availability of a support system.
B. income level and age.
C. self-esteem and self-confidence.
D. mental stability and employment status.

4 A do-not-resuscitate order is written for the client who is near death by:

A. the client.
B. the family.
C. the nurse.
D. the physician.

5 Regardless of the setting, the client's wishes about death should:

A. be kept private.
B. be respected.
C. conform to the cultural norm.
D. be the same as his or her family's wishes.

6 A model of care initiated for clients as they near the end of life, emphasizing quality rather than quantity of life, is known as:

A. hospice.
B. euthanasia.
C. advance directive.
D. home-based care.

7 To provide holistic end-of-life care, it is necessary for the nurse to:

A. control his or her own emotions about death.
B. maintain a sense of detachment.
C. agree with the client's values and beliefs.
D. provide comfort and symptom-management interventions.

8 Respiratory changes to be expected near death include:

A. episodes of tachypnea and coughing.
B. periods of apnea and Cheyne–Stokes respiration.
C. loss of sphincter control and anorexia.
D. emotional distress and crying.

9 Grief before a loss actually occurs is called:

A. dysfunctional.
B. functional.
C. adaptive.
D. anticipatory.

10 The best response for the nurse to help grieving family members express their grief would be:

A. "I know just how you feel."
B. "Things will get better over time."
C. "Tell me how you are feeling."
D. "Let me know if there is anything I can do to help."

Answers for Review Questions, as well as discussion of Care Plan and Critical Thinking Care Map questions, appear in Appendix V.

Jane Souza, a 25-year-old married woman with two children, is involved in a head-on collision. Ms. Souza, who is not wearing a seat belt, is thrown forward against the steering wheel. Her lower legs are trapped under the dashboard. Ms. Souza is transported to the local trauma center. She is conscious, is receiving high-flow oxygen by mask, and has one intravenous line in place.

DATA COLLECTED

Airway is patent, with high-flow oxygen in place. Breathing rate is 36; breath sounds on the right side are decreased (multiple bruises and abrasions on right side of chest); she complains of difficulty breathing. Circulation indicates palpable systolic blood pressure of 80, pulse rate of 120, and palpable pedal pulses. No active external bleeding noted. Skin is pale, cool to the touch, and diaphoretic. Pupils are equal and react to light. Ms. Souza has limited extremity movement because of a broken right arm and an open fracture of the left ankle.

Because of Ms. Souza's respiratory distress, she is intubated and connected to a ventilator with 100% oxygen. An-

other intravenous line is inserted and O-negative blood is given. Her blood pressure continues to decrease, and she is immediately taken to surgery.

CRITICAL THINKING

1 Ms. Souza received blood transfusions in the emergency department. Explain the signs she displayed that resulted in this intervention.

2 Why was she given transfusions?

3 Why was O-negative the blood type of choice?

4 Why did the emergency staff think Ms. Souza had internal bleeding?

PRIORITIES IN NURSING CARE

1 Using Maslow's hierarchy, identify the order in which the emergency staff addressed Ms. Souza's physical needs.

COMMUNICATION

1 Suggest two nursing interventions to assist Ms. Souza's family in coping with this traumatic event.

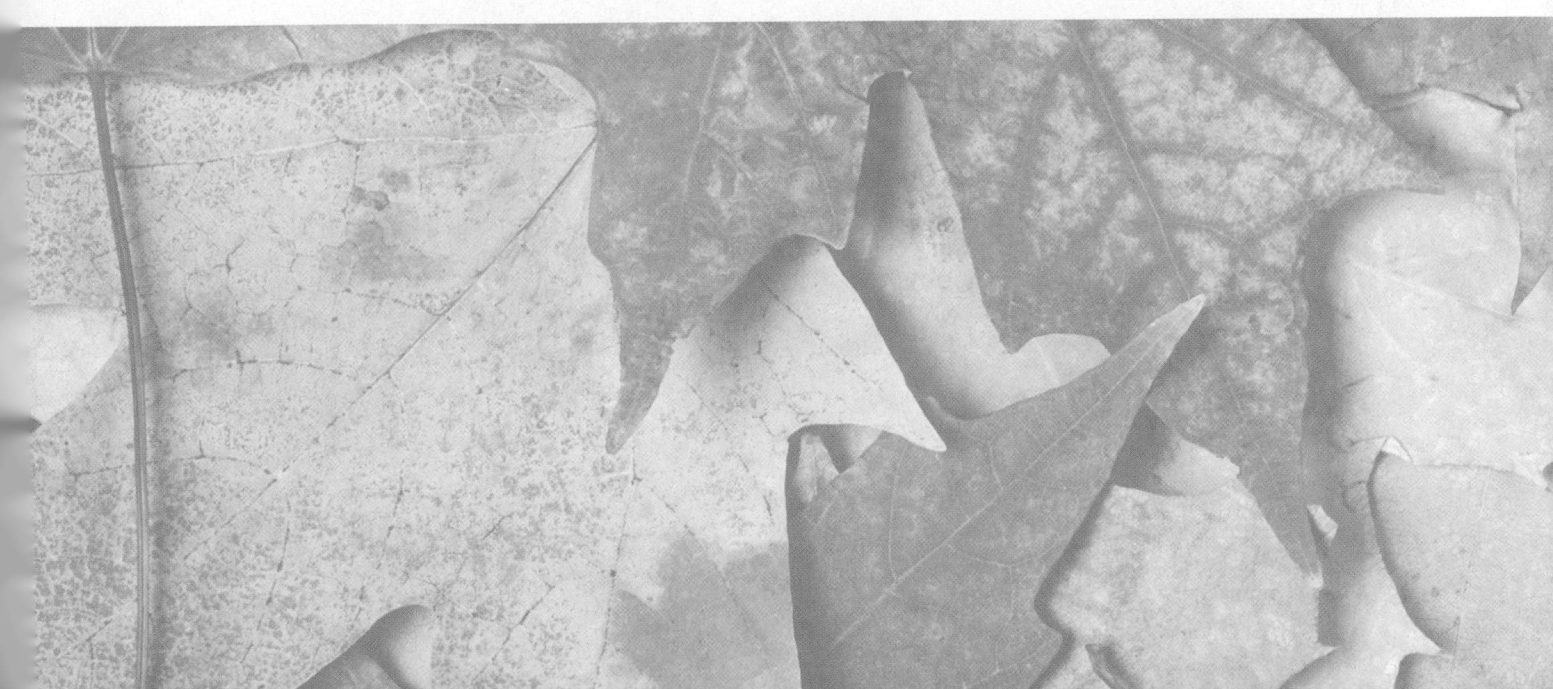

Disrupted Endocrine Function

UNIT III

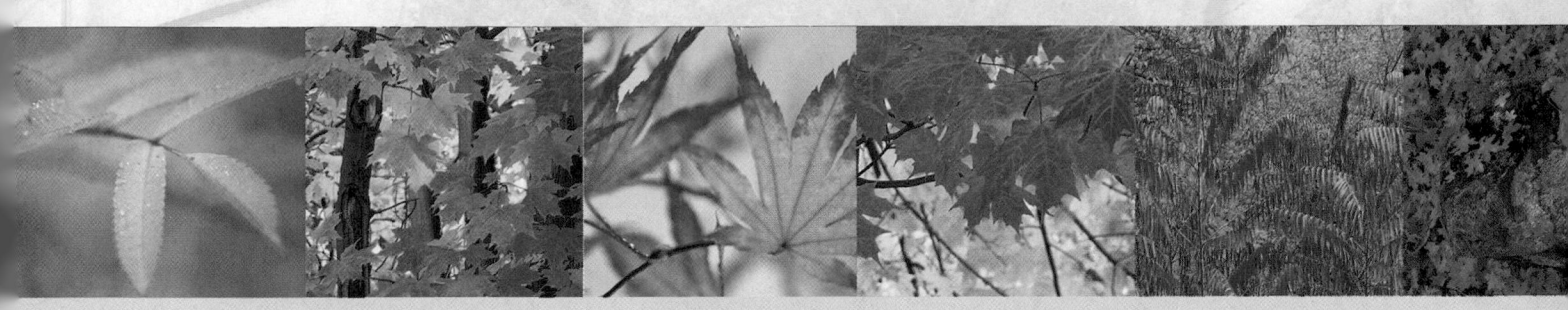

Chapter 15

The Endocrine System and Assessment

BRIEF Outline

Structure and Function of the Endocrine System
- Hypothalamus
- Pituitary Gland
- Thyroid Gland
- Parathyroid Glands
- Adrenal Glands
- Pancreas

Assessment
- Health History
- Physical Examination
- The Older Adult
- Diagnostic Tests

LEARNING Outcomes

After completing this chapter, you will be able to:

- Describe the structure and function of the organs of the endocrine system, including the pancreas.
- Explain the functions of hormones secreted by the endocrine glands.
- Describe the actions of insulin and glucagon.
- Identify subjective and objective assessment data to collect for clients with endocrine disorders.
- Identify nursing responsibilities for common diagnostic tests for clients with endocrine disorders.

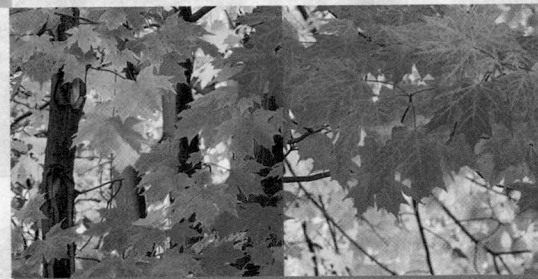

MediaLink

www.prenhall.com/burke
Use the address above to access the free, interactive Companion Website created for this textbook. Get hints, instant feedback, and textbook references to chapter-related NCLEX-style questions. Link to other interesting sites.

Audio Glossary:
Use the Companion Website, or the CD-ROM disk enclosed with your textbook, to hear the pronunciation of key terms in this chapter.

This chapter includes a discussion of the endocrine system and the pancreas. The primary function of the endocrine system is to regulate the body's internal environment. Hormones secreted by endocrine glands regulate growth, reproduction and sex differentiation, metabolism, and fluid and electrolyte balance. The endocrine system helps the body adapt to constant changes in the internal and external environment.

The pancreas produces hormones needed for the metabolism of carbohydrates, proteins, and fats. The pancreatic hormones, insulin and glucagon, are responsible for maintaining blood glucose levels.

Structure and Function of the Endocrine System

The major endocrine organs are the hypothalamus, pituitary gland, thyroid gland, parathyroid glands, thymus, adrenal glands, pancreas, and gonads (reproductive glands) (Figure 15-1 ■). Table 15-1 ■ lists the endocrine organs with their hormones and the primary hormone action. This chapter focuses on the hypothalamus, pituitary gland, thyroid gland, parathyroid glands, and adrenal glands. The pancreas is discussed after the endocrine organs. Specific information about the gonads is presented in Chapters 34 and 35. ⊙

MediaLink ● Endocrine System

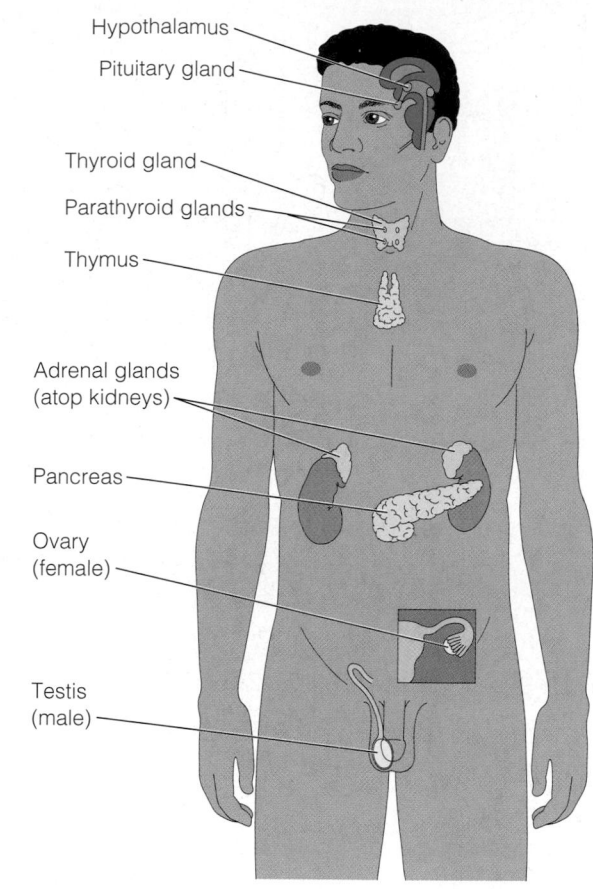

Figure 15-1. ■ Location of the major endocrine glands.

TABLE 15-1

Endocrine Organs, Hormones, and Functions

ORGAN	HORMONE	FUNCTION
Anterior pituitary	Growth hormone (GH)	Promotes growth.
	Thyroid-stimulating hormone (TSH)	Stimulates secretion of thyroid hormone.
	Adrenocorticotropic hormone (ACTH)	Stimulates adrenal cortex to secrete glucocorticoids.
	Melanocyte-stimulating hormone	Controls pigmentation of the skin.
	Follicle-stimulating hormone (FSH)	Stimulates ovary development and egg and sperm production.
	Luteinizing hormone (LH)	Stimulates ovulation and secretion of sex hormones in males and females.
	Prolactin	Stimulates breast milk production.
Posterior pituitary	Antidiuretic hormone (ADH)	Promotes water retention by kidneys.
	Oxytocin	Promotes uterine contraction and release of milk.
Thyroid gland	Thyroid hormone (TH)	Increases metabolic rate.
	Calcitonin	Lowers serum calcium levels.
Parathyroid gland	Parathyroid hormone (PTH)	Increases serum calcium levels.
Adrenal cortex	Glucocorticoids (cortisol)	Stimulates gluconeogenesis and increases blood glucose level; anti-inflammatory response.
	Mineralocorticoids (aldosterone)	Regulates blood volume and electrolytes.
Adrenal medulla	Epinephrine and norepinephrine	Increases sympathetic nervous system response to stress.

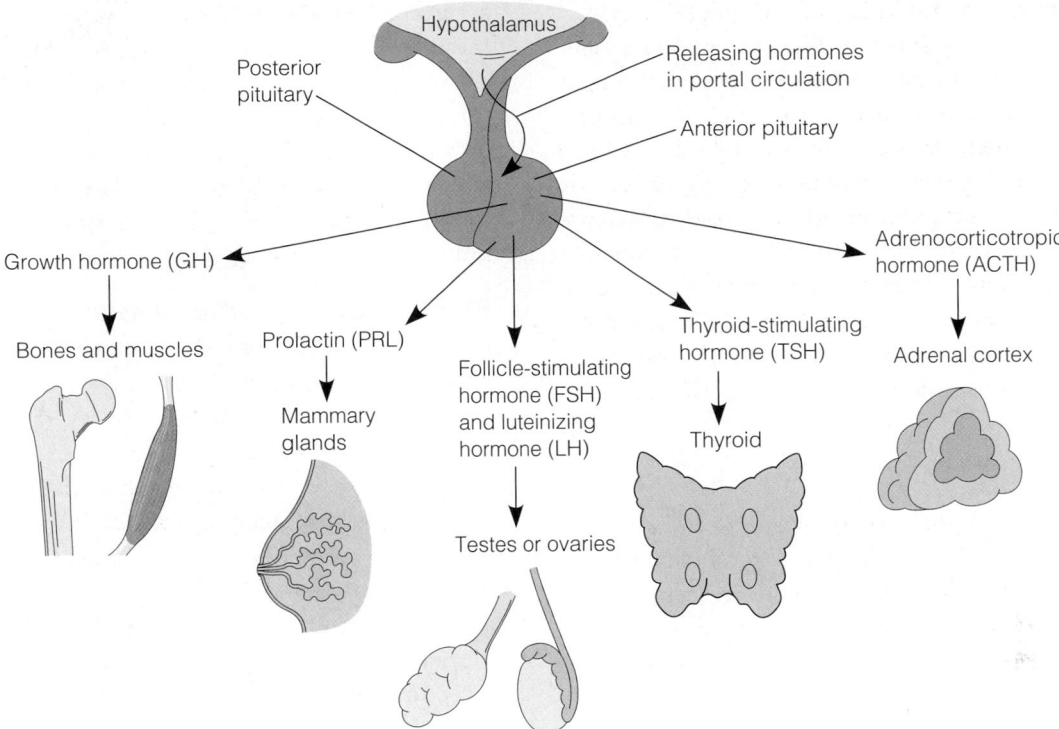

Figure 15-2. ■ Actions of the major hormones of the anterior pituitary.

Hormones are chemical messengers of the body. They act on specific target cells, causing either an increase or decrease in body function. Hormone levels are regulated by a process called *negative feedback.* Negative feedback acts similar to the way the thermostat in a house regulates temperature. When too much hormone is released, the target cell sends back a message to reduce its hormone release. If too little hormone is released, the target cell sends back a message to increase the hormone to the normal level.

HYPOTHALAMUS

The hypothalamus is located in the brain between the cerebrum and the brainstem. The pituitary gland and the hypothalamus are physically attached. The hypothalamus controls anterior pituitary function by regulating temperature, fluid volume, and growth. It also responds to pain, pleasure, hunger, and thirst stimuli.

PITUITARY GLAND

The pituitary gland (*hypophysis*) is located in the skull beneath the hypothalamus of the brain. It is often called the "master gland" because its hormones regulate many different body functions. The pituitary gland has two parts: the anterior lobe (*adenohypophysis*) and the posterior lobe (*neurohypophysis*). The anterior lobe secretes six different hormones

(Figure 15-2 ■). The posterior lobe releases antidiuretic hormone (ADH) and oxytocin.

THYROID GLAND

The thyroid gland is shaped like a butterfly and sits on either side of the trachea. This gland has two lobes connected by a structure called the *isthmus.* The thyroid gland needs an adequate supply of iodine in order to secrete thyroid hormone (thyroxine [T_4] and triiodothyronine [T_3]), which increases metabolism. The thyroid gland also secretes *calcitonin,* a hormone that decreases excess calcium levels in the blood.

PARATHYROID GLANDS

The parathyroid glands (usually four to six) are embedded on the posterior lobes of the thyroid gland. They secrete parathyroid hormone (*PTH,* or *parathormone*). PTH secretion increases when calcium levels in the plasma fall, and it decreases phosphorous levels. Normal levels of vitamin D are necessary for PTH to apply this effect on bone and kidneys.

ADRENAL GLANDS

The two adrenal glands are pyramid-shaped organs that sit on top of the kidneys. Each gland consists of two parts, an outer cortex and an inner medulla.

Adrenal Cortex

The adrenal cortex secretes several different hormones called *corticosteroids*. They are classified into two groups, *glucocorticoids* and *mineralocorticoids,* and are essential to life. *Cortisol,* a glucocorticoid, affects carbohydrate metabolism. Its primary effect is to raise blood glucose levels, making it readily available in times of stress. The primary mineralocorticoid, *aldosterone,* maintains normal salt and water balance through its action on the kidneys. It is released when blood volume or blood pressure falls below normal levels, and acts to save sodium and water, which in turn raises blood volume and pressure. Small amounts of *androgens* (sex hormones) are also released by the adrenal cortex.

Adrenal Medulla

The adrenal medulla produces two hormones (*catecholamines*): epinephrine (also called adrenaline) and norepinephrine (or noradrenaline). Both catecholamines increase heart rate and the force of heart contractions and constrict blood vessels. Epinephrine and norepinephrine are released during times of stress and initiate the *fight-or-flight response.*

PANCREAS

The primary organ involved in diabetes mellitus is the pancreas. It is located behind the stomach between the spleen and the duodenum. The pancreas serves two major functions: (1) Acini cells secrete digestive enzymes into the duodenum, and (2) the *islets of Langerhans* release insulin and glucagon into the bloodstream. To prevent **hyperglycemia** (high blood glucose level) or **hypoglycemia** (low blood glucose level), these hormones must be in balance.

Insulin

Beta cells in the islets of Langerhans produce insulin. Insulin's primary function is to regulate blood glucose levels. This is accomplished through several mechanisms. Insulin eases the active transport of glucose into muscle and fat cells, where it is used as an energy source and for cell functions. It facilitates fat formation, inhibits the breakdown and movement of stored fat, and helps move amino acids into cells for protein synthesis. Glucose unused by the cells is stored in the liver and muscle cells as glycogen. If there is excess glucose at this point, it is converted into fat and stored as adipose tissue. Insulin release increases when blood glucose levels rise and decreases when blood glucose levels fall. When a person eats food, insulin levels rise in minutes, peak in 30 to 60 minutes, and return to baseline in 2 to 3 hours.

Glucagon

Alpha cells in the islets of Langerhans produce glucagon. Glucagon prevents blood glucose from decreasing below a certain level when the body is fasting or is between meals. Glucagon makes new glucose (**gluconeogenesis**), converts glycogen into glucose in the liver and muscles (**glycogenolysis**), and prevents excess glucose breakdown. Usually, glucagon is released when blood glucose falls below about 70 mg/dL. The primary function of glucagon is to decrease glucose oxidation and to increase blood glucose.

Blood Glucose Homeostasis

Normal blood glucose is maintained in healthy people primarily through the balancing actions of insulin and glucagon (Figure 15-3 ■). However, other hormones (known as counterregulatory hormones) can help increase blood glucose levels during periods of hypoglycemia, stress, growth, or increased metabolic demand. Counterregulatory hormones include epinephrine, growth hormone, and cortisol.

Definitions of normal blood glucose levels vary in clinical practice, depending on the laboratory that performs the assay. In this text, normal blood glucose is defined as 70 to 110 mg/dL.

Assessment

Because hormones affect all body systems, manifestations of endocrine dysfunction are often usually nonspecific. This makes assessment of endocrine function more difficult.

HEALTH HISTORY

Ask about changes in energy level and fatigue and how these changes affect the client's activities of daily living. Determine whether the client has become more sensitive to heat or cold. Question about weight loss or gain; diarrhea or constipation; increased appetite, urination, or thirst; and salt cravings.

Inquire about high blood pressure, abnormally fast or slow heart rate, palpitations, or shortness of breath. Ask about vision changes, excessive tearing, or swelling around the eyes. Question if the client experiences any numbness or tingling in lips or extremities, nervousness, hand tremors, change in memory, mood, or sleep patterns. Ask about thinning or loss of hair, dry or moist skin, brittle nails, easy bruising, or slow wound healing.

Obtain a past medical history about taking any hormone replacements such as thyroid, steroids, or insulin. Determine if the client has had previous surgery, chemotherapy, or radiation especially of the neck area, as well as brain surgery or a head injury. Ask about a family history of diabetes mellitus, diabetes insipidus, goiter, obesity, Addison's disease, or infertility. Obtain a sexual history regarding changes in sexual function or secondary

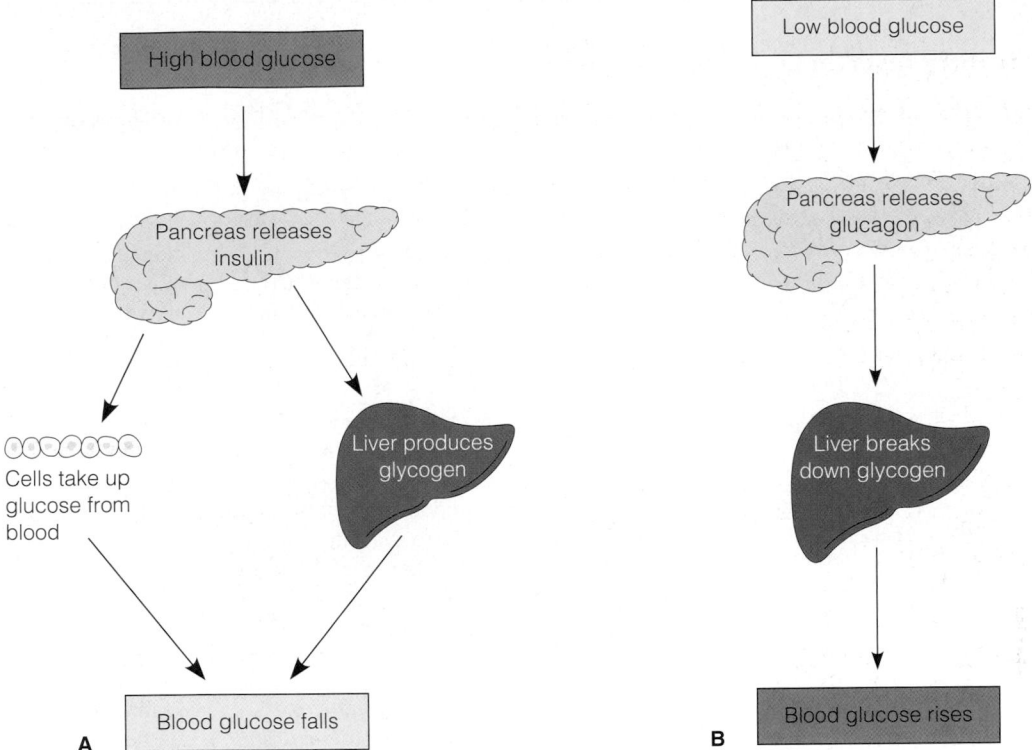

Figure 15-3. ■ Action of insulin and glucagon on blood glucose levels. (**A**) High blood glucose is lowered by insulin release. (**B**) Low blood glucose is raised by glucagon release.

sex characteristics. Ask women about changes in menstruation or menopause.

PHYSICAL EXAMINATION

Begin by assessing the client's general appearance and documenting vital signs, height, and weight. Note extremely short height. Assess skin color, temperature, texture, and moisture. Observe for rough, dry or smooth, flushed skin. Note bronze color over knuckles, purple striae over the abdomen, and bruising. Inspect the lower extremities for lesions and any signs of healing. Assess the texture and condition of hair and nails. Observe for thinning and loss of hair as well as thick or thin brittle nails. Look for excessive hair growth on face, chest, or abdomen.

Inspect the face for shape and symmetry. Inspect the eyes for the presence of **exophthalmos** (forward protrusion of the eyeballs). Determine visual acuity. Inspect the neck for visible signs of masses. Gently palpate the thyroid gland from behind the client. Palpate only one side of the neck at a time (Figure 15-4 ■).

Assess for increased size of hands and feet; trunk obesity and thin extremities. Inspect men for *gynecomastia,* enlargement of the breasts. Evaluate muscle strength and deep tendon reflexes. Assess for Chvostek's sign and Trousseau's sign (see Chapter 7, Figure 7-15 ⚭). Assess ability to sense touch, hot/cold, vibration in the extremities.

Auscultate lungs for adventitious sounds and heart for extra heart sounds. Palpate hands and feet for edema.

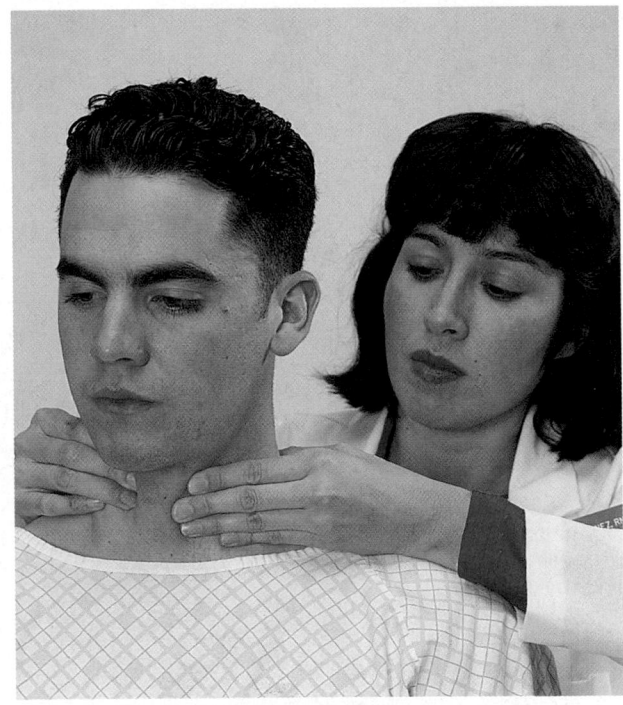

Figure 15-4. ■ Palpating the thyroid gland from behind the client. (*Source:* Lester V. Bergman/Corbis.)

TABLE 15-2

Common Laboratory Tests for Endocrine Disorders

TEST	NORMAL ADULT VALUES	EXPLANATION	NURSING IMPLICATIONS
Pituitary			
Growth hormone (GH)	<5 ng/mL men <10 ng/mL women 1–5 pg/mL	Used to evaluate growth hormone excess or deficiency. Increased values indicate acromegaly.	The client must be fasting, well rested, and not physically or emotionally stressed.
Water deprivation test		Increased level indicates SIADH, decreased level means diabetes insipidus.	Tell client to fast for 12 hours and to withhold fluids and smoking at midnight.
Thyroid			
Thyroid-stimulating hormone (TSH)	2–10 mcg/mL	This is the most sensitive test to evaluate thyroid function by measuring pituitary TSH secretion.	No special preparations are required.
T_3	75–220 ng/dL	Measures triiodothyronine (T_3) and	
T_4	4–12 mcg/dL	thyroxine (T_4) to evaluate thyroid function. Increased level means hyperthyroidism and decreased reflects hypothyroidism.	
Parathyroid			
Serum calcium	9–10.5 mg/dL	This test evaluates parathyroid function and calcium metabolism. It measures serum phosphate. Increased levels in both tests indicate hyperparathyroidism; decreased means hypoparathyroidism.	Fasting not required; however, is part of a chemistry panel in which fasting is required.
Serum phosphate	3–4.5 mg/dL		
Adrenal			
Cortisol	8 A.M. 5–23 mcg/dL 8 P.M. 3–13 mcg/dL	This test measures total serum cortisol, which evaluates adrenal cortex function. Levels are increased in Cushing's syndrome and decreased in Addison's disease.	Assess client for signs of physical stress and report to MD. Explain that two blood samples are drawn—one at 8:00 A.M., the other at 8:00 P.M.
Aldosterone	5–20 mg/dL upright position 8.5 mg/dL supine position	Levels are drawn to diagnose hyperaldosteronism.	Ask client to be in an upright position for 2 hours before test is drawn.
Urinary 17-ketosteroids	6–20 mg/24 hours men 6–17 mg/24 hours women	17-KS are metabolites of testosterone, which are released from adrenal cortex. Levels increase with Cushing's syndrome and decrease in Addison's disease.	Teach client about 24-hour urine collection, which must be iced or refrigerated during collection.
Pancreas			
Fasting blood glucose	70–110 mg/dL	This test measures circulating blood glucose level. Increases are seen in diabetes mellitus, acute pancreatitis; decreased level in Addison's disease.	This test is done fasting.
Glycosylated hemoglobin (Hb A1c)	2.2–4.8%	Test used to measure glucose control during the previous 3 months. Levels increased in newly diagnosed or poorly controlled diabetic. It is not used to diagnose diabetes mellitus.	No fasting is required.

TABLE 15-2

Common Laboratory Tests for Endocrine Disorders (continued)

TEST	NORMAL ADULT VALUES	EXPLANATION	NURSING IMPLICATIONS
Two-hour oral glucose tolerance test (OGTT)	<140 mg/dL	Determines the level of glucose 2 hours after drinking 75 g of glucose. Glucose level should return to pre-meal levels, but in diabetics, the level is > 200 mg/dL.	Client must drink entire 75 g of glucose and not eat anything else until blood is drawn.
Urine glucose Urine ketones	Negative Negative	Estimates the amount of glucose in urine, which should be negative. Measures ketones excreted in urine from incomplete fat metabolism. Positive result means lack of insulin or diabetic ketoacidosis.	Collect a fresh urine sample; stagnant urine may alter test results. Some drugs may interfere with both test results.
Urine test for microalbumin	0.2–1.9 mg/dL	Microalbumin is the earliest indicator for development of diabetic nephropathy. Elevated microalbumin levels increase the risk for end-stage renal disease.	Collect a fresh urine sample and send to laboratory for analysis.

For additional information about assessment techniques, see Chapter 5. ⚭ See Box 15-1 ■ for an example of an endocrine assessment.

THE OLDER ADULT

There is an unclear relationship between aging and endocrine function. Aging causes fibrosis of the thyroid gland and decreases production of T_3 (triiodothyronine), reducing the older adult's metabolic rate and contributing to weight gain. The adrenal cortex decreases in weight but the overall level of cortisol remains the same. The most common endocrine disorders in older adults include thyroid abnormalities and an increased risk for diabetes mellitus.

clinical ALERT

Fatigue, constipation, and mental impairment may be misdiagnosed as normal aging changes rather than being related to endocrine dysfunction.

DIAGNOSTIC TESTS
Laboratory Tests

To diagnose an endocrine disorder, several laboratory tests are used. Table 15-2 ■ lists these tests, their normal values, what the test measures and its significance, and any nursing implications for the test. Other nonspecific laboratory tests are done to give cues about endocrine disorders. A chemistry panel, which includes serum electrolytes such as sodium, potassium, calcium, and phosphate, and blood glucose levels monitor disease progression. For instance, serum sodium and blood glucose levels increase in Cushing's syndrome but decrease in Addison's disease. In diabetics, serum cholesterol and triglyceride levels are drawn to evaluate the risk of developing atherosclerosis.

Imaging Techniques

The imaging techniques used to diagnose endocrine disorders are noninvasive. Table 15-3 ■ summarizes these diagnostic procedures and their nursing implications.

BOX 15-1

DOCUMENTATION OF ENDOCRINE ASSESSMENT

Client: 48-year-old female has an appointment with her family physician to rule out a diagnosis of hyperthyroidism. States eats all the time but has lost 10 lbs in the past 2 months. Has a family history of Graves' disease.

Assessment Note: BP 168/90, P 110, R 26. Alert and oriented but cannot sit still, keeps fidgeting with purse. Hands visibly shake. Has difficulty focusing on interview questions. Appears exhausted. Eyeballs protrude and cannot close eyelids completely. Denies blurry vision. Patchy hair loss with thin, brittle nails noted. Skin warm, smooth, and moist. C/O heart palpitations, denies chest pain. Bowel tones hyperactive.

TABLE 15-3

Imaging Studies

TEST	EXPLANATION AND PURPOSE	NURSING IMPLICATIONS
Magnetic resonance imaging (MRI)	MRI uses a super magnet and radio-frequency signals to elicit a response from hydrogen nuclei. As a result, tumors of the pituitary gland and hypothalamus can be identified.	Assess for presence of metallic implants, because clients with metal implants cannot have an MRI. Inform client of the need to lie motionless during the test. Be sure all metal objects are removed because the magnetic field can be injurious to anyone within the field.
Computed tomography (CT) scan	Specialized radiographic procedures that produce computer-generated images with significantly more detail that standard x-rays allow. May be done with or without contrast media. Abdominal CT is used to detect tumors of the adrenal gland and pancreas.	If contrast dye used, ask about allergies to iodine and seafood. Client must lie still during the procedure.
Thyroid scan	Iodine-125 is injected IV. A scanner passes over the thyroid making a graph of the radiation emitted. "Cold spots," which do not take up the I-125, indicate malignancy.	Ask about allergies to iodine and seafood. Client may need to withhold thyroid drugs or medications containing iodine for weeks before the study. No fasting is needed.
Radioactive iodine (RAI) uptake test	Iodine-131 or I-125 (capsule or liquid form) is given, then the thyroid is scanned three times. Increased uptake indicates Graves' disease; decreased means hypothyroidism.	Client fasts for 8 hours before the test but can eat 1 hour after radioiodine capsule or liquid has been taken. Thyroid drugs or medications containing iodine are held for weeks before the study.

Note: The bibliography listings for this and all chapters have been compiled at the back of the book.

Chapter Review

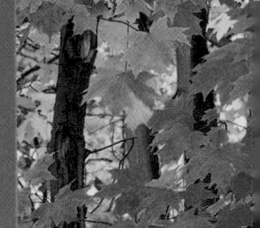

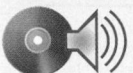 **KEY TERMS** by Topics

Use the audio glossary feature of either the CD-ROM or the Companion Website to hear the correct pronunciation of the following key terms.

Structure and function
hormones, hyperglycemia, hypoglycemia, gluconeogenesis, glycogenolysis

Assessment
exophthalmos

KEY Points

- The endocrine system consists of six major organs, anterior and posterior pituitary, thyroid, parathyroids, adrenal medulla and cortex, pancreas, gonads. The pituitary gland is considered the "master gland" because its hormones regulate numerous body functions.

- Hormone regulation throughout the body is done through a process called negative feedback.

- Blood glucose homeostasis is maintained by the actions of insulin and glucagon.

- Manifestations of endocrine disorders are often nonspecific, making assessment of the endocrine system more difficult.

- Older adults are more prone to thyroid disorders and diabetes mellitus.

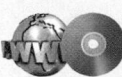 **EXPLORE Media**Link

Additional interactive resources for this chapter can be found on the Companion Website at www.prenhall.com/burke. Click on Chapter 15 and "Begin" to select the activities for this chapter.

For chapter-related NCLEX-style questions and an audio glossary, access the accompanying CD-ROM in this book.

FOR FURTHER Study

For additional information about assessment techniques, see Chapter 5.

See Figure 7-15 for an illustration of a positive Chvostek's sign and Trousseau's sign.

More details about the gonads are presented in Chapters 34 and 35.

NCLEX-PN® Exam Preparation

1 Which one of the following hormones is responsible for promoting water retention by the kidneys?
   A. antidiuretic hormone (ADH)
   B. adrenocorticotropic hormone (ACTH)
   C. epinephrine
   D. aldosterone

2 The nurse is teaching the client about a scheduled thyroid scan. Which of the following points should be emphasized to the client?
   A. "You should fast for eight hours before this test is done."
   B. "It is important to lie very still while the contrast dye is being injected."
   C. "The radioactive dye is harmless to you."
   D. "Two blood samples will be drawn, one in the morning and the other in the evening."

3 When collecting data on a client suspected of having an endocrine disorder, the nurse should observe for which sign?
   A. Kernig's sign
   B. Turner's sign
   C. Cushing's sign
   D. Trousseau's sign

4 What diagnostic test should the nurse anticipate for a client with possible diabetes mellitus?
   A. water deprivation test
   B. glycosylated hemoglobin (Hb A1c)
   C. 17-ketosteroids
   D. serum cortisol

5 When a client experiences an increase in body temperature, this is the function of which endocrine organ?
   A. posterior pituitary gland
   B. pancreas
   C. adrenal medulla
   D. hypothalamus

Answers for Review Questions appear in Appendix V.

Chapter 16

Caring for Clients with Endocrine Disorders

BRIEF Outline

Disorders of the Pituitary Gland
Disorders of the Anterior Pituitary Gland
Disorders of the Posterior Pituitary Gland

Disorders of the Thyroid Gland
Hyperthyroidism
Hypothyroidism

Disorders of the Parathyroid Glands

Disorders of the Adrenal Gland
Cushing's Syndrome
Addison's Disease

Disorders of the Adrenal Medulla

LEARNING Outcomes

After completing this chapter, you will be able to:

- Describe the pathophysiology of the common disorders of the pituitary, thyroid, parathyroid, and adrenal glands.
- Contrast the manifestations resulting from hypersecretion and hyposecretion of the hormones from the pituitary, thyroid, parathyroid, and adrenal glands.
- Identify laboratory and diagnostic tests used to diagnose endocrine disorders.
- Discuss the nursing implications for medications and treatments ordered for clients with endocrine disorders.
- Identify the preoperative and postoperative nursing care for a client undergoing either a subtotal thyroidectomy or an adrenalectomy.
- Use the nursing process to care for clients with disorders of the pituitary, thyroid, parathyroid, and adrenal glands.
- Reinforce teaching guidelines for clients receiving long-term hormonal replacement therapy.

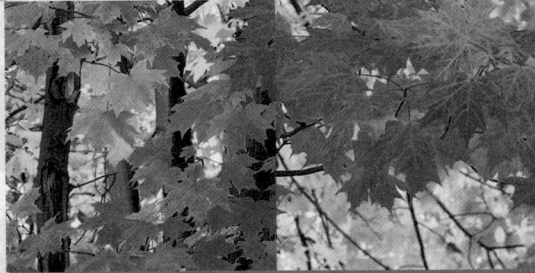

MediaLink

www.prenhall.com/burke
Use the address above to access the free, interactive Companion Website created for this textbook. Get hints, instant feedback, and textbook references to chapter-related NCLEX-style questions. Link to other interesting sites.

Audio Glossary:
Use the Companion Website, or the CD-ROM disk enclosed with your textbook, to hear the pronunciation of key terms in this chapter.

The primary function of the endocrine system is to regulate the body's internal environment. Hormones secreted by endocrine glands regulate growth, reproduction and sex differentiation, metabolism, and fluid and electrolyte balance. The endocrine system helps the body adapt to constant changes in the internal and external environment.

When *hypersecretion* (increase) or *hyposecretion* (decrease) in hormone production occurs, individuals develop an endocrine disorder. Clients with endocrine disorders require care for multiple problems. They often face exhausting diagnostic tests, changes in physical appearance and emotional responses, and permanent alterations in lifestyle. Nursing care focuses on meeting physical and emotional needs and providing education and emotional support for the client and family.

DISORDERS OF THE PITUITARY GLAND

The pituitary gland's hormones affect the thyroid, adrenal cortex, ovary, uterus, mammary glands, testes, and kidneys. Disorders result from an excess or deficient production of one or more of the pituitary hormones.

Disorders of the Anterior Pituitary Gland

Hyperpituitarism (hyperfunction of the pituitary gland) is characterized by excess production and secretion of one or more of its hormones. It most commonly causes oversecretion of growth hormone (GH). **Hypopituitarism** (hypofunction of the anterior pituitary gland) results in a lack of production of one or more of the gland's hormones. Pituitary tumors usually cause both conditions.

PATHOPHYSIOLOGY

Growth hormone, produced by the anterior lobe of the pituitary gland, stimulates the growth of the epiphyseal plates of the long bones and is necessary for skeletal and muscle growth. Excess secretion of GH before puberty and the closure of the epiphyseal plates results in *gigantism*. A person with gigantism becomes abnormally tall, often over 7 feet, but body proportions are normal. This condition is rare today due to early diagnosis and treatment. *Dwarfism* (short stature) occurs from inadequate production of GH during childhood. Usually the dwarf has normal body proportions and intelligence.

Acromegaly (enlargement of bones and connective tissue) develops during adulthood from hypersecretion of GH. Usually, a benign, slow-growing tumor (pituitary adenoma) stimulates the hypersecretion. Because epiphyseal plates close by adulthood, long bones cannot increase in length. However, other bones and connective tissue continue to grow at a very slow rate causing an enlarged forehead and protruding jaw. Overgrowth of tissue in the hands and feet causes clients to buy larger shoes, gloves, and rings. Manifestations can take as long as 10 to 15 years to develop.

INTERDISCIPLINARY CARE

Diagnosis is confirmed by magnetic resonance imaging (MRI) and computed tomography (CT) scans, which show pituitary gland enlargement along with elevated serum growth hormone levels. Acromegaly, caused by a pituitary adenoma, is treated by **transsphenoidal hypophysectomy** (surgical removal of the pituitary gland through an incision in the roof of the mouth) or irradiation of the pituitary tumor. Drug therapy with bromocriptine mesylate (Parlodel) may decrease growth hormone production but does not reduce tumor size.

NURSING CARE

Nursing care of clients with anterior pituitary disorders focuses on helping them cope with body image changes and with anxiety about an unknown future following surgery. (See Chapter 38 ⊂⊃ for nursing care following cranial surgery.) Clients should be taught about the need for lifelong hormone replacement therapy.

Disorders of the Posterior Pituitary Gland

Disorders of the posterior pituitary are caused by too much or too little antidiuretic hormone (ADH). ADH regulates total body water by acting on the kidney to retain or release water. Receptors in the hypothalamus control the release of ADH in response to serum **osmolarity** (concentration of particles in the blood). When serum osmolarity increases (*hyperosmolarity*), ADH secretion increases, and renal water is reabsorbed, which decreases urine output. *Hyposmolarity* suppresses the release of ADH, so urine output increases.

DIABETES INSIPIDUS

Diabetes insipidus (DI) is a condition that results from ADH insufficiency. There are two types: neurogenic and nephrogenic. *Neurogenic DI* can result from damage to the pituitary gland following head injury or cranial surgery. *Nephrogenic DI* occurs when the kidneys fail to respond to ADH secretion. This condition may be due to renal failure.

Deficient supply of ADH causes a urinary output of 5 to 15 liters per day. The client develops *polydipsia* (excessive

> **BOX 16-1**
>
> ### MANIFESTATIONS OF DIABETES INSIPIDUS
>
> - Extreme thirst
> - Polyuria (5–15 L/day)
> - Urine specific gravity < 1.005
> - Very pale urine
> - Weakness
> - Dehydration:
>   - Tachycardia
>   - Poor skin turgor
>   - Dry mucous membranes

thirst). If unable to replace the water loss, the client becomes dehydrated. Additional manifestations are listed in Box 16-1 ■.

INTERDISCIPLINARY CARE

Neurogenic diabetes insipidus is treated by giving additional fluids by mouth or 0.45% normal saline intravenous infusions to replace the lost water. In addition, clients may be given ADH replacement therapy with aqueous vasopressin (Pitressin) or desmopressin (DDAVP). Sodium restriction and thiazide diuretics may be ordered for clients with nephrogenic DI.

NURSING CARE

Priorities in Nursing Care. Nursing care for the client with diabetes insipidus focuses on managing fluid and electrolyte problems.

Deficient Fluid Volume Related to Deficiency of ADH

- Monitor intake and output, urine specific gravity, vital signs, skin turgor, and neurologic function every 1 to 2 hours during the acute phase. Monitor daily weight. *Frequent monitoring alerts the nurse to potential complications.*
- Provide adequate fluids. Be sure client is alert and can reach them. *Client needs to drink extra fluids to reduce or prevent dehydration.*
- Give vasopressin or DDAVP as ordered. *Vasopressin is given IM or SQ. DDAVP is given via nasal spray to replace low ADH levels in neurogenic DI. Monitor for side effects of pounding headache and abdominal cramps.*
- Give thiazide diuretics and low-sodium diet as ordered. *These methods are used to treat nephrogenic DI.*

CONTINUING CARE

Teach the client with DI about the disease process, medications, and the need for follow-up care. Instruct clients who

> **BOX 16-2**
>
> ### MANIFESTATIONS OF SYNDROME OF INAPPROPRIATE ADH (SIADH)
>
> - Headache
> - Anorexia
> - Muscle weakness
> - Decreased urine output
> - Dark yellow, concentrated urine
> - Urine specific gravity > 1.030
> - Weight gain without edema

need long-term ADH replacement therapy in how to self-administer DDAVP intranasally. Teach them the manifestations of water excess from an overdosage of DDAVP.

SYNDROME OF INAPPROPRIATE ADH SECRETION

Syndrome of inappropriate ADH secretion (SIADH) is a condition that results from excess production of ADH. This disorder may be caused by lung tumors, head injury, pituitary surgery, or the use of barbiturates, anesthetics, or diuretics.

Excess production of ADH leads to water retention, hyponatremia (low serum sodium levels), and serum hyposmolarity (excess dilution of the blood). The common manifestations of SIADH are decreased urine output and concentrated urine. Neurologic symptoms appear as brain cells swell. No edema is present because water is distributed between the intracellular and extracellular spaces. Manifestations are found in Box 16-2 ■.

> **clinical ALERT**
>
> Older adults are at an increased risk for developing hyponatremia. Because geriatric clients take many medications and have decreased kidney function, they should be monitored carefully for signs of SIADH.

Interdisciplinary Care

SIADH is treated by correcting the underlying cause and limiting fluid intake. Diuretics such as furosemide (Lasix) are given along with fluid restriction. Clients with severe hyponatremia may receive intravenous hypertonic saline.

NURSING CARE

Excess Fluid Volume Related to Excess Production of ADH

- Monitor intake and output, vital signs, and level of consciousness frequently. *Frequent monitoring alerts the nurse to potential complications.*

- Monitor daily weight and auscultate lungs. *These measures detect the presence of excess fluid buildup.*
- Restrict fluids as ordered. *Fluid restriction prevents further dilution of the plasma and sodium levels.*
- Provide frequent mouth care. *Oral rinses or sucking on hard candy keeps mucous membranes moist.*
- Give diuretics as ordered. *Diuretics will help to decrease fluid volume excess.*
- Institute seizure precautions. *Dangerously low serum sodium levels can lead to seizures.*

CONTINUING CARE

Teach clients with SIADH about the disease process, and the importance of maintaining water restriction at home. They must know how to weigh themselves daily, and they should learn the number of milliliters of fluid in common beverage containers and how to measure urine output. Discuss medication action and side effects as needed, and stress the need for follow-up care.

DISORDERS OF THE THYROID GLAND

Increased or decreased production of thyroid hormone (TH) affects the cardiovascular, gastrointestinal, and neuromuscular systems as well as the metabolic rate. Hyperthyroidism and hypothyroidism are among the most common endocrine disorders.

Hyperthyroidism

Hyperthyroidism (**thyrotoxicosis**) is caused by an excess production of thyroid hormone. It develops more often in women and older adults. The main disorders are Graves' disease and thyrotoxic crisis.

PATHOPHYSIOLOGY AND MANIFESTATIONS

Hyperthyroidism is caused by an autoimmune response, by very large doses of thyroid medication, or by excess secretion of thyroid-stimulating hormone from the pituitary gland. Whatever the underlying cause, increased levels of thyroid hormone increase the metabolic rate. As individuals age, the increased metabolic rate places a strain on the cardiovascular system. If left untreated, this condition can result in cardiac dysrhythmias and eventual heart failure. With increased metabolism of carbohydrates, proteins, and lipids, the person has an increased appetite, yet loses weight. If the condition is prolonged, nutritional deficiencies occur. The multisystem manifestations of hyperthyroidism are shown in Figure 16-1 ■.

Graves' Disease

Graves' disease, the most common cause of hyperthyroidism, is an autoimmune disorder. It develops 10 times more often in women under the age of 40 than in the general population.

Increased production of TH results in a characteristic enlargement of the thyroid gland (Figure 16-2 ■) and *exophthalmos* (Figure 16-3 ■). Often, the sclera is visible above the iris. The upper lids may be retracted, and the person has a characteristic unblinking stare. Exophthalmos is

usually bilateral, but it may involve only one eye. Inability to close the eyelids completely over the protruding eyeballs increases the risk of corneal dryness, infection, and ulceration. The treatment of Graves' disease does not reverse these eye changes.

Thyrotoxic Crisis

Thyrotoxic crisis (thyroid storm) is an extreme state of hyperthyroidism but is rare today. This disorder may result from untreated hyperthyroidism, infection, diabetic ketoacidosis, physical or emotional trauma, or thyroid surgery. Thyroid crisis is a life-threatening condition and requires immediate medical attention.

Oversecretion of TH results in a sudden, rapid rise in metabolic rate. Manifestations include high fever ($>102°F$), tachycardia, and hypertension. Restlessness and tremors are common, progressing to confusion, delirium, coma, and seizures.

Rapid treatment of thyroid crisis is essential to preserve life. The client is admitted to the intensive care unit for close monitoring and treatment. Antithyroid medications such as propylthiouracil (Propyl-Thyracil) are given to reduce thyroid hormone production. An external cooling blanket and acetaminophen are used to lower the severe hyperthermia. Cardiovascular and respiratory status is monitored closely throughout treatment.

clinical ALERT

Do not give aspirin during severe hyperthermia caused by thyroid crisis because it can increase thyroid hormone levels.

INTERDISCIPLINARY CARE

Treatment of hyperthyroidism focuses on reducing the production of TH and preventing or treating complications. Depending on the client's age and physical status, medications, radioactive iodine therapy, or surgery may be used.

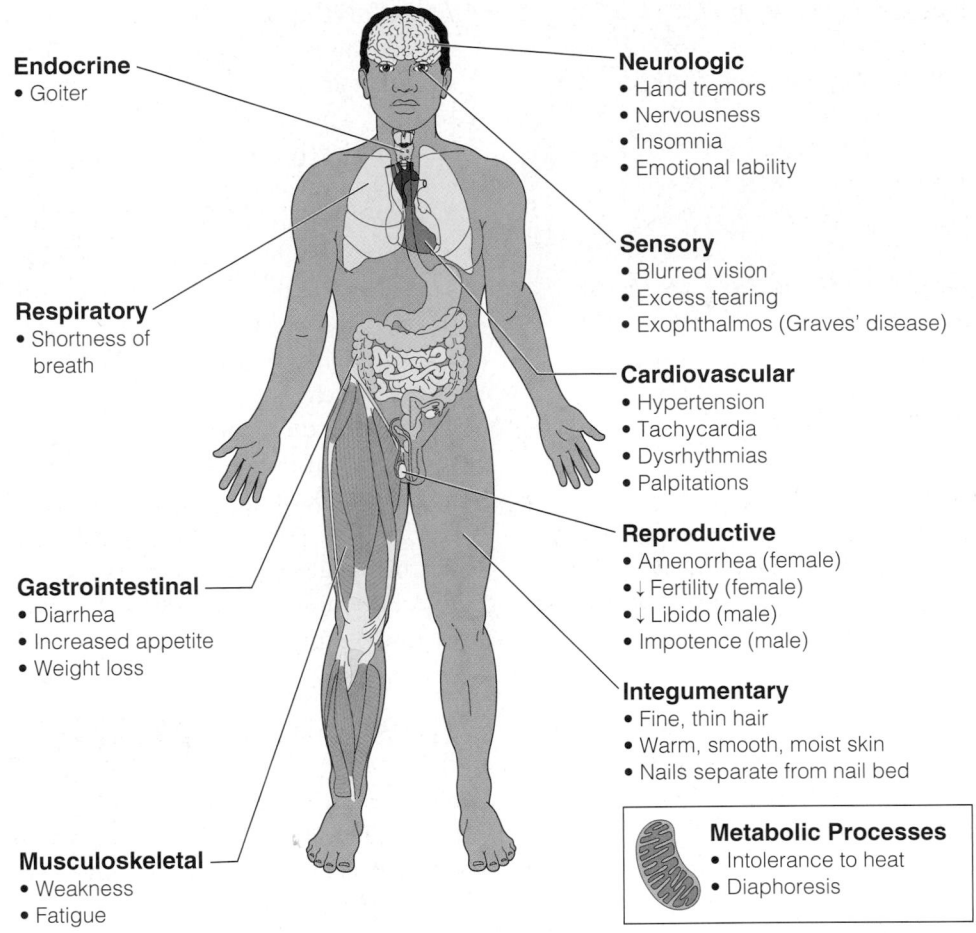

Endocrine
• Goiter

Respiratory
• Shortness of
  breath

Gastrointestinal
• Diarrhea
• Increased appetite
• Weight loss

Musculoskeletal
• Weakness
• Fatigue

Neurologic
• Hand tremors
• Nervousness
• Insomnia
• Emotional lability

Sensory
• Blurred vision
• Excess tearing
• Exophthalmos (Graves' disease)

Cardiovascular
• Hypertension
• Tachycardia
• Dysrhythmias
• Palpitations

Reproductive
• Amenorrhea (female)
• ↓ Fertility (female)
• ↓ Libido (male)
• Impotence (male)

Integumentary
• Fine, thin hair
• Warm, smooth, moist skin
• Nails separate from nail bed

Metabolic Processes
• Intolerance to heat
• Diaphoresis

Figure 16-1. ■ Multisystem effects of hyperthyroidism.

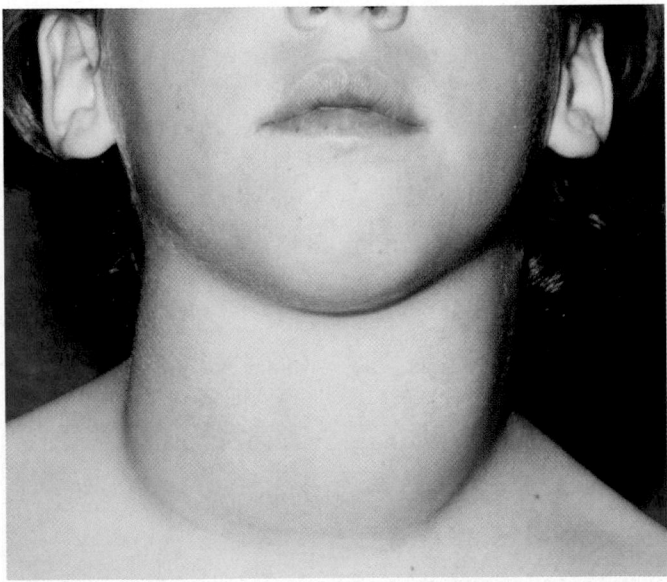

Figure 16-2. ■ Individual with enlargement of the thyroid gland (goiter). (*Source: Courtesy of Lester V. Bergman/Corbis.*)

Hyperthyroidism is diagnosed by a thorough history and physical examination. In addition, the following laboratory tests can confirm a diagnosis: elevated serum T_3 and T_4 levels, decreased TSH levels, and an increased radioactive iodine (RAI) uptake.

Medications

Antithyroid medications that reduce TH production are given to treat hyperthyroidism. Because these drugs do not affect already formed thyroid hormone, therapeutic effects may not be seen for several weeks. The commonly prescribed drugs, their actions, and nursing implications are shown in Table 16-1 ■.

Radioactive Therapy

Radioactive iodine (I-131), which is given orally, is used to destroy thyroid cells so that they produce less thyroid hormone. Treatment is done in an outpatient setting with results seen in about 6 to 8 weeks. After therapy, the client may become hypothyroid and require lifelong thyroid hormone replacement.

Elimination of radioactive iodine from the body takes about 2 to 3 days and is excreted in the urine, saliva, and

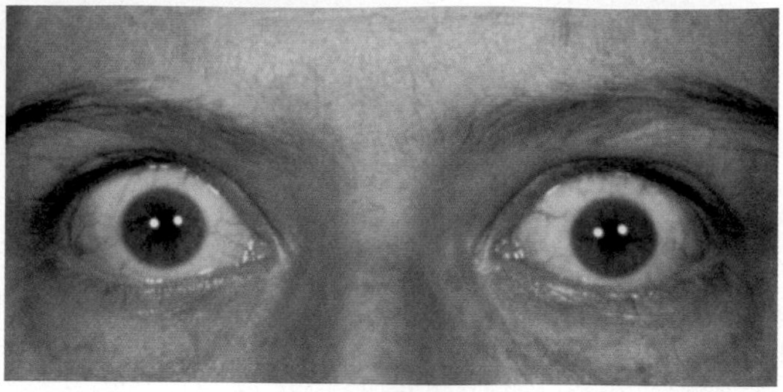

Figure 16-3. ■ Exophthalmos in a client with Graves' disease. This is caused by enlargement of muscle and fatty tissue surrounding the eye, which pushes the eyes outward. (Courtesy of NMSB, Custom Medical Stock Photos, Inc.)

feces. Because the level of radiation emitted is low, no radiation safety precautions are needed. Some clients may experience mouth and throat dryness for 2 to 3 days. Instruct them to take frequent sips of water or ice chips.

Surgery

For clients with large goiters that cause breathing or swallowing problems, and pregnant women who cannot be exposed to radiation therapy, a **subtotal thyroidectomy** (partial removal of the thyroid gland) may be indicated. This surgery leaves enough gland tissue to produce an adequate amount of thyroid hormone. A **total thyroidectomy** (complete removal)

is done to treat cancer of the thyroid, but the client requires lifelong hormone replacement. Before surgery, the client should be in as nearly a *euthyroid* (balanced thyroid) state as possible. This is done by giving antithyroid drugs to reduce hormone levels and iodine preparations to decrease the vascularity and size of the gland.

Following surgery, the client is monitored for five common complications: hemorrhage, respiratory distress, laryngeal nerve damage, tetany, and thyroid storm. The vascularity of the thyroid gland and neck tissues increases the risk of hemorrhage. Respiratory distress can develop from hemorrhage and edema, which compresses the trachea. The laryngeal nerve is located near the thyroid gland and can be damaged during surgery. The parathyroid glands are found in and near the thyroid gland. During surgery they may be damaged or removed accidentally, causing hypocalcemia and tetany. Handling of the thyroid gland during surgery may trigger thyroid storm.

Additional nursing care of the client having a subtotal thyroidectomy is discussed in Box 16-3 ■.

NURSING CARE

Nursing care focuses on the multisystem effects of the disorder. Although each client has different needs, the most common problems are imbalanced nutrition, fatigue, cardiovascular problems, visual deficits, and body image disturbance.

TABLE 16-1

Nursing Implications for Pharmacology: Hyperthyroidism

CLASS/DRUGS	PURPOSE	NURSING IMPLICATIONS	CLIENT TEACHING
Antithyroid Drugs ■ Methimazole (Tapazole) ■ Propylthiouracil (Propyl-Thyracil)	Antithyroid drugs inhibit thyroid hormone production.	Give at the same time each day to maintain stable blood levels. Monitor for itching, rash, fever, nausea, loss of taste, and agranulocytosis. Monitor for hypothyroidism: bradycardia, fatigue, weight gain.	Take at the same time each day. Do not take any drugs with iodine. Report signs and symptoms of hypothyroidism to MD. Carry Medic-Alert card stating condition and medications.
Iodine Sources ■ Potassium iodide, saturated solution (SSKI) ■ Strong iodine solution (Lugol's solution)	Inhibits TH release. Decreases vascularity of thyroid gland to make surgery safer.	Ask about allergies to shellfish. Monitor for hypothyroidism: bradycardia, fatigue, weight gain.	Take at the same time each day. Avoid drugs with iodine and limit iodine-rich foods. Dilute in milk or fruit juice.
Beta-Adrenergic Blockers ■ Propranolol (Inderal)	Relieves thyrotoxicosis, e.g., heat intolerance, palpitations, nervousness, and tremors.	Do not give to clients with asthma or heart disease. Monitor for side effects of bradycardia, fatigue, and weakness.	Teach patient how to check pulse. Notify physician of side effects: bradycardia, fatigue, and weakness.

BOX 16-3	NURSING CARE CHECKLIST

Care of the Client Having a Subtotal Thyroidectomy

Preoperative Care

☑ Review standard preop care in Chapter 9.

☑ Give ordered antithyroid medications and iodine preparations.

Postoperative Care

☑ Review standard postop care in Chapter 9.

☑ Place the client in a semi-Fowler's position; support head and neck with pillows.

☑ Monitor and report the following complications to the physician:

a. *Hemorrhage.* Assess dressing and the back of the neck for bleeding. Assess tightness of dressing. Monitor blood pressure and pulse for symptoms of hypovolemic shock.

b. *Respiratory distress.* Assess respiratory rate, rhythm, depth, and effort. Provide humidification. Have suction equipment, oxygen, and a tracheostomy set available for immediate use.

c. *Laryngeal nerve damage.* Assess for the ability to speak aloud and hoarseness.

d. *Tetany.* Assess for tingling of toes, fingers, and lips; positive Chvostek's and Trousseau's signs. Keep IV calcium gluconate or calcium chloride at the bedside.

e. *Thyroid storm.* Assess for high fever, hypertension, and tachycardia.

ASSESSING

Assessment data collected by the nurse can help determine how much hyperthyroidism is interfering with the client's life and can identify risk factors for complications (Box 16-4 ■).

DIAGNOSING, PLANNING, AND IMPLEMENTING

Priorities in Nursing Care. The nurse must consider the overall effects of hyperthyroidism when planning nursing care for the client with this disorder. The following nursing diagnoses address the most common problems.

Risk for Imbalanced Nutrition: Less than Body Requirements

■ Assess client's daily food intake. Weigh at the same time each day and report losses. *Assessing food intake determines whether food intake is adequate to meet client's needs. The body's inability to meet metabolic demands results in weight loss. Regular monitoring detects continued weight loss.*

BOX 16-4	ASSESSMENT

Assessing Clients with Hyperthyroidism

SUBJECTIVE DATA

■ Any changes in appetite, diet, or weight?

■ Any palpitations, chest pain, or shortness of breath?

■ Complaints of nervousness, fatigue, or insomnia.

■ Any vision changes?

■ Any changes in emotional status?

■ Past medical history:

• Use of thyroid hormones?

OBJECTIVE DATA

■ Blood pressure, pulse, respirations, and temperature.

■ Height and weight.

■ Observe client during interview for nervousness.

■ Assess condition of nails and hair.

■ Inspect neck for visible signs of masses.

■ Inspect eyes for signs of exophthalmos.

■ Palpate the skin for moisture.

■ Monitor and report elevated TSH, T_3, and T_4 levels

■ Encourage client to eat a high-calorie, high-protein diet in six small meals a day. *Increased metabolism causes the body to use protein for energy. Smaller, more frequent meals are easier for clients to increase their daily food intake. This diet can prevent weight loss and muscle breakdown.*

■ Teach client to avoid high-fiber foods and highly seasoned foods that increase peristalsis or cause diarrhea such as apple or prune juice. *Increased gastrointestinal (GI) action and/or diarrhea decreases nutrient absorption.*

Fatigue

The increased metabolic rate robs the client of energy. The client may be unable to perform normal activities of daily living and may have difficulty concentrating.

■ Take pulse and blood pressure before and after an activity. Note any shortness of breath. *This determines how much the client's activity is affecting the cardiovascular and respiratory systems.*

■ Provide rest periods between activity. *Rest is needed to prevent total energy depletion.*

■ Provide back rubs or cool showers as well as a cool, quiet environment. *This promotes relaxation while decreasing nervous energy. A cool, quiet environment reduces stimuli and stressors.*

Risk for Decreased Cardiac Output

■ Monitor blood pressure, pulse rate and rhythm, respiratory rate, and breath sounds. Assess for peripheral edema. *Increased heart rate and cardiac output increase the body's oxygen needs. Stress on the heart may result in hypertension, dysrhythmias, angina, and heart failure. Clients with a preexisting cardiovascular disorder are at a special risk.*

■ Teach relaxation procedures. *Stress increases circulating catecholamines, which further increase cardiac workload.*

Risk for Injury: Corneal Abrasion

If the client is unable to close the eyelids because of exophthalmos, corneal dryness may develop. Without intervention, this could lead to blurred vision or corneal ulceration.

■ Ask the client about feelings of grittiness or eye pain. Assess for incomplete lid closure. *These are signs of corneal abrasion. Prompt intervention is needed to prevent corneal ulceration and loss of visual acuity.*

■ Teach the client measures to prevent eye injury and to maintain visual acuity: using tinted glasses or shields as protection; using artificial tears to moisten the eyes; using cool, moist compresses to relieve irritation; and promptly reporting any pain or changes in vision. *These measures decrease the risk of injury, provide comfort, and decrease periorbital edema.*

clinical ALERT

Teach the client to cover or tape the eyelids shut at night if they do not close and to sleep with the head of the bed elevated.

Disturbed Body Image

Clients with hyperthyroidism often experience an altered body image due to the physical changes found with this disorder. These changes frighten both the client and family members.

■ Encourage the client to discuss feelings and to ask questions about the illness and treatment. Provide reliable information, and clarify misconceptions. *Body image is very important to clients. They need to understand what is causing the physical changes and whether they will last forever.*

■ Explain the effects of the illness on the client's physical and emotional status. *Family members can be sources of support as the client adapts to the illness. They must understand that changes in appearance and behavior may be disease related and can be controlled with treatment.*

EVALUATING

Evaluate the care for the client with hyperthyroidism by collecting data about the client's weight, energy level, resting pulse, and visual acuity. Documentation includes assessment of vital signs, weight, and relief of manifestations such as hand tremors, nervousness, weakness, and diarrhea. Identify and record the client's understanding of teaching related to medications, diet, and need for rest and sleep.

CONTINUING CARE

Clients with hyperthyroidism primarily require self-care at home. Individualized planning and teaching for home care are important nursing responsibilities. Teach clients who are taking oral medications that the condition requires lifelong treatment. After a thyroidectomy, provide information about postoperative wound care. Teach clients the importance of regular follow-up with their health care provider. When teaching, focus on the signs and symptoms of hypothyroidism and hyperthyroidism, and tell clients when to seek medical care.

NURSING PROCESS CARE PLAN
Client with Graves' Disease

Juanita Manuel is a 33-year-old mother of four small children. For the past 3 months, she has been hungry all the time and eating more than usual, but she has lost 15 lbs. Her hands shake, she can feel her heart beating rapidly, and she finds herself laughing or crying for no apparent reason.

Assessment. T, 101°F (38.3°C); BP, 162/86; P, 110; R, 24. Her skin is moist and warm, her hair thin and fine. Her eyeballs protrude, and she cannot close her eyelids completely. Her thyroid is enlarged and she has increased T_3 and T_4 levels. Mrs. Manuel is diagnosed with Graves' disease and is started on the antithyroid medication propylthiouracil, 150 mg orally every 8 hours.

Diagnosis. The following nursing diagnoses are developed for Mrs. Manuel:

■ *Risk for Imbalanced Nutrition: Less than Body Requirements* related to weight loss of 15 lbs.
■ *Risk for Injury: Corneal Abrasion* related to incomplete eyelid closure
■ *Deficient Knowledge* related to a lack of knowledge about the disease process

Expected Outcomes. The expected outcomes for the plan of care are that Ms. Manuel will:

■ Gain at least 1 lb per week.
■ Maintain normal vision and state ways to protect her eyes.
■ State medical treatment and self-care needs.

Planning and Implementation. The following nursing interventions are done for Ms. Manuel:

■ Ask her to record her weight before breakfast daily.
■ Encourage her to eat a high-calorie diet.
■ Teach Ms. Manuel how to apply artificial tears.
■ Tell her to elevate the head of her bed to 45 degrees at night, and tape eye shields over her eyes before sleep.
■ Teach her about Graves' disease, her medications, side effects, and the need for continued medical care.

Evaluation. By her next office visit, Mrs. Manuel had gained 1 lb (0.45 kg). She uses her eyedrops, wears the eye shields, and elevates the head of her bed at night. Mrs. Manuel states, "I'll always take my medicine. I never want to feel like that again!" She also says that she feels less anxious now.

Critical Thinking in the Nursing Process

1. Why are Mrs. Manuel's vital signs abnormal?
2. Why should Mrs. Manuel wear eye shields at night?
3. If Mrs. Manuel tells you that she plans to stop taking her medications, how would you respond to her?

Hypothyroidism

Hypothyroidism occurs when the thyroid gland produces an insufficient amount of thyroid hormone. It is most common in women between the ages of 30 to 60, but the incidence rises with age.

clinical ALERT

Careful evaluation of symptoms is important in the older adult because manifestations of hypothyroidism may be misdiagnosed as normal manifestations of aging.

Thyroid deficiency may be caused by congenital defects in the gland, antithyroid medications, surgical removal of the gland, or iodine deficiency. The main disorders are goiter, Hashimoto's thyroiditis, and myxedema coma.

PATHOPHYSIOLOGY AND MANIFESTATIONS

The underlying problem in hypothyroidism is failure of the thyroid gland. However, certain drugs like lithium carbonate block TH synthesis and lead to hypothyroidism. Hypothyroidism has a slow onset, with manifestations occurring over months or even years. With treatment, the mental and physical symptoms rapidly reverse in clients of all ages. Unfortunately, thyroid hormone replacement may result in hyperthyroidism.

Because reduced thyroid hormone levels decrease metabolic rate and heat production, the rest of the body systems slow. Many of the manifestations are opposite of those in hyperthyroidism (Figure 16-4 ■).

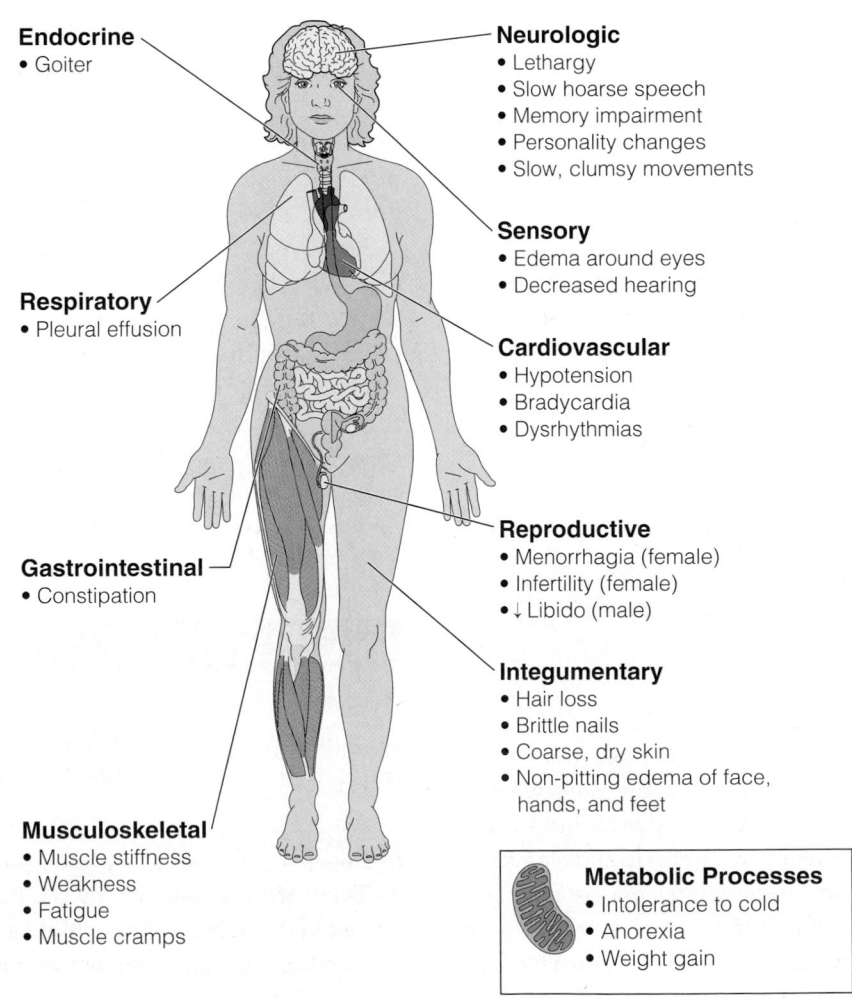

Endocrine
• Goiter

Respiratory
• Pleural effusion

Gastrointestinal
• Constipation

Musculoskeletal
• Muscle stiffness
• Weakness
• Fatigue
• Muscle cramps

Neurologic
• Lethargy
• Slow hoarse speech
• Memory impairment
• Personality changes
• Slow, clumsy movements

Sensory
• Edema around eyes
• Decreased hearing

Cardiovascular
• Hypotension
• Bradycardia
• Dysrhythmias

Reproductive
• Menorrhagia (female)
• Infertility (female)
• ↓ Libido (male)

Integumentary
• Hair loss
• Brittle nails
• Coarse, dry skin
• Non-pitting edema of face, hands, and feet

Metabolic Processes
• Intolerance to cold
• Anorexia
• Weight gain

Figure 16-4. ■ Multisystem effects of hypothyroidism.

TABLE 16-2

Nursing Implications for Pharmacology: Hypothyroidism

CLASS/DRUGS	PURPOSE	NURSING IMPLICATIONS	CLIENT TEACHING
Thyroid Preparations ■ Levothyroxine sodium (Synthroid, Levothroid) ■ Liothyronine sodium (Cytomel)	Increases blood levels of thyroid hormone. Older adults usually require lower doses when treatment is first started.	Give 1 hour before breakfast. Check pulse before giving; call MD when resting pulse > 100. Monitor for side effects of nervousness and weight loss. Monitor for bruising or bleeding if also taking anticoagulants. Check blood glucose levels closely in diabetics. Thyroid drugs alter insulin action. Report C/O chest pain or SOB immediately.	Take each morning before breakfast. Take pulse daily; call physician when resting pulse > 100. Do not take with antacids or iron preparations. Take the medication for the rest of your life. Report unusual weight loss, nervousness, bleeding, chest pain, or SOB. Diabetics need to monitor blood glucose levels. You may need to change insulin dose. Carry Medic-Alert card.

Goiter

When TH production decreases, the thyroid gland enlarges in an attempt to produce more hormone. This enlargement is called a **goiter** (see Figure 16-2). Because iodine is necessary for TH synthesis and secretion, iodine deficiency can result in hypothyroidism. The use of iodized salt has reduced this risk in the United States.

Hashimoto's Thyroiditis

The most common cause of primary hypothyroidism is Hashimoto's thyroiditis. It is classified as an autoimmune disorder because antibodies destroy thyroid tissue. The primary manifestation is the presence of a goiter. It is more common in women between 30 and 50 years old and those with a family history of thyroid disease.

Myxedema Coma

Myxedema coma is a life-threatening form of hypothyroidism requiring immediate medical attention. It may be brought on by exposure to cold temperatures, infection, surgery, trauma, or use of central nervous system depressants (especially narcotics and tranquilizers). This crisis occurs most often in the winter months. Myxedema coma develops frequently in older adults after the age of 60.

The client presents with seizures, lethargy quickly progressing to coma, and hypothermia. Without adequate thyroid hormone, the respiratory and cardiovascular systems shut down, causing bradycardia and decreased respiratory rate. The precipitating cause must be identified immediately to prevent the high mortality rate. Treatment focuses on maintaining a patent airway; stabilizing cardiac function; improving

ventilation; and increasing temperature and TH levels by giving intravenous thyroid hormone (levothyroxine).

INTERDISCIPLINARY CARE

The medical treatment of the client with hypothyroidism focuses on diagnosis, prevention or treatment of complications, and replacement of the deficient thyroid hormone.

Hypothyroidism is diagnosed by a thorough history and physical examination. The presence of hypothyroidism manifestations and a decrease in thyroid hormone, especially T_4, confirms the diagnosis.

Hypothyroidism is treated with thyroid hormone. Drug therapy is started with small doses, which are gradually increased (Table 16-2 ■). When a goiter is large enough to cause respiratory difficulties or dysphagia, a subtotal thyroidectomy may be performed (see Box 16-3).

NURSING CARE

Hypothyroidism affects all organ systems. Nursing care focuses on the most common problems: hypothermia, constipation, activity, and disturbed thought processes.

ASSESSING

Assessment data collected by the nurse can help determine the extent to which hypothyroidism is interfering with the client's life and can identify risk factors for complications (Box 16-5 ■).

BOX 16-5	ASSESSMENT

Assessing Clients with Hypothyroidism

SUBJECTIVE DATA
- Any weight gain or constant constipation?
- Complaints of muscle or joint pain, intolerance to cold, or headaches?
- Any change in memory, attention span, personality?
- Past medical history:
  - Any preexisting goiter?
  - Use of thyroid hormones?

OBJECTIVE DATA
- Blood pressure, pulse, respirations, temperature.
- Height and weight.
- Observe client during interview for sluggishness, memory lapses, decreased attention span, and hoarse voice.
- Inspect neck for visible signs of masses.
- Palpate the skin for dryness and presence of edema.
- Auscultate heart for irregularities and bradycardia.
- Auscultate bowel sounds; decreased bowel sounds indicate decreased peristalsis.
- Monitor and report decreased TSH, T_3, and T_4 levels.

DIAGNOSING, PLANNING, AND IMPLEMENTING

Priorities in Nursing Care. With decreased thyroid levels, care of the client with hypothyroidism focuses on managing the following nursing diagnoses: Hypothermia, Constipation, Activity Intolerance, and Disturbed Thought Processes.

Hypothermia

- Provide extra clothing and blankets to client. *Clients with hypothyroidism often complain of feeling cold. Extra clothing and blankets will increase the client's comfort.*
- Increase room temperature to avoid chilling; avoid drafts. *Chilling increases metabolic rate and puts increased stress on the heart. Warming the room promotes the client's comfort.*

Constipation

- Increase fluid intake to 2,000 mL per day and provide low-calorie liquids. *Reduced appetite, food intake, activity level, and peristalsis contribute to the development of constipation. Adequate fluids are necessary to maintain soft stool.*
- Provide a high-fiber diet. *Diets high in fiber increase fecal mass and assist moving feces through the intestines.*
- Encourage activity as tolerated. *Activity stimulates peristalsis.*
- Give stool softeners and/or laxatives as ordered. *These stimulate bowel elimination, but their use should be limited.*

Activity Intolerance

- Monitor blood pressure, pulse rate and rhythm, and respiratory rate before, during, and after activity level. *Thyroid hormone deficit reduces cardiac and respiratory function. Symptoms of cardiac stress include dyspnea, chest pain, palpitations, and dizziness.*
- Alternate activity with rest periods. Ask the client to report any breathing difficulties, chest pain, heart palpitations, or dizziness. *Activity increases demands on the heart and should be balanced with rest, which decreases oxygen demands.*
- Assist client with activities of daily living (ADLs). *Meeting the needs of the client promotes comfort and well-being.*

Disturbed Thought Processes

- Reorient the client frequently; keep calendar and clock in the room. *Hypothyroidism may slow intellectual processes. Decreased cardiac output reduces cerebral blood flow, resulting in impaired memory. These measures provide orientation to time and day.*
- Remove clutter from room. *Deficiency in thyroid hormone produces clumsy movements. Clutter increases risk for injury.*
- Check on client during the night. *Ensures client safety when they are disoriented.*
- Repeat information as needed. *This allows the client more time to understand the information.*
- Explain to family the relationship between the personality changes and hypothyroidism. *Family will be better able to cope with the client's changes if they understand the reasons.*

EVALUATING

Evaluate the care for the client with hypothyroidism by collecting data about the client's elimination patterns, ability to perform ADLs, temperature, and pulse. Determine the client's understanding of medications, diet, and need for rest and sleep. Documentation includes assessment of vital signs, weight, and relief of manifestations such as hand tremors, nervousness, weakness, and diarrhea. Record effectiveness of client teaching related to medications, diet, and need for rest and sleep.

CONTINUING CARE

The lifelong care required for clients with hypothyroidism can be accomplished at home. Teach the client and family about self-care, compliance with lifelong prescribed medications, and the need for regular follow-up with a health care provider. The older adult may need referrals to social services or community health services, especially if home support is not available.

Because the client may have disturbed thought processes, be sure to include the family in any teaching sessions and to provide written instructions. Instruct them about the signs and symptoms of hypothyroidism, hyperthyroidism, and myxedema coma. Teach the importance of a high-fiber, low-calorie diet with adequate fluid intake. Emphasize the need to balance rest and physical activity, and to avoid extreme cold temperatures and people with infections. Provide instruction about thyroid preparations as presented in Table 16-2.

Cancer of the Thyroid

Although thyroid cancer is relatively rare, with an estimated rate of 23,000 new cases annually, the rate is increasing. The most consistent risk factor is exposure to external radiation to the head and neck during childhood. Thyroid cancer affects women most often between the ages of 25 and 65.

Thyroid cancer appears as a small nodule in the thyroid. If undetected, it may grow and press on the esophagus or trachea, causing difficulty in swallowing or breathing. Diagnosis is made by measuring TH levels, performing a radioisotope scan, and by needle biopsy of the nodule.

The usual treatment is subtotal or total thyroidectomy. A radical neck dissection is performed when lymph nodes are involved. Thyroid-stimulating hormone (TSH) suppression therapy with levothyroxine may be given after surgery. Radioactive iodine therapy, external radiation, and chemotherapy are additional therapeutic options. If the tumor has not metastasized, the 5-year survival rate is 96%. (See nursing care for the client with cancer in Chapter 12. ◯◯)

DISORDERS OF THE PARATHYROID GLANDS

Disorders of the parathyroid glands, hyperparathyroidism and hypoparathyroidism, are not as common as those of the thyroid gland. The main alterations in parathyroid function result in hypercalcemia and hypocalcemia. (See the Hypercalcemia and Hypocalcemia sections in Chapter 7. ◯◯)

Hyperparathyroidism

Hyperparathyroidism results from increased secretion of *parathyroid hormone* (PTH) which regulates normal serum levels of calcium. This disorder occurs frequently in older adults and is three times more common in women. It is classified as either primary or secondary. Primary hyperparathyroidism is the most common and usually results from an adenoma (tumor) in one of the parathyroid glands. Secondary hyperparathyroidism may result from chronic renal failure.

PATHOPHYSIOLOGY AND MANIFESTATIONS

The increase in PTH causes calcium to leave the bones and enter the blood, resulting in *hypercalcemia.* Excess PTH also causes excretion of phosphate leading to *hypophosphatemia.* Many clients with hyperparathyroidism are asymptomatic. When symptoms occur, they affect the musculoskeletal, renal, and gastrointestinal systems. The release of calcium and phosphorus from the bones results in bone decalcification and possible pathologic fractures. Elevated calcium levels alter neural and muscular activity, causing muscle weakness and atrophy. Kidney function is altered, leading to polyuria and renal *calculi* (stones) formation from calcium deposited in the kidney. The manifestations of hyperparathyroidism are summarized in Box 16-6 ■.

INTERDISCIPLINARY CARE

Elevated levels of serum calcium, PTH, and alkaline phosphatase confirm a diagnosis of hyperparathyroidism. Once

the diagnosis is confirmed, bone density studies are conducted to determine whether bone loss has occurred.

Treatment of hyperparathyroidism focuses on decreasing the serum calcium levels. Clients are urged to drink more than 2,000 mL per day and to increase activity. Those with acute hyperparathyroidism are given bisphosphonates such as alendronate (Fosamax) or pamidronate (Aredia) to inhibit bone resorption. Mithramycin (Mithracin), a cytotoxic agent, can reduce calcium levels within 24 to 48 hours.

The main treatment for primary hyperparathyroidism is surgical removal of the parathyroid glands caused by an adenoma. Nursing care of the client after removal of the parathyroid gland affected by the adenoma is essentially the same as that for the client having a thyroidectomy (see Box 16-3).

NURSING CARE

Priorities in Nursing Care. Care focuses on interventions related to impaired physical mobility and risk for injury due to the client's muscle weakness, and altered mentation. The client may also experience pain and altered nutrition

---

BOX 16-6

MANIFESTATIONS OF HYPERPARATHYROIDISM

- *Musculoskeletal:* chronic low back pain; pathologic fractures; muscle weakness; decreased muscle tone
- *Renal:* polyuria; renal calculi
- *Gastrointestinal:* abdominal pain; anorexia; nausea; constipation; peptic ulcers; pancreatitis
- *Cardiovascular:* dysrhythmias; hypertension
- *Central nervous system:* depression; impaired memory; psychosis; stupor; coma

intake. (Nursing care of the client with hypercalcemia is discussed in Chapter 7. ⊘)

CONTINUING CARE

Once the client's condition is stabilized, teach the client and family how to adapt his or her lifestyle at home. Consult a dietitian to discuss a calcium-restricted diet, as well as increased dietary fiber and fluid intake to prevent constipation. The client should contact the health care provider before taking any over-the-counter medications containing calcium.

Teach the client the importance of developing an exercise plan because immobility increases calcium excretion and the risk for kidney stones. Exercise is also important to maintain bone density, even with medications. Discuss safety hazards and injury prevention guidelines. Review the manifestations of hypercalcemia and hypocalcemia, and stress the importance of keeping annual appointments.

Hypoparathyroidism

Hypoparathyroidism results from inadequate secretion of PTH. The usual cause is accidental damage to or removal of the parathyroid glands during a thyroidectomy. The lack of circulating PTH causes hypocalcemia and an elevated blood phosphate level.

PATHOPHYSIOLOGY AND MANIFESTATIONS

Reduced PTH levels impair kidney regulation of calcium and phosphate. Decreased activation of vitamin D leads to lower calcium absorption by the intestines. The low calcium levels increase neuromuscular activity, especially the peripheral motor and sensory nerves.

Clients with mild hypoparathyroidism may be asymptomatic. With more acute disease, neuromuscular manifestations result. **Tetany** (a continuous spasm of muscles) is the primary symptom of hypocalcemia. In severe cases, bronchospasms, laryngeal spasms, convulsions, and even death may occur. Nursing assessments for tetany include Chvostek's sign and Trousseau's sign (see Chapter 7 ⊘). The manifestations of hypoparathyroidism are summarized in Box 16-7 ■.

INTERDISCIPLINARY CARE

Hypoparathyroidism is diagnosed by low serum calcium levels and high phosphorous levels in the absence of renal failure, an absorption disorder, or a nutritional disorder. Tetany usually occurs when serum calcium levels drop below 6 mg/dL.

The first priority for treating hypoparathyroidism is to increase calcium levels. Intravenous calcium gluconate is given immediately to reduce or prevent tetany. Because the client can develop respiratory distress, the nurse must ensure a patent airway. Conscious clients are instructed to breathe in and out of a paper bag. This rebreathing

---

> ### BOX 16-7
>
> ### MANIFESTATIONS OF HYPOPARATHYROIDISM
>
> - *Musculoskeletal:* muscle spasms and tremors, positive Chvostek's and Trousseau's signs
> - *Integumentary:* hair loss; brittle nails; dry, scaly skin
> - *Gastrointestinal:* abdominal cramps
> - *Cardiovascular:* dysrhythmias
> - *Central nervous system:* numbness and tingling in lips, hands, feet; irritability, depression, psychosis

technique increases acid levels in the blood, which temporarily stabilizes calcium levels.

clinical ALERT

Keep oxygen, suctioning equipment, and a tracheostomy set at the bedside.

The client needs a calm environment to prevent excessive neuromuscular irritability. Dim lights, reduced noise, and few visitors are recommended. If the client is at risk for seizures, pad the side rails. Placing the client near the nurses' station decreases the client's anxiety and enables the nurse to provide closer observation.

Long-term therapy includes supplemental calcium with oral calcium salts. The client needs a diet high in calcium but low in phosphorus. Vitamin D therapy is given to increase GI absorption of calcium.

NURSING CARE

Nursing care of the client with hypoparathyroidism must consider the client's risk for injury due to tetany. There may be disturbed thought processes, personality changes, and impaired memory. The client's need for a diet high in calcium must be included. (Nursing care for the client with hypocalcemia is discussed in Chapter 7. ⊘)

CONTINUING CARE

Clients with hypoparathyroidism need instruction for taking calcium and phosphate binders. Teach them the necessity of lifelong medication and follow-up care. Consult a dietitian to identify foods high in calcium and vitamin D and low in phosphorus. Milk and milk products are restricted because they contain high levels of phosphorus. More appropriate foods include spinach, soybeans, and tofu. Review the signs and symptoms of hypocalcemia and hypercalcemia with the client and family. Teach clients to wear a Medic-Alert bracelet identifying condition and medication therapy.

DISORDERS OF THE ADRENAL GLAND

Disorders of the adrenal gland involve either the adrenal cortex, which secretes cortisol and aldosterone, or the adrenal medulla, which releases epinephrine and norepinephrine. Disorders of the adrenal cortex cause physical, psychologic, and metabolic alterations that are potentially life threatening. The most common disorders are Cushing's syndrome, Addison's disease, and pheochromocytoma.

Cushing's Syndrome

Cushing's syndrome is a chronic disorder in which the adrenal cortex produces excessive amounts of the hormone cortisol. Cushing's syndrome is more common in women between the ages of 20 and 50 (Figure 16-5 ■). Several factors may lead to Cushing's syndrome: (1) adrenal tumors causing an increased production of cortisol; (2) a tumor of the pituitary gland increases adrenocorticotropic hormone (ACTH) release, which stimulates the adrenal cortex to produce cortisol; (3) chronic glucocorticoid therapy; and (4) increased release of ACTH from lung or pancreatic tumors.

PATHOPHYSIOLOGY AND MANIFESTATIONS

With excess production of glucocorticoids, there are changes in carbohydrate, protein, and fat metabolism. There are fat deposits in the abdomen, fat pads under the clavicle, a "buffalo hump" over the upper back, and a round "moon" face. Altered protein metabolism leads to muscle weakness and wasting in the extremities. As thinned skin stretches over the abdomen and buttocks, purple *striae* (stretch marks) appear. (Figure 16-6 ■). Glucose metabolism is often altered and diabetes mellitus may occur.

Decreased calcium absorption results in osteoporosis and compression fractures of the vertebrae. Mineralocorticoid release promotes sodium and water retention and potassium loss, leading to hypertension.

The inflammatory and immune responses are delayed, so there is a greater risk for infection. Increased gastric acid secretion may lead to peptic ulcers. Emotional changes range from euphoria to depression. In women, increased androgen levels cause **hirsutism** (excessive facial hair), acne, and menstrual irregularities.

Untreated Cushing's syndrome can lead to multiple complications, including hypernatremia, hypokalemia, hyperglycemia, hypertension, and heart failure. Emotional instability may progress to psychoses. Because of suppressed immunity, severe infections can become life threatening.

INTERDISCIPLINARY CARE

The treatment of Cushing's syndrome includes medication, diet, or surgery. Radiation therapy might be considered for

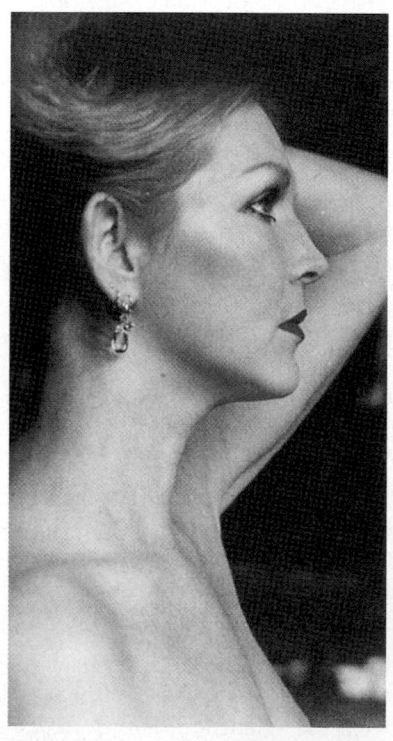 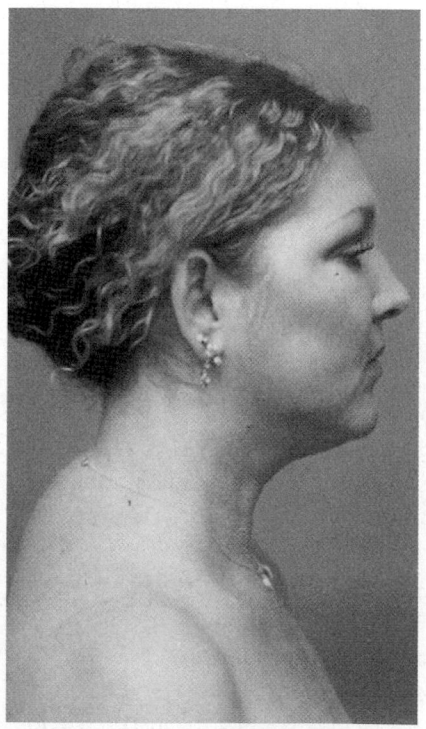

Figure 16-5. ■ A woman before and after developing Cushing's syndrome. In the photo at right, notice the swollen facial features. (*Source:* Courtesy of Dr. Charles Wilson.)

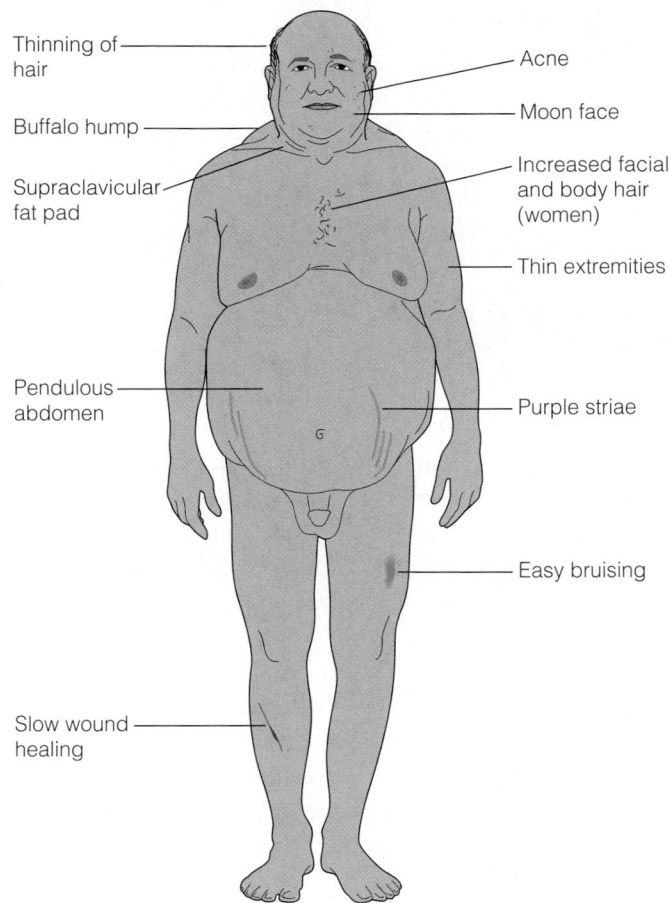

Thinning of hair

Buffalo hump

Supraclavicular fat pad

Pendulous abdomen

Slow wound healing

Acne

Moon face

Increased facial and body hair (women)

Thin extremities

Purple striae

Easy bruising

Figure 16-6. ■ Major clinical manifestations of Cushing's syndrome.

inoperable pituitary gland tumors. The most common treatment is surgery.

Diagnostic Tests

Diagnosis of Cushing's syndrome is confirmed by an increased plasma cortisol level and an elevated 24-hour urine test for 17-ketosteroids and 17-hydroxycorticosteroids. Plasma ACTH levels are elevated when Cushing's syndrome is caused by a pituitary gland tumor. Serum sodium and glucose levels are also elevated in Cushing's syndrome.

Medications

Cushing's syndrome caused by inoperable pituitary or adrenal tumors is treated with medications. Although the drugs control symptoms, they do not cure the disorder. Commonly prescribed drugs include:

- Mitotane (Lysodren)—suppresses activity of the adrenal cortex
- Metyrapone and aminoglutethimide (Cytadren)—inhibit cortisol synthesis by the adrenal cortex.

Clients receiving any of these medications should be monitored closely for side effects of decreased adrenal function, such as anorexia, nausea, vomiting, and diarrhea. They may also cause more serious adverse effects, including hypotension and tachycardia.

Surgery

When an adrenal cortex tumor causes Cushing's syndrome, an *adrenalectomy* may be done. Usually, only one adrenal gland is involved. Removal of both glands, a bilateral adrenalectomy, requires the client to take lifelong corticosteroid and mineralocorticoid replacement therapy. Following an adrenalectomy, the client is cared for in the intensive care unit because of the risk for Addisonian crisis, also known as adrenal crisis.

Surgical removal of the pituitary gland (*hypophysectomy*) is indicated when Cushing's syndrome is the result of a pituitary tumor. (Nursing care for the client having cranial surgery is discussed further in Chapter 38. ⬤⬤)

Radiation Therapy

Radiation therapy is used in clients with an inoperable pituitary tumor causing Cushing's syndrome. Radioactive isotopes may be implanted into the pituitary gland. If the pituitary gland is destroyed, lifelong replacement of pituitary hormones is necessary.

NURSING CARE

The nurse caring for the client with Cushing's syndrome must consider a wide variety of problems. The most common problems are related to fluid and electrolyte balance, injury, infection, and body image. (For additional information about clients with alterations in fluid and electrolyte balance, see Chapter 7. ⬤⬤)

ASSESSING

The nurse must collect assessment data to determine the extent to which Cushing's syndrome is interfering with the client's life. Assessment also identifies risk factors for complications (Box 16-8 ■).

DIAGNOSING, PLANNING, AND IMPLEMENTING

Clients with Cushing's syndrome may need both acute and chronic interventions. When the client is acutely ill, hospitalization may be needed. The priority problems during acute illness include Excess Fluid Volume, Risk for Injury, and Risk for Infection. During the chronic phase, the nurse focuses on client teaching for self-management at home.

Excess Fluid Volume

- Monitor daily weight, and intake and output every 8 hours. *Excess cortisol secretion causes sodium and water retention, which leads to fluid volume excess and weight gain. Body weight and intake and output are accurate indicators of fluid status.*

BOX 16-8	**ASSESSMENT**

Assessing Clients with Cushing's Syndrome

SUBJECTIVE DATA

- Present health status.
- Any changes in weight, increased facial or body hair, poor wound healing, or bruising?
- Presence of back pain, muscle weakness, or fatigue?
- Any changes in memory, ability to concentrate, or sleep patterns?
- Past medical history:
  - Any frequent infections?
  - Use of steroids?

OBJECTIVE DATA

- Vital signs: blood pressure, pulse, respirations, temperature.
- Height and weight.
- Observe client during interview for general body appearance, memory lapses, decreased ability to concentrate.
- Assess for excess body hair and acne; thinning head hair.
- Inspect for thin, fragile skin; bruising; delayed wound healing; purple striae over abdomen; and edema.
- Monitor and report increased serum cortisol, glucose, and sodium levels; and urine 17-ketosteroids.

- Monitor blood pressure, rate and rhythm of pulse, respiratory rate, and breath sounds. Assess for peripheral edema. *Sodium and water retention is manifested by hypertension and a bounding, rapid pulse. Also, there may be crackles, wheezes, and dependent edema.*

clinical ALERT

Limit fluid intake to prevent the risk of fluid overload.

Risk for Injury

The client with Cushing's syndrome has muscle weakness and fatigue, increasing the potential for accidental falls. Excess cortisol increases the likelihood of osteoporosis and risk of pathologic fractures.

- Maintain a safe environment. Keep unnecessary clutter and equipment out of the way and off the floor. Ensure adequate lighting, especially at night. *A well-lit, clutter-free environment reduces the risk of injury.*
- Encourage the client to use assistive devices for ambulation or to ask for help if needed. Encourage the use of nonskid slippers or shoes. *Encouraging the client to use assistive devices and nonslip footwear can decrease injury risk.*
- Provide rest between physical activities. *Rest conserves energy so that the client is less likely to fall from fatigue.*

Risk for Infection

- Place the client in a private room, and limit visitors. *The client with impaired immunity must avoid exposure to infection.*
- Monitor temperature, pulse, and client's feeling of well-being. *Increased temperature and pulse are systemic indicators of infection. Because Cushing's syndrome decreases the inflammatory response, the client may not show the normal manifestations of infection.*

clinical ALERT

A feeling of malaise may be the first indicator of infection.

- Use sterile technique for invasive procedures. *Aseptic technique reduces the risk of infection in the client with an impaired immune system.*
- Assess wounds for pain, color, odor, and drainage. *Excess cortisol decreases protein synthesis, causing delayed wound healing and closure.*

Risk for Impaired Skin Integrity

- Change client's position frequently. *Clients with Cushing's syndrome have thin, fragile skin, which increases the risk for tissue injury. Position changes and massage minimize pressure and improve circulation to keep skin intact.*
- Use mild soap, dry gently and thoroughly, and apply lotion as needed. *Good hygiene promotes healthy skin to prevent bacteria from entering the body.*
- Provide protection by using pillows, pads, foam mattress, and so forth. *These measures increase circulation and reduce tissue pressure.*

Disturbed Body Image

The abnormal fat distribution, moon face, buffalo hump, striae, acne, and facial hair (in women) disrupts the way clients view themselves. They may be unable to perform usual activities because of their negative feelings about their appearance.

- Encourage the client to express feelings about the physical changes. *Understanding the disease and adapting to changes are the first steps in regaining control of one's own body.*
- Spend time with the client and listen carefully. *Each situation affects individuals differently, depending on their coping skills.*

EVALUATING

Collect the following data to evaluate the effectiveness of care for the client with Cushing's syndrome: (1) improved memory, (2) no falls or injuries, (3) normal temperature without signs of infection, (4) no skin breakdown or edema, and (5) coping with physical changes. Documentation includes assessing the client for a decrease in clinical manifestations and the response to interventions. Record client teaching about medications, safety measures at home, fluid restriction, and diet modifications.

CONTINUING CARE

The client with Cushing's syndrome requires education about self-care at home. Teach about safety measures if fatigue, weakness, and osteoporosis are present. Caution the client to avoid extremes of temperature, infections, and emotional stress. Stress can lead to acute adrenal insufficiency, so it is important to teach the client signs and symptoms of urinary tract, upper respiratory, and wound infections. Also, stress the importance of contacting the physician if cuts do not heal.

Instruct the client about prescribed medications, including side effects and adverse reactions. Recommend wearing a Medic-Alert bracelet indicating the client has Cushing's syndrome and listing the medication therapy.

Provide instruction on a diet high in potassium and low in calories, sodium, and carbohydrates. Teach the client and family why fluid intake is restricted. Be sure the client and family understand and are able to perform protective skin measures. Stress the importance of regular visits to the physician.

Addison's Disease

Adrenal cortex hypofunction may be *primary* (Addison's disease) or *secondary,* from lack of pituitary ACTH. **Addison's disease** is the most common form of adrenal cortex insufficiency. It occurs most frequently in women under the age of 60.

PATHOPHYSIOLOGY AND MANIFESTATIONS

In primary Addison's disease, an autoimmune response destroys the client's own adrenal cortex. This leads to reduced levels of glucocorticoids, mineralocorticoids, and androgens. The onset of Addison's disease is slow, and manifestations develop when more than 90% of the gland is destroyed. Manifestations result from elevated ACTH levels and decreased aldosterone and cortisol (Box 16-9 ■). The primary complication of Addison's disease is addisonian crisis.

Addisonian Crisis

Addisonian crisis or adrenal crisis, is a serious, life-threatening response to acute adrenal insufficiency. Major stressors such as surgery, trauma, or severe infections usually precipitate this condition. Addisonian crisis may also occur in clients who are abruptly withdrawn from corticosteroid medications.

The client is monitored for hypotension; rapid, weak pulse; extreme weakness; and confusion resulting from circulatory collapse and shock. Potassium levels can reach

---

BOX 16-9
MANIFESTATIONS OF ADDISON'S DISEASE
■ *Integumentary:* bronze color over knuckles, knees, and elbows
■ *Musculoskeletal:* muscle weakness, joint pain
■ *Cardiovascular:* postural hypotension; weak, irregular pulse
■ *Central nervous system:* dizziness, lethargy, depression
■ *Gastrointestinal:* anorexia, nausea, vomiting, salt craving

dangerously high levels, leading to cardiac dysrhythmias. The client is managed in the intensive care unit for intravenous administration of fluids, glucose, sodium, and glucocorticoids. During the crisis stage, the client is kept warm and quiet. Once the crisis has resolved, the client requires teaching and follow-up.

INTERDISCIPLINARY CARE

The client with Addison's disease requires early diagnosis and treatment. Medical treatment involves cortisol replacement therapy, which can induce Cushing's syndrome.

Diagnostic Tests

Addison's disease is diagnosed through findings of decreased serum levels of cortisol and aldosterone, and urinary 17-ketosteroids. Potassium is increased, and blood glucose and sodium levels are decreased. CT scan and MRI may identify atrophy of the adrenal glands.

Medications

Addison's disease is treated by replacing corticosteroids and mineralocorticoids and by giving a diet high in sodium. Hydrocortisone is given orally to replace cortisol; fludrocortisone (Florinef) is given orally to replace mineralocorticoids. During a crisis such as surgery, serious illness, or trauma, increased doses of corticosteroids and mineralocorticoids are required to prevent Addisonian crisis. Nursing implications and client teaching guidelines for these drugs are presented in Table 16-3 ■.

NURSING CARE

Nursing care of the client with Addison's disease focuses on managing fluid and electrolyte problems, activity intolerance, and altered nutrition.

ASSESSING

Assessment data (Box 16-10 ■) can help determine the extent to which Addison's disease is affecting the client's life and can identify risk factors.

TABLE 16-3

Nursing Implications for Pharmacology: Addison's Disease

CLASS/DRUGS	PURPOSE	NURSING IMPLICATIONS	CLIENT TEACHING
Corticosteroids ■ Cortisone (Cortone) ■ Hydrocortisone (Cortef, Solu-Cortef) ■ Prednisone (Deltasone) ■ Dexamethasone (Decadron) ■ Prednisolone (Delta-Cortef) ■ Methylprednisolone (Solu-Medrol)	Used to replace glucocorticoids in acute and chronic adrenal insufficiency.	Give oral forms of the drug with food to reduce ulcers. Check stools for occult blood; urine for glycosuria. Report increased blood pressure, edema or weight gain, bruising, or weakness (Cushing's syndrome). Assess for impaired wound healing.	Take medications with food; report any gastric distress or dark stools. Never abruptly stop the medication. Take medications for the rest of your life. Eat a diet high in potassium, low in sodium. Weigh yourself daily; report weight gain, edema, or round face (adrenal excess). Use safety measures to avoid accidents. Wear a Medic-Alert bracelet. Avoid exposure to infection; wash hands frequently. Report adrenal insufficiency: dizziness on sitting or standing, nausea and vomiting, pain, thirst, feelings of anxiety, malaise, infections.

BOX 16-10   ASSESSMENT

Assessing Clients with Addison's Disease

SUBJECTIVE DATA

■ Present health status.

■ Describe skin color changes.

■ Presence of anorexia, nausea, vomiting, salt craving.

■ Complaints of muscle weakness, joint pain, dizziness.

■ Feelings of lethargy or depression.

■ Past medical history:

   ● Use of steroids, adrenal surgery, recent infection?

OBJECTIVE DATA

■ Vital signs: blood pressure (standing and sitting), pulse, respirations, temperature.

■ Height and weight.

■ Observe client during interview for lethargy or depression.

■ Test muscle strength.

■ Inspect exposed skin for bronze color.

■ Auscultate pulse for irregularities.

■ Monitor and report decreased serum cortisol, glucose, and sodium levels; and increased potassium levels.

DIAGNOSING, PLANNING, AND IMPLEMENTING

Priorities in Nursing Care. Clients with Addison's disease may require acute and chronic interventions. Acutely ill clients need immediate hospitalization. Nursing care focuses on restoring fluid and electrolyte balance and increasing nutritional intake. During the chronic phase, the client needs support and teaching to manage the disease.

Deficient Fluid Volume

In the client with Addison's disease, fluid volume deficit results from loss of water and sodium often caused by vomiting and diarrhea. During the crisis phase, acute volume deficit may lead to hypotension and hypovolemic shock.

■ Monitor intake and output, and assess for signs of dehydration (dry mucous membranes; thirst; poor skin turgor; sunken eyeballs; scanty, dark urine; and weight loss). *Glucocorticoid and mineralocorticoid depletion causes fluid volume deficit.*

■ Monitor blood pressure (lying, sitting, standing) and strength of peripheral pulses. *Fluid volume deficit may lead to hypotension and a rapid, weak, or thready pulse.*

■ Increase oral fluids to 3,000 mL per day and increase salt intake. *Fluids and sodium are given to manage the fluid volume deficit and hyponatremia characteristic of adrenal insufficiency.*

Activity Intolerance

- Keep client on bed rest and perform ADLs for client. *This prevents stimulation of an overly stressed adrenal cortex.*
- Slowly increase physical activity. *Once adrenal cortex hormones are replaced, the client will be able to regain normal physical activity.*

Imbalanced Nutrition: Less than Body Requirements

- Provide a high-calorie diet in six small meals each day. *A high-calorie diet is used to replace lost weight.*
- Auscultate bowel tones and note presence of diarrhea. *Hyperactive bowel sounds and diarrhea indicate an inability to absorb nutrients.*

EVALUATING

Collect and document the following data to evaluate the effectiveness of care for the client with Addison's disease: (1) no signs of dehydration, (2) activity level increases, and (3) increased dietary intake. Record client teaching about medications, stress reduction measures, increased fluid intake, diet modifications, and manifestations of adrenal hormone excess.

CONTINUING CARE

Educate the client and family about the need for lifelong treatment and self-care. Explain the possible complications that can result from not following the treatment plan. Teach clients that regular follow-up with the health care provider is important, and how to recognize the signs and symptoms that require medical attention.

Discuss the relationship between hormone levels and stress. Teach clients and families how to adjust medication doses during times of physical and emotional stress. Instruct them about the manifestations of adrenal hormone excess and insufficiency.

Teach the client and family how and when to administer corticosteroids and mineralocorticoids. Stress the importance of carrying at all times an emergency kit containing parenteral cortisone and a syringe/needle. Advise the client to wear a Medic-Alert bracelet that identifies both the disease and medication therapy.

Remind the client to increase oral fluid intake and to maintain a diet high in sodium and low in potassium. Stress the importance of not skipping meals.

DISORDER OF THE ADRENAL MEDULLA

Pheochromocytoma is a benign tumor of the adrenal medulla. It occurs in adults between 40 and 50 years old. The tumor erratically produces excessive amounts of catecholamines (epinephrine or norepinephrine), which stimulate the sympathetic nervous system. This leads to a dramatic rise in the systolic blood pressure of 200 to 300 mm Hg and a diastolic greater than 150 mm Hg. Additional symptoms include pounding headache, tachycardia, profuse sweating, flushing, and palpitations. If untreated, this can lead to such life-threatening conditions as myocardial infarction and stroke.

A pheochromocytoma is diagnosed by increased catecholamine levels in the blood or urine, CT scan, and MRI.

Surgical removal of the tumor(s) by adrenalectomy is the treatment of choice.

Nursing care during the acute attack and prior to surgery focuses on stabilizing the client's blood pressure. The client is admitted to the intensive care unit, where constant hemodynamic monitoring and intravenous antihypertensive medications are instituted. Following surgery, the client may require adrenal hormone replacement therapy. Sometimes clients remain hypertensive and require continual follow-up.

Note: The bibliography listings for this and all chapters have been compiled at the back of the book.

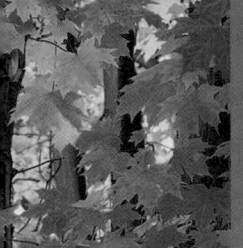

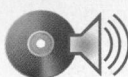 **KEY TERMS** by Topics

Use the audio glossary feature of either the CD-ROM or the Companion Website to hear the correct pronunciation of the following key terms.

Pituitary gland

hyperpituitarism, hypopituitarism, transsphenoidal hypophysectomy, osmolarity, diabetes insipidus

Thyroid gland

thyrotoxicosis, thyrotoxic crisis (thyroid storm), subtotal thyroidectomy, total thyroidectomy, hypothyroidism, goiter, myxedema coma

Parathyroid glands

tetany

Adrenal gland

Cushing's syndrome, hirsutism, Addison's disease, Addisonian crisis, pheochromocytoma

KEY Points

- Hyposecretion of the posterior pituitary gland can result in diabetes insipidus; hypersecretion can lead to syndrome of inappropriate ADH secretion (SIADH).

- Graves' disease is the most common disorder caused by hyperthyroidism and leads to an increased metabolic rate.

- A life-threatening form of hyperthyroidism is thyroid crisis; it requires immediate medical treatment.

- Hypothyroidism develops when the thyroid gland fails to secrete an adequate amount of thyroid hormones.

- The primary symptom of acute hypoparathyroidism is tetany as manifested by positive Chvostek's and Trousseau's signs.

- Excess production of glucocorticoid hormones by the adrenal cortex can result in Cushing's syndrome.

- Addison's disease is an acute deficiency of glucocorticoid, mineralocorticoid, and androgen hormones.

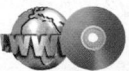 **EXPLORE Media**Link

Additional interactive resources for this chapter can be found on the Companion Website at www.prenhall.com/burke. Click on Chapter 16 and "Begin" to select the activities for this chapter.

For chapter-related NCLEX-style review questions and an audio glossary, access the accompanying CD-ROM in this book.

FOR FURTHER Study

For more information about fluids and electrolytes, hypercalcemia, hypocalcemia, and tetany, see Chapter 7.

Standard preoperative and postoperative care is covered in Chapter 9.

For more information about cancer, see Chapter 12.

For more information about the pancreas, see Chapter 17.

For more information about cranial surgery, see Chapter 38.

Critical Thinking Care Map

Caring for a Client with Hypothyroidism
NCLEX-PN® Focus Area: Psychosocial Adaptation

Case Study: Jane Lee is a 60-year-old retiree. She has gained 10 lbs (4.5 kg) in the past 6 months, even though she is rarely hungry and eats much less than normal. Diagnostic tests reveal decreased serum T_4 level and increased TSH. The medical diagnosis of hypothyroidism is made, and Mrs. Lee is started on levothyroxine 0.05 mg daily.

Nursing Diagnosis: Disturbed Body Image

COLLECT DATA

Subjective	Objective
_____	_____
_____	_____
_____	_____
_____	_____
_____	_____
_____	_____
_____	_____

Would you report this data? Yes/No

If yes, to: _____

Nursing Care

_____
_____
_____
_____
_____
_____
_____
_____
_____
_____

How would you document this? _____

_____
_____
_____

Data Collected (use those that apply)

- Rarely hungry, eats less than normal
- Yellowish, dry skin
- Eyelids will not close
- Weight gain of 10 lbs in past 6 months
- Hoarse voice
- Puffy face
- Always cold
- Slurred speech
- No energy to do housework

Nursing Interventions (use those that apply; list in priority order)

- Teach Mrs. Lee how to increase fluids and fiber in her diet.
- Recommend that Mrs. Lee join a weight reduction class.
- Provide information that helps Mrs. Lee understand why the body changes occurred from hypothyroidism.
- Teach Mrs. Lee about reversible body changes.
- Encourage her to allow her husband and daughter to help with housecleaning and cooking.
- Refer Mrs. Lee for a visual screening.

NCLEX-PN® Exam Preparation

TEST-TAKING TIP Review the basic dietary requirements for specific diseases and illnesses (e.g., high-potassium, low-calorie, low-sodium diet for the client with Cushing's syndrome). Be familiar with the types of foods that contain sodium, calcium, iodine, and other elements.

1 An assessment of your client reveals the following data: enlarged jaw, protruding brow, abnormally large hands and feet. What endocrine disorder should the nurse suspect that this client is experiencing? _____

2 In caring for a client who has had a subtotal thyroidectomy, the nurse should assess for which immediate life-threatening complication?
A. hemorrhage
B. tetany
C. dehydration
D. laryngeal nerve damage

3 A client is diagnosed as having a goiter. This condition is primarily due to:
A. hypothyroidism.
B. hyperthyroidism.
C. hypoparathyroidism.
D. hyperparathyroidism.

4 Which of the following nursing interventions should be implemented for a client with hyperparathyroidism?
A. Provide a high-calorie diet.
B. Increase the room temperature.
C. Reorient the client frequently.
D. Encourage the client to increase activity.

5 For a client diagnosed with Cushing's syndrome, which of these nursing diagnoses should be addressed on the care plan?
A. Deficient Fluid Volume
B. Activity Intolerance
C. Body Image, Disturbed
D. Constipation, Acute

6 Which one of these nursing actions is the highest priority for a client admitted with acute hypoparathyroidism?
A. Provide a quiet, dimly light room.
B. Assess for abdominal cramps.
C. Provide a diet high in calcium.
D. Assess for a patent airway.

7 Which of the following nursing implications should be used when administering potassium iodine (SSKI) to a client with hyperthyroidism? Select all that apply.
A. Do not give with an antacid.
B. Ask about allergies to shellfish.
C. Do not give to clients with asthma.
D. Monitor for itching and rash.
E. Dilute in milk or juice.
F. Monitor for bradycardia.

8 A client newly diagnosed with SIADH is preparing for discharge. Which of the following teaching points should be included in the discharge instructions?
A. Teach the client how to measure urine output.
B. Encourage the client to eat a high-protein diet.
C. Instruct the client on how to take pulse qd.
D. Teach client to avoid crowds.

9 A patient is taking Synthroid (levothyroxine sodium) for 3 months. Which evaluation would indicate a therapeutic response to this drug?
A. decreased appetite
B. decreased diarrhea
C. normal heart rate
D. weight loss of 5 lbs

10 What clinical manifestation should the nurse expect to observe in a client with Addison's disease?
A. multiple bruises
B. postural hypotension
C. peripheral edema
D. shortness of breath.

Answers for Review Questions as well as discussion of Care Plan and Critical Thinking Care Map Questions, appear in Appendix V.

Chapter 17

Caring for Clients with Diabetes Mellitus

BRIEF Outline

Overview of Diabetes Mellitus

Types of Diabetes Mellitus
Diabetes in the Older Adult
Pathophysiology
Interdisciplinary Care

Complications of Diabetes Mellitus

Acute Complications
Chronic Complications
Complementary Therapies

LEARNING Outcomes

After completing this chapter, you will be able to:

- Define diabetes mellitus, and explain the pathophysiology of type 1 and type 2 diabetes mellitus with the related manifestations.

- Identify the diagnostic tests used to diagnose and monitor self-management of diabetes mellitus.

- Discuss the nursing implications for insulin and oral antidiabetic agents ordered for clients with diabetes mellitus.

- Compare and contrast the manifestations and interdisciplinary care of hypoglycemia, diabetic ketoacidosis (DKA), and the hyperosmolar hyperglycemic state (HHS).

- Describe the pathophysiology and interdisciplinary care of chronic complications for clients with type 1 and type 2 diabetes mellitus.

- Reinforce teaching guidelines to clients with diabetes mellitus regarding self-management of medications, diet, exercise, and foot care.

- Identify specific concerns for young, middle-aged, and older adults with diabetes mellitus.

- Use the nursing process to collect data, establish outcomes, provide individualized care, and evaluate responses for the client with diabetes mellitus.

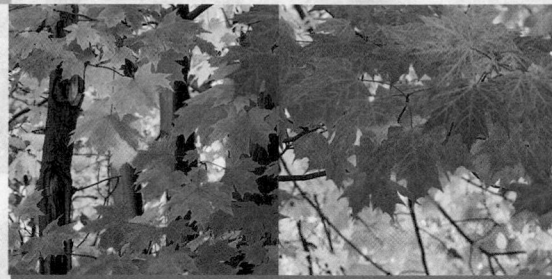

MediaLink

www.prenhall.com/burke
Use the address above to access the free, interactive Companion Website created for this textbook. Get hints, instant feedback, and textbook references to chapter-related NCLEX-style questions. Link to other interesting sites.

Audio Glossary:
Use the Companion Website, or the CD-ROM disk enclosed with your textbook, to hear the pronunciation of key terms in this chapter.

Diabetes mellitus is a common chronic disease of adults. It is not a single disorder but a group of metabolic disorders characterized by hyperglycemia (too much glucose in the blood). This condition is due to an insufficient supply of insulin, ineffective insulin action, or both.

Clients with diabetes mellitus face lifelong changes in lifestyle and health status. Depending on the type of diabetes and the client's age, client needs and nursing care may vary greatly. Nursing care is provided in many settings for the diagnosis and care of the disease and treatment of complications.

Overview of Diabetes Mellitus

The American Diabetes Association estimates that approximately 18.2 million people in the United States have diabetes. Unfortunately, 5.2 million people are undiagnosed. Approximately 1 million new cases are diagnosed each year. It is the sixth leading cause of death in the United States and more than $132 billion are spent annually on health care. Type 2 diabetes is increasing among older adults, African American women, Hispanic women, Native Americans, Asians, and Pacific Islanders. Even more alarming is the rapid increase in type 2 diabetes among children and adolescents, especially those who are obese. Diabetes mellitus cannot be cured, but it can be controlled in order to reduce complications, which most often affect the eyes, kidneys, and the nervous and cardiovascular systems.

The term *diabetes,* or *DM,* when used throughout the chapter, refers to diabetes mellitus.

TYPES OF DIABETES MELLITUS

There are two broad categories of diabetes, type 1 and type 2 (Table 17-1 ■). The type of diabetes that was known as type I diabetes mellitus, juvenile-onset diabetes mellitus, or insulin-dependent diabetes mellitus (IDDM) is now *type 1* diabetes. The type of diabetes that was known as type II non–insulin-dependent diabetes mellitus (NIDDM) or adult-onset diabetes is now known as *type 2 diabetes.*

DIABETES IN THE OLDER ADULT

Older adults may have either type 1 or type 2 DM, but most have type 2. Improved management strategies have increased the survival rates for people with type 1 DM. As older adults are living longer and the incidence of diabetes increases with age, more people over age 65 will develop DM. In addition, those older adults with diabetes tend to develop more severe chronic complications.

Complicating the problem is that over the age of 50, blood glucose levels rise. This makes it more difficult to diagnose older adults with DM. Sometimes people are mistakenly diagnosed with diabetes because they show normal aging changes. The usual physiologic changes of aging may

TABLE 17-1

Classification and Characteristics of Diabetes

CLASSIFICATION	CHARACTERISTICS
Type 1 diabetes	State of absolute insulin deficiency Usually occurs before childhood and adolescence but may occur at any age Autoimmune destruction of beta cells Client prone to developing ketoacidosis Insulin dependent *(If client does not receive insulin, he or she will die.)*
Type 2 diabetes	State of sufficient insulin to prevent ketoacidosis but insufficient to lower blood glucose levels Usually occurs after age 30 Most clients are obese May become *insulin requiring* but not insulin dependent *(If client does not receive insulin, he or she will become ill but will not die.)*
Other types	Occurs from genetic defects or associated with pancreatitis, Cushing's syndrome, infection, or chemical toxins
Gestational	Any degree of glucose intolerance with onset or first recognition of diabetes mellitus during pregnancy

Source: American Diabetes Association. (2004). Diagnosis and classification of diabetes mellitus. *Diabetes Care, 27* (Suppl.), S5–S10.

mask manifestations of a diabetes onset and may also increase the potential for complications. For instance, urinary incontinence may be confused with polyuria. Other symptoms of diabetes such as blurred vision and fatigue are blamed on age. Peripheral vascular disease related to diabetes or cardiovascular disease may be undetected until serious wound healing problems occur. Older adults often have hypertension, requiring treatment with diuretics, which impairs glucose tolerance test results.

The older adult with diabetes has multiple and complex health care problems and needs. Consider the following concerns when working with the older client:

■ Physical limitations due to arthritis and Parkinson's disease as well as confusion can interfere with food preparation, activities of daily living, insulin administration and blood glucose testing, foot care, and hygiene.
■ Lower fixed incomes and rising costs of medications, blood glucose monitoring equipment, visits to the physician, and hospitalization may be a problem. Even though Medicare pays part of the medical expenses, the client is still responsible for part of the cost.
■ Cultural background and ethnic origin may encourage a fatalistic acceptance of illness and its complications.

Chronic illness often interferes with family communication and relationships.

- Vision or hearing deficits may require the nurse to adapt teaching materials and methods.

PATHOPHYSIOLOGY

Although there are various types of diabetes mellitus, the two major types are type 1 diabetes and type 2 diabetes. Both are discussed next.

Type 1 Diabetes Mellitus

Type 1 diabetes usually occurs in children and adolescents, but it may occur at any age. Type 1 DM results from an autoimmune response, which destroys the beta cells of the islets of Langerhans in the pancreas. The end result is that insulin is no longer produced. Insulin deficiency causes **hyperglycemia** (excess glucose in the blood) and a breakdown of body fats and proteins. Without insulin to move glucose into the cells, the cells begin starving so they burn fats and protein for their energy source. During the burning of fats **ketosis** develops, a toxic accumulation of *ketone bodies* (by-products from the burning of fatty acids).

When blood glucose exceeds the level the kidneys can process, glucose spills into the urine, and **glycosuria** (excess glucose in the urine) occurs. The body's state of hyperglycemia and glycosuria cause the three primary manifestations of type 1 DM: polyuria, polydipsia, and polyphagia. Hyperglycemia acts as an **osmotic diuretic,** meaning it draws fluid from the intracellular spaces into the general circulation. This causes **polyuria** (increased urine output). The increased urinary output leads to dehydration. The mouth becomes dry, and thirst sensors are activated, causing the person to drink increased amounts of fluid (**polydipsia**).

Because glucose cannot enter the cell without insulin, energy production decreases. This decrease in energy stimulates hunger, and the person eats more food (**polyphagia**). Despite increased food intake, the person loses weight. Malaise and fatigue accompany the decrease in energy. Manifestations are listed in Box 17-1 ■.

BOX 17-1

MANIFESTATIONS OF TYPE 1 AND TYPE 2 DIABETES MELLITUS

Type 1	Type 2
Polyuria	Polyuria
Polydipsia	Polydipsia
Polyphagia	Recurrent infections
Weight loss	Obesity
Fatigue	Fatigue
Malaise	Blurred vision
	Paresthesias

Heredity plays a key role in the development of diabetes mellitus. The child of a diabetic has a 1 in 20 to 1 in 50 risk. Environmental factors may also trigger DM. Viral infections including mumps and rubella or a chemical toxin found in smoked or cured meats have been linked to type 1 DM.

Type 2 Diabetes Mellitus

Type 2 DM is characterized by hyperglycemia due to insufficient insulin production and insulin resistance. The inadequate insulin supply cannot lower blood glucose levels through the usual uptake of glucose by muscle and fat cells. However, sufficient insulin is produced to prevent the breakdown of fats; therefore, ketosis does not develop. Heredity plays an important role in its transmission. Other risk factors include obesity, increasing age, and belonging to a high-risk ethnic group.

The majority of people with type 2 DM are overweight. Obesity, especially of the upper body, reduces available insulin receptor sites in the cells of skeletal muscles and adipose tissues and leads to insulin resistance. About three-fourths of older adults with type 2 DM are overweight. All older adults with type 2 DM develop insulin resistance. Diabetics who lose weight through diet and exercise can lessen insulin resistance and improve insulin release. Sometimes insulin efficiency can improve enough so that the type 2 diabetic may no longer require oral hypoglycemic agents.

Unfortunately, type 2 diabetes is often undiagnosed for years. People are unaware of its presence until health care is sought for another problem. The hyperglycemia found in type 2 is less severe than that of type 1, so only polyuria and polydipsia are seen. Other manifestations include recurrent infections, blurred vision, fatigue, and paresthesias (see Box 17-1). Accumulated glucose in the tissues provides a breeding ground for bacterial infections. High glucose levels cause a cloudiness of the lens of the eye, leading to blurred vision, as well as destruction of peripheral nerves, resulting in paresthesias. Fatigue results from an inadequate amount of glucose being available to feed the cells.

INTERDISCIPLINARY CARE

Treatment of the client with diabetes focuses on maintaining blood glucose at levels as nearly normal as possible through medications, diet, and exercise.

Diagnostic Tests

Three laboratory tests are used to screen for the presence of diabetes mellitus: a plasma glucose (PG) level, fasting blood glucose (FBG), and an oral glucose tolerance test (OGTT). Although any of the three tests may be used, in the clinical setting the FBG is preferred because it is easier to administer, more convenient, and more economical than the other two.

Diagnostic criteria recommended by the American Diabetes Association include:

1. Classic diabetic symptoms plus *casual* plasma glucose (PG) concentration greater than 200 mg/dL (*casual* is defined as any time of day without regard to when last meal was eaten).
2. Eight-hour *fasting* plasma glucose (FPG also known as FBS) greater than 126 mg/dL (*fasting* is defined as no food or drink intake for 8 hours).
3. Two-hour PG greater than 200 mg/dL during an oral glucose tolerance test (OGTT).

It is usually recommended that the diagnostic test be repeated on a subsequent day to confirm the diagnosis of diabetes mellitus.

Because of the risk for developing multisystem complications, routine screening should be done for any person who meets one or more of the following seven risk criteria:

1. Is obese (>120% of standard body weight)
2. Has a first-degree relative with diabetes
3. Is a member of a high-risk ethnic population (e.g., African American, Hispanic American, Native American, Asian American, Pacific Islander)
4. Has delivered a baby weighing more than 9 lbs or has been diagnosed with gestational diabetes mellitus
5. Is hypertensive (>140/90)
6. Has a high-density lipoprotein (HDL) cholesterol level <35 mg/dL and/or a triglyceride level >250 mg/dL
7. On previous testing, had impaired glucose tolerance or impaired fasting glucose.

Delayed insulin release from the pancreas, decreased tissue sensitivity to insulin, or both lead to decreasing glucose tolerance in older adults. Because of these physiologic changes in persons over age 60, their fasting blood glucose levels may be slightly increased. (The diagnostic tests and normal results used to diagnose diabetes are summarized in Chapter 15, Table 15-2. 🔗)

MONITORING BLOOD GLUCOSE AND KETONES. People with diabetes must monitor their condition daily by testing glucose levels. Two types of tests are available. The first type, direct measurement of blood glucose, is widely used in all types of health care settings and in the home. The second type is urine testing for glucose and ketones. Urine testing is less common today.

Self-Monitoring of Blood Glucose. Self-monitoring of blood glucose (SMBG) allows the person with diabetes to monitor and achieve metabolic control. It is also useful when the person is ill or pregnant or has symptoms of hypoglycemia or hyperglycemia. The American Diabetes Association (ADA) recommends that all diabetics be taught some method of monitoring their blood glucose. SMBG should be done three or more times per day for diabetics taking insulin. For those who do not use insulin, testing is recommended two to three times per week.

Equipment needed for SMBG includes:

- Some type of lancet device to perform a finger stick for obtaining a drop of blood (such as an Autolet, Penlet, or Soft Touch)
- A blood glucose measuring machine (e.g., the Glucometer, the AccuChek, or the Ultra) if the most accurate measurement is desired or recommended
- Test strips that change color when they come into contact with glucose or that can be read by machine (e.g., Glucostix and Chemstrip bG). Usually, the strip is read by comparing its color with a color chart on the side of the container or on an insert.

Blood glucose monitoring machines can provide a single reading or are computerized. They can provide a memory of previous glucose readings to show a pattern of control. Each machine has specific operating instructions that must be followed closely. If the timing of the blood on the strip is not exact, the test will be inaccurate. The machine must be cleaned according to the manufacturer's directions to ensure accuracy. Monitors that use no-wipe technology improve the accuracy of glucose measurement.

A noninvasive system such as the GlucoWatch Biographer is worn as a watch. The device measures the glucose value in the client's perspiration and reports values every 10 minutes for up to 13 hours. When readings are too low or too high, an alarm sounds. Studies have shown the device to be accurate and to provide more information than the traditional finger stick.

Urine Testing for Ketones and Glucose. At one time, urine testing for glucose and ketones was the only available method for evaluating diabetic management. Although inexpensive and noninvasive, it has unpredictable results and cannot be used to detect or measure hypoglycemia.

Urine testing should be done in people with type 1 DM who have unexplained hyperglycemia during illness or pregnancy to monitor for hyperglycemia and ketoacidosis.

To test the urine for ketones:

1. Ask the client to void, discard the urine, and drink a full glass of water.
2. Thirty minutes later, collect a urine sample.
3. For Acidtest tablets: Place the tablet on a white paper towel, place one drop of urine on the tablet, and wait 30 seconds. If the tablet turns any shade from lavender to deep purple, the test is positive for ketones.
4. For Ketostix: Dip the reagent stick into the urine sample. Wait 15 seconds, and compare the color of the pad

at the end of the stick to an accompanying color chart. Purple indicates ketonuria.

To test the urine for glucose:

1. Follow the same procedure to collect a urine sample.
2. Dip the reagent stick into the urine sample, and wait the specified time. Compare the color of the pad on the end of the reagent stick with an accompanying color chart. The glucose is expressed as a percentage (for example, 1/2%, 1%, 2%).

clinical ALERT

Normally, no glucose is found in the urine, so the presence of glucose indicates hyperglycemia.

Medications

The pharmacologic treatment for diabetes mellitus depends on the type of diabetes. People with type 1 DM must have insulin; those with type 2 are usually able to control glucose levels with an oral antidiabetic medication, but they may require insulin when control is inadequate.

INSULIN. Insulin is derived from pork pancreas or made in the laboratory. Synthetically produced insulin comes either from altered pork insulin or through genetic engineering using strains of *Escherichia coli* to form a biosynthetic human insulin. Insulins are available in rapid-acting, short-acting, intermediate-acting, and long-acting preparations. (The common insulins, times of onset, peak, and duration of action are listed in Table 17-2 ■.)

TABLE 17-2

Action of Insulin Preparations

TYPE OF INSULIN	ONSET (HR)	PEAK (HR)	DURATION (HR)
Rapid-Acting			
■ Lispro (Humalog)	0.25	0.5–1.5	4–5
Short-Acting			
■ Regular	0.5–1	2–4	4–6
Intermediate-Acting			
■ NPH	1–2	6–12	18–24
■ Lente	1–3	8–12	18–24
■ Novolin NPH 70/ regular 30	0.5	4–8	Up to 24
Long-Acting			
■ Ultralente	4–6	18–24	36
■ Glargine (Lantus)	1.5	Unclear peak	24

clinical ALERT

Regular and Lantus insulins appear clear. All other insulins appear cloudy.

Insulin is dispensed as 100 U/mL (U-100 insulin) and U-500/mL (U-500 insulin). The standard concentration is 100 U/mL. U-500 insulin is only used in rare cases of insulin resistance when very large doses are needed.

Insulin is given in sterile, single-use, disposable insulin syringes, marked in units per milliliter. This means that in U-100 insulin, there are 100 U of insulin in 1 mL. Common syringe size is either 0.5 mL (50 U) or 1.0 mL (100 U). The advantage of the 0.5-mL size is that the distance between unit markings is greater so that it is easier to measure the dose accurately. Most insulin syringes are manufactured with the needle permanently attached in a 25- to 26-gauge, 0.5-inch size.

All insulins are given parenterally. Only regular insulin may be given by either subcutaneous or intravenous routes; all others are given only subcutaneously. Currently, an inhalation form of insulin is being studied.

Special Injection Products. Special injection products such as insulin pens and jet injectors are available. Insulin pens use an insulin cartridge with a disposable needle. The insulin pen is useful for people who need only one type of insulin or need to travel away from their home. Jet injectors shoot insulin through the skin in the subcutaneous tissue. High cost and bruising limit their use.

Regular insulin can be delivered through a continuous subcutaneous insulin infusion (CSII) device, also called an insulin pump. The CSII device has a small external pump, about the size of a pager, that holds a syringe connected to a subcutaneous needle by tubing. The client places the needle into the subcutaneous tissue, usually the abdomen. This device delivers a constant amount of programmed insulin throughout each 24-hour period. It also delivers a bolus of insulin manually (e.g., before meals). Frequent blood glucose monitoring is necessary to program the amount of insulin to be delivered. The advantages of CSII include more normal glucose control and greater lifestyle flexibility. Disadvantages are an increased risk of ketoacidosis from a malfunctioning pump and infection at the needle insertion site.

Insulin Injection Sites. Recommended injection sites are the upper arm, the abdomen except for a 2-inch circle around the navel (the umbilicus), the anterior lateral part of the thigh, and the buttocks (Figure 17-1 ■). Absorption and peak action of insulin differ according to the site. The most rapid absorption site is the abdomen, followed by the arms, thighs, and buttocks.

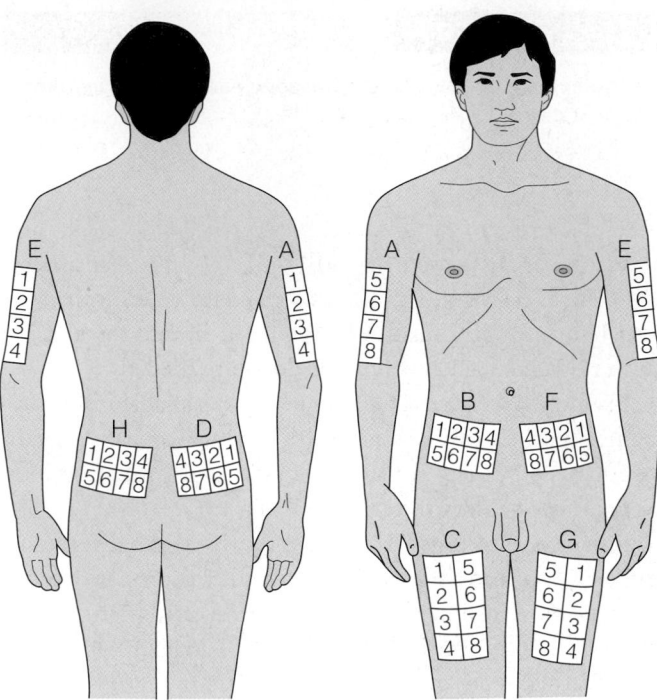

Figure 17-1. ■ Sites of insulin injection.

To administer insulin, gently pinch a fold of skin and inject the needle at a 90-degree angle. If the person is very thin, a 45-degree angle may be required to avoid injecting into muscle. Do not massage the site after giving the injection because this may interfere with absorption. Rotation within injection sites is recommended to give more consistent blood glucose levels and to prevent lipodystrophy. The distance between injections should be about 1 inch. Techniques to minimize painful injections are summarized in Box 17-2 ■.

Lipodystrophy (hypertrophy of subcutaneous tissue) or *lipoatrophy* (atrophy of subcutaneous tissue) may occur if the same

---

BOX 17-2   PROCEDURE CHECKLIST

Techniques to Minimize Painful Injections

☑ Inject insulin at room temperature.

☑ Make sure no air bubbles remain in the syringe before injection.

☑ Wait until alcohol on the skin dries completely before injection.

☑ Teach client to relax muscles in the injection area.

☑ Penetrate the skin with the needle quickly.

☑ Don't change the direction of the needle during insertion or withdrawal.

☑ Don't reuse needles.

Source: American Diabetes Association. (2004). Insulin administration. *Diabetes Care, 27*(Suppl. 1), S106–S107.

---

injection sites are used repeatedly. The use of refrigerated synthetic or pork insulin may trigger the development of tissue hypertrophy or atrophy. These problems rarely occur with the use of human insulins. Lipodystrophy and lipoatrophy alter insulin absorption by delaying its onset. Lipodystrophy usually resolves if the area is unused for a minimum of 6 months.

Mixing Insulins. People who require more than one type of insulin must mix their insulins to avoid multiple injections per dose. In addition, clients often need different doses of insulin throughout the day to provide adequate blood glucose control. The *procedure* for mixing insulins is described in Box 17-3 ■. Additional nursing implications and guidelines for teaching clients insulin administration techniques are listed in Table 17-3 ■.

clinical ALERT

1. Mix only insulins of like concentration (e.g., regular insulin U-100 with NPH insulin U-100).
2. Regular insulin may be mixed with all other types of insulin except Lantus insulin.
3. Do not mix human and pork insulins because they will inactivate each other.

Insulin Regimens. The appropriate insulin dosage is individualized to achieve balance among insulin, diet, and exercise. Most diabetics require two or more insulin injections each day. Usually, they mix short-acting and intermediate-acting insulins. Timing of the injections depends on blood glucose levels, food consumption, exercise, and types of insulin used.

Tight glucose control results in fewer long-term complications. This can be achieved through an intensive insulin regimen (three or four injections per day) (Table 17-4 ■). Whether the client needs one or multiple daily injections, the goal is to avoid daytime hypoglycemia while achieving adequate blood glucose control overnight.

ORAL ANTIDIABETIC AGENTS. Oral antidiabetic agents are used to treat people with type 2 DM (Table 17-5 ■). All clients taking oral antidiabetics must be taught to monitor their blood glucose levels at least two to three times per week.

clinical ALERT

Clients taking sulfonylureas can develop hyperglycemia or hypoglycemia when taken with the following drugs:

Monitor for Hyperglycemia	Monitor for Hypoglycemia
■ Corticosteroids	■ Alcohol
■ Estrogen	■ Coumadin
■ Thiazide diuretics	■ Beta blockers
■ Epinephrine	■ Ranitidine (Zantac)

BOX 17-3	PROCEDURE CHECKLIST

Mixing Insulins: 10 Units of Regular and 20 Units of NPH

☑ Wash hands.

☑ Inspect regular insulin for clarity. *Regular insulin is contaminated if cloudy.*

☑ Gently rotate NPH insulin to mix well. *Shaking insulin creates bubbles and prevents an accurate dose from being withdrawn.*

☑ Wipe off the top of both vials with an alcohol pad. *Prevents contamination of insulin.*

☑ Draw 20 U of air into the syringe, and inject air into the NPH vial. Withdraw needle. *Prepares vial by creating pressure.*

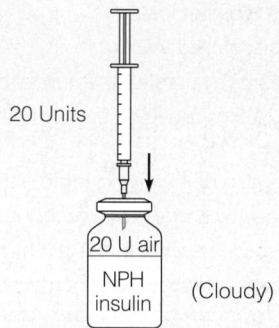

A Injecting air into the NPH vial.

☑ Draw 10 U of air into the syringe, and inject air into the regular vial. *Prepares vial by creating pressure.*

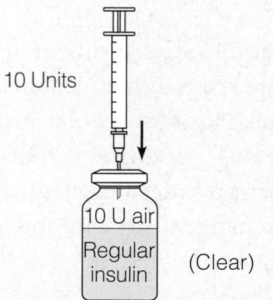

B Injecting air into the regular insulin vial.

Note: Refer to a nursing fundamentals or skills text for more detailed instruction. Check state guidelines and facility policy before performing any procedure.

☑ Invert the regular insulin vial, and withdraw 10 U of regular insulin. Withdraw the needle. *Withdrawing regular insulin first prevents contaminating regular insulin with NPH insulin.*

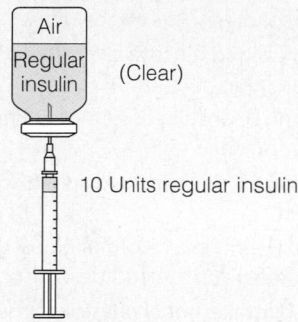

C Withdrawing regular insulin.

☑ Insert the needle into the NPH vial, and carefully withdraw 20 U of NPH insulin. *Accurate dosage is important for effectiveness.*

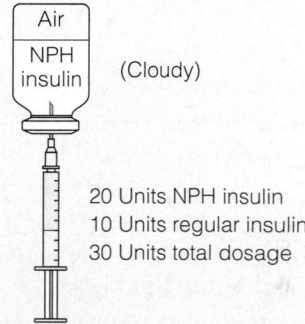

D Withdrawing NPH insulin.

☑ Administer the insulin.

☑ Dispose of the syringe properly and wash hands.

SAMPLE DOCUMENTATION

10/1/06	07:30am Regular insulin 10 units and NPH insulin 20 units given sub-q in right upper arm.
	_____R. Perry, LPN.

Nutrition Therapy

Diabetes management requires a careful balance between nutrient intake, daily expenditure of energy, and the dose and timing of insulin or oral antidiabetic agents. Persons with diabetes must eat a more structured diet in order to prevent hy-

perglycemia. The American Diabetes Association has established the following dietary goals for adults with diabetes:

1. Maintain as near-normal blood glucose levels as possible by balancing food intake with insulin or oral glucose-lowering medications and exercise.

TABLE 17-3

Nursing Implications for Administering Insulin and Client Teaching

NURSING IMPLICATIONS	CLIENT/FAMILY TEACHING
■ Discard vials of insulin whose expiration date has passed.	■ Know the manifestations of diabetes mellitus.
■ Discard any vial that is discolored or contains clumps, granules, or solid deposits on the sides.	■ Store opened insulin vials in a cool place for up to 4 weeks; avoid exposure to extreme temperatures (36° to 46°F) or sunlight.
■ Check client's blood glucose level 30 minutes before giving an insulin injection.	■ Refrigerate unopened extra insulin vials; do not freeze them.
■ When drawing up insulin dose, always check type and dose with another nurse.	■ Refrigerated insulin should be brought to room temperature before using it.
■ If a client's meal is delayed, hold administration of rapid-acting insulin.	■ Demonstrate self-administration of insulin (review procedure checklist in Box 17-3).
■ Monitor and maintain a record of blood glucose readings before each meal and at bedtime or as ordered.	■ Know how to mix two types of insulin.
■ Monitor food intake; notify physician when client eats an inadequate diet.	■ Discard outdated or discolored insulin.
■ Inspect injection sites for signs of lipodystrophy.	■ Keep a regular insulin vial available for emergencies.
■ Monitor for signs and symptoms of hypoglycemia or hyperglycemia and take appropriate action.	■ Check blood glucose before meals, at bedtime, and as prescribed.
	■ If breakfast is delayed, also delay giving rapid-acting insulin.
	■ Know the signs of hypoglycemia and hyperglycemia.
	■ Keep candy or sugar source available to treat hypoglycemia.
	■ Avoid alcoholic beverages to prevent hypoglycemia.
	■ Observe injection site for hardness, dimpling, or sunken areas; develop a plan for rotating injection sites.

2. Achieve optimal serum lipid levels.

3. Provide adequate calories to maintain or attain reasonable weights and to recover from illness.

4. Prevent and treat acute and chronic complications.

Early in the diagnosis of diabetes, clients should be referred to a certified diabetic educator and registered dietitian for meal planning and teaching. The dietary plan should consider food preferences, food habits, age, and other medical conditions (Table 17-6 ■).

MEAL PLANNING. Several different systems for meal planning are available to the person with diabetes. These include the consistent-carbohydrate diabetes meal plan, exchange lists, and calorie counting. Regardless of the system selected, the dietitian must consider the person's usual eating habits, diet history, culture, food values, and special needs. Altering foods and meal patterns is one of the most difficult parts of diabetes management. Careful consideration of individual preferences promotes dietary compliance.

Consistent-Carbohydrate Diabetes Meal Plan. The consistent-carbohydrate diabetes meal plan focuses on counting carbohydrates. Carbohydrates have the greatest effect on postprandial (after-meal) blood glucose levels. In this plan, clients are taught to count carbohydrates so they can administer 1 unit of regular insulin or lispro insulin for every 10 to 15 grams of carbohydrate eaten in a meal. This method provides better glucose control than the traditional exchange list plan and is, therefore, replacing it.

Exchange Lists. The exchange list diet is based on the person's ideal (or reasonable) weight, activity level, age, and occupation. These factors determine the total kilocalories (kcal) that the person may consume each day. After the calories have been determined, the proportions of carbohydrates, proteins, and fats are calculated, using the guidelines established by the American Diabetes Association and the American Dietetic Association (see Table 17-6).

The distribution of foods throughout the day is based on the exchange lists. There are six main exchange lists: bread/starch, vegetable, milk, meat, fruit, and fat. Foods are grouped into each exchange list according to their composition of carbohydrate, protein, fat, and calories. Standard household measurements determine portion sizes. The number of

TABLE 17-4

Insulin Regimens

REGIMEN	INSULIN TYPE*
One injection per day	NPH or NPH with regular before breakfast

One injection of either NPH or NPH with regular is used to cover all meals. This is a simple regimen, it is often difficult to control FBG levels, and afternoon hypoglycemia may result from increases in NPH.

Two injections per day	NPH or NPH with regular or premixed (N and R) before breakfast and dinner

This regimen aims to mimic normal pancreatic function, but the client must have a fairly rigid schedule of food intake and exercise.

Three or four injections per day	R before each meal; NPH at dinner or bedtime

This regimen more closely mimics normal pancreatic function; it allows greater choice in mealtimes and exercise. However, each premeal dose of R must be determined by blood glucose tests.

*Insulin types are abbreviated as follows: NPH = intermediate-acting, R = regular, rapid-acting.

_ _ _ _ _ _ = Regular   _____ = NPH

servings is based on the calorie count needed by the client. A food item on the list can be substituted ("exchanged") for another with very little difference in calories or amount of carbohydrates, proteins, and fats. The meal plan prescribes how many exchanges are allowed for each food group per meal and snacks.

NUTRITIONAL CONCERNS FOR OLDER ADULTS. An obese older adult with type 2 DM may need a diet, exercise, and weight reduction program. To improve compliance with the diet plan, the nurse should consider the following factors: dietary likes and dislikes, eating habits, who prepares the meals, age-related changes in taste and smell, and dental health. Other factors to consider include the age-related decline in calorie needs and reduced physical activity. The older adult who is overweight should reduce calorie intake in order to lose weight. Many older adults live on a fixed income, limiting their diet to canned meat, fruits, and vegetables. Coexisting illnesses and the use of multiple medications decrease appetite and reduce their energy to plan, cook, or eat. Dietary restrictions may cause the older adult to avoid social gatherings. If possible, encourage older adults to eat their meals with others, which may increase their appetite.

Exercise

Exercise is extremely important for diabetic clients. It reduces blood glucose levels by increasing glucose use by the muscles. This potentially decreases the need for insulin. Exercise also decreases cholesterol and triglycerides, reducing the risk of cardiovascular disorders. People with diabetes should consult their primary health care provider before beginning or changing an exercise program. The ability to maintain an exercise program may be affected by fatigue and glucose levels.

The nurse should assess the client's lifestyle before determining the type of exercise program. Lifestyle factors to consider are the client's usual exercise habits, living environment, and community programs. The type of exercise the person usually enjoys is probably the one that he or she will continue throughout life. Whatever exercise the client chooses, it must be done on a regular basis.

Clients with diabetes should follow the recommendations of the American Diabetes Association when exercising: Use proper footwear, inspect the feet daily and after exercise, avoid exercise in extreme heat or cold, and avoid exercise during periods of poor glucose control. The client over age 35 should have an exercise-stress electrocardiogram prior to beginning an exercise program (see Chapter 26). ⚭ General exercise guidelines for clients with type 1 and type 2 diabetes are listed in Box 17-4 ∎.

MediaLink Glipizide

TABLE 17-5

Nursing Implications for Pharmacology: Oral Antidiabetic Agents

CLASS/DRUGS	PURPOSE	NURSING RESPONSIBILITIES	CLIENT TEACHING
Sulfonylureas ■ Glimepiride (Amaryl) ■ Glipizide (Glucotrol, Glucotrol XL) ■ Glyburide (Dia Beta)	Increases release of insulin from pancreas and increases the number and action of receptor cells to maintain blood glucose levels within normal range.	Assess for allergy to sulfonamides. Observe for signs and symptoms of hypoglycemia (sweating, hunger, weakness, dizziness, tremor, tachycardia, anxiety). Test client's blood glucose level before giving drug. Assess for side effects of nausea, heartburn, or diarrhea.	Take at the same time each day. Take 30 minutes before meals, except Glucotrol XL, which must be taken with food. Monitor for hypoglycemia. Test blood glucose level before taking drug.
Biguanides ■ Metformin (Glucophage)	Reduces liver glucose production and improves glucose use in skeletal muscle to maintain blood glucose levels within normal.	Monitor renal function, especially in clients at risk for kidney disease. Monitor glucose levels throughout therapy. Discontinue 48 hours before injection with any radiocontrast dye. Call physician if weakness, drowsiness, or malaise occurs. These are early signs of lactic acidosis.	Take at the same time each day. If a dose is missed, do not double doses. Call physician if weakness, drowsiness, or malaise occurs. These are early signs of lactic acidosis.
Alpha-Glucoside Inhibitors ■ Acarbose (Precose) ■ Miglitol (Glyset)	Slows digestion and absorption of carbohydrates to maintain normal blood glucose levels.	Do not give to clients with intestinal disorders; acarbose will worsen these conditions.	Take with the first bite of a meal. May cause gas and diarrhea; tends to decrease with continued therapy.
Meglitinides ■ Repaglinide (Prandin) ■ Nateglinide (Starlix)	Stimulates pancreas to secrete insulin.	Monitor for hypoglycemia.	Monitor for hypoglycemia.
Thiazolidinediones ■ Rosiglitazone (Avandia) ■ Pioglitazone (Actos)	Increases insulin sensitivity at receptor sites on liver, muscle, and fat cells.	Assess for signs of liver toxicity (e.g., anorexia, jaundice, or dark urine).	Call physician if anorexia, jaundice, or dark urine develops.

Complications of Diabetes Mellitus

The person with diabetes mellitus, regardless of type, is at increased risk for acute and chronic complications involving multiple body systems. Altered blood glucose levels affect the vascular and nervous systems and cause an increased susceptibility to infection. Figure 17-2 ■ shows the progression from early manifestations to acute complications to chronic multisystem complications. A discussion of each of these complications with related interdisciplinary and nursing care follows.

ACUTE COMPLICATIONS

Diabetic ketoacidosis, hyperosmolar hyperglycemic state, and hypoglycemia are the primary acute complications of diabetes mellitus. These can be life threatening and require immediate medical treatment.

Diabetic Ketoacidosis

Diabetic ketoacidosis (DKA) is a life-threatening illness occurring in type 1 diabetics. It is characterized by hyperglycemia, dehydration, and coma. DKA often develops in a client with undiagnosed and untreated diabetes. An individual who is sick, has an infection, omits insulin, or has excessive

TABLE 17-6

Nutrient Recommendations for Adults with Diabetes

NUTRIENT	RECOMMENDED DAILY INTAKE
Calories (kcal)	Amount needed to attain and maintain as close as possible the desired body weight.
Carbohydrates	Individualized, based on client's individual eating habits and glucose and lipid goals.
Sweeteners	Non-nutritive sweeteners such as saccharin (Sweet & Low) or aspartame (Nutrasweet) are safe when consumed within acceptable daily levels by FDA.
Protein	Approximately 15% to 20% of the daily caloric intake; should be from both animal and vegetable sources. Clients with nephropathy need lower protein intake.
Saturated fat and cholesterol	Less than 10% of the daily calories should be from saturated fats, with dietary cholesterol limited to $\leq$ 300 mg/day.
Fiber	20–35 g of dietary fiber each day from a wide variety of food sources.
Sodium	The same as for the general population; no more than 2,400–3,000 mg/day.
Vitamins and minerals	Sufficient to meet daily requirements.
Alcohol	Limit alcohol intake to no more than two alcoholic beverages per day for men. Ingest with a meal to decrease the risk of hypoglycemia and count in the meal plan (one alcoholic beverage equals 90 kilocalories).

Source: American Diabetes Association. (2004). Nutrition principles and recommendations in diabetes. *Diabetes Care,* 27(Suppl. 1), S36–S46.

physical or emotional stress is also at an increased risk for developing DKA.

Without insulin, glucose cannot enter the cell, which stimulates the liver to increase glucose production, leading to hyperglycemia. This excess glucose acts an osmotic diuretic (pulls fluid from extracellular space) causing polyuria and eventually leads to dehydration and sodium and potassium loss.

Because glucose cannot be used for energy, the fat stores break down, resulting in continued hyperglycemia and burning of fatty acids. This causes the formation of ketones. When more ketones are produced than the cell can use and the kidneys can excrete, *ketoacidosis* develops. Ketoacidosis alters acid–base balance, causing metabolic acidosis. The increased buildup of ketones depresses the central nervous system (CNS) leading to coma and death if left untreated (Figure 17-3 ■). The manifestations of DKA are listed in Box 17-5 ■.

TREATMENT OF DIABETIC KETOACIDOSIS. DKA is the most serious metabolic disturbance of people with type 1 diabetes. Hospital admission may be required when the person has a blood glucose of greater than 250 mg/dL and ketones in the urine (**ketonuria**).

DKA is treated with fluids (for dehydration), insulin (to reduce hyperglycemia and acidosis), and correction of electrolyte imbalances. If the client is alert and conscious, fluids may be given orally. Unconscious clients require intravenous fluids. The nurse should be prepared to administer a 0.9% normal saline solution to replace the sodium losses. After 2 to 3 hours, the intravenous (IV) solution is changed to 0.45% normal saline to prevent hypernatremia. When the blood glucose levels reach 250 mg/dL, dextrose is added to prevent hypoglycemia. Potassium may be added to an IV solution if the client's laboratory values show a deficit. Regular insulin is used to treat the client's hyperglycemia. The

BOX 17-4   POPULATION FOCUS

Exercise Guidelines for Clients with Type 1 and Type 2 DM

1. Include a warm-up and cool-down period in your exercise program.
2. Check feet for blisters or other damage before and after exercise.
3. Consume adequate fluids before, during, and after exercise.
4. Monitor blood glucose before and after exercise.
5. Always carry quick-acting carbohydrate (Life-Savers or 5-g glucose tablets).
6. Always carry diabetic ID card and wear ID bracelet.

Type 1

- Exercise within 30–60 minutes of eating.
- Avoid exercise if fasting blood glucose is >250 mg/dL and ketones present in urine.

Type 2

- Exercise at least three to four times per week.
- If taking sulfonylureas, eat a snack before exercising.

Source: American Diabetes Association. (2004). Diabetes mellitus and exercise. *Diabetes Care, 27*(Suppl. 1), S58–S62.

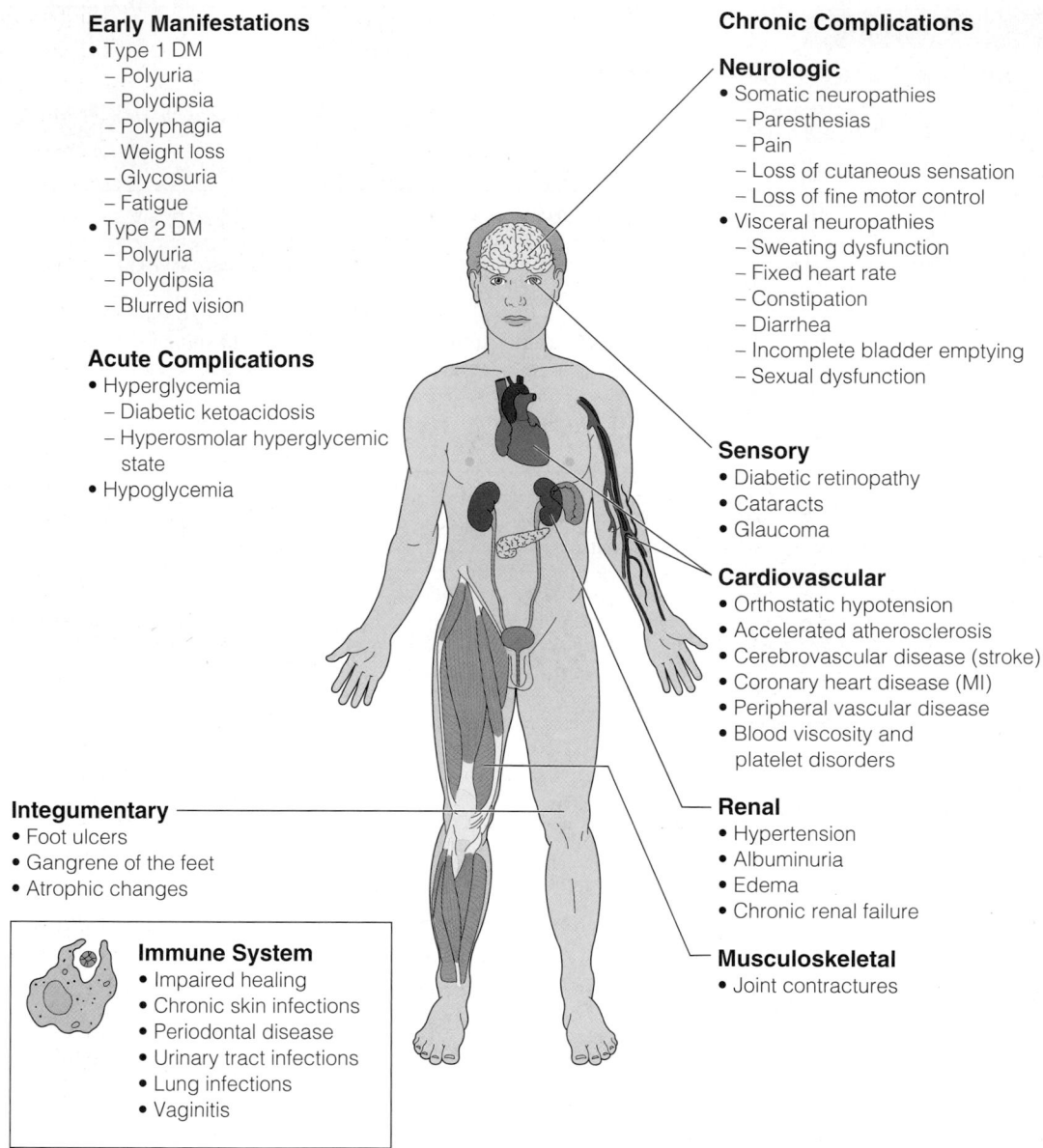

Early Manifestations
- Type 1 DM
  - Polyuria
  - Polydipsia
  - Polyphagia
  - Weight loss
  - Glycosuria
  - Fatigue
- Type 2 DM
  - Polyuria
  - Polydipsia
  - Blurred vision

Acute Complications
- Hyperglycemia
  - Diabetic ketoacidosis
  - Hyperosmolar hyperglycemic state
- Hypoglycemia

Integumentary
- Foot ulcers
- Gangrene of the feet
- Atrophic changes

Immune System
- Impaired healing
- Chronic skin infections
- Periodontal disease
- Urinary tract infections
- Lung infections
- Vaginitis

Chronic Complications

Neurologic
- Somatic neuropathies
  - Paresthesias
  - Pain
  - Loss of cutaneous sensation
  - Loss of fine motor control
- Visceral neuropathies
  - Sweating dysfunction
  - Fixed heart rate
  - Constipation
  - Diarrhea
  - Incomplete bladder emptying
  - Sexual dysfunction

Sensory
- Diabetic retinopathy
- Cataracts
- Glaucoma

Cardiovascular
- Orthostatic hypotension
- Accelerated atherosclerosis
- Cerebrovascular disease (stroke)
- Coronary heart disease (MI)
- Peripheral vascular disease
- Blood viscosity and platelet disorders

Renal
- Hypertension
- Albuminuria
- Edema
- Chronic renal failure

Musculoskeletal
- Joint contractures

Figure 17-2. ■ Multisystem effects of diabetes mellitus.

degree of hyperglycemia and ketosis determines whether insulin is given by the subcutaneous or IV route. Typically, a continuous insulin infusion is started and maintained until the ketoacidosis is resolved.

clinical ALERT

Only regular insulin may be given by the intravenous route.

Hyperosmolar Hyperglycemic State (HHS)

Hyperosmolar hyperglycemic state (HHS) occurs in people with type 2 DM. It is characterized by severely elevated blood glucose levels, extreme dehydration, and an altered level of consciousness. This condition usually develops slowly over several hours to days. It is a serious, life-threatening medical emergency that has a higher mortality rate than DKA. Infection, surgery, and dialysis are a few factors that can trigger HHS.

The state of extreme hyperglycemia leads to osmotic diuresis and results in severe dehydration, especially of the brain. The manifestations result from the effects of hyperglycemia and dehydration (see Box 17-4). Ketosis does not occur like it does in DKA, because the type 2 diabetic has sufficient insulin.

TREATMENT OF HYPEROSMOLAR HYPERGLYCEMIC STATE.

Treatment is similar to that of DKA, namely, correcting fluid and electrolyte imbalances and providing insulin to lower hyperglycemia. Intravenous fluids of 0.9% normal

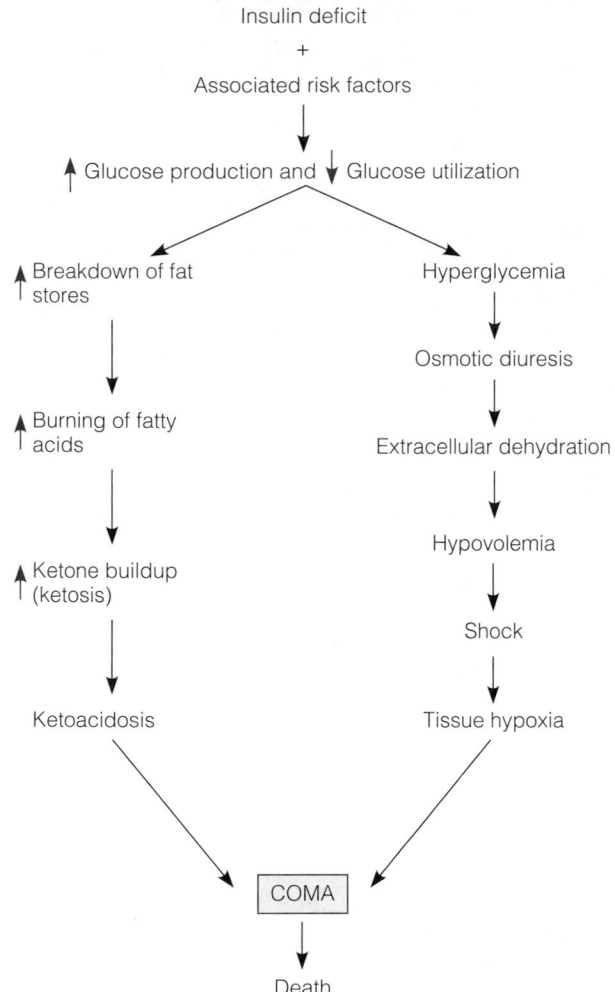

Insulin deficit

+

Associated risk factors

↑ Glucose production and ↓ Glucose utilization

↑ Breakdown of fat stores

Hyperglycemia

↑ Burning of fatty acids

Osmotic diuresis

↑ Ketone buildup (ketosis)

Extracellular dehydration

Ketoacidosis

Hypovolemia

Shock

Tissue hypoxia

COMA

Death

Figure 17-3. ■ Pathophysiology of diabetic ketoacidosis.

saline are given, followed by 0.45% normal saline to correct the fluid and sodium losses. Insulin is administered to reduce the severe hyperglycemia. When blood glucose levels reach 250 mg/dL, the insulin is discontinued because, in contrast to DKA, ketosis is not present.

Whether caring for the client with DKA or HHS, the nurse is responsible for measuring the client's vital signs, monitoring the level of consciousness, monitoring IV infusions, monitoring fluid status through intake and output, and notifying the physician of the client's response to treatment.

Hypoglycemia

Hypoglycemia can occur in people with type 1 DM and people with type 2 DM who are treated with oral antidiabetic agents. It may be caused by too much insulin intake, overdose of oral antidiabetic agents, too little food, or excess physical activity. The onset is sudden, and blood glucose is usually less than 50 mg/dL.

The brain requires a constant supply of glucose, so a hypoglycemic episode alters brain function. The manifesta-

tions of hypoglycemia (Box 17-6 ■) result from activation of the autonomic nervous system (ANS) and from impaired cerebral function. People who experience frequent hypoglycemic episodes during which the blood glucose level drops below 20 mg/dL may develop decreased cerebral function. Severe untreated hypoglycemia may lead to death.

clinical ALERT

As the body ages, the autonomic nervous system becomes less responsive. The elderly may not experience the manifestations caused by the autonomic nervous system.

Some people with long-standing type 1 diabetes may develop hypoglycemia unawareness. The normal compensatory mechanisms, which should raise blood glucose levels, fail. The person does not show any symptoms of hypoglycemia, even though they exist. Because treatment is delayed, the client may experience more frequent and severe episodes of hypoglycemia.

TREATMENT OF HYPOGLYCEMIA. Hypoglycemia may occur at any time, but it most often develops before meals or in the middle of the night. Mild hypoglycemia is usually recognized and self-managed, but severe hypoglycemia requires treatment by health care providers.

Mild Hypoglycemia. When mild hypoglycemia (blood glucose between 60 and 70 mg/dL) occurs, immediate treatment is necessary. People experiencing hypoglycemia should take about 15 g of a rapid-acting sugar. Examples of fast-acting glucose are:

- 3 glucose tablets
- 1/2 cup of fruit juice or regular soda
- 8 oz of skim milk
- 6 to 8 Life-Savers candies
- 2 to 3 tsp of sugar or honey.

clinical ALERT

Do not add sugar to fruit juice, because it causes a rapid rise in blood glucose, which would require additional treatment.

If the manifestations continue, the 15/15 rule should be followed: Wait 15 minutes, then monitor blood glucose; if it remains below 60 mg/dL, eat another 15 g of carbohydrate. This procedure can be repeated until blood glucose levels return to normal. People with diabetes should always carry a rapid-acting carbohydrate source. Clients experiencing frequent hypoglycemic episodes should consult their health care provider.

BOX 17-5

MANIFESTATIONS OF DIABETIC KETOACIDOSIS (DKA) AND HYPEROSMOLAR HYPERGLYCEMIC STATE (HHS)

DKA	HHS
DEHYDRATION (FROM HYPERGLYCEMIA)	**DEHYDRATION**
Thirst	Extreme thirst
Warm, dry skin with poor turgor	Warm, dry skin with poor turgor
Dry mucous membranes	Dry mucous membranes
Rapid, weak pulse	Rapid, weak pulse
Hypotension	Hypotension
Soft eyeballs	
METABOLIC ACIDOSIS (FROM KETOSIS)	**NEUROLOGIC MANIFESTATIONS**
Nausea and vomiting	Depressed level of consciousness to coma
Lethargy to coma	Grand mal seizures
Acetone (fruity, alcohol-like) breath odor	
OTHER MANIFESTATIONS	**OTHER MANIFESTATIONS**
Abdominal pain	Abdominal discomfort may be present
Kussmaul's respirations (rapid, deep respirations; a compensatory response to prevent a further decrease in pH)	Rapid, shallow breathing
LABORATORY FINDINGS	
Blood glucose:	
>250 mg/dL	>600 mg/dL
Blood and urine ketones:	
Positive	Negative
Arterial blood pH:	
<7.3	Normal (7.35–7.45)
Serum osmolality:	
<340 mOsm/L	>340 mOsm/L

BOX 17-6

MANIFESTATIONS OF HYPOGLYCEMIA
CAUSED BY RESPONSES OF THE AUTONOMIC NERVOUS SYSTEM

Hunger	Shakiness
Nausea	Irritability
Anxiety	Rapid pulse
Pale, cool skin	Hypotension
Sweating	

CAUSED BY IMPAIRED CEREBRAL FUNCTION

Strange or unusual feelings	Blurred vision
Headache	Decreasing levels of
Difficulty in thinking	consciousness
Inability to concentrate	Seizures
Change in emotional behavior	Coma
Slurred speech	

LABORATORY FINDINGS

Blood glucose	<50 mg/dL
Blood and urine ketones	Negative
Plasma pH	Normal
Serum osmolality	Normal

Severe Hypoglycemia. Diabetic clients with severe hypoglycemia (blood glucose less than 60 mg/dL) are often hospitalized. If the client is conscious and alert, 10 to 15 g of an oral carbohydrate may be given. When the client is unconscious, 25 to 50 mL of 50% dextrose is given intravenously, followed by intravenous infusion of 5% dextrose in water (D_5W). Intravenous glucose acts the fastest to raise blood glucose levels. When it is unavailable, glucagon 1 mg may be given by the subcutaneous or intramuscular route to stimulate the release of glycogen. Because glucagon has a short action period, a carbohydrate snack is given to prevent a recurrence of hypoglycemia. Glucagon should be included in the client's emergency kit and family members should be taught how and when to administer it.

Other Alterations in Blood Glucose Levels

SOMOGYI EFFECT. **Somogyi effect** is a morning rise in blood glucose to hyperglycemic levels following an episode of nighttime hypoglycemia. The morning hyperglycemia is thought to be caused by the release of counterregulatory hormones.

Clients with Somogyi effect are taught to monitor their blood glucose levels and assess for manifestations of nocturnal hypoglycemia: tremors, night sweats, and restlessness. The treatment focuses on increasing the bedtime snack or decreasing the evening dose of intermediate-acting insulin.

DAWN PHENOMENON. **Dawn phenomenon** is a rise in blood glucose between 5 A.M. and 9 A.M. The exact cause is unknown but may be related to nighttime release of growth hormone. Treatment may include increasing the insulin dose or changing the injection time of the intermediate-acting insulin from dinnertime to bedtime.

CHRONIC COMPLICATIONS

Chronic complications of diabetes mellitus result from consistently high glucose levels in the body. The longer the client has been diagnosed with diabetes, the greater the chance of developing one or more of these complications. The complications are categorized as macrovascular disease and microvascular disease.

In a 1993 landmark study the Diabetes Control and Complications Trial (DCCT), people who kept their blood glucose levels close to normal reduced their risk for development and progression of complications involving the eyes, the kidneys, and the nervous system. This was accomplished by frequent blood glucose monitoring, several daily insulin injections, exercise, and a healthier diet. To prevent long-term complications of diabetes, clients must keep their blood glucose levels within the normal or near-normal range.

Macrovascular Complications

The macrocirculation (the large blood vessels) in people with diabetes undergoes changes due to atherosclerosis. (See Chapter 26 ⚭ for more information about atherosclerosis.) Atherosclerosis has an increased incidence and earlier age of onset in people with diabetes. Macrovascular complications include coronary artery disease, stroke, and peripheral vascular disease.

Atherosclerotic coronary heart disease is a major risk factor in the development of myocardial infarction in the type 2 diabetic. These people also have high cholesterol and triglyceride levels. Coronary heart disease is the most common cause of death in people with type 2 diabetes. Persons who have a myocardial infarction are more prone to develop heart failure as a complication of the infarction. They are also less likely to survive in the period immediately following the infarction. (Myocardial infarction is fully discussed in Chapter 26. ⚭)

Stroke is two to six times more likely to occur in the type 2 diabetic. Although the exact cause is unknown, hypertension plays a major role in its development. The manifestations of impaired cerebral circulation are often similar to hypoglycemia or HHS and warrant immediate medical attention.

Peripheral vascular disease of the lower extremities accompanies both types of diabetes mellitus, but the incidence is greater in type 2 DM. Diabetes-induced arteriosclerosis of the lower legs is usually bilateral, develops at an earlier age, pro-

gresses more rapidly, and develops equally in men and women. Occlusions can form in the large vessels below the knee, causing impaired peripheral circulation. Decreased arterial circulation can lead to lower leg ulcers and **gangrene** (necrosis or tissue death). Gangrene from diabetes is the most common cause of nontraumatic amputations of the lower leg. Manifestations of peripheral vascular disease are summarized in Box 17-7 ■. (Peripheral vascular disease is discussed in Chapter 28. ⚭)

Microvascular Complications

Microvascular complications involve alterations in the microcirculation (the smaller blood vessels and capillaries), especially the eyes, kidneys, and nerves. Microvascular disease is sometimes called microangiopathy.

Diabetic retinopathy is the collective name for the destructive retinal changes that occur in the person with diabetes. Changes in the retinal capillaries cause decreased blood flow to the retina, leading to retinal ischemia and possible retinal hemorrhage or detachment. Retinopathy has two stages: nonproliferative and proliferative. Varying degrees of visual impairment can occur at any stage. Retinopathy is the leading cause of blindness in people between ages 20 and 74. All diabetics have a greater risk for developing cataracts (opacity of the lens) as a result of increased glucose levels within the lens. Yearly eye exams by an ophthalmologist are recommended for these clients.

Diabetic nephropathy is a disease of the kidneys characterized by the presence of albumin in the urine, hypertension, edema, and progressive renal insufficiency. This disorder is the most common cause of renal failure requiring dialysis or transplantation in the United States. Nephropathy occurs in 20% to 30% of people with diabetes mellitus.

Changes in the glomerular capillaries in the kidney result in **glomerulosclerosis** (fibrosis of the glomerular tissue). This condition severely impairs the filtering function of the glomerulus so that albumin is lost in the urine.

The first indication of nephropathy is **microalbuminuria** (small amounts of albumin in the urine). With the presence

---

BOX 17-7

MANIFESTATIONS OF PERIPHERAL VASCULAR DISEASE

- Loss of hair on lower leg, feet, and toes
- Atrophic skin changes: shininess and thinning
- Cool to cold feet
- Legs become red when dependent; legs become white when elevated
- Thick toenails
- Diminished or absent peripheral pulses
- Intermittent claudication—pain with walking
- Pain at rest, usually at night

of microalbuminuria, usually the client progresses to end-stage renal disease or renal failure. (Renal failure is discussed in Chapter 32. ⟨⟨⟩⟩) Because hypertension increases the progression of nephropathy, clients are treated with angiotensin-converting enzyme (ACE) inhibiting drugs such as captopril (Capoten).

Diabetic neuropathy involves disorders of the peripheral nerves and the autonomic nervous system. Diabetic neuropathies cause one or more of the following problems: sensory and motor impairment, postural hypotension, delayed gastric emptying, diarrhea, and impaired genitourinary function. Neuropathies result from thickening of the capillary membrane and destruction of myelin sheath, which impairs nerve conduction.

Peripheral neuropathies are bilateral sensory disorders. Manifestations appear first in the toes and feet and progress upward to involve the fingers and hands. Initial manifestations include **distal paresthesia** (a subjective feeling of numbness or tingling); pain described as aching, burning, or shooting; and a feeling of cold feet. People experience reduced feeling, touch, and position sense, increasing their risk for falls. Foot injuries are common due to impaired temperature and pain sensation. There is no specific treatment for peripheral neuropathy. Collaborative management focuses on controlling the neuropathic pain with tricyclic antidepressants or a topical cream called capsaicin (Zostrix).

Autonomic neuropathies involve numerous organ systems, including:

- *Cardiovascular:* fixed, slightly rapid heart rate and postural hypotension
- *Gastrointestinal:* delayed gastric emptying, resulting in irregular blood glucose control, constipation, and diarrhea
- *Genitourinary:* neurogenic bladder (inability to empty the bladder completely), leading to urinary retention and an increased risk of urinary tract infections; sexual dysfunction in men and women.

THE DIABETIC FOOT. People with diabetes mellitus experience more problems with their feet and subsequent amputations because of macrovascular disease, neuropathy, and infection. Often, they experience some type of foot trauma without knowing it. Because they have lost their perception of pain, an injury may go unattended for days or weeks. Common sources of foot trauma are cracks and fissures caused by dry skin or infections such as athlete's foot, blisters from ill-fitting socks and shoes, ingrown toenails, and direct trauma (cuts, bruises, or burns).

Foot lesions usually begin as a superficial injury, then progress into an ulceration (Figure 17-4 ■). In time, the ulcer extends deeper into muscles and bone and can lead to abscess or osteomyelitis. Infections commonly occur in the traumatized or ulcerated tissue. Dry gangrene is manifested

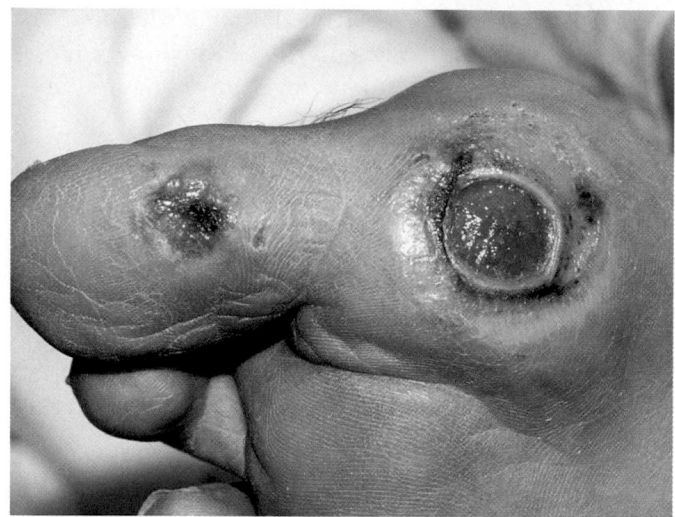

Figure 17-4. ■ Ulceration following trauma to the foot of a person with diabetes. (Courtesy of Harry Przekop/Medichrome/The Stock Shop, Inc.)

by cold, dry, shriveled, and black tissues of the toes and feet. If untreated, the whole foot eventually becomes gangrenous and requires amputation. Treatment consists of bed rest, antibiotics, and debridement. Additional foot care guidelines are discussed later in Box 17-8.

INCREASED SUSCEPTIBILITY TO INFECTION. The person with diabetes has an increased risk of developing frequent bacterial and fungal infections. Normally, glucose is used efficiently throughout the body, but in people with diabetes, glucose accumulates in the epidermal layer of the skin. Moisture tends to collect under the armpits, breasts, groin, or genitalia. The higher-than-normal concentration of glucose in the skin coupled with the moisture creates a perfect breeding area for microorganisms. When the skin appears beefy red to violet red, an infection should be suspected. Fungal infections can develop under the nails, giving them a thick, yellow, crumbly appearance. Treatment focuses on prevention of infection.

Special Concerns

SICK-DAY MANAGEMENT. When the person with diabetes is sick, blood glucose levels increase, even though food intake decreases. The person mistakenly alters or omits the insulin dose or oral antidiabetic agent, causing further problems. Dietary guidelines during illness focus on preventing dehydration and providing nutrition for promoting recovery. The nurse teaches the following sick-day management:

- Monitor blood glucose every 4 hours throughout the illness.
- Test urine for ketones if the blood glucose level is greater than 250 mg/dL.
- Continue to take the usual insulin dose or oral antidiabetic agent.

- Drink 8 to 12 oz of fluid each waking hour.
- Eat 10 to 15 g of carbohydrate every 1 to 2 hours such as:
  - 1/2 cup regular Jell-O
  - 1/2 cup regular soft drink
  - 1/2 cup pure fruit juice
  - 1 whole Popsicle
- Call the physician if you are unable to eat for more than 24 hours or if vomiting and diarrhea last for more than 6 hours.

SURGERY MANAGEMENT. Surgery is a stressor that releases excess counterregulatory hormones, causing hyperglycemia and insulin resistance. Protein stores are decreased. In addition, diet and activity patterns change, and medication types and dosages vary. As a result, surgical clients with diabetes are at a greater risk for postoperative infection, delayed wound healing, fluid and electrolyte imbalances, hypoglycemia, and DKA.

For clients with type 2 DM, oral antidiabetic agents are usually withheld 1 to 2 days before surgery, and clients are given regular insulin. Clients with type 1 DM follow a carefully prescribed insulin regimen to meet their specific needs.

The surgical procedure should be scheduled for early in the morning to decrease the fasting time. If there is no food intake after surgery, intravenous dextrose is given along with subcutaneous regular insulin every 6 hours. Although intake is decreased postoperatively, stress increases insulin requirements. Glucose control is also affected postoperatively by nausea and vomiting, anorexia, and gastrointestinal suction.

During the postoperative period, the client with type 2 DM may continue to require insulin or may resume oral medications, depending on glucose levels. The client with type 1 DM may require reduced insulin as healing progresses and stress-induced hyperglycemia diminishes. Regular blood glucose monitoring is essential, as are assessments for hypoglycemia.

Sometimes postsurgical clients require enteral tube feedings or total parenteral nutrition to meet their dietary needs. Both nutritional supplements contain glucose. Diabetic clients receiving these supplements must be monitored closely for hyperglycemia. Often, they need additional insulin to prevent acute hyperglycemia complications.

PANCREAS TRANSPLANTATION. Surgical management of diabetes involves replacing or transplanting the pancreas, pancreatic cells, or beta cells. Islet cell transplantation has had moderate success. Researchers are investigating transplantation of the tail of the pancreas, which offers promise for long-term glucose control. Before clients can be considered transplant candidates, an extensive physical and emotional evaluation is done.

COMPLEMENTARY THERAPIES

Acupuncture may be used to relieve the chronic pain from peripheral neuropathy. Some diabetics use guided imagery as a means to control or cure diabetes. No scientific evidence supports this technique and it is not harmful as long as clients continue with their diabetic medications, diet, and exercise plan.

Before diabetics take any herbal supplements, they should talk with their health care provider. The following supplements may increase blood glucose levels: ginkgo biloba, glucosamine, and bee pollen. In contrast, basil, chromium, garlic, and ginseng are herbal supplements that may reduce blood glucose levels.

NURSING CARE

Nursing care differs for the person with newly diagnosed diabetes, the person with long-term diabetes, and the person with acute complications. Diabetics require lifelong collaborative care.

ASSESSING

Assessment data collected by the nurse can determine the extent to which DM is affecting the client's life, identify risk factors for complications, and suggest guidelines for medical treatment or self-care (Box 17-8 ■).

DIAGNOSING, PLANNING, AND IMPLEMENTING

Priorities in Nursing Care. Nursing care focuses on maintaining and promoting health status related to nutrition, skin care, and prevention of complications. A primary focus is teaching the client self-management strategies.

Imbalanced Nutrition

- Monitor blood glucose levels regularly and report values below 60 mg/dL or above 200 mg/dL. *Clients with diabetes are at risk for hypoglycemia or hyperglycemia.*
- Monitor percentage of meals and snacks that client eats. *Anorexia, gastric fullness, and abdominal pain can reduce oral intake. To prevent hypoglycemia, the client must consume the amount of food indicated in the diet plan.*
- Identify food preferences, including ethnic/cultural needs. *Clients are more likely to eat food they like and that meets their ethnic/cultural requirements.*
- Provide meals and snacks on time. *Glucose and insulin control is more effective when meals are eaten on time.*
- Give insulin and/or oral antidiabetic agents as ordered. *To prevent hyperglycemia, insulin and/or oral antidiabetic agents must be given on time. Altered times might be necessary when food is delayed or diagnostic procedures are being done.*

BOX 17-8	ASSESSMENT

Assessing for Diabetes Mellitus

SUBJECTIVE DATA

- Present health status:
  - Presence of hyperglycemia manifestations: polyuria, polydipsia, polyphagia.
  - Weight loss or gain; changes in appetite.
  - Changes in vision or speech.
  - Presence of numbness and/or tingling or burning in feet.
  - Presence of slow healing wounds.
  - Pain or burning with urination.
  - Problems of vulvular itching in females.
- Family history of type 1 or type 2 diabetes mellitus.
- Use of insulin or oral antidiabetic medications.
- Any recent surgery.

OBJECTIVE DATA

- Vital signs (blood pressure—standing and lying, pulse, respirations, temperature).
- Weight and height.
- Assess for DKA, HHS, and/or hypoglycemia.
- Assess visual acuity.
- Assess sensations of touch and position, pain, and temperature.
- Observe mental status for signs of confusion or disorientation; slurred speech.
- Observe gait patterns, use of assistive devices for walking, and abnormal wear patterns on shoes.
- Inspect oral cavity for bad breath, bleeding, red gums, and tooth pain.
- Inspect skin for dryness or excessive perspiration; presence of hair on lower extremities; presence of lesions, redness over pressure points, cellulitis, or gangrene.
- Palpate peripheral pulses for decrease or absence.
- Palpate lower extremity for capillary refill, color and temperature of skin, and edema.
- Monitor and report blood glucose levels above or below expected range.

Impaired Skin Integrity

- Teach foot care. Wash feet daily with lukewarm water and mild hand soap; pat dry, especially between the toes. Apply a thin film of lubricating lotion except between the toes. *Proper hygiene decreases the chance of infection.*

clinical ALERT

Teach the diabetic client to always check the water temperature in the shower or bath with a bath thermometer before stepping in to prevent burns.

- Use alternating pressure mattresses, elbow and heel protectors, and foot cradle as ordered. *These devices reduce pressure on the skin to prevent skin breakdown.*
- Encourage fluid intake of at least 2,500 mL/day unless cardiac complications exist. *Adequate fluid intake prevents dry skin and the risk for skin breakdown. However, clients with cardiac disease may develop fluid overload with an excess intake.*
- Discuss the importance of not smoking. *Nicotine in tobacco causes vasoconstriction and decreases blood supply to the feet.*
- If boils, pimples, or skin breakdown occurs, notify the physician immediately. *Immediate intervention is needed to prevent the development of deep wounds and infection.*
- Rotate insulin injection sites. *Site rotation prevents lipodystrophy.*
- Conduct foot care teaching sessions as often as necessary (Box 17-9 ■). *Foot care is a priority in diabetes management to prevent serious problems.*

Risk for Infection

- Assess for manifestations of infection: fever; chills; tachycardia; abnormal breath sounds; vaginal discharge; cloudy, foul-smelling urine; or redness, pain, swelling, or discharge at injury site. *Common infections include urinary tract and nail infections, osteomyelitis, vaginal yeast infections, chronic gingivitis, and pyorrhea. Early diagnosis and treatment can control their severity and decrease complications.*
- Obtain specimens and send for culture and sensitivity test as ordered. *Before antibiotic therapy is begun, specimens must be sent for culture and sensitivity to identify the causative organism and appropriate antibiotic.*
- Use and teach meticulous hand washing. *Hand washing is the best method for preventing the spread of infection.*
- Keep the skin clean and dry, using mild soap and lukewarm water. *Clean, intact mucous membranes are the first line of defense against infection.*
- Provide catheter and perineal care. *Clients with diabetes are prone to developing urinary tract infections.*
- Use meticulous sterile technique when performing wound care or any invasive procedure. *These measures prevent infection in existing wounds or introduction of bacteria into the body.*
- Encourage adequate nutrition and fluid intake. *Maintaining satisfactory food and fluid intake reduces susceptibility to infection.*
- Assist client with oral hygiene. Brush teeth with a soft toothbrush and fluoridated toothpaste at least twice a day and floss. *Proper oral hygiene reduces the risk of periodontal disease.*
- Teach female diabetics the symptoms and preventive measures of vaginitis caused by *Candida albicans:*
  - Symptoms are an odorless, white or yellow, cheeselike vaginal discharge and itching.

BOX 17-9	CLIENT TEACHING

SAMPLE FOOT CARE TEACHING SESSION

Buying and Wearing Shoes and Stockings

- Shoes that allow 1/2 to 3/4 inch of toe room are best; there should be room for toes to spread out and wiggle. The lining and inside stitching should be smooth, and the insole soft. The sole should be flexible and cushion the foot. The heel should fit snugly, and the arch support should give good support.
- Do not wear open-toed shoes, sandals, high heels, or thongs; they increase the risk of trauma.
- Buy shoes late in the afternoon, when feet are at their largest; always buy shoes that feel comfortable and do not need to be "broken in."
- Shoes made of natural materials (leather, canvas) allow perspiration to escape.
- Check the shoes before each wearing for foreign objects, wrinkled insoles, and cracks that might cause lesions.
- Stockings made of wool or cotton allow perspiration to dry.
- Do not wear garters, knee stockings, or panty hose; they may interfere with circulation.
- Wear insulated boots in the winter.

Inspecting the Feet

- Check the feet daily for red areas, cuts, blisters, corns, calluses, or cracks in the skin. Check between the toes for cracks or reddened areas.
- Check the skin of the feet for dry or damp areas.
- Use a mirror to check each sole and the back of each heel.
- If you are unable to inspect the feet daily, be sure that someone else does so.

Care of Toenails

- Cut the toenails after washing, when they are softer and easier to trim.
- Cut the nails straight across with a clipper, and smooth edges and corners with an emery board.
- Do not use razor blades to trim the toenails.
- If you are unable to see well or to reach the feet easily, have someone else trim the nails. If the nails are very thick or ingrown, if the toes overlap, or if circulation is poor, get professional care.

General Information

- Take your shoes off at every visit to your health care provider.
- Never go barefoot. Wear slippers when leaving the bed during the night.
- Do not use commercial corn medicines or pads, chemicals (such as boric acid, iodine, or hydrogen peroxide), or over-the-counter cortisone medications on the feet.
- Do not put heating pads, hot water bottles, or ice packs on the feet. If the feet become cold at night, wear socks or use extra blankets.
- Do not allow the feet to become sunburned.
- Do not put tape on the feet.
- Do not sit with the legs crossed at the knees or ankles or wear constrictive clothing.

- Sexual transmission is unlikely, but discomfort may cause the client to avoid sexual activity. *Diabetes is a predisposing factor for* Candida albicans *vaginitis. Poor personal hygiene and use of clothing that keeps the vaginal area warm and moist increase the risk of vaginitis.*

clinical ALERT

Teach women with DM to take preventive measures such as not douching, wiping from front to back after voiding, wearing cotton underwear, and avoiding tight jeans and nylon pantyhose.

Risk for Injury

- Reduce environmental hazards in the health care facility.
  - Orient the client to new surroundings on admission.
  - Keep the bed at the lowest level with side rails raised if needed.
  - Keep the floors free of objects and wipe up spills immediately.
  - Use a night-light.
  - Teach the client to wear shoes or slippers when getting out of bed.
  - Monitor for side effects of prescribed medications, such as dizziness or drowsiness. *Strange environments increase the risk of falls.*
- Teach about safety in the home and community.
  - Use a night-light, preferably one with a soft, nonglare bulb. (*Note:* Red light is better, because the eyes adjust more quickly.)
  - Turn the head away when switching on a bright light.
  - Avoid looking directly into headlights when driving at night.
  - Conduct a daily foot inspection.
  - Wear shoes and slippers with nonskid soles.
  - Do not use throw rugs.
  - Provide handgrips in the tub and shower and next to the toilet. *Environmental hazards increase the risk of falls or other accidents. Glare is often responsible for falls when visual deficits exist.*

- Assist the client with tasks requiring finger and hand dexterity. *Clients with neuropathies may lose their ability to grip handles of cups or sharp objects.*
- Assist client during ambulation; provide ambulatory aids as needed. Do not rush the client. *These interventions decrease the potential for falls.*
- Advise client to get out of bed slowly. *Autonomic neuropathy can cause postural hypotension. When a client rises too quickly, there is a risk for dizziness and falls.*
- Monitor for DKA in the client with type 1 diabetes and for HHS in the client with type 2 DM. Teach the client and family to recognize and seek care for the manifestations of DKA or HHS. *DKA and HHS can be life threatening, which requires immediate medical treatment.*

clinical ALERT

Monitor frequently the older adult for symptoms of HHS, especially after major surgery.

- Monitor for and teach the client and family to recognize and treat the manifestations of hypoglycemia. The person should carry some form of a rapid-acting sugar source at all times. *Severe hypoglycemia causes a decreased level of consciousness.*
- Recommend that clients wear a Medic-Alert bracelet or necklace identifying themselves as having diabetes. *In case of sudden illness or accident, a Medic-Alert tag alerts health professionals about the client's diagnosis so that appropriate medical attention can be begun.*

Ineffective Coping

- Assess the client's perception of the current situation. *This establishes how the client feels about his or her diagnosis.*
- Assess the client's emotional resources and support sources. *Chronic illness affects all dimensions of a person's life as well as the lives of family members.*
- Provide an atmosphere of trust and support. *A positive emotional environment helps clients feel comfortable about discussing their concerns.*
- Explore with client and family the effects of the diagnosis and treatment on finances, occupation, energy levels, and relationships. *Failure to cope successfully can lead to noncompliance and poor blood glucose control. Common frustrations associated with diabetes are the disease itself, the treatment modalities, and the health care system.*
- Provide information about support groups and community resources. *Support groups offer opportunities for mutual support and problem solving. Community resources may help the client and family with other methods for coping with diabetes.*

EVALUATING

To evaluate the effectiveness of care for a client with DM, collect data related to the presence of chronic complications such as frequent infections, unhealed wounds, decreased vision, altered kidney function, peripheral neuropathy, and hypertension. In addition, identify the frequency with which the client has experienced DKA or HHS, and hypoglycemia. Document the client's vital signs, level of consciousness, skin integrity, and the presence of any acute or chronic complications. Notify the physician of the client's response to treatment. All reinforcement of client teaching related to medications, diet, and self-care must be documented.

CONTINUING CARE

Teaching the client and family involves all aspects of diabetes management. The nurse's role is to reinforce teaching completed by other health care providers such as registered nurses, certified diabetes educators, or dietitians. Because diabetes mellitus is a chronic disease, clients must be able to self-manage their disease at home.

During hospitalization, teaching should begin on admission. Before the actual teaching session starts, the nurse assesses the client's and the family's knowledge and learning needs, educational level, preferred learning methods and style, life experiences, and support systems. In addition, the nurse determines past diabetes management practices and identifies physical, emotional, and sociocultural needs.

It is important for the nurse and client to establish mutual goals based on the assessment data. Responsibility for daily management lies with the client. Family members must understand that their primary role is support. However, they must know how to provide physical care for the client if necessary.

If the client is newly diagnosed, the teaching first focuses on basic skills, then progresses to lifelong management strategies. Clients with a long-standing history of DM should not be overlooked. Often, they need a review of basic management strategies.

Below are some general guidelines for the nurse on teaching clients with diabetes mellitus:

- Listen to questions and provide information about common myths regarding diabetes.
- Present information in small segments.
- Explain medical terms so that the client understands the meaning.
- Be specific about what the client needs to know.
- Repeat and reinforce information as many times as necessary.
- Validate the person's knowledge and skills.
- Adapt teaching to the special needs of the older adult:

■ Diet changes may be difficult to implement. Favorite foods are hard to give up. Balanced meals at regular times may not have been part of the client's lifestyle. Purchasing, storing, and preparing foods may be a problem. Dentures may not fit well. Changes in taste sensation may cause the client to use more salt and sugar. A decreased thirst mechanism may lead to dehydration.

■ Exercise of any type may not have been part of the activities of daily living. Exercise is individualized to accommodate physical limitations caused by arthritis, Parkinson's disease, chronic respiratory diseases, and/or cardiovascular diseases.

■ A chronic illness diagnosis threatens independence and self-worth. After years of taking care of themselves, older adults who have to depend on others may withdraw from social situations. Distance from family or death of a spouse may cause depression.

■ Money to purchase medications and supplies or visit health care providers must be taken out of a fixed income.

■ Visual and fine motor skill deficits can make insulin administration, blood glucose monitoring, food preparation, exercises, and foot care difficult or impossible.

Box 17-10 ■ summarizes the knowledge and skills needed for self-management of DM.

Multiple resources are available to provide information on all aspects of self-management. Most hospitals or outpatient settings offer diabetes educational programs and support groups. Blood glucose screenings are often provided at little or no cost as part of community health promotion activities. Restaurants and airlines provide diabetic meals on request. Encourage clients to explore resources in their own communities.

NURSING PROCESS CARE PLAN
Client with Type 1 Diabetes

James Meligrito, 24 years old, is a first-year nursing student at a local community college. He attends school full time and works 20 hours a week as a campus student security guard. He works from 8 P.M. to 12 midnight, 5 nights a week. Mr. Meligrito dislikes cooking and usually eats "whatever is handy." He was diagnosed with type 1 diabetes mellitus when he was 12. Currently, he takes a total of 32 units of insulin each day, 10 units of NPH, and 6 units of regular insulin each morning and evening. He monitors his blood glucose about three times a week. He feels that he is too busy for a regular exercise program and that he gets

BOX 17-10   CLIENT TEACHING

Teaching for Client Self-Management of Diabetes

The nurse reinforces teaching and skills for clients with DM. The content of a teaching plan includes the following points:

■ Information about how diabetes changes body metabolism.

■ *Dietary plan:* How diet helps keep blood glucose in normal range; why they should eat complex carbohydrates and foods high in fiber but limit the intake of sugar, fat, sodium, and alcohol; how to read food labels for sugar and fat; integrating personal food preferences; eating meals away from home; relationship between diet, exercise, and medication.

■ *Exercise:* How it helps lower blood glucose; the importance of regular exercise program; types of exercise; and integrating personal exercise choices.

■ *Glucose levels:* Self-monitoring of blood glucose; how to perform the tests accurately; how to care for equipment; what to do for high or low blood glucose.

■ *Medications:*
  ■ Insulin type, dosage, mixing instructions (if necessary); times of onset and peak actions; how to get and care for equipment; how to give injections; where to give injections; timing of insulin injections and mealtimes.
  ■ *Oral agents:* Type, dosage, side effects, interaction with other drugs.

■ *Complications:*
  ■ Factors that cause diabetic ketoacidosis or HHS; manifestations of each; what to do when they occur.
  ■ Factors that cause hypoglycemia; manifestations; what to do when they occur.

■ *Safety precautions:* Identify person to contact in an emergency; carrying ID card and rapid-acting glucose; carrying insulin and glucagon kit.

■ *Hygiene:* Skin, dental, foot care.

■ *Vision:* Yearly exam, sources for vision aids such as magnifying sleeve for insulin syringe or large-print instructions.

■ *Sick days:* What to do about food, fluids, and medications.

■ *Communication and follow-up:*
  ■ What signs and symptoms to report; whom to contact; when to report.
  ■ Importance of keeping follow-up appointments.
  ■ Resources such as American Diabetes Association, diabetic education classes, diabetic support groups, weight loss programs, and publications such as *Diabetes Forecast.*

enough exercise in clinicals and in weekend sports activities. He has not seen a health care provider for over a year.

One day during a 6-hour clinical, Mr. Meligrito notices that he is urinating frequently, is thirsty, and has blurred vision. He is very tired but blames all his symptoms on working too much and studying for school. He forgot to take his morning insulin and realizes he must have hyperglycemia but decides that he will be all right until he gets home in the afternoon. Around noon, he complains of abdominal pain, weakness, and a rapid pulse. When he reports his physical symptoms to his clinical instructor, she takes him immediately to the hospital emergency department (ED).

Assessment. In the ED his blood glucose level is 300 mg/dL. Urine shows the presence of ketones. His electrolytes are normal, with a pH of 7.1. Vital signs: T 99°F (37.2°C); P 140; R 28; BP 102/52. An IV of 1,000 mL 0.9% normal saline is started at a rate of 400 mL/hr. He receives 10 units of regular insulin IV. Three hours later, his blood glucose level is 160, with normal vital signs. He is sent home with an appointment the next morning with the hospital's diabetes clinical specialist, Carole Traci.

Diagnosis. The following nursing diagnoses are identified for Mr. Meligrito:

■ *Powerlessness* related to a perceived lack of control of diabetes due to demands on his time
■ *Deficient Knowledge* regarding self-management of diabetes
■ *Ineffective Therapeutic Regimen Management* related to difficulty in modifying his personal habits.

Expected Outcomes. The expected outcomes for the plan of care are that Mr. Meligrito will:

■ Identify those aspects of diabetes that can be controlled and participate in making decisions about self-managing care.
■ Demonstrate an understanding of diabetes self-management through planned medication, diet, exercise, and blood glucose self-monitoring activities.
■ Verbalize ways to modify his personal habits.

Planning and Implementation. Ms. Traci plans and implements the following nursing interventions for Mr. Meligrito during the diabetes education program:

■ Develop short-term and long-term goals for Mr. Meligrito's self-management of control of blood glucose.
■ Discuss Mr. Meligrito's personal habits and ways to modify them.
■ Provide positive reinforcement for increasing his involvement in self-care activities.
■ Review insulin administration, dietary management, exercise, self-monitoring of blood glucose, and healthy lifestyle.

Evaluation. After participating in weekly diabetes classes for 2 months, Mr. Meligrito has increased his understanding of and compliance with managing his diabetes. He states that he finally understands how insulin, food, and exercise affect his body, having previously thought they were "just things I should do when I wanted to." Mr. Meligrito developed a workable meal schedule and weekly grocery list. Mr. Meligrito and a friend have arranged to walk 2 to 3 miles three times a week on a community hiking trail. To gain a sense of control over his illness, Mr. Meligrito has also worked out a schedule that allows time for school, health care, and himself.

Critical Thinking in the Nursing Process

1. What factors caused Mr. Meligrito's diabetic ketoacidosis?
2. Explain why this client received an intravenous infusion of 0.9% NS and intravenous insulin?
3. Consider that you are teaching Mr. Meligrito and another client, Mr. McDaniel (age 75, newly diagnosed with type 2 DM). What components of your teaching plan would be the same and what components would be different?

Note: The bibliography listings for this and all chapters have been compiled at the end of the book.

Chapter Review

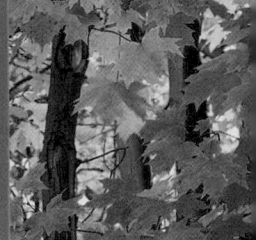

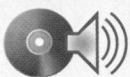 ## KEY TERMS by Topics

Use the audio glossary feature of either the CD-ROM or the Companion Website to hear the correct pronunciation of the following key terms.

Diabetes mellitus

diabetes mellitus, hyperglycemia, keto-sis, glycosuria, osmotic diuretic, polyuria, polydipsia, polyphagia

Complications

diabetic ketoacidosis (DKA), ketonuria, hyperosmolar hyperglycemic state (HHS), hypoglycemia, Somogyi effect, dawn phenomenon, gangrene, diabetic retinopathy, diabetic nephropathy, glomerulosclerosis, microalbuminuria, diabetic neuropathy

KEY Points

- Diabetes mellitus (DM) is a metabolic disorder of the pancreas that results from insulin deficiency.

- The classic manifestations of type 1 diabetes include polydipsia, polyuria, polyphagia, weight loss, and fatigue. Type 2 diabetes is characterized by polyuria, polydipsia, obesity, recurrent infections, and fatigue.

- Diabetes is diagnosed by fasting blood glucose, glycosylated hemoglobin, and oral glucose tolerance test.

- Type 1 diabetes is managed with insulin, diet, and exercise. Type 2 diabetes may be managed with oral antidiabetic drugs, diet, and exercise.

- Diabetic ketoacidosis (DKA) can occur in type 1 DM while hyperosmolar hyperglycemic state develops in type 2 DM; both of which are life-threatening complications.

- DKA is treated with a combination of intravenous fluid and electrolyte solutions, and insulin.

- Clients who develop hypoglycemia must be treated immediately with 15 g of a rapid-acting sugar to prevent prolonged neurologic damage.

- Clients with long-term diabetes have a greater incidence of chronic complications especially affecting vision, the kidneys, renal and nerve function, and lower extremities.

- Nursing management focuses on maintaining normal blood glucose levels, preventing acute and chronic complications, maintaining skin integrity, teaching self-management, and increasing coping skills.

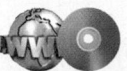 ## EXPLORE MediaLink

Additional interactive resources for this chapter can be found on the Companion Website at www.prenhall.com/burke. Click on Chapter 17 and "Begin" to select the activities for this chapter.

For chapter-related NCLEX-style review questions and an audio glossary, access the accompanying CD-ROM in this book.

FOR FURTHER Study

See Table 15-2 for tests used to diagnose diabetes.

For more information about exercise-stress electrocardiograms and a discussion of myocardial infarctions and atherosclerosis, see Chapter 26.

For more about peripheral vascular disease, see Chapter 28.

For more information on renal failure, see Chapter 32.

Critical Thinking Care Map

Caring for a Client with Diabetes Mellitus
NCLEX-PN® Focus Area: Health Promotion and Maintenance

Case Study: Mrs. Vaughn, age 64, has type 2 diabetes mellitus and is visiting her physician for a 6-month checkup. As she walks to the exam, the nurse notices that she walks with a slight limp. She is helped to remove her shoes, and the nurse notices several red spots over the top of the toes on her right foot and a blister on her left heel. Mrs. Vaughn tells you that she does not know how this happened. "I never saw these red spots on my toes or the blister on my heel." She also says that she bought a new pair of shoes last week and has been wearing them every day.

Nursing Diagnosis: Impaired Skin Integrity

COLLECT DATA

Subjective

_____
_____
_____
_____
_____
_____

Objective

_____
_____
_____
_____
_____
_____

Would you report this data? Yes/No

If yes, to: _____

Nursing Care

_____
_____
_____
_____
_____
_____
_____
_____
_____
_____
_____

How would you document this? _____
_____
_____
_____

Data Collected
(use those that apply)

- Weight 160 lbs
- Red spots on top of the toes on her right foot
- Fasting blood glucose 160 mg/dL
- Blister on the left heel
- Does not complain of any discomfort in her feet
- Says she uses a hot water bottle on her feet at night
- Complains of tingling in both feet

Nursing Interventions
(use those that apply; list in priority order)

- Discuss changes in her diet.
- Cleanse feet with normal saline.
- Discuss the importance of not smoking.
- Apply lubricating lotion to her feet and between the toes.
- Teach her to wear new shoes for a short period of time each day.
- Instruct client in proper foot care.
- Teach her to monitor red areas for signs of skin breakdown.

1 A client is instructed to check his blood glucose before meals and administer insulin according to a sliding scale. The nurse will teach him to use which type of insulin?

A. Humulin N
B. Humulin R
C. Lente
D. Humulin 70/30

2 A client with diabetes mellitus experiences hypoglycemia during the night followed by episodes of hyperglycemia when the blood glucose is assessed in the morning. The nurse recognizes these symptoms as:

A. Somogyi effect.
B. diabetic ketoacidosis.
C. dawn phenomenon.
D. hyperosmolar hyperglycemic state.

3 A female client with a history of diabetes mellitus visits her physician because of flulike symptoms. Which of the following indicates a need for further teaching when she discusses her sick-day care:

A. "I will check my blood glucose every four hours."
B. "I will check my urine ketones if my blood glucose is above 250 mg/dL."
C. "I will hold my daily insulin dose until I stop vomiting."
D. "I will consume ten to fifteen grams of carbohydrates every one to two hours."

4 A client with diabetes mellitus asks if he must stop smoking because diabetes mellitus increases his risk of lung disease. The nurse's response is based on the knowledge that:

A. diabetics are at greater risk for lung cancer.
B. diabetics are at greater risk for emphysema.
C. nicotine in tobacco causes venous vasodilatation.
D. nicotine in tobacco leads to arterial vasoconstriction.

5 A 16-year-old girl is diagnosed with diabetes mellitus. Which of her following statements indicates a need for further instruction?

A. "When my blood sugar is stable, I will be able to stop taking insulin and use pills for my diabetes."
B. "I will rotate my insulin injection sites."
C. My blood glucose should be maintained between 70 and 110 mg/dL."
D. "I will perform foot care and inspect my feet daily."

6 A client with diabetes received Humulin N 40 units at 7:30 A.M. The most likely time the nurse would expect him to experience hypoglycemia is:

A. 9:30 A.M.
B. 11:30 A.M.
C. 12:30 P.M.
D. 1:30 P.M.

7 A client is admitted to the nursing unit with a diagnosis of diabetic ketoacidosis. Which of the following assessment findings should the nurse expect?

A. cool, clammy skin
B. acetone breath odor
C. slurred speech
D. radial pulse 70, bounding

8 The nurse instructs a client to mix Humulin N and Humulin R insulin. List the actions in the sequence in which the client should perform them.

A. Inject air into the Humulin N vial first.
B. Gently rotate Humalin N vial.
C. Withdraw Humulin R insulin first.
D. Wipe off top of both vials with alcohol pad.
E. Inspect Humulin R for clarity.

9 A client is conscious when she arrives in the emergency department with a blood glucose of 50 mg/dL. What nursing intervention should the nurse anticipate doing for this client?

A. Give lispro (Humalog) injection.
B. Give crackers and cheese.
C. Give glucagon injection.
D. Give a half cup regular soda.

10 The nurse instructs a diabetic client on foot care. Appropriate instruction should include which of the following points? Select all that apply.

A. Cut the toenails straight across with a clipper.
B. Have a family member check a heating pad before applying to feet.
C. Apply lotion or oil generously between the toes.
D. Wear closed-toe shoes made of soft leather.
E. If buying a new pair of shoes, shop in early morning.
F. Use a mirror to check your soles every day.

Answers for Review Questions, as well as discussion of Care Plan and Critical Thinking Care Map questions, appear in Appendix V.

Thinking Strategically About...

Jake, a 54-year-old male, was admitted with a diagnosis of type 2 diabetes mellitus, end-stage renal disease, and gangrenous infection of the left foot. Client is receiving hemodialysis 3 times per week. Physician's orders on admission are as follows:

- Bed rest
- Lab in A.M.
  - Chemistry panel (chem. 16)
  - Glycohemoglobin level
  - CBC
- Diet: 1,500-calorie carbohydrate-consistent
- Fluid restriction: 1,200 mL per 24 hours
- Glucoscan a.c. and h.s.
- Sliding scale insulin coverage

A.M. Lab Results

	NORMAL VALUES	CLIENT VALUES
Potassium	(3.6–5.0)	5.6
Chloride	(98–107)	94
Creatinine	(0.7–1.5)	10
Blood urea nitrogen	(7–20)	50
Glucose	(70–110)	328

CRITICAL THINKING

You need to prioritize Jake's care. Outline your plan of care for Jake and provide rationales.

COLLABORATIVE CARE

The lab calls the results to the nursing unit. What should you do about the lab report?

COMMUNICATION

Jake expresses concerns about his self-care when he is discharged. Outline important client teaching points that must be addressed and how you would evaluate Jake's learning and his ability to carry out his self-care.

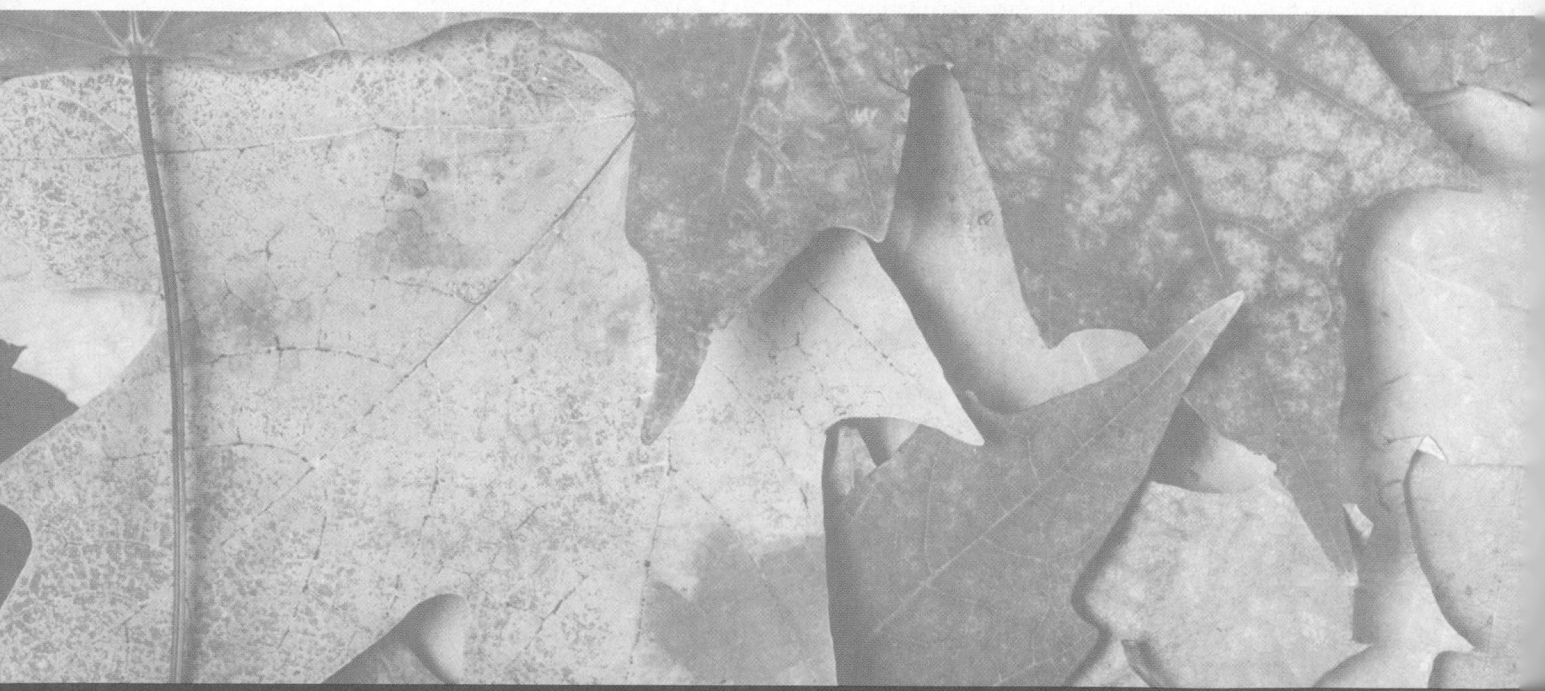

Disrupted Gastrointestinal Function

UNIT IV

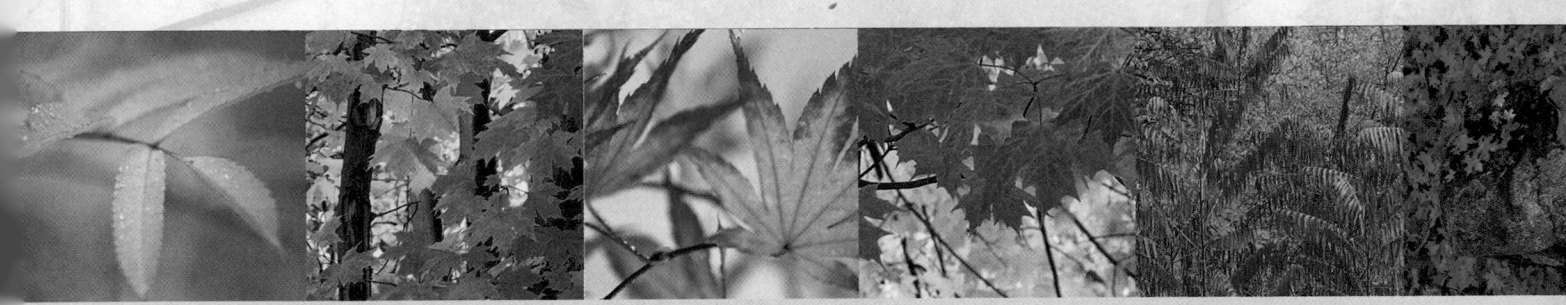

The Gastrointestinal System and Assessment

BRIEF Outline

The Gastrointestinal Tract
Mouth, Pharynx, and Esophagus
Stomach
Small Intestine
Large Intestine
Common Changes Associated with Aging

Accessory Organs of Digestion
Liver and Gallbladder
Pancreas
Nutrients
Metabolism

Assessment
Health History
Physical Examination
Diagnostic Tests

LEARNING Outcomes

After completing this chapter, you will be able to:

- Describe the structure and function of the gastrointestinal (GI) tract and accessory organs of digestion (liver, gallbladder, and pancreas).
- Describe the physiologic processes involved in ingestion, digestion, and elimination of foods and nutrients.
- Identify sources of various nutrients, including vitamins.
- Collect assessment data related to digestion and nutritional status.
- Discuss the nursing implications of diagnostic tests for clients with disorders of nutrition or affecting the GI tract or accessory organs.

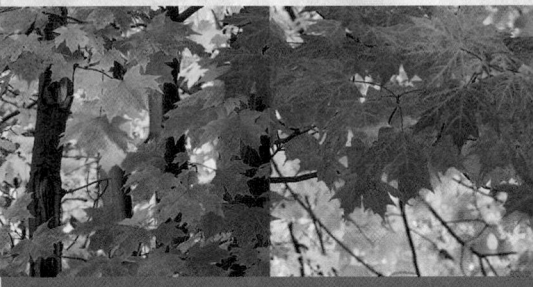

MediaLink

www.prenhall.com/burke
Use the address above to access the free, interactive Companion Website created for this textbook. Get hints, instant feedback, and textbook references to chapter-related NCLEX-style questions. Link to other interesting sites.

Audio Glossary:
Use the Companion Website, or the CD-ROM disk enclosed with your textbook, to hear the pronunciation of key terms in this chapter.

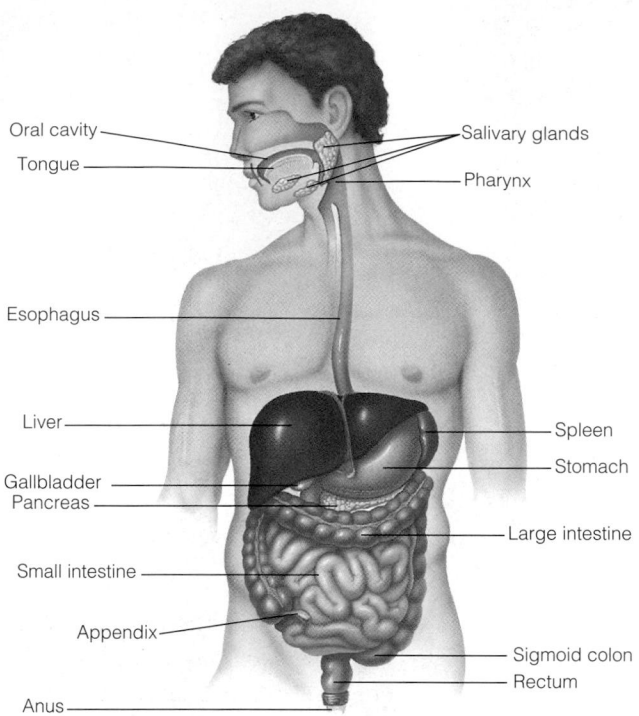

Figure 18-1. ■ Organs of the gastrointestinal tract and accessory digestive organs.

Nutrition is the process of ingesting, absorbing, using, and eliminating food in the body. The digestive organs involved in these processes are the gastrointestinal (GI) tract and the accessory digestive organs. The GI tract includes the mouth, pharynx, esophagus, stomach, small intestine, and large intestine (Figure 18-1 ■). The large intestine is primarily an organ of elimination. The accessory digestive organs include the liver, gallbladder, and pancreas.

The Gastrointestinal Tract

The gastrointestinal tract is a continuous hollow tube. Once foods are ingested, they are broken down into products that can be absorbed as they move through the GI tract.

MOUTH, PHARYNX, AND ESOPHAGUS

The *mouth,* the upper opening of the GI tract, is lined with mucous membranes. In the mouth, the teeth chew and grind food into smaller parts. *Saliva* (produced by the salivary glands) moistens food for tasting, chewing, and swallowing. The digestive process starts in the mouth as enzymes in saliva (*amylase* and *lysozyme*) begin to break down food. The tongue mixes food with saliva, forms the food into a mass (*bolus*), and initiates swallowing. Muscles in the pharynx move food to the esophagus. The esophagus carries food to the stomach through **peristalsis** (alternating waves of contraction and relaxation). The esophagus enters the stomach through the *cardiac* or *lower esophageal sphincter.* This sphincter, normally closed except during swallowing, keeps food in the stomach.

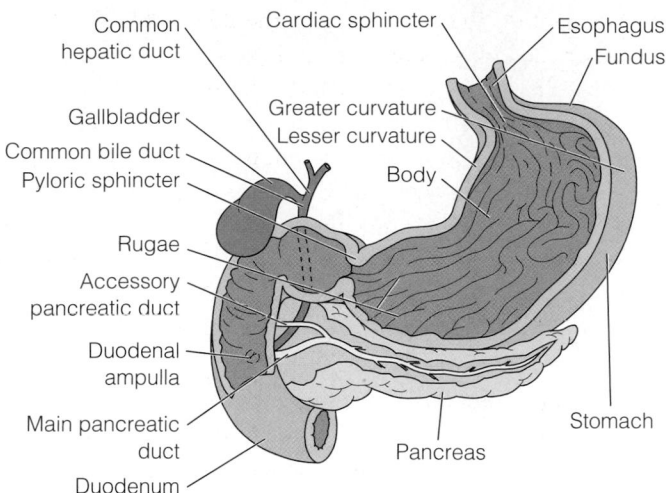

Figure 18-2. ■ Structures of the stomach and duodenum, including the common bile duct, pancreatic duct, pancreas, and gallbladder.

STOMACH

The *stomach,* connected to the esophagus at the upper end and to the small intestine at the lower end, can expand to hold up to 4 L of food and fluid (Figure 18-2 ■). The stomach continues the digestive process. Mechanical digestion in the stomach mixes partially digested food with gastric juices to produce **chyme.** Four to five liters of gastric juices are produced by specialized cells in the stomach lining every day:

■ *Parietal cells* secrete hydrochloric acid and intrinsic factor. Hydrochloric acid is vital to protein digestion; intrinsic factor is necessary for vitamin B_{12} absorption.
■ *Chief cells* produce pepsin, the primary enzyme in gastric juice, which digests protein.
■ *Mucous cells* produce alkaline mucus that protects the lining of the stomach from gastric juices.
■ *Enteroendocrine cells* secrete hormones that help regulate digestion.

The nervous system also controls gastric secretion. Seeing, smelling, or tasting food stimulates the parasympathetic nervous system to send signals via the vagus nerve that increase gastric secretion. Emotions such as anxiety or stress, on the other hand, inhibit gastric secretion and motility.

The *pyloric sphincter* controls emptying of the stomach into the duodenum. The stomach empties completely within 4 to 6 hours after a meal.

SMALL INTESTINE

The small intestine is about 20 ft (6 m) long but only about 1 in. (2.5 cm) in diameter. It hangs in coils in the abdomen, suspended by folds of peritoneal membrane and surrounded by the large intestine. The small intestine has three regions:

the duodenum, the jejunum, and the ileum. The *duodenum* begins at the pyloric sphincter and extends for about 10 in. (25 cm). Pancreatic enzymes and bile from the liver enter the small intestine at the duodenum (see Figure 18-2). The *jejunum,* the middle region, is about 8 ft (2.4 m) long. It connects with the *ileum,* the distal 12 ft (3.6 m) of small bowel, which meets the large intestine at the ileocecal valve.

Food is chemically digested, and most of it is absorbed, as it moves through the small intestine. Enzymes in the small intestine break down carbohydrates, proteins, and fats. Buffers produced by the pancreas neutralize the acid from the stomach. *Microvilli* (tiny cell projections), *villi* (finger-like projections of the mucosa), and deep folds of the mucosal layers increase the surface area of the small intestine to enhance absorption of food. Almost all food products and water, as well as vitamins and minerals, are absorbed through the intestinal mucosa into the blood or lymph. Although up to 10 L of food, liquids, and secretions enter the GI tract each day, less than 1 L reaches the large intestine. Only indigestible fibers, some water, and bacteria enter the large intestine.

Bowel elimination is the end process in digestion. After foods are eaten and broken down into usable elements, nutrients are absorbed and indigestible materials are eliminated.

LARGE INTESTINE

The *large intestine,* or colon, begins at the *ileocecal valve* and terminates at the *anus* (Figure 18-3 ■). It is about 5 ft (1.5 m) long. The first part of the large intestine, the *cecum,* includes the *appendix.* The colon is divided into *ascending, transverse,* and *descending* segments. The descending colon ends at the S-shaped *sigmoid colon.* The sigmoid colon terminates at the rectum.

The *rectum* has transverse folds that help retain feces while allowing flatus to pass. The anorectal junction separates the rectum from the *anal canal,* which terminates at

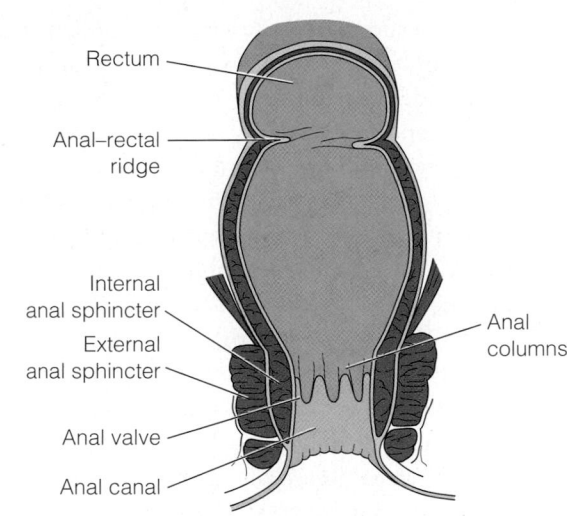

Figure 18-4. ■ Structure of the rectum and anus.

the anus. The *anus,* a hairless, dark-skinned area, is the end of the digestive tract. It has an internal involuntary sphincter and an external voluntary sphincter (Figure 18-4 ■). The sphincters are usually open only during defecation.

The major function of the large intestine is to eliminate indigestible food residue from the body. It absorbs water, salts, and vitamins from the semiliquid chyme that passes through the ileocecal valve, forming it into *feces (stool).* Feces is moved along the intestine by *peristalsis,* waves of alternating contraction and relaxation. Goblet cells lining the large intestine secrete mucus that lubricates the feces, helping it move.

When feces enter the rectum and stretch the rectal wall, the *defecation reflex* causes the walls of the sigmoid colon to contract and the anal sphincters to relax. The reflex can be suppressed by voluntary control of the external sphincter. Defecation can be assisted by closing the glottis and contracting the diaphragm and abdominal muscles to increase intra-abdominal pressure *(Valsalva's maneuver).*

COMMON CHANGES ASSOCIATED WITH AGING

Common changes in gastrointestinal function associated with aging can have a significant effect on nutrition, general health, and well-being. Some are normal consequences of the aging process; other changes, such as periodontal disease and tooth loss, do not result from the aging process itself, but are prevalent in older adults.

Periodontal disease, disease of the supporting structures of the teeth, is a common cause of tooth loss in older adults. It results from poor dental hygiene and environmental factors such as lack of access to fluoridated water supplies. In addition, genetics plays a role in periodontal disease, accounting for a significant portion of people affected. Loosening and loss of teeth affect the older adult's ability to chew food

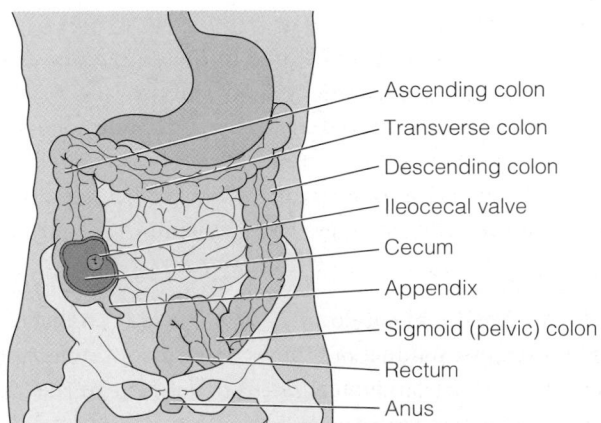

Figure 18-3. ■ Anatomy of the large intestine.

effectively. This, in turn, can lead to nutritional deficiencies as the person limits the intake of foods that are difficult to chew, for example, fresh fruits and vegetables or meat.

The tongue atrophies with aging and the number of taste buds decrease. The resulting alterations in taste can lead to excessive use of salt to make food more flavorful and appealing. Saliva production decreases with aging. The mouth is dry, increasing the risk for irritation of the oral mucosa. The lack of saliva also interferes with the initial digestion of starches, which occurs in the mouth, and with swallowing.

The swallowing mechanism itself also is impacted by age, increasing the time required to initiate and complete a swallow. Esophageal peristalsis slows, and food may remain in the esophagus, causing discomfort. The lower esophageal (cardiac) sphincter tends to relax, increasing gastric reflux and the risk for aspiration.

In the stomach and proximal small intestine, digestive juice secretion may be decreased. As a result, the older adult may experience more food intolerances and a feeling of satiety (fullness) after just a few bites of food. In the small intestine, fats are more slowly absorbed, and other nutrients such as glucose, some B vitamins, vitamin D, and minerals such as calcium and iron are less effectively absorbed. Intestinal peristalsis slows, and less mucous secretion occurs in the large bowel. The rectal wall is less elastic, affecting the ability to expel feces. These changes, along with changes in food intake patterns and lower activity levels common in aging, increase the risk for constipation.

Accessory Organs of Digestion

LIVER AND GALLBLADDER

The liver is the largest gland in the body, weighing about 3 lbs (1.4 kg) in the average-sized adult. It is located in the right side of the abdomen, inferior to the diaphragm and anterior to the stomach (see Figure 18-1). The liver has four lobes: right (the largest), left, caudate, and quadrate. It is encased in a fibrous capsule and covered by a layer of visceral peritoneum.

Each lobe contains many **lobules,** the basic functional units of the liver. Within each lobule, plates of **hepatocytes** (liver cells) are arranged like the spokes of a wheel out from a central vein (Figure 18-5 ■). Each lobule receives oxygen-rich blood from a branch of the hepatic artery and nutrient-rich venous blood from the digestive tract via the portal vein. Arterial and venous blood flows through enlarged capillaries *(sinusoids)* into the central vein. The sinusoids are lined with macrophages called *Kupffer cells,* which remove debris, such as bacteria and aged blood cells, from the blood.

Hepatocytes produce bile and perform many metabolic functions. *Bile* is a greenish, watery solution containing bile

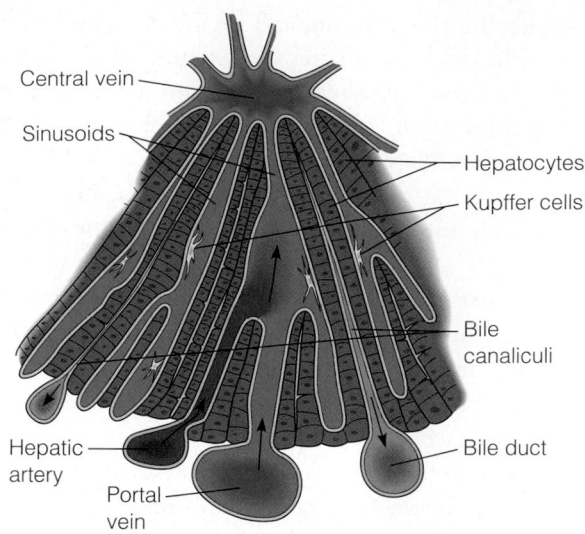

Figure 18-5. ■ A section of a liver lobule with plates of hepatocytes, the central vein, bile duct, portal vein, and hepatic artery.

salts, cholesterol, bilirubin, electrolytes, water, and phospholipids. Bile is necessary to emulsify and absorb fats. The bile flows out through tiny channels called *canaliculi* to the bile ducts.

The liver's primary activities can be categorized as metabolic, hematologic, and digestive. It performs many different functions essential to life:

- Metabolizes carbohydrates, proteins, and fats.
- Eliminates old blood cells, cellular debris, and bacteria.
- Inactivates toxins and foreign substances such as alcohol and drugs.
- Synthesizes plasma proteins and enzymes.
- Metabolizes or inactivates hormones.
- Stores blood, vitamins, and minerals.
- Produces and excretes bile.

Liver cells make from 700 to 1,200 mL of bile every day. When bile is not needed for digestion, the *sphincter of Oddi* (located at the point at which bile enters the duodenum) is closed, and the bile backs up the cystic duct into the gallbladder for storage.

Bile is concentrated and stored in the *gallbladder,* a small sac on the inferior surface of the liver (Figure 18-6 ■). When food containing fats enters the duodenum, hormones stimulate the gallbladder to secrete bile into the cystic duct. The cystic duct joins the hepatic duct to form the common bile duct, from which bile enters the duodenum.

PANCREAS

The pancreas, a gland located between the stomach and small intestine, produces enzymes necessary for digestion. It extends across the abdomen, with its tail next to the spleen and its head next to the duodenum (see Figure 18-1). The body and tail of the pancreas lie behind the stomach and

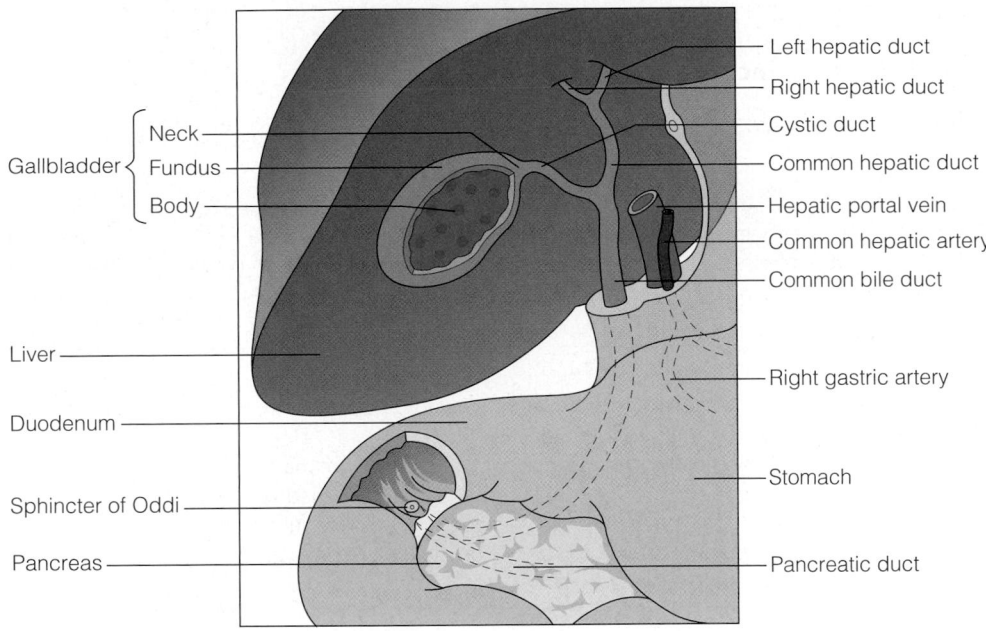

Figure 18-6. ■ The gallbladder, common bile duct, and sphincter of Oddi.

the peritoneal membrane (**retroperitoneal**). The pancreas is actually two organs in one, having both exocrine and endocrine structures and functions. The exocrine portion secretes alkaline pancreatic juice into the pancreatic duct. The pancreatic duct joins with the common bile duct just before it enters the duodenum (see Figure 18-6). The pancreas also has endocrine functions (see Chapter 17). ∞

Every day, the pancreas produces 1 to 1.5 L of pancreatic juice containing bicarbonate to neutralize the acidic chyme as it enters the duodenum. The increased pH promotes digestion in the small intestine. Pancreatic secretion is controlled by the vagus nerve and the hormones secretin and cholecystokinin. Pancreatic juice contains enzymes that can digest all categories of foods: *Lipase* promotes fat breakdown and absorption; *amylase* completes starch digestion; and *trypsin, chymotrypsin,* and *carboxypeptidase* are responsible for half of all protein digestion. *Nucleases,* which digest nucleic acids, are also present in pancreatic juice.

CHANGES ASSOCIATED WITH AGING

The size of the liver decreases with age, and it becomes less able to regenerate. The incidence of gallstones increases with age due to changes in cholesterol metabolism and absorption. Ducts of the pancreas dilate and distend with aging. The effects of these changes on liver and pancreatic function are unclear.

NUTRIENTS

Nutrients are substances in foods that are used by the body for growth, maintenance, and repair. They include carbohydrates, proteins, fats, vitamins, minerals, and water (Table 18-1 ■).

METABOLISM

After nutrients are ingested, digested, absorbed, and transported to the cells, they are metabolized to produce energy. **Metabolism** is the term for biochemical reactions that occur in the cells. Metabolism involves two basic processes. *Catabolism* breaks down complex structures into simpler forms, such as carbohydrates into adenosine triphosphate (ATP)—the fuel for cell processes. *Anabolism* combines simpler molecules to build more complex structures (e.g., amino acids into proteins). Water and carbon dioxide are waste products of metabolism. The energy produced by foods is measured as *kilocalories (kcal)*.

Assessment

In the focused assessment of the gastrointestinal tract, the nurse collects data about the client's nutritional status, the GI system, and its function.

HEALTH HISTORY

Ask the client about any current complaints related to food intake or tolerance, appetite, heartburn, nausea or vomiting, abdominal discomfort, diarrhea, or constipation. Inquire about recent weight changes and any associated factors (such as dieting). Question regarding food allergies or intolerances and their effects. Have the client relate the usual pattern and amount of daily food intake. Ask if the client wears dentures (full or partial) and about any associated problems such as fit or irritation. As indicated, ask specific questions about the teeth, mouth discomfort, and ability to chew and to swallow.

TABLE 18-1

Nutrients, Food Sources, and Function

NUTRIENT	COMMON FOOD SOURCES	FUNCTION	EFFECT OF EXCESS OR DEFICIT
Carbohydrates ■ Composed of simple or complex sugars ■ *Recommended intake:* 125–175 g/day	Simple sugars: milk, sugar cane, sugar beets, honey, fruits Complex starches: grains, legumes, root vegetables	Converted to glucose, used by cells to make ATP Excess glucose converted to glycogen or fat for storage	Excess: obesity, dental caries, elevated serum triglycerides Deficit: tissue wasting (protein breakdown), metabolic acidosis (fat breakdown)
Proteins ■ Composed of amino acids ■ *Recommended intake:* 0.8 g/kg body weight	Complete proteins (contain all the essential amino acids): eggs, milk, milk products, and meat, fish, and poultry Plant (or *complementary*) proteins: legumes, nuts, grains, cereals, and vegetables	Vital for body structure and function *Nitrogen balance* maintained by intake equal to that needed for protein synthesis, preventing breakdown of body proteins	Excess: obesity Deficit: weight loss, tissue wasting, thin, sparse hair, edema, anemia
Fats (Lipids) ■ Composed of triglycerides, phospholipids, sterols ■ *Recommended intake:* 30% or less of total daily caloric intake; saturated fat, 10% or less of total daily caloric intake	Saturated fats: animal fats, cocoa butter, palm and coconut oils; hydrogenated (solid) vegetable fats (stick margarine, vegetable shortening) Unsaturated fats: liquid vegetable oils, soft margarines	Triglycerides: fuel supply, insulation; essential fatty acids help form cell membranes and hormones; carry fat-soluble vitamins A, D, E, and K Phospholipids: cell membranes Sterols: bile, sex hormones, adrenal hormones, vitamin D, and cholesterol	Excess: obesity, increased risk of heart disease Deficit: weight loss; skin lesions
Vitamins ■ Organic, essential nutrients; includes fat-soluble A, D, E, K; water-soluble B complex, C, niacin, biotin, folic acid ■ *Recommended intake:* Varies by specific vitamin	Found in a variety of foods, including fruits, vegetables, grains, and animal products	Specific functions that promote growth, reproduction, maintenance of health	Selected effects of deficits: Nails: iron—soft, spoon-shaped Hair: zinc—dry, dull, sparse Skin: vitamins A, B—flaky, dry; niacin—cracks; vitamin K—easy bruising; vitamin C—delayed healing Eyes: vitamin A—poor night vision; iron—pale conjunctiva Nervous system: thiamine—↓ deep tendon reflexes, peripheral neuropathies, confusion, apathy Musculoskeletal: thiamine—calf pain; vitamin C—joint pain GI: vitamin B complex—*cheilosis*, stomatitis, glossitis
Minerals ■ Inorganic elements; includes sodium, potassium, calcium, magnesium, chloride, phosphorus ■ *Recommended intake:* Varies by mineral	Found in a variety of foods, including fruits, vegetables, grains, and animal products	Specific regulatory functions (see Chapter 7) ⟳	
Water ■ *Recommended intake:* 1,500 to 2,000 mL/day as fluid	Water Other liquids such as fruit juices, milk, coffee, tea, soft drinks Foods such as gelatin	Body structure and form Transport and exchange medium Medium for metabolic reactions within cells Insulation and temperature regulation Lubricant	Deficit: thirst, weakness, weight loss, ↓ BP, orthostatic hypotension, ↑ heart rate, poor skin turgor Excess: ↑ BP, ↑ heart and respiratory rates, shortness of breath, weight gain, edema

TABLE 18-2	
Healthy Weights for Adults	
HEIGHT	**WEIGHT RANGE IN POUNDS**[a]
4'10"	91–119
4'11"	94–124
5'0"	97–128
5'1"	101–132
5'2"	104–137
5'3"	107–141
5'4"	111–146
5'5"	114–150
5'6"	118–155
5'7"	121–160
5'8"	125–164
5'9"	129–169
5'10"	132–174
5'11"	136–179
6'0"	140–184
6'1"	144–189
6'2"	148–195
6'3"	152–200
6'4"	156–205
6'5"	160–211
6'6"	164–216

Note: The higher weights in the ranges generally apply to men; the lower weights more often apply to women.
[a]Without shoes or clothing.

Have the client describe any abdominal pain or discomfort, including its location, timing, and relationship to food intake. Ask about usual bowel habits, and any recent changes that may have occurred, such as increased or decreased frequency of elimination, change in color or consistency of stool, or decreased caliber (size) of stools.

Ask about current medications, including use of over-the-counter drugs such as aspirin, ibuprofen, or other non-steroidal anti-inflammatory drugs (NSAIDs), antacids, or laxatives. Inquire about chronic diseases such as diabetes, inflammatory bowel disease, or peptic ulcer disease. Question regarding any previous surgery of the GI tract or abdomen.

PHYSICAL EXAMINATION

Observe general health status, including skin color and condition, hair, and nails. Obtain height and weight. Compare weight with ideal weight for height using height–weight charts (Table 18-2 ■).

Using a light source, inspect the mouth and teeth, noting the size and furrows of the tongue, condition and moisture of the mucous membranes and gums, and presence and condition of the teeth. Note any redness, irritation, color changes, or bleeding of mucous membranes or gums. Be sure to inspect under the tongue as well. Ask the client to swallow, and observe the swallow reflex.

Inspect the abdomen, noting shape and contour, any visible vessels, striae, or other skin or color changes. Observe for visible peristalsis. Auscultate for bowel sounds, listening in all four quadrants (Figure 18-7 ■). Bowel sounds (clicks or gurgles) normally are heard every 5 to 15 seconds.

Percuss the abdomen in all four quadrants as indicated. Tympany normally is heard over the stomach and much of the bowel. A fecal mass, tumor, or full bladder may cause a dull percussion tone. The percussion tone also is dull over the liver.

Lightly palpate all abdominal quadrants, noting muscle tone or guarding and any areas of tenderness. If the client has complained of abdominal pain, palpate the affected quadrant or area last. See Chapter 5 ⬤⬤ for more information about patient assessment and specific assessment techniques. Box 18-1 ■ presents a sample assessment of a client with a gastrointestinal complaint.

BOX 18-1	

DOCUMENTATION OF GASTROINTESTINAL AND NUTRITIONAL ASSESSMENT

Client: A 25-year-old woman presents at her primary care nurse practitioner's office with complaints of abdominal pain and frequent diarrhea for the past 3 to 4 weeks.

Assessment note: Current complaint of intermittent crampy abdominal pain and frequent diarrhea began gradually about 4 weeks ago. Denies other current or previous symptoms such as anorexia, nausea, vomiting, general malaise, or fever. No known exposure to contaminated food or water; has not traveled out of the region for over 6 months. Having 4 to 6 stools per day; has noticed some blood and mucus in stool. Crampy left lower quadrant abdominal pain is relieved following defecation. Denies previous problems with abdominal pain, diarrhea, or constipation. States she has been healthy all her life and able to maintain normal weight without dieting, but thinks she has lost several pounds since this problem began. Denies chronic diseases or known allergies to food or drugs. No previous surgery.

Appears somewhat anxious and uncomfortable. Color pink, skin warm and dry. Height 65 inches, weight 110 pounds (with clothing; without shoes). BP 106/60, P 84, R 16, T 97.6 F PO. Abdomen flat and symmetrical, no visible veins or striations noted. Active bowel sounds (10–12/min) noted in all quadrants. Tympanic percussion tone throughout. Tender to palpation in left lower quadrant, no guarding.

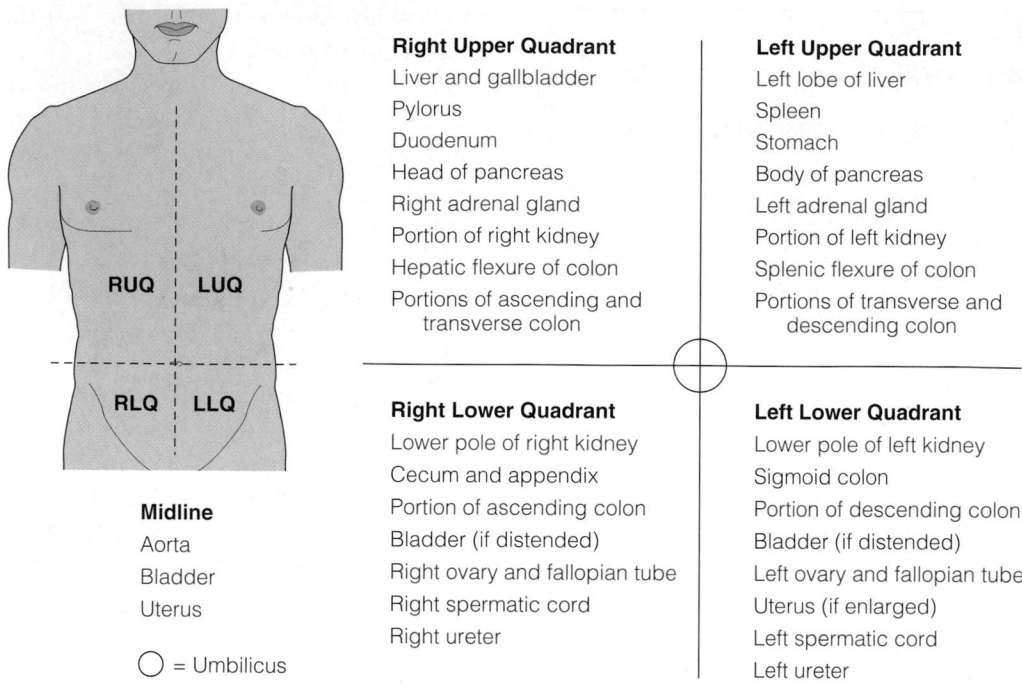

Right Upper Quadrant
Liver and gallbladder
Pylorus
Duodenum
Head of pancreas
Right adrenal gland
Portion of right kidney
Hepatic flexure of colon
Portions of ascending and
   transverse colon

Left Upper Quadrant
Left lobe of liver
Spleen
Stomach
Body of pancreas
Left adrenal gland
Portion of left kidney
Splenic flexure of colon
Portions of transverse and
   descending colon

Right Lower Quadrant
Lower pole of right kidney
Cecum and appendix
Portion of ascending colon
Bladder (if distended)
Right ovary and fallopian tube
Right spermatic cord
Right ureter

Left Lower Quadrant
Lower pole of left kidney
Sigmoid colon
Portion of descending colon
Bladder (if distended)
Left ovary and fallopian tube
Uterus (if enlarged)
Left spermatic cord
Left ureter

Midline
Aorta
Bladder
Uterus

◯ = Umbilicus

RUQ   LUQ

RLQ   LLQ

Figure 18-7. ■ The four quadrants of the abdomen, with the organs located within each quadrant.

DIAGNOSTIC TESTS

A number of laboratory and diagnostic tests commonly are used to evaluate the structure and function of the gastrointestinal tract and the accessory organs of digestion. Some, such as hemoglobin and hematocrit measurements and serum electrolyte levels are general indicators of health and illness; others provide specific information about GI function. The focus of this section is on those tests performed specifically to evaluate the structure and function of the gastrointestinal tract and its accessory organs. Measurements and calculations to evaluate the client's nutritional status are found in Chapter 19. ◗◗

Laboratory Tests

Several laboratory tests commonly are performed to evaluate the gastrointestinal system and the accessory organs of digestion. Table 18-3 ■ lists these tests, their normal values, what the test measures and its significance, and any nursing implications for the test.

Other Diagnostic Tests

Table 18-4 ■ lists special diagnostic procedures that may be used to evaluate the function of the GI tract or for specific disorders, such as gastroesophageal reflux or peptic ulcer disease.

A variety of imaging techniques are used to diagnose gastrointestinal disorders. These procedures range from noninvasive to very invasive. The use of noninvasive ultrasonography has replaced many of the more invasive and uncomfortable procedures in recent years. Diagnostic imaging procedures with their nursing implications are summarized in Table 18-5 ■.

Because the GI tract is a hollow tube accessible at each end (via the mouth and the anus), it can be visualized using a flexible endoscope. Endoscopes are fiber-optic instruments with a lighted lens that allow visual examination of organs and cavities of the body. Endoscopy is increasingly commonly used to evaluate the esophagus, stomach, colon, and peritoneal space. Endoscopy has significantly reduced the use of procedures such as x-rays using contrast media to evaluate the anatomy of the stomach and the colon. Common endoscopic procedures for evaluating the GI tract are outlined in Table 18-6 ■.

Chapter 18 The Gastrointestinal System and Assessment

TABLE 18-3

Common Laboratory Tests for Gastrointestinal Assessment

TEST	NORMAL ADULT VALUES	EXPLANATION	NURSING IMPLICATIONS
Serum albumin and total protein	Total protein: 6.0–8.0 g/dL or 60–80 g/L Albumin: 3.8–5.0 g/dL or 38–50 g/L	Used to assess general nutritional status and liver function.	Requires no special precautions or fasting. Total protein levels lower during pregnancy or prolonged bed rest.
Serologic *H. pylori* testing	No detectable antibody	Positive result indicates presence of antibodies to *H. pylori* bacteria; may or may not indicate current infection with *H. pylori*.	No special precautions or fasting required. .
Stool specimen for ova and parasites	None present	Used to detect the presence of infective organisms.	Avoid contamination of the specimen with urine, use a clean bedpan or collection device; instruct client to avoid mixing stool with urine or toilet tissue.
Liver Function Tests Alanine aminotransferase (ALT) Aspartate aminotransferase (AST) Alkaline phosphatase (ALP) Gamma-glutamyltransferase (GGT) Serum bilirubin	All values are for adults. 10–60 U/L 5–40 U/L Women: 81–234 U/L Men: 98–251 U/L Women: 5–55 U/L Men 5–85 U/L Total: 0.2–1.3 mg/dL Conjugated (direct): 0–0.2 mg/dL	Used to assess liver function, evaluate clients with jaundice, and detect liver disease such as hepatitis, alcoholic cirrhosis.	Fasting is required for the bilirubin, samples for other liver function studies may be drawn without fasting. Water is permitted.
Pancreatic Function Tests Serum amylase Serum lipase	Adult: 25–130 U/L Elderly: 21–160 U/L Adult: 10–140 U/L Elderly: 18–180 U/L	Used to assess pancreatic and salivary gland function and to monitor treatment of pancreatitis.	

TABLE 18-4

Diagnostic Tests for Gastrointestinal Assessment

DIAGNOSTIC TEST	EXPLANATION	NURSING IMPLICATIONS
Gastric analysis	Used to assess hydrochloric acid secretion and for the presence of *H. pylori* in the stomach. The sample is collected via nasogastric tube or during endoscopy. A drug to stimulate gastric acid secretion may be given during the test.	Food, fluids, smoking, chewing gum, and some drugs are withheld for 8–12 hours prior to the test. Insert a nasogastric tube per institutional procedure and collect samples as ordered. Observe for and take precautions to prevent aspiration during tube insertion or during the test. Instruct the client about anticipated discomfort with tube insertion, the duration of the test, and the procedure itself.

(continued)

TABLE 18-4

Diagnostic Tests for Gastrointestinal Assessment (continued)

DIAGNOSTIC TEST	EXPLANATION	NURSING IMPLICATIONS
Urea breath test	Used to detect infection with *H. pylori* bacteria. Radio-tagged urea is administered orally. If *H. pylori* is present, exhaled ammonia and carbon dioxide can be measured.	Food and fluids are withheld for 4 hours prior to the test; use of antacids, bismuth sulfate, antibiotics, and omeprazole (Prilosec) is restricted for 2 weeks before testing.
Ambulatory pH monitoring	Used to diagnose gastrointestinal reflux. A pH electrode inserted through the nose into the esophagus is connected to a data recorder worn on the belt. Recorded data are later analyzed by computer.	Provide instructions per protocol for caring for the electrode and data recorder.
Esophageal manometry	Measures pressures of the esophageal sphincters and esophageal peristalsis.	Food and fluids are withheld for 8 hours prior to testing; some medications may be withheld as well. Insertion of the tube may cause gagging; instruct the client to breathe through the mouth to control. The test takes about an hour to complete.
Paracentesis	An invasive procedure used to detect bleeding, contamination, or infection in the peritoneal cavity.	See Box 21-13 ⬀ for the nursing implications for paracentesis.

TABLE 18-5

Imaging Studies

TEST	EXPLANATION	NURSING IMPLICATIONS
Ultrasonography Abdominal ultrasound Gallbladder ultrasound Liver echogram	Echoes from high-frequency sound waves are used to detect and evaluate abdominal disorders, detect masses, and screen for abdominal aneurysms. Can detect gallstones and evaluate gallbladder emptying. Noninvasive.	Often performed at the client's bedside. Food and fluids are withheld for 8 hours prior to the exam, cleansing enemas or other bowel preparation may be ordered. Advise the client that this test is not painful and generally is completed in 30 minutes or less.
Radiologic Studies	Used to identify the size and location of structures, and, when combined with use of an injected contrast medium, used to study blood flow through vessels and organs.	X-ray studies expose the client to radiation; inquire about possible pregnancy prior to the exam. If contrast is used, inquire about allergies, particularly to iodine, seafood, or contrast media.
Abdominal x-ray (flat plate of the abdomen)	Used to evaluate abdominal pain, detect fluid collections, organ enlargement or rupture, masses, obstruction, or foreign bodies.	No fasting or contrast media is required for this x-ray.
Upper GI series (barium swallow, upper GI with small bowel follow-through)	Uses contrast media (barium), fluoroscopy, and still pictures to assess the structure and peristalsis of the esophagus, stomach, and upper small intestine.	See Box 20-6 ⬀ for the nursing implications for an upper GI or small bowel series. When both an upper GI series and a barium enema are required, the barium enema is scheduled 1 to 2 days before the upper GI to prevent interference with evaluation by retained barium. Monitor for barium excretion following the exam.

TABLE 18-5

Imaging Studies (continued)

TEST	EXPLANATION	NURSING IMPLICATIONS
Barium enema (lower GI series)	Uses contrast media (barium) administered by enema to show the anatomy and movement of the colon.	See Box 20-4 ⚭ for the nursing implications for a barium enema.
Oral cholecystogram	Uses orally ingested contrast media to detect stones or deformity of the gallbladder and to assess its ability to concentrate and excrete bile.	Assess for allergy to iodine, seafood, or other contrast media. Fat intake is restricted the evening before the test. Schedule before barium enema if ordered; may be scheduled on the same day as an upper GI series.
CT scans	Specialized radiographic procedures produce computer-generated images with significantly more detail than standard x-rays. May be done with or without contrast media.	If contrast is used, inquire about allergies (to iodine and seafood in particular), and ensure that the client is well hydrated to reduce the risk of kidney damage.

TABLE 18-6

Endoscopic Studies

TEST	EXPLANATION	NURSING IMPLICATIONS
Upper endoscopy (esophagoscopy, gastroscopy)	Endoscopic examination of the esophagus, stomach, duodenum, and upper jejunum. Used to evaluate disorders such as difficulty swallowing, gastric reflux, and peptic ulcer disease. Also used to locate, diagnose, and control upper GI bleeding.	Requires fasting for 8 hours prior to the procedure. A local anesthetic and conscious sedation are used during the procedure. See Box 19-13 ⚭ for nursing care of the client undergoing upper endoscopy.
Colonoscopy, sigmoidoscopy	Visual examination of the large intestine from the anus to the ileocecal valve (or, in a sigmoidoscopy, the descending colon). Used as a screening examination to detect colorectal cancer and to evaluate chronic constipation, diarrhea, persistent bleeding, abdominal pain. Polyps may be removed during the procedure and tissue samples taken.	Bowel preparation with cathartics and limited food intake occurs 24–48 hours prior to the exam. Conscious sedation is used during the procedure. See Box 20-16 ⚭ for nursing care of the client undergoing colonoscopy.
Endoscopic retrograde cholangiopancreatography	Combines endoscopic and x-ray procedures to evaluate the pancreatic, hepatic, common bile ducts, ampulla of Vater, and gallbladder.	Food and fluids are withheld for at least 8 hours prior to the exam. A local anesthetic and conscious sedation are used. See Box 19-13 ⚭ for nursing care of the client undergoing upper endoscopy.

Note: The bibliography listings for this and all chapters have been compiled at the back of the book.

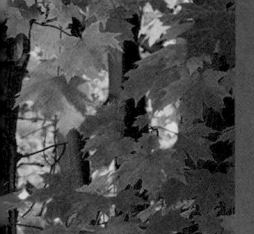

Chapter Review

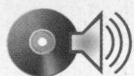 **KEY TERMS** by Topics

Use the audio glossary feature of either the CD-ROM or the Companion Website to hear the correct pronunciation of the following key terms.

Gastrointestinal tract
nutrition, peristalsis, chyme

Accessory organs of digestion
lobules, hepatocytes, retroperitoneal, nutrients, metabolism

KEY Points

- The gastrointestinal system, which includes the mouth, pharynx, esophagus, stomach, and small and large intestines, is a hollow tube that begins at the mouth and ends at the anus.

- Along with the accessory organs of digestion, the liver, gallbladder, and pancreas, the GI tract is vital to maintaining health and nutrition.

- Assessment of the GI system and its function includes gathering information about the client's ability to ingest a variety of foods and maintain a regular pattern of elimination.

- Diagnostic tests to evaluate GI system function include blood tests such as the serum albumin and liver function tests, imaging studies such as ultrasonography and x-rays, and direct examination of organs and tissue via endoscopy.

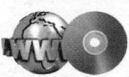 **EXPLORE Media**Link

Additional interactive resources for this chapter can be found on the Companion Website at www.prenhall.com/burke. Click on Chapter 18 and "Begin" to select the activities for this chapter.

For chapter-related NCLEX-style review questions and an audio glossary, access the accompanying CD-ROM in this book.

FOR FURTHER Study

Chapter 5 provides more information about client assessment and specific assessment techniques.

Endocrine functions of the pancreas are discussed in Chapters 15 and 17.

Measurements and calculations for evaluating nutritional status are found in Chapter 19.

Nursing implications for upper GI disorders are discussed in Chapter 19.

Nursing implications for a barium enema are discussed in Chapter 20.

Further information on paracentesis is given in Chapter 21.

NCLEX-PN® Exam Preparation

TEST-TAKING TIP Although it is unlikely that you will be asked to identify normal laboratory values on the NCLEX-PN examination, you will be expected to *apply* knowledge of normal values when responding to questions. For example, how would you expect a serum albumin level of 2.5 g/dL to affect the distribution and availability of a given drug that is highly protein bound?

1 The nurse caring for a client with dry mouth knows that this can affect the client's nutrition because

A. the client needs to drink more water during a meal.
B. digestion begins in the mouth.
C. foods are likely to taste stronger.
D. the client will eat more hard candy to stimulate saliva.

2 A client is admitted with stenosis of the cardiac sphincter. The nurse knows that this will affect the client's

A. ability to swallow.
B. cardiac output.
C. blood pressure.
D. gastric emptying.

3 When assessing the abdomen of a client, the nurse notes dullness to percussion in the lower left quadrant. One possible explanation for this finding is

A. enlargement of the liver.
B. a full bladder.
C. air in the small intestine.
D. a fecal mass in the sigmoid colon.

4 A client scheduled to undergo a colonoscopy asks the nurse just how the test is done. The nurse explains that this test involves

A. instilling a contrast medium into the bowel and taking x-rays.
B. using ultrasonic waves to create and detect an echo off of abdominal structures.
C. Inserting a flexible fiber-optic scope into the colon to visualize its mucous membranes.
D. taking multiple x-ray films that are then analyzed by computer to create a multidimensional image.

5 A client loses a significant portion of the small intestine as a result of a gunshot wound. The nurse caring for the client knows that this is likely to affect

A. the absorption of most nutrients from food.
B. the ability to form a solid stool mass.
C. secretion of hydrochloric acid.
D. conjugation and elimination of bilirubin.

Answers for Review Questions appear in Appendix V.

Chapter 19

Caring for Clients with Nutritional and Upper Gastrointestinal Disorders

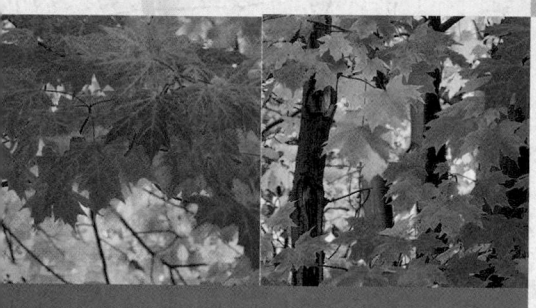

MediaLink

www.prenhall.com/burke
Use the address above to access the free, interactive Companion Website created for this textbook. Get hints, instant feedback, and textbook references to chapter-related NCLEX-style questions. Link to other interesting sites.

Audio Glossary:
Use the Companion Website, or the CD-ROM disk enclosed with your textbook, to hear the pronunciation of key terms in this chapter.

BRIEF Outline

Obesity
Malnutrition
Eating Disorders
Stomatitis
Oral Cancer
Gastroesophageal Reflux Disease
Hiatal Hernia
Esophageal Cancer
Gastroenteritis
Gastritis
Peptic Ulcer Disease
Cancer of the Stomach

LEARNING Outcomes

After completing this chapter, you will be able to:

- Describe the causes, pathophysiology, and manifestations of common nutritional and upper GI disorders.
- Recognize and take appropriate action for common complications of nutritional and upper GI disorders.
- Contribute to assessing, planning, and evaluating care for clients with nutritional and upper GI disorders.
- Implement client-centered nursing care for clients with nutritional and upper GI disorders.

Nutritional disorders and diseases affecting the upper gastrointestinal tract have the potential to affect multiple body systems and all aspects of the client's health. Clients with problems affecting nutrition, eating, or digestion require holistic nursing care that addresses nutritional needs, education, and psychosocial factors.

NUTRITIONAL DISORDERS

Nutritional disorders are major causes of illness and disability. The major nutritional disorders in the world today are obesity and malnutrition. Developmental, sociocultural, psychologic, and physiologic factors contribute to these disorders. Regardless of their cause, nutritional disorders affect many body systems and functions and often lead to serious health problems.

Obesity

Obesity is defined as excess adipose tissue or fat. *Overweight,* in contrast, is body weight greater than ideal for height; the excess weight may be from muscle, bone, or fat. Some people are overweight without being obese, body builders for example. *Morbid obesity* is body weight of more than 100% over ideal weight.

Obesity occurs when excess calories are stored as fat. It is one of the most prevalent, preventable health problems in the United States. Nearly two-thirds of American adults are overweight; approximately one-third of adults are obese, making it the most prevalent health problem in the United States.

PATHOPHYSIOLOGY

Body weight is regulated by a complex set of factors. Overeating and physical inactivity do contribute to obesity, but they are not the entire cause of the problem. Factors such as appetite, hormones, heredity, and social and cultural influences also play a role in body weight.

Appetite is regulated by the central nervous system and by emotional factors. Appetite is stimulated by the hunger center in the hypothalamus in response to stimuli such as low blood sugar. Appetite may have little relationship to hunger: People sometimes eat to relieve depression or anxiety. *Satiety,* a feeling of fullness, counters appetite. The satiety center, also in the hypothalamus, is stimulated by gastric filling, a rise in nutrient levels, and hormones. Several hormones are involved in regulating obesity, including thyroid hormone, insulin, and leptin (a peptide produced by fatty tissue that suppresses appetite and increases energy expenditure). Some studies suggest that leptin resistance is a cause of obesity. There is a strong link between heredity and obesity. A person with one obese parent has a 40% chance of becoming obese; one with two obese parents has an 80% chance.

Physical inactivity is probably the most important factor contributing to obesity. Inactive people may consume fewer calories than active people and continue to gain weight due to lack of energy expenditure. Fat and calorie intake also contribute to obesity: People who eat more fat have a higher body fat content than people who consume less fat and more complex carbohydrates and fiber. When more calories are consumed than are required to meet the body's energy needs, they are stored as fat.

Environmental and sociocultural influences—such as an abundant and readily accessible food supply, rewarding behavior with food, and spending significant amounts of time watching television—play a role in the prevalence of obesity in the United States.

Upper body obesity (or *central obesity*) is associated with a high risk of complications. The waist/hip ratio determines upper body obesity; it is greater than 1 in men and 0.8 in women with upper body obesity. **Lower body obesity** (or *peripheral obesity*) is more common in women than men. In lower body obesity, the waist/hip ratio is less than 0.8. Although it is difficult to treat, lower body obesity carries a lower risk for complications than does upper body obesity.

Complications

Obesity is associated with increased mortality and morbidity. Common complications associated with obesity include:

- Cardiovascular disease, such as high blood pressure, coronary heart disease, and heart failure
- Insulin resistance and type 2 diabetes
- Reduced production of male sex hormones in obese men and an increased risk for menstrual irregularities and polycystic ovarian syndrome (PCOS) in obese women.

Box 19-1 ■ lists other complications associated with obesity.

BOX 19-1

PROBLEMS ASSOCIATED WITH OBESITY

- Cancers of the breast, uterus, prostate, and colon
- Cholecystitis and cholelithiasis
- Coronary heart disease
- Heart failure
- Hiatal hernia
- Hypertension
- Muscle strains and sprains
- Osteoarthritis
- Peripheral vascular disease
- Postoperative complications
- Stress incontinence

INTERDISCIPLINARY CARE

Because obesity is caused by many factors, its treatment is complex. Most experts recommend an individualized program combining exercise, diet, and behavior modification to meet the client's specific needs.

Diagnostic Tests

- *Standard height–weight tables* (see Table 18-2 ⚭) can be used to determine a person's ideal weight.
- *Body mass index (BMI)* is used to determine obesity. It is calculated using the following formula: BMI = weight in kg/height^2 in m. A BMI of 19 to 24 kg/m^2 is considered healthy for adults. A BMI of 25 to 29.9 kg/m^2 is overweight; obesity is a BMI of 30 kg/m^2 or greater.
- *Fat-fold measures* (Figure 19-1 ■) provide an estimate of total body fat and its distribution.
- *Waist/hip ratio* is used to evaluate central obesity. It is calculated by dividing the waist measurement by the hip measurement.

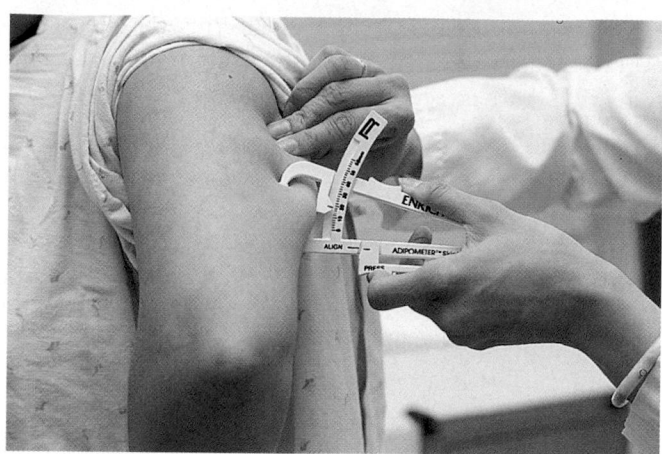

Figure 19-1. ■ With calipers, measure the thickness of a fold of skin on the back of the arm or below the shoulder blade. (Photographer: Elena Dorfman.)

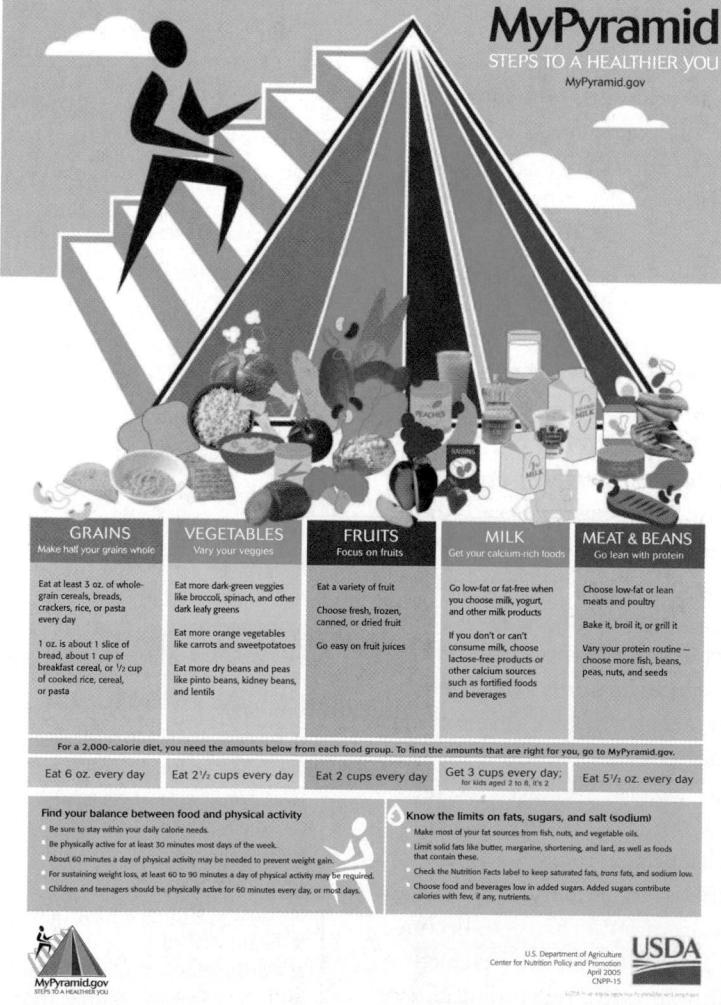

Figure 19-2. ■ The USDA Food Guide Pyramid (*Source:* U.S. Department of Agriculture.)

Other diagnostic tests may be done, such as a *thyroid pro-file* (see Chapter 15 ⃝), *serum glucose* and *cholesterol,* and *lipid profile* (see Chapter 25 ⃝). An *electrocardiogram (ECG)* (Chapter 25 ⃝) may be ordered to evaluate effects of obesity on the heart.

Diet and Exercise

Treatment of obesity focuses on changing both eating and exercise habits. A pound of body fat is equivalent to 3,500 kcal. To lose 1 pound, therefore, a person must increase activity to burn these calories or reduce daily caloric intake by 250 kcal for 14 days.

Exercise is critical to weight loss and maintenance. After consulting their health care providers, clients should engage in aerobic exercise of moderate intensity for at least 30 minutes a day, 4 to 6 days a week. This will reduce *adipose* (fatty) tissue, increase lean body mass (which burns more calories), and promote weight loss and long-term weight control.

The diet should be low in kilocalories and fat and contain adequate nutrients, minerals, and fiber. Selection of foods from all food groups helps ensure adequate nutrient consumption. The new USDA food guide pyramid is a valuable guide (Figure 19-2 ■) to proper nutrition. Whole grains, foods with little or no added sugar, vegetables and fruits, lean protein sources, and use of unsaturated fats are emphasized. Regular meals with small servings are recommended. Weight loss should be gradual, no more than 1 to 2 pounds per week. This usually means a diet of 1,000 to 1,500 kcal per day. Fewer than 1,200 kcal each day may lead to nutritional deficiencies and loss of lean tissue.

Behavior modification is a critical part of successful weight management. Keeping food records and identifying cues that create a desire to eat can help the dieter gain self-control. Weight loss and weight maintenance are separate but related issues. Most dieters regain lost weight within 2 years. Long-term weight management requires a lifelong commitment to changing food and eating habits, activity and exercise routines, and lifestyle. Physical activity has been shown to be key to maintaining weight loss. People who exercise for 60 minutes a day most days of the week have a much greater likelihood of maintaining a healthy weight. Box 19-2 ■ outlines strategies for weight management.

Social support and group programs (Weight Watchers, Overeaters Anonymous, and Take Off Pounds Sensibly) provide weight-loss strategies and peer support. Most programs charge a fee; this may also encourage compliance.

Medications

Drugs may be helpful for people with morbid obesity. However, tolerance, addiction, and side effects may occur.

| BOX 19-2 | **CLIENT TEACHING** |

Behavior Strategies for Weight Loss

Control the Environment

- Purchase low-calorie foods, shopping from a prepared list and on a full stomach.
- Keep all foods in the kitchen or pantry. Store them in opaque containers out of sight.
- Prepare exact portions of food to eliminate leftovers.
- Eat all foods in the same place, avoiding the kitchen.
- Do not eat while watching television or reading.
- Reduce frequency of eating out at restaurants, parties, and picnics.

Control Physical Responses to Food

- Eat a salad or drink a hot beverage before a meal.
- Eat slowly; take small bites and chew each thoroughly. Allow 20 minutes for a meal.
- Put eating utensils or food down between bites.
- Concentrate on the eating process; savor the food.
- Stop eating with the first feelings of fullness.

Control Psychosocial Responses to Food

- Make eating a pleasant experience, using attractive dinnerware and a formal setting.
- Use small plates and cups to make servings of food look larger.
- Concentrate on conversations and socialization during the meal.
- Use nonfood rewards for meeting a goal.
- Acknowledge small successes and improvements in all behavior.
- Substitute other pleasurable activities for eating (e.g., reading, exercise, hobbies).

Make Exercise a Daily Routine

- Make exercise a priority instead of trying to "fit it in" to a daily schedule.
- Try out different types of exercise to find one that is enjoyable.
- Form an exercise group or recruit an exercise "buddy."
- Plan strategies to maintain exercise during inclement weather.
- Wear comfortable and supportive clothing and shoes for exercising.

Appetite suppressants such as sibutramine (Meridia) may be prescribed for limited periods of time (no more than 1 year). Sibutramine, which inhibits the reuptake of serotonin (a neurotransmitter) in the brain, has been shown to produce gradual weight loss when combined with a reduced calorie diet. Phentermine (Adipex-P, Zantryl, others) also acts by altering the appetite center in the hypothalamus. Orlistat (Xenical) has a different mechanism

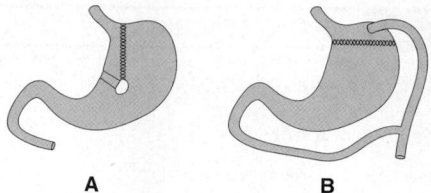

Figure 19-3. ■ Surgical procedures to treat obesity. (**A**) Vertical banding. (**B**) Gastric bypass.

of action: It reduces the absorption of fat from the GI tract, leading to weight loss. It has the added benefit of lowering blood glucose and cholesterol, but its effectiveness in promoting weight loss is questionable. These products must be used in combination with diet and exercise to be successful.

Surgery

Surgery to treat obesity generally is reserved for morbidly obese individuals. Commonly used surgical procedures either restrict stomach capacity, thereby limiting food intake, or both restrict stomach capacity and absorption of nutrients from the stomach and duodenum. In *gastric banding* procedures, the capacity of the stomach is reduced using a band to create a small pouch just below the esophagus. *Vertical banding* is the most common of these procedures. It combines banding with stomach staples to create a pouch that holds no more than about 1 cup of food or less (Figure 19-3A ■).

Surgeries that affect nutrient absorption as well as capacity are more commonly used and, over time, are more effective in maintaining weight loss. In a *gastric bypass* procedure, a small stomach pouch is formed to restrict food intake, and a section of small intestine is attached to the pouch to bypass the lower stomach, duodenum, and upper jejunum (Figure 19-3B ■). The risk of nutritional deficiencies, iron and calcium in particular, due to malabsorption is higher with these surgeries.

NURSING CARE

ASSESSING

Ask about eating habits, and have the client describe food intake for a typical day. Identify activity and exercise patterns for a typical weekday and weekend. Ask about prior weight-loss efforts and discuss whether the client is satisfied with current weight and appearance. Inquire about recent changes in appetite or weight. Ask about any medical problems such as cardiovascular disease and diabetes. Assess height and weight, and compare actual weight to ideal

body weight (see Table 18-2 ◯◯). Using a caliper, obtain fat-fold measurements (see Figure 19-1). Measure waist circumference at the level of the umbilicus.

DIAGNOSING, PLANNING, AND IMPLEMENTING

Priorities in Nursing Care. Overweight and obesity affect both physical and emotional health of the client. Helping the client develop effective weight loss strategies is a priority of nursing care.

Imbalanced Nutrition: More than Body Requirements

- Encourage identification of factors that contribute to excess food intake. *Identifying cues to eating helps the client eliminate or reduce these cues.*
- Establish realistic weight-loss goals. *Success is more likely with small, reasonable goals (losing 1 to 2 pounds per week) and a longer term goal of losing 10% of current body weight.*
- Assess knowledge and provide teaching about well-balanced diet plans. *Knowledge empowers the client to make appropriate diet choices.*
- Help develop an exercise plan that fits into the client's lifestyle and includes enjoyable activities. Encourage 30 minutes of sustained activity daily. *A realistic, enjoyable exercise plan promotes participation and self-esteem.*
- Explore ability and willingness to make changes in daily patterns of diet, exercise, and lifestyle. *This provides assessment data for setting realistic goals with the client.*
- Help identify behavior-modification strategies and support systems to promote weight loss and maintenance. *Lifestyle patterns that motivate the client to continue exercising and eating sensibly promote success. Family and social support are critical to sticking with the plan.*
- Refer the client to a dietitian, nutritional counselor, or weight-loss support program. *Professionals and support groups provide additional resources to help achieve and maintain weight loss.*
- Help plan strategies to deal with "stress" eating or relapses to previous eating patterns. *Overeating or not exercising can cause a sense of failure and lead to further overeating. Identifying strategies ahead of time helps the client accept and deal with relapses.*

Chronic Low Self-Esteem

Obese clients often experience "fat prejudice" in their family, workplace, or community. These experiences, coupled with the difficulty of finding attractive clothing or a chair large enough to sit on, can affect the client's self-esteem. Hospitalized obese clients may be subject to frequent comments about their physical condition.

- Set small goals with the client and offer positive feedback and encouragement. *Small goals provide more opportunities for success. Positive feedback and encouragement help develop self-esteem.*
- Explore the possibility of psychologic counseling with the client. *Many clients benefit from counseling for issues related to self-esteem.*

EVALUATING

To evaluate the effectiveness of nursing care, monitor weight, looking for a slow, progressive weight loss. Ask about eating and exercise patterns. Assess knowledge and willingness to consume a nutritionally sound diet. Discuss the client's sense of success and self-image.

Documenting. Document the client's progress in achieving weight loss goals, as well as any interventions or strategies to overcome barriers.

CONTINUING CARE

The client is ultimately responsible for managing and maintaining weight loss. Teaching and planning must therefore be individualized. Tailor teaching and weight-loss strategies to address coexisting health problems. (For example, teach the overweight client with diabetes about a diabetic, calorie-restricted diet. Develop an individualized exercise program for the overweight client with heart disease.) Provide information about community or hospital-based programs and resources. Discuss strategies for incorporating exercise into the client's daily schedule.

Malnutrition

Malnutrition results from inadequate nutrient intake. It occurs when food and nutrient intake and absorption do not meet the needs for growth, development, or function. Malnutrition can result from lack of major nutrients (carbohydrates, proteins, and fats) or micronutrients (vitamins and minerals). It affects all body systems and increases the risk of disease and death. Malnutrition is common in hospitalized clients, often leading to poor wound healing and lower resistance to infection.

Other groups at risk for malnutrition include the young, poor, elderly, homeless, low-income women, and ethnic minorities. Clients may be undernourished because of poor food choices. Disorders such as *anorexia nervosa* (an eating disorder marked by a disturbed body image and fear of gaining weight) and *bulimia* (episodic binge eating and self-induced vomiting) are serious concerns, especially among teenagers and young adults (see the Eating Disorders section later in this chapter for more information about anorexia and bulimia). Fad diets may also result in nutritional deficien-

---

BOX 19-3

CONDITIONS ASSOCIATED WITH MALNUTRITION

- Aging
- AIDS
- Alcoholism
- Burns, trauma
- Cancer
- Chronic diseases (COPD, renal disease)
- Eating disorders (anorexia, bulimia)
- Gastrointestinal disorders, short bowel syndrome
- Neurologic disorders
- Surgery

---

cies. Gastrointestinal problems such as nausea or vomiting, altered digestion, or impaired absorption can lead to malnutrition, as can other illnesses (Box 19-3 ■).

PATHOPHYSIOLOGY

When food intake does not meet the body's energy needs, it uses glycogen, body proteins, and fats to support metabolism. Glucose and glycogen stores, the energy sources in the body, are depleted within 12 to 24 hours of no food intake. When adequate calories are not available to meet energy needs, the body then turns to its proteins (in muscle and organs) and fats (in subcutaneous tissue). The size of all body compartments is reduced, and metabolically active tissues are lost, decreasing energy expenditure.

In hospitalized clients, the acute stress response to illness or trauma increases the metabolic rate and energy expenditure. This leads to **catabolism** (cell and tissue breakdown), and loss of lean body mass and protein stores. Inadequate protein and calorie intake can lead to *protein–calorie malnutrition (PCM)*. Protein synthesis is impaired, delaying wound healing. Serum albumin levels fall, leading to edema. Immune function is impaired, increasing the risk of infection. The cardiovascular and GI systems also are impaired by malnutrition.

clinical ALERT

Approximately half of all hospitalized adults are malnourished or at risk for PCM. Carefully assess your client's food and fluid intake, and alert the charge nurse or physician when poor appetite, nausea, or NPO status interfere with intake.

MANIFESTATIONS AND COMPLICATIONS

Manifestations of malnutrition vary, depending on the nutrient deficit (see Table 18-1). Weight loss is the most apparent sign. Body mass and skin-fold thickness are reduced.

Malnourished clients may have a wasted appearance, dry and brittle hair, pale mucous membranes, peripheral edema, and a sore, smooth tongue.

In PCM, loss of subcutaneous fat and muscle proteins can impair mobility and increase the risk of skin and tissue breakdown (decubitus or pressure ulcers). Wound healing is impaired. Serum albumin levels fall, with resulting abdominal edema, diarrhea, and impaired absorption of nutrients. The risk of infection increases. Cardiac output drops, increasing the risk for falls.

BOX 19-4 **PROCEDURE CHECKLIST**

Inserting a Nasogastric Tube

- ☑ Gather all supplies.
- ☑ Provide for privacy.
- ☑ Explain the procedure, using nonthreatening terms. Inserting the tube may be uncomfortable, but once the tube is in place, little or no discomfort should be felt. Emphasize the need to follow instructions to swallow during tube insertion.
- ☑ Follow Standard Precautions; wear clean gloves.
- ☑ Place client in Fowler's or high-Fowler's position with a towel or disposable pad on the chest.
- ☑ Occluding one nares at a time, ask the client to breathe. Use the nares with the better airflow for insertion.
- ☑ Measure the tube: Hold the tip of the tube at the client's nose, extend the tube to the tip of the earlobe and then to the tip of the sternum (see photo). If the tube is to be placed in the duodenum, add 8 to 10 inches (20 to 25 cm) to the measurement. Mark the tube.

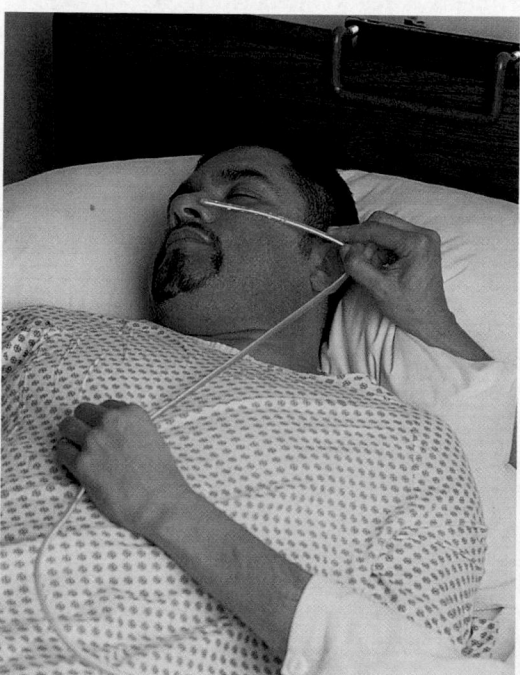

Measuring the appropriate length for nasogastric tube insertion. (Photographer: Elena Dorfman.)

- ☑ Provide a glass of water with a straw if allowed.
- ☑ For a small-bore tube, insert the guidewire or stylet into the tube.
- ☑ Using water-soluble lubricant, lubricate 3 to 4 inches of the tube tip.
- ☑ Gently insert the tube into the selected nares, directing it along the floor of the nares toward the ear. Use a smooth, continuous motion. Have the client tip the head forward, chin to chest, and ask the client to sip and swallow on command. Advance the tube 3 to 4 inches (7 to 10 cm) with each swallow until the point marked on the tube is at the opening of the nares.
- ☑ Pause briefly if the client gags (do not withdraw the tube); have the client take a few breaths through the mouth, then resume advancing the tube. If gagging continues, check the mouth. If the tube is curled in the mouth, withdraw it until the tip is in the oropharynx before resuming.
- ☑ If the client coughs and is unable to speak, withdraw the tube until the tip is in the oropharynx. Have the client tip the head further forward and swallow to prevent this from occurring.
- ☑ Verify that the tube is correctly placed. Withdraw a small amount of fluid from the tube and check the pH of the fluid. If the pH is 5 or lower, the tube is very likely in the stomach. If the pH is 6 or higher, confirm tube placement with an x-ray.
- ☑ Secure the tube with tape.
- ☑ Initiate feeding or gastric suction as ordered.
- ☑ Reposition the client and provide mouth and nose care as indicated.

SAMPLE DOCUMENTATION

4/24/06 1030 8 Fr. Dobbhoff gastric feeding tube inserted via R nares. Small amount green drainage obtained, pH 4. Tolerated procedure well.
_____S. Williams, LPN.

Note: Refer to a nursing fundamentals or skills text for more detailed instruction. Check state guidelines and facility policy before performing any procedure.

INTERDISCIPLINARY CARE

Laboratory studies can provide additional assessment data to evaluate the effects of malnutrition on the client. Clients with PCM have low *serum albumin* levels. On complete blood count (CBC), the *lymphocyte count, hemoglobin,* and *hematocrit* often are decreased due to iron deficiencies. *Serum electrolyte levels* also may be altered.

The goal of treatment is to restore the malnourished client to ideal body weight and replace necessary nutrients and minerals. In severe malnutrition, fluid and electrolyte imbalances are corrected first, then food and nutrients are reintroduced gradually. Oral feedings and supplements are preferred. Small, around-the-clock feedings are generally tolerated best. Energy- and protein-rich foods or commercially available nutritional supplements (Carnation Instant Breakfast, Ensure, etc.) may be ordered. Intravenous solutions may be used to replace fluids and electrolytes. Malnourished clients generally need supplemental vitamins and minerals to restore adequate levels.

Enteral Feedings

Enteral or *tube feedings* may be used to meet all or part of the nutritional needs in clients who are unable to eat. Tube feedings are usually administered through a soft, small-caliber nasogastric or nasoduodenal tube with a weighted tip. Box 19-4 ■ outlines the procedure for inserting a nasogastric tube. Enteral feedings also can be administered through a gastrostomy or jejunostomy tube, discussed under Cancer of the Stomach later in this chapter.

A number of tube-feeding formulas are commercially available. All are nutritionally complete. Some formulas have added fiber to reduce the incidence of diarrhea, a common side effect of enteral feedings. Others have specific formulations for clients with chronic diseases such as chronic obstructive pulmonary disease (COPD) or kidney disease. Formulas may be diluted to half strength for the first day of therapy. If tolerated, they are given at three-fourths strength on the second day and at full strength thereafter. Fluid and electrolyte status are monitored carefully, and additional water is given to meet the client's specific needs. The volume of feedings is gradually increased, with a maximum feeding of 240 to 360 mL every 2 to 4 hours, or 2 L for a 24-hour period, based on the client's caloric needs. Formulas may be administered as a bolus feeding, by continuous drip, or on a cyclic schedule (Box 19-5 ■). To prevent aspiration, elevate the head of the bed at least 30 degrees during feeding and for at least 1 hour after feeding.

Parenteral Nutrition

Total parenteral nutrition (*TPN* or *hyperalimentation*) is intravenous administration of a solution that meets all the client's nutritional needs (except for fiber). TPN is used for both short- and long-term management of nutritional deficiencies when the client is unable to eat or use enteral feedings. Clients who have undergone major surgery or trauma, or who are seriously undernourished, are often candidates for TPN. Many clients are discharged to home with TPN and are monitored by home health nurses.

BOX 19-5	PROCEDURE CHECKLIST

Enteral Feedings

☑ Obtain ordered formula and all supplies. Use Standard Precautions.

☑ Elevate the head of the bed to at least 30 degrees during and for at least 1 hour after the feeding.

☑ Provide mouth care.

☑ Explain the procedure.

☑ Check residual stomach contents prior to intermittent feedings or every 4 hours if continuous. Reinstill the aspirated formula.

☑ Withhold the feeding and notify the charge nurse or physician if more than 100 mL (gastrostomy tube) or 200 mL (nasogastric tube) residual is obtained.

☑ Fill the feeding bag with the ordered amount of formula and water. Clear the tubing of air and/or attach it to a feeding pump.

☑ Attach the tubing to the feeding or gastrostomy tube. Set the flow rate by drip or on the pump and begin feeding.

SAMPLE DOCUMENTATION

4/24/06 1000   340 mL Sustacal with 100 mL water administered via gastric feeding tube. 75 mL residual obtained prior to feeding; reinstilled. Tolerated well with no evidence of aspiration.

_____S. Williams, LPN.

Note: Refer to a nursing fundamentals or skills text for more detailed instruction. Check state guidelines and facility policy before performing any procedure.

BOX 19-6	NURSING CARE CHECKLIST

Parenteral Nutrition

☑ Use aseptic technique at all times. Do not add any medication to the solution or administer medications or other IV solutions through the catheter lumen into which TPN is being administered.

☑ Use an infusion pump to ensure the correct rate of infusion.

☑ Keep accurate intake and output records for clients receiving TPN.

☑ Check blood glucose by finger stick and administer insulin as ordered.

☑ Monitor and record vital signs, including temperature, reporting any changes to the charge nurse or physician.

☑ Carefully assess respiratory status. Report changes to the charge nurse or physician.

☑ Monitor for signs of infection such as fever, malaise, redness, swelling, or drainage at the catheter insertion site. Report these signs if noted.

TPN formulas have high concentrations of dextrose, protein (amino acids), electrolytes, vitamins, minerals, and fat emulsions. They are usually administered through a central vein, such as the subclavian vein. To initiate therapy, the physician usually inserts a triple-lumen catheter that permits medications and other intravenous solutions to be given at the same time. Nursing responsibilities related to TPN are outlined in Box 19-6 ■.

NURSING CARE

ASSESSING

Ask about eating habits and typical food intake for a day. Ask about recent weight changes and factors contributing to weight change. Assess for other factors such as anorexia, nausea, medications, or inability to buy and prepare food for meals. Ask about medical problems such as chronic lung or heart disease, thyroid problems, or kidney disease. Look at psychosocial factors affecting nutrition, such as body image, loneliness, depression, and economic status. Determine food preferences.

Assess height, weight, and fat-fold measurements (see the section on obesity earlier in the chapter). Wearing gloves, evaluate the mouth, looking for inflammation, gum disease, dental caries, or poorly fitting dentures. Assess ability to swallow liquids, semisolid, and solid foods.

On admission and during treatment, monitor serum albumin, serum electrolytes, and the hemoglobin and hematocrit. Report unanticipated changes, and critical values (see Chapter 7 ⌦ for critical electrolyte values).

DIAGNOSING, PLANNING, AND IMPLEMENTING

Priorities in Nursing Care. Nursing care priorities focus on both the interdisciplinary problem of malnutrition, as well as its effects and potential complications, such as increased risk for infection, deficient fluid volume, and skin breakdown.

Imbalanced Nutrition: Less than Body Requirements

■ Monitor and record weight. Note the amount and type of foods eaten at meals and snacks. *This data is important to evaluate the effectiveness of nutritional therapy.*

■ Consult with the dietitian, client, family, and caregivers to plan a nutritionally complete diet. *The best diet plan will not achieve its objective if the client cannot or will not eat it or if the caregivers will not prepare it.*

■ Provide mouth care before and after meals, eliminate foul odors, and offer frequent, small meals including foods the client prefers. *Oral hygiene and a pleasant environment make food more appetizing. Small meals are generally more appealing and less overwhelming to a client with anorexia.*

■ Provide a rest period before and after meals. *Eating requires energy, and the undernourished client may have decreased physical strength.*

Risk for Infection

■ Monitor and record temperature; report any elevation to the charge nurse or physician. Note and report chills, malaise, confusion, local inflammation, or elevated WBC. *Early detection of infection may prevent complications.*

■ Maintain Standard Precautions and sterile technique for procedures as indicated. *Hand washing is the best strategy to prevent the spread of infection. Sterile technique is required for procedures such as changing dressings.*

Risk for Deficient Fluid Volume

The client with malnutrition is at risk for fluid volume deficit due to inadequate fluid intake, concentrated enteral feeding solutions, or hypertonic parenteral nutrition.

■ Monitor oral mucous membranes, skin turgor, urine output and specific gravity, level of consciousness, and laboratory results (see Fluid Volume Deficit section in Chapter 7 ⌦). *Dry mucous membranes, poor skin turgor, decreased urine output, and increased specific gravity may indicate dehydration. Dehydrated clients may have a decreased level of consciousness. Laboratory studies such as serum osmolality, electrolytes, and hematocrit also provide data about fluid balance.*

■ Weigh daily at the same time, on the same scale, and with the same clothing. Monitor intake and output. Document carefully. *Daily weights and intake and output records help monitor fluid balance.*

■ If fluids are allowed, offer them often in small amounts, considering the client's preferences. *Small amounts are tolerated best; frequent drinking promotes adequate intake.*

Risk for Impaired Skin Integrity

■ Frequently assess the skin, noting areas of redness, abrasions, or other lesions. Record and report any abnormal findings or changes from previous assessments to the charge nurse or physician. *Skin integrity depends on adequate nutrition. Early identification of pressure areas or lesions allows intervention to prevent further breakdown or complications.*

■ Turn and reposition every 2 hours. Encourage passive and active range-of-motion exercises. *Pressure areas are at high risk for decreased circulation and breakdown. These measures reduce pressure and promote oxygenation of cells.*

■ Keep skin dry and clean, and minimize shearing forces. Keep linens smooth, clean, and dry. Provide therapeutic beds, mattresses, or pads. *These measures promote comfort and reduce the risk of skin breakdown.*

EVALUATING

Collect the following data to evaluate the effectiveness of nursing interventions for the client with malnutrition: consuming prescribed diet; evidence of weight gain; stable intake and output; laboratory values improving; remains free of infection or skin breakdown.

Documenting. Document weight, food and fluid intake and responses to meals and snacks. Note skin condition, recording and reporting any areas of redness or early tissue breakdown (see Chapter 45 ○○).

CONTINUING CARE

Diet therapy (including enteral or parenteral nutrition) often is continued in the home setting. Box 19-7 ■ lists assessment data to collect when planning for discharge. Box 19-8 ■ describes strategies for older adults with malnutrition.

Teach the client and care providers about the importance of hand washing and proper food and supplement storage. If en-

---

BOX 19-7	ASSESSMENT

Assessing for Discharge: Malnutrition

CLIENT

■ Self-care: ability to perform ADLs independently; obtain, prepare, and eat prescribed diet or manage enteral or parenteral feedings

■ Knowledge: general nutrition; recommended diet or feeding regimen; importance of monitoring weight and intake; indications for seeking medical care

■ Psychosocial: self-concept and body image; support network or significant others; willingness to follow dietary plan for weight gain

■ Home environment: facilities for food storage and preparation; access to clean water for drinking and hand washing; atmosphere conducive to eating

FAMILY AND CAREGIVERS

■ Members of household: responsibilities for obtaining and preparing food; other members with nutritional deficits or special diets

■ Caregivers: availability, willingness, and knowledge to provide nutritional care and support as needed, assist with shopping, transportation, and management of enteral or parenteral feedings

■ Financial resources: income; resources for food, nutritional support, and medical care

COMMUNITY

■ Access to health care resources such as home health agencies or home IV therapy services; access to grocery stores or home-delivered groceries

■ Availability of communal meals or home-delivered meals

■ Financial support options such as Women, Infants, and Children (WIC) programs

---

BOX 19-8	FOCUS ON OLDER ADULTS

Promoting Nutrition in the Older Adult

Changes that occur with aging can affect nutrition and the enjoyment of food in the older adult. The ability to taste salty and sweet flavors declines, and the sense of smell is reduced. Less saliva is produced, making it more difficult to swallow. Increased problems with teeth and gums or ill-fitting dentures affect eating. The lower esophageal sphincter relaxes, increasing the incidence of gastroesophageal reflux and heartburn. Less gastric acid is produced, impairing absorption of some nutrients. Peristalsis and digestion slow, often causing the older adult to feel full after eating small amounts. Medications taken for chronic diseases can lead to anorexia. Functional limitations may impair the ability to shop and cook. Psychosocial issues such as a fixed income, depression, social isolation, and loneliness contribute to the risk of nutritional problems. Older adults who eat alone often do not eat as well as those who share meals with companions.

To promote nutrition in older adults:

■ Suggest congregate meals (usually offered through senior centers) and programs such as Meals-on-Wheels (for people who are homebound and physically unable to prepare meals).

■ Discuss a well-balanced diet that includes whole grains, fresh fruit, and vegetables.

■ Advise clients to avoid processed foods and foods high in fat, to drink adequate fluids, and to exercise regularly.

■ Assist clients to shop wisely to get the most value for their money.

teral or parenteral nutrition will continue at home, instruct the client, family, and caregivers how to (a) prepare and handle enteral or parenteral solutions, (b) add solutions to either the feeding tube or central line, (c) manage infusion pumps, (d) care for the feeding tube or central catheter, and (e) recognize and manage problems and complications. Teach the client how and when to notify the home health agency or health care provider of problems. Document all teaching and the learners' understanding of what has been taught. Assess compliance with the treatment plan on a continuing basis, especially when psychosocial factors contribute to malnutrition.

Eating Disorders

Eating disorders such as *anorexia nervosa* and *bulimia* are characterized by severely disturbed eating behavior and weight management. **Anorexia nervosa** is characterized by an intense fear of weight gain and weight less than 85% of expected for age and height. Clients with **bulimia nervosa**, in contrast, often have normal body weight. This disorder, which is more common than anorexia, is characterized by binge–purge behavior: episodes of binge eating are followed by self-induced vomiting, laxative or diuretic use, or excessive exercise. Table 19-1 ■ compares the manifestations and complications of anorexia and bulimia.

Eating disorders often are difficult to effectively treat. The intense fear of weight gain and disrupted body image cause clients with anorexia to resist increased food intake. A multidisciplinary treatment team approach is necessary, involving nutritional, behavioral, and psychologic therapies. Refeeding of clients with anorexia must be approached slowly to avoid complications of refeeding such as heart failure. Meals are supervised to prevent hiding of food. Antidepressant drugs may be prescribed.

NURSING CARE

Early identification and referral of clients with anorexia and bulimia are important to prevent adverse effects of these disorders on growth and development. Be alert for clients who complain of being overweight, relate a history of dieting, laxative or diuretic use, and significant amounts of exercise when combined with weight less than ideal for height. Imbalanced Nutrition: Less than Body Requirements is the priority nursing diagnosis. Other applicable nursing diagnoses include Disturbed Body Image and Ineffective Family Coping. Consider the following nursing care activities when caring for clients with an eating disorder:

- Monitor weight, using standard conditions. *Weight provides a measurement of the effectiveness of interventions.*
- Monitor food intake during meals and snacks, recording amount consumed. Continue close observation for at least 1 hour after meals; do not allow client to use the bathroom alone. *Monitoring the client during and after meals is important to prevent food hiding or disposal and purging after eating.*

TABLE 19-1		
Manifestations and Complications of Anorexia Nervosa and Bulimia		
	ANOREXIA NERVOSA	**BULIMIA**
Onset and Population	■ Adolescence ■ Women > men	■ Late adolescence or early adulthood ■ Women > men
Manifestations	■ Weight < 85% of normal ■ Disturbed body image ■ Fear of weight gain ■ Refusal to eat, excessive exercise ■ Muscle wasting ■ Skin and hair changes ■ Amenorrhea ■ Low blood pressure, slow pulse ■ Low body temperature ■ Constipation ■ Insomnia	■ Weight normal or greater than normal ■ Binge–purge behavior ■ Scant menses or amenorrhea ■ Lacerations of palate (from induced vomiting) ■ Callous on fingers or back of hand
Complications	■ Electrolyte and acid–base imbalances ■ Low cardiac output, dysrhythmias ■ Anemia ■ Hypoglycemia ■ Osteoporosis ■ Delayed gastric emptying ■ Abnormal liver function	■ Enlarged salivary glands ■ Stomatitis ■ Loss of dental enamel ■ Fluid, electrolyte, and acid–base imbalances ■ Dysrhythmias ■ Esophageal tears, stomach rupture

■ Serve small, frequent, balanced meals, gradually increasing serving size. *Calorie intake is gradually increased to prevent complications of refeeding. "Normal" serving sizes may be overwhelming to the client, reducing appetite and food intake.*

Ongoing treatment of eating disorders is vital. Clients and their families are referred to a multidisciplinary team for continuing care. Stress the importance of continuing treatment and involvement of the whole family for effective care.

UPPER GI DISORDERS

Inflammations of the mouth and oral cancer affect nutrition and the ability to eat. Although oral problems affect many adults, they often are unrecognized and untreated.

Stomatitis

Stomatitis, inflammation of the oral mucosa, is a common problem that affects eating. Clients with stomatitis may experience pain, difficulty eating, and body image disturbances. Stomatitis frequently develops secondarily to conditions such as cancer, dental disease, and acquired immune deficiency syndrome (AIDS).

PATHOPHYSIOLOGY AND MANIFESTATIONS

Stomatitis may be caused by viral infection (herpes simplex) or fungal infection (*Candida albicans*). Clients on prolonged antibiotic therapy are at risk for candidiasis (thrush). Other causes include mechanical trauma (e.g., cheek biting) and irritants such as tobacco. Chemotherapy or radiation therapy also can cause stomatitis. *Aphthous ulcers* (canker sores) are a type of stomatitis. These ulcers are usually less than 1 cm in diameter and can last weeks to months.

The manifestations of stomatitis vary, depending on the cause. Herpes lesions are clustered and painful, usually occurring on the lips and oral mucosa. Candidiasis causes painful white patches with a red base. Other manifestations of stomatitis include red and swollen oral mucosa, pain, and possible ulcerations.

INTERDISCIPLINARY CARE

Treatment is directed at both the cause and the symptoms of stomatitis. Lesions may be cultured or scrapings examined to determine the cause of stomatitis. Table 19-2 ■ lists nursing implications and client teaching for selected drugs used to treat stomatitis.

TABLE 19-2			
Nursing Implications for Pharmacology: Stomatitis			
AGENTS/DRUGS	PURPOSE	NURSING RESPONSIBILITIES	CLIENT TEACHING
Topical Anesthetics/ Anti-Inflammatory Agents ■ Orajel ■ Viscous lidocaine ■ Anbesol ■ Triamcinolone acetonide	Provide temporary pain relief. Triamcinolone has an anti-inflammatory effect.	Assess for adverse or hypersensitivity reactions. Notify the primary care provider if they occur. Provide mouth care after eating and at bedtime.	Apply every 1 to 2 hours or as directed. Brush teeth after eating and at bedtime. Contact primary care provider if symptoms worsen or do not heal within 1 week after starting treatment.
Topical Antifungal Agents ■ Clotrimazole ■ Nystatin	Used to treat candidiasis. Effect is local rather than systemic.	These drugs are contraindicated in pregnancy. Instruct client to dissolve troches or lozenges in mouth. For oral suspension, instruct client to swish the solution throughout the mouth for at least 2 minutes, then either expectorate or swallow as directed.	Use the medication as prescribed. Do not eat or drink for 30 minutes after the medication. Contact your primary care provider if symptoms worsen or do not improve. Brush teeth after eating and at bedtime. Remove dentures at bedtime and cleanse well.

(continued)

TABLE 19-2			
Nursing Implications for Pharmacology: Stomatitis (continued)			
AGENTS/DRUGS	PURPOSE	NURSING RESPONSIBILITIES	CLIENT TEACHING
Antiviral Agent ■ Acyclovir (Zovirax)	Reduces the severity and duration of herpes lesions. May reduce frequency of outbreaks.	Administer with food or on an empty stomach.	Begin taking the medication at the first sign of an outbreak. Take as ordered. Contact your primary care provider if symptoms worsen.

NURSING CARE

Suspect stomatitis in a client who refuses to eat or who complains about mouth pain. Wearing gloves, inspect the mouth and oropharynx. Document any visible lesions, as well as the general condition of mucous membranes, teeth, and gums. Note the client's breath. Foul breath odor may be noted in clients with stomatitis. Assess ability to chew and swallow, as well as food and fluid intake.

Assist with mouth care as needed after eating and at bedtime. If the client is unable to tolerate a toothbrush, use sponge or gauze toothettes or a water pick with gentle pressure. Avoid alcohol-based mouthwashes. Encourage a high-calorie, high-protein diet tailored to the client's likes and dislikes. Offer soft, lukewarm, or cool foods or liquids (eggnog, milkshakes, nutritional supplements, popsicles, and puddings) frequently in small amounts. Avoid spicy or irritating foods. Use straws or feeding syringes as needed to promote intake.

To evaluate the effectiveness of nursing interventions, monitor the client's weight, food intake, comfort, and healing. Assess the client's understanding of the problem and its treatment.

CONTINUING CARE

For discharge, provide clear and easily understood instructions for oral care. Instruct the client to avoid alcohol, tobacco, and spicy or irritating foods. Discuss nutritional needs and strategies to minimize discomfort when eating. Teach the client and family about prescribed medications, including how and when to use and possible side effects. Discuss signs and symptoms to report to the physician.

Oral Cancer

An estimated 30,000 new cases of oral cancer are diagnosed annually in the United States. The incidence is twice as high in men as in women, and it is seen more often in men over 40. The major risk factor for oral cancer is tobacco use (both smoking and smokeless tobacco). Alcohol consumption and prolonged exposure to sunlight also are significant risk factors.

PATHOPHYSIOLOGY AND MANIFESTATIONS

Most oral cancers are squamous cell carcinomas. Tobacco and alcohol damage cells lining the mouth and oropharynx. These damaged cells grow more rapidly to repair the damage, increasing the risk for malignancy. Oral cancer may develop anywhere on the oral mucosa, including the lips, tongue, or pharynx (Figure 19-4 ■). Box 19-9 ■ lists manifestations of oral cancer.

INTERDISCIPLINARY CARE

Biopsy is done to determine whether an oral lesion is benign or malignant. Treatment and the prognosis for cure of oral cancer depend on the stage of the tumor. Additional diagnostic studies such as CT scans or MRI may be done to stage the tumor. (See Chapter 12 ⚭ for more information about staging and grading of cancer.)

Eliminating risk factors (tobacco and alcohol) is vital. Early lesions without cancerous cells may heal when exposure to these substances is eliminated. Early cancers may be treated with radiation therapy (external beam or implants), resection

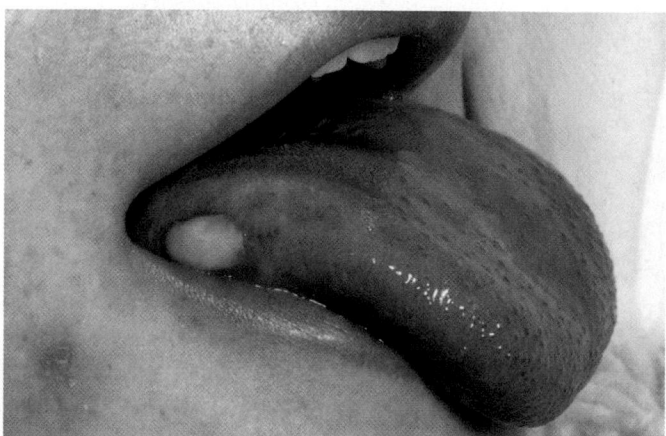

Figure 19-4. ■ Oral cancer. (*Source:* John Radcliffe Hospital/Science Photo Library.)

BOX 19-9

MANIFESTATIONS OF ORAL CANCER

- A sore or lesion in the mouth that does not heal
- *Leukoplakia:* irregular white patches on the lips, tongue, gums, tonsil, or oral mucosa
- *Erythroplakia:* slightly raised, irregular red patches that bleed easily when scraped
- Visible or palpable masses of the lips, cheek, or tongue
- Sore throat or a feeling of something caught in the throat
- Difficulty chewing, swallowing, or moving the jaw or tongue
- Asymmetry of the head, face, jaws, or neck
- Loosening of teeth, or dentures that no longer fit properly
- Swollen lymph nodes
- Blood-tinged sputum

of the tumor, or both. Advanced oral cancers may require extensive surgery such as *radical neck dissection*, a potentially disfiguring procedure. Lymph nodes and some muscles of the neck are removed and a tracheostomy is performed during this procedure. The tracheostomy may be temporary or permanent. (See Chapter 23 ⟳ for nursing care of the client with a tracheostomy.) Chemotherapy is used as adjunctive treatment when the tumor has metastasized beyond the local area.

NURSING CARE

Oral cancer and its treatment can affect airway clearance, food intake and nutrition, communication, and the client's body image. Assess airway patency and respiratory status, particularly if the client has undergone surgery to remove the tumor. Place the client in Fowler's position, and assist with turning, coughing, and using the incentive spirometer. Maintain adequate hydration to help loosen respiratory secretions and promote airway clearance.

Enteral feedings or parenteral nutrition may be necessary for clients with oral cancer. Monitor weight daily and food and nutrient intake. If the client is able to eat, offer a soft, bland diet with enriched foods or dietary supplements. Offer small, frequent feedings, making mealtimes pleasant. Consider a dietary consultation to assess diet and plan appropriate supplements.

Provide a magic slate, flash cards, or picture or alphabet board as needed to facilitate communication. Allow ample time for communication, and do not answer for the client. Observe nonverbal communications to supplement verbal efforts. If the client is unable to speak clearly, use yes/no questions and simple phrases. Keep the call light within easy reach and respond promptly. Alert all staff if the client is unable to respond verbally over the intercom system. Consult with a speech therapist as needed.

Radical surgery of the head or neck can seriously affect the client's body image. Assess coping, self-perception, and responses to surgery. Encourage the client to express feelings regarding body image changes, and provide emotional support.

CONTINUING CARE

Teach all clients about the relationship between alcohol and tobacco use (especially smokeless tobacco) and oral cancer. Provide referrals to smoking cessation classes and Alcoholics Anonymous or alcohol treatment agencies as appropriate. Teach the early signs of oral cancer, demonstrating how to check tissues of the mouth. For clients with oral cancer, teach about the cancer, its treatment, and any specialized care. As needed, teach caregivers how to change dressings and to provide tube or gastrostomy feedings, tracheostomy care, or central line care. Provide referrals to home health agencies as appropriate, and discuss support groups for cancer survivors or clients who have had head and neck surgery. If the client and family have decided not to pursue treatment, support their decision and refer them to cancer support groups or hospice care.

Gastroesophageal Reflux Disease

The esophagus, essential for ingesting food and fluids, may be affected by inflammatory, mechanical, or cancerous disorders. The symptoms of these disorders often mimic other illnesses.

Gastroesophageal reflux is the backward movement of gastric contents into the esophagus. When the reflux of gastric contents causes inflammation and tissue damage to the esophagus, it is known as *gastroesophageal reflux disease (GERD)*. GERD is common, affecting 15% to 20% of adults, many of whom experience daily symptoms.

PATHOPHYSIOLOGY AND MANIFESTATIONS

The lower esophageal sphincter normally prevents gastric contents from entering the esophagus. However, if the sphincter does not function effectively or gastric emptying is delayed, gastric contents may *reflux* (back up) into the lower esophagus. Factors contributing to reflux include increased volume of the stomach following meals, positioning, and increased gastric pressure due to obesity or restrictive clothing. Esophageal peristalsis and alkaline saliva normally clear and neutralize these corrosive gastric fluids, but this process may be impaired during sleep or by impaired esophageal peristalsis. Corrosive gastric fluids lead to tissue inflammation and may cause erosions, ulcers, or *strictures* (narrowing) of the esophagus. The risk of esophageal cancer is increased in clients with GERD.

Heartburn that increases after meals and is aggravated by bending over or lying down is the primary symptom of GERD. The client also may have a sore throat, pain with swallowing, or chest pain.

INTERDISCIPLINARY CARE

Diagnostic tests used to establish the diagnosis of GERD include a barium swallow, upper endoscopy, and ambulatory pH monitoring. See Chapter 18 ◯◯ for more information about these studies. (Nursing care of the client undergoing upper endoscopy is outlined later in Box 19-13 on page 417.)

GERD is managed with a combination of lifestyle changes and medications. Histamine-2 receptor blockers and proton pump inhibitors are often ordered to suppress acid secretion in the stomach and promote esophageal healing. Table 19-4 later in the chapter discusses the nursing implications and client teaching for these drugs.

NURSING CARE

Nursing care for clients with GERD focuses on teaching. Instruct clients to avoid lying down within 3 hours after meals and to elevate the head of the bed on 6-inch blocks or use a foam wedge when sleeping. Discuss the need to avoid using alcohol and tobacco. Provide information about smoking cessation and support groups as needed. Weight loss, smaller meals, and avoiding bending may help to relieve symptoms. Discuss diet changes, such as avoiding acidic foods (such as orange juice), and foods that affect the lower esophageal sphincter or gastric emptying (fatty foods, peppermint, and chocolate).

Hiatal Hernia

A *hiatal hernia* occurs when part of the stomach protrudes through the opening of the diaphragm into the chest cavity. Hiatal hernias usually occur with aging or because of increased intra-abdominal pressure. Most people have no symptoms.

With a *sliding hernia* (the more common type), part of the stomach slides through the opening of the diaphragm when the client reclines and moves back into place when the client stands. With a *paraesophageal hernia,* part of the stomach protrudes through the opening beside the esophagus (Figure 19-5 ■). Upper GI bleeding or erosive esophagitis may complicate hiatal hernias.

The same medical, lifestyle, and pharmacologic interventions used for GERD are usually prescribed for clients with hiatal hernia. If the hernia becomes trapped, impairing blood flow to the hernia, surgery may be necessary. Nursing care for the client undergoing hiatal hernia surgery is similar to that for a client undergoing other abdominal or thoracic surgery. (See Chapter 9 ◯◯ for care of the surgical client.)

Esophageal Cancer

Cancer of the esophagus is relatively uncommon in the United States. Cigarette smoking and alcohol consumption,

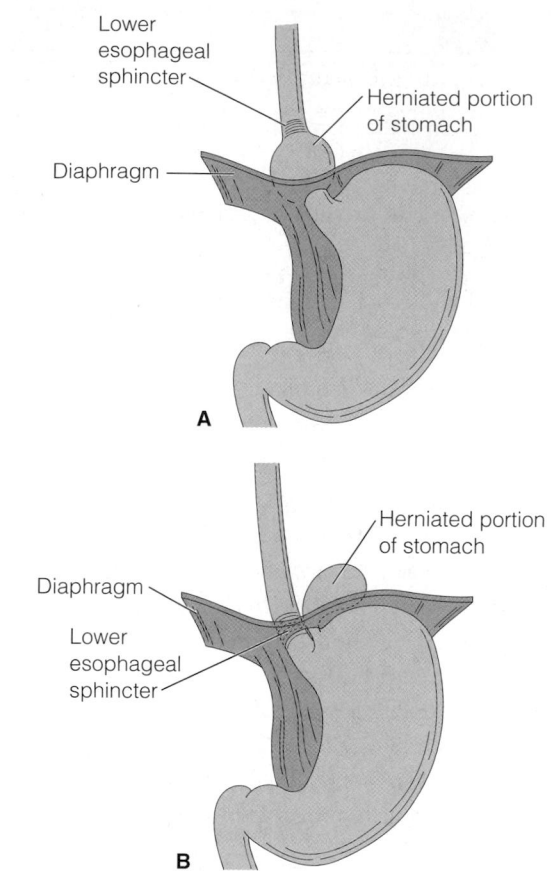

Figure 19-5. ■ Hiatal hernias. (**A**) Sliding. (**B**) Paraesophageal.

particularly in combination, are the major risk factors for esophageal cancer.

Most tumors affect the middle or lower third of the esophagus. The most common symptom, which often does not develop until late in the disease, is **dysphagia** (difficulty or pain in swallowing). Later symptoms include reflux, weight loss, regurgitation, and blood loss.

Treatment may involve surgery, radiation therapy, and/or chemotherapy. (See Chapter 12 ◯◯ for more information about cancer treatments.) Controlling dysphagia is essential; many clients with esophageal cancer are undernourished because of dysphagia. TPN or enteral (tube) feedings may be needed to maintain weight and nutrition (see Boxes 19-5 and 19-6). A gastrostomy tube may be inserted.

Following surgery, the client is at high risk for aspiration and airway problems. Assess level of consciousness and respiratory status at least every hour after surgery. Encourage coughing and deep breathing every 1 to 2 hours and as needed.

Teach the client, family members, and caregivers about the diagnosis and prescribed treatment, including wound care and follow-up care. If tube feedings or TPN will be continued at home, have the client and caregivers demonstrate skills required to perform the procedure. Refer the client to home health services or hospice as indicated.

Gastroenteritis

The stomach and upper intestinal tract (duodenum and jejunum) are responsible for the majority of food digestion. Gastroenteritis, gastritis, peptic ulcer disease, and cancer of the stomach are the major disorders affecting food intake and digestion. Nurses provide both acute care for the hospitalized client and teaching for the client who will manage these conditions at home.

Gastroenteritis is inflammation of the stomach and intestines. It usually is caused by a bacterial, viral, or parasitic infection, or by a toxin. Bacterial and viral infections are often termed *food poisoning,* because contaminated food is often the route of entry. Clients experience diarrhea, abdominal discomfort, and often anorexia, nausea, and vomiting.

PATHOPHYSIOLOGY AND MANIFESTATIONS

Bacterial or viral infection of the GI tract produces inflammation, tissue damage, and symptoms by two primary mechanisms:

1. *Production of enterotoxins.* Many bacteria produce and excrete a toxin that damages and inflames the GI tract. Enterotoxins impair intestinal absorption and can cause electrolytes and water to be secreted into the bowel, leading to diarrhea and fluid loss.
2. *Invasion and ulceration of the mucosa.* Other bacteria invade intestinal mucosa, causing ulceration, bleeding, fluid exudate, and water and electrolyte secretion.

BOX 19-10

MANIFESTATIONS OF GASTROENTERITIS

Gastrointestinal
- Anorexia, nausea, and vomiting
- Abdominal pain and cramping
- Borborygmi (excessively loud, hyperactive bowel sounds)
- Diarrhea

General
- Malaise, weakness, muscle aches
- Dry skin and mucous membranes, poor turgor
- Orthostatic hypotension, tachycardia
- Elevated temperature

Manifestations of bacterial and viral enteritis vary by organism but have several common features (Box 19-10 ■). Excess fluid in the bowel and increased bowel motility cause diarrhea with frequent, watery stools. Lost fluids and electrolytes can lead to dehydration, hypovolemia, and manifestations of fluid and electrolyte or acid–base imbalances.

Severe vomiting may lead to metabolic alkalosis. With diarrhea, metabolic acidosis is more likely. Hypokalemia and hyponatremia may also occur. The specific effects of certain GI infections are summarized in Table 19-3 ■.

INTERDISCIPLINARY CARE

Identifying the cause, managing symptoms, and preventing complications are the primary goals of care. The client's his-

TABLE 19-3

Selected Causes of Gastroenteritis

DISEASE AND ORGANISM	INCUBATION	SOURCE	MANIFESTATIONS
Traveler's diarrhea *Escherichia coli*	24–72 hours	Contaminated food or water	Abrupt onset of diarrhea; vomiting rare
Staphylococcal food poisoning	2–8 hours	Contaminated food—meats and fish, dairy products	Severe nausea and vomiting; abdominal cramping and diarrhea; headache and fever
Botulism *Clostridium botulinum*	1.5–8 days	Improperly preserved foods such as home-canned vegetables, smoked meats, vacuum-packed fish	Diplopia, blurred vision; dry mouth, dysphagia; progressive muscle weakness and paralysis; possible nausea, vomiting, abdominal cramps
Cholera *Vibrio cholerae*	1–3 days	Water or food contaminated by feces; endemic in parts of Asia, Middle East, and Africa	Asymptomatic or severe diarrhea with watery, gray, odorless stool; vomiting; thirst, oliguria, muscle cramps; weakness; dehydration
Hemorrhagic colitis *E. coli O157:H7*	1–3 days	Undercooked beef; unpasteurized milk or apple juice	Severe cramping, watery to grossly bloody diarrhea; fever; complications of acute renal failure and thrombotic thrombocytopenic purpura

(continued)

TABLE 19-3

Selected Causes of Gastroenteritis (continued)

DISEASE AND ORGANISM	INCUBATION	SOURCE	MANIFESTATIONS
Salmonellosis *Salmonella*	8–48 hours	Raw or improperly cooked meat, poultry, eggs, and diary products	Diarrhea with cramping, nausea, and vomiting; low-grade fever, chills, weakness
Shigellosis (bacillary dysentery) *Shigella*	1–4 days	Fecal-contaminated food, fomites (inanimate objects), and vectors (such as fleas)	Watery diarrhea with blood, mucus, and pus; severe abdominal cramping and urgency of defecation; lethargy; dehydration
Giardiasis *Giardia lamblia*	1–3 weeks	Fecal–oral spread through contaminated food or water; direct contact	Diarrhea, mild or severe; anorexia, nausea, vomiting; epigastric pain, cramping; flatulence and belching; may be asymptomatic
Amebiasis *Entamoeba histolytica*	2–4 weeks	Fecal–oral spread through contaminated food or water; direct contact	Usually asymptomatic; diarrhea with blood and mucus; abdominal cramping, tenderness, colic, tenesmus, and flatulence; nausea and vomiting; fever, fatigue, weight loss

tory and symptoms provide valuable clues about the cause. A *stool specimen* may be obtained for culture, ova and parasites, and leukocyte count. See Table 18-3 ⚭ for nursing responsibilities related to collecting a stool specimen.

Fluid and electrolyte replacement is the primary focus of care. Oral rehydration is optimal. An oral glucose–electrolyte solution is often well tolerated in sips, even by the client who is vomiting. Commercial or homemade preparations may be used. Intravenous fluids such as glucose in normal saline, Ringer's, or lactated Ringer's may be ordered when vomiting and diarrhea are severe.

An antidiarrheal drug may be prescribed to promote comfort and reduce fluid loss. Nursing measures related to the use of antidiarrheal agents are outlined in Table 20-2 ⚭.

Gastric lavage and catharsis—to "wash out" the stomach and intestines—may be ordered if botulism is suspected and if the food has been recently ingested. Botulism antitoxin is administered as soon as possible when botulism is suspected. It can prevent paralysis from progressing but does not affect existing paralysis. Epinephrine is kept at the bedside because the antitoxin can cause anaphylaxis. The client is observed closely for signs of respiratory distress. Respiratory support with endotracheal intubation and mechanical ventilation may be required (see Chapter 24 ⚭). The procedure for gastric lavage is outlined in Box 19-11 ■.

clinical ALERT

Antidiarrheal agents are not used when botulism is suspected. To remove the toxin from the bowel, cathartics may be ordered for these clients.

NURSING CARE

Few clients with acute gastroenteritis require hospitalization. Assessment, education, and support of self-care measures are major nursing responsibilities related to these disorders.

Ask about the onset of diarrhea and other symptoms such as nausea, vomiting, and abdominal pain. Inquire about recent travel, changes in diet or water supply, or activities such as picnics or pot-luck meals. Ask about others in the family or household who also may be experiencing symptoms. Ask about the frequency and severity of vomiting and diarrhea and the nature of diarrheal stools. Ask about other manifestations such as abdominal pain or cramping. Inquire about measures taken to relieve the symptoms and the ability to take in and retain fluids.

Emphasize that fluid replacement is more important than eating while diarrhea is severe. Advise use of a glucose–electrolyte solution. (See directions for making a rehydrating solution in the Continuing Care section for diarrhea in Chapter 20 ⚭.) Discuss manifestations of dehydration or hypovolemia that require a physician's care.

Teach the importance of good hand washing to prevent spread of infection to others. Instruct to wash hands thoroughly with soap and running water for at least 10 seconds after each defecation. Wash contaminated clothing and linens separately in hot water and detergent. Emphasize the need to keep toilet areas clean and to maintain good personal hygiene. Advise avoiding rectal contact during sexual activity.

BOX 19-11   PROCEDURE CHECKLIST

Gastric Lavage

☑ Obtain all supplies.

☑ Provide for privacy.

☑ Use standard precautions.

☑ Explain the procedure. Instruct client to report any pain, difficulty breathing, or other problems during the procedure.

☑ Document baseline vital signs, abdominal girth, and bowel sounds.

☑ Place in semi-Fowler's or Fowler's position. If hypotension is present, place in left side-lying position.

☑ Insert a nasogastric (NG) tube (14 to 16 French, unless otherwise indicated) if one is not already in place, and verify placement. (See Box 19-4.)

Closed System Irrigation

Connect irrigating solution to NG tube with Y connector. Attach drainage or suction tube to other arm of connector. Empty the stomach, clamp drain tube or turn off suction, and allow 50 to 200 mL of solution to run into stomach by gravity. Stop solution and allow to drain or suction out. Repeat until ordered amount has been used or desired results are obtained. Measure the drainage, subtracting the amount of irrigant instilled, to obtain gastric output.

Intermittent Open System

Empty the stomach using suction or a 50-mL catheter-tip syringe. Measure and discard the aspirate. Using the syringe, draw up approximately 50 mL of irrigation solution, and instill it using gentle pressure. Withdraw and discard the solution into a measuring container. Continue until the desired amount of irrigant or desired results have been obtained.

☑ Monitor vital signs, respiratory status, and client tolerance during the procedure.

☑ Notify the charge nurse or physician if the procedure is ineffective or the client is unable to tolerate it.

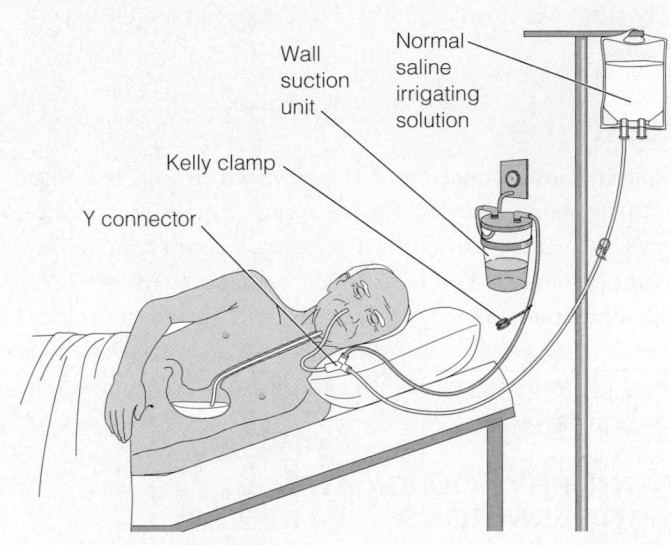

Wall suction unit

Normal saline irrigating solution

Kelly clamp

Y connector

A client with a closed system gastric lavage.

SAMPLE DOCUMENTATION

8/13/06 1630 Gastric lavage with 750 mL normal saline. Irrigant returned clear; no bleeding noted. 50 mL gastric contents returned with irrigant. Tolerated procedure well with no abdominal or respiratory distress.
_____S. Williams, LPN.

Note: Refer to a nursing fundamentals or skills text for more detailed instruction. Check state guidelines and facility policy before performing any procedure.

For specific interventions to manage diarrhea, see Chapter 20 ⨀.

CONTINUING CARE

Teach clients in all settings the following food and water safety measures:

- Maintain proper food temperatures. Promptly refrigerate cooked meats, dairy products, eggs, and egg products.
- Do not drink unpasteurized milk.
- Do not eat raw meat products. Cook hamburger until no redness remains.

- Follow directions precisely when home-canning foods; use a pressure canner when processing nonacidic foods, such as vegetables, mushrooms, meats, and fish.
- Boil home-canned foods for 10 to 15 minutes after opening to destroy any potential toxin.
- Destroy, without touching or tasting, any food that is discolored or comes from a container that has been punctured, is cracked or bulging, or does not have a tight seal.
- When using untreated water, boil, filter, or treat it with water purification tablets.

MediaLink

Video: Gastric Lavage

- Where water is untreated or sanitation is poor, avoid foods that cannot be peeled or cooked.
- When traveling out of the country, consume only bottled water unless local water supplies are clearly safe.

Gastritis

Gastritis, inflammation of the stomach lining, is a common stomach disorder. *Acute gastritis,* the most common form, is usually caused by ingesting irritants such as aspirin, alcohol, caffeine, or foods contaminated with certain bacteria. *Chronic gastritis,* however, leads to progressive and irreversible changes in the gastric mucosa. It is more common in the elderly, chronic alcoholics, and cigarette smokers.

PATHOPHYSIOLOGY AND MANIFESTATIONS

Normally, the stomach is protected from the digestive substances it secretes—namely, hydrochloric acid and pepsin—by the mucosal barrier (Figure 19-6 ■). When this barrier is disrupted, the gastric mucosa becomes irritated and inflamed.

Acute Gastritis

In acute gastritis, a local irritant disrupts the mucosal barrier, allowing gastric juices to come into contact with the

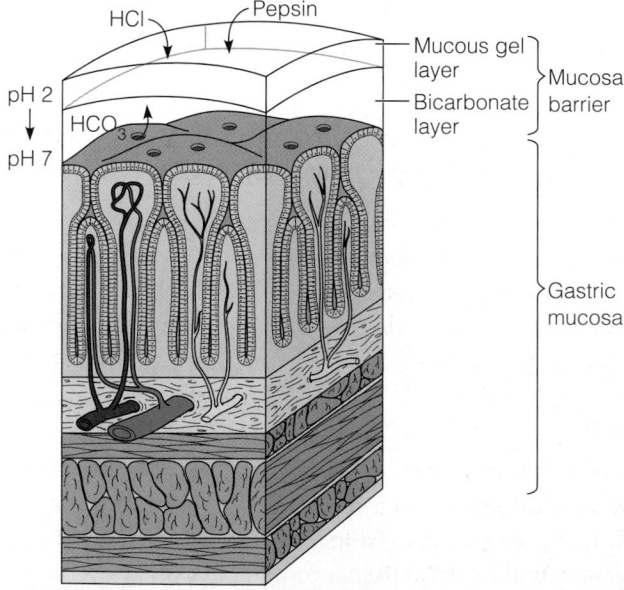

Figure 19-6. ■ The gastric mucosa and the mucosal barrier. The mucous gel and bicarbonate of the mucosal barrier protect the gastric mucosa from damage by gastric secretions.

BOX 19-12

MANIFESTATIONS OF ACUTE AND CHRONIC GASTRITIS

Acute Gastritis
- Anorexia
- Nausea and vomiting
- Abdominal pain or discomfort
- Hematemesis (vomiting blood)
- Melena (black, tarry stool)

Chronic Gastritis
- Vague discomfort after eating
- Anemia
- Fatigue

---

gastric tissue. This causes irritation, inflammation, and superficial erosions. The gastric mucosa rapidly regenerates, and healing occurs within several days.

Acute gastritis often is caused by drugs such as aspirin or other nonsteroidal anti-inflammatory drugs (NSAIDs), corticosteroids, and chemotherapy. Bacterial toxins in contaminated food can cause an abrupt, severe gastritis. Ingestion of a strong alkali (such as ammonia) or acid severely damages the stomach, and may lead to perforation, hemorrhage, and peritonitis. *Erosive* or *stress-induced gastritis* (a severe form of acute gastritis) is a potential complication of conditions such as shock, severe trauma, or major surgery. Decreased blood flow to the gastric mucosa leads to superficial erosions and a significant risk for bleeding.

The client with acute gastritis may have few symptoms. Possible manifestations are listed in Box 19-12 ■. Gastric bleeding may occur, causing **hematemesis** (vomiting of blood) or **melena** (black, tarry stool that contains blood).

---

clinical ALERT

Clients with stress gastritis often have no symptoms until signs of severe bleeding, shock, or an *acute abdomen* (severely painful, rigid, boardlike abdomen) develop.

Chronic Gastritis

Chronic gastritis is a progressive disorder in which the gastric mucosa thins and atrophies, and the mucosal barrier becomes less effective. Chronic gastritis is associated with colonization of the gastric mucosa by *Helicobacter pylori* (*H. pylori*), the bacteria that cause peptic ulcer disease. Chronic alcohol use, cigarette smoking, and exposure to toxins such as lead may also contribute to chronic gastritis.

Chronic gastritis is often asymptomatic until digestion and gastric emptying are affected. The client may complain of vague gastric distress after eating or ulcer-like symptoms. See Box 19-12.

INTERDISCIPLINARY CARE

Acute gastritis is often diagnosed by the client's history and symptoms. It usually is treated in a community-based setting unless severe vomiting or bleeding occurs. Chronic gastritis may require lifelong therapy.

Diagnostic Tests

The following diagnostic tests may be ordered:

- *Gastric analysis* to assess hydrochloric acid secretion. See Table 18-4 ⚭ for more information about gastric analysis.
- *Hemoglobin* and *hematocrit* are used to identify possible anemia due to bleeding.
- *Endoscopy* may be done to inspect the gastric mucosa, evaluate for *H. pylori* infection, and obtain tissue for biopsy. Areas of bleeding may be treated directly. Box 19-13 ■ describes nursing care of the client having an endoscopy.

Medications

Antiemetics and antacids are used in acute gastritis to control gastric distress and vomiting. If nausea and vomiting are severe, intravenous fluids and electrolyte replacement are ordered.

Proton-pump inhibitors such as lansoprazole (Prevacid) or omeprazole (Prilosec), or histamine-2 (H_2)-receptor antagonists (such as cimetidine or famotidine) may be ordered to prevent or treat acute stress gastritis. Sucralfate (Carafate) may also be used. It works locally to prevent acid and pepsin from damaging gastric tissue. These drugs or antacids also may be ordered for the client with chronic gastritis. If *H. pylori* infection is found, treatment to eradicate the infection is initiated (see the section on peptic ulcer disease that follows). Table 19-4 ■ outlines the nursing implications and client teaching for these drugs.

Other Therapies

For *acute gastritis*, 6 to 12 hours of GI tract rest is prescribed. Food and fluids are slowly reintroduced, beginning with clear liquids (broth, tea, gelatin, carbonated beverages), followed by heavier liquids (cream soups, puddings, milk) and finally solid foods.

When acute gastritis results from ingesting a poisonous or corrosive substance (acid or strong alkali), the substance must immediately be diluted and removed. Vomiting is not induced because it might further damage the esophagus

| BOX 19-13 | NURSING CARE CHECKLIST |

Upper Endoscopy

Before the Procedure

☑ Provide routine preoperative care as ordered (see Chapter 9 ⚭).

☑ Assess knowledge and understanding of the procedure, reinforcing teaching as needed. Conscious sedation often is used during the procedure, which requires 20 to 30 minutes to complete.

☑ Remove dentures and check for loose teeth prior to the procedure. Provide mouth care. Remove eyewear, jewelry, hairpins, and combs.

After the Procedure

☑ Provide routine postoperative care as ordered (see Chapter 9 ⚭).

☑ Monitor for evidence of complications: bleeding, abdominal or back pain, dyspnea, dysphagia, or fever.

☑ Withhold all food and fluids until gag and swallow reflexes have returned. Place in semi-Fowler's position with the head to the side to allow drainage of saliva from mouth.

☑ Provide tissues for the client to expectorate into.

☑ Tell the client that a sore throat, hoarseness, abdominal bloating, belching, and flatulence are common after the procedure. Warm saline gargles or throat lozenges may help relieve discomfort.

☑ Ensure that the client is not discharged alone.

☑ Instruct the client to notify the physician immediately if any of the following develop: persistent difficulty swallowing; epigastric, substernal, or shoulder pain; vomiting blood; black, tarry stools; or fever.

and trachea. Instead, *gastric lavage* (irrigation or washing out of the stomach) is performed (see Box 19-11).

Complementary Therapies

Complementary therapies such as herbal remedies or aromatherapy may be appropriate to recommend for clients with gastritis. Refer the client to a health care provider trained in natural and herbal remedies or to an aromatherapist for an individualized treatment plan. Recommendations may include:

- Chamomile tea or the essential oil used in aromatherapy
- Garlic; one clove chopped fine and taken daily at bedtime
- Ginger, powdered, capsules, or made into a tea taken before or after meals
- Mint oil aromatherapy via a diffuser, in a bath, or diluted with a carrier oil and used for a soothing massage.

TABLE 19-4

Nursing Implications for Pharmacology: GERD, Gastritis, and Peptic Ulcer Disease

AGENTS/DRUGS	PURPOSE	NURSING RESPONSIBILITIES	CLIENT TEACHING
Proton Pump Inhibitors ■ Esomeprazole (Nexium) ■ Lansoprazole (Prevacid) ■ Omeprazole (Prilosec) ■ Pantoprazole (Protonix) ■ Rabeprazole (Aciphex)	These drugs significantly reduce gastric acid secretion and the amount of acid in the stomach between and following meals. They are used to heal and prevent recurrence of peptic ulcers and for GERD.	Administer at bedtime or before breakfast. Do not open or crush capsules or tablets. Monitor liver function tests (see Table 18-3) ⟳ and report abnormal results. These drugs may slow the elimination of diazepam, warfarin, and phenytoin; monitor for adverse effects.	Take at bedtime or before breakfast. Take the drug for the full course of therapy, even if you feel better. Don't smoke, drink alcohol, or take aspirin or NSAIDs while taking this drug because they may interfere with healing. Adverse effects are rare with these drugs but should be reported to your physician.
H2-Receptor Blockers ■ Cimetidine (Tagamet) ■ Famotidine (Pepcid) ■ Nizatidine (Axid) ■ Ranitidine (Zantac)	H_2-receptor blockers reduce stomach acid by blocking the acid-stimulating effects of histamine. This reduces the volume and concentration of hydrochloric acid in the stomach.	Should not be taken during pregnancy and lactation. Administer 30 minutes before meals and at bedtime or as ordered. Do not administer antacids within 1 hour before or after these drugs to ensure absorption. When given intravenously, do not mix with other drugs. Administer in 20–100 mL of solution over 15 to 30 minutes.	Take as directed, even after pain and gastric discomfort are relieved. Avoid taking antacids for 1 hour before and 1 hour after taking H_2 blockers. Report any of the following to the physician: diarrhea, confusion, rash, fatigue, malaise, or bruising.
Antacids ■ Aluminum hydroxide (Amphojel, AlternaGEL) ■ Magnesium hydroxide (Milk of Magnesia) ■ Calcium carbonate (Tums) ■ Magnesium hydroxide and aluminum hydroxide (Maalox, Mylanta, Gelusil)	Antacids buffer or neutralize gastric acid, generally by a local action. They help relieve pain and prevent further damage to the gastric mucosa.	Antacids interfere with absorption of many drugs; separate dosage times by at least 2 hours. Monitor for constipation or diarrhea. Notify the physician should either occur; a different antacid may be prescribed. Monitor for electrolyte imbalances in clients taking high doses of antacids.	Do not use sodium bicarbonate as an antacid because of its local and systemic effects. Take as prescribed; to work effectively, the antacid must be in the stomach. Avoid taking the antacid for approximately 2 hours before and after taking other medication. Report diarrhea or constipation to the physician. Continue taking the antacid for the duration prescribed; mucosal healing takes 6–8 weeks.
Sucralfate	Sucralfate creates a protective barrier against gastric juices. It does not neutralize gastric acid or affect its secretion.	Give sucralfate on an empty stomach 1 hour before meals and at bedtime or as ordered. Sucralfate may interfere with absorption of other drugs; separate administration times by at least 2 hours.	This drug has few side effects. Constipation may rarely develop. If you have difficulty swallowing the tablets, an oral suspension is available.

(continued)

TABLE 19-4

Nursing Implications for Pharmacology: GERD, Gastritis, and Peptic Ulcer Disease (continued)

AGENTS/DRUGS	PURPOSE	NURSING RESPONSIBILITIES	CLIENT TEACHING
Bismuth Compounds ■ Bismuth subsalicylate (Pepto-Bismol) ■ Ranitidine bismuth citrate (Tritec)	Bismuth has a local antibiotic effect on *H. pylori;* it also may help prevent the bacteria from adhering to the gastric mucosa.	Do not give bismuth subsalicylate if fecal impaction is suspected. This drug is contraindicated for clients who are allergic to aspirin.	This drug may cause stools to turn dark or appear black. Do not take this drug if you are allergic to aspirin. Do not give this drug to children who have chickenpox or another viral illness.
Misoprostol (Cytotec)	Misoprostol is a synthetic prostaglandin used to prevent ulcers in clients who require long-term NSAID therapy.	Do not give during pregnancy because it may cause abortion of the fetus. Administer with meals and at bedtime.	Stress the importance of avoiding this drug during pregnancy. May cause diarrhea, abdominal pain, spotting, and uterine cramps. Report these effects to the doctor.

NURSING CARE

ASSESSING

Collect data regarding the onset, duration, and nature of the client's symptoms. Ask specifically about foods, fluids, and other substances (such as aspirin or other drugs) that have been taken recently. Inquire about evidence of bleeding in emesis or stools. Note appearance and any visible distress. Assess vital signs, including orthostatic blood pressures. Inspect the abdomen and auscultate bowel sounds. Measure abdominal girth, and lightly palpate for tenderness. Measure and document the color and character of any emesis or stools.

Monitor the results of laboratory and diagnostic testing, particularly the hemoglobin and hematocrit. See Chapter 30 ⬥ for critical values. If acute gastritis is accompanied by vomiting, monitor serum electrolyte values and results of arterial blood gases for acid–base balance. See Chapter 7 ⬥ for normal and critical values of these tests.

DIAGNOSING, PLANNING, AND IMPLEMENTING

Priorities in Nursing Care. The effects of acute gastritis and its manifestations on fluid balance and intravascular volume are the priority nursing care focus for the client. Chronic gastritis, in contrast, affects food and nutrient intake, making possible nutritional deficiencies the priority for nursing care.

Deficient Fluid Volume

Nausea, vomiting, and abdominal distress are the primary manifestations of acute gastritis. Fluid and electrolyte imbalances may develop as a result.

■ Frequently monitor vital signs, including orthostatic vital signs. *Tachycardia and orthostatic hypotension may indicate fluid volume deficit. Electrolyte imbalances may affect heart rate and rhythm, as well as blood pressure.*

■ Monitor and record intake and output. Weigh daily. *Intake and output records and daily weights provide important data about fluid balance.*

■ Provide meticulous skin and mouth care frequently. *Clients with fluid volume deficit are at high risk for impaired skin and mucous membrane integrity.*

■ Report significant changes or deviations from normal laboratory values for electrolytes and acid–base balance. *Significant changes in electrolyte or acid–base balance may occur as a result of vomiting and poor food and fluid intake.*

■ Provide fluids by mouth or parenterally as ordered. *Oral fluids are gradually reintroduced when the client is no longer vomiting. Intravenous fluids restore or maintain hydration until adequate oral intake is resumed.*

■ Administer antiemetic and other medications as ordered to relieve nausea and vomiting. *Medications can help prevent or relieve vomiting and can promote oral intake.*

■ Provide for the safety of clients with orthostatic hypotension: Place the signal light within reach, put up the side rails, instruct the client not to get up or walk without assistance. *Orthostatic hypotension may lead to fainting or falls.*

Imbalanced Nutrition: Less than Body Requirements

The client may become fearful of eating or may reduce food intake to the point of becoming undernourished.

- Monitor and record food and fluid intake and any abnormal losses (such as vomiting). *Careful monitoring provides valuable information about nutritional status.*
- Weigh daily at the same time. *Weight changes occurring over days to weeks are an indicator of nutritional status.*
- Arrange for dietary consultation. *Clients with chronic gastritis may have specific food intolerances and preferences that need to be considered.*
- Provide nutritional supplements between meals or frequent small feedings as needed. *Many clients with chronic gastritis tolerate small, frequent feedings better than three large meals per day.*

EVALUATING

Collect the following data to evaluate the effectiveness of nursing care: indicators of fluid and electrolyte balance, such as thirst, skin turgor, weight, intake and output, mental status, and laboratory values; appetite and food intake; skin condition, color, and other indicators of nutritional status.

Documenting. Document manifestations of the disorder and the response to treatment. Document continuing assessment data, particularly any episodes of vomiting, diarrhea, and the presence of blood in emesis or stool. Note the client's ability to resume normal food and fluid intake.

CONTINUING CARE

Teaching is a vital component of nursing care for clients whose gastritis is managed at home. Teach clients with acute gastritis how to identify and avoid causative factors, manage acute symptoms, reintroduce fluids and foods, and when to contact the physician (unrelieved vomiting, severe weight loss, changes in mental status or lack of urine output).

Teach clients with chronic gastritis how to manage their condition. Provide information on maintaining nutritional status, helpful dietary modifications, known gastric irritants, use of prescribed medications, and complementary therapies. Refer clients to smoking-cessation classes or programs to treat alcohol abuse if appropriate. In all cases, document teaching and referrals.

Peptic Ulcer Disease

A **peptic ulcer** is a break in the mucous lining of the stomach or duodenum where it comes in contact with gastric juice. *Peptic ulcer disease (PUD)* is a chronic health problem that primarily affects adults (often duodenal ulcers in young and middle adults, and gastric ulcers in older adults). Chronic *H. pylori* infection and ingestion of aspirin and other NSAIDs are the major risk factors. Cigarette smoking doubles the risk of PUD.

PATHOPHYSIOLOGY

The mucosal barrier protects the gastric mucosa. It is maintained by (1) bicarbonate secreted by epithelial cells, (2) mucous gel produced in response to prostaglandins, and (3) an adequate blood supply to the mucosa. Ulcers develop when the mucosal barrier is unable to prevent damage by gastric digestive juices.

The mucosal barrier can be impaired by poor circulation, decreased mucus, or reflux of bile or pancreatic enzymes into the stomach or duodenum. Aspirin and other NSAIDs inhibit prostaglandins and mucous gel production.

About three-fourths of the people with PUD have *H. pylori* infection. This bacterium secretes substances that break down mucous gel and also appears to stimulate acid production in the stomach. It also causes an inflammatory response in the lining of the stomach. Cigarette smoking contributes by inhibiting bicarbonate secretion.

Ulcers may develop in the esophagus, stomach, or duodenum. In the stomach, the lesser curvature and area closest to the pylorus are most often affected (Figure 19-7 ■). Ulcers may be superficial or deep, affecting all layers of the mucosa (Figure 19-8 ■).

MANIFESTATIONS AND COMPLICATIONS

Epigastric pain is the classic symptom of PUD. The pain is often described as gnawing, burning, aching, or hunger-like. It occurs when the stomach is empty (2 to 3 hours after meals and in the middle of the night) and is relieved by eating. It may radiate to the back. The client may complain of heartburn or regurgitation and vomiting. Older adults with PUD may have no symptoms or may complain of vague discomfort, chest pain, or dysphagia. Weight loss or anemia may be present.

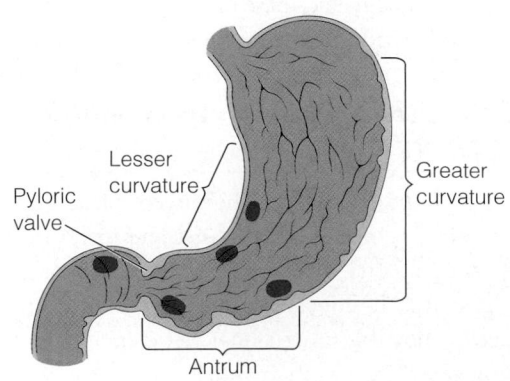

Figure 19-7. ■ Sites commonly affected by peptic ulcer disease.

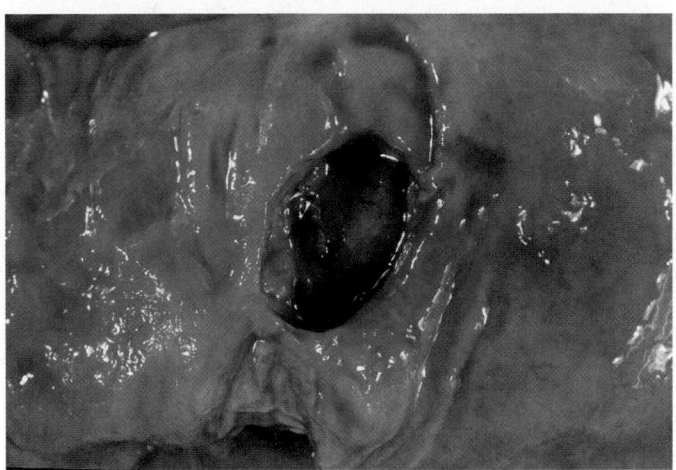

Figure 19-8. ■ A large gastric ulcer. (*Source:* Photo Researchers, Inc.)

Complications

The complications of PUD include hemorrhage, obstruction, and perforation. *Hemorrhage* results from ulceration and erosion into blood vessels of the gastric mucosa. Erosion into small blood vessels may cause slow bleeding and black, tarry stools. Erosion into a larger vessel can lead to sudden, severe bleeding with hematemesis or **hematochezia** (red blood with clots in the stool), and signs of shock. Box 19-14 ■ lists the manifestations of PUD complications.

Peptic ulcer disease can cause *obstruction* of the upper GI tract. This usually occurs gradually. If the obstruction becomes complete, vomiting occurs.

BOX 19-14

MANIFESTATIONS OF PUD COMPLICATIONS

Hemorrhage
- Occult or obvious blood in the stool
- Hematemesis
- Fatigue, weakness, dizziness
- Orthostatic hypotension
- Shock

Obstruction
- Feeling of epigastric fullness
- Nausea and vomiting

Perforation
- Severe upper abdominal pain, radiating to the shoulder
- Rigid, boardlike (acute) abdomen
- Absent bowel sounds
- Signs of shock: diaphoresis, tachycardia, rapid and shallow respirations
- Fever

Perforation of the ulcer through the mucosal wall is the most dangerous complication of PUD. When perforation occurs, gastric or duodenal contents enter the peritoneum, causing inflammation and *peritonitis.* Chemical peritonitis from GI secretions develops immediately; bacterial peritonitis from contamination of the normally sterile peritoneal cavity follows. When an ulcer perforates, the client develops immediate manifestations of an acute abdomen, with pain, guarding, and absent bowel sounds. Signs of shock may be present. Older adults may have less specific manifestations of perforation; pain may be absent. See Chapter 20 ◯◯ for more information about peritonitis and its treatment.

INTERDISCIPLINARY CARE
Treatment of PUD focuses on relieving symptoms, healing ulcers, and preventing complications and ulcer recurrence.

Diagnostic Tests
- *Upper endoscopy* (*gastroscopy*) is done to inspect the mucosa of the upper GI tract and obtain samples for biopsy and *H. pylori* testing. (Review Box 19-13 for nursing care related to an upper endoscopy.)
- A *urea breath test* may be done to detect *H. pylori* infection. (See Table 18-4 ◯◯ for more information about this test.)
- *CBC* to assess for anemia.
- *Stool* for occult blood.

Medications
Drug therapy is used to eradicate *H. pylori* and heal existing ulcers. A combination of a proton-pump inhibitor such as omeprazole (Prilosec) and two antibiotics is commonly prescribed to treat *H. pylori* infection. Metronidazole (Flagyl), clarithromycin (Biaxin), and tetracycline are commonly used antibiotics for this therapy. (See Chapter 10 ◯◯ for nursing responsibilities and client teaching related to antibiotic therapy.)

Proton-pump inhibitors and H_2-receptor antagonists are used to reduce gastric acid production, to promote healing, and to prevent stress gastritis and ulcers in at-risk clients. Agents that protect the mucosa (sucralfate, bismuth, antacids, and prostaglandin analogs) also may be prescribed. Review Table 19-4 for nursing implications and client teaching for drugs used to treat PUD.

Diet
No special diet is prescribed for PUD. Encourage clients to eat a well-balanced diet with meals at regular intervals. Bland or restrictive diets are no longer recommended. Mild alcohol intake is not harmful. Discourage smoking because it slows the rate of healing and increases the frequency of relapses.

Treatment of Complications
Clients with complications of PUD require additional treatment measures.

In *hemorrhage* associated with PUD, restoring and maintaining circulation is the priority of care. Intravenous solutions such as Ringer's solution are administered to restore intravascular volume. Whole blood or red blood cell concentrate (packed cells) may also be given to restore the oxygen-carrying capacity of blood.

When the client is stable, an endoscopy is done to identify and treat the bleeding site. A vasoconstricting agent may be injected at the site or the vessel may be cauterized. Most clients can be discharged within 72 hours following endoscopy for bleeding.

If *obstruction* is suspected, a nasogastric tube is inserted to relieve pressure and vomiting. The obstruction is visualized by endoscopy, and balloon therapy may be used to dilate the obstruction. Surgery may be required to relieve the obstruction.

Perforation requires immediate intervention. The client is kept NPO; intravenous fluids are administered. To minimize peritoneal contamination, gastric contents are removed by nasogastric tube connected to suction. The client is placed in Fowler's or semi-Fowler's position so that peritoneal contaminants will pool in the pelvis. Intravenous antibiotics are given to treat bacterial infection by intestinal flora. Many perforations seal spontaneously, but some require closure by laparoscopic surgery.

Surgery

When drug therapy and lifestyle management cannot control the symptoms or complications of PUD, surgery may be necessary. Acute perforation or massive hemorrhage may require emergency surgery. See the section on gastric cancer that follows for more information about surgical procedures, their complications, and nursing care of the client undergoing gastric surgery.

NURSING CARE

ASSESSING

Collect the subjective and objective data identified in Box 19-15 ■. Ask the client specifically about pain, carefully assessing each episode. Do not make assumptions about cause and severity. Document all complaints of pain, and notify the charge nurse or physician if pain becomes severe or changes in character or timing.

clinical ALERT

Pain may indicate a complication of PUD, or may be related to another process (e.g., coronary heart disease, gallbladder disease).

BOX 19-15	ASSESSMENT

Assessing Clients with Peptic Ulcer Disease

SUBJECTIVE DATA
- Pain: location, character, intensity, duration, and timing; relationship to meals; measures that relieve or aggravate pain
- Complaints of nausea, vomiting, heartburn, indigestion, or abdominal pain
- Color, consistency, and amount of any emesis
- Color and consistency of feces, any recent changes
- Current or previous treatment (prescribed or over-the-counter); compliance with treatment regimen
- Use of tobacco, alcohol, aspirin, NSAIDs, or other medications

OBJECTIVE DATA
- Check vital signs, including orthostatic blood pressures.
- Inspect abdomen, observing shape, contour, and appearance.
- Auscultate bowel sounds in all four quadrants; note frequency.
- Palpate for tenderness and guarding.
- Test any emesis and stool for the presence of occult blood.

If the client is being admitted with a possible complication such as bleeding, obstruction, or perforation, determine the duration and severity of symptoms. Carefully observe the client's general appearance, watching for signs of acute distress. Focus interview questions and physical assessment to collect data quickly.

DIAGNOSING, PLANNING, AND IMPLEMENTING

Priorities in Nursing Care. In the client with uncomplicated PUD, the discomfort associated with the disease and the effects of that discomfort on nutrition are the primary focus for nursing care. When the client is admitted with an acute bleed related to PUD, the effects of resulting hypovolemia on the client are the immediate priority of nursing care.

Pain

- Assess pain, reporting any changes in intensity or character to the charge nurse or physician. *A change in the nature or severity of pain may indicate a complication of PUD or a separate problem.*
- Administer medications as ordered. *Medications for PUD help prevent pain and promote healing. Administration at bedtime helps prevent nighttime ulcer pain that typically occurs between 1:00 and 3:00 A.M.*

- Limit food intake after the evening meal; eliminate bedtime snacks. *Eating before bed can stimulate gastric acid and pepsin production, increasing the chance of nighttime pain.*

Imbalanced Nutrition: Less than Body Requirements

- Assess diet, including pattern of food intake, eating schedule, and foods associated with pain. *This step increases client awareness and identifies whether nutrient intake is adequate.*
- Arrange consultation with a dietitian. *A dietitian can help plan meals that meet the client's nutritional needs and preferences. Foods that increase pain should be avoided. Providing six small meals per day generally helps increase food tolerance and decrease discomfort after meals.*
- Document and report complaints of anorexia, fullness, nausea, vomiting, or symptoms of dumping syndrome. *Problems with gastric emptying may be associated with PUD or surgery to treat PUD. It is important to monitor and report symptoms, because a change in therapy or food intake may be necessary.*

Decreased Cardiac Output

Acute bleeding can cause hypovolemia and a fall in cardiac output.

- Frequently monitor and record vital signs until stable. Closely monitor urinary output. Weigh daily. *Careful monitoring is essential to identify possible shock and to intervene at an early stage.*
- Monitor stools and gastric drainage for overt and occult blood. Assess gastric drainage (vomitus or from a nasogastric tube) to estimate the amount and rate of hemorrhage. *Drainage is bright red with possible clots in acute hemorrhage; dark red or the color of coffee grounds when blood has been in the stomach for a period of time. Hematochezia (stool containing red blood and clots) is present in acute hemorrhage; melena (black, tarry stool) indicates less acute bleeding.*
- Maintain intravenous infusions and assist with blood administration as needed. *Intravenous fluids and blood products are administered to maintain or restore blood volume. Whole blood and packed cells provide additional oxygen-carrying capacity to meet cell needs.*

clinical ALERT

Monitor urine output and report output of less than 30 mL/hr for two consecutive hours. Low urine output may indicate poor renal blood flow due to hypovolemia and decreased cardiac output, and an increased risk for acute renal failure.

- Insert a nasogastric (NG) tube and maintain its position and patency. Initially, measure and record gastric output hourly, then every 4 to 8 hours. *NG suction is used to re-move blood from the GI tract and prevent vomiting and possible aspiration. Gastric output is replaced with a balanced electrolyte solution to maintain homeostasis.*
- Prepare for possible endoscopy. *Endoscopy can identify bleeding sites and allow direct treatment of the erosion.*

clinical ALERT

Frequently monitor hemoglobin and hematocrit in the client admitted with gastrointestinal bleeding and report results that are below the expected level.

- Monitor serum electrolytes, blood urea nitrogen (BUN), and creatinine. Report abnormal findings. *Electrolytes are lost through vomiting, gastric drainage, and diarrhea. Digestion and absorption of blood in the GI tract may cause elevated BUN and creatinine levels.*
- Assess abdomen, including bowel sounds, girth, and tenderness every 4 hours and record findings. *Borborygmi and abdominal tenderness are common in clients with acute GI bleeding. Increased abdominal girth, absent bowel sounds, or extreme tenderness with a rigid, boardlike abdomen may indicate perforation.*
- Maintain bed rest with the head of the bed elevated and side rails up; ensure safety. *Loss of blood volume may cause orthostatic hypotension with syncope or dizziness upon standing.*

EVALUATING

To evaluate the effectiveness of nursing care for a client with peptic ulcer disease, collect data regarding pain, weight, nutritional status (including food intake), fluid balance, and circulation (vital signs, peripheral pulses and capillary refill, mental status, and urinary output). Frequently monitor for and promptly report any manifestation of complications of the disease or gastric surgery.

Documenting. Document continuing assessment data and the effects of interventions (e.g., relief of pain following antacid administration). Document all teaching provided, and the client's understanding of information presented. As indicated, document compliance with prescribed regimen.

CONTINUING CARE

Because PUD is a chronic disease, it is managed primarily by the client at home. Teach clients about treatment measures and counter common misconceptions and myths (e.g., drinking milk or cream every 2 hours "to coat the stomach" is no longer part of the treatment plan and can increase serum cholesterol levels and the risk for heart disease). Provide written and verbal instruction about medications, including the importance of continuing therapy even when symptoms are relieved. Teach clients taking metronidazole to eradicate *H. pylori* infection to avoid alcohol in any form while taking the drug and for a minimum of 48 hours after discontinuing the medication. Discuss the relationship between peptic ulcers and factors such as smoking. If indicated, refer the client to a smoking-cessation clinic. Stress the importance of avoiding aspirin and other NSAIDs, as well as the need to read the labels of over-the-counter medications to identify the presence of aspirin.

Discuss the manifestations of PUD complications, such as abdominal pain or distention, vomiting, black or tarry stools, light-headedness, or fainting. Emphasize the importance of contacting the physician if symptoms of a complication develop.

Reinforce stress and lifestyle management techniques that may help prevent flare-ups. Refer the client to resources for stress management, such as classes, counseling, and formal or informal groups.

NURSING PROCESS CARE PLAN
Client with Peptic Ulcer Disease

Sean O'Donnell is a 47-year-old policeman. He has had "heartburn" and epigastric pain for years but thought it went along with his job. Last year, after becoming weak, light-headed, and short of breath, he was found to be anemic and was diagnosed as having a duodenal ulcer. He took famotidine (Pepcid) and ferrous sulfate for 3 months before stopping both, saying he had "never felt better in his life." Sean has now been admitted to the hospital with active upper GI bleeding.

Assessment. Mr. O'Donnell is alert and oriented, though very apprehensive about his condition. Skin pale and cool; BP 136/78 and pulse 98. Abdomen distended and tender with extremely active bowel sounds. NG tube inserted; 200 mL bright red blood obtained. Laboratory results include hemoglobin 8.2 g/dL and hematocrit 23%. An endoscopy is done to control Mr. O'Donnell's bleeding, and he receives two units of packed red blood cells as well as intravenous fluids to replace his lost blood volume.

Diagnosis. The following nursing diagnoses are identified for Mr. O'Donnell:

- *Deficient Fluid Volume* related to acute upper GI bleeding
- *Impaired Tissue Integrity: Gastrointestinal* related to active peptic ulcer disease
- *Ineffective Therapeutic Regimen Management* related to lack of understanding of the need for continued treatment

Expected Outcomes. The expected outcomes for the plan of care specify that Mr. O'Donnell will:

- Regain homeostasis with stable vital signs and normal hemoglobin and hematocrit.

- Remain free of further bleeding and other potential complications of peptic ulcer disease.
- Demonstrate knowledge and understanding of prescribed treatment measures.
- Identify ways to promote ulcer healing and prevent recurrence.
- State manifestations to report to his primary care provider.

Planning and Implementation. The nurse plans and implements the following interventions for Mr. O'Donnell:

- Monitor and document vital signs, mental status, intake and output, and abdominal assessment every 4 hours until stable, then every 8 hours.
- Maintain intravenous fluids and blood replacement as ordered.
- Monitor laboratory values (hemoglobin, hematocrit, serum electrolytes), reporting abnormal values to the charge nurse or physician as indicated.
- Explain PUD and ulcer healing, clarifying misconceptions.
- Discuss the importance of following the treatment plan to ensure healing and prevent further ulcers from developing.
- Discuss the effect of smoking, aspirin, and NSAIDs on PUD. Provide information about other over-the-counter analgesics.
- Provide written and verbal instructions about prescribed medications.
- With the client, plan a medication schedule that fits his lifestyle.
- Discuss stress-reduction strategies such as exercise, meditation, controlled breathing, and other relaxation exercises.

Evaluation. Mr. O'Donnell is discharged after 72 hours. He has had no further bleeding, and is eating a normal diet. His hemoglobin and hematocrit levels have improved; other blood values are within normal limits. His physician has prescribed omeprazole (Prilosec), amoxicillin, and clarithromycin for 2 weeks to eradicate *H. pylori* infection confirmed during the endoscopy. He will continue to take the omeprazole daily at bedtime for another 6 weeks. He verbalizes an understanding of the need for these medications, when to take them, and what side effects he should report. He had used aspirin and ibuprofen regularly for tension headaches, but says he is willing to try acetaminophen and relaxation techniques to "avoid ending up in here again!" He states that the hardest part of going back to work will be not drinking 6 to 10 cups of coffee a day, as he used to do.

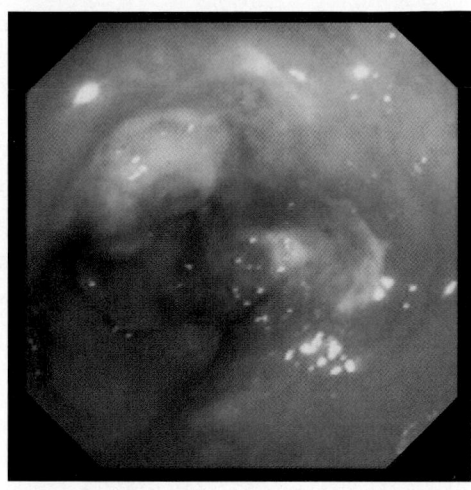

Figure 19-9. ■ Gastric cancer as seen through an endoscope. (*Source:* Photo Researchers, Inc.)

Critical Thinking in the Nursing Process

1. What is the likely reason Mr. O'Donnell developed another peptic ulcer and hemorrhage after having been treated for a previous episode?
2. Discuss the relationship between aspirin and NSAIDs and peptic ulcer disease.
3. What additional lifestyle changes would you recommend for Mr. O'Donnell?

Cancer of the Stomach

Except for skin cancer, cancer of the stomach is the most common cancer in the world, but it is less common in the United States. Its incidence is highest in Hispanics, African Americans, and Asian Americans; men are affected twice as often as women. Chronic *H. pylori* gastritis is the major risk factor for gastric cancer.

PATHOPHYSIOLOGY AND MANIFESTATIONS

Gastric carcinomas usually develop in the distal portion of the stomach. Half of all gastric cancers occur in the antrum or pyloric region (Figure 19-9 ■). Lesions spread by direct extension to tissues surrounding the stomach, particularly the liver. Lymph node involvement and metastasis occur early due to the rich blood and lymphatic supply to the stomach. Metastatic lesions are often found in the liver, lungs, ovaries, and peritoneum.

Early symptoms of gastric cancer are vague (early satiety, anorexia, indigestion, and possibly vomiting). There may also be ulcer-like pain, typically occurring after meals and unrelieved by antacids. As the disease progresses, weight loss occurs, and the client may be *cachectic* (very thin and malnourished).

INTERDISCIPLINARY CARE

An abdominal mass may be palpable in the client with gastric cancer, and there may be occult blood in the stool. The diagnosis is confirmed with an endoscopy and biopsy of the lesion.

Surgery

When gastric cancer is diagnosed before metastases develop, a partial or total gastrectomy is done. A *total* **gastrectomy** (removal of the entire stomach) is rarely done because of its impact on digestion and nutrition. Extensive gastric cancer, however, may require it. In a total gastrectomy, an **anastomosis** (surgical connection) connects the esophagus to the duodenum or jejunum (Figure 19-10C ■). More commonly, surgery involves *partial gastrectomy,* removal of a portion of the stomach, usually the distal half to two-thirds (Figures 19-10A and B ■). Nursing care of the client having gastric surgery is outlined in Box 19-16 ■.

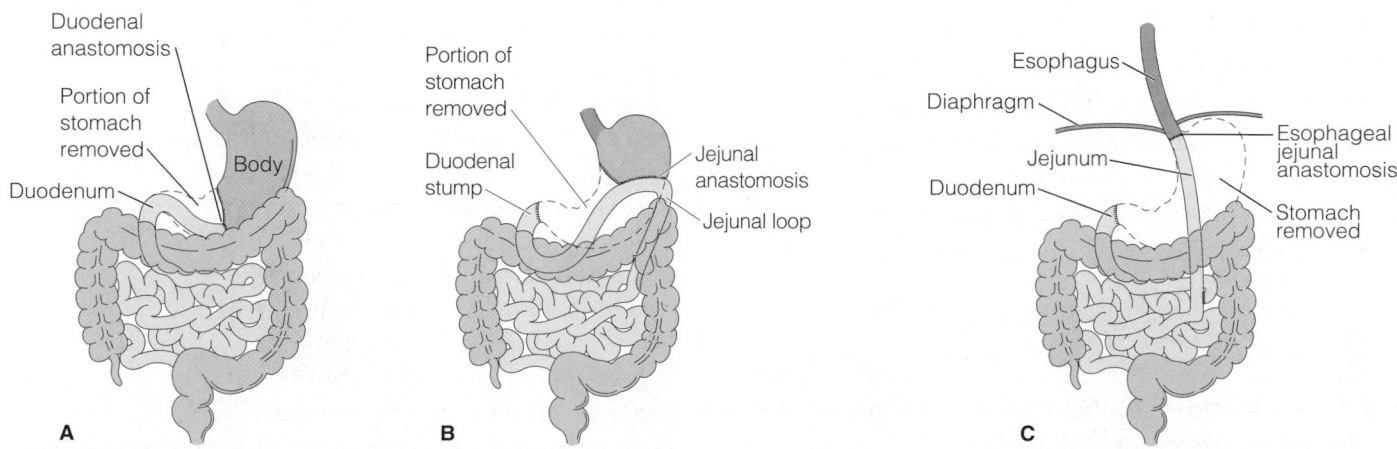

Figure 19-10. ■ Partial and total gastrectomy procedures. (**A**) Partial gastrectomy with anastomosis to the duodenum. (**B**) Partial gastrectomy with anastomosis to the jejunum. (**C**) Total gastrectomy with anastomosis of the esophagus to the jejunum.

Gastric Surgery

Before Surgery

☑ Provide routine preoperative care and teaching (see Chapter 9). ◖◗

After Surgery

☑ Provide routine postoperative care as outlined in Chapter 9. ◖◗

☑ Assess position and patency of NG tube, connecting it to low suction. Unless contraindicated, gently irrigate with sterile normal saline if tube becomes clogged.

☑ Assess color, amount, and odor of gastric drainage, noting any changes, the presence of clots, or bright bleeding. Chart all assessments and notify the charge nurse or physician of clots or bright bleeding.

☑ Monitor bowel sounds and abdominal girth.

☑ Maintain intravenous fluids while nasogastric suction is in place.

☑ Resume oral food and fluids as ordered. Initial feedings are clear liquids, progressing to full liquids and then frequent small feedings of regular foods. Monitor bowel sounds and for abdominal distention frequently during this period.

☑ Begin discharge planning and teaching. Consult with a dietitian for diet instructions and menu planning; reinforce teaching. Teach the client how to recognize and prevent potential postoperative complications, such as infection, dumping syndrome, postprandial hypoglycemia, or pernicious anemia.

Complications of Surgery

Dumping syndrome is the most common problem following a partial gastrectomy. After pyloric resection or bypass, concentrated chyme may enter the small bowel rapidly. Water is pulled from the vascular system into the intestine, decreasing blood volume and dilating the intestine. Early symptoms of dumping syndrome occur within 5 to 30 minutes after eating; they include nausea and possible vomiting, epigastric pain, cramping, **borborygmi** (loud, hyperactive bowel sounds), and diarrhea. Systemic symptoms from decreased blood volume include tachycardia, orthostatic hypotension, dizziness, flushing, and diaphoresis. The rapid entry of undigested carbohydrates into the jejunum stimulates the pancreas to release excess insulin, and the client develops symptoms of hypoglycemia 2 to 3 hours later.

Dumping syndrome is managed primarily by altering dietary intake to delay gastric emptying and allow smaller boluses of undigested food to enter the intestine. Meals are small and more frequent. Liquids and solids are taken at separate times instead of together. Proteins and fats in the diet are increased, because they exit the stomach more slowly than carbohydrates; carbohydrates, especially simple sugars, are reduced. The client is taught to rest in a recumbent or semirecumbent position for 30 to 60 minutes after meals.

After gastric surgery, clients are at risk for nutritional deficiencies because of reduced absorption and inability to eat large meals. Nearly 50% of clients who undergo gastric surgery experience significant weight loss due to insufficient calorie intake.

Other Treatments

Radiation, chemotherapy, or both may be used to reduce the risk of spread of the cancer. For the client with more advanced disease, treatment is palliative and may include surgery and chemotherapy. These clients may require a gastrostomy or jejunostomy feeding tube. Gastrostomy tubes are inserted into the stomach through a stoma in the epigastric region (Figure 19-11 ■). The tube may initially be

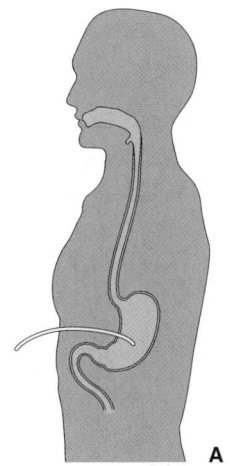

A

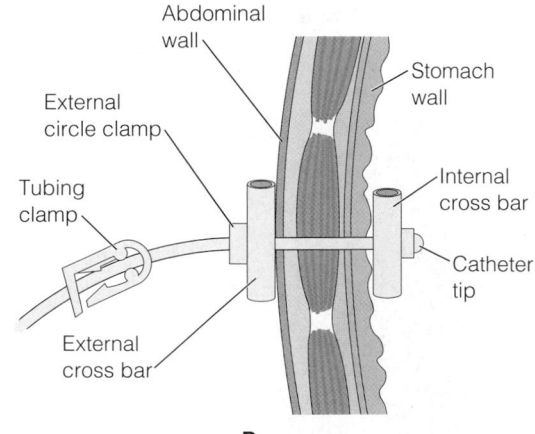

B

Figure 19-11. ■ **(A)** Gastrostomy tube placement. **(B)** The tube is held in place by cross bars.

BOX 19-17	NURSING CARE CHECKLIST

Gastrostomy Tube

Nursing Care

☑ Use Standard Precautions.

☑ Assess tube placement by aspirating stomach contents and checking the pH of aspirate (see Box 19-4 for expected pH readings for the stomach and small intestine).

☑ Inspect skin around the stoma for healing, redness, swelling, and any drainage. If drainage is present, note the color, amount, consistency, and odor. Document findings and report to charge nurse or physician.

☑ Assess the abdomen for distention, bowel sounds, and tenderness; document.

☑ Until the stoma is well healed, use sterile technique for dressing changes and site care. Clean technique is appropriate for use once healing is complete.

☑ Cleanse the site with antiseptic swabs or soap and water. A well-healed stoma site may be cleansed in the shower with the tube clamped or plugged. Allow to air dry. Apply a protective barrier cream as needed.

☑ Redress the wound using a stoma dressing or folded 4 × 4 gauze pads.

☑ Irrigate the tube with 30 to 50 mL of water; clean the tube inside and out as indicated or ordered. A special brush may be used to clean the inside of soft gastric tubes.

☑ Provide mouth care or remind the client to do so.

☑ If the client is to be discharged with a gastrostomy tube, teach the client and family how to care for the tube and administer feedings. Refer to a home health agency or visiting nurse for support and reinforcement of learning.

connected to low suction or plugged. Tube feedings may be restarted shortly after the procedure. Box 19-17 ■ describes nursing care of the client with a gastrostomy tube.

Because gastric cancer is often advanced by the time of diagnosis, the prognosis is poor. The 5-year survival rate of all clients treated for gastric carcinoma is 10%.

NURSING CARE

Nursing and home care for the client with gastric cancer depend on the stage of the disease and the treatment planned. If surgery is performed, provide pre- and postoperative care as outlined in Box 19-17. Imbalanced Nutrition: Less than Body Requirements is a priority nursing diagnosis for clients with gastric cancer because of the effects of the cancer, surgery, and other treatments such as chemotherapy or radiation therapy. Total parenteral nutrition may be necessary to maintain weight and nutrition. Refer to home health services as needed for assistance with dressing changes, tube feedings, or TPN.

Because disease is usually advanced at the time of diagnosis, provide grief counseling and refer the client and family to cancer support groups or hospice services as appropriate.

Note: The bibliography listings for this and all chapters have been compiled at the back of the book.

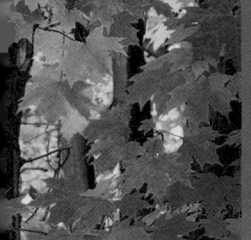

Chapter Review

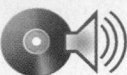 **KEY TERMS** by Topics

Use the audio glossary feature of either the CD-ROM or the Companion Website to hear the correct pronunciation of the following key terms.

Nutritional disorders

obesity (upper body, lower body), malnutrition, catabolism, enteral, total

parenteral nutrition, anexoria nervosa, bulimia nervosa

Disorders of the mouth and esophagus

stomatitis, gastroesophageal reflux, dysphagia

Disorders of the stomach and upper intestinal tract

gastroenteritis, gastritis, hematemesis, melena, peptic ulcer, hematochezia, gastrectomy, anastomosis, borborygmi

KEY Points

- Nutritional disorders such as obesity and malnutrition are major causes of illness and disability. These disorders may be caused by a wide variety of factors, including diseases or their effects, problems of access to adequate food and nutrients, or by eating disorders such as anorexia nervosa. Upper body obesity is associated with a higher risk for cardiovascular disease. Protein-calorie malnutrition (PCM) is now recognized as a major problem in hospitalized clients.

- Tobacco and alcohol use contribute to a number of upper GI disorders, including GERD, oral and esophageal cancers, and peptic ulcer disease. Encourage all clients to stop smoking or using smokeless tobacco and to consume alcohol in moderate amounts if at all to reduce their risk of these disorders.

- Both esophageal and gastric cancer often are diagnosed late in the disease because their symptoms may be vague. Encourage all clients with complaints of dysphagia, a sensation of gastric fullness, or heartburn to seek medical evaluation.

- Gastroenteritis is usually caused by a food- or water-borne pathogen. The symptoms, duration, and treatment of gastroenteritis depend on the organism; however, most cases of gastroenteritis are self-limiting and require no treatment other than supportive care.

- While acute gastritis is generally benign and self-limited, stress gastritis can lead to unexpected gastric hemorrhage. Chronic gastritis, especially when associated with *H. pylori* infection, is a risk factor for gastric cancer.

- *H. pylori* infection also is the primary cause of peptic ulcer disease. Effectively treating the infection can reduce or eliminate the risk of future exacerbations of PUD.

- Promptly report a change in the nature of abdominal pain in a client with PUD, especially if the pain is accompanied by vomiting, guarding of the abdomen, or a change in bowel sounds. These manifestations could indicate an obstruction or perforation into the peritoneal cavity.

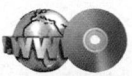 **EXPLORE Media**Link

Additional interactive resources for this chapter can be found on the Companion Website at www.prenhall.com/burke. Click on Chapter 19 and "Begin" to select the activities for this chapter.

For chapter-related NCLEX-style review questions and an audio glossary, access the accompanying CD-ROM in this book.

FOR FURTHER Study

For further information on fluid volume deficit and critical electrolyte values, see Chapter 7.

For more information on care of the surgical client, see Chapter 9.

For nursing responsibilities and client teaching related to antibiotic therapy, see Chapter 10.

For more information about the staging and grading of cancer and cancer treatments, see Chapter 12.

For specific interventions to manage diarrhea, see Chapter 20.

For more information on the liver, gallbladder, and pancreas, see Chapter 21.

See Chapter 23 for information about nursing care of the client with a tracheostomy.

For more information on critical hemoglobin and hematocrit values, see Chapter 30.

For more information on diagnostic tests, see Chapter 25.

Critical Thinking Care Map

Caring for a Client with Altered Nutrition
NCLEX-PN® Focus Area: Prevention and Health Maintenance

Case Study: Sam Elliott has gained 30 pounds since retiring 2 years ago, and now the most active thing he does each day is "walk to the end of the driveway to get the mail." He reports having juice, oatmeal, a muffin, and coffee with cream for breakfast and meeting friends midmorning for doughnuts and coffee. Lunch is usually a bologna-and-cheese sandwich with chips and a root beer. He has cheese, crackers, and wine before a dinner of meat, potatoes, vegetables, and dessert. He tells the nurse, "I have never had to diet. I just don't know how to get this weight off."

Nursing Diagnosis: Imbalanced Nutrition: More than Body Requirements

COLLECT DATA

Subjective	Objective
_____	_____
_____	_____
_____	_____
_____	_____
_____	_____
_____	_____

Would you report this data? Yes/No
If yes, to: _____

Nursing Care

_____
_____
_____
_____
_____
_____
_____
_____
_____
_____
_____

How would you document this? _____
_____
_____
_____

Data Collected
(use those that apply)

- Height 5'10" (178 cm)
- Easily fatigued
- Weight 201 lbs (91.2 kg)
- "Needs to lose weight"
- Shortness of breath with activity
- LDL 180 mg/dL
- BP 138/90
- Fasting blood glucose 103 mg/dL
- Reports feeling hungry most of the time
- Cholesterol 240 mg/dL
- Stool negative for occult blood

Nursing Interventions
(use those that apply; list in priority order)

- Instruct client to lose 30 pounds in 60 days.
- Discuss Food Guide Pyramid.
- Discuss role of exercise in weight loss and control.
- Instruct client to jog 45 minutes a day.
- Suggest food substitutions that will reduce fat intake.
- Provide a list of local support groups and weight-loss programs.
- Instruct client to exercise at least three times a week, gradually increasing time.

NCLEX-PN® Exam Preparation

1 Which of the following would be an expected finding when assessing a client who has central or upper body obesity?

A. weight 190 lbs, height 5'10"
B. serum cholesterol 180 mg/dL
C. waist circumference 38", hip circumference 37"
D. The client's parents are obese.

2 When planning care for a client who has a diagnosis of malnutrition, the nurse would include which of these goals?

A. Will gain 1 to 2 lbs per week.
B. Will consume a 1,500-kcal diet.
C. Will state need to exercise 60 minutes five times per week.
D. Will limit intake of unsaturated fats and whole-grain carbohydrates.

3 When planning care for a client who has stomatitis, the nurse should give priority to which of these treatment measures?

A. Encourage consumption of raw fruits and vegetables.
B. Administer viscous lidocaine prior to each meal.
C. Assess the client's gag reflex.
D. Encourage the client to use a mouthwash after each meal.

4 During the initial assessment, the nurse notes a small, painless, dark-colored lesion on the client's tongue. He states that the sore has been in his mouth for several months. Which of the following interventions should be the next priority?

A. Document findings and notify the health care provider.
B. Tell the client to report any changes in the size or color of the lesion.
C. Prepare the client for a biopsy of the lesion.
D. Immediately notify the charge nurse.

5 The nurse reinforcing teaching for a client with gastroesophageal reflux disease includes which of the following in her instructions? (Choose all that apply.)

A. Avoid lying down for several hours after eating.
B. Use of alcohol and tobacco in moderation is allowed.
C. Stop taking the prescribed proton-pump inhibitor once symptoms are relieved.
D. Raise the head of the bed on 6-inch blocks.
E. Peppermint and chocolate candies can help relieve symptoms.

6 A 58-year-old male is admitted with the diagnosis of esophageal cancer with erosion to the middle portion of the esophagus. Which of the following is most important to immediately report?

A. aspiration pneumonia
B. bright bleeding from the mouth
C. weight loss
D. difficulty swallowing

7 During the insertion of a nasogastric tube, the client begins to gag. The nurse should

A. withdraw the tube completely.
B. briefly halt the insertion.
C. have the client sip water to assist the tube to advance.
D. check for placement.

8 The client is receiving enteral feedings of Ensure (240 mL/can) at a rate of 60 mL/hr. The nurse anticipates that each can of the formula will run for _____ hours.

9 The physician has prescribed an antibiotic for a client with a peptic ulcer. The client asks you why this type of medication is being given. The appropriate response is:

A. "This medication will help reduce the gastric acid in your stomach."
B. "The antibiotic will help to rid the stomach of the *H. pylori* bacteria."
C. "It will increase the production of mucus in the stomach."
D. "It is used only as a prophylactic to prevent colonization of bacteria in the stomach."

10 When developing a teaching plan for a client who has undergone a partial gastrectomy, which of the following would the nurse include related to preventing dumping syndrome?

A. diet low in protein and fats
B. taking a walk before each meal
E. eating three meals a day
D. resting in a semirecumbent position after eating

Answers for Review Questions, as well as discussion of Care Plan and Critical Thinking Care Map questions, appear in Appendix V.

INTEGRATING CULTURAL DIVERSITY IN CLIENT EDUCATION

Judith Lightfoot, a 29-year-old Native American, comes in to see the nurse about her diet for diabetes. While the nurse and Judith are talking, Judith says, "I really can't follow the diabetic diet you gave me. You see, on our Indian reservation everybody shares what we have. We don't have much food at our house, so if I have special food I can't save it for the week. I need to share it with anybody in the house who is hungry. Of course, that means that some days we don't have anything to eat. But things usually work out. It is part of our culture to be generous with what we have and we will worry about tomorrow when the time comes."

When a client is from a different culture, the nurse should be alert for cultural barriers that may interfere with the treatment regimen or effective client education. Initial assessment is necessary to determine whether the client understands the language being spoken. If necessary, an interpreter should be obtained to serve as translator. When interpreters are not available at an agency, a telephone translator service may be an option. In some cases, a bilingual family member can help. Children should be avoided as interpreters, since the child may not be able to translate medical information adequately, and in some cultures getting information from a child is not acceptable (Davidhizar & Brownson, 2000).

Differences in Dialect

It is important for nurses to be aware that there can be significant contrasts within cultural groups. For example, there are 10 Hispanic/Latino groups, more than 20 Asian American/Pacific Islander groups, and more than 500 Native American tribal groups. In addition, census-defined African Americans may come from non-African countries such as Haiti, Jamaica, and Panama. Significant differences in language and dialects within a culture may exist. Thus, even though an interpreter may speak the language of the client—for example, Spanish—communication may not be clear.

Differences in Communication Variables

It is important to assess not only language but also the essential elements of communication of the language including dialect, style (language and social situations), volume (silence), use of touch, context of speech (emotional tone), and kinetics (gesture, stance, and eye behavior). If the nurse always associates a soft voice with timidity, lack of assertiveness, and incompetence, the cultural reasons for this behavior may be ignored. If the nurse always associates loudness with aggressiveness, while in the client's culture loudness has a different meaning, behavior may be misinterpreted.

Even when individuals speak the same language, communication may be difficult. The meaning of words and how facts are presented may vary based on life experiences and cultural context. For example, "That person is a real dog" may have a positive meaning in one cultural setting while having a negative meaning in another.

Differences in Gender and Family Member Roles

Gender and gender roles can significantly influence attitudes about health and health education. Taboos related to sexual behavior have special significance for client education. In male-dominated societies (Arab, Hispanic, and many Asian societies), information and decision making must be given to the male. Women are expected to be modest and submissive. Thus, education about sexual matters needs to take into account who should be present in the room and who is appropriate (Davidhizar & Brownson, 2000).

Literacy/Educational Handouts

Many English-speaking people have difficulty understanding medical terminology. If English is a second language, medical terminology is even more challenging. When written instructions are used, the language, the literacy, and the reading level of the client should be evaluated. Written handouts should match the client's reading level.

Nursing Implications

- *Before teaching, assess the client's understanding of English.* If the nurse and the client do not speak the same language, an interpreter may be necessary in order to provide effective teaching. If the client and family can speak English but either speaks English as a second language or is from another culture, the nurse should be aware that there may be obstacles to communication.

- *Match client education materials to the literacy level of the client.* If a client is from another culture, both literacy level and understanding of medical terminology should be assessed. Select appropriate educational materials that can be understood.

Self-Reflection Questions

1. Are you an effective teacher?

2. If your client cannot understand English, what translating services are available to assist in client teaching?

3. What teaching materials are available that can assist in client education?

Chapter 20

Caring for Clients with Bowel Disorders

BRIEF Outline

Diarrhea
Constipation
Irritable Bowel Syndrome
Fecal Incontinence
Malabsorption
Appendicitis
Peritonitis
Inflammatory Bowel Disease
Colorectal Cancer
Bowel Obstruction
Hernia
Diverticular Disease
Hemorrhoids
Anorectal Lesions

LEARNING Outcomes

After completing this chapter, you will be able to:

- Discuss the pathophysiology, manifestations, and management of bowel absorption and elimination disorders.
- Provide appropriate nursing care and teaching related to measures used to manage bowel disorders.
- Effectively care for the client undergoing intestinal surgery.
- Discuss the care of clients with a colostomy or ileostomy.
- Contribute to assessment, planning, and evaluation of nursing care for clients with disorders of bowel absorption and elimination.

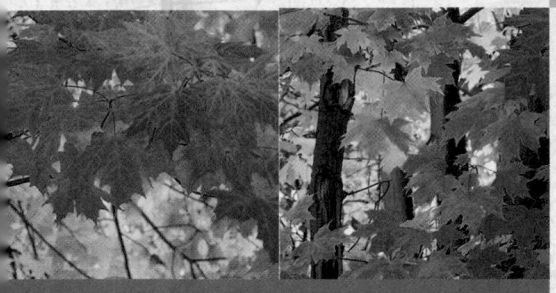

MediaLink

www.prenhall.com/burke
Use the address above to access the free, interactive Companion Website created for this textbook. Get hints, instant feedback, and textbook references to chapter-related NCLEX-style questions. Link to other interesting sites.

Audio Glossary:
Use the Companion Website, or the CD-ROM disk enclosed with your textbook, to hear the pronunciation of key terms in this chapter.

Inflammation, obstructions, disorders of absorption, or changes in structure can alter bowel elimination. Some disorders can severely impair the client's health, cause intense pain, or require surgical intervention. Nursing care focuses on meeting the client's physiologic needs, providing emotional support, and teaching about lifestyle changes.

DISORDERS OF INTESTINAL MOTILITY AND ABSORPTION

"Normal" patterns of defecation vary widely, from two to three stools per day to as few as three stools per week. Few body functions respond as readily to both internal and external factors as the process of defecation. Factors such as food and bacteria directly affect the GI tract and the number and consistency of stools. Indirect factors (psychologic stress or voluntary postponement of defecation) also affect elimination patterns.

Diarrhea

Diarrhea is an increase in the frequency, volume, and water content of stool. Diarrhea is a symptom, not a primary disorder. Causes of diarrhea include bacterial toxins, infections, malabsorption syndromes, medications, systemic diseases, and psychogenic factors (e.g., pretest diarrhea).

PATHOPHYSIOLOGY
Diarrhea can result either from impaired water absorption or from increased water secretion into the bowel. Impaired water absorption occurs when the rate of peristalsis increases, or when the absorptive surface of the bowel decreases. Increased water secretion into the bowel may occur by osmosis, from infection (e.g., cholera, *Escherichia coli*), from unabsorbed fat, and from some drugs. Inflammatory disorders cause plasma, blood, and mucus to accumulate in the bowel.

MANIFESTATIONS AND COMPLICATIONS
Clients with diarrhea may have several large, watery stools per day or very frequent small stools containing blood, mucus, or pus. The manifestations depend on the cause, duration, and severity of the diarrhea, as well as the area of bowel affected.

clinical ALERT

Immediately report bloody diarrhea to the charge nurse or physician because it may indicate bleeding or hemorrhage in the gastrointestinal tract. GI bleeding can lead to significant blood loss and hypovolemic shock.

Diarrhea can have devastating results because water and electrolytes are lost in the stool. Clients, particularly very young or older, debilitated clients, can become dehydrated. Hypovolemic shock may occur with rapid fluid losses. Potassium, magnesium, and bicarbonate loss may lead to electrolyte deficiencies and metabolic acidosis. (See Chapter 7 ⬤ for further discussion of the effects of these imbalances.)

INTERDISCIPLINARY CARE
Care of the client with diarrhea focuses on identifying and treating the underlying cause. The diarrhea itself may need to be treated for client comfort and to prevent complications.

Diagnostic Tests
■ A *stool specimen* may be ordered to look for blood, pus, mucus, or excess fat (*steatorrhea*). Microscopic examination is done to identify blood cells and parasites. Because parasites may not be in the stool at all times, a series of three stool specimens, spaced 2 to 3 days apart, is obtained when parasitic infection is suspected.
■ *Stool culture* is ordered when an infection is suspected.
■ Blood is drawn to assess for fluid, electrolyte, and acid–base imbalances.
■ A *sigmoidoscopy* is done to allow direct examination of the bowel mucosa. The preparation and teaching for a client undergoing sigmoidoscopy are outlined in Box 20-1 ■.

Dietary Management
Fluid replacement is most important for clients with diarrhea. If the client is able to take oral fluids, a glucose-balanced electrolyte solution is used (e.g., Pedialyte, Gatorade). Solid food is withheld during the first 24 hours of acute diarrhea to provide bowel rest. Then frequent, small meals can be added. Milk and milk products are added last. Raw fruits and vegetables, fried foods, bran, whole-grain cereals, condiments, spices, coffee, and alcoholic beverages are avoided during recovery. Clients with chronic diarrhea may need to eliminate certain foods and nonfood substances that can aggravate diarrhea (Table 20-1 ■). These clients need a diet that is high in calories and nutritional value. Vitamin supplements may be necessary, particularly the fat-soluble vitamins (A, D, E, and K). Parenteral nutrition (see Chapter 19 ⬤) may be required. A balanced electrolyte intravenous solution may be required to replace fluid losses.

Medications
Antidiarrheal medications may not be used until the cause of diarrhea has been identified, because they could worsen or prolong the disease. Opium derivatives and absorbents

BOX 20-1	NURSING CARE CHECKLIST

Sigmoidoscopy

Before the Procedure

☑ Verify a signed informed consent for the procedure has been obtained.

☑ Withhold food and fluids as ordered. Clear liquids may be allowed.

☑ Administer enemas or rectal suppositories as ordered.

Client and Family Teaching

Before the Procedure

☑ The procedure takes approximately 15 minutes.

☑ You may be positioned in the knee–chest position or on the left side.

☑ Breathe deeply and slowly as the scope is inserted and advanced.

☑ Air may be injected into the bowel to improve visualization.

☑ Specimens of stool or tissue may be obtained during the procedure.

After the Procedure

☑ Report any abdominal pain, fever, chills, or rectal bleeding.

☑ If a polyp is removed, avoid heavy lifting for 7 days, and avoid high-fiber foods for 1 to 2 days.

TABLE 20-1	
Foods That May Aggravate Chronic Diarrhea	
FOODS	REASON
Milk, ice cream, yogurt, soft cheeses, cottage cheese	Contain lactose, which requires the enzyme lactase to digest; lactase deficiency common
Apple juice, pear juice, grapes, honey, dates, nuts, figs, fruit-flavored soft drinks	Contain fructose, which can draw fluid into the bowel when consumed in large quantities
Table sugar	Contains sucrose, which requires the enzyme sucrase to digest
Apple juice, pear juice, sugarless gums and mints	May contain sorbitol, a sugar that is not absorbed and can pull fluid into intestine
Antacids	Magnesium-containing antacids increase peristalsis and can draw fluid into the bowel
Coffee, tea, cola drinks, over-the-counter analgesics	Contain caffeine, which can increase peristalsis

such as Pepto-Bismol are commonly used to treat acute diarrhea (Table 20-2 ■). Opium derivatives also may be used with caution for clients with chronic diarrhea. A potassium supplement may also be prescribed.

NURSING CARE

Nursing care of the client with diarrhea is directed toward identifying the cause, relieving the symptoms, preventing complications, and, if the cause is infectious, preventing the spread of infection to others.

ASSESSING

The client's history and physical examination often provide enough information to identify the cause of diarrhea. Box 20-2 ■ provides assessment data to collect from clients with complaints of diarrhea.

DIAGNOSING, PLANNING, AND IMPLEMENTING

Priorities in Nursing Care. While the diarrhea itself is a priority nursing care focus, the effects of the diarrhea on fluid balance and skin integrity also are of importance in planning and implementing nursing care.

Diarrhea

■ Monitor and record the frequency and characteristics of bowel movements. *This provides a measure of the effectiveness of treatment.*

■ Measure abdominal girth and auscultate bowel sounds every shift as indicated. *These indicate the effectiveness and possible complications of treatment such as constipation.*

■ Administer antidiarrheal medications as prescribed. *These medications promote comfort and prevent excess fluid loss.*

■ Limit food intake for acute diarrhea, slowly reintroducing solid foods in small amounts. *Limiting food allows the bowel to rest and lets the mucosa heal.*

Risk for Deficient Fluid Volume

■ Record intake and output; weigh daily; assess skin turgor, mucous membranes, and urine specific gravity every 8 hours. *These assessments help monitor fluid volume status.*

■ Monitor vital signs, including orthostatic vitals, every 4 to 8 hours. *A drop in blood pressure of more than 10 mm Hg on moving from lying to sitting or from sitting to standing indicates orthostatic hypotension and possible fluid volume deficit. The pulse rate typically increases as well.*

TABLE 20-2

Nursing Implications for Pharmacology: Antidiarrheal Medications

AGENT/DRUGS	PURPOSE	NURSING IMPLICATIONS	CLIENT TEACHING
Absorbants and Protectants ■ Kaolin and pectin (Kaopectate) ■ Charcoal ■ Bismuth subsalicylate (Pepto-Bismol)	Absorbant preparations act in the intestines to bind substances that can cause diarrhea. They are safe drugs that are generally available over the counter. Bismuth sub-salicylate is used to prevent and treat traveler's diarrhea because it has an antimicrobial effect as well.	Assess for contraindications, such as chronic inflammatory bowel disease. If fever is present, check with physician before giving the drug. Give at least 1 hour before or 2 hours after other oral medications; they may interfere with the absorption of other drugs. Observe for potential constipation while using these drugs.	Take at the onset of diarrhea and after each loose stool. Do not use any of these drugs for more than 48 hours. If diarrhea persists, contact your doctor. Chew bismuth tablets, rather than swallowing them whole, for maximal effectiveness. This medication may cause the tongue and stool to darken. If you are allergic to aspirin, do not use bismuth subsalicylate; avoid taking aspirin while taking bismuth subsalicylate.
Opium and Opium Derivatives ■ Camphorated tincture of opium (paregoric) ■ Tincture of opium (laudanum, opium tincture) ■ Difenoxin (Motofen) ■ Diphenoxylate (Lomotil, Logen, others) ■ Loperamide hydrochloride (Imodium)	Opium and related drugs act on the CNS to slow peristalsis and allow more water absorption. They also decrease the sensation of a full rectum and increase anal sphincter tone. Paregoric and tincture of opium are controlled prescription drugs. Opium derivatives have few narcotic or abuse-promoting effects and are more commonly used.	Assess for contraindications and drug interactions prior to giving these drugs. Administer paregoric undiluted with water. Observe for increased effects of other CNS depressants, such as alcohol, narcotic analgesics, or barbiturate sedatives. Report abdominal distention to the charge nurse or physician.	Take as recommended at the onset of diarrhea and after each loose stool. These drugs may be habit forming; use for no more than 48 hours. Avoid using alcohol and over-the-counter cold preparations while taking these drugs. These drugs may cause drowsiness; avoid driving or operating machinery while taking them.
Synthetic Hormone ■ Octreotide acetate (Sandostatin)	Octreotide stimulates fluid and electrolyte absorption from the GI tract and slows intestinal motility. It is primarily used to treat chronic diarrhea associated with certain tumors and HIV disease.	Do not use solution if it is discolored or has particulates. Administer room temperature solution slowly by SC injection. Refrigerate vials for long-term storage; use room temperature solution within 24 hours.	Rotate injection sites, using the hips, thighs, or abdomen. Administer between meals and at bedtime to minimize nausea and diarrhea. Do not use this medication if you are pregnant.

■ Remind the client to ask for help when getting up. *The client with orthostatic hypotension may become dizzy or light-headed on rising.*

■ Provide fluid and electrolyte replacement solutions as indicated. Ensure ready access to fluids. Assist the debilitated client with fluid intake. *If tolerated, oral fluids are encouraged to prevent dehydration. Fluids may be replaced intravenously if necessary. A fluid intake of 3,000 mL or more per day may be necessary to replace losses.*

Risk for Impaired Skin Integrity

■ Provide good skin care. Frequently reposition, and protect pressure areas. *Poorly hydrated skin is at increased risk for breakdown.*

■ Assist with perianal cleaning as needed. Use warm water and soft cloths. Apply protective ointment. *These measures help prevent tissue irritation, trauma, and breakdown.*

BOX 20-2	ASSESSMENT

Assessing Clients with Diarrhea

SUBJECTIVE DATA

- Frequency, character, and timing (day or night, relationship to meals) of stools.
- Onset and duration of diarrhea; any related events such as recent travel, changes in diet, possible exposure to contaminated food or water.
- Abdominal or rectal pain or cramping, associated nausea, vomiting, or anorexia.
- Chronic conditions such as inflammatory bowel disease, diabetes, or other chronic diseases.
- Current medications, including any used to relieve diarrhea.

OBJECTIVE DATA

- Vital signs, including orthostatic vitals (blood pressure and pulse) and strength of peripheral pulses.
- General appearance, nutritional status, apparent distress.
- Inspect mucous membranes for color, moisture; assess skin color, temperature, moisture, and turgor.
- Observe for abdominal distention or scaphoid (concave, hollowed) appearance; auscultate bowel sounds; lightly palpate for tenderness.
- Inspect feces for color, consistency, presence of blood, mucus, pus, or steatorrhea (bulky, foul-smelling stool).

LABORATORY TESTS

- Complete blood count (CBC), including white blood cells (WBC), hemoglobin, and hematocrit.
- Serum electrolytes, osmolality, and acid–base balance.
- Stool analysis results.

EVALUATING

To evaluate the effectiveness of nursing interventions for clients with diarrhea, collect data related to stool frequency, nutritional status, weight, fluid volume status, and skin integrity. Monitor laboratory results, particularly serum electrolytes and serum osmolality, and acid–base balance, on a continuing basis.

Documenting. Document the number and characteristics of stools, complaints of abdominal pain or cramping, physical assessment data, and treatment measures initiated throughout the client's care. Note compliance with fluid and dietary intake recommendations. Document teaching provided and reinforced, as well as the client's (and, as appropriate, the family's) understanding of information presented.

CONTINUING CARE

Teach about the causes of diarrhea and preventive measures such as food and water safety. Discuss measures to prevent the spread of bacteria, especially good hand washing after every bowel movement. Stress the importance of seeking medical intervention if diarrhea continues or is severe or prolonged. Instruct clients planning travel outside the United States or to wilderness areas on how to purify water for drinking and cooking.

Discuss the importance of maintaining fluid intake to replace lost water and electrolytes. Encourage use of Gatorade or a similar product rather than water for fluid replacement. A solution of 1 quart (1 L) of water, 1 teaspoon (5 mL) each of table salt and baking soda, 4 teaspoons (20 mL) of granulated sugar, and desired flavoring (such as lemon extract or juice) can be made at home to replace water and electrolytes.

Explain that food intake is not vital or recommended during episodes of acute diarrhea. If an antidiarrheal drug is used, review its precautions and limitations. For the client with chronic diarrhea, provide information on foods to avoid (see Table 20-1) and foods to include to maintain adequate nutritional status.

Constipation

Constipation is defined as infrequent or difficult passage of stools. Clients may complain of constipation when they have less than one stool per day, even if feces are of normal consistency and are not difficult to expel. The term *constipation* is appropriate only when the client has two or fewer bowel movements weekly, or when defecation is excessively difficult or requires straining.

Constipation affects older adults more often than younger people. Although intestinal transit times slow somewhat with aging, more significant factors include general health, diet, medications, and activity levels (Box 20-3 ■).

PATHOPHYSIOLOGY AND MANIFESTATIONS

Acute constipation may be due to an organic cause such as a tumor or partial bowel obstruction. Lifestyle and psychogenic factors (such as ignoring the urge to defecate or feeling the need to defecate on schedule) are the most frequent causes of chronic constipation. In older adults, habitual use of laxatives can lead to constipation when laxatives are withdrawn. Other common causes of constipation are listed in Table 20-3 ■. The client with significant constipation may develop a *fecal impaction* (hardened stool). Small amounts of watery mucus or liquid stool may pass around the impaction. The client has a full sensation in the rectal area and abdominal cramping.

INTERDISCIPLINARY CARE

On examination, the abdomen may appear distended, and bowel sounds may be reduced. Digital examination of the rectum in the client with an impaction reveals a palpable hard or putty-like fecal mass. Simple or chronic constipation is best treated with education and modification of diet and exercise routines.

BOX 20-3   FOCUS ON OLDER ADULTS

Constipation in the Older Adult

Slowed peristalsis, decreased activity levels, reduced food and fluid intake, and decreased sensory perception contribute to a higher incidence of constipation in the older adult. Chronic diseases, mobility problems, and medications also increase their risk of constipation.

Because cultural influences and advertising lead many older adults to believe that a daily bowel movement is important for health, the older adult may come to rely on laxatives, suppositories, or enemas to facilitate movement of soft stool every 2 to 3 days.

When assessing the older adult, focus on bowel patterns and factors contributing to actual or perceived constipation. Ask about normal elimination patterns (frequency, timing, size, and consistency). Assess dietary patterns, including types and amounts of foods and fluids normally consumed. Evaluate medications (including over-the-counter) for their effects on elimination. Discuss daily activity patterns and the ability to respond to the urge to defecate.

Teach about normal bowel patterns and expected changes that occur with aging. Discuss the following preventive measures:

- Increase dietary fiber intake to provide bulk and keep stools soft and easy to expel. Fresh fruits and vegetables, whole grains, high-fiber breakfast cereals, and unprocessed bran added to other foods are good sources of dietary fiber.

- Drink 6 to 8 glasses of water per day (unless contraindicated). Drinking a cup of warm water after breakfast may help stimulate the urge to defecate.

- Remain physically active to promote bowel function and maintain muscle tone. Good abdominal muscle tone helps expel feces.

- Respond to the urge to defecate when it is felt. Delaying defecation may contribute to constipation.

- Do not use laxatives, suppositories, or enemas on a regular basis. Only bulk-forming agents (FiberCon, Citrucel, or Metamucil) are safe for long-term use. It is important to drink at least 6 to 8 glasses of water daily when using any laxative.

- Report to your primary care provider any change in bowel habits such as constipation or diarrhea; abdominal pain, black or bloody stools; nausea or anorexia, weakness, or unexplained weight loss.

Diagnostic Tests

If constipation is acute or does not resolve, diagnostic studies such as *serum electrolytes* and *thyroid function tests* may be ordered. A *barium enema* or *flexible colonoscopy* may be done to identify structural lesions of the colon. (See Chapter 18 ⊙⊙ for more information about diagnostic tests used to identify bowel problems and the section on colon cancer later in this chapter for nursing care related to a colonoscopy.) Nursing care for clients having a barium enema is outlined in Box 20-4 ■. Table 20-4 ■ provides nursing implications for commonly prescribed bowel preparations used to cleanse the bowel before colonoscopy or barium enema.

TABLE 20-3

Common Causes of Constipation

FACTOR	RELATED CAUSE
Activity	Lack of exercise; impaired mobility; bed rest
Dietary	Highly refined, low-fiber foods; inadequate fluid intake
Drugs	Antacids containing aluminum or calcium salts; narcotic analgesics; many antidepressants, tranquilizers, and sedatives; antihypertensives; iron salts
Large bowel	Diverticular disease, inflammatory disease, tumor, obstruction; changes in rectal or anal structure or function
Systemic	Advanced age; pregnancy; neurologic conditions (such as stroke); endocrine and metabolic disorders (such as hypothyroidism)
Psychogenic	Voluntary suppression of urge; perceived need to defecate on schedule; depression
Other	Chronic laxative or enema use

Dietary Management

Foods that have a high fiber content are recommended. Review Box 20-3 for recommended foods and strategies.

clinical ALERT

Bulk-forming agents, such as methylcellulose, are the only safe laxatives for long-term use. They increase the bulk of the feces and draw water into the bowel to soften it. At least 6 to 8 glasses of water should be consumed daily when using these (or any) laxatives.

Medications

Laxatives and cathartics were among the earliest drugs. Milder preparations are generally known as *laxatives; cathartics* have a stronger effect. Most laxatives are appropriate only for short-term use. Cathartics and enemas interfere with normal bowel reflexes and should not be used for simple constipation. Commonly ordered laxatives are listed in Table 20-4.

clinical ALERT

Laxatives should *never* be given if a bowel obstruction or impaction is suspected, nor to people with abdominal pain of unknown cause. Administering laxatives or cathartics when the bowel is obstructed may damage the bowel and lead to perforation.

BOX 20-4	NURSING CARE CHECKLIST

Barium Enema

Before the Procedure

☑ Verify signed consent for the procedure has been obtained.

☑ Withhold food and fluids as ordered (usually liquids only the day before and NPO for 8 hours before the procedure).

☑ Administer laxatives, enemas, or suppositories as ordered the evening before and morning of the procedure.

Client and Family Teaching

Before the Procedure

☑ Do not eat or drink anything for 8 hours before the exam.

☑ The procedure takes approximately 1 hour.

☑ You will be asked to turn to different positions during this procedure.

☑ You will feel a full sensation and the urge to defecate as the barium is instilled.

☑ The bowel will be examined as it fills with barium, and x-rays will be taken.

☑ You will expel the barium in the bathroom.

After the Procedure

☑ You will be given a laxative to help expel the barium.

☑ Your stools may be white for the next 1 to 2 days.

Enemas

Significant or chronic constipation or a fecal impaction may require the administration of an enema. They may also be prescribed to prepare the bowel for diagnostic testing or examination. They are never used when there may be obstruction or risk of perforation. The following types of enemas may be prescribed:

- A *saline enema* using 500 to 2,000 mL of warmed normal saline solution is the least irritating to the bowel.
- *Tap-water enemas* use 500 to 1,000 mL of water to soften feces and irritate the bowel mucosa, stimulating peristalsis and evacuation.
- *Soap-suds enemas* consist of a tap-water solution to which soap is added as a further irritant.
- *Phosphate enemas* (e.g., Fleet) use a hypertonic saline solution to draw fluid into the bowel and irritate the mucosa, leading to evacuation.
- *Oil-retention enemas* instill mineral or vegetable oil into the bowel to soften the fecal mass. The instilled oil is retained overnight or for several hours before evacuation.

Excess enema use, especially of tap-water or phosphate enemas, can impair bowel function and cause fluid and electrolyte imbalances.

TABLE 20-4

Nursing Implications for Pharmacology: Cathartics and Laxatives

AGENT/DRUGS	PURPOSE	NURSING IMPLICATIONS	CLIENT TEACHING
Bowel Preparation Cathartics **Magnesium Citrate** ■ Citrate of magnesia ■ Citro-Nesia ■ Citroma **Polyethylene Glycol and Electrolytes** ■ Colyte ■ GoLYTELY ■ X-Prep	These laxatives often are used as bowel preparation prior to colon x-ray studies or colonoscopy. They promote bowel evacuation by drawing fluid into the bowel. As fluid accumulates, it distends the colon and stimulates peristalsis, causing diarrhea, which rapidly cleans the bowel. Electrolytes may be added to the solution to minimize electrolyte imbalance with their use.	Chill the solution to enhance palatability. Administer in early evening to reduce sleep disturbance. Evacuation begins within 1 hour and continues until stool is clear and free of solid mater. *Magnesium Citrate* ■ Administer on an empty stomach followed by a full glass of water. *Polyethylene Glycol* ■ Administer 8 ounces of solution every 10 minutes.	Expect some degree of abdominal cramping. Do not eat solid food 3 to 4 hours prior, nor within 2 hours of, ingesting polyethylene glycol solution. Do not use this medication for routine treatment of constipation.
Laxatives **Bulk-Forming Agents** ■ Bran ■ Calcium polycarbophil (FiberCon) ■ Methylcellulose (Citrucel)	Bulk-forming agents contain indigestible vegetable fiber. This natural fiber creates bulk and draws water into the intestine, softening the stool mass.	Mix the agent with a full glass of cool liquid just prior to administering. Do not administer to clients with possible impaction or bowel obstruction.	These agents may be mixed with water, milk, or fruit juice. Take in the morning or with meals. To reduce the risk of impaction, do not take at bedtime.

TABLE 20-4

Nursing Implications for Pharmacology: Cathartics and Laxatives (continued)

AGENT/DRUGS	PURPOSE	NURSING IMPLICATIONS	CLIENT TEACHING
■ Psyllium hydrophilic mucil-loid (Metamucil, Effer-Syllium)			With these and all laxatives, drink at least 6 to 8 glasses of water daily.
Stool Softeners ■ Docusate (Colace, Surfak, Doxidan, others)	Stool softeners draw water into the stool and form an emulsion of fat and water, softening the stool. They are used to prevent straining and reduce the discomfort of expelling hard stools.	Administer with ample fluids. Stool softeners may affect drug absorption. Do not give within 1 hour of other oral medications. Do not crush or open caplets; a liquid form is available for clients who have difficulty swallowing.	Do not use for longer than 1 week. Take in the morning or evening; avoid taking it at the same time as other medications.
Osmotic and Saline Laxative/Cathartics ■ Lactulose (Cholac, Heptalac, others) ■ Sorbitol ■ Magnesium hydroxide (Milk of Magnesia) ■ Magnesium citrate ■ Polyethylene glycol (Klean-Prep)	These laxatives contain poorly absorbed salts or carbohydrates that draw water into the intestine to increase stool volume, decrease its consistency, and stimulate peristalsis. These drugs also may stimulate peristalsis by irritating the bowel mucosa. They are used to relieve acute constipation and should be limited to acute, short-term use; chronic use may suppress normal bowel reflexes.	Assess for contraindications, such as bowel obstruction, fluid or electrolyte imbalances, heart failure, or renal failure. Administer with a full glass of liquid, preferably in the morning to avoid sleep disturbance. Monitor fluid and electrolyte status; skin turgor; mucous membranes; intake and output; daily weight; and serum electrolytes.	Do not use these drugs on a regular basis to treat or prevent constipation. Notify your doctor if you develop abdominal pain, bloody stool, excessive skin or mucous membrane dryness, rapid weight loss, dizziness, or other unusual symptoms. These agents work in 3 to 6 hours; take them in the morning to avoid sleep disturbance.
Irritant or Stimulant Laxatives ■ Bisacodyl (Dulcolax, Bisco-Lax, Carter's Liver Pills, Theralax, others) ■ Phenolphthalein (Evac-U-Gen, Evac-U-Lax, Feen-A-Mint, Phenolax, others) ■ Cascara sagrada ■ Senna (Senna laxative, Fletcher's Castoria) ■ Castor oil	These laxatives stimulate intestinal motility and secretions. They cause watery stool, often accompanied by abdominal cramping and pain. They are used as a secondary measure to relieve constipation and for bowel preparation prior to diagnostic testing.	Assess for contraindications such as abdominal pain and cramping, nausea and vomiting, anal or rectal fissures. Food may affect absorption; give on an empty stomach. Do not crush enteric-coated bisacodyl tablets. This may hasten their dissolution in the stomach, leading to gastric distress.	Do not use this type of laxative, even in over-the-counter preparations, for initial treatment of constipation. Do not use for more than 1 week because these drugs can be habit forming. Do not use if you are pregnant or lactating. Laxatives that contain phenolphthalein may turn urine pink or red. Stop taking the drug and contact your doctor if you develop difficulty breathing, dizziness or light-headedness, or a rash.
Lubricants ■ Mineral oil	Mineral oil forms an oily coat on feces, preventing water reabsorption, and softening stool. Mineral oil reduces absorption of the fat-soluble vitamins A, D, E, and K and may damage the liver and spleen; pneumonia may develop from aspiration of oil droplets into the lungs.	Do not give with wetting agents or stool softeners, because these may increase systemic absorption and the effects of the mineral oil. Administer in the evening before bedtime to reduce the effect on vitamin absorption and minimize the risk of aspiration. Assess the manifestations of vitamin deficiency.	Long-term use of mineral oil is not recommended. Do not use mineral oil if you have hemorrhoids or rectal lesions; oil leakage may cause itching and interfere with healing. Suck on a lemon or orange slice after taking mineral oil to reduce the oily aftertaste.

NURSING CARE

In many cases, nursing care measures can relieve constipation and help prevent it from recurring.

Constipation

- Assess and document pattern of defecation, including time of day, amount, and stool consistency. *Information about bowel habits helps identify physiologic versus perceived constipation. Whether real or perceived, constipation disrupts daily activities and life satisfaction.*
- Assess diet, fluid intake, and activity. Evaluate for other contributing factors, such as use of narcotic analgesics, prescribed bed rest, painful hemorrhoids, and perianal surgery. *These provide clues about possible causes of constipation. The client may require a bulk laxative or stool softener while contributing factors are present.*
- Assess abdominal shape and girth, bowel sounds, and tenderness. If impaction is suspected, examine the rectum digitally, using a lubricated, gloved finger. *Constipation may cause abdominal distention, reduced bowel sounds, and some abdominal tenderness. Digital removal of stool impacted in the rectum may be required.*
- Provide additional fluids to maintain an intake of at least 2,500 mL per day. *Adequate hydration facilitates normal bowel elimination.*
- Encourage drinking of a glass of warm water before and after breakfast. Provide time and privacy following breakfast for bowel elimination. *Warm water provides mild stimulation of bowel peristalsis. Privacy helps encourage a pattern of natural elimination.*
- Consult with the dietitian to increase dietary fiber (unless contraindicated). Provide foods such as natural bran, prunes, or prune juice. *Natural fiber adds bulk to the stool and has a mild stimulant effect.*
- Encourage activity. *Activity stimulates peristalsis and strengthens abdominal muscles, facilitating elimination.*
- If indicated, obtain an order for a stool softener, laxative, or enema. *Pharmacologic agents may be necessary to relieve acute constipation. Clients with restricted mobility or diet restrictions may need a bulk-forming laxative to prevent constipation.*

CONTINUING CARE

Education is key, because the measures to relieve constipation are often the same as those to prevent it. Discuss the importance of maintaining a diet high in natural fiber, including foods such as fresh fruits, vegetables, whole-grain products, and bran. Encourage reduced consumption of meats and refined foods, which are low in fiber and can be constipating. Stress the need to maintain a high fluid intake, particularly when hot weather or exercise increases fluid loss. Discuss the relationship between exercise and bowel regularity. Encourage the client to engage in some form of exercise, such as walking, daily.

Provide information about the range of normal bowel habits. Encourage the client to respond to the urge to defecate when it occurs. Suggest setting aside a time, usually following a meal, for elimination. Discuss restricting the use of laxatives and enemas, and stress that bulk-forming laxatives are the only safe preparations for long-term use. Teach the client that straining to have a bowel movement can lead to hemorrhoids and tissue damage. Suggest abdominal massage to reduce discomfort and promote elimination.

Irritable Bowel Syndrome

Irritable bowel syndrome (IBS) is a motility disorder characterized by alternating periods of constipation and diarrhea. It affects up to 20% of people in Western civilization.

PATHOPHYSIOLOGY AND MANIFESTATIONS

Central nervous system (CNS) regulation of the motor and sensory functions of the bowel is altered in IBS. Intestinal motility can be affected by eating, stress, hormones, and drugs. Motility of both the small and large intestine increases in response to stimulation by food intake, hormones, and physiologic and psychologic stress in clients with IBS. In addition, sensory responses to the movement of chyme through the bowel are exaggerated. Excess mucus may be secreted in the colon as well.

Stress may increase the manifestations of irritable bowel syndrome but does not cause them. The client with IBS may experience a change in the frequency or consistency of stools, straining, urgency, or a sensation of incomplete evacuation. Other manifestations of the disorder are listed in Box 20-5 ■.

BOX 20-5

MANIFESTATIONS OF IRRITABLE BOWEL SYNDROME

- Abdominal pain and tenderness:
  - Often in right lower quadrant
  - Intermittent and colicky or dull and continuous
  - May be relieved by defecation
- Alternating constipation and diarrhea; stool may contain mucus
- Abdominal bloating and flatulence
- Possible nausea, vomiting

INTERDISCIPLINARY CARE

The diagnosis of irritable bowel syndrome is based on the client's history, the pattern of symptoms and elimination, and physical examination.

Diagnostic Tests

A *stool specimen* is examined for occult blood, WBCs, and ova and parasites (to rule out infectious causes). *Sigmoidoscopy* or *colonoscopy* may be done to visually examine the bowel mucosa and measure pressures within the large bowel. See Chapter 18 and Boxes 20-1 and 20-16 for nursing implications and care of clients undergoing these procedures.

A *small-bowel series* (also known as an upper GI series with small-bowel follow-through) and barium enema may be ordered. For the small-bowel series, the client is given an oral barium preparation, and the small intestine is examined under fluoroscopy. The entire GI tract may demonstrate increased motility. Box 20-6 ■ outlines nursing care of the client undergoing a small-bowel series.

Treatment

Management is directed toward relieving the symptoms and reducing or eliminating precipitating factors. Stress reduction, exercises, or counseling may benefit the client. Regular use of bulk-forming laxatives can help reduce bowel spasm and reestablish a normal pattern of elimination. Antidepressant medications, particularly selective serotonin reuptake inhibitors such as sertraline (Zoloft) and fluoxetine (Prozac), may help relieve abdominal pain and spasm.

Although no specific diet is recommended, reduced milk intake may benefit some clients. Restricting gas-forming foods, fruits and berries, or caffeinated drinks may also be helpful. Some clients benefit from limiting their intake of sugars such as lactose (milk sugar), fructose (fruit sugar), or sorbitol (see Table 20-1). Addition of dietary fiber reduces the incidence of both loose diarrheal stools and hard, constipated stools.

NURSING CARE

When clients with irritable bowel syndrome are seen in the acute care setting, the disorder usually is a secondary condition. The previous sections on diarrhea and constipation provide selected nursing interventions for clients experiencing these manifestations.

When teaching, emphasize that the symptoms are real, believed, and not "all in the mind." Discuss related factors, such as stress, anxiety, and depression. Assist the client to explore any relationship between mental stress and bowel manifestations. Teach stress- and anxiety-reduction techniques, such as exercise and progressive relaxation. Refer to a counselor for assistance in dealing with psychologic factors.

Help identify possible dietary influences on elimination patterns, and suggest changes such as increased water and fiber intake that may help relieve symptoms. Encourage changes in exercise and dietary patterns and use of stress-reduction techniques to gradually eliminate the need for prescribed medications.

Stress the importance of notifying the primary care provider if symptoms change, because the manifestations of irritable bowel syndrome may mask symptoms of an organic problem, such as a tumor.

Fecal Incontinence

Fecal incontinence, the loss of voluntary control of defecation, is an infrequent but distressing problem. Clients often do not reveal this problem when discussing health concerns. Physiologic and psychologic factors, as well as age-related changes, can contribute to fecal incontinence (Box 20-7 ■). Factors that interfere with either sensory or motor control of the rectum and anal sphincters (e.g., spinal cord injury or disease) are the most common causes. Relaxation of pelvic floor muscles can make it difficult to retain stool when the defecation reflex occurs.

INTERDISCIPLINARY CARE

Management of fecal incontinence is directed at its cause. Medications to relieve diarrhea or constipation may be ordered.

BOX 20-6	NURSING CARE CHECKLIST

Small-Bowel Series

Before the Procedure

☑ A low-residue diet may be ordered for 48 hours before the study; a tap-water enema or cathartic may be administered the evening before.

☑ Instruct to avoid food, fluids, and smoking for at least 8 hours before the examination.

☑ Withhold medications affecting bowel motility for 24 hours before study unless prescribed.

Client and Family Teaching

☑ The test requires several hours to complete. Bring reading material or other materials to occupy time.

☑ The barium is instilled through a weighted tube inserted into the small bowel.

☑ Increase your fluid intake for at least 24 hours after the procedure to facilitate evacuation of the barium. A laxative may be prescribed.

☑ Stool will be chalky white for up to 72 hours after the exam. Normal stool color will return on complete evacuation of barium.

SELECTED CAUSES OF FECAL INCONTINENCE
- Diarrhea
- Stool impaction
- Pelvic floor relaxation or loss of sphincter tone
- Tumors
- Local trauma (obstetric tears, anorectal injury, or surgery)
- Spinal cord injury, head injury, stroke
- Degenerative neurologic disease
- Diabetic neuropathy
- Depression or dementia

Dietary changes, ample fluids, and regular exercise may be helpful. Kegel exercises to improve sphincter and pelvic floor muscle tone may help. A bowel training program to establish a regular pattern of elimination is often effective. The client is taught to establish a regular time of day for elimination, usually 15 to 30 minutes after breakfast. A stimulant, such as a cup of coffee or a rectal suppository, may be given to prompt defecation.

NURSING CARE

For the alert client, fecal incontinence can lead to a loss of self-esteem and social isolation.

Bowel Incontinence
- Teach caregivers to place the client on a toilet or commode and provide for privacy at a certain time of day. *Placing the client in a normal position to defecate at a consistent time of day helps reestablish a pattern of stool evacuation.*
- If necessary, insert a glycerin suppository 15 to 20 minutes before placing on the toilet or commode. *This helps to stimulate evacuation. Once a regular elimination pattern is established, it may be possible to discontinue suppository use.*
- Maintain a caring, nonjudgmental manner. Provide room odor control with deodorizer tablets, sprays, or other devices. *These measures help the client feel accepted and help reduce embarrassment when caregivers or visitors enter the room.*

Risk for Impaired Skin Integrity
- Clean skin thoroughly with soap and water after each bowel movement. Apply a skin barrier cream or ointment. *Irritation of perianal and perineal skin by fecal material can lead to tissue breakdown and pressure ulcers. Toilet tissue may increase irritation and is less effective than soap and water for removing fecal material.*

- If incontinence pads or briefs are used, check frequently for soiling, and change promptly when soiled. *Although these help protect bedding and clothing, they can contribute to skin breakdown if they are not checked and changed frequently.*

CONTINUING CARE

Managing fecal incontinence is challenging for both the client and caregivers. Stress that incontinence is never normal (i.e., not a result of aging) and often is treatable. Provide teaching as for constipation (Box 20-3). Provide bowel training instructions. Stress the importance of good skin care.

Malabsorption

Malabsorption is ineffective intestinal absorption of nutrients. It commonly occurs with disorders of the small intestine.

PATHOPHYSIOLOGY AND MANIFESTATIONS

Two major causes of malabsorption are celiac disease and lactose intolerance. *Celiac disease* (or nontropical sprue) is a hereditary disorder characterized by sensitivity to *gluten* (a cereal protein found in wheat, rye, barley, and oats). In celiac disease, absorption of nutrients, particularly fats, is impaired. *Lactose intolerance* is caused by deficient lactase, the enzyme required to digest milk and milk products. Lactase deficiency affects up to 90% of Asians and 75% of African Americans and Native Americans, as well as many Jewish Americans and Hispanics (Kasper et al., 2005).

Resection of the small intestine (*short bowel syndrome*) also can lead to malabsorption. The severity of the disorder depends on the amount and location of bowel resected. Whatever the cause, manifestations result from impaired absorption of food and nutrients (see Box 20-8 ■).

INTERDISCIPLINARY CARE

With any malabsorptive disorder, the first focus is finding the cause. *Stool samples* are examined for fat content. A D-*xylose absorption test* or *xylose tolerance test* is used to evaluate intestinal absorption. A *lactose breath test* or a *lactose tolerance test*

MANIFESTATIONS OF MALABSORPTION
- Anorexia
- Abdominal bloating
- Diarrhea; loose, bulky, foul-smelling stools
- Steatorrhea (fatty stools)
- Weight loss
- Weakness, general malaise
- Muscle cramps, bone pain
- Abnormal bleeding, anemia

BOX 20-9

SELECTED DIETARY SOURCES OF GLUTEN

- Bread, cereal, pasta products, desserts, and pastries made with wheat, rye, oats, or barley
- Breaded meats, meatloaf, soy protein meat substitutes
- Malt, Postum, Ovaltine, other beverage mixes, beers and ales, some whiskeys, root beer
- Commercial salad dressings, ketchup and mustard; gravy, white sauce; nondairy creamer

may be ordered. Numerous laboratory tests for nutrient deficiencies may be ordered to evaluate the effects of malabsorption. (See Table 18-1 ⬭ for the manifestations of selected nutrient deficiencies.)

Treatment focuses on the underlying disorder. A gluten-free diet is ordered for clients with celiac disease (Box 20-9 ■). Clients with lactose intolerance may need to eliminate all milk and milk products. Lactase enzyme preparations may be given to improve milk tolerance. Frequent, small, high-calorie, high-protein feedings are prescribed for short bowel syndrome. All clients may require vitamin and mineral supplements.

NURSING CARE

Nursing care focuses on the effects of the disorder on nutrition and on bowel elimination. Document nutritional status, including weight, fat-fold measurements, laboratory values, and dietary intake. Supplement intake with enteral feedings as ordered. Maintain central lines and total parenteral nutrition, if required. Assess intake and output, daily weights, skin turgor, and condition of mucous membranes to monitor hydration. For diarrhea, document the number and character of stools. Administer antidiarrheal medications as ordered. Provide good skin care of the perianal region.

Discuss day-to-day management of the disorder, including the recommended diet and medication regimen. Provide a detailed list of foods to include and to eliminate from the diet. Teach to read labels and lists of ingredients to identify hidden sources of the nutrient to which they are sensitive.

Emphasize the importance of adequate fluid intake, increasing intake for hot weather or increased exercise. Teach to regularly monitor weight and report changes. Address manifestations that should be reported to the physician. Refer to a dietitian or counselor for additional dietary teaching and coping strategies.

INFLAMMATORY DISORDERS

The gastrointestinal tract is constantly exposed to the external environment, making it particularly vulnerable to inflammation and infection. Most pathogens that affect it are ingested in food or water. Gastroenteritis, a general term for infection of the GI tract, is discussed in Chapter 19. ⬭ Acute disorders such as appendicitis and peritonitis occur when bacteria normally residing in the GI tract infect damaged or normally sterile tissue.

Appendicitis

Appendicitis (inflammation of the appendix) is the most common reason for emergency abdominal surgery in the United States. The appendix is in the right lower quadrant region at *McBurney's point* (Figure 20-1 ■). Its function is not fully understood, but it regularly fills with and empties digested food. Appendicitis is most common in adolescents and young adults and is slightly more common in males than females.

PATHOPHYSIOLOGY

The appendix can become obstructed by a *fecalith* (hard mass of feces). As a result, the appendix becomes distended with fluid secreted by bowel mucosa. This increases pressure within the appendix and impairs its blood supply. This leads to inflammation, edema, ulceration,

and infection of the tissue. Within 24 to 36 hours, the appendix becomes necrotic and perforates if treatment is not initiated.

Appendicitis is classified by the stage of the process. In *simple appendicitis,* the appendix is inflamed but intact. In *gangrenous appendicitis,* the appendix has areas of tissue necrosis and microscopic perforations. With a *perforated appendix,* the appendix has ruptured, contaminating the peritoneal cavity with its contents.

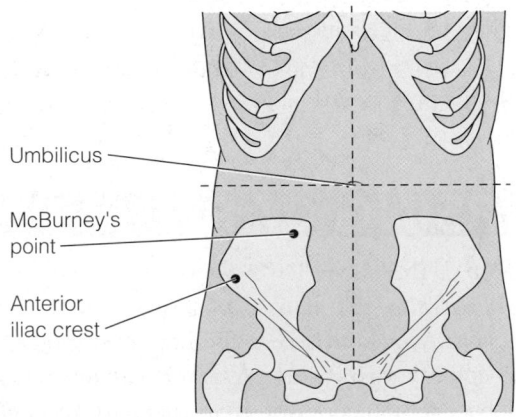

Umbilicus

McBurney's point

Anterior iliac crest

Figure 20-1. ■ McBurney's point, located midway between the umbilicus and the anterior iliac crest in the right lower quadrant.

MANIFESTATIONS AND COMPLICATIONS

Generalized or upper abdominal pain often is the initial symptom of acute appendicitis. The pain gradually intensifies and localizes in the right lower quadrant of the abdomen. It is aggravated by moving, walking, or coughing. Localized and rebound tenderness are noted at McBurney's point. *Rebound tenderness* is demonstrated by relief of pain during palpation followed by pain on release of pressure. Extension of the right hip increases the pain. Less acute pain and local tenderness may delay diagnosis in pregnant women and older adults. The client may have a low-grade fever, anorexia, nausea, and vomiting.

Perforation is the major complication of acute appendicitis. Perforation is manifested by increased pain and a high fever. It can result in a small, localized abscess, local peritonitis, or significant generalized peritonitis.

INTERDISCIPLINARY CARE

Because the acutely inflamed appendix can perforate within 24 hours, prompt diagnosis and treatment are important. The client is admitted to the hospital, and intravenous fluids are initiated. Oral food and fluids are withheld until a diagnosis is confirmed.

Diagnostic Tests

Diagnostic testing and preoperative treatment are limited. The *white blood count (WBC)* is elevated in appendicitis. An *abdominal ultrasound* may be done to confirm the diagnosis if symptoms are atypical. See Chapter 18 ⚭ for more information about and nursing responsibilities for abdominal ultrasound.

Surgery

The treatment of choice for acute appendicitis is an *appendectomy,* surgical removal of the appendix. The appendectomy may be performed through a **laparotomy** (surgical opening of the abdomen) or by **laparoscopy** (exploration of the abdomen using an endoscope). *Laparoscopic appendectomy* requires three very small incisions, and recovery is rapid. Antibiotic therapy is initiated prior to surgery and continues for at least 48 hours postoperatively.

NURSING CARE

Assessment of the client with suspected appendicitis focuses on describing the pain, as well as its onset, severity, and duration. Ask about recent food or fluid intake, allergies, and current medications. Ensure that informed consent has been obtained prior to surgery. If time allows, teach postoperative turning, coughing, deep breathing, and pain management. Report WBC results as soon as available.

clinical ALERT

Withhold all food and fluids from the client with suspected appendicitis, because surgery is the treatment of choice. Do not administer laxatives or enemas or apply heat to the abdomen because these measures may cause perforation of the appendix.

Ineffective Tissue Perfusion: Gastrointestinal

Inflammation and edema of the appendix interfere with its blood supply, increasing the risk for tissue necrosis and rupture.

- Monitor for signs of perforation and peritonitis preoperatively. *A primary goal of care is to prevent complications. Perforation may be signaled by a sudden relief of pain as the appendix ruptures, followed by increased generalized pain and abdominal distention.*
- Monitor vital signs. *An elevated pulse and rapid shallow breathing may indicate perforation of the appendix with infection and peritonitis. The temperature may be elevated. If sepsis develops, the blood pressure may fall.*
- Maintain intravenous fluids until the client is able to drink adequate amounts postoperatively. *Intravenous fluids help maintain fluid and electrolyte balance and vascular volume.*
- Postoperatively, monitor wound, abdominal girth, and pain. *Swelling of the wound, increased abdominal girth, or increased pain may indicate infection or peritonitis.*

Pain

- Assess pain, including its character, location, severity, and duration. Report any unexpected changes in description of pain. *Careful pain assessment can provide important clues about diagnosis and possible complications. For example, generalized abdominal pain with guarding of abdominal muscles may indicate peritonitis.*
- Administer prescribed analgesics. *Preoperatively, pain medication can be given after a diagnosis is established. Postoperatively, provide analgesics to promote comfort and enhance mobility.*
- Assess effectiveness of medication after administration. If pain is not relieved, contact the charge nurse or physician. *Pain unrelieved by analgesics may indicate a complication.*
- Provide alternative methods of pain relief, including distraction, therapeutic touch, massage, meditation, or visualization. *These techniques can enhance comfort and the effectiveness of analgesics.*

CONTINUING CARE

Following an uncomplicated appendectomy, the client is usually dismissed from the acute-care setting either the day of surgery or the day following surgery. Teach wound or incision care. Instruct to report swelling, redness, drainage, bleeding, or warmth at the operative site to the surgeon. If a dressing is present, teach proper hand washing and dressing change procedures. Instruct the client to report any fever or increased abdominal pain.

Discuss activity restrictions. Heavy lifting may be restricted for up to 6 weeks. Depending on the surgery, driving and return to work may be allowed within 1 to 2 weeks. Community health or home health care nurses may be required if the client has a preexisting illness or has trouble performing activities of daily living (ADLs) and self-care.

Peritonitis

Peritonitis is inflammation of the peritoneum, a double-layered membrane that lines the walls and organs of the abdominal cavity. It is a serious complication of many acute abdominal disorders. Peritonitis results when the normally sterile, potential space between the layers of the peritoneum is contaminated. A perforated appendix or gastric ulcer, traumatic injury such as a gunshot wound, or contamination during abdominal surgery can lead to peritonitis.

PATHOPHYSIOLOGY

Perforation of a peptic ulcer (see Chapter 19 ⊙), rupture of the appendix, or contamination of the abdominal cavity by bowel contents during surgery allows chemicals and bacteria from the GI tract to enter the normally sterile peritoneal cavity. *Chemical peritonitis* develops immediately following perforation of a peptic ulcer, as gastric juices (hydrochloric acid and pepsin) enter the peritoneal cavity. *Bacterial peritonitis* results when bacteria that are normally confined within the bowel enter the peritoneal cavity. Normal inflammatory and immune defense mechanisms may effectively eliminate small numbers of bacteria or localize the infection. Massive or continued contamination, however, leads to generalized inflammation of the peritoneal cavity. The inflammatory process causes a fluid shift into the peritoneal space (*third-spacing*). Peristalsis slows or stops (**paralytic ileus**) due to the inflammation.

MANIFESTATIONS AND COMPLICATIONS

The signs and symptoms of peritonitis depend on the severity and extent of the infection, as well as the age and general health of the client. Both abdominal and systemic manifestations are present (Box 20-10 ■). The client often presents with evidence of an *acute abdomen*. An acute abdomen is characterized by an abrupt onset of severe pain, often accompanied by boardlike abdominal muscle rigidity.

clinical ALERT

The older, chronically debilitated, or immunosuppressed client may have few of the classic signs of peritonitis. Increased confusion and restlessness, decreased urinary output, and vague abdominal complaints may be the only manifestations.

BOX 20-10

MANIFESTATIONS OF PERITONITIS

Abdominal
- Diffuse or localized pain, usually severe
- Tenderness with rebound
- Boardlike rigidity or guarding of abdominal muscles
- Diminished or absent bowel sounds
- Progressive distention
- Anorexia, nausea, and vomiting

Systemic
- Fever, malaise
- Tachycardia, tachypnea
- Restlessness, confusion
- Oliguria

Complications of peritonitis may be life threatening and either localized or systemic. Formation of an *abscess* is the most common complication. *Septicemia,* the presence of pathogens in the blood, may develop. Without prompt treatment, shock may result from hypovolemia or sepsis. Shock (see Chapter 13 ⊙) requires immediate, aggressive treatment to prevent multiple organ failure and death. *Adhesions* or bands of scar tissue may develop after peritonitis and subsequently cause a bowel obstruction.

INTERDISCIPLINARY CARE

Care of the client with peritonitis focuses on identifying and treating both the peritonitis and its cause.

Diagnostic Tests

The WBC is significantly elevated in peritonitis. *Blood cultures* are obtained to identify possible *bacteremia* (bacterial invasion of the blood), which often precedes septicemia. A *paracentesis* may be done to obtain peritoneal fluid for analysis. (See Box 21-13 ⊙ for nursing care of a client having a paracentesis.)

Management

Intestinal decompression is initiated to relieve abdominal distention. A nasogastric or long intestinal tube (Figure 20-2 ■) is inserted and connected to continuous drainage. Suction is maintained and the client is NPO until peristalsis returns (bowel sounds are heard and flatus is being passed). Intravenous fluids and electrolyte replacements are provided. Total parenteral nutrition is given until oral intake resumes. The client is placed on bed rest in Fowler's position to help localize the infection and to make breathing easier. Oxygen is often ordered.

A broad-spectrum antibiotic is prescribed until the infecting organism has been identified. Then antibiotic therapy is modified to the specific organism(s). (Nursing implications for the use of common antibiotics are outlined in Table 10-5. ⊙) The client may receive narcotic analgesics and sedatives to promote comfort and rest.

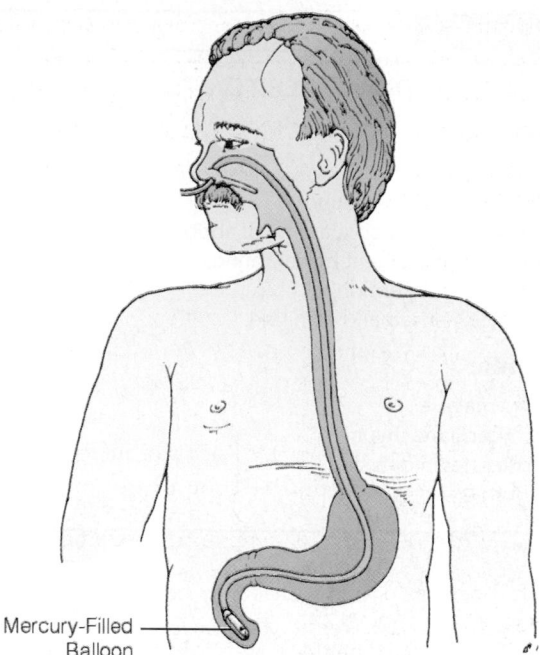

Mercury-Filled
Balloon

Figure 20-2. ■ An intestinal tube is advanced in increments of 1 to 2 inches every hour. Suction is applied after the balloon or weighted tip passes the pyloric valve.

Surgery

A laparotomy may be done to close a perforation, remove damaged and inflamed tissue, or remove an abscess. *Peritoneal lavage* (washing of the peritoneal cavity with warm isotonic fluid) may be done during surgery. Peritoneal lavage may be continued for up to 3 days after surgery. The solution is infused into the upper portion of the peritoneal cavity and removed via drains in the pelvis. Careful attention to fluid and electrolyte status and strict aseptic technique are necessary.

Clients who have had laparotomy for peritonitis often return from surgery with drains such as a Jackson-Pratt. In some cases, the incision may be left unsutured. The abdomen may be closed temporarily with mesh containing a nylon zipper or Velcro to allow repeated exploration of the abdomen and drainage of infectious sites.

NURSING CARE

Peritonitis is a serious illness. Clients require intensive nursing and medical interventions to recover fully.

ASSESSING

Nursing assessment of clients with peritonitis focuses on monitoring their current status, progress of recovery, and identifying possible complications. Continuing assessments for clients with peritonitis are listed in Box 20-11 ■.

| BOX 20-11 | **ASSESSMENT** |

Assessing Clients with Peritonitis

SUBJECTIVE DATA

- Pain: type or character, location, severity.
- Anxiety and coping.

OBJECTIVE DATA

- Assess mental status and level of consciousness every 4 to 8 hours. Report changes to the charge nurse or physician.
- Check vital signs (including temperature and measurements such as central venous pressure as ordered) hourly or as indicated.
- Check urine output every 1 to 2 hours. Report output of less than 30 mL/hr.
- Assess drainage from gastrointestinal tube and surgical drains such as Jackson-Pratt every 4 hours or as ordered. Record color, odor, and type of drainage; report changes.
- Assess intake (intravenous and oral) every 8 hours or as indicated.
- Weigh daily. Report changes.
- Assess skin turgor, color, temperature, mucous membrane color, and moisture every 8 hours.
- Measure abdominal girth with the same measuring tape at the umbilicus every 8 hours.

LABORATORY TESTS

- Monitor WBC, hemoglobin and hematocrit, serum osmolality and electrolytes, and liver and renal function tests (see Chapters 18 and 31 ⊂⊃).

DIAGNOSING, PLANNING, AND IMPLEMENTING

Priorities in Nursing Care. Supporting the client and managing responses to the acute inflammatory process are the priorities for nursing care of the client with peritonitis.

Pain

- Place in Fowler's or semi-Fowler's position with the knees and feet elevated. *This position helps minimize stress on abdominal structures and facilitate respirations, promoting comfort.*
- Administer analgesics as ordered on a routine basis or using patient-controlled analgesia (PCA). Frequently evaluate response to analgesics. *Routine administration of analgesics helps maintain pain control, facilitating healing and movement. Decreasing effectiveness of the medication may indicate a complication.*
- Teach and assist to use alternative pain management techniques along with analgesics. *Meditation, visualization, massage, and progressive relaxation augment analgesics and increase comfort.*

Deficient Fluid Volume

- Record vital signs, intake and output, weight, moisture of skin and mucous membranes as indicated. Measure or estimate fluid losses through abdominal drains and on dressings. *Fluid losses occur through third-spacing, gastrointestinal suction, and drainage from surgical wounds and drains. This can lead to hypovolemia.*
- Monitor laboratory values, such as hemoglobin and hematocrit, urine specific gravity, and serum electrolytes. Report changes to the physician. *These values provide information about the client's fluid and electrolyte status.*
- Maintain intravenous fluids and electrolytes as ordered. *Gastrointestinal drainage may be replaced milliliter for milliliter with a balanced electrolyte solution. In addition, fluid intake must be maintained intravenously while the client is NPO.*
- Provide good skin care and frequent oral hygiene. *Fluid loss increases the risk of skin breakdown and ulceration of mucous membranes.*

Ineffective Protection

- Monitor for signs of infection, including fever, tachycardia, redness and swelling around incisions and drain sites, increased or purulent drainage, and cloudy, malodorous, or scant urine. *Surgical interventions and stress on immune defenses increase the risk for further infection.*
- Obtain cultures of purulent drainage from any site. *Early identification allows appropriate intervention to be instituted.*
- Practice meticulous hand washing before and after providing care. Use strict aseptic technique for dressing changes and wound or peritoneal irrigations. *Hand washing reduces transient bacteria on the skin and remains the most important method of controlling infection. Interruption of the skin barrier increases the risk for infection.*
- Maintain fluid balance and adequate nutrition through either enteral or parenteral feedings, as indicated. *Adequate nutrition and fluid balance are necessary for optimal immune system function.*

Anxiety

- Assess the client's and family's anxiety level and coping skills. *This provides a basis on which to plan interventions.*
- Present a calm, reassuring manner. Encourage the client and family to express their concerns; listen carefully, and acknowledge their validity. *This helps establish trust.*
- Minimize changes in caregiver assignments. *Consistency of nursing care and care providers helps reduce anxiety. Complex wound care and irrigation procedures are best performed by people who are very familiar with prescribed techniques.*
- Explain all treatments, procedures, tests, and examinations. Reinforce and clarify information provided by physicians. *Understanding what is being done helps reduce anxiety and promote acceptance.*
- Teach and assist with relaxation techniques such as meditation, visualization, and progressive relaxation. *These measures promote positive coping skills and reduce physical manifestations of anxiety.*

EVALUATING

Collect the following data to evaluate the effectiveness of nursing care for the client with peritonitis: level of pain and effectiveness of analgesics; weight, urine output, and other indicators of fluid volume status; temperature, wound healing and drainage, and other indicators of infection; and indicators of anxiety and effective coping.

Documenting. Document continuing assessment data, including subjective complaints of pain and the effect of analgesia in relieving pain. Document the type and amount of drainage from nasogastric or intestinal tubes and wound drains. Note wound healing (as appropriate), drainage from the incision, and any foul odor on dressings or of drainage.

CONTINUING CARE

Teaching is vital throughout hospitalization and prior to discharge. Assessment data collected prior to discharge helps individualize teaching to the client and family (Box 20-12 ■).

BOX 20-12	ASSESSMENT

Assessing for Discharge: Peritonitis

CLIENT

- Self-care: ability to independently perform ADLs; to manage wound care and medications; to prepare and eat a nutritionally sound diet
- Knowledge: wound care needs and medications, diet recommendations and activity limitations, follow-up care; signs of complications to report to physician
- Psychosocial: ability to cope with continued care needs and economic effects; acceptance of altered body image and roles/relationships
- Home environment: access to clean running water, hand washing and cooking facilities; clean area in which to perform wound care

FAMILY AND CAREGIVERS

- Members of household: ability and willingness to assist with ADLs, wound care, central line management, and other care needs
- Financial resources: income; resources for dressings, supplies, food supplements; effect of extended recovery period on roles and relationships, stability of family unit

Begin teaching for home care prior to discharge. Provide verbal and written instructions for wound care, dressing changes, and irrigation procedures. Allow the client and family members to practice and demonstrate procedures before discharge. Include information on where to obtain necessary supplies. Discuss medications, including the name and purpose of the drug and potential adverse effects and their management.

Describe the signs and symptoms of further infection (redness, heat, swelling, purulent drainage, chills, and fever) and other potential complications. Emphasize the need to report adverse responses promptly to the primary care provider. Reinforce instructions about activity restrictions. Discuss the importance of consuming a diet with adequate calories and protein to promote healing and optimal immune function. Provide a referral to home health services for assessment, wound care, and further teaching, as needed.

Inflammatory Bowel Disease

Ulcerative colitis and Crohn's disease are two conditions categorized as *inflammatory bowel disease (IBD)*. These conditions are similar in many ways:

- Their cause is unknown, although autoimmunity (see Chapter 11 🔗) and lifestyle factors are thought to play a role.
- Both affect primarily young adults and also may affect older adults.
- Both are chronic and recurrent.
- Diarrhea is the predominant symptom of each.
- Both may have associated manifestations, such as arthritis.

Ulcerative colitis and Crohn's disease also differ from one another in several ways: Ulcerative colitis tends to affect the large bowel in a continuous pattern, whereas Crohn's disease primarily affects the small intestine in a patchy pattern. Table 20-5 ■ compares the manifestations and complications of ulcerative colitis and Crohn's disease.

ULCERATIVE COLITIS

Ulcerative colitis is a chronic inflammatory bowel disorder of the mucosa and submucosa of the colon and rectum. It affects primarily the young, although it also is seen in people between ages 50 and 70. It is more common in whites than in people of color.

Ulcerative colitis is thought to be an *autoimmune disorder*, in which the individual's own antibodies attack the colon. Factors such as infection, diet, and environment (e.g., smoking) may contribute to development of ulcerative colitis. Stress and psychologic factors affect, but do not cause, ulcerative colitis.

Pathophysiology

Ulcerative colitis usually begins in the rectal area. It may progress proximally along the colon, involving the bowel in a continuous pattern. The mucosa becomes inflamed and edematous and bleeds easily. The mucosa ulcerates, sloughs, and is lost in the feces. As scar tissue forms, the bowel wall thickens and shortens. In most people, only the rectum and sigmoid colon are affected. Less commonly, the entire colon may be involved.

Manifestations and Complications

A gradual onset of diarrhea with intermittent rectal bleeding and mucus is common. In its most common form, acute attacks of colitis last 1 to 3 months and occur at intervals of months to years. Diarrhea is the chief symptom. In mild cases, the client may have fewer than 4 stools per day with intermittent rectal bleeding and mucus, and few systemic manifestations. Clients with severe ulcerative colitis may have more than 6 to 10 bloody stools per day, extensive

TABLE 20-5		
Manifestations and Complications of Inflammatory Bowel Disease		
	ULCERATIVE COLITIS	**CROHN'S DISEASE**
Manifestations	■ 5 to 30 stools per day ■ Blood and mucus in stool ■ Left lower quadrant crampy abdominal pain; relieved by defecation ■ Weight loss ■ Anemia, low serum protein levels ■ May have systemic symptoms	■ Diarrhea common but less severe ■ No obvious blood or mucus in stool ■ Right lower quadrant or central abdominal pain, cramping or steady ■ Significant weight loss ■ Anemia, multiple nutrient deficits ■ Fever, general malaise, fatigue
Complications	Toxic megacolon, perforation, massive hemorrhage Colon cancer	Obstruction, fistula or abscess formation, malabsorption Colon cancer

colon involvement, dehydration, and malnutrition. Rectal inflammation causes fecal urgency and *tenesmus* (straining). Left lower quadrant cramping relieved by defecation is common. Systemic manifestations include fatigue, anorexia, and weakness. Clients with severe disease may develop a related arthritis.

Complications of ulcerative colitis include *colon perforation,* the leading cause of death in these clients. *Toxic megacolon* is characterized by paralysis of the colon with significant distention, usually in the transverse segment of the large bowel. Manifestations of toxic megacolon include fever, tachycardia, hypotension, dehydration, abdominal tenderness, and cramping. An acute decrease in diarrhea stools may signal toxic megacolon. Clients with ulcerative colitis have a high risk for developing colon cancer.

CROHN'S DISEASE

Crohn's disease (*regional enteritis*) is a chronic, relapsing inflammatory disorder of the GI tract. Crohn's disease usually begins between ages 10 and 30. Genetic and environmental factors, infectious agents, and autoimmune processes may contribute to its development. It is more common in urban settings, among residents of the northern United States, and among Ashkenazi Jews (Kasper et al., 2005).

Crohn's disease can affect any part of the GI tract from the mouth to the anus, but it usually affects the distal portion of the small intestine and the ascending colon.

Pathophysiology

Crohn's disease causes inflammatory lesions of the bowel mucosa that may extend into all layers of the bowel wall. These inflammatory lesions are localized, surrounded by normal gut. Ulcers and deep fissures develop, and fistulas may form between loops of bowel or between the bowel and other organs. Inflammation and scarring cause the bowel to narrow and become partially or fully obstructed (Figure 20-3 ■). Over time, the bowel wall thickens and loses flexibility, and looks somewhat like a rubber hose. Malabsorption and malnutrition may develop because inflammation and ulcers prevent absorption of nutrients, especially vitamin B_{12} and bile salts.

Manifestations and Complications

Most people with Crohn's disease experience continuous or episodic diarrhea. Stools are liquid or semiformed and typically do not contain blood. Clients have abdominal pain and tenderness, and a mass may be palpable in the right lower quadrant. Many clients with Crohn's disease develop lesions of the rectum and anus, such as fissures, ulcers, fistulas, and abscesses. Systemic manifestations such as fever, malaise, and fatigue are common.

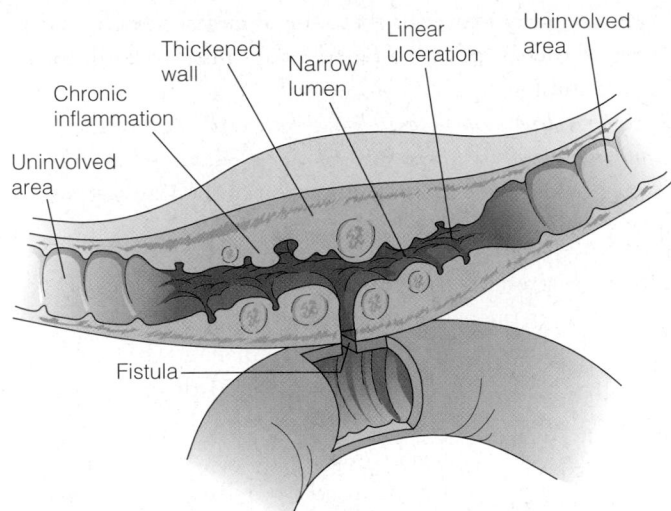

Figure 20-3. ■ An illustration of the major characteristics of Crohn's disease in the small intestine, and a potential complication (fistula formation).

Intestinal obstruction, abscess, and fistula are so common that they are considered part of the disease process. Intestinal obstruction causes abdominal distention, cramping pain, borborygmi, and sometimes nausea and vomiting. When an abscess forms, the client develops chills and fever, a tender abdominal mass, and leukocytosis. Fistulas may be asymptomatic, particularly if they occur between loops of small bowel. A fistula between the small bowel and colon may increase diarrhea, weight loss, and malnutrition. When a fistula involves the bladder, recurrent urinary tract infections occur. Long-standing Crohn's disease increases the risk of cancer of the small intestine or colon by five to six times.

INTERDISCIPLINARY CARE

Treatment of IBD is supportive, directed toward managing symptoms and controlling the disease process. Supportive care measures include rest, stress reduction, drugs, and nutritional support. When the disease does not respond to treatment or complications develop, surgery may be required.

Diagnostic Tests

Diagnostic testing is used to establish the diagnosis of IBD.

- A *stool specimen* is examined for blood and mucus and is sent for culture to rule out infectious causes.
- *Complete blood count (CBC), serum albumin level,* and serum levels of multiple vitamins are drawn to evaluate nutritional status.
- *Sigmoidoscopy* or *colonoscopy* is performed to visualize the bowel mucosa and collect tissue for biopsy. (Nursing implications of these tests are presented in Boxes 20-1 and 20-16.) Harsh bowel preparations are avoided

because they may exacerbate the disease. Instead, a clear liquid diet is ordered for 2 to 3 days prior to endoscopic examination.

- *Upper GI series with small-bowel follow-through* and a *barium enema* (see Boxes 20-6 and 20-4, respectively) may be done for x-ray examination of the GI tract.

Medications

Drugs are prescribed to terminate acute attacks of IBD and reduce the frequency of relapse. Locally acting and systemic anti-inflammatory drugs are used to manage IBD.

Sulfasalazine (Azulfidine) and related drugs are poorly absorbed from the GI tract and act as local anti-inflammatory agents on the bowel mucosa. For an acute episode, corticosteroids may also be used to reduce inflammation (Table 20-6 ■). Immunosuppressive drugs may be pre-scribed to maintain remission for some clients with in-flammatory bowel disease.

Antidiarrheal agents, such as loperamide and diphenoxy-late, may be given to slow GI motility and reduce diarrhea. These drugs are not given during acute attacks of ulcerative colitis because they may cause toxic megacolon.

Dietary Management

A well-balanced diet is recommended. Dietary supplements such as Ensure may be added to promote weight gain and nutritional status. Lactose intolerance is common in clients with IBD, so milk and milk products may be eliminated. When the disease primarily affects the colon, increasing di-etary fiber may reduce diarrhea. Clients with obstruction or small-bowel narrowing, however, need a low-roughage diet (no raw fruits and vegetables, popcorn, nuts, etc.).

TABLE 20-6

Nursing Implications For Pharmacology: Inflammatory Bowel Disease

AGENT/DRUGS	PURPOSE	NURSING IMPLICATIONS	CLIENT TEACHING
Local Anti-Inflammatory Agents ■ Sulfasalazine (Azulfidine) ■ Mesalamine (Rowasa) ■ Olsalazine (Dipentum)	These drugs have a local anti-inflammatory effect on intestinal mucosa. The drug inhibits prostaglandin pro-duction in the bowel. Prostaglandin is an important mediator of the inflammatory process; blocking its produc-tion reduces inflammation. These drugs may be adminis-tered by rectal suppository, by enema, or by mouth.	Do not give to clients who are preg-nant or allergic to sulfonamides or salicylates. Suppositories or retention enemas may be administered at bedtime. Give oral forms with a full glass of water. Monitor for adverse effects: a. Rash, dermatitis, hives, or pruritus b. Bleeding, easy bruising, fever c. Low blood cell counts d. Changes in urine output or renal function studies e. Evidence of hepatitis or myocarditis Teach clients how to administer the drug by enema or suppository as ap-propriate.	Take oral preparations after meals to decrease GI effects. Drink at least 2 quarts of fluid per day. Use sunscreen to prevent sunburns. Do not take aspirin, vitamin C, or any other over-the-counter medications containing aspirin or vitamin C without consulting with your doctor. Oral contraceptives may be less effective; use alternative methods of contraception. Notify your doctor if you develop a rash or hives, sore throat or mouth, bleeding gums, joint pain, easy bruising, or fever.
Corticosteroids ■ Methylpred-nisolone (Medrol, Solu-Medrol) ■ Prednisone	Glucocorticoids have potent anti-inflammatory effects and are used to treat acute episodes of IBD. They can be given by enema, by mouth, or by IV infusion. Because of their multiple and significant side effects, they are used for short periods only.	Notify the physician if the client has peptic ulcer disease, glaucoma or cataracts, diabetes, or a psychiatric dis-order. Monitor vital signs, weight, and intake and output during therapy. Assess for edema. Administer in the morning as ordered. Give oral forms with meals. Monitor for adverse effects: a. Infection b. Hyperglycemia c. Hypokalemia d. Fluid retention e. Peptic ulcers or gastritis f. Mental status changes	Take as prescribed, do not take additional doses. Do not stop the drug abruptly. Notify your doctor if you develop adverse effects. Take with food or meals. Monitor weight. Contact your doctor if you gain more than 5 pounds. Moderate salt intake and avoid high-sodium foods and snacks. Increase intake of foods high in potassium, such as fruits, vegeta-bles, and lean meats. Carry a card or wear a tag identify-ing corticosteroid use.

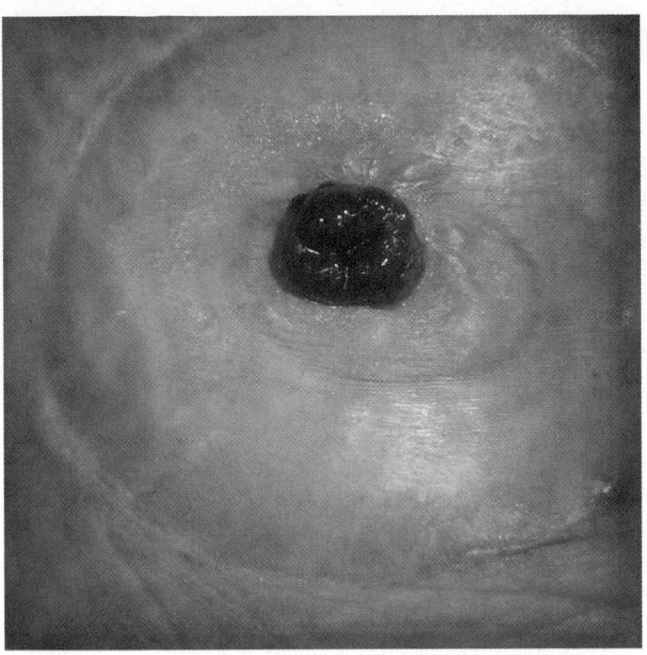

Figure 20-4. ■ A healthy appearing stoma. (Courtesy of Carol Williams.)

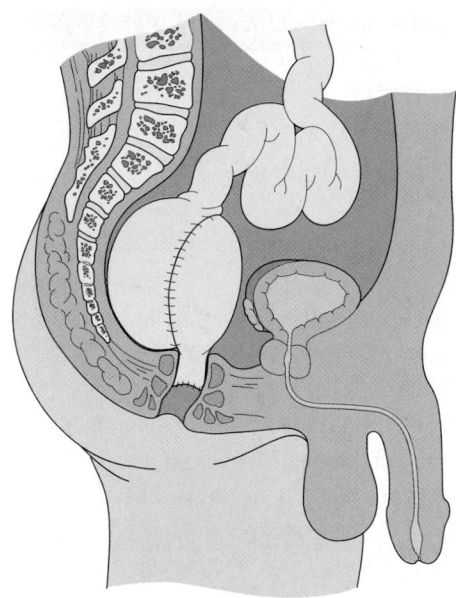

Figure 20-6. ■ Ileoanal anastomosis with reservoir.

During an acute exacerbation, the client is usually kept NPO. Total parenteral nutrition (TPN) is administered to maintain nutritional status. As the episode resolves, an elemental diet that contains all essential nutrients in a residue-free formula (e.g., Ensure) may be ordered. These measures reduce intestinal motility and allow the bowel to rest.

Surgery

Surgical removal of the colon cures ulcerative colitis. Most clients, however, choose surgery only when other treatments are ineffective or manifestations of the disease interfere with ADLs. Surgery may also be indicated for complications of Crohn's disease, such as bowel obstruction, fistulas, or abscesses.

Clients with ulcerative colitis may undergo a total **colectomy**, surgical removal of the colon. When the colon is

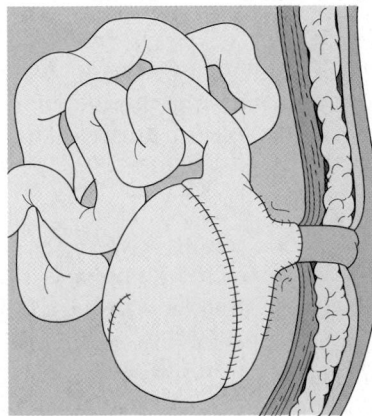

Figure 20-5. ■ Kock's (continent) ileostomy.

removed, the terminal ileum may be brought to the surface of the abdomen to form an **ostomy**, an opening that allows elimination of fecal material. The surface opening of the ostomy is called a *stoma* (Figure 20-4 ■). The precise name of the ostomy depends on the location of the stoma (e.g., an **ileostomy** is an ostomy made in the ileum of the small intestine). A permanent ileostomy may allow feces to drain directly (and constantly) through the stoma. The surgeon may create an internal pouch from the terminal ileum to collect feces until the client drains it with a catheter (Figure 20-5 ■). A nipple valve prevents leakage of the stool between catheterizations.

A pouch formed from the terminal ileum also may be sutured to the anal canal (Figure 20-6 ■). This procedure allows more normal bowel elimination and helps preserve body image. The client may return from surgery with a temporary ileostomy, which is later closed.

Nursing care of the client having bowel surgery is outlined in Box 20-13 ■. Nursing care of the client with an ostomy is described later in this chapter in Boxes 20-17 through 20-19.

NURSING CARE

ASSESSING

Assessment for clients with IBD focuses on their current health status, presence of complications, and psychosocial factors related to the disease. Assessment data to collect for clients with inflammatory bowel disease are listed in Box 20-14 ■.

BOX 20-13	NURSING CARE CHECKLIST

Bowel Surgery

Before Surgery

☑ Provide routine preoperative care and teaching as outlined in Chapter 9. ∞

☑ Assess understanding and clarify information as indicated.

☑ Reinforce preoperative teaching: pain management, expected tubes, turning, coughing, and deep breathing after surgery.

☑ Insert a nasogastric tube if ordered preoperatively.

☑ Perform bowel preparation procedures as ordered.

After Surgery

☑ Provide routine care for the surgical client (see Chapter 9). ∞

☑ Monitor bowel sounds and abdominal distention.

☑ Assess nasogastric tube position and patency; connect to low suction. If the tube becomes clogged, gently irrigate with sterile normal saline.

☑ Assess color, amount, and odor of drainage from surgical drains and the ostomy (if present), noting any changes or the presence of clots or bright bleeding. Initial ostomy drainage may be bright red and then become dark and finally clear or greenish yellow during the first 2 to 3 days. Report significant changes in color, amount, or odor.

☑ Frequently assess respiratory status including rate, depth, and lung sounds.

☑ Encourage frequent turning, coughing, and deep breathing. Provide a pillow or blanket to splint the abdominal incision or assist the client to splint the incision.

☑ If an abdominoperineal resection has been performed, alert all personnel to avoid rectal temperatures, suppositories, or other rectal procedures.

☑ Maintain intravenous fluids as ordered.

☑ Provide antacids, H$_2$-receptor blockers, and antibiotic therapy as ordered.

☑ Reintroduce oral intake with clear liquids, gradually progressing to frequent small feedings of regular foods. Monitor bowel sounds and abdominal distention frequently during this period.

☑ Encourage ambulation to stimulate peristalsis.

☑ Begin discharge planning and teaching. Consult with a dietitian for diet instructions and menu planning; reinforce teaching. Teach about potential complications, such as abdominal abscess or bowel obstruction, their manifestations, and prevention.

BOX 20-14	ASSESSMENT

Assessing Clients with Inflammatory Bowel Disease

SUBJECTIVE DATA

■ Disease history: onset, course, and severity; precipitating and relieving factors, including timing and circumstances.

■ Current manifestations: abdominal pain or cramping, timing, character (constant or intermittent), factors that aggravate or relieve it; number of stools per day, blood or mucus in the stool; tenesmus; abdominal distention, anorexia, nausea, vomiting; general malaise, fatigue; joint pain or other symptoms; recent weight changes.

■ Previous surgeries or treatments for the disease; date of most recent colonoscopy.

■ Current medications, usual diet and current food intake.

■ Knowledge and understanding of the disease; ability to deal with the ostomy and drainage devices (if present); effect on roles, family relationships, sexuality; ability to cope with disease and its effects.

OBJECTIVE DATA

■ General appearance, including apparent state of health or distress, weight for height; skin color and condition.

■ Vital signs, including orthostatic vital signs if indicated.

■ Weight, height, fat-fold measurements.

■ Inspect abdomen, noting shape, presence of surgical scars or stomas, and any apparent distention; auscultate bowel sounds; palpate for tenderness, guarding, or masses.

DIAGNOSTIC TESTS

■ Monitor CBC (including hemoglobin and hematocrit), serum albumin, serum osmolality and electrolytes.

■ Obtain stool specimen and report results when available.

DIAGNOSING, PLANNING, AND IMPLEMENTING

Priorities in Nursing Care. Measures to manage diarrhea and its effects on the client's health and well-being are the highest priority for nursing care of the client with IBD. Among nursing care priorities are the psychosocial effects of frequent diarrhea as well.

Diarrhea

■ Monitor the appearance (including presence of mucus and occult or bright bleeding) and frequency of bowel movements using a stool chart. *The severity of diarrhea often correlates well with the severity of the disease and the need for fluid replacement. Large amounts of bright or dark blood may indicate a complication of the disease.*

- Administer anti-inflammatory and antidiarrheal medications as ordered. *Anti-inflammatory medications can reduce the severity and manifestations of the disease. Unless contraindicated, antidiarrheals reduce fluid loss and increase comfort.*
- Assess perianal area for irritated or denuded skin from the diarrhea. Use or provide gentle cleansing agents (Peri-Wash, Tucks, or cotton balls saturated with witch hazel) and zinc oxide–based cream to use after bowel movements. *Digestive enzymes in the stool are very corrosive to the skin.*

Risk for Deficient Fluid Volume

- Maintain accurate intake and output records, including emesis and diarrheal stools. *The client with IBD can experience significant fluid losses during an acute exacerbation of the disease. Accurate records help determine fluid replacement needs.*
- Document vital signs every 4 hours. *Elevated pulse and respiratory rates may indicate fluid volume deficit.*
- Weigh daily. Assess for other indications of fluid deficit. *Weight loss may indicate dehydration from persistent diarrhea. Warm, dry skin; poor skin turgor; dry, shiny mucous membranes; weakness; lethargy; and complaints of thirst are manifestations of dehydration.*
- Maintain fluid intake by mouth or intravenously as indicated. *Adequate fluid replacement is vital. If enteral supplements or TPN is ordered, additional fluids may be necessary to meet the client's needs.*
- Provide good skin care. *A fluid deficit increases the risk for skin breakdown.*

Imbalanced Nutrition: Less than Body Requirements

- Carefully monitor food intake. *Accurate assessment of food intake provides a way to estimate the client's calorie intake in relation to nutritional needs.*
- Provide a high-calorie, high-protein diet with nutritional supplements as ordered. Consider food preferences as allowed. Arrange for dietary consultation. *Calories and protein are important to replace lost nutrients and meet metabolic needs. Nutritional supplements help restore losses and promote intake. A dietary consultant can design a diet to meet the client's specific needs and food preferences.*
- Provide parenteral nutrition as necessary. *Parenteral nutrition can help reverse nutritional deficits and promote weight gain when the client is unable to consume adequate amounts of food.*
- Engage family members, especially the primary food preparer, in dietary teaching. *Families can reinforce teaching, encourage intake, and help the client follow the recommended diet.*
- Monitor hemoglobin and hematocrit, serum electrolytes, and serum albumin levels. *Laboratory values provide information about specific nutrient losses as well and the client's overall nutritional status.*

Disturbed Body Image

The inability to control, or even predict, fecal elimination, can interfere with the client's body image and self-concept.

- Encourage discussion about the effect of the disease or treatment on the client's feelings, self-perception, and relationships (including intimate). Accept the client's feelings and perceptions; do not discount them. *This demonstrates understanding and acceptance, and gives the client an opportunity to express his or her thoughts and feelings.*
- Discuss possible effects of treatment options openly and honestly. Encourage the client to make choices and decisions about care. *Open discussion allows the client to make more informed decisions and increases the client's sense of control.*
- Involve the client in care. Teach coping strategies (odor control, dietary modifications, etc.), and support their use. *This encourages and facilitates independence and healthy adaptation to the disease.*
- Provide care in an accepting, nonjudgmental manner. *Acceptance of the client despite potential embarrassment about odors or diarrhea enhances self-esteem.*
- Arrange for interaction with others who have IBD or ostomies. *People who have experienced a similar problem can understand the client's feelings better.*

EVALUATING

Collect data related to the following to evaluate the effectiveness of nursing interventions for the client with IBD: number of diarrheal stools per day, maintenance of skin integrity, hydration status, weight, ability to consume an adequate diet, and apparent coping with current situation.

Documenting. Document continuing assessment data and response to treatment, as well as food and fluid intake and output. Note teaching provided and the client's and family's understanding and acceptance of information.

CONTINUING CARE

Teaching is a vital component of care for the client with IBD, because it is the client who manages the disease on a day-to-day basis. Teach about the disease process, short- and long-term effects, and the relationship of stress to exacerbations of the illness. Talk about risks and benefits of various treatment options. Present information on stress management. Provide information about prescribed medications (names, desired effects, adverse reactions and their management, and schedules for tapering doses if ordered). Discuss manifestations of potential complications and their management. Discuss the increased risk for colorectal cancer and the need for periodic medical follow-up.

Give verbal and written instructions about the recommended diet, and refer to a dietitian as necessary. Emphasize the need to consume a diet of good nutritional value, and note any specific restrictions (e.g., milk and milk products with lactose intolerance). Discuss use of nutritional supplements as needed. Emphasize the need to maintain a fluid intake of at least 2 to 3 quarts per day to replace fluids lost through the stool. Instruct to drink more fluid in hot weather, during exercise or strenuous work, or when feverish. Explain possible indications of malabsorption and impaired nutrition, self-care measures, and when to seek medical intervention. If home parenteral nutrition is planned, teach catheter care and troubleshooting, as well as TPN administration. Have the client and a family member demonstrate catheter care techniques and initiation of feedings prior to discharge.

If surgery is planned, instruct about the surgery and follow-up care. Contact an enterostomal therapy (ET) nurse to meet with the client and family. Teach ostomy care as indicated. Provide resources for obtaining ostomy supplies. Discuss the use of enteric-coated and timed-release drugs that may not be absorbed adequately before elimination through an ileostomy. Provide a list of local ostomy support groups, such as the Foundation for Colitis and Ileitis and the United Ostomy Association. Refer for home care as needed after discharge.

NURSING PROCESS CARE PLAN
Client with Ulcerative Colitis

Cortez Lewis is 42 years old and has had ulcerative colitis for 18 years. She has been treated with prednisone and sulfasalazine. During her most recent exacerbation, she had abdominal pain, cramping, frequent bloody diarrhea stools, and a 20-lb (9-kg) weight loss. A recent colonoscopy showed that her colon is extensively involved. On admission, Mrs. Lewis states, "I'm tired of fighting this disease. I am a prisoner in my home because of the diarrhea." She is admitted for a total colectomy and ileostomy.

Assessment. The nursing assessment on admission reveals that Mrs. Lewis weighs 115 lbs (52.2 kg). Her vital signs are BP 104/72; T 98°F (36.6°C); P 72; R 20. Her skin is cool and pale. Her hemoglobin and hematocrit are low, as is her serum albumin at 2.4 g/dL (normal: 3.5 to 5 g/dL).

Diagnosis. The following nursing diagnoses are established for Mrs. Lewis:

- *Imbalanced Nutrition: Less Than Body Requirements* related to impaired absorption
- *Risk for Deficient Fluid Volume* related to abnormal fluid losses
- *Risk for Impaired Tissue Integrity* related to drainage from ileostomy

- *Pain* related to surgical intervention
- *Risk for Sexual Dysfunction* related to presence of ileostomy
- *Risk for Situational Low Self-Esteem* related to presence of ileostomy

Expected Outcomes. The expected outcomes are that Mrs. Lewis will:

- Tolerate prescribed diet.
- Maintain adequate fluid balance, as demonstrated by assessment data, vital signs, and laboratory results.
- Demonstrate appropriate ostomy care.
- Report pain at 3 or less on a scale of 1 to 10.
- Verbalize feelings about sexuality and discuss issues with her husband.
- Return to work and social activity 6 weeks following surgery.

Planning and Implementation. The nurses plan and implement the following nursing interventions for Mrs. Lewis:

- Discuss dietary modifications related to ileostomy, including foods to avoid and the need to limit high-fiber foods and to chew them well.
- Teach the importance of maintaining a high fluid intake and how to assess its adequacy. Review manifestations of dehydration.
- Teach to empty and change either a one-piece or two-piece ostomy pouch.
- Teach to assess her stoma and peristomal skin with each pouch change.
- Refer to the local United Ostomy Association.
- Provide names of local medical supply companies that sell ostomy appliances.

Evaluation. On discharge, Mrs. Lewis is independently caring for her ileostomy appliance. The ET nurse has given her written and verbal instructions on ileostomy care. Mrs. Lewis verbalizes her understanding of the recommended diet and medications that should be avoided (timed-release forms). The ET nurse has also discussed sexual aspects of having an ileostomy and has given Mrs. Lewis a booklet, "Sex and the Female Ostomate," available through the United Ostomy Association.

Critical Thinking in the Nursing Process

1. Why is the client with an ileostomy at risk for dehydration? What assessments can Mrs. Lewis use at home to monitor her fluid volume status?
2. Why would Mrs. Lewis's hemoglobin and hematocrit be low on admission?
3. What suggestions would you provide to the client with an ileostomy who is concerned about the bag being visible under her clothing or leaking?

STRUCTURAL AND OBSTRUCTIVE DISORDERS

Colorectal Cancer

Colorectal cancer, malignancy of the colon or rectum, is the second leading cause of cancer deaths in Western countries. In the United States, about 145,000 new cases of colorectal cancer were diagnosed in 2005, and 56,300 people died from this disease. The specific cause of colorectal cancer is unknown. A number of risk factors have been identified (Box 20-15 ■), but only about one-fourth of clients diagnosed with colorectal cancer fall into a high-risk group. Therefore, screening for the disease is important. Recent studies suggest that people who use aspirin or another nonsteroidal anti-inflammatory drug on a regular basis and women on hormone replacement therapy have a lower rate of colorectal cancer (American Cancer Society, 2005).

PATHOPHYSIOLOGY

Nearly all colon cancers begin as *polyps,* benign precancerous lesions of the large intestine. The tumor typically grows undetected in the rectum or sigmoid colon (the regions of the bowel most frequently affected, as illustrated in Figure 20-7 ■). By the time symptoms occur, the disease often has spread into deeper layers of the bowel tissue and adjacent organs. Colorectal cancer spreads by direct extension to involve the entire bowel wall. It may extend into neighboring structures (liver or genitourinary tract). It may "seed" other areas of the peritoneal cavity through the bowel wall or during surgery. Metastasis to regional lymph nodes is common, although sometimes distal nodes contain cancer cells while regional nodes remain normal. Cancerous cells may also spread through the lymphatic or circulatory system to the liver, lungs, brain, bones, and kidneys.

MANIFESTATIONS AND COMPLICATIONS

Bowel cancer usually grows slowly. There may be 5 to 15 years of growth before symptoms occur. Manifestations depend on

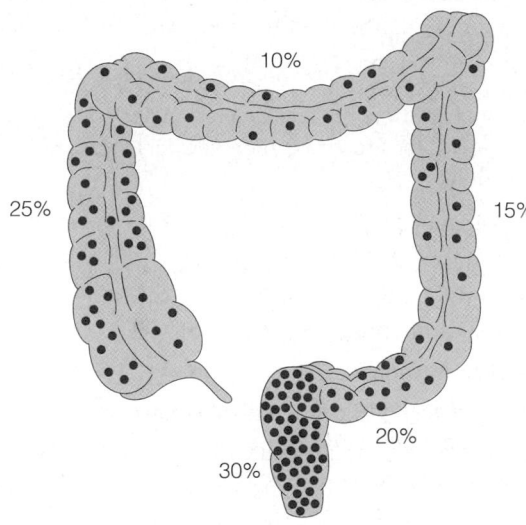

Figure 20-7. ■ The distribution and frequency of colorectal cancer.

tumor location, type and extent, and complications. Bleeding with defecation is often what prompts clients to seek care. A change in bowel habits is another early symptom. In advanced disease, pain, anorexia, and weight loss occur, and a palpable abdominal or rectal mass may be present. Occasionally, anemia from occult bleeding is the presenting symptom.

The prognosis for colon cancer depends most on the stage of the disease at diagnosis and initial treatment. More than half of all people diagnosed with colorectal cancer survive 10 years.

Bowel obstruction due to tumor growth is the primary complication associated with colorectal cancer. Bowel wall perforation and tumor spread to adjacent organs may also occur.

INTERDISCIPLINARY CARE

Because colorectal cancer is often a silent disease and treatment at an early stage has a high cure rate, the American Cancer Society recommends routine screening of all people beginning at age 50:

- Annual *digital rectal examination*
- Annual *fecal occult blood test (FOBT)* or *fecal immunochemical test (FIT)*
- Flexible *sigmoidoscopy* every 5 years; flexible *colonoscopy* every 10 years.

Screening exams are initiated earlier and performed more frequently for clients with IBD, a history of polyps, or a strong family history of colorectal cancer.

Diagnostic Tests

The client with suspected colorectal cancer may undergo extensive diagnostic procedures:

- *Barium enema* may detect the presence and location of a tumor.

BOX 20-15

Risk Factors for Colorectal Cancer

- Age over 50 years
- Personal or family history of colorectal cancer
- Polyps of rectum or colon
- Inflammatory bowel disease
- Smoking, alcohol consumption
- Physical inactivity (possibly)
- Obesity
- High-saturated-fat, low-fiber diet; inadequate fruit and vegetable intake

BOX 20-16   NURSING CARE CHECKLIST

Colonoscopy

Client Preparation

☑ Verify signed consent for the procedure has been obtained.

☑ Withhold food and fluids as ordered. Intake is limited to clear liquids for 1 to 2 days, then NPO for 8 hours before the procedure.

☑ Administer or instruct the client to perform bowel preparation procedures as ordered.

☑ Administer sedation as ordered.

Client and Family Teaching

Before the Procedure

☑ Explain dietary restrictions and their purpose.

☑ The procedure takes 30 minutes to 1 hour. You will be sedated but able to breathe on your own.

☑ The scope is inserted through the anus to visualize the entire large bowel.

☑ Air may be instilled into the bowel during the procedure.

☑ A biopsy may be taken. Polyps may be removed.

☑ Discomfort is minimal.

After the Procedure

☑ Report any abdominal pain, chills, fever, rectal bleeding, or purulent discharge.

☑ If a polyp has been removed, avoid heavy lifting for 7 days, and avoid high-fiber foods for 1 to 2 days.

■ *Sigmoidoscopy* or *colonoscopy* is done to detect and visualize tumors, and to collect tissue for *biopsy.* See Box 20-16 ■ for nursing care of the client undergoing colonoscopy. Tumors typically appear as raised, red, centrally ulcerated, bleeding lesions.

■ *Complete blood count (CBC)* is done to evaluate for anemia.

■ *Carcinoembryonic antigen (CEA,* a protein found in colorectal cancers) levels are measured. CEA levels are used primarily to predict prognosis and to detect tumor recurrence following surgery.

■ *Chest x-ray* is obtained to detect tumor metastasis to the lung. *Computed tomography (CT) scans, magnetic resonance imaging (MRI),* or *ultrasound examinations* may identify involvement of other organs.

Surgery

Surgical resection of the tumor, adjacent colon, and regional lymph nodes is the treatment of choice for colorectal cancer. Small, localized tumors may be excised by laser endoscopy, eliminating the need for abdominal surgery. Most clients with colorectal cancer undergo a *colectomy* (surgical resection of the colon with anastomosis of remaining bowel). Most tumors of the ascending, trans-

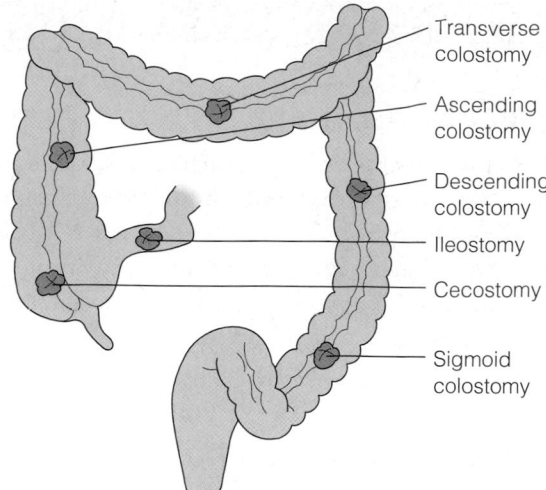

Figure 20-8. ■ The location of different types of colon and small intestinal ostomies.

verse, descending, and sigmoid colon can be resected. Whenever possible, the anal sphincter is preserved and **colostomy** (ostomy made in the colon) is avoided. Tumors of the rectum, however, usually require an *abdominoperineal resection,* in which the sigmoid colon, rectum, and anus are removed through both abdominal and perineal incisions. A permanent colostomy is created for elimination of feces. Nursing care of the client having bowel surgery was described in Box 20-13.

A colostomy may be created if the bowel is obstructed by the tumor or as a temporary measure to promote healing of anastomoses. Colostomies take the name of the portion of the colon from which they are formed (Figure 20-8 ■). In a *double-barrel colostomy,* created to allow bowel healing, two separate stomas are created (Figure 20-9 ■). The distal colon

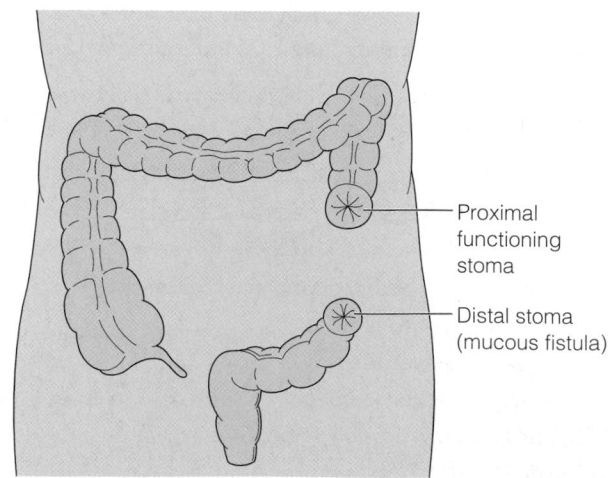

Figure 20-9. ■ A temporary, double-barrel colostomy. The proximal stoma expels feces; the distal stoma expels mucus from the distal colon.

BOX 20-17	NURSING CARE CHECKLIST

Ileostomy or Colostomy

Before Surgery

☑ Contact enterostomal therapy nurse to mark stoma placement and to provide initial teaching about ostomy care and appliances.

☑ Discuss concerns about surgery and the ostomy.

☑ Refer to an ostomy support group as needed or desired.

☑ Provide preoperative bowel preparation as ordered (cathartics, enemas, preoperative antibiotics).

After Surgery

☑ Assess stoma location and appearance. A healthy stoma appears pink or red and moist (see Figure 20-4). It should protrude approximately 2 cm from the abdominal wall. Report dark or white color, prolapse, or *retraction* (indentation) of the stoma to the charge nurse or physician.

☑ Position a collection bag or drainable pouch over the stoma. (Application of ostomy pouches is described in Box 20-18 ■.) Monitor and record color and consistency of ostomy output.

☑ Empty a drainable pouch or replace the colostomy bag when it is no more than one-third full. Measure the drainage, and record as output.

☑ Assess skin surrounding the stoma, and protect with caulking agents, such as Stomahesive or karaya paste, and a skin barrier wafer as needed. Change the bag or pouch if leakage occurs or the client complains of burning or itching skin.

☑ A small needle hole high on the colostomy pouch will allow flatus to escape. For odor control, this hole may be closed with a Band-Aid and opened only while the client is in the bathroom.

☑ Report abnormal assessment findings such as a rash, purulent drainage, ulcerated skin, or bulging around the stoma to the charge nurse or physician.

☑ Prior to discharge, teach ostomy care, pouch management, skin care, and irrigation (as indicated). Allow time for practice.

☑ Emphasize the importance of adequate fluid intake, particularly for clients with an ileostomy or proximal colostomy.

☑ Discuss dietary concerns. A low-residue diet (Table 20-7 ■) may initially be recommended. Foods that may cause excessive odor or gas (e.g., vegetables such as asparagus or cabbage, dried beans, beer and carbonated drinks, or dairy products) are typically avoided, as are foods that can cause a blockage (e.g., popcorn, corn, nuts, caraway seeds, cucumbers, celery, fresh tomatoes, and berries).

TABLE 20-7	
Low-Residue Diet	
FOOD GROUP	**ALLOWED**
Breads and cereals	Products made from refined flours (e.g., white bread) or finely milled grains
Desserts	Gelatins, puddings; ice cream without fruit or nuts
Fruits	Juices and strained fruits; cooked or canned fruits; bananas
Meats and other proteins	Roasted, baked, or broiled meat, poultry, or fish; smooth peanut butter; cream and mild cheeses; milk
Potatoes, rice, and pasta	Peeled potatoes; white rice; most pasta products
Vegetables	Juices and strained vegetables; cooked or canned vegetables
Other	Coffee, tea, carbonated beverages; cream sauce and plain gravy

is not removed, but feces are diverted through the proximal stoma. Small amounts of mucus may be expelled from the distal stoma. A double-barrel colostomy usually is temporary but may be permanent. Nursing care of the client with a colostomy is outlined in Box 20-17 ■.

Adjunctive Therapy

Radiation and chemotherapy often are used in conjunction with surgery to treat colorectal cancers. Pre- or postoperative radiation therapy is used to reduce the recurrence of rectal tumors in the pelvic area. Chemotherapeutic agents are also used postoperatively as adjunctive therapy for colorectal cancer. (Further discussion about radiation and chemotherapy and their nursing implications is included in Chapter 12. 🔗)

NURSING CARE

Nursing care for the client with colorectal cancer is aimed at providing emotional support, teaching, and addressing the surgical client's needs.

ASSESSING

Nursing assessment of the client with colorectal cancer focuses on the effects of the disease and its treatment on the client's ability to function and maintain ADLs.

■ Subjective: Ask about onset of symptoms and current manifestations (including pain); treatment (current and previous); effect of disease and its treatment on ADLs and ability to maintain usual life roles.

BOX 20-18   PROCEDURE CHECKLIST

Changing a One- or Two-Piece Ostomy Pouch

Before the Procedure

☑ Collect all supplies.

☑ Provide for privacy.

☑ Explain the procedure.

Procedure

☑ Use Standard Precautions.

☑ Remove soiled pouch (and the skin barrier flange if present).

☑ Empty the pouch; discard in a plastic bag. Save the tail closure (clamp).

☑ Rinse and reuse pouch from a two-piece system if desired.

☑ Cleanse skin and stoma with warm water and skin cleanser or mild soap. Rinse and pat dry.

☑ Assess stoma and skin condition.

☑ Use a measuring guide or previous pattern to check size of stoma. Trace stoma size onto the back of the pouch flange, and cut the opening no more than 1/8 inch larger than stoma.

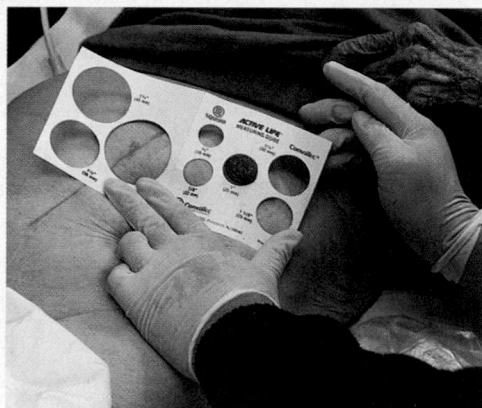

A guide to measure the stoma.

☑ Apply skin prep to peristomal skin and allow to dry.

☑ Remove backing from pouch or flange.

☑ Apply a bead of skin barrier paste around the base of stoma or around the opening of the pouch or flange. Allow the paste to air dry for 1 to 2 minutes.

☑ Center the pouch or flange over the stoma, and press to adhere.

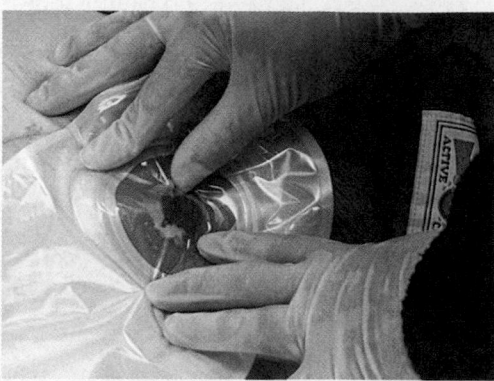

Applying a disposable pouch.

☑ For a two-piece pouch, snap the pouch onto skin barrier flange.

☑ Place deodorizing tablets or a few drops of liquid pouch deodorizer in the pouch. Apply clamp.

☑ "Picture frame" the pouch with tape for extra security as needed.

SAMPLE DOCUMENTATION

11/12/06 1930	Ileostomy pouch changed. 250 mL yellowish brown liquid stool emptied. Stoma bright pink, moist; skin pink and intact with no evidence of breakdown or excoriation.
	_____Karen Leah, LPN.

Note: Refer to a nursing fundamentals or skills text for more detailed instruction. Check state guidelines and facility policy before performing any procedure.

- Objective: general appearance; vital signs; abdominal assessment (see Chapter 18 ⬤) and appearance of any incisions or ostomies, type of fecal output from ostomy.
- Laboratory data: CBC, hemoglobin and hematocrit, serum electrolytes and albumin; CEA level if done.

DIAGNOSING, PLANNING, AND IMPLEMENTING

Pain

The client with colorectal cancer may experience pain from surgical incisions, "phantom" rectal pain, and tumors pressing on nerves and other organs. Postoperatively, patient-controlled analgesia (PCA) and regularly administered analgesics are used to manage pain. If the tumor is inoperable, continuous analgesia delivery (CAD) systems may also be used. (See Chapter 8 ⚭ for more information on caring for clients with pain.)

- Assess frequently for pain, using a standard pain scale. Document intensity, location, and character of the pain. *Pain is a subjective experience; careful assessment improves pain management. Controlling pain facilitates healing and recovery.*
- Assess the effectiveness of pain medications and monitor for adverse effects. *The prescribed dose may need to be increased or decreased based on the client's response.*
- Assess abdomen for distention, tenderness, and bowel sounds; incision for inflammation or swelling; and drainage catheters and tubes for patency. *Poorly controlled pain may indicate an infection, impaired tube drainage, or a complication such as bleeding, peritonitis, or paralytic ileus.*
- Administer analgesics prior to an activity or procedure. *The analgesic can help prevent discomfort with movement or ambulation.*
- Provide nonpharmacologic relief measures, such as positioning, diversion, guided imagery, and relaxation techniques. *These techniques can enhance the effects of analgesia.*
- Splint incision with a pillow, and teach how to self-splint when coughing and deep breathing. *Splinting the incision reduces discomfort associated with muscle contraction and allows more effective coughing and deep breathing.*

Anticipatory Grieving

- Work to develop a trusting relationship with the client and family. Demonstrate respect for cultural, spiritual, and religious values and beliefs. *Providing support during the initial stages of grieving can improve physical recovery, psychologic coping, and eventual adaptation. This increases your effectiveness in helping clients work through the grieving process.*
- Encourage expression of fears and concerns and discussion about the potential impact of loss on individual family members, as well as family structure and function. *Sharing concerns with one another provides support and helps family members develop coping strategies.*
- Help the client and family identify strengths, support systems, and successful coping mechanisms used in past experiences. *These resources can help in dealing with the current situation.*
- Refer to cancer support groups, social services, or counseling as appropriate. *These provide additional resources for support in the grieving process.*

Risk for Sexual Dysfunction

Sexual function may be impaired by surgery, radiation therapy, chemotherapy, or medications prescribed after surgery.

In addition, clients with an ostomy may feel undesirable and fear rejection. They may be concerned about odors or pouch leakage during sexual activity.

- Provide opportunities for client and family to express their feelings about the ostomy. *By doing this, the nurse acknowledges that feelings of anger and depression are normal responses to this change in body function.*
- Provide consistent, secure colostomy care. *An accepting attitude and consistent care that controls odor and leakage instill confidence in the client.*
- Encourage expression of sexual concerns within the client's comfort zone. Provide reassurance that sexual function often improves with healing. *Sexuality is a very private concern, and most people will discuss it only with someone they trust. Many people think an initial decrease in libido means that sexual activity will never be possible again.*
- Refer to social services or a family counselor for further interventions. *Clients are often discharged from acute care settings before concerns about sexual activity begin to surface. Ongoing counseling provides a continuing resource.*
- Arrange for a visit by a member of the United Ostomy Association. *A person who is living successfully with an ostomy is a valuable source of information and support, and often can address questions the client hesitates to ask.*

EVALUATING

To evaluate the effectiveness of care for the client with colorectal cancer, monitor pain levels and the effectiveness of analgesia and other measures to promote comfort. Assess emotional and psychologic responses to the disease and treatment measures (such as colostomy, chemotherapy, etc.). Assess learning and understanding of the disorder, planned treatment, and care of incisions and ostomies.

Documenting. Document the client's and family's responses to teaching and treatment measures, as well as continuing assessment data. If an ostomy is created, document stoma appearance, fecal output, and teaching related to ostomy care.

CONTINUING CARE

Primary prevention of colorectal cancer is an important nursing issue. Teach all clients about American Cancer Society dietary recommendations, including decreasing intake of fat, refined sugar, and red meats and increasing intake of dietary fiber, fresh fruits, and vegetables.

Stress the importance of regular health examinations, including screening by digital rectal exam, fecal occult blood tests, and colonoscopy after age 50. Also stress the need to seek medical treatment if blood is noted in or on the stool. Teach clients that a change in bowel habits may be a warning sign for bowel cancer.

BOX 20-19	PROCEDURE CHECKLIST

Colostomy Irrigation

Before the Procedure

☑ Collect all supplies.

☑ Provide for privacy.

☑ Explain the procedure.

☑ If ambulatory, place client on toilet or commode. Position client confined to bed on right side with bedpan in front.

Procedure

☑ Follow Standard Precautions.

☑ Fill irrigation or enema bag with prescribed amount of warm water or saline. Clear the tubing of air.

☑ Remove ostomy pouch and discard.

☑ Attach an irrigation sleeve over stoma using the belt. Place the bottom of sleeve into the toilet, commode, or bedpan.

☑ Lubricate the cone and insert tip into the stoma. Hold securely to prevent backflow of water.

☑ Instill irrigating solution into the colon from a height of no greater than 12 to 18 inches.

☑ Allow fluid and feces to flow into the toilet or bedpan. Allow about 15 minutes for drainage.

☑ Cleanse the bottom of the sleeve, clamp, and allow client to resume activities.

☑ After approximately 30 to 45 minutes, drain the sleeve and remove.

☑ Clean the stoma and peristomal skin.

☑ Apply a clean ostomy pouch.

After the Procedure

☑ Wash and dry all equipment before storing. Irrigation sleeves are reusable.

SAMPLE DOCUMENTATION

11/12/06 0930	Colostomy irrigated with 500 mL NS. Moderate amount of formed brown stool returned with irrigant. Tolerated procedure well with minimal abdominal cramping and no pain. Stoma pink and moist; skin intact without signs of breakdown.

_____ Mary Alaha, LPN.

Note: Refer to a nursing fundamentals or skills text for more detailed instruction. Check state guidelines and facility policy before performing any procedure.

Teach about various tests and preparation for diagnostic procedures including bowel preparation and food and fluid restrictions. Discuss postprocedure care and potential adverse effects.

Teach care of the ostomy and possible complications to report. (See Boxes 20-18 and 20-19 ■.) Provide a list of resources for ostomy supplies. Refer to the local ostomy association or group. Discuss management of adverse effects if radiation and chemotherapy are planned.

If the cancer is advanced, provide information about pain and symptom management. Discuss the hospice philosophy and available services. Provide referrals as needed.

See the Critical Thinking Care Map at the end of this chapter for an opportunity to apply the nursing process for a client with colorectal cancer.

Bowel Obstruction

A _bowel obstruction_ occurs when intestinal contents fail to move through the bowel. An obstruction can occur in any portion of the intestinal tract. The small intestine (especially the ileum) is the most common site.

PATHOPHYSIOLOGY

A bowel obstruction may be either mechanical or functional. With a _mechanical obstruction_, the bowel is obstructed by a physical barrier like scar tissue or a tumor. _Adhesions_ (bands of scar tissue) are the most common cause of mechanical bowel obstruction. Adhesions usually result from previous abdominal surgery or inflammation. They may cause partial or complete obstruction. Tumors, a twisted bowel, or loops of bowel trapped within a hernia also may cause mechanical bowel obstruction (Figure 20-10 ■). With _functional obstruction (paralytic ileus),_ the bowel lumen remains patent, but peristalsis stops. Paralytic ileus is common in acutely ill clients. It is associated with gastrointestinal surgery, peritoneal inflammation, and certain drugs such as narcotic analgesics.

When obstruction occurs, gas and fluid collect in the bowel proximal to the obstruction, stretching its lumen. Extracellular fluid and electrolytes are drawn into the bowel, producing further distention. This increases pressure within the bowel, which may lead to ischemia and necrosis of the bowel wall. Hypovolemia and shock may result from fluid trapping within the intestine.

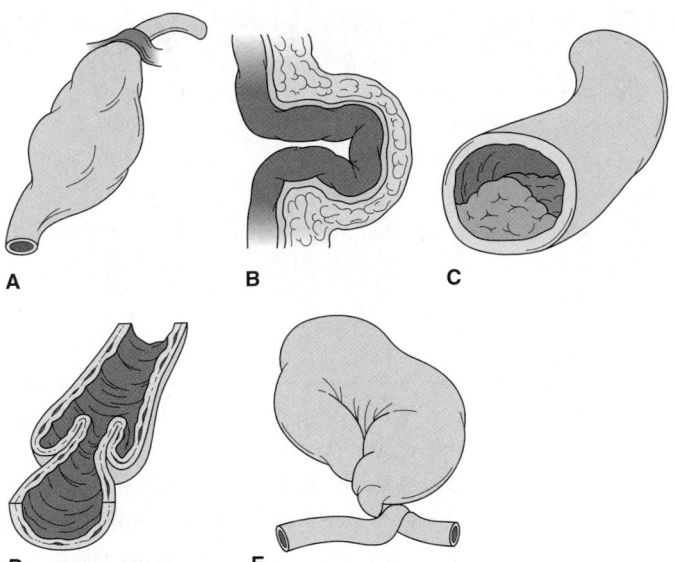

Figure 20-10. ■ Selected causes of mechanical bowel obstruction. **(A)** Adhesions, **(B)** incarcerated (irreducible) hernia, **(C)** tumor, **(D)** intussusception (telescoping of the bowel); **(E)**, volvulus (twisting of the bowel).

MANIFESTATIONS AND COMPLICATIONS

The manifestations of a small-bowel obstruction depend on how fast the obstruction develops and where it occurs (Box 20-20 ■). Cramping or colicky abdominal pain that becomes progressively more severe is common. Vomiting also is common, particularly with obstructions of the small intestine. The vomitus may smell like feces. Early in the obstructive process, bowel sounds are hyperactive and loud (borborygmi); they may be high pitched. As the obstructive process continues and with functional obstruction, few or no bowel sounds are heard. The abdomen becomes distended and tender.

Hypovolemic shock with multiple organ failure and death can result from bowel obstruction. The mortality rate for small-bowel obstruction is approximately 10% (mostly in older adults). Strangulation of the bowel significantly increases the risk of death.

INTERDISCIPLINARY CARE

Management of the client with a bowel obstruction focuses on relieving the obstruction and providing supportive care. Restoration and maintenance of fluid and electrolyte balance is vital to prevent complications.

Diagnostic Tests

Abdominal x-rays are used to confirm the diagnosis of a bowel obstruction. In addition to plain films, contrast media may be used. Evaluation for iodine or seafood allergies prior to the exam is important, because the contrast medium used may contain iodine.

Gastrointestinal Decompression

Most partial and functional small-bowel obstructions are successfully treated with gastrointestinal decompression using a nasogastric tube or long intestinal tube. An intestinal tube (see Figure 20-2) may be inserted through the nose or via gastrostomy. A balloon or weighted tip draws the tube from the stomach into the intestine by peristalsis. Low suction removes fluid and gas until peristalsis resumes or the obstruction is relieved.

Surgery

Surgery may be required to relieve mechanical bowel obstruction. Prior to surgery, a nasogastric or intestinal tube is inserted to relieve vomiting and distention and to prevent aspiration. Intravenous fluids and electrolytes are given to restore fluid and electrolyte balance. Intravenous antibiotics are administered prophylactically. Nursing care of the client having bowel surgery was described in Box 20-13.

NURSING CARE

ASSESSING

Nurses can help identify bowel obstructions early in older adults, homebound clients, or long-term care residents, thus significantly reducing morbidity. Assess all clients who complain of abdominal pain or who stop eating. Inspect the abdomen for distention, listen for bowel sounds, and notify the charge nurse or physician of abnormal findings.

In clients with a suspected or confirmed bowel obstruction, frequent assessment for complications such as fluid and electrolyte imbalance, acid–base imbalances, hypovolemic shock, perforation, and peritonitis is necessary. Monitor laboratory data and report abnormal or unexpected values. Promptly report the client whose abdomen becomes quiet, rigid or boardlike to the touch, and extremely painful and/or tender.

BOX 20-20

MANIFESTATIONS OF BOWEL OBSTRUCTION

- Abdominal pain: cramping or colicky; may be intermittent; increasing intensity; tenderness to palpation; severe, continuous pain may indicate bowel ischemia and possible perforation
- Vomiting; may smell of feces
- Borborygmi and high-pitched, tinkling bowel sounds; diminished or absent bowel sounds
- Abdominal distention; visible peristaltic waves
- Signs of hypovolemia and shock: orthostatic hypotension, tachycardia, tachypnea; decreased urine output

DIAGNOSING, PLANNING, AND IMPLEMENTING

Priorities in Nursing Care. Nurses provide care for clients undergoing nonsurgical treatment for bowel obstruction as well as those who require surgery to relieve the obstruction. Preventing complications of obstruction and surgery are the priority areas of focus for nursing care.

Deficient Fluid Volume

The obstructive process draws body fluids into the bowel and often causes vomiting. As a result, the client is at risk for a fluid volume deficit.

- Monitor vital signs and central venous pressure (CVP) hourly. *Tachycardia, a drop in blood pressure, and tachypnea may indicate hypovolemia. The CVP is an effective measurement of fluid volume status.*
- Measure urine output hourly and nasogastric output every 2 to 4 hours. Maintain intravenous fluids and blood replacement as ordered. *Urine output of less than 30 mL/hr indicates decreased cardiac output and hypovolemia. Nasogastric output is measured as a guideline for fluid replacement. Intravenous fluids are given to meet current needs and replace losses.*
- Measure abdominal girth every 4 to 8 hours. Mark the area to be measured on the abdomen. *A reference mark allows consistent, accurate measurements. Increased abdominal girth indicates increasing intestinal distention.*
- Notify the charge nurse or physician of changes in status. *Changes can indicate the need for immediate surgery.*

Ineffective Breathing Pattern

Abdominal distention from a bowel obstruction can place pressure on the diaphragm. Pain from abdominal surgery may lead to shallow breathing. Aspiration of GI contents during vomiting is also a risk in the client with bowel obstruction.

- Assess respiratory rate, pattern, and lung sounds every 2 to 4 hours. Monitor pulse oximetry levels. *Diminished breath sounds or crackles in the lung bases indicate poor ventilation. Tachypnea, shortness of breath, dyspnea, or fall in pulse oximetry readings (<90% to 92%) may indicate respiratory compromise. Notify the charge nurse or physician.*
- Elevate the head of the bed. *This reduces pressure on the diaphragm.*
- Provide a pillow or folded bath blanket to use in splinting the abdomen while coughing postoperatively. *The ease and effectiveness of coughing are improved when abdominal muscles and incisions are splinted.*
- Maintain the patency of nasogastric or intestinal suction. *Suction prevents further abdominal distention or aspiration of intestinal contents during vomiting.*

- Encourage use of incentive spirometry or other assistive devices. *Assistive devices help the client open distal airways and prevent atelectasis.*
- Contact respiratory therapy as indicated. *Additional measures to maintain pulmonary status may be available.*
- Provide good oral care at least every 4 hours. *Dehydration and nasogastric suction lead to dry mouth and throat, increasing the risk of bacterial growth. Many respiratory infections are the result of aspirated organisms.*

EVALUATING

To evaluate the effectiveness of nursing care, collect continuing assessment data related to the obstruction itself (abdominal girth, bowel sounds, pain and tenderness), fluid volume status (vital signs, weight, intake and output, skin and mucous membrane temperature and moisture, skin turgor), and potential complications such as atelectasis (respiratory assessment including breath sounds over all lung fields).

Documenting. Document continuing assessment data; intake and output; amount, color, and odor of nasogastric drainage; vomitus; or stool. If surgery has been performed, document appearance of the wound, and the type, color, and amount of any drainage noted on the dressing or from wound drains. Monitor bowel sounds on a continuing basis, and document when they return and when the client begins to pass flatus.

CONTINUING CARE

Instruct the client and family about wound care, activity level after discharge, return to work, and any other recommended restrictions or procedures. If a temporary colostomy has been created, teach the client and family about its care. For the client with recurrent obstructions, discuss cause, early identification of symptoms, and preventive measures.

Hernia

A *hernia* is a protrusion of an organ or structure through a defect in the muscular wall of the abdomen. Hernias may contain loops of bowel or other internal organs. They may be congenital or acquired. Acquired hernias are associated with weakening of the normal musculature. They may be related to surgery, trauma such as heavy lifting, or gradual increases in intra-abdominal pressure caused by pregnancy, obesity, or ascites.

PATHOPHYSIOLOGY AND MANIFESTATIONS

Hernias are classified by their location (Figure 20-11 ■). Most hernias occur in the groin and are known as *inguinal hernias*.

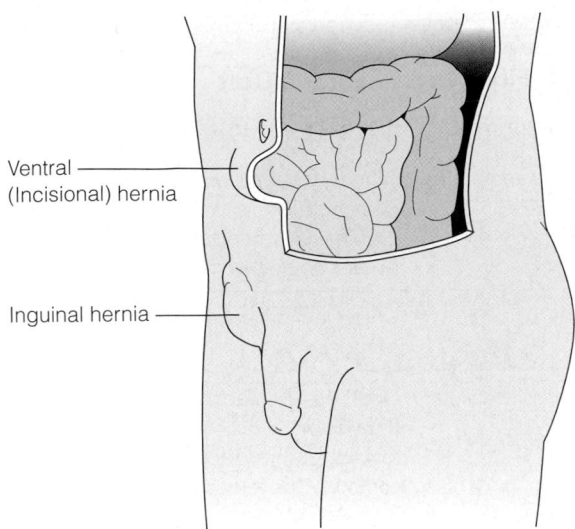

Ventral (Incisional) hernia

Inguinal hernia

Figure 20-11. ■ An abdominal wall (ventral or incisional) hernia and an inguinal hernia.

Inguinal hernias are usually caused by incomplete closure of the tract that develops as the testes descend into the scrotum before birth. They often do not become apparent until increased intra-abdominal pressure causes abdominal contents to enter the channel in adulthood. In older adults, weakness of the posterior inguinal wall can also lead to an inguinal hernia. Inguinal hernias often produce no symptoms and are discovered during routine physical examination. A lump, swelling, or bulge in the groin may be noted with lifting or straining. The client may complain of pain that radiates into the scrotum.

Umbilical and ventral (*incisional*) hernias occur in the abdominal wall. *Umbilical hernias* may be congenital or acquired; pregnancy, obesity, and ascites are common risk factors. *Ventral hernias* result from inadequate healing of a surgical incision.

If a hernia is *reducible,* contents of the sac return to the abdominal cavity when intra-abdominal pressure is reduced (as with lying down) or with manual pressure. When the contents of a hernia cannot be returned to the abdominal cavity, it is said to be *irreducible* or *incarcerated.* Contents of an incarcerated hernia are trapped, usually by a narrow opening to the hernia. *Obstruction* occurs when the lumen of the bowel contained within the hernia becomes occluded, much like the crimping of a hose.

A *strangulated hernia* occurs when the blood supply to tissue within the hernia is compromised. This can lead to infarction (necrosis) of affected bowel with severe pain and perforation. Manifestations of a strangulated hernia include abdominal pain and distention, nausea, vomiting, tachycardia, and fever.

INTERDISCIPLINARY CARE

The diagnosis of a hernia is made by examining the client in a supine and sitting or standing position. A bulge may be seen or felt when the client coughs or bears down. No laboratory or diagnostic testing is usually required, unless bowel obstruction or strangulation is suspected.

All types of hernia are surgically repaired (*herniorrhaphy*) unless specific contraindications to surgery exist. Heavy lifting and heavy manual labor are restricted for approximately 3 weeks after surgery. When surgery is not an option, the client may be taught to reduce the hernia by lying down and gently pushing down against the mass. A binder or truss may be worn to prevent or control the protrusion.

NURSING CARE

The client undergoing a herniorrhaphy has few acute nursing care needs apart from preoperative assessment and immediate postoperative care. Operative nursing care is similar to care of a client with an appendectomy.

Risk for Ineffective Tissue Perfusion: Gastrointestinal

- Assess comfort. Notify the primary care provider if the hernia becomes painful or tender. Promptly report an acute increase in abdominal, groin, perineal, or scrotal pain. *Pain or tenderness of the hernia may indicate incarceration. An abrupt increase in pain may indicate bowel ischemia due to strangulation. Rapid identification of the problem is vital to prevent major complications such as peritonitis.*
- Assess bowel sounds and abdominal distention at least every 8 hours. *A change in bowel sounds—either cessation of sounds or hyperactive, high-pitched sounds—and increasing abdominal girth may indicate obstruction.*
- If signs of possible obstruction or strangulation occur, place the client in the supine position with the hips elevated and knees slightly bent. Keep NPO, and begin preparations for surgery. *This position helps relax abdominal muscles and may facilitate reduction of the hernia. Strangulation or obstruction require immediate surgical intervention.*

CONTINUING CARE

Most teaching related to hernias is done during routine health examinations. Teach clients what hernias are and the risk factors for their development. Reassure clients that surgical intervention is generally without complications, even in older adults, and carries a lower risk than not repairing the hernia. Teach clients how to reduce hernias if necessary, and stress the importance of seeking immediate medical intervention if signs of strangulation or obstruction occur. When surgery is planned, instruct the client to notify the physician should he or she develop an upper respiratory infection and cough, because forceful coughing is not recommended postoperatively. Reinforce postoperative teaching about pain management and activity restrictions following surgery.

Diverticular Disease

Diverticula are acquired saclike projections of bowel mucosa through the muscular layer of the colon (Figure 20-12 ▪). They occur most often in the sigmoid colon. Diverticular disease affects millions, but few people have symptoms. A diet of highly refined and fiber-deficient foods is a major risk factor for diverticula. Other risk factors include aging, a sedentary lifestyle, and postponing bowel movements.

PATHOPHYSIOLOGY AND MANIFESTATIONS

Diverticula form when increased pressure within the bowel causes the mucosa to herniate through defects in the wall. *Diverticulosis* is the presence of diverticula. Diverticulosis is usually asymptomatic. Clients may experience episodic left lower quadrant pain, constipation, and diarrhea.

Diverticulitis is inflammation and perforation of a diverticulum, usually in the sigmoid colon. The process is similar to that which occurs when appendicitis develops. Infection occurs when undigested food becomes trapped in a diverticulum, and its blood supply is impaired, allowing bacterial invasion. Perforation results from ischemia and necrosis of the mucosa.

Pain is a common manifestation of diverticulitis. It is usually left sided and may be mild to severe and either steady or cramping. Constipation or diarrhea, nausea, vomiting, and low-grade fever may occur. Complications include hemorrhage, peritonitis, abscess or fistula formation, and bowel obstruction.

INTERDISCIPLINARY CARE

Management of diverticular disease ranges from no prescribed intervention to surgical resection of affected colon.

TABLE 20-8	
High-Fiber, High-Residue Diet	
FOOD GROUP	RECOMMENDED FOODS
Cereals and grains	Wheat or oat bran; cooked whole-grain cereals; dry cereals such as bran flakes, corn flakes, shredded wheat; whole-grain breads or crackers; brown rice
Fruits	Unpeeled raw apples, peaches, and pears; oranges
Vegetables	Dried beans (black, red, pinto, or kidney), lima beans; broccoli; peas; corn; squash; raw vegetables such as carrots, celery, and tomatoes; potatoes with skins

In addition to the history and physical exam, a *flexible sigmoidoscopy* or *colonoscopy* or a *CT scan* may be performed to establish the diagnosis. See Chapter 18 ⚭ and Boxes 20-1 and 20-16 for more information about these tests.

A diet high in fiber is prescribed for clients with diverticulosis (Table 20-8 ▪). The client generally is advised to avoid foods with small seeds (such as popcorn, caraway seeds, figs, or berries), which could obstruct diverticula.

Bowel rest and antibiotic therapy are prescribed during an acute episode of diverticulitis. The client initially may be NPO with intravenous fluids and total parenteral nutrition. Feeding is resumed gradually, progressing from clear liquids to a soft, low-roughage diet with daily added psyllium seed to soften stool and increase its bulk. The high-fiber diet is resumed following full recovery. Surgery may be required if the client develops an abscess or peritonitis. Review Box 20-13 for nursing care of the client having bowel surgery.

NURSING CARE

The nurse's role for diverticulosis is mainly educational. Teach clients in all settings about the benefits of a high-fiber diet in preventing diverticular disease, bowel cancer, and other disorders. In residential or foster care settings, work with dietary staff and care providers to increase the amount of fiber in residents' diets, unless contraindicated.

Emphasize the importance of maintaining a high-fiber diet to reduce the incidence of complications of diverticulosis. Discuss how to increase dietary fiber, and refer to a dietitian as needed. Provide instruction about complications of the disease and their manifestations.

For the client with acute diverticulitis, explain prescribed treatment and food and fluid limitations. Explain

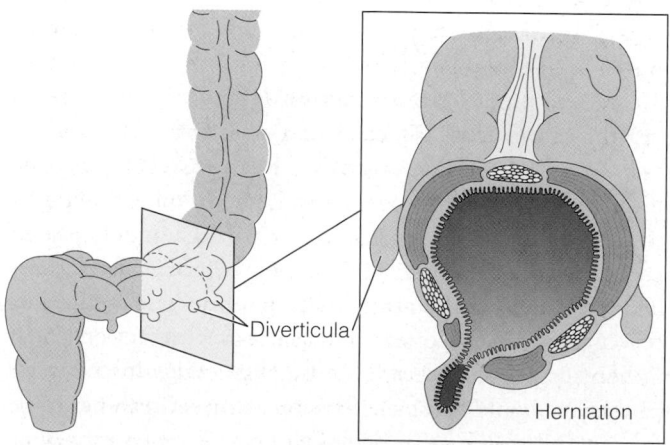

Figure 20-12. ▪ Diverticula of the colon.

why dietary fiber is limited during acute inflammation but increased for chronic management. Provide discharge instruction for clients undergoing surgery. Refer to community health care agencies as needed.

ANORECTAL DISORDERS

Anorectal conditions include hemorrhoids, as well as lesions such as fissures, abscess, fistulas, and pilonidal disease.

Hemorrhoids

When pressure on the veins of the anus and anal canal is increased or venous return is impaired, the veins weaken and distend, forming **hemorrhoids** (or *piles*). Virtually all adults have hemorrhoids, usually asymptomatic.

Straining to defecate is the most common cause of hemorrhoids. Pregnancy increases intra-abdominal pressure and also is an important cause of hemorrhoids. Contributing factors include prolonged sitting, obesity, chronic constipation, and a low-fiber diet.

Internal hemorrhoids develop above the mucocutaneous junction of the anus (Figure 20-13 ■). They rarely cause pain, and usually present with bright red bleeding that is unmixed with stool. It can vary from streaks on toilet tissue to enough to color the water in the toilet. The client may experience a feeling of incomplete stool evacuation. As they enlarge, hemorrhoids may *prolapse* or protrude through the anus.

External hemorrhoids develop below the mucocutaneous junction. Bleeding is rare with external hemorrhoids. Anal irritation, a feeling of pressure, and difficulty cleaning the anal region may be manifestations of external hemorrhoids.

"Normal" hemorrhoids are not painful. Prolapsed hemorrhoids may become strangulated, leading to thrombosis (clotting). Thrombosed hemorrhoids cause extreme pain.

Internal hemorrhoids associated with portal hypertension and liver disease may rupture and bleed profusely.

INTERDISCIPLINARY CARE

Management of hemorrhoids is conservative unless complications occur. Internal hemorrhoids are diagnosed by *anoscopic* exam. A sigmoidoscopy or colonoscopy may be done to rule out colorectal cancer, which can produce similar manifestations.

A high-fiber diet and increased water intake to increase stool bulk, improve its softness, and reduce straining is effective for most clients with internal or external hemorrhoids. Bulk-forming laxatives (e.g., Metamucil) or stool softeners like docusate sodium may be prescribed. Suppositories and local ointments (e.g., Preparation H, Nupercaine) have an anesthetic and astringent effect that reduces discomfort and irritation of surrounding tissues. They have little or no effect on the hemorrhoid itself. Warm sitz baths, bed rest, and local astringent compresses may be recommended to shrink edematous prolapsed hemorrhoids after digital reduction.

Prolapsed or thrombosed hemorrhoids may require additional treatment. *Sclerotherapy* involves injecting a chemical irritant into tissues surrounding the hemorrhoid to cause inflammation and scarring. *Rubber band ligation* involves placing a rubber band snugly around the hemorrhoid and surrounding mucosa, causing the tissue to necrose and slough within 7 to 10 days. Repeat treatments may be necessary. In *hemorrhoidectomy,* hemorrhoids are surgically excised.

NURSING CARE

Most clients with hemorrhoids are treated in outpatient settings. Nurses have frequent opportunities to teach preventive measures for hemorrhoids. Stress the importance of dietary fiber, liberal fluid intake, and regular exercise to maintain stool bulk, softness, and regularity. Discuss the need to respond to the urge to defecate rather than postpone it. Discuss constipation management, including use of bulk-forming laxatives. Stress that stool softeners should be used only for short-term relief. Discuss appropriate use of over-the-counter preparations for hemorrhoid symptom relief.

Discuss signs of possible complications, such as chronic bleeding, prolapse, and thrombosis. Discuss the link between manifestations of hemorrhoids and colorectal cancer. Urge the client to seek medical care for persistent, unresolved, or progressive symptoms.

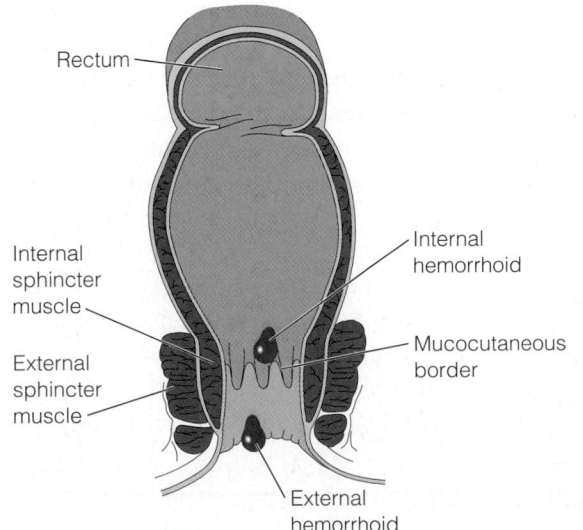

Figure 20-13. ■ The location of internal and external hemorrhoids.

BOX 20-21   NURSING CARE CHECKLIST

Perianal Surgery (Postoperative)

☑ Monitor vital signs and urinary output every 4 hours.

☑ Inspect rectal dressing every 2 to 3 hours; observe closely for bleeding.

☑ Assist to position of comfort, usually side-lying.

☑ Provide analgesics as ordered and before first bowel movement.

☑ Apply ice packs over rectal dressing as ordered.

☑ Assist with sitz bath three to four times per day, providing a rubber ring or donut device for comfort.

☑ Provide a flotation pad for sitting.

☑ Give stool softeners as ordered.

☑ Encourage fluid intake of at least 2,000 mL per day.

Client and Family Teaching

☑ Take sitz bath after each bowel movement for 1 to 2 weeks after surgery.

☑ Drink at least 2 quarts of fluid per day.

☑ Eat adequate dietary fiber, and exercise moderately.

☑ Take stool softeners as prescribed.

☑ Report to the physician the following symptoms: rectal bleeding, continued pain on defecation, a temperature greater than 101°F (38.3°C), purulent rectal drainage.

When a hemorrhoidectomy is performed, the client requires more direct nursing care. Postoperative care of the client with perianal surgery is outlined in Box 20-21 ■. Anal packing may be left in place for 24 hours after surgery. Closely observe for bleeding when it is removed. Postoperative pain can be significant because of rich innervation of the anal region and possible muscle spasms.

Anorectal Lesions

ANAL FISSURE

An *anal fissure* is an ulcer on the anal margin. Irritating diarrheal stools, childbirth trauma, habitual cathartic use, and anal intercourse may cause anal fissures. Tissues surrounding the fissure become chronically inflamed. Pain and small amounts of bright red bleeding occur with defecation. Anticipated pain may lead to constipation, which further aggravates symptoms. Treatment involves increased fluid and dietary fiber intake, as well as bulk-forming laxatives. A topical agent such as hydrocortisone cream may be prescribed.

ANORECTAL ABSCESS

Bacterial invasion of tissue around the anus can lead to *anorectal abscess*. Pain, which may be aggravated by sitting or walking, is the primary manifestation of an anorectal abscess. External swelling, redness, heat, and tenderness are apparent on examination. If the abscess does not drain spontaneously, an incision and drainage (I&D) is performed. Anorectal abscesses rarely resolve with antibiotic therapy alone.

ANORECTAL FISTULA

A *fistula* is a tunnel or tubelike tract with openings at each end. Anorectal fistulas have one opening in the anal canal and the other usually in skin around the anus. A fistula may develop spontaneously or result from an anorectal abscess or Crohn's disease. Drainage is intermittent or constant and may be purulent. It may be accompanied by local itching, tenderness, and pain with defecation. The fistula may heal spontaneously, or a *fistulotomy* may be performed. The primary opening of the fistula is closed, and the tract is opened to allow healing by secondary intention, from the inside out.

PILONIDAL DISEASE

Pilonidal disease is an acute abscess or chronic draining sinus in the sacrococcygeal area. Beneath the abscess or sinus is a cyst that often contains hair tufts. Pilonidal disease usually affects young hirsute (hairy) males; it is probably caused by trapping of hair in deep tissues. It may be congenital. The cyst is generally asymptomatic unless it becomes infected. Infection causes pain, tenderness, redness, heat, and swelling of the affected area. Purulent discharge may be noted. Pilonidal disease is treated with incision and drainage. The sinus tract and underlying cyst are excised and closed.

NURSING CARE

Teach the client with a perianal lesion to maintain a high-fiber diet and liberal fluid intake to decrease discomfort with defecation. Stress the importance of responding to the urge to defecate to prevent constipation.

Following surgical treatment of any of these disorders, teach the client to avoid soiling the dressing with urine or feces during elimination. Instruct to keep the perianal region clean and dry, gently cleansing the area with soap and water after a bowel movement. Encourage sitz baths for cleaning and comfort. Suggest taking an analgesic prior to defecation, but caution that some analgesics may promote constipation. Teach signs and symptoms of infection or other possible complications to report to the physician.

Note: The bibliography listings for this and all chapters have been compiled at the back of the book.

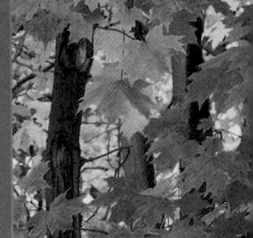

Chapter Review

 **KEY TERMS** by Topics

Use the audio glossary feature of either the CD-ROM or the Companion Website to hear the correct pronunciation of the following key terms.

Disorders of motility and absorption
diarrhea, constipation, malabsorption

Inflammatory disorders
appendicitis, laparotomy, laparoscopy, peritonitis, paralytic ileus, ulcerative colitis, Crohn's disease, colectomy, ostomy, ileostomy

Structural and obstructive disorders
colostomy, diverticulitis, hemorrhoids

KEY Points

- Diarrhea is a manifestation of many bowel disorders. When prolonged or severe, diarrhea can lead to serious fluid and electrolyte imbalances, as well as excoriation of perianal tissues.

- Constipation, another disorder of bowel motility, often is a functional disorder caused by inadequate fluid intake, lack of dietary fiber, or voluntary retention of stool. Encourage all clients (unless specifically contraindicated) to consume generous amounts of water and a diet high in fiber.

- Most laxatives are appropriate for short-term use (1 week or less) only. Bulk-forming laxatives may be used for longer periods if necessary.

- Clients with early manifestations of appendicitis need to be evaluated promptly to reduce the risk of perforation of the inflamed appendix and contamination of the peritoneal cavity.

- A rigid, boardlike abdomen and severe abdominal pain usually indicate acute inflammation of the peritoneum and a need for immediate medical intervention.

- Rectal bleeding may indicate hemorrhoids (a common, benign condition) or colorectal cancer. All clients with rectal bleeding should undergo testing (e.g., colonoscopy) for colorectal cancer.

- Advise all clients over the age of 50 to undergo yearly digital rectal exam and testing for occult blood in the stool. A colonoscopy should be done at age 50 and every 5 to 10 years thereafter. Clients with inflammatory bowel disease have a significantly increased risk for colorectal cancer and should begin screening exams at an earlier age.

- Early manifestations of a bowel obstruction include high-pitched, tinkling bowel sounds. Later manifestations include absent bowel sounds, abdominal distention, and possible vomiting.

- A warm sitz bath is an appropriate nursing measure for clients with an anorectal disorder such as hemorrhoids (unless contraindicated by specific procedures performed).

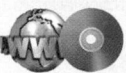 **EXPLORE MediaLink**

Additional interactive resources for this chapter can be found on the Companion Website at www.prenhall.com/burke. Click on Chapter 20 and "Begin" to select the activities for this chapter.

For chapter-related NCLEX-style review questions and an audio glossary, access the accompanying CD-ROM in this book.

FOR FURTHER Study

For more information on fluid imbalances, see Chapter 7.

See Chapter 8 for more information on caring for clients in pain.

For information on providing routine care for the surgical client, see Chapter 9.

For nursing implications for common antibiotics, see Table 10-5.

Autoimmunity is discussed further in Chapter 11.

For more information on radiation and chemotherapy, see Chapter 12.

For an in-depth discussion of shock, see Chapter 13.

See Chapters 18 and 31 for more information about diagnostic tests used to identify bowel problems.

For more about parenteral nutrition, see Chapter 19.

Nursing care for the client having paracentesis is given in Box 21-13.

Critical Thinking Care Map

Caring for a Client with Colorectal Cancer

NCLEX-PN® Focus Area: Reduction of Risk Potential

Case Study: William Cunningham is a 65-year-old man who has noticed small amounts of blood in his stools for the past 3 months. His physician finds a palpable mass on digital rectal exam, and orders a colonoscopy. A large rectal lesion is found; biopsy shows it to be adenocarcinoma. Mr. Cunningham is scheduled for an abdominoperineal resection and sigmoid colostomy.

Nursing Diagnosis: Risk for Impaired Skin Integrity

COLLECT DATA

Subjective	Objective
_____	_____
_____	_____
_____	_____
_____	_____
_____	_____
_____	_____

Would you report this data? Yes/No

If yes, to: _____

Nursing Care

_____

_____

_____

_____

_____

_____

_____

_____

How would you document this? _____

_____

_____

_____

Data Collected
(use those that apply)

- Sense of pressure in rectum
- Intermittent constipation
- BP 118/78; T 98.4°F (36.9°C); P 82; R 18
- Height 5'10" (178 cm), weight 185 lbs (84 kg)
- States, "I really don't want a colostomy, but if that is what it takes to keep me well, I'm ready to get it over with."

Nursing Interventions
(use those that apply; list in priority order)

- Provide analgesia as ordered, evaluating its effectiveness.
- Frequently assess stoma and peristomal skin condition.
- Discuss foods that cause odor and gas.
- Teach colostomy care.
- Maintain consistent nursing personnel assignment to facilitate trust.
- Refer to the local United Ostomy Association.
- Provide a list of local resources for ostomy supplies.
- Provide for privacy when teaching and discussing concerns about ostomy.

NCLEX-PN® Exam Preparation

1 The first priority for a nurse admitting a client with severe diarrhea to an acute medical unit would be to:

A. prevent skin breakdown.

B. assess the client's fluid volume status.

C. administer an antidiarrheal medication.

D. obtain a thorough client history.

2 An elderly client complains that her bowels move only two or three times a week. The most appropriate response by the nurse would be:

A. "You should start using a laxative to ensure a daily movement. I'll write down some safe laxatives for you."

B. "Reducing the amount of fiber in your diet may help. I'll give you a low-residue diet plan."

C. "Let's talk to the doctor about getting you scheduled for a colonoscopy to evaluate your large intestine."

D. "That pattern may be normal for you. Tell me about your stool—is it hard or difficult to expel?"

3 A client comes to the walk-in clinic complaining of abdominal pain that started about 2 hours previously. In his assessment, the nurse notes tenderness in the right lower quadrant, and checks for rebound. Rebound tenderness is characterized by:

A. relief of pain with palpation followed by pain when pressure is released.

B. intensification of pain when the area is palpated.

C. a rigid, boardlike abdomen that is extremely tender.

D. pain in the affected quadrant when the opposite quadrant is palpated.

4 A client with irritable bowel syndrome states, "If it wasn't for my job I wouldn't be here." Your best response would be:

A. "I think you should discuss this with a trained counselor."

B. "Usually, this disease is related to stress. I'll get an educational video for you to watch."

C. "You must have some strong feelings about your job. Do you want to talk about it?"

D. "I will ask the physician for an antianxiety medication."

5 A client has been admitted with severe diarrhea. The nurse bases his decision on whether to administer the prescribed antidiarrheal medication on the understanding that antidiarrheal medication:

A. should not be used until the cause of diarrhea has been determined.

B. should be administered upon manifestation of diarrhea to prevent losses of fluids and electrolytes.

C. should be withheld until stool cultures and samples have been obtained.

D. should not be administered until fluid and electrolyte status have been established.

6 The nurse is teaching a client with newly diagnosed ulcerative colitis about her prescription for sulfasalazine (Azulfidine). Which of the following does the nurse include in teaching? (Choose all that apply.)

A. Take this pill with a small sip of water at least an hour before meals.

B. Use sunscreen while you are taking this drug to prevent sunburns.

C. If you use oral contraceptives, use additional protection while taking this drug.

D. A skin rash is a common side effect of this drug; it will abate with time.

E. While you are using this drug, use aspirin, not acetaminophen for pain relief.

7 When a client is prescribed a low-residue diet, which of the following menu choices indicates an understanding of the diet?

A. steak, baked potato, carrot sticks, lemon meringue pie

B. steamed fish, baked potato, green beans, fresh fruit cup

C. broiled chicken breast, mashed potatoes, whipped squash, angel food cake

D. fried chicken, mashed potatoes, corn, angel food cake

8 The nurse caring for a client with a possible bowel obstruction would immediately report which of the following?

A. hypoactive bowel sounds

B. a flat, soft abdomen

C. fecal-smelling nasogastric tube drainage

D. increased pain with a rigid, boardlike abdomen

9 A client recovering from bowel surgery is asking for regular food. The nurse's most appropriate response would be:

A. "When you start passing gas and your bowel is working again, it will be safe to start eating again."

B. "When you no longer require narcotic pain medication, it will be safe to reintroduce food."

C. "The IV fluids you are receiving are adequate nourishment."

D. "When you are able to ambulate, introducing food will be considered."

10 The nurse talking to a community group includes which of the following in her discussion of colorectal cancer?

A. When you have reached the age of 50, you should have an annual digital rectal exam and a flexible sigmoidoscopy or colonoscopy every 5 years.

B. People with inflammatory bowel disease need a flexible sigmoidoscopy or colonoscopy every 5 years after age 50 for early detection of polyps.

C. When you have reached the age of 50, you need to have a lab test called carcinoembryonic antigen (CEA) to determine the need for colonoscopy.

D. When you have reached the age of 50, you need to have annual checks due to the rapid growth of bowel tumors.

Answers for Review Questions, as well as discussion of Care Plan and Critical Thinking Care Map questions, appear in Appendix V.

Chapter 21

Caring for Clients with Gallbladder, Liver, and Pancreatic Disorders

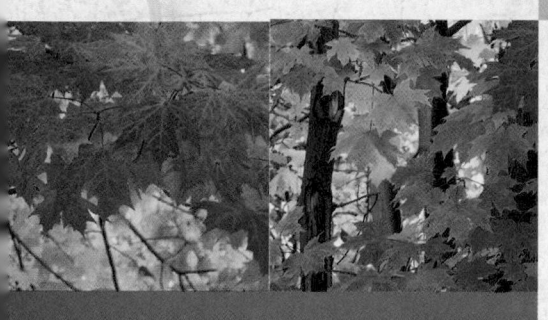

BRIEF Outline

Gallbladder Disorders
Cholelithiasis and Cholecystitis
Cancer of the Gallbladder

Liver Disorders
Hepatitis
Cirrhosis
Cancer of the Liver
Liver Trauma

Exocrine Pancreatic Disorders
Pancreatitis
Cancer of the Pancreas

LEARNING Outcomes

After completing this chapter, you will be able to:

- Describe the pathophysiology, manifestations and effects, and management of common disorders of the gallbladder, liver, and exocrine pancreas.

- Discuss nursing implications for dietary and pharmacologic interventions related to the gallbladder, liver, and exocrine pancreas.

- Provide appropriate nursing care for the client who has surgery of the gallbladder, liver, or pancreas.

- Use the nursing process to assess, plan, provide, and evaluate care for clients with disorders of the gallbladder, liver, or exocrine pancreas.

Disorders of the accessory digestive organs—the gallbladder, liver, and exocrine pancreas—may present as solitary problems or may be related to other disease processes. One organ's functioning frequently affects that of another. Inflammation or obstruction of ducts and impairment of the multiple functions of the gallbladder, liver, and exocrine pancreas are some of the problems that can adversely affect a person's health. Review Chapter 18 🔗 for the normal structure and function of the gallbladder, liver, and pancreas.

Clients who have a disorder of the gallbladder, liver, or exocrine pancreas may experience severe pain, altered body image, and a host of metabolic and nutritional disturbances. Nursing care addresses the client's and family's physiologic and psychosocial needs through attention to individualized care planning.

GALLBLADDER DISORDERS

Altered bile flow through the ducts of the liver, gallbladder, and common bile duct is common, often leading to inflammation and other problems of the affected organs.

Cholelithiasis and Cholecystitis

Cholelithiasis, the formation of stones (*calculi*) within the gallbladder or biliary duct system, is the most common disorder of the gallbladder. Gallstones also are the most common cause of obstructed bile flow. Risk factors for cholelithiasis include middle age, female gender, obesity, pregnancy, and use of oral contraceptives or estrogen therapy (Box 21-1 ■).

clinical ALERT

Certain very low calorie diets increase the risk for gallstones. Ask clients with symptoms of gallbladder disease about their current diet and any recent changes.

PATHOPHYSIOLOGY

Most gallstones are formed in the gallbladder, prompted by the interaction of abnormal bile composition, ineffective bile flow, and inflammation of the gallbladder. Gallstones usually contain cholesterol, bile pigments, and small amounts of other materials, such as calcium salts. Several factors raise the level of cholesterol in bile: obesity, a high-calorie, high-cholesterol diet, and drugs that lower blood cholesterol levels. Ironically, very low calorie diets and fasting also raise bile cholesterol concentration and reduce its flow in the biliary system.

Gallstones usually form in the gallbladder and may migrate into the ducts, causing ductal inflammation (*cholangitis*). It often is this migration and resulting inflammation that cause the manifestations of cholelithiasis.

Cholecystitis is inflammation of the gallbladder. It usually results from stones obstructing the cystic or common bile duct (Figure 21-1 ■). The obstruction causes increased pressure and ischemia of the gallbladder, as well as chemical irritation from the bile. The gallbladder becomes acutely inflamed as a result. The inflammation causes edema and further obstruction of bile flow. Ischemia can lead to necrosis and perforation of the gallbladder. Chronic cholecystitis is caused by repeated attacks of acute cholecystitis. Chronic cholecystitis may be asymptomatic.

If the common bile duct is obstructed, bile backs up into the liver and possibly the pancreas, producing jaundice, pain, possible hepatic damage, pancreatitis (discussed later in this chapter), or sepsis.

BOX 21-1	ASSESSMENT

Risk Factors for Gallstones

- Age
- Family history
- Race or ethnicity: Native American, Northern European heritage
- Obesity, high blood cholesterol levels
- Rapid weight loss; very low calorie diets
- Female gender, oral contraceptive use
- Biliary stasis: pregnancy, fasting, prolonged total parenteral nutrition
- Disorders: cirrhosis, small intestinal disorders, sickle cell anemia

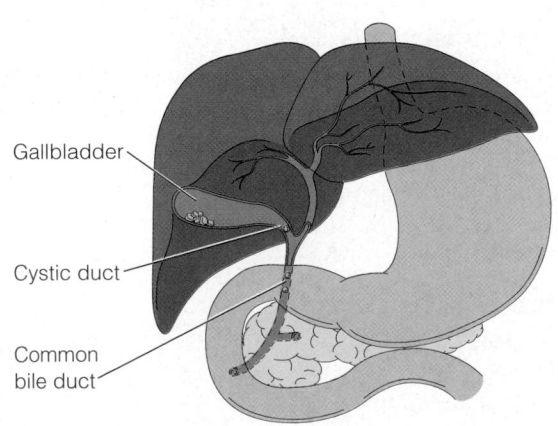

Figure 21-1. ■ Common locations of gallstones.

MANIFESTATIONS AND COMPLICATIONS

Cholelithiasis often is asymptomatic. When symptoms do develop, they often relate to movement of a stone through the bile ducts or inflammation of the gallbladder and bile ducts.

Early manifestations of cholelithiasis often are vague, including mild gastric distress after eating a large or fatty meal. When stones obstruct the cystic or common bile duct, pressure increases behind the stone. This causes **biliary colic,** a severe, steady pain in the right upper quadrant or epigastric region of the abdomen. The pain often begins suddenly following a meal, and may radiate to the back or right shoulder.

Cholecystitis is classified as either acute or chronic. *Acute cholecystitis* is characterized by severe epigastric or upper right quadrant pain radiating posteriorly to the scapular region. This spasmodic pain results from contraction of the ducts and is usually initiated by a high-fat meal. This pain lasts longer than biliary colic, continuing for 12 to 18 hours, and often is accompanied by anorexia, nausea, and vomiting. *Chronic cholecystitis* generally has a more moderate presentation. See Box 21-2 ■ for the manifestations of acute and chronic cholecystitis.

Bile duct obstruction can lead to reflux (backflow) of bile into the liver, with resulting jaundice, pain, and possible liver damage. Pancreatitis can result from obstruction of the common bile duct.

Perforation of the gallbladder and peritonitis are possible complications of cholecystitis. Other complications include infection, fistula formation, and cancer.

BOX 21-2

MANIFESTATIONS OF CHOLELITHIASIS AND CHOLECYSTITIS

Cholelithiasis
- Epigastric fullness, gastric distress following a meal
- Biliary colic: severe, steady right upper quadrant or epigastric pain; often follows a meal

Acute Cholecystitis
- Epigastric or right upper abdominal pain; may radiate to back
- Pain precipitated by high-fat meal
- Right upper quadrant guarding and tenderness
- Nausea and vomiting
- Fever
- Possible jaundice

Chronic Cholecystitis
- Fatty food intolerance
- Belching
- Vague gastric symptoms
- Pain after eating

INTERDISCIPLINARY CARE

Diagnostic Tests

Gallstones often are diagnosed through a right upper quadrant *abdominal ultrasound.* This test is noninvasive and requires no special preparation; see Chapter 18 ⚭ for more information about this and other diagnostic tests. An *oral cholecystogram* may be performed in nonacute situations. *Gallbladder scans,* also called liver-biliary scans, use nuclear medicine techniques to assess acute cholecystitis. Laboratory tests may show elevated white blood cell (WBC), serum bilirubin, alkaline phosphatase, alanine transaminase (ALT), and aspartate transaminase (AST) levels.

Medications

Clients who refuse surgery or for whom surgery would pose a high risk (e.g., a frail older adult) may be treated with oral bile acids to dissolve stones. Ursodiol (Actigall) or chenodiol (Chenix) may be used to treat small cholesterol stones. These drugs work by reducing the cholesterol content of gallstones, gradually dissolving the stone. Nurses need to monitor liver enzymes and watch for possible diarrhea in clients taking these drugs. Several years of therapy may be required, and stones frequently recur after treatment is stopped. Cholestyramine (Questran) is a drug that binds with bile salts to promote their excretion. It may be given to clients with jaundice and resulting severe itching. If infection is suspected, antibiotics may be prescribed. Parenteral narcotic analgesics such as morphine may be necessary to relieve the pain of acute cholecystitis.

Dietary Management

Because dietary fat stimulates gallbladder contraction, clients are usually placed on a low-fat diet. Examples of foods to avoid are listed in Box 21-3 ■. Clients who are obese are encouraged to lose weight to reduce surgical risks. All food and fluids may be withheld during an attack of acute cholecystitis; total parenteral nutrition may be used to maintain the client's nutritional status.

BOX 21-3

HIGH-FAT FOODS TO AVOID IN CHOLELITHIASIS
- Whole milk products (e.g., cheese, cream, ice cream)
- Deep-fried foods and pastries (e.g., donuts, French fries, batter-fried fish)
- Avocados
- Sausage, bacon, hot dogs
- Gravies made with fat or cream
- Most nuts
- Snack foods (e.g., potato chips, tortilla chips)
- Peanut butter
- Chocolate

Other Therapies

Extracorporeal shock wave lithotripsy (ESWL), a procedure in which stones are fragmented by shock waves, may be used in conjunction with drug treatment. After treatment, the nurse monitors for possible biliary colic, nausea, and possible transient hematuria. *Percutaneous cholecystostomy,* drainage of the gallbladder, may be performed to delay or eliminate the need for surgery in high-risk clients.

Surgery

Most clients with symptomatic gallbladder disease are treated with *laparoscopic cholecystectomy.* This minimally invasive surgery allows a hospital stay of 24 hours or less, and the client often is able to return to work within a week. See Box 21-4 ■ for nursing care of the client having laparoscopic cholecystectomy.

clinical ALERT

During laparoscopic cholecystectomy, the abdomen is inflated with carbon dioxide. This can cause shoulder pain after surgery. Carefully assess the client's pain and provide adequate analgesia. Inform the client that as the gas is absorbed, the pain will be relieved.

Nursing care for clients who require a traditional cholecystectomy is similar to that required by any client having abdominal surgery. (See Chapter 9 ∞ for more information about care of the surgical client.) Coughing, deep breathing, and early ambulation are vital to prevent respiratory complications because of the upper abdominal incision.

Clients may return from surgery with a T-tube (Figure 21-2 ■). Inserted after common bile duct exploration, a T-tube keeps the duct open and promotes bile flow until edema

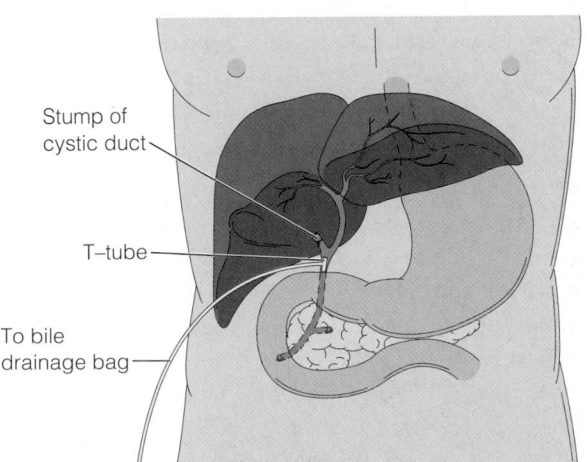

Figure 21-2. ■ T-tube placement in the common bile duct. Bile flows by gravity into a collection device placed below the level of the abdomen.

Stump of cystic duct

T–tube

To bile drainage bag

BOX 21-4   NURSING CARE CHECKLIST

Laparoscopic Cholecystectomy

Before Surgery

☑ Reinforce preoperative teaching, including the procedure, postoperative care, and pain management.

☑ Provide routine preoperative care as outlined in Chapter 9. ∞

After Surgery

☑ Monitor vital signs every 15 minutes for 2 hours or until stable, then every 4 hours until discharge.

☑ Provide routine postoperative care.

☑ Assess location and severity of pain; provide analgesia as needed.

☑ Assist out of bed and with ambulation as ordered.

☑ Reinforce and provide postoperative and discharge teaching:

   ☑ Wound care

   ☑ Pain management

   ☑ Diet and activity

   ☑ Medications

   ☑ Follow-up appointments and care.

decreases. Excess bile is collected in a drainage bag secured below the surgical site. Nursing care of a client with a T-tube is outlined in Box 21-5 ■.

BOX 21-5   NURSING CARE CHECKLIST

T-Tube Care

☑ Connect T-tube to a sterile container; keep the tube below the level of the surgical wound.

☑ Monitor color and consistency of drainage; record amount on output record. Up to 500 mL of drainage is expected in the first 24 hours after surgery, decreasing to under 200 mL in 2 to 3 days; thereafter, drainage is minimal. Initial drainage may be blood tinged, changing to green-brown. Report excessive drainage to the charge nurse or physician immediately (after 48 hours, drainage greater than 500 mL is considered excessive).

☑ Place in Fowler's position to promote drainage.

☑ Assess skin for bile leakage during dressing changes; apply a protective skin barrier if necessary.

☑ Teach client how to manage tube when turning, ambulating, and performing activities of daily living.

☑ Clamp the T-tube only as ordered by the physician.

☑ If indicated, teach the client care of the T-tube, how to clamp it, and signs of infection.

Complementary and Alternative Therapies

Goldenseal, an herb, has been used to treat cholecystitis. It stimulates bile and bilirubin secretion, and inhibits the growth of many of the bacteria known to infect the gallbladder. Studies have shown goldenseal to be effective in relieving all manifestations of cholecystitis. It is contraindicated for use during pregnancy and lactation, however, because it can stimulate the uterus.

NURSING CARE

ASSESSING

Assessment data to collect on clients with suspected gallbladder disease is outlined in Box 21-6 ■.

DIAGNOSING, PLANNING, AND IMPLEMENTING

Priorities in Nursing Care. For most clients with gallbladder disease, the priority of nursing care is managing the symptoms of the disorder and promoting comfort.

BOX 21-6	ASSESSMENT

Assessing Clients with Gallbladder Disease

SUBJECTIVE DATA
- Pain: location, character, radiation; frequency and timing, relationship to meals and foods; aggravating factors, relief measures and their effectiveness.
- Nausea and vomiting; relationship to pain, meals, foods.
- Epigastric upset or heartburn.
- Usual diet and effect of symptoms on diet.
- Previous diagnosis of gallbladder disease and its treatment.

OBJECTIVE DATA
- Observe:
  - General appearance; apparent nutritional status
  - Color, consistency, and amount of any emesis
  - Color and consistency of feces
  - Color of skin and sclera, presence of jaundice.
- Inspect abdomen for distention.
- Auscultate bowel sounds.
- Palpate abdomen (especially right upper quadrant) for tenderness and guarding.

LABORATORY DATA
- Monitor WBC, serum bilirubin, and liver function tests (see Chapter 18 ⬥).

Acute Pain

- Teach clients to avoid fat in their diets. (See Box 21-3 for foods to avoid.) *Fat initiates gallbladder contractions and is a stimulus for pain.*
- Administer narcotic analgesics as ordered for severe pain. *Severe pain can cause muscle spasm and increased GI symptoms. Parenteral analgesia may be required.*
- Place in Fowler's position. *Fowler's position decreases pressure on the inflamed area and may help relieve pain.*

Nausea

- Monitor complaints of nausea. Document amount, color, and consistency of any emesis. Monitor food and fluid intake. *Nausea may result from cholecystitis or be caused by pain. Nausea increases the risk of a nutritional deficit; vomiting can lead to fluid volume deficit.*
- Administer prescribed antiemetics. *Giving antiemetic medication before meals and procedures helps promote food intake and prevent vomiting.*
- Promptly remove noxious items and odor-producing substances (e.g., food, commodes). *The sight or smell of food and noxious substances can stimulate or aggravate nausea.*
- Provide oral care and clean bedding (as needed) after each emesis. *This reduces nausea stimuli.*
- Withhold food and fluids during episodes of nausea and vomiting. Offer cold, low-fat or fat-free foods and foods with little odor in small quantities when the client is able to eat. *Attempting to eat when nauseous may precipitate vomiting. Cold, low-fat foods are better tolerated, as are small quantities rather than large meals.*

Risk for Impaired Gas Exchange

The incision used for an open or traditional cholecystectomy is high on the abdomen and disrupts many of the muscles of respiration. Clients who require traditional cholecystectomy often are obese, and may be experiencing complications of cholecystitis before surgery. The location of the incision and the client's preoperative condition increase the risk for respiratory complications following surgery.

- Assist the client who has had an open (traditional) cholecystectomy to turn, deep breathe, and cough at least every 2 hours; use incentive spirometry every hour while awake, and ambulate at least four times daily. *These interventions help expand the lungs and prevent accumulation of secretions in the lungs following a traditional cholecystectomy. Clients may have difficulty ventilating all lung areas because of the high abdominal incision.*
- Assist with splinting the incision during coughing and deep breathing. *Splinting the incision with a blanket or pillow reduces the discomfort of deep breathing and coughing.*

■ Monitor temperature every 4 hours; promptly report elevations to the charge nurse or physician. *An elevated temperature may indicate infection.*

EVALUATING

To evaluate the effectiveness of nursing interventions, collect data related to level of comfort, ability to consume the ordered diet and fluids, respiratory status, and freedom from infection.

Documenting. Document the client's manifestations and responses to treatment measures. Note diagnostic tests, procedures, or surgery if performed, and continuing assessment data following the procedure. Document teaching provided and reinforced, and the client's and family's apparent understanding of instructions.

CONTINUING CARE

Clients with cholelithiasis may manage their disease at home with medical interventions, or they may require prompt surgical intervention. Reinforce teaching about the disease, prescribed medications, diagnostic procedures, and treatment options. Discuss the relationship of food intake to episodes of acute cholecystitis, and the importance of maintaining a low-fat, low-kilocalorie diet if indicated. Explain the role of bile and the function of the gallbladder in terms that the client and family can understand.

Provide preoperative teaching, discussing what to expect before and after surgery. Discuss measures to reduce discomfort, promote healing, and prevent complications.

After surgery, prepare the client for discharge and home care. Discuss pain control, monitoring for and preventing infection, and T-tube care. Include instructions about activities, diet, and returning to work. Inform about signs or symptoms to report to the physician.

Refer the client to a dietitian to review low-fat foods; include the person preparing foods. Most clients start with a low-fat diet and gradually add fatty foods as tolerated. Refer the client to home care services as indicated.

NURSING PROCESS CARE PLAN
Client with Cholelithiasis

Joyce Red Wing is a 44-year-old member of the Chickasaw tribe. Recently, she has noticed a dull pain in her upper abdomen that gets worse after eating fatty foods; the pain is accompanied by nausea. She remembers having similar pain after the birth of her last child. The diagnosis of cholelithiasis is made, and Ms. Red Wing is admitted for a laparoscopic cholecystectomy.

Assessment. Ms. Red Wing's admission history reveals that her usual diet consists of fatty foods, particularly tacos or fried bread and biscuits with gravy for breakfast. She reports "not wanting to eat much of anything lately." She states she has never had surgery before and hopes "everything goes well." She has a good understanding of the procedure to be done. Physical assessment findings: T 100°F (37.7°C); BP 130/84; P 88; R 20. Weight 130 lbs (59 kg), a 5-pound weight loss from her usual; 5'3" (160 cm) tall. Abdomen tender to palpation in the upper right quadrant. No jaundice, chills, or other evidence of complications noted.

Diagnosis. The following nursing diagnoses are identified for Ms. Red Wing:

■ *Anxiety* related to concerns about surgery
■ *Acute Pain* related to surgery
■ *Deficient Knowledge: Low-Fat Diet* related to lack of nutritional information

Expected Outcomes. The expected outcomes specify that Ms. Red Wing will:

■ Verbalize reduced anxiety related to undergoing surgery.
■ Maintain adequate pain control postoperatively.
■ Follow prescribed diet postoperatively.

Planning and Implementation. The following interventions are planned and implemented:

■ Teach about the gallbladder and the function of bile.
■ Discuss pre- and postoperative care, including plans for discharge, pain management, wound care, activities, and follow-up.
■ Provide analgesia as needed.
■ Review specific high-fat foods to avoid and ways to maintain weight.

Evaluation. Ms. Red Wing is discharged the morning following surgery. She has no signs of infection and is able to care for her incisions. She identifies the importance of eating a low-fat diet and keeping her weight stable, as well as gradually resuming activities. Ms. Red Wing states that she "is glad it is over, but it wasn't as bad as I thought it would be at first." She has an appointment to see her surgeon in 1 week.

Critical Thinking in the Nursing Process

1. What is the rationale for a low-fat diet with cholelithiasis? Discuss nutritional practices as they relate to cholelithiasis and Ms. Red Wing's culture.
2. Why would it be important to place Ms. Red Wing in Fowler's position after surgery?
3. List five areas to cover in predischarge teaching for Ms. Red Wing.

Cancer of the Gallbladder

Gallbladder cancer is rare, primarily affecting people over 65. Women are more likely to develop the disorder. Clients with cancer of the gallbladder complain of intense pain in the right upper quadrant of the abdomen; a mass may be palpated in the region. Jaundice and weight loss usually accompany the pain. Most gallbladder cancers metastasize via the blood, lymph system, or through direct extension; the liver is most commonly affected. Most cancers of the gallbladder cannot be treated surgically unless they are found at an early stage incidental to another surgical procedure. Most clients with primary cancer of the gallbladder die within 1 year.

LIVER DISORDERS

Because of the liver's many essential functions, when it is impaired by inflammation, cell damage, or cancer, all other body systems are affected. The liver is vulnerable to inflammation, damage, and tumor growth because it is constantly exposed to a large amount of blood that may contain pathogens, drugs, toxins, and possibly malignant cells from elsewhere in the body.

Hepatitis

Hepatitis is inflammation of the liver. It usually is caused by a virus, but also may be caused by alcohol, toxins (such as drugs), or gallbladder disease. Acute and chronic forms of hepatitis exist. Cirrhosis, discussed in the next section, is a possible consequence of hepatic cell damage resulting from hepatitis.

PATHOPHYSIOLOGY

One of the primary functions of the liver is the metabolism and elimination of bilirubin (a breakdown product of hemoglobin). The liver also is vital to the metabolism of carbohydrates, proteins, and fats, as well as most drugs and alcohol. The inflammation of hepatitis disrupts these vital liver functions. Although the underlying pathology of hepatitis varies, its effects and manifestations are similar. Much depends on the degree of liver damage and the client's health status at the time.

Viral Hepatitis

At least six different viruses (designated by letters of the alphabet) can cause hepatitis. Hepatitis A virus (HAV) and hepatitis B virus (HBV) are the most common, although the incidence of hepatitis C (HCV) is increasing. Viral infection causes liver cell injury and necrosis. The liver cell damage may be directly caused by the virus or may occur as a result of the body's immune response to the virus. The manifestations of viral hepatitis are similar for all types, but other characteristics of the disease vary. Table 21-1 ■ compares the onset, incubation, mode of transmission, and other characteristics of the more common types of viral hepatitis.

Hepatitis A causes epidemics and sporadic cases of hepatitis. Transmitted by the fecal–oral route, it frequently occurs in crowded, unsanitary living conditions. Contaminated food, water, or shellfish often are responsible for outbreaks of hepatitis A.

Hepatitis B is usually transmitted by blood transfusion or contaminated needles, but also may be spread by sexual contact and from an infected mother to her fetus. *Carriers* can transmit HBV while having no symptoms of the disease. The risk of liver cancer is significant in clients infected with hepatitis B. Health care workers are at risk for hepatitis B. Following Standard Precautions and obtaining hepatitis B immunization are important preventive strategies.

Hepatitis C is nearly always transmitted by blood and contaminated needles. This type of viral hepatitis affects African Americans and Mexican Americans more frequently than whites. It often leads to chronic liver disease, and is the most common indication for liver transplant. A vaccine has been developed, but is not commonly administered.

The *hepatitis delta virus (HDV)* causes infection only in people who have active hepatitis B. It causes more severe infection than hepatitis B alone, and may lead to *fulminant hepatitis* with widespread liver necrosis and failure.

Hepatitis E is rare in the United States, occurring more commonly in underdeveloped areas of southeast Asia, parts of Africa, and Central America. Transmitted by water contaminated by feces, it primarily affects young adults. Pregnant women are particularly vulnerable to the devastating effects of hepatitis E whereas the disease is generally mild and self-limiting in nonpregnant adults.

Chronic Hepatitis

Chronic hepatitis, a chronic infection of the liver, may lead to cirrhosis, liver cancer, or liver failure and the need for a liver transplant. It may develop with HBV, HCV, and HDV infections. Its manifestations often are mild and nonspecific, such as general malaise and fatigue, and an enlarged liver.

TABLE 21-1

Types of Viral Hepatitis

	HEPATITIS A (HAV)	HEPATITIS B (HBV)	HEPATITIS C (HCV)	HEPATITIS D (HDV OR DELTA HEPATITIS)	HEPATITIS E (HEV)
Incubation (In Weeks)	2–6	8–24	5–12	3–13	3–6
Onset	Abrupt	Slow	Slow	Abrupt	Abrupt
Transmission	Fecal–oral	Blood and body fluids; perinatal	Blood and body fluids	Blood and body fluids; possible perinatal	Fecal–oral
Communicable	1 week before onset; minimal after onset of jaundice	1–2 months before symptoms; when HBsAg present in blood	When HCV present in blood	When HDVAg present in blood	Rarely spread person to person
Carrier State	No	Yes	Yes	Yes	Yes
Possible Complications	Rare	Chronic hepatitis, cirrhosis, liver cancer	Chronic hepatitis, cirrhosis, liver cancer	Chronic hepatitis, cirrhosis, fulminant hepatitis	May be severe in pregnant women
Laboratory Findings	Anti-HAV antibodies	Positive HBsAg; anti-HBV antibodies	Anti-HCV antibodies	Positive HDVAg early; anti-HDV antibodies later	Anti-HEV antibodies
Prevention	Hepatitis A vaccine (primary dose + booster in 6–12 months)	Hepatitis B vaccine (HBV) (primary dose + second 1–2 months later + third 2–5 months after second)	None	HBV vaccine	None
Prophylaxis	Standard immune globulin before or within 2 weeks of exposure	Hepatitis B immune globulin (HBIG) within 1–2 days of exposure; second dose 28–30 days after exposure	None	See hepatitis B prophylaxis	None

Noninfectious Hepatitis

Alcoholic hepatitis is acute or chronic inflammation of the liver caused by alcohol. While it often is reversible, alcoholic hepatitis can lead to necrosis of liver cells. It is the most common risk factor for cirrhosis (discussed in the next section of this chapter) in the United States. Many drugs (e.g., acetaminophen and tetracyclines) and other toxins (such as poisonous mushrooms, heavy metals, and carbon tetrachloride) can damage the liver, leading to inflammation and necrosis (*toxic hepatitis*). Interruption of normal bile flow due to cholelithiasis and blockage of the bile duct also can lead to inflammation of the liver, a condition known as *hepatobiliary hepatitis.*

MANIFESTATIONS

The manifestations of hepatitis range from asymptomatic infection to a rapidly fatal disease. The course of acute viral hepatitis generally follows three phases.

The *preicteric* (before jaundice) or *prodromal phase* may have an abrupt or insidious onset. The **icteric** (*jaundice*) *phase* of the disease develops after 5 to 10 days. Early manifestations may worsen when jaundice develops, then begin to improve. **Jaundice** occurs when serum bilirubin levels are high, causing the skin, mucous membranes, and sclera of the eyes to appear yellow. The *posticteric* or *convalescent phase* is characterized by an increasing sense of well-being, return of appetite, and the disappearance of

BOX 21-7	

MANIFESTATIONS OF ACUTE VIRAL HEPATITIS

Preicteric or Prodromal Phase

- "Flulike" symptoms: malaise, fatigue, headache, muscle aches, nasal discharge, sore throat.
- Gastrointestinal: anorexia, nausea, vomiting, diarrhea, or constipation.
- Joint pain.
- Mild and constant right upper abdominal pain.

Icteric Phase

- Jaundice.
- Pruritus.
- Clay-colored stools, dark urine.

Posticteric or Convalescent Phase

- Well-being improves, energy increases.
- Jaundice resolves.

BOX 21-8	**POPULATION FOCUS**

People Who Should Be Vaccinated For Hepatitis B

- People at risk for sexual transmission: homosexual or bisexual men, prostitutes, people with multiple partners or recently diagnosed sexually transmitted disease
- Injection drug users
- Male prison inmates
- People on hemodialysis
- Health care workers
- Clients and staff of institutions for the developmentally disabled
- High-risk populations: Alaska Natives, Pacific Islanders, and immigrants from HBV endemic areas
- Household members and partners of HBV carriers
- International travelers to HBV endemic areas
- Recipients of certain blood products such as clotting factors

jaundice. Box 21-7 ■ summarizes the manifestations of each phase of hepatitis.

INTERDISCIPLINARY CARE

There is no specific treatment for hepatitis. Prevention, early identification of the disease, and teaching are vital.

Diagnostic Tests

- Blood is drawn to assess for *viral antigens* (e.g., hepatitis B surface antigen [HBsAg]) or *antibodies* to the viral agents that cause hepatitis (see Table 21-1).
- *Liver function tests* (see Chapter 18) ⬤⬤ are measured. Serum levels of these enzymes increase when the liver is inflamed or damaged.
- *Serum bilirubin* levels also are measured. Total bilirubin usually is elevated, as are both direct (conjugated) and indirect (unconjugated) bilirubin levels. Unconjugated bilirubin rises because the liver does not effectively metabolize it; conjugated bilirubin increases because excretion is impaired.
- *Prothrombin time* may be prolonged if the liver is not able to manufacture the protein needed for blood coagulation.

Prevention

Vaccines and immune globulin injections are available to prevent hepatitis A and B. Vaccines are recommended for people who are at increased risk for exposure to the disease. Immune globulin is used for postexposure prophylaxis, to prevent the disease after known or suspected contact with the virus. Table 21-1 lists recommended immunizations.

Hepatitis A vaccine is recommended for adults traveling internationally, homosexual men, drug users, and people with clotting disorders, hepatitis C, or an occupational risk. It also is recommended for children over the age of 2 who live in areas where the incidence of hepatitis A is high.

When exposure to hepatitis A virus has occurred, illness often can be prevented by a single dose of immune globulin (IG) given within 2 weeks of exposure. IG is recommended for people in close contact with someone who has hepatitis A, for child care workers where a case of hepatitis A has been identified, and for restaurant patrons where a food handler has developed hepatitis A.

Hepatitis B vaccine is recommended for all infants, adolescents who have not been immunized, and adults at risk for exposure to hepatitis B. All health care workers including nurses should be vaccinated. Box 21-8 ■ summarizes who should receive hepatitis B vaccine.

Following exposure to hepatitis B, both hepatitis B vaccine and hepatitis B immune globulin (HBIG) are given to prevent infection. With perinatal exposure, infants are given both HBIG and the vaccine within 24 hours of birth.

Treatment

There currently is no cure for viral hepatitis. Clients are encouraged to get adequate rest, maintain nutritional intake, and avoid strenuous activity, alcohol, and agents that are toxic to the liver. Bed rest is necessary only when symptoms are severe. Intravenous fluids may be given if nausea and vomiting interfere with intake. Interferon may be ordered for clients with hepatitis B or C. Potential complementary therapies for hepatitis B and C are discussed in Box 21-9 ■. In most cases, clinical recovery takes 3 to 16 weeks.

BOX 21-9	COMPLEMENTARY THERAPIES

Hepatitis

Herbalists in Europe have used milk thistle to treat liver disease for more than 2,000 years. Silymarin is believed to be the active ingredient in milk thistle. Silymarin helps prevent complications and promote more rapid recovery. It also benefits clients who have liver damage due to toxins, cirrhosis, and alcoholic liver disease. It appears that silymarin:

- Promotes liver cell growth
- Is a powerful antioxidant
- Blocks toxins from entering and damaging liver cells
- Reduces inflammation in the liver.

Licorice root also may be used by herbalists to treat hepatitis. Licorice root has both antiviral and anti-inflammatory effects, but long-term use may lead to hypertension and affect fluid and electrolyte balance.

Other herbal remedies may help relieve the adverse effects of interferon (flulike symptoms, fatigue, dizziness, anorexia, nausea, diarrhea, and cough). These include ginger for nausea and St. John's wort for depression. Refer clients interested in complementary therapies for hepatitis to a certified herbalist.

NURSING CARE

ASSESSING

Clients with acute hepatitis often present with classic manifestations of hepatitis. However, clients who have chronic hepatitis may have more vague manifestations. Assessment data to collect for clients with confirmed or suspected hepatitis are presented in Box 21-10 ■.

DIAGNOSING, PLANNING, AND IMPLEMENTING

Priorities in Nursing Care. For most clients, hepatitis is a self-limiting disease that requires little treatment beyond supportive care (rest, a balanced diet). The primary focus for nursing care is preventing transmission of the disease to others. Standard Precautions, which treat all body fluids as potentially contaminated, are adequate to prevent spread of the disease to others. Because hepatitis A is spread via the fecal–oral route, careful handling of feces and meticulous hand washing are vital.

Risk for Infection (Transmission)

- Use Standard Precautions and meticulous hand washing. *One of the most important goals when caring for clients with acute viral hepatitis is preventing the spread of infection. Proper aseptic technique can stem transmission of the viruses.*
- For clients with hepatitis A, use Standard Precautions and contact isolation if fecal incontinence is present. *The fecal–oral route is the primary mode of transmission of hepatitis A.*

- Encourage at-risk clients to obtain hepatitis A or hepatitis B immunizations, or both. *Prevention is a key strategy for reducing the incidence and long-term consequences of viral hepatitis.*

Activity Intolerance

- Encourage client to rest as needed to relieve fatigue. *Fatigue and possible weakness are common in clients with hepatitis. Adequate rest promotes optimal immune function and recovery.*
- Plan nursing care activities that promote rest, allowing gradual resumption of activities. *As the client recovers, fatigue and activity tolerance improve.*

Imbalanced Nutrition: Less Than Body Requirements

- Encourage the client to eat smaller, more frequent meals. *Clients with hepatitis often experience significant anorexia and possible nausea. Smaller meals are frequently better tolerated.*
- Help the client select a palatable diet with adequate calories. Suggest supplements such as Ensure as needed to maintain intake. Low-fat diets are sometimes better tolerated. *Sufficient energy is required for healing.*

BOX 21-10	ASSESSMENT

Assessing Clients with Hepatitis

SUBJECTIVE DATA

- Known or possible exposure to hepatitis virus: recent travel; close contact with someone who has hepatitis; a high-risk occupation or behaviors; eating where a food handler has been diagnosed with hepatitis; injection drug use.
- Recent flulike illness.
- Anorexia, nausea, vomiting; change in bowel habits; color of feces and urine.
- Pain: location and character, frequency and timing, aggravating factors.
- Change in color of skin or sclera; itching.
- History of hepatitis vaccine or prophylaxis.

OBJECTIVE DATA

- Observe:
  - General appearance; apparent nutritional status
  - Color of skin and sclera, presence of jaundice
  - Color and consistency of feces; color of urine.
- Inspect abdomen for distention.
- Auscultate bowel sounds.
- Palpate abdomen for tenderness.

LABORATORY DATA

- Monitor serum bilirubin and liver function tests (see Chapter 18 ⊙).

- Encourage eating more food at times when nausea and anorexia are minimal. *Many clients with acute hepatitis are nauseated in the afternoon and evening hours.*
- If nausea and vomiting persist, give intravenous fluids as ordered. Monitor fluid and electrolytes, and assess for signs of dehydration. *Prompt assessment of fluid and electrolyte imbalance allows early treatment to maintain homeostasis.*

EVALUATING

To evaluate the effectiveness of nursing care, collect data such as the following:

- Household members remain free of infection.
- Client can verbalize appropriate measures to prevent spreading the disease.
- Client gets adequate rest.
- Weight remains stable.

Documenting. Document continuing assessment data, including trends in serum bilirubin and liver function tests. Document teaching provided to the client and family, as well as their understanding and apparent willingness to comply with precautions. If prophylactic measures are provided or immunizations administered, note the date and time administered. Report to the local health department cases of hepatitis A among food handlers, child care workers, and others at high risk for spreading the disease to the public.

CONTINUING CARE

Most clients with acute viral hepatitis are cared for at home and in community-based settings. Teach the client, family members, and members of the household how to prevent spread of the disease. Recommend prophylactic treatment and immunization for household contacts and others at risk for contracting the disease. Instruct the client with hepatitis A not to prepare food for other members of the family until he or she is no longer infectious. Include instructions for cleaning eating utensils and soiled linens. Emphasize the importance of not sharing toothbrushes, razors, or dirty needles, and the need to abstain from sexual activity until the client is no longer infectious. Stress the importance of avoiding hepatotoxins, such as alcohol and acetaminophen, until the liver is fully healed. Discuss the need to undergo follow-up evaluations and the importance of following diet and activity recommendations for the full period of recovery.

Cirrhosis

Cirrhosis is a chronic liver disease that destroys the structure and function of liver lobules. Because the liver performs so many functions, cirrhosis has devastating effects and often leads to death.

Alcoholic liver disease (*Laënnec's* or *alcoholic cirrhosis*) is the most common type of cirrhosis. Cirrhosis also may result from chronic hepatitis B or C, toxic liver damage from drugs or chemicals (*postnecrotic cirrhosis*), heart failure, or from obstructed bile flow (*biliary cirrhosis*).

PATHOPHYSIOLOGY

In cirrhosis, hepatocytes (functional liver cells) are destroyed, disrupting the metabolic functions of the liver. Lost cells are replaced by scar tissue that forms constrictive bands within liver lobules (see Figure 18-5 ⬤⬤) and disrupts blood and bile flow within the liver. Impaired blood flow through the liver increases pressure in the portal venous system, leading to portal hypertension (Figure 21-3 ■).

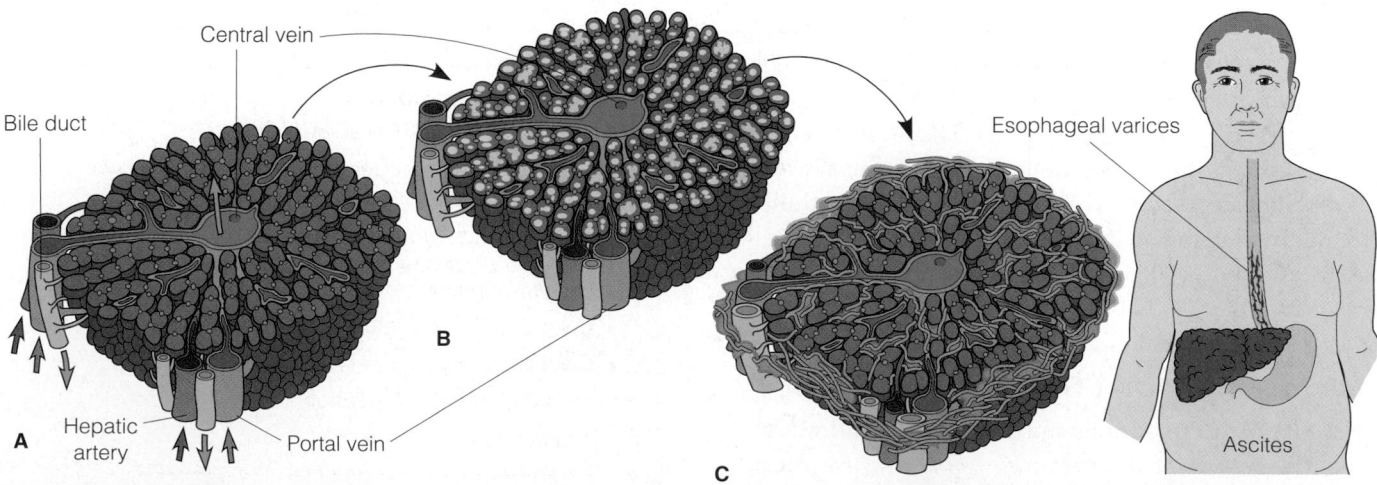

Figure 21-3. ■ Portal hypertension in cirrhosis. (**A**) The portal vein, which drains capillaries of the gut, provides the majority of the liver's blood supply. (**B**) In cirrhosis, cellular necrosis leads to fibrosis and scarring. Isolated liver cells continue to regenerate, forming nodules among the fibrous scar tissue. (**C**) The nodules and scar tissue interfere with blood flow through the liver, increasing pressure and congestion in the portal venous system. Shunting of blood into lower pressure vessels leads to esophageal varices, hemorrhoids, and visible surface veins. The increased pressure also contributes to ascites.

Obstructed bile outflow damages liver cells. Loss of functioning liver lobules ultimately leads to liver failure.

MANIFESTATIONS AND COMPLICATIONS

The manifestations and complications of cirrhosis result both from impaired liver function and from altered blood flow through the portal venous system. Early in the course of the disease, the liver is enlarged and tender. The client may complain of right upper quadrant pain. Other early signs include weight loss, weakness, and anorexia. Bowel function may be disrupted. As the disease progresses, symptoms of liver failure and portal hypertension develop (Figure 21-4 ■).

Portal hypertension is elevated blood pressure in the portal vein that carries venous blood from the gut through the liver. Higher pressure forces fluid out of the vessels, contributing to the formation of ascites. Blood is shunted from vessels of the portal system into lower pressure vessels, resulting in congestion of veins in the esophagus, rectum, and abdomen.

Ascites is an accumulation of serous fluid in the peritoneal cavity. Portal hypertension is the primary cause of ascites, because fluid is forced out of capillaries by high pressure within the vessels. Impaired liver function affects the production of plasma proteins (such as albumin), reducing plasma osmotic pressure (see Chapter 7 ⬤). This allows fluid to escape from blood vessels, leading to ascites and peripheral edema. Fluid and electrolyte imbalances also contribute to edema and ascites.

Splenomegaly (enlargement of the spleen) develops as blood is shunted from the portal system into the splenic vein. Splenomegaly can lead to anemia and low platelet and WBC counts. Low platelets (*thrombocytopenia*) and decreased clotting factor production by the liver lead to increased risk for bleeding. Infection is a risk due to low WBC counts (*leukopenia*).

Esophageal varices are enlarged, overdistended veins in the distal esophagus that result from portal venous congestion. Clients with esophageal varices are at high risk for bleeding. Even high-roughage foods (like bacon) can lead to hemorrhage of these fragile vessels. *Upper gastrointestinal bleeding* is a frequent complication of cirrhosis. Bleeding, which can be massive, may result from varices, gastritis, or peptic ulcer.

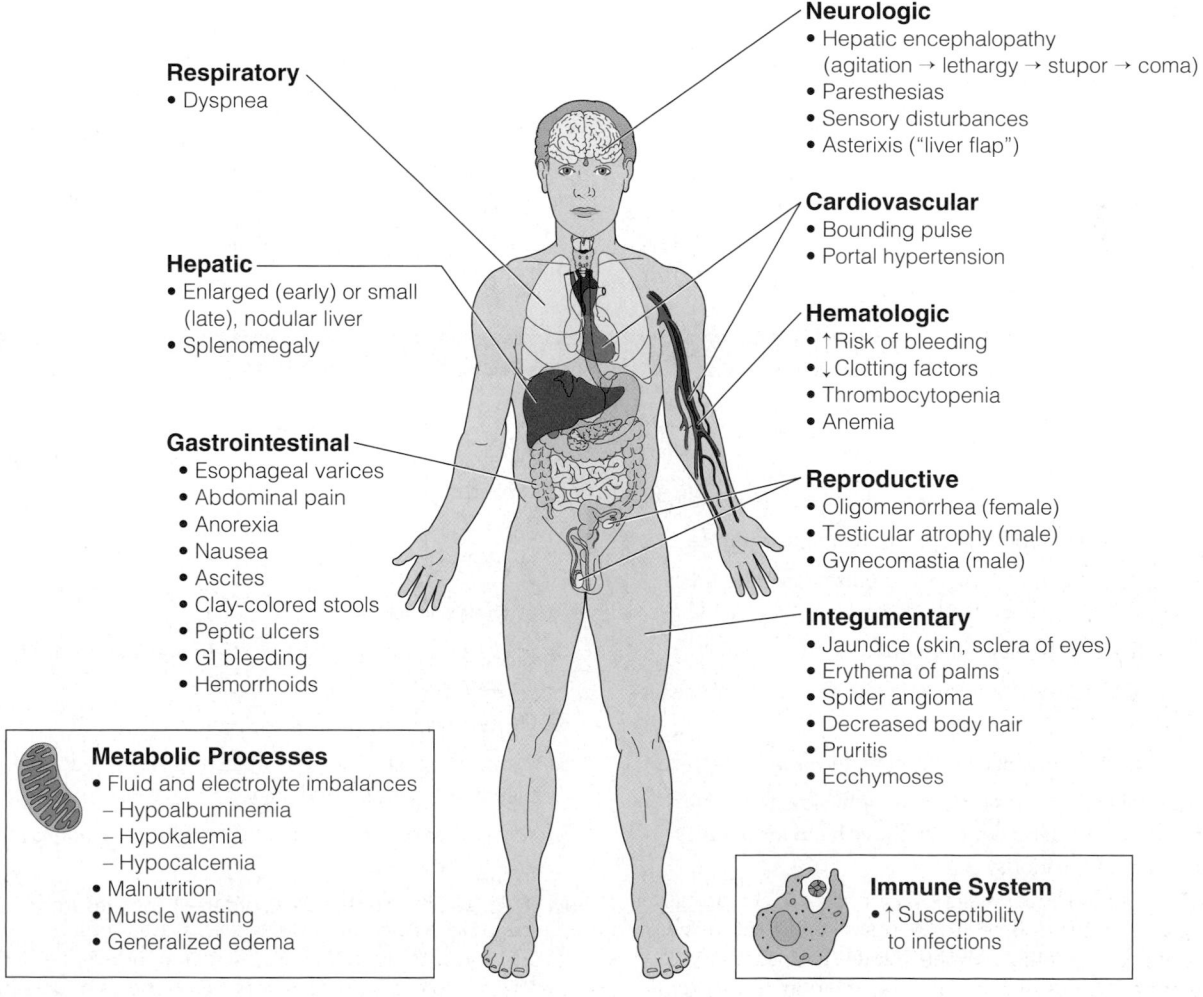

Neurologic
• Hepatic encephalopathy
  (agitation → lethargy → stupor → coma)
• Paresthesias
• Sensory disturbances
• Asterixis ("liver flap")

Respiratory
• Dyspnea

Cardiovascular
• Bounding pulse
• Portal hypertension

Hepatic
• Enlarged (early) or small
  (late), nodular liver
• Splenomegaly

Hematologic
• ↑Risk of bleeding
• ↓Clotting factors
• Thrombocytopenia
• Anemia

Gastrointestinal
• Esophageal varices
• Abdominal pain
• Anorexia
• Nausea
• Ascites
• Clay-colored stools
• Peptic ulcers
• GI bleeding
• Hemorrhoids

Reproductive
• Oligomenorrhea (female)
• Testicular atrophy (male)
• Gynecomastia (male)

Integumentary
• Jaundice (skin, sclera of eyes)
• Erythema of palms
• Spider angioma
• Decreased body hair
• Pruritus
• Ecchymoses

Metabolic Processes
• Fluid and electrolyte imbalances
  – Hypoalbuminemia
  – Hypokalemia
  – Hypocalcemia
• Malnutrition
• Muscle wasting
• Generalized edema

Immune System
• ↑Susceptibility
  to infections

Figure 21-4. ■ The multisystem effects of cirrhosis.

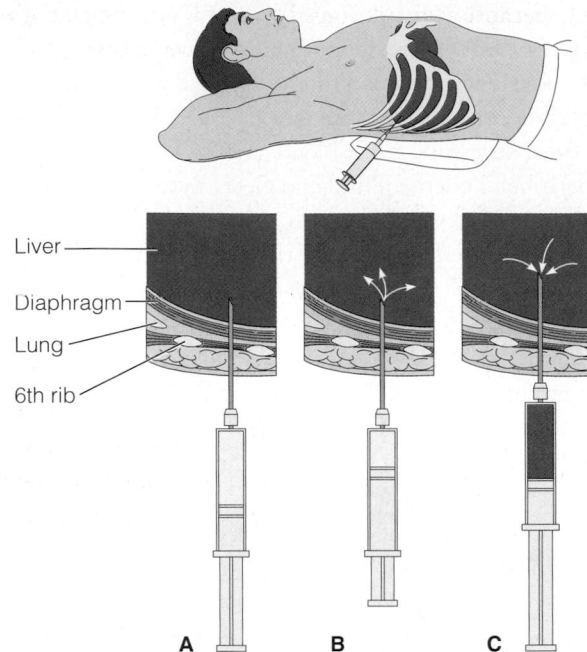

Liver

Diaphragm

Lung

6th rib

A   B   C

Figure 21-5. ■ Liver biopsy. (**A**) The client exhales completely and holds breath, bringing the liver and diaphragm to their highest position. The needle is inserted between the 6th and 7th ribs. (**B**) A small amount of saline is injected to clear the needle of blood and tissue. (**C**) A tissue sample is aspirated into the needle. The needle is then withdrawn and pressure is applied to the site.

As the liver is progressively destroyed, its ability to metabolize proteins is impaired. Ammonia and toxic nitrogenous wastes accumulate in the blood. These substances affect the central nervous system. **Hepatic encephalopathy** is characterized by altered levels of consciousness, cognition,

and motor function. *Hepatorenal syndrome* (renal failure associated with end-stage liver disease) also may develop. Its cause is unknown, and treatment generally is ineffective.

INTERDISCIPLINARY CARE

The goals of cirrhosis treatment are to prevent further liver damage and manage the effects and complications of cirrhosis. Holistic care that addresses physiologic, psychosocial, and spiritual needs is important. It is vital to include the family in the plan of care, particularly if alcohol abuse is the cause.

Diagnostic Tests

A number of laboratory and diagnostic tests may be ordered:

- *Liver function tests* (see Chapter 18 ⊕) are elevated in cirrhosis, although not to the extent seen in hepatitis.
- A *complete blood count (CBC)* is done to evaluate possible anemia, leukopenia, and thrombocytopenia.
- *Blood chemistries,* including serum electrolytes and glucose, protein, albumin, and ammonia levels are done to evaluate liver function and its effects.
- *Coagulation studies* are ordered to evaluate the client's risk for bleeding.
- An *abdominal ultrasound* is performed to evaluate liver size, identify nodules, and detect ascites. See Chapter 18 ⊕ for more information about abdominal ultrasound.
- *Liver biopsy* (Figure 21-5 ■) may be ordered to determine the type and severity of cirrhosis. Nursing implications for the procedure are found in Box 21-11 ■.
- An *upper endoscopy* may be done to assess for esophageal varices. (See Box 19-13 ⊕ for nursing care related to upper endoscopy.)

BOX 21-11   **NURSING CARE CHECKLIST**

Liver Biopsy

Before the Procedure

☑ Verify informed consent for the procedure has been obtained.

☑ Reinforce teaching about the procedure and its purpose.

☑ Keep NPO as ordered, usually 4 to 6 hours before the procedure.

☑ Assess and record baseline vital signs.

☑ Review prothrombin time (PT) and platelet count; administer vitamin K as ordered.

☑ Have the client empty bladder immediately before the test.

☑ Place client in supine position on far right side of bed; turn head to left and extend right arm above head for better visualization of the biopsy site.

During the Procedure

☑ Help client hold breath following expiration to keep diaphragm and liver high in the abdominal cavity during needle insertion (see Figure 21-5).

☑ Obtaining biopsy tissue usually requires only 10 to 15 seconds.

☑ Some pain or discomfort may be experienced during the procedure.

After the Procedure

☑ Apply direct pressure to the site immediately after the needle is removed.

☑ Position client on right side.

☑ Frequently assess site and vital signs for evidence of bleeding; report immediately.

☑ Advise that pain may occur in the right shoulder as the anesthetic loses effect.

☑ Keep NPO for 2 hours (or as ordered), then resume usual diet.

☑ Instruct to avoid coughing, lifting, or straining for 1 to 2 weeks.

Medications

Substances that are toxic to the liver, such as alcohol and acetaminophen, are avoided. Drugs metabolized by the liver, including barbiturates and sedatives and hypnotics, also are avoided. Doses of other drugs may need to be adjusted, because impaired liver function may alter their metabolism and subsequent excretion.

Several groups or classes of drugs commonly are prescribed for clients with cirrhosis. *Diuretics* are prescribed to reduce edema and ascites. Spironolactone (Aldactone), a potassium-sparing diuretic, or the potent loop diuretic furosemide (Lasix) may be used. *Medications to reduce ammonia absorption* from the bowel frequently are used, particularly when blood ammonia levels are high. Two drugs used for this purpose are lactulose and neomycin (see Table 21-2 ■).

Beta-adrenergic blockers such as propranolol or nadolol (Corgard) may be given to reduce portal hypertension. *Vitamin K* is given to promote clotting. *Platelets* and other blood products such as *fresh frozen plasma* or *salt-poor albumin* may be administered to restore blood cells and replenish plasma proteins. *Histamine-2 antagonists* or *antacids* are ordered to manage associated gastritis and upper gastrointestinal bleeding. *Oxazepam*

(Serax) is an anti-anxiety/sedative drug that is not metabolized by the liver and may be used to treat acute agitation.

Dietary and Fluid Management

Abstinence from alcohol is vital for clients with cirrhosis. Dietary support also is essential. The diet should be palatable and include adequate protein and calories. If serum ammonia levels are high or the client has signs of hepatic encephalopathy, dietary protein is restricted. Sodium intake is restricted to less than 2 g/day. Fluids may be limited as needed to control ascites, edema, and heart failure. Clients who are NPO may require total parenteral nutrition. Vitamin and mineral supplements are ordered as indicated, particularly thiamine, folate, and B_{12}. The fat-soluble vitamins, A, D, and E, may need to be given in a water-soluble form. Clients with alcohol-induced cirrhosis may also need a magnesium supplement.

Surgical Procedures

Various surgical procedures may be used to manage the effects and complications of cirrhosis. *Liver transplant* is the only definitive treatment, and is not appropriate for all clients with cirrhosis (e.g., clients who continue to abuse

---

TABLE 21-2

Nursing Implications for Pharmacology: Cirrhosis

AGENTS/DRUGS	PURPOSE	NURSING RESPONSIBILITIES	TEACHING
Diuretics ■ Spironolactone (Aldactone) ■ Furosemide (Lasix)	Spironolactone is a potassium-sparing diuretic that reduces ascites by increasing urine output and decreasing aldosterone levels. Furosemide is a loop diuretic that promotes the excretion of potassium. These drugs may be given in combination.	Monitor vital signs and serum electrolytes and osmolality. Report changes to the charge nurse or physician. Weigh daily. Monitor and record intake and output.	Take diuretics in the morning and early afternoon to avoid sleep disruption caused by increased urine output. Report increases in weight or edema to your physician. Keep scheduled appointments for laboratory testing and with your physician.
Laxatives ■ Lactulose (Cephulac, Chronulac)	Lactulose inhibits ammonia absorption from the bowel and promotes its excretion in feces. It also is an osmotic laxative that pulls water into the bowel lumen, softening stool and stimulating peristalsis. The drug may be given orally or rectally.	Assess bowel sounds and abdominal girth. Maintain accurate stool chart. Adjust dose to achieve two to three soft stools per day as ordered. Monitor electrolytes and hydration status.	Mix with fruit juice, water, or milk to make more palatable. Drink adequate fluids. Report diarrhea to your physician. If this drug causes nausea, take it with a soda or crackers. Do not stop the medication.
Anti-Infective Agents ■ Neomycin sulfate (Neo Tabs)	Neomycin sulfate is a gastrointestinal antibiotic that is used to destroy intestinal bacteria and decrease ammonia production in the bowel. It may be given as an oral or rectal preparation.	Assess and monitor hearing, kidney, and neurologic functions before and during treatment. Monitor intake and output. Monitor blood urea nitrogen (BUN) and creatinine levels. Monitor digitalis levels as indicated.	Report dizziness, tinnitus (ringing in ears), hearing loss, headaches, tremors, or visual alterations immediately. Keep follow-up appointments. Maintain fluid intake; avoid dehydration.

| BOX 21-12 | NURSING CARE CHECKLIST |

Liver Transplant

Before Surgery

☑ Reinforce preoperative teaching provided by the transplant team.

☑ Provide psychologic support.

☑ Provide routine preoperative care and teaching as outlined in Chapter 9. ∞

☑ Prepare the client for returning from surgery to the intensive care unit.

After Surgery

☑ Provide routine postoperative care as indicated by postoperative day (see Chapter 9). ∞

☑ Manage pain and promote respiratory function through coughing, deep breathing, incentive spirometry, and early ambulation.

☑ Administer drugs to prevent rejection (e.g., cyclosporine A, corticosteroids, and azathioprine) as ordered.

☑ Carefully monitor for infection because these drugs suppress the immune response.

☑ Monitor renal function and blood glucose levels.

☑ Monitor for signs of rejection: increasing temperature (an early sign), discomfort over transplant site, anorexia, decreased bile drainage from drain, arthralgia (joint pain), abnormal liver function tests (see Chapter 18 ∞ for normal levels). Promptly report abnormal assessment data to the charge nurse or physician.

☑ Provide discharge teaching:

  ☑ Avoid infections, recognizing signs of infection, and the importance of reporting all fevers.

  ☑ Recognize signs of rejection.

  ☑ Follow verbal and written instructions and a schedule for all prescribed medications. Stress importance of reporting adverse effects and maintaining regular follow-up appointments.

  ☑ Prepare for potential body image changes associated with steroid use and for the psychologic effects of receiving a transplanted organ.

alcohol). Nursing care of the client having a liver transplant is outlined in Box 21-12 ■.

Paracentesis (removal of fluid from the peritoneal cavity) may be done if ascites is severe (Figure 21-6 ■). Excess fluid in the peritoneal cavity puts pressure on the diaphragm, increasing the work of breathing. Removing this fluid improves breathing, but fluid will reaccumulate unless the underlying cause of ascites is corrected. Albumin may be given after paracentesis; it increases the intravascular oncotic pressure and slows the development of ascites. Nursing implications for paracentesis are listed in Box 21-13 ■.

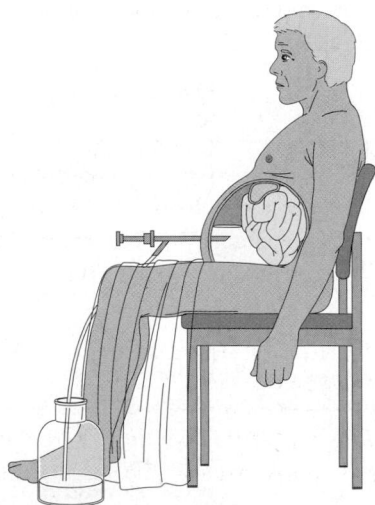

Figure 21-6. ■ Position of the client during paracentesis.

| BOX 21-13 | NURSING CARE CHECKLIST |

Paracentesis

Before the Procedure

☑ Verify informed consent for the procedure has been obtained.

☑ Reinforce teaching and clarify questions about the procedure.

☑ Weigh the client, and obtain baseline vital signs.

☑ Have client void immediately prior to the test to avoid bladder puncture.

☑ Place in a sitting position, either on the side of the bed or in a chair, with the feet supported.

During the Procedure

☑ Explain procedure. Following cleansing and local anesthesia, a needle or trocar is inserted through a small abdominal incision to withdraw fluid. The trocar is connected to tubing and a collection bottle; specimens may be sent to laboratory.

☑ Monitor blood pressure.

After the Procedure

☑ Put a small dressing over the puncture site; monitor drainage.

☑ Send specimens with completed requisitions to the laboratory for analysis as ordered.

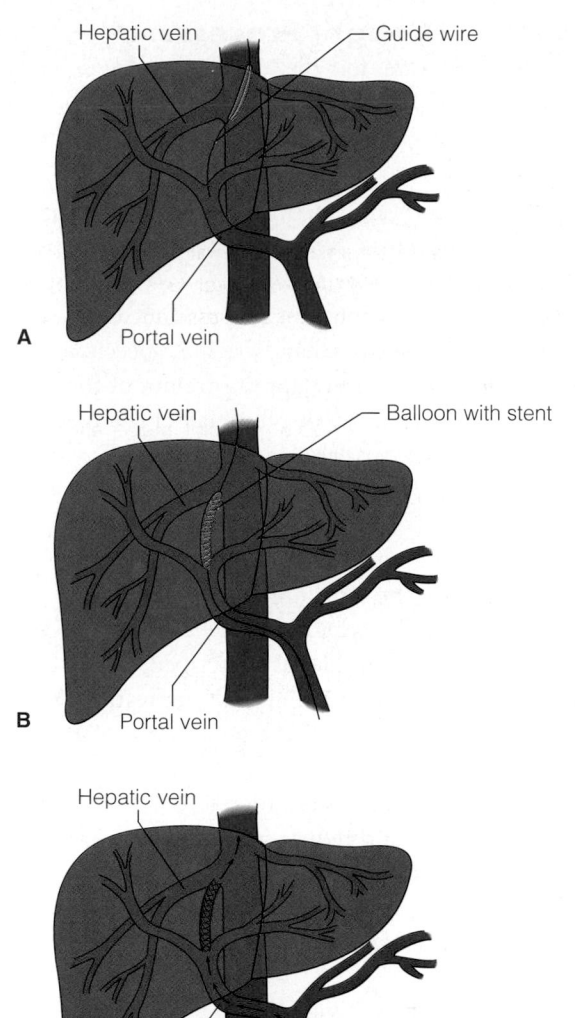

Figure 21-7. ■ Transjugular intrahepatic portosystemic shunt (TIPS). (**A**) A catheter inserted via the internal jugular vein is guided into the hepatic vein. From there, a new route connecting the hepatic and portal veins is created through liver tissue. (**B**) An expandable metal stent is positioned between the portal and hepatic veins. (**C**) The catheter and guidewire are removed, leaving the stent in place.

A *transjugular intrahepatic portosystemic shunt (TIPS)* may be used to relieve portal hypertension for some clients. The shunt directs venous blood from the portal vein to the hepatic vein, allowing it to bypass the liver (Figure 21-7 ■). It can be inserted in a vascular catheterization lab, avoiding the need for surgery. Following the procedure, observe the client closely for evidence of bleeding, either at the insertion site (the jugular vein) or internally. Monitor vital signs, color, and level of consciousness frequently, and report changes to the charge nurse or physician.

Bleeding esophageal varices, a potentially life-threatening complication of cirrhosis, may be treated with *endoscopic*

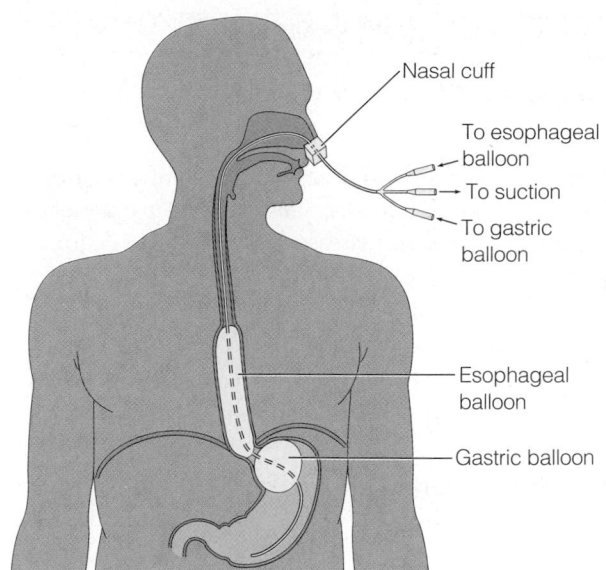

Figure 21-8. ■ A triple-lumen nasogastric (Sengstaken–Blakemore) tube used to control bleeding esophageal varices.

sclerotherapy or *endoscopic band ligation.* Once the varices have been identified, a sclerosing agent is injected into the enlarged vessel, causing an inflammatory reaction and clotting. In band ligation, the bleeding vessel is obstructed with a latex band or clip. (Review Box 19-10 🔗 for nursing care of clients having an upper endoscopy.) In an acute situation, a multiple-lumen gastrointestinal tube such as a Sengstaken–Blakemore tube may be inserted to *tamponade* (place pressure on) the bleeding varices (Figure 21-8 ■).

NURSING CARE

Nursing care of the client with cirrhosis presents many challenges because liver dysfunction affects many body systems. Psychosocial and spiritual aspects of care are as vital as the physical care needs of the client.

ASSESSING

Clients with cirrhosis may have vague symptoms or be acutely ill with bleeding, respiratory distress, or neurologic manifestations of hepatic encephalopathy. The extent of assessment data collected depends on the situation (Box 21-14 ■).

DIAGNOSING, PLANNING, AND IMPLEMENTING

Priorities in Nursing Care. The priority nursing care focus for clients with cirrhosis may vary, depending on the stage of the disease, its effects on other body systems, and the presence of complications.

BOX 21-14	ASSESSMENT

Assessing Clients with Cirrhosis

SUBJECTIVE DATA

- Risk factors for cirrhosis: alcohol use (amount per day or week, duration), chronic hepatitis, exposure to drugs or toxic chemicals, gallbladder disease.
- Current manifestations such as anorexia, nausea, indigestion; malaise; upper right abdominal pain; change in bowel habits; color of feces and urine.
- Change in color of skin or sclera; itching.
- History of complications such as ascites, upper GI bleeding, or mental changes.
- Current diet and fluid intake.

OBJECTIVE DATA

- General appearance; apparent nutritional status.
- Level of consciousness, mental status, and cognition.
- Color of skin and sclera, ecchymoses (bruising) or spider nevi (branching, dilated capillaries resembling a spider); dryness of skin, evidence of scratching.
- Color and consistency of feces, presence of frank blood or melena; color of urine.
- Color and consistency of emesis; evidence of GI bleeding.
- Inspect abdomen for distention, ascites, dilated, visible veins.
- Auscultate bowel sounds.
- Palpate abdomen for tenderness.

LABORATORY DATA

- Monitor liver function tests, CBC and platelets, serum electrolytes, glucose, and ammonia levels. Report significant or unexpected changes.

Excess Fluid Volume

- Weigh daily. Monitor intake and output. *Impaired salt and water regulation caused by cirrhosis can lead to problems such as peripheral edema, ascites, and heart failure. Changes in daily weight are an accurate indicator of fluid balance, as is monitoring intake and output.*
- Assess for neck vein distention and peripheral edema. *Neck vein distention and peripheral edema are indicators of excess fluid.*
- Measure abdominal girth daily. With the client supine, position the measuring tape around the abdomen at the level of the umbilicus. Mark the skin with indelible marker. *This ensures consistent, accurate measurements about the presence and amount of ascites.*
- Provide a low-sodium diet (500 to 2,000 mg/day) and restrict fluids as ordered. *Sodium causes water retention, which clients with cirrhosis need to avoid.*

Disturbed Thought Processes

The priority of care for the client who is experiencing manifestations of high serum ammonia levels and hepatic encephalopathy is preserving safety and implementing measures to reduce its effects.

- Avoid unnecessary medications that can affect the central nervous system (CNS). *Careful use of medications can help avoid worsening manifestations of encephalopathy.*
- Assess level of consciousness and mental status. Monitor for changes in behavior, handwriting, speech, and development of *asterixis* (a flapping tremor of the hands). Notify the charge nurse or physician of changes. *Accumulated nitrogenous waste products affect the CNS and thinking processes. Early identification of problems allows prompt intervention—subtle changes in neurologic functioning are important!*
- If possible, have the same nurses care for client. *Consistent care may allow early recognition of neurologic changes.*
- Provide a low-protein diet as prescribed; teach the family the importance of maintaining diet restrictions. *Nitrogenous by-products from dietary protein increase serum ammonia levels.*
- Administer medications as ordered to prevent gastrointestinal bleeding and reduce gastrointestinal production of nitrogenous waste products. Give laxatives and stool softeners as needed to avoid constipation. *These measures help decrease ammonia production in the bowel and serum ammonia levels.*
- Orient to time, place, and person; provide simple explanations for care at the client's level of understanding. Maintain a calm environment; minimize external stimuli. *These measures help prevent agitation and anxiety when thinking is impaired.*

Ineffective Protection

The client with esophageal varices is at significant risk for massive hemorrhage and hypovolemic shock.

- Monitor vital signs. *Increased pulse and decreasing blood pressure may indicate hemorrhage.*
- Institute bleeding precautions. (See Box 21-15 ■ for specific interventions.) *Preventive measures can decrease the incidence of active bleeding.*
- Monitor coagulation studies and platelet count. *The results determine the need to continue bleeding precautions and to administer vitamin K as ordered.*

Risk for Suffocation

Clients with a Sengstaken–Blakemore or other multiple-lumen nasogastric tube (see Figure 21-8) to control bleeding esophageal varices have special care needs. These clients usually are in intensive care units for close monitoring.

BOX 21-15

BLEEDING PRECAUTIONS

- Prevent constipation.
- Avoid rectal temperatures or enemas.
- Avoid injections; if needed, use small-gauge needle and apply pressure.
- Assess for bruises or purpura (hemorrhage into the skin).
- Apply pressure to bleeding sites.
- Apply direct pressure to venipuncture sites for at least 5 minutes.
- Use only a soft toothbrush.
- Avoid blowing nose.
- Assess oral cavity for bleeding gums.
- Administer H_2-blockers or antacids as ordered to prevent gastrointestinal bleeding.

- Secure and maintain the original position of the tube. Use soft wrist restraints as needed to prevent the client from pulling on the tube. *If the tube is dislodged while the esophageal balloon is inflated, the airway can be obstructed.*

clinical ALERT

Keep a large syringe or scissors at the bedside to rapidly deflate the balloons should the tube become displaced, obstructing the airway.

- Place in Fowler's position. Suction the oropharynx as needed. *The esophageal balloon impairs the ability to swallow oral secretions. Elevating the head of the bed reduces the risk of aspiration and promotes gas exchange.*
- Monitor and release balloon pressures as ordered. *The gastric balloon helps keep the distal end of the tube in the stomach, preventing the esophageal balloon from obstructing the airway. The inflated balloons place pressure on gastric and esophageal tissues; they may be periodically deflated to reduce the risk of tissue necrosis.*

clinical ALERT

Always deflate the esophageal balloon before deflating the gastric balloon.

- Frequently check the nares for tissue damage. Keep the nasal cuff (a small piece of foam) in place. *Pressure sores can develop on the nares through which the tube is inserted.*

Ineffective Breathing Pattern

- Place in high-Fowler's position with feet elevated; assist to chair as tolerated. Avoid supine position when possible. *The sitting position permits full expansion of the lungs*

and allows gravity to pull fluid and abdominal organs away from the diaphragm.

- Monitor respirations, lung sounds, and oxygen saturation levels. Report abnormal findings or changes in status. *Continuing respiratory assessments are important to prevent problems from impaired ventilation and oxygenation.*
- Administer oxygen as ordered. *Oxygen therapy may be necessary to prevent hypoxia.*

Impaired Skin Integrity

- Use warm water rather than hot water when bathing. *Hot water can dry the skin further and increase itching.*
- Avoid soap for bathing, apply an emollient or lotion without alcohol to moisten skin, and do not rub the skin. *These measures help prevent dry skin and pruritus.*
- Apply mittens or mitts to hands as needed to prevent scratching. *Clients with encephalopathy may not understand why they should not scratch.*
- Turn at least every 2 hours, use an alternating pressure mattress, and assess skin for breakdown. *Position changes relieve pressure and promote tissue oxygenation.*

EVALUATING

To evaluate the effectiveness of nursing care, collect data related to outcomes for the identified nursing diagnoses. For example:

- Are the weight and abdominal girth stable?
- Is behavior and mental status normal for the client?
- Has the client remained free of bleeding?
- Is the client's respiratory status improved?
- Has the skin remained intact?

Documenting. Document continuing assessment data, including mental status, respiratory effort, abdominal girth, daily weight, and intake and output. Note any diagnostic or therapeutic procedures performed, and the client's response to and recovery from these procedures. Document teaching provided to the client and family, and their apparent understanding and acceptance of information and prescribed care measures (e.g., alcohol avoidance, dietary restrictions).

CONTINUING CARE

Home care for the client with cirrhosis requires a coordinated team effort that includes the client, family, physician, nurses, and social services. Box 21-16 ■ outlines assessment data to consider in planning for discharge.

Include family members in all teaching, particularly when alcohol abuse and hepatic encephalopathy are considerations. Consistently reinforce teaching; repeat explanations as needed. Reinforce teaching about the prescribed diet and any fluid restrictions. If necessary, refer to a dietitian for

BOX 21-16 **ASSESSMENT**

Assessing for Discharge: Cirrhosis

CLIENT

- Self-care: ability to perform ADLs; to prepare and eat the prescribed diet
- Knowledge: understanding of disease and its progression; preventing complications; diet and fluid restrictions; toxins to avoid; when to contact the physician
- Psychosocial: support network and significant others; willingness to abstain from alcohol and other drugs; ability to cope with long-term effects or with liver transplant; evidence of grieving
- Home environment: factors affecting the client's ability to abstain from alcohol (e.g., roommates, type and location of housing)

FAMILY AND CAREGIVERS

- Members of household: ability and willingness to help with food preparation, family responsibilities, and care
- Availability of and referral to home health and social services
- Support groups and Alcoholics Anonymous meetings or other alcohol treatment options

diet planning. Provide written and verbal instructions about all medications and when to contact the physician. Teach follow-up care and any home care considerations following procedures such as liver biopsy or TIPS placement. Stress the importance of avoiding all substances toxic to the liver, including alcohol and over-the-counter medications containing acetaminophen. If the client is in end-stage liver disease, refer for hospice care as appropriate.

NURSING PROCESS CARE PLAN
Client with Alcoholic Cirrhosis

Richard Wright is a 48-year-old man who has alcoholic cirrhosis. He is admitted to the hospital with ascites and malnutrition. He has had three previous admissions for cirrhosis, the most recent being 6 months ago.

Assessment. Mr. Wright is lethargic but responds appropriately to verbal stimuli. He complains of "spitting up blood the past week or so" and says, "I just don't feel hungry." He has lost 20 lbs (9 kg) since his previous admission. He is jaundiced and has petechiae and ecchymoses on his arms and legs. His admitting nurse notes 3+ pitting edema of his ankles and feet. His abdomen is distended and tight, with distended superficial veins. Vital signs are: T 100°F (37.7°C); BP 110/70; P 110; R 24.

Laboratory test results include RBC 4.0 million/mm^3, WBC 3,700/mm^3, platelets 75,000/mm^3; elevated serum ammonia, total bilirubin, and serum sodium levels; low serum potassium, total protein, and albumin levels.

The diagnosis of alcohol-induced cirrhosis with gastritis is made. Mr. Wright is started on Aldactone, Riopan, lactulose, an 800-mg sodium, low-protein diet, and fluid restriction of 1,500 mL/day.

Diagnosis. The following nursing diagnoses are identified for Mr. Wright:

- *Excess Fluid Volume* related to electrolyte imbalance and low serum albumin
- *Imbalanced Nutrition: Less than Body Requirements* related to anorexia and possible alcohol abuse
- *Disturbed Thought Processes* related to high ammonia levels
- *Ineffective Protection* related to low platelets and malnutrition

Expected Outcomes. The expected outcomes for the plan of care specify that:

- Abdominal girth will decrease by 1 to 2 cm per day; peripheral edema will decrease to no more than 1+.
- Weight will increase by 1 lb (0.45 kg) per week while losing excess fluid.
- Will be alert and oriented to time, place, and person.
- No further active bleeding will occur.

Planning and Implementation. The following nursing interventions are implemented:

- Weigh daily before breakfast.
- Consult dietitian to plan a low-salt, low-protein, high-calorie diet.
- Frequently assess mental status; promptly report changes.
- Measure abdominal girth every shift.
- Institute bleeding precautions.
- Keep head of bed elevated; assist to chair with legs elevated tid as tolerated.
- Refer to home health and community agencies for discharge follow-up.

Evaluation. Mr. Wright is discharged after 7 days. His weight has decreased by 4 lbs, but decreased peripheral edema (now 1+) and abdominal girth indicate that this is due to loss of excess fluid. He does not experience any further bleeding. His serum ammonia levels return to normal. Lactulose will be continued on discharge.

Mr. Wright and his teenage children have made contact with Alcoholics Anonymous and Al Anon; they also have appointments to meet with a psychiatric social worker and primary caregiver.

Critical Thinking in the Nursing Process

1. Why was Mr. Wright lethargic on admission? Why does bleeding into the gastrointestinal tract increase serum ammonia levels?
2. Discuss the relationship between portal hypertension, low serum protein levels, and ascites.
3. Outline a 1-day meal plan for Mr. Wright that is low in protein, high in calories, and low in salt.

Cancer of the Liver

Primary liver cancer is uncommon in the United States, but metastases to the liver from other primary sites are relatively frequent. The prognosis for primary hepatic cancer is poor, in part because the disease often is not diagnosed before it reaches an advanced stage. Metastases to the lungs are common.

Most primary liver cancers arise from the liver's **parenchymal** (essential, functional) cells; about 10% develop in the bile duct. Regardless of where the cancer develops, the progress of the disease is similar. Chronic hepatitis B or hepatitis C and alcohol-induced cirrhosis are the primary risk factors for liver cancer in the United States.

Manifestations of liver cancer include malaise, painful mass in the right upper quadrant, epigastric fullness, weight loss, anorexia, and fever. Clients may present with ascites, jaundice, or signs of liver failure. Liver biopsy establishes the diagnosis. Magnetic resonance imaging (MRI), ultrasound, and computed tomography (CT) scans can aid in diagnosis, as can tests for serum markers such as alpha-fetoprotein (AFP).

Partial *hepatectomy* (resection and removal of a portion of the liver) is possible when the cancer is limited and has not spread beyond the liver. Liver transplantation is a potential option. Radiation therapy is used to shrink the tumor, decreasing pressure on surrounding organs and reducing pain. Chemotherapy may be used as adjunctive treatment for liver cancer.

Preventive nursing care focuses on teaching about the causes of liver cancer and their prevention. Avoiding alcohol, particularly in excess, also is a preventive measure. For the client with liver cancer, pain control is a priority. Refer clients with inoperable liver cancer to hospice services and cancer support groups.

Liver Trauma

Liver trauma can be caused by blunt trauma or penetrating injury to the abdomen. Automobile crashes, stab or gunshot wounds, and iatrogenic sources, such as liver biopsy, are possible causes of liver trauma. Because the liver is highly vascular, hemorrhage is a significant risk in liver trauma.

Preventing and treating hypovolemic shock are priorities of care for clients with liver trauma. (See Chapter 13 for more information about hypovolemic shock.) Intravenous fluids and blood products may be given to maintain blood volume and cardiac output. Surgery may be necessary to locate and control bleeding. Postoperative nursing care focuses on preventing pulmonary complications and monitoring for signs of infection or additional bleeding. Keeping family members informed is an important aspect of care, especially until the client's condition stabilizes.

EXOCRINE PANCREATIC DISORDERS

The pancreas is both an exocrine and an endocrine gland. As an exocrine gland, it produces enzymes that empty through ducts into the small intestine. As an endocrine gland, it produces hormones that enter the bloodstream directly. Disorders of the exocrine pancreas affect the secretion of digestive enzymes and may affect its endocrine functions as well. (*Diabetes mellitus,* a disorder of the endocrine pancreas, is discussed in Chapter 17.)

Pancreatitis

Pancreatitis (inflammation of the pancreas) may be either acute or chronic. *Acute pancreatitis* usually develops in middle life; gallstones and alcoholism are the primary risk factors for acute pancreatitis. Alcoholism also is the primary risk factor for *chronic pancreatitis,* a disease that

eventually leads to pancreatic insufficiency. Clients with pancreatitis often are acutely ill, and they may require lifelong treatment.

PATHOPHYSIOLOGY

Acute Pancreatitis

Acute pancreatitis occurs when the pancreas is damaged or the duct is blocked, allowing pancreatic enzymes to accumulate within the pancreas itself. Pancreatic duct obstruction by a gallstone or spasm of the sphincter of Oddi (associated with alcohol use) can obstruct the outflow of pancreatic enzymes. When this happens, a self-destructive process known as *autodigestion* begins.

In the milder form of acute pancreatitis, *interstitial edematous pancreatitis,* the pancreas becomes inflamed and

---

BOX 21-17

MANIFESTATIONS OF PANCREATITIS

Acute Pancreatitis

- Acute severe epigastric pain; may radiate to back
- Nausea, vomiting
- Abdominal distention, decreased bowel sounds
- Low-grade fever
- Tachycardia, hypotension
- Cool, clammy skin
- Elevated WBC, serum amylase, and lipase
- Low serum calcium and magnesium

Chronic Pancreatitis

- Persistent or recurring episodes of upper abdominal pain radiating to the back
- Anorexia, nausea, vomiting, weight loss
- Flatulence and constipation
- Steatorrhea (fatty, frothy, foul-smelling stools)
- Elevated serum amylase and lipase
- Elevated glucose levels

---

edematous. This process often is self-limiting and clients recover completely.

The more severe form, *necrotizing pancreatitis,* is an acute inflammatory process. Pancreatic tissue bleeds and becomes necrotic, and secondary bacterial infection can lead to abscess formation. Clients with necrotizing pancreatitis may recover completely, have recurrent attacks, or develop chronic pancreatitis.

MANIFESTATIONS AND COMPLICATIONS. The onset of acute pancreatitis is often sudden. The client experiences continuous severe epigastric and abdominal pain. This pain commonly radiates to the back and is relieved somewhat by sitting up and leaning forward. The onset of pain often occurs after a fatty meal or excessive alcohol consumption. Other manifestations are listed in Box 21-17 ■.

Clients with acute pancreatitis may develop hypovolemic shock (see Chapter 13 ⚭) due to vasodilation and a fluid shift into the small bowel (see Chapter 7 ⚭). Bleeding into the retroperitoneal space may occur, as evidenced by bruising in the flanks (*Turner's sign*) or around the umbilicus (*Cullen's sign*). A *pancreatic pseudocyst* (a collection of blood, fluid, and pancreatic secretions in the abdominal cavity) may develop. If the pseudocyst ruptures, peritonitis results. *Pancreatic abscess* (a collection of secretions and necrotic products within the pancreas) may be fatal. These complications usually occur 2 to 3 weeks after the onset of pancreatitis.

Chronic Pancreatitis

Chronic pancreatitis, which leads to gradual destruction of the pancreas, may follow acute pancreatitis or may have no identified cause. Alcoholism is the primary risk factor for chronic pancreatitis in the United States; worldwide, malnutrition is the major risk factor. In chronic pancreatitis, small ducts of the pancreas are blocked by calcified proteins. This initiates an inflammatory process in which normal pancreatic tissue is destroyed and replaced by fibrous scar tissue. Chronic pancreatitis is progressive and irreversible. It ultimately leads to pancreatic insufficiency, which in turn leads to malabsorption and, if endocrine function of the pancreas is affected, diabetes mellitus. The manifestations of chronic pancreatitis are listed in Box 21-17.

Malabsorption, malnutrition, and peptic ulcer disease are the primary complications of chronic pancreatitis. In addition, chronic pancreatitis increases the risk for pancreatic cancer and narcotic addiction (due to frequent episodes of severe pain).

INTERDISCIPLINARY CARE

Diagnostic Tests

- Laboratory tests may be ordered to confirm the diagnosis of pancreatitis. See Table 18-3 ⚭ for normal values of tests of pancreatic function, and Table 21-3 ■ for changes in laboratory results related to pancreatic dysfunction.
- *Abdominal x-ray* or *abdominal ultrasound* may show inflammatory changes or the presence of gallstones in acute pancreatitis.
- *CT scans* help differentiate acute and chronic pancreatitis.
- *Endoscopic retrograde cholangiopancreatography (ERCP)* is used to diagnose chronic pancreatitis.
- *Percutaneous fine-needle aspiration biopsy* may be done to distinguish between chronic pancreatitis and pancreatic cancer.

Treatment

Treatment of acute pancreatitis focuses on eliminating its causes (such as gallstones or alcohol abuse), minimizing additional damage to the pancreas by reducing pancreatic secretions, relieving pain, and preventing complications. The client initially is given nothing by mouth. A nasogastric tube may be inserted and connected to suction, and intravenous fluid therapy or total parenteral nutrition (TPN) is initiated (see Chapter 19 ⚭). These measures decrease pancreatic enzyme production while maintaining hydration and nutrition. Oral food and fluids are resumed when serum amylase levels return to normal, bowel sounds are present, and pain has disappeared. Intake begins with clear liquids and progresses to a low-fat diet as tolerated.

Parenteral narcotic analgesics may be required for pain relief. Antibiotics may be ordered to prevent or treat infection. Once the acute episode resolves, a laparoscopic cholecystectomy is done to reduce the risk of future episodes.

TABLE 21-3

Laboratory Tests for Pancreatic Disorders

TEST	SIGNIFICANCE
Serum amylase Critical value > 500 IU/L Serum lipase Critical value > 600 IU/L	Elevated in acute pancreatitis and acute episodes of chronic pancreatitis; may be elevated in pancreatic cancer
Urine amylase	Elevated in acute pancreatitis
Serum calcium Critical value < 6 mg/dL Serum magnesium Critical value < 1 mg/dL	Decreased in acute pancreatitis
White blood cells (WBCs)	Elevated in acute pancreatitis
Carcinoembryonic antigen (CEA) Normal value < 5 ng/mL	Elevated in pancreatic cancer

Treatment for chronic pancreatitis includes pain management, nutritional support, and replacement of deficient enzymes and hormones. Narcotic analgesics are avoided if possible, because the risk of addiction is high. Octreotide (Sandostatin) is a synthetic hormone that suppresses pancreatic enzyme secretion. It may be used to relieve the pain of chronic pancreatitis. Alcohol is forbidden; it may precipitate an attack. Pancreatic enzyme supplements (Table 21-4 ■) are given to manage *steatorrhea* (fat in stools).

Omeprazole (Prilosec), ranitidine (Zantac), or a similar drug is prescribed to reduce gastric acidity (which stimulates pancreatic enzyme production). Diabetes resulting from chronic pancreatitis is treated (see Chapter 17). ⚭ Surgery may be performed to drain persistent pseudocysts or to dilate an obstructed duct.

NURSING CARE

ASSESSING

Assessment data focus on identifying the onset of symptoms and risk factors for pancreatitis. Ask the client to describe the pain: its onset, intensity using a standardized pain scale (see Chapter 8), ⚭ character (steady, boring, stabbing, radiating), duration, relieving and aggravating factors, and any associated symptoms such as sweating, nausea, or vomiting. Ask about any history of previous attacks or a history of gallbladder disease. Inquire about alcohol use (number of drinks per day or per week, most recent alcohol consumption). Ask about food intake for the day prior to the onset of the pain.

Observe for nonverbal cues of pain: restlessness or rigid stillness; tense facial features; clenched fists; rapid, shallow breathing; tachycardia; diaphoresis. Listen for bowel sounds and gently palpate the abdomen for tenderness. Report assessment data to the charge nurse or physician.

DIAGNOSING, PLANNING, AND IMPLEMENTING

Priorities in Nursing Care. Relieving the acute, severe pain often associated with acute or chronic pancreatitis is the priority for nursing care.

Acute Pain

- Administer ordered narcotic analgesics on a regular schedule or teach the client to use patient-controlled analgesia (PCA). Assess the effectiveness of analgesia. *Severe, established pain is difficult to control. Unrelieved pain may increase secretion of pancreatic enzymes.*
- Maintain nothing by mouth (NPO) status and nasogastric tube patency as ordered. *Gastric secretions stimulate*

TABLE 21-4

Nursing Implications For Pharmacology: Chronic Pancreatitis

AGENTS/DRUGS	PURPOSE	NURSING RESPONSIBILITIES	CLIENT TEACHING
Pancreatic Enzyme Replacement			
■ Pancrelipase (Lipancreatin)	Pancrelipase promotes starch and fat digestion by replacing the pancreatic enzymes protease, amylase, and lipase. It improves nutrition and decreases the number of bowel movements.	Monitor frequency and consistency of stools. Weigh every other day. Record weights. Administer with meals. Monitor for side effects: Rash, hives, respiratory difficulty, hematuria, gout, or joint pain.	Take the drug with meals or snacks. If medicine is enteric coated, do not crush, chew, or mix with foods such as milk or ice cream. Be sure to follow prescribed diet.

pancreatic secretion, aggravating pain. Withholding food and maintaining nasogastric suction reduce gastric secretions and help relieve nausea and vomiting.

- Maintain client on bed rest in a calm, quiet environment. *Reducing physical movement and mental stimulation decreases metabolic rate, gastrointestinal secretion, and resulting pain.*
- Provide comfort measures:
  - Provide oral and nasal care every 1 to 2 hours.
  - Assist to a comfortable position, such as side-lying with knees flexed and head elevated 45 degrees.
  - Encourage relaxation techniques and guided imagery to decrease pain.
  - Explain all procedures and care; listen carefully to concerns and evaluation of pain relief.

  The client who is NPO needs frequent mouth care for comfort. Inflammation and stretching of the peritoneum causes pain. Sitting up, leaning forward, or lying in a fetal position tends to decrease the pain. Alternative pain relief measures help reduce anxiety and help the client gain a sense of control (see Chapter 8 on pain). 🔗
- Ask the family and visitors to avoid bringing food into the client's room. *The sight of food may stimulate pancreatic secretions.*

Risk for Imbalanced Nutrition: Less than Body Requirements

- Weigh daily at the same time. *Decreasing weight may indicate poor nutritional status.*
- Maintain stool chart; include frequency, color, odor, and consistency of stools. *Pancreatitis affects fat absorption, so undigested fats are excreted in the stool. Steatorrhea may indicate an increase in the severity of pancreatitis.*
- Regularly assess bowel sounds. *Nasogastric suction usually is discontinued within 24 to 48 hours after the return of bowel sounds indicates that the client is regaining bowel motility.*
- Administer intravenous fluids and TPN as prescribed. *Inflammation increases metabolism and nutritional needs. TPN may be ordered to maintain nutritional status while the client is NPO (see Chapter 19).* 🔗
- When eating resumes, provide small, frequent feedings and a high-carbohydrate, low-protein, low-fat diet. Avoid caffeine (coffee, tea, colas), spicy foods, or gas-producing foods. *Small, frequent feedings are better tolerated. A low-protein, low-fat diet minimizes pancreatic enzyme secretion, reducing inflammation and pain. Caffeine and spicy or gas-producing foods may increase pancreatic secretion and pain.*

Risk for Injury

- Assess vital signs (including orthostatic blood pressures), peripheral pulses, skin color, temperature, and turgor every 1 to 2 hours until stable, then every 4 hours. Record data and report abnormal findings to the charge nurse or physician. *Frequent assessment of cardiovascular and fluid volume status is important because fluid losses associated with vomiting, diaphoresis, third-space shifts, and nasogastric suction can affect cardiac output and tissue perfusion.*
- Monitor respiratory status including breath sounds. Encourage to cough and deep breathe hourly. *Abdominal pain causes shallow respirations and impaired ventilation, increasing the risk of atelectasis (see Chapter 24* 🔗 *) or pneumonia. Coughing and deep breathing improve ventilation and mobilize secretions.*
- Measure urine output hourly; maintain accurate intake and output. Report output of less than 30 mL/hr to the charge nurse or physician. *A drop in urine output may be an early indication of decreased cardiac output, which increases the risk of acute renal failure.*
- Frequently assess mental status, level of consciousness, and behavior. *Impaired mental status may indicate poor cerebral oxygenation, alcohol withdrawal, or other complications of acute pancreatitis.*

EVALUATING

When evaluating the effectiveness of nursing care for a client with acute pancreatitis, collect data such as pain level, weight, ability to resume eating, and stability of cardiovascular and respiratory status.

Documenting. Document continuing assessment data and measures employed to relieve pain and their effects. Document client and family teaching about the disorder, and their apparent understanding of teaching.

CONTINUING CARE

When appropriate, teach the client and family members about the disease and how to prevent further attacks. Discuss specific risk factors and needs, such as these:

- Alcohol abstinence is vital to prevent future attacks of acute or chronic pancreatitis. (Refer as needed to community agencies, support groups such as Alcoholics Anonymous, or individual counseling.)
- Smoking and stress stimulate the pancreas and should be avoided.
- Possible treatment for gallstones if appropriate, including options such as laparoscopic cholecystectomy.
- Instruct to take pancreatic enzymes and insulin as ordered. Refer to a diabetes educator as appropriate.
- Advise to maintain a low-fat diet and to avoid crash dieting or binge eating, which can bring on attacks. Discuss foods to avoid, such as spicy foods, caffeinated beverages, and gas-forming foods. Refer to a dietitian or nutritionist as needed for diet planning and teaching.

- Instruct to report signs of infection promptly (a fever of 102°F [38.8°C]) or higher, pain, rapid pulse, malaise) to the physician. An abscess may form months after the initial attack, necessitating further intervention.
- Refer to a community or home health agency as needed for home care.

Cancer of the Pancreas

While cancer of the pancreas is not common, its incidence is increasing in the United States. Older adults, African Americans, and men have a greater risk of developing pancreatic cancer. Smoking is a major risk factor for pancreatic cancer. Its incidence is twice as high in smokers as in non-smokers. The prognosis for pancreatic cancer is poor because the disease often is advanced at the time of diagnosis. More than 98% of people diagnosed with pancreatic cancer die of the disease.

Early manifestations of pancreatic cancer include anorexia, nausea, weight loss, flatulence, and dull epigastric pain. The pain increases in severity as the tumor grows. Cancer of the head of the pancreas, the most common site, often obstructs bile flow through the common bile duct, causing jaundice, clay-colored stools, dark urine, and pruritus. Late manifestations include a palpable abdominal mass and ascites.

With early diagnosis, surgery may be done to resect the tumor. If the head of the pancreas is affected, a pancreato-duodenectomy *(Whipple's procedure)* is done to remove the head of the pancreas, the duodenum, the distal third of the stomach, a portion of the jejunum, and part of the common bile duct. The common bile duct is then sutured to the end of the jejunum, and the remaining pancreas and stomach are sutured to the side of the jejunum (Figure 21-9 ■). Radiation and chemotherapy are often used in addition to surgery.

Postoperative nursing care of the client undergoing Whipple's procedure is similar to that of the client undergoing intestinal surgery (see Chapter 20). The client with pancreatic cancer has multiple problems that require nursing care. (Chapter 12 discusses nursing care for clients with cancer.) The nursing diagnoses and interventions discussed for

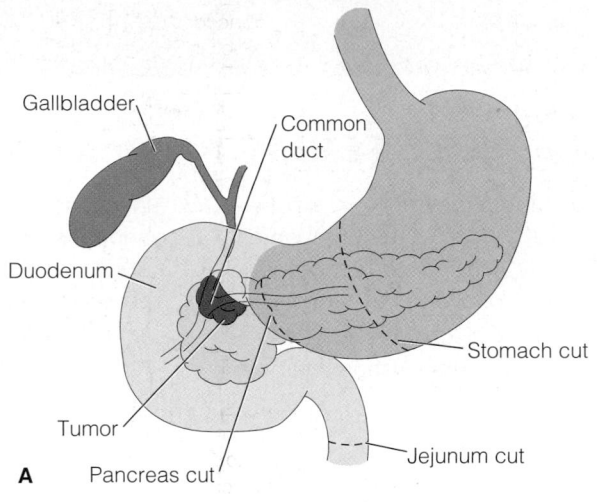

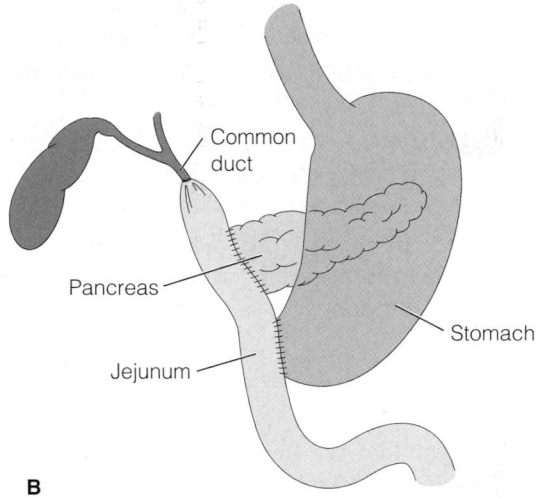

Figure 21-9. ■ Whipple's procedure. (**A**) Areas of resection. (**B**) Appearance following resection.

the client with pancreatitis are also appropriate for the client with pancreatic cancer.

Note: The bibliography listings for this and all chapters have been compiled at the back of the book.

Chapter Review

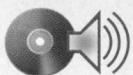 **KEY TERMS** by Topics

Use the audio glossary feature of either the CD-ROM or the Companion Website to hear the correct pronunciation of the following key terms.

Gallbladder Disorders
cholelithiasis, cholecystitis, biliary colic

Liver Disorders
hepatitis, icteric, jaundice, cirrhosis, portal hypertension, ascites, esophageal varices, hepatic encephalopathy, paracentesis, parenchymal

Exocrine Pancreatic Disorders
pancreatitis

KEY Points

- Alcohol abuse is a significant risk factor for the liver and pancreatic disorders discussed in this chapter. Prevention, early identification, and treatment of alcohol abuse reduces the risk of these disorders.

- Hepatitis usually is a viral disease and therefore cannot be cured at this time. Preventing the spread of hepatitis is an important nursing responsibility.

- Some types of viral hepatitis, most notably hepatitis B and C, can lead to a carrier state in which the infected client has no symptoms of the disease, but can spread it to others.

- Hepatitis B and C also can become chronic and ultimately lead to liver failure.

- The complications of cirrhosis, including portal hypertension, ascites, esophageal varices, and hepatic encephalopathy affect multiple body systems.

- Bleeding from esophageal varices may be massive, and requires prompt control to maintain cardiac output.

- Acute pancreatitis often develops as a complication of gallstones, whereas chronic pancreatitis is more frequently related to alcohol abuse.

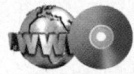 **EXPLORE MediaLink**

Additional interactive resources for this chapter can be found on the Companion Website at www.prenhall.com/burke. Click on Chapter 21 and "Begin" to select the activities for this chapter.

For chapter-related NCLEX-style review questions and an audio glossary, access the accompanying CD-ROM in this book.

FOR FURTHER Study

For further study about plasma osmotic pressure, see Chapter 7.

Chapter 8 provides information on pain scales.

See Chapter 9 for more information about care of the surgical client.

Chapter 12 discusses nursing care for clients with cancer.

See Chapter 13 for more information about hypovolemic shock.

For more on diabetes mellitus, see Chapter 17.

See Chapter 18 for the normal structure and function of the gallbladder, liver, and pancreas, and information about diagnostic tests for gallbladder, liver, and pancreatic disorders.

Figure 18-5 shows a liver lobule.

See Chapter 19 for nursing care related to upper endoscopy (Box 19-13).

Chapter 20 discusses care of the client undergoing intestinal surgery.

For more information about impaired ventilation, see Chapter 24.

Caring for a Client with Pancreatitis

NCLEX-PN® Focus Area: Physiologic Adaptation

Case Study: Rose Schliefer, 59 years old, is home following a 2-month hospitalization for acute pancreatitis. The pancreatitis was caused by gallstones. Mrs. Schliefer spent 3 weeks in intensive care and underwent surgery for the gallstones and to drain a pseudocyst. At discharge she was on a soft, low-protein, low-fat diet and was able to walk in the hall. She has been referred for home health services.

Nursing Diagnosis: Imbalanced Nutrition: Less than Body Requirements

COLLECT DATA

Subjective

_____
_____
_____
_____
_____
_____

Objective

_____
_____
_____
_____
_____
_____

Would you report this data? Yes/No

If yes, to: _____

Nursing Care

_____
_____
_____
_____
_____
_____
_____
_____
_____
_____
_____

How would you document this? _____
_____
_____
_____

Data Collected
(use those that apply)

- Thin, appears anxious and tired
- States she lost 30 lbs (13.6 kg) in the hospital
- Weight 102 lbs (46 kg), height 66 in. (168 cm)
- Vital signs within normal limits
- Well-healed upper abdominal scar and two stab wounds on sides of abdomen noted; scabs present on stab wounds
- Skin cool and dry, poor turgor
- Alert and oriented, responds appropriately
- Blood glucose 80 mg/dL
- States main problems are lack of energy and lack of appetite
- Family expresses concern about ability to provide care

Nursing Interventions
(use those that apply; list in priority order)

- Explain causes of fatigue.
- Help Mrs. Schliefer develop activity goals and identify steps to achieve goals.
- Plan daily rest periods, especially before meals.
- Discuss dietary restrictions and how to adapt to usual diet.
- Assist family to plan six small meals a day.
- Obtain a shower chair.
- Assist family to identify and divide responsibilities for care.
- Encourage client to identify strengths and concerns.

NCLEX-PN® Exam Preparation

1 A client diagnosed with cholelithiasis requests medication for pain relief. Which of the following medications is the physician most likely to prescribe?

   A. acetaminophen (Tylenol)

   B. morphine sulfate

   C. codeine

   D. ibuprofen (Motrin)

2 A client returns to his room following an open cholecystectomy. He has a T-tube in place attached to a drainage bag. The nurse would report which of the following assessments to the charge nurse or physician?

   A. There is less than 50 mL output from the T-tube each 8-hour shift.

   B. Client experiences nausea and vomiting 30 minutes after eating.

   C. T-tube drainage decreases after 24 hours.

   D. Client requires pain medication every 4 to 6 hours.

3 A client will manage her cholelithiasis at home using medical interventions. The nurse reinforces which of the following in discharge teaching?

   A. Sleep in prone position to decrease pain.

   B. Report episodes of pain that occur before meals.

   C. Use a heating pad for pain relief.

   D. Adhere to a low-fat, low-calorie diet.

4 A client who was diagnosed with hepatitis A (HAV) states he was told by the nursing assistant that his disease could be transmitted only through blood contact. The appropriate action by the nurse would be to:

   A. provide the correct information to the client and nursing assistant.

   B. take no further action because the information is correct.

   C. remove all precautions because hepatitis A cannot be transmitted.

   D. place a sign on the client's door stating "Blood Precautions."

5 A client is diagnosed with hepatitis B (HBV). Which of the following information, if obtained during the admission assessment, would indicate a risk factor?

   A. She ate in a restaurant 2 weeks ago.

   B. She uses barrier protection during sexual intercourse.

   C. She is an intravenous drug user.

   D. She has never received a blood transfusion.

6 A client with cirrhosis is scheduled for discharge. The LPN/LVN recognizes the need for further teaching if the client states:

   A. "I will use a soft toothbrush for oral hygiene."

   B. "I will maintain a low-protein diet."

   C. "I will report increased difficulty breathing to my physician."

   D. "I will limit alcohol intake to two servings per day."

7 The nurse evaluates a 54-year-old client with cirrhosis for improvement in her ascites. Which of the following assessment findings may indicate improvement? (Choose all that apply.)

   A. weight loss of 3 pounds in the past 72 hours

   B. abdominal girth 2 cm less than previous measurement

   C. urinary output 30 mL/hr

   D. tea-colored urine

   E. complains of increasing shortness of breath

8 A 45-year-old client with liver disease is prescribed lactulose (Chronulac) 30 mL every 6 hours. The LPN/LVN explains that the action of this medication is to:

   A. promote diuresis.

   B. decrease ammonia absorption.

   C. decrease fat metabolism.

   D. promote reabsorption of potassium.

9 A client is admitted to the nursing unit with a diagnosis of acute pancreatitis. The client complains of severe pain. Place the following nursing activities to promote client comfort in the order in which the nurse would do them.

   A. Insert the ordered nasogastric tube and connect to low intermittent suction.

   B. Administer prescribed parenteral narcotic analgesic.

   C. Place an NPO sign over the client's bed and notify dietary services.

   D. Place in a side-lying position with knees flexed and elevate the head of the bed 45 degrees.

   E. Promote rest by darkening the room and placing a sign on the door to limit visitors.

10 The nurse is caring for a client with acute pancreatitis. Which nursing assessment should receive the highest priority?

   A. Assess intake and output.

   B. Assess cardiovascular status and fluid volume status.

   C. Assess bowel sounds and fecal output.

   D. Assess mental status.

Answers for Review Questions, as well as discussion of Care Plan and Critical Thinking Care Map questions, appear in Appendix V.

Thinking Strategically About ...

Jamie Lynn, a 19-year-old college student, presents at the emergency department complaining of general lower abdominal pain that started the previous evening. The pain has localized to the right lower quadrant and became severe about 6 hours ago. She reports anorexia for the past two days. She complains of nausea and has vomited twice today.

DATA COLLECTED

Physical assessment data for Ms. Lynn include: T 102.6°F (39.2°C); P 96; R 24; BP 110/70. Her skin is warm to the touch. Her abdomen is flat, with marked tenderness in the right lower quadrant. Guarding is present throughout. Her WBC is 15,400/mm^3. The diagnosis of acute appendicitis with possible perforation is made.

Intravenous fluids are started to prevent and/or correct fluid and electrolyte imbalance and to combat dehydration. Intravenous antibiotics are also started. Ms. Lynn is transferred to surgery for an exploratory laparotomy. In surgery,

Ms. Lynn's ruptured appendix is removed and her peritoneal cavity is flushed with warmed saline before her incision is closed.

CRITICAL THINKING

1 Ms. Lynn's WBC was 15,400/mm^3. How does this compare with a normal WBC?

2 Why was Ms. Lynn's WBC elevated?

3 What elements would be important to include in a teaching plan for Ms. Lynn's home care?

MANAGEMENT OF NURSING CARE

1 What nursing care is indicated when a patient presents with an acute abdomen, as did Ms. Lynn?

2 What nursing care would be indicated for Ms. Lynn post-operatively?

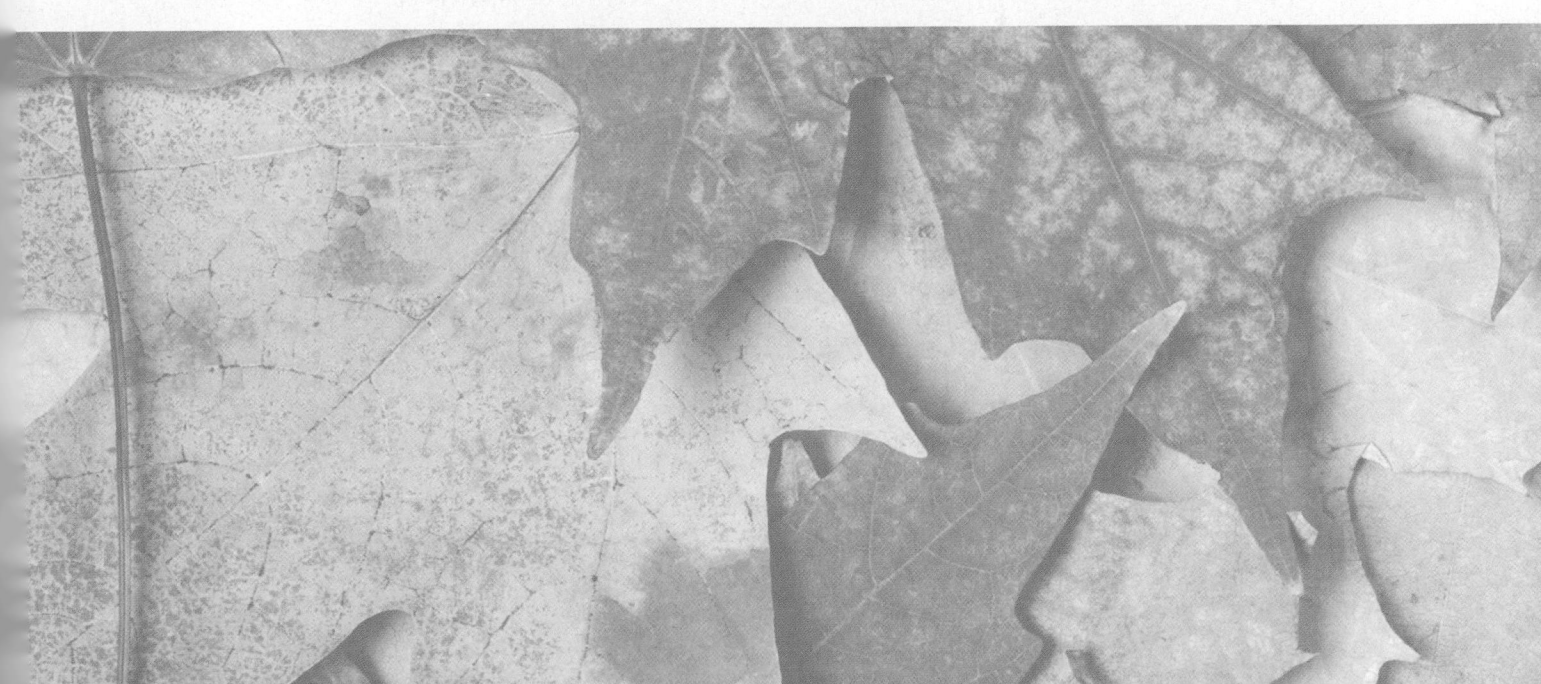

Disrupted Respiratory Function

UNIT V

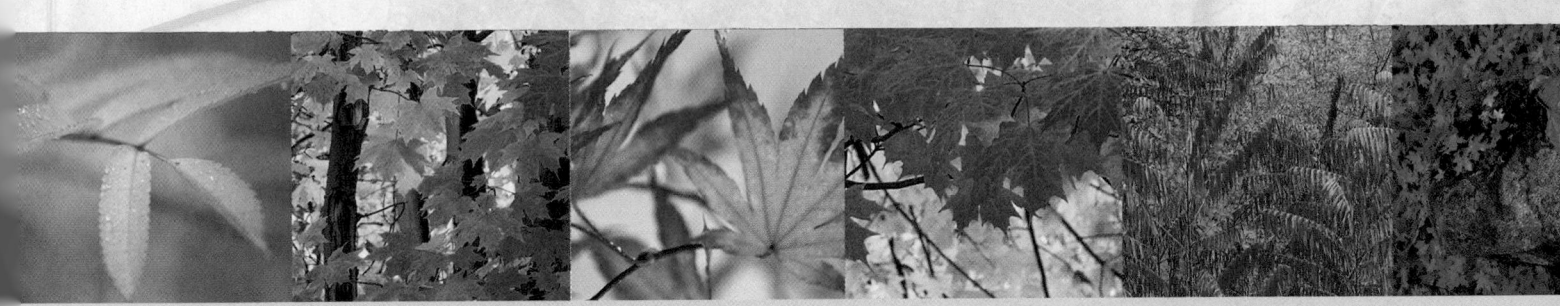

Chapter 22

The Respiratory System and Assessment

BRIEF Outline

Structure and Function of the Upper Respiratory System
- The Nose and Sinuses
- The Pharynx
- The Larynx

Structure and Function of the Lower Respiratory System
- The Lungs
- Bronchi and Alveoli
- Pulmonary Circulation
- The Pleura
- Rib Cage and Intercostal Muscles
- Mechanics of Respiration
- Factors Affecting Respiration

Respiratory Changes Associated with Aging

Assessment
- Subjective Data
- Physical Examination
- Diagnostic Tests

LEARNING Outcomes

After completing this chapter, you will be able to:
- Describe the structure and functions of the respiratory tract.
- Explain the mechanics of respiration.
- Describe assessment and data collection for respiratory function.
- Provide appropriate nursing care and teaching for clients undergoing diagnostic tests and procedures related to the respiratory system.

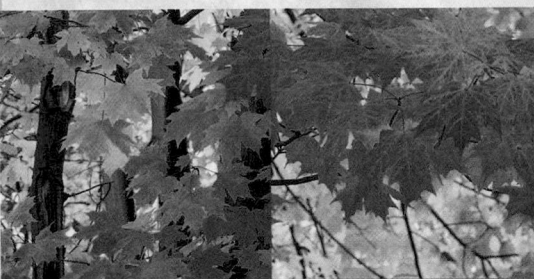

MediaLink

www.prenhall.com/burke
Use the address above to access the free, interactive Companion Website created for this textbook. Get hints, instant feedback, and textbook references to chapter-related NCLEX-style questions. Link to other interesting sites.

Audio Glossary:
Use the Companion Website, or the CD-ROM disk enclosed with your textbook, to hear the pronunciation of key terms in this chapter.

The primary function of the respiratory system is to provide the cells of the body with oxygen and to eliminate carbon dioxide (a waste product of cellular metabolism).

Structure and Function of the Upper Respiratory System

Air moves into the lungs and carbon dioxide moves out of the body through the upper respiratory tract. The upper airway cleans, humidifies, and warms air. An open upper airway is needed for effective breathing.

THE NOSE AND SINUSES

The respiratory system begins at the *nose* (Figure 22-1A ■). Cartilage and the facial bones give the nose structure. The nostrils (*nares*) are two cavities in the nose, separated by the *nasal septum.* They open into the nasal portion of the pharynx. Nasal hairs just inside the nares filter air as it enters the nose. The air is warmed by mucous membranes lining the nares. Mucous membranes contain scent receptors and cells that secrete thick mucus. The mucus traps dust and bacteria and contains an enzyme that destroys bacteria. The mucus and trapped debris are moved to the pharynx and then swallowed. Ridges within each nasal cavity (called *turbinates*) help trap heavier particles of debris.

The *sinuses* are openings in the facial bones (Figure 22-1B). Sinuses lighten the skull, assist in speech, and produce mucus that drains into the nasal cavities and helps trap debris.

THE PHARYNX

The *pharynx* (throat) is a passageway for both air and food. It is divided into three regions: the nasopharynx, oropharynx, and laryngopharynx.

The *nasopharynx* starts at the nose. Air, mucus, and trapped debris move through the nasopharynx, where the *tonsils* and *adenoids* (masses of lymphoid tissue in the back wall of the nasopharynx) trap and destroy infectious agents.

The *eustachian tubes* also open into the nasopharynx, connecting it with the middle ear.

The *oropharynx* lies behind the oral cavity. It carries both air and food. During swallowing, the soft palate (see Figure 22-1A) rises to prevent food from entering the nasopharynx. The lining of the oropharynx protects it from damage by friction and from chemicals in food and fluids.

The *laryngopharynx,* a passageway for both food and air, connects the oropharynx to the larynx.

THE LARYNX

The *larynx* (voice box) connects the laryngopharynx with the trachea and routes air and food into the proper passageway. The larynx is protected by cartilages that help keep it open (see Figure 22-1A). The inlet to the larynx (the *epiglottis*) is open when air is moving through it; during swallowing, the epiglottis tips down to cover the opening of the larynx. The larynx also contains the vocal cords, which help produce speech. If anything other than air enters the larynx, a cough reflex is initiated to expel the foreign substance before it can reach the lungs.

clinical ALERT

The cough reflex does not work if the person is unconscious.

Structure and Function of the Lower Respiratory System

The lower respiratory system includes the lungs and the bronchi. Its function is to provide oxygen to the cells of the body and to eliminate carbon dioxide, a waste product of metabolism. This process, called **respiration**, includes:

■ *Ventilation* (breathing): Air moves into and out of the lungs.

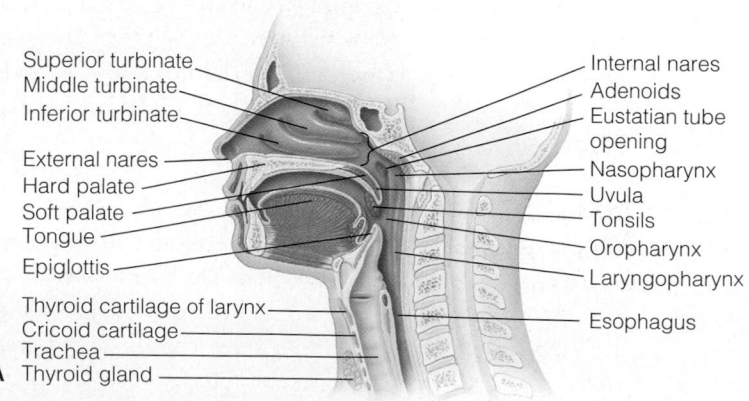

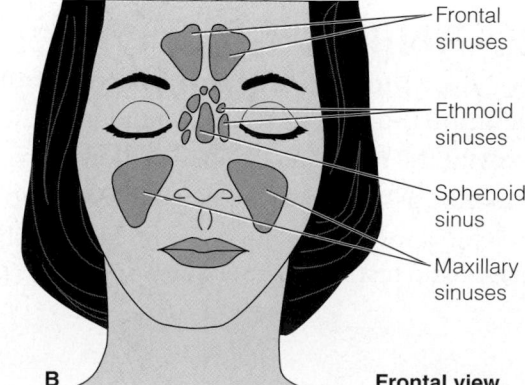

Figure 22-1. ■ **(A)** Structures of the upper respiratory system. **(B)** The sinuses.

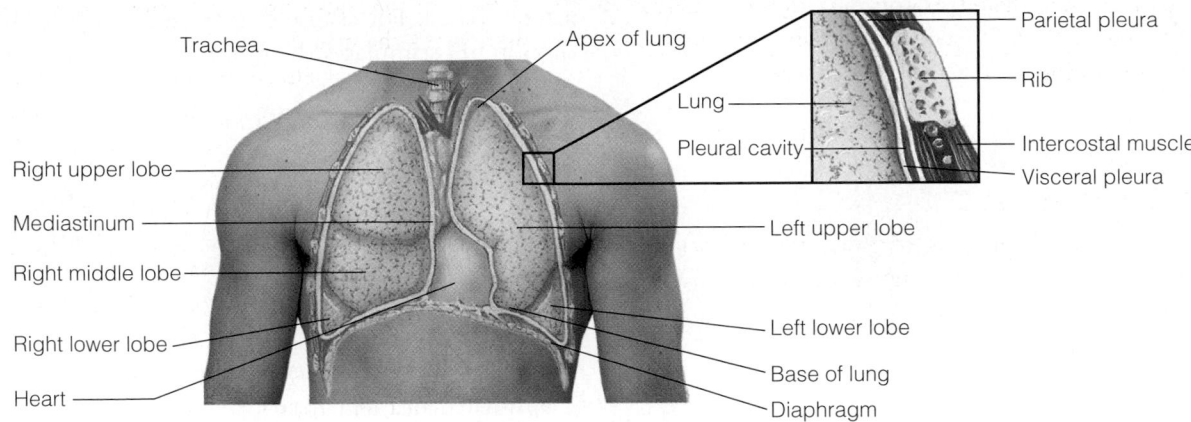

Figure 22-2. ■ The lower respiratory system, showing the lungs and layers of the visceral and parietal pleura.

- *External Respiration:* Oxygen and carbon dioxide are exchanged between the alveoli and the blood.
- *Gas Transport:* Blood transports oxygen and carbon dioxide to and from the lungs and the cells of the body.
- *Internal Respiration:* Oxygen and carbon dioxide are exchanged between the blood and the cells.

THE LUNGS

The lungs fill both sides of the chest, separated by the mediastinum. The heart, great blood vessels, bronchi, trachea, and esophagus sit in the *mediastinum* (Figure 22-2 ■). The *apex* of each lung is just below the clavicle, and the *base* of each lung rests on the diaphragm. The lungs are soft and spongy, composed of elastic connective tissue.

The right lung has three lobes; the left is smaller, with only two lobes. Each lobe is further divided into segments.

BRONCHI AND ALVEOLI

The trachea divides into *right* and *left mainstem bronchi.* The mainstem bronchi enter the lungs at the *hilus.* The bronchi branch into smaller bronchi, then into smaller and smaller *bronchioles,* ending in the tiny *alveoli* (Figure 22-3 ■). During inspiration, air moves through these passageways to the alveoli, where gas exchange occurs.

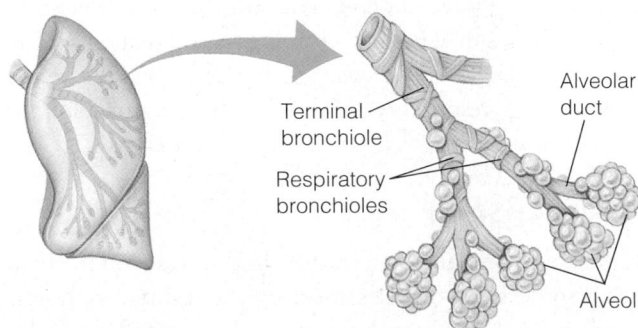

Figure 22-3. ■ The functional tissue of the lungs, including the respiratory bronchioles and alveoli.

Each lung has millions of alveoli, providing a huge area for gas exchange. Alveoli have extremely thin walls, made of a single layer of cells over a very thin connective tissue (basement) membrane. The outer surface of the alveolus is covered with pulmonary capillaries. Oxygen and carbon dioxide easily diffuse across the walls of the alveoli and capillaries. The alveoli contain cells that secrete *surfactant,* a detergent-like substance that helps keep them open.

PULMONARY CIRCULATION

The pulmonary circulation includes the pulmonary arteries, which deliver oxygen-poor blood to the lungs, and the pulmonary veins, which return oxygenated blood to the heart. In the lungs, the vessels branch into a pulmonary capillary network that surrounds the alveoli. Vessels enter and exit the lungs at the hilus.

THE PLEURA

The *pleura* is a double-layered membrane that covers the lungs (see Figure 22-2). The *parietal pleura* lines the chest wall and mediastinum. The *visceral pleura* covers the outer lung surfaces. The layers of the pleura hold the lungs out to the chest wall, sliding against one another during breathing. The potential space between the layers of the pleura contains a small amount of serous fluid to lubricate and reduce friction during breathing. There is a slight negative pressure in the pleural space.

RIB CAGE AND INTERCOSTAL MUSCLES

The lungs are protected by the rib cage and the intercostal muscles. There are 12 pairs of ribs. The spaces between the ribs (the *intercostal spaces*) are named for the rib immediately above (e.g., the space between the third and fourth ribs is the third intercostal space). The *intercostal muscles* between the ribs, along with the diaphragm, are *inspiratory muscles.*

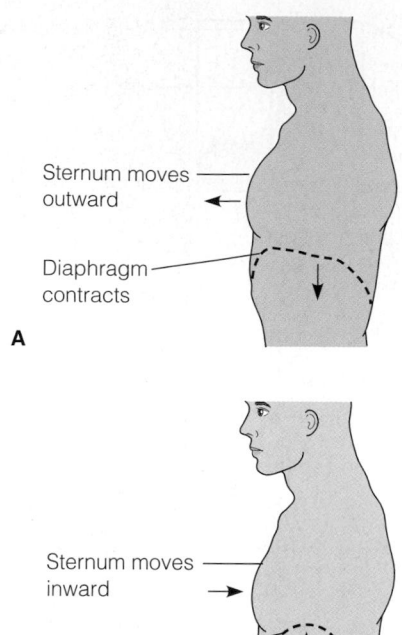

Figure 22-4. ■ **(A)** During inspiration, the diaphragm contracts and flattens, and the intercostals muscles contract, moving the chest wall up and outward. This increases the volume of the chest cavity. **(B)** During expiration, the muscles relax, the diaphragm rises, and the lungs recoil.

MECHANICS OF RESPIRATION

Ventilation, air movement into and out of the lungs, has two phases: *inspiration,* as air flows into the lungs, and *expiration,* when gases flow out of the lungs. The two phases make up a breath, and normally occur 12 to 20 times per minute. Inspiration lasts about 1 to 1.5 seconds; expiration lasts about 2 to 3 seconds.

During inspiration, the diaphragm contracts and flattens out and the intercostal muscles contract to increase the size of the chest cavity (Figure 22-4A ■). The lungs stretch and their volume increases. This reduces pressure within the lungs to slightly less than atmospheric pressure. Air rushes into the lungs as a result.

Expiration is primarily passive. The inspiratory muscles relax, the diaphragm rises, the ribs descend, and the lungs recoil (Figure 22-4B). Pressures in the chest cavity increase, compressing the alveoli. The pressure within the lungs is higher than atmospheric pressure, and gases flow out of the lungs.

FACTORS AFFECTING RESPIRATION

Breathing is controlled by respiratory centers in the brain and by chemoreceptors in the brain, aortic arch, and carotid arteries. These centers and receptors respond to changes in the amount of oxygen, carbon dioxide, and hydrogen ions in

arterial blood. For example, increased carbon dioxide or a drop in pH stimulates the respiratory centers, and the respiratory rate increases.

Other factors affect ventilation and the work of breathing:

- *Airway resistance* is created by friction as gases move through the airways. Resistance is increased by airway constriction or edema, excess mucus, or by tumors that narrow the airways. As resistance increases, gas flow decreases.
- **Compliance** is the *distensibility* (stretchiness) of the lungs. It depends on both lung tissue and the rib cage.
- *Elasticity* is the tendency of lung tissue to return to its uninflated size and shape.

clinical ALERT

A balloon is a good example of compliance and elasticity. When a balloon is brand new, it is very elastic and not very compliant—it takes a lot of work to begin inflating it (poor compliance). When the air is released, it returns to its previous shape (good elasticity). After it has been blown up a few times, it becomes increasingly compliant, and easier to inflate. However, it does not return to its original shape, because some of its elasticity has been lost.

- Alveoli contain a liquid film that creates *surface tension,* drawing the walls of the alveolus closer together. *Surfactant* reduces this surface tension, prevents the alveoli from collapsing between breaths, and reduces the work of breathing.

RESPIRATORY CHANGES ASSOCIATED WITH AGING

Aging commonly leads to both structural and functional changes of the respiratory system. Cartilage that connects the ribs to the sternum and spinal column calcifies, decreasing the mobility of the rib cage. The anterior-posterior diameter of the chest increases as well. Muscles of respiration become weaker. The cough and laryngeal reflexes are less effective. The overall size of the lungs is reduced, and alveoli are less elastic (less able to fully recoil on expiration). This loss of elasticity increases the residual volume of the lungs and reduces vital capacity. As a result of these changes, the client is at greater risk for developing respiratory infections and being unable to effectively clear secretions from the alveoli and airways.

Assessment

Nursing assessment of respiratory function is vital in clients with disorders and diseases affecting the respiratory system, as well as in clients at risk for respiratory complications resulting from other disorders. It is a particularly important component when assessing older adults.

SUBJECTIVE DATA

Collect information from the client (or family, if necessary) about the current complaint or presenting condition. Ask about the onset and duration of symptoms, as well as their effect on the client's ability to maintain activities of daily living (ADLs). Specifically inquire about the following as appropriate:

- Nasal congestion, difficulty breathing through one nares; nosebleeds
- Sore throat, difficult or painful swallowing
- Change in voice quality
- Difficult or painful breathing; ability to breathe when lying down
- Chest wall pain; effect of deep breathing, coughing, or movement on pain
- Presence of cough, including timing, severity, productivity of mucus
- If present, amount, color, consistency of sputum.

Ask about exposure to infectious conditions such as colds or influenza. Inquire about any chronic respiratory conditions, such as asthma, chronic bronchitis, emphysema, or chronic obstructive pulmonary (lung) disease (COPD or COLD). In addition, ask about heart failure. Discuss potential occupational exposure to chemicals, smoke, asbestos, coal dust, animal droppings, or other substances known to have possible respiratory consequences. Inquire about previous respiratory problems such as pneumonia or tuberculosis.

Obtain other relevant information such as allergies to medications or environmental allergens, smoking history, and exposure to cigarette smoke in the environment. Ask about use of other substances such as chewing tobacco, marijuana, cocaine, or injected drugs. Determine the extent of alcohol consumption, if any.

PHYSICAL EXAMINATION

Begin assessing the client with a respiratory disorder by observing the client's apparent state of health, color, and ease of breathing. Note the respiratory rate and pattern. (See Chapter 5 ⏺ for descriptions of abnormal breathing patterns.) Observe for nasal flaring, use of accessory muscles of respiration (muscles of the neck, shoulders, abdomen), and any signs of difficult or painful breathing. Listen to the client's speech for hoarseness or pausing to breathe or cough.

Inspect mucosa of the nares (using an otoscope with a nasal speculum), the mouth, and the oropharynx, being sure to check under the tongue and between the cheeks and gums. Inspect the neck for position of the trachea and any apparent growths. Observe chest movement for equality with respirations. Look for **barrel chest**, an increased anterior-posterior (AP) chest diameter.

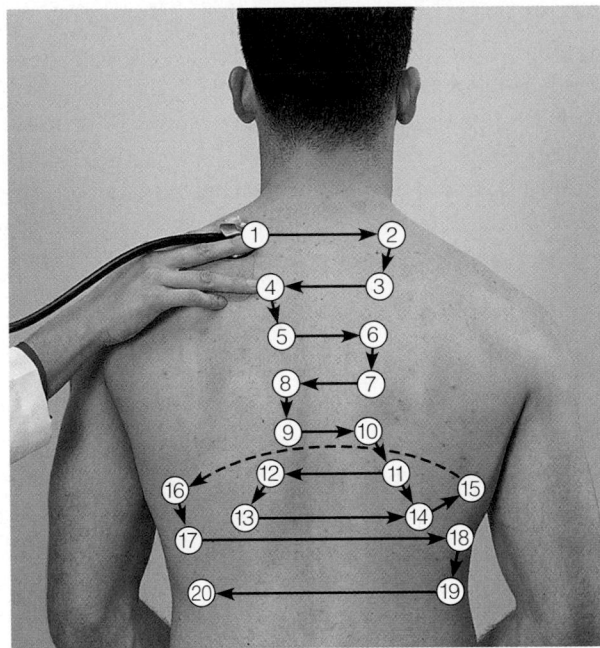

Figure 22-5. ■ Sequence for lung auscultation on the back.

Palpate the lips for nodules. Assess salivary glands and cervical and supraclavicular lymph nodes for swelling or tenderness. Lightly palpate the chest for tenderness and equality of respiratory movement.

Using the diaphragm of the stethoscope, auscultate the anterior, posterior, and lateral thorax for breath sounds (Figure 22-5 ■). Note the presence and quality of breath sounds, as well as any abnormal (**adventitious**) breath sounds (e.g., wheezes, crackles) and their location. An example of documentation of a respiratory assessment is presented in Box 22-1 ■.

BOX 22-1

DOCUMENTING RESPIRATORY ASSESSMENT

Joanna Speisla, 72 years old, presents at the local urgent care clinic with complaints of "the flu."

Relates 4-day history of chills, fever, headache, and sore throat. Developed a cough within past 24 hours; initially dry, now productive of thick, yellow-green sputum. States her general health is good. Denies history of serious or chronic heart or lung disease. Allergic to penicillin.

Appears in good general health, although acutely ill at this time. Does not appear to be in acute respiratory distress; no nasal flaring or use of accessory muscles noted. Color good, skin very warm and dry. Coughing frequently; productive of small to moderate amounts of thick yellow sputum. No unusual odor noted. BP 134/86; P 92, reg; R 24, reg; T 101.5°F PO. Nasal mucosa pink and moist. Oropharynx red, no patches or blisters noted. No cervical lymphadenopathy noted. Good breath sounds noted throughout all lung fields; no adventitious sounds heard. ---------S. Wagner, LPN

DIAGNOSTIC TESTS

A number of diagnostic tests are used to evaluate respiratory function. Some, such as the complete blood count with white blood cell count differential (CBC with diff), are not specific to assessment of the respiratory system, but provide very useful information. This section focuses on those tests that are used primarily to evaluate the upper and lower respiratory system and diagnose disorders of these systems.

Laboratory Tests

The primary laboratory tests used to evaluate the respiratory system and diagnose disorders affecting it are pulse oximetry, arterial blood gases (ABGs), cultures of nasal or throat swabs, analysis and culture of sputum, and tissue biopsy.

PULSE OXIMETRY. Pulse oximetry, a noninvasive test, often is used to evaluate and monitor oxygen saturation (SaO_2) of blood in clients with respiratory disorders. SaO_2 is the percentage of arterial hemoglobin that is saturated, or combined with oxygen. Normally, the SaO_2 is 95% or higher; lower values indicate impaired lung ventilation and/or gas exchange. The pulse oximeter sensor is applied to a fingertip, the forehead, nose, or earlobe in adults (Figure 22-6 ■). The sensor emits light, evaluating oxygen saturation by measuring the amount of red and infrared light absorbed by hemoglobin.

ARTERIAL BLOOD GASES. Normal arterial blood gas values are presented in Table 7-12, and a suggested series of steps to use to evaluate the results are outlined in Box 7-15 . The nurse often is responsible for applying pressure to the site for a period of 2 to 5 minutes following arterial puncture. This is necessary because arteries, unlike veins, are high-pressure vessels that may

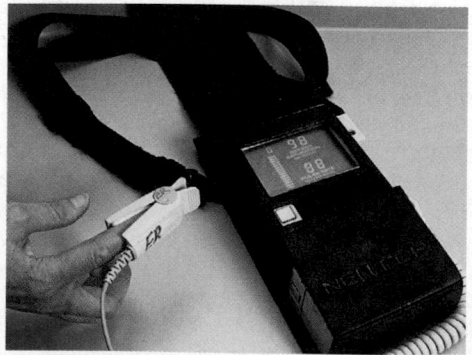

Figure 22-6. ■ Sensor probe placed on the finger for oxygen saturation analysis, and a microprocessing unit with digital display.

bleed into the tissue following puncture. It also is important for the nurse to promptly report ABG results to the charge nurse or physician, particularly when values are abnormal or outside of the expected range for the client.

SERUM ALPHA₁-ANTITRYPSIN. Serum levels of alpha₁-antitrypsin (AAT) may be obtained to identify a deficiency of this protein as a contributing factor to emphysema and COPD. The normal level of AAT in adults is 150 to 350 mg/dL. Inflammatory processes and exercise increase blood levels. A fasting specimen is collected in clients with elevated serum cholesterol or triglyceride levels.

SPUTUM AND TISSUE SPECIMENS. When infection of the upper or lower respiratory system is suspected, nasal or throat swabs or a sputum specimen are obtained for culture of pathogens. Culture requires 24 to 48 hours for bacterial growth; some pathogens, such as the tuberculosis bacillus, require longer to grow. For this reason, a sputum smear may be analyzed by Gram staining or for acid-fast bacillus. Nursing responsibilities for obtaining a throat swab are outlined in Box 22-2 ■; Box 22-3 ■ details the steps for obtaining a sputum specimen. Tests often performed on sputum specimens are outlined in Table 22-1 ■, along with normal or expected results and specific nursing responsibilities.

Tissue for biopsy, or microscopic examination, may be obtained by needle aspiration of a lymph node, during fiberoptic examination of the larynx or bronchi, or during surgery and tumor resection. Biopsy is performed when a tumor is suspected to identify the degree of tumor cell differentiation (staging) from normal cells and to detect the spread of tumor cells beyond the primary site. See Chapter 12 for more information about cancer, biopsy, staging, and grading.

Imaging Techniques

The chest x-ray and other radiologic studies such as CT scans are important diagnostic tools for detecting and evaluating respiratory disorders. Table 22-2 ■ presents imaging studies that may be used to diagnose respiratory conditions.

X-rays and CT scans are used with or without injected contrast media to identify the size and location of structures. They are also used to study blood flow through vessels and organs of the respiratory system. Ventilation-perfusion scans, which evaluate both lung ventilation (air movement) and perfusion (blood flow), are used to assess regional ventilation and pulmonary blood supply.

| BOX 22-2 | PROCEDURE CHECKLIST |

Obtaining a Throat Swab

☑ Obtain a sterile cotton swab or throat swab kit.

☑ Identify the client, explain the procedure, and provide for privacy.

☑ Place the client in a sitting position if possible.

☑ Use Standard Precautions.

☑ Ask the client to open the mouth, extend the tongue, and say "ah."

☑ Quickly swab the tonsils, reddened areas of the oropharynx, and any exudate.

☑ Insert the swab into the specimen container. Avoid contaminating the outside of the container or the swab.

☑ Label the container.

☑ Send the specimen and requisition to the laboratory.

SAMPLE DOCUMENTATION

10/27/06 Oropharynx red, patches of white exudate noted on tonsils and oropharynx. Throat swab (oropharynx, tonsils, and exudate) obtained and sent to lab for culture.
_____J. Doene, LPN.

Note: Refer to a nursing fundamentals or skills text for more detailed instruction. Check state guidelines and facility policy before performing any procedure.

| BOX 22-3 | PROCEDURE CHECKLIST |

Obtaining a Sputum Specimen

Before the Procedure

☑ Gather all supplies.

☑ If possible, obtain specimen before starting oxygen and/or antibiotic therapy.

☑ Unless otherwise specified, obtain specimen early morning, just after awakening.

☑ Increase fluid intake prior to obtaining specimen to help liquefy secretions.

Procedure

☑ Use Standard Precautions.

☑ Provide for privacy.

☑ Provide mouth care to reduce contamination by oral flora.

☑ Instruct to cough deeply several times, expectorating mucus into container.

☑ To obtain specimen by suctioning:

  ☑ Use aseptic technique.

  ☑ Attach sterile mucous trap between suction catheter and tubing.

  ☑ Perform tracheal suctioning.

  ☑ Detach and close mucous trap. Clear suction catheter and tubing, and dispose of suction equipment appropriately.

☑ Close container securely using aseptic technique.

☑ Label container (name and other identifying data, time and date, and any special conditions).

☑ Enclose container in clean plastic bag, and send to laboratory.

After the Procedure

☑ Provide mouth care.

☑ Document the time and date the specimen was obtained, and note its color, consistency, and odor.

SAMPLE DOCUMENTATION

8/13/06   Specimen of moderate amount thick
0630   green odorless sputum obtained by deep coughing. Sent for culture and sensitivity.
_____S. Hamilton, LVN.

Note: Refer to a nursing fundamentals or skills text for more detailed instruction. Check state guidelines and facility policy before performing any procedure.

TABLE 22-1

Sputum Analysis

TEST	NORMAL ADULT VALUES	EXPLANATION	NURSING RESPONSIBILITIES
Culture and sensitivity (C&S)	No pathogens present	Sputum is placed in or on an appropriate growth medium. If pathogens are present, they are microscopically identified. When combined in sensitivity testing, the specimen is grown in or on media containing disks of various antibiotics to identify those drugs that inhibit bacterial growth.	Obtain sputum from the bronchi (see Box 22-3). ⚭ If possible, collect the specimen in the early morning. Use Universal or Standard Precautions and sterile or aseptic technique when collecting the specimen.
Gram stain	Negative for pathogens	Gram stain is applied to a smear of the specimen to differentiate organisms by their staining qualities (gram-positive or gram-negative).	
Acid-fast stain	Negative for mycobacteria	Used to identify the presence of mycobacteria in the specimen (e.g., *Mycobacterium tuberculosis*). Provides more rapid results than culture when TB is suspected (cultures of *M. tuberculosis* require weeks to grow).	Three sputum specimens collected in the early morning are advised when tuberculosis is suspected.
Cytology	No abnormal cells detected	Microscopic examination of sputum obtained by collection or during bronchoscopy for the presence of abnormal (cancer) cells.	See above. May require several specimens.

TABLE 22-2

Imaging Studies

DIAGNOSTIC STUDY	EXPLANATION AND PURPOSE	NURSING IMPLICATIONS
X-ray of the head and neck	Used to detect abnormalities of the sinuses, larynx, or other tissues of the head and neck.	If contrast is injected, ask about allergies (specifically including to iodine or seafood) before the exam; ensure good hydration before and after the exam to reduce the risk of kidney damage.
Chest x-ray	Used to evaluate the appearance of the lungs, mediastinum, chest wall, and diaphragm. Detects masses, abscesses, and lung disorders such as pneumonia, obstructive lung disease, and atelectasis.	Although these studies are noninvasive, they expose the client to potentially damaging radiation. Ask women of childbearing age about possible pregnancy before the exam.
Computed tomography (CT) scan of the head and neck or chest	Specialized radiographic procedures that produce computer-generated images with significantly more detail than standard x-rays allow. May be done with or without contrast media, although contrast is used when a CT scan is done to identify vessel abnormalities such as pulmonary embolism.	If contrast is used, inquire about allergies (to iodine and seafood in particular), and ensure that the client is well hydrated to reduce the risk of kidney damage.
Ventilation-perfusion scan	These procedures involve inhalation of a radioactive gas to evaluate lung ventilation and injection of a radiologic contrast medium to evaluate perfusion of the lungs. They are used to detect pulmonary emboli, evaluate chronic lung disease, and assess the function of lung transplants.	Assess for allergy to iodine or radiologic contrast media. Explain the procedure, and address fears about exposure to radioactivity (the amount is small and no special precautions are required). Obtain an accurate weight before the procedure.

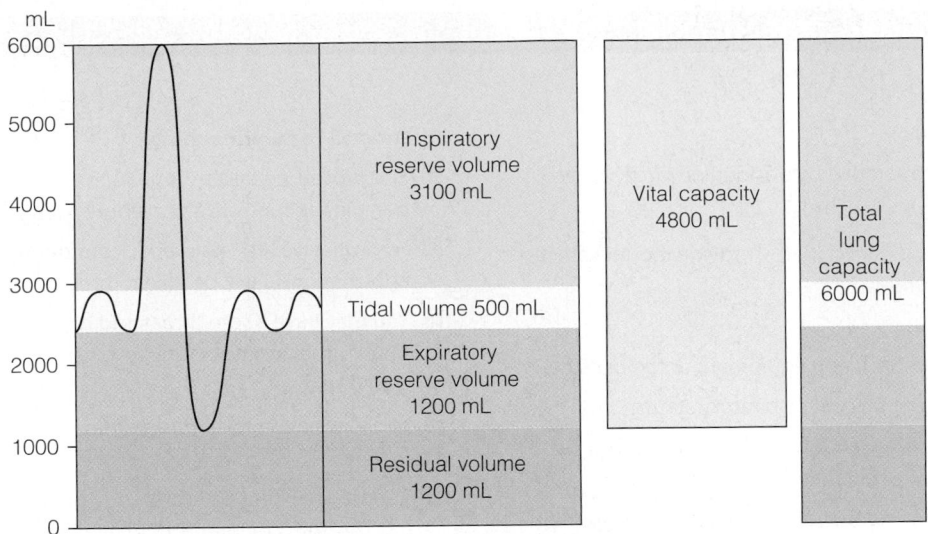

Figure 22-7. ■ The relationship of lung volumes and capacities. Volumes shown are for an average adult male.

Pulmonary Function Tests

Lung volume and capacity are measured with *pulmonary function tests (PFTs)*. Lung volume and capacity (Figure 22-7 ■) are affected by sex, age, weight, and health status. PFTs are performed in a pulmonary function laboratory. After teaching and preparation, a nose clip is applied and the client breathes into a spirometer or body plethysmograph, a device for measuring and recording lung volume in liters versus time in seconds. The client is instructed to breathe in a specific manner for these tests; for example, to inhale as deeply as possible, then exhale as much air as possible. Because bronchodilators, smoking, and caffeine interfere with test results, bronchodilators are withheld for 4 to 6 hours prior to the test, and the client is encouraged not to smoke or drink caffeinated beverages before the test.

The *total lung capacity (TLC)* is the total volume of the lungs at their maximum inflation. It is calculated by adding the (1) *tidal volume (Vt)*, the air (about 500 mL) exchanged during normal quiet breathing; (2) *inspiratory reserve volume (IRV)*, the air (about 2,100 to 3,100 mL) that can be inhaled over and above a normal inspiration; (3) *expiratory reserve volume (ERV)*, the air (about 1,200 mL) that can be forced out following a normal exhalation; and (4) *residual volume (RV)*, the air (about 1,200 mL) remaining in the lungs after maximal exhalation. The *vital capacity (VC)*, about 4,500 to 4,800 mL in healthy adults, is the sum of the Vt, IRV, and ERV. About 150 mL of air remains in the airways with each breath, never reaching the alveoli. This is called *anatomic dead space volume.*

Clients with asthma or other restrictive lung diseases may use a peak expiratory flow rate (PEFR) meter on a day-to-day basis to monitor airway constriction. These inexpensive meters provide a guide for self-care and use of medications.

Direct Visualization

Direct or indirect laryngoscopy may be used to identify and evaluate laryngeal tumors. A fiberoptic laryngoscope is used for direct laryngoscopy; mirrors are used to visualize the larynx in indirect laryngoscopy. General or local anesthesia is used for laryngoscopy. If local anesthesia is used, the client receives sedation to promote relaxation before the procedure. Dental prostheses (dentures, partial plates, bridges, etc.) are removed prior to the procedure. All food and fluids are withheld after the procedure until the gag reflex returns.

In fiberoptic bronchoscopy, a flexible bronchoscope is used to visualize the trachea, bronchi, and selected bronchioles. This procedure is done to identify tumors or other structural disorders, obtain tissue for biopsy or sputum for examination, or perform therapeutic procedures such as removing a foreign body. Nursing responsibilities related to bronchoscopy are outlined in Box 22-4 ■.

Note: The bibliography listings for this and all chapters have been compiled at the back of the book.

BOX 22-4 | **NURSING CARE CHECKLIST**

Bronchoscopy

Before the Procedure

☑ Provide routine preoperative care as outlined in Chapter 9.

☑ Reinforce teaching.

☑ Remove dentures and partial plates; provide mouth care just prior to the procedure.

After the Procedure

☑ Keep resuscitation and suction equipment at the bedside.

☑ Closely monitor vital signs and respiratory status.

☑ Maintain NPO status until cough and gag reflexes have returned.

☑ Provide emesis basin and tissues for expectorating sputum and saliva.

☑ Monitor color and character of respiratory secretions. Sputum may be blood tinged for several hours; notify physician if sputum is grossly bloody.

Client and Family Teaching

☑ The procedure takes about 30 to 45 minutes, and may be done in the room, in a procedure room, or in surgery.

☑ You will have little pain or discomfort. You will receive an anesthetic. You will be able to breathe, but not talk.

☑ You may have a sore throat and hoarse voice after the procedure. Throat lozenges or warm saline gargles can help relieve sore throat.

☑ You may have a fever during the first 24 hours after the procedure.

☑ Report persistent cough, bloody or purulent sputum, wheezing, shortness of breath, difficulty breathing, or chest pain to your doctor.

Chapter Review

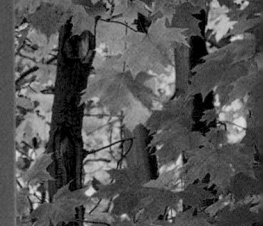

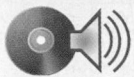 **KEY TERMS** by Topics

Use the audio glossary feature of either the CD-ROM or the Companion Website to hear the correct pronunciation of the following key terms.

Lower respiratory system
respiration, ventilation

Assessment
adventitious, barrel chest

KEY Points

- A patent airway and unobstructed airflow are vital to sustain life and function.

- The upper respiratory system provides a passageway for air to the lungs, cleaning, humidifying, and warming the air that passes through it. Mucus and lymphoid tissue in the upper airway trap dust and bacteria, reducing the risk of lower airway contamination.

- The lungs and bronchi of the lower respiratory system work together with the pulmonary vessels in the process of respiration, which includes ventilation (breathing) and gas exchange in the alveoli.

- Assessment of respiratory function is important in most clients and vital in people with respiratory disorders.

- Respiratory function is evaluated through diagnostic tests such as arterial blood gases, pulmonary function tests, x-rays, and direct visualization of tissues of the respiratory tract.

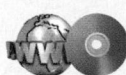 **EXPLORE MediaLink**

Additional interactive resources for this chapter can be found on the Companion Website at www.prenhall.com/burke. Click on Chapter 22 and "Begin" to select the activities for this chapter.

For chapter-related NCLEX-style review questions and an audio glossary, access the accompanying CD-ROM in this book.

FOR FURTHER Study

See Chapter 5 for descriptions of abnormal breathing patterns.

Normal ABG values are presented in Table 7-12, and suggestions for interpreting ABG results are given in Box 7-15.

Chapter 12 gives more information about cancer, biposy, staging, and grading.

NCLEX-PN® Exam Preparation

TEST-TAKING TIP   When preparing for the NCLEX-PN® examination and initial nursing licensure, think about how you will apply knowledge of normal anatomy and physiology to assessing and planning care for your clients. For example, understanding the physiology and mechanics of breathing is important to recognize how a fractured rib or pneumothorax can affect the client's ability to breathe and effectively oxygenate the blood and tissues.

---

1 When caring for a client admitted following a motor vehicle wreck, the nurse knows that which of the following could interfere with effective respiration. (Choose all that apply.)

   A. facial injuries with possible fractures

   B. rib fractures

   C. a concussion

   D. torn knee cartilage

   E. a cardiac contusion

2 The nurse caring for a client who is in a coma positions the client on his side with his head elevated to help prevent aspiration because

   A. the esophageal sphincter relaxes in comatose clients.

   B. the cough reflex is lost in comatose clients.

   C. the client will gag frequently on oral secretions.

   D. this position facilitates mouth care and feeding.

3 A client scheduled for a ventilation-perfusion scan asks the nurse if this procedure poses a risk of radiation exposure to her children. The nurse's response is based on the knowledge that

   A. special precautions must be taking during and following the procedure to protect health care workers from radiation exposure.

   B. no radioactive substances are used in this diagnostic procedure.

   C. because this procedure studies the circulation of blood through pulmonary vessels, all radioactivity is internal and excreted via the urine.

   D. although the client inhales a gas tagged with a radioactive ion, no special precautions are required to protect others.

4 The physician has ordered a serum alpha$_1$-antitrypsin level on a client. The nurse explains that this is

   A. to determine whether the dose of her prescribed drug is within the therapeutic range.

   B. to evaluate the amount and efficacy of surfactant within the alveoli.

   C. a protein that is necessary to help preserve the normal structure of the lungs.

   D. an enzyme that, when levels are excessively high, is associated with early onset emphysema.

5 The nurse is providing instructions to a client scheduled for pulmonary function tests. Which of the following does the nurse include?

   A. Use your bronchodilator inhaler as needed the day of the test.

   B. Avoid smoking the morning of the test.

   C. Do not eat or drink anything for 12 hours before the test.

   D. This test, although painful, is vital to predict your future care needs.

Answers for Review Questions appear in Appendix V.

Chapter 23

Caring for Clients with Upper Respiratory Disorders

BRIEF Outline

Upper Respiratory Infections and Inflammations
- Rhinitis
- Influenza
- Sinusitis
- Pharyngitis and Tonsillitis
- Epiglottitis
- Laryngitis

Pertussis

Epistaxis

Nasal Trauma or Deviated Septum

Laryngeal Obstruction or Trauma

Sleep Apnea

Benign Laryngeal Tumors

Laryngeal Cancer

LEARNING Outcomes

After completing this chapter, you will be able to:

- Describe common disorders affecting the upper respiratory tract and their manifestations.
- Discuss the nursing implications for diagnostic tests, medications, and treatments ordered for clients with upper respiratory disorders.
- Provide care for clients having surgery involving the upper respiratory system.
- Identify nursing care needs for the client with a tracheostomy.

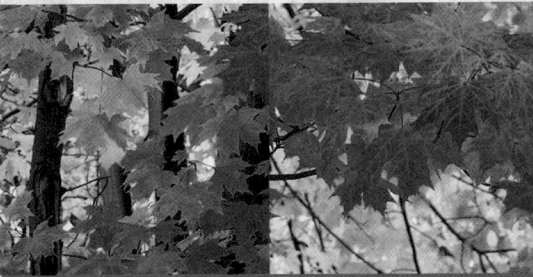

MediaLink

www.prenhall.com/burke
Use the address above to access the free, interactive Companion Website created for this textbook. Get hints, instant feedback, and textbook references to chapter-related NCLEX-style questions. Link to other interesting sites.

Audio Glossary:
Use the Companion Website, or the CD-ROM disk enclosed with your textbook, to hear the pronunciation of key terms in this chapter.

Upper respiratory disorders may affect the nose, sinuses, pharynx, tonsils, and larynx. They range from minor colds to life-threatening conditions such as laryngeal obstruction. When swelling, bleeding, or secretions affect breathing, the client may become frightened and anxious. Nursing care focuses on managing the airway and symptoms, communicating effectively, and providing psychologic support for the client and family.

Upper Respiratory Infections and Inflammations

The upper respiratory tract is constantly exposed to infectious and inflammatory agents in the environment. Most upper respiratory infections (URIs) and inflammations are minor illnesses. However, complications may result. In the frail older adult, the risk of serious problems following a URI can be significant.

PATHOPHYSIOLOGY AND MANIFESTATIONS

Most upper respiratory infections are caused by easily spread viruses. When the virus or an allergen enters the airway, it may cause acute inflammation of the upper airway, including the sinuses, pharynx, or larynx. The airway mucosa swells and secretes clear, yellow, or greenish exudate. A bacterial infection may develop following the viral infection. URIs occur more frequently during the fall and winter.

Rhinitis

Rhinitis, inflammation of the nasal cavities, is the most common upper respiratory disorder.

Acute viral rhinitis (the common cold) is highly contagious. Most adults experience two to four colds each year. More than 200 strains of virus can cause the common cold, including rhinovirus, respiratory syncytial virus, and adenovirus. These viruses are spread by hand-to-hand contact and by inhaling the virus. The virus can be spread to others for a few days *before* and *after* symptoms appear.

Allergic rhinitis (hay fever) results from an allergic response to substances such as plant pollens, mold, or animal dander. Allergic rhinitis tends to occur seasonally. Histamine and other immune mediators are released in response to contact with the allergen. This causes vasodilation and increased leakiness of capillaries in the mucosa (Table 23-1 ■). The sinuses may become congested, causing a headache. Chronic allergies may lead to postnasal drip and snoring.

Influenza

Influenza (flu) is a highly contagious viral respiratory disease. It often occurs in epidemics. Yearly outbreaks of influenza affect about 48 million Americans each winter. Influenza and its complications (primarily bacterial pneumonia) cause about 20,000 deaths yearly. Older adults with influenza have an increased risk of complications (Box 23-1 ■).

TABLE 23-1			
Manifestations and Course of Rhinitis and Influenza			
	ACUTE VIRAL RHINITIS	**ALLERGIC RHINITIS**	**INFLUENZA**
Local Manifestations	Nasal mucosa red, swollen, and congested Clear, watery secretions with **coryza** (runny nose) Sneezing and coughing	Nasal mucosa pale, swollen, and congested Thin, watery nasal discharge Itchy, watery eyes Sneezing	Coryza Sore throat Dry, nonproductive cough; may become productive Substernal burning
Systemic Manifestations	Low-grade fever Headache Malaise Muscle ache	Headache	Chills and fever Headache Malaise Muscle ache Fatigue and weakness
Course and Possible Complications	Lasts few days to 2 weeks Mild and self-limited Secondary infections (e.g., sinusitis, otitis media) may follow	Occurs with exposure to allergens (pollen, mold, animal dander) Chronic congestion may cause snoring, postnasal drip	Abrupt onset 1- to 2-week duration Cough and fatigue may last several weeks Secondary infections (sinusitis, otitis media, pneumonia, bronchitis) may follow

BOX 23-1   FOCUS ON OLDER ADULTS

Influenza in Older Adults

Older adults who get influenza have a high risk of developing pneumonia. Respiratory function changes with aging: The cough is less effective and residual lung volume increases. These changes increase the risk for pneumonia. Pneumonia is a serious complication of influenza that may be fatal. (See Chapter 24 ⬳ for more information about pneumonia.)

Reye's syndrome is a rare but potentially fatal complication of influenza. It is more likely to affect children but also has been identified in older adults. It usually develops within 2 to 3 weeks after the influenza. Although Reye's syndrome is associated with the use of aspirin in children, there is no evidence linking aspirin and Reye's syndrome in adults. Clients with Reye's syndrome often develop liver failure and brain dysfunction.

BOX 23-2

MANIFESTATIONS OF ACUTE PHARYNGITIS

Viral Pharyngitis

- Gradual onset
- Low-grade fever
- Sore throat
- Mild hoarseness
- Headache
- Throat bright pink to red

Streptococcal Pharyngitis

- Abrupt onset
- Fever of 101°F (38.3°C) or higher
- Severe sore throat
- Dysphagia
- Malaise, muscle aches
- Tender, enlarged cervical lymph nodes
- Throat bright red
- Patches of creamy exudate may be seen on oropharynx and tonsils

Influenza viruses are transmitted by airborne droplet and direct contact. The incubation period is short, and the manifestations develop rapidly (see Table 23-1). Fever and acute manifestations last up to a week; cough and fatigue may persist for several weeks.

Sinusitis

Sinusitis is an inflammation of the mucous membranes of the sinuses (see Figure 22-1B). Sinusitis is usually caused by a bacterial infection, and often follows a URI.

When drainage from the sinuses is obstructed, mucous secretions caught in the sinus cavity become a bacterial growth medium. This infection causes an inflammatory and immune response, leading to more swelling and pressure. Sinusitis may become chronic if the infection is not adequately treated. Clients who smoke, have allergies, or habitually use nasal sprays also may develop chronic sinusitis.

Sinusitis causes pain and tenderness across the infected sinuses, headache, fever, and malaise. The pain usually increases with leaning forward. Pain also may be referred to the upper teeth. The nasal mucous membrane is red and swollen in clients with sinusitis. The client may complain of nasal congestion, purulent nasal discharge, bad breath, fever, malaise, and fatigue. Symptoms often worsen after awakening and then become less severe in the afternoon and evening as secretions drain.

Sinus infection may spread to surrounding structures, causing complications such as abscess or cellulitis, meningitis, sepsis, or hearing loss.

Pharyngitis and Tonsillitis

Pharyngitis (acute inflammation of the throat) is common. It is usually viral but may also be bacterial. *Group A beta-hemolytic Streptococcus* (strep throat) is the most common bacterial cause. Streptococcal infection also may cause **tonsillitis** (acute inflammation of the tonsils). Streptococcal infections usually occur between late fall and spring, especially in cold climates. Pharyngitis and tonsillitis are contagious and are spread by droplet nuclei. Incubation varies from a few hours to several days.

Pharyngitis causes pain and fever. Throat discomfort may vary from scratchiness to pain and **dysphagia** (difficulty swallowing). The manifestations of acute viral and bacterial pharyngitis are listed in Box 23-2 ▪.

In tonsillitis, the tonsils are bright red and swollen with white exudate. The uvula may also be red and swollen. Cervical lymph nodes are usually tender and enlarged. The client with tonsillitis complains of a sore throat, difficulty swallowing, general malaise, fever, and *otalgia* (pain in the ear). The infection may extend to the ear through the eustachian tubes, causing acute otitis media. (See Chapter 40 ⬳ for more information about otitis media and its potential complications.)

Peritonsillar abscess (*quinsy*) is a potential complication of tonsillitis. In a peritonsillar abscess, pus forms behind the tonsil, causing marked swelling and deviation of the uvula toward one side. The client may be unable to swallow anything but liquids. Drooling and contraction of the muscles used in chewing may also occur.

Rare but serious complications of streptococcal pharyngitis and tonsillitis include acute glomerulonephritis and rheumatic fever. These potential complications are caused by an abnormal immune response to the bacteria. They can develop 1 to 5 weeks after the acute infection. (See Chapter 32 ⬳ for more information about acute glomerulonephritis, and Chapter 27 ⬳ for more information about rheumatic fever.)

Epiglottitis

Acute epiglottitis (inflammation of the epiglottis) is uncommon. It is, however, a medical emergency. Clients with epiglottitis have difficulty swallowing food (*odynophagia*) and have manifestations of pharyngitis. The epiglottis appears red, swollen, and edematous.

clinical ALERT

Constantly monitor clients with epiglottitis for signs of respiratory distress: nasal flaring, restlessness, **stridor** (a high-pitched, harsh sound heard during inspiration), use of accessory muscles, and decreased oxygen saturation measurements. Do not insert a nasal or oral airway because this can cause spasm and total airway obstruction. Nasotracheal intubation may be necessary to maintain the airway. Be prepared for emergency intubation of the client at any time.

Epiglottitis is frightening for both the client and the nurse. Maintain a calm, reassuring manner to help relieve anxiety.

Laryngitis

Laryngitis (inflammation of the larynx) is common. Laryngitis may occur alone or with other disorders of the upper respiratory tract. It is commonly associated with viral URI and may also occur in clients with bronchitis, pneumonia, or other respiratory infections. Excessive use of the voice, sudden changes in temperature, or exposure to dust or pollutants can also cause laryngitis. It is more common in the winter and in colder climates.

In laryngitis, the mucous membrane lining the larynx becomes inflamed and the vocal cords may be swollen. The primary manifestation of laryngitis is a change in the voice. Hoarseness or *aphonia* (complete loss of the voice) may occur. Clients complain of a sore, scratchy throat and may have a dry, harsh cough.

INTERDISCIPLINARY CARE

Most acute URIs are self-limiting, and clients are encouraged to provide self-care. Rarely is hospitalization required, unless a complication occurs. Medical management focuses on establishing an accurate diagnosis, providing symptomatic relief, and preventing complications. Bacterial URIs such as sinusitis and streptococcal pharyngitis are treated to speed recovery and reduce the risk of complications.

In long-term care facilities, URIs can spread rapidly and have devastating effects on the frail older adult population. Box 23-3 ■ outlines measures to help control the spread of URIs in long-term care and other group living facilities.

Diagnostic Tests

A *throat swab* is obtained when streptococcal pharyngitis is suspected. Nurses are often responsible for obtaining the

---

| BOX 23-3 | NURSING CARE CHECKLIST |

Controlling URIs in Long-Term Care

☑ Post visual alerts asking people with symptoms of a respiratory infection to notify health care personnel.

☑ Discourage people who are ill from visiting residents.

☑ Reassign health care personnel with influenza symptoms or confirmed cases to nondirect care activities for 5 days after the onset of symptoms.

☑ Provide tissues or masks to residents and visitors with upper respiratory symptoms.

☑ Provide hand washing supplies and alcohol-based hand rub dispensers by sinks and in handy locations.

☑ Encourage people who are coughing to sit at least 3 feet away from others.

☑ Ensure that health care personnel know and follow Standard Precautions (see Appendix I). ⚭

☑ Move residents with influenza symptoms to a private room.

☑ If private rooms are not available, place residents with similar symptoms in one area (particularly for meals, activities).

☑ Provide annual influenza vaccine to all residents and personnel unless contraindicated by allergy or health status (Centers for Disease Control and Prevention, 2005).

---

culture (Box 22-2). ⚭ Tests such as the LA antigen and ELISA allow rapid identification of the bacteria (in as little as 10 minutes), but are not highly sensitive. If the test is positive, treatment for strep throat is started. If the test is negative, the swab is cultured to determine if streptococcus is present. (See Chapter 22 ⚭ for more information about throat and sputum cultures.)

A *complete blood count (CBC)* may be done. The white blood cell (WBC) count is usually normal or low in viral infections and elevated in bacterial infections. A *chest x-ray* may be done to rule out complications such as pneumonia.

Nasal swabs or *radiologic studies* (x-ray or computed tomography [CT] scan) may be ordered if sinusitis is suspected. CT scans are more sensitive than x-rays in detecting the inflammatory changes of sinusitis.

Medications

INFLUENZA. Yearly immunization with influenza vaccine is the most important measure to reduce the risk of influenza. *Polyvalent* influenza virus vaccine (containing antigens of several viral strains) is about 85% effective in preventing influenza infection for up to a year. Although the vaccine is readily available and inexpensive, only about a third of people at risk get the vaccine each year. The vaccine should be given annually to:

■ People over the age of 50

- Residents of nursing homes
- Pregnant women
- Adults and children with chronic heart or lung disorders or chronic metabolic diseases (e.g., diabetes)
- Health care workers
- Family members of at-risk clients.

Because the vaccine is produced in eggs, it should not be given to people with an allergy to eggs. About 5% of those vaccinated may develop low-grade fever, malaise, or muscle aches after vaccination. Serious adverse reactions include anaphylaxis (an acute allergic response) and Guillain–Barré syndrome, an acute neurologic disorder that can cause temporary paralysis. An intranasal vaccine is available, but is recommended for use only in healthy people between the ages of 5 and 55 years.

Several drugs are available to prevent or shorten the duration of influenza in unvaccinated people who are exposed to the virus. Amantadine (Symmetrel) and rimantadine (Flumadine) also may be used to prevent influenza or decrease symptoms. Zanamivir (Relenza), oseltamivir (Tamiflu), and ribavirin (Virazole) reduce the severity and duration of influenza. These drugs attack the virus itself, reducing its spread in the body.

BACTERIAL INFECTIONS. Bacterial infections such as sinusitis, strep pharyngitis, and tonsillitis are treated with antibiotics. Treatment is continued for at least 10 days. The client is no longer contagious after 24 hours of antibiotic therapy.

Antibiotics also are used to treat sinusitis. Antibiotic therapy is continued for a full 2 weeks; a longer course may be prescribed to prevent relapse. If the client's sinusitis does not improve, hospitalization and intravenous antibiotic therapy may be required.

RHINITIS. A number of drugs, many available without prescription, provide symptomatic relief of viral URIs. Mild decongestants may help relieve the manifestations of coryza and nasal congestion. Oral or topical (nasal spray) decongestants are also prescribed for clients with sinusitis to reduce mucosal edema and promote sinus drainage. See Box 23-4 ■ for how to administer nose drops. Topical nasal steroids may be used after antibiotic

therapy has been initiated, in the later stages of treating subacute or chronic sinusitis, and for prophylaxis of recurrent problems.

clinical ALERT

Decongestant nasal sprays should be used for no more than 3 to 5 days. When used for a longer time, they can cause *rebound congestion*, which causes the client to use the spray more frequently and in larger doses.

Decongestants and antihistamines help relieve the manifestations of allergic rhinitis. Many decongestants and antihistamines are available without a prescription, including long-acting nonsedating antihistamines. Inhaled steroids or cromolyn, a mast cell stabilizer, may be prescribed if nonprescription drugs are ineffective. (See Table 23-2 ■.)

clinical ALERT

Pseudoephedrine, a popular over-the-counter decongestant, is an ingredient used to manufacture *methamphetamine*, a drug of abuse. Alert clients that they may need to ask at a pharmacy for these drugs, because in some states they no longer are kept on shelves accessible to the public.

Warm salt-water gargles, throat lozenges, or mild analgesics may be used for sore throat. Over-the-counter analgesics such as aspirin, acetaminophen, or NSAIDs help relieve fever and muscle ache. Antitussives may decrease cough and promote rest. Systemic mucolytic agents such as guaifenesin help liquefy secretions and promote sinus drainage.

Complementary Therapies

Complementary therapies and practices are appropriate for treating many URIs. Herbal remedies such as echinacea and garlic have antiviral and antibiotic effects. Taken at the first sign of infection, echinacea may reduce the duration and symptoms of a common cold or influenza. The recommended dose of echinacea varies, depending on the part of the plant used in the preparation. It should not be used for longer than 2 weeks. Echinacea is contraindicated for women who are pregnant or lactating. It should not be used by people who have an autoimmune disease such as multiple sclerosis or rheumatoid arthritis.

Aromatherapy with essential oils such as basil, cedarwood, eucalyptus, frankincense, lavender, marjoram, peppermint, or rosemary can reduce congestion, enhance comfort, and promote recovery from a URI. Caution clients that these essential oils should be used only for inhalation and must not be taken internally.

BOX 23-4	NURSING CARE CHECKLIST

Administering Nose Drops

To administer nose drops:

☑ Tilt the client's head backward and to the side on which the drops are to be instilled.

☑ Have the client remain in position for 5 minutes to allow the drops to reach the posterior nares.

TABLE 23-2

Nursing Implications For Pharmacology: Upper Respiratory Infections

CLASS/DRUGS	PURPOSE	NURSING RESPONSIBILITIES	CLIENT TEACHING
Decongestants ■ Phenylephrine (Neo-Synephrine, others) ■ Phenylpropanolamine (Comtrex, Ornade, Triaminic, others) ■ Pseudoephedrine (Sudafed, Actifed, others)	Decongestants constrict blood vessels, reducing inflammation and edema of nasal mucosa and relieving nasal congestion. Very effective when applied topically (by nasal spray) due to rapid onset of action. Duration of effect is short, followed by vasodilation and rebound congestion. May be habit forming.	Assess for contraindications such as high blood pressure or chronic heart disease. These drugs constrict blood vessels, increasing the blood pressure and heart rate. Do not give the drug if the client is taking antihypertensive medications or a monoamine oxidase (MAO) inhibitor.	Do not use more than the recommended dose. Check with your doctor before taking these drugs if you are taking any prescription medications or are being treated for high blood pressure or heart disease. Do not use nasal sprays for more than 3–5 days. Increase fluid intake to relieve mouth dryness. These drugs may cause nervousness, shakiness, or difficulty sleeping. Stop the drug if these effects occur.
Antihistamines ■ Brompheniramine (Dimetane, others) ■ Chlorpheniramine (Chlor-Trimeton, others) ■ Clemastine (Tavist) ■ Dexchlorpheniramine (Dexchlor, others) ■ Triprolidine (Actidil, Myidil) Nonsedating ■ Cetirizine (Zyrtec) ■ Fexofenadine (Allegra) ■ Loratadine (Claritin)	Antihistamines are widely available without prescription. They are frequently combined with decongestants in over-the-counter cold and allergy preparations. Other than the nonsedating forms, most antihistamines cause some drowsiness.	Before giving or recommending these drugs, ask about possible contraindications, such as: a. Acute asthma or chronic respiratory disease b. Glaucoma (increased intraocular pressure) c. Impaired gastrointestinal function or obstruction d. An enlarged prostate gland or other urinary tract obstruction e. Heart disease.	Do not drive or operate machinery while taking antihistamines that are known to be sedating. Stop the drug and notify your doctor immediately if you become confused or very drowsy or sleepy, or you experience chest tightness, wheezing, bleeding, or easy bruising. Do not use alcohol or other CNS depressants while taking antihistamines. Hard candy, gum, ice chips, and liquids help relieve mouth dryness caused by antihistamines.

Surgery

Clients with sinusitis, tonsillitis, or peritonsillar abscess may require surgery. *Irrigation* of an infected sinus (*antral lavage*) can be performed in the physician's office under local anesthesia. The sinus is irrigated with saline solution to wash out purulent exudate and promote drainage. *Endoscopic sinus surgery* may be performed to relieve obstruction of the opening to the sinus and restore ventilation and drainage of the sinus. Nasal packing is left in place for 24 to 48 hours following surgery. On discharge, the client is instructed to:

■ Use a humidifier or normal saline spray.

■ Avoid blowing the nose, straining, lifting, and strenuous exercise for a week.

■ Sneeze with the mouth open.

■ Avoid smoking, air pollutants, and nasal trauma.

■ Notify the physician for a temperature greater than 101°F, severe pain, or excessive bleeding.

Tonsillectomy (surgical removal of the tonsils) is done to treat recurrent or chronic infections, enlarged tonsils that may obstruct the airway, peritonsillar abscess, or malignancy. The most significant postoperative complication of tonsillectomy is hemorrhage. If hemorrhage develops, the client returns to surgery, where the bleeding vessel is *ligated* (tied off). A peritonsillar abscess may be drained by *needle aspiration* or by *incision and drainage (I&D)* under local anesthesia. Tonsillectomy follows the I&D, either immediately or 6 weeks later.

NURSING CARE

Education is the primary nursing role in caring for most clients with acute or chronic URIs. Self-care is appropriate for most clients with viral infections. Unless the problem is recurrent or a complication occurs, medical treatment is rarely required. Clients need to be able to recognize the difference between acute, self-limiting disorders and those that require medical treatment.

ASSESSING

Assessment data collected by the nurse help determine the effects of an upper respiratory problem on the client's life, can identify risk factors for complications, and can suggest whether the problem is appropriate for self-care or for medical treatment. Box 23-5 ■ lists subjective and objective data to collect.

DIAGNOSING, PLANNING, AND IMPLEMENTING

Priorities in Nursing Care. Nursing care for clients with significant manifestations or complications of URI focuses on maintaining airway clearance, breathing patterns, and adequate rest.

BOX 23-5	ASSESSMENT

Assessing Clients with Upper Respiratory Infections

SUBJECTIVE DATA

- **Pain:** location (nose, face, throat, or chest); character, timing (frequency, duration), aggravating factors, and relief measures.
- **Cough:** type (dry or productive), timing.
- **Sputum and/or Nasal Drainage:** amount, color, odor.
- Shortness of breath or *dyspnea* (difficult or labored breathing).
- Difficulty swallowing or smelling, or altered taste.
- **Past Medical History:** known allergies, chronic respiratory problems; surgery or trauma of the upper respiratory tract; chronic diseases, such as diabetes or heart disease; smoking history and/or exposure to environmental pollutants or allergens.

OBJECTIVE DATA

- Observe for difficulty breathing, pausing while talking, hoarseness, and cough; respiratory rate and depth.
- Inspect nares and oropharynx for color, moisture; presence of swelling, exudate, or postnasal drainage.
- Percuss (lightly tap) over frontal and maxillary sinuses for tenderness.
- Auscultate lung sounds.

Ineffective Breathing Pattern

- Monitor respiratory rate and pattern for changes from baseline. *Tachypnea or rapid, shallow respirations may result from fever and muscle ache. Shallow respirations may lead to decreased ventilation of alveoli or to atelectasis (lack of ventilation of an area of lung).*
- Pace activities to allow rest periods. *Tachypnea increases the work of breathing and is fatiguing.*
- Elevate the head of the bed. *The upright position reduces the work of breathing and improves lung expansion.*

Ineffective Airway Clearance

- Monitor the effectiveness of cough and ability to remove airway secretions. *Fatigue and general malaise may decrease the ability to cough effectively and move secretions. Changes in the respiratory system associated with aging also affect the older adult's ability to maintain a clear airway effectively.*
- Following tonsillectomy, position with head to the side for drainage of secretions from the mouth and pharynx. Leave the nasopharyngeal airway in place until the client can swallow and the gag reflex returns. *This prevents aspiration and maintains the airway.*
- Apply an ice collar as ordered. *The ice collar reduces swelling and provides a mild analgesic effect.*
- Immediately report excessive bleeding (large amounts of bright red drainage, choking on drainage, or vomiting of bright red blood) to the charge nurse and physician. *The client may need to return to surgery to stop the hemorrhage.*
- Maintain adequate hydration. Assess mucous membrane moisture and skin turgor. *Fever, rapid respiratory rate, and decreased fluid intake may lead to dehydration and thick, sticky secretions that are more difficult to expectorate.*
- Increase the humidity of inspired air with a bedside humidifier. *Increasing the water content of inhaled air helps loosen secretions and soothe mucous membranes.*
- Teach the client how to cough effectively. Administer analgesic medications as ordered. *The huff technique of coughing increases the cough's effectiveness and spares energy. (See Chapter 24 ⬭ for client teaching of this technique.) Relieving muscle ache increases the ability to cough effectively.*

Disturbed Sleep Pattern

- Assess sleep using subjective and objective information. *Decreased ability to rest increases fatigue and prolongs recovery time.*
- Place in a semi-Fowler's or Fowler's position for sleep. *Elevating the head of the bed decreases the work of breathing and may allow better rest.*
- Provide antipyretic and analgesic medications at bedtime or shortly before. *These medications promote comfort by reducing fever and relieving muscle aches.*

- If necessary, request a cough suppressant medication for nighttime use. *Cough suppressants are not recommended during the day because coughing promotes airway clearance, but at night they may allow the client to rest.*

Impaired Verbal Communication

- Encourage the client with laryngitis to rest the voice and to use alternate methods of communicating such as writing. *Resting the voice speeds recovery and decreases throat discomfort.*
- Instruct to use throat lozenges or sprays, or to gargle with a warm antiseptic solution. *These measures soothe the throat.*
- If the client smokes, encourage quitting. *Cigarette smoke is an irritant that increases the risk for laryngitis and delays healing.*

EVALUATING

To evaluate the effectiveness of care for a client with an URI, collect data such as the rate and ease of breathing, ability to manage symptoms, knowledge of appropriate medication use, and absence of complications.

Documenting. Document initial assessment data and teaching, as well as follow-up assessments and understanding of information presented.

CONTINUING CARE

Because many URIs are appropriately treated at home, planning and teaching for home care are vital.

Encourage rest during the acute phase of the illness. Stress the importance of staying well hydrated. Teach clients to use disposable tissues to cover the mouth and nose while coughing or sneezing to prevent airborne spread of URIs. Instruct the client to blow the nose with both nostrils open to prevent infected matter from being forced into the eustachian tubes. Remind clients to wash hands frequently, especially after coughing or sneezing, to help prevent spreading the disease to others. Clients can limit their incidence of URIs by avoiding exposure to crowds. Teach the client that although becoming chilled or going out in the rain does not cause colds and influenza, physical or psychologic stress does make the body more susceptible to URIs. Maintaining good general health and stress-reduction activities supports the immune system and helps prevent acute URIs.

Teaching about influenza focuses on prevention. Stress the importance of yearly influenza vaccination for clients in high-risk groups and their families. Teach clients how the disease is spread, including how to reduce risk by avoiding crowds and people who are ill.

Discuss appropriate use of over-the-counter medications for relief of manifestations (see Table 23-2). Teach clients to limit their use of nasal decongestants to every 4 hours for only a few days at a time. Suggest that clients avoid using aspirin or acetaminophen unless needed to relieve muscle aches and promote rest, because these medications may actually prolong acute viral URIs. Encourage warm saline gargles or throat lozenges for symptomatic relief of sore throat.

Help the client with allergic rhinitis identify possible allergens and strategies to avoid contacting them. Discuss the possible benefits of skin testing to identify allergens and, if necessary, immunotherapy to reduce the allergic response.

Stress the importance of completing the entire course of prescribed antibiotics for bacterial infections. Discuss the prescribed antibiotic and help develop a schedule that helps the client remember to take all doses. If the course of therapy will be prolonged, discuss measures to prevent superinfections such as vaginitis or oral thrush. Unless contraindicated, suggest that the client eat 8 ounces daily of yogurt containing live bacterial cultures while on antibiotics.

Teach about possible complications of influenza and other URIs and their manifestations. Emphasize that complications should be reported promptly to the physician.

NURSING PROCESS CARE PLAN
Client with Upper Respiratory Infection

Monica Wunderman is a 27-year-old woman who was recently treated for tonsillitis caused by group A *Streptococcus*. She presents to the emergency department (ED) 10 days later appearing acutely ill. She states that her throat is so sore that she has difficulty swallowing even liquids. Barbara Ironhorse, the ED nurse, completes an assessment of Ms. Wunderman.

Assessment. T 102°F (38.8°C). On inspection of her mouth, an acutely swollen and reddened area of the soft palate is noted. Yellow exudate is present. CBC reveals an elevated WBC of 16,000/mm^3. A diagnosis of peritonsillar abscess is made. Needle aspiration of the abscess is performed.

Diagnosis. The following nursing diagnoses are identified for Ms. Wunderman:

- *Pain* related to swelling
- *Risk for Ineffective Airway Clearance* related to pain and swelling
- *Deficient Fluid Volume* related to fever and difficulty in swallowing fluids

Expected Outcomes. The expected outcomes for the plan of care are that Ms. Wunderman will:

- Experience minimal or no pain.
- Maintain a patent airway as demonstrated by normal respiratory rate and rhythm.
- Maintain optimal fluid intake as evidenced by ability to consume fluids and semiliquid foods, appearance of moist mucous membranes, normal skin turgor, and a decrease in temperature.

Planning and Implementation. Ms. Ironhorse implements the following interventions to prepare Ms. Wunderman for home care:

- Advise to drink ice-cold fluids, because they may be easier to swallow and may provide a local analgesic effect. Instruct to avoid citrus juices, hot or spicy foods, and rough-textured foods for 1 week.
- Teach pain-relief measures such as applying an ice collar as desired and gargling with warm saline solution every 1 to 2 hours for the first 24 to 48 hours after aspiration of the abscess.
- Instruct to take all medications as prescribed.

Evaluation. When Ms. Ironhorse contacts Ms. Wunderman by telephone 2 days after her visit to the ED, she reports complete relief of symptoms. She is afebrile, takes fluids without difficulty, and has had no problems with her breathing. She has not experienced any pain.

Critical Thinking in the Nursing Process

1. Describe common manifestations of upper respiratory infections and measures to promote comfort.
2. Describe common pharmacologic interventions for these clients.
3. While Ms. Wunderman developed a complication that required medical intervention, many clients present in the emergency department or urgency care clinics with uncomplicated URI. What can nurses do to reduce this unnecessary use of emergency departments and urgency care clinics?

Pertussis

Pertussis, or *whooping cough,* is an acute, highly contagious upper respiratory infection. Although once thought to have been virtually eliminated from the United States, its incidence is increasing among all ages. Adolescents have the highest incidence, but it also affects adults and young children.

PATHOPHYSIOLOGY AND MANIFESTATIONS

Pertussis is caused by infection with *Bordetella pertussis,* a gram-negative rod that is spread by respiratory droplets.

(See Chapter 10 ⬤ to review the spread of infection.) The bacteria attach to cells in the nasopharynx, where they multiply and spread to respiratory tissues. The infection itself is generally symptom free; however, toxins produced by the bacteria damage respiratory mucosa and paralyze the cilia. This impairs respiratory clearance, increasing the risk for pneumonia. These toxins also stimulate an inflammatory response and inhibit immune defenses.

Pertussis often has a predictable pattern, with symptoms of upper respiratory infection beginning 7 to 10 days after exposure. Within 1 to 2 weeks, the cough increases, with frequent *paroxysms* (bursts) of coughing that may end with an audible whoop of rapid inspiration. The whoop occurs less frequently in adolescents and adults than in young children. Coughing episodes may precipitate vomiting, and can interfere with eating and sleeping. This stage of the disease can last up to 6 weeks, and is followed by gradually decreasing frequency and severity of coughing.

INTERDISCIPLINARY CARE

Nasopharyngeal secretions are cultured to establish the diagnosis of pertussis. Blood tests for antibodies to the bacteria also may be used to identify this disease. The primary preventive strategy for pertussis is active immunization, routinely administered to infants and young children.

Adolescents and adults are treated with erythromycin, the antibiotic of choice. Trimethoprim-sulfamethoxazole (TMP-SMZ, Bactrim, Septra) may be used as an alternative to erythromycin. (See Chapter 10 ⬤ for more information about these antibiotics.)

NURSING CARE

Nurses are instrumental in educating clients about and promoting immunization of vulnerable populations. Nurses also can help identify people with pertussis by recommending that clients with persistent, severe cough that disrupts sleep or causes vomiting have a nasopharyngeal culture.

Clients usually remain in the community during treatment, rarely requiring hospitalization.

clinical ALERT

When hospitalization is required for pertussis, place the client in respiratory isolation for 5 days after antibiotic therapy is started to prevent spread of the disease to other patients.

The primary nursing role is teaching about the disorder and measures to prevent its spread to others. Teach respiratory isolation measures to be used until the client is no longer communicable (5 days after the start of antibiotic therapy). Discuss control of respiratory secretions and measures to maintain food and fluid intake and rest. Teach about the prescribed antibiotic, its potential adverse effects, and measures to reduce them, such as taking erythro-mycin with meals to reduce gastric distress. Stress the importance of prophylactic antibiotic therapy for all household contacts of an infected person. Pertussis is a reportable disease; contact the local county health department when a case is identified.

UPPER RESPIRATORY TRAUMA OR OBSTRUCTION

Epistaxis

The nose has a rich blood supply. **Epistaxis,** or nosebleed, may begin in many ways: trauma (picking the nose or getting hit), drying of nasal mucous membranes, local or systemic infection, substance abuse (e.g., cocaine), arteriosclerosis, and hypertension. Nosebleed may result from bleeding disorders, severe liver disease, or treatment with an anticoagulant or antiplatelet medication. In adults, men have more nosebleeds than women.

PATHOPHYSIOLOGY AND MANIFESTATIONS

Ninety percent of all nosebleeds arise from a rich vascular area in the anterior nasal septum. These vessels are the most susceptible because of their location. Posterior nosebleed may also be caused by trauma, but more often occurs secondary to systemic disorders such as hypertension or diabetes. Posterior epistaxis tends to be more severe and occurs more frequently in the older adult.

INTERDISCIPLINARY CARE

The goal of treatment for epistaxis is to identify and control the source of bleeding. Anterior bleeding can usually be managed by simple first-aid measures, such as pressure (pinching the nose toward the septum) for 5 to 10 minutes and applying ice packs to the nose and forehead to cause vasoconstriction. The sitting position decreases blood flow to the head and reduces venous pressure. Having the client lean forward reduces drainage of blood into the nasopharynx and lessens the chance the client will swallow it. The client should spit out the blood. This allows a better estimate of the amount of bleeding and prevents nausea and vomiting resulting from swallowed blood. If applying pressure does not control the bleeding, pharmacologic interventions, nasal packing, or surgery may be necessary.

Medications and Nasal Packing

Topical vasoconstrictors such as cocaine (0.5%), phenylephrine (Neo-Synephrine) (1:1000), or adrenaline (1:1000) may be applied by nasal spray or on a cotton swab held against the bleeding site. The bleeding vessel may be cauterized using a chemical such as silver nitrate or Gelfoam.

If bleeding cannot be controlled with pressure and local medications, quarter-inch petroleum gauze may be used to pack the nasal cavity. Anterior nasal packs generally are left in place for 24 to 72 hours. Posterior nasal packing (Figure 23-1 ■) remains in place longer, up to 5 days, and is very uncomfortable for the client. It can significantly interfere with respirations, leading to hypoxemia. Supplemental oxygen is given while posterior packing is in place. Discomfort is managed with narcotic analgesics. Complications such as dysrhythmias, hypertension, myocardial infarction, and toxic shock syndrome are risks associated with posterior packing. A Foley catheter or inflatable nasal balloon may be used as an alternative to posterior packing.

Surgery

Chemical or surgical cautery procedures may be used to seal bleeding vessels and, in the case of posterior epistaxis, as an alternative to nasal packing. The resulting scab must be left undisturbed until the mucosa has healed, or further bleeding may occur. Some clients with posterior bleeding require surgery to tie off the bleeding artery. These procedures may

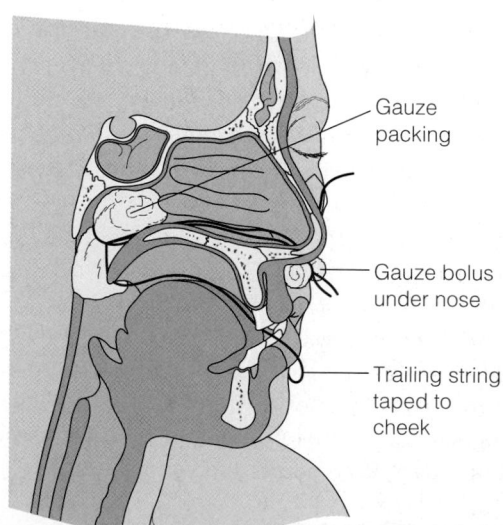

Figure 23-1. ■ Posterior nasal packing. Ties exiting through the nose and mouth are used to stabilize the packing in position and remove it when it is no longer needed.

be done endoscopically, under conscious sedation or local or general anesthesia. Following surgery, the client is carefully monitored for bleeding or respiratory complications.

NURSING CARE

Nosebleeds can be frightening, particularly when they occur spontaneously, without preceding trauma. Support, reassurance, and education are important roles for nurses caring for clients with epistaxis.

ASSESSING

In clients with epistaxis, data collection occurs while measures to stop the bleeding are implemented. Subjective data include information about when the nosebleed started, how long it has continued, and measures that have been taken to stop the bleeding. The client's medical history, including chronic diseases and current medications, may provide clues. Objective data to obtain include the client's vital signs and the extent of bleeding. Inspect the oropharynx using a penlight and tongue depressor for further evidence of bleeding.

DIAGNOSING, PLANNING, AND IMPLEMENTING

Priorities in Nursing Care. The priorities of nursing care for the client with epistaxis are reducing the client's anxiety and helping the client to maintain an open airway.

Anxiety

- Maintain an attitude of calm encouragement. *This reassures the client that the nosebleed is not life threatening. If epistaxis has occurred spontaneously, the client may fear that it indicates a major health problem.*
- Have the client pinch the nares together at the bridge of the nose. *Ninety percent of nosebleeds originate in the front of the nose where direct pressure usually stops the bleeding. Having the client put pressure on the nose provides focus and helps restore a sense of control. This reduces anxiety.*
- Encourage to breathe slowly and deeply through the mouth. *Controlled mouth breathing maintains lung ventilation and reduces anxiety.*
- Assess the client with nasal packing frequently for adequate oxygenation (e.g., mental status, oxygen saturation measurements). Maintain supplemental oxygen as ordered. *Cerebral hypoxia produces a sense of apprehension and fear.*

Risk for Aspiration

The highly anxious client who has blood draining into the nasopharynx is at risk for aspirating blood into the trachea.

The client with nasal packing is unable to breathe through the nose, increasing the risk of aspirating food or fluids when eating.

- Position upright with the head forward. Provide a basin into which the client can expectorate blood. *This reduces the risk of aspiration and nausea from swallowed blood.*
- Apply ice or a cold compress to the nose. *Cold constricts blood vessels and reduces bleeding.*
- Place the client with nasal packing with the head elevated and on one side when asleep. *This position reduces the risk of aspiration of oral secretions.*

Evaluating

To evaluate care for the client with epistaxis, check for additional bleeding (be sure to check the oropharynx for blood running down the throat). Evaluate the client's understanding of instructions, including when to return for removal of nasal packing and measures to prevent future nosebleeds.

Documenting. Document the circumstances preceding the nosebleed, assessment data, and the time and measures required to control bleeding. Document teaching provided regarding home care measures, follow-up care, and prevention of future episodes.

CONTINUING CARE

Following an episode of epistaxis, teaching focuses on measures to prevent further nosebleeds. Advise the client to avoid strenuous exercise for several days or weeks, depending on the severity of the nosebleed and its treatment. Instruct clients not to blow the nose or do things like heavy lifting or bending that could increase pressure and dislodge the crust. Caution to sneeze with the mouth open to avoid increasing pressure in nasal vessels.

Suggest lubricating nasal mucosa with petroleum jelly, a water-soluble lubricant, or bacitracin ointment to reduce the risk of spontaneous bleeding in clients with anterior nose bleeds. Recommend using a humidifier or vaporizer to minimize dryness of the mucous membranes. Instruct clients not to blow the nose forcefully or pick the nose. Encourage the client who has experienced spontaneous epistaxis to seek medical evaluation for possible underlying problems such as hypertension or bleeding disorder.

Nasal Trauma or Deviated Septum

The nose is the most commonly broken bone of the face. A *nasal fracture* (broken nose) usually results from a sports injury or from trauma related to violence or motor vehicle wrecks.

PATHOPHYSIOLOGY AND MANIFESTATIONS

One or both sides of the nose may be broken. A fracture that involves only one side of the nose rarely causes displacement or deformity. It is usually not serious, although swelling can obstruct the airway. Bilateral fractures are more common. Complex fractures may involve other nasal structures and frontal bones of the face as well as soft tissue. The manifestations of bilateral nasal fracture are listed in Box 23-6 ■.

Hematoma, infection or abscess, perforation or deviation of the septum, and leakage of cerebrospinal fluid (CSF) may complicate nasal fractures. The client with a nasal fracture may also have fractures of other facial bones, particularly when facial trauma is severe.

In a deviated nasal septum, the septal cartilage bulges or deviates to one side. It causes some degree of nasal obstruction. Few symptoms accompany mild deviation. Partial obstruction of airflow through the affected side may cause noisy breathing or snoring. Pain from sinus obstruction or infection may occur with major deviation. Dry nasal mucosa and nosebleeds may occur. The defect may be severe enough to cause cosmetic deformity.

INTERDISCIPLINARY CARE

The major goals of treatment for nasal fractures are to maintain a patent airway and prevent deformity. X-rays of the head and face are done to identify the fracture and to assess for other facial fractures. The nasal cavity is examined to rule out septal hematoma. If a cerebrospinal fluid (CSF) leak is suspected, additional diagnostic tests such as a CT scan may be performed.

Simple reduction of a nasal fracture may be done in the emergency room using local anesthesia. An external splint may then be applied for 7 to 10 days to maintain proper alignment until healing takes place. Ice may be gently applied to the face and nose to control edema and bleeding. Nasal packing may be used to control epistaxis.

Complex nasal fractures, fractures that do not heal properly, or a persistent CSF leak may require surgical repair of the fracture or realignment of the nasal bones. The most common procedure used is rhinoplasty with concurrent septoplasty.

Rhinoplasty (surgical reconstruction of the nose) is done to relieve airway obstruction and repair visible deformity of the nose following fracture. Using an intranasal incision, the framework of the nose is reshaped. Prosthetic implants may assist in reshaping the nose. Rhinoplasty is usually an outpatient procedure. Following surgery, nasal packing is left in place for up to 72 hours to minimize bleeding and provide tissue support. A plastic splint molded to the shape of the nose is removed in 3 to 5 days. The splint protects the reshaped nose and helps to control swelling. Most swelling and bruising subside within 10 to 14 days; normal sensation may take several months to return.

Septoplasty or submucous resection (SMR) may be done to correct septal deviation. The procedures are done using local anesthesia. In these procedures, the deviated portion of nasal cartilage is removed; bone also may be removed if necessary. Following the procedure, the nares on both sides are packed to prevent bleeding and provide support to the septum.

NURSING CARE

Nursing care for clients with nasal fracture focuses on airway management; controlling pain, bleeding, and swelling; and providing necessary teaching.

ASSESSING

Ask the client with a suspected nasal fracture how and when the injury occurred. Carefully observe respiratory status and call for help immediately if the airway is compromised. Inquire about pain, bleeding, and difficulty breathing. Inspect the nose and face for apparent deformity, swelling, and *ecchymosis* (bruising). Gently palpate the nose for *crepitus* (a grating sound or sensation).

DIAGNOSING, PLANNING, AND IMPLEMENTING

Priorities in Nursing Care. The primary risk in nasal trauma or with a deviated septum is impaired airway clearance due to swelling or obstruction of the nasal passage.

Ineffective Airway Clearance

- Monitor for signs of respiratory distress such as tachypnea, dyspnea, shortness of breath, tachycardia, and use of accessory muscles. Monitor oxygen saturation levels. *Swelling and deformity may obstruct the airway. If the fracture is malpositioned during healing, resulting deformity can also impair nasal airway clearance. Abnormal signs and declining oxygen saturation levels may indicate airway obstruction.*
- Have suction equipment available. *Suctioning of the oropharynx may be necessary to remove blood and secretions and maintain a clear airway. Avoid suctioning the nasopharynx; this could cause additional tissue trauma.*

- Monitor cough effectiveness and ability to manage airway secretions. *Pain, edema, and nasal bleeding may affect the client's ability to cough effectively.*
- Maintain adequate hydration. *Decreased fluid intake or active bleeding may cause dehydration and increase the viscosity of secretions, making them harder to spit out.*

Risk for Infection

- Assess for evidence of a CSF leak (clear fluid leaking from the ear or nose). If noted, test drainage for glucose. CSF will test positive for glucose on a dextrostrip. Report to the charge nurse or physician. *A CSF leak indicates a higher risk for ascending infection and meningitis.*
- Avoid suctioning if possible. *Suction catheters could cause additional trauma and introduce microorganisms.*
- Monitor vital signs every 4 hours. *A rise in temperature may indicate infection.*
- Administer antibiotics as ordered. *Antibiotics are often prescribed to prevent infection because nasal mucosa are populated with many bacteria.*

EVALUATING

Evaluate the effectiveness of nursing care by collecting data related to patency of the airway, comfort, and absence of infection. As the fracture heals, evaluate the position of the nasal septum and appearance of the nose.

Documenting. Document the circumstances of the injury, initial and continuing assessment data, including the client's ability to maintain a clear airway, and treatment measures instituted. Document teaching for home care, instructions for follow-up, and the client's apparent understanding of information.

CONTINUING CARE

When a nasal fracture is suspected, the client should seek medical evaluation and treatment as soon as possible. Encourage the client to elevate the head of the bed with blocks and apply ice or cold packs to the nose for 20 minutes four times a day to reduce swelling. Inform the client that while swelling will subside within days, bruising may persist for several weeks. Reassure that the final cosmetic outcome following a nasal fracture cannot be determined until swelling has subsided.

Instruct the client who has a CSF leak to rest in bed with the head elevated or in a recliner chair. Fluids may be restricted; with the client, explore ways to distribute allowed fluids throughout the day. Instruct to avoid straining, blowing the nose, sneezing, or vigorous coughing. Discuss manifestations of infection, including stiff neck, headache, and fever. Instruct the client to contact the physician immediately if these manifestations occur.

Laryngeal Obstruction or Trauma

Laryngeal obstruction is a life-threatening emergency. The larynx is the narrowest part of the upper airway. It can be partially or fully obstructed by aspirated food or foreign objects.

PATHOPHYSIOLOGY AND MANIFESTATIONS

Laryngospasm (spasm of the muscles of the larynx) or *laryngeal edema* due to inflammation, injury, or anaphylaxis also can obstruct the larynx. The most common cause of obstruction in adults is ingested meat that lodges in the airway (the "café coronary"). Risk factors for food aspiration include ingesting large boluses of food and not chewing them enough, consuming excess alcohol, and wearing dentures. Laryngospasm may be caused by repeated or traumatic attempts at intubation, chemical irritation of the airway, or hypocalcemia. An acute type I allergic response may cause anaphylaxis and severe laryngeal edema. (See Chapter 11 ⚭ for more information about allergic responses.)

The manifestations of laryngeal obstruction include coughing, choking, gagging, obvious difficulty breathing with use of accessory muscles, and inspiratory stridor. As the airway is obstructed, signs of asphyxia are seen. Respirations are labored and noisy with wheezing and stridor. The client may become *cyanotic* (blue). Respiratory arrest and death may result without prompt intervention.

Trauma to the larynx can occur in motor vehicle wrecks or assaults (e.g., blows to the neck or attempted strangulation). Trauma may cause laryngeal or tracheal cartilage fractures and loss of airway patency. Soft tissue injuries can cause swelling that impairs the airway further. The client with laryngeal trauma may have *subcutaneous emphysema* (air under the skin), a change in the voice, dysphagia, inspiratory stridor, *hemoptysis* (bloody sputum), and a cough.

INTERDISCIPLINARY CARE

The goal of treatment is to maintain an open airway. If airway obstruction is partial and the client is able to cough and breathe, diagnostic tests such as x-rays or ultrasound may be done to locate the foreign body. An endotracheal tube may be inserted to maintain the airway that is in spasm or for laryngeal edema. For the client in anaphylaxis, epinephrine is given to reduce laryngeal edema and relieve obstruction.

clinical ALERT

When airway obstruction is complete, the Heimlich maneuver must be performed immediately to clear the obstruction. Perform the maneuver by administering forceful thrusts to the upper abdomen or lower chest, continuing until the obstruction is relieved or more definitive care can be given (Figure 23-2 ■).

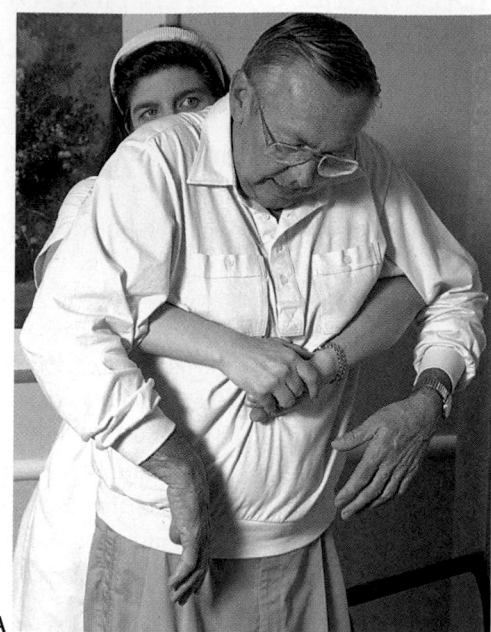

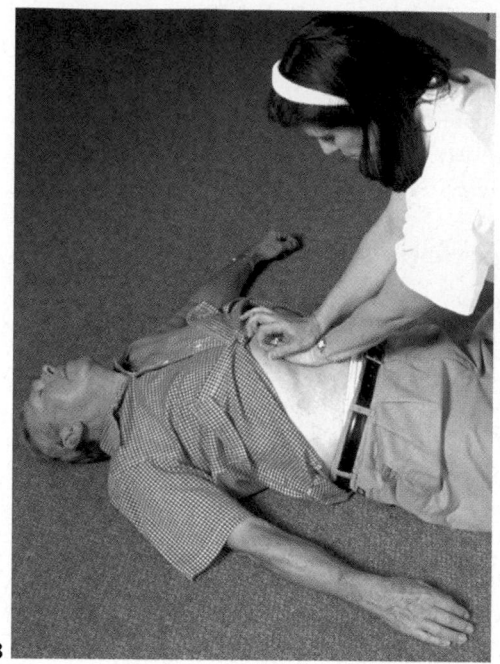

A   **B**

Figure 23-2. ■ (**A**) The Heimlich maneuver performed on a conscious victim who is sitting or standing. (**B**) The Heimlich maneuver performed on an unconscious victim.

NURSING CARE

Closely monitor clients at risk for laryngeal obstruction (e.g., newly extubated clients and clients receiving medications that may cause anaphylaxis, such as intravenous antibiotics or radiologic dyes) for manifestations of obstruction, including dyspnea, nasal flaring, tachypnea, anxiety, wheezing, and stridor. Laryngeal obstruction is a medical emergency requiring immediate intervention to open the airway and prevent brain damage or death. Suction the airway as needed; small aspirated foreign bodies may be removed by suctioning. Be prepared to assist with emergency intubation or tracheotomy as needed. If obstruction is complete, initiate a cardiopulmonary arrest procedure (code).

Client and family teaching focuses on preventing aspiration and teaching techniques to relieve obstruction. Clients who wear dentures should be cautioned to take small bites and to chew carefully before swallowing. Discuss the relationship between excess alcohol intake and food aspiration. Promote training of the general public in cardiopulmonary resuscitation (CPR) and the Heimlich maneuver. The more people who are adequately trained in emergency procedures, the more likely it is that emergency procedures will be initiated in a timely manner. Advise clients with a known risk for anaphylaxis (such as people with a previous anaphylactic response and those allergic to bee venom) to wear a Medic-Alert tag and carry a bee-sting kit to prevent severe laryngeal edema.

Sleep Apnea

Sleep apnea, the temporary absence of breathing during sleep, is common. Sleep apnea affects men more than women, and is more common in older adults. Obesity, enlarged tonsils, and the use of alcohol or sedatives before sleep contribute to sleep apnea.

Obstructive sleep apnea is the most common form. The upper airway is obstructed as muscles of the pharynx relax and the tongue falls back (Figure 23-3 ■). In *central sleep*

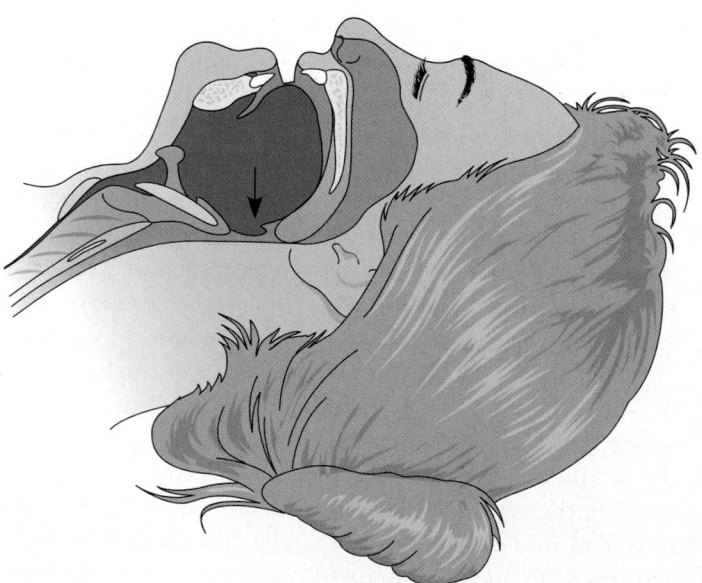

Figure 23-3. ■ In obstructive sleep apnea, the pharynx is obstructed by the soft palate and tongue.

apnea, no effort to breathe is seen; the respiratory muscles remain relaxed.

Common manifestations of sleep apnea include loud snoring, frequent nighttime waking, daytime sleepiness, headache, and irritability. Other problems may follow, such as hypertension, morning headache, irritability, and impotence. Clients may show personality changes, impaired memory, and inability to concentrate.

Sleep apnea is diagnosed in a sleep laboratory. The treatment plan includes measures to reduce airway obstruction, prevent apneic episodes, and provide psychologic support. Weight loss often is the first intervention

prescribed. Strict avoidance of alcohol and hypnotic medications also is vital.

Continuous positive airway pressure (CPAP) therapy is often prescribed for sleep apnea. The client wears a tightly fitting nasal mask. An air compressor blows air into the back of the throat, preventing the airway from collapsing.

Nursing care for clients with sleep apnea focuses on teaching the client and family how to use respiratory equipment and other management measures. Discuss the relationship of obesity, alcohol, and sedatives to the syndrome and provide instruction and referral to programs such as Weight Watchers and Alcoholics Anonymous.

UPPER RESPIRATORY TUMORS

Tumors of the upper respiratory tract are relatively uncommon. They can, however, obstruct the airway and interfere with breathing. The larynx is the upper airway structure most often affected by tumors.

Benign Laryngeal Tumors

Benign tumors may develop on the vocal cords of the larynx, particularly in clients who chronically shout, project, or vocalize in a very high or low tone. Vocal cord nodules are often called "singer's nodules"; cheerleaders and public speakers may also develop them. Cigarette smoking and chronic irritation from pollution contribute to their development. Hoarseness and a breathy voice are manifestations of vocal cord nodules.

Correcting the underlying problem (e.g., voice training or quitting smoking) may correct benign tumors. If necessary, the tumors may be surgically removed.

If surgery is performed, observe closely for signs of airway obstruction, such as labored breathing or inspiratory stridor. Apply cold packs to the neck area to reduce the risk of swelling. To prevent aspiration, do not give food or fluids until the cough and gag reflexes have returned.

When teaching the client and family, stress the importance of voice rest. Refer clients, particularly singers, to a speech therapist for voice training. Emphasize the need to keep the voice within its normal range to reduce vocal cord stress. Talk to the client about quitting smoking, particularly if the client is also a singer.

Laryngeal Cancer

Cancer of the larynx is uncommon, but can be devastating. If found early, it can be cured, especially when it is limited to the vocal cords. The disease usually affects older adults; men are affected more often than women. Laryngeal cancer is more common in African Americans than in whites (Box 23-7 ■).

The two major modifiable risk factors for laryngeal cancer are prolonged use of tobacco and alcohol. Other modifiable risk factors include poor nutrition and occupational exposure to wood dust, paint fumes, chemicals, and asbestos.

PATHOPHYSIOLOGY AND MANIFESTATIONS

Changes in laryngeal mucosa occur when it is continually subjected to noxious irritants such as cigarette smoke. White, patchy precancerous lesions known as *leukoplakia* develop first, followed by the appearance of red, velvety patches called *erythroplakia,* a later stage of tumor development. Laryngeal cancer spreads both by direct invasion of surrounding tissues and by metastasis.

Laryngeal cancer may occur in any of the three areas of the larynx: the glottis, the supraglottis, and the subglottis. Lesions of the true vocal cords or *glottis* are more common than cancers of other areas of the larynx (Figure 23-4 ■). Fortunately, these cancers tend to be slow growing.

The primary manifestation of *glottic* cancer is a change in the voice; the tumor prevents complete closure of the vocal cords during speech. The *supraglottic* (above the glottis) area includes the epiglottis and false vocal cords. A tumor may be large before manifestations such as painful swallowing, a sore throat, or a feeling of a lump in the

| BOX 23-7 | POPULATION FOCUS |

Laryngeal Cancer

Laryngeal cancer is about 50% more common in African Americans than it is in whites. Teach African American clients how to reduce their risk for laryngeal cancer by stopping smoking, abstaining from alcohol or drinking only moderately, and managing other risk factors (exposure to fumes, etc.). Discuss the early manifestations of laryngeal cancer, and stress the importance of seeking treatment promptly.

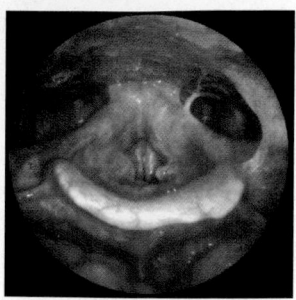

Figure 23-4. ■ Cancer of the larynx. Most lesions form along the edges of the glottis. (*Source:* Phototake NYC.)

throat develop. As the tumor grows, difficulty breathing, foul breath, a palpable lump in the neck, and pain that radiates to the ear may occur. *Subglottic* tumors (below the vocal cords) are the least common laryngeal cancers and often have no early symptoms. As the tumor enlarges, manifestations of airway obstruction develop. Common manifestations of laryngeal cancer are summarized in Box 23-8 ■.

INTERDISCIPLINARY CARE

Most small cord lesions can be cured with early diagnosis and treatment. Left untreated, however, 90% of clients die within 3 years. Treatment (surgical removal, radiation, chemotherapy) is determined by the stage of the cancer. (See Chapter 12 ⬤ for a discussion of cancer staging.)

Diagnostic Tests

Direct or indirect *laryngoscopy* is performed when the client has manifestations of laryngeal cancer. (See Chapter 22 ⬤ for the nursing implications for laryngoscopy.) Suspicious lesions are biopsied. Other diagnostic tests may include x-rays of the head, neck, and chest, as well as CT or magnetic resonance imaging (MRI) scan. A needle biopsy of enlarged lymph nodes helps confirm the diagnosis. A barium swallow may be done to evaluate swallowing and tumor extension into the esophagus.

BOX 23-8

MANIFESTATIONS OF LARYNGEAL CANCER

- Hoarseness or voice change that lasts more than 2 weeks
- Persistent cough
- Persistent sore throat
- Difficult or painful swallowing
- Dyspnea
- Foul breath
- Palpable lump in neck
- Persistent earache
- Unintended weight loss

Radiation

Radiation therapy is often the treatment of choice for early laryngeal cancer. Radiation disrupts the DNA of the cell, causing it to die. External beam radiation may be used, or implants of radioactive seeds may be inserted directly into the tumor or near the tumor site. Radiation therapy is often combined with surgery, but it may be used alone in the early stages of laryngeal cancer or when the client refuses (or is not a candidate for) surgery. In advanced cancer, it may be used in combination with chemotherapy to avoid total laryngectomy, or following laryngectomy to treat cervical lymph nodes.

Chemotherapy

Chemotherapy is not the treatment of choice, although it may be used to treat tumors that have metastasized beyond the head and neck or for tumors that are too large to be surgically removed. A multiple-drug treatment regimen often is used to maximize effectiveness. (See Chapter 12 ⬤ for more information about chemotherapy.)

Surgery

Surgery may be performed to remove the tumor and maintain an open airway. The type and extent of surgery are determined by the size, site, and invasiveness of the tumor. Carcinoma *in situ* and vocal cord polyps may be treated on an outpatient basis, using a laser to vaporize the tumor. The voice is preserved, although total voice rest is prescribed, with only whispering allowed for at least a week following surgery.

Laryngectomy, removal of the larynx, may be necessary for some clients. With a *partial laryngectomy* (removal of one-half or more of the larynx), the client is able to resume normal speaking, breathing, and swallowing. A **tracheostomy** (a surgical opening into the trachea) tube may be inserted to maintain the airway in the early postoperative period, but it is usually removed within about a week and the stoma is allowed to heal.

In *total laryngectomy,* the entire larynx is removed, along with the surrounding tissues; normal speech is lost, and a permanent tracheostomy is created. The tracheostomy tube inserted during surgery may be left in place for several weeks and then removed, leaving a natural stoma, or it may be left in place permanently. Because the trachea and the esophagus are permanently separated by this surgery (Figure 23-5 ■), there is no risk of aspiration during swallowing.

If cervical lymph nodes contain cancer cells, a *modified* or *radical neck dissection* may be done along with total laryngectomy. In a radical neck dissection, cervical lymph nodes, the sternocleidomastoid muscle, internal jugular vein, cranial nerve XI (spinal accessory), and submaxillary salivary gland

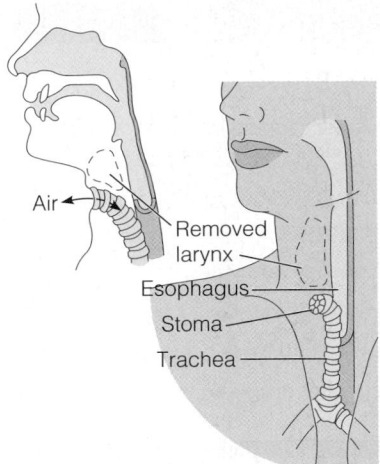

Figure 23-5. ■ Following a total laryngectomy, the client has a permanent tracheostomy. No connection between the trachea and esophagus remains.

are removed on the tumor side of the neck. After surgery, the client may have difficulty lifting and turning the head because of muscle loss. The shoulder on the affected side drops. Postoperative neck exercises can help reduce shoulder drop and increase range of motion on the affected side.

Box 23-9 ■ outlines nursing care for the client having a total laryngectomy.

clinical ALERT

Maintaining a patent airway and controlling bleeding are priorities of care for any client undergoing neck surgery, and particularly for the client who has had a laryngectomy.

Speech Rehabilitation

Various techniques may be used to restore speech after a total laryngectomy. A surgical procedure, the *tracheoesophageal puncture (TEP)*, is the usual method used to restore speech. TEP creates a small *fistula* (passage) between the posterior tracheal wall and the anterior esophagus (Figure 23-6 ■). A small, one-way valve in the fistula allows the client to force air from the lungs into the mouth by covering the tracheostomy stoma with a finger. The air creates vibration and sound, and the client uses the tongue, lips, teeth, and palate to articulate the words. The one-way valve prevents food from entering the trachea.

Several *speech generators* are available for the laryngectomy client. One type is held against the neck; it transmits

---

BOX 23-9	NURSING CARE CHECKLIST

Total Laryngectomy

Before Surgery

☑ Provide routine preoperative care and teaching (see Chapter 9). ⏺⏺

☑ Assess anxiety level and provide psychologic support.

☑ Discuss postoperative communication strategies. Emphasize that total laryngectomy results in a loss of speech and that the client will breathe through a permanent stoma in the neck.

After Surgery

☑ Provide routine postoperative care (see Chapter 9). ⏺⏺

☑ Monitor respiratory status at least every 1 to 2 hours, including airway patency; respiratory rate, depth, and pattern; and lung sounds.

☑ Monitor oxygen saturation levels. Report levels of less than 95% (or established parameters) to the charge nurse or physician.

☑ Place the call light within easy reach at all times; answer the call light promptly.

☑ Encourage family members to stay with the client whenever possible.

☑ Encourage deep breathing and coughing.

☑ Elevate the head of the bed.

☑ Maintain humidification of inspired gases.

☑ Suction tracheostomy using sterile technique as needed.

☑ Provide tracheostomy care per protocol and as needed (see Box 23-10 ■).

☑ Teach to support the head when moving in bed.

☑ Assist out of bed and with ambulation as soon as allowed after surgery.

☑ Teach to protect the stoma from particulate matter in the air with a gauze square or other stoma protector.

☑ Maintain fluid intake with intravenous fluids and/or enteral feedings until able to take adequate amounts of food and fluids orally.

☑ Prior to initiating feeding, assist to begin performing mouth rinses.

☑ When able to resume oral intake, begin with soft foods, not liquids.

☑ Reassure the client that choking is not possible, because there is no connection between the esophagus and trachea.

☑ Provide for privacy during initial attempts at eating.

☑ Encourage the client and family members to express their fears and anxieties.

BOX 23-10   PROCEDURE CHECKLIST

Tracheostomy Care

☑ Gather all supplies

☑ Provide for privacy. Explain the procedure and provide for communication (e.g., eye blinking or raising a finger to indicate distress).

☑ Place in semi-Fowler's or Fowler's position.

☑ Use Standard Precautions and sterile technique as indicated.

☑ Assess lung sounds; suction as needed using sterile technique.

☑ Wearing clean gloves, remove the tracheostomy dressing.

☑ Wearing sterile gloves, use sterile applicators or gauze 4 × 4s moistened with normal saline to clean the incision.

☑ If the tracheostomy tube has an inner cannula that can be removed for cleaning, remove the tube and soak it in sterile saline.

☑ Cleanse the tracheostomy tube flange (collar) in the same manner as the incision.

☑ Clean the inner cannula using a small brush or cotton-tipped applicators. Rinse thoroughly in normal saline and tap it gently to remove excess liquid.

☑ Suction the outer cannula using sterile technique.

☑ Replace the inner cannula into the tracheostomy tube.

☑ Replace the dressing. Do not cut the dressing or use a cotton-filled dressing because fibers may be aspirated into the respiratory tract.

☑ Apply clean tracheostomy ties.

☑ Once the clean ties are secured, remove the old ties.

☑ Assess breathing and tolerance of the procedure.

☑ Dispose of supplies and used solutions. Wash hands.

SAMPLE DOCUMENTATION

5/31/06 0830	Trach care provided. Suctioned for moderate amount of thin, yellow sputum. Lung sounds clear after suctioning. Incision clean, no evidence of inflammation. Healing well. Tolerated procedure well. _____J. Doene, LPN.

Note: Refer to a nursing fundamentals or skills text for more detailed instruction. Check state guidelines and facility policy before performing any procedure.

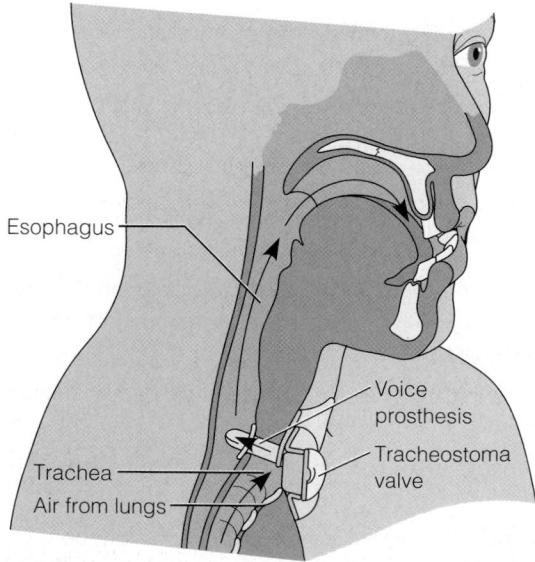

Figure 23-6. ■ The tracheoesophageal prosthesis allows air from the trachea to be diverted through the prosthesis into the esophagus and oropharynx, producing speech when the tracheostomy stoma is occluded. A one-way valve prevents food from entering the trachea.

vibrations to the neck and into the mouth. Muscles of the mouth and tongue form vibrations into words (Figure 23-7A ■). Another device delivers a tone into the mouth through a plastic tube (Figure 23-7B). The lips, tongue, and mouth muscles then form the sound into words.

Esophageal speech uses swallowed air and controlled belching to create sound and form words. The client uses muscles of the mouth and tongue normally involved in speech. This form of speech takes practice, and many clients are unable to resume speaking fluently.

NURSING CARE

ASSESSING

Nurses can help to identify clients at risk for or with early manifestations of laryngeal cancer. Because manifestations of the disease often do not occur until the cancer is advanced, obtaining good subjective data from the client is vital. Box 23-11 ■ lists assessment data to collect.

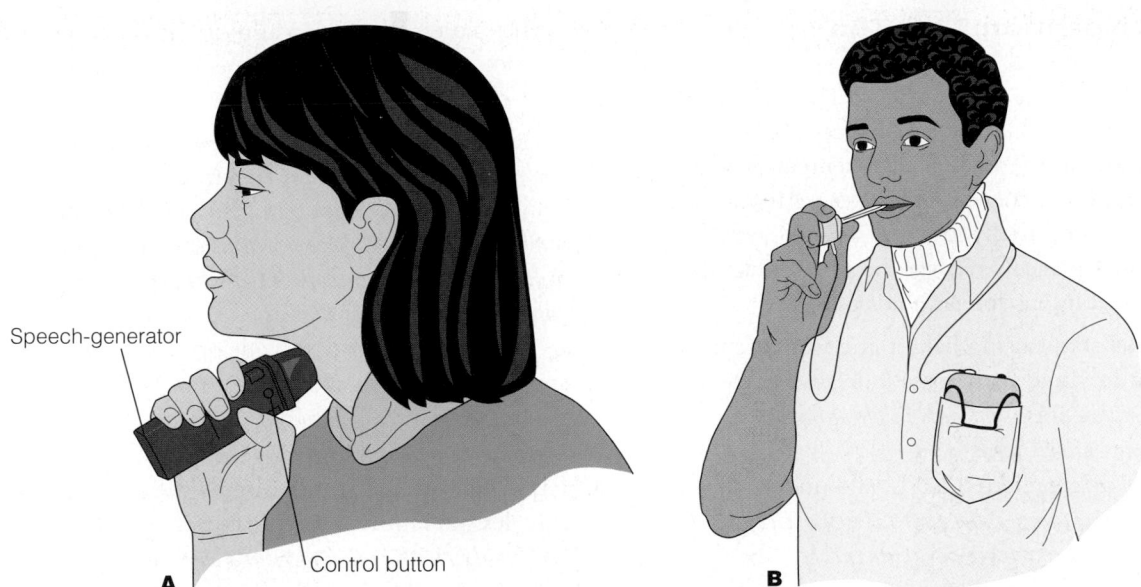

Figure 23-7. ■ **(A)** The client holds the vibrating tip of the speech generator against the throat, using the mouth to form words. **(B)** A plastic tube on the handpiece of the speech aid device produces an audible tone. The client holds the tube against the roof of the mouth when forming words.

DIAGNOSING, PLANNING, AND IMPLEMENTING

Priorities in Nursing Care. The client with laryngeal cancer has multiple nursing care needs. The risk for impaired verbal communication exists, whether or not a total laryngectomy is planned. Clients may experience dysphagia

that interferes with swallowing and nutrition before treatment. Radiation, chemotherapy, or surgery also may interfere with nutrition. The diagnosis of cancer is frightening for most clients, no matter what the potential for cure is with treatment. Problems related to communication, nutrition, and anticipatory grieving are included in this section. Nursing care specific to the client undergoing a laryngectomy is given in Box 23-9. Nursing care of the client with a tracheostomy is reviewed in Box 23-10.

Impaired Verbal Communication

Removing the larynx results in voice loss. Before surgery, discuss alternate methods of communication, both short and long term, with the client and family members. Ultimately, the choice is the client's; some may choose to forego laryngectomy to avoid voice loss when the chance for long-term success and cancer cure is minimal.

- Before surgery, assess for additional obstacles to communication. *Hearing loss, illiteracy, previous stroke, or weakness may affect the ability to use alternate communication strategies.*
- Provide alternate ways to communicate (pencil and paper, Magic Slate, an alphabet board) and encourage practice. *Having the client choose what to practice helps reduce anxiety and increases the sense of control.*
- Encourage the client to consult a speech therapist before surgery if possible. *The client may be a candidate for esophageal speech, TEP, or a speech generator.*
- Assess frequently. Place the call bell at hand when leaving. *The presence and availability of a caring nurse decrease anxiety and promote communication.*

BOX 23-11   ASSESSMENT

Assessing Clients with Laryngeal Cancer

SUBJECTIVE DATA

- Recent and/or persistent voice changes (hoarseness, breathiness); difficulty or pain with swallowing; persistent sore throat, cough, or ear pain; difficulty breathing; sensation of a lump in the throat.
- Recent unintended or unexplained weight loss.
- Smoking history: packs smoked per day; number of years smoked. Alcohol consumption: amount per day or week; number of years of alcohol use.
- Chronic diseases; occupation.

OBJECTIVE DATA

- General appearance: apparent health, skin color.
- Difficulty breathing or swallowing, hoarseness, changes in voice quality, and cough.
- Inspect neck for asymmetry or masses; mouth and oropharynx for white or red patches.
- Palpate lips, cheeks, and tongue for masses; neck for symmetry, masses, lymph node enlargement, and tenderness.

Imbalanced Nutrition: Less Than Body Requirements

Large tumors may affect the ability to eat. The client with cancer often requires additional calories because of the effects of the disease. After surgery, enteral or parenteral feedings often are ordered until the client is able to eat. After a total laryngectomy, the client initially loses the senses of taste and smell. The client may partially recover the sense of taste but may complain that eating no longer holds pleasure.

- Assess nutritional status using height and weight charts, reported weight loss, and body mass indicators such as skin folds. *A complete assessment aids in planning to meet current and anticipated calorie needs.*
- Evaluate current diet, preferred foods, and understanding of nutrition. *Providing a diet that takes the client's preferences into account will encourage adequate intake.*
- Monitor intake and output and food consumption. *Monitoring food and fluid intake is necessary to determine if the client is consuming adequate calories and fluids for healing.*
- Weigh daily. *The daily weight provides a measure of both nutritional status and fluid balance.*
- Contact the dietitian for further evaluation, planning, and education. *A professional can identify nutritional needs and help plan a diet to meet them.*
- Encourage experimentation with foods of different textures and temperatures. *Cold foods or foods with a soft texture are easier to swallow.*
- Encourage frequent, small meals rather than three large meals per day. *The client who has difficulty swallowing is likely to consume more food this way.*
- Recommend liquid supplements such as Ensure as needed to increase calorie intake. Provide information about where to obtain supplements. *Liquid dietary supplements provide balanced nutrition and added calories. They are available in major supermarkets.*
- Provide mouth care prior to meals and supplemental feedings. For the client with stomatitis or esophagitis related to radiation or chemotherapy, provide a topical anesthetic such as viscous lidocaine before eating. *Bad breath or a foul taste in the mouth suppresses appetite. Inflamed mucosa may make eating uncomfortable. A topical anesthetic can relieve discomfort and promote food intake* (see the Stomatitis section in Chapter 19). ⨂
- Provide an antiemetic 30 minutes before eating if nausea is a problem. *An antiemetic can relieve nausea and make eating possible.*

Anticipatory Grieving

The client with laryngeal cancer faces the diagnosis of cancer, the prospect of mutilating surgery, and loss of both a body part and an important function, speech. Loss of speech affects social interactions, one's career, and the ability to get help when necessary. A radical neck dissection changes the appearance and function of the neck, altering body image and self-concept.

- Provide opportunities for the client and family members to express feelings of grief, anger, or fear about the diagnosis of cancer, the impending surgery, and the anticipated loss of speech. *The client needs the opportunity (and permission) to grieve anticipated losses in order to move toward coping and acceptance of the loss.*
- Be calm and supportive. Provide privacy and emotional support for the client and family to work through the grieving process. *It is important for the client and family to know that their feelings of loss are real and accepted by caregivers.*
- Help the client and family discuss the potential impact of the loss on family structure and function. *Discussion helps family members to understand and support one another.*
- Refer the client and family for counseling as appropriate. *Counseling may be necessary to prevent a sense of defeat and hopelessness.*
- Help the client and family identify additional resources for coping, such as strategies they have used in the past to deal with crises. *This identifies strengths they can use to deal with the present situation.*

EVALUATING

Collect the following data to evaluate the effectiveness of nursing interventions for the client with laryngeal cancer:

- Airway remains patent; experiences no difficulty breathing.
- Communicates care needs effectively.
- Anxiety remains within a manageable level.
- Maintains weight.
- Demonstrates willingness to participate in speech therapy.

Documenting. Document continuing assessment data, as well as procedures and nursing care performed. Note the client's and family's responses to the surgery, the resulting voice loss, presence of the tracheostomy (if performed), and, if radical neck surgery was performed, weakness and disfigurement of the neck. Document teaching provided and the client's and family's ability to demonstrate care measures taught (e.g., protecting the tracheostomy stoma, suctioning and cleaning the tracheostomy, care of the incision).

CONTINUING CARE

In the community, teach about the risk factors and early warning signs of laryngeal cancer, so it can be recognized and treated early. After diagnosis of laryngeal cancer, provide information and clarify treatment options, discussing the risks and benefits of each. Stress the importance of early intervention to reduce the risk of local spread and metastasis.

If a total laryngectomy is the treatment of choice, discuss options for communication after surgery. Present the options realistically. Clients may have difficulty manipulating the tracheoesophageal puncture device for speech; only about 30% of clients master esophageal speech.

Teach the client undergoing radiation therapy about the treatments, care of the skin and secretions during therapy, and expected side effects. (See Chapter 12 🔗 for further discussion about managing the effects of radiation therapy.)

Assess the client's and family's resources and ability to provide home care following surgery (Box 23-12 ■).

Teach the client and family members how to care for the tracheostomy and provide the opportunity for redemonstration of care. The client uses clean technique rather than sterile technique in providing stoma care. Once the stoma is fully healed, the tracheostomy tube may no longer be needed. Teach the following:

- Use a humidifier or vaporizer in the home to add humidity to inspired air.
- Increase fluid intake to maintain mucosal moisture and loosen secretions.
- Shield the stoma with a stoma guard (such as a gauze square) to prevent particles from entering the lower respiratory tract.
- Promptly remove secretions from skin surrounding the stoma to prevent irritation and skin breakdown.
- Protect the stoma with a cupped hand or washcloth while showering or bathing; don't submerge the neck or head.
- Do not participate in water sports. All other activities are allowed, but lifting may be more difficult because of the inability to hold the breath (the Valsalva maneuver).

Encourage the client to work with a physical therapist to regain function and mobility of the neck and shoulder if a radical neck dissection has been done.

Both the client and family need emotional and motivational support through this trying time. Provide referral to local support groups such as a laryngectomy club or lost cord club. Encourage the client to discontinue the use of cigarettes and alcohol. Discuss ways to achieve good nutrition. If the client and family are having difficulty adjusting to the diagnosis of cancer and the effects of treatment, provide referral to counseling. (See the Critical Thinking Care Map at the end of this chapter.)

Note: The bibliography listings for this and all chapters have been compiled at the back of the book.

| BOX 23-12 | **ASSESSMENT** |

Assessing for Discharge: Laryngeal Cancer

CLIENT

- Self-care: ability to perform ADLs independently, care for tracheostomy, manipulate TEP device or electronic speech device
- Knowledge: treatment plan; dealing with adverse effects of radiation or chemotherapy; preventing respiratory infections; using communication techniques; maintaining nutritional status; indications for seeking medical intervention
- Motivation: smoking cessation, abstinence from alcohol consumption
- Home environment: access to clean water for hand washing and tracheostomy care; indoor pollutants such as cigarette smoke, dust, and allergens such as pets

FAMILY

- Caregivers: availability and willingness to provide care as needed; ability to assist with shopping, transportation, and caring for dependents; willingness to avoid smoking inside the home
- Financial resources: income; availability of sick leave; impact of diagnosis and treatment options on career and income; resources for drugs, medical supplies, and medical care required

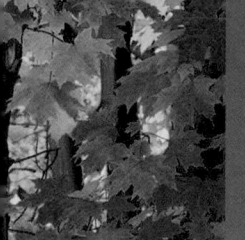

Chapter Review

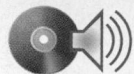 KEY TERMS by Topics

Use the audio glossary feature of either the CD-ROM or the Companion Website to hear the correct pronunciation of the following key terms.

URIs and Inflammations
rhinitis, coryza, influenza, sinusitis, pharyngitis, tonsillitis, dysphagia, stridor, laryngitis, tonsillectomy

Pertussis
pertussis

Trauma or Obstruction
epistaxis, rhinoplasty, laryngospasm, sleep apnea

Tumors
laryngectomy, tracheostomy

KEY Points

- A patent airway and unobstructed airflow are vital to sustain life and function. While upper airway disorders often are minor, many can potentially affect airway patency and become life threatening.

- Most upper respiratory infections are relatively minor and appropriate for self-care.

- While many decongestants and antihistamines are available without a prescription, these drugs are not appropriate for all people. They may cause drowsiness, increased blood pressure, or problems for people who have glaucoma, intestinal problems, or urinary retention.

- Bacterial complications such as pneumonia, sinusitis, and peritonsillar abscess may follow viral URIs. These complications do require medical treatment, often antibiotic therapy.

- Acute epiglottitis and laryngeal spasm, edema, or obstruction are medical emergencies that require immediate treatment to maintain an open airway and sustain life.

- Most nosebleeds occur in the anterior portion of the nose and can be controlled by putting pressure and ice on the nose. Older adults are at risk for posterior nosebleeds. Posterior nosebleeds are more difficult to control and often require medical treatment.

- The primary risk factors for laryngeal cancer are smoking and excess alcohol use. Discuss these lifestyle factors with all clients, especially those who have other risk factors for laryngeal cancer.

- Persistent hoarseness or voice change is a common manifestation of laryngeal cancer. Prompt clients to seek medical assessment if this occurs. Stress that with early intervention, laryngeal cancer is curable and the ability to speak is preserved.

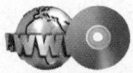 EXPLORE MediaLink

Additional interactive resources for this chapter can be found on the Companion Website at www.prenhall.com/burke. Click on Chapter 23 and "Begin" to select the activities for this chapter.

For chapter-related NCLEX-style review questions and an audio glossary, access the accompanying CD-ROM in this book.

FOR FURTHER Study

For more information on care and teaching of the surgical client, see Chapter 9.

See Chapter 10 to review the spread of infection, and for more information about antibiotics.

See Chapter 11 for more information about allergic responses.

For more information on cancer staging, chemotherapy, and radiation therapy, see Chapter 12.

Stomatitis is discussed in Chapter 19.

For more about pneumonia and about the huff technique of coughing, see Chapter 24.

For discussion of rheumatic fever, see Chapter 27.

For further study about acute glomerulonephritis, see Chapter 32.

For more information about otitis media and other ear disorders, see Chapter 40.

Critical Thinking Care Map

Caring for a Client with Total Laryngectomy
NCLEX-PN® Focus Area: Reduction of Risk Potential

Case Study: David Tom is a 61-year-old divorced man with two grown children. He has smoked two packs of cigarettes daily since high school. He drinks three or four cocktails every evening. Mr. Tom was recently diagnosed with laryngeal cancer after he sought care for a sore throat and hoarseness that had persisted for a few months. He has been admitted to the surgical care unit from the intensive care unit (ICU) 2 days post–total laryngectomy.

Nursing Diagnosis: Risk for Ineffective Airway Clearance

COLLECT DATA

Subjective _____

_____

_____

_____

_____

_____

Objective _____

_____

_____

_____

_____

_____

Would you report this data? Yes/No

If yes, to: _____

Nursing Care

_____

_____

_____

_____

_____

_____

_____

_____

_____

_____

How would you document this? _____

_____

_____

Data Collected (use those that apply)

- PB 146/84; P 92 and regular; R 18; T 100°F (37.7°C) per rectum
- Tracheostomy tube present
- O$_2$ per tracheostomy collar
- Oxygen saturation 94%
- Rates pain in neck and right shoulder at 6 on a scale of 1 to 10
- Continuous tube feeding per nasogastric tube
- Two Hemovac wound drains in the right neck draining 15 and 35 mL serosanguineous fluid
- Complains that head "feels heavy"
- Ambulatory within the room without assistance
- Using Magic Slate to communicate

Nursing Interventions (use those that apply; list in priority order)

- Assess respiratory rate, lung sounds, and cough effectiveness every 2 hours.
- Monitor quantity, color, and odor of secretions.
- Encourage to deep breathe and cough hourly.
- Assess pain at least every 2 to 3 hours and administer analgesics as ordered.
- Up at bedside and ambulating at least four times per day.
- Provide written information as requested.
- Monitor intake, output, and daily weight.
- Arrange for a dietary consultation to determine calorie needs.

NCLEX-PN® Exam Preparation

TEST-TAKING TIP The NCLEX-PN is a timed test. Pace yourself. Be aware of your remaining time. Use all of the time allotted, if needed. You will have 5 hours to complete the test.

1 After teaching a client about the antihistamine Chlor-Trimeton, which statement indicates that further instruction is necessary?

A. "I'm not going to drive today. My sister will pick me up."
B. "I will stop at the grocery store for a bag of hard peppermint candy."
C. "I'm going to a wine-tasting party tonight."
D. "I'll call my doctor if I have trouble breathing."

2 To most effectively anticipate the needs of a client who has undergone a tonsillectomy, the nurse would plan to:

A. apply a warm compress to the neck.
B. place the patient in a supine position.
C. remove the nasopharyngeal airway immediately.
D. place a humidifier by the bedside.

3 A client presents at the urgent care clinic with complaints of a severe cough that interferes with her ability to eat and drink, and often causes her to vomit. The client has manifestations of dehydration and talking stimulates paroxysms of coughing during which she has difficulty catching her breath. Recognizing these as classic manifestations of pertussis, the nurse

A. administers a narcotic cough suppressant.
B. initiates respiratory isolation precautions.
C. obtains a sputum specimen for culture.
D. alerts coworkers that anyone not vaccinated for pertussis as an infant should avoid contact with the client.

4 A resident of a nursing home will be receiving an influenza injection. Which information would be the most important for the care of this client?

A. allergy history
B. name of insurance company
C. medical history
D. respiratory status

5 The nurse understands that the most important intervention for the client with a noncomplicated upper respiratory viral infection is:

A. obtaining throat cultures.
B. teaching self-care.
C. monitoring vital signs.
D. antibiotic medication teaching.

6 In teaching a client about laryngitis, it is important to focus on:

A. resting the voice.
B. effective coughing techniques.
C. increased fluids.
D. use of a cough suppressant at bedtime.

7 A client presents to the emergency department with severe bleeding from the anterior nasal septum. All of the following nursing actions are appropriate. Place them in order of priority.

A. Apply ice packs to the nose.
B. Give the client an emesis basin into which she can spit the blood.
C. Pinch the nose toward the septum.
D. Ask what precipitated the incident.
E. Inquire about current medications.

8 Which of these statements, if made by a client diagnosed with sleep apnea, would indicate an understanding of this condition?

A. "I'm going to sleep on my back for the next 2 weeks."
B. "I would like to see the dietitian about my weight."
C. "Please ask the doctor to order a sleeping pill for me."
D. "I won't snore so loud if I drink a glass of wine before bedtime."

9 A client at a blood pressure clinic tells the nurse that his voice has been hoarse for "about a month now." He denies sore throat or difficulty swallowing. The appropriate response by the nurse is:

A. "Since you don't also have a sore throat, it really isn't anything to worry about."
B. "Persistent hoarseness is a sign of voice strain. You should rest your voice for a couple of weeks and see if it improves."
C. "Try using warm salt-water gargles three to four times a day. This sounds like persistent laryngitis."
D. "Persistent hoarseness can be an early sign of laryngeal cancer. Please tell your doctor about this."

10 A client who has had a total laryngectomy and permanent tracheostomy is afraid to eat for fear of choking. The nurse's response is based on the knowledge that:

A. choking is a significant risk following total laryngectomy.
B. choking can be prevented by closing the tracheostomy stoma with a finger while swallowing.
C. the trachea and esophagus are separate, so choking is not a risk.
D. oral intake should begin with water only until the client learns to swallow without choking.

Answers for Review Questions, as well as discussion of Care Plan and Critical Thinking Care Map questions, appear in Appendix V.

Chapter 24

Caring for Clients with Lower Respiratory Disorders

BRIEF Outline

Acute Bronchitis; Pneumonia; Tuberculosis
Lung Abscess and Empyema
Asthma
Chronic Obstructive Pulmonary Disease
Cystic Fibrosis
Atelectasis and Bronchiectasis
Occupational Lung Disease and Sarcoidosis
Lung Cancer
Pulmonary Embolism
Pulmonary Hypertension and Cor Pulmonale
Pleuritis and Pleural Effusion
Pneumothorax and Hemothorax
Chest and Lung Trauma
Respiratory Failure
Acute Respiratory Distress Syndrome

LEARNING Outcomes

After completing this chapter, you will be able to:

- Describe the pathophysiology of common lower respiratory system disorders.
- Relate manifestations of lower respiratory system disorders to the normal structure and function of the lungs and thoracic cage.
- Discuss nursing implications for medications and treatments used for lower respiratory system disorders.
- Provide appropriate care for a client having thoracic surgery.
- Use the nursing process to assess, plan, and implement individualized care for clients with lower respiratory system disorders.
- Reinforce teaching and learning for clients with lower respiratory system disorders and their families.

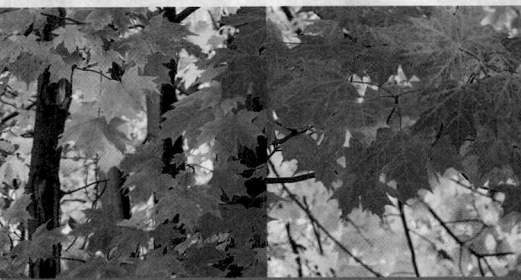

MediaLink

www.prenhall.com/burke
Use the address above to access the free, interactive Companion Website created for this textbook. Get hints, instant feedback, and textbook references to chapter-related NCLEX-style questions. Link to other interesting sites.

Audio Glossary:
Use the Companion Website, or the CD-ROM disk enclosed with your textbook, to hear the pronunciation of key terms in this chapter.

Disorders of the lower respiratory system are common, affecting people in the community and in acute-care and long-term care facilities. Lower respiratory system disorders have both local and systemic effects. Local effects include cough, excess mucous production, **dyspnea** (difficulty breathing), **hemoptysis** (bloody sputum), and chest pain. Systemic effects may include fever, anorexia and malaise, **cyanosis** (a bluish-gray skin color), edema, clubbing of fingers and toes, and other manifestations of impaired gas exchange.

INFECTIOUS AND INFLAMMATORY DISORDERS

The lower respiratory system is protected from infection by a number of defenses. If an organism makes it past the upper respiratory tract, it is usually trapped in mucus of the lower respiratory tract. *Cilia* (small hairs) that line the airways and the cough reflex then push the mucous-trapped organism out. Organisms that make it past all of these barriers usually are killed rapidly in the alveolus by the immune defenses of the body. When these defenses are impaired, the risk of infection increases. For example, chronic lung disease impairs the mucous and ciliary responses to invasion. Older adults have a higher risk than others of lower respiratory infections (Box 24-1 ■). Even in healthy clients, pathogens can enter the lungs, causing an infectious or inflammatory response.

Acute Bronchitis

Bronchitis (inflammation of the bronchi) can be either acute or chronic. Acute bronchitis is relatively common among adults. Chronic bronchitis is a component of chronic obstructive pulmonary disease (COPD) and is discussed in that section of this chapter.

PATHOPHYSIOLOGY AND MANIFESTATIONS

Acute bronchitis typically follows an upper respiratory infection (URI). People with impaired defense mechanisms and smokers have a higher risk for bronchitis. Viruses, bacteria, and toxic gases or chemicals can cause bronchitis. The inflammatory response leads to vasodilation and edema of the bronchial linings. Mucus production increases, stimulating the cough reflex.

BOX 24-1	FOCUS ON OLDER ADULTS

Lower Respiratory Tract Infections in Older Adults

Changes associated with aging and disease affect respiratory function and airway clearance, increasing the risk of infections. The number of cilia decreases, and the cough weakens. Gag and cough reflexes diminish. Residual volume increases, and vital capacity decreases. The older adult is at risk for dehydration, leading to thick, sticky mucus that is difficult to expectorate. Immune function declines with aging. Limited mobility, a smoking history, surgery, multiple medications, malnutrition, and chronic diseases also may increase older adults' risk for respiratory infections.

The cough is initially nonproductive, but later becomes productive. The cough often occurs in *paroxysms* (uncontrollable bursts), and may be aggravated by cold, dry, or dusty air. Substernal chest pain is common. Other symptoms include fever and general malaise.

INTERDISCIPLINARY CARE

Acute bronchitis usually is diagnosed by the history and examination. A *chest x-ray* may be ordered to rule out pneumonia, because the manifestations can be similar. Treatment includes rest, increased fluid intake, and mild analgesics to relieve fever and malaise. An antibiotic such as erythromycin or penicillin may be prescribed. An expectorant cough medication is recommended for daytime, and a cough suppressant at night to facilitate rest.

NURSING CARE

Clients with acute bronchitis are rarely hospitalized, so nursing care focuses on teaching. Advise that bed rest is not often necessary. Activities of daily living (ADLs) can be maintained with adequate rest. Instruct to increase fluid intake. Discuss the use and effects of ordered drugs. Stress the importance of smoking cessation. Instruct to contact primary care provider if symptoms do not improve within a week or if they become worse.

Pneumonia

Pneumonia is inflammation of the respiratory bronchioles and alveoli. It is a leading cause of death in the United States, particularly among older adults and people with debilitating diseases. Pneumonia may be either infectious or noninfectious. Bacteria, viruses, fungi, protozoa, and other microbes can lead to infectious pneumonia. Noninfectious causes include aspiration of gastric contents and inhalation of toxic or irritating gases.

PATHOPHYSIOLOGY AND MANIFESTATIONS

In most cases, microbes responsible for infectious pneumonia initially colonize the nasal or oral pharynx. From there, they enter the lungs when secretions from the pharynx are aspirated. *Streptococcus pneumoniae* (pneumococcal pneumonia) is the most common pathogen causing infectious pneumonia;

TABLE 24-1

Features of Infectious Pneumonias

TYPE	ONSET	RESPIRATORY MANIFESTATIONS	OTHER MANIFESTATIONS
Pneumococcal or lobar pneumonia	Abrupt	Cough productive of purulent or rust-colored sputum Chest pain Decreased breath sounds and crackles over affected area Possible dyspnea and cyanosis	Chills and fever
Bronchopneumonia	Gradual	Cough, scattered crackles Minimal dyspnea and shortness of breath	Low-grade fever
Legionnaires' disease	Gradual	Dry cough Dyspnea	Chills and fever Malaise, headache Muscle and joint pain Confusion
Viral pneumonia	Sudden or gradual	Dry cough	Flulike symptoms
Atypical pneumonia	Gradual	Dry, hacking, nonproductive cough	Fever, headache Muscle and joint pain
Pneumocystis carinii pneumonia	Abrupt	Dry cough Tachypnea and shortness of breath Respiratory distress	Fever

others include *Haemophilus influenzae,* some gram-negative bacteria, and the influenza virus.

Pneumonia is classified by its cause (acute bacterial or viral) or by its location (lobar or bronchial) (Table 24-1 ■).

Acute Bacterial Pneumonia

When bacteria invade the lungs, an inflammatory response follows. Inflammation causes the alveoli to become edematous and fill with fluid. Blood cells and bacteria collect in the alveoli and respiratory bronchioles, leading to *consolidation* (solidification) of lung tissue. The lower lobes of the lungs are usually affected because of gravity. Consolidation of a large portion of an entire lung lobe is known as *lobar pneumonia. Bronchopneumonia* is patchy consolidation involving several lobules. Eventually, macrophages digest and remove the fluid, bacteria, and damaged cells from the infected lung.

The onset of bacterial pneumonia typically is acute, with shaking chills, fever, and cough productive of rust-colored or purulent sputum. Chest pain (aching or sharp and localized) is common. Diminished breath sounds and fine crackles are heard over the affected lung area. If the involved area is large, respiratory distress is evident. The older adult may have fewer respiratory symptoms, presenting with fever, tachypnea, and altered mental status.

The most common complication of pneumococcal pneumonia is *pleuritis* (pleurisy), painful inflammation of the adjacent pleura. Pneumonias can cause extensive lung damage, leading to necrosis, abscess, and *empyema* (a collection of pus in the pleural cavity).

Pneumocystis carinii Pneumonia

The majority of people with acquired immunodeficiency syndrome (AIDS) develop pneumonia caused by *Pneumocystis carinii,* a common parasite. Most people with intact immune systems are immune to *P. carinii,* but it is an *opportunistic* organism that can cause an infection when the immune system is suppressed.

Infection with *P. carinii* causes affected alveoli to thicken, become edematous, and fill with foamy, protein-rich fluid. Gas exchange is severely impaired as the disease progresses. Respiratory distress can be significant. (See also Chapter 11. ⬤⬤)

Legionnaires' Disease

Legionnaires' disease is an acute bronchopneumonia caused by a gram-negative bacterium, *Legionella pneumophila.* This bacterium commonly is found in warm, standing water. Legionnaires' disease tends to occur in sporadic outbreaks. People at risk for Legionnaires' disease include smokers, older adults, and people with chronic diseases or impaired immune systems. The disease has a relatively high mortality rate of up to 31% in previously healthy people.

Symptoms of Legionnaires' disease develop 2 to 10 days following exposure. Its onset is gradual, with dry cough, shortness of breath, and general symptoms such as malaise, anorexia, headache, chills and fever, and muscle and joint pain.

Atypical Pneumonia

Pneumonia caused by *Mycoplasma pneumoniae* is called atypical pneumonia, because its presentation and course differ from other bacterial pneumonias. It typically is mild, with symptoms that tend to mimic influenza, leading many people to refer to it as "walking pneumonia." Young adults (college students, military recruits) have the highest incidence of atypical pneumonia. It is highly contagious. Fever, headache, muscle aches, and malaise are the usual symptoms; the cough associated with atypical pneumonia is dry, hacking, and nonproductive.

Viral Pneumonia

Influenza virus and adenovirus are the organisms usually responsible for viral pneumonia. Cytomegalovirus (CMV) pneumonia is increasing in frequency, particularly among people with HIV disease. Viral pneumonia often affects older adults and people with chronic diseases. It typically is mild, and characterized by flulike symptoms with headache, fever, fatigue, malaise, dry cough, and muscle aches.

Aspiration Pneumonia

Aspiration of gastric contents into the lungs causes a chemical and bacterial pneumonia known as *aspiration pneumonia.* The risk for aspiration pneumonia is highest during emergency surgery and when cough and gag reflexes are depressed or swallowing is impaired. Older adults and clients receiving tube feedings are also at risk for aspiration pneumonia. Vomiting may not be obvious; silent regurgitation of gastric contents may occur if the level of consciousness is reduced. The low pH of gastric juice causes severe inflammation in the lungs. Pulmonary edema and respiratory failure may result.

INTERDISCIPLINARY CARE

With early diagnosis and treatment, most clients with pneumonia recover fully. However, pneumonia has a significant mortality, especially among the old and weak.

Diagnostic Tests

- *Sputum Gram stain* and *culture and sensitivity* are done to identify the organism and appropriate antibiotic therapy. It is important to obtain sputum for culture from the lower respiratory tract, not the mouth and nasal passages (Box 22-3). ⊙⊙
- *Complete blood count (CBC)* with *white blood cell (WBC) differential* shows an elevated WBC count with more immature WBCs in an acute bacterial pneumonia.
- *Arterial blood gases (ABGs)* may be done to evaluate gas exchange. See Chapter 7 ⊙⊙ for more information about ABGs.
- *Pulse oximetry* is used to monitor arterial oxygen saturation. An SaO_2 of less than 95% may indicate impaired gas exchange or ventilation.

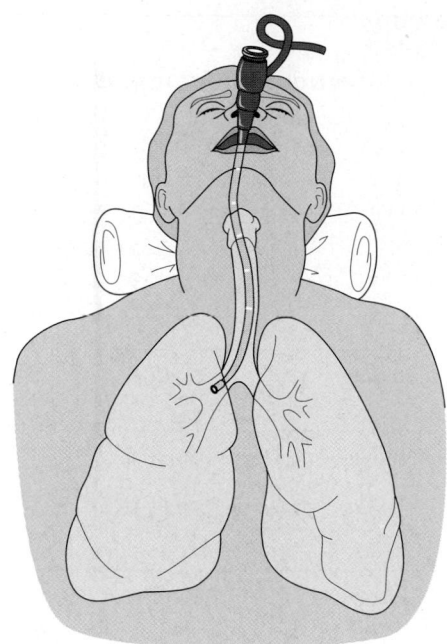

Figure 24-1. ■ Fiberoptic bronchoscopy.

- *Chest x-ray* helps identify the extent and pattern of lung involvement. Fluid, consolidated lung tissue, and *atelectasis* (areas of alveolar collapse) can be identified.
- *Fiberoptic bronchoscopy* may be done to obtain a sputum specimen or remove secretions from the bronchi (Figure 24-1 ■). Nursing care for the client undergoing a bronchoscopy is summarized in Box 22-4 ⊙⊙.

Immunization

Pneumococcal vaccine is recommended for people over age 65, for immunocompromised people, and for those with chronic cardiac or respiratory conditions, diabetes mellitus, alcoholism, or other chronic diseases. Annual influenza vaccine is also recommended for vulnerable populations such as those just listed, health care workers, and residents of long-term care facilities.

Medications

Medications used to treat pneumonia may include antibiotics to eradicate causative organisms and bronchodilators to reduce bronchospasm and improve ventilation. Bronchodilators and their nursing implications are discussed in more detail in the section of this chapter on asthma.

An agent to "break up" mucus or reduce its viscosity may be prescribed. Guaifenesin, a common ingredient in expectorant cough syrups, helps to liquefy mucus, making it easier to expectorate.

Oxygen Therapy

Oxygen may be ordered when pneumonia interferes with gas exchange. The *nasal cannula* delivers 24% to 45% oxygen (room air is 21% oxygen) with flow rates of 2 to 6 liters per minute (Figure 24-2 ■). A *simple face mask* can deliver

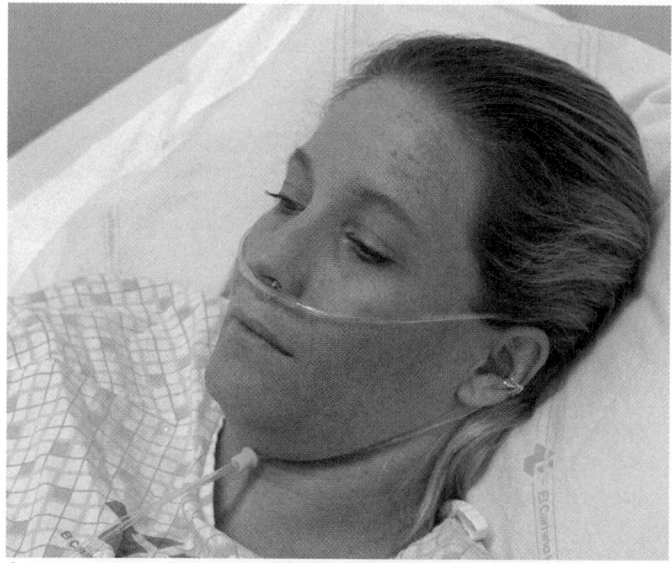

A

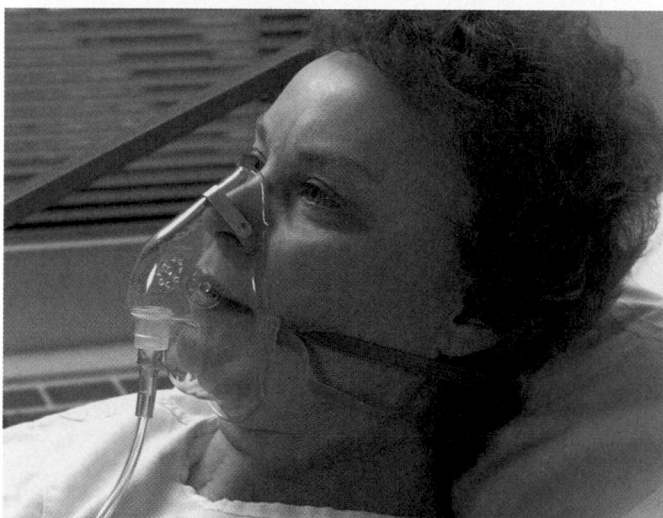

B

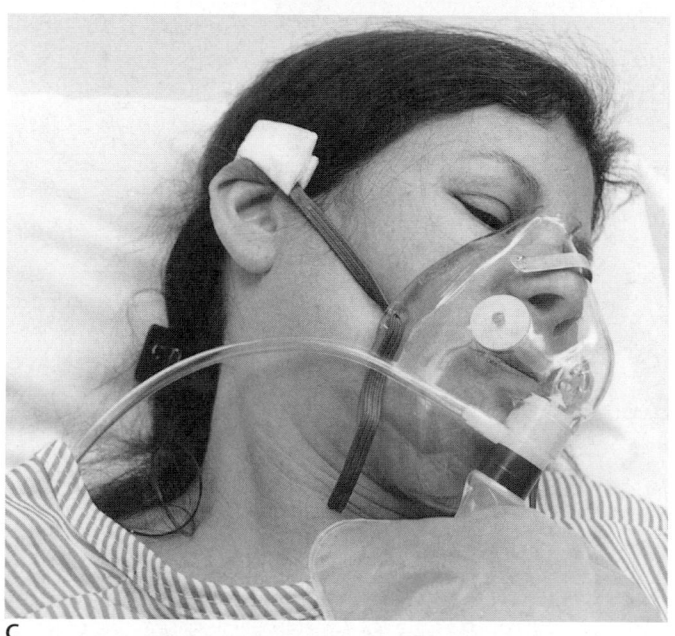

C

Figure 24-2. ■ **(A)** Nasal cannula. **(B)** Simple face mask. (*Source:* NMSB, Custom Medical Stock Photos, Inc.) **(C)** Nonrebreather mask.

40% to 60% oxygen. Up to 100% oxygen can be delivered by the *nonrebreather mask,* the highest concentration possible without mechanical ventilation. When the amount of oxygen delivered must be carefully regulated, a *Venturi mask* is used. The percentage of oxygen delivered by Venturi mask can be precisely regulated, from 24% to 50%. A severely hypoxic client may require intubation and mechanical ventilation. Endotracheal intubation and mechanical ventilation are discussed in the section on respiratory failure.

Other Therapies

Increasing fluid intake to 2,500 to 3,000 mL/day helps liquefy secretions, making them easier to cough up and expectorate. If oral intake is inadequate, intravenous fluids and nutrition may be required.

When mucous secretions are thick and viscous or the cough is weak, percussion, vibration, and postural drainage may be ordered. *Percussion* is done by rhythmically striking or clapping the chest wall with cupped hands (Figure 24-3 ■). Cupping traps air between the palm and the skin, causing

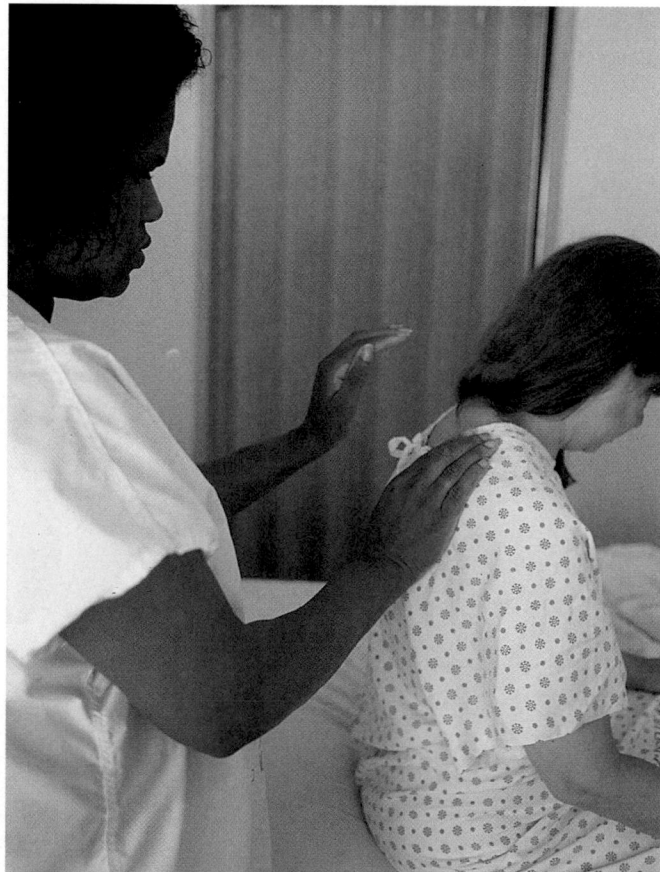

Figure 24-3. ■ Percussing the upper posterior chest. Note the cupped position of the nurse's hands.

vibrations that loosen respiratory secretions. The trapped air also provides a cushion, preventing injury. A mechanical percussion device also may be used. The breasts, sternum, spinal column, and kidney areas are avoided during percussion.

Vibration helps loosen and move secretions into larger airways. Vibrations are produced by tensing and vibrating the arm muscles while keeping firm pressure on the chest wall with the hands.

Percussion and vibration are performed along with postural drainage. *Postural drainage* uses gravity to help remove secretions from a particular lung segment. The client is positioned with the lung area to be drained above the trachea or mainstem bronchus. Drainage of all lung segments requires a variety of positions (Figure 24-4 ■);

however, few clients need all segments drained. Postural drainage should be done before meals to avoid nausea and vomiting.

NURSING CARE

ASSESSING

Collecting assessment data is important not only to monitor the progress of clients with pneumonia, but also to identify possible manifestations of pneumonia in clients with other problems. Nurses often identify clients in the community, long-term care, and acute care settings who are at risk for pneumonia. Box 24-2 ■ outlines assessment data related to pneumonia.

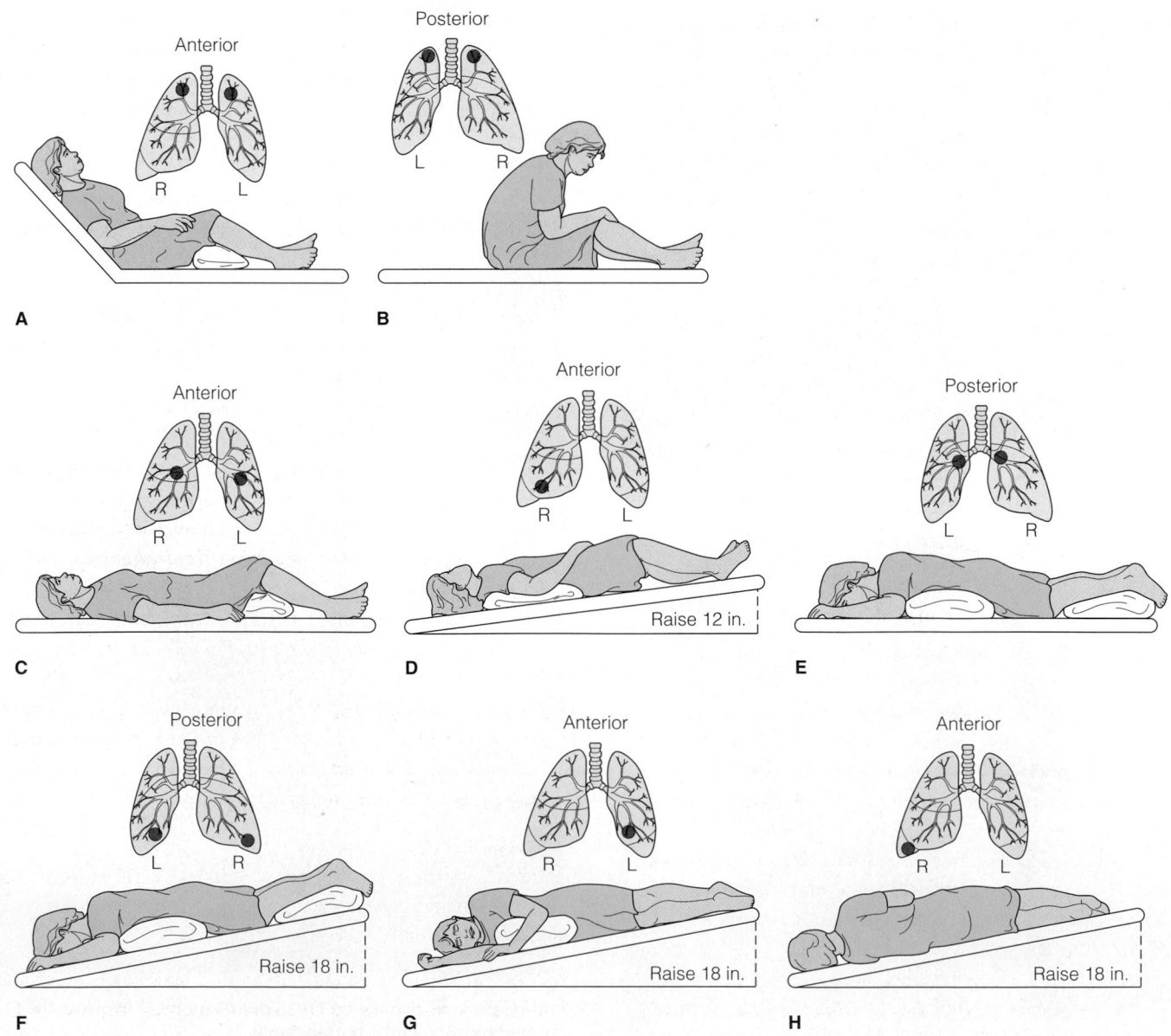

Figure 24-4. ■ Positions for postural drainage.

Assessing Clients with Pneumonia

SUBJECTIVE DATA

- Chest pain (location, character, timing, duration); shortness of breath or difficulty breathing; cough (timing, productive or nonproductive); type and amount of sputum
- History of chronic diseases; allergies, asthma, or other respiratory conditions; heart failure; medications used
- Smoking history or exposure to environmental or occupational pollutants; use of alcohol and/or other drugs such as heroin, cocaine, or marijuana

OBJECTIVE DATA

- Vital signs including temperature and apical pulse
- Skin color
- Level of consciousness and mental status
- Respiratory rate and depth, O_2 saturation, dyspnea, cough; lung sounds including any adventitious sounds such as:
  - *Crackles:* short, discrete, crackling, or bubbling sounds
  - *Wheezes:* musical sounds caused by narrowed airways due to inflammation, constriction, or excessive mucus
  - *Friction rub:* a loud, dry, creaking sound caused by inflammation of the pleura

Laboratory Tests

- WBC, ABGs, sputum smear, and culture

DIAGNOSING, PLANNING, AND IMPLEMENTING

Priorities in Nursing Care. The priority of nursing care for clients with pneumonia is its effects on the client's ability to maintain open airways and on the exchange of gases in the alveoli.

Ineffective Airway Clearance

Airway inflammation, edema, and secretions interfere with air movement and airway clearance in clients with pneumonia.

- Assess respiratory status, including vital signs, breath sounds, and cough and sputum at least every 4 hours. *The client with acute pneumonia can quickly develop respiratory distress; frequent assessment allows early intervention.*
- Notify the physician if oxygen saturation falls below 92% or ordered level. *Airway obstruction can interfere with alveolar ventilation and gas exchange, leading to tissue hypoxia.*
- Place in Fowler's position. Encourage frequent position changes, sitting at the bedside, and ambulation as allowed. *These measures promote lung expansion and facilitate the movement of secretions.*
- Assist to cough, deep breathe, and use the incentive spirometer. *Coughing and deep breathing help clear airways.*
- Provide at least 2,500 to 3,000 mL of fluid per day. *A liberal fluid intake helps liquefy secretions, promoting their clearance.*

- Assist with pulmonary hygiene measures, such as postural drainage, percussion, and vibration. *These techniques help mobilize and clear secretions.*
- Administer ordered medications, and monitor their effects. *If the ordered medications are ineffective or have adverse effects, a different drug may need to be prescribed.*
- Administer oxygen as ordered. *Oxygen promotes alveolar gas exchange.*

Ineffective Breathing Pattern

Chest pain can lead to rapid and shallow breathing that causes fatigue and does not fully ventilate all areas of the lungs.

- Place in an upright or semi-upright position. *This position promotes lung expansion and ventilation as well as comfort.*
- Provide for periods of rest. *Rest reduces fatigue and the work of breathing.*
- Assess and document chest pain. Provide analgesics as ordered. *Adequate pain relief allows better lung ventilation.*
- Reassure the client who is experiencing respiratory distress. *Hypoxia and respiratory distress cause anxiety. Anxiety increases the respiratory rate and fatigue, and decreases ventilation.*
- Teach use of slow abdominal breathing. *This promotes lung expansion.*
- Teach relaxation techniques, such as visualization and meditation. *These techniques help reduce anxiety and slow breathing.*

Activity Intolerance

- Assess for any increase in pulse, respirations, dyspnea, diaphoresis, or cyanosis with activity. *These findings may indicate limited activity tolerance.*
- Assist with self-care activities as needed. *Assistance with ADLs reduces the client's energy demands.*
- Schedule activities, planning for rest periods. *Rest periods minimize fatigue and improve activity tolerance.*
- Provide assistive devices, such as an overhead trapeze. *Assistive devices help reduce the energy required to move and change positions.*
- Enlist support persons to help minimize stress and anxiety. *Stress and anxiety increase metabolic demands and can decrease activity tolerance.*
- Provide emotional support and reassurance that strength and activity level will return to normal when pneumonia has resolved. *The client may be concerned that fatigue will continue after the acute infection is resolved.*

Evaluating

To evaluate the effectiveness of nursing care, reassess the client's respiratory status, ability to clear secretions, and ability to gradually increase activity levels.

Documenting. Document continuing assessment data and the client's responses to treatment (such as improving O_2 saturation levels with decreasing supplemental oxygen, ability to tolerate activities). Note teaching provided to the client and family, as well as their apparent understanding and acceptance of instructions.

CONTINUING CARE

Teaching focuses on prevention of pneumonia as well as its treatment. Discuss the benefits of immunizations against influenza and pneumococcal pneumonia with clients in high-risk groups. Pneumococcus vaccine usually provides immunity to pneumococcal pneumonia. Annual influenza vaccine helps prevent pneumonia, because viral infection often precedes pneumonia.

Many clients with pneumonia are managed in the community, unless their respiratory status is significantly compromised. Stress the importance of taking ordered medications and completing the entire prescription. Provide information about side effects and their management. Teach to identify adverse effects that should be reported to the primary care provider.

Instruct to limit activities and increase rest to conserve energy. Encourage to maintain fluid intake to keep mucus thin for easier expectoration. Explain that small, frequent meals reduce the energy demand for eating and may be better tolerated. Recommend that the client and household members avoid smoking to prevent further irritation of the lungs. Complementary therapies (Box 24-3 ■) may be used to relieve chest congestion and promote comfort.

Tell the client and family to report increasing shortness of breath, difficulty breathing, temperature, fatigue, headache, sleepiness, or confusion to the physician as these may indicate worsening condition. Stress the importance of keeping all follow-up appointments to ensure cure of the disease.

Tuberculosis

Tuberculosis (TB) is a chronic, recurrent infectious disease that usually affects the lungs. Tuberculosis also can involve other organs. This disease, caused by *Mycobacterium tuberculosis,* is an important health problem worldwide. It is common in the developing countries of Asia, Africa, the Middle East, and Latin America.

In the United States, TB usually affects immigrants, people with HIV, and disadvantaged populations, such as the homeless. People with altered immune function, including older adults, are at particular risk for tuberculosis. Some strains of tuberculosis have become resistant to the drugs used to treat the disease.

PATHOPHYSIOLOGY

M. tuberculosis is a slow-growing, slender, rod-shaped, acid-fast organism. It has a waxy outer capsule that increases its resistance to destruction. It is transmitted by *droplet nuclei,* airborne droplets produced when an infected person coughs, sneezes, speaks, or sings. Infection develops when a susceptible host breathes in droplet nuclei and the contaminated particle evades the normal defenses of the upper respiratory tract to reach the alveoli. A small, poorly ventilated or crowded environment and prolonged exposure increase the risk of infection. The risk also is increased by impaired immune function.

Pulmonary Tuberculosis

Droplet nuclei containing the bacillus implant in an alveolus or respiratory bronchiole, usually in an upper lobe. An immune response brings WBCs to the site. These cells phagocytize and isolate the bacteria but cannot destroy them. A sealed-off colony of bacilli, called a *tubercle,* is formed.

Usually, scar tissue forms around the tubercle, and the bacilli remain isolated. These lesions can be seen on x-ray. If the immune system is impaired, primary tuberculosis can progress, destroying lung tissue. A previously healed lesion may be reactivated. This is known as *reactivation tuberculosis.* It occurs when the immune system is suppressed by age (Box 24-4 ■), disease, or immunosuppressive drugs. About 5% of infected people develop active primary disease; another 5% develop reactivation tuberculosis at a later time (Figure 24-5 ■).

MANIFESTATIONS. Manifestations of pulmonary tuberculosis develop gradually. They include fatigue, weight loss, anorexia, low-grade afternoon fever, and night sweats. The

---

BOX 24-3	COMPLEMENTARY THERAPIES

Pneumonia and Bronchitis

The aromas of cedarwood and frankincense or inhaling the steam of water containing eucalyptus or sage may help relieve chest congestion. Massaging the chest with lavender also may help. Licorice root can be used to relieve congestion and as a cough suppressant. Licorice interacts with some drugs used to treat high blood pressure and heart disease and should be used with caution. Its use is contraindicated during pregnancy. Tea tree oil (applied topically or a few drops on a handkerchief) has anti-infective properties and may be used together with conventional treatment of pneumonia.

BOX 24-4	FOCUS ON OLDER ADULTS

Tuberculosis in Older Adults

Up to 30% of newly diagnosed tuberculosis affects people over age 65. Most cases are due to reactivation of dormant bacteria as cell-mediated immunity declines with aging. Living in long-term care facilities also increases the risk for tuberculosis.

Presenting symptoms of tuberculosis in an older adult may be vague, such as coughing, weight loss, anorexia, or periodic fevers. Yearly tuberculin skin testing with purified protein derivative (PPD) is recommended for long-term care residents.

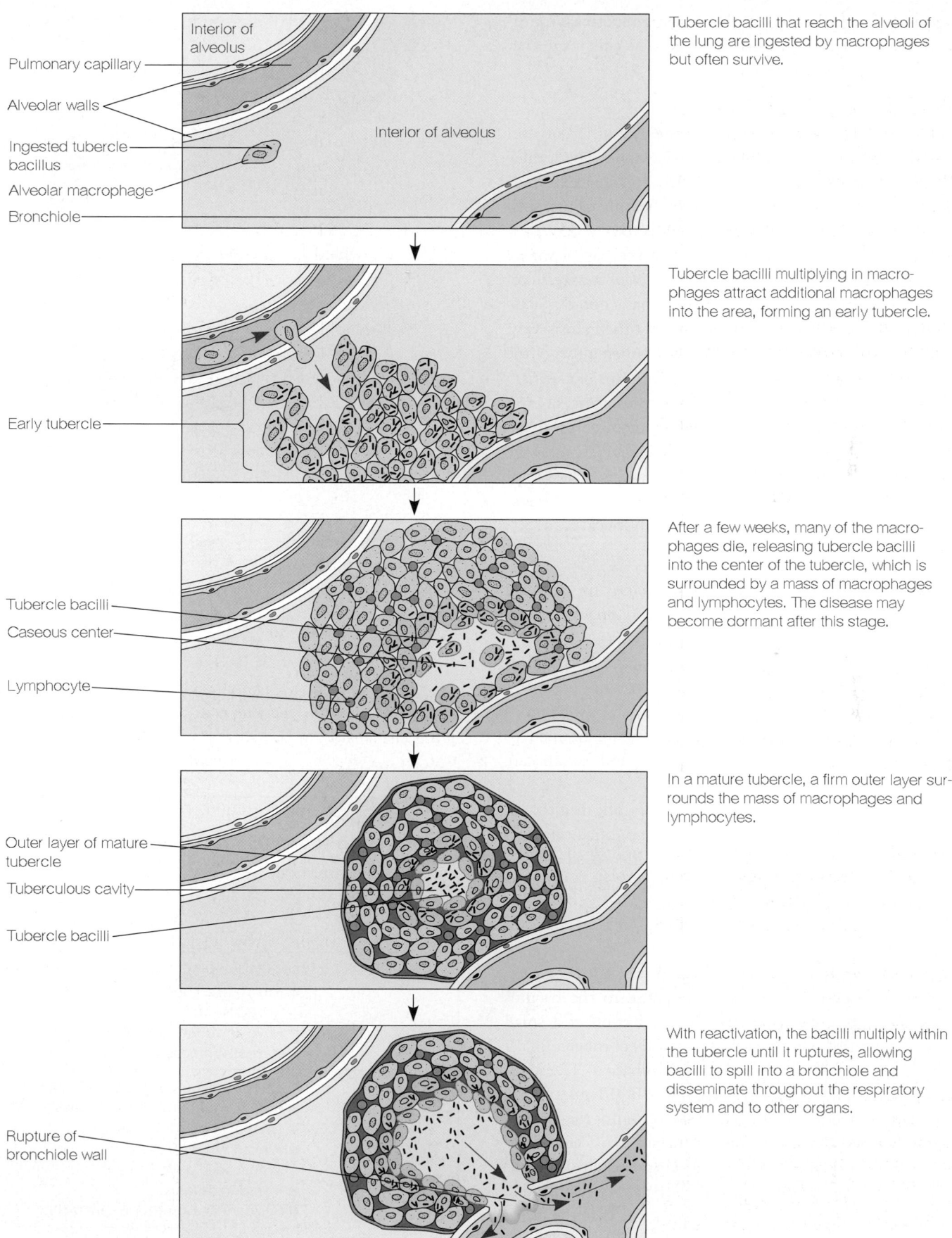

Tubercle bacilli that reach the alveoli of the lung are ingested by macrophages but often survive.

Tubercle bacilli multiplying in macrophages attract additional macrophages into the area, forming an early tubercle.

After a few weeks, many of the macrophages die, releasing tubercle bacilli into the center of the tubercle, which is surrounded by a mass of macrophages and lymphocytes. The disease may become dormant after this stage.

In a mature tubercle, a firm outer layer surrounds the mass of macrophages and lymphocytes.

With reactivation, the bacilli multiply within the tubercle until it ruptures, allowing bacilli to spill into a bronchiole and disseminate throughout the respiratory system and to other organs.

Figure 24-5. ■ The pathogenesis of tuberculosis.

cough is dry initially and later becomes productive of purulent or blood-tinged sputum. It is often at this stage that the client seeks medical attention.

Extrapulmonary Tuberculosis

Colonies of *M. tuberculosis* can develop in other organs. These distant sites may be active or dormant. The kidney and genitourinary tract are common sites for extrapulmonary tuberculosis. The large, weight-bearing joints, such as the hips and knees, are most often affected by *tuberculous arthritis. Miliary tuberculosis* occurs when the bacilli spread throughout the body via the blood. *Tuberculosis meningitis* results when tuberculosis spreads to the subarachnoid space.

The manifestations of extrapulmonary tuberculosis vary, depending on the organ system affected. Tuberculosis of the genitourinary tract may present with symptoms of a urinary tract infection (see Chapter 32), 🔗 prostatitis or epididymitis in men, or pelvic inflammatory disease in women. Headache of increasing severity and behavior changes are early manifestations of tuberculosis meningitis. The symptoms of miliary tuberculosis are generalized, with chills and fever, weakness, malaise, and progressive dyspnea.

INTERDISCIPLINARY CARE

Interdisciplinary care for tuberculosis focuses on (1) early detection, (2) effective treatment, and (3) preventing its spread to others.

Clients with active tuberculosis rarely need hospitalization. With appropriate treatment, they become noninfective to others fairly rapidly. When a client with tuberculosis is hospitalized, respiratory isolation is maintained to reduce the risk of infecting other clients and health care workers.

Tuberculosis is a potential threat to public health. As such, it must be reported to local and state public health departments. The client's contacts are then identified and examined. People who share living or work environments should receive testing and prophylactic treatment.

Screening

The *tuberculin test* is used to screen for tuberculosis. People exposed to TB develop an immune response to the bacillus within 3 to 10 weeks after infection. Injection of a small amount of purified protein derivative (PPD) of tuberculin activates this response, causing local inflammation. The Mantoux test is commonly used to screen for TB; 0.1 mL of PPD is injected intradermally into the dorsal aspect of the forearm (Figure 24-6 ■). The test is read within 48 to 72 hours, and recorded as the diameter of induration (raised area) in millimeters. The area of induration is used to determine infection (Table 24-2 ■). A positive response indicates that the client has developed an immune response to the bacillus; it does *not* mean that the client has active TB or is currently infectious.

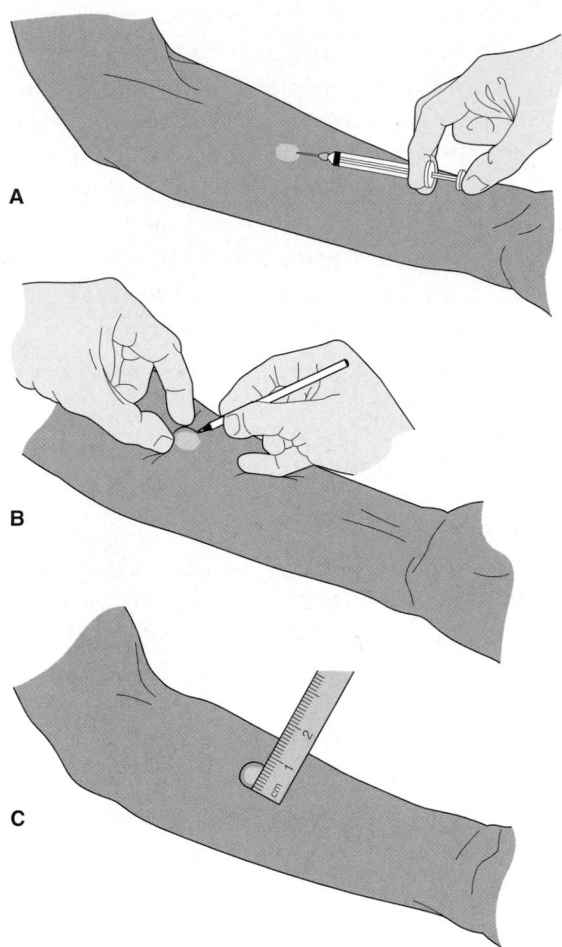

Figure 24-6. ■ (**A**) Intradermal injection of PPD. (**B**) A local inflammatory response to PPD. (**C**) Measuring induration produced by the inflammatory response.

TABLE 24-2	
Interpreting Tuberculin Test Results	
AREA OF INDURATION	**SIGNIFICANCE**
<5 mm	Negative response
5–9 mm	Positive for people who: ■ Are in close contact with someone who has active TB ■ Have an abnormal chest x-ray ■ Have HIV infection
10–15 mm	Positive for people with other risk factors: ■ Born in a high-incidence country ■ Low socioeconomic status ■ African American, Hispanic, Asian American in poverty areas ■ Injection drug use ■ Resident in a long-term care facility
>15 mm	Positive for all people

Diagnostic Tests

- A series of three consecutive early morning sputum specimens are sent for *acid-fast bacilli smear* and *culture* (see Box 22-3). Use personal protective devices when obtaining sputum specimens that may carry TB. Collect the specimens in a room equipped with airflow control devices, ultraviolet (UV) light, or a combination of these. If airflow or UV protection is not available, wear a special mask that can filter the droplet nuclei.
- *Chest x-ray* is used to diagnose and evaluate TB.
- *Fiberoptic bronchoscopy* and bronchial washing may be used to obtain culture specimens if necessary. Review Box 22-4 ⚭ for nursing care of the client undergoing fiberoptic bronchoscopy.

Medications

Antituberculosis drugs are used to prevent and treat tuberculosis. Clients with a recent skin test conversion from negative to positive are started on prophylactic treatment, especially when other risk factors are present. Daily isoniazid (INH) for 6 to 12 months is commonly used to prevent active TB.

The tuberculosis bacillus readily becomes drug resistant when only one anti-infective agent is used. Active disease is always treated with at least two antibacterial medications. Because the organism is protected by the tubercle, 6 or more months of treatment are required to eliminate it. Three antitubercular drugs may be used for the first 2 months of treatment. All three drugs are given daily by mouth. For the remainder of the treatment period, the drugs may be given twice weekly. (See Table 24-3 ■.)

Antitubercular medications have many undesired effects. Most are toxic to the liver. Warn clients to avoid alcohol and other liver toxins (such as acetaminophen) while taking these drugs. Report manifestations of adverse effects to the physician.

Compliance with the prescribed regimen may be a problem. Medications often are given under direct supervision, with a public health nurse watching the client take and swallow the drug.

NURSING CARE

Tuberculosis presents a greater threat to public health than it does to the individual. When the treatment regimen is followed, more than 90% of clients become noninfective within 3 months. Relapse is uncommon; the main cause of treatment failure is noncompliance.

ASSESSING

Nurses in community-based care settings often identify early manifestations of tuberculosis, therefore it is vital to collect and attend to data that may indicate active disease.

Ask the client about fatigue, weight loss, night sweats, and respiratory symptoms such as difficulty breathing, cough, bloody sputum, or chest pain. Inquire about known exposure to TB, the most recent tuberculin test and its results, as well as the client's living circumstances and use of alcohol and/or recreational drugs.

Obtain vital signs, including temperature, and assess the client's general appearance, respiratory rate, and lung sounds. Monitor laboratory data (including sputum for acid-fast bacillus and liver function tests) and chest X-ray results.

DIAGNOSING, PLANNING, AND IMPLEMENTING

Priorities in Nursing Care. In most cases, tuberculosis presents a lower risk to the affected client than spread of the disease does to public health and safety. Risk for infection of vulnerable populations and teaching the client and others how to minimize this risk are the priorities of nursing care.

Risk for Infection

- Place in a private room with ventilation that prevents air in the room from circulating into the hallway or other rooms (a negative flow room). *A negative-flow room with frequent fresh-air exchanges reduces droplet nuclei in the room and prevents their spread to other areas.*
- Use Standard Precautions and TB isolation as recommended by the Centers for Disease Control and Prevention (CDC). Wear a mask and gown when caring for clients who do not cover mouth when coughing. *These measures are important to prevent the spread of TB to others.*
- Use personal protective devices (HEPA-filtered respirator) during care to protect against occupational exposure to TB. *Surgical masks do not filter droplet nuclei; protective devices capable of filtering bacteria and particles smaller than 1 micron are necessary.*
- Discuss the importance of respiratory isolation during initial treatment. Instruct to avoid crowds and close physical contact, and to maintain ventilation in living facilities during the first 3 weeks of treatment. *These measures help protect others when sputum is still likely to contain bacilli.*
- Place a mask on the client when transporting within the facility for diagnostic or treatment procedures. *Covering the mouth during transport reduces air contamination and the risk to visitors and personnel.*
- Communicate the diagnosis to all personnel in contact with the client. *This allows personnel to take appropriate precautions.*
- Assist visitors to mask prior to entering the room. *Providing appropriate masks or respirators reduces the risk of infection.*

TABLE 24-3

Nursing Implications for Pharmacology: Antituberculosis Drugs

DRUG	ACTION	NURSING RESPONSIBILITIES	CLIENT AND FAMILY TEACHING
Isoniazid (INH, Laniazid, Nydrazid)	Isoniazid is used alone to prevent tuberculosis, and in combination with rifampin, ethambutol, or both to treat active disease.	Give 1 hour before or 2 hours after eating if tolerated; may be given with meals to reduce GI effects. Report adverse effects: a. Numbness and tingling of the extremities b. Abnormal liver function studies or jaundice c. Rash, drug fever, anemia, or abnormal bleeding. Monitor responses to other medications, because INH may interfere with their metabolism, causing toxicity.	Take as ordered for the entire course of treatment. Take on an empty stomach; take with meals if nausea and vomiting occur. Call your doctor if you develop anorexia and jaundice (yellowing of skin and eyes). Take pyridoxine as ordered to prevent neurologic effects. Avoid alcohol and other liver toxins while taking INH. Call your doctor if you develop a rash, fever, bruising, bleeding gums, or fatigue. Use birth control while taking INH; this drug may harm the fetus.
Rifampin (RMP, Rifadin, Rimactane)	Rifampin is commonly used in combination with INH and other antitubercular drugs. It is relatively low in toxicity. Rifampin increases the rate of metabolism of many drugs, decreasing their effectiveness.	Give on an empty stomach. Report abnormal CBC, liver function studies, and renal function studies to the physician. Monitor the effectiveness of drugs administered concurrently.	Rifampin causes sweat, urine, saliva, and tears to turn red-orange. This is not harmful, but may permanently stain soft contact lenses. Do not take aspirin with rifampin. Report fever, flulike symptoms, fatigue, sore throat, or unusual bleeding to your doctor. If you use oral contraceptives, use supplemental birth control while taking this drug.
Pyrazinamide (PZA, Tebrazid)	Pyrazinamide often is given during the first 2 months of treatment. It is toxic to the liver. It also increases serum uric acid levels, but rarely causes gout.	Give with meals to reduce GI side effects. Report changes in liver function studies and serum uric acid levels to the physician.	Call your doctor if you develop anorexia, nausea, vomiting, jaundice, or a painful, red, hot, swollen joint. Avoid using alcohol or other liver toxins while taking this drug.
Ethambutol (EMB, Myambutol)	Ethambutol reduces bacterial resistance to other drugs. It is reversibly toxic to the optic nerve. Signs include decreased visual and color acuity. This drug may be safe for use in pregnancy.	Schedule eye exams as recommended during treatment. Give with meals to reduce GI effects. Report changes in liver and renal function tests and neurologic status to the physician.	Monitor vision daily by reading newspapers and looking at the same blue object. Notify your doctor if changes in vision or color perception occur.
Streptomycin (SM)	Streptomycin is a highly effective antibiotic. Resistance may develop if it is used alone. It must be given parenterally because it is not absorbed in the GI tract. It also has toxic effects on the kidneys and ears.	Inject deep IM into a large muscle mass, rotating sites. Report significant changes in urine output, weight, and renal function studies to the physician. Maintain fluid intake of 2,000–3,000 mL/day. Assess hearing and balance often. Schedule audiometric testing as indicated.	Drink at least 2½–3 quarts of fluid daily. Weigh yourself on the same scale at least twice a week; report significant weight gain to your doctor. Call your doctor if your hearing declines, or you develop dizziness or ringing or buzzing sensations in the ear.

- Teach to cough and expectorate into tissues, then personally dispose of tissues in a closed bag. *This reduces potential contact with the bacilli by others.*
- Teach to collect sputum specimens, stepping outside to do so if necessary. *This reduces the risk of exposure to health care personnel, allows rapid dilution of droplet nuclei produced, and exposes them to UV light (which kills the bacteria).*

Deficient Knowledge: Tuberculosis and Treatment Regimen

- Assess knowledge, learning ability and interest, developmental level, and obstacles to learning. *Assessment allows teaching tailored to the client's needs and abilities.*
- Include significant others in teaching. *This allows clarification and reinforcement of teaching and learning.*
- Use teaching strategies and learning aids such as written and visual materials appropriate for age, level of education, and intellect. *Teaching tailored to the client is more effective and results in better learning.*
- Teach about TB and its treatment, including:
  - Nature of tuberculosis
  - Purpose of treatment and ordered follow-up
  - Preventing TB spread to others
  - Importance of maintaining good general health by eating a well-balanced, nutritious diet, balancing rest and exercise, and avoiding exposure to infection
  - Names, doses, purposes, and side effects of prescribed drugs
  - Importance of avoiding alcohol and other liver toxins while taking antituberculosis drugs
  - Fluid intake needs of 2½ to 3 quarts of fluid per day
  - Symptoms to report to the physician: chest pain, hemoptysis, or difficulty breathing; manifestations of drug toxicity (see Table 24-3).

  This information is necessary for the client to effectively manage TB and its treatment.
- Document teaching and learning. Reinforce as needed. *Several teaching–learning sessions may be needed due to the amount and complexity of information.*

Ineffective Therapeutic Regimen Management

- Assess self-care abilities and support systems. *Assessment helps predict the ability to follow the ordered regimen.*
- Help identify barriers or obstacles to managing the ordered treatment. *Identifying potential barriers allows planning for solutions.*
- Assist to develop a plan for managing treatment. *A plan increases the sense of control and ownership and considers personal, cultural, and lifestyle factors.*

- Provide clear, written instructions at the client's level of literacy, knowledge, and understanding. *Written directions provide support and reinforcement.*
- Refer to smoking cessation programs, alcohol treatment and Alcoholics Anonymous, drug treatment and Narcotics Anonymous, and other support groups as appropriate. *Counseling, support groups, and other community resources provide additional assistance and support in managing TB and its treatment.*
- For homeless clients, arrange shelter placement or other housing and ongoing follow-up by easily accessed health care providers. *Active intervention for necessary services helps ensure compliance with treatment.*
- Refer to public health department for management and follow-up as indicated. *Public health follow-up often is required to prevent the spread of TB to other people.*

EVALUATING

To evaluate the effectiveness of nursing care for a client with TB, collect data related to the client's knowledge and understanding of TB and its treatment, ability and willingness to follow instructions for preventing the spread of TB to others, and compliance with the ordered treatment.

Documenting. Document continuing assessment data, including assessments related to potential adverse effects of prescribed drugs. Document teaching (including reinforcement of teaching) and the client's understanding of information presented and willingness to comply with the prescribed treatment regimen.

CONTINUING CARE

Tuberculosis is a public health problem that requires a focus on the community as well as on the individual. Teach community members and people with TB how to reduce its spread:

- Cover the mouth when coughing or sneezing.
- Use disposable tissues to contain respiratory secretions.

Because the client with TB may be infective long before the disease is diagnosed, teach these measures to all people. Encourage people at high risk for TB to have regular screening. Discuss prophylactic treatment for people in close contact with a client who has active TB.

Explain the effect, dose, and timing for all medications. Emphasize the importance of long-term therapy to cure TB. Discuss precautions and possible side effects of the drugs that should be reported to the health care provider:

- Isoniazid (INH) may cause numbness, tingling, or burning in the extremities. Pyridoxine (vitamin B_6) often is ordered to prevent this effect.

- Avoid alcohol while taking INH or rifampin because these drugs may affect the liver. Report nausea, anorexia, jaundice, a change in urine or stool color, or pain in the upper right quadrant.
- Rifampin may change the color of saliva, tears, and urine.
- Streptomycin can affect hearing and balance; promptly report any changes.
- Ethambutol may affect vision and color perception. Use caution when driving or walking in unfamiliar areas. Promptly report any vision changes.

Refer to community services and agencies as appropriate. See the Critical Thinking Care Map at the end of this chapter for an opportunity to use the nursing process to plan care for a client with tuberculosis.

Lung Abscess and Empyema

Lung abscess and empyema are potential complications of pneumonia and other respiratory infections. A *lung abscess* is local lung destruction or necrosis and pus formation. Aspiration pneumonia is the most common cause of lung abscess. *Empyema* is pus in the pleural cavity. Bacterial pneumonia, rupture of a lung abscess, and infection due to chest trauma are the major causes of empyema.

Manifestations of these disorders typically develop about 2 weeks after the initiating event (aspiration, pneumonia, etc.). Signs of an acute infection with chills and fever, pleuritic chest pain, malaise, and anorexia develop. The cough may be productive of foul-smelling, purulent, and even blood-streaked sputum. Breath sounds are diminished, and crackles may be heard in the region of the abscess. Rupture and drainage of an abscess into a bronchus is a frightening complication.

Intravenous antibiotic therapy is ordered. Postural drainage may be done to relieve obstruction and promote drainage. In some cases, bronchoscopy is used to drain an abscess. A chest tube may be used to drain an empyema. See the section on pneumothorax for further discussion of chest tubes.

Most clients recover fully with appropriate treatment. Nursing care needs relate primarily to maintaining a patent airway and adequate gas exchange. When teaching, emphasize the importance of completing the prescribed antibiotic therapy. Antibiotic therapy may be continued for up to 1 month or more. Stress the need to contact the physician if symptoms do not improve or if they become worse: Infection from lung abscess can spread to lung and pleural tissue, and also via the blood, causing systemic sepsis.

Emerging Respiratory Infections

Recent years have seen the emergence of newly identified respiratory infections as well as the use of infectious microbes as weapons.

Severe acute respiratory syndrome (SARS) is a lower respiratory illness caused by a newly identified virus called SARS-associated coronavirus (SARS-CoV). This virus spreads primarily by close human contact. It also may be spread during some medical procedures and by touching a surface infected with the virus and subsequently touching the eyes, nose, or mouth. While most coronaviruses cause only mild respiratory illnesses, most people with SARS develop severe pneumonia. It typically begins with flulike symptoms, including high fever, headache and muscle aches, cough, and shortness of breath. The mortality rate during an outbreak in 2003 was approximately 9%. Intensive and supportive medical care is the primary treatment for SARS.

Inhalation anthrax is a relatively new potential threat in the United States. While it rarely affects humans in nature, the infectious agent, *Bacillus anthracis,* has been identified as a potential biologic weapon. Inhalation anthrax causes initial flulike symptoms, with malaise, dry cough, and fever. Severe dyspnea, stridor, and cyanosis develop abruptly, along with inflammation and enlargement of lymph nodes in the mediastinum and thorax. The client may develop septic shock or meningitis. Blood cultures and chest x-ray are used to diagnose inhalation anthrax. Fortunately, the antibiotic ciprofloxacin (Cipro) is effective for both prevention and treatment of inhalation anthrax.

In both of these emerging infections, intensive and supportive nursing care is required. The nursing diagnoses and interventions identified for pneumonia and respiratory failure may be appropriate for clients with SARS or inhalation anthrax. Contact and airborne precautions are implemented in addition to Standard Precautions for clients with SARS. The CDC recommends hand washing, gown, gloves, eye protection, and a respirator to prevent SARS transmission in health care settings.

OBSTRUCTIVE AND RESTRICTIVE LUNG DISORDERS

Many diseases affect the airways and airflow. Airflow decreases when (1) secretions obstruct the airway; (2) airway walls are edematous or swollen; (3) smooth muscle of the airways constricts, reducing their size; (4) the lungs lose elasticity, making exhalation more difficult; and (5) supportive tissue is lost, allowing airways to collapse.

Decreased airflow increases the work of breathing and causes air trapping in the lungs. Inhaled air mixes with trapped air, and less oxygen is available for gas exchange in the alveoli.

Asthma

Asthma is a chronic inflammatory disorder of the airways characterized by recurrent episodes of wheezing, breathlessness, chest tightness, and coughing. Although it is more common in children than adults, about 5% of adults have asthma. It is becoming more common and is causing an increasing number of deaths.

PATHOPHYSIOLOGY

During symptom-free periods, there is little airway inflammation in clients with asthma. A variety of factors can trigger an acute inflammatory response, including allergens, environmental pollutants such as tobacco smoke and smog, and workplace pollutants. Respiratory infection is a common stimulus, as is exercise in cold, dry air for clients with exercise-induced asthma. Emotional stress can trigger an attack. Drugs such as aspirin and other NSAIDs, sulfites (used as preservatives), and beta blockers can prompt an attack in some clients.

When a trigger occurs, an *acute* or *early response* develops. Inflammatory mediators (e.g., histamine, prostaglandins) are released, leading to bronchoconstriction and increased capillary permeability. This, in turn, causes edema and increased mucus production, further narrowing airways. Airflow is reduced, and the work of breathing increases. The sequence of events is outlined in Figure 24-7 ■.

The *late phase response* develops 4 to 12 hours after exposure to the trigger, prolonging the attack. Activation of inflammatory cells (e.g., basophils and eosinophils) damages the airway epithelium, produces mucosal edema, impairs airway clearance, and prolongs bronchoconstriction. Air is trapped distal to the narrowed airways, distending alveoli. Trapped air mixes with inspired air, reducing available oxygen for gas exchange. Blood flow is reduced to distended alveoli, further impairing gas exchange. Hypoxemia develops.

MANIFESTATIONS AND COMPLICATIONS

The frequency and severity of attacks vary. Some clients have infrequent, mild attacks, while others have nearly continuous symptoms.

An attack of asthma may develop abruptly or slowly. It is characterized by chest tightness, difficulty breathing, wheezing, and cough. Expiration is prolonged. Associated symptoms include tachypnea, tachycardia, anxiety, and apprehension. Use of accessory muscles of respiration, intercostal retractions, and distant breath sounds may be present during a severe attack. Severe dyspnea may allow the client with asthma to speak only one or two words between breaths.

Respiratory failure can develop, marked by inaudible breath sounds, reduced wheezing, and an ineffective cough.

clinical ALERT

Respiratory failure is a medical emergency requiring prompt treatment to preserve life. Immediately report manifestations of impending respiratory failure.

Status asthmaticus is severe, prolonged asthma that does not respond to routine treatment. Without aggressive treatment, status asthmaticus can lead to respiratory failure. The client may require intubation and mechanical ventilation.

INTERDISCIPLINARY CARE

Asthma is diagnosed by the client's history and manifestations. Diagnostic tests are used to identify possible triggers and to evaluate respiratory function during and between acute attacks. *Peak expiratory flow rate (PEFR)* assesses airflow restriction and the effectiveness of treatment. Clients with asthma use inexpensive PEFR meters to monitor airflow and the need for treatment on a continuing basis. *Pulse oximetry* and *arterial blood gases* evaluate oxygenation during an acute attack. *Skin testing* may be done to identify specific allergens that may trigger asthma attacks.

Treatment focuses on controlling symptoms and preventing acute attacks. When an acute episode occurs, therapy focuses on restoring airflow and alveolar ventilation.

Preventive Measures

Asthma attacks often can be prevented by avoiding allergens and other triggers. Modifying the home environment (e.g., controlling dust, removing carpets, covering mattresses and pillows to reduce dust mites, and installing air filtering systems) may help. Pets may need to be removed from

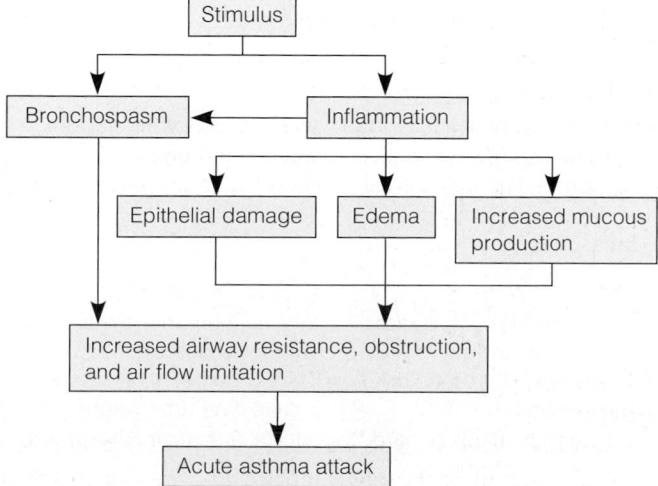

Figure 24-7. ■ The sequence of an acute episode of asthma.

the household. Eliminating tobacco smoke in the house is also important. For exercise-induced asthma, wearing a mask that retains humidity and warm air when exercising in cold weather may prevent an attack. Early treatment of respiratory infections is vital.

Medications

Drugs are used to prevent and control asthma symptoms, reduce the frequency and severity of attacks, and reverse airway obstruction. Drugs used for long-term control are taken daily. These include anti-inflammatory agents, long-acting bronchodilators, and leukotriene modifiers. Quick-relief medications used to relieve bronchoconstriction and airflow obstruction include rapid-acting bronchodilators, anticholinergic drugs, and systemic corticosteroids (Table 24-4 ■). Complementary and alternative therapies may help treat and control asthma, as outlined in Box 24-5 ■.

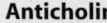

TABLE 24-4			
Nursing Implications for Pharmacology: Asthma Drugs			
DRUG	**ACTION**	**NURSING RESPONSIBILITIES**	**CLIENT AND FAMILY TEACHING**
Beta-Adrenergic Agonists ■ Epinephrine ■ Isoproterenol (Isuprel) ■ Metaproterenol (Alupent, Metaprel) ■ Terbutaline (Brethine) ■ Isoetharine (Bronkosol) ■ Albuterol (Proventil) ■ Bitolterol (Tornalate) ■ Pirbuterol (Maxair) ■ Salmeterol (Serevent)	These drugs stimulate sympathetic nervous system (SNS) receptors in the lungs, causing bronchodilation. Given orally, parenterally, or by metered-dose inhalers (MDIs), they are used to prevent and treat acute attacks. Their side effects include nervousness, irritability, tachycardia, and dysrhythmias, particularly when given parenterally or by mouth.	Use with caution in clients with hypertension, cardiovascular disease, hyperthyroidism, or diabetes. When given by MDI, wait 1–2 minutes between puffs to allow airways to dilate, permitting the second dose to reach distal airways. Chart response. Desired effect is reduced dyspnea and wheezing; anxiety, irritability, insomnia, and tremor are common side effects.	Use your inhaler or nebulizer as instructed. If you are taking this drug with another medication by inhalation, use this drug first to open airways. Rinse your mouth after using inhalers to reduce systemic effects. Keep a log of your use; if drug becomes less effective, or you need it more often, contact your doctor. Report irregular pulse and other side effects to your doctor.
Methylxanthines ■ Theophylline (Bronkotabs, Theo-Dur, others) ■ Aminophylline (Somophyllin)	Methylxanthines, which are related to caffeine, are primarily used to prevent nocturnal asthma in adult clients. Theophylline has a narrow margin of safety and a high risk for toxicity.	Monitor therapeutic blood levels (10–20 μg/mL). Monitor for manifestations of toxicity: anorexia, nausea, vomiting, restlessness, insomnia, dysrhythmias, and seizures. Give with meals or a full glass of water or milk. Aminophylline is incompatible with many other intravenous drugs; administer in a separate line or flush the line with normal saline before and after giving any other drug.	Theophylline is ineffective to treat an acute asthma attack; do not delay other treatment by using these drugs. Check with your doctor before taking any over-the-counter drugs or other prescription drugs while taking theophylline. Do not smoke while you are taking this drug. Report adverse effects to your doctor.
Anticholinergics ■ Atropine ■ Ipratropium bromide (Atrovent)	Anticholinergics dilate the bronchi. Atropine is used infrequently because it tends to dry secretions and has other side effects. Ipratropium bromide is available as an inhaler and has fewer side effects than atropine.	Assess for possible contraindications to the drug, including glaucoma, an enlarged prostate, or urinary retention. Provide ice chips, fluids, or hard candy to relieve dry mouth.	Take no more than the ordered number of doses per day. If the drug becomes less effective over time, notify your doctor. A dosage adjustment may be needed.

TABLE 24-4

Nursing Implications for Pharmacology: Asthma Drugs (continued)

DRUG	ACTION	NURSING RESPONSIBILITIES	CLIENT AND FAMILY TEACHING
Corticosteroids ■ Beclomethasone dipropionate (Vanceril, Beclovent) ■ Triamcinolone acetonide (Azmacort) ■ Flunisolide (AeroBid) ■ Dexamethasone sodium phosphate (Decadron Phosphate Respihaler)	These are potent anti-inflammatory drugs used to prevent and treat acute episodes. They reduce the frequency and severity of attacks and allow lower doses of other drugs. Giving these drugs by inhalation reduces systemic side effects.	Give inhaler doses after bronchodilators to improve transit of the drug to distal airways. Report common side effects: sore throat, hoarseness, and oropharyngeal *Candida albicans* infection.	Rinse your mouth after taking the drug; use good oral hygiene to reduce the risk of fungal infections. Do not use these drugs to treat an acute attack. The desired effect may not be noticed for several weeks. Call your doctor if you gain weight, retain fluid, or have muscle weakness, mood changes, or an appearance change.
Mast Cell Stabilizers ■ Cromolyn sodium (Intal, NasalCrom) ■ Nedocromil (Tilade)	These drugs reduce inflammatory airway responses and prevent airway constriction in response to cold air. They have a wide margin of safety.	Report potential adverse effects of wheezing and bronchoconstriction.	Use these drugs only to prevent asthma attacks; do not use to treat an acute attack. Several weeks may be required before a beneficial effect is noted.
Leukotriene Modifiers ■ Zafirlukast (Accolate) ■ Zileuton (Zyflo)	Leukotriene modifiers interfere with airway inflammation, improving airflow and decreasing asthma symptoms. They are used to prevent asthma attacks; they are not used to treat an acute attack.	Give at least 1 hour before or 2 hours after meals. These drugs affect warfarin metabolism. Monitor for bleeding. Monitor liver enzymes, because these drugs may be toxic to the liver.	Take as ordered on an empty stomach. Call your doctor if you notice a change in color of stools or urine, or if jaundice develops.

NURSING CARE

ASSESSING

Good nursing assessment is vital to determine the effects of an acute asthma attack, initiate early interventions when needed, and evaluate the effectiveness of treatment.

BOX 24-5   COMPLEMENTARY THERAPIES

Asthma

Herbal preparations such as atopa belladonna (the natural form of atropine, an anticholinergic drug that blocks bronchoconstriction), capsaicin, quercetin, and grape seed extract may be helpful in managing and relieving symptoms of asthma. These preparations may interact with prescribed therapies. Stress the importance of discussing all herbal preparations with the physician and consulting with a qualified herbalist before taking any herbal preparation.

Other complementary therapies such as biofeedback, yoga, breathing techniques, acupuncture, homeopathy, and massage also have been found to help control and relieve asthma symptoms.

Box 24-6 ■ summarizes assessment data to collect for clients with asthma.

DIAGNOSING, PLANNING, AND IMPLEMENTING

Priorities in Nursing Care. This section focuses on the priority nursing care needs for a client experiencing an acute attack of asthma.

Ineffective Airway Clearance

■ Frequently assess respiratory status (see Box 24-6). Notify the charge nurse or physician of significant changes. *Respiratory status can change rapidly during an acute asthma attack.*

clinical ALERT

Slow, shallow respirations; faint breath sounds; decreased wheezing; and an ineffective cough may indicate exhaustion and possible respiratory failure. Immediate intervention is vital.

BOX 24-6	ASSESSMENT

Assessing Clients with Asthma

SUBJECTIVE DATA

- Complaints of cough, shortness of breath, difficulty breathing, fatigue, apprehension
- History of asthma, allergies; known exposure to a trigger
- Current medications, effectiveness, when last used

OBJECTIVE DATA

- Respiratory status, including PEFR, oxygen saturation, ability to converse without pausing for breath; dyspnea; nasal flaring, chest expansion, use of accessory muscles, presence of retractions; lung sounds throughout chest, adventitious sounds; presence and effectiveness of cough, sputum production
- Vital signs, skin color
- Level of consciousness and mental status
- State of anxiety, apprehension

Diagnostic Tests

- PEFR, O_2 saturation, ABGs

- Assess skin color and temperature and level of consciousness (LOC) every 1 to 2 hours or as indicated. *Cyanosis; cool, clammy skin; and changes in LOC (such as agitation, lethargy, or confusion) indicate worsening hypoxia.*
- Report abnormal or significant changes in oxygen saturation levels and ABG results. *Oxygen saturation and ABG values indicate the effectiveness of gas exchange and treatment.*
- Place in Fowler's, high Fowler's, or orthopneic (with head and arms supported on the over-bed table) position. *These positions reduce the work of breathing and increase lung expansion.*
- Administer oxygen as ordered. If a mask is used, monitor for feelings of claustrophobia or suffocation. *Supplemental oxygen reduces hypoxemia. Although the mask is very effective for delivering oxygen, it may increase anxiety.*
- Administer nebulizer treatments and provide humidification as ordered. *Bronchodilators and other drugs are given by nebulizer; humidity helps loosen secretions.*
- Assist with chest physiotherapy, including percussion and postural drainage. *Percussion and postural drainage facilitate airway clearance.*
- Increase fluid intake. *Increasing fluids helps thin secretions.*
- Monitor effects of prescribed medications. *Medications used to improve airway status and facilitate breathing also may have significant adverse effects.*

Fatigue

- Assist with ADLs as needed. *This allows energy conservation.*
- Provide rest periods between activities and treatments. *Rest helps prevent fatigue and reduce oxygen demands.*

- Assist with breathing and relaxation techniques to control breathing pattern. *Pursed-lip breathing helps keep airways open; abdominal breathing improves lung expansion. Relaxation techniques reduce anxiety and help slow the respiratory rate.*

Anxiety

An acute asthma attack causes significant anxiety with a fear of suffocation. Hypoxia contributes to the sense of anxiety.

- Help identify coping skills that have been successful in the past. *Coping skills can help the client regain control.*
- Provide physical and emotional support. Remain present during periods of acute anxiety. Schedule time with the client every 1 to 2 hours, and reassure about a prompt response to the call light. *The severely anxious client may fear that he or she will die if someone is not on hand. Reassurance of readily available assistance and the presence of the nurse reduces anxiety.*
- Listen actively to concerns; do not deny or negate the fear of dying or of being unable to breathe. *Active listening promotes trust and helps the client express concerns.*
- Provide clear, concise directions and explanations. Avoid presenting too much information. *Anxiety interferes with learning. Explanations may need to be repeated frequently.*
- Reduce excessive stimuli, and maintain a calm demeanor. *This promotes rest.*
- Allow supportive family members to remain with the client. *Significant others provide additional support and can help reduce anxiety.*
- Assist with relaxation techniques such as guided imagery, muscle relaxation, and meditation. *These techniques help reduce anxiety and restore a sense of control.*

Ineffective Therapeutic Regimen Management

- Assess understanding of asthma and prescribed treatment. Reinforce teaching as indicated. *Assessment helps identify misperceptions about asthma and its management that may contribute to acute attacks.*
- Discuss the effect of asthma and its management on lifestyle. *Discussion can help identify conflicts between lifestyle and the treatment regimen.*
- Help identify factors that contributed to the acute attack. *Awareness of contributing factors helps identify ways to prevent future attacks.*
- Assist to identify ways to integrate daily treatment into lifestyle. *Asthma management can impact significant others as well as the client, for example, eliminating smoking and pets in the household, removing carpets, and measures to reduce dust mites.*

- Provide verbal and written instructions. *Written instructions reinforce learning and allow future reference.*
- Refer to counseling, support groups, or self-help organizations. *Services such as these can help with required lifestyle changes and the demands of treatment.*

Evaluating

To evaluate the effectiveness of nursing care, collect data related to:

- Respiratory status and breathing pattern
- Fatigue and activity tolerance
- Anxiety level
- Knowledge and understanding of measures to prevent future asthma attacks.

BOX 24-7	CLIENT TEACHING

Using A Metered-Dose Inhaler

- Firmly insert the metered-dose inhaler (MDI) canister into holder.
- Shake vigorously for 3 to 5 seconds.
- Exhale slowly and completely.
- Close lips around mouthpiece or hold mouthpiece directly in front of mouth.
- Press and hold canister down once while inhaling deeply and slowly for 3 to 5 seconds (see figure).

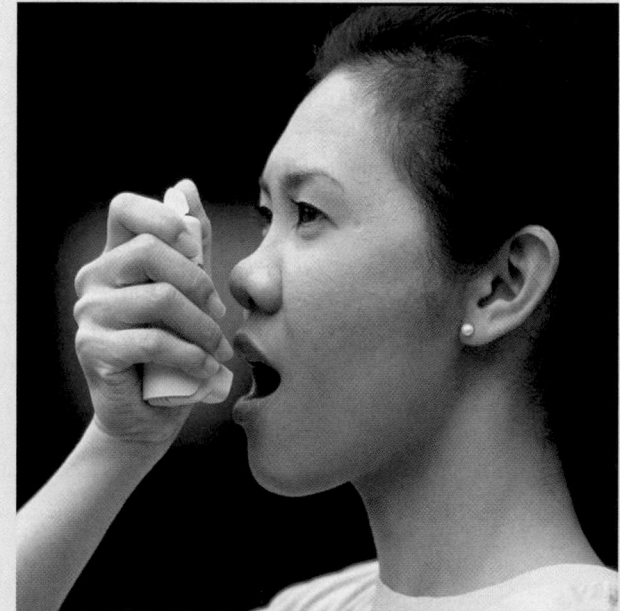

(*Source:* NMSB, Custom Medical Stock Photos, Inc.)

- Hold breath for 10 seconds. Release pressure on container and remove from mouth, then exhale.
- Wait 20 to 30 seconds (or as directed) before repeating for a second puff.
- Rinse mouth after using inhaler.
- Rinse mouthpiece at least once a day.

Documenting. Document initial and continuing assessment data, specifically noting response to treatment measures. Document all teaching provided, and the client's and family's apparent understanding and acceptance of teaching.

CONTINUING CARE

Teach about PEFR monitoring and using readings to manage use of short-acting inhalers. Provide information about all prescribed drugs verbally and in writing, including:

- The drug name, its frequency, dose, and how to use it
- The desired effect and purpose of the drug
- Potential adverse effects and their management, including those that should be reported to the physician
- Potential interactions with other medications (including over-the-counter medications and herbal preparations) or with foods
- What to do if the medication becomes less effective or is needed with increasing frequency over time.

See Box 24-7 ■ for teaching related to using a metered-dose inhaler (MDI).

If specific triggers for asthma attacks have been identified, help identify ways to avoid these triggers. Because exercise, particularly in cold weather, often triggers an attack, instruct to warm up slowly before exercise and wear a mask to retain air warmth and humidity while exercising. If necessary, help identify alternate indoor exercises. Discuss measures to prevent respiratory infections and support immune function, including adequate rest, good nutrition, and stress management. Recommend yearly influenza vaccine and immunization against pneumococcal pneumonia. Help identify stress management techniques to incorporate into lifestyle. Refer to a local or regional agency for further teaching and support as needed. See Box 24-8 ■ for home care resources.

BOX 24-8	POPULATION FOCUS

Home Care Resources for Clients with Asthma

American Lung Association
800-LUNG-USA (800-586-4872)
www.lungusa.org

Asthma and Allergy Foundation of America
202-466-7643
www.aafa.org

Asthma Information Center
http://my.webmd.com/medical_information/
condition_centers/asthma

National Heart, Lung, and Blood Institute
www.nhlbi.hih.gov/health/public/lung/index

MediaLink Video: Metered-Dose Inhaler

Chronic Obstructive Pulmonary Disease

Chronic obstructive pulmonary disease (COPD) is characterized by chronic and progressive obstruction of airflow in the lungs. It usually affects middle and older adults. Smoking is the most common cause of COPD. Other risk factors are secondhand smoke exposure, air pollution, occupational pollutants, and family history of COPD.

COPD affects more than 11 million Americans. It affects whites more often than blacks, and men more frequently than women, although its incidence in blacks and in women is increasing. Not only is it a leading cause of death, it is second only to heart disease as a cause of disability and lost work time.

PATHOPHYSIOLOGY AND MANIFESTATIONS

In COPD, the airways are narrowed and gradually obstructed by inflammation, excess mucous production, and loss of elastic tissue and alveoli. Two different processes, chronic bronchitis and emphysema, cause these airway and lung tissue changes (Figure 24-8 ■). Alveolar ventilation is impaired, as is gas exchange between the alveoli and the blood.

By the time COPD is diagnosed, the client may have had a productive cough, dyspnea, and exercise intolerance for as long as 10 years. The cough usually occurs in the mornings ("smoker's cough"). Dyspnea becomes worse as the disease progresses. Periodic episodes of increased sputum and difficulty breathing are common, often caused by respiratory infection.

Chronic Bronchitis

Chronic bronchitis is a chronic inflammatory airway disorder that causes excessive secretion of thick, tenacious mucus and a productive cough lasting 3 or more months. Inhaled irritants, primarily cigarette smoke, lead to a chronic inflammatory process in the bronchial mucosa. Narrowed air-

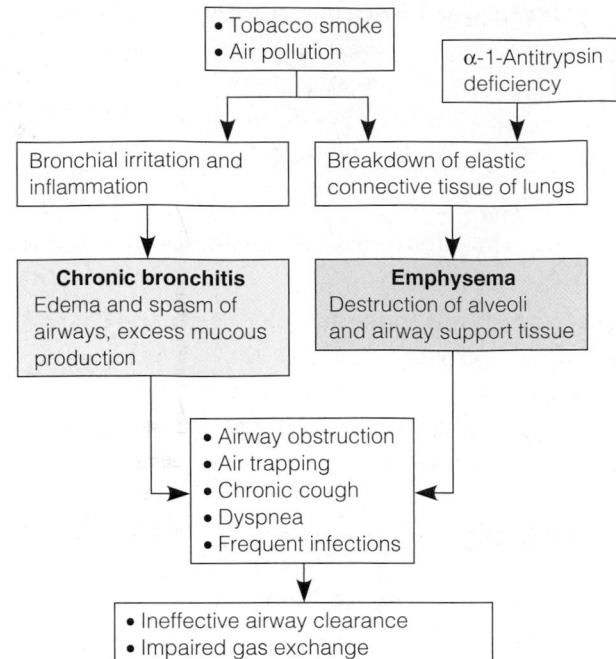

Figure 24-8. ■ The process of COPD.

ways due to mucosal edema and excess secretions obstruct airflow. Expiratory airflow is affected first. Ciliary function is impaired, so normal defense mechanisms cannot clear mucus and inhaled pathogens. Recurrent infection is common. The manifestations of chronic bronchitis are listed in Table 24-5 ■. The client also frequently develops manifestations of right-sided heart failure with distended neck veins, edema, and an enlarged heart. (See Chapter 27 ◯◯ for more information about heart failure.)

Emphysema

Emphysema is destruction of alveolar walls leading to large, abnormal air spaces in the lungs. As in chronic bronchitis, cigarette smoking is its major cause. Deficiency of alpha$_1$-antitrypsin, an enzyme that normally prevents lung tissue destruction, also causes emphysema.

TABLE 24-5		
Manifestations of Chronic Bronchitis and Emphysema		
	CHRONIC BRONCHITIS	**EMPHYSEMA**
Onset	After age 35; recurrent respiratory infections	After age 50; progressive shortness of breath
Cough	Persistent; productive of copious, thick sputum	Absent or mild, nonproductive
Appearance	Often obese Edema and cyanosis Distended neck veins	Thin and *cachectic* (malnourished) Barrel chest Use of accessory muscles of respiration
Chest auscultation	Wheezing and rhonchi	Distant or diminished breath sounds

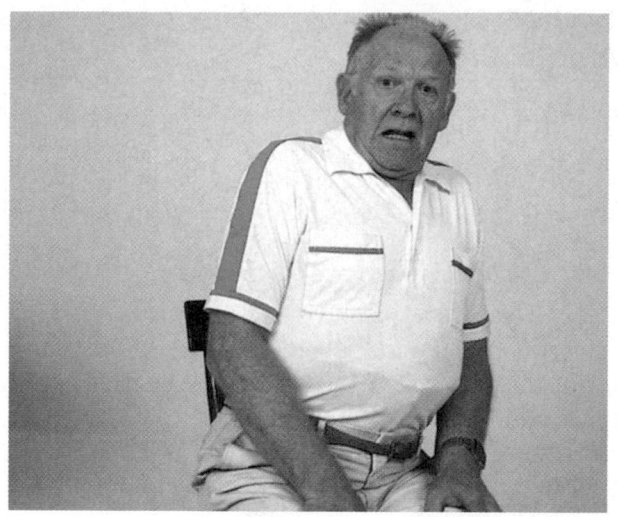

Figure 24-9. ■ Typical appearance of a client with emphysema.

When alveolar walls are destroyed, air spaces enlarge and the surface area for gas exchange decreases. Think about an apple and an equal size bunch of grapes: the skin (surface area) of the apple is much smaller than the combined surface area of all the grapes in the cluster.

The alveoli become less elastic and airways tend to collapse during exhalation. This causes air trapping in the lungs. Over time, the anterior–posterior chest diameter increases, and the client develops a **barrel chest** (Figure 24-9 ■). Expiration is prolonged. The client often is thin, uses accessory muscles of respiration, and frequently assumes a position of sitting and leaning forward. The manifestations of emphysema are summarized in Table 24-5.

INTERDISCIPLINARY CARE

Avoiding—never starting or stopping—smoking is the only way to prevent COPD and to slow its progression. Early in the disease, airway obstruction can be reversed and disability minimized. Treatment focuses on reducing symptoms and maintaining optimal function.

Diagnostic Tests

The following tests are used to help diagnose COPD, assess the client's status, and monitor the effectiveness of treatment:

- *Pulmonary function testing* is used to evaluate lung ventilation and function. See Chapter 22 ⚭ for more information about pulmonary function tests.
- *Serum alpha$_1$-antitrypsin* levels may be drawn to screen for a deficiency of this enzyme.
- *ABGs* are drawn to evaluate the effect of COPD on gas exchange. During an acute episode, a low Po_2 (hypoxemia), high Pco_2 (hypercapnia), and low pH (respiratory acidosis) may be seen. (See Chapter 7 ⚭ for more information about ABGs.)

> **clinical ALERT**
>
> Clients with COPD may have chronic hypercapnia. This reduces the effect of Pco_2 and pH on the respiratory drive; instead, breathing is driven by a drop in arterial oxygen levels. These clients may develop sleep apnea and respiratory arrest when given oxygen, because their drive to breathe is suppressed.

- *Pulse oximetry* is used to measure oxygen saturation of the blood. These levels may be used to continuously assess the need for supplemental oxygen.
- Other diagnostic tests may include *ventilation/perfusion scanning,* a *chest x-ray,* or a *computed tomography (CT) scan* of the chest (see Chapter 22). ⚭

Medications

Medications are used to help manage COPD symptoms and slow progression of the disease.

Immunization against pneumococcal pneumonia and yearly influenza vaccine are recommended. A broad-spectrum antibiotic is ordered if infection is suspected. A bronchodilator such as ipratropium (Atrovent) or theophylline may be ordered. Theophylline also improves cardiac and respiratory muscle function. Review the nursing implications for bronchodilators as outlined in Table 24-4 ⚭. Corticosteroids may be given to reduce inflammation and edema of the airways. Cough suppressants and sedatives are avoided. Alpha$_1$-antitrypsin may be given when this enzyme is deficient.

Oxygen Therapy

Clients with COPD may need home oxygen therapy. Oxygen may be used intermittently, at night, or continuously. Home oxygen is available as liquid oxygen, compressed gas cylinders, or oxygen concentrators. During an acute episode, oxygen and ventilatory assistance using a continuous positive airway pressure (CPAP) mask or mechanical ventilation may be required. CPAP is discussed in Chapter 23 ⚭; mechanical ventilation is discussed later in this chapter. Careful observation is vital when oxygen is given without ventilatory support, because the drive to breathe may be inhibited, leading to respiratory arrest.

Other Therapies

Smoking cessation is vital. Nicotine chewing gum or patches may be prescribed, and referral made to a clinic, group, or counselor. Clients are advised to avoid other airway irritants and allergens. When air pollution is significant, the client may need to remain indoors. Air filtering systems or air conditioning may be useful.

Increased fluid intake, effective cough, percussion, and postural drainage help clear secretions. A liberal fluid intake keeps secretions thin. Forceful coughing is often less effective than leaning forward and repeatedly "huffing," with relaxed breathing between huffs. Percussion and postural drainage help clear secretions when they are thick or tenacious. Breathing exercises slow the respiratory rate and reduce fatigue. *Pursed-lip breathing* helps slow respirations and keep airways during exhalation by keeping positive pressure in the airways. *Abdominal breathing* helps reduce the work of accessory muscles of respiration. (See Box 24-10.)

A lung transplant or lung reduction surgery may be done in end-stage COPD. Lung reduction surgery reduces the volume of the lung, reshapes it, and improves elastic recoil. It improves pulmonary function and exercise tolerance, and reduces dyspnea. (See Box 24-12, page 566, for nursing care of the client with lung surgery.)

NURSING CARE

ASSESSING

Clients with COPD need careful and frequent assessment (Box 24-9 ■).

BOX 24-9   ASSESSMENT

Assessing Clients with COPD

SUBJECTIVE DATA
- Complaints of shortness of breath, difficulty breathing; onset and duration; fatigue; cough, amount and character of sputum
- Recent respiratory infection
- Smoking history; history of chronic lung disease, asthma, pneumonia, allergies
- Current medications, effectiveness, when last used; home oxygen

OBJECTIVE DATA
- Respiratory status, including PEFR, oxygen saturation; dyspnea, chest expansion, nasal flaring, use of accessory muscles; cough, sputum produced; lung sounds throughout chest, adventitious sounds such as wheezes, fine or coarse crackles
- Vital signs including apical pulse and capillary refill; neck vein distention
- Skin color; clubbing of nails
- Level of consciousness and mental status
- Level of anxiety, apprehension
- Height and weight; general nutritional status

Diagnostic Tests
- Pulmonary function tests, ABGs, O$_2$ saturation

DIAGNOSING, PLANNING, AND IMPLEMENTING

Priorities in Nursing Care. Because of the obstructive nature of COPD, airway clearance is a high-priority nursing problem. This chronic disease affects all areas of life as it progresses, making psychosocial issues a concern in planning nursing care.

Ineffective Airway Clearance

- Frequently assess respiratory status (see Box 24-9), skin color, and mental status. Report changes such as diminished breath sounds, ineffective cough, increasing cyanosis, or altered mental status to the charge nurse or physician. *Changes may indicate a decline in the client's condition.*
- Report oxygen saturations of less than 95% (or identified parameters). *Decreasing oxygen saturation levels may indicate airway obstruction and impaired alveolar ventilation.*
- Encourage fluid intake of at least 2,000 to 2,500 mL/day unless contraindicated. *Adequate fluid intake helps keep secretions thin.*
- Place in Fowler's, high Fowler's, or orthopneic position. Encourage activity to tolerance. *An upright position improves lung ventilation. Activity helps mobilize secretions and prevent them from pooling.*
- Assist to cough at least every 2 hours while awake. *Coughing helps mobilize secretions and maintain open airways.*
- Provide tissues and a paper bag to dispose of sputum. *This infection control measure reduces the spread of respiratory organisms to others.*
- Assist with percussion and postural drainage as needed. *Percussion helps loosen secretions in airways; postural drainage facilitates movement of these secretions out of the respiratory tract.*
- Provide rest periods between treatments and procedures. *Rest conserves energy and reduces fatigue.*
- Give expectorant and bronchodilator medications as ordered. *Using expectorants and bronchodilators before coughing, percussion, and postural drainage improves airway clearance.*
- Provide humidified oxygen as ordered. *Oxygen helps maintain blood and tissue oxygenation. Humidification decreases the drying effects of oxygen on respiratory tissues.*
- Prepare for transfer to intensive care if condition is deteriorating. *Respiratory failure is a possible complication of COPD that requires aggressive intervention to preserve life.*

Imbalanced Nutrition: Less than Body Requirements

- Obtain diet history, weight and height, and skinfold measurements. *These data are used to evaluate nutritional status.*
- Observe and document food intake, including types and amounts consumed. *This provides information about the possible need for supplements.*

- Monitor serum albumin and electrolyte levels. *These values provide information about nutritional status.*
- Consult with a dietitian to plan meals and supplements. *High-protein, high-calorie foods help maintain nutrition and reduce fatigue.*
- Provide frequent, small feedings with between-meal supplements. *Frequent, small meals help maintain intake and reduce fatigue associated with eating.*
- Assist to choose preferred foods from menu; encourage family members to bring food from home if allowed. *Providing food preferences encourages eating.*
- Keep snacks at bedside. *Snacks provide additional caloric intake.*
- Provide mouth care before meals. *This improves appetite.*

Compromised Family Coping

- Assess interactions and the effect of the illness on the family. *Assessment helps identify effective and disruptive behaviors.*
- Help identify strengths for coping with the situation. *Identifying strengths helps the client and family regain a sense of control.*
- Encourage expression of feelings. Avoid judging the feelings as "good" or "bad," "right" or "wrong." *Active listening without judging promotes trust.*
- Help identify family members' behaviors and attitudes that may hinder effective treatment, such as continuing to smoke in the house when the client is present. *Family members may be unaware of the effect of their behavior on the client's ability to change habits and cope with a disabling disease.*
- Encourage participation in care. *This helps develop skills for use at home.*
- Refer to available support groups, pulmonary rehabilitation programs, and community agencies or services such as home health, homemaker services, or Meals-on-Wheels as appropriate. *Support groups, community services, and structured rehabilitation programs provide additional support and enhance coping abilities.*

Decisional Conflict: Smoking

- Encourage to express feelings; acknowledge concerns, values, and beliefs. *This demonstrates acceptance of the client's right to make the decision. The nurse needs to avoid imposing personal values and beliefs about smoking on the client.*
- Help plan a course of action for quitting smoking. *When the client develops the plan, he or she has more ownership and interest in making it work.*
- Demonstrate respect for decisions and the right to choose. *Respect supports self-esteem and ability to cope.*
- Refer to a counselor or other professional as needed. *Counselors or other people trained to assist with smoking cessation can help with the decision and plan.*

EVALUATING

To evaluate the effectiveness of nursing care, collect assessment data related to airway clearance and respiratory status, nutritional status and diet intake, demonstrated coping behaviors by the client and family, and a commitment to smoking cessation. Continuously monitor oxygen saturation to help evaluate the effectiveness of medical management.

Documenting. Document continuing assessment data and the client's response to treatment and care measures. Note teaching provided, and the client's and family's understanding and acceptance of information. Document referrals made, including to a nutritionist, smoking cessation resources, and home care services.

CONTINUING CARE

Teach the client with COPD effective coughing and breathing techniques (Box 24-10 ■), how to prevent exacerbations, and management of the treatment regimen.

Advise client to maintain a fluid intake of at least 2 to 2½ quarts of fluid daily. Instruct to avoid respiratory irritants such as cigarette smoke (primary and secondary), other smoke sources, dust, aerosol sprays, air pollution, and

---

BOX 24-10	CLIENT TEACHING

Breathing and Coughing Techniques
Pursed-Lip Breathing
1. Inhale through nose with mouth closed.
2. Exhale slowly through pursed lips, as though whistling or blowing out a candle. Exhale twice as long as inhalation.

Diaphragmatic or Abdominal Breathing
1. Place one hand on abdomen, the other on the chest.
2. Inhale, concentrating on pushing abdominal hand outward while chest hand remains still.
3. Exhale slowly, while abdominal hand moves inward and chest hand remains still.

Controlled Cough Technique
1. After using bronchodilator, inhale deeply, and hold breath briefly.
2. Cough twice, first to loosen mucus, then to expel secretions.
3. Inhale by sniffing to prevent mucus from moving back into deep airways.
4. Rest.

Huff Cough Technique
1. Inhale deeply while leaning forward.
2. Exhale sharply with a "huff" sound. This helps keep airways open while mobilizing secretions.

very cold, dry air. Teach to avoid large crowds and people with known infections to prevent infection. Instruct to obtain yearly influenza immunization. Discuss an exercise program, and encourage a balance of rest and activity as tolerated. Aerobic physical exercise (e.g., walking for 20 minutes at least three times weekly) improves exercise tolerance. Activities that strengthen the muscles used for breathing and ADLs, such as swimming and golf, also are helpful. Stress the importance of maintaining food intake, eating small frequent meals, and using nutritional supplements as needed. If a salt-restricted diet is ordered, teach about foods to avoid and suggest seasonings to improve taste without salt.

Instruct to promptly report early signs of infection or exacerbation of the disease to the physician: fever, increased sputum, purulent (green or yellow) sputum, upper respiratory infection, increased shortness of breath or difficulty breathing, decreased activity tolerance or appetite, increased need for oxygen.

Reinforce teaching about prescribed medications, including purpose, use, and expected effects. Instruct to avoid over-the-counter medications unless approved by the physician. Teach about other treatment measures, such as home oxygen, percussion, postural drainage, and nebulizer treatments. If special equipment is required, be sure to discuss its use, cleaning, and maintenance.

Finally, advise clients with COPD to wear an identification band and carry a list of their medications at all times.

NURSING PROCESS CARE PLAN
Client with COPD

Anna "Happy" Mercurio is an 83-year-old widow who lives with her two grown sons. During the past 15 years, she has become more short of breath and has developed a chronic cough. Ten years ago, emphysema was diagnosed. She is in the hospital with possible pneumonia and an acute exacerbation of COPD.

Assessment. Mrs. Mercurio denies smoking but says that her husband and two sons have been smokers "for practically their whole lives." She reports that she now must rest after just a few minutes of activity. Her cough is productive of moderate to large amounts of sputum, particularly in the mornings. Her dyspnea and sputum became worse 2 days ago; this morning, she was unable to get dressed without resting.

Mrs. Mercurio's skin is very warm and dry, her color dusky. She pauses frequently while talking to catch her breath. Respiratory rate 36, fairly shallow. Frequent cough productive of large amounts of thick, tenacious green sputum. Vital signs:

P 115, irregular; BP 186/60; T 102.4°F (39°C). Weight 96 lbs (43.6 kg), height 5′3″ (160 cm). Appears barrel-chested with moderate kyphosis. Chest hyperresonant to percussion. Distant breath sounds with scattered wheezes and rhonchi throughout lung fields. Chest x-ray shows patchy infiltrates. Laboratory results include high RBC count, low serum albumin, and oxygen saturation of 83%.

Admitting orders include sputum for culture; intravenous penicillin G, 2 million units every 4 hours; ipratropium (Atrovent) inhaler, 2 puffs every 6 hours; beclomethasone (Vanceril) inhaler, 2 puffs every 6 hours; bed rest with bathroom privileges; oxygen per nasal cannula at 2 L continuously; regular diet.

Diagnosis. The following nursing diagnoses are identified for Mrs. Mercurio:

- *Ineffective Airway Clearance* related to pneumonia and COPD
- *Impaired Gas Exchange* related to lung disease
- *Risk for Impaired Spontaneous Ventilation* related to oxygen therapy and respiratory muscle fatigue
- *Impaired Home Maintenance* related to activity intolerance

Expected Outcomes. The expected outcomes specify that Mrs. Mercurio will:

- Expectorate secretions effectively.
- Return to her previous level of respiratory function.
- Maintain oxygen saturation greater than 92%.
- Maintain spontaneous respirations without excess fatigue.
- Express willingness to allow help with household tasks.

Planning and Implementation. The following interventions are planned and implemented:

- Assess respiratory status and level of consciousness every 1 to 2 hours until stable, then at least every 4 hours.
- Monitor O_2 saturation continuously.
- Increase fluid intake to at least 2,500 mL/day.
- Provide bedside humidifier.
- Keep head of bed elevated to at least 30 degrees.
- Provide mouth care after inhaler treatments.
- Provide uninterrupted rest periods after respiratory therapy and other procedures.
- Refer to home health for nursing follow-up.
- Refer to social services for assistance with home maintenance.

Evaluation. Mrs. Mercurio's condition gradually improves. At discharge, she is able to provide self-care with less fatigue and dyspnea. She is using oxygen only at night, admitting that it is just for security. Although scattered wheezes are present, her sputum is thinner, white, and easily expectorated. She will continue oral penicillin V for an additional 10 days at home. She will continue to use Atrovent and Vanceril inhalers at home. Mrs. Mercurio's sons have agreed to smoke only in the garage or outside. A home health nurse will visit three times weekly. A housekeeper will clean and do laundry weekly. Mrs. Mercurio is glad to go home and grateful for the help she will receive.

Critical Thinking in the Nursing Process

1. Mrs. Mercurio had long-term exposure to secondhand smoke. How does secondhand smoke contribute to lung disease in adults and children?
2. The nursing care plan included the nursing diagnosis "Risk for Impaired Spontaneous Ventilation related to oxygen therapy and respiratory muscle fatigue." Review the respiratory drive and describe how chronic hypercapnia affects this process.
3. The client with COPD is at high risk for developing respiratory failure. What are the assessment findings of respiratory failure that you should report to the charge nurse or physician?

Cystic Fibrosis

Cystic fibrosis (CF) is an inherited disorder of childhood that causes excess mucous secretion. Its most damaging effects are to the lungs. Today, many people with CF live into adulthood.

PATHOPHYSIOLOGY AND MANIFESTATIONS

The genetic defect of CF causes excess mucous production in the lungs. Thick mucus plugs small airways and impairs normal airway clearing mechanisms. This leads to *atelectasis,* infection, *bronchiectasis,* and airway dilation. The lungs become scarred and stiff. Over time, COPD, *pulmonary hypertension* (increased pressures in the pulmonary vascular system), and right heart failure develop. The other primary features of CF are lack of pancreatic enzymes and impaired digestion, and increased sodium and chloride in sweat.

The signs and symptoms of CF include dyspnea, chest congestion, and a chronic cough productive of large amounts of thick, sticky sputum. A barrel chest and clubbing of the fingers and toes may be seen. Digestive problems cause abdominal pain and *steatorrhea* (bulky, foul-smelling stool).

INTERDISCIPLINARY CARE

Treatment goals for CF include preventing or treating respiratory complications and maintaining adequate nutrition.

A *pilocarpine iontophoresis sweat chloride test* is used to diagnose CF. Pilocarpine and a small electric current are used to increase sweating. The sweat is collected and analyzed.

Dornase alfa, an enzyme that helps liquefy mucus in CF, is given to improve airway clearance. This drug is given by aerosol. Prophylactic antibiotics often are given to prevent recurrent respiratory infections.

Chest physiotherapy with percussion, vibration, postural drainage, and coughing is essential for airway clearance. Oxygen therapy may be necessary. A liberal fluid intake helps liquify mucous secretions. Lung transplantation currently is the only definitive treatment for CF. Single-lung, double-lung, and heart–lung transplants have been successful in CF clients.

NURSING CARE

Nursing care for the client with CF is similar to that for COPD. The genetic component of CF and the client's age are important considerations. Many adults with CF are just entering their productive years and face a shortened life span.

Reinforce teaching for respiratory care techniques, including percussion, postural drainage, and controlled cough techniques. Stress the importance of avoiding respiratory irritants, such as cigarette smoke and air pollution. Discuss prevention of respiratory infection by maintaining immunizations, good general health, and avoiding large crowds and infected people.

Discuss the genetic transmission of CF. Refer for genetic testing if desired. Help sort through the impact of CF on future pregnancies and generations. Remember that the risk of CF may present an ethical dilemma about future pregnancies for clients and their families. Provide support as needed.

Atelectasis

Atelectasis is partial or total lung collapse and airlessness. It may be acute or chronic. The usual cause of atelectasis is obstruction of the airway to affected area of lung. It may affect a small segment of a lung or an entire lobe. Atelectasis also may result from compression of the lung (e.g., a tumor) or an inability to keep alveoli open. The manifestations of atelectasis include absent or diminished breath sounds over the affected area, tachycardia, tachypnea, and dyspnea.

Prevention is the primary treatment for atelectasis. Clients with risk factors such as COPD, smokers undergoing surgery, and clients on prolonged bed rest, need vigorous chest physiotherapy to keep airways open. Frequent respiratory assessment is important for early detection and treatment. Position on the unaffected side, with the involved side up to promote drainage. Move frequently, and encourage coughing and deep breathing. Encourage oral fluids to help liquefy secretions.

Bronchiectasis

Bronchiectasis is permanent dilation and destruction of large airways. It is usually due to repeated respiratory infections. Inflammation and airway obstruction weaken and dilate bronchial walls, causing secretions to pool and further infection and inflammation.

Bronchiectasis causes a chronic cough productive of large amounts of sputum. Other manifestations include hemoptysis, recurrent pneumonia, wheezing and shortness of breath, malnutrition, right-sided heart failure, and cor pulmonale (see the section of this chapter on pulmonary vascular disorders).

Treatment is similar to that for COPD. Antibiotics are ordered at the first sign of infection and may be used prophylactically. Inhaled bronchodilators also may be ordered. Chest physiotherapy is a vital part of care. Percussion and postural drainage help mobilize secretions. Oxygen may be ordered. If lung destruction is local, the affected segment may be surgically removed.

Nursing care of the client with bronchiectasis is much the same as for COPD. Airway clearance is a primary problem, as is ineffective breathing pattern. Teaching is vital to help the client and family manage the disease and prevent progression.

INTERSTITIAL LUNG DISORDERS

Many lung diseases damage the interstitial or connective tissue of the lung. Occupational lung diseases and sarcoidosis fall into this group of disorders. Toxic drugs and radiation also cause interstitial damage.

PATHOPHYSIOLOGY AND MANIFESTATIONS

In these disorders (Table 24-6 ■), inflammation damages the alveoli and interstitial tissue of the lung. Normal lung tissue is replaced by fibrotic (scar) tissue. As a result, the lungs become stiff and noncompliant (difficult to inflate).

The onset of interstitial lung disease may be acute or gradual. A dry cough and dyspnea on exertion are common symptoms of interstitial lung diseases. Respirations are often rapid and shallow. Fine inspiratory crackles at the lung bases may be heard. Clubbing of the fingers and toes may develop.

Occupational Lung Disease

Occupational lung diseases are directly related to inhaling noxious substances in the work environment. There are two major classifications:

1. *Pneumoconioses,* caused by inhaling *inorganic* dusts and particulates
2. *Hypersensitivity pneumonitis,* allergic responses to inhaled organic dusts.

When a noxious substance is inhaled, the body's response depends on the size of the particles, whether it is organic or inorganic, where it lands in the respiratory tract, and the individual. Normal lung defenses attempt to remove foreign

TABLE 24-6		
Common Interstitial Lung Disorders		
DISORDER	**CAUSE**	**HIGH-RISK POPULATION**
Pneumoconioses ■ Silicosis ■ Asbestosis ■ Black lung disease	Inorganic dusts ■ Silica ■ Asbestos ■ Coal	 Hard rock miners, foundry workers, sandblasters, pottery makers, granite cutters People involved in mining, milling, manufacturing, and application of asbestos products Coal miners
Hypersensitivity pneumonitis	Organic dusts	People exposed to cotton dust, moldy sugar cane fiber; farmers; people who raise birds
Sarcoidosis	Unknown	Young adults; African Americans

matter; however, these defenses may be impaired by smoking, alcohol, or allergic reactions.

The inhaled substance and resulting inflammatory response damage the alveoli and interstitial tissue of the lung. The normally elastic fibers of the lung are replaced by scar tissue, leaving the lungs stiff and noncompliant. Lung volumes decrease, the work of breathing increases, and gas exchange is impaired, leading to hypoxemia.

Sarcoidosis

Sarcoidosis is a chronic, systemic disease of unknown cause. Lesions develop in the lungs, lymph nodes, liver, eyes, skin, and other organs. These lesions may heal or cause scarring. It can cause significant lung damage and eventual disability. Manifestations of sarcoidosis vary, depending on the organ system affected. When the lungs are involved, pulmonary hemorrhage and cardiac and respiratory failure are risks.

INTERDISCIPLINARY CARE

Prevention is important for all occupational lung diseases. Containing dust and wearing personal protective devices that limit the amount of inhaled particles are essential for people who work in industries with known risks.

Diagnostic testing shows restricted ventilation, with reduced vital capacity and total lung capacity. Gas exchange is affected, leading to low oxygen saturation and hypoxemia, especially with exercise. The chest x-ray shows interstitial lung damage. A bronchoscopy may be done to obtain tissue for biopsy. Specialized lung scans can show the extent of scarring.

Management of interstitial lung disease includes measures to identify and remove the cause, reduce inflammation, prevent progression, and support current lung function. Treatment is nonspecific. Anti-inflammatory drugs, such as corticosteroids, may reduce the inflammatory response and slow the progression of the disease. Generally, care is supportive, similar to that for clients with COPD.

NURSING CARE

Nursing care for clients with interstitial lung diseases is much the same at that for a client with COPD.

Activity intolerance is a common problem. The client's ability to perform ADLs may be significantly impaired. Nursing measures to reduce energy use and provide rest are essential. Caregiver role strain, either actual or potential, must be considered when the client with severe disability is being cared for at home.

Ineffective coping may also be a priority nursing diagnosis. Many occupational lung diseases develop after 20 to 30 years of exposure to the hazardous material. Clients who began working after high school may develop signs of disease in their 40s and face the possibility of changing occupations or becoming disabled. The resulting role strain affects all family members.

CONTINUING CARE

Teach clients at risk for occupational lung diseases how to reduce this risk. Nurses in industrial and public health settings should be alert to potential dangers. Teach workers about measures to reduce dust in their work area and the use of personal protective devices such as masks. Educate children of people with occupational lung disease about the risks associated with the occupation.

Teach how to avoid further lung damage, for example, avoid respiratory irritants such as cigarette smoke and heavy air pollution. Recommend influenza and pneumococcal pneumonia immunizations. Yearly tuberculin testing is recommended for clients with silicosis.

Teach pulmonary hygiene measures, such as maintaining fluid intake, coughing, and deep-breathing exercises. If oxygen therapy is ordered, teach about its use and care of the equipment. Always include teaching about the use and effects of any ordered medications.

If corticosteroid therapy is prescribed, stress the importance of taking the medication as prescribed and not stopping it abruptly. Include information about managing the side effects of corticosteroids by limiting sodium and increasing potassium in the diet, taking the medication with food or milk to minimize gastric irritation, and identifying early signs of infection. See Chapter 11 ⚭ for more information about corticosteroid drugs.

LUNG CANCER

Lung cancer is the leading cause of cancer deaths in the United States, causing an estimated 163,000 deaths in 2005. It has a grim prognosis: Most people with lung cancer die within 1 year of the diagnosis.

Cigarette smoking is the most important cause of lung cancer. About 85% of lung cancer is related to smoking. The disease is 10 to 30 times more common in smokers than nonsmokers. The more the person smokes and the longer the person smokes, the greater the risk. Other risk factors for lung cancer are radiation exposure and inhaled irritants, asbestos in particular.

PATHOPHYSIOLOGY

Most primary lung tumors arise in the cells lining the airways. These tumors differ by cell type, incidence, presentation, and manner of spread (Table 24-7 ■).

Lung cancer tends to be aggressive and locally invasive, and metastasize widely. Tumors begin as mucosal lesions that grow to obstruct the bronchi or invade adjacent tissue. Tumors frequently spread via the lymph system to nodes

and other organs. Lung cancer usually is well advanced when diagnosed, with tumor cells in lymph nodes and distant metastasis.

MANIFESTATIONS AND COMPLICATIONS

Initial symptoms often are blamed on smoking or chronic bronchitis. In addition to manifestations of the tumor and cancer (Box 24-11 ■), lung cancers often produce hormone-like substances that cause indirect symptoms. These are known as *paraneoplastic syndromes* or manifestations.

Lung cancer metastasizes to the lymph nodes, brain, bones, liver, and other organs. Confusion, impaired balance,

---

TABLE 24-7

Lung Cancer Cell Types

	CELL TYPE	LOCATION AND MANIFESTATIONS	SPREAD
	Small-cell (oat cell) carcinoma 20–25% of all lung cancers	Central mass; may cause endocrine symptoms (SIADH, Cushing's syndrome) or thrombophlebitis	Aggressive; distant metastasis common at diagnosis
	Adenocarcinoma 20–40% of all lung cancers	Peripheral mass; few symptoms	Early metastasis to CNS, bone, adrenal glands
	Squamous cell carcinoma 30–32% of all lung cancers	Central mass in large bronchi; cough, dyspnea, atelectasis, wheezing	Spreads by local invasion
	Large-cell carcinoma 10–15% of all lung cancers	Large peripheral lesion; may cause gynecomastia or thrombophlebitis	Early metastasis

BOX 24-11

MANIFESTATIONS OF LUNG CANCER

Local
- Cough, hemoptysis
- Wheezing and dyspnea
- Chest pain, hoarseness or dysphagia

General
- Anorexia, weight loss
- Fever

Paraneoplastic
- Fluid and electrolyte imbalances
- Cushing's syndrome
- Peripheral neuropathy, muscle weakness
- Thrombophlebitis
- Anemia, disseminated intravascular coagulation (DIC)

headache, and personality changes may be symptoms of brain metastasis. Tumor spread to the bone causes bone pain, pathologic fractures, and possible spinal cord compression. When the liver is affected, symptoms may include jaundice, anorexia, and upper right quadrant pain.

Superior vena cava syndrome, partial or complete obstruction of the superior vena cava, is a potential complication. Symptoms such as edema of the neck and face, headache, dizziness, vision changes, and syncope may develop abruptly or gradually. Veins of the upper chest and neck are dilated, and the skin is flushed or cyanotic. Laryngeal edema may cause dyspnea.

INTERDISCIPLINARY CARE

Prevention of lung cancer should be a primary goal for all health care providers. Reducing tobacco use will have a greater positive effect on the death rate from lung cancer than treatment advances.

Diagnostic Tests
- *Chest x-ray* often shows the first evidence of lung cancer.
- Malignant cells may be identified by *sputum cytology.* This test requires a sputum sample on arising.
- A *CT scan* is used to evaluate tumor size and location.
- *Bronchoscopy* may be done to visualize the tumor and obtain a specimen for biopsy. A cable-activated instrument is used to obtain a biopsy specimen. (See Box 22-4 for nursing care of the client undergoing bronchoscopy.)
- A *percutaneous needle biopsy* or aspiration of pleural fluid by *thoracentesis* may be done if the tumor is in the periphery of the lung (see Box 24-15, page 572).

Medications
Combination chemotherapy is the primary treatment for some types of lung cancer. It is used as an adjunct to surgery or radiation for other types. It may lengthen survival when metastases are present. (See Chapter 12 ⬭ for more information about chemotherapy.)

Other medications that may be ordered include bronchodilators to reduce airway obstruction and antibiotics to treat infection. Analgesics are ordered after surgery and for pain management in advanced cancers.

Surgery
Surgery is the only real chance for a cure in most lung cancers. At the time of diagnosis, however, most tumors are beyond the stage at which they can be completely removed. The goal of surgery is to remove all tumor cells, including involved lymph nodes.

The type of surgery depends on the location and size of the tumor, as well as the client's health status (Table 24-8 ■). As much functional lung as possible is preserved. Nursing care of the client having lung surgery is outlined in Box 24-12 ■.

TABLE 24-8

Types of Lung Surgery

PROCEDURE	DESCRIPTION	USED FOR
Laser bronchoscopy	Bronchoscopy used to guide laser to resect tumor	Tumors localized in a main bronchus
Thoracotomy	Incision into the chest wall	Gain access to the lung for surgery
Wedge resection	Removal of a small section (wedge) of lung tissue	Small, peripheral lesions
Segmental resection	Removal of a single bronchovascular segment of a lobe	Localized peripheral lung tumors
Lobectomy	Removal of a single lung lobe	Tumors confined to a single lobe
Pneumonectomy	Removal of an entire lung	Tumors throughout a lung, in the main bronchus, or fixed to the hilum

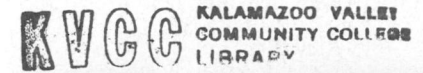

BOX 24-12 **NURSING CARE CHECKLIST**

Lung Surgery

Before Surgery

☑ Provide routine preoperative care and teaching (see Chapter 9). ⦾

☑ Obtain baseline assessment data, particularly respiratory and cardiovascular status.

☑ Reinforce teaching, allowing time to practice breathing and coughing techniques.

☑ Establish a way to communicate if an endotracheal tube will be in place after surgery.

☑ Introduce to intensive care unit and policies if client will return there after surgery.

After Surgery

☑ Assess and provide routine postoperative care (Chapter 9). ⦾

☑ Frequently assess respiratory status (color, rate and depth, chest expansion, lung sounds, and oxygen saturation). Promptly report changes to the charge nurse or physician.

☑ Assist with coughing, postural drainage, and incentive spirometry. Suction as needed while intubated.

☑ Maintain chest tube drainage system. Initially measure output hourly, then every 2 to 4 or 8 hours as indicated. Notify physician if output exceeds 70 mL/hr and/or is bright red, warm, and free flowing.

☑ Assist to move in bed and ambulate as soon as possible.

Radiation Therapy

Radiation therapy is used alone or in combination with surgery or chemotherapy. Before surgery, it is used to shrink tumors. When surgery is not an option, radiation therapy may be the treatment of choice. Complications such as superior vena cava syndrome may be treated with radiation. (Radiation therapy is discussed further in Chapter 12. ⦾)

Other Therapies

Pleural effusion is a frequent complication of lung cancer. As fluid collects, the lung cannot fully expand and ventilation is impaired. A *thoracentesis* may be done to remove the excess pleural fluid. (See Box 24-15 on page 572 for nursing care related to a thoracentesis.)

NURSING CARE

ASSESSING

Obtain complete respiratory assessment data. Include smoking history and the duration of current symptoms. Obtain data related to both respiratory and cardiovascular status, especially if surgery is anticipated. Review laboratory and diagnostic test results, and report abnormal values to the charge nurse or physician.

Assess for concerns related to lung function, the cancer itself, and the planned treatment.

DIAGNOSING, PLANNING, AND IMPLEMENTING

Priorities in Nursing Care. The effects of the tumor and of surgery on breathing and gas exchange are the highest priorities for nursing care related to physiologic function. Because lung cancer frequently cannot be cured, its psychologic and emotional effects on the client and family also are high priorities for caring.

Ineffective Breathing Pattern

■ Assess and document respiratory status at least every 4 hours; more frequently as indicated. *Early identification of altered respiratory function is important to maintain tissue oxygenation.*

■ Report abnormal oxygen saturation levels and blood gas results to the charge nurse or physician. *Changes in blood oxygen levels may indicate respiratory compromise.*

■ Elevate the head of the bed to 60 degrees. *Elevating the head of the bed promotes lung expansion.*

■ Assist to turn, cough, deep breathe, and use incentive spirometer. Help splint the chest with a pillow or blanket when coughing. *These measures promote airway clearance.*

■ Administer oxygen as ordered. *Supplemental oxygen improves alveolar oxygenation and gas exchange.*

■ Suction as needed. *Pharyngeal suctioning may be required when the client is unable to clear secretions by coughing.*

■ Assist with percussion and postural drainage as ordered. *Percussion and postural drainage help clear airways and maintain effective respirations.*

■ Provide reassurance and emotional support. *Relief of anxiety promotes a more effective breathing pattern.*

Activity Intolerance

Loss of functional lung tissue due to the tumor or surgery affects the ability to maintain normal activities.

■ Document responses to activity, including pulse, respiratory rate, dyspnea, and fatigue. *Tachycardia, tachypnea, dyspnea, or fatigue with activities is a sign of activity intolerance.*

■ Plan rest periods interspersed with activities and procedures. *Rest periods reduce oxygen demands and fatigue.*

■ Assist to increase activities gradually. *Gradual increases in activity improve exercise tolerance.*

■ Teach energy conservation measures, such as sitting while showering and dressing and wearing slip-on shoes. *These measures reduce oxygen demand and promote independence.*

■ Keep frequently used objects within easy reach. *This helps conserve energy.*

- Encourage to remain as active as possible. *Maintaining activity levels improves physical and emotional well-being.*
- Allow family members to provide assistance as needed. *This helps the client conserve energy and allows the family to feel useful.*

Pain

- Assess and document pain. *Remember that pain is subjective; however, reluctance to cough or move may indicate unreported pain.*
- Provide analgesics as needed to maintain comfort. *Adequate pain relief promotes postoperative recovery and coping. Good pain management is vital to improve recovery from surgery and to allow a peaceful death for the terminal cancer client.*
- For cancer pain, maintain a continuous medication schedule using opiates, NSAIDs, and other drugs as ordered. *Addiction is not a concern for the terminal cancer client; adequate pain relief that does not allow "breakthrough" pain is vital.*
- Use adjunctive pain relief measures, such as massage, positioning, distraction, and relaxation techniques. *These techniques promote relaxation and enhance pain relief.*
- Encourage activities that distract from pain such as reading, television, and social interactions. *Distraction helps the client focus away from the pain.*
- Allow significant others to remain with the client. *Physical presence provides emotional support.*

Anticipatory Grieving

- Spend time with the client and family. *Time is necessary to develop a trusting, therapeutic relationship.*
- Answer questions honestly; do not deny the probable outcome of the disease. *Honesty reinforces reality and promotes a sense of control over decisions to be made.*
- Encourage expression of feelings, fears, and concerns. *Open communication helps promote understanding and acceptance.*
- Assist to understand the grieving process and to accept responses as normal. *Explanation enhances understanding of the grieving process and the ability to cope.*
- Help identify strengths and effective coping measures. *Past successes in coping with crises can help with the present situation and help the client develop a sense of control.*
- Encourage use of other support systems, such as spiritual and social groups. Refer to support groups, social services, and hospice care as indicated. Provide American Cancer Society literature and information as appropriate. *These support systems can help the client and family cope with the diagnosis.*
- Discuss advance directives (the living will and durable power of attorney for health care). *These documents give more control over treatment when the client is no longer able to express his or her own wishes.*

EVALUATING

Collect data related to the client's respiratory status, ability to complete ADLs and other activities, pain control, and acceptance of the probable outcome of the disease to evaluate the effectiveness of nursing care.

Documenting. Document continuing assessment data, particularly during the early postoperative period if surgery has been performed. Assess for and document any adverse responses to other cancer treatments such as chemotherapy and radiation therapy (see Chapter 12). Note the client's and family's response to the diagnosis and treatment plan. Document any referrals provided, such as home health care or hospice.

CONTINUING CARE

Provide honest information about lung cancer, the expected outcome, and planned treatment. Do not promote false hope.

Stress the importance of stopping smoking, especially if surgery has been done. The client with lung cancer may have difficulty recognizing the need to stop smoking. Include information about the effects of nicotine and the tars in cigarette smoke on healing and already compromised lung tissue (Box 24-13 ■).

BOX 24-13	**CLIENT TEACHING**

Cigarette Smoking

Tobacco was first used in religious ceremonies and to offer friendship. At one time, it was thought to help cure many common diseases. Tobacco is now known as the leading preventable cause of illness in the world.

Cigarette smoke contains about 4,000 chemicals, including nicotine. Nicotine is highly addictive, producing a feeling of well-being. Tar, the particulate matter in cigarette smoke, causes most of its ill effects in the lungs. Smoke paralyzes cilia, reducing clearance of tars from the bronchial tree.

To help the client quit smoking:

- Help identify barriers and obstacles to quitting.
- Teach about nicotine's addictive properties.
- Explain that withdrawal may cause anxiety, irritability, headache, and insomnia.
- Help develop a plan with a target date to quit and ways to deal with obstacles, withdrawal symptoms, and the temptation to resume smoking.
- Offer self-help material at an appropriate reading level.
- Refer to a counselor, physician, or smoking-cessation clinic.
- Reassure that relapse is common. Continue to provide support and encouragement, helping avoid further relapses.

In addition, help prevent children and teens from starting to smoke:

- Provide education programs to help them avoid smoking.
- Reduce minors' access to tobacco, especially cigarettes and chewing tobacco (often the first product used by teenage boys).

Provide information about planned treatments, explaining expected effects and usual side effects of each. Help identify ways to cope with noxious effects. If surgery has been done, discuss activities and exercises to improve strength and regain function. Stress the need to continue coughing and deep-breathing exercises at home. Provide information about symptoms to report to the physician: fever, increasing dyspnea, cough, increased or purulent sputum, redness, pain, swelling, or incisional drainage.

Discuss medication use, including desired and adverse effects and interactions with other drugs or foods. Teach how to use analgesics and other pain relief measures.

Provide information about hospice services, home health, cancer support groups, and American Cancer Society services.

PULMONARY VASCULAR DISORDERS

The cardiovascular and respiratory systems are closely linked. A good match of airflow and blood flow is essential to maintain gas exchange and oxygen delivery to all body tissues and organs. Disorders previously discussed in this chapter affect airflow; this section discusses disorders that affect blood flow to the lungs.

Pulmonary Embolism

A **pulmonary embolism** is blockage of a pulmonary artery that disrupts blood flow to the lung. *Thromboemboli,* or blood clots, are the most common pulmonary emboli. Tumors, bone marrow fat, amniotic fluid, and foreign matter also can become emboli. Because a large pulmonary embolism can be fatal, prevention is the best treatment.

PATHOPHYSIOLOGY

Most pulmonary emboli begin as clots in the deep veins of the legs or pelvis. The risk factors are those for deep venous thrombosis (DVT): impaired venous blood flow, blood vessel damage, and altered coagulation. Prolonged immobility is the primary risk factor; others are discussed in Chapter 28 ⬤.

Deep venous thrombosis may not be suspected until pulmonary embolism occurs. When the clot breaks loose from the vein wall, it travels through vessels that become gradually larger until it reaches the right side of the heart and enters the pulmonary artery. The pulmonary arteries and arterioles become smaller and smaller, and the clot is trapped, obstructing blood flow. No blood flows through capillaries beyond the occlusion, so no gas exchange occurs in that portion of the lung. A large clot can obstruct blood flow to a major part of the lung, causing sudden death.

Manifestations

The symptoms of a pulmonary embolism depend on its size and location (Box 24-14 ■). Small emboli may go unnoticed; larger emboli cause manifestations similar to a myocardial infarction (heart attack).

Fat emboli may occur after a long bone fracture (e.g., the femur) that releases bone marrow fat. Fat emboli cause a sudden onset of dyspnea, tachypnea, tachycardia, confusion, delirium, and decreased level of consciousness. *Petechiae* may be seen on the chest and arms.

INTERDISCIPLINARY CARE

Preventive measures include elastic stockings (TED hose), pneumatic compression devices, anticoagulation therapy, and early ambulation to prevent venous stasis. Elevating the legs of immobilized clients and leg exercises also help prevent venous stasis and pulmonary emboli.

Treatment of a pulmonary embolism is supportive. Oxygen is given, and analgesics may be ordered to relieve pain and anxiety. Pulmonary artery and wedge pressures are monitored with a balloon (Swan–Ganz) catheter. The client is monitored for dysrhythmias.

Diagnostic Tests

Plasma D-dimer levels are specific to the presence of a thrombus; elevated levels indicate formation of a blood clot. When a pulmonary embolism is suspected, a *ventilation-perfusion scan* may be ordered to evaluate blood flow in the pulmonary circulation (Figure 24-10 ■). *Pulmonary angiography* uses a contrast media to evaluate pulmonary circulation. This procedure has a higher risk than the lung scan. Other diagnostic tests may include chest x-ray, ECG to rule out myocardial infarction, and coagulation studies.

Medications

A thrombolytic drug (e.g., streptokinase, urokinase, or t-PA) may be given to disintegrate a large pulmonary embolus and restore pulmonary blood flow. The primary risk of

---

BOX 24-14

MANIFESTATIONS OF PULMONARY EMBOLISM
- Abrupt onset of dyspnea, chest pain
- Anxiety, apprehension
- Cough
- Tachycardia, tachypnea
- Diaphoresis
- Cyanosis

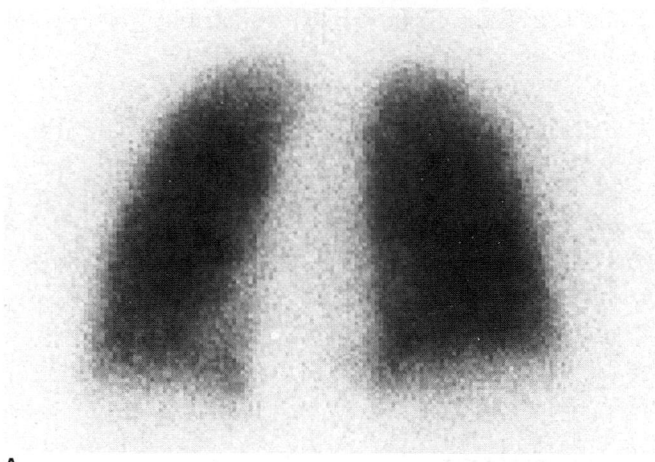

A

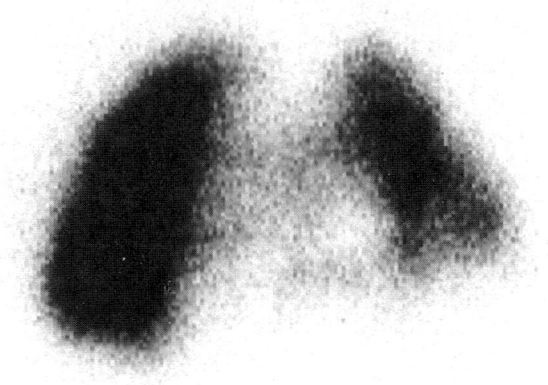

B

Figure 24-10. ■ (A) A normal lung scan showing perfusion of all areas of the lungs. (B) A lung scan showing impaired blood flow to the right lung due to pulmonary embolus. (Courtesy of University of California Davis Medical Center.)

thrombolytic therapy is bleeding, particularly intracranial bleeding. See Chapter 26 ⬭ for more information about thrombolytic therapy and its nursing implications.

Anticoagulants are ordered to prevent further clotting and embolization. Low-dose heparin is given to prevent DVT. When pulmonary embolus has occurred, an intravenous heparin infusion is ordered. The activated partial thromboplastin time (APTT) or PTT is monitored, and the client is assessed for signs of abnormal bleeding. Heparin is continued until oral anticoagulant (warfarin) therapy is fully effective, 5 to 7 days after its initiation. Anticoagulants are continued for 2 to 3 months or longer. Bleeding is a risk for any client taking anticoagulants. (See Table 28-5 ⬭ for nursing implications of anticoagulants.)

Surgery

An umbrella-like filter may be inserted into the inferior vena cava of clients who have recurrent pulmonary emboli. This device traps large emboli while allowing blood to flow through the vena cava (Figure 24-11 ■).

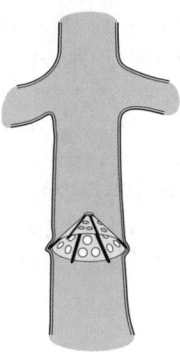

Figure 24-11. ■ Example of a vena caval filter to prevent emboli from reaching the lungs.

NURSING CARE

When a pulmonary embolus occurs, the client has urgent nursing care needs and may be transferred to intensive care for close observation and monitoring.

ASSESSING

Because pulmonary embolism can be a medical emergency, assessment often is very focused. Inquire about chest pain, shortness of breath and other manifestations. Ask about risk factors such as recent diagnosis of venous thrombosis, surgery, childbirth, or malignancy.

Objective assessment data include level of consciousness; vital signs including heart and respiratory rate; skin color and temperature; heart and breath sounds; oxygen saturation; and neck vein distention.

clinical ALERT

A large pulmonary embolus may cause cardiac and respiratory arrest. Immediately initiate cardiopulmonary resuscitation (CPR) procedures if the client is unresponsive and pulse and respirations are absent.

DIAGNOSING, PLANNING, AND IMPLEMENTING

Priorities in Nursing Care. Prevention of DVT and pulmonary embolism is a priority of nursing care for all clients at risk. When pulmonary embolism does occur, maintaining effective gas exchange is of highest priority.

Risk for Ineffective Tissue Perfusion: Cardiopulmonary

- Encourage early ambulation following surgery or illness.
- Apply elastic stockings or pneumatic compression devices as ordered.

- Assist with leg exercises.
- Discourage using pillows under the knees. *These measures promote venous return from the legs, reducing venous stasis and the risk for DVT and pulmonary emboli.*

Impaired Gas Exchange

- Frequently assess respiratory status, including rate, depth, effort, and lung sounds. *Maintaining optimal ventilation facilitates gas exchange in well-perfused areas of the lung.*
- Report changes in level of consciousness, mental status, and skin color to the charge nurse or physician. *A change in LOC or mental status and/or cyanosis may indicate hypoxemia.*
- Place in Fowler's or high-Fowler's position. *This position promotes lung expansion and ventilation.*
- Start oxygen by nasal cannula or mask as ordered. *Supplemental oxygen increases alveolar and arterial oxygenation.*
- Report low oxygen saturation levels and abnormal arterial blood gas results. *ABGs and pulse oximetry are used to assess gas exchange and the effect of interventions.*
- Maintain bed rest. *Bed rest reduces oxygen demands.*

Decreased Cardiac Output

A large pulmonary embolus can affect cardiac output and tissue perfusion.

- Assess vital signs every 15 to 30 minutes initially, then every 2 to 4 hours as indicated. *Frequent assessment is important during the early, unstable period following pulmonary embolus.*
- Record hourly urine output. *Decreased urine output may indicate impaired renal perfusion.*
- Assess skin color, temperature, and capillary refill. *These assessments are used to evaluate tissue perfusion.*
- Monitor cardiac rhythm. *Monitoring allows early detection and treatment of dysrhythmias.*
- Assess for and report neck vein distention and peripheral edema. *Right-sided heart failure may result from pulmonary embolism due to increased pulmonary pressures.*
- Maintain intravenous and arterial lines. *The client may be unstable and critically ill, requiring immediate interventions to maintain life.*
- Provide frequent skin care. *Impaired peripheral perfusion and tissue oxygenation increase the risk of skin breakdown.*
- Instruct to report chest pain or other symptoms. *Decreased cardiac output and an increased workload may cause angina.*

Anxiety

- Reassure and provide emotional support. Accept fear of dying, and reassure that treatment usually restores respiratory function. *The fear of death is very real; reassurance helps relieve excess anxiety.*

- Remain with the client as much as possible. *This helps reduce anxiety.*
- Explain procedures and treatments, using short, simple sentences. *Simple explanations reduce fear of the unknown.*
- Reduce environmental stimuli, and use a calm, reassuring manner. *These measures help reduce anxiety in both the nurse and the client.*
- Allow family members to remain present as much as possible. *Calm, supportive family members provide further reassurance.*
- Administer morphine as ordered. *Morphine reduces both pain and anxiety.*

EVALUATING

To evaluate the effectiveness of nursing care for the client who is at risk for a pulmonary embolism, collect assessment data related to ambulation, manifestations of deep venous thrombosus, and respiratory status on a continuing basis. For the client who experiences a pulmonary embolism, frequently evaluate mental status, respiratory status, and cardiovascular status, reporting significant changes to the physician or charge nurse. Assess the client's return to previous health status after resolution of the acute event.

Documenting. Document measures instituted to prevent DVT and pulmonary embolism (e.g., leg exercises, ambulation, application of elastic hose or pneumatic compression devices) in all clients at risk. Document assessment data related to DVT, including complaints of calf or leg pain, swelling, redness, warmth, or a positive Homan's sign. Regularly document respiratory assessment data, noting any changes from previous findings. If a pulmonary embolism develops, document initial subjective and objective assessment data, emergency care measures instituted, and the client's response to treatment. Document personnel notified, including the physician. Note diagnostic tests performed. If the client is transferred to an acute care facility or critical care unit, document the transfer.

CONTINUING CARE

Teach clients to reduce the risk for DVT and pulmonary embolism:

- On automobile trips, stop every 1 to 2 hours for a brief stretch and walk to restore venous circulation.
- During long flights, get up every hour or so, and do leg exercises while seated.
- Do not cross legs.
- Exercise regularly (e.g., walking).
- Wear elastic hose when standing for prolonged periods. Avoid hose that bind around the knee or thigh.

Teach about prescribed anticoagulants, including symptoms of bleeding to report to the physician. Instruct to use a soft toothbrush and avoid taking aspirin (unless prescribed) and other over-the-counter drugs without the doctor's approval. Stress the importance of wearing an identification bracelet or tag to alert medical personnel about anticoagulant use.

Pulmonary Hypertension and Cor Pulmonale

Arterial pressure in the pulmonary system normally is low (25/8) compared with the systemic BP (120/80). **Pulmonary hypertension** is an abnormal elevation of the pulmonary arterial pressure. It can develop with no obvious cause, or may occur as a result of chronic lung disease or another problem. Long-standing pulmonary hypertension can lead to *cor pulmonale,* with right ventricular hypertrophy and failure. COPD is the usual cause of cor pulmonale.

Manifestations of pulmonary hypertension include increasing dyspnea, fatigue, angina, and syncope (fainting or light-headedness) with exertion. Clients with cor pulmonale have a chronic productive cough, progressive dyspnea, wheezing, and signs of right heart failure (peripheral edema and distended neck veins). The skin is warm, moist, and dusky red.

Supplemental oxygen and drugs such as calcium channel blockers may be ordered for pulmonary hypertension. Rapid-acting direct vasodilators such as inhaled nitric oxide may be ordered. Salt and water intake may be restricted. Bilateral lung or heart–lung transplant may be done for primary pulmonary hypertension.

Nursing care is supportive, focusing on the underlying lung disease. *Impaired Gas Exchange* is a significant problem, as are problems such as *Activity Intolerance, Anxiety, Fatigue,* and others. See nursing assessment and interventions for COPD and for heart failure.

Provide information about pulmonary hypertension and cor pulmonale as appropriate. Include the disease process, and manifestations to report to the physician, including change in activity tolerance, increased edema, and signs of respiratory infection or exacerbation. Discuss the importance of planned rest periods between activities and ways to conserve energy, such as using a shower chair. Stress the importance of not smoking due to its effects on the lungs and blood vessels. As always, teach about the purpose, use, and effects of medications.

PLEURAL DISORDERS AND TRAUMA

A closed chest cavity with negative pressure in the pleural space (the potential space between the visceral and parietal pleura) is necessary for breathing. (Review the mechanics of breathing in Chapter 22. ⬭) Excess fluid, air, or blood in the pleural space interferes with lung expansion and breathing. Chest and lung injury can result from penetrating or blunt trauma or inhalation injury. Assessment of airway, breathing, and circulation (ABCs) is vital in these disorders.

Pleuritis

Pleuritis (pleurisy) is inflammation of the pleura that covers the lung surface and lines the inner chest wall. Pleuritis usually results from another process, such as a viral infection, pneumonia, or rib injury.

The onset of pleuritis is often abrupt, with characteristic *pleuritic* pain. Pleuritic pain is sharp or stabbing and usually very localized. Deep breathing, coughing, and movement aggravate the pain. Breathing is rapid and shallow, and breath sounds are diminished. A *pleural friction rub* or harsh, grating sound, may be heard over the affected area.

Treatment of pleuritis includes analgesics and NSAIDs to relieve the pain. Codeine may be ordered to relieve pain and suppress the cough.

Nursing care focuses on promoting comfort. Positioning and splinting the chest while coughing can be helpful. Wrapping the chest with 6-inch-wide elastic bandages may help relieve pain; care must be taken, however, to ensure that the lungs are still fully ventilated.

Advise that pleuritis usually lasts only a short time and resolves spontaneously. Instruct to report symptoms such as increased fever, productive cough, difficulty breathing, or shortness of breath to the physician. Discuss appropriate use of and precautions when taking NSAIDs and recommended analgesics.

Pleural Effusion

Pleural effusion is a collection of excess fluid in the pleural space. Pleural effusions result from respiratory disorders (e.g., pneumonia, lung cancer, or trauma) or from systemic diseases such as heart failure or kidney disease.

A large pleural effusion presses on lung tissue, causing dyspnea and shortness of breath. Breath sounds are diminished or absent, and the affected area may sound dull when percussed. Chest wall movement may be limited.

When pleural effusion interferes with breathing, a *thoracentesis* may be done to remove the fluid. A large needle is inserted into the pleural space to remove the excess fluid

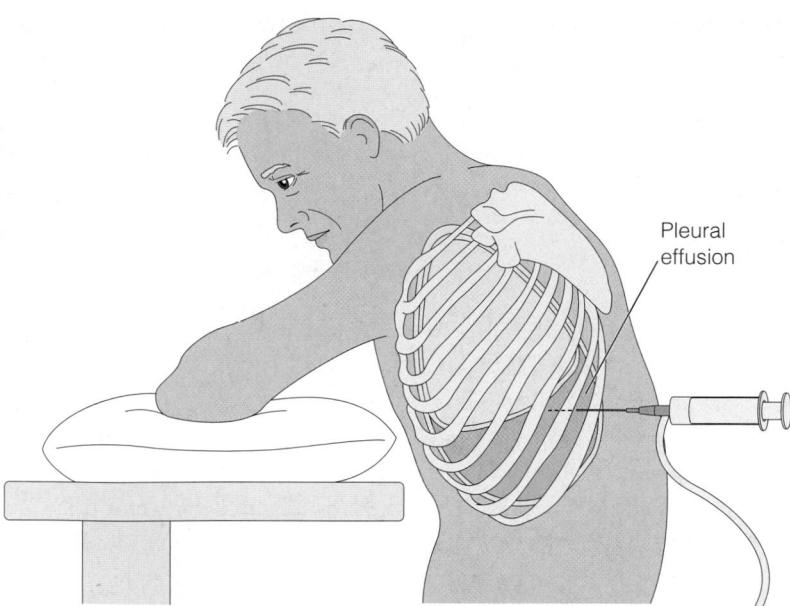

Pleural
effusion

Figure 24-12. ■ Thoracentesis. A needle is inserted between the ribs into the pleural space to withdraw excess pleural fluid.

(Figure 24-12 ■). Thoracentesis may be done at the bedside. Local anesthesia is used. The procedure requires less than 30 minutes to complete. Nursing care for the client undergoing a thoracentesis is outlined in Box 24-15 ■.

Nursing care focuses on supporting respiratory function and assisting with procedures such as thoracentesis. With a large pleural effusion, diagnoses of Impaired Gas Exchange and Activity Intolerance are high-priority nursing problems. Following thoracentesis, it is important to monitor for complications such as pneumothorax.

Teaching focuses on symptoms of recurrent effusion or complications after thoracentesis that should be reported to the physician. Instruct to report increasing dyspnea or shortness of breath, cough, hemoptysis, or pleuritic pain.

Pneumothorax

Accumulation of air in the pleural space is called **pneumothorax.** Pneumothorax can occur without apparent cause, due to chronic lung disease, or as a result of trauma.

BOX 24-15 **NURSING CARE CHECKLIST**

Thoracentesis

Before the Procedure

☑ Verify a signed consent for this procedure has been obtained.

☑ Reinforce teaching.

☑ Administer cough suppressant if ordered.

☑ Bring supplies to the client's room: thoracentesis tray, sterile gloves, local anesthetic, antiseptic solution, dressing, and an extra over-bed table or Mayo stand.

☑ Position client sitting on side of bed, leaning forward with arms and head supported on an anchored over-bed table.

☑ Advise that pressure may be felt when the needle is inserted, but no pain should be experienced.

During the Procedure

☑ Support and assist client to remain still and in position during the procedure.

☑ Provide psychologic support as needed.

☑ Monitor respirations, pulse, and color, informing the physician of any changes.

After the Procedure

☑ Apply dressing to puncture site.

☑ Position client on unaffected side for 1 hour.

☑ Label any specimens (name, date, source, and diagnosis); send to laboratory for analysis.

☑ Record vital signs, breath sounds, and cough and assess for bleeding or crepitus at puncture site every 15 minutes × 4, every 30 minutes × 2, then every 2 to 4 hours or as indicated.

☑ Obtain chest x-ray.

☑ Allow resumption of normal activities after 1 hour if no complications develop.

TABLE 24-9

Types of Pneumothorax

	TYPE	PATHOPHYSIOLOGY	MANIFESTATIONS
Normal lung — Pleural space	Spontaneous	Rupture of a bleb (blister) on lung surface allows air from lungs into pleural space. ■ *Primary* occurs in previously healthy people, usually young men. Smoking is a risk factor. ■ *Secondary* affects people with COPD and other chronic lung diseases.	Abrupt onset Pleuritic chest pain Shortness of breath Tachypnea, tachycardia Unequal chest movement Decreased breath sounds on affected side Hyperresonant percussion tone
Puncture wound through chest wall	Traumatic	Result of chest trauma. ■ *Open* due to penetrating trauma that allows air from outside to enter pleural space. ■ *Closed* occurs when torn visceral pleura allows air from lung to enter pleural space; rib fracture a common cause. ■ *Iatrogenic* due to laceration of visceral pleura during a procedure such as central line insertion.	Pain Dyspnea Tachypnea, tachycardia Decreased chest movement Absent breath sounds on affected side Air movement through an open wound
Mediastinal shift to unaffected side — Wound in chest wall allows air to enter pleural space but not to escape	Tension	Air enters pleural space through chest wall or from lungs but is unable to escape. Air accumulates rapidly, causing collapse of lung on affected side. Heart, great vessels, trachea, and esophagus shift toward unaffected side.	Hypotension, shock Severe dyspnea Tachypnea, tachycardia Decreased chest wall movement Absent breath sounds on affected side Trachea deviates toward unaffected side

PATHOPHYSIOLOGY

When the pleura is breached, air enters the pleural space. Pressure in the pleural space is no longer negative, and the lung on the affected side collapses. A small portion of the lung or the entire lung may be affected, depending on the amount and rate of air accumulation. Table 24-9 ■ illustrates and summarizes the major types of pneumothorax.

When a bleb on the lung surface ruptures (*spontaneous pneumothorax*), air moves freely into and out of the pleural space. As a result, the pneumothorax often is small. A gunshot wound or stab wound to the chest causes a *traumatic open pneumothorax (sucking chest wound)* that allows air to move freely through the chest wall. In a *tension pneumothorax,* injury to the chest wall or lungs allows air into the pleural space but prevents it from escaping. Air accumulates rapidly, and the lung on the affected side collapses. The heart, great vessels, and trachea shift to the unaffected side of the chest, placing pressure on the opposite lung.

clinical ALERT

Tension pneumothorax is a medical emergency requiring immediate intervention to maintain the airway, breathing, and circulation.

MANIFESTATIONS

The manifestations of spontaneous pneumothorax depend on the size of the pneumothorax, extent of lung collapse, and any underlying lung disease. *Primary pneumothorax* typically affects tall, slender young adult men who are otherwise healthy. *Secondary pneumothorax* occurs in people with preexisting lung disease, usually COPD. Both primary and secondary pneumothorax are heralded by an abrupt onset of pleuritic chest pain and shortness of breath. Tachypnea and tachycardia develop, and there is less chest wall movement on the affected side. Breath sounds are diminished on the affected side. Clients with secondary pneumothorax have a higher risk of developing severe hypoxemia and respiratory failure as a result of pneumothorax.

Although the manifestations of traumatic pneumothorax are similar, they may be unrecognized due to the presence of other injuries. If a penetrating wound is present, air can be heard and felt moving into and out of the wound. In tension pneumothorax, additional manifestations of deviation of the trachea toward the unaffected side, hypotension and possible shock, and distended neck veins are seen.

INTERDISCIPLINARY CARE

Diagnostic Tests

Often pneumothorax can be diagnosed simply by its manifestations. Oxygen saturation is measured to determine its effect on gas exchange. A chest X-ray is obtained to determine the size and extent of the pneumothorax.

Treatment

Treatment of pneumothorax depends on its severity. In a small simple pneumothorax, air is gradually reabsorbed, and the lung reexpands. With a larger pneumothorax, the air is removed from the pleural space to allow the collapsed lung to reexpand. A *thoracentesis* may be done by inserting a needle into the pleural space to withdraw air. Review Box 24-15 for nursing care of a client having a thoracentesis. A catheter with a one-way valve may be inserted into the pleural space. The one-way valve allows air to leave the pleural space but prevents it from entering.

Chest Tubes

The usual treatment for pneumothorax is *chest tubes* connected to a closed-drainage system. The drainage system has a one-way valve or a "water seal" that prevents air from entering the chest cavity during inspiration and allows air to escape during expiration. Applying low suction to the system helps reestablish negative pressure, allowing the lung to reexpand.

Several closed-drainage systems are available. Some use water to prevent air from entering the pleural space and to regulate suction (Figure 24-13 ■). Others are "dry" systems that include a mechanical one-way valve to prevent air entry and a suction regulator. Chest tube drainage collects in a graduated chamber that allows easy measurement. To ensure system function, it is important to prevent damage and maintain the integrity of all tubes and connections. Box 24-16 ■ outlines nursing care for a client with chest tubes.

NURSING CARE

Restoring ventilation and gas exchange is the highest priority of care for the client with a pneumothorax.

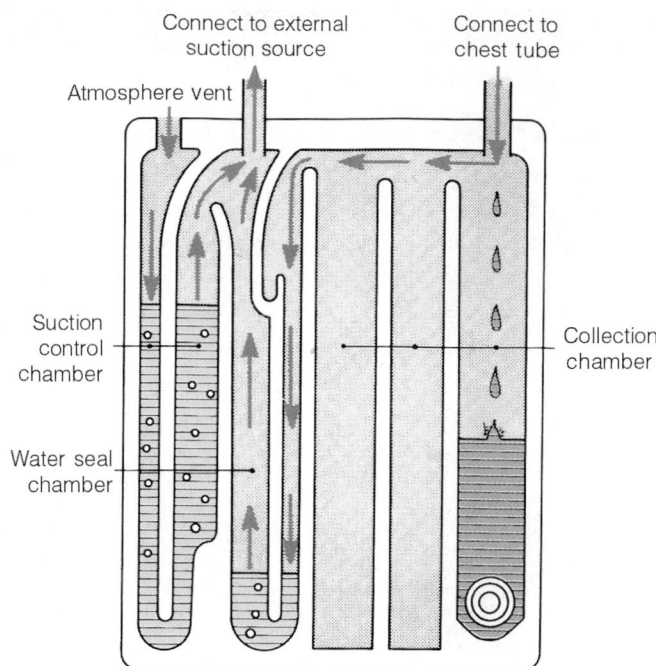

Figure 24-13. ■ A closed chest drainage system.

ASSESSING

Collect assessment data from clients with risk factors for pneumothorax, such as chest or abdominal trauma (e.g., motor vehicle crash or fall from a height), COPD, or procedures such as central line insertion or thoracentesis. Assess clients with known pneumothorax for the effect of treatment measures. Ask about chest pain or difficulty breathing. Inquire about previous history of pneumothorax or chronic lung disease. Obtain smoking history.

Assess respiratory status, including dyspnea, rate and depth of respirations, chest wall movement, and lung sounds. Note level of consciousness and skin color. Observe neck veins for distention and position of trachea.

clinical ALERT

Immediately notify the physician if the trachea is displaced toward one side. This could indicate tension pneumothorax, a medical emergency that requires immediate treatment.

DIAGNOSING, PLANNING, AND IMPLEMENTING

Priorities in Nursing Care. The priority for nursing care of the client with pneumothorax is the effect of the condition on gas exchange and tissue oxygenation.

BOX 24-16	NURSING CARE CHECKLIST

Chest Tubes

Before the Procedure

☑ Verify a signed consent for the procedure has been obtained.

☑ Reinforce teaching. Local anesthesia will be used; pressure may be felt during insertion. Breathing will improve when the chest tube is in place.

☑ Gather supplies as indicated: thoracostomy tray, local anesthetic, sterile gloves, drainage system, sterile water to fill water seal and suction chambers.

☑ Position as ordered for the procedure.

During the Procedure

☑ Assist as needed. Provide physical and psychologic support.

☑ Notify physician of changes in respiratory rate and effort, pulse, and color.

After the Procedure

☑ Document vital signs, breath sounds, oxygen saturation, color, and respiratory effort at least every 4 hours.

☑ Maintain closed system. Tape all connections; secure chest tube to chest wall.

☑ Keep collection device below chest level.

☑ Check tubes frequently for kinks or loops.

☑ If water seal system is used:

   ☑ Frequently check water seal chamber. The water level should fluctuate with respiratory effort; if it does not, the system may not be patent or intact. Periodic air bubbles in the water seal chamber are normal and indicate that trapped air is being removed from the chest.

   ☑ Keep the device upright.

   ☑ Add water to the suction control chamber as needed.

☑ Measure drainage every 8 hours, marking the level on the drainage chamber. Do not empty the chamber. Report drainage that is cloudy, in excess of 70 mL/hr, or red, warm, and free flowing.

☑ When chest tube is removed, immediately apply sterile occlusive dressing.

Impaired Gas Exchange

When the lung collapses, gas exchange no longer occurs in the affected part of the lung.

- Document vital signs, oxygen saturation, and respiratory status at least every 4 hours. *Frequent assessment is necessary to monitor response to impaired lung function and treatment.*
- Place in Fowler's or high Fowler's position. *This position facilitates lung expansion.*
- Administer oxygen as ordered. *Supplemental oxygen improves blood oxygen levels.*
- Provide emotional support. *Dyspnea and hypoxemia are frightening and produce anxiety.*
- Assist with frequent position changes and ambulation. *Movement promotes lung ventilation.*
- Provide rest. *Rest conserves energy and reduces oxygen demands.*

Risk for Injury

- Assess chest tube and drainage system at least every 2 hours. *The system must remain patent and intact to function effectively. Inadvertent removal of a chest tube or damage to the closed-drainage system allow air and pathogens to enter the chest cavity.*
- Secure chest tubes to chest wall and prevent tension on the tubes during care and ambulation. *Chest tubes are minimally secured with a suture and can be dislodged during activity.*
- Secure drainage tubing to sheet or gown. *Looping the drainage tubing prevents direct pressure on the chest tube itself.*

- Prevent kinking or occlusion of chest or drainage tube during repositioning. *This maintains the patency of the tubing.*
- Teach to keep drainage system below the level of the chest when sitting or ambulating. Suction usually can be disconnected during ambulation. *Ambulation promotes lung ventilation and reexpansion. Keeping the system lower than the chest promotes drainage.*
- Observe insertion site for redness, swelling, pain, or drainage. Report fever or signs of infection to the physician. *Disruption of skin integrity increases the risk for infection.*
- Immediately reconnect any disrupted connections. *A closed system is vital to prevent air from entering the pleural space.*
- If the tube is inadvertently removed, promptly seal the wound with a sterile occlusive dressing. If a sterile dressing is not available, use other occlusive material such as foil or plastic wrap. Tape dressing on three sides only. *An occlusive dressing taped on three sides allows air to escape through the wound but prevents air from entering the wound on inhalation.*

EVALUATING

Frequently assess respiratory status and oxygenation to evaluate the effectiveness of nursing care.

Documenting. Document continuing respiratory assessment data, including the amount of drainage and functioning of the closed chest drainage system. Document all teaching provided. Note if referral to a smoking cessation program has been made, and the client's responsiveness to quitting smoking.

CONTINUING CARE

Clients who have had a spontaneous pneumothorax have a 50% risk of recurrence. Stress the importance of quitting smoking to reduce the risk. Advise avoiding activities that can increase the risk, such as mountain climbing, flying in unpressurized aircraft, scuba diving, and possibly contact sports.

Instruct to gradually increase exercise and activity to previous levels. Stress the importance of follow-up care and monitoring. Advise to report the following to the physician: upper respiratory infection; fever, cough, or difficulty breathing; sudden, sharp chest pain; or redness, pain, swelling, tenderness, or drainage from the chest tube puncture wound.

Hemothorax

Hemothorax, blood in the pleural space, usually results from chest trauma or surgery. When blood collects in the pleural space, pressure on the affected lung impairs ventilation and gas exchange.

Hemothorax causes symptoms similar to those of a pneumothorax. Lung sounds are decreased. A dull percussion tone is heard over the collection of blood, usually at the lung base. Chest x-ray is used to confirm the diagnosis of hemothorax.

Thoracentesis or chest tubes are used to remove blood from the pleural space. With significant hemorrhage (e.g., following trauma or surgery), the blood may be collected for reinfusion.

Nursing care focuses on maintaining respirations, gas exchange, and cardiac output. In a large, slow-developing hemothorax, respiratory status is the primary concern. Nursing diagnoses and interventions are similar to those for pneumothorax. When hemothorax develops rapidly and hemorrhage is significant, shock is a risk (see Chapter 13). ⬯

Chest and Lung Trauma

Trauma, or injury due to an external source, can affect the chest wall as well as the lung itself. Chest wall injuries (including fractured ribs, flail chest, and underlying damage to lung tissue), smoke inhalation, and near-drowning are commonly seen.

RIB FRACTURE

Simple rib fracture, usually of a single rib, is the most common chest wall injury. This usually is a minor injury. In older adults or people with chronic lung disease, however, it can lead to problems such as pneumonia, atelectasis, and respiratory failure. If the fracture is displaced, bone can tear the pleura and cause pneumothorax.

A rib fracture causes pain on inspiration and coughing. Bruising may be seen over the fracture site. *Crepitus* (a grating sensation) may be felt with breathing. Breath sounds are diminished, especially in the bases, because of splinting.

Flail Chest

When two or more adjacent ribs are broken in several places, part of the chest wall becomes free-floating. This is a *flail chest.* The flail segment moves inward during inspiration and moves outward with expiration. This is called *paradoxic movement* (Figure 24-14 ■). Flail chest affects lung expansion and increases the work of breathing. The lung under the flail segment often is damaged.

In addition to paradoxic chest movement, flail chest causes pain and dyspnea. Chest expansion is unequal, and crepitus is present. Breath sounds are diminished, and crackles may be heard.

PULMONARY CONTUSION

Pulmonary contusion, or lung tissue injury, frequently occurs with chest trauma. When the chest is rapidly compressed and

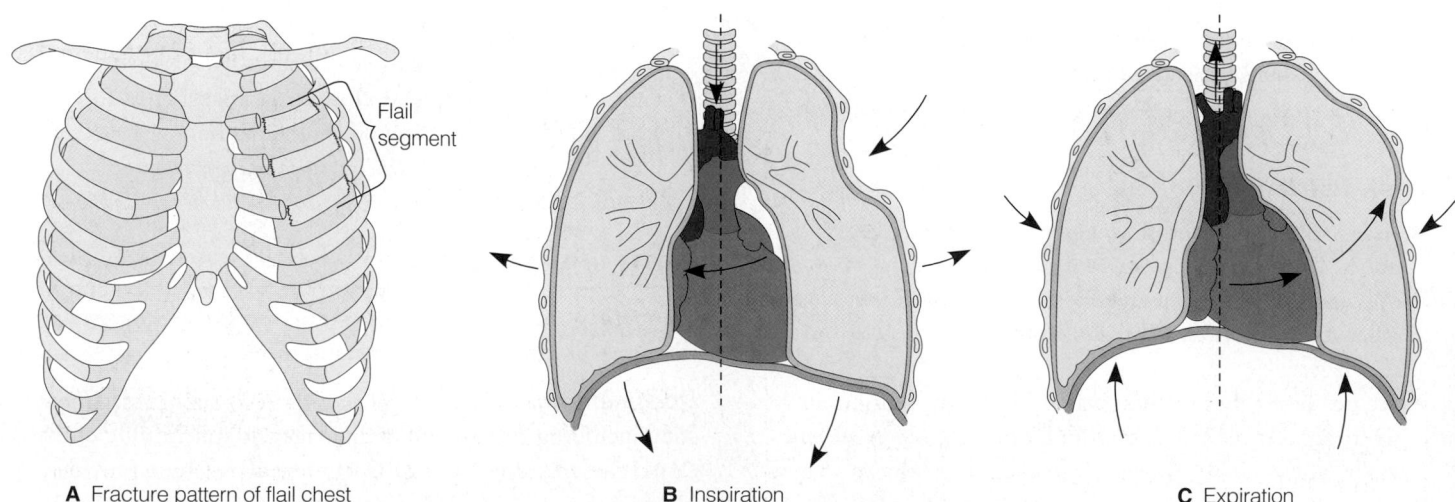

A Fracture pattern of flail chest   **B** Inspiration   **C** Expiration

Figure 24-14. ■ Flail chest with paradoxic chest wall movement.

then decompressed (e.g., being thrown forward against the steering wheel then back in a motor vehicle crash), alveoli and pulmonary vessels rupture, causing tissue hemorrhage and edema. After the initial injury, inflammation further impairs breathing and gas exchange.

Manifestations of pulmonary contusion include shortness of breath, restlessness, apprehension, and chest pain. Copious sputum, possibly blood tinged, is present. Tachycardia, tachypnea, dyspnea, and cyanosis develop as well.

SMOKE INHALATION

Smoke inhalation is the leading cause of death in burn injury. Smoke inhalation is common when a burn occurs in a closed space, and is suspected with burns on the face or upper torso or singed nasal hairs.

Smoke inhalation can lead to burns of airways, carbon monoxide or cyanide poisoning, and lung damage from noxious gases. Manifestations of smoke inhalation include dyspnea, wheezes or crackles, and possibly ashlike material in sputum. Carbon monoxide is a colorless, odorless gas that binds readily with hemoglobin, reducing its ability to carry oxygen to cells of the body. The manifestations of carbon monoxide poisoning are listed in Box 24-17 ■. Survivors of severe carbon monoxide poisoning may have permanent neurologic damage. Cyanide inhalation can be fatal; other toxic chemicals can cause bronchospasm and edema of the airways and alveoli.

NEAR-DROWNING

Aspiration and oxygen deprivation are the primary problems in near-drowning. Significant hypoxemia and loss of consciousness can occur within 3 to 5 minutes of immersion; death can occur within 5 to 10 minutes. Immersion in very cold water may prolong survival.

The near-drowning victim who aspirates either fresh or salt water can develop pulmonary edema and respiratory failure. Freshwater drowning also causes blood cell hemolysis and electrolyte imbalances. In near-drowning, inhaled microorganisms and debris can lead to pneumonia.

Manifestations of near-drowning include altered consciousness, restlessness, and apprehension. The client may be hypothermic and complain of headache or chest pain. Other signs include vomiting, cyanosis, apnea, tachypnea, and wheezing. Pink froth may be seen in the mouth and nose. Shock and cardiac arrest may occur.

INTERDISCIPLINARY CARE

Diagnostic tests to determine injury and lung function include:

- *Serum electrolytes* and *ABGs* to evaluate fluid and electrolyte and acid–base balance and oxygenation
- *Carboxyhemoglobin* if carbon monoxide poisoning is suspected
- *Chest x-ray* to evaluate chest wall injury and lung damage
- *Bronchoscopy* for suspected pulmonary contusion or smoke inhalation.

Simple rib fractures typically heal uneventfully. Analgesia is ordered to facilitate breathing, coughing, and movement. An intercostal nerve block may be done. Rib belts, binders, and taping of ribs are *not* recommended, because they can interfere with ventilation. With a flail chest, however, taping may be done to stabilize the chest wall.

Initial treatment of inhalation injury is removing the victim from the fire or water and providing effective cardiopulmonary resuscitation (CPR). Immediate restoration of effective breathing and circulation is key to preserving life. Oxygen is given as soon as available.

clinical ALERT

When the victim is hypothermic, resuscitation is continued until the body temperature is about 90°F (32°C). "Not dead until warm and dead" is a basic rule in hypothermia.

All clients with inhalation injury need supplemental oxygen. Coughing and suctioning are important to remove secretions and debris. Percussion and postural drainage may be done.

Intubation and mechanical ventilation may be ordered for flail chest, pulmonary contusion, and inhalation injuries because these clients often are critically ill. Intubation and mechanical ventilation are discussed in the next section of this chapter.

NURSING CARE

Priorities in Nursing Care. Promoting effective airway clearance and gas exchange are the nursing care priorities for clients with chest and lung trauma.

BOX 24-17

MANIFESTATIONS OF CARBON MONOXIDE POISONING

Low Levels

- Headache, dizziness
- Dyspnea
- Nausea
- "Cherry-red" skin and mucous membranes

Higher Levels

- Confusion, irritability, hallucinations
- Visual disturbance
- Hypotension
- Seizures, coma

Ineffective Airway Clearance

- Frequently assess respiratory status. Note the amount, color, and consistency of sputum. *The client often is unstable; frequent assessment is necessary to rapidly detect changes.*
- Elevate head of bed. *This promotes alveolar ventilation.*
- Instruct to cough, deep breathe, and change position every 1 to 2 hours. Encourage to use incentive spirometer. Assist with percussion and postural drainage as needed. *These measures help remove secretions and debris, and prevent atelectasis or pneumonia following chest trauma.*
- Teach to splint affected area with a blanket or pillow when coughing. *Splinting improves ventilation and reduces pain.*
- Suction as needed. *Suctioning may be required when cough is ineffective or when intubated.*
- Stabilize endotracheal tube with tape and ties. *Stabilizing the tube prevents its displacement into a mainstem bronchus, which could result in ventilation of only one lung.*
- Report decreased breath sounds, increased adventitious sounds; pink, frothy or purulent sputum; chills or fever; or changes in vital signs or mental status. *Changes in respiratory status, vital signs, or mental status may indicate a complication such as pulmonary edema or pneumonia.*

Impaired Gas Exchange

- Report changes in skin color, oxygen saturation, and arterial blood gases. *Alveolar damage and pulmonary edema can significantly impair gas exchange.*
- Assess for anxiety or apprehension, restlessness, confusion or lethargy, or complaints of headache. *These may indicate hypoxia or hypercapnia.*
- Monitor intake and output; weigh daily. Maintain ordered fluid restriction. *Fluid volume excess can increase pulmonary edema and further impair with gas exchange.*
- Maintain oxygen and mechanical ventilation as ordered. *Oxygen and/or mechanical ventilation improve gas exchange.*
- Administer sedation as needed. *Sedation may be required to maintain effective mechanical ventilation.*
- Provide frequent mouth care. *Oxygen dries mucous membranes. Mouth care promotes comfort and helps prevent damage.*
- Restrict activity and allow periods of uninterrupted rest. *These measures reduce oxygen consumption.*

Pain

- Frequently assess pain, using a pain scale. *Pain interferes with lung expansion and coughing.*
- Provide analgesics as ordered or on a schedule. *Regular analgesia controls pain more effectively than prn doses.*
- Assess for respiratory depression related to narcotic analgesia. *Although pain control is important to maintain ventilation, narcotics can depress the respiratory center.*

Ineffective Tissue Perfusion: Cerebral

Inhalation injury can affect cerebral perfusion and oxygenation. Increased intracranial pressure (ICP) may develop after near-drowning.

- Frequently monitor neurologic status. Report changes promptly. *Change in level of consciousness or behavior is the earliest sign of increased ICP.*
- Place in Fowler's position. Keep the head in a neutral position. *Elevating and keeping the head straight promotes blood and CSF circulation.*
- Maintain effective ventilation and oxygenation. *Hypercapnia and hypoxemia increase cerebral edema.*

EVALUATING

To evaluate the effectiveness of nursing care for the client who has experienced pulmonary trauma, collect respiratory assessment data on a continuing basis. If the client experienced smoke inhalation or near-drowning, frequently assess neurologic and cardiovascular status as well.

Documenting. Document continuing assessments, including neurologic, respiratory, cardiovascular, and pain status. Note the effectiveness of analgesia and other measures to relieve pain, and the client's ability to effectively ventilate all areas of the lungs. Document all teaching, including that related to identification and reporting of potential complications. Note teaching of the client and family about safety measures to prevent pulmonary trauma.

CONTINUING CARE

The most effective treatment for chest trauma and lung injury is prevention. Teach use of seat belts with shoulder restraints to help prevent lung and chest injuries in motor vehicle crashes.

A working smoke detector (with functioning batteries) could prevent most deaths from smoke inhalation. Instruct to regularly check smoke detectors and replace batteries yearly. Encourage families to develop a fire escape plan and to use fire drills to rehearse the plan. Smoldering cigarettes are a leading cause of house fires; help develop a plan to stop smoking. Teach to drop and roll should clothing catch fire. (Fire rises, increasing the risk of respiratory injury when standing.)

To prevent drowning, life preservers and flotation vests or jackets need to be worn, not stored in the boat hold. These devices are designed to keep the head above water. Encourage to always wear life vests when boating, water-skiing, or wind-surfing. Wet suits help prevent hypothermia in very cold water. Advise never to swim alone, when fatigued, or immediately after a meal. Advise to cover or fence swimming pools, hot tubs, and ponds to prevent inadvertent entry and drowning. Just as alcohol and driving do not mix, neither do alcohol and boating or other water sports.

A population well trained in effective CPR provides the best second line of defense. Rapid restoration of breathing is essential to prevent brain damage. Encourage everyone to be trained and maintain current CPR certification. Work with communities to increase the number of trained individuals. Refer to local chapters of the American Red Cross or the American Heart Association for classes.

For a minor chest wall injury, discuss pain control and its importance in preventing complications. Teach to splint the rib cage during coughing. Stress the importance of coughing and deep breathing. Explain the reasons to avoid taping or wrapping the chest continuously. Describe complications to report to the physician: chills and fever, productive cough, purulent or bloody sputum, shortness of breath or difficulty breathing, and increasing chest pain. Emphasize the importance of avoiding respiratory irritants, such as cigarette smoke and pollutants.

A large pulmonary contusion can lead to long-term respiratory compromise. This can require changes in activities and possibly occupation.

CRITICAL RESPIRATORY CONDITIONS

Respiratory Failure

Many of the conditions discussed in this chapter can lead to **respiratory failure.** In respiratory failure, the lungs are unable to oxygenate blood and remove carbon dioxide to meet the body's needs, even at rest. COPD is the usual cause of respiratory failure. Other lung diseases, trauma, neuromuscular disorders, and heart disease can also lead to respiratory failure.

PATHOPHYSIOLOGY AND MANIFESTATIONS

Respiratory failure is not a disease; it results from severe respiratory dysfunction. Blood oxygen levels are very low; the PO_2 may be less than 50 to 60 mm Hg (hypoxemia). Carbon dioxide levels rise as the lungs are unable to eliminate it. Tissue hypoxia and high PCO_2 levels (hypercapnia) lead to acidosis. See Chapter 7 ∞ to review acid–base balance.

The manifestations of respiratory failure are caused by hypoxemia and hypercapnia (Box 24-18 ■). Hypercapnia causes vasodilation and depresses the central nervous system. As carbon dioxide levels increase, the respiratory center may be depressed. When this occurs, the usual carbon dioxide stimulus to breathe is lost, and low blood oxygen levels provide the only stimulus to breathe. Providing oxygen without mechanical ventilation may remove any drive to breathe, with dire results.

The prognosis for acute respiratory failure depends on the underlying disease. Acute respiratory failure due to an uncomplicated drug overdose usually resolves quickly and completely. Respiratory failure due to chronic lung disease often has a prolonged course and less favorable outcome.

Acute Respiratory Distress Syndrome

Acute respiratory distress syndrome (ARDS) is a severe form of acute respiratory failure. ARDS is characterized by noncardiac pulmonary edema and progressive hypoxemia that does not respond to oxygen therapy. It can follow direct or indirect lung injury. Smoke inhalation and near-drowning are direct lung injuries that may lead to ARDS; shock and sepsis cause indirect lung damage and can precipitate ARDS.

PATHOPHYSIOLOGY

A massive unregulated systemic inflammatory response damages the lungs. This damage occurs rapidly, often within 24 hours of the initial insult. Damage to the alveolar–capillary membrane allows plasma and blood cells to leak into the interstitial space and alveoli. Alveolar surfactant is inactivated, and the cells that produce it are damaged. Alveoli collapse, the work of breathing increases, and gas exchange is impaired. Hypoxemia develops and the PCO_2 rises.

MANIFESTATIONS

The manifestations of ARDS usually develop 24 to 48 hours after the initial insult. Dyspnea and tachypnea are initial

---

BOX 24-18

MANIFESTATIONS OF RESPIRATORY FAILURE

Due to Hypoxemia
- Dyspnea, tachypnea
- Cyanosis
- Restlessness, anxiety, confusion
- Tachycardia, dysrhythmias
- Hypertension
- Metabolic acidosis

Due to Hypercapnia
- Dyspnea, respiratory depression
- Headache, drowsiness, coma
- Tachycardia, hypertension
- Heart failure
- Respiratory acidosis

MediaLink

ARDS

symptoms. Breath sounds are initially clear. Increasing respiratory distress and *refractory hypoxemia* (low oxygen saturation and PO_2 levels that do not improve with supplemental oxygen) develop. As respiratory failure progresses, the client may become agitated and confused or lethargic.

The prognosis for ARDS varies. Many clients recover fully. However, sepsis and multiple organ dysfunction syndrome (MODS) may develop. When this occurs, the prognosis is poor.

INTERDISCIPLINARY CARE

Treatment of respiratory failure and ARDS focuses on the underlying cause or disease process, as well as supporting ventilation and correcting hypoxemia and hypercapnia.

Diagnostic Tests

Diagnostic tests include *arterial blood gases (ABGs)*. The arterial PO_2 may be less than 50 to 60 mm Hg, and the PCO_2 often is high, usually more than 50 mm Hg. The pH is low, indicating acidosis. In ARDS, *chest x-ray* shows diffuse infiltrates and a "white-out" pattern as lung tissue collapses and fibrosis develops. *Ventilation-perfusion scans* and *exhaled carbon dioxide ($ETCO_2$)* are used to evaluate alveolar ventilation and gas exchange.

Medications

Bronchodilators may be given to reverse airway spasm and constriction. Infection is treated with antibiotics. Corticosteroids and NSAIDs may be ordered to reduce airway edema and inflammation. Surfactant therapy may be ordered for clients with ARDS. Other drugs used to treat ARDS may include inhaled nitric oxide and drugs to block the inflammatory response.

Clients on mechanical ventilation often require sedation to reduce anxiety and analgesics to relieve pain. Benzodiazepines such as midazolam (Versed) provide sedation, and intravenous analgesics such as morphine relieve pain. These drugs also reduce the respiratory drive, facilitating mechanical ventilation. Occasionally, a neuromuscular blocking agent may be given to paralyze the respiratory muscles and

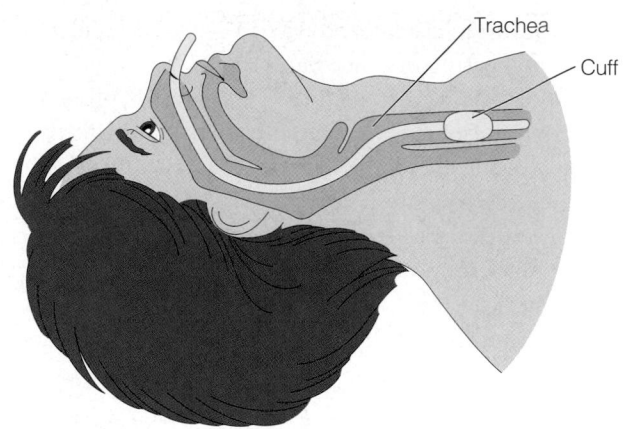

Figure 24-15. ■ Nasal endotracheal intubation.

allow the ventilator to control the client's respirations. These clients require intensive care management.

Oxygen Therapy

Oxygen therapy is vital to treat the hypoxemia of acute respiratory failure. Clients with chronic COPD may need only 1 to 3 liters by nasal cannula; higher flow rates often are necessary for other clients. High oxygen concentrations (40% to 60% or higher) are used only for short periods to avoid oxygen toxicity. Oxygen toxicity reduces lung compliance, increasing the work of breathing. A tight-fitting mask with continuous positive airway pressure (CPAP) may be used to improve alveolar ventilation and allow lower oxygen concentrations.

Airway Management

Clients who need mechanical ventilation are intubated with an endotracheal tube (ETT) extending from the mouth or nose into the trachea (Figure 24-15 ■). Most ETTs have an air-filled or foam cuff just above the end of the tube that prevents air from escaping back into the upper airways during ventilation. A tracheostomy may be done if mechanical ventilation is needed for more than 3 or 4 weeks (see Table 24-10 ■). Box 24-19 ■ outlines nursing care for the client with an ETT.

TABLE 24-10		
Advantages and Disadvantages of Endotracheal Airways		
AIRWAY	**ADVANTAGES**	**DISADVANTAGES**
Oroendotracheal	Rapidly inserted Larger endotracheal tube can be used	Uncomfortable Difficult to stabilize Can interfere with mouth care
Nasoendotracheal	Better tolerated Easier to stabilize	Smaller tube may be difficult to clear of secretions Risk of pressure necrosis of nares Risk of otitis media (can impair eustachian tube drainage)
Tracheostomy	More comfortable Easily stabilized Allows oral food intake	Requires surgical procedure

BOX 24-19   NURSING CARE CHECKLIST

Endotracheal Tube (ETT)

☑ Frequently assess respiratory status. Report changes to charge nurse or physician.

☑ Monitor vital signs, skin color, LOC, and mental status at least every 4 hours.

☑ Secure ETT with tape and/or ties. Mark tube placement in relation to the mouth or nose. Notify charge nurse or physician if the tube becomes displaced.

☑ Provide oral and nasal care every 2 hours; assess oral and nasal mucosa for redness and irritation. Move oral ETT to opposite side of mouth every 8 hours.

☑ Using sterile technique, suction ETT as needed to remove secretions. Using clean technique, suction oropharynx as needed.

☑ Closely monitor ETT cuff pressure, maintaining recommended pressure.

☑ Provide humidified air or oxygen.

☑ Ensure that all ventilator alarms are in "on" position.

☑ Establish communication using hand signals, eye movement, a note pad, Magic Slate, or picture board.

TABLE 24-11

Modes of Ventilator Operation

MODE	DESCRIPTION
Control	Ventilator controls rate, volume or pressure, and flow rate of all breaths.
Assist-control	Client can trigger ventilator with inspiratory effort; breaths will be delivered at a preset rate if client fails to breathe.
Synchronized intermittent mandatory ventilation (SIMV)	Ventilator delivers a set number of mandatory breaths (synchronized with client's breathing) per minute; client can breathe on own between ventilator-assisted breaths.
Positive end-expiratory pressure (PEEP)	Used together with other ventilator modes; positive pressure is maintained in airways throughout respiratory cycle.
Pressure support ventilation (PSV)	Pressurized inspiratory flow supports inspiratory effort, reducing work of breathing.

Endotracheal intubation increases the risk for infection because the defenses of the upper airway are bypassed. ETTs pass through the larynx, so talking is not possible. Enteral or parenteral nutrition is required, because eating is not possible when an ETT is in place. A nasogastric feeding tube, gastrostomy, or jejunostomy may be used for enteral nutrition. See Chapter 19 ⊂⊃ for more information about enteral feedings.

When the ETT is removed, the client is placed on humidified oxygen and closely observed for respiratory distress (nasal flaring, dyspnea, wheezing, anxiety, decreased oxygen saturation levels). Reintubation may be necessary. Sore throat and a hoarse voice are common following extubation. Oral intake is restarted slowly, with careful assessment of swallowing.

Mechanical Ventilation

Clients with respiratory failure may require mechanical ventilation. *Positive-pressure ventilators* are commonly used in acute respiratory failure. These ventilators work by pushing air into the lungs. They may be cycled by the volume of air delivered (e.g., set to deliver 500 mL of air with each breath) or by pressure within the airways (set to cycle off when a certain airway pressure is reached). Positive-pressure ventilation increases lung volume and reduces the work of breathing and oxygen demand.

TYPES, MODES, AND SETTINGS. Positive-pressure ventilators can be set for a number of different modes or patterns of ventilation (Table 24-11 ■). In addition to the mode of operation, four other settings are used when a volume-cycled ventilator is used:

■ The rate or number of breaths per minute

■ The tidal volume, or milliliters of air delivered with each breath

■ Oxygen concentration of delivered air (FIO_2)

■ Positive end-expiratory pressure (PEEP).

For most adults, the *rate* is initially set between 12 and 15 breaths per minute. It is adjusted based on the PCO_2. If the PCO_2 falls below 40 mm Hg, the client is being hyperventilated so the rate is reduced. An increased PCO_2, above 40 mm Hg, indicates hypoventilation; in this case, the rate is increased.

The *tidal volume (Vt)* setting controls the amount of air delivered with each breath. For adults, the tidal volume is set at 500 to 750 mL, depending on the client's size. Excess tidal volumes can cause lung trauma.

The oxygen percentage of delivered air can be adjusted. The FIO_2 is set at the lowest possible level to maintain the PO_2 and oxygen saturation at desired levels. For most clients, the goal is to maintain an oxygen saturation of greater than 90%.

When oxygen concentrations of 50% or higher cannot maintain the PO_2 or oxygen saturation within the desired range, *PEEP* is added to improve oxygenation. PEEP prevents airway pressure from falling below a preset level, even at the end of expiration.

COMPLICATIONS. Although endotracheal intubation and mechanical ventilation can be life saving, they also carry a risk for injury.

The intubated client may develop pressure necrosis of the nose, lip, or trachea. Less saliva is produced, and mouth care can be difficult. If the tube is dislodged, ventilation of one or both lungs may be affected. Infection is a significant risk; sterile technique must be used when suctioning to avoid introducing bacteria into the respiratory tract. Condensed moisture in ventilator tubing is always drained toward the ventilator (away from the client) to further reduce the risk of infection. Secretions often become thick and tenacious, increasing the risk of atelectasis.

Mechanical ventilation can cause *barotrauma* (lung injury due to pressure). Pneumothorax and subcutaneous emphysema may result. Decreased cardiac output is a risk. GI bleeding is another potential complication. Many of these complications can be prevented by careful ventilator management and ETT care.

WEANING. *Weaning* is the process of removing the ventilator. Clients who require mechanical ventilation for a brief period may be taken off the ventilator and extubated rapidly. A more gradual weaning process is used if mechanical ventilation has been prolonged. The client is closely monitored during weaning. Vital signs, respiratory rate, dyspnea, oxygen saturation, and arterial blood gases are frequently assessed. If the oxygen saturation or PO_2 falls below specified limits, mechanical ventilation may be restarted.

Terminal weaning, gradual withdrawal of mechanical ventilation from a client who is not expected to survive, may be done for a terminal illness or irreversible condition. The client is moved to a quiet room or even home prior to removing the ventilator. Family members are encouraged to stay throughout the process. Ventilator support is gradually withdrawn, while analgesia and sedation are given to maintain comfort.

Other Therapies

A pulmonary artery catheter is inserted to monitor pressures and cardiac output. Fluid replacement is carefully monitored to avoid either hypovolemia or fluid overload. Enteral or parenteral feeding is provided to maintain nutritional status. The client with ARDS may be placed in the prone position to improve oxygenation.

NURSING CARE

Clients in respiratory failure often are critically ill. They need both intensive medical care and intensive nursing care.

ASSESSING

Frequent monitoring and assessment are critical. Obtain subjective data such as complaints of dyspnea and a history of COPD or acute pneumonia. Identify any recent episode of shock, sepsis, or other critical condition.

Carefully assess respiratory status, including rate, depth, and ease of breathing (retractions, use of accessory muscles, nasal flaring). Auscultate breath sounds for depth, equality, and adventitious sounds. Assess mental status, including level of consciousness and level of anxiety. Obtain complete vital signs, including apical pulse and oxygen saturation. Document color of skin and mucous membranes, peripheral pulses, and capillary refill.

DIAGNOSING, PLANNING, AND IMPLEMENTING

Priorities in Nursing Care. Clients in respiratory failure have multiple nursing care needs. Both the failure and its treatment can affect the client's ability to maintain spontaneous respirations and to effectively clear secretions of airways. Hypoxemia produces intense apprehension and air hunger; when it is necessary to insert an endotracheal airway, the client loses the ability to communicate easily. Anxiety is common and can be intense.

Impaired Spontaneous Ventilation

- Assess vital signs and respiratory status every 15 to 30 minutes. Report changes. *The client in respiratory failure is critically ill; frequent assessment is vital to detect changes and evaluate interventions. Respiratory failure increases the work of breathing and can lead to fatigue and inadequate ventilation. This may occur before mechanical ventilation is established or during the weaning process.*
- Promptly report changes in arterial blood gases and oxygen saturation. *These are important indicators of gas exchange and respiratory status.*
- Administer oxygen as ordered. Observe closely for respiratory depression. *Supplemental oxygen may suppress the respiratory drive.*
- Place in Fowler's position. *Fowler's position improves lung ventilation and decreases the work of breathing.*
- Promote rest. Assist with care, space procedures and activities, and allow uninterrupted rest periods. *Rest reduces oxygen and energy demands.*
- Unless intubated and mechanically ventilated, avoid sedatives and respiratory depressant drugs. *These medications can further depress the respiratory drive, worsening respiratory failure.*
- Prepare for endotracheal intubation and mechanical ventilation:
    - Obtain intubation tray with sterile endotracheal tubes and laryngoscope with a variety of adult blades.

- Set up endotracheal suction and bring sterile catheter and glove kits and sterile normal saline to bedside.
- Notify respiratory therapy department to set up ventilator.
- Request portable chest x-ray to verify tube placement when procedure completed.

The client with respiratory failure may require emergency intubation and mechanical ventilation to sustain respirations.

- Explain procedure, reassuring client that this is a temporary measure to reduce the work of breathing and allow rest. Instruct that endotracheal tubes interfere with talking, and establish a way to communicate. *Thorough explanations help relieve anxiety.*

Ineffective Airway Clearance

- Frequently assess respiratory status. *Increasing respiratory rate, crackles and rhonchi, frequent coughing, setting off of ventilator alarms, and increasing restlessness or anxiety may indicate ineffective airway clearance and a need for suctioning.*
- Suction as needed to maintain patent airway. Box 24-20 ■ outlines the steps for endotracheal suctioning. *Suctioning removes secretions the client is unable to clear.*

BOX 24-20 PROCEDURE CHECKLIST

Endotracheal Suctioning

Before the Procedure

☑ Use Standard Precautions.

☑ Obtain all supplies.

☑ Identify client; provide for privacy.

☑ Explain procedure. Suctioning is not painful, but is uncomfortable. During suctioning, breathing will be difficult. This lasts only a brief time (up to 10 seconds). Suctioning causes coughing, helping to clear the lungs.

☑ Establish a way to communicate during suctioning (e.g., raising a finger if unable to tolerate suctioning).

Procedure

☑ Regulate suction to no more than −80 to −120 mm Hg of suction.

☑ Open sterile saline, leaving cap loosely in place.

☑ Put on personal protective wear.

With an In-Line Catheter

☑ Attach catheter to suction tubing.

☑ Adjust the oxygen (FIO_2) to 100%; allow three breaths.

☑ Manipulating catheter through plastic shield (to maintain sterility), insert the catheter with no suction until resistance is met; slowly withdraw catheter while applying suction.

☑ Apply suction for no more than 10 seconds (count seconds or watch clock—the time passes quickly), then allow rest for three to five breaths. Repeat as needed for a total of no more than three times.

☑ Disconnect suction tubing from catheter, clear tubing, and turn off suction.

With a Separate Catheter-and-Glove Kit

☑ Open suction catheter/glove kit. Remove saline cup, and fill with sterile saline.

☑ Put on sterile gloves. Attach catheter to suction tubing, keeping dominant hand sterile; lubricate catheter with sterile saline.

☑ Use nondominant hand to adjust oxygen (FIO_2) to 100%; allow three breaths.

☑ Using nondominant hand, disconnect ventilator tubing from endotracheal tube.

☑ Holding suction catheter with dominant (sterile) hand and suction control valve with nondominant hand, insert catheter, with no suction, until resistance is met. Apply suction while slowly withdrawing catheter.

☑ Suction for no more than 10 seconds. Reconnect ventilator, and allow rest for three to five breaths; clear suction tubing with sterile saline.

☑ Repeat as needed for a total of three times.

☑ Reconnect ventilator.

☑ Clear suction tubing; turn off and disconnect catheter, discarding it with the gloves.

☑ Provide three additional breaths at 100% oxygen, then readjust to previous ordered level.

After the Procedure

☑ Assess lung sounds and tolerance of the procedure.

SAMPLE DOCUMENTATION

6/15/06 2100	Suctioned via endotracheal tube for moderate amount of thick, grayish sputum. Tolerated procedure well. Good breath sounds noted in all lung fields; scattered coarse crackles cleared with suctioning. _____ S. Evans, LVN.

Note: Refer to a nursing fundamentals or skills text for more detailed instruction. Check state guidelines and facility policy before performing any procedure.

- Obtain specimen for culture if sputum appears purulent or becomes odorous. *Sputum culture and sensitivity are done to identify pathogens and appropriate antibiotics to treat infection.*
- Perform percussion, vibration, and postural drainage as ordered. *These techniques help loosen secretions and move them into larger airways, where they can be cleared.*
- Firmly secure endotracheal or tracheostomy tube. Prevent tension on tube during turning, positioning, transferring, or getting out of bed. If necessary, loosely restrain hands. *These measures help prevent displacement or inadvertent removal of the endotracheal tube or tracheostomy.*
- Maintain fluid intake. Monitor intake and output. Weigh daily. *Adequate hydration helps liquefy secretions but preventing fluid overload is important for lung function.*

Risk for Injury

The client in respiratory failure is at risk for injury due to altered level of consciousness, endotracheal intubation, and mechanical ventilation.

- Assess frequently, including a head-to-toe assessment. *Frequent assessment allows early identification of potential problems.*
- Maintain low pressure in the ETT cuff. *Low cuff pressures reduce the risk of damage to the trachea.*
- Do not bypass or turn off any ventilator alarms. *The intubated client cannot call out for help. The client who has received a neuromuscular blocker cannot breathe without ventilator support and cannot use the call bell.*
- Report changes such as increasing air leak around ETT cuff and decreased breath sounds or chest movement. *These may indicate tracheal necrosis, migration of the ETT into the right mainstem bronchus, pneumothorax, or atelectasis.*
- Turn and reposition frequently, stabilizing the ETT while moving. *Frequent position changes help prevent skin and tissue breakdown due to pressure.*
- Keep skin and linens clean, dry, and wrinkle-free. Protect bony prominences with padding. *Because the client may not perceive pain and pressure or move voluntarily, good skin care is mandatory.*
- Perform passive range-of-motion (ROM) exercises every 4 to 8 hours. *These exercises maintain joint flexibility and help prevent contractures associated with long-term immobility.*
- Keep side rails up and use soft restraints as needed. *These measures help prevent falling, inadvertent disconnection of the ventilator, or pulling out of the ETT.*
- Administer H_2-blockers and antacids as ordered. *Stress gastritis and GI hemorrhage are common, preventable complications of mechanical ventilation.*

Decreased Cardiac Output

- Monitor vital signs every 1 to 2 hours. *Positive-pressure ventilation decreases cardiac output; applying PEEP further reduces cardiac output. This drop can increase tissue damage and cause dysrhythmias. Frequent assessment allows early detection of decreased cardiac output.*
- Measure urinary output hourly; report if less than 30 mL/hr. *A fall in urine output is an early sign of decreased cardiac output.*
- Assess level of consciousness every 2 to 4 hours. *A change in LOC may indicate cerebral hypoxia.*
- Report changes in hemodynamic pressures to the charge nurse or physician. *Changes in hemodynamic pressures may indicate a drop in cardiac output.*
- Weigh daily. *Daily weight is the best indicator of fluid status; decreased cardiac output may cause fluid retention.*
- Provide frequent skin care, keeping skin clean and dry and protecting pressure points. *Tissue hypoxia increases the risk of skin breakdown, infection, and sepsis.*
- Maintain intravenous fluids as ordered. *Intravenous fluids are given to maintain vascular volume and prevent dehydration.*

Anxiety

- Stay with the client as much as possible. *The presence of a caregiver provides reassurance that help is readily available.*
- Explain all monitors, procedures, unusual sounds, and machinery. *Understanding the equipment and the meaning of beeps, buzzers, and alarms reduces anxiety.*
- Provide a simple means of communicating, such as a slate, picture board, or alphabet board. If a muscle-paralyzing drug has been given, use methods such as looking to the right for "yes" and left for "no." Reassure that the ability to speak will return once the ETT is removed. *The inability to speak and call out for help is frightening. Providing an alternate means of communication helps reduce anxiety.*
- Encourage family members to visit frequently and remain with the client if possible. Assist family to provide as much care as possible. *Family visits help reduce anxiety and feelings of abandonment. Allowing family members to participate in care helps reduce their anxiety as well as the client's.*
- Provide distraction with radio or television if allowed. *Distraction helps reduce the focus on machines and unusual sounds of monitors and alarms.*
- Reassure clients that intubation and mechanical ventilation are temporary measures and that they will be able to breathe independently again. *Clients may fear continued dependence on mechanical ventilation.*
- Provide sedation and antianxiety medications as needed, especially when a neuromuscular blocker has been used. *The client whose voluntary muscles have been paralyzed remains mentally alert.*

EVALUATING

To evaluate the effectiveness of nursing care for the client with respiratory failure, collect assessment data related to breathing, respiratory status, and cardiac output; freedom from injury, tissue damage, and complications of immobility; and level of anxiety.

Documenting. Frequently document continuing assessment data, including respiratory rate, breath sounds, ease of respirations, equality of chest movement, and measures of cardiac output. Note ventilator settings and changes in laboratory data such as ABGs in response to changes in ventilator settings. When the client is being weaned from a ventilator, note the heart and respiratory rate and ease as indicators of tolerance for lack of ventilator support. Following extubation, document respiratory rate and ease. Promptly report any signs of respiratory distress such as nasal flaring, stridor, or intercostal retractions.

CONTINUING CARE

Prior to discharge, discuss factors that precipitated respiratory failure and measures to prevent it in the future. Discuss the importance of avoiding respiratory irritants. Encourage to remain indoors with an air filter or air conditioning when pollution levels are high, obtain influenza and pneumonia immunizations, and avoid exposure to cigarette smoke. Teach effective coughing and measures such as percussion, vibration, and postural drainage.

For the client with ARDS, explain that ARDS did not result from their actions, but results from serious illness. Reassure that clients who survive the initial insult of ARDS generally recover without significant long-term adverse effects. Advise that recovery may be prolonged, however. Stress the importance of avoiding cigarette smoking.

Note: The bibliography listings for this and all chapters have been compiled at the back of the book.

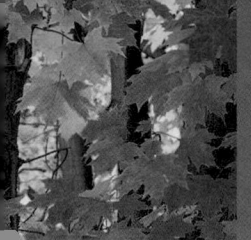

Chapter Review

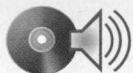 **KEY TERMS** by Topics

Use the audio glossary feature of either the CD-ROM or the Companion Website to hear the correct pronunciation of the following key terms.

Lower Respiratory Disorders
dyspnea, hemoptysis, cyanosis

Infectious and Inflammatory Disorders
bronchitis, pneumonia, tuberculosis

Obstructive Airway Disorders
asthma, chronic obstructive pulmonary disease (COPD), atelectasis

Pulmonary Disorders
pulmonary embolism, pulmonary hypertension, pleural effusion, pneumothorax, hemothorax

Critical Respiratory Conditions
respiratory failure, acute respiratory distress syndrome (ARDS)

KEY Points

- Effective lung ventilation and gas exchange can be affected by infectious diseases, airway restriction, structural changes of the lung tissue or chest wall, acute or chronic inflammatory disorders, and tumors.

- Pneumonia remains a leading cause of death, particularly in older adults. It interferes with gas exchange in the alveoli. It may be caused by bacteria, viruses or other infectious organisms, or by aspiration of gastric contents.

- Tuberculosis (TB) is a chronic infectious disease that can remain asymptomatic and undetected for years. A combination of antituberculosis drugs is given for 6 to 12 months to treat active TB. Controlling the spread of TB and promoting compliance with therapy are primary nursing responsibilities.

- Asthma is a chronic inflammatory airway disease that often can be controlled with medications and by avoiding triggers for acute attacks. Acute asthma can cause severe airway restriction, interfering with ventilation of alveoli and gas exchange.

- Chronic obstructive pulmonary disease (COPD) is a progressive disorder that gradually destroys lung tissue and obstructs airflow. Cigarette smoking is the primary risk factor for COPD.

- Cigarette smoking is the primary risk factor for lung cancer. Lung cancer often is advanced by the time it is diagnosed, so its prognosis is poor. Surgery offers the best hope for cure.

- Prevention of venous stasis and deep venous thrombosis (DVT) is the best treatment for pulmonary embolism. Elastic hose, early ambulation, and leg exercises are nursing care measures to prevent DVT.

- Pneumothorax (air in the pleural space) and hemothorax (blood in the pleural space) interfere with lung expansion and ventilation. Chest tubes are inserted to restore negative pressure in the pleural space.

- Respiratory failure is the inability of the lungs to exchange oxygen and carbon dioxide to meet the needs of the body. Clients often require intensive care management with endotracheal intubation and mechanical ventilation.

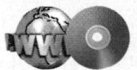 **EXPLORE MediaLink**

Additional interactive resources for this chapter can be found on the Companion Website at www.prenhall.com/burke. Click on Chapter 24 and "Begin" to select the activities for this chapter.

For chapter-related NCLEX-style review questions and an audio glossary, access the accompanying CD-ROM in this book.

FOR FURTHER Study

Chapter 7 provides more information on ABGs and acid–base balance.

For care of the client having surgery, see Chapter 9.

For more about nursing implications of corticosteroid drugs, and for more information about *Pneumocystis carinii* pneumonia, see Chapter 11.

See Chapter 12 for more information about chemotherapy and radiation therapy.

For in-depth discussion of shock, see Chapter 13.

See Chapter 19 for more information about enteral feedings.

Chapter 26 provides more information on thrombolytic therapy.

See Chapter 27 for more information about heart failure.

For discussion of deep venous thrombosis and of methods for measuring arterial pressure, see Chapter 28.

Tuberculosis of the genitourinary tract is discussed further in Chapter 32.

Critical Thinking Care Map

Caring for a Client with Tuberculosis
NCLEX-PN® Focus Area: Physiologic Integrity, Reduction of Risk Potential

Case Study: Harry Facée, a 53-year-old man, arrives at a community clinic in a large metropolitan city. He complains of aching chest pain that has lasted for the past few days and says that now his sputum is bloody. He is afraid he might have lung cancer, so he feels he should see a doctor.

Nursing Diagnosis: Risk for Noncompliance

COLLECT DATA

Subjective	Objective
_____	_____
_____	_____
_____	_____
_____	_____
_____	_____
_____	_____
_____	_____

Would you report this data? Yes/No

If yes, to: _____

Nursing Care

_____
_____
_____
_____
_____
_____
_____
_____
_____
_____

How would you document this? _____
_____
_____
_____

Data Collected
(use those that apply)

- Homeless for past 10 years; uses shelters only during very cold or wet weather
- Complains of chronic cough that now is productive of pink sputum
- Often wakes up drenched with sweat in the middle of the night
- Complains of increasing fatigue
- Vital signs: BP 152/86; P 92; R 20; and T 100.2°F (37.8°C)
- Clean; answers questions appropriately and intelligently
- Very thin, almost emaciated
- Sputum Gram stain positive for acid-fast bacillus

Nursing Interventions
(use those that apply; list in priority order)

- Provide verbal and written information about tuberculosis.
- Teach about prescribed medications, possible adverse effects, and importance of completing the entire prescribed regimen.
- Emphasize importance of continued follow-up.
- Teach and demonstrate sputum and droplet control measures.
- Refer to local incentive shelter program for directly observed medical therapy and meals.

NCLEX-PN® Exam Preparation

1 The nurse collecting a history from a client with chronic bronchitis would expect to find that the client:

A. worked in a cotton mill for 25 years.
B. smoked cigarettes for 40 years.
C. received a pacemaker at the age of 55.
D. had a father who died of lung cancer.

2 Your client had a tuberculin skin test with a positive result. The husband is concerned that he may also have TB. You explain that a positive skin test indicates that:

A. the client has active TB and the husband should immediately start prophylactic treatment.
B. the client has developed antibodies to TB; further testing is necessary to determine if the disease is active.
C. tuberculosis is a bloodborne disease and the husband does not have to worry.
D. the husband definitely has contracted the disease and should begin medications.

3 The nurse is caring for a client with acute asthma. When reporting to the next shift, it is most important for the nurse to describe:

A. medication effectiveness.
B. intake and output results.
C. lung assessment findings.
D. level of consciousness.

4 When teaching use of a metered-dose inhaler (MDI), the nurse instructs her client to:

A. take quick shallow breaths in rapid succession while holding the canister down.
B. use the inhaler containing the anti-inflammatory drug first, then the bronchodilator.
C. use the anti-inflammatory drug as needed to treat acute episodes of wheezing.
D. rinse the mouth after using the inhaler to reduce systemic absorption of the drug.

5 Which of the following statements best represents a nurse's understanding of use of supplemental oxygen in clients with COPD?

A. Because oxygen is flammable, the client should not smoke.
B. Oxygen is used only at night for clients with COPD.
C. Oxygen is never used for clients with COPD because they may become dependent on it.
D. The client needs to be closely monitored for signs of respiratory depression.

6 Which of these statements by the client would indicate that further instruction in preventing atelectasis is needed?

A. "It is too painful to walk in the hallway today."
B. "I need to drink extra water for lunch."
C. "I don't need any pain medication right now."
D. "I would like to have a laxative before I go to sleep."

7 When assisting with a thoracentesis, the nurse knows that the physician will insert the needle into the:

A. thoracic cavity.
B. pleural space.
C. mediastinum.
D. visceral space.

8 A client with a chest tube trips while ambulating, accidentally pulling his chest tube out of the chest. The first thing the nurse should do is:

A. call the physician.
B. place an occlusive dressing over the wound.
C. reinsert the tube.
D. empty the collection device.

9 The nurse teaching a group of high school students about preventing lung damage evaluates his teaching as effective when the students (Choose all that apply):

A. develop plans to form a cooperative exercise group.
B. verbalize the importance of smoke detectors.
C. organize a clinic for pneumococcal pneumonia vaccinations.
D. start a smoking prevention campaign for their peers.
E. develop a program to supply low-cost flotation devices to local boaters.

10 The nurse caring for a client with COPD recognizes which of the following as an early sign of possible respiratory failure?

A. restlessness and tachypnea
B. deep coma
C. hypotension and tachycardia
D. decreased urine output

Answers for Review Questions, as well as discussion of Care Plan and Critical Thinking Care Map questions, appear in Appendix V.

Thinking Strategically About...

After coughing up bloody sputum, James Mueller, 68 years old, sees his physician. A chest x-ray shows a mass in his right lung. He is admitted for diagnostic tests.

DATA COLLECTED

In the nursing history, Mr. Mueller describes himself as "pretty healthy," except for a smoker's cough. He has a 50 pack-year smoking history (one pack per day for 50 years, since age 18). He says he quit after a small heart attack 3 years ago but started again after 4 months. His cough has become productive and he admits he is more short of breath than usual with activity.

Vital signs are BP 162/86; P 78, regular; R 20; and T 98.4°F (36.9°C). Color is good, skin warm and dry. Wheezes are noted in right chest; good breath sounds throughout. A sputum specimen sent for cytology is positive for small-cell bronchogenic cancer. The CT scan shows a central mass with mediastinal and subclavicular lymph node involvement. A small mass is also seen on Mr. Mueller's lumbar spine. After talking with his physician and an oncologist, and discussing the information with his family, Mr. Mueller decides on a trial course of chemotherapy.

COORDINATION OF INTERDISCIPLINARY CARE

After 3 months of chemotherapy, Mr. Mueller's tumor has not regressed, and a liver scan shows further metastasis. After discussion with his family, Mr. Mueller decides to stop treatment. The Muellers are referred to hospice for end-of-life care. With these services, Mr. Mueller is able to remain at home. His pain is managed with oral morphine sulfate (Roxanol). Mr. Mueller dies at home with his family at his side 9 months after his diagnosis of lung cancer.

1 What are the major focuses of hospice end-of-life care?

2 What kinds of services might be included with hospice end-of-life care?

CRITICAL THINKING

1 What causes the toxic side effects of chemotherapy?

2 How could the nurse help if a client decided to stop cancer treatment but the family disagreed with the decision?

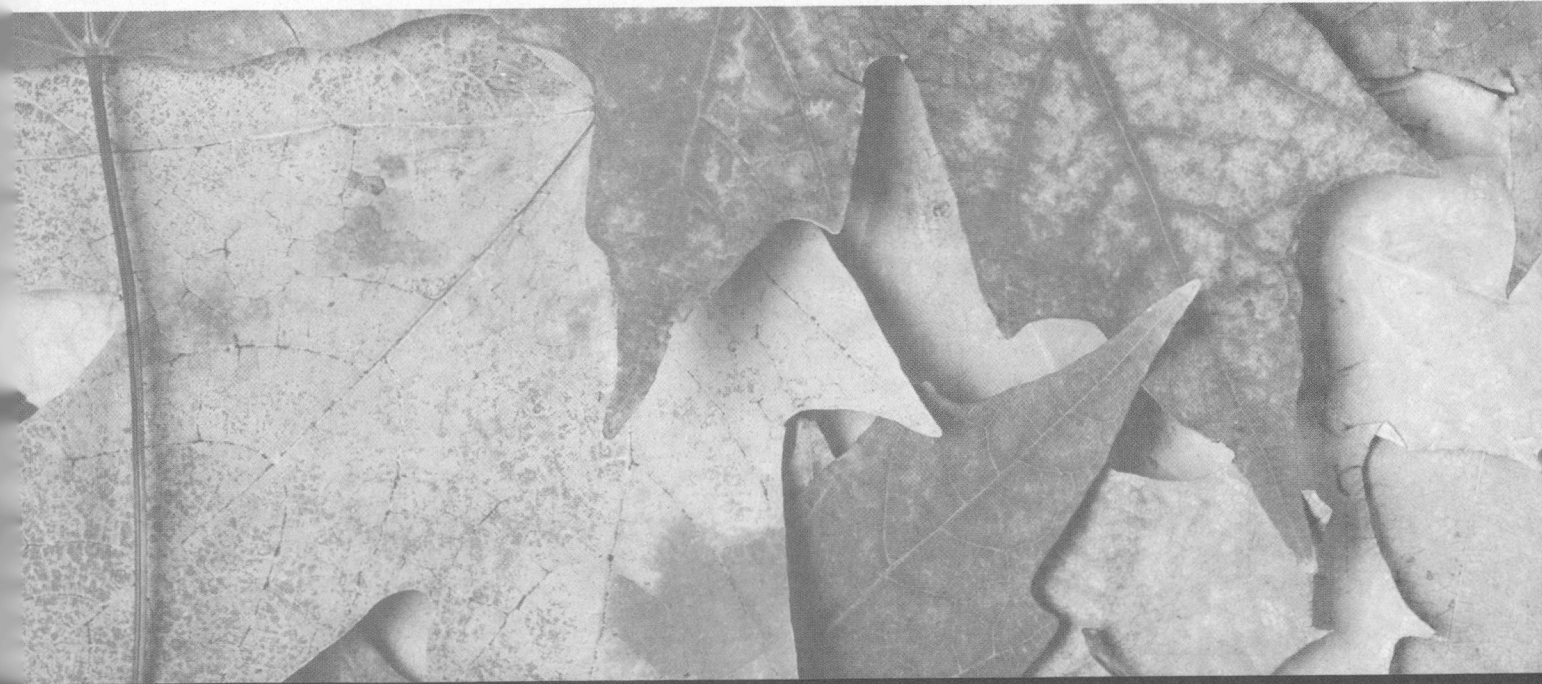

Disrupted Cardiovascular Function

UNIT VI

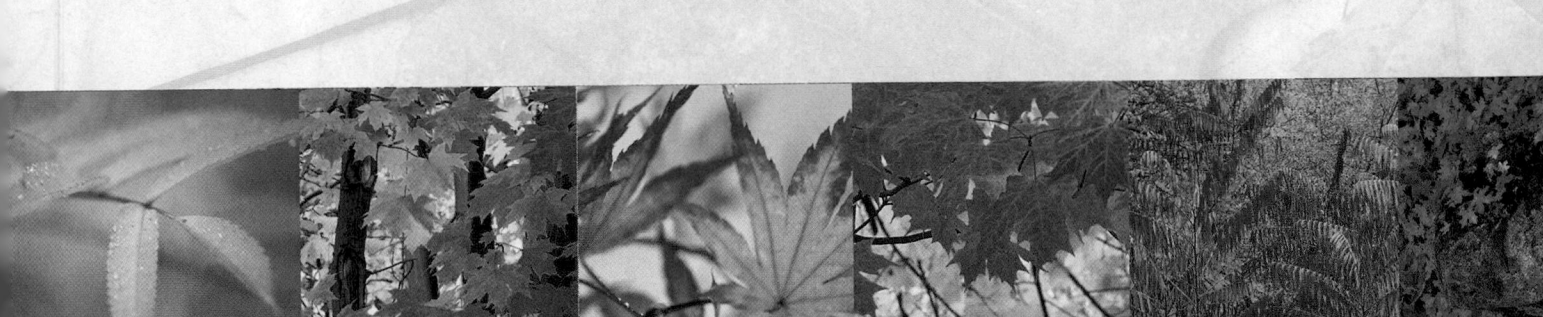

Chapter 25

The Cardiovascular System and Assessment

BRIEF Outline

The Heart
Structure of the Heart
Conduction System
Cardiac Cycle
Cardiac Output

The Peripheral Vascular System
Arteries and Veins
Arterial Circulation

Assessment
Health History
Physical Examination
The Older Adult
Diagnostic Tests

LEARNING Outcomes

After completing this chapter, you will be able to:

- Describe the structure and function of the heart and vascular systems.
- Discuss the mechanical and electrical properties of the heart.
- Identify subjective and objective assessment data to collect for clients with cardiovascular disorders.
- Identify nursing responsibilities for common diagnostic tests and monitors for clients with cardiovascular disorders.

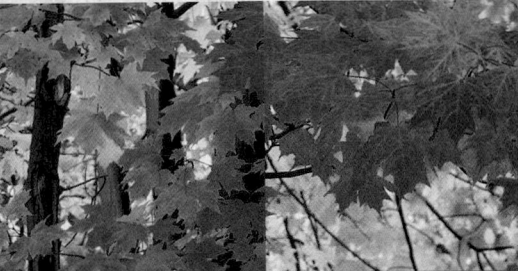

MediaLink

www.prenhall.com/burke
Use the address above to access the free, interactive Companion Website created for this textbook. Get hints, instant feedback, and textbook references to chapter-related NCLEX-style questions. Link to other interesting sites.

Audio Glossary:
Use the Companion Website, or the CD-ROM disk enclosed with your textbook, to hear the pronunciation of key terms in this chapter.

The heart, blood, and blood vessels, collectively known as the cardiovascular system, work together as a fuel delivery and waste removal system for the body. The heart, a simple pump, pushes blood through a system of blood vessels to deliver oxygen and glucose to the cells and tissues. Waste products such as carbon dioxide and other by-products of metabolism are, in turn, taken back to the liver, lungs, and kidneys for disposal. Cardiovascular disorders affect this distribution system, reducing the fuel available to the cells and leading to accumulated waste products in the tissues.

The Heart

The heart, a hollow, cone-shaped organ approximately the size of an adult's fist, weighs less than 1 lb. It is located behind the sternum and between the lungs in the thoracic cavity, slightly to the left of midline (Figure 25-1 ■). The heart is a double pump: The right side receives blood from the body and pumps it to the lungs; the left side receives blood from the lungs and pumps it to the body.

STRUCTURE OF THE HEART

The heart is covered by the *pericardium*. The pericardium encases the heart and anchors it to surrounding structures. It has two layers: The *parietal pericardium* is the outermost layer, and the *visceral pericardium* (also called the *epicardium*) adheres to the heart surface. The small space between these layers contains serous lubricating fluid that cushions the heart as it beats. The epicardium is the outermost layer of the heart wall. The middle layer is the *myocardium,* or heart muscle, and the innermost layer, the *endocardium,* lines the inside of the heart's chambers and great vessels (Figure 25-2 ■).

The heart has four hollow chambers: two upper *atria* and two lower *ventricles.* A septum (or wall) separates the two sides of the heart; *atrioventricular (AV) valves* separate the atria from the ventricles. The flaps of these valves are an-

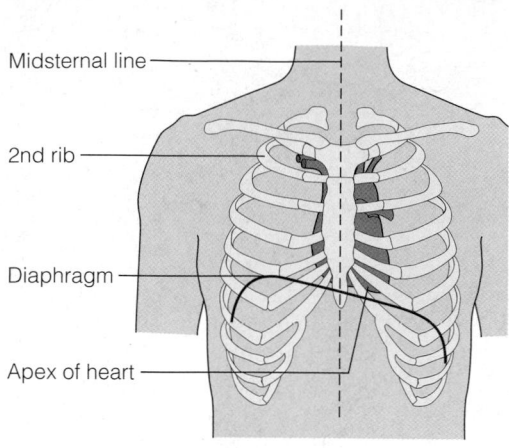

Figure 25-1. ■ Location of the heart within the chest cavity.

chored to the muscles of the ventricles by the chordae tendineae. These structures prevent the backflow of blood during contraction of the higher pressure ventricles.

The *right atrium* receives deoxygenated blood from the veins of the body via the *superior* and *inferior venae cavae.* The right atrium is separated from the right ventricle by the *tricuspid valve.* When open, deoxygenated blood flows through this valve into the *right ventricle,* which then pumps it through the *pulmonary artery* to the lungs (Figure 25-3 ■).

The *left atrium* receives freshly oxygenated blood from the lungs through the *pulmonary veins.* The *left ventricle,* separated from the left atria by the *bicuspid* or *mitral valve,* pumps this freshly oxygenated blood out the *aorta* to the systemic circulation.

The ventricles are connected to their great vessels by the *semilunar valves.* On the right, the *pulmonary valve* joins the right ventricle with the pulmonary artery. On the left, the *aortic valve* joins the left ventricle to the aorta.

The AV valves close as the ventricles start to contract, producing the first heart sound, or S_1 ("lub"). As the ventricles

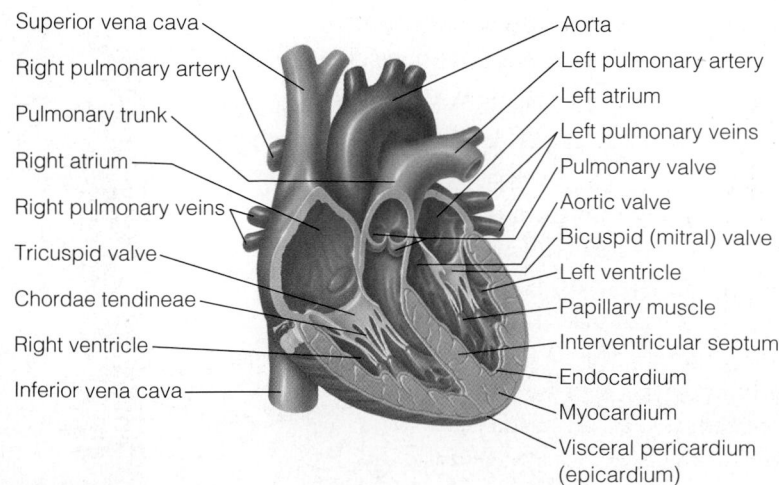

Figure 25-2. ■ The internal anatomy of the heart.

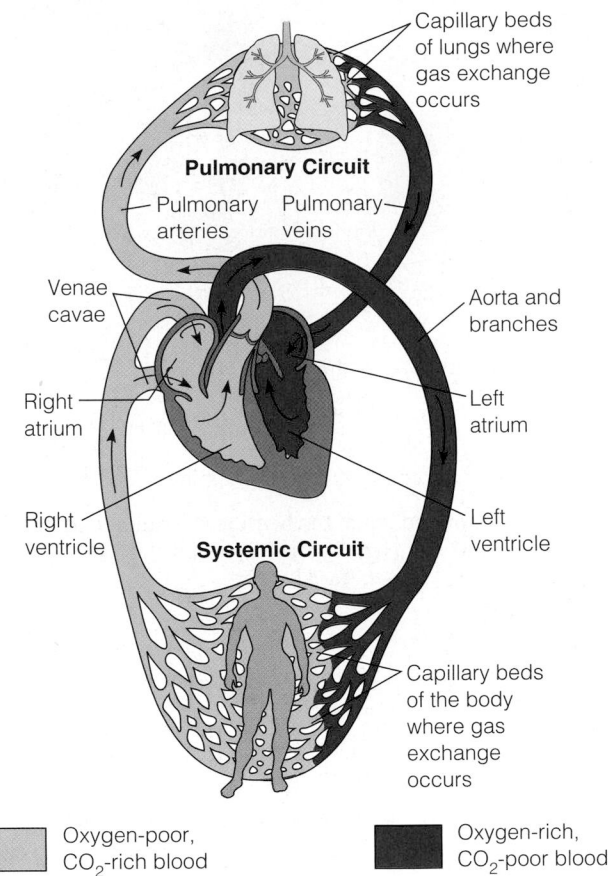

Figure 25-3. ■ Pulmonary and systemic circulation.

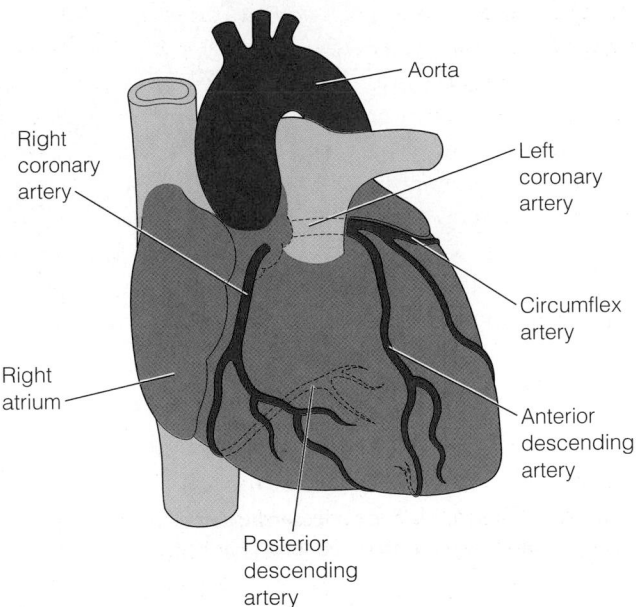

Figure 25-4. ■ The coronary arteries.

start to relax after contraction, the semilunar valves close, producing the second heart sound, or S_2 ("dup").

The *coronary circulation* supplies blood to the heart muscle. The *left* and *right coronary arteries* originate at the base of the aorta and branch out to encircle the myocardium (Figure 25-4 ■). The coronary arteries fill with oxygen-rich blood during ventricular relaxation. Then, after the blood perfuses the heart muscle, the *cardiac veins* drain the blood into the coronary sinus, which empties into the right atrium of the heart.

CONDUCTION SYSTEM

Cardiac muscle is unique. Unlike skeletal muscle tissue, cardiac muscle can generate an electrical impulse and contraction independent of the nervous system. The heartbeat is controlled by specialized cells within the myocardium known as the *conduction system.* The structures of the cardiac conduction system include the sinoatrial node, internodal pathways, atrioventricular node, bundle of His, right and left bundle branches, and Purkinje fibers (Figure 25-5 ■).

The *sinoatrial (SA) node,* located in the wall of the right atrium, acts as the "pacemaker" of the heart, usually generating an impulse 60 to 100 times per minute. This impulse travels through the *internodal pathways* to the *atrioventricular*

(AV) node at the junction between the atria and ventricles. The impulse is slowed as it moves through the AV node, slightly delaying its transmission to the ventricles. It then passes through the *bundle of His* and continues down the interventricular septum through the *right* and *left bundle branches* and out to the *Purkinje fibers* in the ventricular muscle walls.

The electrical impulse, or *action potential,* generated by pacemaker cells is caused by the movement of ions across cell membranes. At rest, myocardial cells are *polarized,* or have a negative charge. The action potential causes the cell membrane to become more positive. This is known as *depolarization.* The action potential and depolarization cause the muscle to contract. With each beat, the heart muscle

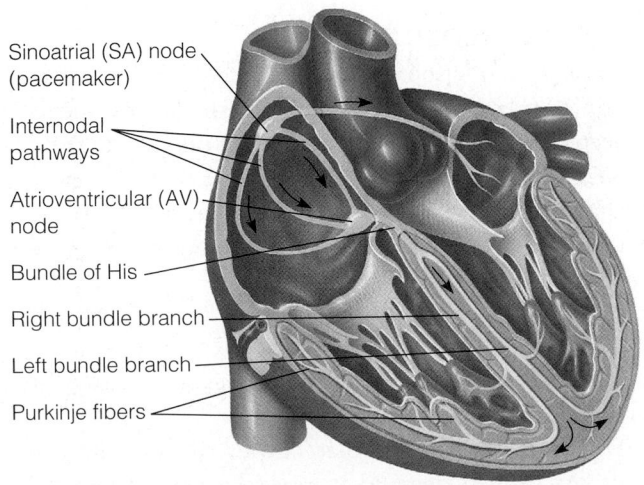

Figure 25-5. ■ The cardiac conduction system.

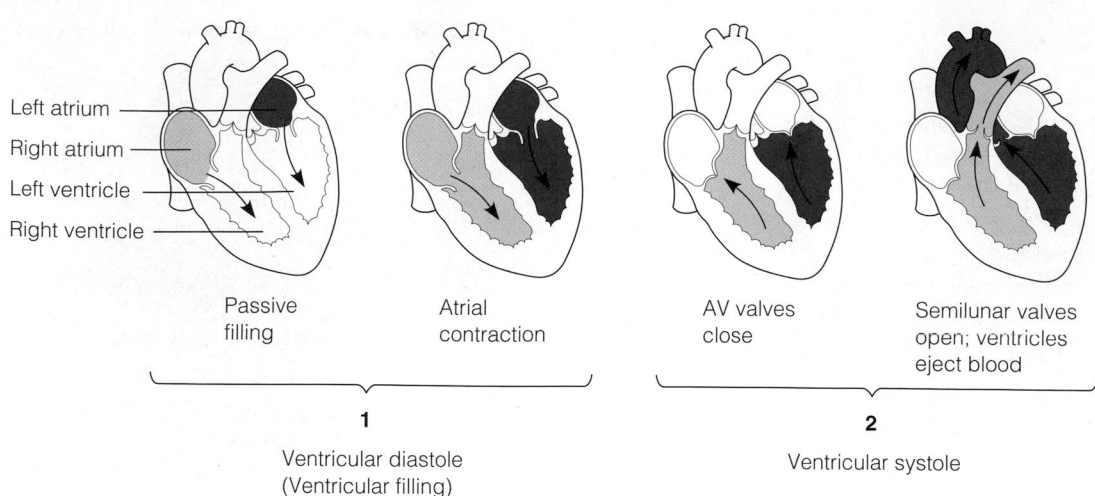

Left atrium
Right atrium
Left ventricle
Right ventricle

Passive filling | Atrial contraction | AV valves close | Semilunar valves open; ventricles eject blood

1 | **2**
Ventricular diastole (Ventricular filling) | Ventricular systole

Figure 25-6. ■ The cardiac cycle. Ventricular filling occurs during diastole (1); blood is pumped out of the heart to the pulmonary and systemic circulation during ventricular systole (2).

contracts to its fullest potential (the *all-or-nothing response*). *Repolarization* begins immediately after depolarization, returning the cell to its resting state. For a brief period during and after repolarization, the cell resists stimulation. This is known as the *refractory period.* It protects the heart muscle from going into spasm or tetany (continuous contraction). This electrical activity produces the waveforms represented on ECG strips.

CARDIAC CYCLE

The contraction and relaxation of the heart constitute one heartbeat and is called the cardiac cycle (Figure 25-6 ■). Ventricular filling occurs during **diastole,** when the ventricles are relaxed. Toward the end of diastole, the atria contract, pumping additional blood into the ventricles. During ventricular **systole,** the ventricles contract, ejecting blood into the pulmonary and systemic circuits. Normally, the complete cardiac cycle occurs about 70 to 80 times per minute (the *heart rate*).

CARDIAC OUTPUT

With each contraction, a certain volume of blood (approximately 70 mL in an adult), called the **stroke volume (SV),** is ejected from the heart. The **cardiac output (CO)** is the amount of blood pumped by the ventricles in 1 minute. Cardiac output indicates how well the heart is functioning as a pump. It is calculated by multiplying the stroke volume by the heart rate (HR):

$$CO = HR \times SV$$

The average adult cardiac output ranges from 4 to 8 liters per minute (L/min).

The heart regulates cardiac output to meet the body's needs. As oxygen demand increases, oxygen supply must also increase. *Cardiac reserve* is the ability of the heart to in-

crease CO and blood pressure to meet the demand. Cardiac output is determined by four major factors: heart rate, preload, afterload, and contractility.

Heart rate is affected by activity level, the autonomic nervous system, and hormones. Increased heart rates increase cardiac output; however, very rapid heart rates allow less time for ventricular filling and may reduce stroke volume and cardiac output. If the heart rate is too slow, cardiac output falls simply because the heart contracts less often.

Preload is the amount of blood in the ventricles prior to contraction. The blood in the ventricles stretches the muscle fibers, causing them to contract more forcefully. Preload is affected by venous return. If blood volume is low (e.g., due to hemorrhage or dehydration), it falls. To a certain point, the greater the blood volume, the greater the force with which the ventricle contracts. Beyond a certain volume, however, the heart contracts less effectively. This is called *Starling's law of the heart.*

Afterload is the force the ventricles must develop to push blood into the circulation. The right ventricle pushes blood into the low-pressure pulmonary system. The left ventricle ejects its blood into the systemic circulation. Systemic arterial pressures are much higher than pulmonary pressures; therefore, the left ventricle has to work much harder than the right ventricle.

Contractility is the natural ability of the cardiac muscle fibers to shorten during systole. Contractility is necessary to move blood into the circulation. Poor contractility reduces the ability of the ventricle to eject blood, decreasing stroke volume. The *ejection fraction,* or percentage of blood in the ventricle that is ejected with each contraction, is affected by the interaction of preload, afterload, and contractility.

The Peripheral Vascular System

The **peripheral vascular system** is a network of blood vessels that carry blood to peripheral tissues and then return it to the heart. This network includes arteries, veins, and capillaries.

ARTERIES AND VEINS

Arteries carry blood away from the heart. Oxygenated blood leaves the left ventricle via the *aorta.* Major arteries branch off the aorta and into successively smaller arteries. These eventually divide into *arterioles.* Arterioles feed into beds of hairlike *capillaries* within the organs and tissues.

In the capillary beds, oxygen and nutrients are exchanged for metabolic wastes, and deoxygenated blood begins its journey back to the heart through *venules.* Venules join onto veins, which in turn join larger and larger veins. *Veins* carry blood toward the heart. Peripheral veins empty into the *superior* and *inferior venae cavae,* and then into the right atrium.

Blood Vessel Structure

The structure of blood vessels reflects their different functions within the circulatory system. Except for the capillaries, blood vessel walls have three layers: the tunica intima, the tunica media, and the tunica adventitia (Figure 25-7 ■). The innermost layer, the *tunica intima,* or *endothelium,* has a slick surface to assist blood flow. The middle layer, or *tunica media,* contains smooth muscle. This layer is thicker and more elastic in arteries than it is in veins. It allows arteries to expand and contract, maintaining blood flow to the capillaries between heartbeats. *Constriction* (narrowing) and *dilation* (widening) of the arterioles is the major factor controlling blood pressure. The *tunica adventitia,* or outermost layer, is connective tissue that protects and anchors the vessel. Veins have a thicker tunica adventitia than do arteries.

The pressure in the veins is much lower than in the arteries. Veins have thinner walls, a larger lumen, and greater capacity than arteries. Many have valves that help move blood against gravity back to the heart. Skeletal muscle contraction helps: When skeletal muscles contract against veins, the valves open, and blood is propelled toward the heart. Changes in abdominal and thoracic pressure that occur with breathing also propel blood toward the heart.

The tiny capillaries, which connect the arterioles and venules, contain only one thin layer of tunica intima. This allows gases and nutrients to escape the blood vessels and reach tissue cells. Waste products from metabolism enter the capillaries for elimination. Capillaries are found in interwoven networks.

ARTERIAL CIRCULATION

Arterial circulation is maintained by a balance of blood flow, peripheral vascular resistance, and blood pressure. *Blood flow* is the amount of blood transported.

Peripheral vascular resistance (PVR) is the force opposing blood flow. PVR is determined by three factors:

1. *Blood viscosity (thickness):* The greater the viscosity of the blood, the greater its resistance to moving and flowing.
2. *Vessel length:* The longer the vessel, the greater the resistance to blood flow.
3. *Vessel diameter:* The smaller a vessel is, the more friction is produced, and the greater the resistance is to blood flow.

Blood pressure (BP) is the force exerted by blood against the walls of the arteries. The *systolic* pressure is the force exerted as the heart contracts (systole). The *diastolic* pressure reflects the force exerted when the heart is filling

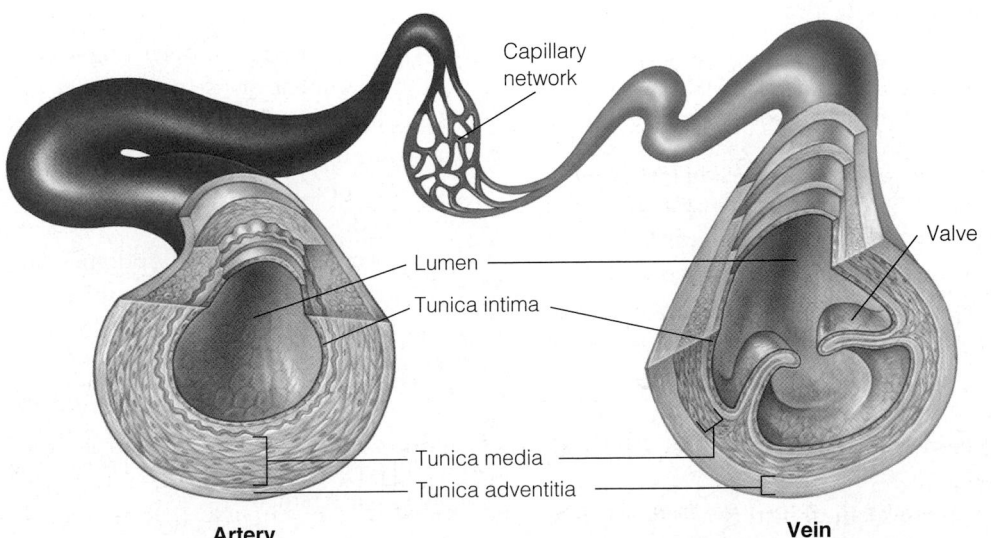

Artery   **Vein**

Figure 25-7. ■ Structure of arteries, veins, and capillaries.

(diastole). The average adult BP is 120/80 mm Hg. The blood pressure is regulated mainly by cardiac output (CO) and peripheral vascular resistance (PVR). A number of factors affect CO and PVR:

- Sympathetic nervous system (SNS) stimulation increases cardiac output and constricts arterioles, increasing blood pressure. Pressure-sensitive receptors (*baroreceptors*) and *chemoreceptors* in the aortic arch, carotid sinus, and other large vessels stimulate the SNS.
- Parasympathetic stimulation causes dilation of arterioles, lowering the blood pressure.
- The kidneys help regulate BP. A fall in BP stimulates the renin–angiotensin–aldosterone mechanism, causing vasoconstriction and salt and water retention. Antidiuretic hormone (ADH) from the pituitary gland promotes water retention, increasing blood volume, cardiac output, and blood pressure.
- Temperatures affect peripheral resistance: Cold causes vasoconstriction; warmth produces vasodilation.
- Many chemicals, hormones, and drugs affect cardiac output or peripheral vascular resistance.

Other factors that affect cardiac output, peripheral vascular resistance, and BP include diet (e.g., sodium and calcium intake), race, gender, age, weight, time of day, position, exercise, and emotional state.

Assessment

HEALTH HISTORY

Focused assessment of the client with cardiovascular disease begins by asking about current symptoms. Inquire about the presence of chest pain and its duration.

clinical ALERT

If the client is experiencing acute chest pain or shortness of breath, complete only a brief, focused assessment on the acute symptoms. Notify the charge nurse or physician. Complete assessment data collection once the acute symptoms have been relieved and the client is resting comfortably.

Ask about past episodes of chest or leg pain and its relationship to activity. Inquire about shortness of breath, and determine how many pillows the client uses to sleep (clients with heart failure may be unable to sleep lying flat). Ask about recent changes in energy level or fatigue, as well as recent weight gain.

Obtain the client's past medical history and family health history, focusing on previous episodes of heart disease, circulation problems, or blood disorders. Inquire about the presence or a family history of diabetes and high blood pressure.

Ask the client to identify all medications (including prescription, over-the-counter, and natural or herbal preparations) currently being taken and the purpose of each drug. This information often helps identify the presence of a medical problem not previously mentioned, or may help the nurse relate current symptoms to an adverse drug effect or interaction.

Lifestyle factors have a significant effect on the risk for heart disease. Inquire about diet and usual alcohol intake (average number of mixed drinks, beers, or glasses of wine per day). Have the client describe usual patterns of exercise and physical activity. If the client smokes, ascertain at what age the client started smoking and the number of packs of cigarettes per day smoked or type of tobacco product used. Ask about use of illicit drugs such as cocaine.

PHYSICAL EXAMINATION

The focused physical examination for the client with cardiovascular disease begins by assessing the client's general appearance. Observe for apparent general health, facial expression, and body type. Assess skin color and temperature; evaluate hair distribution, particularly on the lower extremities. Observe for taut, shiny, thin-appearing skin and areas of discoloration on the lower extremities as well. Note any wounds or ulcerations, and assess for healing. Evaluate skin turgor.

Obtain the blood pressure on both arms (unless contraindicated), an apical pulse, and the respiratory rate. Note any evidence of neck vein distention. Palpate peripheral pulses on upper and lower extremities, noting their strength and equality. Note capillary refill on both the upper and lower extremities. Observe and palpate the lower extremities for the presence of edema. Measure the circumference of the calves if they appear unequal or if the client complains of lower extremity pain. Note any heat, tenderness, or redness of the extremities.

Observe the ease of breathing, noting any asymmetry of chest movement or use of accessory muscles of respiration. Auscultate breath sounds throughout all lung fields, noting any diminished or adventitious breath sounds. Note the presence of a cough, and, if present, describe any sputum produced.

Inspect the chest and abdomen for visible pulsations. Palpate for the location of the apical impulse (point of maximal impulse or PMI). Auscultate the heart, noting the rate and rhythm and any irregularities. Report any abnormal heart sounds such as a gallop or murmur.

For more information about assessment techniques, see Chapter 5 ⬤. See Box 25-1 ■ for an example of a cardiovascular assessment.

THE OLDER ADULT

Physical changes commonly associated with aging may affect cardiovascular assessment in the older adult. Subcutaneous

BOX 25-1

DOCUMENTATION OF CARDIOVASCULAR ASSESSMENT

Client: 72 y.o. black male admitted to rule out myocardial infarction following acute episode of chest pain. No evidence of infarction; undergoing diagnostic testing. Has type 2 diabetes and peripheral vascular disease.

Assessment note: Alert and oriented. Appears moderately anxious but in no acute distress. Denies pain, shortness of breath at this time. Vital signs stable. Skin color and turgor good, no cyanosis of oral mucosa or nail beds noted. Skin warm and dry on trunk and upper extremities; cool, dry, and shiny bilaterally below the knees. Several areas of darker pigmentation noted over both shins and medial ankles. No edema or ulcerations noted. Peripheral pulses strong (3+) and equal upper extremities; weak (2+) and equal lower extremities. Upper extremity capillary refill immediate, slower (>3 seconds) lower extremities. Breathing relaxed, chest movement equal. Good breath sounds throughout lung fields with no crackles or rhonchi noted. Apical pulse basically regular with an occasional early beat noted (<1–2 per minute). Clear S_1, S_2.

tissue is lost with aging, causing the skin to appear paler and thinner. Skin turgor may be more accurately assessed over the sternum than on the arms. Less hair may be noted on the ex-

tremities. Thinning of capillary walls and loss of tissue support may lead to easy bruising, petechiae, and bleeding into subcutaneous tissues. Varicose veins and tortuous, irregular veins are more commonly seen in aging.

Many older adults experience occasional early heartbeats, although the rate remains basically regular. Although many older adults become more sedentary, regular exercise such as walking, swimming, and weight training is encouraged. The heart rate does not respond as rapidly to exercise and physical activity, requiring longer warm-up and cooldown periods.

An increased incidence of chronic diseases and medication use in older adults increases the risk of drug interactions that may affect the cardiovascular system. Changes in the heart rate and its regularity may occur. Some medications may increase the risk for orthostatic hypotension (a drop in blood pressure occurring with changes in position) and falls.

DIAGNOSTIC TESTS

Laboratory Tests

Several laboratory tests commonly are performed to evaluate the cardiovascular system. Table 25-1 ■ lists these tests,

TABLE 25-1

Common Laboratory Tests for Cardiovascular Disease

TEST	NORMAL ADULT VALUES	EXPLANATION	NURSING IMPLICATIONS
Lipid Profile: ■ Total cholesterol ■ Triglycerides ■ High-density lipoproteins (HDL) ■ Low-density lipoproteins (LDL) ■ Very low-density lipoproteins (VLDL)	140–199 mg/dL <200 mg/dL 60 mg/dL <100 mg/dL (desirable) 25–50% of total triglycerides	Performed to evaluate risk for atherosclerosis and coronary heart disease. Lower levels or total cholesterol and triglycerides are better. Higher levels of HDL help remove excess cholesterol from the blood and are desirable. LDL and VLDL promote cholesterol buildup in arteries; lower levels are better.	These tests should be performed fasting. Instruct the client to refrain from eating or drinking (sips of water are allowed) for 12 hours prior to testing, and to avoid alcohol intake for 24 hours prior to testing.
C-reactive protein	<0.5 mg/dL	A sensitive measure of inflammation; may help predict coronary heart disease.	No special precautions or preparation required.
Serum Cardiac Markers ■ Creatine phosphokinase (CK or CPK) ■ CK-MB ■ cT_nT ■ cT_nI	Male: 12–80 U/L Female: 10–70 U/L 0–3% of total CK <0.2 mcg/L <3.1 mcg/L	Cardiac markers are proteins released from dead or damaged heart muscle cells. CK is a protein in heart and skeletal muscle; CK-MB is a subset of CK found in heart muscle. Cardiac muscle troponins, cT_nT and cT_nI, are sensitive indicators of heart muscle damage.	Fasting is not required but some drugs may interfere with test results. Serial levels of these enzymes often are obtained, necessitating blood draws every 12 to 24 hours for several days.
Serum Cardiac Hormones ■ Atrial natriuretic factor (ANF) or hormone (ANH) ■ B-type natriuretic peptide (BNP)	20–27 pg/mL 34–42 pg/Ml	These hormones are released by the heart muscle in response to changes in blood volume. Increased blood levels indicate heart failure.	These tests are performed fasting. Unless contraindicated, withhold cardiac drugs for 24 hours before testing.

BOX 25-2

ELECTROCARDIOGRAM

An electrocardiogram (ECG) is a "picture" of the heart's electrical activity. Electrodes placed on different parts of the body allow different views of the heart's electrical activity, much like turning while holding a camera provides different views of the scenery.

A standard 12-lead ECG includes recordings of 6 limb leads and 6 precordial leads. The *limb leads* provide a view of the inferior and lateral walls of the heart. The *precordial leads* (chest or V leads) provide a view of the anterior, septal, lateral, and posterior walls of the heart.

ECG waveforms show the direction of electrical flow. Current moving toward the positive electrode causes an upward (positive) waveform; current moving away from it produces a downward (negative) waveform. When no electrical activity is occurring, a straight line, called the *isoelectric line*, is seen.

ECG waveforms are recorded on paper marked at intervals that represent time and voltage or amplitude (see first figure). Each small box represents 0.04 second. Five small boxes make one large box, equivalent to 0.20 second. Five large boxes represent 1 full second.

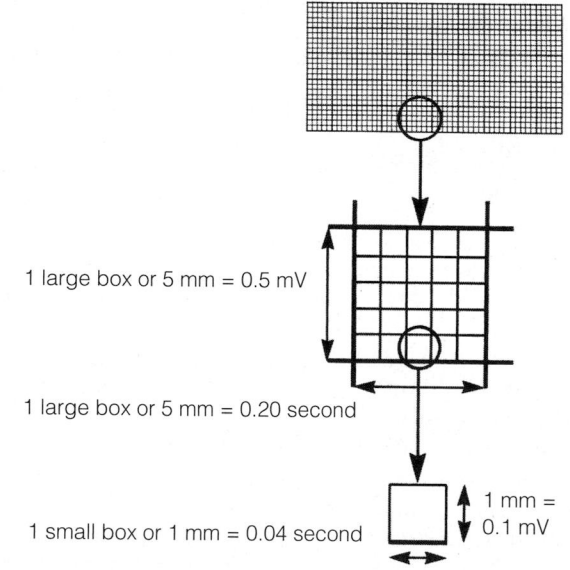

1 large box or 5 mm = 0.5 mV

1 large box or 5 mm = 0.20 second

1 small box or 1 mm = 0.04 second

1 mm = 0.1 mV

The P, Q, R, S, and T waves represent the cardiac cycle (see second figure). The P *wave* shows the SA node impulse and atrial depolarization. It precedes the QRS complex and is normally smooth, round, and upright. The PR *interval* is the time required for the impulse to travel to the AV node and the bundle branches. It is measured from beginning of P wave to beginning of QRS complex. The PR interval is normally 0.12 to 0.20 second.

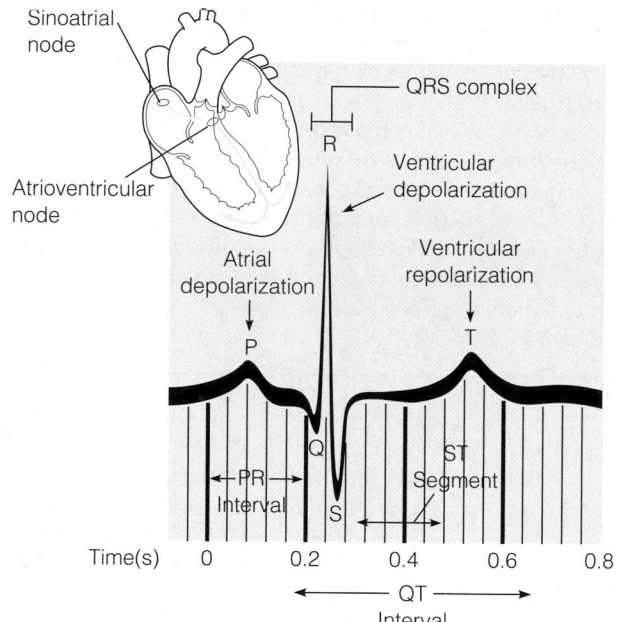

The *QRS complex* indicates ventricular depolarization. It occurs rapidly, lasting from 0.06 to 0.10 second. The *ST segment*, the period from the end of the QRS complex to the beginning of the T wave, is normally isoelectric. The T wave represents ventricular repolarization; it is smooth and rounded, and points in the same direction as the QRS complex. The *QT interval*, measured from the beginning of the QRS to the end of the T wave, indicates the total time for ventricular depolarization and repolarization. Its duration varies with gender, age, and heart rate; usually, it is 0.32 to 0.44 second long. The *U wave* is not normally seen but may show repolarization of the terminal Purkinje fibers.

their normal values, what the test measures and its significance, and any nursing implications for the test.

Electrocardiography

The **electrocardiogram (ECG)** is a record of the heart's electrical activity detected by electrodes placed on the skin (Box 25-2 ■). ECG waveforms and patterns are used to detect dysrhythmias, myocardial damage or enlargement, and the effects of drugs.

Electrocardiography may be used on a continual or intermittent basis, depending on the client's needs. Table 25-2 ■ summarizes ECG studies used in diagnosing heart problems, along with their nursing implications.

Imaging Techniques

Imaging techniques used to diagnose cardiovascular disease range from noninvasive to very invasive. These diagnostic procedures and their nursing implications are summarized in Table 25-3 ■.

Electrophysiology Studies

Cardiac electrophysiology (EP) studies are used to diagnose (and sometimes treat) abnormal cardiac rhythms. EP procedures are invasive procedures performed in an electrophysiology laboratory. Electrode catheters inserted into the heart through the brachial or femoral vein are used to evaluate the conduction system of the heart and locate sites where

TABLE 25-2

Diagnostic Electrocardiographic Studies

DIAGNOSTIC TEST	PURPOSE	NURSING IMPLICATIONS
12-Lead ECG (resting ECG)	Used to evaluate the heart rhythm, conduction through the electrical pathways of the heart, and the size and position of the heart in the chest cavity. Can reveal areas of ischemia, injury, or infarction (tissue necrosis).	Noninvasive. Very tense muscles (for example, a highly anxious client) and movement can interfere with results. Note current medications because some drugs affect the ECG.
Stress electrocardiography (treadmill testing)	Monitors the ECG during exercise on a treadmill or stationary bicycle to detect asymptomatic coronary heart disease (CHD). During exercise, the workload of the heart increases; this increased workload may cause myocardial ischemia and angina in clients with CHD.	The client's ECG, heart rate, and blood pressure are monitored continuously during testing. Stress testing may cause a cardiac emergency. A physician is present or immediately available during stress testing and emergency resuscitation supplies are kept in the immediate area.
Pharmacologic stress testing	Used when physical exercise is not possible (e.g., for clients with orthopedic problems). A vasodilator drug is administered which may cause ischemia in areas of the heart affected by CHD, much like exercise does.	
Continuous cardiac monitoring (telemetry, Holter monitoring)	Electrodes placed on the client's chest are connected to a monitoring system for continuous monitoring of the heart rate and rhythm to detect and diagnose abnormal heart rhythms. ECG signals may be displayed on a bedside monitor, central monitoring station, or recorded in a portable unit for later evaluation (*Holter monitoring*). Ambulatory monitors may record continuously for a 24- to 72-hour period or allow the client to record cardiac activity intermittently when symptoms are experienced (such as chest pain or palpitations).	Provide teaching about the purpose of monitoring. Apply electrodes to clean, dry skin, removing hair as appropriate. Instruct the client how to replace the electrodes (if appropriate) and about care of the skin and recording or telemetry unit. Caution the client to avoid getting the telemetry or recording unit wet. Instruct the client when it is appropriate to contact the nurse or physician.

TABLE 25-3

Imaging Studies

DIAGNOSTIC STUDY	EXPLANATION AND PURPOSE	NURSING IMPLICATIONS
Sonography (Doppler Studies, Echocardiography)	Echoes from high-frequency sound waves are used to study the structure and movement of organs (e.g., the heart) and the flow of blood within a vessel.	
Transthoracic echocardiogram (TTE)	A transducer lubricated with conductive gel held against the chest wall transmits and receives the ultrasonic impulses. A computer converts the impulses to an image of the heart walls, chambers, and their movements.	Noninvasive; performed at the client's bedside. Conductive gel may be cold. Provide a washcloth or wash the chest wall following the exam for comfort.
Transesophageal echocardiogram (TEE)	A flexible transducer mounted on an endoscope provides a more direct view of the heart by avoiding the interference of chest wall structures.	The client is sedated and the throat anesthetized to allow passage of the endoscope into the esophagus. Monitor breathing, cough, and gag reflexes following the exam. Keep NPO until the gag reflex returns and the client is fully awake.
Stress echocardiogram	This test combines a resting TTE, exercise on a treadmill or stationary bicycle with continuous ECG monitoring, and a repeat TTE immediately following exercise to evaluate the effect of exercise on cardiac function.	Although noninvasive, requires monitoring as for a stress ECG (see Table 25-2).

(*continued*)

TABLE 25-3

Imaging Studies (continued)

DIAGNOSTIC STUDY	EXPLANATION AND PURPOSE	NURSING IMPLICATIONS
Vascular ultrasound (Doppler imaging, duplex scans)	These are noninvasive procedures that provide information about the structure of and blood flow through major blood vessels. Conductive gel is applied over the vessel to be studied, and a handheld transducer is maneuvered over the vessel. Blood pressures at various locations of the extremity are taken when used to evaluate peripheral circulation.	Explain the test and its purpose. Monitor blood pressures as indicated. Wash the extremity following the exam for comfort.
Radiography (X-Ray Studies) Chest and abdominal x-rays	Used to identify the size and location of structures, and, when combined with use of an injected contrast medium, used to study blood flow through vessels and organs. Used to evaluate the size and position of the heart and to identify abnormalities of major blood vessels such as the aorta (e.g., an abdominal aortic aneurysm).	If contrast is injected, ask about allergies (specifically including iodine or seafood) before the exam; ensure good hydration before and after the exam to reduce the risk of kidney damage. While these studies are noninvasive, they expose the client to potentially damaging radiation. Ask women of childbearing age about possible pregnancy before the exam.
Angiography	This is an invasive procedure that combines x-rays and fluoroscopy (a radiographic image displayed on a screen) with injection of a contrast agent into the vessel to illuminate blood flow through the vessel, and evaluation of its patency and structure. May also be used to treat cardiovascular disease, e.g., insertion of a stent into a partially blocked vessel to restore blood flow. Risks associated with insertion of the catheter into a high-pressure artery include (1) bleeding from the insertion site and (2) clot formation at the insertion site and impaired blood flow to the extremity.	See Box 26-3 ☍☍ for a nursing care checklist for the client undergoing a coronary angiography procedure. **clinical ALERT** Closely monitor the client, the insertion site, and the extremity after the procedure. Immediately report evidence of bleeding, pain, or a pale, pulseless extremity to the charge nurse and physician.
Cardiac catheterization	Used to detect abnormalities in the chambers and valves of the heart; often done together with coronary angiography. A catheter inserted into the chambers of the heart (via a large vein to access the right side of the heart, or the femoral or brachial artery to access the left side of the heart) is used to measure pressures within the chambers of the heart, cardiac output, and the oxygen content and saturation of the blood. Contrast agents injected into the heart outline structures of the heart.	Nursing care for the client undergoing a cardiac catheterization is similar to that for coronary angiography (see above and Box 26-3 ☍☍).
Computed tomography (CT) scans	Specialized radiographic procedures that produce computer-generated images with significantly more detail than standard x-rays allow. May be done with or without contrast media, although contrast is used when a CT scan is done to identify vessel abnormalities such as an aneurysm.	If contrast is used, inquire about allergies (to iodine and seafood in particular), and ensure that the client is well hydrated to reduce the risk of kidney damage.
Electron beam computed tomography (EBCT)	A noninvasive imaging study that can detect calcium deposits in coronary arteries. Calcium deposits indicate atherosclerosis, and can predict coronary heart disease in people with no symptoms. May be used as an alternative to stress testing for diagnosing coronary heart disease.	Ask women of childbearing age about possible pregnancy.

TABLE 25-3

Imaging Studies (continued)

DIAGNOSTIC STUDY	EXPLANATION AND PURPOSE	NURSING IMPLICATIONS
Magnetic Resonance Imaging (MRI)	MRI uses a supermagnet and radio-frequency signals to elicit a response from hydrogen nuclei. As a result, blood flow can be studied, and diseased tissue can be differentiated from healthy tissue. ■ *Cardiac MRI* shows thickness of the heart walls, size of the chambers, valve function, and coronary vessel flow. ■ *MRI angiography* is noninvasive, and is used to evaluate vessel structure and blood flow.	The client is not exposed to radiation during an MRI. Ask about implanted metal (e. g., a joint prosthesis) or electronic devices such as pacemakers or automatic defibrillators. Provide teaching because the experience can be frightening.
Radionuclear Scans	Used to evaluate blood flow to the heart muscle. A radioactive substance is injected intravenously, and the heart is scanned with a radiation detector. Ischemic or infarcted heart muscle cells do not take up the substance normally, creating an image on the scan.	The amount of radioisotope injected is very small; no special radiation precautions are required during or after the scan. Increased fluid intake is encouraged after the scan to speed elimination of the substance from the body.

abnormal rhythms originate. Nursing care for the client undergoing EP studies is similar to that for coronary angiography (see Box 26-3 ⬤⬤).

Other Diagnostic Tests

The *ankle-brachial index* is a noninvasive test that has been shown to be highly indicative of atherosclerosis. Blood pressure cuffs (up to four) are placed at intervals on the extremity. Each cuff is inflated, and a Doppler device is used to measure the systolic pressure distal to the cuff, until the entire extremity has been evaluated. The ankle-brachial index is calculated by dividing the systolic pressure at the ankle by the brachial systolic pressure. An index of greater than 1.0 is considered normal.

Note: The bibliography listings for this and all chapters have been compiled at the back of the book.

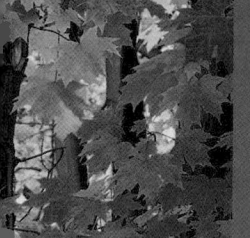

Chapter Review

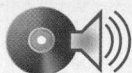 **KEY TERMS** by Topics

Use the audio glossary feature of either the CD-ROM or the Companion Website to hear the correct pronunciation of the following key terms.

The heart
diastole, systole, stroke volume (SV), cardiac output (CO), contractility

The peripheral vascular system
peripheral vascular system, peripheral vascular resistance (PVR), blood pressure (BP)

Assessment
electrocardiogram (ECG)

KEY Points

- The heart is a simple pump: The right side receives blood from the veins and pumps it into the low-pressure pulmonary system; the left side receives blood from the lungs, and pumps it to the higher pressure systemic circulation.

- The myocardium, or heart muscle, receives its blood supply through the coronary arteries. The left and right coronary arteries originate at the base of the aorta; the left coronary artery supplies blood to most of the left ventricle.

- Electrical impulses, usually generated by the sinoatrial (SA) node, travel through conduction pathways in the heart, causing the muscle to contract.

- The cardiac output is the amount of blood pumped by the heart in 1 minute; it can be calculated by multiplying the stroke volume (amount ejected during systole) by the heart rate. Cardiac output is affected by heart rate, preload (amount of blood in the ventricles prior to contraction), afterload (determined primarily by peripheral vascular resistance), and the contractility of the heart muscle.

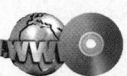 **EXPLORE Media**Link

Additional interactive resources for this chapter can be found on the Companion Website at www.prenhall.com/burke. Click on Chapter 25 and "Begin" to select the activities for this chapter.

For chapter-related NCLEX-style review questions and an audio glossary, access the accompanying CD-ROM in this book.

FOR FURTHER Study

For more information about assessment techniques, see Chapter 5.

See Box 26-3 for a nursing care checklist for the client undergoing a coronary angiography procedure.

NCLEX-PN® Exam Preparation

1 The nurse caring for a client with pericarditis recognizes that this disorder affects which layer of the heart?

A. the innermost layer
B. the heart muscle layer
C. the middle layer
D. the outermost layer

2 A client with mitral valve stenosis is admitted to the medical unit. The nurse knows that this disorder will affect

A. blood flow from the right atrium to the right ventricle.
B. blood flow from the left atrium to the left ventricle.
C. blood flow from the right ventricle to the lungs.
D. blood flow from the left ventricle to the body.

3 Ventricular systole corresponds with which waveform on the ECG?

A. the P wave
B. the QRS complex
C. the T wave
D. the S-T segment

4 Which of the following factors have a significant effect on peripheral vascular resistance? (Select all that apply.)

A. the number of capillaries
B. length of blood vessels
C. blood vessel diameter
D. the position of the body
E. viscosity of the blood
F. age of the client

5 The nurse is teaching a client about an upcoming echocardiogram. Which information below is accurate?

A. The test provides information about the size and movement of the heart and its structures.
B. This test is noninvasive and simply requires external electrodes to be placed on the arms, legs, and chest.
C. Dye will be injected during this test to illuminate the structures of the heart and blood flow through its chambers and valves.
D. This test is noninvasive but does expose the client to a magnetic field.

Answers for Review Questions appear in Appendix V.

Chapter 26

Caring for Clients with Coronary Heart Disease and Dysrhythmias

BRIEF Outline

Coronary Heart Disease
Angina Pectoris
Acute Myocardial Infarction
Cardiac Dysrhythmias
Sudden Cardiac Death

LEARNING Outcomes

After completing this chapter, you will be able to:

- Describe the causes, pathophysiology, effects, and manifestations of coronary heart disease and heart rhythm disruptions.

- Discuss nursing implications for drugs commonly prescribed for clients with coronary heart disease or dysrhythmias.

- Describe nursing care for clients undergoing invasive procedures or surgery of the heart.

- Use the nursing process to collect assessment data, contribute to care planning, and provide individualized nursing care for clients with coronary heart disease and dysrhythmias.

- Provide and reinforce appropriate teaching for clients with coronary heart disease or dysrhythmias and their families.

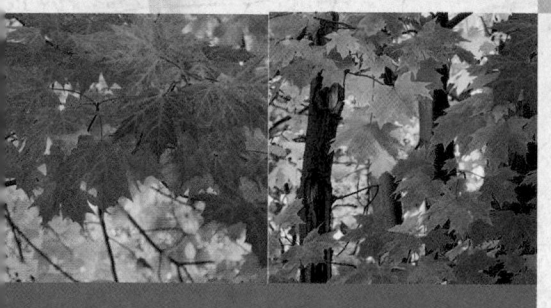

MediaLink

www.prenhall.com/burke
Use the address above to access the free, interactive Companion Website created for this textbook. Get hints, instant feedback, and textbook references to chapter-related NCLEX-style questions. Link to other interesting sites.

Audio Glossary:
Use the Companion Website, or the CD-ROM disk enclosed with your textbook, to hear the pronunciation of key terms in this chapter.

Cardiovascular disease (CVD) is the leading cause of death and disability in the United States. Approximately 21 million people are affected by heart disease and more than 700,000 people die from it each year. Public education efforts aimed at reducing fat intake, increasing exercise, and lowering stress levels have made people more aware of risk factors for heart disease, and the incidence of new cases has fallen.

In this chapter, you will learn about the causes and effects of two major heart disorders: impaired blood flow to the heart muscle itself (*coronary heart disease*) and abnormal heart rhythms, or *dysrhythmias*. The following chapter, Chapter 27, ⬤⬤ discusses caring for clients with disorders that affect the structure and function of the heart.

Nurses need to know about heart disease and its causes to teach and care for clients appropriately. This chapter provides the beginning nurse with the tools necessary to effectively care for clients with coronary heart disease and dysrhythmias.

Coronary Heart Disease

Coronary heart disease (CHD), or coronary artery disease (CAD), is the leading cause of death for both men and women in the United States. Of the more than 1 million people who have heart attacks each year, about 460,000 die. Nearly half of the deaths occur before the client reaches the hospital. CHD is caused by narrowing of the coronary arteries that supply blood to the heart muscle. *Atherosclerosis* is the primary cause of this narrowing and obstructed blood flow. Clients with CHD may have no symptoms, may experience episodic chest pain (*angina pectoris*), or may have a *myocardial infarction* resulting from complete obstruction of blood flow to part of the heart muscle (Figure 26-1 ■).

Both men and women are affected by CHD. In women, however, it often develops later in life because of the heart-protective effects of estrogen. After menopause, women's risk is equal to that of men.

RISK FACTORS

While the cause of atherosclerosis is unknown, *risk factors* for CHD have been identified (Table 26-1 ■). Some risk factors for CHD (*age, gender, race,* and *heredity*) cannot be changed. More than 50% of heart attack victims are *age 65 or older*. *Men* are affected at an earlier age than women. *Blacks* have a higher incidence of high blood pressure, and tend to develop atherosclerosis earlier in life. A *family history* of CHD is a risk factor for both men and women. Educating women about CHD is important, because many do not realize that their risk after menopause is just as high as men's risk.

Lifestyle risk factors can be controlled or completely eliminated. *Cigarette smoking* is a major risk factor, increasing the risk of heart disease by three to four times that of a

TABLE 26-1		
Risk Factors for Coronary Heart Disease		
	MODIFIABLE	
NONMODIFIABLE	**PHYSIOLOGIC**	**LIFESTYLE**
Age	High blood pressure	Cigarette smoking
Gender	Diabetes mellitus	Obesity
Race/ethnic background	High blood lipids	Physical inactivity
Heredity	Metabolic syndrome: abdominal obesity, hyperlipidemia, hypertension, insulin resistance, clotting and inflammation tendencies High homocystine levels Women: premature menopause	Diet high in saturated fats Women: oral contraceptive use, hormone replacement therapy

nonsmoker. People who quit smoking reduce their risk almost immediately, no matter how long they have smoked. *Obesity* (body weight more 30% over ideal) and fat distribution affect the risk for CHD. Central or abdominal obesity is associated with abnormal blood lipids and a higher risk of CHD.

Physical inactivity, or a sedentary lifestyle, is associated with higher risk. People who maintain a regular program of physical activity are less likely to develop CHD than sedentary people.

Physiologic risk factors such as high blood pressure (hypertension), diabetes, and elevated blood lipid and cholesterol levels can usually be controlled through medication, weight control, and diet. Two additional physiologic risk factors have recently been identified: metabolic syndrome and high homocystine levels.

Hypertension, which affects more than 50 million people in the United States, is a systolic blood pressure greater than 140 mm Hg or a diastolic blood pressure greater than 90 mm Hg. Controlling blood pressure decreases the risk of heart disease, stroke, and renal failure. *Diabetes* affects both small and large blood vessels. It also is associated with a higher incidence of high blood lipids, high blood pressure, and obesity—all risk factors in their own right.

High blood lipids (hyperlipidemia) increase the risk for CHD. Lipoproteins carry cholesterol in the blood. LDL (low-density lipoprotein) is the primary carrier of cholesterol. High levels of LDL (remember **LDL** = *Less* healthy) promote atherosclerosis because LDL deposits cholesterol on the artery walls. In contrast, high-density lipoprotein, HDL (remember **HDL** = *Highly* healthy), helps clear cholesterol from the arteries, transporting it to the liver for

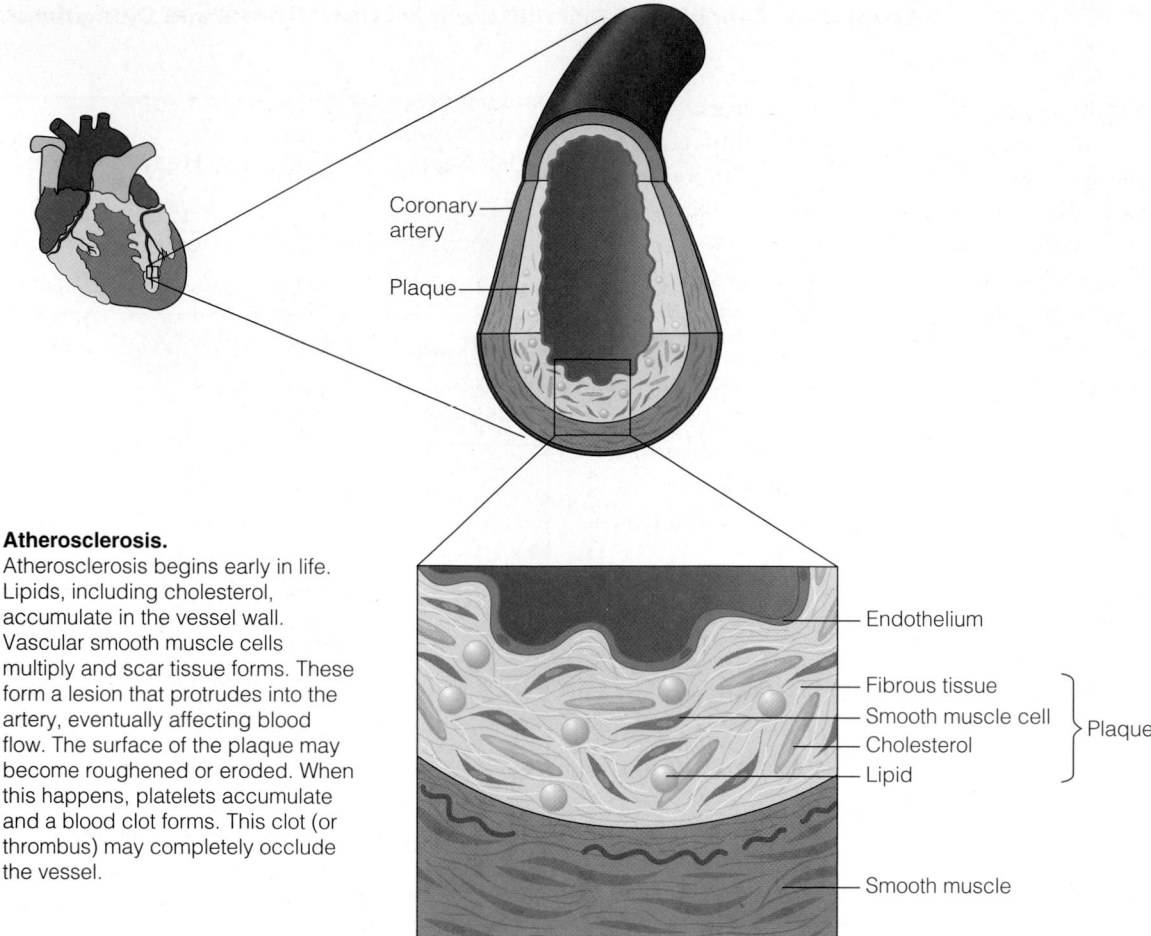

Atherosclerosis.
Atherosclerosis begins early in life. Lipids, including cholesterol, accumulate in the vessel wall. Vascular smooth muscle cells multiply and scar tissue forms. These form a lesion that protrudes into the artery, eventually affecting blood flow. The surface of the plaque may become roughened or eroded. When this happens, platelets accumulate and a blood clot forms. This clot (or thrombus) may completely occlude the vessel.

Angina pectoris.
Angina is characterized by episodes of chest pain. When the heart muscle needs more oxygen than partially occluded vessels can supply, the cells become ischemic. Lactic acid produced by ischemic cells stimulates nerve endings, causing pain. The pain subsides when cells again receive enough oxygen to meet their needs.

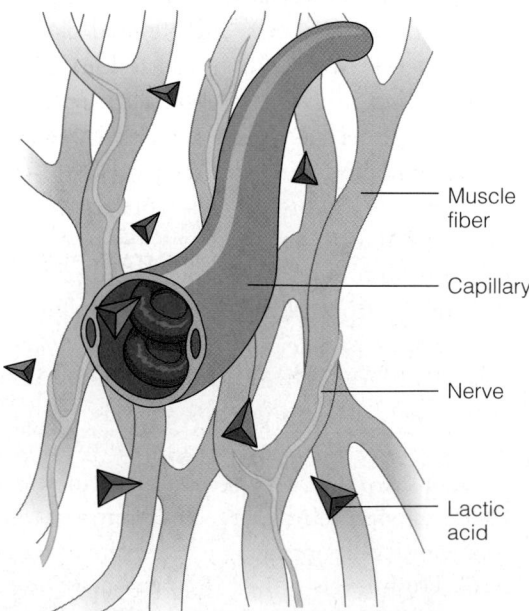

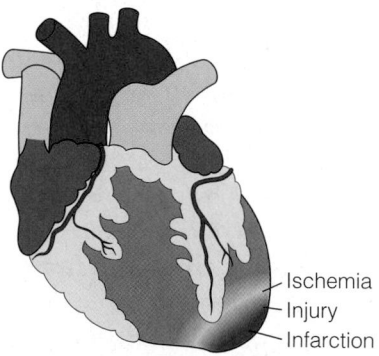

Myocardial infarction.
Myocardial infarction occurs when a coronary artery is completely obstructed, interrupting blood supply to the heart muscle. Affected tissue becomes ischemic and eventually dies (*infarcts*) if the blood supply is not restored. Surrounding the area of infarction, there is an area of tissue injury. Surrounding the injured tissue is an area of ischemic but undamaged tissue.

Figure 26-1. ■ Coronary heart disease. Most cases of coronary heart disease are due to atherosclerosis, occlusion of the coronary arteries by fibrous, fatty plaque. Clients with coronary heart disease may experience angina pectoris or myocardial infarction. Risk factors for coronary heart disease include age, heredity, smoking, obesity, high serum cholesterol levels, hypertension, and diabetes mellitus. Other factors, such as stress and lack of exercise, also contribute to the risk of CHD.

TABLE 26-2		
Classification of Cholesterol and LDL Levels		
	TOTAL CHOLESTEROL (MG/DL)	LDL CHOLESTEROL (MG/DL)
OPTIMAL		<100
DESIRABLE	<200	<130 (Near optimal)
BORDERLINE HIGH	200–239	120–159
HIGH	≥240	160–189
VERY HIGH		≥190

excretion. HDL levels above 35 mg/dL reduce the risk of CHD. Table 26-2 ■ lists optimal and desired levels of total cholesterol and LDL as identified by the National Heart, Lung, and Blood Institute (2002). Triglycerides, used for fat storage by the body, also contribute to the development of CHD when elevated.

Metabolic syndrome is a group of related risk factors occurring in the same person: hyperlipidemia, hypertension, abdominal obesity, insulin resistance, and a tendency toward clotting and inflammation. High blood levels of *homocystine,* an amino acid, also have recently been linked with CHD. Stress is a risk factor for CHD, although it is unclear how it contributes to developing CHD.

PATHOPHYSIOLOGY

Atherosclerosis is the primary cause of coronary heart disease. Atherosclerosis is a disease in which lesions called *atheromas* (or *plaque*) develop in the lining of medium and large arteries. These lesions protrude into the artery and may affect blood flow through the artery. The cause of atherosclerosis is unknown. The process of lipid and cholesterol accumulation is thought to start with inflammation. Smooth muscle cells and connective tissue proliferate within the wall of the blood vessel, contributing to plaque growth. As the plaque develops, it gradually occludes the vessel lumen and impairs the vessel's ability to dilate in response to increased oxygen demands. Atheromas often develop where arteries divide, curve, or become narrow.

When a coronary blood vessel is significantly occluded, the cells it supplies become **ischemic,** without enough blood and oxygen to meet their metabolic needs. Ischemic CHD generally is divided into two categories: *chronic ischemic heart disease,* which includes stable angina and asymptomatic myocardial ischemia, and *acute coronary syndromes* such as unstable angina and myocardial infarction (heart attack).

INTERDISCIPLINARY CARE

Management of CHD focuses on reducing plaque buildup and maintaining adequate coronary blood flow.

Diagnostic Tests

The total serum cholesterol and a lipid panel are obtained to evaluate serum lipid levels. Serum C-reactive protein levels, an indicator of inflammation, are measured as well. See Chapter 25, Table 25-1, ⬭ for normal levels of tests and related nursing responsibilities.

The ankle-brachial index is a noninvasive test of peripheral vascular disease that also may predict CHD. Other diagnostic tests, such as treadmill testing (ECG stress test) and electron beam computed tomography (EBCT) also may be done to evaluate the risk for CHD and identify myocardial ischemia. These tests are explained in Tables 25-2 and 25-3. ⬭

Risk Factor Management

DIET. A low-fat, low-cholesterol diet is suggested to help control blood lipid levels and promote weight loss. The National Cholesterol Education Program recommends reducing total intake to 25% to 35% of the total daily calories. Saturated fats should make up less than 7% of total calories, with the majority of remaining fat intake comprised of monounsaturated fats. Much saturated fat is found in whole-milk products and in red meats. Eating nonfat dairy products, fish, and poultry as primary protein sources can lower cholesterol levels. Monounsaturated fats, found in olive, canola, and peanut oils, and omega-3 fatty acids found in certain cold-water fish, such as tuna, salmon, and mackerel, help reduce total serum cholesterol, LDL, and triglyceride levels. Several programs that combine diet, exercise, and other therapies have been proven to reduce atherosclerotic deposits. These programs are quite restrictive, however, and require significant commitment to follow (Box 26-1 ■).

BOX 26-1	COMPLEMENTARY THERAPIES

Coronary Heart Disease (CHD)

The *Pritikin diet* is basically vegetarian, high in complex carbohydrates and fiber, low in cholesterol, and extremely low in fat (<10% of daily calories). Egg whites and limited amounts of nonfat dairy or soy products are allowed. The Pritikin program requires 45 minutes of walking daily and recommends multivitamin supplements, including vitamins C and E and folate.

The *Ornish diet* also is vegetarian, although egg whites and a cup of nonfat milk or yogurt per day are allowed. No oil or fat is permitted, even for cooking. Two ounces of alcohol a day are permitted. The Ornish program also calls for stress reduction, emotional social support systems, daily stretching, and walking for an hour three times a week.

MediaLink Atorvastatin

TABLE 26-3

Nursing Implications for Pharmacology: Cholesterol-Lowering Drugs

CLASS/DRUGS	PURPOSE	NURSING RESPONSIBILITIES	CLIENT TEACHING
Statins ■ Atorvastatin Ca (Lipitor) ■ Fluvastatin (Lescol) ■ Pravastatin (Pravachol) ■ Simvastatin (Zocor)	Lower total serum cholesterol and LDL levels.	Monitor serum cholesterol and liver enzyme levels. Report elevated liver enzymes to the physician. Assess for muscle pain and tenderness; report to physician if present. Monitor for clients taking digitalis for toxicity.	Inform your doctor if you are taking other medications or using natural remedies. Promptly report muscle pain, tenderness, or weakness; skin rash, hives, or color changes; abdominal pain, nausea, vomiting. Do not use these drugs if you are pregnant or intend to become pregnant.
Nicotinic acid ■ Niacin (Nicobid, Nicolar, Niaspan, others)	Lowers VLDL, LDL, triglyceride, and total cholesterol levels; raises HDL levels.	Give with meals and a cold beverage to minimize GI effects. Monitor blood glucose, uric acid levels, and liver function tests; report abnormal levels to the physician.	This drug often causes flushing of the face, neck, and ears; these effects diminish over time, but are aggravated by alcohol use. Change positions slowly to reduce the risk of injury. Report dizziness or weakness to your doctor.
Bile acid sequestrants ■ Cholestyramine (Questran) ■ Colestipol (Colestid) ■ Colesevelam (Welchol)	Lower LDL levels by binding with bile acids in the intestine. Primarily used in combination drug treatment.	Mix powders with 4 to 6 ounces of water or juice. Administer as ordered with meals.	Drink ample amounts of fluid to reduce the risk of constipation. Do not omit doses. Promptly report back or abdominal pain, nausea/vomiting, or black or bloody stools to your doctor.

MEDICATIONS. Drug therapy to lower total cholesterol and LDL levels is now the standard of care for clients at risk for coronary heart disease. Cholesterol-lowering drugs should be used together with dietary changes to reduce saturated and total fat intake. The statins, such as atorvastatin (Lipitor), pravastatin (Pravachol), and simvastatin (Zocor) are widely prescribed for this purpose. These drugs inhibit cholesterol synthesis in the liver. They are very effective in lowering LDL levels; some also increase HDL levels to a certain extent. Headache and gastrointestinal (GI) effects are the most common side effects of these drugs. Myalgias (muscle aches) or skin rashes may also develop. Liver function tests and muscle enzymes are monitored during therapy to assess for possible toxic effects.

If a combination of diet and a statin drug do not lower serum cholesterol and LDL levels to desired goals, a different class of cholesterol-lowering drugs may be added to the treatment plan. Niacin or nicotinic acid (Niacor, Nicobid, Nicolar) lowers LDL levels and raises HDL levels. Nicotinic acid is available without a prescription. Flushing, or "hot flashes," and pruritus are common side effects of niacin therapy. Cholestyramine (Questran) and colestipol (Colestid)

bind with bile acids and cholesterol in the intestine, promoting their excretion in the feces. These drugs may have GI side effects, such as constipation, gas, and abdominal cramping.

Nursing implications for drugs used to lower serum cholesterol levels are summarized in Table 26-3 ■.

NURSING CARE

Strongly encourage all clients to stop all forms of tobacco use. Discuss the effects of smoking on the body and the benefits of quitting. Resource materials to help clients stop smoking are available from the American Heart Association, the American Lung Association, and the American Cancer Society. Refer to a smoking cessation program to increase the likelihood of success in quitting.

Discuss the role of diet in CHD and obesity. Help assess food intake and patterns of eating to identify areas that can be improved. Refer to a dietitian for diet planning and further teaching. Encourage to make dietary changes gradually but progressively, maintaining a well-balanced low-fat diet.

Advise to avoid fad diets for weight loss. Suggest American Heart Association and other cookbooks that offer low-fat recipes to encourage healthier eating.

Discuss the physical and psychosocial benefits of regular exercise. Help the client identify favorite forms of exercise and schedule exercise periods of 30 to 45 minutes of continuous aerobic activity (i.e., walking, running, bicycling, swimming) four to six times a week. Walking provides many benefits and is an easily accessible and low-cost form of exercise. Encourage identification of an "exercise buddy" to help maintain motivation.

Discuss the importance of controlling high blood pressure, diabetes, and elevated blood lipid levels. Refer clients to their primary care provider for treatment as needed, and provide teaching about specific diseases and/or prescribed treatments.

Stress is a normal part of every person's life. Assist the client to identify and develop stress-management techniques such as physical exercise or meditation. It is important to emphasize that relaxation techniques require practice.

Angina Pectoris

Angina pectoris is chest pain that occurs when there is a temporary imbalance between myocardial blood supply and demand. Angina often occurs in a pattern: Exercise brings on the pain; rest relieves the pain.

PATHOPHYSIOLOGY

Atherosclerosis and coronary heart disease often lead to angina. Obstruction of a coronary artery reduces blood flow to the part of the heart normally supplied by that vessel. Although the heart muscle may still receive enough blood and oxygen to meet its needs at rest, anything that further reduces blood flow or increases the oxygen demand of the heart muscle can cause angina. Exercise increases myocardial oxygen demand. The obstructed vessel is unable to provide an adequate supply, and cells are deprived of oxygen. Inadequate oxygen causes cells to switch from aerobic metabolism (a very efficient process that requires oxygen) to anaerobic metabolism (a very inefficient process that occurs in the absence of oxygen). Lactic acid and other substances that stimulate nerve fibers are released, causing pain.

Three types of angina have been identified:

1. *Stable angina* is the most common and predictable form of angina. It occurs with a known amount of activity or stress. Stable angina is relieved by rest and nitrates.
2. *Unstable angina* occurs with increasing frequency, severity, and duration. Pain is unpredictable and may occur at rest. Clients with unstable angina are at risk for myocardial infarction.

BOX 26-2

MANIFESTATIONS OF ANGINA

- Chest Pain
  - Substernal or precordial (across the chest)
  - May radiate to neck, arms, shoulders, or jaw
  - Tight, squeezing, constricting, or heavy
  - Precipitated by exercise or activity, strong emotion, stress, cold, heavy meal
  - Relieved by rest, nitroglycerin
- Shortness of breath, pallor, anxiety, and fear

---

3. *Prinzmetal's angina* is atypical angina that occurs without an identified precipitating cause, usually at the same time each day, often waking the client from sleep. It is caused by coronary artery spasm.

Progression of the disease is marked by a change from stable angina to unstable angina. This change may herald an impending myocardial infarction.

The cardinal manifestation of angina is chest pain. The pain typically is precipitated by an identifiable event, such as physical activity, strong emotion, stress, eating a heavy meal, or exposure to cold. The classic sequence of angina is activity–pain, rest–relief. Anginal pain usually lasts less than 15 minutes and is relieved by rest. The manifestations of angina are summarized in Box 26-2 ■.

INTERDISCIPLINARY CARE

Angina is diagnosed by the client's symptoms, past medical history and family history, and physical assessment. Laboratory tests may confirm the presence of risk factors, such as abnormal blood lipids or the presence of diabetes mellitus.

Diagnostic Tests

Common diagnostic tests to determine the extent of coronary heart disease and angina include electrocardiography, stress testing, nuclear medicine studies, and coronary angiography. These tests and their nursing implications are summarized in Chapter 25, Tables 25-2 and 25-3. ⬯

ELECTROCARDIOGRAPHY. A resting ECG may be normal in clients with angina. However, characteristic changes are seen during anginal episodes. During periods of myocardial ischemia, the ST segment is depressed, and the T wave may flatten or invert (Figure 26-2 ■). These changes reverse when adequate blood flow is restored. *Stress electrocardiography* also is used to help diagnose angina and to identify clients at risk. In coronary heart disease, the increased cardiac workload caused by exercise or administration of a vasodilator drug may cause myocardial ischemia and angina. ECG changes associated with ischemia are noted if myocardial ischemia occurs.

MediaLink Angina

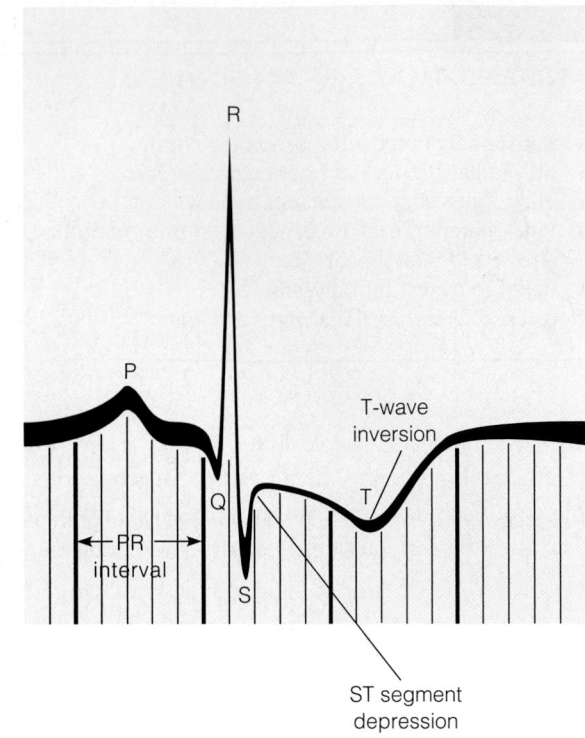

Figure 26-2. ■ ECG changes during an episode of angina. Note the ST-segment depression and T-wave inversion characteristic of myocardial ischemia.

IMAGING STUDIES. Electron beam computed tomography (EBCT) testing usually reveals calcium deposits indicative of coronary heart disease in the client with angina. Clients with variant angina, however, may have no evidence of calcium deposits. An *echocardiogram* may be performed following exercise stress testing to evaluate chest wall movement. *Radionuclear scanning* may be performed. Ischemic or infarcted cells of the myocardium may appear as a "cold spot" on the scan. *Coronary angiography* is the "gold standard" for evaluating the coronary arteries. Narrowing of a vessel by more than 50% is considered significant; most lesions that produce symptoms obstruct more than 70% of the vessel. Nursing care of the client undergoing a coronary angiogram is summarized in Box 26-3 ■.

Medications

Sublingual nitroglycerin (NTG) is the drug of choice to treat acute anginal attacks, acting within 1 to 2 minutes. Rapid-acting NTG is also available as a buccal spray in a metered-dose system. *Longer acting nitroglycerin preparations* include oral tablets, ointment, and transdermal patches. In these forms, NTG is used to prevent attacks of angina, not to treat an acute attack. Headache, nausea, dizziness, and hypotension are common adverse effects of NTG preparations.

Beta blockers (e.g., propranolol and atenolol) and *calcium channel blockers* (e.g., diltiazem and nifedipine) are used to prevent angina (Table 26-4 ■). These drugs act too slowly

---

| BOX 26-3 | NURSING CARE CHECKLIST |

Coronary Angiography and Percutaneous Transluminal Coronary Angioplasty

Before the Procedure

☑ Assess knowledge and understanding of the procedure. Reinforce teaching and provide additional information as needed.

☑ Provide routine preoperative care as ordered (see Chapter 9). ⚭

☑ Administer ordered cardiac medications with a small sip of water prior to the procedure unless contraindicated.

☑ Document and report any allergies to iodine, radiographic dyes, or seafood.

☑ Record height, weight, and vital signs. Record equality and amplitude of peripheral pulses; mark their locations.

☑ Explain that client will remain awake during the procedure, which lasts 1 to 2 hours. Sedation may be given, and a local anesthetic will be used where the catheter is inserted. A sensation of warmth (a "hot flash") and a metallic taste may be experienced as the dye is injected. A rapid pulse or a few "skipped beats" also are common during the procedure.

After the Procedure

☑ Provide routine postoperative care (see Chapter 9). ⚭

☑ Monitor vital signs, distal pulses, color, movement, sensation, temperature, and capillary refill of affected extremity as ordered, usually every 15 minutes for the first hour, every 30 minutes the next hour, hourly for 8 hours, and then every 4 hours.

☑ Monitor cardiac rhythm continuously. Report dysrhythmias, ECG changes, or chest pain to the charge nurse or physician.

☑ Maintain bed rest with the affected extremity extended and the head of the bed elevated no more than 30 degrees.

☑ Keep a pressure dressing in place over arterial access sites. Place a 5-lb. sandbag over the access site for 6 hours or as ordered. Check frequently for bleeding (if the access site is in the groin, check for bleeding under the buttocks).

☑ Unless contraindicated, encourage liberal fluid consumption.

☑ Administer medications as ordered.

☑ Monitor intake, output, and laboratory values. Report abnormal values to the physician.

TABLE 26-4

Nursing Implications for Pharmacology: Antianginal Drugs

CLASS/DRUGS	PURPOSE	NURSING RESPONSIBILITIES	CLIENT TEACHING
Nitrates ■ Nitroglycerin (Nitropaste, Nitro-Dur, Nitro-Bid, Nitrol, Transderm-Nitro, Nitrogard, Nitrodisc, Tridil) ■ Isosorbide dinitrate (Isordil) ■ Isosorbide mononitrate (Ismo)	Nitrates dilate blood vessels, increasing blood flow to the myocardium and reducing the workload of the heart. Sublingual nitroglycerin (NTG) tablets and buccal spray are used to prevent and treat acute angina. Oral and transdermal forms are used to reduce the frequency and severity of anginal attacks.	Administer sublingual NTG at the onset of chest pain. In some cases, tablets may be left at the bedside for prompt treatment of angina. Wear gloves when applying nitroglycerin ointment to prevent absorbing the drug through your skin. Measure dose carefully and spread evenly in a 2-by-3 inch area. Remove nitroglycerin patches or ointment at night to help prevent tolerance to the drug. Help the client identify events that precipitate anginal attacks.	Use only rapid-acting forms to treat acute anginal attacks, taking the drug at the onset of chest pain. Dissolve tablets under the tongue; do not swallow the tablet. If chest pain is not relieved within 5 minutes, take a second dose. After 5 minutes more, a third dose may be taken. If pain continues, seek medical help immediately. Keep NTG tablets in original container and protect them from heat, light, and moisture. Refill your prescription every 6 months and throw away unused tablets. Apply ointment or transdermal patches to a hairless area; spread ointment evenly; do not rub or massage. Remove the old patch or residual ointment before bedtime; apply a fresh dose in the morning. Rotate sites. If you are using long-acting NTG, keep a supply of rapid-acting NTG to treat acute angina.
Beta Blockers ■ Atenolol (Tenormin) ■ Metoprolol (Lopressor) ■ Propranolol (Inderal) ■ Nadolol (Corgard)	Beta blockers decrease cardiac workload by blocking sympathetic nervous system stimulation. They are frequently used to prevent angina and to treat hypertension.	Record heart rate and BP before giving. Withhold the drug if the heart rate is below 50 bpm or the BP is below identified levels. Notify the charge nurse or physician. Assess for possible contraindications to beta blockers, such as asthma or COPD. These drugs should not be abruptly discontinued, but gradually withdrawn when necessary.	Beta blockers do not work immediately; keep a supply of fast-acting NTG for acute chest pain. Do not abruptly stop taking this drug. Talk to your doctor about discontinuing its use. Take and record your pulse daily. Do not take the drug and notify your doctor if your heart rate is below 50 bpm. Have your BP checked frequently. Report a slow or irregular pulse, swelling or weight gain, or difficulty breathing to your doctor.
Calcium Channel Blockers ■ Nifedipine (Procardia) ■ Diltiazem (Cardizem) ■ Verapamil (Calan) ■ Bepridil (Vascor) ■ Felodipine (Plendil) ■ Isradipine (DynaCirc) ■ Nicardipine (Cardene) ■ Nimodipine (Nimotop)	Calcium channel blockers are used to control angina, hypertension, and dysrhythmias. They reduce cardiac workload and increase blood flow to the myocardium. They are often ordered for clients with coronary artery spasm (Prinzmetal's angina).	Record BP and heart rate before giving the drug. Withhold drug if the heart rate is below 50 bpm. Notify the charge nurse or physician if withheld. Nifedipine may be given by withdrawing the liquid from the capsule with a syringe and squirting the dose under the tongue (discard the needle first!). Immediately report manifestations of toxicity (nausea, generalized weakness, decreased cardiac output, hypotension, dysrhythmias).	Take your pulse before taking the drug. Do not take the drug and notify physician if your heart rate drops below 50 bpm. For acute angina, keep a fresh supply of rapid-acting NTG available (e.g., sublingual tablets). Calcium channel blockers will not work fast enough to relieve an acute attack.

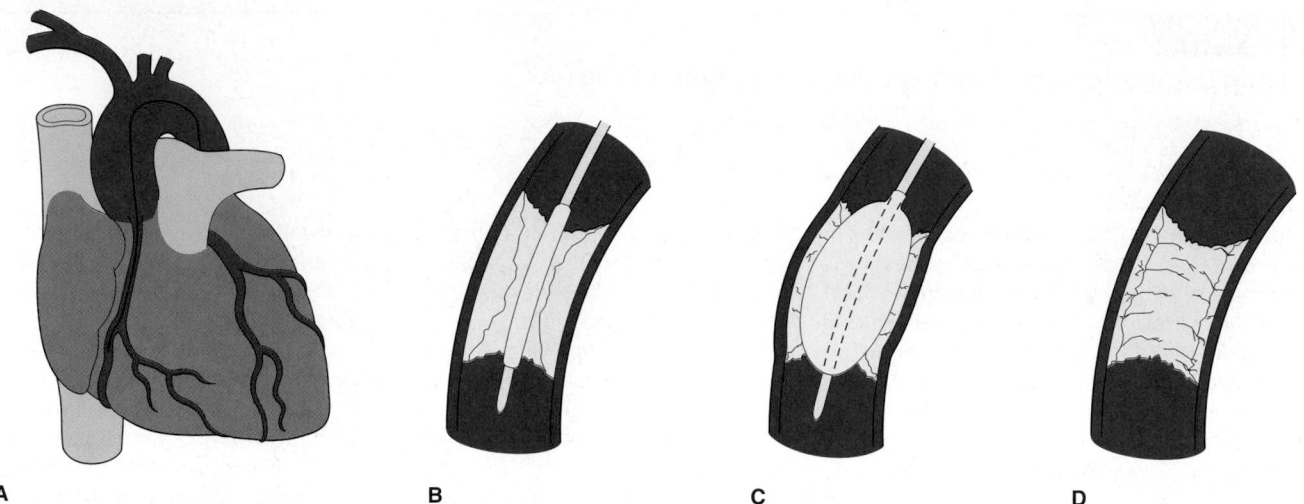

Figure 26-3. ■ PTCA. **(A)** The balloon catheter is threaded into the affected coronary artery. **(B)** The balloon is positioned across the area of obstruction. **(C)** The balloon is then inflated, flattening the plaque against the arterial wall **(D)**.

to treat acute attacks of angina; they are used for long-term prophylaxis. Beta blockers may significantly slow the heart rate, and are contraindicated for clients with asthma or severe chronic obstructive pulmonary disease (COPD) (see Chapter 24) ⊙⊙ because they may cause severe bronchospasm in these clients.

The client with angina, particularly unstable angina, is at risk for myocardial infarction because of significant narrowing of the coronary arteries. Low-dose aspirin (81 mg/day) is often prescribed to reduce the risk that clots will form in narrowed arteries, causing a myocardial infarction.

Surgery and Revascularization Procedures

Clients with severe or unstable angina may undergo surgery or a *percutaneous coronary revascularization (PCR)* procedure to restore blood flow to the myocardium.

Percutaneous transluminal coronary angioplasty (PTCA) is an invasive procedure used to increase blood flow to heart muscle. PTCA is performed in the cardiac catheterization laboratory under local anesthesia. Using the femoral artery, a small balloon-tipped catheter is threaded into the obstructed coronary artery. The balloon is positioned across the area of narrowing (Figure 26-3 ■). The balloon is inflated to reduce the narrowing and increase blood flow through the obstructed area. An intracoronary stent usually is inserted at the same time. The stent remains in the artery as a prop after the balloon is deflated (Figure 26-4 ■). *Atherectomy* procedures, another type of PCR, actually remove plaque from an identified blood vessel lesion. Nursing care for the client having a PCR procedure is similar to care for clients undergoing coronary angiogram (see Box 26-3).

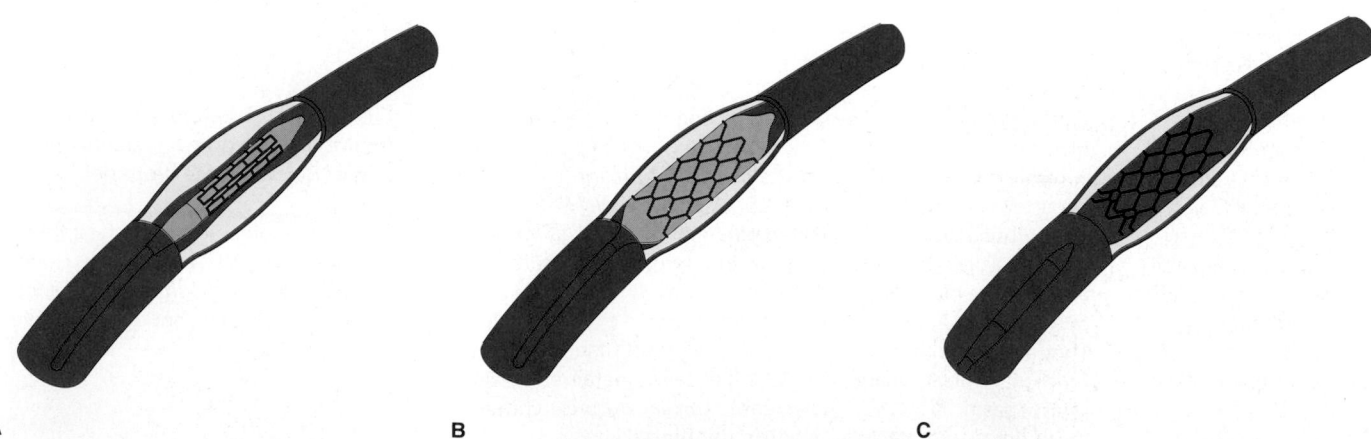

Figure 26-4. ■ Placement of an intracoronary stent. **(A)** The stent is fitted over the balloon-tipped catheter. **(B)** The stent is positioned in the area of narrowing and expanded with balloon inflation. **(C)** The balloon is deflated and removed, leaving the stent in place.

clinical ALERT

Although PCR procedures are common and generally very safe, complications such as myocardial infarction, bleeding, or formation of a hematoma at the catheter insertion site may occur. Closely monitor the client for complaints of chest or extremity pain. Frequently check color, temperature, and pulses on the affected extremity. Keep pressure dressing in place as ordered, and check for evidence of bleeding (look in the groin and feel under the buttocks if the femoral artery was used for access). Immediately report pain, changes in vital signs or extremity perfusion, or evidence of excess bleeding to the physician.

In a *coronary artery bypass graft (CABG),* a vein or arterial graft is used to "bypass," or bridge, the coronary artery obstruction and provide blood to the ischemic portion of the heart. The internal mammary artery (IMA) in the chest and the saphenous vein from the leg are the most popular vessels used for cardiac bypass grafts. The distal end of the IMA is sutured to the coronary artery distal to the obstruction (Figure 26-5 ■). When the saphenous vein is used, it is removed from the leg, reversed so that its valves do not interfere with blood flow, then grafted to the aorta and the coronary artery, distal to the occlusion. This provides a bridge for blood flow past the obstruction.

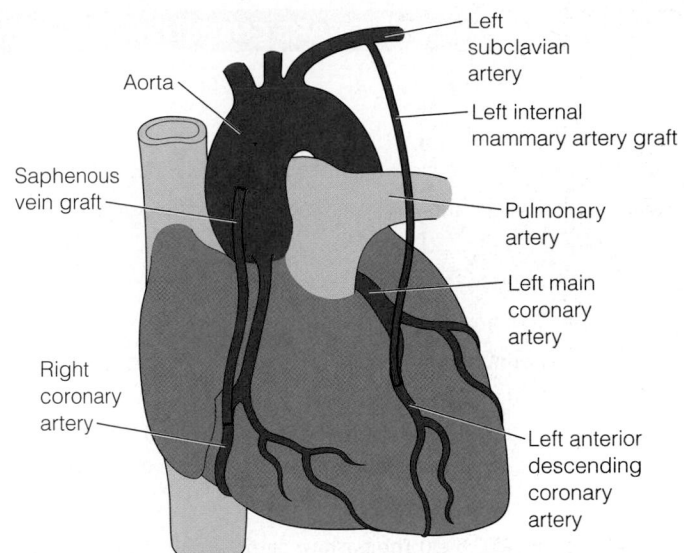

Figure 26-5. ■ CABG using the internal mammary artery and a saphenous vein graft.

Although CABG is a relatively safe procedure, the heart is usually stopped during surgery to make it easier to work on. The *cardiopulmonary bypass pump,* or *heart–lung machine,* is used to maintain blood flow to the rest of the organs during surgery (Figure 26-6 ■). The body temperature is lowered

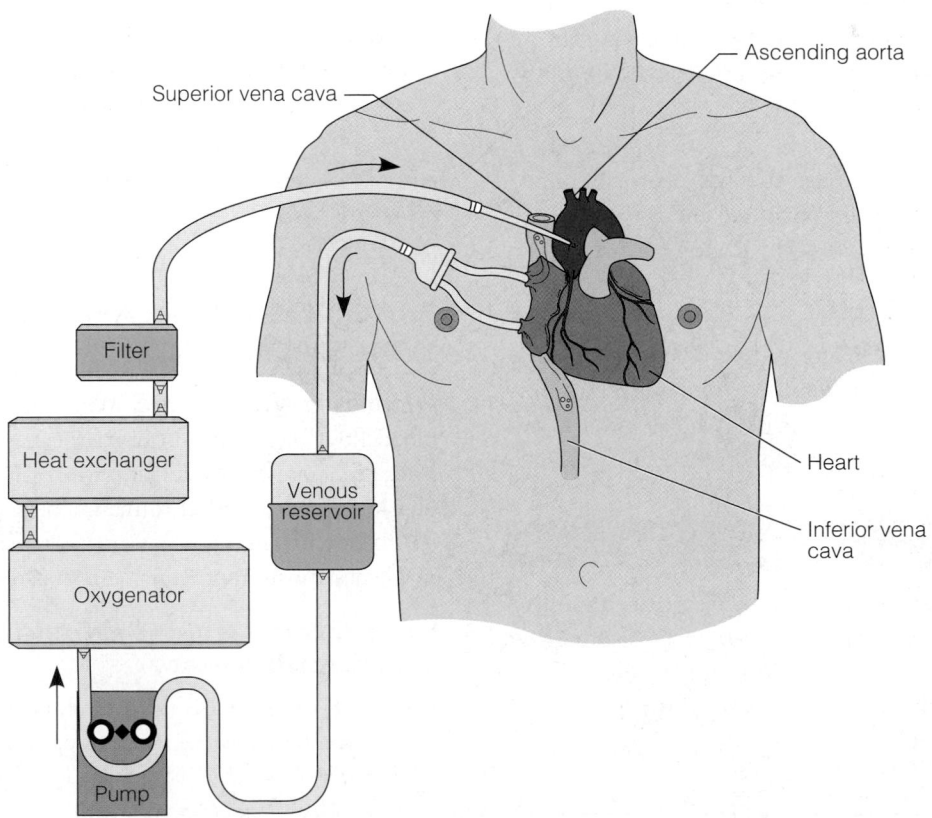

Figure 26-6. ■ A diagram of a cardiopulmonary bypass pump. Venous blood is removed from the venae cavae, pumped through the oxygenator, and returned to the body via the ascending aorta.

BOX 26-4	NURSING CARE CHECKLIST

Cardiac Surgery

Before Surgery

☑ Provide routine preoperative care as outlined in Chapter 9. ⬭

☑ Teach the client and family what to expect after surgery, including:

  ☑ Returning to the cardiac recovery unit

  ☑ Tubes, drains, and general appearance

  ☑ Monitoring equipment (cardiac monitor, hemodynamic monitoring) and alarms

  ☑ Respiratory support (ventilator, endotracheal tube, suctioning, communication while intubated) and exercises

  ☑ Incisions and dressings

  ☑ Activity and diet progression

After Surgery

☑ Provide routine postoperative care as ordered (Chapter 9). ⬭

☑ Monitor vital signs including temperature, oxygen saturation, and hemodynamic measurements every 15 minutes until stable, then hourly. Report significant changes to the physician.

☑ Assess heart sounds and respiratory status at least every 4 hours. Monitor arterial blood gas (ABG) results. Report changes.

☑ Assess skin color and temperature, peripheral pulses, and level of consciousness with vital signs. Report changes.

☑ Monitor cardiac rhythm continuously; document rhythm every shift. Document and report any changes as they occur.

☑ Record intake and output hourly. Report urine output of under 30 mL/hr for 2 consecutive hours.

☑ Record chest tube output hourly. Monitor hemoglobin and hematocrit values. Report excessive blood loss or falling values to the surgeon immediately.

☑ Institute rewarming as needed (per orders or if temperature is below 96.8°F or 36°C), using warmed intravenous fluids or transfusions, warmed blankets, and other prescribed measures.

☑ Manage analgesia (PCA or by schedule) as ordered. Document effectiveness. Report anginal pain immediately to the physician.

☑ Note endotracheal tube (ETT) placement on chest x-ray; secure it in place. Insert an oral airway as needed to prevent biting and obstruction of the ETT.

☑ Maintain ventilator settings as ordered. Suction as needed. Hyperoxygenate before and after suctioning.

☑ After extubation, teach and assist with use of the incentive spirometer. Assist the client to splint the chest incision when coughing.

☑ Maintain a sterile dressing for the first 48 hours, then leave the incision open to the air. Use Steri-Strips as needed to maintain wound approximation.

☑ Monitor serum electrolytes and other lab values; report significant changes.

☑ Encourage the client and family to participate in care and decision making.

---

during surgery. Once the procedure has been completed, cardiopulmonary bypass is discontinued and the client is rewarmed. Nursing care for the client having cardiac surgery is outlined in Box 26-4 ■.

Minimally invasive coronary artery surgery uses several small incisions to access the affected coronary arteries. Another revascularization procedure, *transmyocardial laser revascularization,* uses a laser to drill tiny holes into the myocardial muscle itself to provide blood to ischemic muscle.

NURSING CARE

Clients with angina are frequently treated in community-based settings; the primary nursing care focus is education. In an acute or long-term care setting, nursing care focuses on reducing the workload of the heart and improving its blood and oxygen supply.

ASSESSING

Assessment of the client with angina focuses on collecting data related to risk factors, the nature of the client's pain

and associated manifestations, and measures the client is currently using to manage this condition. See Box 26-5 ■ for focused assessment data to collect.

DIAGNOSING, PLANNING, AND IMPLEMENTING

Priorities in Nursing Care. Maintaining adequate coronary blood flow and perfusion of the heart muscle is the highest priority of care for the client with CHD and angina. Because physical activity is vital to maintaining heart health, care for the client with angina focuses on improving the supply of blood to the heart instead of reducing the workload of the heart.

Ineffective Tissue Perfusion: Cardiopulmonary

■ If short-acting NTG is ordered, keep it at the bedside so it can be taken at the onset of pain. *Immediate treatment can restore blood flow to the heart muscle and reduce the intensity and duration of anginal pain.*

■ Start oxygen at 4 to 6 L/min per nasal cannula unless contraindicated. *Supplemental oxygen reduces myocardial hypoxia.*

BOX 26-5   ASSESSMENT

Assessing Clients with Angina Pectoris

SUBJECTIVE DATA

- Pain: location, character (heavy, burning, tight, squeezing), intensity, radiation; timing (relationship to activity, meals, or other factors), duration; aggravating and relieving factors; associated manifestations
- History of angina or other heart disease, previous or current treatment measures
- Risk factors: family history of CHD; history of hypertension, diabetes, high blood cholesterol levels; smoking and alcohol intake, use of other recreational drugs; perceived stress levels and techniques used to manage stress; for women, age of menopause, use of hormone replacement therapy or oral contraceptives

OBJECTIVE DATA

- Frequency and duration of angina; effectiveness of relief measures (oxygen, NTG, rest)
- Vital signs and ECG tracing during anginal episode
- Laboratory data: cardiac enzyme levels, serum cholesterol and glucose; hemoglobin and hematocrit (particularly following PCR or surgery).

- Space activities to allow rest between them. *Activity increases cardiac work and may precipitate angina. Spacing of activities allows the heart to recover.*
- Instruct the client to take a sublingual NTG tablet before engaging in activities that precipitate angina (e.g., climbing stairs, sexual intercourse). *This prophylactic dose of NTG helps maintain cardiac perfusion when increased work is anticipated, preventing ischemia and chest pain.*
- Encourage risk factor management, e.g., losing weight, making dietary changes (reducing fat, cholesterol, and kilocalorie intake), reducing stress, and others as indicated. *Managing risk factors can slow the process of atherosclerosis and preserve myocardial perfusion.*
- Encourage the client to implement and maintain a progressive exercise program under the supervision of his or her primary care provider. *Exercise slows the atherosclerotic process and helps develop collateral circulation to the heart muscle.*
- Refer the client who smokes to a smoking cessation program. *Nicotine causes vasoconstriction and increases the heart rate, decreasing myocardial perfusion and increasing cardiac workload.*

Risk for Ineffective Therapeutic Regimen Management

- Assess knowledge and understanding of angina. *Assessment allows teaching and interventions to be tailored to the needs of the client.*

- Teach about angina and atherosclerosis as needed. *Denial or exaggerated fear may be strong in clients with angina pectoris. Teaching helps the client understand that angina can be managed, pain controlled, and disease progress slowed.*
- Provide written and verbal instructions about prescribed medications and their use. *Written instructions reinforce teaching and are available to the client for future reference.*
- Stress the importance of taking chest pains seriously while maintaining a positive attitude. *Chest pain is a warning and necessitates appropriate response.*
- Refer to a cardiac rehabilitation program or other organized activities and support groups for clients with coronary artery disease. *Programs such as these help the client develop strategies for risk factor management, maintain a program of supervised activity, and gain coping skills.*

EVALUATING

When evaluating the effectiveness of nursing care for the client with angina, collect data regarding the onset, duration, and management of anginal episodes. Use subjective and objective data to evaluate knowledge, understanding, and willingness to follow physician's orders and manage risk factors.

Documenting. Document the frequency and duration of anginal episodes, as well as precipitating factors. Document teaching provided and the client's understanding of the disease, risk factors, and the prescribed treatment plan.

CONTINUING CARE

Clients with stable angina often manage their pain effectively, continuing to live active and productive lives. Discuss the relationship between modifiable risk factors and angina. Provide information about risk factor management, as well as the disease process. Emphasize the relationship between reduced blood flow to the heart muscle and pain. Discuss the use of prescribed medications. Instruct to take NTG prophylactically, before activities that tend to cause chest pain. Advise taking NTG at the first indication of pain rather than waiting to see whether the pain develops. Emphasize the importance of seeking immediate medical assistance if three NTG tablets over 15 to 20 minutes do not relieve the pain. Instruct to call 911 or go to the emergency department immediately rather than contacting the physician.

Teach safe medication storage, especially for NTG. Because nitroglycerin is affected by heat and light and has a short shelf life, instruct the client to store it in a cool, dry, dark place and to keep no more than a 6-month supply on hand. Advise to always carry a few tablets but not the whole supply, because body warmth (transmitted through a shirt or pants pocket) causes tablets to deteriorate more rapidly. If an NTG patch or ointment is prescribed, teach how to apply it. Explain the rationale for removing the patch or ointment at night.

Stress the importance of not discontinuing medications abruptly, particularly beta blockers. Review their adverse effects, and instruct when to notify the physician.

When cardiac surgery is anticipated, provide general preoperative teaching (see Chapter 9), ⚭ as well as specifics related to the planned surgery. Reinforce instructions about respiratory care, activity, and pain management. Reinforce the importance of being an active participant in rehabilitation. Before discharge, teach about ordered medications, the manifestations of an infection, pain management, diet, and activity. Discuss post-hospital cardiac rehabilitation.

See the Critical Thinking Care Map at the end of this chapter for an opportunity to apply what you have learned about caring for a client undergoing cardiac surgery.

Acute Myocardial Infarction

In an **acute myocardial infarction (AMI or MI),** cells in an area of cardiac muscle *necrose* (die) due to lack of blood and oxygen. It is a life-threatening event: If circulation to the affected cardiac muscle is not rapidly restored, functional muscle is lost and the heart may be unable to maintain an effective cardiac output. This can lead to cardiogenic shock and death. Most deaths from AMI occur within the first hour following the onset of manifestations, often before the client reaches the hospital.

Approximately 1.1 million Americans experience an AMI annually, nearly half of which are fatal. AMI rarely occurs in clients without preexisting coronary heart disease. While no specific cause has been identified, the risk factors for AMI are those for coronary heart disease: age, gender, heredity, smoking, obesity, hyperlipidemia, hypertension, diabetes, stress, and sedentary lifestyle.

PATHOPHYSIOLOGY

AMI occurs when a coronary artery becomes occluded, blocking blood flow to a portion of cardiac muscle for a prolonged period of time. Occlusion is usually caused by development of a *thrombus* (clot) in an area of atherosclerotic narrowing. The occlusion blocks blood flow to myocardium distal to the obstruction.

When the cells are deprived of oxygen and nutrients for more than 20 to 45 minutes, they are irreversibly damaged, leading to cellular death and tissue necrosis. Intracellular enzymes are released as cells die. This necrotic tissue (*infarct*) is surrounded by an area of injured and ischemic tissues. These injured cells may be *stunned* or *hibernating,* and often contract ineffectively. Because of this, cardiac output falls.

If blood flow is restored, the injured and ischemic tissue recovers and heals. The infarcted tissue, however, no longer conducts electrical energy and ceases to contract. Collateral vessels connected to the smaller arteries in the coronary system dilate to maintain blood flow to the cardiac muscle when a larger coronary artery is occluded. In clients who remain active, collateral vessels develop and enlarge to meet the demand for blood flow as larger coronary arteries progressively narrow. Good collateral circulation can reduce the size of an infarction.

MI usually affects the left ventricle because it is the major "workhorse" of the heart; its muscle mass is greater, as are its oxygen demands.

AMIs are described according to the area of the heart that is damaged. Occlusion of the left anterior descending (LAD) artery damages the *anterior* portion of the left ventricle; occlusion of the left circumflex artery (LCA) causes *lateral* damage. *Right ventricular, inferior,* and *posterior* AMIs involve occlusions of the right coronary artery (RCA) and posterior descending artery (PDA). (See Figure 25-4 on page 595.) ⚭

AMIs may also be classified as either transmural or subendocardial. A *transmural* infarction affects all layers of the heart (the endocardium, myocardium, and epicardium). A *subendocardial* infarction involves only the inner layer of the heart, and does not extend through the myocardium and epicardium.

Manifestations

Pain is a classic manifestation of AMI. Chest pain is often described as crushing and severe; the client may call it a pressure, heavy, or squeezing sensation, or complain of chest tightness or burning. The pain begins in the center of the chest (in the substernal region), and may radiate to the shoulders, neck, jaw, or arms. It lasts more than 15 to 20 minutes and is not relieved by rest or NTG. The client often experiences a sense of impending doom and death. Typical signs and symptoms of AMI are listed in Box 26-6 ■.

BOX 26-6

MANIFESTATIONS OF ACUTE MYOCARDIAL INFARCTION
- Chest pain: substernal or precordial; may radiate to neck, shoulder, or arm
- Tachycardia
- Shortness of breath, dyspnea
- Cool, clammy skin
- Diaphoresis (profuse perspiration)
- Anxiety
- Feeling of impending doom
- Nausea and vomiting
- Possible dysrhythmias

BOX 26-7	POPULATION FOCUS

Heart Disease in Women and Older Adults

Heart disease—myocardial infarction in particular—is the leading cause of death for women and older adults. In fact, more women than men die of heart disease every year. Women with symptoms of an acute myocardial infarction are likely to delay seeking treatment for several hours—an average of an hour longer than men. After an MI, the death rate for women is three times that of men, both in the hospital and within the first year.

Women and older adults are more likely than men to have a "silent" or unrecognized heart attack. Many women having an AMI experience epigastric pain and nausea, causing them to believe their pain is due to heartburn. Chest pain in women often occurs during mental stress or while resting. Shortness of breath is common, as is fatigue and weakness of the shoulders and upper arms.

Older people may seek treatment for vague complaints of difficulty breathing, confusion, fainting, dizziness, abdominal pain, or cough. Many older adults who experience AMI do not complain of chest pain. When these clients seek care with vague symptoms and a history of cardiovascular problems, an AMI should be suspected.

When teaching women and older adults about heart disease, emphasize the importance of seeking immediate medical care for manifestations of AMI. With prompt treatment, survival in both groups is improved.

Women and older adults may not have the "typical" manifestations of AMI, increasing the risk that they will not seek treatment. As with men, the most common symptom of AMI in women is chest pain or discomfort. Upper abdominal pain also may occur. Women and older adults may experience other common manifestations of AMI without chest pain, particularly shortness of breath, nausea/vomiting, and back or jaw pain. Box 26-7 ■ focuses on AMI in women and older adults.

Cocaine-Induced MI

In recent years, acute MI associated with cocaine intoxication has been reported. Cocaine stimulates the heart rate, increases its contractility, and causes vasoconstriction and hypertension. As a result, the workload of the heart increases. Cocaine also increases the risk of dysrhythmias. The client with cocaine-induced MI may have an altered level of consciousness, confusion and restlessness, seizure activity, tachycardia, hypotension, increased respiratory rate, and respiratory crackles.

Complications

The risk of complications associated with MI is related to the size and location of infarcted tissue.

clinical ALERT

Promptly report manifestations such as a significant change in heart rate or rhythm, chest pain, increasing shortness of breath, a change in mental status, pallor or cyanosis, or cool, clammy skin to the charge nurse or physician. These signs and symptoms may indicate a complication that can jeopardize the client's chances for recovery.

DYSRHYTHMIAS. Dysrhythmias, disruptions of the electrical conduction system of the heart and/or its rhythm, are the most frequent complication. Sinus tachycardia (heart rate greater than 100 bpm) is common. The heart rate may slow sufficiently due to bradycardia or heart blocks to produce symptoms such as shortness of breath, dizziness, and altered mental status. Premature atrial contractions (PACs) and atrial fibrillation may occur. Premature ventricular contractions (PVCs) are common, particularly in the first few hours following an AMI. Frequent PVCs (more than 6 per minute), couplets, short bursts of ventricular tachycardia, and early PVCs (R on T wave) are treated with drugs to reduce the risk of ventricular fibrillation. The risk of V-fib is greatest the first hour after AMI; it is a frequent cause of sudden cardiac death associated with acute MI. (See the section on dysrhythmias and Table 26-6 on page 627 for more information about dysrhythmias.)

PUMP FAILURE. AMI reduces myocardial contractility and ventricular filling. Heart failure may develop, particularly when large portions of the left ventricle are affected. With loss of 20% to 30% of the left ventricular muscle, the client may develop manifestations of left-sided heart failure, including dyspnea, fatigue, weakness, and respiratory crackles on auscultation. Heart failure and its manifestations are discussed in greater depth later in Chapter 27. ⚭

If more than 40% of the left ventricle is infarcted, **cardiogenic shock**, impaired tissue perfusion due to pump failure, results. The client is hypotensive and has signs of impaired tissue perfusion, such as low urinary output, decreased level of consciousness, and cool, clammy skin. Perfusion of the heart muscle itself also is affected, further increasing tissue damage. See Chapter 13 ⚭ for a more extensive discussion of shock.

OTHER COMPLICATIONS. *Pericarditis* (inflammation of the pericardium) may develop after an AMI, usually within 2 to 3 days. Chest pain associated with pericarditis is sharp and stabbing, aggravated by movement or deep breathing. A pericardial friction rub may be noted on auscultation of heart sounds.

Approximately 10% of clients experience *extension* or *expansion* of the MI within 10 to 14 days. The client may have continuing chest pain, unstable vital signs, or worsening heart failure. Because the scar tissue that replaces necrotic muscle is thinner than the ventricular muscle mass, a *ventricular aneurysm* may develop or rupture may occur. A ventricular aneurysm is an outpouching of the ventricular wall. *Myocardial rupture* is often fatal, and may occur between days 4 and 7 after an AMI, when the injured tissue is soft and weak.

INTERDISCIPLINARY CARE

Rapid assessment and early diagnosis are vital in an MI. "Time is muscle"—the quicker the artery is reopened (medically or surgically) and blood flow restored, the more myocardium can be saved and fewer complications develop. The American Heart Association (AHA) recommends definitive treatment be initiated within 1 hour of arrival at the emergency center.

The major problem is delay in seeking medical care after the onset of chest pain or other cardiac symptoms. Up to 44% of clients with symptoms of MI wait more than 4 hours before seeking treatment.

Laboratory Tests

The principal laboratory tests ordered when an MI is suspected are *serum cardiac markers* (see Table 25-1 ⊕ on page 599). Serum levels of cardiac markers are ordered on admission and for 3 succeeding days. Serial blood levels are used to establish the diagnosis and to evaluate the extent of myocardial damage. The serum creatine kinase (CK) and cardiac-specific troponins are most specific for diagnosis of AMI. CK levels rise rapidly following AMI; it is detectable in the serum within 3 to 6 hours, peaks within 12 to 24 hours, and then declines during the next 48 to 72 hours. The peak CK level indicates the size of the AMI: The greater the amount of infarcted tissue, the higher the CK level. The CK-MB isoenzyme is the most sensitive indicator of AMI. Cardiac muscle troponins remain in the blood for 10 to 14 days, so they can help diagnose AMI when treatment is delayed by several days (Table 26-5 ■).

Diagnostic Tests

Electrocardiography, echocardiography, and myocardial nuclear scans are the most common diagnostic tests performed for a suspected AMI. Ischemic or necrotic cardiac cells do not respond normally to electrical stimulation, altering ECG waveforms (Figure 26-7 ■). The location of myocardial damage can be identified on the 12-lead ECG. Characteristic changes in the ECG with an acute MI include:

- Inversion of the T wave
- Depression or elevation of the ST segment
- Formation of a Q wave.

Echocardiography is used to diagnose AMI and complications such as ventricular aneurysm. *Myocardial perfusion imaging scans* may be done to localize an AMI and evaluate the extent of the infarction.

Medical Management

The focus of medical management for the client with AMI is on restoring blood flow to the heart muscle, reducing the workload of the heart, and preventing or promptly treating complications. The client is monitored continuously from entry into the medical system. Care is provided in the intensive coronary care unit for the first 24 to 48 hours, after which less intensive monitoring (e.g., telemetry) may be required. An intravenous line is established to allow rapid administration of emergency drugs. Oxygen is administered

TABLE 26-5			
Cardiac Marker Changes in AMI			
MARKER	CHANGES OCCURRING IN AN MI		
	Appears	*Peaks*	*Duration*
Creatine kinase (CK or CPK)	3–6 hours	12–24 hours	24–48 hours
CK M-bands (CK-MB)	4–8 hours	18–24 hour	72 hours
Cardiac-specific troponin T (cT$_n$T)	2–4 hours	24–36 hours	10–14 days
Cardiac-specific troponin I (cT$_n$I)	2–4 hours	24–36 hours	7–10 days

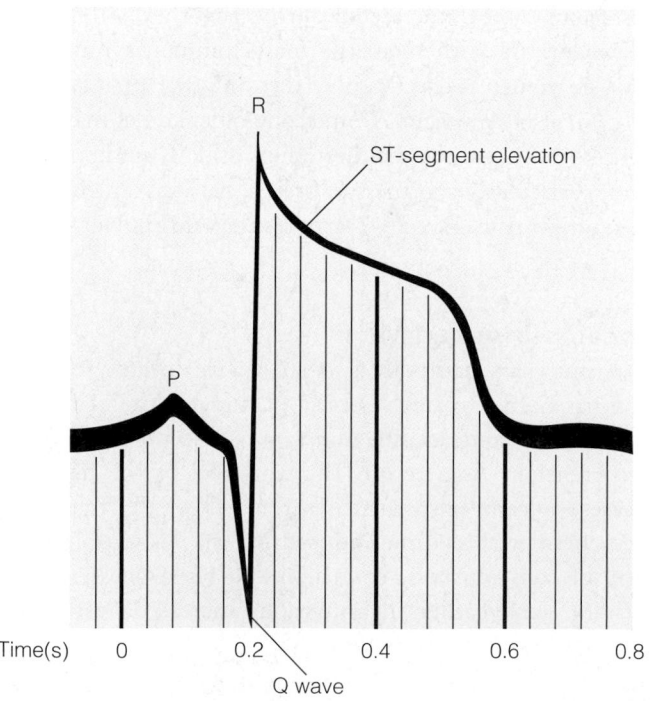

Figure 26-7. ■ ECG changes noted with acute myocardial infarction. Note the deep Q wave and significant elevation of the ST segment characteristic of AMI.

BOX 26-8	NURSING CARE CHECKLIST

Fibrinolytic Therapy

Before the Infusion

☑ Obtain subjective and objective assessment data.

☑ Ask about possible contraindications to fibrinolytic therapy: duration of symptoms, recent surgery or trauma (including prolonged CPR), bleeding disorders or any active bleeding, stroke, peptic ulcers, diabetic retinopathy, and uncontrolled hypertension.

☑ Reinforce teaching about the purpose of therapy, bleeding risk, and the need to remain still during and after the infusion.

During the Infusion

☑ Assess vital signs, peripheral pulses, and the infusion site every 15 minutes for the first hour, every 30 minutes for the next 2 hours, and then hourly until the intravenous catheter is discontinued. Record all data.

☑ Remind the client to keep the extremity still and straight.

☑ Maintain continuous cardiac monitoring. Keep antidysrhythmic medications and the emergency cart readily available.

After the Infusion

☑ Frequently assess vital signs, distal pulses, and infusion site for bleeding.

☑ Maintain bed rest for 6 hours. Reinforce the need to keep the extremity straight and immobile. Avoid injections for 24 hours after catheter removal.

☑ Assess puncture sites for bleeding. When the intravenous catheter is removed, hold direct pressure over the site for at least 30 minutes. Apply pressure dressings to venous or arterial punctures if needed. Perform routine care in a gentle manner to avoid undue bruising or injury.

☑ Assess body fluids, including urine, vomitus, and feces, for evidence of bleeding. Regularly monitor level of consciousness and neurologic function. Assess surgical sites for bleeding. Monitor hemoglobin and hematocrit levels. Report any bleeding or changes in neurologic status to the physician.

☑ Report manifestations of reocclusion, including ECG changes, chest pain, or dysrhythmias.

---

by nasal cannula at 2 to 6 L/min to improve oxygenation of the myocardium and other tissues.

Bed rest with bedside commode is ordered initially to reduce the cardiac workload. After 12 to 24 hours, activities are gradually increased. A quiet, calm environment with limited outside stimuli, such as television and telephone, is preferred. Visitors are limited to close family members for short periods of time. A low-fat, low-cholesterol, reduced-sodium diet is allowed. Small, frequent feedings are often recommended. Drinks containing caffeine and very hot and cold foods may be limited.

Medications

Pain relief is vital in treating the client with an acute MI. Pain stimulates the sympathetic nervous system, increasing the heart rate and blood pressure and, in turn, myocardial workload. *Morphine sulfate* is the drug of choice for pain and sedation. It is given intravenously in small doses until pain is relieved. *Intravenous* or *sublingual NTG* frequently is ordered to relieve pain and improve blood flow to the myocardium. It is important to assess frequently for pain relief and possible adverse effects of analgesia, such as excessive sedation. Antianxiety agents, such as diazepam (Valium), may also be given to promote rest.

Fibrinolytic agents, drugs that dissolve or break up blood clots, are used to treat acute MI. These drugs activate the *fibrinolytic (fibrin* = a key component of blood clots; *lysis* = break down or destroy) system to destroy the clot, restoring blood flow to the obstructed artery. When given within the first 6 hours of MI symptoms, fibrinolytics limit infarct size, reduce heart damage, and improve the chances of survival. These drugs also can cause multiple complications; up to 5% of clients receiving them experience serious bleeding. Fibrinolytic therapy is contraindicated in clients with known bleeding disorders, history of stroke, uncontrolled hypertension, pregnancy, or recent trauma or surgery. Nursing care of the client receiving fibrinolytic agents is outlined in Box 26-8 ■.

Aspirin, a platelet inhibitor, is given to clients with suspected MI in the emergency department. It is chewed for buccal absorption. This initial dose is followed by a daily dose of one regular or baby aspirin tablet by mouth. Heparin, an anticoagulant, also may be prescribed following an MI. Antidysrhythmic medications are used as needed to treat or prevent dysrhythmias. Beta blockers such as propranolol (Inderal), atenolol (Tenormin), and metoprolol (Lopressor) may be given to decrease the heart rate and reduce cardiac work and myocardial oxygen demand. Angiotensin-converting enzyme (ACE) inhibitors also may be ordered. These drugs reduce ventricular remodeling following AMI, reducing the risk of heart failure. Intravenous nitroglycerin is a vasodilator that both reduces cardiac work and increases coronary blood flow.

Revascularization Procedures

For many clients, an immediate or early revascularization procedure (PCR) such as angioplasty with stent placement is performed to restore blood flow to the infarcted section of heart muscle. In some cases, surgery may be performed. These procedures and related nursing care are covered in more depth in the preceding section on angina.

Other Invasive Procedures

Clients with large AMIs and pump failure may require invasive devices to temporarily take over the function of the heart, allowing the injured myocardium to heal. The *intra-aortic balloon pump (IABP)* temporarily supports cardiac function by decreasing myocardial workload and oxygen demand and increasing coronary artery perfusion. The balloon inflates during diastole, increasing perfusion of the coronary and renal arteries, and deflates just prior to and during systole, allowing blood to flow past it (Figure 26-8 ■). The inflation–deflation series is triggered by the ECG pattern. As the heart muscle recovers, IABP is gradually decreased, until the client no longer requires mechanical assistance.

Ventricular assist devices (VADs) can temporarily take partial or complete control of cardiac function. VADs may be used for clients with acute MI and cardiogenic shock, following surgery requiring cardiopulmonary bypass, or while awaiting heart transplant.

Cardiac Rehabilitation

Cardiac rehabilitation is a planned program of activity and exercises, psychologic support, and education for clients who have had an MI. The goal of cardiac rehabilitation is to improve quality of life by reducing risk factors for heart disease. It begins with admission to the hospital. This is followed by 3 to 6 months of a supervised outpatient program. The final phase of cardiac rehabilitation is a lifetime maintenance program of minimally supervised (or even unsupervised) physical fitness and risk factor reduction.

An interdisciplinary team works with the client in cardiac rehabilitation to:

- Assess previous activity and exercise habits.
- Gradually increase activity and exercise in a planned manner.
- Evaluate and monitor the client's responses to increasing activity levels.
- Teach the client to monitor his or her tolerance of activity.

The initial assessment and teaching may be done while the client is in the hospital. Activity is gradually increased as tolerated. Subjective complaints of fatigue, shortness of breath, chest pain, and dizziness are used to evaluate the client's ability to tolerate increased activity, as are objective data including vital signs and ECG changes. The outpatient phase of the program begins within 3 weeks following discharge. Teaching emphasizes risk factor reduction and progressive, regular exercise. Issues such as returning to work and resumption of sexual activity are discussed during this

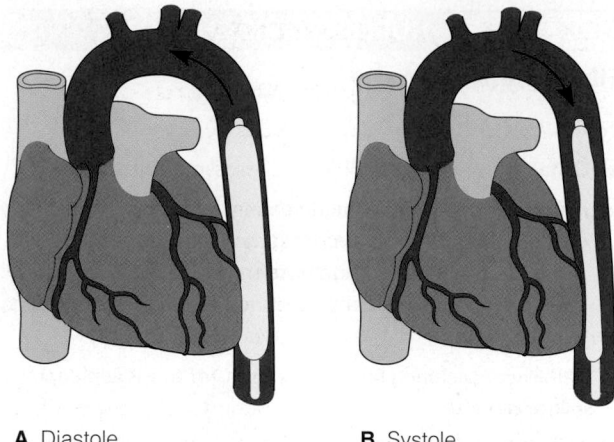

A Diastole   **B** Systole

Figure 26-8. ■ The intra-aortic balloon pump. **(A)** The balloon inflates during diastole to help perfuse coronary, renal, and cerebral arteries. **(B)** During systole, the balloon is deflated, allowing blood to freely flow past it.

phase. The final, maintenance phase of cardiac rehabilitation may be indefinite, continuing for the remainder of the client's lifetime.

NURSING CARE

ASSESSING

The client who experiences an AMI requires immediate and ongoing assessment. Initially, assessments may be done hourly or more frequently as necessary. Once stable, the client is assessed every 4 hours and if the condition changes. Uninterrupted rest periods are important however, so data are collected when the client is awake or in conjunction with other procedures. The ECG is continuously monitored, and laboratory results (cardiac markers in particular) are reported to the physician. Subjective and objective assessment data are outlined in Box 26-9 ■.

DIAGNOSING, PLANNING, AND IMPLEMENTING

Priorities in Nursing Care. Reducing the workload of the heart to protect injured muscle cells from further damage is a priority of care for the client with AMI. Pain stimulates the sympathetic nervous system, increasing the heart rate and its contractility—and, consequently, its workload. Eliminating pain and maintaining cardiac output and tissue perfusion are of highest priority in the client with AMI.

Pain

- Assess for verbal and nonverbal signs of pain. Document characteristics and intensity of pain, using a standard

BOX 26-9	ASSESSMENT

Assessing Clients with Myocardial Infarction

SUBJECTIVE DATA

- Pain: onset, location, character (heavy, burning, tight, squeezing), intensity (on a standardized pain scale), radiation (arms, shoulders, neck, jaw); timing (intermittent or continuous), duration; aggravating and relieving factors; associated manifestations (shortness of breath, nausea, apprehension)
- Effectiveness of pain relief measures (oxygen, nitroglycerin, analgesia, rest)
- History of angina or other heart disease, previous or current treatment measures
- Risk factors: family history of CHD; history of hypertension, diabetes, high blood cholesterol levels; smoking and alcohol intake, use of other recreational drugs; activity just prior to or at onset of pain
- Expressions of denial or disbelief; acceptance of activity restrictions; readiness for learning and activity progression

OBJECTIVE DATA

- Vital signs; BP, pulse and respiratory rate changes with activity
- Heart and lung sounds; dyspnea and its relationship to activity
- Skin color, temperature, and moisture; capillary refill; oxygen saturation levels
- Urine output
- Level of consciousness; anxiety or fear
- Cardiac rhythm; any abnormal rhythms or waveforms
- Central venous pressure, pulmonary artery pressure, or cardiac output as ordered
- Vital signs and ECG tracing during chest pain
- Laboratory data: cardiac enzyme levels

Ineffective Tissue Perfusion

- Report increased heart rate and changes in heart rhythm, blood pressure, and respiratory rate to the charge nurse or physician. *Damage to the heart muscle affects the pumping ability of the ventricles. The heart rate increases when cardiac output falls, increasing the workload of the heart.*
- Report changes in level of consciousness; decreased urine output; moist, cool, pale, mottled, or cyanotic skin; dusky or cyanotic mucous membranes and nail beds; diminished to absent peripheral pulses; delayed capillary refill. *These are manifestations of decreased tissue perfusion. A change in level of consciousness is often the first manifestation of altered perfusion because brain tissue and cerebral function depend on a continuous supply of oxygen.*
- Auscultate heart and breath sounds. Note abnormal heart sounds (e.g., an S_3 or S_4 gallop or murmur) or adventitious lung sounds. *Abnormal heart or lung sounds may indicate impaired cardiac function.*
- Monitor ECG rhythm continuously. Report dysrhythmias. *Dysrhythmias can further impair cardiac output and tissue perfusion.*
- Administer antidysrhythmic medications as needed. *Dysrhythmias affect tissue perfusion by altering cardiac output.*

clinical ALERT

Dysrhythmias are the most frequent complication following AMI, often developing within the first 24 hours. Prompt recognition and treatment of dysrhythmias is vital; however, remember to treat the client, not the monitor. Assess the client's response to the dysrhythmia before initiating treatment.

pain scale. *Frequent monitoring allows early intervention and reduces the risk of further tissue damage.*

- Administer oxygen at 2 to 6 L/min per nasal cannula. *Supplemental oxygen increases oxygen supply to the myocardium, decreasing ischemia and pain.*
- Provide for physical and psychologic rest. Provide information and emotional support. *Rest decreases cardiac workload and sympathetic nervous system stimulation. Information and emotional support help reduce anxiety and promote psychologic rest.*
- Administer 2 to 4 mg morphine by intravenous push for chest pain as ordered. *Morphine decreases pain and anxiety, and reduces the workload of the heart.*
- Reassess for relief of chest pain. Report continued pain to the charge nurse or physician. *The goal of pain management in an MI client is complete relief of pain.*

Ineffective Coping

- Establish an environment of caring and trust. Encourage the client to express feelings. *A trusting nurse–client relationship provides a safe environment for the client to discuss feelings of helplessness, powerlessness, anxiety, and hopelessness.*
- Accept denial as a coping mechanism, but do not reinforce it. *Denial may initially help decrease anxiety by diminishing the perceived threat to health. Prolonged denial, however, can interfere with acceptance of reality and cooperation, possibly delaying treatment and hindering recovery.*
- Note aggressive behaviors, hostility, or anger. Document any failure to comply with treatments. *These behaviors may indicate anxiety and denial.*
- Help identify positive coping skills used in the past (e.g., problem-solving skills, verbalization of feelings, asking for help, prayer). Reinforce positive coping behaviors. *Previously successful coping behaviors can help the*

client deal with the current situation. These familiar methods can decrease feelings of powerlessness.

- Allow the client to make decisions about care, as possible. *Participating in care planning gives a sense of control and the opportunity to use positive coping skills.*
- Provide privacy for the client and significant other to share their questions and concerns. *Privacy allows the client and partner the opportunity to share their feelings and fears, offer support and encouragement to one another, relieve anxiety, and establish effective coping methods.*

Fear

- Acknowledge the client's perception of the situation. Allow him or her to verbalize concerns. *The sudden change in health status brings on anxiety and fear of the unknown. Verbalizing these fears may help the client cope with the changes and allow the health care team to provide information and correct misconceptions.*
- Encourage questions, and provide consistent, factual answers. Repeat information as needed. *Accurate and consistent information can reduce fear and help develop realistic expectations. Anxiety and fear decrease the ability to concentrate and retain information; information may need to be repeated.*
- Administer antianxiety medications as ordered. *These medications promote rest and relaxation and decrease feelings of anxiety, which may act as barriers to restoration of health.*
- Teach nonpharmacologic methods of stress reduction (e.g., relaxation methods, mental imagery, music therapy, breathing exercises, meditation, massage). *Stress management techniques may help reduce tension and anxiety, provide the client with a sense of control, and enhance coping skills.*

EVALUATING

To evaluate the effectiveness of nursing care for the client with an MI, collect data such as the following:

- Pain level and relief with prescribed analgesic
- Evidence of adequate tissue perfusion: level of consciousness, urine output, heart and lung sounds, skin color and temperature, peripheral pulses, ECG rhythm
- Acceptance of diagnosis, involvement in care, and participation in care planning
- Expressions or nonverbal evidence of fear and anxiety.

Documenting. Document the location, frequency, and intensity of pain and the client's response to pain relief measures. Note level of anxiety. Record vital signs and assessment data, and note any changes that occur with activity. Document ECG rhythm per protocol and when any changes occur. Record any medications given to treat dysrhythmias or other complications of AMI, and the response to treatment. Document all teaching with the client's apparent understanding or acceptance of the information presented.

CONTINUING CARE

Teaching and planning for home care begin with admission to the coronary care unit and continue through the hospital stay and after discharge into the rehabilitation period. The emphasis is on restoring optimal health and reducing the risk of future cardiac events.

Assessing readiness to learn is an important first step. The client in strong denial may not believe that the information being taught has any relevance. Evaluate ability to learn, assessing knowledge base, physiologic and psychologic health, health beliefs, and expectations of the health care system.

Teach about CHD and myocardial infarction. Explain the purpose of prescribed dietary changes and activity restrictions. Discuss prescribed medications, including their purposes and side effects. Encourage the client to ask questions. Reinforce teaching with written materials.

Provide referral to a cardiac rehabilitation program. Emphasize the importance of complying with the medical regimen and cardiac rehabilitation program and of keeping follow-up appointments. Provide telephone numbers of resource personnel who are available to respond to questions and concerns after the client's discharge.

Provide information about community resources, such as the local chapter of the American Heart Association. Encourage family members to learn CPR in the event of an emergency, and provide information about other community agencies that offer CPR classes.

NURSING PROCESS CARE PLAN
Client with Acute Myocardial Infarction

Betty Williams, a 62-year-old psychologist, is admitted to the emergency department complaining of severe substernal chest pain. She thought the pain, which started after lunch, was indigestion. She describes the pain as "like someone sitting on my chest." The pain radiates to her jaw and left arm, and is accompanied by a "choking feeling," severe shortness of breath, and diaphoresis. The pain is unrelieved by rest, antacids, or three sublingual NTG tablets (gr 1/150).

After inserting an intravenous catheter and beginning oxygen at 6 L/min per nasal cannula, a 12-lead ECG and cardiac enzymes are obtained. Mrs. Williams's pain is relieved by intravenous morphine sulfate. Based on her history, assessment, and ECG, an acute anterior wall MI is diagnosed. Intravenous alteplase (t-PA) is administered followed by intravenous infusions of heparin. Mrs. Williams is transferred to the coronary care unit (CCU).

Assessment. Mrs. Williams's medical history includes type 2 diabetes, angina, and hypertension. She has smoked cigarettes for 45 years, averaging 1½ to 2 packs per day. Her father died at age 42 of MI, and her paternal grandfather died at age 65 of MI. Mrs. Williams is currently taking tolbutamide (Orinase) and metoprolol (Lopressor).

On admission to the CCU, Mrs. Williams is alert and oriented to time, place, and person; P 118; BP 172/92; R 24; T 99.6°F (37.5°C). Auscultation reveals an S_4 and fine crackles in the bases of both lungs. The ECG shows sinus tachycardia with occasional PVCs. Her skin is cool and slightly diaphoretic. Capillary refill is less than 3 seconds, and peripheral pulses are strong and equal. Her nail beds are pink.

A triple-lumen central line is in place, with nitroglycerin, t-PA, and heparin infusions controlled by infusion pumps. A solution of 5% dextrose in ¼ normal saline solution is infusing in a peripheral intravenous line. Mrs. Williams states, "The pain is better since the nurse in the ER gave me a shot. But it has been coming and going. I would rate it a 4 right now, but it was terrible before. The doctor told me that this drug I'm getting will quickly open up the artery that is blocked. I hope it works! Do many people get this drug?"

Diagnosis. The CCU nurses formulate the following nursing diagnoses for Mrs. Williams:

- *Pain* related to cardiac muscle ischemia and infarct
- *Anxiety* related to change in health status
- *Ineffective Protection* related to the risk of bleeding secondary to fibrinolytic therapy
- *Risk for Injury* related to altered cardiac rate and rhythm

Expected Outcomes. The expected outcomes of the plan of care specify that Mrs. Williams will:

- Verbalize relief of chest pain.
- Verbalize a reduced anxiety and fear.
- Exhibit no signs of internal or external bleeding.
- Maintain an adequate cardiac output.

Planning and Implementation. The following interventions are planned and implemented:

- Instruct to report any chest pain. Titrate NTG infusion for chest pain; stop infusion if systolic BP drops below

100 mm Hg. Administer 2 to 4 mg morphine intravenously for chest pain unrelieved by nitroglycerin infusion.

- Encourage verbalization of fears and concerns. Answer questions honestly, and correct any misconceptions about disease process, therapeutic interventions, or prognosis.
- Explain that the t-PA will dissolve the clot that is obstructing blood flow to the heart muscle, thus limiting heart damage.
- Explain the need for frequent assessment.
- Assess for evidence of internal or intracranial bleeding: back or abdominal pain, headache, decreased level of consciousness, dizziness, bloody secretions or excretions, or pallor. Test all stools, urine, and vomitus for occult blood. Notify physician immediately of any abnormal findings.
- Continuously monitor ECG.
- Immediately treat dysrhythmias or other cardiac emergencies per unit protocol.

Evaluation. Mrs. Williams's chest pain is relieved with the morphine, NTG infusion, and fibrinolytic therapy. She states that she feels "much better now that the pain is gone. I was afraid it would just get worse." No indication of bleeding problems are noted, and while her PVCs increase with reperfusion therapy, she experiences no significant dysrhythmias. Mrs. Williams remains in CCU for 2 days and is transferred to the floor.

Critical Thinking in the Nursing Process

1. You are admitting Mrs. Williams to the medical unit from CCU. What assessment data will you obtain? What nursing diagnoses and interventions will you anticipate as part of Mrs. Williams's care at this point in her recovery?
2. Two days after her initial therapy, Mrs. Williams complains of palpitations. You notice frequent PVCs on the ECG monitor. What do you do?
3. Mrs. Williams states, "I have been smoking for over 45 years, and I am not going to stop now! Besides, it calms me down when I am feeling anxious." How would you respond to this statement?

CARDIAC RHYTHM DISORDERS

Cardiac Dysrhythmias

The heart contracts in response to electrical stimulation of its cells. In the normal heart, this produces a coordinated, rhythmic contraction that pushes blood into the circulation. The normal heart rhythm is *normal sinus rhythm (NSR)*. Impulses originate in the sinoatrial (SA or sinus) node and travel

through normal conduction pathways without delay. The rate is between 60 and 100 bpm. Changes from this rhythm can affect the heart's ability to pump blood effectively to body tissues. See Chapter 25 ⊕ for more information about the conduction pathways and normal rhythms of the heart.

A **cardiac dysrhythmia** is a disturbance or irregularity in the electrical system of the heart. Cardiac dysrhythmias

BOX 26-10

ECG RHYTHM ANALYSIS

Interpreting an ECG strip is a skill that takes practice. Use a consistent, systematic method to determine the heart rhythm. A suggested sequence of steps follows:

1. *Determine rate.* Assess the heart rate using one of the following to determine number of beats per minute (bpm):
   - Count the number of R waves in a 6-second strip and multiply by 10.
   - Count the number of large boxes between two consecutive R waves, and divide 300 (the number of large boxes in 1 minute) by this number. For example, there are 6 large boxes between two R waves; $300 \div 6 = 50$ bpm.
   - Memorize the following sequence: 300, 150, 100, 75, 60, 50. One large box between complexes equals a rate of 300; two = 150; three = 100, and so on.
2. *Determine regularity.* Measure the interval from one R wave to the next R wave, then evaluate successive R to R intervals for their regularity. Irregular rhythms may be *irregularly irregular* (if there is no pattern to the irregularity) or *regularly irregular* (if a consistent pattern can be identified).
3. *Assess P waves.* All the P waves should look alike in size and shape.
4. *Assess P to QRS relationship.* There should be one P wave before every QRS complex and one QRS complex following every P wave.
5. *Measure PR interval and QRS complex.* To determine the duration of any interval, count the number of small boxes from the beginning of the interval to the end, and multiply by 0.04 second. The normal PR interval is 0.12 to 0.20 second; the normal QRS complex lasts 0.06 to 0.10 second.
6. *Identify abnormalities.* Note any ectopic (abnormal) beats, deviation of the ST segment above or below the baseline, and abnormalities in waveform shape and duration.

may be benign or life threatening. Changes in heart rhythm occur due to "normal" events such as exercise or fear, as well as to pathologic changes. Any dysrhythmia can affect cardiac output. The effect of the dysrhythmia determines the need for treatment. Box 26-10 ■ lists steps for heart rhythm analysis.

PATHOPHYSIOLOGY

Dysrhythmias develop due to two mechanisms: altered formation of impulses or altered conduction of the impulse through the heart.

Abnormalities of impulse formation are caused by changes in *automaticity*, the ability of the heart to generate an electrical impulse and contraction without input from the nervous system. Impulses may develop more rapidly or more slowly than normal, or may originate outside the SA node. These are called *ectopic beats.*

An impulse may be blocked or delayed as it moves through the conduction pathways of the heart. This is known as *heart block.* In some cases, an impulse is delayed in one area of the heart but conducted normally through the rest. This pattern of normal and slow conduction, known as *reentry phenomenon,* is responsible for many dysrhythmias.

Cardiac rhythms are classified according to the site of impulse formation or the site and degree of conduction block (Table 26-6 ■). In *supraventricular rhythms,* impulses form above the ventricles. *Ventricular rhythms* originate in the ventricles and may be fatal. *AV conduction blocks* result from impaired impulse transmission from the atria to the ventricles. See Box 26-11 ■ for a discussion of dysrhythmias in older adults.

Supraventricular Rhythms

Supraventricular (*supra* = above or over) rhythms arise above the ventricles. They may originate in the sinus node, the atria, or within the atrioventricular (AV) node. Conduction of the impulse through the ventricles usually is unaffected, so the QRS complex appears normal.

SINUS TACHYCARDIA. In *sinus tachycardia,* the heart rate is greater than 100 bpm. Tachycardia is a normal response to

BOX 26-11   FOCUS ON OLDER ADULTS

Dysrhythmias in Older Adults

Aging affects the heart and the cardiac conduction system, increasing the risk for dysrhythmias, even when no other evidence of heart disease is found. Older adults are more likely to experience ectopic beats during exercise. AV blocks also are more common in people over the age of 65.

Assessing dysrhythmias in older adults focuses on the effect on function.

- Inquire about episodes of dizziness, light-headedness, fainting, palpitations, chest pain, or shortness of breath.
- Ask about the relationship of symptoms to food intake and caffeine-containing beverages.
- Evaluate other contributing factors such as heart disease, medications, smoking, or alcohol intake.
- Inquire about falls, particularly those occurring without apparent reason.

Teach older adults to reduce their risk for dysrhythmias and their consequences by:

- Taking medications (including over-the-counter drugs) as ordered.
- Eliminating caffeine intake.
- Stopping smoking and eliminating alcohol intake if appropriate.
- Engaging in regular exercise.
- Contacting their primary care provider for symptoms such as dizziness, fainting, frequent palpitations, shortness of breath, unexplained falls, or chest pain.

TABLE 26-6

Characteristics, Causes, and Management of Selected Cardiac Rhythms

RHYTHM/ECG APPEARANCE	CHARACTERISTICS AND MANIFESTATIONS	MANAGEMENT
Supraventricular Rhythms		
Normal sinus rhythm (NSR)	Regular; rate 60–100 bpm. All waveforms and intervals normal	None; normal heart rhythm
Sinus tachycardia	Regular; rate > 100 bpm. Other characteristics as for NSR	Treated only if symptomatic or if client at risk for MI
Sinus bradycardia	Regular; rate < 60 bpm. Other characteristics as for NSR	Treated only if symptomatic; may give atropine or require pacemaker
Premature atrial contractions (PACs)	Irregular, an ectopic atrial beat occurring earlier than expected	Usually require no treatment
Atrial flutter	Usually regular with saw-tooth appearance of P waves. Atrial rate 240+ bpm; ventricular rate < 150 bpm	Synchronized cardioversion; medication to slow ventricular response

(continued)

TABLE 26-6

Characteristics, Causes, and Management of Selected Cardiac Rhythms (continued)

RHYTHM/ECG APPEARANCE	CHARACTERISTICS AND MANIFESTATIONS	MANAGEMENT
Atrial fibrillation 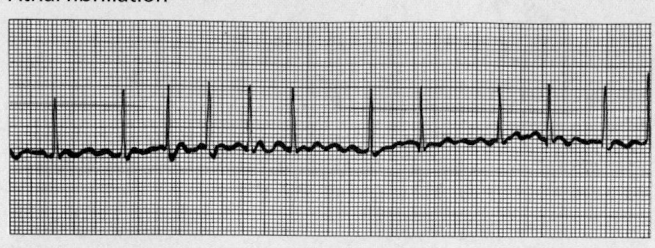	Irregularly irregular; no identifiable P waves; variable ventricular rate	Synchronized cardioversion; medication to slow ventricular rate; anticoagulants to reduce risk of stroke
Ventricular Rhythms Premature ventricular contractions (PVCs) 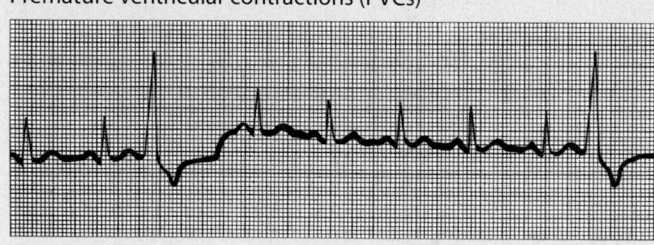	Irregular; ectopic ventricular beat interrupts normal rhythm; ectopic QRS wide and bizarre	Abstain from nicotine, caffeine; medication if symptomatic or if result of recent AMI
Ventricular tachycardia (VT or V-tach) 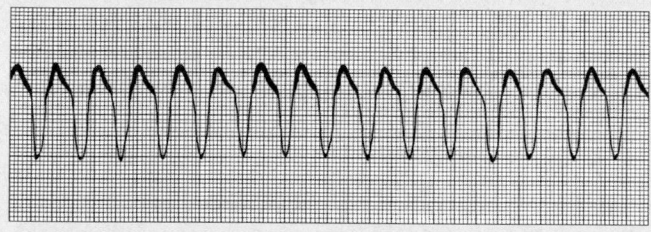	Regular; rate 100–250 bpm; no identifiable P waves, QRS wide and bizarre	Treated if symptomatic; intravenous drugs; cardioversion or defibrillation if unconscious or unstable
Ventricular fibrillation (V-fib) 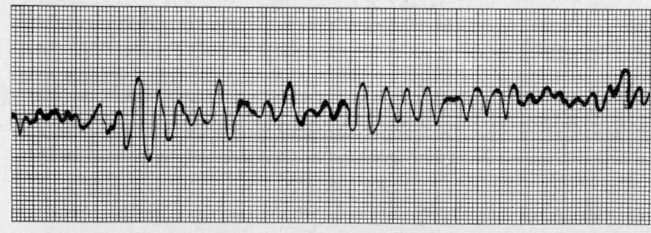	Grossly irregular; rate too rapid to count; no P waves, QRS bizarre and variable	Immediate defibrillation necessary to preserve life
AV Conduction Blocks First-degree AV block 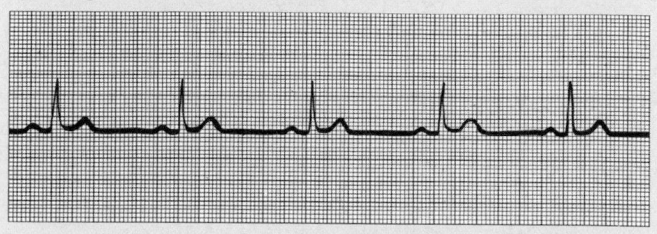	Regular; rate usually 60–100 bpm; PR interval > 0.21 sec	No treatment necessary

TABLE 26-6

Characteristics, Causes, and Management of Selected Cardiac Rhythms (continued)

RHYTHM/ECG APPEARANCE	CHARACTERISTICS AND MANIFESTATIONS	MANAGEMENT
Second-degree AV block 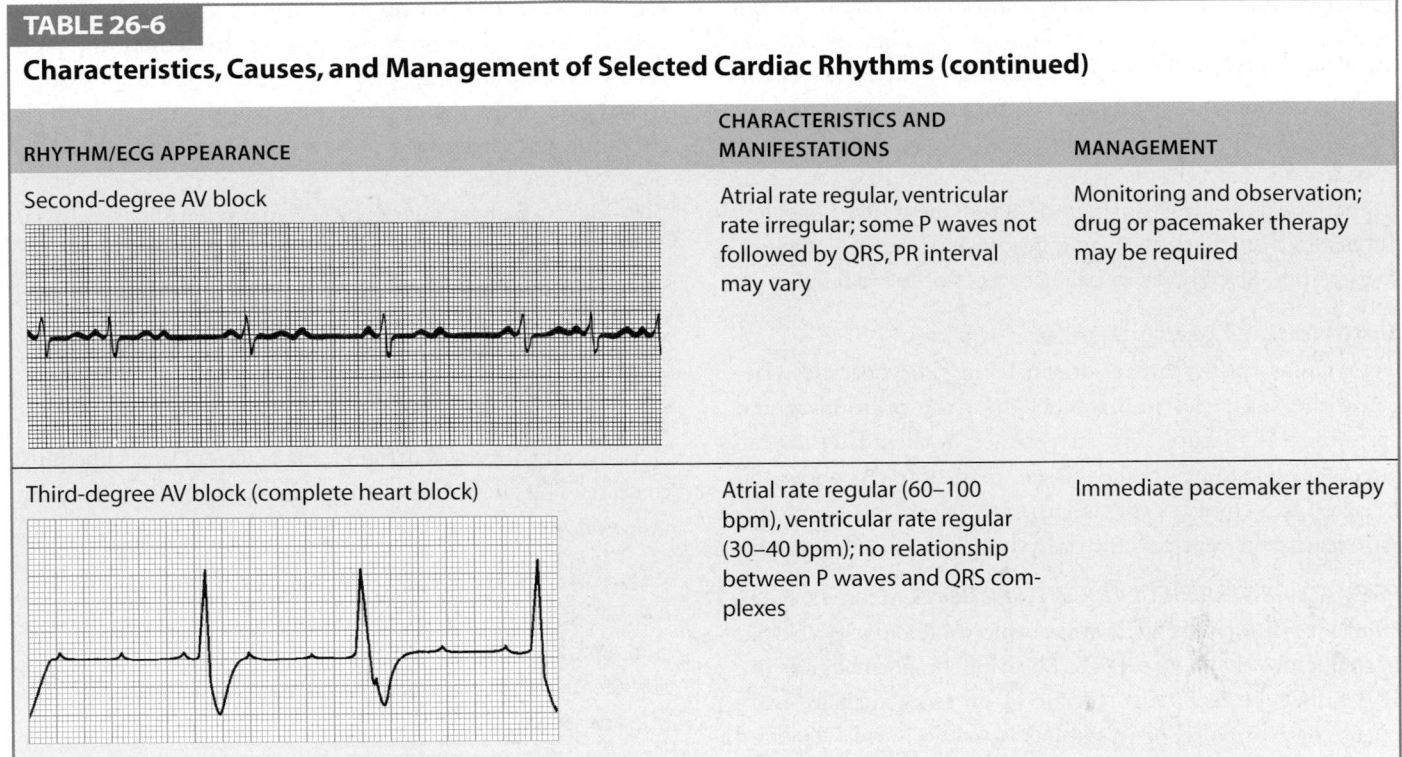	Atrial rate regular, ventricular rate irregular; some P waves not followed by QRS, PR interval may vary	Monitoring and observation; drug or pacemaker therapy may be required
Third-degree AV block (complete heart block)	Atrial rate regular (60–100 bpm), ventricular rate regular (30–40 bpm); no relationship between P waves and QRS complexes	Immediate pacemaker therapy

conditions that increase the body's demand for oxygen and nutrients, such as exercise. Other causes of sinus tachycardia include anxiety, pain, fever, hypoxia, hyperthyroidism, caffeine intake, and some drugs. Sinus tachycardia may be an early warning sign of cardiac problems such as heart failure.

The client with sinus tachycardia has a rapid pulse rate and may complain of a "racing" heart or shortness of breath. Clients with heart disease may experience chest pain.

SINUS BRADYCARDIA. *Sinus bradycardia* is a heart rate less than 60 bpm. It may be normal in some clients (e.g., clients with athletic heart syndrome) and during sleep. Bradycardia also may be caused by pain, increased intracranial pressure, hypothermia, heart disease, and certain drugs.

Clients with sinus bradycardia may be asymptomatic or may have manifestations of decreased cardiac output, such as decreased level of consciousness, syncope (faintness), or hypotension.

PREMATURE ATRIAL CONTRACTIONS. A *premature atrial contraction (PAC)* is an ectopic atrial beat that occurs earlier than the next expected sinus beat. PACs are usually asymptomatic and benign, but they may initiate supraventricular tachycardia in some people. PACs are common in older adults, and may occur without an obvious cause. Frequent PACs may cause heart palpitations or a fluttering sensation in the chest.

Supraventricular tachycardia (SVT) is usually characterized by a sudden onset and abrupt cessation. It may be caused by sympathetic nervous system stimulation and stressors such as fever, sepsis, and hyperthyroidism. Manifestations of SVT include complaints of palpitations and a "racing" heart, anxiety, dizziness, dyspnea, chest pain, diaphoresis, and fatigue.

ATRIAL FLUTTER. *Atrial flutter* is a very rapid and regular atrial rhythm. Causes include sympathetic nervous system stimulation due to anxiety, caffeine, and alcohol intake; thyrotoxicosis; and heart disease.

Clients with atrial flutter may complain of palpitations or a fluttering sensation in the chest or throat. If the ventricular rate is rapid, cardiac output falls, causing decreased level of consciousness, hypotension, decreased urinary output, and cool, clammy skin.

ATRIAL FIBRILLATION. *Atrial fibrillation* is a common dysrhythmia characterized by disorganized atrial activity without discrete atrial contractions. Extremely rapid impulses bombard the AV node, causing an irregularly irregular ventricular response. Atrial fibrillation may occur suddenly and recur, or it may become chronic. It is common in clients with heart failure.

Manifestations of atrial fibrillation include irregular pulses of variable strength. The client may have hypotension, shortness of breath, fatigue, and angina. Clients with extensive heart disease may develop syncope or heart failure.

Atrial fibrillation increases the risk of forming thromboemboli (blood clots). Stroke (brain attack) is a risk because these clots may travel to the brain.

JUNCTIONAL DYSRHYTHMIAS. *Junctional dysrhythmias* originate in the AV node or bundle of His. They include escape rhythms, which occur when sinus and atrial pacemakers fail, ectopic beats (premature junctional contractions or PJCs), and junctional tachycardia. While the QRS typically appears normal, the P wave may be inverted or occur immediately before, during, or after the QRS complex. Junctional dysrhythmias may be caused by drug toxicity, hypoxemia, electrolyte imbalance, AMI or heart failure.

Ventricular Dysrhythmias

Ventricular dysrhythmias originate in the ventricles. Because the ventricles pump blood into the pulmonary and systemic vasculature, any disturbance in their rhythm can affect cardiac output and tissue perfusion. A wide and bizarre QRS complex (greater than 0.12 sec) is a characteristic feature of ventricular dysrhythmias.

PREMATURE VENTRICULAR CONTRACTIONS. *Premature ventricular contractions (PVCs)* are ectopic ventricular beats that occur before the next expected beat of the normal rhythm. PVCs may be isolated or occur in patterns such as every other beat, in pairs, or in triplets (three in a row). Isolated PVCs often are benign. They may be triggered by anxiety or stress, tobacco, alcohol, or caffeine. Benign PVCs are common in older adults. In people with heart disease, PVCs are common. Frequent PVCs may signal an increased risk for lethal dysrhythmias.

Clients experiencing PVCs may complain of feeling their hearts "skip a beat" or of palpitations. The early beat may be heard on auscultation; it is felt as a "missed" beat on palpation of peripheral pulses.

VENTRICULAR TACHYCARDIA. *Ventricular tachycardia (VT; V-tach)* is three or more consecutive PVCs. VT may occur in short bursts, or "runs," or it may persist for longer periods. The rate is greater than 100 bpm, and the rhythm is usually regular. Myocardial ischemia and infarction are the most common causes of VT, although it also may occur with other heart diseases or in the absence of heart disease. It may be associated with anorexia nervosa, metabolic disorders, and drug toxicity.

Short bursts of VT may cause a sensation of fluttering in the chest, palpitations, and brief shortness of breath. Cardiac output drops with sustained VT, causing severe hypotension, a weak or nonpalpable pulse, and loss of consciousness. Allowed to continue, VT can deteriorate into ventricular fibrillation at any time. Sustained VT is a medical emergency that requires immediate intervention to preserve life.

VENTRICULAR FIBRILLATION. *Ventricular fibrillation (V-fib)* is defined as extremely rapid, chaotic ventricular depolarization that causes the ventricles to quiver and stop contract-

ing; the heart does not pump. This is known as **cardiac arrest,** a medical emergency requiring immediate intervention with cardiopulmonary resuscitation (CPR) measures. Death will follow the onset of V-fib within 4 minutes if the rhythm is not recognized and terminated, with a return to a perfusing rhythm.

V-fib is usually triggered by severe myocardial ischemia or infarction. It occurs without warning 50% of the time. It is the terminal event in many disease processes or traumatic conditions. V-fib also may be caused by digitalis toxicity, electrolyte and acid–base imbalances, certain drugs, mechanical stimulation (as with the insertion of cardiac catheters or pacing wires), and electric shock.

Clinically, loss of ventricular contraction causes the pulse to cease. The client loses consciousness and stops breathing (*cardiopulmonary arrest*).

Atrioventricular Conduction Blocks

Conduction defects that cause delayed or blocked transmission of sinus impulses through the AV node are called *atrioventricular (AV) conduction blocks.* AV blocks vary from benign to severe.

FIRST-DEGREE AV BLOCK. *First-degree AV block* is a benign conduction delay that poses no immediate threat and requires no treatment. There are no clinical manifestations except a prolonged PR interval. Causes of first-degree block include myocardial infarction, digitalis therapy or toxicity, complications from cardiac surgery, chronic heart disease, or drug effects.

SECOND-DEGREE AV BLOCK. In *second-degree AV block,* some atrial impulses are totally blocked at the AV node, prevented from reaching the ventricles. Two types of second-degree block are recognized. *Type I,* also known as Mobitz I or Wenckebach, is characterized by a repeating pattern in which PR intervals become progressively longer until one QRS complex is not conducted or is dropped. It is usually asymptomatic, unless the heart rate slows and cardiac output falls.

Type II, also called Mobitz II, is characterized by a regular pattern of nonconducted impulses; usually, two atrial impulses occur for every one that is transmitted to the ventricles. Type II heart block is usually associated with acute myocardial infarction. Its manifestations depend on the ventricular rate and cardiac output.

THIRD-DEGREE AV BLOCK. *Third-degree AV block (complete heart block)* occurs when atrial impulses are completely blocked at the AV node and not conducted to the ventricles. Atrial and ventricular rhythms are completely independent of one another. The ventricular impulse is slow at a rate of 30 to 40 bpm, while the normal atrial rate of 60 to 100 bpm continues.

Third-degree block is frequently caused by an acute myocardial infarction. Other heart diseases, drugs, and electrolyte imbalances also can precipitate it. Cardiac output falls, leading to light-headedness, confusion, and syncope (fainting). Third-degree AV block is life threatening and requires immediate treatment to restore the cardiac output.

INTERDISCIPLINARY CARE

Although many dysrhythmias pose little risk, others, such as ventricular fibrillation, are life threatening and require immediate intervention. Early recognition is vital. Clients at risk for dysrhythmias often are cared for in cardiac intensive care or other specialty units that allow constant monitoring of the ECG and client's status.

Diagnostic Tests

Diagnostic tests commonly ordered for clients with dysrhythmias include serum cardiac markers (CK, cardiac troponins), serum electrolytes (sodium, potassium, chloride, calcium, and magnesium), and, as appropriate, serum drug levels (e.g., digitalis levels). Cardiac electrophysiology (EP) studies may be done to locate the focus of persistent dysrhythmias. See Chapter 25 ◯◯ for more information about EP studies. Nursing care of the client undergoing an EP study is similar to that provided for clients undergoing angiography (see Box 26-3).

Cardiac Monitoring

Cardiac monitoring allows continuous observation of the client's cardiac rhythm. Different types of ECG monitoring are employed for different situations.

CONTINUOUS CARDIAC MONITORING. Electrodes placed on the client's chest are connected to a monitoring system. The heart rate and rhythm are visually displayed on a bedside monitor and a central monitoring station. Alarms on the monitors warn of potential problems such as very rapid or very slow heart rates. Box 26-12 ■ describes how to initiate cardiac monitoring.

PORTABLE CARDIAC MONITORING. Distance ECG monitoring (telemetry) is frequently used on medical–surgical or cardiac units. Telemetry allows the client to engage in activities

---

BOX 26-12	PROCEDURE CHECKLIST

Initiating Cardiac Monitoring Checklist

☑ Gather supplies.

☑ Provide for privacy.

☑ Explain the reason for ECG monitoring, reassuring the client that it allows immediate treatment of abnormal rhythms if necessary. Explain alarms, their purpose, and possible causes such as loose or disconnected lead wires and other mechanical problems. Activity is permitted within ordered restrictions while on the monitor.

☑ Follow Standard Precautions.

☑ Check equipment for damage (i.e., fraying, bent, or broken wires). Connect lead wires to cable, and secure the connections.

☑ Select electrode sites on the chest wall, considering lead to be monitored, skin condition, and any incisions or catheters.

☑ Clean sites with soap and water, and dry thoroughly. Alcohol may be used to remove skin oils; allow the skin to dry for 60 seconds after use.

☑ Peel backing from a fresh electrode; check to ensure that the pad is moist with conductive gel.

☑ Apply electrode pads, pressing firmly to ensure contact.

☑ Attach leads and position cable with sufficient slack for comfort. Place telemetry unit (if used) in gown pouch or pocket.

☑ Assess ECG tracing on the monitor, adjusting settings as needed.

☑ Set ECG monitor alarm limits as indicated, typically at 20 bpm higher and lower than the baseline rate. Turn alarms on, and leave on at all times. Assess immediately if an alarm is triggered.

☑ Remove and apply new pads every 24 to 48 hours and as needed. Clean gel residue from previous site, and document skin condition. Use a different site if skin appears irritated or blistered. Time and date pads with every change.

☑ Save ECG strips according to unit policy, and when the rhythm or the client's condition changes. Note date, time, client, and monitor lead on each strip. Notify the charge nurse or physician of significant changes in heart rhythm.

SAMPLE DOCUMENTATION

12/8/06	Placed on cardiac monitor, lead 2.
1430	Monitor shows NSR at 75/min with no ectopy noted. Resting comfortably. S. Craven, LPN.

Note: Refer to a nursing fundamentals or skills text for more detailed instruction. Check state guidelines and facility policy before performing any procedure.

while being monitored. Ambulatory or Holter monitoring may be used in community settings to diagnose infrequent dysrhythmias or dysrhythmias associated with activities.

Medications

Antidysrhythmic drugs may be used to treat acute dysrhythmias or to manage chronic conditions. The overall goal of therapy is to maintain an effective cardiac output by stabilizing cardiac rhythm.

Many different classes of drugs are used to treat cardiac dysrhythmias. Table 26-7 ■ identifies common antidysrhythmic drugs, their class, and the nursing implications in caring for the client receiving an antidysrhythmic drug.

clinical ALERT

All antidysrhythmic drugs can also *cause* dysrhythmias. Closely monitor all clients receiving cardiac drugs for dysrhythmias.

Cardioversion/Defibrillation

Cardioversion (or defibrillation) is used to treat rhythms that affect cardiac output and the client's welfare. An electrical shock is administered to depolarize all cells of the heart at the same time. This often stops the abnormal rhythm and allows the sinus node to resume control of the rhythm.

TABLE 26-7

Nursing Implications for Pharmacology: Antidysrhythmic Drugs

CLASS/DRUGS	PURPOSE	NURSING RESPONSIBILITIES	CLIENT TEACHING
Class IA ■ Quinidine ■ Procainamide (Procan, Pronestyl) ■ Disopyramide (Norpace)	Used to treat symptomatic or frequent PVCs, supraventricular or ventricular tachycardias, and to prevent ventricular fibrillation	Obtain baseline vital signs, cardiac rhythm, and physical assessment. Monitor ECG. Notify the physician of new dysrhythmias. Notify the physician immediately if manifestations of toxicity develop: ■ Signs of heart failure ■ Changes in ECG complex ■ Skin rash or flulike symptoms ■ Urinary retention ■ Neurologic effects such as confusion, dizziness, agitation ■ Shortness of breath ■ Altered liver function tests. Use an infusion pump to administer intravenous infusions. Monitor dose and its effectiveness.	Take the drug exactly as ordered. Do not skip or double doses. Check with your doctor if you miss a dose. Take and record your pulse rate daily before rising. Count pulse for 1 full minute. Bring the record to each office or clinic appointment. Report the following to your doctor: irregular pulse rate or rhythm, dizziness, eye pain, vision changes, skin rashes, wheezing or other respiratory problems, behavior changes.
Class IB ■ Lidocaine ■ Tocainide (Tonocard) ■ Phenytoin (Dilantin) ■ Mexiletine (Mexitil)	Primarily used to treat ventricular dysrhythmias, including PVCs and ventricular tachycardia		
Class IC ■ Flecainide (Tambocor) ■ Propafenone (Rythmol) ■ Moricizine (Ethmozine)	Usually reserved for serious ventricular dysrhythmias		
Class II: Beta Blockers ■ Esmolol (Brevibloc) ■ Propranolol (Inderal, others) ■ Acebutolol (Sectral)	Used to prevent SVT and possibly V-fib. May cause bronchospasm, so are contraindicated for clients with asthma or COPD		
Class III ■ Sotalol (Betapace) ■ Amiodarone (Cordarone) ■ Bretylium (Bretylol) ■ Dofetilide (Tikosyn)	Primarily used to treat V-tach and V-fib		
Class IV: Calcium Channel Blockers ■ Verapamil (Calan, Isoptin) ■ Diltiazem (Cardizem, Dilacor)	Used to manage supraventricular tachycardias		
Miscellaneous Drugs to Treat Dysrhythmias ■ Adenosine (Adenocard) ■ Digoxin (Lanoxin) ■ Ibutilide fumarate (Corvert)	Used to treat atrial dysrhythmias		

MediaLink Lidocaine

MediaLink Amiodarone

MediaLink Digoxin

Synchronized cardioversion delivers an electrical current synchronized with the client's rhythm to prevent ventricular fibrillation. It is used to treat rhythms that are not life threatening, such as supraventricular tachycardia and atrial fibrillation. It is usually an elective procedure, and the client is sedated prior to cardioversion. Anticoagulants may be given before the procedure to reduce the risk of thromboembolism.

Defibrillation is an emergency treatment that delivers an electrical charge without regard to the cardiac cycle. Early defibrillation improves survival of clients experiencing V-fib. External defibrillation may be performed by any health care provider who has been trained in the procedure. Initiate CPR and the cardiac arrest (code) procedure when V-fib is recognized. Remove nitroglycerin patches from the client's chest in preparation for defibrillation, but leave monitor pads in place. Conductive gel pads are applied to the chest wall at the apex and base of the heart, and an electrical shock is delivered by *automated external defibrillator (AED)* or manually (Figure 26-9 ■). The cardiac rhythm is evaluated after each shock is delivered. After successful defibrillation, the client is transferred to the critical care unit for monitoring and therapy to prevent further episodes of V-fib.

AUTOMATIC IMPLANTABLE CARDIOVERTER–DEFIBRILLATOR.
The *automatic implantable cardioverter–defibrillator (AICD)* recognizes life-threatening changes in heart rhythm and automatically delivers an electric shock to convert the rhythm back into a normal rhythm. Electrodes surgically placed on

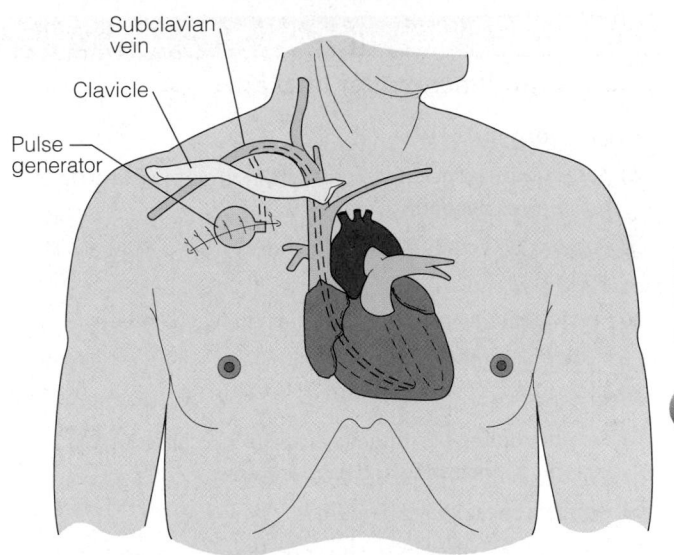

Figure 26-10. ■ A permanent pacemaker with a transvenous electrode into the right ventricle.

the heart are attached to an implanted cardioverter–defibrillator device. The AICD is used for clients with recurrent ventricular tachycardia and people who have survived cardiac arrest not associated with an acute myocardial infarction. When V-tach or V-fib occur, the AICD delivers a shock to convert the rhythm.

Pacemakers

Pacemakers may be used to treat AV blocks. *Temporary pacemakers* have an external generator attached to an electrode threaded intravenously into the right ventricle or to temporary pacing wires implanted during cardiac surgery. *Permanent pacemakers* have an implanted pulse generator attached to electrodes that are sewn directly onto the heart or passed into the heart via the subclavian or jugular vein (Figure 26-10 ■).

Pacemakers have both sensing and pacing functions. *Sensing* detects the heart's own beats. When the pacemaker senses a heart rate within preset limits, it provides no electrical stimuli. *Pacing,* or the delivery of an electrical pulse to stimulate the heart to contract, occurs when the client's heart rate falls outside the programmed limits. Pacing is detected on the ECG strip (Figure 26-11 ■) by the

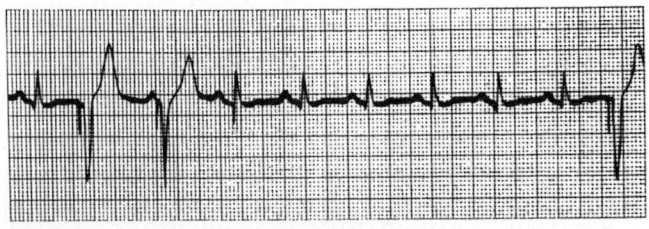

Figure 26-11. ■ Ventricular pacing. Note the presence of pacer spikes prior to the wide, ventricular QRS complexes, and the absence of spikes when the client's natural rhythm resumes.

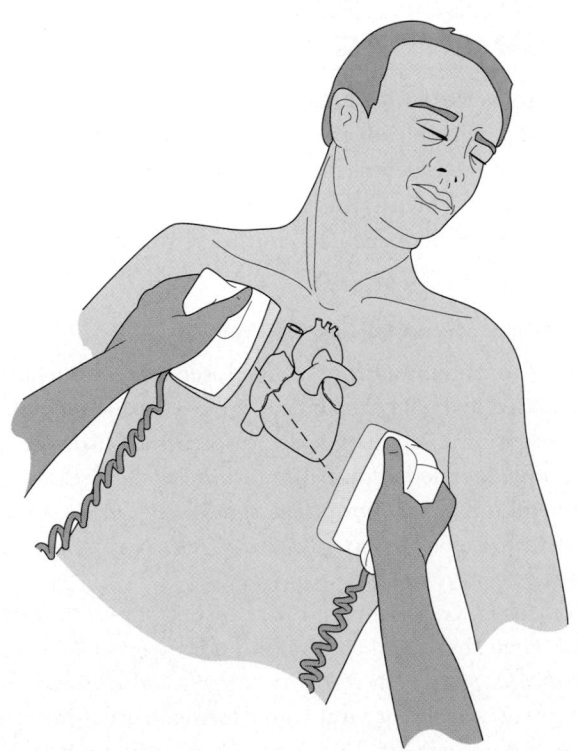

Figure 26-9. ■ Placement of paddles or pads for defibrillation.

MediaLink

Defibrillation

BOX 26-13	NURSING CARE CHECKLIST

Permanent Pacemaker Implant

Before Surgery

☑ Assess knowledge and understanding; reinforce and clarify teaching as needed.

☑ Position ECG monitor electrodes away from potential incision sites.

☑ Provide routine preoperative care and teaching (see Chapter 9). ⦵

After Surgery

☑ Provide routine postoperative care (see Chapter 9), ⦵ including monitoring and incision care.

☑ Obtain a chest x-ray as ordered.

☑ Administer analgesia and position for comfort. Restrict movement of affected arm and shoulder for 24 hours.

☑ After 24 hours, assist with gentle ROM exercises at least tid.

☑ Monitor pacemaker function and cardiac rhythm. Report pacemaker problems such as failure to pace or hiccups to the physician.

☑ Report dysrhythmias to the charge nurse or physician.

☑ Document date of insertion, pacemaker model and type, and settings.

☑ Provide a pacemaker identification card including manufacturer's name, model number, mode of operation, rate parameters, and expected battery life. Instruct to carry the card at all times, and to wear a Medic-Alert bracelet or tag.

☑ Teach about the pacemaker, its function, how to take and record the pulse rate, and usual battery replacement procedure.

☑ Instruct to report the following to the physician: pulse rate 5 or more bpm slower than preset pacemaker rate; fever; signs of pacemaker malfunction, such as dizziness, fainting, fatigue, weakness, chest pain, or palpitations.

☑ Notify all care providers of the pacemaker.

presence of a pacing spike before the P wave (atrial pacing) or QRS complex (ventricular pacing). Box 26-13 ■ outlines nursing care for the client having a permanent pacemaker implant.

Surgery

Surgical *ablation* (removal of a part or pathway) may be used when the site of an ectopic focus can be identified. The affected tissue may be excised (cut out) or destroyed by freezing with liquid nitrogen, laser, or an electric current.

NURSING CARE

ASSESSING

It is vital to assess the client before treating any suspected dysrhythmia. What appears to be ventricular tachycardia on the monitor may be a client tapping the electrode pad or brushing the teeth. Apparent asystole on the monitor may be a sleeping client whose electrode patch has come loose. Similarly, a heart rate of 52 bpm may be normal for some clients and not affect their functioning at all. Compare the present rhythm with previous rhythm recordings and report significant changes.

Ask about the presence of chest pain, shortness of breath, or palpitations. Inquire about dizziness or feeling light-headed, faint, or nauseated. Obtain vital signs and an ECG monitor strip. Assess skin color, temperature, and moisture; level of consciousness and mental status; heart sounds and peripheral pulses; respiratory status; and anxiety level. Check electrode placement, leads, the monitor cable, and connections.

clinical ALERT

Remember: Treat the client, not the monitor!

Monitor laboratory results, including serum electrolytes, hemoglobin and hematocrit, cardiac markers, and drug levels. Report abnormal results to the charge nurse or physician.

DIAGNOSING, PLANNING, AND IMPLEMENTING

Priorities in Nursing Care. Although many dysrhythmias are benign, with no adverse effects, others such as ventricular tachycardia or ventricular fibrillation can seriously affect cardiac output. Maintaining an adequate cardiac output to ensure delivery of oxygen and nutrients to the body's cells is the highest priority of care.

Decreased Cardiac Output

■ Assess for manifestations of decreased cardiac output: decreased level of consciousness; tachycardia; tachypnea; hypotension; diaphoresis; decreased urine output; cool, clammy, mottled skin; pallor or cyanosis; decreased peripheral pulses. *Manifestations of decreased cardiac output may indicate the client is not tolerating the dysrhythmia and needs immediate treatment.*

■ Monitor ECG rhythm and post ECG strip every shift and when rhythm changes occur. *Documenting ECG rhythms helps evaluate status and the effect of treatment.*

■ Frequently monitor vital signs during acute dysrhythmias and treatment. *Vital signs are an indicator of the effect of the dysrhythmia and treatment on cardiovascular status.*

- Monitor lab values, especially serum electrolytes and drug levels as ordered. Report abnormal values to the charge nurse and physician. *Electrolyte imbalances can cause dysrhythmias. Serum drug levels need to be within the therapeutic range for optimal effectiveness.*

- Maintain intravenous access with an intravenous infusion or saline lock. *Many drugs used to treat dysrhythmias are administered intravenously. In an emergency, an existing intravenous site facilitates rapid treatment of the dysrhythmia.*

- On recognizing ventricular fibrillation, begin emergency procedures. Call for help. Begin CPR until a defibrillator is available. Initiate advanced cardiac life support (ACLS) protocols. Defibrillate as soon as possible. Assist the code team as needed. *V-fib is a medical emergency requiring immediate treatment to preserve life.*

- After a cardiac arrest, transfer to critical care. *The period immediately following resuscitation is critical, and the client needs careful monitoring.*

Risk for Ineffective Tissue Perfusion: Cerebral

- Monitor level of consciousness and orientation to time, place, and person. *A change in mental status may indicate lack of adequate blood and oxygen supply to cells of the brain.*

- Assess neurologic status indicators such as respirations, movement, grip strength, and papillary reaction to light. *Changes in neurologic signs may indicate significant ischemia of the brain.*

- Initiate oxygen therapy if not currently in place. *Supplemental oxygen increases the oxygen saturation of the blood and its delivery to the tissues, including the brain. This helps preserve cellular metabolism and function.*

- Lower the head of the bed to no greater than 15 degrees if possible. *Lowering the head of the bed supports and improves cerebral blood flow.*

- Unless contraindicated (e.g., if the client is vomiting), maintain supine position with the head straight (in alignment with the body). *Alignment of the head and neck with the body facilitates blood flow to and from the brain through major vessels in the neck.*

- Promote rest with a quiet environment to the extent possible. *Reducing environmental stimuli reduces mental activity and the metabolic needs of brain cells.*

Anxiety

- Notify family of significant changes in the client's condition or cardiac arrest, providing up-to-date information. Prepare family members for visits by explaining interventions such as invasive tubes, a ventilator, or additional equipment. *Concern for the family and significant others is part of holistic nursing. Family members need information, honest communication, and compassionate care.*

Preparing the family for changes in the client's condition and plan of care helps them to cope with a difficult situation.

EVALUATING

To evaluate the effectiveness of care for a client with a dysrhythmia, collect data related to cardiac output and cerebral perfusion. For example, evaluate level of consciousness and mental status, skin color and temperature, vital signs, oxygen saturation, and urinary output. Monitor cardiac rhythm, promptly reporting increased or significant dysrhythmias or unresponsiveness to treatment measures. Monitor laboratory data such as arterial blood gas results and serum electrolytes.

Documenting. Document mental status, vital signs, and other assessment data during episodes of dysrhythmia, noting changes from previous status. Document cardiac rhythms, as well as the effect of activities. Record treatment measures and their effects on the dysrhythmia and client's status. Note the client's perception of the situation and apparent level of anxiety. If family members are notified of a significant or critical dysrhythmia, document the time and their response or presence.

CONTINUING CARE

Dysrhythmias can have a significant physical and psychologic impact. The client and family may fear sudden cardiac death. Teaching focuses on coping strategies and specific treatments. Involve both the client and the family in teaching. Teach about prescribed drugs, including their desired and potential adverse or toxic effects. Stress the importance of follow-up visits with the cardiologist, and schedule them, if possible.

Teach clients with a pacemaker or an AICD about the device and how it works, how to take their pulse, signs of infection or other complications, resumption of and any limitations to activities, and safety issues. Stress the importance of promptly reporting problems to the physician, and attending follow-up appointments. In some states driving is prohibited for clients with AICDs; address the impact of this on lifestyle. Inform the client that magnetic interference can damage the AICD or cause it to discharge. Procedures such as magnetic resonance imaging (MRI) and equipment such as arc welders, radar, and theft prevention equipment can damage the AICD and should be avoided.

Encourage the client and family to learn and maintain current training in CPR. Refer to the American Heart Association or the American Red Cross for training.

Sudden Cardiac Death

Sudden cardiac death is defined as death occurring within 1 hour of the onset of cardiac symptoms. It usually is caused by ventricular fibrillation and cardiac arrest. Cardiac arrest occurs when effective circulation ceases. Nearly half of cardiac arrest victims die before reaching the hospital.

BOX 26-14	PROCEDURE CHECKLIST

Cardiopulmonary Resuscitation (CPR) Checklist

☑ Assess for responsiveness; shake and ask "Are you okay?"

☑ Call for help. Dial 911 (if outside the health care facility) or initiate the institutional cardiac arrest procedure.

☑ Open the airway using the head tilt–chin lift maneuver: Simultaneously press down on the client's forehead with one hand to tilt the head back. Lift the chin forward using the fingers of the other hand under the bony part of the chin (part A of the accompanying figure).

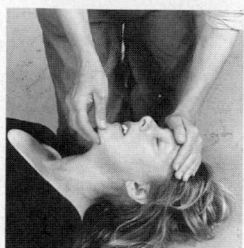

A

☑ Check for breathing. With the ear next to the client's mouth and nose, *look* for the chest to rise and fall with respirations, *listen* for exhalation, and *feel* for the flow of air.

☑ If not breathing, give two full breaths using a pocket mask, mouth shield, or bag-valve mask (see part B of the figure). Observe for chest rise and fall during ventilation.

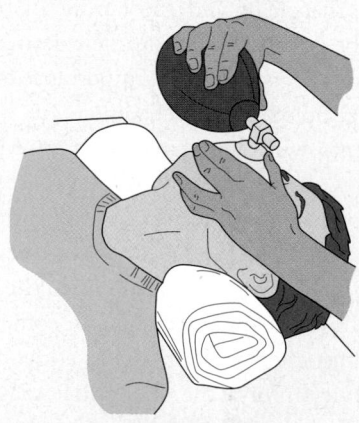

B

☑ Check for a carotid or femoral pulse. (Take less than 10 seconds to check the pulse.)

☑ If pulse is present, continue rescue breathing at 8 to 10 breaths per minute. Recheck the carotid pulse every 2 minutes.

☑ If pulse is absent, analyze rhythm and defibrillate, or if AED is unavailable begin chest compressions. Place the client on a firm surface. Place the heel of one hand on the center of the chest between the nipples and the other hand on top of the hand on the sternum with the fingers either extended or interlocked (see part C of the figure).

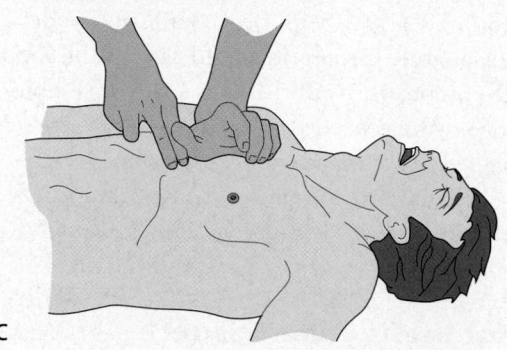

C

☑ With the arms straight, the shoulders directly over the hands, and elbows locked, press straight down to depress the sternum 1½ to 2 inches (part D of the figure). Release pressure completely between compressions but do not lift the hands from the chest.

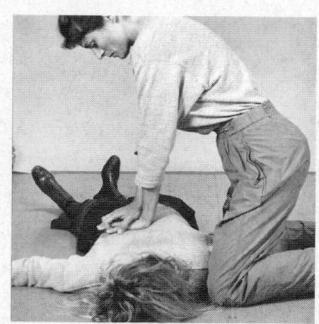

D

☑ Compress the chest hard and fast, at a rate of approximately 100 times per minute. With one- and two-rescuer CPR, provide 2 breaths after each 30 compressions. Assess the pulse after 5 complete cycles of 30 compressions and 2 breaths; continue CPR until help arrives.

Note: Refer to a nursing fundamentals or skills text for more detailed instruction. Check state guidelines and facility policy before performing any procedure.

Coronary heart disease is the most common cause of sudden cardiac deaths in the United States. Other causes include electrocution, pulmonary embolism, and rapid blood loss from a ruptured aortic aneurysm. Ventricular fibrillation is the most common dysrhythmia causing sudden cardiac death; asystole or cardiac standstill also leads to sudden death. The risk of sudden cardiac death is highest in the first 6 to 18 months following an acute myocardial infarction (AMI) or other major cardiac event.

Effective CPR must be instituted within 2 to 4 minutes of cardiac arrest to prevent permanent brain damage. CPR is a mechanical means of maintaining tissue perfusion and oxygenation using ventilation and external cardiac compressions. All health care providers need to be proficient in CPR or basic cardiac life support (BCLS). A review of CPR procedures is provided in Box 26-14 ■. ACLS incorporates electrical and drug treatment in addition to mechanical compressions.

CPR can be traumatic, causing injuries to the skin, thorax, upper airway, abdomen, lungs, heart, and great vessels. These complications can be minimized by using appropriate CPR techniques.

Because most instances of sudden cardiac death result from ventricular fibrillation, the American Heart Association recommends early defibrillation when appropriate. Automated external defibrillators (AEDs) are easy to use (Figure 26-12 ■). The device senses the heart rhythm through two electrodes placed on the chest, and delivers a shock when necessary. A shock can be delivered simply by pressing the "shock" button on the device.

The client who survives sudden cardiac death and family members have significant teaching needs to recognize and reduce the risk of subsequent events.

If the cause of cardiac arrest is identified, teach risk factor reduction. For example, if a myocardial infarction precipitated the cardiac arrest, teach the risk factors for MI and ways to reduce them. If the cause of cardiac arrest is unknown, explain diagnostic studies and discuss possible interventions such as the AICD. Stress the importance of carrying a card at all times listing all medications and the client's health care provider. In all cases, teach recognition of early manifestations or warning signs of cardiac arrest. All family members should become proficient in performing CPR.

To reduce death rates from cardiac arrest, teach community members how to perform effective CPR and the importance of early intervention. Work with community and emergency services agencies to provide and train community members to use the AED as well.

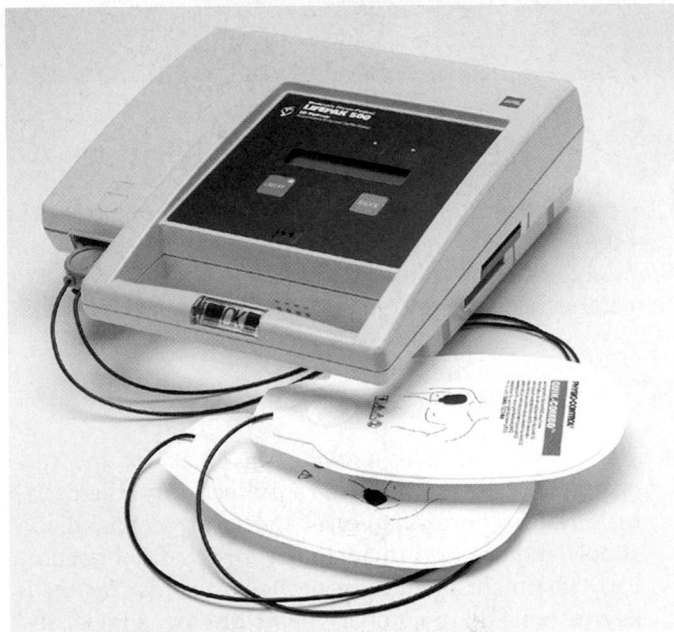

Figure 26-12. ■ An automatic external defibrillator for emergency resuscitation. (Courtesy of Medtronic Physiocontrol.)

ADVANCE DIRECTIVES

Unless otherwise stipulated by the client, family, or an advance directive, all resuscitative measures necessary (CPR, respiratory, and pharmacologic support) are used to treat cardiac arrest. *Advance directives* allow clients to make treatment decisions regarding care before a medical emergency occurs. The living will and the durable power of attorney for health care are two forms of advance directives.

Through an advance directive, a client may request that no or limited resuscitation procedures be used if cardiac arrest occurs. Without an advance directive, this decision falls to family members. A *"no code"* or *do-not-resuscitate (DNR)* order limits the use of resuscitative measures. Caring for clients with DNR orders does not mean withdrawing care. Nurses continue to provide optimal care for the clients and family.

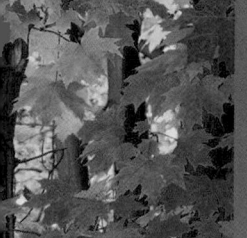

Chapter Review

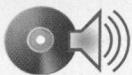 **KEY TERMS** by Topics

Use the audio glossary feature of either the CD-ROM or the Companion Website to hear the correct pronunciation of the following key terms.

Coronary heart disease
atherosclerosis, angina pectoris, acute myocardial infarction (AMI or MI), cardiogenic shock

Rhythm disorders
cardiac dysrhythmia, cardiac arrest, cardioversion

KEY Points

- The coronary arteries provide the "fuel" for the myocardium. These arteries often are affected by atherosclerosis. Narrowing of the vessel affects myocardial blood supply and can lead to angina or myocardial infarction. Early treatment of atherosclerosis and its risk factors is key to preventing coronary heart disease, angina, and acute myocardial infarction.

- Angina is caused by myocardial ischemia, a temporary imbalance between myocardial oxygen supply and demand. Angina often indicates an increasing risk for myocardial infarction.

- Myocardial infarction results from total blockage of the blood supply to a part of the myocardium. Unless blood flow is restored within a few hours, the affected myocardium will infarct and die. This affects function of the heart muscle and cardiac output.

- The cardiac conduction system, which controls the heart's rhythm, can be affected by disease, drugs, or electrolyte imbalances, leading to dysrhythmias. Dysrhythmias may originate in the atria, AV nodal tissue, or the ventricles. Disruption of the conduction pathways can lead to heart blocks.

- Most dysrhythmias are benign, having little effect on function; others are more serious and can lead to excessively slow, fast, or irregular rhythms that affect cardiac output and tissue perfusion. Timely recognition and treatment of these rhythms is vital.

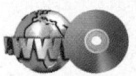 **EXPLORE Media**Link

Additional interactive resources for this chapter can be found on the Companion Website at www.prenhall.com/burke. Click on Chapter 26 and "Begin" to select the activities for this chapter.

For chapter-related NCLEX-style review questions and an audio glossary, access the accompanying CD-ROM in this book.

FOR FURTHER Study

For nursing measures related to pain, see Chapter 8.

For routine preoperative and postoperative care, see Chapter 9.

For further information about cardiogenic shock, see Chapter 13.

Asthma and COPD are discussed in Chapter 24.

See Table 25-1, 25-2, and 25-3 for information on diagnostic tests for coronary heart disease.

Figure 25-4 shows the coronary arteries.

For information on disorders that affect the structure and function of the heart, see Chapter 27.

For more information about fibrinolytic therapy, see Chapter 28.

Caring for a Client after Coronary Artery Bypass Surgery

NCLEX-PN Focus Area: Coping and Adaptation

Case Study: John Clements, 50 years old, had emergency triple bypass surgery 3 days ago. His initial recovery has been uneventful, and he has transferred from the cardiac recovery unit to the cardiac unit for the remainder of his hospital stay.

Nursing Diagnosis: Ineffective Role Performance

COLLECT DATA

Subjective	Objective
_____	_____
_____	_____
_____	_____
_____	_____
_____	_____
_____	_____
_____	_____

Would you report this data? Yes/No

If yes, to: _____

Nursing Care

_____
_____
_____
_____
_____
_____
_____
_____
_____
_____
_____

How would you document this? _____
_____
_____
_____

Data Collected (use those that apply)

- History of progressive angina for 4 years
- Anterior wall myocardial infarction 2 years ago; treated with immediate fibrinolytic therapy and percutaneous balloon angioplasty
- BP 138/72, P 86, regular, R 24, T 99.1°F PO
- Faint crackles left lung base
- Strong family history of CHD (father died age 51, brother died age 48 of myocardial infarctions)
- Does not smoke, uses alcohol occasionally
- Enjoys "good Southern-style cooking" and watching TV; rarely exercises other than dancing with wife and friends about once a month
- Incision clean and dry, healing well
- Color good; O_2 sats 95% on 4 L O_2 per cannula
- Bowel sounds active, taking regular diet in small amounts
- Usually works 50 to 60 hours per week at own contracting business
- States, "I have got to get back to work! You just can't sit around in my business—you have to make sure that the work is getting done on time."

Nursing Interventions (use those that apply; list in priority order)

- Teach about the heart and coronary heart disease; exercise and activities; lifestyle modifications, including diet and stress management.
- Discuss emotional reactions to CHD and sexual activity after discharge.
- Provide analgesics as needed for comfort.
- Ambulate at least four times per day for increasing distances.
- Encourage use of incentive spirometer every 1 to 2 hours.
- Encourage rest before and after activity/exercise.
- Provide information about community resources for emotional support.
- Help identify coping strategies for concerns about role in business.

NCLEX-PN® Exam Preparation

1 The nurse is teaching a client whose physician has prescribed atorvastatin (Lipitor) to be taken daily. Which of the following is vital to include in the teaching?

   A. Report any change in the color of your skin or sclera to your doctor.

   B. Always take this drug with a meal.

   C. Reduce the amount of fat in your diet to less than 20% of your calories.

   D. If your muscles become sore, increase the amount of exercise you do.

2 A client asks the nurse how he can distinguish between angina and chest pain associated with a myocardial infarction. An accurate response by the nurse would be:

   A. "Chest pain associated with myocardial infarction is relieved by nitroglycerin."

   B. "Chest pain associated with angina is unrelieved by nitroglycerin."

   C. "Chest pain associated with angina is relieved by rest."

   D. "Chest pain associated with myocardial infarction is relieved by rest."

3 The nurse caring for a client who has undergone a percutaneous coronary revascularization procedure identifies which of the following as the highest priority nursing diagnosis?

   A. Ineffective Coping as evidenced by poor compliance with diet and exercise regimen

   B. Disturbed Body Image related to presence of a coronary artery stent

   C. Impaired Tissue Integrity related to catheterization of the brachial artery

   D. Risk for Impaired Tissue Perfusion: peripheral related to disruption of the femoral artery

4 A male client has experienced a myocardial infarction. The nurse assesses him for signs of complications. Which of the following would concern the nurse MOST?

   A. B/P 138/84, P 72

   B. B/P 90/50, urinary output 20 mL/hr

   C. P 92, urinary output 50 mL/hr

   D. B/P 150/70, P 100

5 Which of the following would the nurse identify as an expected finding in a client who was admitted for an acute MI 24 hours ago?

   A. CK 240 U/L

   B. Hct 30%

   C. blood glucose 210 mg/dL

   D. BUN 45 mg/dL

6 Teaching for a client with a diagnosis of acute myocardial infarction should include which of the following?

   A. Take nitroglycerin sublingually every 5 minutes until chest pain disappears.

   B. Call 911 immediately if chest pain occurs.

   C. Avoid all stress.

   D. Adjust diet to low cholesterol, low fat, low sodium.

7 A client who is being monitored by telemetry has a rhythm in which all ECG waveforms appear normal and have expected relationships to one another. The heart rate is 104 bpm. The nurse correctly charts this as

   A. normal sinus rhythm.

   B. sinus bradycardia.

   C. sinus tachycardia.

   D. sinus arrhythmia.

8 The nurse observing the central monitor in a progressive coronary unit notes that one of the clients has abruptly developed a rhythm that appears to be ventricular tachycardia. What should the nurse do first?

   A. Initiate a cardiac arrest response (Code 99, Code Blue).

   B. Notify the physician.

   C. Assess the client.

   D. Document the time the dysrhythmia started.

9 In preparing a client who has experienced dysrhythmias for discharge, the nurse should

   A. reassure the client and families that dysrhythmias rarely recur.

   B. encourage the client and family to become trained in cardiopulmonary resuscitation (CPR).

   C. provide resources for obtaining an automatic external defibrillator unit.

   D. stress the low incidence of adverse effects associated with antidysrhythmic drugs.

10 When initiating cardiac monitoring for a client on a progressive cardiac unit, the nurse should (select all that apply):

   A. inform the client of the reason for monitoring.

   B. check equipment, wires, and leads for damage.

   C. apply electrode pads to each shoulder and at the 6th intercostal space, midaxillary line bilaterally.

   D. select electrode sites that are free of irritation or incisions.

   E. discuss reasons for limiting visitors during cardiac monitoring.

Answers for Review Questions, as well as discussion of Care Plan and Critical Thinking Care Map questions, appear in Appendix V.

Chapter 27

Caring for Clients with Cardiac Disorders

BRIEF Outline

Heart Failure
Rheumatic Fever and Rheumatic Heart Disease
Infective Endocarditis
Myocarditis
Pericarditis
Valvular Heart Disease
Cardiomyopathy

LEARNING Outcomes

After completing this chapter, you will be able to:

- Compare and contrast the causes, pathophysiology, effects, and manifestations of common cardiac disorders.
- Identify nursing responsibilities for common diagnostic tests and monitors for clients with heart disease.
- Discuss nursing implications for drugs commonly prescribed for clients with heart disease.
- Describe nursing care for clients undergoing invasive procedures or surgery of the heart.
- Use the nursing process to collect assessment data, contribute to care planning, and provide individualized nursing care for clients with disorders of the heart.
- Provide and reinforce appropriate teaching for clients with heart disorders and their families.

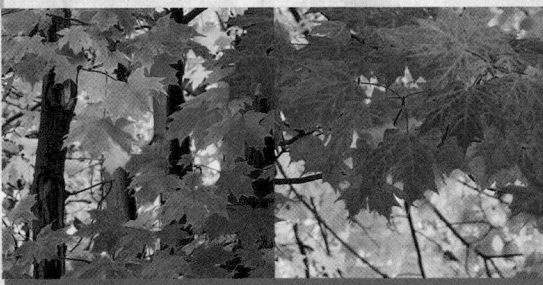

MediaLink

www.prenhall.com/burke
Use the address above to access the free, interactive Companion Website created for this textbook. Get hints, instant feedback, and textbook references to chapter-related NCLEX-style questions. Link to other interesting sites.

Audio Glossary:
Use the Companion Website, or the CD-ROM disk enclosed with your textbook, to hear the pronunciation of key terms in this chapter.

Disorders of the heart muscle or its structures affect its ability to effectively pump blood to meet the needs of the cells of the body. When the heart is unable to function effectively, other organ systems may fail because their fuel supply is impaired. In this chapter, you will learn about heart failure, a common chronic disease with potentially devastating effects, and about other disorders of the heart that can lead to heart failure. In addition, you will learn how to apply the nursing process in caring for clients with heart disease.

DISORDERS OF CARDIAC FUNCTION

Heart Failure

Heart failure is defined as the inability of the heart to function as a pump to meet the needs of the body. Heart failure may result from any condition that (1) impairs effective contraction of the heart muscle, (2) chronically increases the workload of the heart, or (3) acutely increases the workload of the heart (Table 27-1 ■). Hypertension and coronary heart disease with myocardial ischemia and myocardial infarction (MI) are the leading causes of heart failure in the United States.

The incidence of heart failure increases significantly with age; 10% or more of people age 75 or older are affected (Box 27-1 ■). African Americans, who have a high incidence of hypertension, also have a significant risk of developing heart failure. Heart failure generally is a progressive disease, with the client experiencing declining heart function and more frequent episodes of failure. Box 27-2 ■ shows the American Heart Association classification for heart failure.

PATHOPHYSIOLOGY

When the cardiac output drops, *compensatory mechanisms* are activated to maintain blood flow to body tissues. The sympathetic nervous system (SNS) is stimulated. As a result, the heart rate and stroke volume increase. SNS stimulation also causes arteries and veins to constrict, increasing venous return to the heart. Increased venous return increases ventricular filling and myocardial stretch (preload), increasing the force of contraction. Blood flow is redistributed to the brain and the heart to maintain perfusion of these vital organs.

A fall in cardiac output also activates the renin–angiotensin–aldosterone system, which produces additional vasoconstriction and salt and water retention. Salt and water retention increase the blood volume to help restore cardiac output.

The chambers of the heart dilate to accommodate the additional fluid volume. Initially, this leads to more effective contractions. Cardiac muscle cells enlarge, leading to *ventricular hypertrophy.*

Although all of these responses may initially help maintain cardiac output, their long-term effects hasten the deterioration of cardiac function. Heart failure occurs when these mechanisms no longer maintain a cardiac output that meets the metabolic needs of the body.

The rapid heart rate, salt and water retention, increased preload, and arterial vasoconstriction increase the workload of the heart. The ventricles continue to dilate to accommodate the excess fluid, but the heart eventually loses its ability to contract forcefully. The heart muscle may become so large that the coronary blood supply is inadequate, causing myocardial ischemia.

TABLE 27-1
Selected Causes of Heart Failure

IMPAIRED FUNCTION	INCREASED WORKLOAD	NONCARDIAC CONDITIONS
Coronary heart disease	Hypertension	Volume overload
Cardiomyopathies	Valve disorders	Hyperthyroidism
Rheumatic fever	Anemias	Fever, infection
Infective endo-carditis	Congenital heart defects	Pulmonary embolus

BOX 27-1   FOCUS ON OLDER ADULTS

Cardiac Function

Aging affects cardiac function. Ventricular walls become stiffer, affecting filling. The response to exercise and sympathetic stimulation is slowed, and cardiac reserve is reduced. Other health problems (e.g., arthritis) often contribute to a more sedentary lifestyle, further decreasing the heart's ability to respond to stress. Salt intake often increases with aging as taste decreases. Limited mobility or visual acuity may cause the older adult to rely on high-sodium foods like canned soups and frozen meals. Teach older adults how to adapt to changes in cardiovascular function:

- Allow longer warm-up and cooldown periods during exercise.
- Engage in regular exercise such as walking 3 to 4 times a week.
- Rest with feet elevated (e.g., in a recliner) when fatigued.
- Maintain adequate fluid intake.
- Reduce sodium intake by using herbs and other flavorings; read food labels for sodium content.

BOX 27-2

HEART FAILURE CLASSIFICATION
A—High risk for heart failure, but no current structural or functional damage

B—Structural heart disease, but no symptoms of heart failure

C—Structural heart disease with current or prior symptoms of heart failure

D—Advanced heart disease with symptoms of heart failure at rest despite treatment

In normal hearts, the **cardiac reserve** allows the heart to adjust its output to meet the metabolic needs of the body. Clients with heart failure have very little cardiac reserve. At rest, they may be unaffected; however, any stressor (e.g., exercise, illness) taxes their ability to meet the demand for oxygen and nutrients.

Heart failure is often classified by the primary pumping chamber affected. Clients may have manifestations of *left-sided* and/or *right-sided failure.* The effects of heart failure on cardiac output and venous congestion are referred to as *forward* and *backward effects.* Heart failure also may be classified as either *acute* or *chronic.* Finally, when heart failure results from acute excessive demands placed on the heart, such as fluid overload, hyperthyroidism, or fever, it may be referred to as *high-output failure.*

Left-Sided Heart Failure
Although either side of the heart can fail, the left ventricle is affected more often than the right because of its high workload and oxygen demand. Left-sided heart failure results from ventricular muscle damage or overloading. As left ventricular function deteriorates, cardiac output falls (*forward effect*). Impaired emptying of the left ventricle leads to increased pressures on the left side of the heart and in the pulmonary vascular system (*backward effects*). Increased pressures in this normally low-pressure system push fluid from the blood vessels into interstitial tissues and the alveoli (Figure 27-1 ■).

The manifestations of left-sided heart failure result from pulmonary congestion and decreased cardiac output (Box 27-3 ■). Fatigue, activity intolerance, and dyspnea on exertion (DOE) are common early manifestations. **Orthopnea** (breathing difficulty while lying down) may prompt the client to sleep propped up on two or three pillows or in a recliner. Inspiratory crackles (rales) and wheezes may be heard in lung bases.

ACUTE PULMONARY EDEMA. **Acute pulmonary edema,** accumulation of fluid in the interstitial spaces and alveoli of the lungs, may occur with severe left-ventricular failure. The client in pulmonary edema has acute and severe dyspnea,

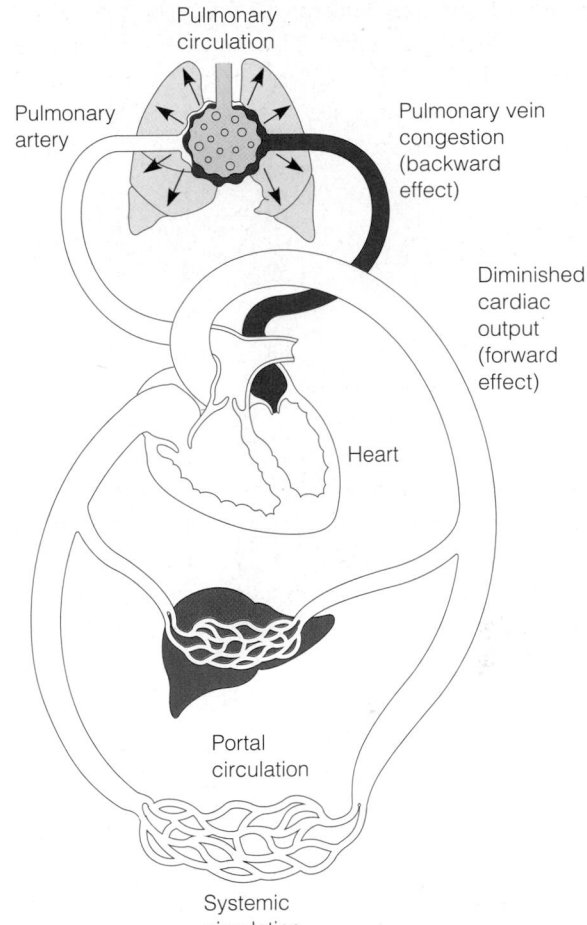

Figure 27-1. ■ The forward and backward effects of left-sided heart failure.

shortness of breath, and anxiety. The skin is cool, clammy, and cyanotic. A productive cough with pink, frothy sputum is also present. If cerebral hypoxia occurs, the client may be confused or lethargic. Crackles are heard throughout the

BOX 27-3

MANIFESTATIONS OF HEART FAILURE

Left-Sided	Right-Sided
Forward Effects	*Forward Effects*
Activity intolerance	Fatigue
Fatigue	Activity intolerance
Weakness	
Dizziness and syncope	
Backward Effects	*Backward Effects*
Shortness of breath	Jugular vein distention
Dyspnea, orthopnea	Peripheral edema
Cough	Anorexia, nausea
Tachycardia	Abdominal distention, ascites
Crackles in lung bases	Liver, spleen enlargement, tenderness

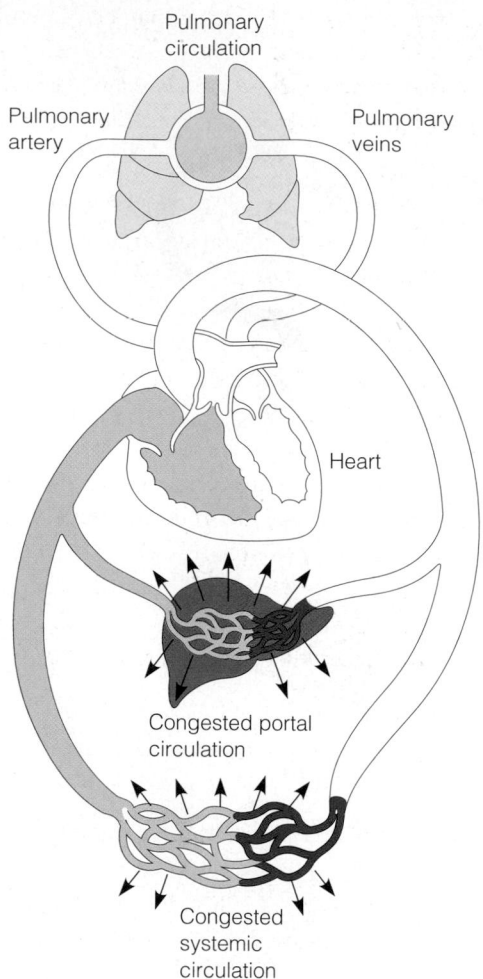

Figure 27-2. ■ The effects of right-sided heart failure.

lung fields. As the condition worsens, breathing becomes more labored and lung sounds harsher. Pulmonary edema is a medical emergency: The client is "drowning" as a result of fluid in the alveolar and pulmonary spaces and must be treated immediately.

Right-Sided Heart Failure

The most common cause of right ventricular failure is left ventricular failure. Increased pressures in the pulmonary system or damage to the right ventricle impair blood flow into the pulmonary circulation. The right ventricle and atrium become distended, and blood accumulates in the systemic venous system. Increased venous pressures lead to abdominal organ congestion and peripheral tissue edema (Figure 27-2 ■).

Fluid collects in dependent tissues because of the effects of gravity. Edema develops in the feet and legs of an upright client and in the sacrum of one who is reclining. Congestion of vessels in the abdomen can lead to right upper quadrant pain, anorexia, and nausea. Distended jugular veins may be visible even when the client is standing (see Box 27-3).

Biventricular Failure

When both ventricles fail to function adequately, the client has manifestations of both right- and left-sided or *biventricular* heart failure. **Paroxysmal nocturnal dyspnea (PND),** a frightening condition in which the client awakens at night acutely short of breath, may occur. PND occurs when edema fluid that has accumulated during the day is reabsorbed into the circulation at night, causing fluid overload and pulmonary congestion. The client in severe heart failure may be dyspneic at rest as well as with activity, signifying little or no cardiac reserve.

Acute and Chronic Failure

Acute heart failure occurs as a result of acute damage to the heart muscle, for example, resulting from a large acute myocardial infarction. *Chronic heart failure,* in contrast, develops gradually as the result of a long-standing or progressive condition such as hypertension or valve disease.

INTERDISCIPLINARY CARE

The main goals of care for the client with heart failure are to reduce cardiac workload, improve cardiac pumping ability, and control fluid retention. The focus is on improving activity tolerance and decreasing mortality and morbidity.

Diagnostic Tests

Diagnostic tests are used to diagnose heart failure and evaluate its effects. Cardiac hormones, atrial natriuretic factor and B-type natriuretic peptide, are released from the heart muscle and are involved in fluid regulation. Their blood levels increase in heart failure but do not change in other cardiac disorders, making them valuable indicators of heart failure. *Serum electrolytes* are measured to evaluate fluid and electrolyte status, as well as the effects of treatment. The *chest x-ray* may show pulmonary vascular congestion and cardiomegaly if the heart has hypertrophied or dilated. An *echocardiogram* is done to evaluate left ventricular function and assess for ventricular dilation and hypertrophy. The *ECG* shows changes associated with ventricular enlargement, and may show dysrhythmias, myocardial ischemia, or infarction.

Hemodynamic Monitoring

Hemodynamic monitoring may be used to assess cardiovascular function and the client's response to treatment. A multilumen catheter inserted through a central vein into the right side of the heart and pulmonary artery is used to measure central venous pressure, pulmonary artery pressures, and cardiac output. These pressures and the cardiac output are used to evaluate fluid balance, ventricular function, and the effects of interventions (e.g., drug therapy). The arterial blood pressure can be measured using a peripheral arterial line.

The pressure within a vessel is converted into an electrical signal. The electrical signal is then recorded on graph paper

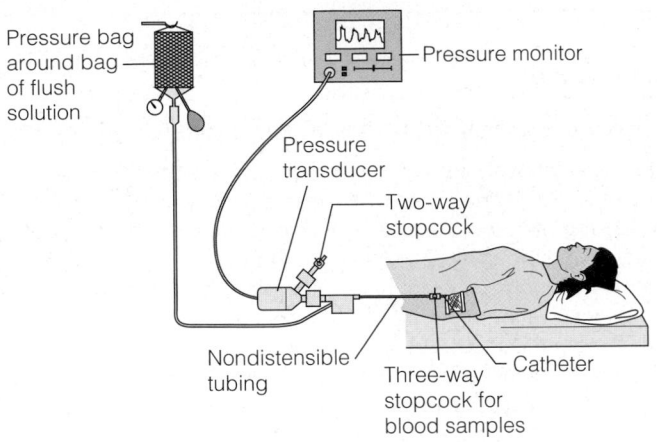

Figure 27-3. ■ A hemodynamic monitoring setup.

and displayed on a monitor (Figure 27-3 ■). Although hemodynamic monitoring provides valuable information to help manage heart failure, it has some risks. The presence of an invasive catheter increases the risk of infection, bleeding,

and thrombus formation. The lung may be punctured during insertion of the catheter into the subclavian vein, causing a pneumothorax. Dysrhythmias may develop as the catheter passes through the right ventricle.

Pharmacology

Clients with heart failure typically receive multiple medications to reduce cardiac work and improve cardiac function. The main drug classes used to treat heart failure are the angiotensin-converting enzyme (ACE) inhibitors, diuretics, **inotropic** medications (drugs that increase the strength of the heart's contractions), and direct vasodilators (Table 27-2 ■). Complementary treatment with hawthorn is discussed in Box 27-4 ■.

Morphine sulfate is a drug of choice for treating acute pulmonary edema. Morphine relieves anxiety, improves breathing, and also is a venous vasodilator. It reduces venous return and lowers left atrial pressure. Potent loop diuretics such as furosemide (Lasix) or bumetanide are administered intravenously to promote rapid diuresis.

TABLE 27-2

Nursing Implications For Pharmacology: Heart Failure

CLASS/DRUGS	PURPOSE	NURSING RESPONSIBILITIES	CLIENT TEACHING
Angiotensin-Converting Enzyme (ACE) Inhibitors ■ Enalapril maleate (Vasotec) ■ Lisinopril (Prinivil, Zestril) ■ Captopril (Capoten) ■ Moexipril (Univasc) ■ Ramipril (Altace) ■ Fosinopril (Monopril) ■ Quinapril (Accupril) ■ Trandolapril (Mavik)	ACE inhibitors block the effect of the renin–angiotensin–aldosterone system, reducing vasoconstriction and sodium and water retention. The result is decreased cardiac workload and reduced edema.	Avoid discontinuing these agents abruptly. Give captopril 1 hour before meals. Maintain bed rest and monitor BP for 3 hours following the initial dose because significant hypotension can develop. Monitor serum potassium levels during treatment because hyperkalemia may develop.	Do not stop taking your drugs without talking to your doctor. Keep follow-up medical appointments. Avoid sudden position changes; for example, rise from bed slowly. Report easy bruising and bleeding, sore throat, or fever, weight gain of 2 lbs or more per day, edema, dizziness, or skin rash. Immediately report swelling of the face, lips, or eyelids, itching, or breathing problems.
Diuretics ■ Hydrochlorothiazide (HydroDIURIL) ■ Chlorothiazide (Diuril) ■ Furosemide (Lasix) ■ Ethacrynic acid (Edecrin) ■ Bumetanide (Bumex) ■ Spironolactone (Aldactone) ■ Triamterene (Dyrenium) ■ Amiloride (Midamor) ■ Acetazolamide (Diamox)	Diuretics act on different portions of the kidney tubule to promote sodium and water excretion. With the exception of the potassium-sparing diuretics—spironolactone, triamterene, and amiloride—diuretics also promote potassium excretion, increasing the risk of hypokalemia.	Monitor fluid volume status: BP, intake and output, weight, skin turgor, edema. Assess for volume depletion, particularly with loop diuretics (furosemide, ethacrynic acid, and bumetanide): dizziness, orthostatic hypotension, tachycardia, muscle cramping. Notify the charge nurse or physician of abnormal serum electrolyte values.	Report abdominal pain, jaundice, dark urine, abnormal bleeding or bruising, flulike symptoms, signs of electrolyte imbalance, or dehydration (Chapter 7) 🔗 to your doctor. Monitor your blood pressure, pulse, and weight daily. Report changes in your weight of 2 lbs or more per day. Avoid making sudden position changes. You may feel dizzy, light-headed, or faint.

(continued)

TABLE 27-2

Nursing Implications For Pharmacology: Heart Failure (continued)

CLASS/DRUGS	PURPOSE	NURSING RESPONSIBILITIES	CLIENT TEACHING
		Administer intravenous furosemide slowly, no more than 20 mg/min. Notify the physician if the client is on an aminoglycoside antibiotic. When given concurrently with furosemide or ethacrynic acid, there is an increased risk of ototoxicity and hearing loss.	Drink at least 6 to 8 glasses of water per day. Take your diuretic when it will be the least disruptive to your lifestyle. Take with meals to decrease GI symptoms. Unless you are taking a potassium-sparing diuretic, increase intake of potassium-rich foods. Limit salt intake.
Positive Inotropic Agents *Digitalis Glycosides* ■ Digoxin (Lanoxin)	Improve myocardial contractility, increasing stroke volume and cardiac output. Greater cardiac output improves renal perfusion, decreasing renin secretion and cardiac work. Slow heart rate and reduce oxygen consumption.	Assess apical pulse before giving digitalis. Hold the drug and notify the physician if HR < 60 bpm. Record HR on medication record. Assess serum electrolytes and digoxin levels. Hypokalemia increases the risk of digitalis toxicity. Report manifestations of digitalis toxicity: anorexia, nausea, vomiting, abdominal pain, weakness, vision changes (diplopia, blurred vision, halos seen around objects), and dysrhythmias.	Take your pulse before each dose. Do not take the digitalis if your pulse is <60. Notify your doctor immediately. Call your doctor if you develop palpitations, weakness, loss of appetite, nausea, vomiting, abdominal pain, blurred or colored vision, double vision. Avoid antacids and laxatives; they decrease the absorption of digoxin. Include high-potassium foods in your diet: orange or tomato juice, bananas, raisins, dates, figs, prunes, apricots, spinach, cauliflower, and potatoes.
Sympathomimetic Agents ■ Dopamine (Inotropin) ■ Dobutamine (Dobutrex) **Phosphodiesterase Inhibitors** ■ Amrinone (Inocor) ■ Milrinone (Primacor)	These drugs improve the force of ventricular contraction. Sympathomimetic drugs are given intravenously, adjusting the dose to obtain maximal effect. Phosphodiesterase inhibitors also cause vasodilation, reducing cardiac workload.	Use an infusion pump to administer these drugs. Frequently monitor vital signs and hemodynamic measurements. Titrate the drug to maintain the BP and heart rate. Avoid discontinuing these agents abruptly. Change solutions and tubing every 24 hours.	Notify the nursing staff if you experience abdominal pain or notice a skin rash or bruising.

BOX 27-4 COMPLEMENTARY THERAPIES

Heart Failure

The dried fruit of the hawthorn (also known as English hawthorn, maybush, or whitethorn) or a tincture or liquid extract of the fruit or leaf may benefit the client with heart failure. Hawthorn increases coronary blood flow and has positive inotropic effects. Therapeutically, it increases cardiac output; decreases the blood pressure, cardiac workload, and oxygen consumption; and acts like an ACE inhibitor. Advise clients to consult their health care provider before taking hawthorn or using it in conjunction with prescribed drugs.

DIGITALIS. Digitalis has a positive inotropic effect on the heart, increasing the strength of myocardial contraction. Digitalis has a *narrow therapeutic index;* in other words, therapeutic levels are very close to toxic levels. Early manifestations of digitalis toxicity include anorexia, nausea and vomiting, headache, alterations in vision, and confusion. A number of dysrhythmias are also associated with digitalis toxicity. Low serum potassium levels increase the risk of digitalis toxicity, as do low magnesium and high calcium levels. Older adults are at particular risk for digitalis toxicity.

Diet and Activity

Clients in heart failure are generally put on a restricted sodium diet to minimize sodium and water retention. An intake of 1.5 to 2 g of sodium per day, a moderate restriction, is recommended. Activity may be limited to bed rest during acute episodes of heart failure to reduce cardiac workload and allow the heart to recompensate. Activity is gradually increased as the client's condition improves and is encouraged to tolerance to improve cardiovascular performance.

Surgery

Heart transplant is the primary treatment for end-stage heart failure. In most cases, the client's diseased heart is removed, leaving portions of the atria intact. The donor heart is sutured to the remaining atrial walls (Figure 27-4 ■). In a "piggyback transplant," the client's heart is left in place and the donor heart is sutured to it. The client then has two functioning hearts, although most of the work is performed by the donor heart. Although cardiac transplantation benefits many clients with end-stage heart disease, it is limited by the availability of donor hearts. Transplanted organs typically are obtained from young accident victims with no evidence of cardiac trauma. Ventricular assist devices are often used as a bridge to transplantation. Mechanical heart transplants are in development.

Nursing care of the heart transplant client is similar to the care of any cardiac surgery client. Infection and rejection are major postoperative concerns. Immunosuppressive drugs are given to prevent rejection of the transplanted organ (see Chapter 11). ⚭ Although immunosuppressive drugs help prevent rejection, they also leave the client with impaired defenses against infection. Rejection of the transplanted heart can occur at any time. Acute rejection is the most common type, and is a leading cause of death within the first year after surgery. Because immunosuppressive drugs may mask symptoms of rejection, clients are routinely monitored with tissue biopsies of the transplanted organ.

Another surgical procedure, *dynamic cardiomyoplasty,* involves wrapping a skeletal muscle graft around the heart to lend support to the failing myocardium. This procedure, however, has not been shown to improve either survival or quality of life.

NURSING CARE

Heart failure impacts quality of life, interfering with such day-to-day activities as self-care and role performance. Reducing the oxygen demand of the heart is a major nursing care goal. This includes providing both physical and psychologic rest, as well as administering and monitoring multiple drugs to reduce cardiac work, improve contractility, and manage symptoms.

ASSESSING

Clients with heart failure require frequent and careful nursing assessment. Box 27-5 ■ outlines assessment data to be collected by the nurse.

DIAGNOSING, PLANNING, AND IMPLEMENTING

Priorities in Nursing Care. The client experiencing acute heart failure may be critically ill because the heart is unable to meet the needs of the cells for blood and oxygen. As the heart becomes less effective as a pump, vessels and tissues become congested with fluid. Congestion of the pulmonary circulation can impair gas exchange, compounding the client's condition. Decreased Cardiac Output and Fluid

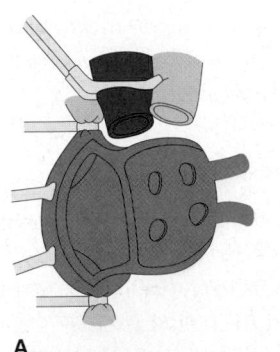
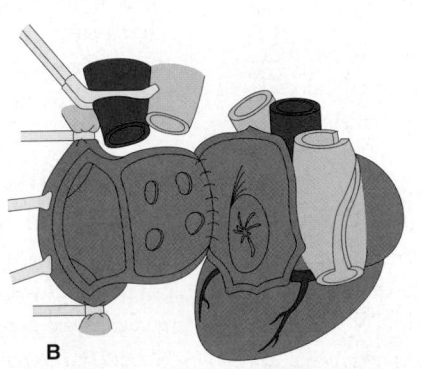
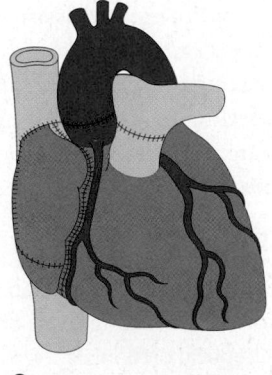

A   **B**   **C**

Figure 27-4. ■ Cardiac transplantation. **(A)** The heart is removed, leaving the posterior walls of the atria intact. The donor heart is sutured to the atria **(B)** and the great vessels **(C)**.

BOX 27-5	ASSESSMENT

Assessing Clients with Heart Failure

SUBJECTIVE DATA

- Shortness of breath, level of activity, number of pillows used to sleep; swelling of legs and feet; weight changes; appetite, nausea, abdominal discomfort
- History of MI or other heart disease, recent stressors such as upper respiratory infection; previous or current treatment; current medications
- Risk factors: family history of heart disease; history of hypertension, diabetes, high blood cholesterol levels; smoking and alcohol intake
- Understanding of disease and treatment, compliance with activity prescriptions; current diet and use of salt

OBJECTIVE DATA

- Vital signs at rest and changes with activity; cardiac rhythm; any dysrhythmias

- Dyspnea and its relationship to activity; oxygen saturation levels
- Skin color, temperature, and moisture; capillary refill; extent and degree of dependent edema; presence of neck vein distention
- Heart and lung sounds; presence of S_3 or S_4 heart sounds; presence and extent of crackles or wheezes on auscultation of lungs
- Intake and output; daily weight
- Level of consciousness; anxiety or fear
- Central venous pressure, pulmonary artery pressure, or cardiac output as ordered
- Cardiac rhythm, dysrhythmias
- Laboratory test results: atrial natriuretic factor (ANF) and B-type natriuretic peptide (BNP) levels; serum electrolytes; serum drug levels (e.g., digitalis levels); arterial blood gases (ABGs)

Volume Excess are the highest priority nursing diagnoses for the client in acute failure.

Decreased Cardiac Output

- Auscultate heart and breath sounds regularly. *An S_3 or an S_4 may be heard in heart failure. Crackles are often heard in the lung bases; increasing crackles, dyspnea, and shortness of breath indicate worsening failure.*
- Report manifestations of decreased cardiac output: changes in mental status; decreased urine output; cool, clammy skin; tachycardia, diminished pulses; pallor or cyanosis; dysrhythmias. *These are manifestations of decreased tissue perfusion.*
- Administer oxygen as needed. *This improves oxygenation of the blood, decreasing the effects of hypoxia and ischemia.*
- Administer medications as ordered. *Drugs are used to decrease the cardiac workload and increase the effectiveness of contractions.*
- Encourage rest, explaining its purpose. Keep the head of the bed elevated to reduce the work of breathing. Provide a bedside commode, and assist with personal needs. *These measures reduce cardiac workload.*
- Maintain a quiet environment, allow the client to express fears and feelings, and explain the reasons for medical and nursing care. *These measures reduce anxiety and decrease oxygen consumption.*

Excess Fluid Volume

- Immediately notify the physician if the client develops air hunger, an overwhelming sense of impending doom or panic, tachypnea, orthopnea, or a cough productive of pink, frothy sputum. *Acute pulmonary edema, a medical emergency, can develop rapidly, requiring immediate intervention to preserve life.*
- Monitor intake and output. Notify the physician if urine output drops to less than 30 mL/hr. *Intake and output*

records help evaluate the effectiveness of treatment. A drop in urine output may indicate reduced cardiac output.

- Weigh daily. *Weight is an accurate measure of fluid status; 1 liter of fluid is equal to 1 kg or 2.2 lbs of weight.*
- Place in Fowler's or high Fowler's position, with the head of bed elevated to 45 degrees. *Elevating the head of the bed reduces venous return to the heart, decreasing its work. It also improves lung expansion.*
- Report decreased urine output, vital sign changes, distended neck veins, peripheral edema, weight gain, increased dyspnea, or dysrhythmias to the charge nurse or physician. *These may indicate progressive worsening of the client's condition.*
- Administer diuretics and other medications as ordered. *Diuretics increase sodium and water excretion.*
- Restrict fluids as ordered. Encourage the client to help choose the time and type of fluid consumed. Schedule the majority of intake during the morning and afternoon. Offer ice chips and frequent mouth care; provide hard candies if allowed. *Involving the client increases the sense of control. Ice chips, hard candies, and mouth care relieve dry mouth and thirst and promote comfort.*

Activity Intolerance

- Assess vital signs and heart rhythm before and after activity. *Tachycardia, dysrhythmias, changes in blood pressure, diaphoresis, pallor, or complaints of increasing dyspnea, chest pain, excessive fatigue, or palpitations indicate activity intolerance. Instruct to rest if these manifestations are noted.*
- Organize nursing care to allow for rest periods. *Grouping care activities as much as possible allows adequate time to "recharge."*

- Assist as needed with self-care. Encourage independent performance of activities of daily living (ADLs) within prescribed limits. *Assisting with ADLs helps meet care needs while reducing the cardiac workload. Involving the client promotes a sense of control and reduces helplessness.*
- Plan and implement progressive activity plan. Employ passive and active range-of-motion (ROM) exercises as appropriate. Consult with physical therapist on activity plan. *Progressive activity slowly increases exercise capacity by strengthening and improving cardiac function without strain. Progressive activity also helps prevent skeletal muscle atrophy. ROM exercises prevent complications of immobility in bedridden or severely compromised clients.*
- Encourage small, frequent meals rather than three heavy meals per day. *Small, frequent meals provide continuing energy resources and decrease the work required to digest a large meal.*

EVALUATING

Collect data such as the following to evaluate the effectiveness of nursing care:

- Vital signs, urine output, and degree of dyspnea at rest and during activity
- Presence or absence of abnormal heart or lung sounds and edema
- Ability to tolerate gradually increased activity levels.

Documenting. Document assessment findings, noting any changes that occur with activity. Record treatment measures implemented and the client's response to treatment. Include subjective data such as statements of improved ease of breathing in documentation. Note referrals made (e.g., to a dietitian) and teaching provided, as well as the client's apparent understanding and acceptance of instruction.

CONTINUING CARE

The chronic and progressive nature of heart failure requires that the client and family actively participate in managing the disease. When planning for discharge care, carefully assess the client's and family's understanding of heart failure, prescribed medications, diet and activities, and symptoms to report to physician. Explain heart failure and its effects on the client's life. This helps the client understand the reasons for ordered treatments. Discuss the warning signs of impending failure and when to contact the physician. Teach about prescribed drugs and their potential adverse effects. Stress the importance of the medications in managing heart failure. Provide verbal and written information regarding each specific medication to encourage compliance. Instruct to keep regular follow-up appointments to monitor disease progression and the effects of therapy.

Lifestyle changes are important, although they may be the most difficult to achieve. Teach the client and family about the prescribed diet. Give practical suggestions for reducing salt intake. The American Heart Association (AHA) has written materials and recipes that may make adjusting to a low-sodium diet easier to tolerate. Refer to a dietitian for further teaching and diet planning as needed. Discuss the importance of family support for dietary restrictions and avoiding exposure to cigarette smoke.

Encourage exercise within prescribed limits to strengthen the heart muscle and improve aerobic capacity. Box 27-6 ■ provides activity guidelines for clients with heart failure.

Provide referrals to a home health agency and community agencies, such as local cardiac rehabilitation programs, heart support groups, or the AHA, as needed for further nursing evaluation and care, education, and psychosocial support.

BOX 27-6	CLIENT TEACHING

Activity Guidelines for Clients with Heart Failure

- Perform as many activities as independently as you can.
- Space meals and activities. Eat six small meals a day. Allow rest periods during the day.
- Perform all activities at a comfortable pace; rest for 15 minutes if you get tired.
- Stop any activity that causes chest pain, shortness of breath, dizziness, excessive weakness, or sweating. Rest. Notify your doctor if your activity tolerance changes and if symptoms continue after rest.
- Avoid straining. Do not lift heavy objects. Eat a high-fiber diet and drink plenty of water to prevent constipation. Use bulk-forming laxatives or stool softeners, as allowed, to avoid constipation and straining.
- Begin a graded exercise program. Walking is good exercise. Plan to walk twice a day at a comfortable, slow pace for the first couple of weeks, and then gradually increase the distance and pace. Below is a suggested schedule:

Week 1	200 to 400 yards (1/4 mile)	Twice a day, slow leisurely pace
Week 2	¼ mile	15 min, minimum of 3 times per week
Week 3	½ mile	30 min, minimum of 3 times per week
Week 4	1 mile	30 min, minimum of 3 times per week
Week 5	1½ mile	30 min, minimum of 3 times per week
Week 6	2 miles	40 min, minimum of 3 times per week

NURSING PROCESS CARE PLAN
Client with Heart Failure

One year ago, Arthur Jackson, 67 years old, had an anterior MI followed by coronary artery bypass surgery. On discharge, he was started on digoxin, furosemide, Coumadin, and a potassium chloride supplement. He has now been admitted to the medical intensive care unit (MICU) after developing severe shortness of breath, a productive cough, and no appetite for 1 week. He is diagnosed with heart failure.

Assessment. On entering his room, Mr. Jackson's nurse, Myumi Takashi, notices that he is sitting in the bedside recliner in high Fowler's position. He says, "Lately, this is the only way I feel fairly comfortable." He states that he gets short of breath working in his garden and complains of his shoes and belt being too tight. On questioning, Mr. Jackson insists that he takes his medications regularly. He admits to a fondness for bacon and Chinese food and sheepishly says he snacks between meals "even though I need to lose weight."

Mr. Jackson's vital signs are BP 95/72 mm Hg; AP 124, irregular; R 28 and labored; and T 97.5°F (36.5°C). The ECG shows atrial fibrillation. An S_3 is heard on auscultation. He has crackles and diminished breath sounds in the bases of both lungs. Neck veins distended, 3+ pitting edema of ankles and feet, and abdominal distention are noted. Skin is cool and diaphoretic. Chest x-ray shows cardiomegaly and pulmonary infiltrates.

Diagnosis. Ms. Takashi identifies the following nursing diagnoses for Mr. Jackson:

- *Excess Fluid Volume* related to impaired cardiac pump and salt and water retention
- *Activity Intolerance* related to imbalance between oxygen supply and demand
- *Deficient Knowledge* regarding diet and fluid restrictions

Expected Outcomes. The expected outcomes specify that Mr. Jackson will:

- Demonstrate weight loss, and decreased edema, jugular venous distention, and abdominal distention.
- Achieve improved activity tolerance.
- Verbalize understanding of diet and fluid restrictions.

Planning and Implementation. Ms. Takashi plans and implements the following interventions for Mr. Jackson:

- Take hourly vital signs until stable.
- Weigh daily. Record intake and output (I&O).
- Restrict fluids to 1,500 mL/24 hr (as ordered by physician); 600 mL day shift, 600 mL evenings, 300 mL at night.
- Auscultate breath and heart sounds every 4 hours and as necessary.
- Monitor oxygen saturation levels. Notify physician if below 94%.
- Place in high Fowler's position to maintain comfort.
- Teach about all medications and how to take and record his pulse daily.
- Design an activity plan that incorporates preferred activities and scheduled rest periods throughout the day.
- Instruct on a sodium-restricted diet. Allow choices for meals within allowed limits.
- Consult dietitian to assist Mr. and Mrs. Jackson in planning a low-sodium diet.

Evaluation. Mr. Jackson is transferred to the medical unit after 2 days in MICU. He has lost 8 lbs. His respirations are unlabored at rest, and his edema is significantly reduced. He is able to sleep in low Fowler's with only one pillow. The dietitian is helping Mr. and Mrs. Jackson develop a realistic eating plan to limit sodium, sugar, and fats. Mr. Jackson is relieved to know that he can still enjoy Chinese food that is prepared without monosodium glutamate (MSG) or added salt. The physical therapist has designed a progressive activity plan with Mr. Jackson for both in-hospital and at-home activity. Mr. Jackson's knowledge about his medications is assessed and reinforced. Mr. Jackson is discharged 5 days after his admission.

Critical Thinking in the Nursing Process

1. Design an exercise plan for Mr. Jackson to follow after discharge.
2. Mr. Jackson tells you, "Talk to my wife about my medications—she's Tarzan and I'm Jane now." How would you respond?
3. Nine months later, Mr. Jackson is admitted to the hospital complaining of abdominal pain and weakness. Blood work shows his serum potassium level to be 2.4 mEq/dL. What subjective information will you gather to help determine what has led to this problem?

INFLAMMATORY CARDIAC DISORDERS

Any layer of the heart—the endocardium, myocardium, or pericardium—can become inflamed, damaging the heart valves, heart muscle, or pericardium. Manifestations of inflammation may range from very mild to life threatening. This section discusses rheumatic heart disease, endocarditis, myocarditis, and pericarditis.

Rheumatic Fever and Rheumatic Heart Disease

Rheumatic fever is a systemic inflammatory disease caused by an abnormal immune response to infection by group A beta-hemolytic streptococci (usually streptococcal pharyngitis or strep throat). While children between ages 5 and 15 have the highest incidence, rheumatic fever may affect people of any age. Rheumatic fever can damage the heart valves, and often leads to mitral and aortic valve disorders (discussed in the next section of this chapter).

PATHOPHYSIOLOGY

Rheumatic fever results from an abnormal immune response to the *Streptococcus* bacterium or its toxins. Antibodies produced to attack the invading bacteria (the antigen) appear to also attack connective tissues of the heart, blood vessels, joints, and subcutaneous tissues, initiating an inflammatory response.

Any layer of the heart may be affected in acute rheumatic fever; usually all three are involved. The valves become red and swollen, and small inflammatory lesions develop on the leaflets. As the inflammation resolves, scarring occurs, causing deformity. Myocarditis and pericarditis associated with rheumatic fever are generally mild and have no long-term effects.

Rheumatic heart disease (RHD) is slowly progressive valve deformity that can occur following acute or repeated attacks of rheumatic fever. Valve leaflets become rigid and deformed, resulting in stenosis or regurgitation of the valve. In **stenosis,** the valve leaflets fuse, obstructing forward blood flow. In **regurgitation,** the valve fails to close properly, allowing blood to flow back through it. Valves on the left side of the heart, the mitral valve in particular, are most often affected.

Manifestations

Manifestations of rheumatic fever typically follow the initial streptococcal infection by about 2 to 3 weeks (Box 27-7 ■). About 50% of clients with rheumatic fever develop some form of rheumatic heart disease.

INTERDISCIPLINARY CARE

The diagnosis of rheumatic fever is based on the client's history and physical examination. Laboratory testing helps establish the diagnosis.

- The *WBC count* is elevated, as is the *erythrocyte sedimentation rate (ESR)*, a general indicator of inflammation.
- A positive *C-reactive protein (CRP)* indicates active inflammation.
- The *antistreptolysin-O (ASO)* titer is a streptococcal antibody test that rises within 2 months of the disease's onset and is found in most clients with rheumatic fever.
- In severe carditis associated with rheumatic fever, the *cardiac enzymes* are elevated.

In addition to laboratory testing, an *echocardiogram* is done to evaluate the structures (including valves) and function of the heart.

Management of rheumatic heart disease focuses on treating the primary infection, managing its manifestations, and preventing complications and recurrences of the disease. In clients with acute carditis, treatment focuses on decreasing myocardial work. Although bed rest is not necessary, activity is limited during the acute phase, then gradually increased after about 4 to 5 weeks.

Antibiotics are prescribed to eliminate the streptococcal infection. Joint pain and fever are treated with aspirin, ibuprofen, or another nonsteroidal anti-inflammatory drug (NSAID); corticosteroids may be used for severe pain.

NURSING CARE

Nurses have a significant role in identifying clients at risk for rheumatic heart disease and teaching for primary prevention. Identify risk factors for streptococcal infections. These include crowded living conditions, poor nutrition, immunodeficiency, and poor access to health care.

ASSESSING

Ask about recent sore throat or "strep throat" and treatment. Other subjective data include complaints of chest pain, shortness of breath, fatigue, weakness, fever, or joint pain. Obtain objective data such as heart rate and heart sounds, respiratory rate, and ease of breathing.

BOX 27-7

MANIFESTATIONS OF RHEUMATIC FEVER

- Fever
- Migratory joint pain and inflammation
- Rash on trunk and proximal extremities
- Chest pain or discomfort
- Tachycardia, shortness of breath
- Cardiac friction rub, S_3, S_4, possible murmur
- Involuntary muscle spasms, difficulty concentrating

---

clinical ALERT

Auscultate heart sounds every shift and as necessary. Notify the physician if a pericardial friction rub or a new murmur appears. A friction rub may be produced by an inflamed pericardium; it also causes chest pain and discomfort. A change in heart sounds, a newly developed heart murmur in particular, may indicate further valve damage and a risk for complications such as clot formation and embolization or heart failure.

Observe for joint redness, swelling, or heat, and the presence of a rash on trunk or extremities. Note mental status and any abnormal muscle movements. Monitor the results of laboratory and other diagnostic tests, reporting significant changes to the charge nurse or physician.

DIAGNOSING, PLANNING, AND IMPLEMENTING

Priorities in Nursing Care. Nursing care for clients with rheumatic fever and carditis generally is supportive, with a focus on teaching for self-care and preventing complications. Pain and Activity Intolerance are the highest priority nursing diagnoses.

Pain

- Report increased chest pain to the charge nurse or physician. *Increased chest pain may indicate development of pericarditis or increased carditis.*
- Administer anti-inflammatory drugs as ordered. Give aspirin and other NSAIDs with food, milk, or antacids to minimize gastric irritation. Report tinnitus (a symptom of aspirin toxicity), vomiting, or GI bleeding. *Anti-inflammatory drugs are given to control inflammation. The dose of aspirin and NSAIDs may be high, and the drugs are given around the clock rather than as needed.*
- Provide warm, moist compresses for local pain relief. *Direct application of moist heat may help relieve the pain associated with inflamed joints.*

Activity Intolerance

- Explain the importance of activity limitations. Instruct to avoid or stop any activity that causes dyspnea or shortness of breath. *Activities are limited for 4 to 6 weeks to decrease the stress on the heart.*
- Encourage visits from friends and family members and diversional activities, such as reading, playing games, watching television, listening to the radio or favorite music cassettes, and so on. *Diversionary activities help reduce boredom when activity is limited.*
- Monitor activity tolerance (vital signs, fatigue, shortness of breath) as activity is gradually increased. *The client may require bed rest or limited activity for a longer period of time to allow carditis to resolve and prevent permanent heart damage.*

EVALUATING

To evaluate the effectiveness of nursing care, collect data such as the client's reports of pain and discomfort, vital signs at rest and with activity, and response to increasing activity levels.

Documenting. Document and notify the physician of any new symptoms or changes in heart or breath sounds. Note the client's response to activity, as well as teaching about the disorder, activity restrictions, and continuing care.

CONTINUING CARE

Rheumatic fever is preventable. Prompt treatment of streptococcal throat infections helps decrease the spread of this pathogen and the risk of rheumatic fever. Manifestations of strep throat include a red, fiery-looking throat, pain on swallowing, enlarged and tender cervical lymph nodes, fever in the range of 101 to 104°F (38.3 to 40.0°C), and headache. Emphasize the importance of finishing the complete course of prescribed antibiotics to eradicate the pathogen.

To prevent recurrence of rheumatic fever, emphasize the importance of continuing antibiotic prophylaxis as ordered. Teach the client with chronic RHD about the importance of antibiotic prophylaxis for any invasive procedure (e.g., dental care, endoscopy, or surgery) to prevent bacterial endocarditis. Preventive dental care and good oral hygiene help discourage gingival infections and are important.

clinical ALERT

The client with chronic RHD is at significant risk for developing infective endocarditis (see the next section of this chapter). Discuss and provide written information about the signs and symptoms of infective endocarditis, and stress the importance of notifying the primary care physician if symptoms develop.

Instruct the client with rheumatic carditis to limit salt intake to reduce the workload of the heart. A high-carbohydrate, high-protein diet is usually recommended to promote healing and to combat weakness and fatigue. Teach the early manifestations of heart failure. Provide instructions about prescribed medications, including dosage, signs of adverse or allergic reactions, and possible drug interactions. Assess the need for home health care, and provide a referral as needed.

Infective Endocarditis

Endocarditis, inflammation of the endocardium, is an infectious process that usually affects clients with underlying heart disease. Lesions develop on deformed valves, on valve prostheses (artificial valves), or in areas of the heart where tissue has been damaged. Bacteria often enter through invasive procedures or devices, such as intravenous catheters, indwelling urinary catheters, dental procedures, or during heart surgery. The left side of the heart, the mitral valve in particular, is the most common site of infection. Intravenous drug use is also a risk factor; in these individuals, the right side (the tricuspid valve) is often involved.

TABLE 27-3

Classifications of Infective Endocarditis

	ACUTE INFECTIVE ENDOCARDITIS	SUBACUTE INFECTIVE ENDOCARDITIS
Onset	Sudden	Gradual
Usual Organism	*Staphylococcus aureus*	*Streptococcus viridans;* others
Risk Factors	Intravenous drug use, sepsis	Previous heart or valve damage or deformity; dental work, invasive procedures
Pathologic Processes	Rapid valve destruction	Valve destruction with regurgitation; embolization of friable vegetations
Presentation	Abrupt onset with spiking fever and chills; manifestations of heart failure	Gradual onset of febrile illness with cough, dyspnea, arthralgias, abdominal pain

Endocarditis is frequently classified by its onset and disease course (Table 27-3 ■). *Acute endocarditis* has an abrupt onset and is a rapidly progressive, severe disease. *Staphylococcus aureus* is the usual infective organism in acute endocarditis. In contrast, *subacute endocarditis* has a more gradual onset. It is more likely to occur in clients with preexisting heart disease. *Streptococcus viridans* is the most common organism causing subacute endocarditis.

PATHOPHYSIOLOGY

Organisms in the bloodstream attach to the endocardial lining of the heart and become enmeshed in deposits of fibrin and platelets. This covering "protects" the bacteria from quick removal by the immune system. These vegetations develop on heart valve leaflets, varying in size and shape. *Friable* (easily broken, fragile) vegetations can break off, traveling through the bloodstream to other organs. When they lodge in small vessels, they may cause hemorrhages, infarcts, or abscesses. The vegetations prevent normal valve closure, causing regurgitation of blood through the valve and heart murmurs.

Manifestations and Complications

Infective endocarditis generally causes elevated temperature (above 101.5°F or 39.4°C) and flulike symptoms. The client may have a cough, shortness of breath, and complain of joint pain. Acute staphylococcal endocarditis presents with sudden and more severe manifestations, including a high fever. Heart murmurs are common.

Peripheral manifestations of endocarditis may include *petechiae* (small, purplish-red spots) on the trunk, conjunctiva, and mucous membranes; *splinter hemorrhages* (red streaks under the fingernails or toenails); small, painful growths on the fingers and toes; or small, purplish-red lesions on the palms of the hands and soles of the feet. Complications of infective endocarditis include heart failure, and infarctions of other organs (lungs, brain, kidneys, or bowel) from embolization of vegetative fragments.

clinical ALERT

Immediately report manifestations of complications of infective endocarditis, such as an abrupt change in mental status, vision, or other neurologic signs, a new heart murmur, or an abrupt onset of a respiratory distress with dyspnea, tachycardia, cough, or cyanosis.

INTERDISCIPLINARY CARE

Prevention of infective endocarditis is key; education of clients at high risk for the disease is essential. Teaching the public about the risks of intravenous drug use, including endocarditis, can also help reduce the incidence of this frightening disease. The management priorities for infective endocarditis are to eradicate the infecting organism and minimize valve damage and complications of the disease.

There are no definitive tests for infective endocarditis. A *CBC* and *blood cultures* are done. *Echocardiography* is performed to identify vegetations and evaluate valve function.

Pharmacology

To prevent infective endocarditis, antibiotics are commonly prescribed prior to high-risk procedures for clients with preexisting heart disease or damage. Table 27-4 ■ lists

TABLE 27-4

Indications for Antibiotic Prophylaxis to Prevent Endocarditis

CONDITIONS	PROCEDURES
Rheumatic heart disease	Dental procedures, including cleaning
Prosthetic heart valves	
Previous episodes of infective endocarditis	Surgery
	Bronchoscopy or cystoscopy
Congenital heart conditions	Urinary catheterization
Mitral valve prolapse	Incision and drainage of infected tissue

conditions and procedures for which prophylactic antibiotic therapy is recommended.

Antibiotics are prescribed to eradicate the infecting organism from the blood and heart lesions. Because the fibrin covering that protects organisms from the immune system also protects them from the antibiotic, an extended course of multiple intravenous antibiotics is required. Intravenous drug therapy is continued for 2 to 4 weeks.

Some clients with infective endocarditis require surgery to repair or replace damaged valves. The most common indication for surgery is valvular regurgitation that causes heart failure. When the infection has not responded to antibiotic therapy within 7 to 10 days, the infected valve may be replaced to help eliminate the organism.

NURSING CARE

Nursing care of the client with infective endocarditis focuses on managing its manifestations, administering antibiotics, and educating the client and family members. Preventing and identifying complications promptly is also a nursing priority.

ASSESSING

Subjective data collected for the client with infective endocarditis include information about risk factors such as previous heart damage or surgery, recent dental work or other invasive procedures, and intravenous drug use. Ask about current symptoms such as persistent fatigue and activity intolerance, or shortness of breath. Obtain vital signs, including temperature and apical pulse; observe ease of breathing and auscultate breath sounds; and assess for other manifestations such as petechiae or splinter hemorrhages. Monitor laboratory results, particularly results of blood cultures and serum antibiotic levels. Report results to the physician.

DIAGNOSING, PLANNING, AND IMPLEMENTING

Priorities in Nursing Care. Effectively treating the infectious process, maintaining heart function, and preventing complications are the priorities for nursing care of the client with infective endocarditis.

Risk for Imbalanced Body Temperature

- Record temperature every 2 to 4 hours. Notify physician if above 101.5°F (39.4°C). *Body temperature usually returns to normal within 1 week of antibiotic therapy. Continuing fever may indicate a need to modify the treatment regimen.*
- Obtain blood cultures as ordered before giving the first dose of antibiotics. *Blood cultures can identify the causative*

organism and direct the choice of antibiotic. Initial blood cultures must be obtained before antibiotic therapy is started to obtain enough organisms for culture. Follow-up cultures are used to assess the effectiveness of therapy.

- Administer anti-inflammatory or antipyretic agents as prescribed. *Fever may be treated with aspirin, ibuprofen, or acetaminophen.*
- Administer antibiotics as ordered; obtain peak and trough drug levels as indicated. *Intravenous antibiotics are given for 2 to 6 weeks to eradicate the pathogen. Peak and trough levels evaluate the adequacy of the dose to maintain a therapeutic blood level.*

Risk for Ineffective Tissue Perfusion

- Notify the charge nurse or physician of manifestations of altered organ perfusion:
  - *Brain:* altered level of consciousness, numbness or tingling in extremities, hemiplegia, visual disturbances, or manifestations of stroke
  - *Kidneys:* decreased urine output, hematuria, elevated blood urea nitrogen (BUN) or creatinine
  - *Lungs:* dyspnea, hemoptysis, shortness of breath, diminished breath sounds, restlessness, sudden chest or shoulder pain
  - *Heart:* chest pain radiating to jaw or arms, tachycardia, anxiety, tachypnea, hypotension
  - *Bowel:* abdominal pain, tenderness, guarding; decreased or absent bowel sounds, nausea, vomiting
  Embolization of vegetative lesions can affect tissue perfusion. Vegetations from the left heart may lodge in vessels of the brain, kidneys, or peripheral tissues, causing infarction or abscess. Emboli from the right side of the heart can lead to manifestations of a pulmonary embolism.
- Assess skin color and temperature, quality of peripheral pulses, and capillary refill. *Assessment of peripheral tissue perfusion is important to reduce the risk of tissue necrosis and possible extremity loss.*

Evaluating

To evaluate care for the client with infective endocarditis, collect assessment data such as that noted in the Assessing section.

Documenting. Document assessment data, including subjective information such as complaints of shortness of breath or fatigue. Note subjective and objective assessments following activity, as well as the extent of activity tolerated by the client.

CONTINUING CARE

The client with infective endocarditis needs education and support throughout the course of the disease, as well as teaching to prevent future recurrences. In basic terms,

Preventing Endocarditis

- Teach the function of the heart valves and the effects of endocarditis. Define endocarditis, and explain why the client is at risk.
- Stress the importance of notifying care providers of valve disease, heart murmur, or valve replacement before undergoing any invasive procedures.
- Encourage good oral and dental hygiene and regular dental checkups. Discuss the importance of preventing oral trauma (e.g., gentle toothbrushing, properly fitting dentures, and avoiding use of toothpicks, dental floss, and high-flow water devices).
- Encourage pneumococcal vaccine and annual influenza immunizations.

teach the client what is happening in the heart and the reasons for the symptoms. Emphasize that infective endocarditis, although serious and frightening, can usually be treated effectively with intravenous antibiotics. Stress the importance of promptly reporting any unusual manifestation, such as a change in vision, sudden pain, or weakness, so that treatment can be promptly implemented. Explain the rationale for all treatments and procedures, including activity restrictions, to reduce anxiety and enhance cooperation. Describe the manifestations of heart failure, and instruct the client to notify his or her care provider if these manifestations develop.

Client and family education is also extremely important to prevent recurrences of infective endocarditis. Box 27-8 ■ outlines a teaching plan for clients at risk.

Clients who acquire infective endocarditis from intravenous drug use need additional teaching about the risks of intravenous drug injection. Refer the client and significant others as appropriate to a drug or substance abuse treatment program or facility.

Myocarditis

Myocarditis is an inflammatory disorder of the heart muscle that may be caused by infection (viral, bacterial, protozoal), an immune response, radiation, chemical poisons, drugs, or burns. Myocarditis can occur at any age, and it is more common in men than women. Clients whose immune system is suppressed—those with acquired immunodeficiency syndrome (AIDS) in particular—are at risk. Factors that alter immune response—such as malnutrition, alcohol use, immunosuppressive drugs, radiation, stress, and advanced age—increase the risk for myocarditis.

The client with myocarditis may be asymptomatic or have nonspecific symptoms such as fever, fatigue, general malaise, dyspnea, palpitations, and arthralgias. Often, there is a history of recent nonspecific illness or upper respiratory infection. Manifestations of heart failure, including tachycardia, dysrhythmias, and an S_3 and S_4 may be present. A heart murmur, pericardial friction rub, cardiomegaly, and ECG abnormalities may be noted. The long-term effects of the disease depend on the extent of damage to the heart muscle. While many clients recover fully, others may develop progressive heart failure and cardiomyopathy.

Care for the client with myocarditis focuses on treating the inflammatory process to prevent further damage to the heart muscle. Bed rest and activity restrictions are ordered during the acute stage to reduce myocardial work. Oxygen is administered to clients with signs of cardiac dysfunction. If the cause is infectious, antimicrobial therapy is prescribed. Corticosteroids or other immunosuppressive agents (see Chapter 11) ◯◯ may be given to reduce inflammation. Digoxin may be ordered to manage heart failure.

Nursing care is directed at decreasing myocardial work and increasing oxygen supply. Encourage strict bed rest to reduce physical activity. Emotional rest also is indicated, because anxiety increases myocardial oxygen demand. Closely monitor vital signs, heart rhythm, and pump effectiveness during the acute phase of the illness. Consider the following nursing diagnoses for the client with myocarditis:

- *Decreased Cardiac Output* related to impaired cardiac muscle function
- *Fatigue* related to the inflammatory process and inadequate cardiac output
- *Anxiety* related to possible long-term effects of the disorder
- *Excess Fluid Volume* related to compensatory mechanisms for decreased cardiac output.

Explain all procedures, tests, and treatments to decrease anxiety and cardiac workload. Teach the early manifestations of heart failure to report to the physician. Stress the importance of following the treatment regimen, including activity restrictions, any dietary modifications (such as a low-salt diet if signs of heart failure are present), and medications. Emphasize that adhering to the treatment plan can reduce the risk of long-term consequences, such as cardiomyopathy.

Pericarditis

Pericarditis is inflammation of the pericardium, the outermost layer of the heart. Acute pericarditis is usually viral. Pericarditis is a frequent complication of end-stage kidney disease. Pericarditis also may follow a myocardial infarction or open heart surgery.

PATHOPHYSIOLOGY

Damage to pericardial tissue triggers an inflammatory response. The inflammatory response causes fluid and exudate to collect in the pericardial space. Accumulation of a large volume of fluid and exudates may interfere with cardiac filling. The inflammatory process often resolves without long-term consequences. In some cases, scar tissue and adhesions may form between the pericardial layers. Fibrosis and scarring of the pericardium can restrict the heart's ability to function effectively.

Manifestations and Complications

Classic manifestations of acute pericarditis include chest pain, a pericardial friction rub, and fever. The onset of chest pain is often abrupt. It is usually sharp and may radiate to the back or neck. The pain may be steady or intermittent, and is aggravated by deep breathing, coughing, movement, or swallowing. The client often sits upright and leans forward to reduce the discomfort.

A **pericardial friction rub** is the characteristic sign of pericarditis. It is a leathery, grating sound produced by the inflamed pericardial layers rubbing against the chest wall or pleura. The rub is best heard at the left lower sternal border with the client sitting up or leaning forward. It may be constant, or it may disappear and then reappear hours later. A low-grade fever (below 100°F [38.4°C]) is often present. Dyspnea and tachycardia are common.

A *pericardial effusion,* an abnormal collection of fluid between the pericardial layers, may develop in pericarditis. If the fluid collects gradually, the pericardial sac stretches to accommodate it. Heart function is not affected, although heart sounds may be muffled. In contrast, a rapid buildup of pericardial fluid (as little as 100 mL) does not allow the sac to stretch and can compress the heart, interfering with myocardial function. This is known as **cardiac tamponade.** It is a medical emergency that is fatal if it is not aggressively treated.

In cardiac tamponade, cardiac output is critically reduced. A hallmark sign of cardiac tamponade is a *paradoxical pulse,* in which the systolic blood pressure drops more than 10 mm Hg during inspiration. Peripheral pulses weaken or disappear as well during inspiration. The increased pressure in the chest cavity during inspiration further interferes with cardiac output, causing paradoxical pulse. Other manifestations of cardiac tamponade include muffled heart sounds, dyspnea and tachypnea, tachycardia, and a narrowed pulse pressure.

INTERDISCIPLINARY CARE

Although it is uncomfortable, acute pericarditis is usually self-limiting, and will resolve with or without treatment. However, close observation is important to detect early manifestations of increasing effusion or cardiac tamponade.

In acute pericarditis, *cardiac enzymes* may be slightly elevated. Acute pericarditis produces characteristic changes on

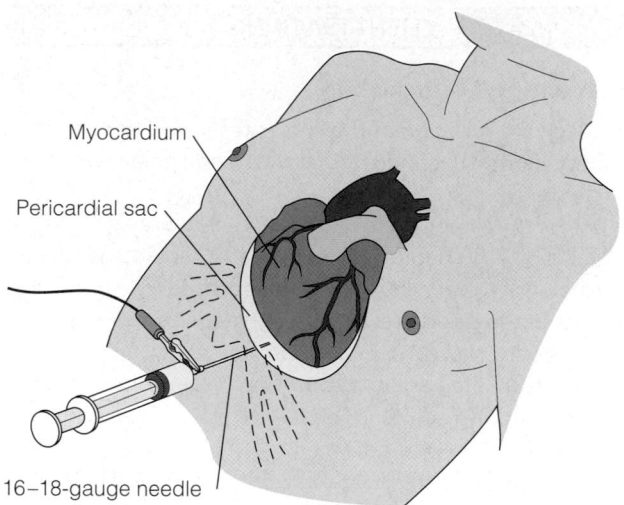

Figure 27-5. ■ Pericardiocentesis.

the *electrocardiogram. Echocardiography* is used to evaluate for pericardial effusion or restricted heart motion. A *computed tomography (CT) scan* or *magnetic resonance imaging (MRI)* may also be used to identify pericardial effusions.

Aspirin, acetaminophen, or NSAIDs are ordered to reduce fever and inflammation and to promote comfort. If heart function is affected, activity may be restricted.

Pericardiocentesis

Pericardiocentesis may be done to remove fluid from the pericardial sac (Figure 27-5 ■). The physician inserts a large (16- to 18-gauge) needle into the pericardial sac and withdraws excess fluid. Pericardiocentesis may be done as an emergency procedure for cardiac tamponade. Nursing implications for the client undergoing pericardiocentesis are outlined in Box 27-9 ■.

NURSING CARE

Priorities in Nursing Care. The nursing care focus for the client with pericarditis is on promoting comfort and closely monitoring for manifestations of cardiac tamponade or other complications.

Pain

■ Assess chest pain on a standardized scale; note quality and radiation of the pain. Ask about factors that aggravate or relieve the pain. *Assessing the severity, quality, and characteristics of chest pain help differentiate the pain of pericarditis from angina.*

■ Administer NSAIDs on a regular basis as prescribed with food. *NSAIDs are ordered to reduce fever, inflammation, and pericardial pain. They are most effective when given on a regular schedule. Administering the drugs with food helps decrease GI distress.*

BOX 27-9	NURSING CARE CHECKLIST

Pericardiocentesis

Before the Procedure

☑ Gather all supplies.

☑ Reinforce teaching about the procedure, clarifying information and answering questions. Provide emotional support.

☑ Verify informed consent for the procedure has been obtained.

☑ Provide for privacy.

☑ Obtain baseline vital signs.

☑ Initiate cardiac monitoring and obtain a baseline rhythm strip.

☑ Have emergency resuscitation equipment at the bedside.

☑ Administer oxygen as ordered.

During the Procedure

☑ Follow Standard Precautions.

☑ Position at a 45- to 60-degree angle. Place a dry towel to catch blood or fluid.

☑ Assist with the aspiration as directed.

☑ Notify physician of changes in cardiac rhythm, vital signs, level of consciousness, and urine output.

After the Procedure

☑ Monitor vital signs and cardiac rhythm every 15 minutes for first hour, every 30 minutes next hour, then hourly for 24 hours.

☑ Record fluid removed as output on the intake and output record.

☑ If indicated, send aspirated fluid for culture and sensitivity and laboratory analysis.

☑ Assess heart and breath sounds.

☑ Document the procedure and the client's response.

- Maintain a quiet, calm environment. Provide position changes, back rubs, heat/cold therapy, diversional activity, and emotional support. *Supportive interventions convey caring, enhance the effects of the medication, and decrease the perception of pain.*

Ineffective Breathing Pattern

The pain of pericarditis increases with respiratory movement, leading the client to breathe shallowly.

- Assess respiratory rate and effort, and auscultate breath sounds every 4 hours. Report adventitious or diminished breath sounds. *Congestion or atelectasis may result from decreased ventilation of peripheral alveoli due to shallow respirations.*

- Assist to use the incentive spirometer at least every 2 hours. Provide pain medication before respiratory therapy treatments, as needed. *Deep breathing and the incentive spirometer help ensure alveolar ventilation and prevent atelectasis. Analgesia prior to painful treatments promotes comfort and facilitates participation.*

- Administer oxygen as needed. *Supplementary oxygen promotes optimal gas exchange and tissue oxygenation.*

- Place in Fowler's or high Fowler's position. *Elevating the head of the bed reduces the work of breathing and decreases pericardial chest pain.*

Risk for Decreased Cardiac Output

- Assess vital signs hourly during acute inflammatory processes. *Frequent assessment allows early identification of manifestations of decreased cardiac output, such as tachycardia, hypotension, or changes in pulse pressure.*

- Assess heart sounds and peripheral pulses, and observe for neck vein distention and pulsus paradoxus every hour.

clinical ALERT

Promptly notify the physician of distant, muffled heart sounds, new murmurs or extra heart sounds, decreasing quality of peripheral pulses, and distended neck veins. Immediately report altered level of consciousness; decreased urine output; cold, clammy, mottled skin; delayed capillary refill; and weak peripheral pulses. *Acute pericardial effusion and tamponade interfere with cardiac filling and pumping, causing venous congestion, decreased cardiac output, and impaired organ and tissue perfusion.*

- If emergency pericardiocentesis and/or surgery is needed to remove pericardial fluid, prepare the client for the procedure, providing appropriate explanations and reassurance. Observe for adverse effects during pericardiocentesis. *Emotional support and explanations reduce anxiety and promote a caring atmosphere.*

CONTINUING CARE

Stress the importance of continuing anti-inflammatory medications as ordered. Teach about prescribed drugs, including dose, desired and possible adverse effects, and interactions with other drugs or food. Instruct to take anti-inflammatory medications with food, milk, or antacids to minimize gastric distress, and to contact the physician if unable to tolerate the drug. Tell clients taking NSAIDs to monitor their weight at least weekly, because these drugs may cause fluid retention. Encourage to maintain a fluid intake of at least 2,500 mL/day to minimize the risk of kidney damage. Advise to avoid aspirin while taking other NSAIDs because it may interfere with their activity. Instruct to avoid over-the-counter preparations containing aspirin, as well.

If an activity restriction is ordered, suggest measures to maintain this restriction. Emphasize that activity will be gradually increased once the inflammatory process has resolved.

The client may be at risk for recurrence of pericarditis. Teach manifestations that may indicate recurrent pericarditis, and stress the importance of promptly reporting these to the physician.

DISORDERS OF CARDIAC STRUCTURE

Valvular Heart Disease

Proper functioning of the heart valves is necessary to ensure one-way blood flow through the heart and vascular system. **Valvular heart disease** interferes with blood flow to and from the heart. Rheumatic heart disease is the most common cause of valvular disease, especially in older adults. Valve disorders also can result from endocarditis or after myocardial infarction, due to damaged papillary muscles. Congenital heart defects may affect heart valves, often with no symptoms until adulthood. Changes in the heart that occur with normal aging also may lead to valvular disease.

PATHOPHYSIOLOGY AND MANIFESTATIONS

There are two major types of heart valve disorders: stenosis and regurgitation. *Stenosis* occurs when valve leaflets fuse together and are unable to open or close fully. The valve opening narrows, impairing the forward flow of blood. *Regurgitant valves* (also called *incompetent valves*) do not close completely. This allows *regurgitation,* or backflow of blood, through the incompletely closed valve into the area it just left.

Valve disorders affect pressures and blood flow both in front of and behind the affected valve. Stenosis increases the work of the chamber behind the affected valve as the heart attempts to push blood through the narrowed opening. Excess blood volume behind regurgitant valves causes the chamber to dilate. Blood volume and pressures are reduced in front of the diseased valve, because flow is impeded through a stenotic valve and backflow occurs through a regurgitant valve. These changes can lead to pulmonary complications or heart failure. The heart muscle hypertrophies as the heart attempts to maintain cardiac output.

The valves on the left side of the heart (mitral and aortic) are subjected to higher pressures, increasing their risk of damage. Blood flow through the heart becomes turbulent as blood moves or attempts to move through damaged valves; the result is a murmur, one of the characteristic manifestations of valvular disease (Table 27-5 ■).

TABLE 27-5

Characteristics of Common Heart Murmurs

MURMUR	TIMING	LOCATION	CONFIGURATION	QUALITY
Mitral stenosis	Diastole	Apex—5th intercostal space (ICS), midclavicular line (MCL)	S_2 S_1	Continuous rumble, increasing toward end of diastole
Mitral regurgitation	Systole	Apex	S_1 S_2	Continuous throughout systole (holosystolic)
Aortic stenosis	Systole	Right sternal border, 2nd ICS	S_1 S_2	Crescendo–decrescendo, continuous
Aortic regurgitation	Early diastole	3rd ICS, left sternal border	S_2 S_1	Decrescendo, continuous

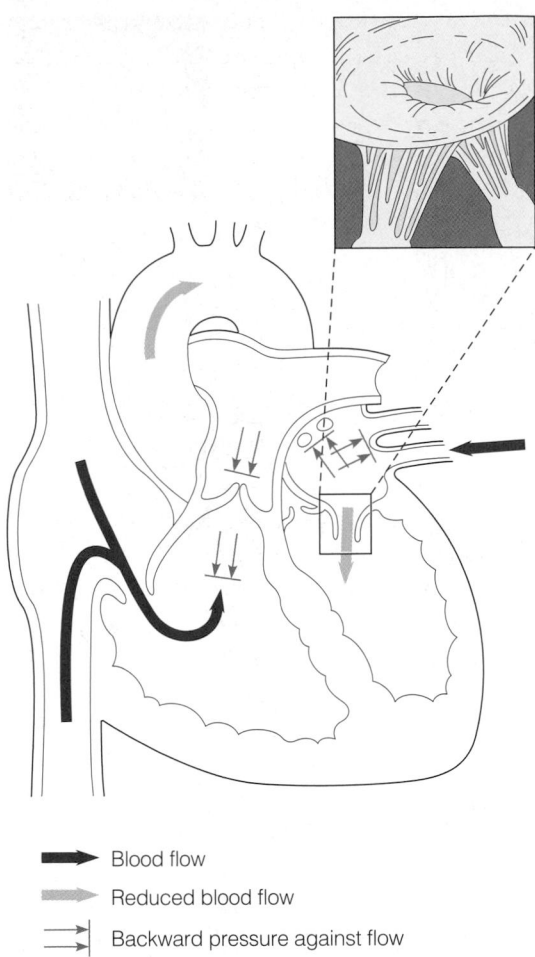

  → Blood flow

  → Reduced blood flow

  → Backward pressure against flow

Figure 27-6. ■ Mitral stenosis.

Mitral Stenosis

Mitral stenosis is narrowing of the mitral valve that obstructs blood flow from the left atrium into the left ventricle during diastole. Mitral stenosis is usually caused by rheumatic heart disease.

The narrowed mitral opening impairs left ventricular filling and cardiac output. It also causes the left atrium to dilate and hypertrophy. High atrial pressures are reflected back into the pulmonary system (Figure 27-6 ■). Increased pressure in the pulmonary system increases the workload of the right ventricle, causing it also to dilate and hypertrophy. Eventually, right-sided heart failure occurs. Chronic atrial distention often leads to atrial dysrhythmias such as atrial fibrillation. Thrombi may form in the left atrium and become emboli to the brain, coronary arteries, kidney, spleen, and extremities—potentially devastating complications.

Dyspnea on exertion (DOE) is typically the earliest manifestation of mitral stenosis. Others include cough, hemoptysis, frequent respiratory infections such as bronchitis and pneumonia, paroxysmal nocturnal dyspnea, orthopnea, weakness, fatigue, and palpitations. As the stenosis increases, manifes-

tations become more severe. Signs of right heart failure, such as distended neck veins and peripheral edema, may develop. The client with severe mitral stenosis may be cyanotic.

> ### clinical ALERT
>
> Women with mitral stenosis may be asymptomatic until they become pregnant. The increased circulating volume (30% more in pregnancy) can precipitate sudden pulmonary edema and heart failure, threatening the lives of the mother and fetus.

On auscultation, a diastolic murmur characterized as low pitched and rumbling may be heard in the apical region. It is heard best with the bell of the stethoscope. The murmur may be accompanied by a palpable *thrill* (a palpable tremor or vibration). Crackles may be noted in the lungs.

Mitral Regurgitation

Mitral regurgitation or *insufficiency* allows blood to flow back into the left atrium during systole because the valve does not close completely. Rheumatic heart disease is a common cause of mitral regurgitation. Only a portion of the blood in the ventricle is ejected into the systemic circulation during systole; the rest returns to the left atrium through the deformed valve. This is added to the blood from the pulmonary system (Figure 27-7 ■). The left atrium dilates to accommodate the extra volume; the left ventricle dilates to compensate for increased preload and low cardiac output.

Clients with mitral regurgitation may experience fatigue, weakness, exertional dyspnea, and orthopnea. In severe or acute mitral regurgitation, manifestations of left heart failure may develop, including pulmonary congestion and edema. With high pulmonary pressures, right-sided heart failure may develop as well.

The murmur of mitral regurgitation is usually loud, high pitched, and rumbling. It may be described as "cooing" or "sea gull–like" or have a musical quality. It is heard best at the apex of the heart and often is accompanied by a palpable thrill.

Mitral Valve Prolapse

Mitral valve prolapse (MVP) is a form of mitral insufficiency that occurs when the posterior cusp of the mitral valve flops back into the left atrium during systole. It is probably congenital and is commonly found in young women between the ages of 14 and 30. Its incidence declines with age. Most clients with MVP are asymptomatic. Chest pain, usually related to fatigue rather than exertion, is the most common symptom of MVP. Dysrhythmias can cause palpitations, light-headedness, and syncope. A high-pitched late systolic murmur, sometimes described as a "whoop" or "honk," may be present.

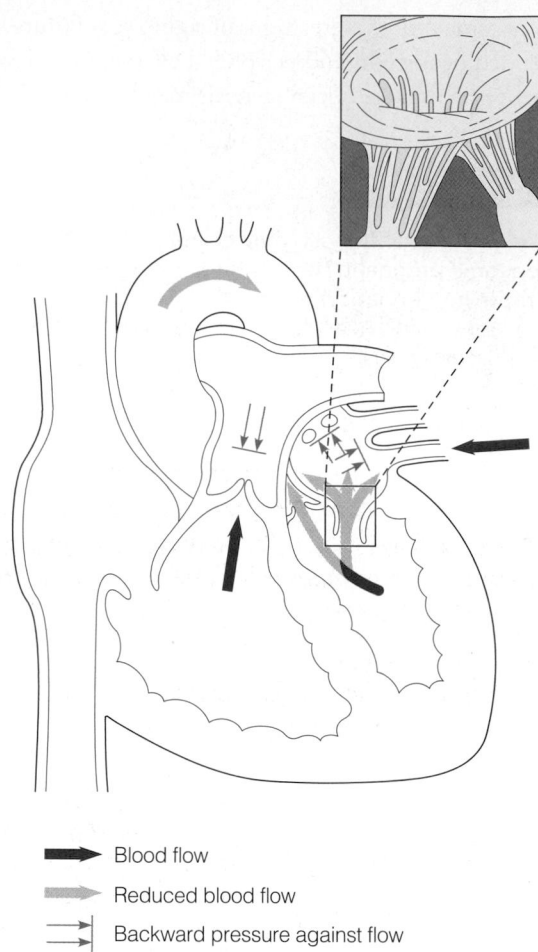

Figure 27-7. ■ Mitral regurgitation.

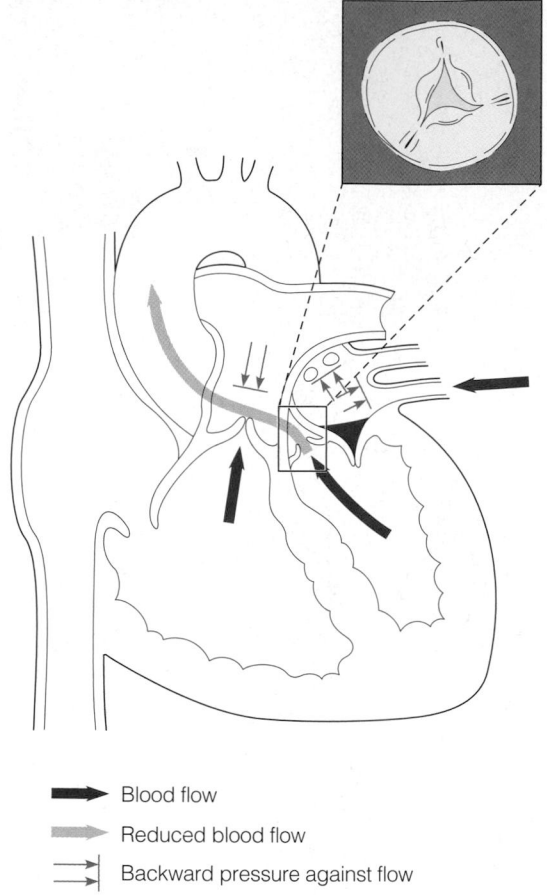

Figure 27-8. ■ Aortic stenosis.

Aortic Stenosis

Aortic stenosis obstructs blood flow from the left ventricle into the aorta during systole. Aortic stenosis is more common in males (80%) than females. It may be *idiopathic* (unknown cause), congenital, or related to rheumatic heart disease. The older adult may develop aortic stenosis from changes associated with aging.

As aortic stenosis progresses, the left ventricle has to work harder to eject blood through the narrowed opening. The ventricle hypertrophies to maintain the cardiac output (Figure 27-8 ■). Because of the extra work, myocardial oxygen needs increase. The increased oxygen consumption can lead to myocardial ischemia. Increased pressures in the left heart are reflected back to the pulmonary vascular system; congestion and pulmonary edema may result.

Manifestations of aortic stenosis usually develop after age 50. They include dyspnea on exertion, angina, and exertional syncope (light-headedness with activity). The pulse pressure narrows as stoke volume and cardiac output fall. Clients with aortic stenosis are at risk for sudden cardiac death.

A harsh systolic murmur can be heard in the second intercostal space to the right of the sternum. A palpable thrill

is often noted. As the condition becomes more severe, S_3 and S_4 heart sounds may be heard.

Aortic Regurgitation

In *aortic regurgitation* or *insufficiency,* the aortic valve fails to close completely, allowing blood to flow back into the left ventricle from the aorta during diastole (Figure 27-9 ■). Rheumatic heart disease is the most common cause of aortic regurgitation.

Blood from the aorta causes volume overload of the left ventricle. The ventricle dilates, and stroke volume increases. Over time, the left ventricle hypertrophies, and cardiac output falls. Eventually, pulmonary congestion and possibly right heart failure develop from increased pressures on the left side of the heart. Unlike many other valve disorders, exercise reduces regurgitation and improves heart function in this disorder.

People with mild to moderate aortic regurgitation may complain of palpitations, especially when flat or in a left-lying position. The heartbeat is visible as a throbbing pulse in the arteries of the neck. Sometimes the force of contraction causes a head bob and shakes the whole body. Other manifestations include dizziness, exercise intolerance, fatigue, exertional dyspnea, and angina. Angina often occurs

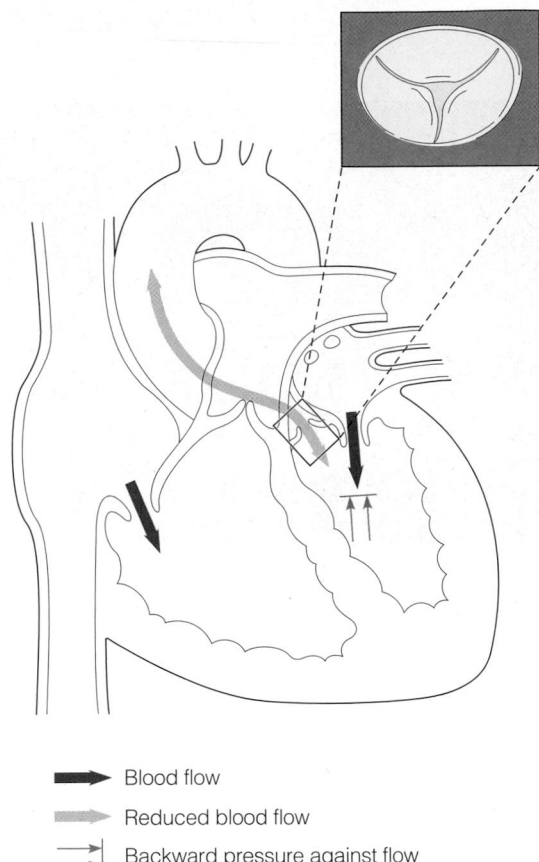

Blood flow
Reduced blow flow
Backward pressure against flow

Figure 27-9. ■ Aortic regurgitation.

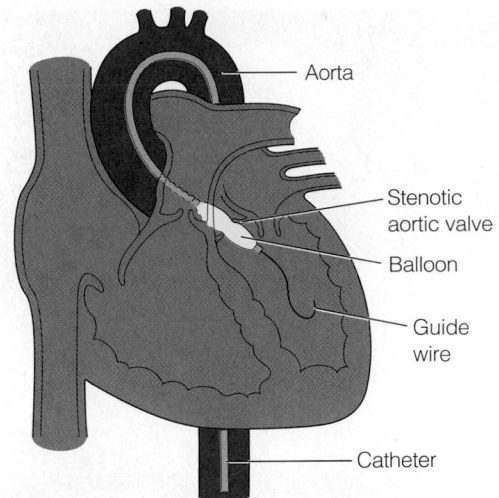

Figure 27-10. ■ Balloon valvuloplasty. The balloon catheter is positioned across the stenosed valve. The balloon is then inflated to increase the size of the valve opening.

at night and may not respond to common treatments. The pulse pressure often is widened.

The murmur of aortic regurgitation is heard in diastole as blood flows back into the left ventricle from the aorta. It is described as a "blowing," high-pitched sound heard most clearly at the third left intercostal space. It may be associated with a thrill. An S_3 and S_4 may be heard. Because the heart is enlarged, the apical impulse is displaced to the left.

INTERDISCIPLINARY CARE

Valvular disease may be asymptomatic for many years. The initial indication often is a heart murmur heard during a routine physical examination. *Echocardiography* is used to diagnose valvular disease. *Cardiac catheterization* is used to assess the effects of valve disease on heart function.

Asymptomatic clients and those with mild manifestations often require no treatment. They are closely observed for signs of disease progression. Valve damage increases the risk for infective endocarditis because the deformed valve alters blood flow through the heart, allowing bacteria to colonize heart tissues. Antibiotics are given prophylactically prior to any dental work, invasive procedures, or surgery (see Table 27-4). Manifestations of heart failure are treated with diet and medications (see the preceding section

on heart failure). When medical treatment no longer controls the disease, surgery is considered.

Percutaneous Balloon Valvuloplasty

Stenotic valve disease may be treated with *percutaneous balloon valvuloplasty*. A balloon catheter is inserted into the femoral vein or artery, and advanced to the stenotic valve. The balloon is then inflated for approximately 90 seconds to divide the fused leaflets and enlarge the valve opening (Figure 27-10 ■). Nursing care of the client with a balloon valvuloplasty is similar to that of the client following percutaneous coronary revascularization (see Box 26-3). ⚭

Surgery

Surgery to repair or replace the diseased valve may be required to restore valve function, relieve symptoms, and prevent complications. *Valvuloplasty* is a general term for reconstruction or repair of a heart valve. Methods include "patching" the perforated portion of the leaflet, resecting excess tissue, removing vegetations or calcification, and other techniques. A *commissurotomy* may be done to open stenotic valves.

Severely damaged valves may be replaced. Many different prosthetic heart valves are available, including mechanical and biologic tissue valves (Figure 27-11 ■). Biologic tissue valves (from animal tissue or a human cadaver) allow more normal blood flow and are less likely to cause clots to form than mechanical ones. Mechanical prosthetic valves are more durable, but require lifetime anticoagulation to prevent clot formation on the valve. Both biologic and mechanical valves increase the risk of emboli and endocarditis, although the incidence of these complications is fairly low. Nursing care of the client having valve surgery is similar to that for other types of open heart surgery (see Box 26-4). ⚭

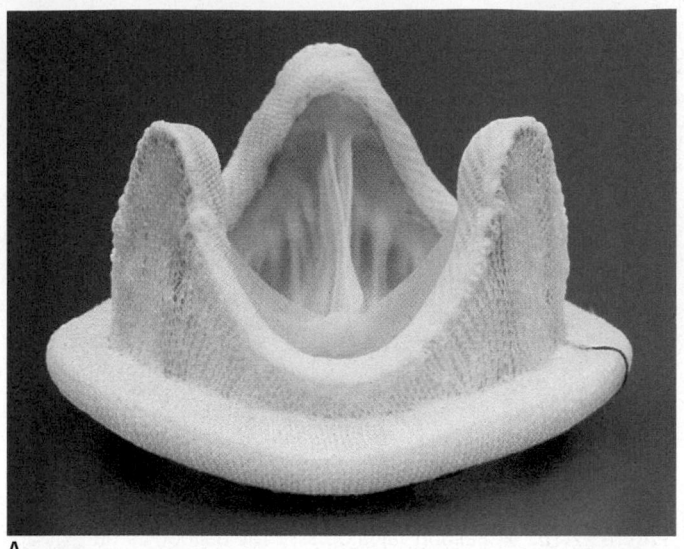

A

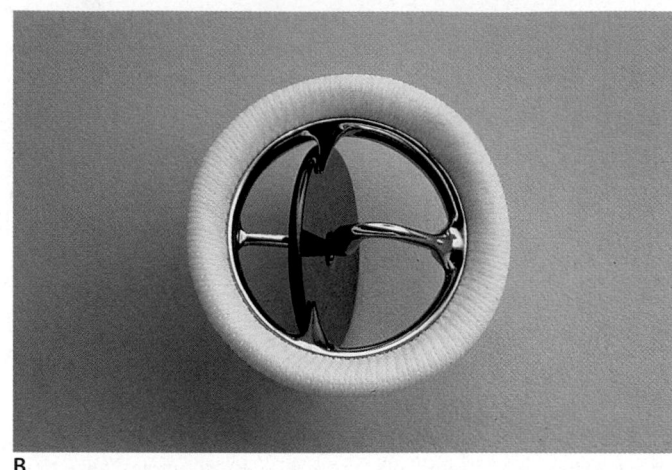

B

Figure 27-11. ■ Prosthetic heart valves. (**A**) Carpentier–Edwards biologic aortic valve prosthesis. (Courtesy of Edwards Lifesciences.) (**B**) Medtronic Hall prosthetic valve. (Courtesy of Medtronic Inc., Minneapolis, MN.)

NURSING CARE

Priorities in Nursing Care. Nursing care focuses on maintaining the cardiac output, managing manifestations of the disorder, teaching about the disease and its treatment, and preventing complications.

Decreased Cardiac Output

- Monitor vital signs and hemodynamic pressures, reporting changes. *A drop in systolic blood pressure and increasing pulse rate may indicate decreased cardiac output.*
- Assess indicators of cardiac output every 8 hours, including level of consciousness, neck vein distention, respiratory effort and lung sounds, urine output, skin color and temperature, peripheral edema, and peripheral pulses and capillary refill. Notify the physician of significant changes. *Decreased cardiac output impairs tissue and organ perfusion, producing clinical manifestations.*
- Monitor intake and output; weigh daily, reporting any gain of 3 to 5 lbs (1 to 2 kg) within 24 hours. *Fluid retention may indicate decreased cardiac output; 2.2 lbs (1 kg) of weight is equal to 1 liter of retained fluid.*
- Maintain fluid restriction as ordered. *Fluid intake may be restricted to minimize cardiac workload.*
- Elevate head of the bed, and administer oxygen as ordered. *These measures facilitate lung ventilation and improve oxygenation.*
- Monitor pulse oximetry. *Pulse oximetry allows assessment of oxygenation.*
- Promote physical, emotional, and mental rest. *Physical and psychologic rest decrease the cardiac workload.*
- Administer medications as ordered. *Diuretics, ACE inhibitors, and direct vasodilators are often ordered to reduce or*

redistribute excess fluid volume and reduce the cardiac workload.

Activity Intolerance

- Obtain vital signs before and during activities. *An increased heart rate, change in BP, diaphoresis, or complaints of shortness of breath, fatigue, or chest pain may indicate poor tolerance of the level of activity.*
- Encourage gradual increases in activity/self-care as tolerated. *Progressive activity prevents sudden stress on the heart and helps improve exercise tolerance.*
- Provide assistance as needed. Suggest using a shower chair, sitting while brushing hair or teeth, and so on. *Energy-saving techniques reduce cardiac workload.*

Ineffective Protection

Anticoagulant therapy may be ordered to reduce the risk of clotting with valve disorders or an artificial valve. This increases the risk for bleeding and hemorrhage.

- Test stools and emesis for occult blood. *Bleeding in the GI tract may not be visible.*
- Caution to avoid using aspirin or other NSAIDs. Instruct to read ingredient labels on over-the-counter drugs; many contain aspirin. *Aspirin and other NSAIDs interfere with clotting and may increase the risk of bleeding.*
- Instruct to use a soft-bristled toothbrush and an electric razor, and to clean fragile skin gently. *These measures reduce the risk of bleeding from skin nicks and cuts or the gums.*
- Monitor hemoglobin, hematocrit, and platelet counts. Notify the charge nurse of significant changes. *Low hemoglobin and hematocrit may indicate blood loss. Platelet counts below 50,000/mm³ significantly increase the risk of bleeding.*

CONTINUING CARE

Preventing rheumatic fever is important to prevent heart valve disorders. Early treatment of strep throat usually prevents rheumatic fever. Teach individual clients, families, and communities the importance of timely and effective treatment of strep throat. Emphasize the importance of completing the full prescription of antibiotics to prevent development of resistant bacteria.

Explain all tests and procedures, including corrective surgery, to increase understanding and decrease anxiety. Discuss symptom management, including activity restrictions or lifestyle changes related to the valve disease. Advise to schedule rest periods to prevent fatigue. Teach about diet restrictions to control heart failure; arrange a consultation with the dietitian for teaching and menu planning. Provide information about prescribed medications, including their purpose, desired and possible adverse effects, scheduling, and possible interactions with other drugs. Refer the client and family to community resources prior to discharge. Emphasize the importance of keeping follow-up appointments to monitor the disease and treatment. Emphasize the importance of notifying all health care providers about valve disease or surgery so that antibiotics can be given before any procedure that might cause infection.

Instruct the client and family to report increasing severity of symptoms, particularly of heart failure and pulmonary edema, to the doctor. The treatment regimen may need to be modified or surgery considered to repair or replace the diseased valve. Advise to report neurologic changes and other symptoms of emboli so anticoagulant therapy can be adjusted. Instruct to notify the physician of manifestations of bleeding, such as joint pain, easy bruising, black and tarry stools, bleeding gums, or blood in the urine or sputum.

Cardiomyopathy

Cardiomyopathy affects the structure and function of the heart muscle. Cardiomyopathies are a diverse group of disorders that often lead to heart failure. In many cases, the cause is unknown. Cardiomyopathy also may be related to another disease or condition, such as chronic alcohol abuse, myocardial ischemia, or a viral infection. Cardiomyopathies are categorized by their effects on the heart (Table 27-6 ■).

Dilated cardiomyopathy is the most common type of cardiomyopathy. The heart chambers dilate, and ventricular contraction is impaired. Manifestations develop gradually. Heart failure may develop years after the onset of dilation and pump failure. Dysrhythmias are common, increasing the risk of sudden cardiac death. The prognosis of dilated cardiomyopathy is grim; most clients get progressively worse and die within 2 years of the onset of symptoms.

Hypertrophic cardiomyopathy is characterized by hypertrophy and decreased compliance of the left ventricle. The interventricular septum tends to hypertrophy to a greater extent than the free wall of the ventricle. This impairs left ventricular filling and outflow. This may be a hereditary disorder. Sudden cardiac death may be the first sign of the disorder; manifestations can occur suddenly during or after physical

---

TABLE 27-6

Classifications of Cardiomyopathy

	DILATED	HYPERTROPHIC	RESTRICTIVE
Description	Ventricles dilate; ventricular contraction is impaired	Left ventricular hypertrophy interferes with filling and outflow	Rigidity of ventricular walls interferes with filling
Manifestations	Heart failure Cardiomegaly Dysrhythmias S_3 and S_4 heard on auscultation	Dyspnea Anginal pain Syncope Dysrhythmias Possible sudden death	Dyspnea on exertion Fatigue Heart failure S_3 and S_4 on auscultation

activity. Frequent manifestations include dyspnea, angina, and syncope.

Restrictive cardiomyopathy is the least common form of cardiomyopathy. Rigidity of the ventricular walls impairs filling, resulting in decreased ventricular size, and decreased cardiac output. The manifestations of restrictive cardiomyopathy are those of heart failure and decreased tissue perfusion. The prognosis is poor.

Medical management of cardiomyopathy focuses on minimizing heart failure, treating dysrhythmias, and preventing sudden cardiac death. Strenuous physical exertion, which may precipitate dysrhythmias and/or sudden cardiac death, is restricted. Dietary and sodium restrictions may help diminish the manifestations.

Without definitive treatment, clients with cardiomyopathy will develop end-stage heart failure. Cardiac transplant is the definitive treatment for dilated cardiomyopathy; without transplant, survival time is limited. Transplantation is not used to treat restrictive cardiomyopathy, because the underlying disease process will eventually also affect the transplanted organ. Obstructive hypertrophic cardiomyopathy may be surgically treated by resecting excess muscle away from the aortic valve outflow tract.

Nursing goals for clients with cardiomyopathies are to prevent complications, assist the client to conserve energy while encouraging self-care, and support coping skills. If surgery is done, nursing care is similar to that for any client undergoing open heart surgery or cardiac transplant (see Box 26-4). ⊂⊃

Client and family teaching focus on self-care measures such as activity restrictions, dietary changes, and drugs used to reduce symptoms and/or prevent complications. Educate about the disease process, its ultimate outcome, and treatment options. Teach clients who are undergoing invasive procedures for diagnosis or treatment about the procedure, including preparation and care following the procedure. If heart transplant is an option, provide information about the procedure and initiate preoperative teaching.

Note: The bibliography listings for this and all chapters have been compiled at the back of the book.

Chapter Review

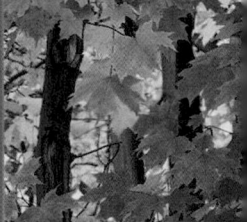

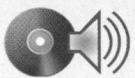 **KEY TERMS** by Topics

Use the audio glossary feature of either the CD-ROM or the Companion Website to hear the correct pronunciation of the following key terms.

Disorders of Cardiac Function
heart failure, cardiac reserve, orthopnea, acute pulmonary edema, paroxysmal nocturnal dyspnea (PND), inotropic

Inflammatory Cardiac Disorders
rheumatic fever, stenosis, regurgitation, endocarditis, myocarditis, pericarditis, pericardial friction rub, cardiac tamponade

Disorders of Cardiac Structure
valvular heart disease, cardiomyopathy

KEY Points

- Heart failure, inability of the heart to meet the body's needs for fuel and oxygen, is caused by impaired pumping of the heart. It usually is caused by extensive heart muscle damage from myocardial infarction, but also can result from inflammatory, congenital, or valve disorders.

- Any layer of heart tissue can be affected by infection or inflammation. Inflammatory disorders can lead to either structural damage or impaired cardiac function.

- Prophylactic antibiotic therapy is an important measure to prevent infective endocarditis in clients with previous heart damage or deformity.

- Pericarditis generally is a mild, self-limited disorder characterized by chest pain and a pericardial friction rub. It can, however, lead to pericardial effusion and possible cardiac tamponade, a medical emergency. Frequent assessment and prompt intervention for manifestations of muffled heart sounds and pulsus paradoxus are vital to survival of the client with cardiac tamponade.

- The aortic and mitral valves are more likely to be affected by valve disorders because of the high pressures on the left side of the heart. When these valves are affected by either stenosis or regurgitation, heart failure is likely to develop.

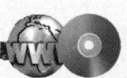 **EXPLORE MediaLink**

Additional interactive resources for this chapter can be found on the Companion Website at www.prenhall.com/burke. Click on Chapter 27 and "Begin" to select the activities for this chapter.

For chapter-related NCLEX-style review questions and an audio glossary, access the accompanying CD-ROM in this book.

FOR FURTHER Study

For nursing measures related to fluid and electrolyte imbalance, see Chapter 7.

For more about immunosuppresive drugs, see Chapter 11.

For further information about cardiac surgery, see Chapter 26.

Critical Thinking Care Map

Caring for a Client with Mitral Stenosis

NCLEX-PN® Focus Area: Reduction of Risk Potential

Case Study: Larry Schain, 68 years old, saw his physician after experiencing flulike symptoms for 2 weeks, along with increasing fatigue and shortness of breath. Laboratory testing and an echocardiogram confirmed a diagnosis of subacute bacterial endocarditis.

Nursing Diagnosis: Risk for Injury

COLLECT DATA

Subjective	Objective
_____	_____
_____	_____
_____	_____
_____	_____
_____	_____
_____	_____

Would you report this data? Yes/No

If yes, to: _____

Nursing Care

_____
_____
_____
_____
_____
_____
_____
_____
_____
_____

How would you document this? _____
_____
_____
_____

Data Collected
(use those that apply)

- History of rheumatic fever as a child
- Has had a heart murmur "for as long as I remember."
- BP 112/68, P 106, regular, R 24, T 102.6°F PO
- Loud (4 to 5/6) rumbling diastolic murmur heard over entire chest wall
- Had his teeth cleaned by dental hygienist 2 months ago
- Does not smoke; uses alcohol occasionally
- Retired, but generally very active; enjoys gardening
- Now gets short of breath walking from bedroom to kitchen
- Petechiae noted on trunk and back
- Color gray; O_2 sats 91%
- States he has lost 5 pounds during past 2 weeks and has no appetite
- Lives in his own home with his wife; school-age grandchildren live nearby
- Wife seems unconcerned; states, "he just has the flu, nothing serious."

Nursing Interventions
(use those that apply; list in priority order)

- Provide information about the heart and its structures and about endocarditis.
- Discuss prophylactic antibiotic therapy for clients with valve damage.
- Discuss prescribed outpatient intravenous antibiotic therapy.
- Teach intravenous catheter care.
- Provide analgesics as needed for comfort.
- Encourage gradually increasing activity.
- Discuss symptoms of complications to report to the physician.
- Encourage rest before and after activity/exercise.
- Provide information about community resources for emotional support.
- Help identify coping strategies for concerns about role in business.
- Schedule appointments for intravenous antibiotic infusions.

1 A client develops left-sided heart failure. An appropriate nursing diagnosis is:

A. Activity Intolerance.
B. Ineffective Airway Clearance.
C. Deficient Fluid Volume.
D. Pain.

2 A client develops right-sided heart failure. Which of the following symptoms would the nurse expect to find?

A. pulmonary edema
B. edematous legs and ankles
C. decreased heart rate
D. increased urinary output

3 The nurse is to administer digoxin (Lanoxin) 0.25 mg PO. The client's apical pulse is 48. The appropriate nursing action is to:

A. check the digoxin level and administer the drug if the level is <2 ng/mL.
B. hold the drug and recheck the apical pulse in 1 hour.
C. hold the drug and notify the physician.
D. administer the drug and report the apical pulse when the physician makes rounds.

4 A man who has been diagnosed with congestive heart failure is prescribed a low-fat, low-cholesterol, and low-sodium diet. Which of the following food items, if chosen by the client, indicates a need for further teaching?

A. baked chicken, green beans, sliced carrots
B. macaroni and cheese, smoked turkey leg, broccoli
C. grilled fish, baked potato, tossed salad
D. turkey bacon, egg white omelet, wheat toast, apple

5 A priority nursing goal for a client diagnosed with rheumatic heart disease includes:

A. determining the etiology of the disease.
B. encouraging visits from friends and family.
C. enforcing prescribed activity limitations.
D. assessing for signs of recurring streptococcal infection.

6 The nurse caring for a client with bacterial endocarditis knows that this disease

A. generally is mild and self-limiting.
B. affects the muscle layer of the heart.
C. often leads to end-stage heart failure requiring cardiac transplant.
D. usually affects clients with previous heart or valve damage.

7 A female client is diagnosed with pericarditis. The nurse expects which of the following assessment findings?

A. peripheral edema
B. wheezing breath sounds
C. absence of chest pain
D. pericardial friction rub

8 The nurse caring for a client with acute pericarditis assesses carefully for manifestations of cardiac tamponade, including

A. a distinct line of demarcation and pallor of the lower extremities.
B. a loud systolic murmur accompanied by a palpable thrill.
C. muffled heart sounds and an ausculatory gap in the blood pressure.
D. an irregularly irregular pulse of variable intensity.

9 A client is diagnosed with mitral stenosis. Discharge teaching should include all but which of the following?

A. how to auscultate heart for murmurs twice per day
B. signs and symptoms of heart failure
C. Notify physician of temperature elevation >100°F for more than 2 days.
D. Report signs and symptoms of activity intolerance to the physician.

10 Following replacement of a stenosed mitral valve with a mechanical heart valve, the nurse identifies which of the following as a high-priority nursing diagnosis?

A. Disturbed Sleep Pattern related to sound of mechanical valve
B. Ineffective Protection related to anticoagulant therapy
C. Decreased Cardiac Output related to impaired blood flow through heart valves and chambers
D. Ineffective Tissue Perfusion: Cardiopulmonary related to disruption of the coronary arteries

Answers for Review Questions, as well as discussion of Care Plan and Critical Thinking Care Map questions, appear in Appendix V.

Chapter 28

Caring for Clients with Peripheral Vascular Disorders

BRIEF Outline

Hypertension
Aneurysm
Peripheral Atherosclerosis
Arterial Thrombus or Embolism
Buerger's Disease
Raynaud's Phenomenon
Venous Thrombosis
Venous Insufficiency
Varicose Veins

LEARNING Outcomes

After completing this chapter, you will be able to:

- Relate physiology of the peripheral vascular system to common disorders affecting the peripheral vascular system.
- Describe the pathophysiology of common peripheral vascular disorders.
- Identify subjective and objective assessment data to collect for clients with peripheral vascular disorders.
- Explain the nursing implications of drugs used to treat clients with peripheral vascular disorders.
- Describe pre- and postoperative care for clients having vascular surgery.
- Reinforce client and family teaching to promote and maintain health in clients with common peripheral vascular disorders.
- Use the nursing process to provide individualized care to clients with peripheral vascular disorders.

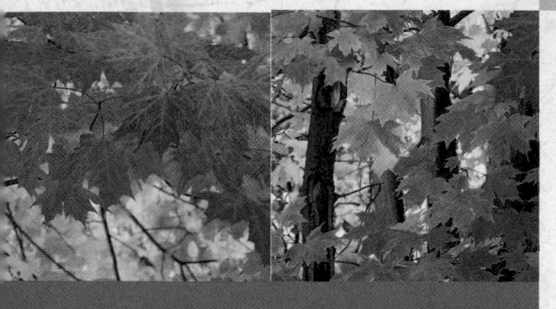

MediaLink

www.prenhall.com/burke
Use the address above to access the free, interactive Companion Website created for this textbook. Get hints, instant feedback, and textbook references to chapter-related NCLEX-style questions. Link to other interesting sites.

Audio Glossary:
Use the Companion Website, or the CD-ROM disk enclosed with your textbook, to hear the pronunciation of key terms in this chapter.

Nursing care for clients with peripheral vascular disorders focuses on relieving pain, improving peripheral circulation, preventing tissue damage, and promoting healing. A holistic approach to caring is important to address the emotional, social, and economic effects of these often chronic and potentially disabling disorders.

Several processes can affect blood vessels and interfere with peripheral blood flow: constriction, obstruction, inflammation, and spasm. When conditions such as aneurysms and varicose veins occur, the structure of the vessel itself is altered.

Hypertension

In adults, **hypertension** is defined as a blood pressure higher than 140 mm Hg systolic or 90 mm Hg diastolic on three separate readings several weeks apart. Hypertension is common, affecting about 50 million people in the United States. People over age 40 are primarily affected by this disorder; 71% of people age 80 and older are hypertensive. Box 28-1 ■ discusses hypertension in older adults. African Americans are more commonly affected than Caucasians: More than 35% of black adults are hypertensive, whereas less than 25% of whites and Hispanics have hypertension.

Hypertension is often called the "silent killer," because it has few symptoms. Its impact is significant because persistent high blood pressure can lead to brain attack (stroke), coronary heart disease, and chronic renal failure. The recognition and treatment of hypertension have significantly

---

BOX 28-2

RISK FACTORS FOR HYPERTENSION

Risk Factors That Can Be Changed

- Mineral intake
  - High sodium intake
  - Low potassium, calcium, and magnesium intake
- Obesity
- Insulin resistance
- Excess alcohol consumption
- Smoking
- Physical and/or emotional stress

Risk Factors That Cannot Be Changed

- Family history
- Age
- Race

---

improved in the past two decades. Approximately 65% of people with hypertension are effectively treated.

Hypertension is classified both by its cause and its course. **Primary** (or *essential*) **hypertension** has no identified cause, although risk factors have been identified (Box 28-2 ■). **Secondary hypertension** results from a known cause, such as kidney disease (see the section that follows).

PATHOPHYSIOLOGY

Peripheral vascular resistance is the primary factor in determining the blood pressure. In hypertension, the resistance to blood flow is increased, primarily due to constriction of the arterioles. Disruption of the physiologic mechanisms that regulate blood pressure is the underlying cause of hypertension:

- Overactivity of the sympathetic nervous system (SNS) leads to vasoconstriction and increased cardiac output.
- Overactivity of the renin–angiotensin–aldosterone system contributes to vasoconstriction, affects the excretion of salt and water, and can cause permanent changes in the arterioles.
- Other chemical mediators such as atrial natriuretic factor also affect blood vessel constriction and salt and water excretion.
- Finally, insulin resistance reduces the effects of natural vasodilator substances, affects kidney function, and increases SNS activity.

Blood volume and peripheral resistance increase as a result, leading to increased blood pressure. This increases the workload of the left ventricle. As a result, left ventricular muscle mass increases. More blood flow and oxygen are required to meet the needs of the heart, increasing the risk for coronary heart disease and heart failure. Sustained increases in blood pressure increase the rate of atherosclerosis, also increasing the risk for stroke. Blood

---

BOX 28-1   **FOCUS ON OLDER ADULTS**

Hypertension

Until recently, a gradual increase in blood pressure was thought to be normal with aging. It is now recognized that blood pressure control is as important in older adults as in the rest of the population. Changes associated with aging that can affect older adults include the following:

- *Isolated systolic hypertension* is common. It increases the risk of stroke and death due to cardiovascular disease. It develops as blood vessels become more rigid. Their ability to expand and contract decreases, and peripheral vascular resistance (PVR) increases.

- An *auscultatory gap* (temporary disappearance of sounds when measuring the blood pressure) is common. This gap can lead to inaccurate blood pressure (BP) readings if the cuff is not first inflated above the systolic pressure (see Box 28-5).

- The reflexes that maintain BP with position changes diminish. This can lead to a temporary fall in BP. When assessing for orthostatic hypotension, allow 2 to 5 minutes after position changes before measuring the blood pressure. Instruct older clients to change positions slowly, especially when rising from bed or a chair.

TABLE 28-1

Effects of Hypertension

ORGAN	EFFECT
Eyes	Retinopathy: narrowed blood vessels, hemorrhages, fluid leakage, and swelling of the optic nerve
Heart	Coronary heart disease: angina and myocardial infarction Left ventricular hypertrophy Heart failure Dysrhythmias
Vascular system	Peripheral vascular disease Aneurysms
Brain	Brain attack (stroke) Cerebral edema and changes in brain tissue
Kidneys	Renal insufficiency Renal failure

vessels in the kidneys are affected, leading to an increased risk for renal disease.

The classifications of blood pressure and stages of hypertension are:

Normal	<120/<80
Prehypertension	120–139/80–89
Stage 1	140–159/90–99
Stage 2	≥160/≥100

MANIFESTATIONS AND COMPLICATIONS

People with hypertension usually have no symptoms other than an increased blood pressure. They may complain of vague headaches or occasional dizziness. Hypertension is usually advanced when symptoms develop. These may include morning headache, blurred vision, unsteadiness, depression, and nocturia.

Without treatment, hypertension affects other organs and can lead to premature death (Table 28-1 ■).

Hypertensive Crisis

Clients with hypertension may experience *hypertensive crisis,* a rapid increase in systolic pressure to greater than 240 mm Hg and/or diastolic pressure to greater than 120 mm Hg. *Malignant hypertension* is a diastolic pressure greater than 130 mm Hg. Hypertensive crisis requires immediate treatment (within 1 hour) to prevent irreversible damage to the brain, kidneys, and heart. Clients may have manifestations such as headache, confusion, blurred vision, restlessness, and motor and sensory deficits.

clinical ALERT

Frequently monitor blood pressure (every 5 to 30 minutes) during a hypertensive emergency.

INTERDISCIPLINARY CARE

Hypertension is diagnosed by blood pressure readings. The BP is measured after resting for at least 5 minutes and avoiding caffeine and smoking for at least 30 minutes.

No specific diagnostic tests are ordered to diagnose hypertension. Laboratory tests such as urinalysis and blood chemistries (including electrolytes, glucose, and cholesterol levels) are done to identify secondary hypertension and to provide baseline data before treatment is started.

Hypertension treatment focuses on lowering the blood pressure to less than 140 mm Hg systolic and 90 mm Hg diastolic. Treatment is directed at reducing the risk of damage to the cardiovascular system and other target organs. Developing a plan of care that the client can and will follow is vital to prevent long-term complications. Although primary hypertension cannot be cured, it can be controlled with lifestyle management and medications (Table 28-2 ■).

TABLE 28-2

Recommended Follow-Up and Treatment for Hypertension

STAGE	FOLLOW-UP RECOMMENDATION	TREATMENT RECOMMENDATION
Normal (<120/<80)	Recheck in 2 years	Lifestyle modification
High-normal (120–139/80–89)	Recheck within 1 year	Lifestyle modification; medication if diabetes or kidney disease present
Stage 1 (140–159/90–99)	Confirm within 2 months	Medication plus lifestyle modification
Stage 2 (160–179/100–109)	Refer for evaluation and/or treatment within 1 month; evaluate and treat within 1 week if >180/>110	Medication plus lifestyle modification

Source: Adapted from National Institutes of Health, National Heart, Lung, and Blood Institute. (2004). *The seventh report of the Joint National Committee on prevention, detection, evaluation, and treatment of high blood pressure.* NIH Publication No. 04-5230.

BOX 28-3

THE DASH DIET

- Whole grains—7 to 8 servings daily
- Vegetables—4 to 5 servings daily
- Fruits—4 to 5 servings daily
- Nonfat/low-fat milk—2 to 3 servings daily
- Lean meat (including fish and poultry)—2 or fewer servings daily
- Nuts, seeds, and dry beans—4 to 5 servings weekly

Calories—2000 per day

Lifestyle Modifications

Lifestyle modifications to reduce blood pressure include weight loss, dietary changes, restricted alcohol use and cigarette smoking, increased physical activity, and stress reduction.

DIET. Dietary changes include limiting sodium and fat in the diet and promoting weight loss if overweight. Foods high in sodium, such as processed foods, canned fruits and vegetables, carbonated beverages, snack foods, and fast foods are avoided (see Box 7-6 in Chapter 7). ⬭ These foods are often high in fats as well, contributing to weight gain. High-sodium, high-fat foods should be replaced with foods higher in potassium and lower in fat (such as fresh fruit and vegetables, freshly cooked meats, and whole grains). The DASH (Dietary Approaches to Stop Hypertension) diet has documented benefits in reducing blood pressure (Box 28-3 ■). Calories are limited to achieve the goal of weight and body mass within normal limits.

ALCOHOL AND SMOKING. Alcohol intake is limited to no more than 1 ounce of ethanol per day. This translates to 24 ounces of beer, 10 ounces of wine, or 2 ounces of whiskey. Women and lighter weight people should reduce this limit by half. Because both smoking and hypertension increase the risk of heart disease, clients are strongly urged to quit. Smoking, which constricts the blood vessels and increases peripheral vascular resistance, reduces the benefits of some antihypertensive medications such as propranolol (Inderal).

PHYSICAL ACTIVITY. Regular exercise (such as walking, cycling, jogging, or swimming) decreases blood pressure and contributes to weight loss, stress reduction, and feelings of overall well-being. At least 30 minutes of continuous aerobic exercise most days of the week (5 or more) is recommended. Exercises that oppose one muscle group to another (isometric), however, can raise systolic blood pressure severely and may not be appropriate.

STRESS REDUCTION. Stress constricts blood vessels, raising the blood pressure. Regular, moderate exercise is the treat-

---

BOX 28-4 | **COMPLEMENTARY THERAPIES**

Hypertension

Stress management is an important part of the lifestyle changes recommended for clients with hypertension. All of the following may help reduce stress:

- Animal-assisted therapy
- Aromatherapy with ylang-ylang, clary sage, lavender, or marjoram
- Biofeedback
- Massage
- Meditation
- Qigong, a Chinese discipline of breathing and mental exercises that may be combined with arm movements (similar to t'ai chi)
- T'ai chi
- Yoga
- Herbal supplements such as garlic and hawthorn

---

ment of choice for reducing stress in the hypertensive client. Other stress reduction techniques may also benefit the client (Box 28-4 ■).

Medications

One or more of the following drug classes may be used to treat hypertension: diuretics, beta-adrenergic blockers, centrally acting sympatholytics, vasodilators, angiotensin-converting enzyme (ACE) inhibitors, angiotensin II receptor blockers (ARBs), and calcium channel blockers. Diuretics, ACE inhibitors, and ARBs reduce circulating blood volume. Diuretics often are used to treat systolic hypertension in older adults, and generally are more effective in treating hypertension in blacks. Hydrochlorothiazide (HydroDIURIL) has been proven to be effective in treating hypertension in about 50% of clients, and has the added benefit of reducing the risk for coronary heart disease. Beta blockers reduce cardiac output. Centrally acting sympatholytics and vasodilators reduce peripheral resistance. Calcium channel blockers produce vasodilation. No one primary antihypertensive drug is used to treat hypertension. A combination of drugs or a trial with a different category of antihypertensives is often used. Nursing implications for administering antihypertensive drugs (other than diuretics) are outlined in Table 28-3 ■. (See also Table 7-4 ⬭ for the nursing implications of diuretics.)

Treatment of clients with other risk factors for coronary heart disease is more aggressive to reduce the risk of an AMI, heart failure, or stroke. When the client's average blood pressure is greater than 200/120, immediate treatment is vital. Parenteral medications are given to reduce the blood pressure rapidly and prevent long-term consequences of the emergency.

TABLE 28-3

Nursing Implications for Pharmacology: Hypertension

CLASS/DRUGS	MECHANISM OF ACTION	NURSING IMPLICATIONS	CLIENT AND FAMILY TEACHING
Angiotensin-Converting Enzyme (ACE) Inhibitors ■ Benazepril (Lotensin) ■ Captopril (Capoten) ■ Enalapril (Vasotec) ■ Fosinopril (Monopril) ■ Lisinopril (Zestril) ■ Moexipril (Univasc) ■ Quinapril (Accupril) ■ Ramipril (Altace) ■ Others **Angiotensin II Receptor Blockers (ARBs)** ■ Eprosartan (Teveten) ■ Irbesartan (Avapro) ■ Candesartan (Atacand) ■ Losartan (Cozaar) ■ Valsartan (Diovan)	ACE inhibitors inhibit the renin–angiotensin system, stimulate vasodilation, and may reduce sympathetic nervous system activity. These drugs have relatively few side effects in clients with essential hypertension.	Give 1 hour before meals to increase absorption; tablets may be crushed. Report abnormal laboratory values to the primary care provider. Take blood pressure before each dose. If hypotension occurs, keep flat with legs elevated. Monitor for rash or hives. Report peripheral edema.	Report peripheral edema, infection, persistent cough, or difficulty breathing to your health care provider. Change position (lying to sitting and sitting to standing) slowly to prevent dizziness and possible falls. Do not skip doses or stop taking drugs, this could cause your blood pressure to rise significantly.
Beta-Adrenergic Blockers ■ Atenolol (Tenormin) ■ Labetalol (Normodyne) ■ Metoprolol tartrate (Lopressor) ■ Nadolol (Corgard) ■ Penbutolol (Levatol) ■ Propranolol (Inderal) ■ Timolol (Blocadren) ■ Others	Beta blockers block sympathetic input to the heart. This reduces heart rate and cardiac output. They also interfere with the renin–angiotensin system, blocking vasoconstriction. Beta blockers can have serious side effects and should not be taken by clients with asthma, COPD, or heart block.	Assess blood pressure and apical pulse before giving; notify the charge nurse if they are not within established limits. Monitor for hypotension if client is also taking a diuretic. Carefully monitor diabetic clients for hypoglycemia.	Take your pulse and blood pressure daily. Change positions slowly to prevent dizziness and possible falls. Report fatigue, lethargy, or impotence to your doctor. If diabetic, check blood glucose more frequently; this medication may block hypoglycemia symptoms. Do not stop taking the drug unless instructed to by your doctor.
Centrally Acting Sympatholytics ■ Clonidine (Catapres) ■ Guanabenz (Wytensin) ■ Guanfacine (Tenex) ■ Methyldopa (Aldomet)	These drugs slow the heart rate and reduce vasoconstriction, lowering the blood pressure. They may be given in combination with a diuretic.	Administer PO; tablets may be crushed. Methyldopa may be given IV over 30 to 60 minutes; do not give subq or IM. Apply transdermal forms to dry, hairless, intact skin on the chest or upper arm. Report rash to physician. Report abnormal laboratory values to the primary care provider. Record baseline BP, pulse, and weight; assess VS before giving drug. Report peripheral edema or other side effects to the physician.	Relieve dry mouth by sipping water or chewing sugarless gum. Use unsalted crackers, noncola beverages, or dry toast to relieve nausea. Change positions slowly to prevent dizziness and possible falls. Do not stop taking or skip doses of this drug. The drug may darken your urine. Report depression or difficulty thinking to your doctor. Side effects tend to diminish over time. Do not drive if the drug causes drowsiness.

TABLE 28-3

Nursing Implications for Pharmacology: Hypertension (continued)

CLASS/DRUGS	MECHANISM OF ACTION	NURSING IMPLICATIONS	CLIENT AND FAMILY TEACHING
Vasodilators ■ Hydralazine (Apresoline) ■ Minoxidil (Loniten)	Vasodilators reduce blood pressure by relaxing vascular smooth muscle and decreasing peripheral vascular resistance.	Administer PO with meals or food; tablets may be crushed. Assess BP and pulse before giving the drug. Monitor bowel movements. Monitor for heart failure, fluid retention, and angina.	Change positions slowly to prevent dizziness and possible falls. Eat dry toast or unsalted crackers to relieve nausea. Report muscle, joint aches, and fever to your doctor. Tearing and nasal congestion may occur. Headache, palpitations, and rapid pulse should stop in about 10 days. Do not stop this drug unless your doctor approves. Report black, tarry stools or red blood in stools to your doctor.
Alpha-Adrenergic Blockers ■ Doxazosin (Cardura) ■ Prazosin (Minipress) ■ Terazosin (Hytrin)	Alpha-adrenergic blockers promote vasodilatation, lowering blood pressure. They also reduce LDL and VLDL levels. Doxazosin and terazosin may cause tachycardia and palpitations, and other unwanted side effects. For these reasons, they are primarily used in acute situations.	Maintain safety during position changes; severe hypotension may develop. Give first dose at bedtime to reduce risk of fainting ("first-dose syncope"). Assess apical pulse and BP immediately before each dose and every 15 to 30 minutes thereafter until stable.	Use sips of water or sugarless gum to relieve dry mouth. Eat dry toast or unsalted crackers to relieve nausea. You may experience nasal congestion. Do not expect full benefit for 3–4 weeks. Change positions slowly to prevent dizziness and possible falls. Do not stop the drug without contacting your doctor.
Calcium Channel Blockers ■ Amlodipine (Norvasc) ■ Diltiazem (Cardizem) ■ Felodipine (Plendil) ■ Isradipine (DynaCirc) ■ Nicardipine (Cardene) ■ Nifedipine (Procardia) ■ Verapamil (Isoptin)	Calcium channel blockers relax arterial smooth muscle, causing vasodilatation.	If given parenterally, monitor heart rhythm continuously. Assess apical pulse and BP before giving. Notify charge nurse if outside identified limits. Monitor frequency and consistency of stools. Assess lungs for crackles and wheezes. Monitor intake and output. Assess extremities for peripheral edema.	Take BP and pulse daily. Change positions slowly to prevent dizziness and possible falls. Drink 6 to 8 glasses of water daily, and increase fiber in diet. Do not abruptly stop taking medications. Report difficulty breathing or chest pain to your doctor.

MediaLink Doxazosin

NURSING CARE

ASSESSING

Obtaining accurate blood pressure measurements is key when assessing clients with hypertension. Inaccurate readings often occur because of inappropriate cuff size or incorrect technique. Box 28-5 ■ gives guidelines that help ensure accurate blood pressure readings.

DIAGNOSING, PLANNING, AND IMPLEMENTING

Priorities in Nursing Care. The priority of nursing care for the vast majority of clients with hypertension is teaching.

BOX 28-5 | NURSING CARE CHECKLIST

Accurate Blood Pressure Measurement

☑ Choose blood pressure cuff that is the correct size: The cuff width should be about 40% of the circumference of the arm (or thigh) (see figure).

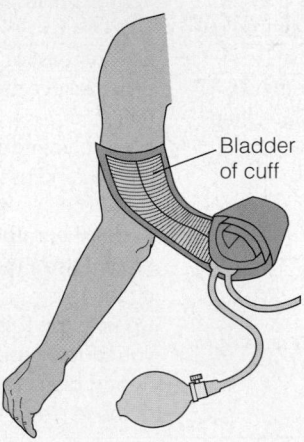

Bladder of cuff

☑ Position the cuff on the extremity with the center of the bladder directly over the artery.

☑ While palpating the artery (brachial if using the upper arm, radial if using the forearm, and popliteal if using the thigh), inflate the cuff until the pulse is no longer felt. Note the pressure and rapidly deflate the cuff. Wait approximately 1 to 2 minutes.

☑ Position the stethoscope over the artery and inflate the cuff to 30 mm Hg above the level at which the pulse was no longer felt. Slowly deflate the cuff at a rate of 2 to 3 mm Hg per second.

☑ Note the systolic reading where the first clear tapping sound (Korotkoff sound) is heard. Note the diastolic reading when the sounds change from distinct, crisp sounds to muffled sounds. In some facilities, a third reading is noted at the point where the last sound is heard.

☑ If possible, measure the pressure on both arms. If there is a difference of more than 5 to 10 mm Hg in the pressures, use the arm with the higher pressure reading for subsequent measurements because it more accurately reflects the systemic blood pressure.

Hypertension is a chronic disease that requires continuing management to prevent its complications. This responsibility falls primarily to the client.

Ineffective Health Maintenance

- Explain the physiology and significance of the blood pressure. *Many people do not understand the significance of the blood pressure and its effects on the body.*
- Emphasize the importance of adhering to prescribed treatment. *Keeping the blood pressure within normal levels reduces the risk for target organ damage.*
- Discuss lifestyle changes with all clients at risk for or with hypertension. *Lifestyle changes may help reduce the risk of hypertension and its consequences. These changes alone will not control stage 2 hypertension but may lower the amount of medication needed to maintain blood pressure within appropriate levels.*
- Discuss the relationship between sodium intake and blood pressure. Refer to dietary services for teaching about a low-sodium diet. Provide opportunities to choose low-sodium foods from simulated menus. *Knowledge and practice help clients understand and take control of their disease.*
- Discuss weight-loss strategies and a low-fat diet. If appropriate, refer the client to an approved weight-loss program (*Weight Watchers, Overeaters Anonymous, Diet Workshop*). *Many overweight clients "diet" frequently without a good understanding of nutrition. Teaching and the support of*

a weight-loss program help the client learn to make more appropriate food choices.
- Help identify realistic and appropriate lifestyle changes such as increasing exercise, stopping smoking, reducing alcohol intake, and controlling stress. *A plan that fits with the client's lifestyle is more likely to succeed. Family support is vital for maintaining lifestyle changes.*
- Help identify strengths and weaknesses in maintaining health. *Anticipating potential difficulties allows the client and family to plan strategies to overcome these hurdles.*

EVALUATING

When evaluating the effectiveness of nursing care related to hypertension, collect data to assess the client's knowledge and understanding of the disease and its treatment. Inquire about continued compliance with recommended diet, exercise, smoking cessation, and other lifestyle changes.

Documenting. Document the response to immediate treatment, if provided. Document teaching provided and referrals made (e.g., to a dietitian for dietary teaching, weight management program, or smoking cessation program), and the client's apparent understanding and acceptance of instructions.

CONTINUING CARE

Hypertension is primarily managed in community settings with regular visits to the primary care provider or hyper-

BOX 28-6	ASSESSMENT

Assessing for Discharge: Hypertension

CLIENT

- **Self-Care:** ability to prepare and eat low-sodium, low-fat, low-cholesterol diet; to engage in aerobic exercise; to manage medications
- **Knowledge:** understanding of disease, prescribed drugs, diet and activity recommendations, lifestyle changes, recommendations for follow-up care
- **Psychosocial:** support network and significant others; ability to cope with lifestyle changes (e.g., smoking cessation, limiting alcohol intake, and stress reduction)
- **Home Environment:** cooking and food storage to allow less reliance on prepared foods; exposure to secondhand smoke

FAMILY AND CAREGIVERS

- Ability and willingness to support lifestyle changes and risk factor reduction
- Financial resources for prescribed medications

COMMUNITY

- Availability of blood pressure clinics, smoking-cessation programs, alcohol treatment programs; safe environment for exercise

tension clinic to monitor treatment. Because the client is primarily responsible for managing this chronic disease, careful assessment of the resources for home care is important (Box 28-6 ■).

Stress the importance of taking medications as ordered. Discuss common side effects and their management. Inform the client that initial drug side effects may be unpleasant, but these effects diminish within 2 to 3 weeks of starting the medication. Review symptoms that should be reported to the primary care provider.

Help clients develop a realistic, regular exercise program that can be continued for life. Aerobic exercise such as walking, swimming, or cycling increases stamina and endurance, reduces stress, and helps manage obesity. Isometric activities (such as weight lifting) should be avoided unless approved by the physician, because they increase blood pressure.

Discuss the impact of stress on blood pressure. Teach stress reduction techniques such as meditation, relaxation, or deep breathing. Discuss the vasoconstrictive effects of anger and hostility, and help identify ways to diffuse these emotions. Explore alternative coping mechanisms to use during stressful situations.

Emphasize the need for regular follow-up care, even if progress is slow or if they have been unable to adhere to the plan. Comparing hypertension to diabetes, another chronic disease that requires lifelong management, may help the client and family understand the importance of continued care and follow-up.

NURSING PROCESS CARE PLAN
Client with Hypertension

Margaret Spezia is a married, 49-year-old Italian American woman with eight children, currently ranging in age from 3 to 18 years. During her annual physical examination 2 months ago, her blood pressure was found to be 146/98. Mrs. Spezia was instructed to reduce her cholesterol intake, to avoid salty foods, and not to add any salt to her foods either at the table or during cooking. An exercise program of short, daily walks was suggested for exercise and to reduce stress. She returns for follow-up.

Assessment. Lisa Christos, the clinic nurse, obtains a nursing history. Mrs. Spezia reveals that between raising their children and working part-time, she rarely gets enough rest. Although her husband has a steady job, money is tight. She admits to a steady weight gain during the past 18 years. There is no known family history of hypertension. Physical assessment data include the following: height 5'3" (160 cm); weight 225 lbs (102 kg); T 99°F (37.2°C); P 100, regular; R 16; BP 170/110 (sitting). Skin cool and dry; capillary refill 3 seconds in upper extremities. Total serum cholesterol 245 mg/dL (normal adult value <200 mg/dL). All other blood and urine studies within normal limits.

Captopril (Capoten), 25 mg by mouth twice daily, and hydrochlorothiazide, 50 mg by mouth daily, are ordered. She is placed on a low-cholesterol, no-added-salt diet.

Diagnosis. The following nursing diagnoses are identified:

- *Imbalanced Nutrition: More than Body Requirements* related to excess food intake
- *Ineffective Health Maintenance* related to lifestyle behaviors
- *Deficient Knowledge* related to lack of information about prescribed treatment

Expected Outcomes. The expected outcomes for the plan of care specify that Mrs. Spezia will:

- Lower blood pressure to less than 150 systolic and 90 diastolic within 1 week.
- Incorporate in her diet low-sodium and low-fat foods from a list provided.
- Develop a plan for regular exercise.
- Verbalize how prescribed medications, dietary restrictions, exercise, and follow-up visits will help her control her hypertension.

Planning and Implementation. The following nursing interventions are planned and implemented:

- Teach how and when to monitor her blood pressure.
- Instruct to withhold medications and contact the clinic if BP is less than 90 mm Hg systolic or 60 mm Hg diastolic.
- Provide written and verbal instructions including the name, dose, action, and side effects of antihypertensive medications.
- Help develop an exercise plan that includes a daily 15-minute walk and possible swimming classes at local YWCA.
- Discuss a realistic weight-loss goal and plan.
- Refer for dietary consultation and teaching about fat and sodium restrictions and weight loss.
- Teach stress-reducing techniques.

Evaluation. When Mrs. Spezia returns to the clinic 1 week later, her blood pressure is 142/88. She has lost 1.5 lbs and says her oldest daughter is encouraging her to join a weight-reduction program. Mrs. Spezia is walking about 20 minutes a day at a local mall. She has met with the dietitian to discuss ways to replace salt with herbs and spices. She has a list of low-fat, low-sodium foods and recommended cookbooks. Mrs. Spezia verbalizes the importance of taking her medications as ordered and managing her stress. She tells Ms. Christos, "I just can't believe that I feel better already. I've actually lost some weight—and I want to keep going. I think I can stick with this plan, even though it's like learning to cook all over again."

Critical Thinking in the Nursing Process

1. Identify factors that contributed to Mrs. Spezia's hypertension. Which were modifiable and which were not?
2. What are the reasons for reducing sodium and fat in Mrs. Spezia's diet?

3. When Mrs. Spezia returns to the clinic for a follow-up exam 6 weeks later, she admits to Ms. Christos that she has difficulty remembering to take her blood pressure medications consistently. What suggestions could Ms. Christos provide?

Secondary Hypertension

Secondary hypertension is an elevated blood pressure that can be related to an identified disorder. Although secondary hypertension accounts for only 5% of all identified cases of high blood pressure, it is important that the nurse be aware of this disorder. Elevated blood pressure readings in a young client with few identified risk factors should trigger additional diagnostic testing for unidentified disease processes.

Kidney disease is a leading cause of secondary hypertension. Kidney disease disrupts regulation of the renin–angiotensin–aldosterone system and can lead to salt and water retention. Coarctation (narrowing) of the aorta also is a common cause of secondary hypertension. The aortic narrowing reduces blood flow to the kidneys and peripheral vascular system, triggering responses that raise the blood pressure. Other conditions that can lead to secondary hypertension include pregnancy (about 10% of pregnant women are hypertensive), endocrine or neurologic disorders, or use of stimulant drugs (e.g., cocaine, amphetamines).

Diagnostic testing to identify secondary hypertension includes obtaining blood chemistries (electrolytes, glucose, lipids), urinalysis and renal function studies (see Chapter 31 ⚭ for further information), and other diagnostic tests as indicated. Secondary hypertension is primarily treated by addressing the underlying disorder. Antihypertensive drugs may be prescribed to manage the blood pressure during disease treatment.

DISORDERS OF THE AORTA

Aneurysm

An **aneurysm** is weakness and localized dilation of a blood vessel wall. Aneurysms usually affect the aorta and arteries, because of the high pressure within these vessels. Most aneurysms are caused by arteriosclerosis or atherosclerosis. Trauma and congenital weakness of a vessel also may cause an aneurysm to form.

PATHOPHYSIOLOGY

Aneurysms are commonly classified by their shape and location (Figure 28-1 ■). *Fusiform aneurysms* involve the entire circumference of the vessel. They generally grow slowly but

progressively. Their length and diameter vary considerably from client to client. *Saccular aneurysms* involve only a portion of the vessel. They are more often associated with congenital malformations or syphilis than with arteriosclerosis. *Berry aneurysms* are a common type of congenital saccular aneurysm found in a section of cerebral arteries (the circle of Willis) in the brain. *Aortic dissection* (also called a *dissecting aneurysm*) develops due to weakening of the medial layer of the aorta. Blood leaks into the vessel wall, separating the intimal (innermost) layer of the artery from the adventitia (outermost layer). Aortic dissection usually occurs in the ascending aorta.

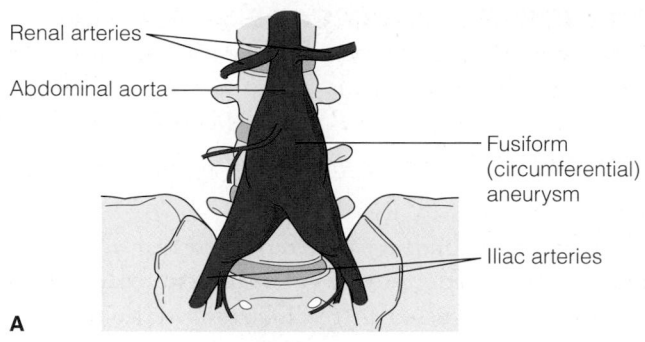

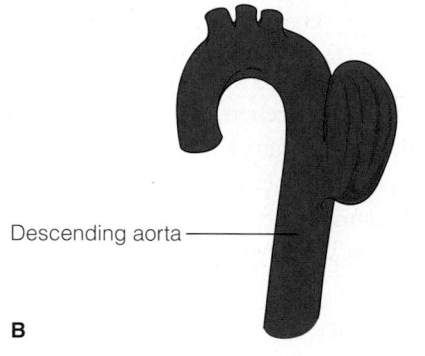

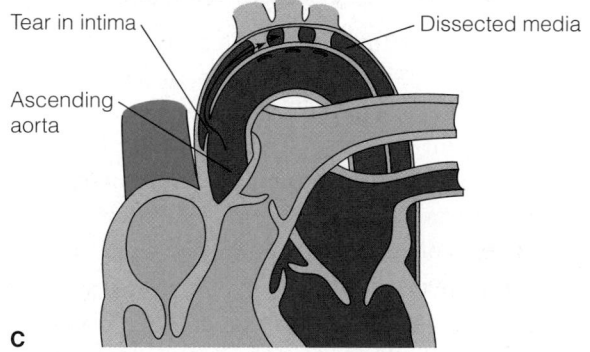

Figure 28-1. ■ Aortic aneurysms. **(A)** Fusiform aneurysm of the abdominal aorta. **(B)** Saccular aneurysm of the descending thoracic aorta. **(C)** Dissecting aneurysm of the ascending thoracic aorta.

Aneurysms often have no symptoms and are discovered during a routine physical examination. When manifestations occur, they are due to the pressure of the aneurysm on adjacent tissues and organs (Table 28-4 ■).

Thoracic Aortic Aneurysms

Thoracic aortic aneurysms frequently cause no symptoms. Substernal (anginal), neck, or back pain may occur. Pressure on the trachea, esophagus, laryngeal nerve, or superior vena cava may cause difficulty breathing, stridor, cough, difficult or painful swallowing, hoarseness, edema of the face and neck, and distended neck veins. Aneurysms of the thoracic aorta tend to enlarge progressively and may rupture, causing death.

Abdominal Aortic Aneurysms

Abdominal aortic aneurysms are associated with arteriosclerosis, hypertension, smoking, and increasing age. Most abdominal aortic aneurysms are found in adults over age 70.

Most clients with abdominal aneurysms are asymptomatic, but on examination have a pulsating mass in the mid and upper abdomen and a bruit over the mass. The client may complain of mild to severe midabdominal or lower back pain. The degree of pain commonly indicates the severity (and urgency) of the problem. Pain may be an indication of an impending rupture.

Emboli may form due to sluggish blood flow within the aneurysm and travel to the lower extremities. The aneurysm may also rupture and lead to death due to hemorrhage and hypovolemic shock.

Aortic Dissections

Dissection is a life-threatening emergency caused by a tear in the inner layer of the aorta and bleeding into the middle layer. This *dissects* or splits the vessel wall, forming a blood-filled channel between its layers. Dissection can occur anywhere along the aorta, but is most common in the ascending aorta where pressures are high.

TABLE 28-4			
Manifestations and Complications of Aortic Aneurysms			
TYPE OR LOCATION	**THORACIC**	**ABDOMINAL**	**DISSECTING**
Manifestations	Chest, back, or neck pain Dyspnea, cough Hoarseness, dysphagia Distended neck veins, edema of face and neck	Pulsating abdominal mass Abdominal or lower back pain Cool, pale, or cyanotic lower extremities	Sudden, severe chest pain Decreased blood pressure in upper extremities Absent radial pulses
Complications	Rupture and hemorrhage	Emboli to lower extremities Rupture and hemorrhage	Hemorrhage Renal failure, cardiac tamponade, sepsis

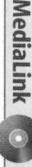

MediaLink   Video: Radial

POPULATION FOCUS

Clients with Marfan Syndrome

Marfan syndrome is a connective tissue disorder with three distinctive features: (1) long, thin extremities, hyperextensible joints, and other skeletal deformities; (2) impaired vision; and (3) cardiovascular defects, including mitral valve prolapse and weakness of the aorta with frequent aortic dissection and rupture. Marfan syndrome affects about 1 in 10,000 people. It is inherited as an autosomal dominant trait.

There is no cure for Marfan syndrome, so teaching is vital. Severe physical and emotional stress and pregnancy increase the risk of aortic dissection and cardiac complications. Encourage to avoid vigorous physical exertion and the physical stress of pregnancy. Teach measures to reduce the risk of endocarditis (see Chapter 22). Scoliosis and kyphosis are common; refer for physical therapy and bracing as needed. Stress the importance of regular eye examinations and immediate care if symptoms of retinal detachment develop (see Chapter 40). Discuss the genetic nature of Marfan syndrome: Each child has a 50% risk of being affected. Encourage consideration of alternatives such as adoption. Make referrals as appropriate.

Hypertension is a major risk factor for aortic dissection. Clients with a genetic disorder called **Marfan syndrome** are at risk for aortic dissection (Box 28-7 ■).

The primary symptom of aortic dissection is sudden, excruciating pain. Pain often is described as a ripping or tearing sensation. It is usually located in the area of dissection (e.g., anterior chest if thoracic, back if abdominal). Blood pressure may initially rise, but it falls rapidly and is often inaudible because the dissection occludes blood flow. Peripheral pulses are also absent.

INTERDISCIPLINARY CARE

Aneurysms often are detected by a *chest* or *abdominal x-ray*. An *abdominal ultrasound* is done when an abdominal aneurysm is suspected. A *CT scan* or *MRI* may be ordered to measure the aneurysm size.

Medications

Clients with aortic aneurysms often are treated with antihypertensive medications to lower blood pressure. Anticoagulant therapy (discussed in the following section) may be started to prevent emboli from forming or after surgical repair of an aneurysm.

Surgery

Surgery is done to repair aneurysms that are tender to palpation or enlarging. The client's general health and surgical risk are considered, unless immediate surgery is necessary to preserve life. In most cases, the aneurysm is excised and replaced with a synthetic fabric graft (Figure 28-2 ■). Nursing care of the client having surgery on the aorta is outlined in Box 28-8 ■.

NURSING CARE

Nurses most often care for clients with an aneurysm before and after surgical repair or treatment of an expanding or ruptured aneurysm. Clients are often highly anxious because of the urgent nature of their disorder. Managing anxiety levels is an important component of nursing care. Establish trust through active listening. Acknowledge the fears and concerns of the client and family. Use a calm demeanor, appropriate and reassuring manner, and factual

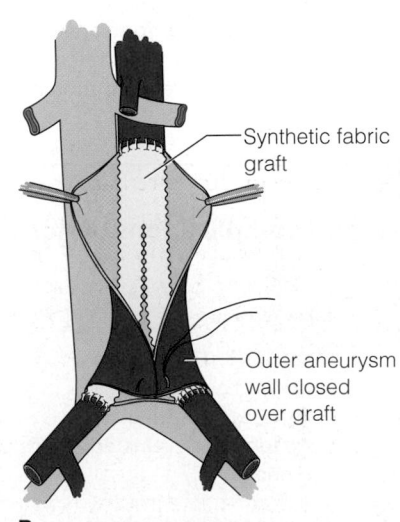

Figure 28-2. ■ Repair of an abdominal aortic aneurysm. (**A**) The aneurysm is exposed and clamped above and below the vessel dilation. (**B**) A synthetic graft is used to replace the aneurysm. The arterial wall is then sutured around the graft.

BOX 28-8	NURSING CARE CHECKLIST

Surgery of the Aorta

Before Surgery

☑ Provide routine preoperative care and teaching as time permits (see Chapter 9). ∞

☑ Orient to intensive care unit. Describe anticipated equipment, tubes, sights and sounds, and postoperative communication. Allow time for questions and to clarify information.

☑ Immediately report changes in blood pressure in upper and lower extremities, peripheral pulses, pain, abdominal girth, and sensation and movement of lower extremities.

☑ Maintain bed rest with legs flat. Instruct to avoid holding breath while moving or defecating.

☑ Report absent peripheral pulses; pale, cyanotic, or cool extremities; diffuse abdominal pain; or an increase in groin, lumbar, or lower extremity pain.

After Surgery

☑ Provide general postoperative care (see Chapter 9). ∞

☑ Monitor chest tube drainage and status as needed (see Chapter 24). ∞

☑ Frequently assess for bleeding. Immediately report signs of graft leakage such as:

   a. Bruising of scrotum, perineum, or penis; hematoma at incision

   b. Increased abdominal girth

   c. Weak or absent peripheral pulses; impaired movement or sensation of extremities

   d. Decreased blood pressure, increased pulse; low urine output (<30 mL/hr)

   e. Increased abdominal, back, or groin pain

   f. Drop in hematocrit, hemoglobin, and red blood cell levels

☑ Maintain intravenous fluids and administer blood as ordered.

☑ Report evidence of complications:

   a. *Lower extremity embolism:* pain and numbness, diminished pulses, and pale, cool, or cyanotic skin

   b. *Bowel ischemia:* blood in stools, diarrhea, severe abdominal pain, and abdominal distention

   c. *Impaired renal function:* output less than 30 mL/hr, fixed specific gravity, increasing BUN and serum creatinine levels

   d. *Spinal cord ischemia:* lower extremity weakness and paraplegia

---

explanations to keep clients calm and prevent any additional stress, which might worsen hypertension.

The nursing diagnoses and interventions described for clients with peripheral vascular disease (see the next section of this chapter) are also appropriate for the client with an aortic aneurysm: Anxiety, Pain, and Ineffective Tissue Perfusion.

CONTINUING CARE

Small or asymptomatic aneurysms often are treated conservatively. Teach measures to control hypertension, discussing diet, stress reduction, alcohol, smoking, and medications. Stress the importance of keeping blood pressure within normal limits to slow growth of the aneurysm. Emphasize the necessity of following the prescribed treatment to prevent complications.

After surgery, provide verbal and written instructions about preventing and recognizing infection, caring for the incision, taking medications to control blood pressure and prevent blood clotting, and recognizing complications. Discuss the importance of regular rest. Suggest ways to prevent constipation and straining at stool (such as increasing fluid and fiber in the diet). Instruct to avoid prolonged sitting, lifting heavy objects, exercising strenuously, and having sexual intercourse until approved by the physician (usually 6 to 12 weeks). Provide information about return appointments. Refer to a home health agency or community health service as necessary for continuing care after discharge.

PERIPHERAL ARTERIAL DISORDERS

Peripheral arterial blood flow is essential to provide oxygen and nutrients to tissues and cells. This blood flow can be affected by arterial wall defects, compression of the blood vessel, or vasospasm. Arterial disorders may be either acute or chronic. Atherosclerosis is the most common chronic peripheral arterial disorder. Other arterial disorders include arterial embolism or thrombus, thromboangiitis obliterans (Buerger's disease), Raynaud's phenomenon, and aneurysms.

Peripheral Atherosclerosis

Arteriosclerosis is a common arterial disorder characterized by thickening, loss of elasticity, and calcification of arterial walls. *Atherosclerosis* is a form of arteriosclerosis in which the arterial walls thicken and harden due to deposits of fat and fibrin (see Chapter 26). ⬭ In the peripheral circulation, arteriosclerosis and atherosclerosis decrease the blood supply to tissues, leading to peripheral vascular disease (PVD). PVD usually affects the lower extremities.

Peripheral arterial disease is more common in people over the age of 50 and is seen in men more than in women. Risk factors include a high-fat diet, hypertension, diabetes mellitus, smoking, obesity, and stress (see Chapter 26). ⬭

PATHOPHYSIOLOGY

As peripheral arteries thicken and harden because of plaque deposits, the vessel lumen narrows. Plaque tends to form at arterial *bifurcations* (where the artery divides into two smaller arteries). Peripheral plaque deposits usually affect the femoral arteries, the common iliac arteries, and the abdominal aorta. Blood flow and oxygen delivery to the distal tissues decrease. If the occlusion develops slowly, **collateral circulation** often develops (growth of small blood vessels to maintain tissue perfusion), but it is usually not adequate to supply tissue needs. Few symptoms are seen until 60% or more of the blood supply to the tissues is occluded.

MANIFESTATIONS

Pain is the primary symptom of peripheral arterial disease. One type of pain, called **intermittent claudication,** is usually described as a cramping or aching sensation in the calves of the legs or the arch of the foot. It develops with exercise such as walking, and is relieved by rest.

Rest pain, in contrast, occurs during periods of inactivity. It is a gnawing, aching, or burning sensation in the lower legs, feet, or toes. Rest pain often occurs at night. It increases when the legs are elevated and decreases when the legs are dependent (e.g., hanging over the side of the bed). Clients often complain that the legs feel cold or numb as well as painful.

The skin is pale when the legs are elevated but often dark red (*dependent rubor*) when the legs are dependent. The skin is often thin and shiny, with areas of discoloration and hair loss. The toenails may be thickened. In addition, areas of skin breakdown may be present. These may lead to ulcerations or gangrene.

Peripheral pulses often are decreased or absent. A **bruit** (a harsh or musical sound caused by turbulent blood flow) may be heard over large affected arteries, such as the femoral artery and the abdominal aorta.

The complications of peripheral arteriosclerosis include gangrene and amputation of one or both lower extremities.

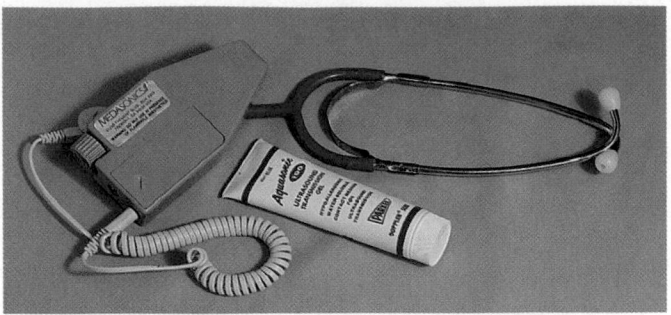

Figure 28-3. ■ A Doppler (ultrasound) stethoscope. (Photographer: Elena Dorfman.)

INTERDISCIPLINARY CARE

Management of clients with peripheral vascular disease focuses on maintaining or improving the blood supply to tissues and relieving symptoms.

Diagnostic Tests

- *Segmental blood pressures* are used to compare blood pressure measurements between the upper and lower extremities and within different portions of an extremity (e.g., the ankle and the thigh). Normally blood pressure readings should be similar when the client is supine. In PVD, the blood pressure may be lower in the legs than in the arms.
- *Exercise stress testing* (see Table 25-2) ⬭ can help identify the client's functional limitations related to PVD.
- *Doppler ultrasound studies* are done to evaluate blood flow. Low-intensity sound waves directed at the affected vessel strike moving RBCs and bounce back to the transducer–receiver (Figure 28-3 ■). Blood flow within the vessel can be evaluated by an audible sound or a graphic recording.
- *Transcutaneous oximetry* is performed to evaluate tissue oxygenation.
- *Angiography* or *magnetic resonance angiography* is performed if surgery is planned to locate and determine the extent of arterial obstruction. See Table 25-3 ⬭ and Box 26-3 ⬭ for nursing implications of angiography.

Conservative Therapy

Smoking cessation is vital in managing peripheral vascular disorders. Nicotine causes vasoconstriction, further decreasing blood supply to the extremities. Continued smoking increases the risk for ulcerations, gangrene, and amputation.

Exercise (e.g., walking for 30 to 45 minutes twice a day) is prescribed for clients with PVD. Exercise improves collateral circulation and is an effective stress management strategy. The client is taught to rest when pain develops (intermittent claudication), resuming activity when the pain is relieved.

Weight reduction improves activity tolerance. A low-fat, low-cholesterol diet is prescribed for clients with atherosclerosis.

BOX 28-9 | COMPLEMENTARY THERAPIES

Peripheral Vascular Disease

To Improve Circulation
- Aromatherapy with rosemary or vetiver
- Biofeedback
- Healing touch
- Herbs: ginkgo, garlic, cayenne, hawthorn, bilberry
- Imagery
- Magnets
- Massage
- Therapeutic touch
- Yoga

To Reduce Stress
- Aromatherapy with juniper, lavender, vetiver, ylang-ylang, or jasmine
- Breathing exercises
- Counseling
- Meditation
- Yoga

Other measures to prevent vasoconstriction and improve blood flow include keeping extremities warm and protecting them from injury, and managing stress. Complementary therapies for PVD are outlined in Box 28-9 ■.

Medications

Medications may be prescribed to reduce the risk of clotting in partially obstructed blood vessels. Aspirin, clopidogrel (Plavix), and cilostazol (Pletal) inhibit platelet aggregation, reducing the risk for clot formation. Cilostazol also acts as a vasodilator, increasing blood flow. Pentoxifylline (Trental) is another drug that may be used to improve peripheral blood flow.

Revascularization

Clients with severe intermittent claudication, rest pain, or gangrenous lesions may have a revascularization procedure to restore peripheral blood flow. Nonsurgical procedures include percutaneous transluminal angioplasty, placement of a stent, and *atherectomy* (removal of the obstructing plaque). See Box 26-3 ⚭ for nursing care of the client having a nonsurgical revascularization procedure. Surgical procedures include *endarterectomy* to remove occlusive plaque and bypass grafts. The risks associated with surgery are greater (infection, embolization, acute myocardial infarction, and stroke) than the risks associated with nonsurgical procedures. Nursing care is similar to that provided for clients undergoing surgery of the aorta (see Box 28-8).

NURSING CARE

ASSESSING

Assessment of the peripheral vascular system may focus on the chief complaint (such as swelling or pain in the legs), or may be a part of a full cardiovascular assessment (Box 28-10 ■).

BOX 28-10 | ASSESSMENT

Assessing Clients with Peripheral Vascular Disease

SUBJECTIVE DATA
- Pain: onset, relationship to activities, characteristics, severity, precipitating and relieving factors
- Other manifestations: burning, numbness, or tingling in limbs or digits; leg fatigue or cramps; ankle swelling and when it occurs; effect of temperature or position on symptoms
- Medical and family history of cardiovascular disorders, peripheral vascular disease, stroke, hypertension, hyperlipidemia, blood clots, or other chronic illnesses (e.g., diabetes); previous surgery or evaluation of blood vessels; current medications
- Usual diet, including caffeine and alcohol consumption; smoking history (in pack years) or other tobacco use; activity level, exercise habits and exercise tolerance.

OBJECTIVE DATA
- Vital signs
- Capillary refill on upper and lower extremities; strength and equality of peripheral pulses (brachial, radial on upper extremities; femoral, popliteal, posterior tibial, and dorsalis pedis pulses on lower extremities—see figure)

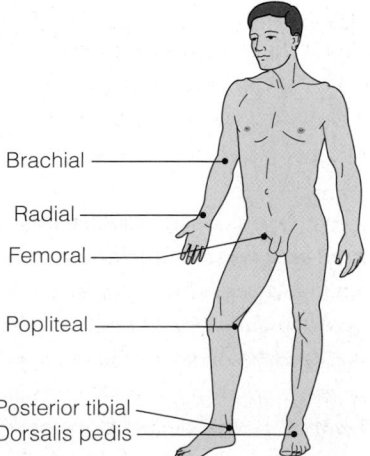

Brachial
Radial
Femoral
Popliteal
Posterior tibial
Dorsalis pedis

- Presence and degree of edema
- Skin color, temperature, texture and hair distribution on trunk, upper and lower extremities; any skin lesions or ulcers

DIAGNOSING, PLANNING, AND IMPLEMENTING

Priorities in Nursing Care. Peripheral vascular disease impairs peripheral blood flow. Managing the effects of chronic diseases such as arteriosclerosis may mean lifetime changes in activities and diet. In all cases, acute or chronic, nurses intervene to help promote blood flow and protect tissues from damage.

Ineffective Tissue Perfusion: Peripheral

■ Assess peripheral pulses, color, temperature, and capillary refill every 4 hours and as needed. If pulses cannot be felt, use a Doppler device to assess pulses. *Continuing assessment is important to detect changes in blood flow that could affect tissue integrity.*

■ Instruct client to keep extremities in a dependent position. *Gravity helps maintain arterial blood flow to distal tissues.*

■ Keep extremities warm using lightweight blankets, socks, and slippers. Do not use electric heating pads or hot water bottles. *Warmth helps prevent vasospasm and promotes arterial flow. Sensation of affected extremities may be decreased; avoid electric heating pads and hot water bottles to reduce the risk of burns.*

■ Avoid raising the knee gatch, placing pillows under the knees, or positioning with 90-degree hip flexion. *These positions may further impair peripheral blood flow.*

■ Encourage frequent position changes and remind the client to avoid crossing legs. *Changing position promotes blood flow. Leg crossing may compress arteries, leading to further compromise of circulation.*

clinical ALERT

Immediately report an extremity that has become cool or cold, pale or cyanotic, and in which pulses are very weak or absent. These are signs of complete obstruction of arterial blood flow. Immediate intervention is necessary to save the limb.

Pain

■ Assess pain level using a pain scale at least every 4 hours and more often if needed. Immediately report acute or very severe pain accompanied by a pale, cold extremity. *The pain scale helps evaluate the severity of pain and the effectiveness of relief measures. Very severe acute pain and a pale, cold extremity may indicate an arterial thrombus or embolism. Immediate treatment is vital to save the extremity.*

■ Keep extremities warm, using socks, slippers, or light blankets. *Cooling causes vasoconstriction and increases pain.*

■ Explain the relationship between smoking and pain, and assist the client in developing a plan for smoking cessa-

tion. *Smoking causes vessel constriction and spasm, increasing the pain of PVD.*

■ Provide time to discuss issues related to pain. Assist to refocus on positive aspects of life rather than on the pain. *Expressing concerns about pain reduces anxiety and may help relieve pain.*

■ Teach stress reduction and pain relief measures such as relaxation, meditation, and guided imagery. *Stress increases vasoconstriction and pain. Many nonpharmacologic techniques may be used to relieve stress and minimize pain.*

Impaired Skin Integrity

■ Assess skin of extremities at least every 8 hours and more often if needed. Report changes to the charge nurse or physician. *Clients may be unaware of accidental injury or skin damage. Early identification helps prevent complications.*

■ Provide meticulous leg and foot care daily, using mild soaps and moisturizing lotions. *Proper skin care helps prevent drying and cracking, reducing the risk of skin breakdown and infection. Once the skin is broken, the warm, moist, dark tissues of the injured extremity provide an excellent medium for bacterial growth.*

■ Use a foot or bed cradle to prevent linens from rubbing against or putting pressure on extremities. *A cradle provides warmth while avoiding pressure on injured or damaged tissues.*

Evaluating

To evaluate the effectiveness of nursing care for a client with peripheral vascular disease, collect data such as strength and equality of peripheral pulses and capillary refill; skin color, temperature, and condition of extremities; reports of pain and its relief; and evidence of bleeding.

Documenting. Document subjective data such as complaints of pain, its relationship to position or activity, or unusual sensations in the affected extremity. Regularly document strength and equality of peripheral pulses, color, temperature, and movement of affected extremities, skin condition, and any changes that occur in response to treatment.

CONTINUING CARE

Teach measures such as exercise to help manage peripheral vascular disease. Stress the importance of smoking cessation. Provide a referral to smoking-cessation classes and encourage the client to discuss alternative methods of nicotine withdrawal with physicians. Teach care of the legs and feet, as described in Box 28-11 ■.

Provide information about progressive exercise and its benefits for peripheral circulation. Discuss stress reduction, medications, and ways to keep the extremities warm. Provide a list of resources such as support groups, public health services, and other community agencies.

Leg and Foot Care for Clients with Peripheral Vascular Disease

- Keep legs and feet clean, dry, and comfortable.
  - Wash legs and feet daily using a mild soap and warm water.
  - Pat dry with a soft towel; do not rub, and be sure to dry between toes.
  - Apply lotion that does not contain alcohol to dry, scaly skin.
  - Use powder on feet and between toes.
  - Buy shoes in the afternoon (when feet are largest). Never buy shoes that are uncomfortable. Be sure the toes have adequate room.
  - Wear a clean pair of cotton socks each day.
- Prevent accidents and injuries to the feet.
  - Always wear shoes or slippers when getting out of bed.
  - Walk on level ground and avoid crowds, if possible.
  - Do not go barefoot.
  - Inspect legs and feet daily. Use a mirror to examine the backs of your legs and the bottoms of your feet.
  - Have a professional foot care provider trim toenails and care for corns, calluses, ingrown toenails, or athlete's foot.
  - Always check the temperature of bath water before stepping into the tub.
  - Use sunblock on your legs and the tops of your feet.
  - Report increased pain, cuts, bruises, blistering, redness, or open areas on your legs or feet to your health care provider.
- Improve blood supply to the legs and feet.
  - Do not cross your legs when sitting or in bed.
  - Do not wear garters or knee stockings.
  - Do not go swimming in cold water.
  - Do not smoke cigarettes or inhale passive smoke.
  - Walk until you develop pain, stop for 3 minutes, then resume walking until fatigued. Do this eight times a day.
  - Take medications as prescribed.

If surgery is planned, provide preoperative teaching as outlined in Chapter 9. ⚭ Discuss expected postoperative measures such as anticoagulant drugs, diet and activity restrictions, and risk factor reduction strategies. Prior to discharge, teach the signs and symptoms of postoperative wound infection and other manifestations that should be reported to their physician. Stress the importance of regular follow-up care.

OLDER ADULTS AND PVD

Blood vessels thicken and become less compliant with age. These changes reduce oxygen delivery to tissues, and impair the removal of carbon dioxide and waste products. Impaired vision may make it more difficult for an older adult to provide careful and safe foot care. Long-standing smoking addiction is difficult to break. The client who lives alone may resist walking. Home and community safety are additional concerns. It is often helpful to arrange periodic visits by a community health or home health nurse. Encourage the client to join a support group for stopping smoking, changing eating habits, and taking part in regular activity.

Arterial Thrombus or Embolism

An acute arterial thrombus or embolism may develop, often as a complication of another disease, occluding blood flow through the artery.

Atherosclerotic changes in blood vessels can cause a **thrombus,** or blood clot, to develop. If the blood clot breaks away from the vessel wall and moves, it becomes an **embolus.** Foreign matter such as fat, bacteria, amniotic fluid, and air bubbles also may become emboli. An embolus eventually lodges in a vessel that is too small to allow it to pass through. Both thrombi and emboli block blood flow through the affected vessel to distal tissues. When arterial flow is interrupted, tissue necrosis and gangrene may result. Manifestations of arterial occlusion by a thrombus or embolus are listed in Box 28-12 ■. A clear line between normal and pale, cold skin may be noted with an embolus.

Buerger's Disease

Buerger's disease (thromboangiitis obliterans) is an occlusive disease of small and medium-sized peripheral arteries. Affected vessels become inflamed, spastic, and thrombotic. It usually affects a leg or foot, although either the upper or lower extremities can be affected.

Buerger's disease primarily (95%) affects men under the age of 40 who smoke. It is more commonly seen in people of Asian or Eastern European descent. Cigarette smoking is the single most significant cause. There also may be a genetic link.

The course of the disease is intermittent, with episodes of pain and impaired blood flow, and periods of remission. It may be dormant for weeks, months, or years. As the disease progresses, arteries become more widely involved, and episodes are more intense and longer. The risk of tissue ulceration and gangrene increases.

BOX 28-12

MANIFESTATIONS OF ARTERIAL THROMBOSIS OR EMBOLUS

- Pain in the affected area; may be sudden or insidious
- Numbness or tingling of affected extremity
- Coldness of the extremity
- Pallor or mottling of the skin
- Absent pulses distal to the blockage
- Muscle weakness or spasms
- Possible paralysis

MANIFESTATIONS

Pain in the involved extremity is the major symptom of Buerger's disease. The client complains of cramping pain in the instep of the foot or the calves of the legs that is relieved by rest (intermittent claudication), or of rest pain in the fingers and toes. Smoking, cold, and emotional distress often trigger burning pain.

The involved digits and/or extremities are pale, and cool or cold to the touch. The skin may be shiny and thin, and the nails are often thick and malformed. Distal pulses often are either difficult to locate or absent, even when a Doppler device is used (Figure 28-3). *Rubor* (redness) is intense when the extremity is dependent.

Raynaud's Phenomenon

Raynaud's phenomenon is characterized by spasms of the small arteries and arterioles of the extremities. The arterial spasms limit blood flow to the fingers and, on occasion, to the toes, ears, or nose. Raynaud's phenomenon is often secondary to another disorder. When the cause is unknown (*idiopathic*), it is known as *Raynaud's disease.* In either case, it almost always affects women between the ages of 15 and 45. A genetic predisposition may have some part in this disease.

MANIFESTATIONS

The signs and symptoms of Raynaud's occur intermittently, often following exposure to cold or work-related vibration. The attacks tend to become more frequent and prolonged. Raynaud's has been called the blue–white–red disease. Vasospasm causes the fingers to first turn blue, then white as blood flow is severely limited, and finally very red as the fingers are warmed and the spasm resolves. Numbness, stiffness, decreased sensation, and aching pain may accompany the color changes.

INTERDISCIPLINARY CARE

Immediate diagnosis and treatment are necessary to save the limb affected by an acute arterial occlusion such as a thrombus or embolus. The diagnosis generally can be made through physical examination; in some cases angiography may be done to localize the obstruction. Fibrinolytic therapy may be administered to break up the clot or embolus, and anticoagulant therapy initiated to prevent further clot formation (see Chapter 26 ⚭ for nursing care related to fibrinolytic therapy). Surgery may be done to remove an obstruction, thrombus, or embolus. Acute arterial embolus requires emergency surgery to restore blood flow and prevent gangrene.

The diagnosis and management of chronic arterial disorders such as Buerger's disease and Raynaud's disease are similar to that for peripheral vascular disease (see the preceding section).

Smoking cessation is vital in all types of peripheral vascular disease. Attacks of Buerger's disease increase in severity and duration with continued smoking. Regular exercise is an important disease management strategy as well; walking for 30 or more minutes several times a day is recommended. The extremities should be kept warm to reduce the incidence of vasospasm. Clients with Raynaud's disease are taught to keep the hands warm, wearing gloves when outside in cold weather and when handling cold items (e.g., frozen foods). Measures to avoid injury to the hands and feet are taught (see Box 28-11 for foot care for clients with PVD).

Amputation is necessary if blood flow cannot be restored and tissue necrosis has occurred. As much healthy tissue as possible is saved, so only part of a limb or digit may be amputated. A below-the-knee amputation is sometimes done for gangrene of the lower leg or for foot pain that cannot be relieved.

NURSING CARE

Nursing assessment and care for the client with Buerger's disease or Raynaud's disease are similar to that provided for the client with peripheral atherosclerosis. Assessment data to be collected on a continuing basis include complaints of pain and its relationship to activity or other factors (such as cold or position changes). Regular assessment of the strength and equality of peripheral pulses, color and temperature of the affected extremity, and condition of the skin is vital for clients with acute or chronic peripheral arterial disorders.

Teaching for continuing care is a vital nursing activity for these clients, because the client is primarily responsible for managing the disorder. Refer to a smoking cessation program or support group. A cardiovascular rehabilitation program may be appropriate to promote physical activity and provide continuing support.

In addition to the nursing diagnoses and interventions identified in the section on peripheral atherosclerosis, Ineffective Protection is an appropriate focus for nursing care of the client with an acute arterial occlusion.

Ineffective Protection

Fibrinolytic drugs or anticoagulants may be given to dissolve or prevent clots. These drugs interfere with normal clotting, increasing the risk for bleeding.

- Report evidence of bleeding, such as excessive bleeding from incisions or injection sites, bleeding from gums or nose, hematuria, or multiple bruises, petechiae, purpura, or ecchymoses. *Rapid identification and treatment of bleeding can prevent significant blood loss.*

■ Report abnormal hemoglobin and hematocrit levels, and activated partial thromboplastin time (APTT), prothrombin time (PT), and INR values greater than the target therapeutic range. *Low hemoglobin and hematocrit levels may indicate undetected bleeding. APTT and PT times are prolonged by anticoagulant therapy. The therapeutic range is from 1.5 to 2 times normal.*

VENOUS DISORDERS

Because the pressure is lower and blood flow is slower in the veins than in the arteries, blood can stagnate or pool. As a result, clots may form, leading to inflammation and obstruction of the vessel. Repeated episodes can lead to chronic venous insufficiency. Three of the most common disorders of venous circulation are venous thrombosis, venous insufficiency, and varicose veins.

Venous Thrombosis

Venous thrombosis occurs when a blood clot (*thrombus*) forms on the wall of a vein and partially or completely blocks blood flow back to the heart. Because inflammation often accompanies the clot, the term *thrombophlebitis* often is used (*thrombo* = clot; *phlebo* = vein; *-itis* = inflammation). Either deep or superficial veins may be affected. **Deep venous thrombosis (DVT)** is a common complication of immobility or surgery.

A number of risk factors have been identified for venous thrombosis (Box 28-13 ■). There is an increased risk in people with impaired heart function, older clients, and people with certain cancers. The major complications of thrombophlebitis are chronic venous insufficiency and pulmonary embolism.

PATHOPHYSIOLOGY

Small, localized clots may develop in small veins. In larger veins, extensive thrombi may form. Three pathologic factors, called *Virchow's triad,* are associated with thrombosis: *venous stasis* (sluggish blood flow), increased blood coagulability, and vessel wall injury.

Damage to the lining of a vein attracts platelets to the area, especially if venous stasis is present, and a clot or thrombus develops. The thrombus may partially or totally block blood flow through the vein. Venous blood returns to the heart through collateral vessels. The thrombus may break loose or fragment, becoming an embolus. Emboli from venous clots tend to lodge in the vessels of the pulmonary vascular system.

Deep Venous Thrombosis

The deep veins of the legs, especially in the calf, and of the pelvis provide the best environment for thrombus formation (Figure 28-4 ■). Most thrombi originate in the vessels of the calf.

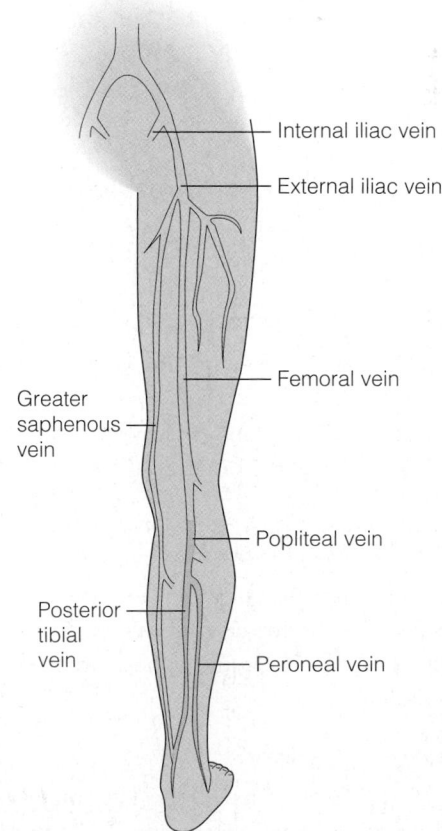

Figure 28-4. ■ Common locations of deep venous thrombosis.

BOX 28-13

RISK FACTORS FOR VENOUS THROMBOSIS

■ Previous venous thrombosis
■ Prolonged immobility, leg paralysis
■ Major general surgery or trauma
■ Myocardial infarction, heart failure
■ Cancer of the breast, pancreas, prostate, or ovary
■ Pregnancy or childbirth
■ Estrogen therapy, oral contraceptives, especially in women who smoke
■ Obesity

MANIFESTATIONS OF DEEP AND SUPERFICIAL VENOUS THROMBOSIS

Deep Venous Thrombosis (DVT)

■ Dull, aching pain, tenderness in affected extremity
■ Pain aggravated by walking
■ Increased calf size
■ Cyanosis
■ Positive Homans' sign
■ Slightly elevated temperature; general malaise

Superficial Venous Thrombosis (SVT)

■ Dull, aching pain over affected vein
■ Redness and warmth along affected vein
■ Palpable cordlike structure

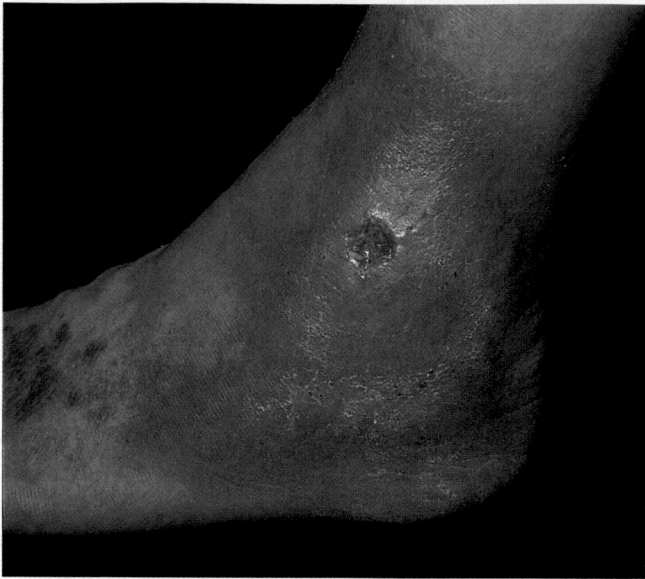

Figure 28-5. ■ Chronic venous insufficiency. Note the discoloration of the ankle and the stasis ulcer. (*Source:* Camera M.D. Studios, Carroll H. Weiss, Director, 8290 N.W. 26th Place, Sunrise, FL 33322.)

MANIFESTATIONS. Deep venous thrombosis may cause calf pain and muscle tenderness. The client may experience dull, aching pain in the leg, particularly when walking. The calf is enlarged and the affected leg may be slightly cyanotic. An elevated temperature and general malaise may be present. A *positive Homans' sign* (pain in the calf when the foot is dorsiflexed) may be noted, but it is not specific to DVT.

COMPLICATIONS. Pulmonary embolism is a serious, potentially fatal complication of DVT. Most pulmonary emboli arise in the proximal leg veins (above the knee). Pulmonary embolism is discussed in Chapter 24.

Superficial Venous Thrombophlebitis

Thrombophlebitis of the arm veins is a common complication of trauma to the vein wall caused by venous catheters, repeated venous punctures, or intravenous solutions that irritate and inflame the vein. Superficial venous thrombi are also found in pregnant or postpartum women, but the cause is unknown.

The clinical manifestations of superficial and deep venous thrombosis are listed in Box 28-14 ■.

Venous Insufficiency

Chronic **venous insufficiency** is *stasis* (stagnation) of venous blood flow in the lower extremities. Chronic venous insufficiency often results from venous thrombosis and incompetent venous valves.

PATHOPHYSIOLOGY

Following DVT, large veins of the legs may remain occluded, increasing pressure in the smaller vessels. This increased pressure distends the veins, preventing closure of

the valves. The valves also may be damaged by DVT. When valves in the veins of the legs become *incompetent* and fail to close, the muscle-pumping action on veins during activity cannot move blood back to the heart. The blood collects and stagnates in the lower leg. This further increases pressure in the veins, leading to congestion and edema of leg tissue. Edema develops in the lower leg, and the leg and foot become darkly colored. Subcutaneous tissue changes make the leg and foot feel hard or firm to palpation.

As the congestion worsens, the body is unable to provide adequate oxygen and nutrients to the cells. Eventually, cells begin to die, forming venous stasis ulcers (Figure 28-5 ■). As the condition worsens, the ulcers enlarge. The impaired circulation also increases the risk of wound infection.

MANIFESTATIONS

Skin around stasis ulcers appears shiny, atrophic, and cyanotic. The color of the skin is brownish. Scar tissue commonly forms, causing the affected area of the leg to feel hard and somewhat leathery to the touch, but even the slightest trauma to the area can lead to serious tissue breakdown.

INTERDISCIPLINARY CARE

Prevention is important to reduce the complications of venous thrombosis (see below). When thrombosis develops, treatment is started to prevent further clots from forming, to treat inflammation, and, in some cases, to dissolve existing clots.

Diagnostic Tests

- *Duplex venous ultrasonography* is used to visualize the vein and blood flow through it.
- *Plethysmography* is often used in conjunction with Doppler ultrasonography to measure the volume of fluid passing through the veins.
- *Magnetic resonance imaging (MRI)* also may be used to detect DVT, particularly in the pelvic veins or venae cavae.
- *Ascending contrast phlebography (or venography)* uses a contrast medium injected into the veins of the leg to identify the location and extent of thrombophlebitis. It is the most accurate diagnostic test for venous thrombosis.

The nursing implications for commonly used diagnostic tests are outlined in Table 25-3.

Medications

Nonsteroidal anti-inflammatory agents (NSAIDs) such as indomethacin (Indocin) or naproxen (Naprosyn) are used to reduce inflammation in clients with thrombophlebitis. Anticoagulant therapy is use to prevent and to treat DVT.

ANTICOAGULANTS. Low-molecular-weight (LMW) heparin is given to clients undergoing orthopedic and other surgeries and to people on prolonged bed rest to prevent venous thrombosis. Anticoagulants are ordered for clients with deep venous thromboses to prevent expansion of the clot and possible pulmonary embolism.

Anticoagulation is started with intravenous or subcutaneous heparin. If a heparin infusion is ordered, an infusion pump should always be used, and the dose should be checked every hour. Anticoagulation is monitored using a blood test, the *activated partial thromboplastin time (APTT)*. The heparin dosage is adjusted so that the APTT is 1.5 to 2 times the normal value. LMW heparin is administered subcutaneously once or twice per day, and does not require the close laboratory monitoring of unfractionated heparins. LMW heparins also are more effective and have lower risk of bleeding, making them the drug of choice.

Oral warfarin is initiated while the client continues to receive heparin. This overlap of therapy is important because the full anticoagulant effect of warfarin is delayed. The *prothrombin time (PT)* or *International Normalized Ratio (INR)* are used to assess the effect of warfarin on clotting. The dosage is adjusted to achieve a PT that is 1.5 to 2.5 times greater than the normal value or an INR of 2.0 to 3.0.

Once this level is achieved, a maintenance dose of warfarin is continued for 2 to 4 months. Anticoagulant treatment (Table 28-5 ■) may be extended if a complication such as pulmonary embolus has occurred. Regular follow-up is important to monitor coagulation.

FIBRINOLYTICS. Fibrinolytic (thrombolytic) drugs dissolve blood clots in the body. They may be used to destroy venous thrombi and prevent additional damage to venous valves. Fibrinolytic therapy, however, increases the risk of bleeding and hemorrhage. Box 26-8 ⚭ reviews nursing care related to fibrinolytic drugs.

Conservative Therapy

Whenever possible, prevention is key. Elastic stockings and pneumatic compression devices are ordered for postoperative clients, people who are immobile for long periods, and for clients who cannot tolerate anticoagulants. Leg exercises

---

TABLE 28-5

Nursing Implications for Pharmacology: Anticoagulants

DRUGS	MECHANISM OF ACTION	NURSING IMPLICATIONS	CLIENT AND FAMILY TEACHING
Heparin sodium	Heparin (also called *unfractionated heparin*) interferes with normal clotting, preventing the formation of new clots and the extension of existing clots.	May be given by intravenous or subcutaneous routes. Check dose with a second licensed person before giving. SC: Administer deep into SC tissue, rotating sites in the lower abdomen. Do not aspirate or massage. IV: Use an infusion pump for continuous infusions; do not mix with other drugs. Report signs of bleeding: bleeding gums, nosebleed, bruising; black, tarry stools; hematuria. Test stools for occult blood. Monitor APTT, platelet count, hemoglobin, and hematocrit. Report results outside the expected range.	Report any unusual bleeding or bruising to your health care provider. Do not take any drugs containing aspirin or NSAIDs while on heparin therapy. Avoid activities that increase your risk of injury. Use a soft toothbrush and electric razor while you are receiving heparin. Tell all health care providers that you are on heparin therapy, and carry an identification card with you at all times.

(continued)

TABLE 28-5

Nursing Implications for Pharmacology: Anticoagulants (continued)

DRUGS	MECHANISM OF ACTION	NURSING IMPLICATIONS	CLIENT AND FAMILY TEACHING
Low-molecular-weight heparins ■ Ardeparin (Normiflow) ■ Dalteparin (Fragmin) ■ Enoxaparin (Lovenox) ■ Tinzaparin (Innohep)	LMW heparins (a shorter form of the heparin molecule) produce the same anticoagulant effect as heparin with less adverse effects. Their response is more predictable, reducing the frequency of laboratory testing.	Assess for and report evidence of active bleeding, history of bleeding disorders, sensitivity to heparin, sulfites, or pork. Check dose with a second licensed person before giving. Administer deep into SC tissue, rotating sites in the abdominal wall, thigh, or buttocks. Do not aspirate or massage. Monitor for masked or hidden bleeding. Bleeding may occur despite normal PT and APTT results. Teach subcutaneous injection technique. Have client and family return demonstration of SC injection.	Administer subcutaneously as taught. Take the medication as directed by your physician. Note where administered, and rotate sites as directed. Do not rub the site after the injection to minimize bruising. Do not take aspirin, NSAIDs, or other over-the-counter drugs unless recommended by your doctor. Promptly report excessive bruising or bleeding, chest pain, difficulty breathing, itching, rash, or swelling to your doctor. Keep appointments with your doctor and for lab testing as scheduled.
Warfarin (Coumadin)	Interferes with synthesis of clotting factors, preventing clot formation. Requires 3–5 days to reach effective levels.	Give at the same time each day. Report signs of bleeding: bleeding gums, nosebleed, bruising; black, tarry stools; hematuria. Test stools for occult blood. Monitor PT or INR, CBC, and liver function studies. Report results outside the expected range. Drug interactions are common; monitor carefully when new drugs are added to medication regimen or other drugs are discontinued.	Take the drug as ordered. If you miss a dose, take it as soon as you remember that day. Do not double your dose. Limit your intake of foods rich in vitamin K (asparagus, beans, broccoli, brussel sprouts, cabbage, cauliflower, cheeses, fish, greens, milk, pork, rice, spinach, turnips, yogurt). Report any unusual bleeding or bruising to your doctor. Do not drink alcohol or take drugs containing aspirin or NSAIDs. Use a soft toothbrush and electric razor. Tell all health care providers that you are taking an anticoagulant, and carry an identification card with this information with you at all times. Keep all follow-up appointments for lab work and with your doctor.

and early ambulation are ordered after surgery to minimize venous stasis. Teach clients not to cross their legs, to wear loose-fitting garments, and to incorporate exercise into their daily schedule.

Warm, moist compresses are applied over a superficial venous thrombosis to relieve symptoms. Clients with DVT may be placed on bed rest until the symptoms of tenderness and edema resolve.

The legs are elevated, with the knees slightly flexed, above the level of the heart to promote venous return and discourage venous pooling. Elastic antiembolism stockings (compression stockings or TED hose) or pneumatic compression devices are often ordered to simulate the muscle-pumping mechanism that promotes blood return to the heart. When permitted, ambulation is encouraged with the caution to avoid prolonged standing or sitting that may contribute to venous stasis.

Stasis Dermatitis and Stasis Ulcer Care

Stasis dermatitis may be treated with wet compresses with boric acid, Burow's solution, or isotonic saline four times daily, for 1-hour intervals. Following the wet compress, topical ointments (such as 0.5% hydrocortisone cream) are applied. Other topical agents such as zinc oxide ointment or broad-spectrum antifungal agents may also be ordered.

Stasis ulcers may be treated with saline compresses or a semirigid boot applied to the foot and lower leg. This device may be made of Unna's paste or Gauzetex bandage. Bony

MediaLink Warfarin

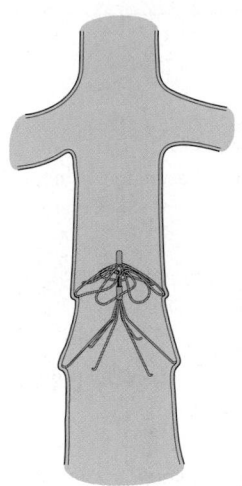

Figure 28-6. ■ A vena caval filter to trap emboli from the pelvis and lower extremities.

prominences must be well padded. The boot is changed every 1 to 2 weeks, depending on the amount of drainage from the ulcer. This device often allows ambulatory treatment. Once the ulcer is healed, a heavy elastic stocking is worn to promote adequate venous return and to prevent ulcer recurrence.

Surgery

Surgery may be done to remove a venous thrombus or to prevent complications such as a pulmonary embolism. A venous

thrombectomy may be done to remove the clot. A filtering device may be inserted into the inferior vena cava via the femoral or jugular vein. This umbrella-like device captures venous thrombi, preventing pulmonary emboli (Figure 28-6 ■).

NURSING CARE

Nurses play a vital role in identifying clients at risk for venous thrombosis, preventing it from occurring, and collecting data to evaluate the effectiveness of treatment.

ASSESSING

Assessment for problems of venous circulation is not limited to clients with diagnosed venous thrombosis, but also includes all clients who are at risk. Box 28-15 ■ outlines subjective and objective assessment data related to venous circulation. (See Table 28-6 ■ for assessment of peripheral edema.)

DIAGNOSING, PLANNING, AND IMPLEMENTING

Priorities in Nursing Care. Preventing venous thrombosis is an important nursing care responsibility. Early ambulation of post-surgical clients, encouraging frequent leg exercises,

---

BOX 28-15 | **ASSESSMENT**

Assessing Clients with Venous Thrombosis

SUBJECTIVE DATA

- Describe any leg pain, including characteristics, intensity, timing (with activity, when standing or sitting for prolonged periods, at rest), aggravating and relieving factors, and any associated manifestations.
- Inquire about ankle swelling, its timing (end of day, after sitting or standing for prolonged periods), extent, effect of temperature; use of support stockings.
- Past history of cardiovascular disorders, peripheral vascular disease, blood clots, or chronic conditions; heart or vascular surgery; cancer.
- Diet, exercise, and smoking history; occupational factors such as prolonged standing or sitting.

OBJECTIVE DATA

- Skin of extremities, particularly legs and feet: color, texture, and hair distribution; presence of ulcers (particularly over the medial malleolus) or irritation; healing.
- Venous pattern on hands, arms, and legs.
- Note edema; grade as 1+ to 4+ (see Table 28-6) if present.

- Palpate calves for tenderness, warmth, swelling; presence of cords.
- If indicated, check Homans' sign: Dorsiflex the foot while holding knee flat or slightly flexed (see figure). Calf pain with dorsiflexion of the foot (positive Homans' sign) may indicate venous thrombosis.

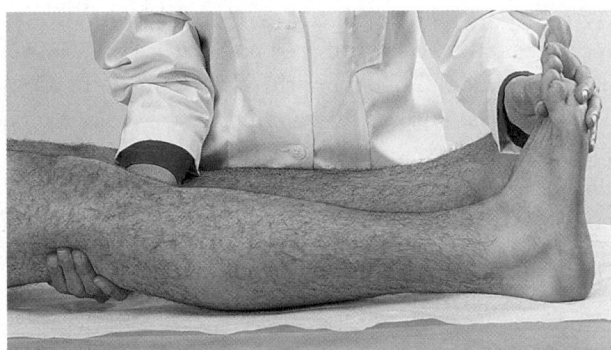

(Photographer: Richard Tauber.)

- Measure leg circumference at forefoot, above ankle, calf, and midthigh.

TABLE 28-6
Evaluating Edema

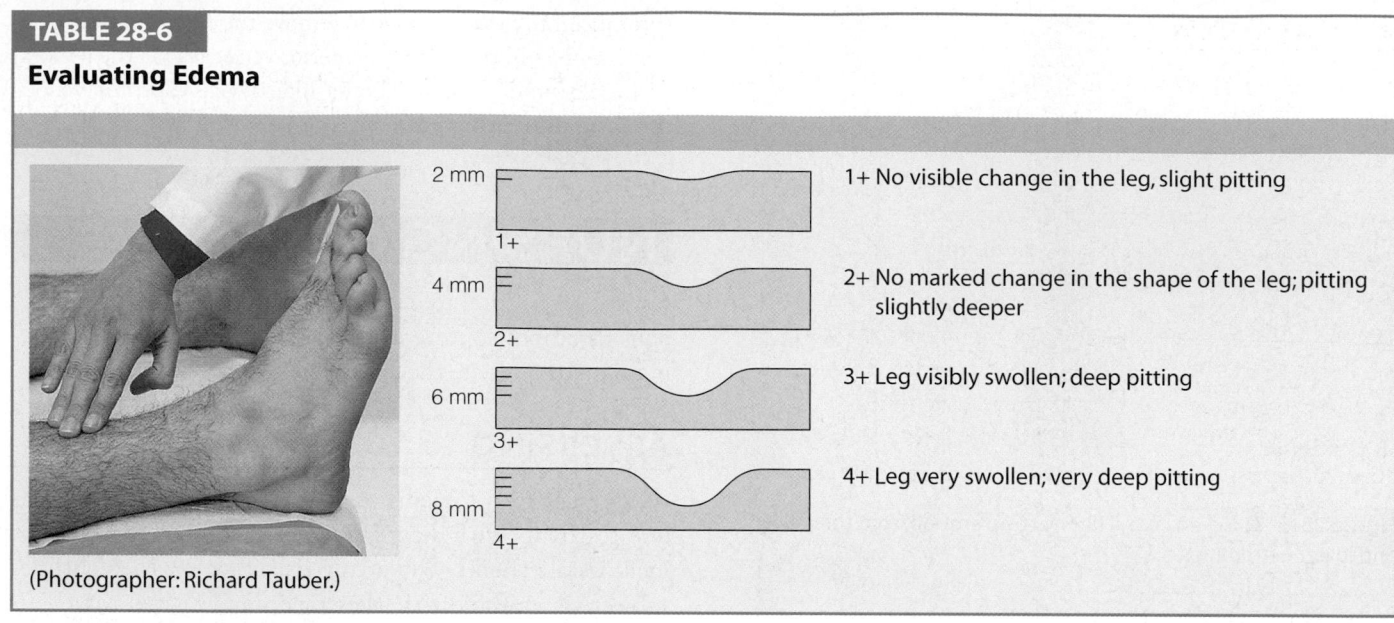

2 mm / 1+	1+ No visible change in the leg, slight pitting
4 mm / 2+	2+ No marked change in the shape of the leg; pitting slightly deeper
6 mm / 3+	3+ Leg visibly swollen; deep pitting
8 mm / 4+	4+ Leg very swollen; very deep pitting

(Photographer: Richard Tauber.)

positioning, and maintaining ordered devices such as compression hose (TED stockings) and pneumatic compression devices are nursing care measures that help maintain peripheral circulation and prevent DVT.

Ineffective Tissue Perfusion: Peripheral

- Assess peripheral pulses, skin integrity, capillary refill, and color of the extremities at least every 8 hours. Report changes promptly. *Swelling from obstructed venous blood flow can impair arterial circulation to the tissues, increasing the risk for ischemia and necrosis.*
- Measure calf and thigh diameter on the affected extremity on admission and daily thereafter. Report increases. *As venous thrombosis resolves, the diameter will decrease. Increased diameters may indicate further inflammation.*
- Elevate legs, keeping knees slightly flexed. Avoid flexing hips more than 60 degrees. *Elevation promotes venous return and reduces peripheral edema. Knee flexion promotes comfort.*
- Apply antiembolic stockings or pneumatic compression devices as ordered, removing them for short periods (30 to 60 minutes) during daily hygiene. *Antiembolic stockings and pneumatic compression devices promote venous return to the heart by gently compressing the extremity.*
- Encourage frequent position changes. *Position changes help prevent further venous stasis and other complications of immobility.*
- Administer and monitor the effectiveness of anticoagulants or thrombolytic drugs as ordered. Monitor laboratory values (APTT, INR, and PT) before giving prescribed anticoagulants. Promptly report values outside the expected range. *Monitoring is vital to evaluate the effectiveness of therapy and prevent complications of treatment.*

Pain

- Regularly assess pain. Immediately report increased pain. *Venous thrombosis causes pain that is not affected by exercise or relieved by elevating the leg. Increased pain may indicate extension of the inflammation and clot.*
- Apply warm, moist heat to affected extremity at least four times daily, using warm, moist compresses or an aqua-K pad. *Heat dilates the vessels and promotes the reabsorption of edema fluid, thus improving circulation and reducing pain.*
- Maintain bed rest; explain the reason. *Using leg muscles during ambulation increases inflammation and pain.*

Impaired Skin Integrity

- Assess skin of the affected leg and foot at least every 8 hours and more often as needed. *Careful, frequent assessment allows early detection of signs of potential skin breakdown and early intervention to prevent further problems.*
- Use mild soaps, solutions, and lotions to clean the affected leg and foot daily. Avoid harsh soaps or alcohol-based solutions. Pat dry. *Gentle cleansing with mild agents helps maintain skin integrity, prevent excessive drying and itching, and prevent infection.*
- Use egg crate mattresses or sheepskin as needed. *Egg crate mattresses and sheepskin distribute the weight more equally and prevent skin breakdown and discomfort.*
- Encourage active or perform passive range-of-motion (ROM) exercises at least every 8 hours. *ROM exercises help preserve joint function, promote circulation, and prevent skin breakdown.*
- Assist with progressive ambulation as ordered. *Daily increases in activity improve circulation and increase stamina and endurance.*

EVALUATING

To evaluate the effectiveness of nursing care for venous thrombosis or venous insufficiency, assess the client's comfort, peripheral circulation (especially of the legs), and skin condition. Monitor for evidence of excessive bruising or bleeding (e.g., bleeding gums, occult blood in urine or stool), and monitor laboratory results for the client receiving anticoagulant therapy.

Documenting. Document continuing assessment data and the client's participation in activities as ordered. Document teaching about the disorder, its prevention, and, if ordered, continuing LMW or anticoagulant therapy. Document the client's (or family's) ability to safely and effectively administer LMW heparin by subcutaneous injection.

CONTINUING CARE

Clients who have experienced an episode of venous thrombosis or who have venous insufficiency often will manage their treatment after discharge. Explain the disease process and course of treatment, including:

- Ordered laboratory tests, their purposes and frequency
- Prescribed medications, including dosage, time of day to take the drug, and side effects that should be reported
- Any continuing order for heat application or wound care, including precautions to avoid burns and infection, and symptoms to report to the health care provider
- Activity restrictions and their duration
- Measures to prevent future episodes of venous thrombosis
- The importance of follow-up visits.

Reinforce teaching with written instructions, and have the client demonstrate injection technique or wound care before discharge.

Teach the following measures to reduce the risk of complications:

- Elevate legs while resting and during sleep.
- Walk as much as possible, and avoid sitting or standing for long periods of time.
- When sitting, do not cross your legs or put pressure on the back of the knees (such as when sitting on the side of the bed).
- Do not wear anything that constricts your legs (knee-high hose, garters, or girdles).
- Wear elastic hose as prescribed. Put on the hose after the legs have been elevated. The elastic hose should be tighter over the feet than at the top of the leg, and the tops should not cut into the legs.
- Keep skin on feet and legs clean, soft, and dry. Follow guidelines for care of the legs and feet (see Box 28-11).

Varicose Veins

Varicose veins are irregular, tortuous veins with poorly functioning (incompetent) valves. *Varicosities* may develop in veins anywhere in the body. In the rectum they are called hemorrhoids; when they develop in the esophagus, they are known as varices. They commonly affect the lower extremities. The long saphenous vein of the leg is most often affected by varicosities (Figure 28-7 ■). Varicose veins affect about one in five people in the world. They are more common in women over the age of 35, perhaps because of venous stasis that occurs during pregnancy. People who stand for long periods at work (waiters, beauticians, nurses) are also prone to develop varicose veins.

PATHOPHYSIOLOGY AND MANIFESTATIONS

Increased pressure that stretches the vessel wall is the major factor leading to varicose veins. Standing increases pressure in the leg veins and decreases venous return to the heart. Blood collects in the leg veins, stretching the vessel wall. As the vessels stretch, their valves cannot close properly and become incompetent. Prolonged standing, obesity, venous thrombosis, and increased pressure on the veins of the abdomen (from pregnancy or an abdominal tumor) contribute to varicose vein development.

Some clients are asymptomatic, but most complain of one or more of the manifestations listed in Box 28-16 ■. The menstrual cycle tends to increase symptoms in women.

Varicose veins can lead to venous insufficiency, stasis dermatitis, and stasis ulcers. The skin above the ankles may be thin and discolored. Venous thrombosis may develop in varicose veins, especially in pregnant or postpartal clients, postoperative clients, or clients taking oral contraceptives.

INTERDISCIPLINARY CARE

Treatment for varicose veins usually is conservative, focused on reducing discomfort. Surgery may relieve major symptoms of the disease, but there is no real cure for varicose veins.

Diagnostic Tests

Doppler ultrasonography may be done to identify the location of incompetent valves. See Table 25-3 ⬤ for more information about Doppler ultrasound testing. The *Trendelenburg*

BOX 28-16

MANIFESTATIONS OF VARICOSE VEINS
- Severe, aching leg pain
- Leg fatigue or heaviness
- Itching of the affected leg
- Heat in the affected leg after prolonged standing
- Visibly dilated veins in the leg

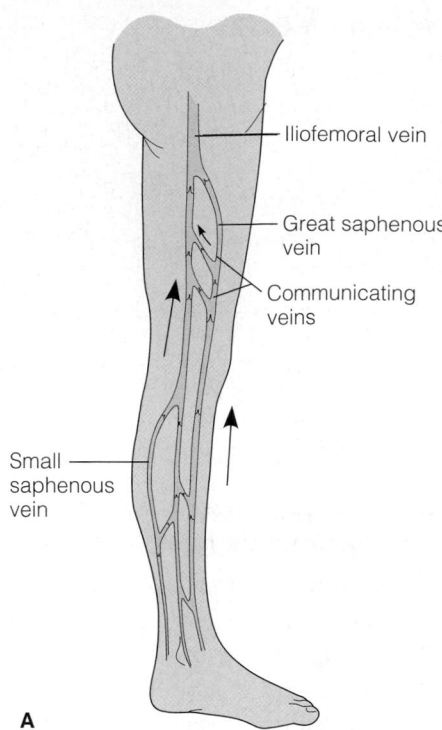

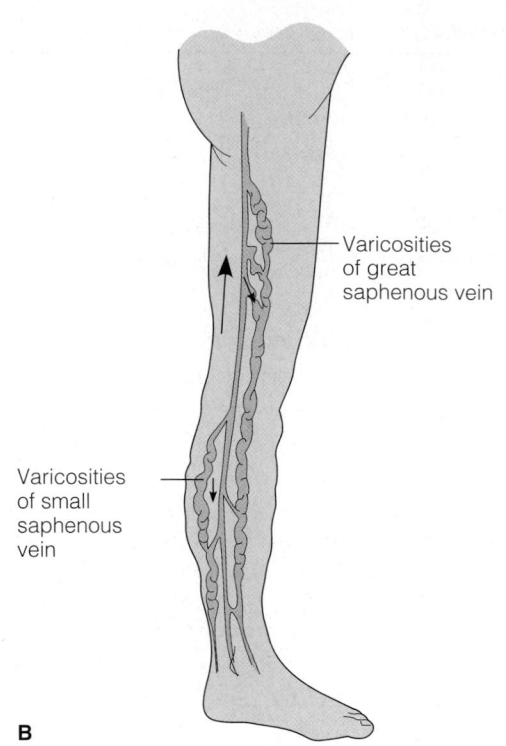

Figure 28-7. ■ **(A)** Normal leg veins. **(B)** Varicose veins.

test may be done to differentiate between incompetent valves in the deep veins of the leg versus incompetent superficial leg vein valves. For this test, the leg is elevated and a tourniquet is applied just above the knee. The varicosities are then observed while the client stands. The veins remain flat when the valves of the deep veins are involved, but distend rapidly when the valves of the superficial veins are affected.

Conservative Therapy

Most clients are managed conservatively with measures to improve venous circulation and relieve the pressure on vein walls and valves. Properly fitted antiembolism (elastic) stockings compress veins, helping move blood back to the heart. Regular, daily walking is an important part of treatment. Prolonged sitting and standing are avoided. The legs are elevated for specified periods of time throughout the day.

Surgery

Two surgical techniques are generally used to treat varicose veins: compression sclerotherapy and vein stripping. In *compression sclerotherapy,* a sclerosing (hardening) agent is injected into the varicosed vein. A compression dressing is then applied to compress and obliterate the vein. Venous blood is rerouted through healthy vessels. In *vein stripping,* the varicose veins are surgically removed. Pressure bandages are applied and the legs are elevated to reduce edema. Ambulation is gradually increased, but sitting and standing are forbidden during the recovery period.

NURSING CARE

Nurses rarely interact with clients whose primary diagnosis is varicose veins, except when surgery is planned. Through teaching and referral, however, nurses can be instrumental in helping clients slow their development and minimize the symptoms of varicose veins.

Ineffective Tissue Perfusion: Peripheral

■ Assess peripheral pulses, capillary refill, skin temperature, and degree of edema. *Assessment helps determine the effects of impaired venous return on blood flow to and perfusion of the extremities.*

■ Apply properly fitted support or antiembolic stockings. Remove stockings daily for 30 to 60 minutes. Inspect and clean the skin while stockings are off. *Antiembolic stockings exert pressure on the veins of the lower extremities, promoting venous return to the heart. During ambulation, they assist the blood-pumping action of the muscles. Because elastic stockings can impair blood flow through small superficial vessels, they should be removed at least once daily for 30 minutes or more.*

■ Wrap the leg(s) with ace bandages as directed if sclerotherapy or vein stripping has been done. Assess pulses, color, temperature, and capillary refill distal to wrappings. Frequently inspect the wrappings, and rewrap as needed to prevent skin irritation or obstruction of blood flow to or from the extremity. *Ace bandages compress the leg from ankle to thigh, obliterating the sclerosed veins, and minimizing the risk of bleeding or edema following surgery. Wrinkled or excessively tight bandages can impair skin integrity or interfere with arterial blood flow.*

- Assist with or instruct to exercise legs at regular intervals. *Exercise (e.g., ROM and Buerger–Allen exercises) promotes normal blood flow and venous return. Walking is excellent exercise and is encouraged.*

- Position with legs elevated when supine. When sitting, use a recliner-type chair to elevate the legs and reduce the angle of hip flexion. Change position frequently. *Leg elevation and limited hip flexion promote venous return and minimize pressure on lower extremity veins.*

CONTINUING CARE

Most clients with varicose veins provide self-care at home. Emphasize the importance of daily walks. Teach technique for applying antiembolism stockings. Instruct to elevate legs for specified periods of time throughout the day. Help identify strategies to avoid prolonged periods of standing or sitting. If the client's job requires prolonged standing, encourage to wear elastic stockings. Teach calf and thigh muscle tightening and relaxation exercises to perform while standing. Encourage clients whose job requires extensive sitting to work on incorporating frequent activity into the job.

Provide referrals for home health services as needed for clients recovering from surgery. In some instances, temporary placement in an extended care facility may be necessary before returning home.

Note: The bibliography listings for this and all chapters have been compiled at the back of the book.

Chapter Review

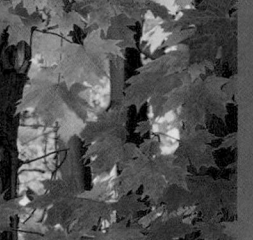

 **KEY TERMS** by Topics

Use the audio glossary feature of either the CD-ROM or the Companion Website to hear the correct pronunciation of the following key terms.

Hypertension
hypertension, primary hypertension, secondary hypertension

Disorders of the aorta
aneurysm, Marfan syndrome

Arterial disorders
arteriosolerosis, collateral circulation, intermittent claudication, bruit, thrombus, embolus

Venous disorders
venous thrombosis, deep venous thrombosis (DVT), venous insufficiency, varicose veins

KEY Points

- Hypertension is a leading, often undiagnosed, cause of cardiovascular disability and mortality. Few people with hypertension have symptoms of the disorder, yet it can lead to heart failure, stroke, and chronic renal failure.

- Encourage all clients to regularly monitor their blood pressure, reduce their salt intake, stop smoking, limit alcohol intake, exercise regularly, and reduce stress.

- Stress the importance of continuing treatment for hypertension; this disease can be managed but cannot, at this time, be cured.

- Both arterial and venous disorders can affect circulation to the extremities.

- Arterial disorders are characterized by cool, pale, hairless skin, diminished peripheral pulses, and often by pain from ischemic tissues.

- Venous disorders are more often characterized by rubor, edema, and brown, leathery skin.

- Peripheral vascular disorders increase the risk of skin trauma and breakdown. Provide meticulous foot and skin care for clients with peripheral vascular disorders, and protect from injury.

- Encourage all clients with peripheral vascular disease to engage in regular activity as approved by their primary care provider.

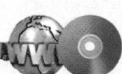 **EXPLORE MediaLink**

Additional interactive resources for this chapter can be found on the Companion Website at www.prenhall.com/burke. Click on Chapter 28 and "Begin" to select the activities for this chapter.

For chapter-related NCLEX-style review questions and an audio glossary, access the accompanying CD-ROM in this book.

FOR FURTHER Study

For more information about foods high in sodium, see Box 7-6. For nursing implications for diuretics, see Table 7-4 in Chapter 7.

For in-depth discussions about surgery, see Chapter 9.

For more information about pulmonary embolism, see Chapter 24.

For more information on diagnostic tests for peripheral vascular disease, see Tables 25-2 and 25-3.

For more discussion about atherosclerosis, its causes, and treatment, see Chapter 26.

Urinalysis and renal function studies are covered in Chapter 31.

Critical Thinking Care Map

Caring for a Client with Buerger's Disease
NCLEX-PN® Focus Area: Reduction of Risk Potential

Case Study: Jeffrey Fang, a 34-year-old computer programmer, develops leg cramps when he climbs the two flights of stairs to his office each day. The cramps began about 2 months ago, and have become so painful during the last week that he cannot walk more than about 50 feet without resting and he is now taking the elevator to his office. Mr. Fang makes an appointment with his primary care provider.

Nursing Diagnosis: Ineffective Tissue Perfusion: Peripheral

COLLECT DATA

Subjective	Objective
_____	_____
_____	_____
_____	_____
_____	_____
_____	_____
_____	_____

Would you report this data? Yes/No

If yes, to: _____

Nursing Care

_____
_____
_____
_____
_____
_____
_____
_____
_____

How would you document this? _____
_____
_____
_____

Data Collected
(use those that apply)

- Has smoked more than two packs of cigarettes a day for 20 years
- Calf pain with activity progressing during past 2 months
- Must rest frequently when walking
- Anxious about seriousness of symptoms
- Weak peripheral pulses in right leg
- Absent pedal and posterior tibial pulses in left foot
- Third, fourth, and fifth toes of left foot pale
- Relates numbness and tingling of toes of left foot
- Right foot pink and warm; left foot cool to touch
- Skin on left leg shiny and thin; hairless below knee
- Moderate amount of evenly distributed hair on right leg

Nursing Interventions
(use those that apply; list in priority order)

- Assess pain at rest and during activity using a scale of 0 to 10.
- Mutually determine most effective methods of managing pain.
- Instruct to walk for at least 30 minutes two or three times per day.
- Teach the importance of smoking cessation.
- Teach foot care measures.
- Provide time to discuss issues that contribute to anxiety.
- Encourage questions about the disease and its management.

NCLEX-PN® Exam Preparation

1   When assessing a bedridden client with a total arterial occlusion, the nurse can expect to find:

   A. palpable pulses in the area below the occlusion.

   B. cyanosis or mottling of the area above the occlusion.

   C. cyanosis or mottling of the area below the occlusion.

   D. extreme pallor, cold, and pain in the area below the occlusion.

2   When the client's extremity is affected by peripheral arteriosclerosis, blood flow to the extremity can be enhanced by:

   A. placing the affected extremity in a dependent position.

   B. elevating the affected extremity.

   C. wrapping the affected extremity with an elastic bandage.

   D. range-of-motion exercises to the affected extremity.

3   You are admitting a client diagnosed with thrombophlebitis. Which of the following medications should you prepare to administer?

   A. heparin

   B. Coumadin

   C. aspirin

   D. nonsteroidal anti-inflammatory drug

4   The nurse can educate the client with Raynaud's disease by offering the following information:

   A. Elevate the extremities above the heart during an episode.

   B. Wear support hose during cold weather.

   C. Practice relaxation techniques to reduce stress.

   D. Avoid any activities that involve repetitive movement.

5   You are caring for a client with Raynaud's disease. Signs and symptoms characteristic of Raynaud's include:

   A. persistent mottling of the hands and feet.

   B. consistent pain and numbness in the feet.

   C. periodic cyanosis and pallor of the hands and feet.

   D. alternating periods of vasodilation and vasoconstriction.

6   The nurse is caring for a client who has recently been diagnosed with stage 2 hypertension. When educating the client about hypertension it is important to emphasize that such clients commonly:

   A. experience severe headaches.

   B. have no symptoms other than an increased blood pressure.

   C. experience symptoms of kidney failure.

   D. experience visual disturbances.

7   When educating a client with stage 2 hypertension about how to manage his or her hypertension, the nurse should stress:

   A. adhering to medication schedules.

   B. the short-term aspect of managing hypertension.

   C. making all recommended lifestyle changes.

   D. engaging in range-of-motion exercises.

8   A 70-year-old male comes to the clinic complaining of severe headaches and dizziness and also states that he recently fell and bumped his head. When reviewing the client's medication history, the nurse should note that the client is taking:

   A. Cardizem.

   B. Inderal.

   C. digoxin.

   D. Coumadin.

9   Your 54-year-old female client has recently been diagnosed with stage 2 hypertension. She states that she cannot understand why smoking is bad for her because it usually helps her to relax. The nurse responds by stating that smoking affects blood pressure because nicotine:

   A. stimulates blood vessels.

   B. increases the pulse rate.

   C. constricts blood vessels.

   D. dilates blood vessels.

10   Which of the following is a symptom of a dissecting aneurysm of the ascending aorta?

   A. sudden, excruciating pain

   B. paralysis of the lower extremities

   C. diminished or absent peripheral pulses

   D. cyanosis

Answers for Review Questions, as well as discussion of Care Plan and Critical Thinking Care Map questions, appear in Appendix V.

Thinking Strategically About...

Mrs. Opal Hipps is a 75-year-old widow who lives alone with her dog Chester. She retired from her job as a postal clerk 10 years ago and now spends a lot of time reading and watching television. Over the past week she developed a vague aching pain in her right leg. Last night it became more severe, especially in her right calf. She noticed that her right lower leg seemed larger than the left, and her calf was very tender and felt warm to the touch. Mrs. Hipps is admitted to the hospital with deep venous thrombosis in the right leg. She is placed on bed rest and intravenous heparin is started. Michael Cookson is her admitting nurse. He implements the following interventions: elevation of legs; application of intermittent, warm, moist compresses to the right leg; and application of antiembolic stockings. Mr. Cookson also assists Mrs. Hipps to arrange for a neighbor to care for Chester.

DATA COLLECTED

Mrs. Hipps tells Mr. Cookson, "This business about a blood clot really has me worried." She also says she is worried about who will care for her dog while she is in the hospital. Objective data includes: height 5'1" (157 cm); weight 149 lbs. (68 kg); T 99.2°F (37.3°C); vital signs within

normal limits. Her left leg is warm, pink, and supple with good skin turgor. Her right calf is warm, red, dry, and tender to touch. Femoral and popliteal pulses are strong bilaterally. Right pedal and posterior tibial pulses are difficult to locate, and the diameter of the right calf is 0.5 inch (1.27 cm) larger than that of the left.

CRITICAL THINKING

1 What were the risk factors that contributed to Mrs. Hipps's development of venous thrombosis?

2 What effect does heat have on deep venous thrombosis?

MANAGEMENT OF CARE

1 Mrs. Hipps was started on warfarin (Coumadin), which is an oral anticoagulant, prior to discharge. What nursing interventions will the nurse provide related to the anticoagulant therapy?

2 What are the nursing implications indicated when caring for a client wearing antiembolic stockings?

3 Knowing that use of the leg muscles will prevent venous stasis, what ideas could be suggested to Mrs. Hipps to prevent future episodes of venous thrombosis?

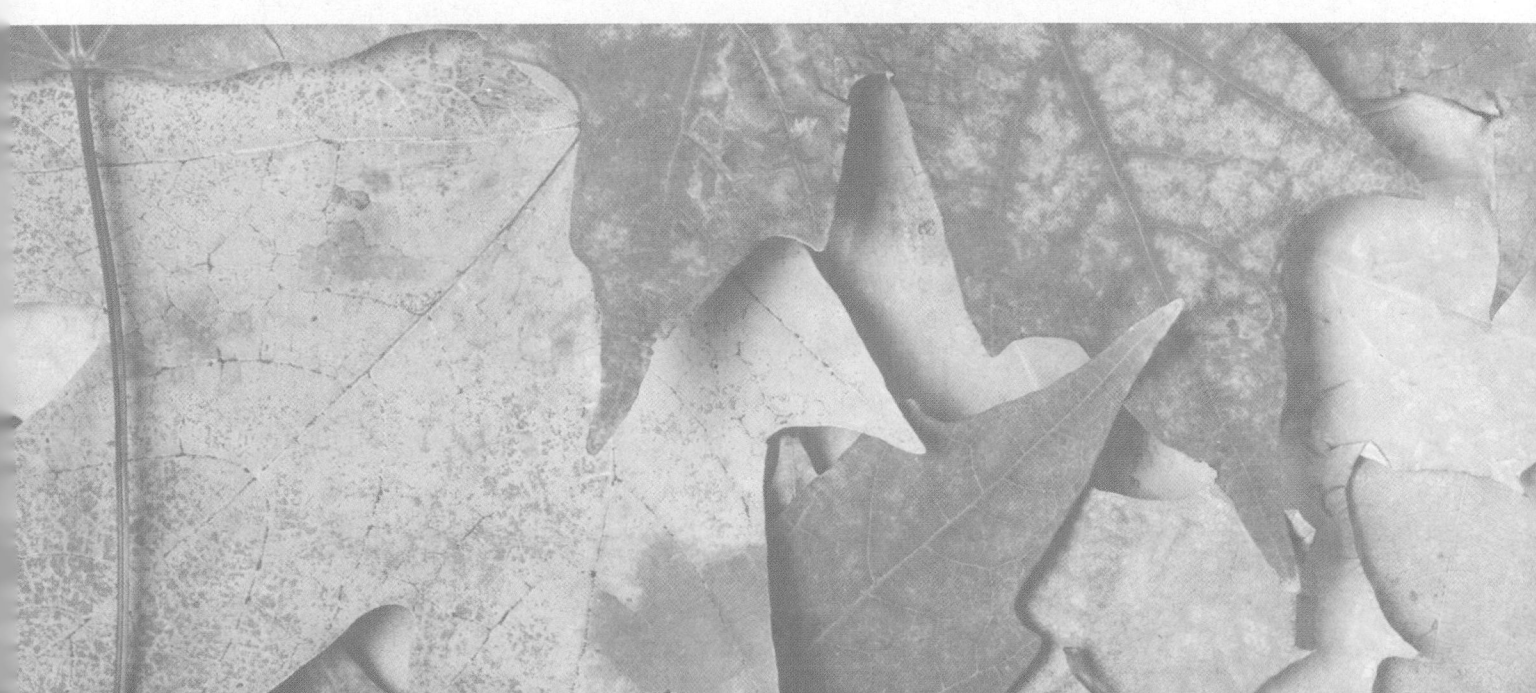

Disrupted Hematologic and Lymphatic Function

UNIT VII

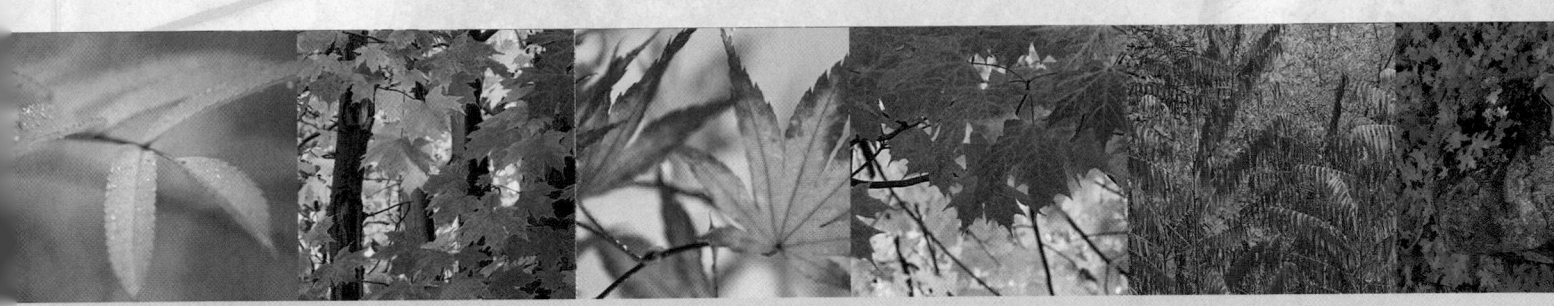

Chapter 29

The Hematologic and Lymphatic Systems and Assessment

BRIEF Outline

Structure and Function of the Hematologic and Lymphatic Systems

The Blood and Blood Cells

Hemostasis

The Lymphatic System

Assessment

Health History

Physical Examination

Diagnostic Tests

LEARNING Outcomes

After completing this chapter, you will be able to:

- Describe the cells of the hematologic system with their functions.
- Identify and describe the structures and functions of the lymphatic system.
- Collect subjective and objective assessment data related to the hematologic and lymphatic systems.
- Provide appropriate nursing care for clients undergoing diagnostic tests to evaluate the hematologic and lymphatic systems.

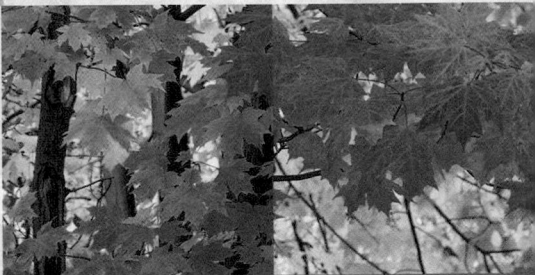

MediaLink

www.prenhall.com/burke

Use the address above to access the free, interactive Companion Website created for this textbook. Get hints, instant feedback, and textbook references to chapter-related NCLEX-style questions. Link to other interesting sites.

Audio Glossary:

Use the Companion Website, or the CD-ROM disk enclosed with your textbook, to hear the pronunciation of key terms in this chapter.

Structure and Function of the Hematologic and Lymphatic Systems

THE BLOOD AND BLOOD CELLS

Blood transports oxygen and nutrients to cells, essential substances (such as hormones and other chemical messengers) to cells and tissues, and waste products away from tissues for removal from the body. Blood is made up of **plasma,** a clear yellow, protein-rich fluid, and the cells suspended in it: *red blood cells* (erythrocytes), *white blood cells* (leukocytes), and platelets (or *thrombocytes*).

A number of body systems are involved in forming blood. Many of the plasma proteins are formed in the liver. Blood cells are formed in bone marrow. All blood cells begin as *stem cells,* or *hemocytoblasts.* Stem cells then differentiate (mature) into the different types of blood cells (red blood cells, platelets, and several kinds of white cells) (Figure 29-1 ■).

This chapter provides an overview of each type of blood cell and its function, as well as a review of the organs and function of the lymphatic system.

Red Blood Cells

Red blood cells (RBCs) and the hemoglobin they contain are vital for transporting oxygen to body tissues. They also help carry carbon dioxide from the tissues to the lungs for excretion.

Red blood cells (**erythrocytes**) are shaped like *biconcave disks* (Figure 29-2 ■). The shape of the RBC increases its surface area for gas exchange and allows it to change shape as it moves through very small capillaries. RBCs are formed in bone marrow through a process known as *erythropoiesis.* Tissue hypoxia stimulates the kidneys to release a hormone, *erythropoietin,* that stimulates the bone marrow to produce RBCs. The complete sequence from stem cell to RBC (see Figure 29-1) takes from 3 to 5 days.

RBCs contain **hemoglobin,** an oxygen-carrying protein. Hemoglobin consists of *heme* molecules within a protein structure. Heme contains iron, which binds with oxygen. Hemoglobin molecules are synthesized within the RBC.

RBCs have a life span of about 120 days. Old or damaged RBCs are destroyed by phagocytes in the spleen, liver, bone marrow, and lymph nodes. The process of RBC destruction is called **hemolysis.** The amino acids and iron from destroyed RBCs are saved and reused by the body. This iron circulates in the bloodstream as *transferrin.* It is not immediately reused, it is stored in the liver, spleen, and bone marrow as *ferritin.* Most of the heme unit is converted to *bilirubin,* an orange-yellow pigment that is removed from the blood by the liver and excreted in the bile.

Normal RBC laboratory values often differ by gender (Table 29-1 ■). Other terms used to describe RBCs include *normocytic* (normal size), *microcytic* (smaller than normal), or *macrocytic* (larger than normal); and *normochromic* (normal color) or *hypochromic* (decreased color).

TABLE 29-1		
Laboratory Values Related to Red Blood Cells		
LABORATORY TEST	**NORMAL VALUE**	**MEASURES**
Red Blood Cell (RBC) count ■ Men ■ Women	 4.2–5.4 million/mm^3 3.6–5.0 million/mm^3	Number of circulating RBCs in one cubic millimeter (mm^3) of blood
Reticulocyte count	1–1.5% of total RBC	Number of immature RBCs in 1 mm^3 of blood
Hemoglobin (Hgb) ■ Men ■ Women	 14–16.5 g/dL 12–15 g/dL	Amount of hemoglobin in 100 mL (1 dL) of blood
Hematocrit (Hct) ■ Men ■ Women	 40–50% 37–47%	Packed volume of RBCs in 100 mL of blood; reported as a percentage
Mean corpuscular volume (MCV)	85–100 μm^3/cell	Average volume of individual RBCs
Mean corpuscular hemoglobin (MCH)	31–35 g/dL	Weight of the hemoglobin in an average RBC
Mean corpuscular hemoglobin concentration (MCHC)	33.4–35.5%	Average concentration (percent) of hemoglobin within RBC

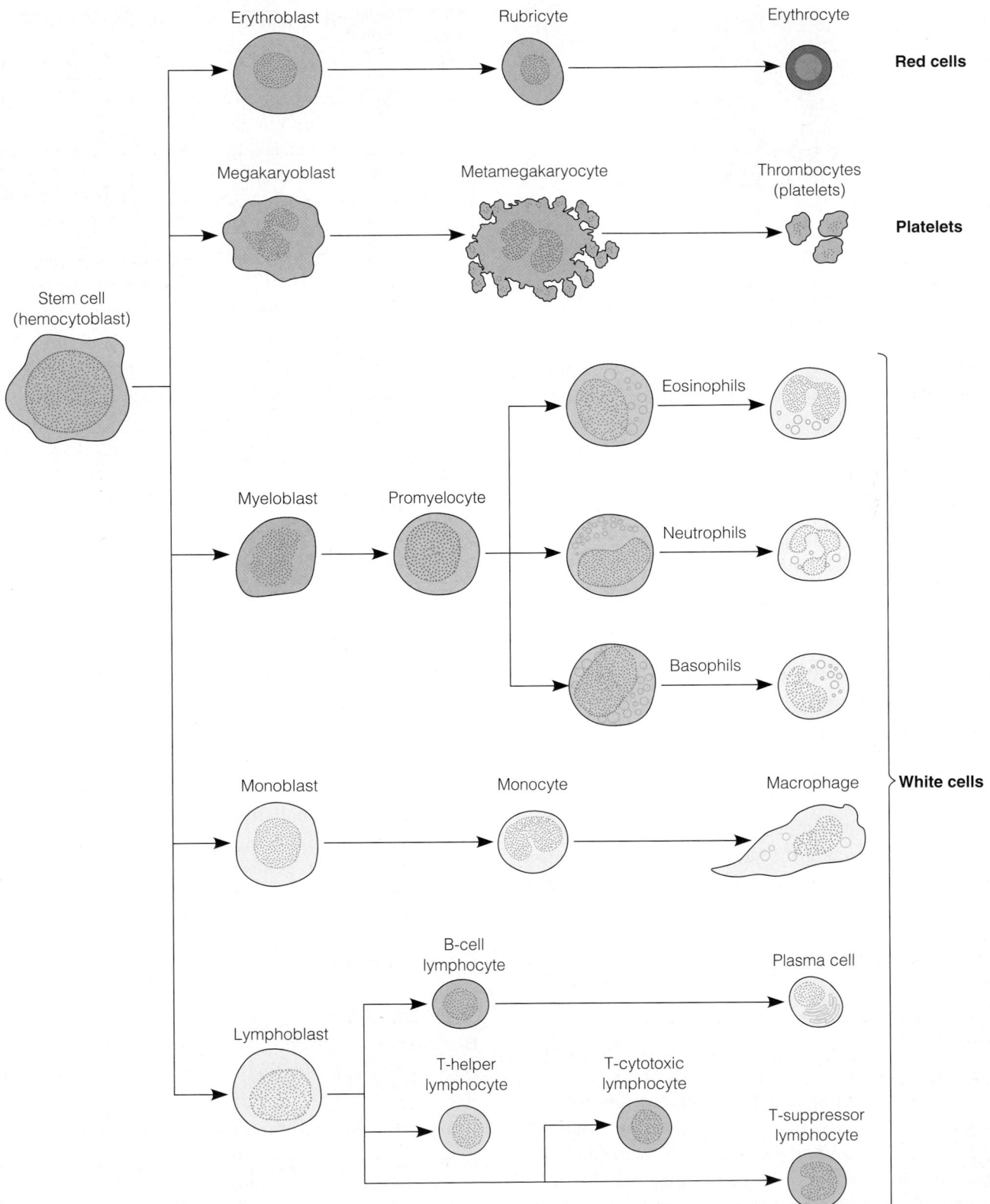

Figure 29-1. ■ The formation of different types of blood cells from the stem cell. The stem cell differentiates into one of five types of blast (immature) cells, which then mature into red blood cells (erythrocytes), platelets (thrombocytes), or white blood cells (leukocytes).

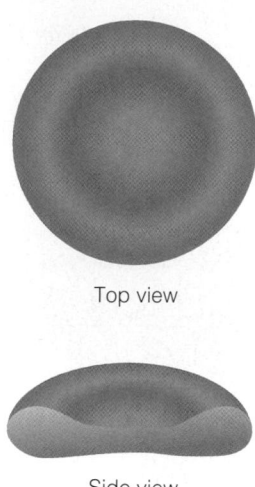

Top view

Side view

Figure 29-2. ■ Top and side views of a red blood cell. Note the distinctive concave shape.

TABLE 29-2

Normal White Blood Cell Count and Differential

LABORATORY TEST	NORMAL VALUES
WBC count	5,000–10,000/mm^3
Differential WBC count	
Neutrophils	60–70% (3,000–7,000/mm^3)
Eosinophils	1–3% (50–400/mm^3)
Basophils	0.3–0.5% (25–200/mm^3)
Lymphocytes	20–30% (1,000–4,000/mm^3)
Monocytes	3–8% (100–600/mm^3)

White Blood Cells

White blood cells (WBCs), also called **leukocytes,** are part of the body's defense against infection and disease. On average, there are 5,000 to 10,000 WBCs per cubic millimeter of blood. WBCs make up about 1% of total blood volume. *Leukocytosis* is a higher than normal WBC count; in *leukopenia,* the WBC count is lower than normal.

WBCs originate from stem cells in the bone marrow (see Figure 29-1). Unlike RBCs, which remain within blood vessels, WBCs use the circulation to move to where they are needed, and can migrate into other tissues. There are three major types of WBCs: granulocytes, monocytes, and lymphocytes.

Granulocytes are the most plentiful WBCs, accounting for 60% to 80% of the total leukocytes. Their cytoplasm looks granular and their nuclei have multiple lobes, giving them a distinctive appearance. Granulocytes play a key role in protecting the body from harmful microorganisms during acute inflammation and infection. There are three types of granulocytes:

1. *Neutrophils* make up 60% to 70% of circulating WBCs. They are also called *polymorphonuclear leukocytes* (*PMNs* or *polys*). Neutrophils are *phagocytic,* that is, responsible for engulfing and destroying foreign matter. They are the first cells to arrive at a site of invasion. Neutrophils have a life span of about 10 hours and must constantly be replaced. *Segmented neutrophils* are mature cells; *bands* are immature neutrophils.
2. *Eosinophils* make up 1% to 3% of WBCs. Their numbers increase during allergic reactions and during infestations with parasites.
3. *Basophils* make up 0.3% to 0.5% of total WBCs and are believed to be a part of the hypersensitivity and stress responses.

Monocytes are the largest of the WBCs and make up approximately 3% to 8% of the total WBC count. Monocytes migrate into body tissues such as the skin, subcutaneous tissue, lungs, and liver. There they mature into *macrophages.* Both monocytes and macrophages are phagocytic cells.

Lymphocytes account for 20% to 30% of WBCs. Although they are small and nondescript, lymphocytes are the primary effectors and regulators of specific immune responses. *B lymphocytes (B cells)* are involved in forming antibodies, whereas *T lymphocytes (T cells)* take part in cell-mediated immunity. A third type of lymphocyte, *natural killer cells (NK cells),* also provides immune surveillance and resistance to infection. Normal laboratory values for WBCs are outlined in Table 29-2 ■.

Platelets and Coagulation

Platelets are an essential part of the body's clotting mechanism. They are small fragments of cytoplasm without nuclei that contain many granules. Most platelets are stored in the spleen before being released into the circulation. There are about 250,000 to 400,000 platelets in each milliliter of blood. An excess of platelets is *thrombocytosis.* Platelets live approximately 10 days in circulating blood.

HEMOSTASIS

Hemostasis, or blood clotting, is a complex process the body uses to stop bleeding. There are five stages in hemostasis:

1. *Vessel spasm:* Damage to a blood vessel causes it to spasm. This spasm, which lasts more than a minute, constricts the vessel and reduces blood flow.
2. *Formation of the platelet plug:* Platelets adhere to the damaged vessel wall and to one another, forming a platelet plug. Von Willebrand's factor is necessary for platelets to adhere to one another. The platelet plug is stabilized by fibrin.
3. *Clot formation:* Coagulation occurs as fibrin forms a meshwork that cements blood components together

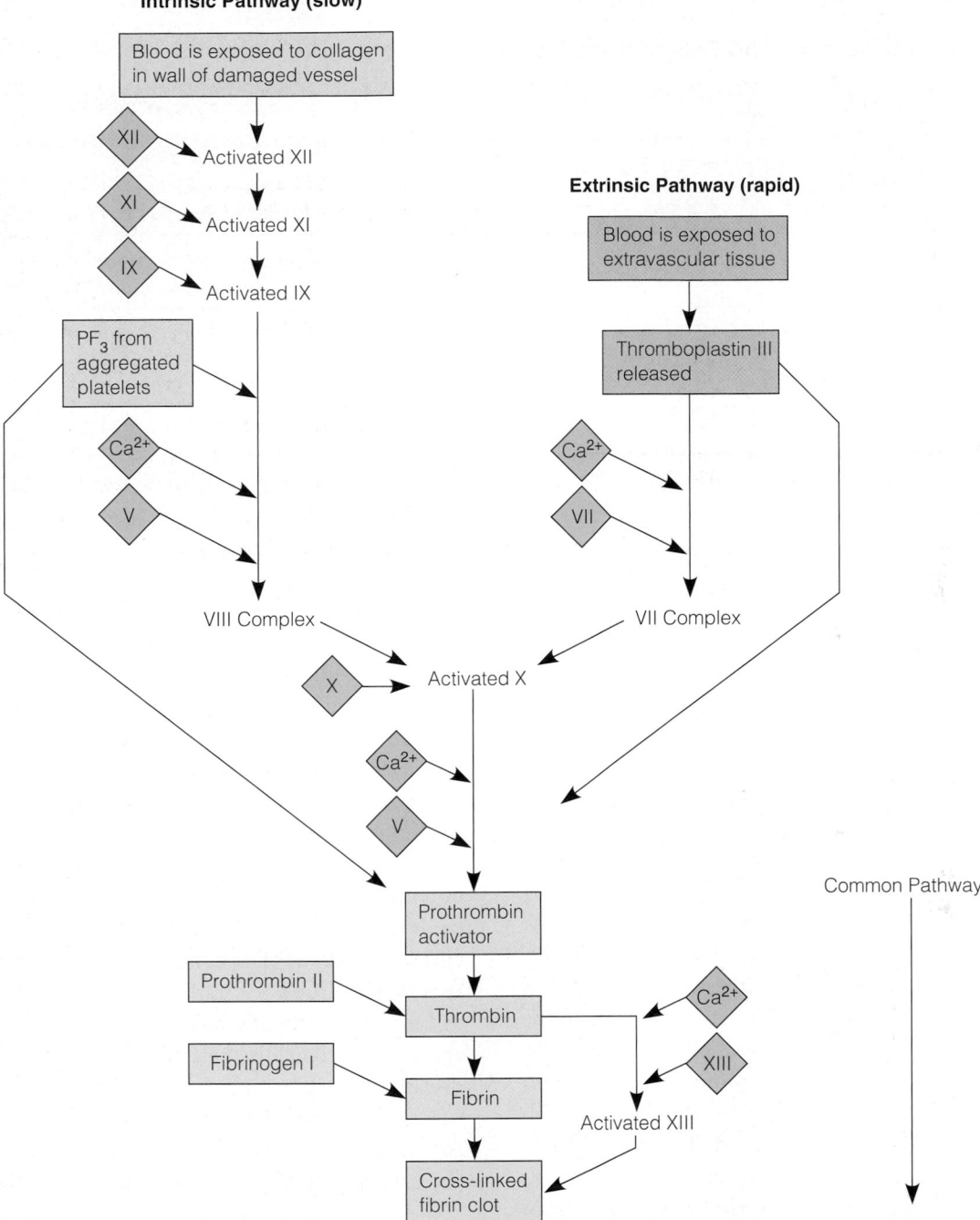

Figure 29-3. ■ Both the slower intrinsic pathway (on the left) and the more rapid extrinsic pathway (on the right) are necessary to form a stable blood clot.

into an insoluble clot. The process involves two different clotting pathways. The *intrinsic pathway* is activated by vessel injury; the *extrinsic pathway* is activated by blood leaking out of the vessel into the tissues (Figure 29-3 ■). The final outcome is fibrin clot formation. Each clotting factor is activated in sequence; activation of one clotting factor activates another in turn. A deficiency of one or more factors interrupts blood clotting.

4. *Clot retraction:* After about 30 minutes, platelets trapped within the clot begin to contract. This pulls the broken portions of the ruptured blood vessel closer together. At the same time, platelets release growth factors that stimulate cell division and tissue repair in the damaged vessel.

5. *Clot dissolution:* A process called *fibrinolysis* removes the clot after tissue has been repaired. Fibrinolysis begins within a few days of clot formation and continues until the clot is dissolved.

TABLE 29-3		
Laboratory Values: Platelets and Coagulation Studies		
STUDY	NORMAL VALUE	MEASURES
Platelets	150,000 to 300,000/mm^3 or $150-300 \times 10^9$/L	The number of circulating platelets in the blood.
Bleeding time	2–9.5 minutes	Used to screen for disorders caused by platelet dysfunction.
Coagulation studies		Measure time required for clotting; used to detect and evaluate clotting disorders, thrombolytic, and anticoagulant therapy
Prothrombin time (PT or protime)	10–13 seconds (varies by laboratory)	Evaluates the extrinsic clotting pathway; prolonged in Coumadin therapy
INR (International Normalized Ratio)	2–3.5	Used to evaluate Coumadin therapy (see Chapter 28 for therapeutic values)
Activated partial thromboplastin time (APTT, PTT)	25–35 seconds	Evaluates the intrinsic clotting pathway; prolonged in heparin therapy
Thrombin time (TT)	24–35 seconds	Evaluates conversion of fibrinogen to fibrin.

Table 29-3 ■ presents normal values for platelets and routinely performed coagulation studies.

THE LYMPHATIC SYSTEM

The **lymphatic system** (Figure 29-4 ■), including the lymphatic vessels, lymph nodes, and lymphoid organs such as the spleen, has several functions. Excess tissue fluid, called *lymph,* returns to the heart through low-pressure lymphatic vessels. Lymph nodes assist the immune system by removing foreign matter, infectious organisms, and tumor cells from lymph. The largest lymphoid organ is the spleen, located in the upper left quadrant of the abdomen. The spleen filters the blood, produces lymphocytes (a type of WBC active in the immune response), and stores blood and platelets. Other lymphoid organs, such as the thymus and lymphoid tissue in the skin, respiratory, and gastrointestinal systems, are important partners in the immune system, helping protect the body from infection.

Assessment

Nurses play an important role in identifying many of the manifestations of hematologic and lymphatic system disorders. Assessment of these systems generally is conducted as part of the general survey of the client's health or concurrently with focused cardiovascular system assessment. However, unless the nurse specifically focuses on these systems, early manifestations of disorders can be missed or attributed to dysfunction of a different body system.

HEALTH HISTORY

Ask the client about recent changes in energy level and ability to maintain usual daily activities, including recreational activities and sports. Inquire about any pain, burning or tingling sensations, changes in skin color or temperature, or swelling (edema). Ask about bleeding or easy bruising, dizziness, fatigue, or changes in lymph nodes (swelling, pain or tenderness, warmth). Have the client relate usual diet, including protein, vitamin, and mineral intake. Ask about current medications, and use of tobacco, alcohol, and other recreational drugs.

Obtain the client's medical history, specifically asking about any chronic diseases, cancer or kidney disease, or HIV disease. Ask about surgeries, blood transfusions, and exposure to radiation or chemicals (during medical procedures, environmental exposure, or occupational exposure). Inquire about family history of cancer, anemia, or blood disorders.

PHYSICAL EXAMINATION

Assessment of the hematologic and lymphatic systems begins with inspection of the color of the skin and mucous membranes for pallor or cyanosis. Inspect oral mucous membranes, and the skin of the trunk and extremities for erythema, red streaks, or lesions such as petechiae, bruising, or purpura (purple rashes caused by blood leaking into the skin). Obtain the vital signs, including temperature and apical pulse. Palpate skin temperature, for capillary refill, and for edema of the extremities (see Figure 5-3). ◐ Palpate lymph nodes for swelling and tenderness (Figure 5-6). ◐ Lightly palpate the upper left quadrant of the abdomen for tenderness.

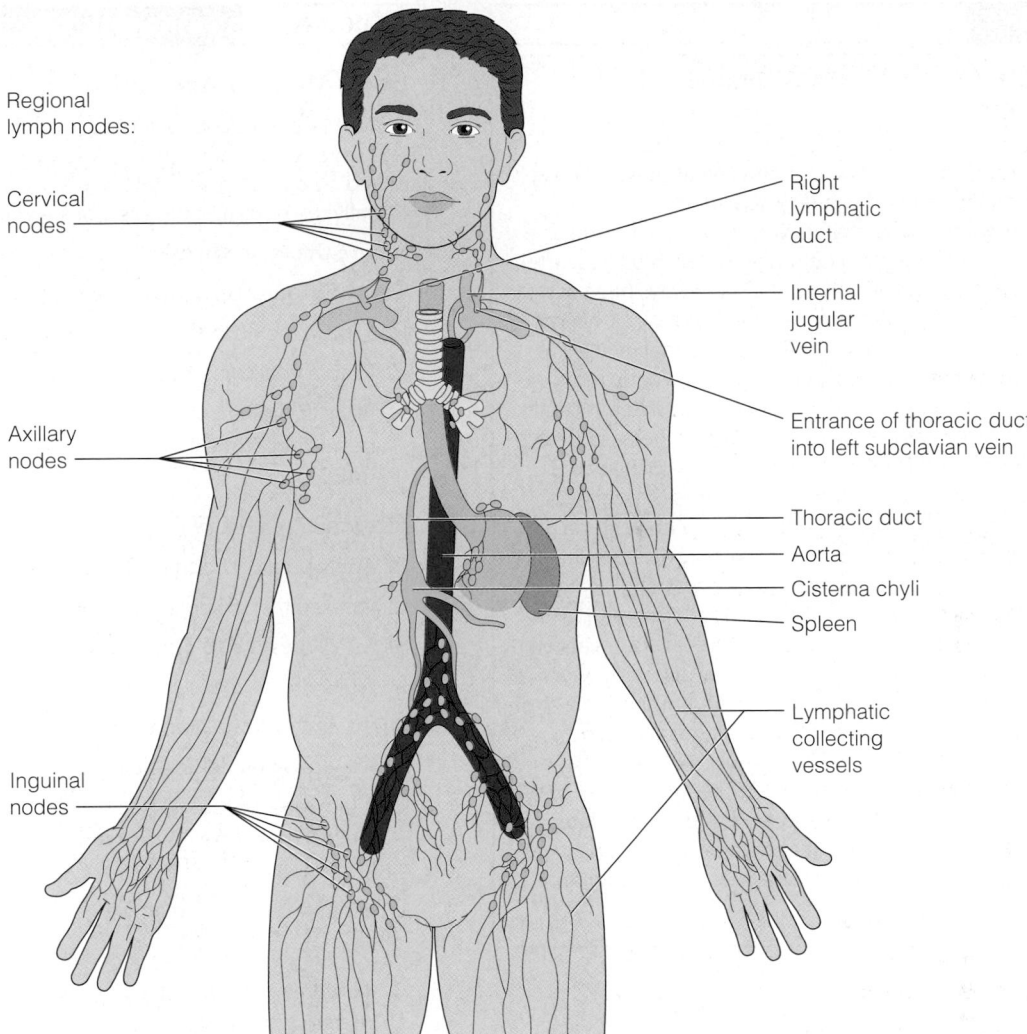

Regional
lymph nodes:

Cervical
nodes

Axillary
nodes

Inguinal
nodes

Right
lymphatic
duct

Internal
jugular
vein

Entrance of thoracic duct
into left subclavian vein

Thoracic duct

Aorta

Cisterna chyli

Spleen

Lymphatic
collecting
vessels

Figure 29-4. ■ The lymphatic system.

Box 29-1 ■ presents an example of documentation of assessment of the hematologic system.

DIAGNOSTIC TESTS

A number of laboratory and diagnostic tests can be done to identify disorders of the blood or lymph systems.

Laboratory Tests

■ The *complete blood count (CBC)* is often performed as a routine screening examination. The CBC includes the red blood cell (RBC) count, the hemoglobin and hematocrit, and red blood cell indices (see Table 29-1); the white blood cell (WBC) count, and, if ordered, WBC differential (see Table 29-2); and the platelet count (see Table 29-3).

■ *Clotting studies* or a *coagulation profile* (see Table 29-3) are performed to evaluate clotting and bleeding disorders, and often are ordered prior to major surgeries (such as heart surgery, joint replacements). These tests also are used to monitor thrombolytic (fibrinolytic) and anticoagulant therapy.

■ *Coombs' test* is used to diagnose hemolytic anemias and investigate transfusion reactions. The expected results are no detected antibodies to RBCs (indirect Coombs') or no detected RBC antigen–antibody complexes (direct Coombs').

■ *Hemoglobin electrophoresis* is performed when sickle cell anemia or another genetically linked anemia is suspected. In this test, blood is examined for the presence of hemoglobin S, an abnormal form of the hemoglobin molecule. None is detected in the blood of people without sickle cell trait or disease (see Chapter 30). ◯◯

■ Tests of body iron stores are performed to evaluate iron deficiency anemia. Table 29-4 ■ outlines commonly used tests of iron stores with their expected results.

■ *Schilling's test* (vitamin B_{12} test) may be ordered to detect pernicious anemia in clients with vitamin B_{12} deficiency. This timed test evaluates the body's ability to absorb vitamin B_{12} from the GI tract. In this test, both an oral dose of radioactively tagged vitamin B_{12} and an intramuscular vitamin B_{12} injection are administered,

BOX 29-1

DOCUMENTATION OF HEMATOLOGIC ASSESSMENT

Client: Janet Hinman, 54 years old, presents at her primary care physician's office with complaints of fatigue that is significantly affecting her usual daily activities.

Assessment Note: States that during the past 3 months she has experienced increasing fatigue, and now must rest after only 30 minutes or so of activity. She has always been active, working out at a fitness center several days a week, hiking, and skiing, but now is unable to walk more than a few blocks without resting and has had to significantly reduce her normal workouts to 15–20 minutes or less. Admits that she bruises more easily than normal. Denies increased incidence of infections. Denies other symptoms such as sore mouth, cracking of lips, extremity numbness or tingling. States she eats well, following a low-fat, low-cholesterol diet; has no known allergies or history of chronic diseases. Taking no medications on a regular basis; uses occasional acetaminophen or ibuprofen for headache or minor discomfort. No known family history of heart or blood disorders or cancer.

BP 122/64, P 86, R 22, T 97.6 F PO. Color pale; skin warm and dry. Conjunctiva and oral mucous membranes pale and moist. Scattered petechiae noted in oral mucous membranes, on trunk and back. Multiple bruises of varying age noted on extremities. Pulses strong, equal, and regular on all 4 extremities. Capillary refill ~3 seconds. No edema noted. No lymphadenopathy noted of cervical nodes. Active bowel sounds all 4 quadrants; slight tenderness noted to light palpation upper left quadrant.

BOX 29-2 NURSING CARE CHECKLIST

Bone Marrow Aspiration

Bone marrow studies are used to diagnose aplastic anemia, leukemias, and other cancers. A sample of bone marrow is obtained by inserting a needle or biopsy instrument into a bone (usually the posterior iliac crest or sternum).

Before the Procedure

☑ Verify signed consent for the procedure has been obtained.

☑ Explain the purpose and procedure of the test.

☑ Record vital signs. Have the client void.

☑ Place in supine position if sternum or anterior iliac crest will be used, in prone position if posterior iliac crest is to be used.

After the Procedure

☑ Apply pressure to the puncture site for 5 to 10 minutes.

☑ Assess vital signs; report changes from baseline.

☑ Apply dressing to puncture site. Monitor for bleeding and infection.

Client and Family Teaching

☑ The procedure takes about 20 minutes.

☑ A local anesthetic will be used; you will feel some pain during insertion. Take deep breaths to help relieve pain during this time.

☑ It is important to remain very still during the procedure.

☑ The site of the aspiration may ache for several days.

☑ Report any unusual bleeding, drainage, or symptoms of infection immediately.

followed by collection of a 24-hour urine specimen. (See Box 31-3 🔗 for a nursing care checklist when collecting a 24-hour urine specimen.) The expected result is excretion of 10% or more of the radioactively tagged vitamin B_{12} within 24 hours.

Bone Marrow Aspiration

In many hematologic disorders, it is necessary to aspirate and analyze bone marrow to establish the diagnosis. See

Box 29-2 ■ for nursing care of the client undergoing a bone marrow aspiration. Once obtained, the bone marrow is analyzed for the different types of cells it contains. Normally, there are up to 15 different types of cells present. (See Figure 29-1 for the different types of mature blood cells

TABLE 29-4

Serum Iron Tests

TEST	EXPECTED VALUE	NURSING IMPLICATIONS
Iron	50–175 µg/dL (9–31 µmol/L)	Antibiotics, estrogen and testosterone, oral contraceptives, aspirin, and ethanol affect results.
Total iron-binding capacity	250–420 µg/dL (45–73 µmol/L)	
Ferritin	Men: 16–300 ng/mL (16–300 µg/L) Women: 10–160 ng/mL (10–160 µg/L)	Results affected by oral contraceptives and nuclear medicine studies.
Transferrin	200–375 mg/dL (2.0–3.75 g/L)	Pregnancy, hormone therapy, oral contraceptives, and some drugs affect levels.

and their immature forms that would be expected in bone marrow.) The number, appearance, and development of the various blood cell types are analyzed to diagnose hemolytic blood disorders, tumors, leukemias, and, in some cases, infectious diseases.

In adults, bone marrow may be obtained from the posterior superior iliac crest, anterior iliac crest, or sternum. The aspiration may be painful for the client, despite the use of local anesthesia. Evaluate pain level following the test, and provide analgesics as needed. The site may be sore for up to 3 or 4 days after the aspiration. Continued pain should be reported to the physician. Following the aspiration, monitor for bleeding, and report excess drainage or bleeding.

Biopsy

When a hematologic or lymphatic malignancy is suspected, bone marrow or tissue from a lymph node is microscopically examined for the presence of abnormal cells. Nursing care for a lymph node biopsy is similar to that provided for the client undergoing bone marrow aspiration, although the risk of bleeding and discomfort following the procedure generally is less. (For more information about tissue biopsy, see Chapter 12. ∞)

Imaging Studies

Although it currently is rarely performed, a *lymphangiogram* may be done to evaluate lymphatic vessels and lymph nodes when the client has unexplained edema of one extremity or when lymphoma, Hodgkin's disease, or another cancer is suspected. In this examination, radiologic contrast media is injected into a lymphatic vessel in the affected extremity. X-ray films are then taken at periodic intervals to evaluate the lymphatic vessels and nodes. Determine any allergies to iodine or seafood prior to the test, and notify the physician if present. No special preparations are necessary for this test. It is contraindicated for pregnant women (because of the exposure to radiation).

Note: The bibliography listings for this and all chapters have been compiled at the back of the book.

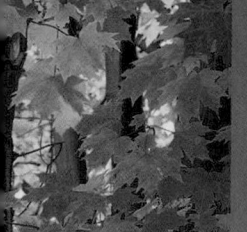

Chapter Review

 **KEY TERMS** by Topics

Use the audio glossary feature of either the CD-ROM or the Companion Website to hear the correct pronunciation of the following key terms.

Hematologic system
plasma, erythrocytes, hemoglobin, hemolysis, leukocytes, platelets, hemostasis

Lymphatic system
lymphatic system

KEY Points

- Blood is the transport medium for oxygen, nutrients, and other substances in the body.
- The primary function of RBCs is to transport oxygen to the cells.
- The primary function of WBCs is to fight infection, destroy foreign matter, and eliminate damaged or abnormal cells in the body. WBCs are an integral part of the immune system and necessary for its functioning.
- Platelets and clotting factors work together in the process of blood clotting and the control of bleeding.
- The lymphatic system also is involved in the immune response.
- Blood tests to evaluate the number and types of cells present, their size and shape, and the ability of the blood to clot are the primary diagnostic tests used to evaluate the hematologic system. Aspiration of bone marrow may be necessary to provide additional information about blood formation.

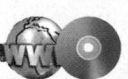 **EXPLORE MediaLink**

Additional interactive resources for this chapter can be found on the Companion Website at www.prenhall.com/burke. Click on Chapter 29 and "Begin" to select the activities for this chapter.

For chapter-related NCLEX-style review questions and an audio glossary, access the accompanying CD-ROM in this book.

FOR FURTHER Study

See Figure 5-3 for more information about assessing for edema.

Figure 5-6 shows the lymph nodes of the head and neck.

For more information about tissue biopsy, see Chapter 12.

For more information about sickle cell trait and disease, see Chapter 30.

Chapter 31 provides more information about 24-hour urine specimens.

NCLEX-PN® Exam Preparation

1 The nurse notes that a client's hemoglobin is 11.5 g/dL and her hematocrit is 30%. The nurse knows that these levels:

A. are within normal limits for a woman.

B. will affect the client's ability to transport oxygen to her cells.

C. significantly increase the client's risk for abnormal clotting.

D. increase the client's risk for infection.

2 A client with renal failure has low erythropoietin levels. As a result, the nurse would expect which of the following in the CBC? (Choose all that apply.)

A. a low RBC count

B. a high hemoglobin level

C. a low hematocrit

D. a high WBC count

E. increased numbers of immature RBCs in the blood

3 When evaluating the WBC differential, the nurse knows that normally the most plentiful type of WBC in circulating blood is the:

A. eosinophil.

B. monocyte.

C. lymphocyte.

D. neutrophil.

4 The nurse caring for a client with a diagnosis of thrombocytopenia (low thrombocyte levels) knows that this disorder will affect the client's:

A. ability to form blood clots.

B. ability to fight infection.

C. energy level.

D. nutritional status.

5 Following a bone marrow aspiration, the nurse appropriately plans to:

A. significantly increase the client's fluid intake to restore blood volume.

B. withhold all analgesics to allow accurate assessment of mental status.

C. carefully monitor the site for signs of excess bleeding.

D. warn the client to remain on bed rest for 24 hours following the procedure.

Answers for Review Questions appear in Appendix V.

Chapter 30

Caring for Clients with Hematologic and Lymphatic Disorders

BRIEF Outline

Anemia
Polycythemia
Leukemia
Multiple Myeloma
Agranulocytosis
Thrombocytopenia
Hemophilia
Disseminated Intravascular Coagulation
Lymphangitis and Lymphedema
Infectious Mononucleosis
Malignant Lymphoma

LEARNING Outcomes

After completing this chapter, you will be able to:

- Describe the pathophysiology and manifestations of common hematologic and lymphatic disorders.
- Discuss interdisciplinary care of clients with hematologic or lymphatic disorders, including diagnostic tests and commonly prescribed medications.
- Relate the nursing implications for selected treatment measures for clients with hematologic or lymphatic disorders.
- Provide individualized nursing care for clients with hematologic or lymphatic disorders.
- Identify continuing care needs for clients with hematologic or lymphatic disorders.

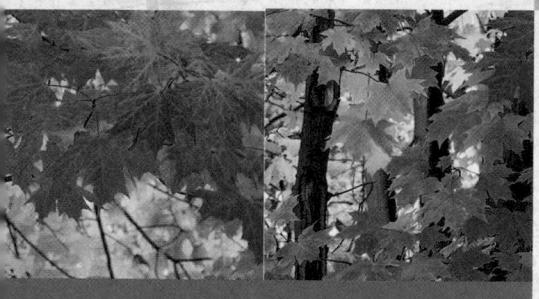

MediaLink

www.prenhall.com/burke
Use the address above to access the free, interactive Companion Website created for this textbook. Get hints, instant feedback, and textbook references to chapter-related NCLEX-style questions. Link to other interesting sites.

Audio Glossary:
Use the Companion Website, or the CD-ROM disk enclosed with your textbook, to hear the pronunciation of key terms in this chapter.

RED BLOOD CELL DISORDERS

Disorders affecting the red blood cells affect the body's ability to carry oxygen to the tissues. As a result, the client often experiences manifestations such as fatigue and activity intolerance. In general, when there are too few red blood cells, the disorder is known as *anemia*. An excess of red blood cells is known as *polycythemia* or erythrocytosis.

Anemia

Anemia is a condition in which the hemoglobin concentration or the number of circulating RBCs is decreased. Anemia typically is caused by either impaired RBC formation or excessive loss or destruction of RBCs (Table 30-1 ■). Hemorrhage or chronic bleeding (e.g., from a bleeding ulcer) can lead to anemia, as can nutritional problems that interfere with the body's ability to form red blood cells.

PATHOPHYSIOLOGY AND MANIFESTATIONS

Anemia reduces the oxygen-carrying capacity of the blood, leading to tissue hypoxia. As tissue oxygenation decreases, the body attempts to restore adequate oxygen delivery. The heart and respiratory rates rise. Blood is redistributed to vital organs, causing pallor of the skin, mucous membranes, nail beds, and conjunctiva. Tissue hypoxia may cause angina, fatigue, dyspnea on exertion, and night cramps. The kidneys release increased amounts of erythropoietin, which stimulates the bone marrow, causing bone pain. Poor oxygen delivery to the brain can cause headache, dizziness, and dim vision. The severity of the manifestations of anemia (Figure 30-1 ■) depends on the cause and severity of the disorder. For example, rapid blood loss causes immediate symptoms, whereas the person with slowly developing anemia may have no symptoms until the condition is advanced or if the oxygen needs of the body increase (e.g., during exercise or infection).

Blood Loss Anemia

Red blood cells and hemoglobin are lost from the body with acute or chronic bleeding. With acute bleeding, the risk of hypovolemia and shock is greater than the risk of anemia. Chronic bleeding, however, often leads to anemia. The symptoms of the anemia may actually alert the client and care provider to the bleeding problem. In blood loss anemia, RBCs are normal in size, shape, and color, but their numbers are reduced. The RBC, hemoglobin, and hematocrit fall.

Nutritional Anemias

Nutritional anemias result when a lack of one or more necessary nutrients for RBC formation disrupts RBC development or hemoglobin synthesis. The nutrient deficiency may be due to a poor diet, impaired absorption of the nutrient, or an increased need for the nutrient. The most common nutritional anemias are iron deficiency anemia, vitamin B_{12} deficiency (pernicious) anemia, and folic acid deficiency anemia.

IRON DEFICIENCY ANEMIA. Iron deficiency anemia is caused by an inadequate supply of iron for RBC formation. It is the most common type of anemia. The body cannot make hemoglobin without iron. Iron deficiency leads to fewer

TABLE 30-1		
Selected Types and Causes of Anemia		
CLASSIFICATION	**CAUSE**	**EXAMPLES**
Blood loss	Acute or chronic bleeding	Trauma Internal bleeding Complications of pregnancy
Nutritional	Decreased RBC or hemoglobin production	Iron deficiency anemia Pernicious or vitamin B_{12} anemia Folic acid deficiency anemia
Hemolytic	Defective hemoglobin synthesis	Sickle cell disease Thalassemia
	Increased hemolysis	Immune reactions Chemical or physical agents
Aplastic (bone marrow failure)	Suppression of bone marrow function	Leukemias Chemical or physical agents

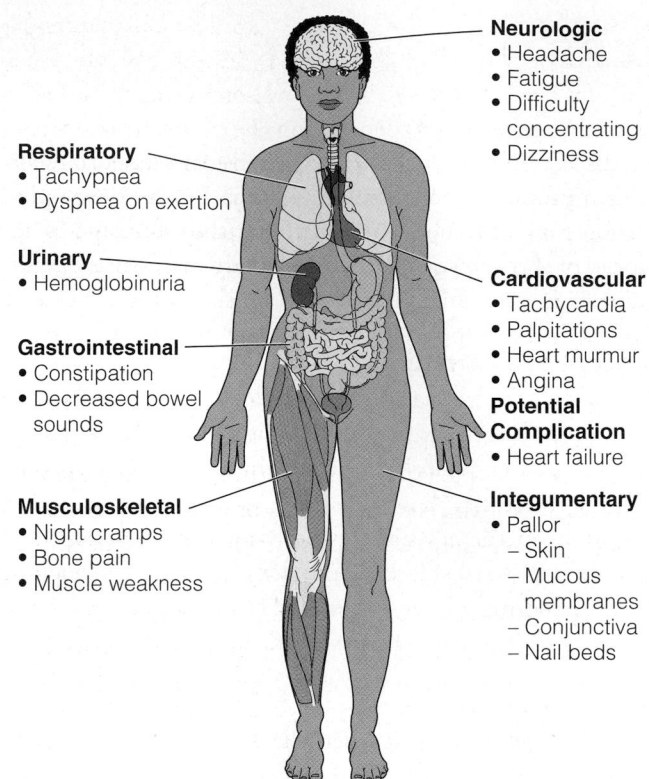

Respiratory
• Tachypnea
• Dyspnea on exertion

Urinary
• Hemoglobinuria

Gastrointestinal
• Constipation
• Decreased bowel sounds

Musculoskeletal
• Night cramps
• Bone pain
• Muscle weakness

Neurologic
• Headache
• Fatigue
• Difficulty concentrating
• Dizziness

Cardiovascular
• Tachycardia
• Palpitations
• Heart murmur
• Angina

Potential Complication
• Heart failure

Integumentary
• Pallor
  – Skin
  – Mucous membranes
  – Conjunctiva
  – Nail beds

Figure 30-1. ■ The multisystem effects of anemia.

RBCs, microcytic (small) RBCs, and hypochromic (pale) RBCs. The RBCs also may be malformed.

In adults, iron loss due to bleeding is the usual cause of iron deficiency anemia. Menstrual blood loss is the common cause in adult females. Chronic, occult (hidden) blood loss may occur from disorders such as bleeding ulcers, gastrointestinal inflammation, hemorrhoids, and cancer.

Inadequate iron intake (less than 1 mg/day) or impaired iron absorption also can lead to iron deficiency anemia. This is common in older adults. Women may develop anemia during pregnancy and lactation because the need for iron is higher.

In addition to the manifestations shown in Figure 30-1, chronic iron deficiency can cause brittle, spoon-shaped nails; *cheilosis* (cracks at the corners of the mouth); a smooth, sore tongue; and *pica* (a craving to eat unusual substances, such as clay or starch).

VITAMIN B₁₂ DEFICIENCY (PERNICIOUS) ANEMIA. Vitamin B$_{12}$ is required for RBC formation and maturation. The usual cause of vitamin B$_{12}$ deficiency is impaired absorption of the nutrient from the GI tract. This is known as *pernicious anemia*. *Intrinsic factor*, a substance secreted by the gastric mucosa, binds with dietary vitamin B$_{12}$ so it can be absorbed by the body.

Vitamin B$_{12}$ deficit interferes with maturation of red blood cells. Great numbers of large, immature RBCs move into the circulation. These cells are fragile and incapable of carrying oxygen in adequate amounts.

Clients with pernicious anemia may develop a smooth, sore, beefy red tongue and diarrhea. Because vitamin B$_{12}$ is important for neurologic function, *paresthesias* (altered sensations, such as numbness or tingling) in the extremities and problems with *proprioception* (the sense of one's position in space) also may develop.

FOLIC ACID DEFICIENCY ANEMIA. Like vitamin B$_{12}$, folic acid is required for normal production and maturation of red blood cells. Folic acid is absorbed from the intestines and is found in green, leafy vegetables; fruits; cereals; and meats. Folic acid deficiency produces an anemia characterized by fragile, megaloblastic (big and immature) cells.

Folic acid deficiency anemia is more common among people who are chronically malnourished (e.g., older adults, alcoholics, and drug users). People receiving total parenteral nutrition (TPN) may develop folate deficiency. Pregnant women, whose folic acid requirements are increased, and clients with certain malabsorption disorders also are at risk.

The manifestations of folic acid deficiency anemia develop gradually. In addition to the symptoms common to anemia, gastrointestinal manifestations such as glossitis, cheilosis, and diarrhea often develop.

Anemia of Chronic Disease

Clients with chronic diseases such as AIDS, rheumatoid arthritis, inflammatory bowel disease, chronic hepatitis, and chronic renal failure often have mild to moderate anemia. This type of anemia is common. Its severity often depends on the severity of the underlying disease. Abnormal immune responses with increased RBC destruction, and impaired bone marrow function and iron metabolism contribute to the anemia of chronic disease.

Manifestations of this type of anemia are similar to those of iron-deficiency anemia. Symptoms often are mild, because the anemia develops gradually and physical activity often is limited by the underlying disease.

Hemolytic Anemias

Hemolytic anemias are characterized by the premature destruction of RBCs. RBCs may be destroyed because the cell itself is improperly formed (*intrinsic*) or because it has been damaged by an outside source (*acquired*). Intrinsic causes include defects in the cell membrane or hemoglobin structure and function, and inherited enzyme deficiencies. External causes of hemolytic anemia include drugs, bacterial and other toxins, and trauma.

SICKLE CELL DISORDERS. Sickle cell disorders are genetically transmitted, inherited as an autosomal recessive trait

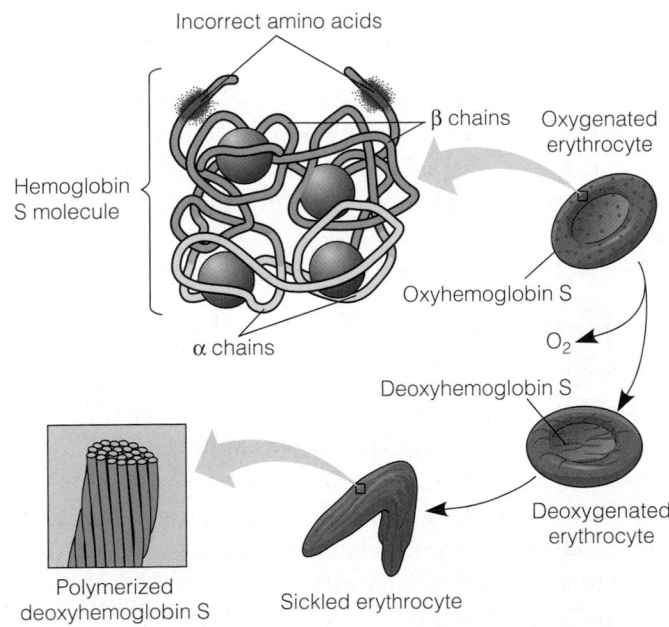

Key:

	Male	Female
Normal	■ (gray square)	● (gray circle)
Sickle cell trait	◨ (half square)	◓ (half circle)
Sickle cell anemia	□ (white square)	○ (white circle)

Figure 30-2. ■ The inheritance pattern for sickle cell anemia.

(Figure 30-2 ■). In disorders with an autosomal recessive inheritance pattern, a person must inherit the abnormal gene from both parents for the disorder to be fully expressed.

Sickle cell disorders are characterized by abnormal hemoglobin, hemoglobin S (HbS), in the RBCs. This abnormal hemoglobin affects how RBCs respond to stress. When blood oxygen levels fall, the cells deform, become sickle shaped, and obstruct small blood vessels (Figure 30-3 ■). Although the shape returns to normal when normal oxygen levels are restored, repeated episodes of sickling damage RBC membranes. The damaged RBCs break down (hemolysis), leading to anemia. Events likely to trigger a sickling event include hypoxia, low temperatures, excessive exercise, anesthesia, dehydration, infections, or acidosis. Box 30-1 ■ provides more information about sickle cell disorders.

Sickling is usually marked by an abrupt onset of intense pain, often in the abdomen. The acute pain also may occur in the chest, back, or joints. The client also has manifestations of anemia and may become jaundiced as bilirubin is released when red blood cells are destroyed.

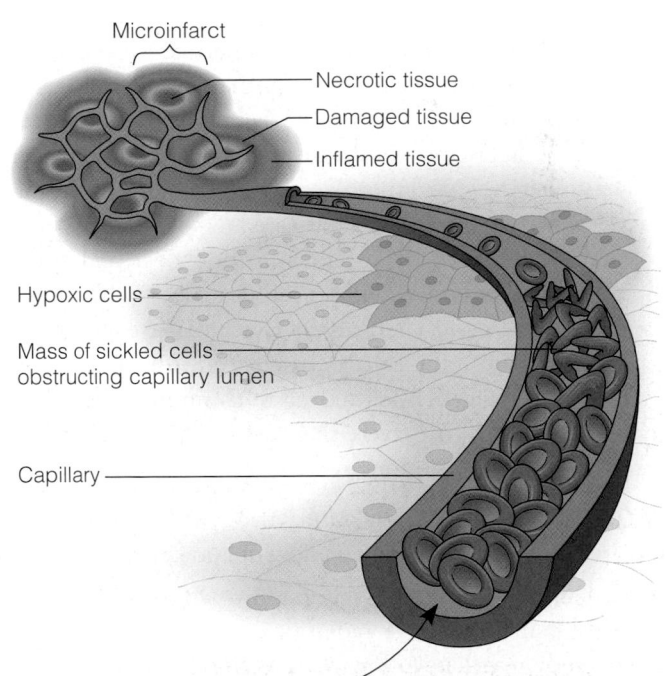

Figure 30-3. ■ Pathophysiology illustrated: sickle cell anemia. Sickle cell anemia is caused by an inherited defect in hemoglobin (Hb) synthesis. When sickle cell hemoglobin (HbS) is oxygenated, it has the same globular shape as normal hemoglobin. However, when HbS is not bound with oxygen, it becomes insoluble and crystallizes into rodlike structures. Clusters of these rods form long chains that bend the erythrocyte into the characteristic crescent shape of the sickle cell.

Sickle cell disease is characterized by episodes of acute painful crises. Sickling crises are triggered by conditions that affect the oxygen supply, increase the oxygen demand, or change the pH. As a sickle cell crisis begins, sickled RBCs cling to capillary walls and each other, obstructing blood flow and causing cellular hypoxia. The crisis accelerates as hypoxia and acidic waste products cause further sickling and cell damage. Sickle cell crises cause small infarctions in joints and organs. Repeated crises slowly destroy organs and tissues. The spleen and kidneys are especially prone to sickling damage.

BOX 30-1	**POPULATION FOCUS**

Sickle Cell Disorders

Inherited sickle cell disorders include sickle cell anemia, sickle cell trait, and related disorders. In *sickle cell anemia,* abnormal hemoglobin (hemoglobin S) is formed within red blood cells.

Sickle cell anemia usually affects people of African descent. About 8% of African Americans have inherited the HbS gene from a parent. They have *sickle cell trait.* They have few symptoms. Each child of a person with sickle cell trait has a 50% risk of inheriting the HbS gene (see Figure 30-2). If both parents have sickle cell trait, each child has a 25% risk of inheriting the HbS gene from both parents. These children are likely to develop sickle cell anemia. Hispanics from the Caribbean and Central and South America also may have the HbS gene.

Sickled cells obstruct blood vessels, causing tissue ischemia (see Figure 30-3). Every organ of the body can be damaged, especially the spleen, bone marrow, lung, eye, and head of the femur and humerus. Good general health maintenance through nutrition, exercise, and avoiding smoking and excess alcohol intake are important to prevent sickling crises.

Sickle cell anemia is chronic, unpredictable, and recurrent, leading to psychosocial stress. The risk of passing the disease to offspring compounds this stress. Genetic counseling is recommended.

THALASSEMIA. Thalassemia is an inherited disorder also caused by abnormal hemoglobin synthesis. It commonly affects people of Mediterranean, Asian, or African descent. Depending on the form of the disorder and whether the person has inherited one or both defective genes, the client may have few symptoms or severe disease.

Manifestations of thalassemia include liver and spleen enlargement from increased red cell destruction. The RBCs are small and fragile; their distinctive bull's-eye appearance has caused them to be called *target cells.* Stress on the bone marrow to produce RBCs can lead to thinning of bones and fractures. People with severe thalassemia may require blood transfusions to sustain life.

ACQUIRED HEMOLYTIC ANEMIA. Acquired hemolytic anemia results when RBCs are damaged by outside factors, such as:

- Mechanical trauma (prosthetic heart valves, severe burns, hemodialysis, or radiation)
- Antibody reactions following infection
- Immune responses (transfusion reactions)
- Drugs, toxins, chemical agents, or venoms.

The manifestations of acquired hemolytic anemia depend on the extent of hemolysis. The spleen enlarges as it removes large numbers of damaged or destroyed RBCs. Bilirubin released from the hemoglobin of damaged RBCs can cause jaundice. In severe cases, bones may become deformed or develop pathologic fractures.

Aplastic Anemia

In *aplastic anemia,* the bone marrow fails to produce RBCs. The cause is usually unknown. Aplastic anemia may follow injury to stem cells in bone marrow caused by radiation or certain chemicals. Benzene, arsenic, nitrogen mustard, certain antibiotics (especially chloramphenicol), and chemotherapeutic drugs can cause aplastic anemia. Aplastic anemia also is associated with some viral infections such as mononucleosis, hepatitis C, and HIV.

People with aplastic anemia usually have *pancytopenia;* that is, they have decreased numbers of red blood cells, white blood cells, and platelets. Signs and symptoms of aplastic anemia may develop gradually or suddenly. These include fatigue, pallor, progressive weakness, dyspnea with exertion, headache, tachycardia, and ultimately heart failure. Platelet deficiency may cause bleeding problems. A deficiency of white blood cells increases the risk of infection.

Myelodysplastic Syndrome

Myelodysplastic syndrome (MDS or *myelodysplasia*) is a group of stem cell disorders characterized by abnormal appearing bone marrow and ineffective blood cell production. MDS is primarily a disorder of older adults. Exposure to environmental toxins such as radiation and benzene and cancer treatment with radiation and chemotherapy are identified risk factors for MDS, although it may develop in people with no known risk factors.

Anemia is the primary manifestation of MDS. The client may be asymptomatic or may complain of weakness and fatigue, dyspnea, and pallor. The spleen may be enlarged, and some clients with MDS develop skin lesions.

INTERDISCIPLINARY CARE

Diagnostic Tests

When anemia is suspected, the following diagnostic tests may be ordered:

- A *complete blood count (CBC)* to determine the RBC count, hemoglobin, and hematocrit.
- *Iron levels* and *total iron-binding capacity tests* to identify iron deficiency. If iron deficiency anemia is present, the serum iron concentration will be low, and the total iron-binding capacity will be high.
- *Serum ferritin* is low in iron deficiency anemia. Ferritin is an iron-storage protein produced by the liver, spleen, and bone marrow.
- *Sickle-cell screening test* is ordered to identify hemoglobin S if sickle cell anemia is suspected.
- *Hemoglobin electrophoresis* is done to identify abnormal forms of hemoglobin when a genetic anemia such as sickle cell anemia or thalassemia is suspected.
- *Schilling's test* is ordered to diagnose pernicious anemia.

TABLE 30-2			
Nursing Implications for Pharmacology: Anemia			
DRUG/CLASS	**ACTION**	**NURSING IMPLICATIONS**	**CLIENT AND FAMILY TEACHING**
Iron Sources ■ Ferrous sulfate (Feosol, Fer-in-sol) ■ Ferrous gluconate (Fergon, Ferralet, Fertinic) ■ Iron dextran injection (Imferon) ■ Iron polysaccharide	Iron preparations are used to treat iron deficiency anemias. They are usually taken by mouth and are absorbed from the gastrointestinal tract.	Assess for drug interactions and GI bleeding. Give with orange juice to improve absorption. Administer elixirs through a straw to prevent staining of teeth. Use Z-track technique when administering parenteral iron (see Box 30-2). Report manifestations of iron toxicity: nausea, diarrhea, or constipation. Monitor hemoglobin and RBC counts.	Take with food (not milk) to reduce gastric distress. Stools may be dark green or black; this is harmless. Increase fluid and fiber intake to decrease constipation. A delayed reaction to iron dextran injection can occur. Report fever, chills, malaise, muscle and joint aches, nausea or vomiting, dizziness, or backache to your primary care provider.
Vitamin B$_{12}$ Sources ■ Cyanocobalamin (Kaybovite [oral], Anacobin [parenteral], Bedoz)	Cyanocobalamin is used to treat vitamin B$_{12}$ deficiencies and pernicious anemia. It is rapidly absorbed and is stored in the liver. Intrinsic factor is required for absorption from the GI tract.	Do not expose injection to light. Do not mix in a syringe with other medications. Administer injections IM or deep SC to decrease local irritation. Monitor hemoglobin, RBC, reticulocyte counts, and potassium levels.	The burning sensation that may occur with injection is temporary. Avoid alcohol, which interferes with absorption. If used to treat pernicious anemia, the medication must be taken for life.
Folic Acid Sources ■ Folic acid (Folvite, novofolacid)	Folic acid is used to treat folic acid deficiency and resulting anemia. Synthetic folic acid is absorbed from the GI tract and stored in the liver.	Do not mix folic acid with other medications in the same syringe. Report hypersensitivity response of skin rash.	Large doses may darken the urine. Excess alcohol intake increases folic acid requirements.

■ *Bone marrow examination* may be done to diagnose aplastic anemia. Nursing care for a client having a bone marrow study is described in Box 29-2.

Medications

Drugs used to treat anemia depend on the type of anemia. Iron replacement is prescribed for clients with iron deficiency anemia. Supplemental iron may be given orally or intramuscularly. Vitamin B$_{12}$ is given by injection to clients with pernicious anemia. Folic acid supplements are ordered for clients with a folic acid deficiency or sickle cell anemia to meet the increased demands of the bone marrow. Hydroxyurea may be prescribed for clients with severe sickle cell disease. This drug promotes fetal hemoglobin production. Fetal hemoglobin reduces sickling and painful crises. Aplastic anemia may be treated using immunosuppressive therapy or androgens (e.g., testosterone) to stimulate blood cell production. Nursing implications for iron, vitamin B$_{12}$,

and folic acid are found in Table 30-2 ■. Box 30-2 ■ reviews Z-track technique to administer iron dextran solution.

Dietary Modifications

Dietary modifications may be ordered for nutritional deficiency anemias, such as iron deficiency anemia or folic acid deficiency anemia. Meats, poultry, and fish provide iron that is readily absorbed. The iron contained in vegetables and grains is less readily absorbed, but accounts for most of the daily iron intake. Selected dietary sources of iron, vitamin B$_{12}$, and folic acid are outlined in Box 30-3 ■.

Blood Transfusion

When anemia is due to a major blood loss, such as from trauma or major surgery, blood transfusions may be given to replace red blood cells. If the bleeding is acute (hemorrhage), whole blood may be given. If the blood loss is chronic, packed red cells may be given. Clients with severe anemia from other causes (such as sickle cell

BOX 30-2	PROCEDURE CHECKLIST

Z-Track Technique Checklist

Before the Procedure

☑ Verify medication order, including drug, dose, route, and time.

☑ Gather all supplies. After drawing the correct dosage into the syringe, draw an additional 0.2 mL of air into the syringe and change the needle.

☑ Identify client and provide for privacy.

☑ Position appropriately for the site to be used (prone or side-lying).

Procedure

☑ Follow Standard Precautions.

☑ Identify and cleanse the site.

☑ Using the nondominant hand, pull skin laterally approximately 1 in. (2.5 cm).

☑ Holding the skin taut, administer the medication and withdraw the needle. Release the skin and apply direct pressure to the injection site.

☑ Document the medication administration, site, and client response.

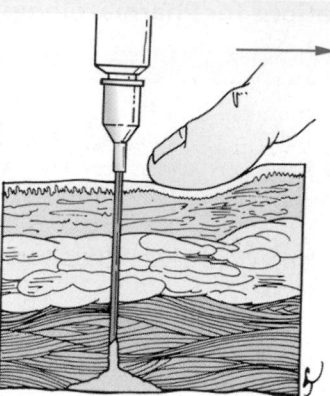

Z-Track Injection

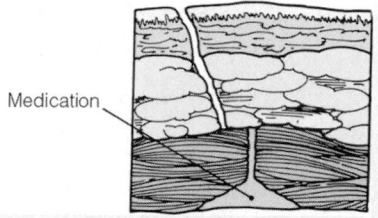

Medication

SAMPLE DOCUMENTATION

12/20/07 1 mL Imferon given R ventral
0900   gluteal site using Z-track
           technique. Tolerated well.
           _____J. Meyer, LPN

Note: Refer to a nursing fundamentals or skills text for more detailed instruction. Check state guidelines and facility policy before performing any procedure.

BOX 30-3	

DIETARY SOURCES OF IRON, FOLIC ACID, AND VITAMIN B$_{12}$

Iron

- Beef, beef liver, pork, ham, chicken, turkey, tuna, shrimp, clams, tofu
- Dried beans, green beans, green peas, spinach, broccoli
- Potatoes, whole grains, brown rice

Folic Acid (Folate)

- Asparagus, okra, spinach and other greens, broccoli
- Green beans and other legumes, dried beans
- Fortified grain products (corn flakes, oatmeal, pasta)

Vitamin B$_{12}$ (Cobalamin)

- Meat, poultry, eggs
- Fish and shellfish
- Milk and cheese

anemia or aplastic anemia) also may require blood transfusions. See Chapter 13 ∞ for more information about blood transfusions.

clinical ALERT

Members of the Jehovah's Witness faith do not accept blood and blood products. Alternatives to blood transfusion include intravenous solutions to increase blood volume and colony-stimulating factors to increase RBC production. Oxygen-carrying blood substitutes are in the process of being developed.

NURSING CARE

Unless anemia is related to acute blood loss, treatment is usually provided in community-based settings. Nurses in these settings play an important role in identifying clients with anemia, monitoring their status and treatment, and providing appropriate teaching.

ASSESSING

Assessment data can reveal manifestations of anemia, as well as provide clues about potential causes of anemia. Assessment data related to anemia are outlined in Box 30-4 ■.

DIAGNOSING, PLANNING, AND IMPLEMENTING

Priorities in Nursing Care. Nursing care priorities for the client with anemia are determined by the acuity of the situation. When anemia is the result of acute hemorrhage, restoring blood volume is of highest priority. When anemia develops gradually, its effects on the client's ability to maintain his or her normal and desired activities are of higher priority.

Activity Intolerance

Inadequate oxygen delivery to the tissues can lead to weakness, fatigue, and shortness of breath with activity.

■ Monitor vital signs, especially heart and respiratory rates, before and after activity. *Vital signs are an objective measure of activity tolerance. Heart and respiratory rates should remain within normal limits during and after normal activities.*

■ Discontinue activity and allow rest for complaints of chest pain, shortness of breath, palpitations, or dizziness;

BOX 30-4	**ASSESSMENT**

Assessing Clients with Anemia

SUBJECTIVE DATA

■ Complaints of fatigue, headache, difficulty concentrating, shortness of breath, palpitations, or dizziness; chest pain, muscle cramps, or aching bone pain; sore mouth or tongue, cracking at corners of lips.

■ Reports of obvious bleeding (excessive menstrual flow, rectal bleeding, or vomiting blood) or black or tarry stools.

OBJECTIVE DATA

■ Vital signs, including orthostatic blood pressure if bleeding is suspected

■ Inspect skin, mucous membranes, nail beds, and conjunctiva for color, condition, presence of petechiae or ulcers; mouth and lips for *glossitis* (inflammation of the tongue), a beefy, red tongue, and *cheilosis* (cracking at the corners); incisions and dressings for acute bleeding.

■ Observe for dyspnea or shortness of breath.

■ Auscultate heart, breath, and bowel sounds.

■ Check stool and vomitus for occult blood.

■ Laboratory reports for RBC, hemoglobin, and hematocrit levels.

---

tachycardia that does not return to normal within 4 minutes of resting; rapid or labored respirations. *These signs and symptoms indicate intolerance of the activity.*

■ Help identify ways to conserve energy during activities of daily living (ADLs), e.g., sitting to shower, spacing activities throughout the day. *Reducing energy use allows greater independence while avoiding excess fatigue or shortness of breath.*

■ Help prioritize activities and distribute tasks among family members. *This allows the client to conserve energy while relieving concerns that necessary tasks are being performed.*

■ Help plan a schedule of balanced rest and activity during the day and 8 to 10 hours of sleep at night. *Rest decreases oxygen demand and reduces fatigue.*

■ Instruct not to smoke. *Smoking is a vasoconstrictor that further increases the workload of the heart and impairs tissue oxygenation.*

Impaired Oral Mucous Membrane

■ Assess condition of lips and tongue daily. *Glossitis and cheilosis increase the risk for bleeding and infection. These conditions also may cause pain and discomfort with eating, interfering with oral intake.*

■ Use a mouthwash of saline, saltwater, or half-strength peroxide and water to rinse mouth every 2 to 4 hours. *This cleans and soothes oral mucous membranes.*

■ Provide frequent oral hygiene (after meals and at bedtime) with a soft-bristle toothbrush or sponge. *Removing food debris promotes comfort and reduces the risk of infection. A soft toothbrush is less likely to cause irritation or bleeding of the oral mucosa.*

■ Instruct to avoid alcohol-based mouthwashes. *Alcohol is drying and will aggravate cracking of the mucous membranes.*

■ Apply a petroleum-based lubricating jelly or ointment to lips after oral care. *A lubricating ointment helps to retain moisture, facilitate healing, and protect the lips from other drying agents.*

■ Instruct to avoid hot, spicy, or acidic foods. *These foods may irritate and dry damaged mucous membranes.*

■ Encourage soft, cool, bland foods. *Foods that are soothing to the mucous membranes promote comfort and help maintain adequate intake.*

■ Encourage four to six small, high-protein, nutritionally balanced meals daily. *Small, frequent meals reduce fatigue. High-protein, well-balanced meals promote healing.*

Self-Care Deficit

■ Assist with ADLs, such as bathing, grooming, and eating. *Assistance decreases energy expenditures and tissue requirements for oxygen.*

■ Instruct to rest between activities such as bathing and dressing. *Rest reduces oxygen demand and cardiac workload, promoting independence and self-esteem.*

■ Listen to and acknowledge concerns about inability to maintain self-care. *Dependence on others for ADLs may signify a loss of control and lead to a loss of self-esteem.*

EVALUATING

To evaluate the effectiveness of nursing care, assess the client's ability to independently perform ADLs, and gradually increase level of activity. Assess skin and oral mucous membrane condition, and ability to consume the recommended diet.

Documenting. Document continuing assessment data, as well as teaching provided. Note the client's apparent understanding of information and willingness to comply with the treatment plan.

CONTINUING CARE

Clients with anemia are primarily managed in the home and community-based health care settings. Assess the client's ability to independently perform ADLs; to prepare and consume the recommended diet, including financial resources for purchasing recommended foods; and to fill prescriptions and manage ordered medications.

Teach about the type of anemia, its causes, effects, and treatment. Provide a list of foods that should be included in the diet. Refer to a dietitian or nutritionist for further teaching as indicated. Discuss ordered medications, including dose, how and when to take the drug, and anticipated side effects and their management. Stress the importance of keeping scheduled follow-up appointments with the health care provider.

Refer the client with an inherited form of anemia for genetic counseling, and discuss the risks of transmitting the condition to offspring. With clients who have sickle cell disease, discuss measures to prevent and treat sickling crises. Provide information about when to contact the primary care provider or seek treatment in the emergency department. Provide contacts for local support groups and national organizations, including:

American Sickle Cell Anemia Association (*www.ascaa.org*)
The Sickle Cell Information Center (*www.scinfo.org*)

Polycythemia

Polycythemia (also called *erythrocytosis*) is an abnormally high red blood cell count with high hematocrit. When the hematocrit is greater than 50%, the blood becomes more viscous or "sticky."

PATHOPHYSIOLOGY AND MANIFESTATIONS

Secondary polycythemia is the most common form of the disorder. It usually develops as a result of chronic hypoxemia or due to excess production of erythropoietin. Decreased tissue

oxygenation stimulates erythropoietin production, which in turn stimulates the bone marrow to produce more RBCs. People who live at high altitudes, where low atmospheric oxygen pressures reduce the amount of oxygen available to the tissues, have a gradual increase in RBCs to adapt to the reduced oxygen. People who have chronic lung disease or who are heavy smokers also often develop polycythemia. Excess erythropoietin production may be due to kidney disease or malignancy.

Polycythemia vera is a primary type of polycythemia in which the production of all blood cells (red, white, and platelets) is increased. Its cause is unknown. Polycythemia vera is relatively rare, and usually affects people over the age of 50. In polycythemia vera, the RBC count increases. The number of WBCs and platelets also increases, although to a lesser degree than for RBCs. The hematocrit and blood volume increase as well. The liver and spleen become congested with RBCs. The client is at risk for thrombosis and infarction.

The onset of polycythemia vera is insidious. Its symptoms are related to excess blood volume, increased blood viscosity, and changes in cerebral blood flow. The client may complain of headaches, dizziness, tinnitus, and blurred vision. Hypertension often develops. Ruddy or dusky cyanosis of the face is common, as is pruritus. The client may develop heart failure, thrombophlebitis, and thrombosis in distal arteries. Gangrene of fingers or toes is a potential complication.

INTERDISCIPLINARY CARE

The *RBC count* and *hematocrit* are elevated in polycythemia. In polycythemia vera, *WBC* and *platelet counts* also are increased. *Erythropoietin levels* are high in secondary polycythemia, but low in polycythemia vera.

Treatment of polycythemia focuses on reducing blood viscosity and volume and relieving symptoms. Phlebotomy, removal of 300 to 500 mL of blood through a vein, can be done repeatedly to keep blood volume and viscosity within normal levels. In some cases, chemotherapy drugs may be used to suppress the bone marrow in clients with polycythemia vera.

NURSING CARE

Nursing care focuses on teaching the importance of maintaining adequate hydration and preventing blood stasis: elevating the legs when sitting, using support stockings, and complying with treatment measures. To smokers, emphasize the importance of smoking cessation. Instruct to immediately report symptoms of thrombosis such as pallor or pain in an extremity, chest or abdominal pain, and any abnormal bleeding.

WHITE BLOOD CELL DISORDERS

Leukemia

Leukemia (literally, "white blood") is a group of malignant disorders of WBCs. In leukemia, the usual ratio of greater numbers of red blood cells than white blood cells is reversed. Bone marrow is gradually replaced by immature, abnormal cells. Eventually, these abnormal cells spill into the circulation and invade other organs such as the liver, spleen, and lymph nodes. If the disease is not treated, leukemic cells replace all normal blood cells, leading to death.

Although leukemia is often considered a childhood disease, it affects many more adults than children each year. It is more common in people over age 50.

The cause of most leukemias is unknown. Identified risk factors include exposure to chemicals such as benzene, genetic factors, viruses, immune disorders, certain cancer drugs, and exposure to large doses of radiation. Its incidence is higher in people who have been treated with radiation or chemotherapy, people living near sites of radiation testing, survivors of atomic bombing sites, radiologists, and people with Down syndrome or other genetic abnormalities.

Leukemias are classified by their onset and duration (acute or chronic) and by the type of abnormal cells (myelogenous or lymphocytic). *Acute leukemia* has an abrupt onset and progresses rapidly. Leukemic cells are immature or undifferentiated (see Chapter 12 ∞ for more information about cell differentiation in malignancy). These immature cells are often referred to as *blasts*. The onset and progression of *chronic leukemia* is more gradual. Leukemic

cells are abnormal and appear mature. *Myelocytic* (or *myeloblastic*) *leukemias* involve myeloid stem cells in the bone marrow. These are the cells that normally become granulocytes (see Figure 29-1). Myelocytic leukemias interfere with the maturation of all blood cells, including RBCs and platelets. *Lymphocytic* or *lymphoblastic leukemias* involve immature lymphocytes in the bone marrow, spleen, lymph nodes, CNS, and other tissues. Table 30-3 ■ compares the four major types of leukemia.

PATHOPHYSIOLOGY

Leukemia begins with the malignant transformation of a single stem cell. Leukemic cells proliferate slowly, but do not become functional WBCs. The bone marrow becomes almost totally filled with leukemic cells. These cells proliferate slowly, but have an extended life span and are unable to function as normal WBCs. They cannot combat infection or maintain immune function. Because cells that produce RBCs and platelets are crowded out, severe anemia and bleeding result.

Leukemic cells leave the bone marrow and infiltrate other tissues such as the central nervous system, testes, skin, GI tract, and the lymph nodes, liver, and spleen. Death usually results from internal hemorrhage and infections.

MANIFESTATIONS

The manifestations of leukemia result from anemia, infection, and bleeding. Anemia causes pallor, fatigue, tachycardia, malaise, lethargy, and dyspnea. Infection, due to impaired WBC function, causes fever; night sweats; ulcers

---

TABLE 30-3

Major Classifications of Leukemia

CLASSIFICATION	CHARACTERISTICS	MANIFESTATIONS	TREATMENT
Acute myelocytic leukemia (AML)	Common in older adults; may affect children and young adults; strongly associated with toxins, genetic disorders, and treatment of other cancers	Fatigue, weakness; fever; anemia; headache, bone and joint pain; abnormal bleeding and bruising; recurrent infection; lymph node, liver, and spleen enlargement	Chemotherapy; stem cell transplant (SCT)
Chronic myelocytic leukemia (CML)	Primarily affects adults; early course is slow and stable, progressing to aggressive phase in 3–4 years	Early: weakness, fatigue, dyspnea on exertion; possible spleen enlargement Later: fever, weight loss, night sweats	Interferon-alpha; chemotherapy, SCT
Acute lymphoblastic leukemia (ALL)	Primarily affects children and young adults; leukemic cells may infiltrate CNS; 70% cure rate in children with aggressive treatment	Recurrent infections; bleeding; pallor, bone pain, weight loss, sore throat, fatigue, night sweats, weakness	Chemotherapy; SCT or bone marrow transplant (BMT)
Chronic lymphocytic leukemia (CLL)	Primarily affects older adults; insidious onset and slow, chronic course	Fatigue; exercise intolerance; enlarged lymph nodes and spleen; recurrent infections, pallor, edema, thrombophlebitis	Often requires no treatment; chemotherapy, BMT

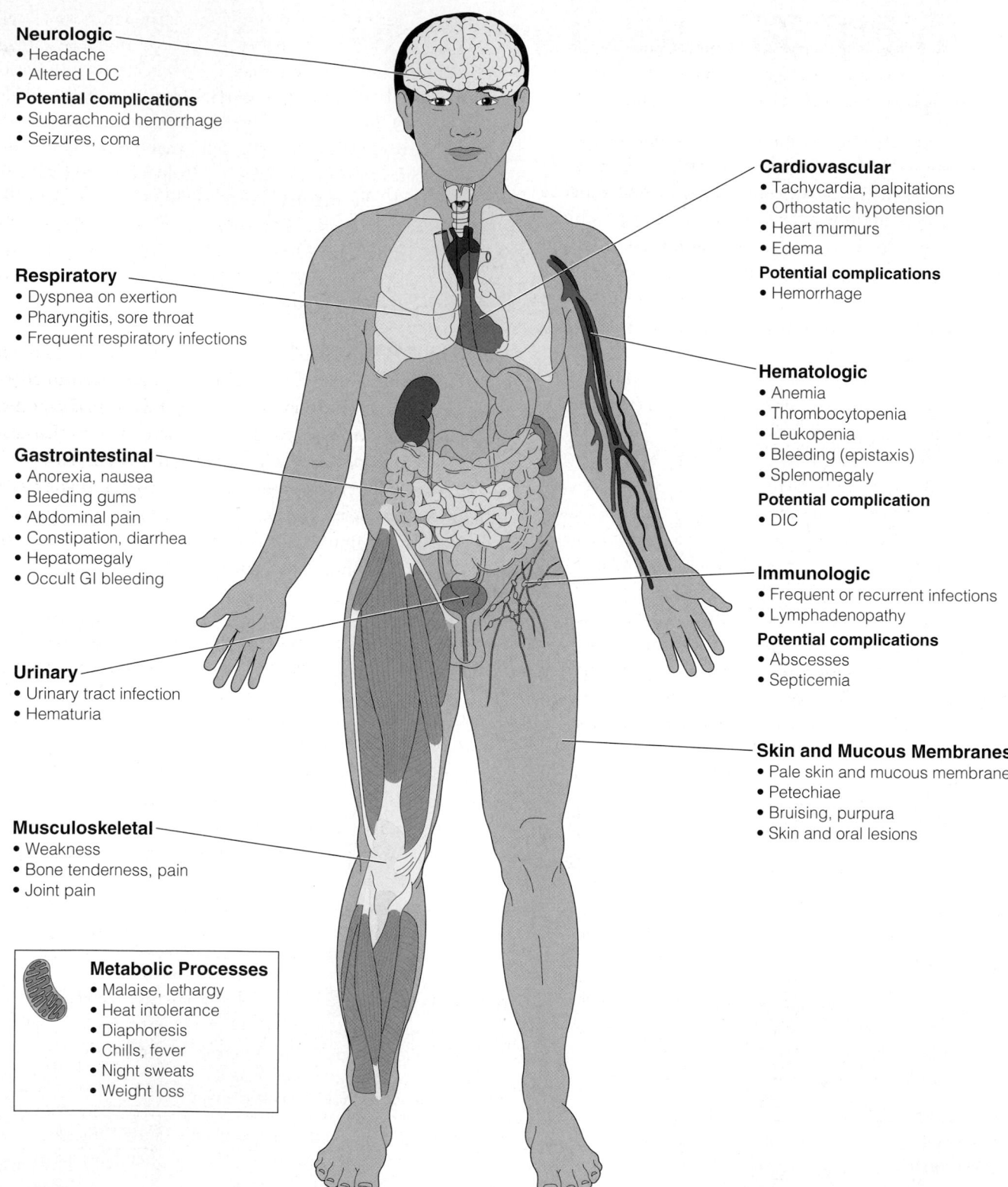

Neurologic
- Headache
- Altered LOC

Potential complications
- Subarachnoid hemorrhage
- Seizures, coma

Respiratory
- Dyspnea on exertion
- Pharyngitis, sore throat
- Frequent respiratory infections

Gastrointestinal
- Anorexia, nausea
- Bleeding gums
- Abdominal pain
- Constipation, diarrhea
- Hepatomegaly
- Occult GI bleeding

Urinary
- Urinary tract infection
- Hematuria

Musculoskeletal
- Weakness
- Bone tenderness, pain
- Joint pain

Metabolic Processes
- Malaise, lethargy
- Heat intolerance
- Diaphoresis
- Chills, fever
- Night sweats
- Weight loss

Cardiovascular
- Tachycardia, palpitations
- Orthostatic hypotension
- Heart murmurs
- Edema

Potential complications
- Hemorrhage

Hematologic
- Anemia
- Thrombocytopenia
- Leukopenia
- Bleeding (epistaxis)
- Splenomegaly

Potential complication
- DIC

Immunologic
- Frequent or recurrent infections
- Lymphadenopathy

Potential complications
- Abscesses
- Septicemia

Skin and Mucous Membranes
- Pale skin and mucous membrane
- Petechiae
- Bruising, purpura
- Skin and oral lesions

Figure 30-4. ■ The multisystem effects of leukemia.

of the mouth and pharynx; and respiratory, urinary tract, and skin infections. Septicemia may develop. *Thrombocytopenia* (low platelet count) increases the risk of bleeding, leading to bruising, petechiae, and hematomas, as well as overt and hidden bleeding into organs. As leukemic cells infiltrate other organs, pain and other symptoms may occur. The manifestations of leukemia are summarized in Figure 30-4 ■.

INTERDISCIPLINARY CARE

Treatment for leukemia focuses on achieving remission or cure and relieving symptoms. Cure is more likely in children than adults. The prognosis for each type of leukemia differs.

Diagnostic Tests

Laboratory tests that may be ordered include:

- *CBC with WBC differential* and *platelet count.* The RBC, hemoglobin, and hematocrit typically are low. The platelet count also may be low. The WBC count tends to be high, with abnormal cells.
- The *bone marrow* is examined to look for abnormal cells. See Box 29-2 for nursing care of the client undergoing a bone marrow aspiration.

Chemotherapy

Systemic chemotherapy is used to destroy leukemic cells and produce remission. Chemotherapy interferes with the proliferation of cells in the bone marrow. A combination of chemotherapy drugs is usually used to treat leukemia. Combining drugs reduces drug resistance, reduces toxicity from high doses of single agents, and interrupts cell growth at various stages of the cell cycle. Cancer treatment with chemotherapy is discussed in greater detail in Chapter 12. 🔗

Radiation Therapy

Radiation therapy may be used to shrink enlarged lymph nodes and destroy leukemic cells in the central nervous system (CNS). Radiation damages the cell DNA so that it is unable to reproduce and multiply. Although normal cells are affected, they are better able to recover from the damage caused by the radiation than are cancer cells. Radiation therapy is discussed in greater detail in Chapter 12. 🔗

Biologic Therapy

Biologic agents such as interferons and interleukins may be used to treat some leukemias. These agents have multiple effects, including moderating immune function and slowing abnormal cell proliferation and growth. Side effects of interferon therapy include flulike symptoms, persistent fatigue and lethargy, weight loss, and muscle and joint pain.

Colony-stimulating factors (CSFs) regulate the growth and differentiation of blood cells. They often are given to clients whose bone marrow function is suppressed due to chemotherapy or leukemic changes. They also are given to stimulate stem cell development prior to harvesting bone marrow for autologous transplant. Bone pain is a common side effect of these agents. Clients also may experience fevers, chills, anorexia, muscle aches, and lethargy. See Table 30-4 ■ for the nursing implications for colony-stimulating factors.

Bone Marrow Transplantation

Bone marrow transplantation (BMT) may be used along with chemotherapy or radiation to treat some types of leukemia. There are two major categories of BMT. In *allogenic BMT,* the bone marrow of a healthy donor is infused

TABLE 30-4			
Nursing Implications for Pharmacology: Colony-Stimulating Factors			
DRUG/CLASS	ACTION	NURSING IMPLICATIONS	CLIENT AND FAMILY TEACHING
Erythropoietin ■ Epoetin alfa (Epogen, Procrit)	Epoetin alfa mimics the action of the hormone erythropoietin in stimulating RBC production. It is used to restore and maintain RBC counts during chemotherapy, renal failure, or zidovudine therapy for HIV disease.	Administer parenterally (IV or SC). Do not shake and do not mix with other drugs. Use only one dose per vial. Monitor BP during treatment; report elevations. Monitor hemoglobin and hematocrit levels.	This drug will be given 3 times per week by injection. Keep all scheduled appointments and BP checks. If you have high blood pressure, take your medication and follow your diet closely. This drug can increase your blood pressure. Headache is common while taking this drug. If it becomes severe, contact your doctor.
Granulocyte Colony-Stimulating Factor ■ Filgrastim (Neupogen)	Filgrastim acts on cells in the bone marrow to increase neutrophil (granulocyte) production. It also enhances the immune function of mature neutrophils. It is used to improve neutrophil counts during chemotherapy, after BMT, and in chronic neutrophilia.	Administer parenterally (IV or SC). Use only one dose per vial. Store refrigerated. Can be allowed to reach room temperature for up to 6 hours before giving. Report elevated WBC and neutrophil counts. Monitor temperature every 4 hours.	This drug is given by injection; you may be taught how to give it to yourself. Bone pain is a common side effect of this drug. Report it to your doctor if you need analgesics for pain relief. Keep all scheduled appointments.

(continued)

TABLE 30-4

Nursing Implications for Pharmacology: Colony-Stimulating Factors (continued)

DRUG/CLASS	ACTION	NURSING IMPLICATIONS	CLIENT AND FAMILY TEACHING
Granulocyte–Macrophage Colony-Stimulating Factor			
■ Sargramostim (Leukine)	Sargramostim stimulates bone marrow production of granulocytes and monocytes/macrophages. It also increases the function of mature WBCs. It is given after BMT to stimulate WBC production.	Administer parenterally by IV infusion or SC injection. Give within 6 hours of reconstitution. Slow IV infusion to half rate if dyspnea develops. Notify physician if dyspnea worsens.	Immediately contact the nurse if you develop difficulty breathing or palpitations during the infusion. Keep all scheduled appointments.
Thrombopoietic Growth Factor			
■ Oprelvekin (Neumega)	Oprelvekin (interleukin-11) increases platelet production. It may be given during chemotherapy to treat resulting thrombocytopenia.	Administer by SC injection. Use reconstituted solution within 3 hours. Causes sodium and water retention; immediately report manifestations of fluid overload. Report hypokalemia and cardiac dysrhythmias.	You may be taught how to give this drug to yourself. Keep all scheduled appointments. Report any of the following to your doctor: shortness of breath, swelling of arms or legs, chest pain, fatigue or weakness, irregular heartbeat, blurred vision.

into the client with the illness; in *autologous BMT,* the client is infused with his or her own bone marrow.

ALLOGENIC BMT. Prior to an allogenic BMT, high doses of chemotherapy and/or total body irradiation are given to eliminate leukemic cells. Then new marrow from a donor (often a sibling with a closely matched tissue type) is infused through a central venous line.

Following allogenic BMT, the client is at risk for *graft-versus-host disease (GvHD).* In GvHD, immune cells in the donated bone marrow identify the recipient's body tissue as foreign. Consequently, T lymphocytes in the donated marrow attack the liver, skin, and gastrointestinal tract, causing skin rashes and sloughing, diarrhea, gastrointestinal bleeding, and liver damage. The disorder is treated with antibiotics, steroids, and, if necessary, other drugs to suppress the immune response.

AUTOLOGOUS BMT. In an autologous bone marrow transplant, about 1 liter of the client's own bone marrow is withdrawn, treated to kill any tumor cells, and then frozen for storage. Massive doses of chemotherapy and/or radiation are then given to destroy tumor cells in the client's body. These high doses destroy any remaining bone marrow and the client's immune system. The stored bone marrow then is thawed and infused through a central venous catheter. The infused bone marrow gradually restores bone marrow and immune function. In an alternative to autologous BMT, stem cells may be harvested from peripheral blood and then reinfused.

During autologous BMT, the client is hospitalized in a private room for at least 6 to 8 weeks. The risk of death due to immunosuppression is a major stressor. Complications that may occur are malnutrition, infection, and bleeding.

Stem Cell Transplant

Stem cell transplant (SCT) is an alternative to BMT. Prior to SCT, the client is treated in a similar manner to clients undergoing BMT. A donor with tissue closely matched to that of the recipient is treated with colony-stimulating factors for several days to increase the concentration of stem cells in circulating blood. Blood is then removed from the donor (a process very similar to blood donation), processed, and administered to the recipient. Stem cells in the donated blood replace the client's blood cell lines with cells that develop from the donated stem cells. The risks for SCT, including infection, GvHD, and other complications, are similar to those for BMT.

NURSING CARE

ASSESSING

In all settings, it is important to recognize the manifestations of leukemia. This is particularly important when working with groups at higher risk (e.g., older adults and children). Assessment data related to manifestations of the disease or the current status of the client with leukemia are outlined in Box 30-5 ■.

DIAGNOSING, PLANNING, AND IMPLEMENTING

Priorities in Nursing Care. Leukemia can be both a chronic and a life-threatening disease. It directly affects a key part of the body's defenses, the immune system. Treatment may require toxic chemotherapy drugs, radiation, or bone marrow transplant. All of these therapies have undesirable side effects. Nursing care focuses on the physical and psychosocial effects of the disease and its treatment.

BOX 30-5	ASSESSMENT

Assessing Clients with Leukemia

SUBJECTIVE DATA

- Complaints of general malaise, fatigue, fever, night sweats; sore mouth or throat, bleeding gums; palpitations, shortness of breath with exercise; anorexia, nausea, constipation, or diarrhea; abdominal pain, headache, bone or joint pain; weight loss, changes in mentation.

OBJECTIVE DATA

- Vital signs, including temperature and orthostatic blood pressure.
- Mental status.
- Inspect skin, mucous membranes, nail beds, and conjunctiva for color, condition, petechiae or lesions, excessive or obvious bruising; check mouth for inflammation, lesions, or bleeding gums.
- Respiratory: apparent dyspnea or shortness of breath; rate and lung sounds.
- Cardiac: auscultate for dysrhythmias, abnormal heart sounds.
- Abdomen: bowel sounds; palpate for tenderness (particularly right upper quadrant); check stool and vomitus for occult blood.
- Laboratory reports for CBC (including RBC, WBC and differential, platelets), hemoglobin, and hematocrit levels.

Risk for Infection

- Institute infection precautions, including the following:
  - If prescribed, maintain protective isolation.
  - Use good hand washing, and remind all care providers and visitors to do the same.
  - Assist to maintain good daily hygiene.
  - Restrict visitors with colds, flu, or infections.
  - Provide oral hygiene after every meal.
  - As much as possible, avoid invasive procedures such as injections, intravenous catheters, catheterizations, and rectal and vaginal procedures. When necessary to perform these procedures, use strict aseptic technique. *These precautions minimize the client's exposure to bacterial, viral, and fungal pathogens.*
- Promptly report evidence of infection: fever, chills, sore throat, cough, chest pain, burning on urination, purulent drainage, and itching and burning in vaginal or rectal areas. *Early detection of infection allows prompt treatment and is vital when the immune system is suppressed.*
- Monitor vital signs and oxygen saturation at least every 4 hours. Promptly report increased pulse or respiratory rate, restlessness, hypotension, or changes in oxygen saturation. *The client with leukemia may not show typical manifestations of infection such as fever. It is important to be alert for other manifestations of infection or sepsis.*

- Report decreasing WBC levels to the charge nurse or physician. *The risk for infection increases as the WBC count declines.*
- Explain the precautions and restrictions to the client and family. Advise that strict precautions are usually temporary. *Understanding increases compliance and thereby lowers the risk of infection.*

Imbalanced Nutrition: Less than Body Requirements

- Regularly monitor weight. *Continued weight loss or a weight below the normal range for height and age may indicate malnutrition. Maintaining adequate nutrition is vital during cancer treatment.*
- Implement measures to promote food and fluid intake, such as:
  - Provide oral hygiene before and after meals; use a soft toothbrush or sponges as necessary.
  - Experiment with food and liquids that have different textures and tastes to identify those best tolerated.
  - Increase liquid intake with meals.
  - Minimize intake of milk and milk products, which makes mucus more tenacious.
  - Encourage to sit upright when eating.
  - Ensure a clean and odor-free environment.
  - Provide medications for pain or nausea 30 minutes before meals, as needed.
  - Provide rest periods before meals.
  - Offer small, frequent meals six times a day. Encourage to avoid very sweet, rich, or greasy foods.
  - Use commercial supplements, such as Ensure.
  - Avoid painful or unpleasant procedures immediately before or after meals.

  Measures to reduce mouth inflammation, sore throat, nausea, and other effects of the disease and its treatment help promote food and fluid intake. Small, frequent meals are often better tolerated, especially high-protein, high-kilocalorie foods.

Impaired Oral Mucous Membrane

- Frequently assess mouth for swelling, lesions, or bleeding. Report complaints of mouth pain or difficulty swallowing to the charge nurse or physician. Culture oral lesions as ordered. *The client with leukemia is at risk for bacterial, viral (especially herpes simplex), and fungal (especially* Candida*) infections of the oral mucosa.*
- Provide a 1:1 solution of hydrogen peroxide and water or warm saline as a mouth rinse for use every 2 to 4 hours. Apply petroleum jelly to the lips as needed to prevent dryness and cracking. *These measures promote healing and comfort and help prevent infection.*
- Encourage use of a soft-bristle toothbrush or sponge to clean the teeth and gums. *Soft-bristle brushes reduce trauma to the gums and mucous membranes of the mouth.*

- Administer drugs as ordered to treat infections or relieve pain. *Topical antifungal agents such as nystatin may be ordered for* Candida *infections. Topical anesthetics such as lidocaine may be prescribed to promote comfort.*
- Instruct to avoid alcohol-based mouthwashes, citrus fruit juices, spicy foods, foods that are either very hot or very cold, alcohol, and crusty foods. Encourage bland, cool foods and cool liquids. *Avoiding food and liquids that irritate the mucosa increases comfort and oral intake.*

Ineffective Protection

Bleeding due to decreased platelets is a common cause of death in leukemia.

- Monitor level of consciousness (LOC) and vital signs every 4 hours and report changes such as hypotension or tachycardia to the charge nurse or physician. *A change in LOC or tachycardia can be early signs of bleeding; hypotension is a later sign.*
- Promptly report manifestations of bleeding:
  - Increased petechiae, bruising, or hematoma formation
  - Obvious bleeding from gums, nose; prolonged bleeding from puncture sites
  - Bright red or coffee-grounds emesis; rectal bleeding or tarry stools
  - Hematuria (blood in the urine)
  - Vaginal bleeding
  - Changes in neurologic status: headache, visual changes, altered mental status, decreasing LOC, seizures
  - Complaints of epigastric pain, absent bowel sounds, increasing abdominal girth, abdominal rigidity
  Prompt reporting allows early treatment of bleeding or hemorrhage. Bleeding into the abdomen or intracranial bleeding may not be readily apparent, and identified only by changes in neurologic status or abdominal assessment data.
- Avoid invasive rectal, vaginal, or urinary tract procedures, and parenteral injections if possible. *Invasive procedures can damage mucous membranes and tissues, increasing the risk of bleeding.*
- Apply pressure to puncture sites for 3 to 5 minutes; apply pressure to arterial blood gas sites for 15 to 20 minutes. *Pressure prevents prolonged bleeding by prompting hemostasis and clot formation.*
- Instruct to avoid straining to have a bowel movement and forceful coughing, sneezing, or blowing of the nose. *Avoiding these activities reduces the risk of external or internal bleeding.*

Anticipatory Grieving

Grieving is an emotional response to the losses associated with a life-threatening illness such as leukemia. See Chapter 14 ⚭ for more information about loss and grieving.

- Use therapeutic communication skills to allow open discussion of losses as well as permission to grieve. *Encouraging discussion about the meaning of the loss helps to decrease some of the anxiety associated with loss.*
- Accept the client's and family's responses to the diagnosis without making judgments. *People respond to stress and grieving in many different ways. Denial, anger, bargaining, and depression are common. Demonstrating acceptance of responses and behaviors promotes trust.*
- Assist to identify ways of managing past stressful situations. In addition, help identify effective coping strategies; sources of strength; reactions to changing family roles; and spiritual or cultural influences on grief reactions. *Grieving is a normal response to a real or potential loss that begins at the time of diagnosis. Identifying resources and strategies that have been successfully used in the past helps the client and family members use these resources during the early crisis of dealing with the diagnosis.*
- Identify agencies, groups, and organizations that may help with the grieving process, and make referrals as indicated. Consider self-help groups, cancer support groups, single-parent groups, and bereavement groups. *A support group that includes others who are anticipating or have experienced a similar loss can decrease the client's feelings of isolation.*

EVALUATING

When evaluating the effectiveness of nursing care for the client with leukemia, look at data that demonstrate freedom from infection (e.g., no fever, vital signs within normal limits). Evaluate weight, food intake, and the integrity of oral mucous membranes. Assess for evidence of bleeding. Finally, look at data that demonstrate coping with the diagnosis, such as talking about the disease and its potential effect on lifestyle and family relationships.

Documenting. Throughout the client's care, document continuing assessment data, indicators of complications, and responses to treatment. Document teaching provided to the client and the family, as well as their apparent understanding and acceptance of information. Note psychologic responses of the client and family, and indicators of their ability or inability to cope with the diagnosis and treatment plan.

CONTINUING CARE

Because leukemia is a chronic disease requiring long-term management, most required care is provided by the client and family members. Teaching is vital to prepare for discharge.

Reinforce teaching about leukemia and its effects, the function of bone marrow, and potential complications. Discuss cancer as a chronic illness that often can be cured or controlled. Provide information about planned treatment, including chemotherapy, radiation, and/or bone marrow transplantation. Discuss the rationale for each type of treatment and techniques to manage the undesirable side effects of the treatment.

Encourage a balance of activity with rest to reduce fatigue. Discuss measures to maintain weight and nutrition: Eat several small, bland meals each day; maintain an ample fluid intake by drinking 4 to 6 glasses of water daily. Instruct to report any continued weight loss, loss of appetite, or an inability to eat for 24 hours. Refer to a dietitian for further teaching and diet planning.

Discuss the importance of measures to prevent infection: Wash hands frequently, especially after using the toilet and before preparing foods or eating; bathe daily; avoid using perineal powders or sprays that could dry mucous membranes; brush teeth using a soft-bristle toothbrush after meals and see a dentist regularly; avoid crowds and contact with people who are ill. Instruct to regularly inspect skin and mucous membranes for signs of bleeding or infection. Instruct to report signs of infection such as fever, chills, burning on urination, foul-smelling urine, vaginal or rectal discharge, or skin lesions to the health care provider. Advise to avoid immunizations unless specifically ordered by the oncologist.

Discuss measures to reduce the risk of bleeding or injury: Avoid contact sports or strenuous exercise if platelet count is low; use an electric razor for shaving; avoid using rectal or vaginal suppositories, vaginal tampons, or enemas to minimize trauma to mucous membranes; increase fiber in the diet, and drink ample water to maintain soft stool and prevent straining. Advise to avoid over-the-counter drugs that increase the risk of bleeding, such as aspirin and preparations containing aspirin, and NSAIDs. Instruct to report any bleeding (nosebleeds, rectal bleeding, vomiting blood, excessive menstrual periods, blood in the urine, bleeding gums, bruises, or collections of blood under the skin) or changes in behavior to the health care provider.

The client and family may need help with physical care, finances, and transportation after discharge. Provide referrals to social services, support groups, home care services if needed, and other agencies that can provide needed services (such as local chapters of the American Cancer Society, which can provide hospital beds and transportation for outpatient cancer treatment).

See the Critical Thinking Care Map at the end of this chapter for an opportunity to use the nursing process to plan care for a client with acute myelocytic leukemia.

Multiple Myeloma

Multiple myeloma is a malignancy in which plasma cells multiply uncontrollably and infiltrate bone marrow, lymph nodes, and other tissues. *Plasma cells* are B-cell lymphocytes that develop to produce antibodies (*immunoglobins*).

The incidence of multiple myeloma is much higher in African Americans than Caucasians. It affects men more often than women, and its incidence increases with age. Multiple myeloma rarely occurs before age 40.

PATHOPHYSIOLOGY AND MANIFESTATIONS

As myeloma cells proliferate, they replace the bone marrow and infiltrate the bone itself. The bone is weakened by these abnormal cells, and may break without trauma (a *pathologic fracture*). Myeloma cells also secrete abnormal immunoglobins. These abnormal proteins are ineffective as antibodies to maintain B-cell or humoral immunity (see Chapter 11). ⚭ They also increase the viscosity of the blood and damage kidney tubules.

The disease develops slowly. Bone or back pain is the most common symptom. As the disease progresses, the pain becomes more severe. Pathologic fractures occur, particularly in weight-bearing bones such as the vertebrae, pelvis, and femur. Vertebral fractures may compress the spinal cord, causing neurologic symptoms. The client becomes more susceptible to infections and develops signs of anemia and bleeding tendencies. Kidney damage may cause manifestations of renal failure (see Chapter 32). ⚭

INTERDISCIPLINARY CARE

Laboratory and diagnostic tests are ordered to confirm the diagnosis of multiple myeloma.

- Urine samples usually are positive for *Bence Jones proteins,* abnormal proteins produced by plasma cells in some forms of multiple myeloma.
- The *CBC* reveals moderate to severe anemia.
- *Bone marrow studies* show excessive immature plasma cells.
- *Bone x-rays* reveal punched-out holes in the bone, particularly in the vertebrae, ribs, skull, pelvis, femurs, clavicles, and scapulae.

There is no cure for multiple myeloma. Treatment focuses on symptom relief (*palliative*). The disease course typically is chronic and progressive; death usually occurs within 2 to 5 years of the diagnosis.

Chemotherapy, radiation therapy, and medications are used to decrease the tumor size and reduce bone pain. Pain is controlled with analgesics. Blood transfusions are used to treat anemia, and infections are controlled with antibiotics. Braces or splints may be ordered as needed to maintain mobility.

NURSING CARE

Clients with multiple myeloma require nursing care similar to that required by clients with leukemia. Pain and the risk for pathologic fractures are additional nursing care considerations discussed in this section.

Chronic Pain

- Assess pain, including location, onset, duration, precipitating factors, and effective relief measures. *Assessment provides baseline data for evaluating the effectiveness of pain relief measures.*
- Assist into the position of greatest comfort. *A client who is weak and uncomfortable may need assistance with repositioning.*
- Support position with pillows. *The client may have painful bony prominences and require the support of many pillows for comfort.*
- Teach effective use of prescribed analgesics. Involve the family as needed to help ensure that pain is relieved. *Taking analgesics on a regular schedule and before pain becomes severe increases their effectiveness.*
- Teach use of nonpharmacologic methods of pain control, including relaxation or guided imagery. *Nonpharmacologic pain management strategies augment the effectiveness of analgesics.*
- Provide for uninterrupted rest periods. *Rest promotes muscle relaxation and emotional equilibrium, increasing the ability to manage pain.*
- Report unrelieved pain to the physician. *Because of the chronic and increasing nature of cancer pain, different or additional medications may be necessary. See Chapter 8 for more information about cancer pain management.*

Impaired Physical Mobility

- Reposition carefully and gently. *Fractures may occur during common activities such as turning or repositioning. Gentle handling reduces the risk of pathologic fracture.*
- Change position at least every 2 hours; more frequently as needed. *Repositioning promotes comfort and minimizes the risk of skin breakdown.*
- Provide a trapeze to assist in repositioning. *A trapeze enables the client to assist with repositioning and promotes self-care.*
- Place needed items close at hand. *This reduces the need to reach for objects and the risk of falling.*
- Place bed in low position, use side rails as indicated, and place the call bell within reach. Keep halls and pathways free of clutter, remove scatter rugs, and provide adequate lighting, a nonslippery floor, and nonskid soles on shoes. *These safety measures reduce the risk for falling and injury.*

CONTINUING CARE

As with leukemia, clients with multiple myeloma must be actively involved in their disease management. Teach signs and symptoms that indicate complications and the need to seek medical help. These complications include infection, pathologic fractures, bleeding, and severe anemia. Infection is the leading cause of death for clients with multiple myeloma. Discuss hospice services with the client and family. Although clients qualify for hospice services during the last 6 months of life, many do not seek services until death is imminent. Hospice services provide pain management, emotional support, and respite services for caregivers.

Agranulocytosis

Agranulocytosis (also called *neutropenia*) is a decrease in granulocytes. In agranulocytosis, both the total granulocyte count and the number of neutrophils are significantly reduced. Impaired WBC formation in the bone marrow is the usual cause of agranulocytosis. Chemotherapy used in cancer treatment and other drugs can suppress bone marrow function. Increased cell destruction also can lead to low WBC levels.

> ### clinical ALERT
>
> Decreased neutrophil counts greatly increase the risk of infection. Protect the client by providing a private room, using excellent hand washing technique, and limiting visitors.

Fatigue, weakness, sore throat, stomatitis, *dysphagia* (difficult or painful swallowing), and fever and chills are the usual symptoms of agranulocytosis. It is diagnosed by the WBC count. The neutrophil count is less than 1,500 cells/mm^3; it may be less than 500/mm^3 when the condition is severe.

Any drug suspected of causing agranulocytosis is discontinued and infections are treated. Filgrastim (Neupogen), a drug that stimulates the growth and development of WBCs in bone marrow, may be given, particularly when neutropenia is associated with chemotherapy. This drug, which is given parenterally, is generally safe. Many clients develop bone pain while taking this drug. (See Table 30-4.)

PLATELET AND COAGULATION DISORDERS

Both adequate numbers of platelets and all of the proteins involved in the clotting cascade (see Chapter 29) ∞ are necessary for the body to form stable clots and to achieve hemostasis. In this section, the focus is on three disorders that

can interfere with effective clotting and lead to excessive bleeding. In the first, thrombocytopenia, the primary problem is a lack of platelets. In hemophilia, lack of one or more clotting factors interferes with clotting. The third disorder presented, disseminated intravascular coagulation, is characterized by abnormal clotting that depletes both platelets and clotting factors, resulting in bleeding.

Thrombocytopenia

Thrombocytopenia is a platelet count of less than 100,000 platelets per milliliter of blood. It is the most common cause of abnormal bleeding. If the number of circulating platelets falls below 20,000/mL, spontaneous bleeding (internal and external) is likely. Thrombocytopenia can result from decreased platelet production, increased destruction of platelets, or accumulation of platelets in the spleen. *Immune* (or *idiopathic*) *thrombocytopenia purpura* is the most common form of thrombocytopenia. It typically affects young adults (ages 20 to 40); women are affected more frequently than men.

PATHOPHYSIOLOGY

In immune thrombocytopenia purpura (ITP), platelets are destroyed much more rapidly than normal. It is an autoimmune disorder in which platelets are destroyed by the body's immune system. Antibodies are developed to proteins in the platelet cell membrane; when these antibodies adhere to the platelet, the spleen identifies the platelet as a foreign cell, and destroys it.

Immune thrombocytopenia may be an acute or a chronic condition. Acute ITP is seen in children and is often preceded by a viral infection. Chronic ITP affects adults and has no known precipitating factors.

MANIFESTATIONS

The manifestations of ITP are caused by abnormal bleeding, particularly into the skin and mucous membranes. **Purpura** (hemorrhage into the tissues), *ecchymoses* (bruises), and **petechiae** (small, flat, purple, or red spots on the skin or mucous membranes) develop on the anterior chest, arms, and neck. Other bleeding may occur as well: *epistaxis* (nosebleed), *menorrhagia* (prolonged and heavy menstrual periods), hematuria, and gastrointestinal bleeding. Spontaneous bleeding into the brain can be fatal. Associated symptoms such as headache, weight loss, and fever also may occur.

INTERDISCIPLINARY CARE

Diagnostic Tests

Thrombocytopenia is diagnosed by its manifestations and diagnostic test results. A *CBC with platelet count* is ordered; the platelet count is decreased to less than 100,000/mL. A *bone marrow examination* may be ordered to evaluate platelet production. Tests for abnormal antibodies, called *antinuclear antibodies (ANA),* are done to assess for autoimmunity.

Medications

Corticosteroids such as prednisone are given to suppress the immune response and the antibodies targeted for the platelets.

Immunosuppressive drugs such as cyclosporine also may be used. See Chapter 11 for more information about immunosuppressant therapy.

Treatments

Platelet transfusions may be needed to restore the platelet count and prevent bleeding. Platelets are prepared from fresh whole blood; one unit contains 30 to 60 mL of platelet concentrate.

clinical ALERT

Platelets must be administered as soon as they are obtained from the blood bank. As with whole blood, platelets are typed and cross-matched to the individual.

Plasma exchange therapy, also known as plasmapheresis, may be done to remove circulating autoantibodies. In this treatment, the client's plasma is removed and replaced with fresh frozen plasma.

Surgery

A *splenectomy* (surgical removal of the spleen) may be necessary. The spleen is the site of platelet destruction and antibody production. This surgery often leads to remission or even cure of the disorder.

NURSING CARE

Nursing care for the client with thrombocytopenia focuses on the risk for injury resulting from bleeding. Although the client faces many challenges related to the disorder and its treatment, protecting the client from consequences of abnormal bleeding is of highest priority.

Ineffective Protection

- Monitor level of consciousness (LOC) and vital signs every 4 hours and report changes such as hypotension or tachycardia to the charge nurse or physician. *A change in LOC or tachycardia can be an early sign of bleeding; hypotension is a later sign.*
- Promptly report manifestations of bleeding:
  - Increased petechiae, bruising, purpura, or hematoma formation
  - Obvious bleeding from gums, nose; prolonged bleeding from puncture sites
  - Bright red or coffee-grounds emesis; rectal bleeding or tarry stools
  - Hematuria (blood in the urine)
  - Vaginal bleeding
  - Changes in neurologic status: headache, visual changes, altered mental status, decreasing LOC, seizures

- Complaints of epigastric pain, absent bowel sounds, increasing abdominal girth, abdominal rigidity. *Prompt reporting allows early treatment of bleeding or hemorrhage. Bleeding into the abdomen or the head may not be readily apparent, and identified only by changes in neurologic status or abdominal assessment data.*
- Avoid invasive rectal, vaginal, or urinary tract procedures, and parenteral injections if possible. *Invasive procedures can damage mucous membranes and tissues, increasing the risk of bleeding.*
- Apply pressure to puncture sites for 3 to 5 minutes; apply pressure to arterial blood gas sites for 15 to 20 minutes. *Pressure prevents prolonged bleeding by prompting hemostasis and clot formation.*
- Instruct to avoid straining to have a bowel movement and forceful coughing, sneezing, and blowing of the nose. *Avoiding these activities reduces the risk of external or internal bleeding.*

CONTINUING CARE

Discuss the need to continue treatment to maintain remission of this chronic disease; also discuss the risks and benefits of long-term corticosteroid or immunosuppressant therapy. Respond to questions about splenectomy. While surgery is an invasive treatment, most people experience partial or complete remission of the disease following surgery. Teach measures to avoid injury and bleeding.

Hemophilia

Hemophilia is not a single disease but a group of hereditary clotting factor deficiencies. Lack of a clotting factor disrupts blood coagulation, leading to persistent and sometimes severe bleeding. Although it usually is considered a disease of children, hemophilia may be diagnosed in adults.

PATHOPHYSIOLOGY AND MANIFESTATIONS

In hemophilia, the first steps of hemostasis, vasoconstriction and the platelet plug, occur normally. The third step,

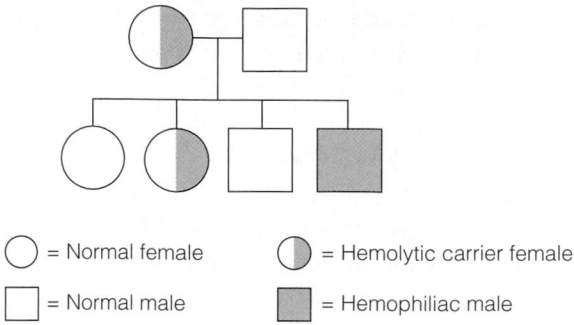

= Normal female   = Hemolytic carrier female
= Normal male   = Hemophiliac male

Figure 30-5. ■ The inheritance pattern for hemophilia A and B. Both are X-linked recessive disorders; females may carry the trait, but only males develop the disorder.

blood clotting, is disrupted by lack of a specific factor required in the clotting cascade. *Hemophilia A* is the most common type of hemophilia. It is caused by a deficiency in factor VIII. *Hemophilia B* (also called *Christmas disease*) is less common. It is caused by a deficiency in factor IX. The clinical manifestations of hemophilia A and B are the same. Both are transmitted from mother to son as sex-linked recessive disorders on the X chromosome (Figure 30-5 ■).

People with hemophilia A or B experience hemorrhages into body tissues. Severe clotting factor deficiencies can lead to spontaneous bleeding episodes. Bleeding of the mouth, gums, lips, and tongue are common, as is hematuria. Bleeding into joints (*hemarthrosis*) causes severe pain and can affect joint structure and function.

Von Willebrand's disease is a common hereditary bleeding disorder classified as one of the hemophilias that is usually seen in adults. It is caused by a deficiency of von Willebrand (vW) factor; factor VIII is often lacking as well. This clotting disorder affects both men and women. Von Willebrand's disease causes less severe bleeding than hemophilia A or B. It is often diagnosed when surgery or a dental extraction causes prolonged bleeding. A comparison of the types of hemophilia is found in Table 30-5 ■.

INTERDISCIPLINARY CARE

Treatment of hemophilia focuses on preventing and/or treating bleeding, primarily by replacing deficient clotting

TABLE 30-5			
Comparison of Types of Hemophilia			
TYPE	DEFICIENCY	CHARACTERISTICS	TREATMENT
Hemophilia A (classic hemophilia)	Factor VIII	Most common form of hemophilia; transmitted from mother with defective gene to sons	Factor VIII concentrate or cryoprecipitate
Hemophilia B (Christmas disease)	Factor IX	Less common; transmitted from mother with defective gene to sons	Factor IX concentrate
von Willebrand's disease	vW factor	Most common hereditary bleeding disorder; affects both males and females	Cryoprecipitate, factor VIII products, or DDAVP

factors. Treatment varies, depending on the clotting defect and the severity of the illness.

Diagnostic Tests

- The *platelet count* is measured; it frequently is within normal limits.
- Coagulation studies, including the *APTT, bleeding time,* and *prothrombin time* are done as screening tests for hemophilia. They often demonstrate prolonged bleeding times.
- *Clotting factor assays* are done to identify specific clotting factor deficiencies.

Medications

Replacement of clotting factors is treatment for hemophilia. They may be given on a regular basis, as a prophylactic measure before surgery and dental procedures, and to control bleeding. Clotting factors may be given in the form of fresh frozen plasma, cryoprecipitates, or concentrates. They may be given intravenously, and may be self-administered. Fresh frozen plasma replaces all clotting factors (including both factor VIII and factor IX) except platelets. People who were treated for hemophilia between 1978 and 1985 have a high incidence of HIV disease, because donated blood was not routinely tested. Rigorous screening of donors, testing of donated blood, and heat treating of blood products have significantly reduced this risk. Factor VIII prepared by recombinant DNA does not contain human plasma, so it carries no risk of infectious disease. It is, however, very expensive.

Desmopressin acetate (DDAVP) also may be used to treat mild hemophilia and von Willebrand's disease. This drug stimulates the body to release vW factor, helping promote clotting.

NURSING CARE

The priority for nursing care for the client with hemophilia is protection from injury and minimizing the risk for bleeding. Assessment of the client is similar to that for a client with leukemia.

Risk for Injury

- Monitor for signs of bleeding, including hematomas, ecchymoses, purpura, and obvious oozing or bleeding. *Careful assessment is necessary to identify hidden or occult bleeding.*
- Notify the charge nurse or physician at the first sign of bleeding. *Prompt intervention decreases the risk of hemorrhage.*
- If bleeding occurs, apply gentle pressure until bleeding stops; apply ice; or apply a topical agent to stop bleeding as ordered. *These measures reduce bleeding until definitive treatment can be given.*

- Avoid giving intramuscular injections, rectal temperatures, and enemas. *These can cause tissue trauma, leading to bleeding.*
- Use safety measures such as a soft-bristle toothbrush and electric razor in personal care. *Use of a soft-bristle toothbrush and electric razor minimize the risk of skin and mucous membrane trauma that may result in bleeding.*
- Protect from injury as needed:
  - Pad side rails of the bed if restless or confused.
  - Assist with ambulation and activities as needed to prevent falling.
  - Provide adequate lighting, especially at night.
  - Keep halls and pathways free of obstruction; make no unnecessary changes in furniture arrangements.
  - Encourage client to wear shoes with nonskid soles when ambulating.

These measures help prevent accidental falls or tissue trauma from bumping into objects.

Risk for Ineffective Therapeutic Regimen Management

- Assess knowledge and reinforce teaching about disorder and its treatments. *Teaching based on current level of knowledge and understanding is more effective than use of standardized teaching plans.*
- Provide emotional support, and express confidence in self-care abilities. *Support and confidence are necessary to incorporate a care regimen into the client's lifestyle.*
- Provide opportunities to learn and practice administering clotting factors and topical hemostatic preparations under supervision. *Practice helps with mastery of psychomotor skills and confidence in the ability to perform self-care.*

CONTINUING CARE

Clients with bleeding disorders need to know how to prevent bleeding, how to treat it at home, and how to administer prescribed drugs. Teach to:

- Recognize and immediately report manifestations of internal bleeding: pallor, weakness, restlessness, headache, disorientation, pain, swelling.
- Apply cold packs and immobilize the joint for up to 24 to 48 hours if hemarthrosis occurs.
- Request a prescription for analgesia if pain is severe. Avoid aspirin, which increases the risk of continued bleeding.
- Ensure a safe home environment. For example, pad sharp furniture edges, leave on a light at night, do not use scatter rugs, and wear gloves when working in the house or yard.
- Use only electric razors.
- Wear a Medic-Alert bracelet in case of accident.

- Practice good dental hygiene to maintain dental health. If dental procedures are necessary, discuss the need for prophylactic clotting factor with dentist and physician.
- Avoid activities that increase the risk of injury, such as contact sports or racquetball.
- Consider physical demands of the job and risk for injury when planning a career or seeking employment.
- Follow safer sex practices.
- Prepare and administer intravenous medications.

Refer clients with hemophilia or a family history of hemophilia who wish to have a family for genetic counseling.

Disseminated Intravascular Coagulation

Disseminated intravascular coagulation (DIC) is a complex disorder characterized by simultaneous blood clotting and hemorrhage. It is a complication of other disorders, such as shock, sepsis, or other conditions listed in Box 30-6 ■. This critical condition has a mortality rate of 50% to 80%.

PATHOPHYSIOLOGY

DIC is a complex process in which the intrinsic and/or extrinsic clotting cascades are activated. Widespread clotting occurs within small blood vessels. Clotting obstructs small blood vessels in the organs, leading to tissue ischemia, infarction, and necrosis. The widespread clotting activates the fibrinolytic pathway that normally breaks down existing clots. Fibrinolytic products interfere with platelet function. Clotting factors are depleted by the abnormal coagulation process, leading to bleeding. Thus, in the client with DIC, both intravascular clotting and hemorrhage are occurring at the same time.

MANIFESTATIONS

Bleeding is the most obvious manifestation of DIC. The bleeding ranges from oozing blood following an injection

---

> **BOX 30-6**
>
> **RISK FACTORS FOR DISSEMINATED INTRAVASCULAR COAGULATION**
>
> - Hypovolemic or septic shock
> - Infection and sepsis
> - Malignancy
> - Obstetric complications
> - Trauma
> - Liver disease
> - Hematologic or immune disorders
> - Acute respiratory distress syndrome
> - Venomous snakebite

> **BOX 30-7**
>
> **MANIFESTATIONS OF DISSEMINATED INTRAVASCULAR COAGULATION**
>
> - Petechiae, purpura, ecchymoses
> - Bleeding from wounds
> - Tachycardia, hypotension
> - Cold, mottled fingers and toes
> - Tachypnea
> - Obvious or occult blood in vomitus and/or stool
> - Abdominal distention
> - Hematuria
> - Oliguria, renal failure
> - Anxiety, confusion
> - Decreased level of consciousness

to frank hemorrhage from every body orifice. Clotting leads to symptoms of tissue ischemia. The manifestations of DIC are listed in Box 30-7 ■.

> **clinical ALERT**
>
> Promptly report abnormal bleeding (e.g., oozing from injection sites, nosebleed) in critically ill clients because it may be an early sign of DIC.

INTERDISCIPLINARY CARE

Clotting studies are ordered to establish the diagnosis of DIC. Treatment focuses on treating the underlying disease and interrupting the clotting/bleeding process. If liver function is intact, it can restore depleted clotting factors in 24 to 48 hours.

Fresh frozen plasma and platelet concentrates are given to control bleeding. Heparin also may be ordered. Heparin interferes with the clotting cascade and may prevent depletion of clotting factors due to uncontrolled clotting. It is used when bleeding is not controlled by plasma and platelets, and when the client is at risk for tissue necrosis and gangrene.

NURSING CARE

Ineffective Tissue Perfusion

Tiny blood clots forming within blood vessels impair perfusion of body tissues.

- Assess peripheral pulses and warmth and capillary refill of extremities. Monitor level of consciousness and mental status. Assess bowel sounds and monitor urine output. Promptly report changes to the charge nurse or physician.

Early treatment of impaired circulation is important to preserve organ function.

- Carefully turn from side to side at least every 2 hours. *Frequent position changes help relieve pressure, maintain tissue perfusion, and preserve skin integrity. Position changes also provide an opportunity to assess tissue integrity and check for bleeding.*
- Discourage from crossing the legs; do not use the knee Gatch on the bed. *These positions can impair blood flow and tissue perfusion of the legs.*
- Minimize tape use. *Tape can damage the skin, causing bleeding.*

Impaired Gas Exchange

Microclots in the pulmonary vascular system can interfere with gas exchange.

- Report oxygen saturation levels and ABGs outside of established limits to the physician. *Oxygen saturation levels and ABGs are objective measures of gas exchange.*
- Administer oxygen as ordered. *Supplemental oxygen helps maintain adequate gas exchange and relieve dyspnea.*
- Place in semi-Fowler's or Fowler's position. *Elevating the head of the bed improves lung ventilation and gas exchange.*
- Maintain bed rest. *Bed rest reduces oxygen demands and improves pulmonary circulation for better gas exchange.*
- Encourage deep breathing and coughing. *Coughing and deep breathing help maintain airway patency, facilitating alveolar ventilation.*

Pain

- Assess pain using a pain scale. Document location, severity, and character of all reported pain. Promptly notify the charge nurse or physician of new or different pain, or if its intensity changes. *The pain scale provides an objective assessment of pain. Changes in the location or severity of pain may indicate tissue ischemia or bleeding into tissues.*
- Handle extremities gently. *Gentle handling minimizes trauma and pain.*

- Apply cool compresses to painful joints. *Application of cold decreases pain perception and may reduce bleeding into joint tissues.*

Fear

DIC is a frightening complication of critical illness.

- Allow client and family to verbalize concerns. *This helps identify concerns and questions.*
- Answer questions truthfully. *Providing truthful answers establishes trust and helps the client and family understand what is happening.*
- Help identify coping strategies. *Past effective coping methods may provide skills to manage the current crisis.*
- Provide emotional support. *The presence of a caring nurse may help reduce the fear and anxiety associated with the crisis.*
- Maintain a calm environment. *A calm, quiet environment and evidence that the staff is in control of the situation help relieve fears and promote rest.*
- Respond promptly to calls for help. *Prompt responses help develop a trusting relationship and reduce anxiety.*
- Teach relaxation techniques. *Relaxation techniques can reduce muscle tension and help the client gain a sense of control.*

CONTINUING CARE

The client with DIC may have continuing effects of the disorder after the crisis is resolved. Clotting in small peripheral vessels may lead to ulcerations and poor wound healing. Teach the client and family about proper foot care (see Chapter 28), ⚭ and any special care needs such as wound care or dressing changes. Heparin therapy may continue in the home setting. Teach administration of the medication, and provide a referral to home health care or home intravenous management services as appropriate. Discuss manifestations of excessive bleeding to be reported to the physician.

LYMPHATIC SYSTEM DISORDERS

Lymphoid tissues are connective tissues that contain many lymphocytes, the WBCs primarily responsible for specific immune responses. **Lymphadenopathy** is swelling and enlargement of the lymph nodes. It may occur in response to infections, inflammation, or cancers.

Lymphangitis and Lymphedema

Lymphangitis is inflammation of the lymph vessels. It is usually caused by a bacterial infection. Clients with lymphangitis develop painful red streaks following the lymph vessels and extending up an arm or leg. If lymph nodes also

become inflamed, it is called *lymphadenitis.* The lymph nodes are swollen and may be tender. Fever, malaise, and chills also accompany lymphangitis or lymphadenitis.

Lymphedema is edema caused by obstruction of lymph vessels. Obstruction of the lymph vessels from surgical removal of lymph nodes (as is done in a radical mastectomy), scarring of lymph nodes following radiation, or invasion of lymph nodes by tumor may cause lymphedema. Clients who live in the tropics may develop *elephantiasis,* a type of lymphedema caused by filaria, a nematode worm.

The affected extremity is swollen and edematous (Figure 30-6 ■). Early in the course of the disorder, the edema is soft

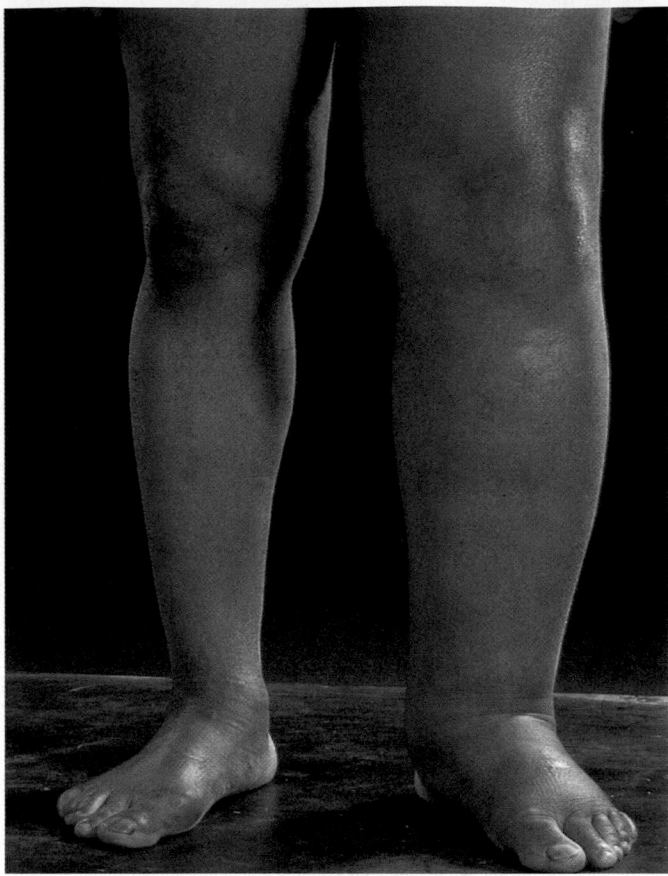

Figure 30-6. ■ Severe lymphedema of the lower extremity. (*Source:* NMSB, Custom Medical Stock Photos, Inc.)

and pitting. With time, the edematous tissue becomes hard to the touch (*brawny edema*). The skin appears thick and hardened and may resemble an orange peel. The edema may worsen in warm weather and (if the legs are affected) after standing for long periods.

INTERDISCIPLINARY CARE

Interdisciplinary care for clients with lymphatic system disorders focuses on relieving edema, maintaining skin integrity in the affected extremity, and preventing or treating infection.

For lymphangitis, moist heat is applied and the affected extremity is elevated and immobilized. Meticulous skin and wound care are vital. Antibiotics are prescribed to treat the infection. Penicillin G is often used because streptococcal bacteria are common causative organisms.

Lymphedema is often chronic and requires longer term treatment. Measures such as the following are ordered:

■ Elevate the extremity, especially during sleep.
■ Use elastic stockings, elastic bandages, or pneumatic pressure devices.
■ Provide meticulous skin hygiene.
■ Remain on bed rest.
■ Restrict dietary sodium.

Occasionally, surgery may be performed to relieve pain, remove cancerous tissue, or treat repeated episodes of lymphangitis in the affected extremity.

NURSING CARE

The nursing care focus for clients with lymphatic system disorders is the same as the interdisciplinary care focus: relieving edema, maintaining skin integrity, and preventing infection.

Measure the circumference of the affected extremity daily or as ordered. Maintain intake and output records, and weigh daily. Report changes to the charge nurse or physician. Restrict sodium intake and help choose low-sodium foods.

Apply antiembolic stockings and intermittent pressure devices as ordered. Remove stockings and pressure devices at least once each shift to inspect the underlying skin for redness, irritation, dryness, or breakdown. Document findings. Elevate extremities while seated or in bed. Keep skin clean and dry, especially between toes. Use protective devices such as egg crate foam, sheepskin, pillows, or padding to reduce the risk of skin breakdown.

CONTINUING CARE

Teach how to apply and use intermittent pressure devices and/or elastic stockings. Instruct to wear elastic stockings during waking hours and to remove them while sleeping. Emphasize the importance of inspecting the skin at least daily for signs of breakdown or cracking.

Teach skin care to promote its integrity, prevent breakdown, and reduce the risk for infection. Help develop a schedule and plan for elevating the affected extremity that interferes as little as possible with daily schedules. Discuss other prescribed measures such as any activity restriction, dietary sodium restriction, and diuretic therapy. Provide a list of high-sodium foods to avoid, and refer to a dietitian for further teaching about salt-restricted diets. If the client is taking a potassium-wasting diuretic, provide a list of foods that are high in potassium (see Box 7-12 in Chapter 7). ∞

Provide information about contacts for questions, and make referrals as needed. The client may face long years of self-management and may need assistance with health care management, meals, and housework.

Infectious Mononucleosis

Infectious mononucleosis is an acute infectious disease caused by the Epstein–Barr virus (EBV). This disease, which primarily affects young adults, is usually benign and self-limiting. It appears to be transmitted by saliva; hence, it is often called the "kissing disease."

When the virus enters the body, it invades B cells in the lymphoid tissues of the oropharynx. The infection causes increased lymphocyte production and swelling of lymph glands. The manifestations begin with headache, malaise, and fatigue. Most clients with infectious mononucleosis have fever, sore throat, and enlargement and pain in the cervical lymph nodes. Enlargement of the spleen occurs in about half of all people with the illness.

Laboratory findings include increased lymphocytes and monocytes; about one-fifth of the cells are atypical in form. The WBC count increases and remains high for 4 to 8 weeks. Platelet counts are often low during the illness.

Recovery occurs in 2 to 3 weeks. However, weakness and lethargy may last for up to 3 months. Treatment includes bed rest and analgesics to relieve the symptoms.

Malignant Lymphoma

Malignant lymphomas are cancerous tumors of lymphoid tissue. They are characterized by lymphocyte proliferation and progressive, painless enlargement of the lymph nodes.

PATHOPHYSIOLOGY AND MANIFESTATIONS

Lymphomas are classified as Hodgkin's disease (or Hodgkin's lymphoma) and non-Hodgkin's lymphomas.

Hodgkin's Disease

Hodgkin's disease is one of the most curable of all cancers. It is characterized by painless, progressive enlargement of one or more lymph nodes and the presence of *Reed–Sternberg cells* in the affected node. It usually affects people between the ages of 15 and 35 or over age 50. It is more common in men than women. The cause of Hodgkin's disease is unknown, but it may be linked to viral infection (Epstein–Barr virus). The lymph nodes of the neck or above the clavicle often are the first affected. If untreated, it spreads via the lymphatic system to nodes throughout the body.

The most common manifestation of Hodgkin's disease is an enlarged lymph node that is not painful or tender. The node or nodes are firm but movable. Other common symptoms are listed in Box 30-8 ■.

BOX 30-8

MANIFESTATIONS OF HODGKIN'S DISEASE
- One or more painless, enlarged lymph nodes
- Fever
- Night sweats
- Pruritus
- Weight loss
- Fatigue
- Malaise

Non-Hodgkin's Lymphoma

Non-Hodgkin's lymphomas are more common than Hodgkin's disease. Unlike Hodgkin's disease, multiple lymph nodes and lymphoid tissue in other body tissues are involved. Non-Hodgkin's lymphomas tend to occur in older adults. They also are more common in people whose immune system has been suppressed by HIV disease or immunosuppressive drugs (e.g., people who have had an organ transplant).

The first symptom of non-Hodgkin's lymphoma often is an enlarged lymph node. The client may, however, have symptoms such as abdominal pain, nausea, vomiting, or bloody diarrhea. Involvement of other organs can lead to symptoms of urinary tract obstruction or infection, neurologic symptoms, shortness of breath, cough, or chest pain. Systemic manifestations such as weight loss, fatigue, and night sweats also may be present. The prognosis for non-Hodgkin's lymphoma is not as good as it is for Hodgkin's disease.

INTERDISCIPLINARY CARE

Diagnostic Tests and Staging

A *chest x-ray* and *chest* and *abdominal CT scans* are done to identify enlarged lymph nodes. The diagnosis of lymphoma is made based on *biopsy* of tissue from the enlarged node or tissue mass. If Reed–Sternberg cells are present, the diagnosis of Hodgkin's disease is confirmed. For both Hodgkin's disease and non-Hodgkin's lymphoma, the *Ann Arbor staging system* is used to determine the extent and severity of the disease and to estimate the prognosis. For Hodgkin's disease, the newer *Cotswold Staging Classification System* may be used. These systems use the number and location of involved lymph nodes to stage the disease. In stage I disease, only one lymph node region, lymphoid organ, or site outside the lymphatic system is involved. Stages II and III are used to identify the involvement of additional lymph node regions, organs, or extralymphatic sites. Stage IV indicates widely spread disease. An A indicates no systemic manifestations; a B is used to indicate the presence of systemic symptoms such as fever, night sweats, and weight loss.

Chemotherapy

Combination chemotherapy is used to treat both Hodgkin's disease and non-Hodgkin's lymphoma. The choice of drug combination depends on the stage of the disease as well as the client's age and general condition. Chemotherapy results in complete remission in more than 75% of clients with Hodgkin's disease who do not have systemic symptoms.

Radiation Therapy

Radiation therapy is used to treat both Hodgkin's disease and non-Hodgkin's lymphoma. It is the primary treatment for early Hodgkin's; it is combined with chemotherapy to treat later stages and non-Hodgkin's lymphomas. Therapy usually

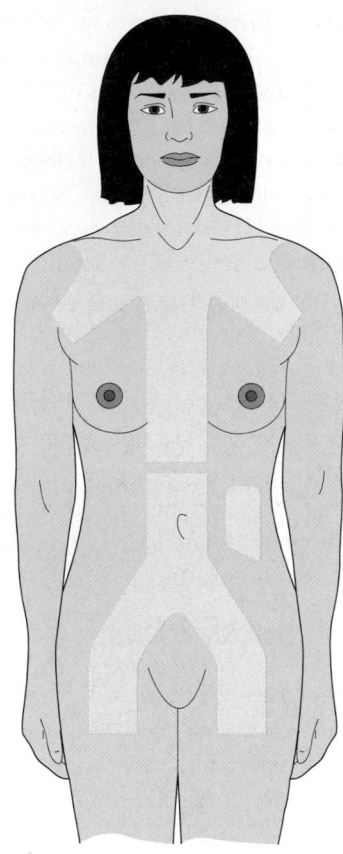

Figure 30-7. ■ Areas of radiation for total nodal radiation therapy.

involves external radiation of the involved lymph node region. If the disease is advanced, total nodal irradiation may be done (Figure 30-7 ■). This may cause permanent sterility.

NURSING CARE

Nursing care of the client with malignant lymphoma involves providing physical and emotional support throughout the course of treatment. The client is at risk for infection because cancerous lymphocytes are less effective in mounting an immune response. Nutritional status also must be considered due to the effects of the disease and treatment on appetite and food tolerance. See Risk for Infection and Imbalanced Nutrition: Less than Body Requirements in the Nursing Care section for leukemia for nursing activities to address these problems.

Risk for Impaired Skin Integrity

Pruritus and night sweats (symptoms of lymphoma) increase the risk for skin lesions. Radiation therapy also can damage the skin.

- Discuss measures to relieve itching:
  - Use cool water and a mild soap to bathe.
  - Blot (rather than rub) dry skin; apply plain cornstarch or nonperfumed lotion or powder to the skin unless

contraindicated (lotions and powders may not be allowed if undergoing radiation therapy).
  - Use lightweight cotton blankets and clothing.
  - Maintain adequate humidity and a cool room temperature.
  - Wash bedding and clothes in mild detergent, and put them through a second rinse cycle.

Pruritus is aggravated by excessive warmth, excessive dryness, rough fabrics, fatigue, and stress. These interventions reduce mechanical or chemical irritation of the skin.

Nausea

- Administer ordered antiemetics before chemotherapy is started. *Premedication with an antiemetic can prevent nausea and reduce the psychological association between chemotherapy and nausea.*
- Teach measures to prevent or relieve nausea and vomiting:
  - Eat soda crackers and suck on hard candy.
  - Eat soft, bland foods that are cold or at room temperature.
  - Avoid unpleasant odors, and get fresh air.
  - Do not eat immediately before chemotherapy.
  - Use distraction or progressive muscle relaxation when nauseated.

Crackers and hard candy often relieve queasiness. Foods that are hot, warm, salty, sweet, or have strong odors often increase nausea. Alternative methods of relieving nausea may be effective.

Fatigue

- Assess complaints of malaise (a vague feeling of body weakness or discomfort) and fatigue (a pervasive, drained feeling that cannot be eliminated). *Malaise and fatigue are subjective experiences.*
- Encourage expression of feelings about the disease and its impact on lifestyle and roles. *Discussion may help the client identify lifestyle priorities.*
- Encourage enjoyable but quiet activities, such as reading, listening to music, or doing puzzles. *Enjoyable activities such as these help conserve energy and decrease fatigue.*
- Help establish priorities, and include rest periods or naps when scheduling daily activities. *This helps the client maintain control and self-esteem while conserving energy.*
- Encourage client to delegate some responsibilities to others. *Delegating responsibilities helps conserve energy while allowing others to be more involved in care and decision making.*
- Encourage a diet high in carbohydrates and fluids. *A high-carbohydrate diet helps maintain energy stores, while increased fluid intake promotes excretion of waste products that may cause malaise and fatigue.*

Disturbed Body Image

- Collect subjective data related to body image by asking questions such as these:
  - What do you like the most/least about your body?
  - What do you understand about your disease?
  - How do you feel about this illness?
  - How do you think your illness or treatment will affect you?
  - Has the illness changed the way you believe others will respond to you?

  A person's image of his or her body is based on past and present experiences. It includes both the physical body and emotional responses to that body. Body image changes constantly.

- Assess for objective signs of altered body image, such as refusal to touch or look at a body part or to look in a mirror; refusal to discuss body changes; refusal to participate in self-care or rehabilitation; increasing dependence on others; signs of grieving (weeping, despair, anger); hostility toward healthy people; or withdrawal from social contacts. *Although there is no one response to an altered body image, clients may demonstrate any of the above signs.*

- Teach ways to cope with *alopecia* (hair loss). Discuss using wigs, scarves, hats, and caps during hair loss and regrowth. Teach scalp care using baby shampoo or mild soap, a soft brush, and mineral oil to reduce itching. Emphasize the importance of using sunscreen and covering the head to prevent sunburn. If eyelashes and eyebrows are lost, teach methods of protecting the eyes, such as eyeglasses and caps with wide brims. Discuss and refer to resources (such as the American Cancer Society or insurance) for financial assistance to buy wigs. *Alopecia may range from thinning of hair to total hair loss. Regrowth usually begins 2 to 3 months after treatment ends. New hair may be softer, more curly, and slightly different in color.*

- Assess knowledge of the effects of illness and treatment on sexuality and reproduction. Provide information and clarify misconceptions as needed. Encourage the client and significant other to verbalize concerns. Discuss options such as storing sperm in a sperm bank prior to undergoing radiation therapy. Refer for counseling as indicated. *Sexual function often is altered by the disease and the effects of treatment. This may include temporary or permanent sterility, changes in menstruation, and changes in libido (sexual desire).*

- Encourage participation in support groups. *Support groups are often effective in helping the client and family deal with loss and altered body image.*

CONTINUING CARE

Teach about lymphoma, its treatment, and the side effects of treatments. Topics that are appropriate for the client with leukemia are also appropriate for the client with a malignant lymphoma. In addition, teach the client and family to:

- Care for the skin and avoid scratching to reduce the risk of infection.
- Report new or different symptoms that may indicate extension of the disease.
- Use complementary pain management strategies as well as prescribed drugs to promote comfort. See Chapter 8 ⚭ for more information about cancer pain management.
- Plan activities of daily living to ensure adequate rest and exercise.
- Eat a well-balanced diet.

Refer to the local chapter of the American Cancer Society for information, financial assistance, and counseling. Clients with malignant lymphomas may obtain a list of state and local agencies that offer information about the disease and financial assistance from the Leukemia Society of America.

NURSING PROCESS CARE PLAN
Client with Hodgkin's Disease

Albin Quito, age 28, is a nurse manager in a large teaching hospital. Lately, he has noticed that he is more tired than usual, often wakes up at night covered with sweat, and just does not feel well. He attributed his symptoms to "a touch of the flu" and to his busy work schedule. Yesterday morning, he noticed a large swollen area on the right side of his neck. He made an appointment with his primary health provider. At that appointment, a large cervical lymph node was found, and blood was drawn. A biopsy of the node and a computed tomography (CT) scan of the chest were scheduled.

Assessment. David Herzog, the clinic nurse, obtains a nursing assessment on Mr. Quito. His physical exam is normal, with the exception of the enlarged node, which is not painful to touch. When Mr. Quito is weighed, he says that he has lost 7 lbs (3.2 kg) in the past 2 months. Test results include mild anemia and an increased neutrophil count. Reed–Sternberg cells are found in the lymph node biopsy. The physician makes the diagnosis of Hodgkin's disease and tells Mr. Quito that his prognosis is very good. After learning about treatment options, Mr. Quito decides to undergo radiation therapy.

Diagnosis. Mr. Herzog identifies the following nursing diagnoses:

- *Anxiety* related to malignancy and uncertainty about ability to continue working in his present position
- *Risk for Infection* related to impaired immunologic function
- *Fatigue* related to the effects of the cancer and planned treatment

Expected Outcomes. The expected outcomes in the plan of care specify that Mr. Quito will:

- Verbalize a decrease in anxiety.
- Remain free of infection.
- Use methods to preserve energy.

Planning and Implementation. The following nursing interventions are planned and implemented:

- Encourage to discuss treatment schedule with supervisor to plan release time.
- Encourage to join a support group for people with cancer.
- Provide information about illness and radiation therapy.
- Discuss ways to decrease the risk of infection.
- Discuss energy management strategies such as:
  - Take a short nap once or twice a day to provide total body rest.
  - Do not overexert during weekends.
  - Maintain a well-balanced diet.

Evaluation. When Mr. Quito returns to begin radiation, he brings his friend Nancy. He asks Mr. Herzog to discuss his treatment with her. Mr. Quito says, "I am still really scared, but being able to talk about this with Nancy will help a lot." Mr. Quito has made arrangements for a leave of absence from work, with the understanding that his job will be held for him. He states that he will have some money problems but is working them out. He also says he feels that taking a nap is silly but he'll try it. They have found a cancer support group and plan to attend the next meeting.

Critical Thinking in the Nursing Process

1. Review radiation and chemotherapy in Chapter 12. How do each of these treatments work to kill malignant cells?
2. What information will you give Mr. Quito about preventing infection while he is at home?
3. How might the psychologic and socioeconomic effect of the diagnosis of cancer differ in a young adult versus an older adult?

Note: The bibliography listings for this and all chapters have been compiled at the back of the book.

Chapter Review

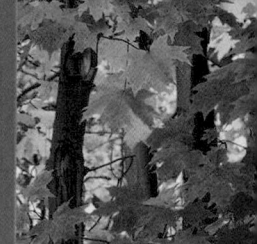

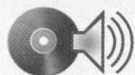 **KEY TERMS** by Topics

Use the audio glossary feature of either the CD-ROM or the Companion Website to hear the correct pronunciation of the following key terms.

Red blood cell disorders
anemia, polycythemia

White blood cell disorders
leukemia, bone marrow transplantation (BMT), stem cell transplant (SCT), multiple myeloma, agranulocytosis

Platelet and coagulation disorders
thrombocytopenia, purpura, petechiae, hemophilia

Lymphatic system disorders
lymphadenopathy, malignant lymphomas

KEY Points

- Because blood is the transport medium for oxygen, nutrients, and other substances, disorders that affect the blood often have widespread effects on other organs and systems.

- Anemia (lack of RBCs and hemoglobin) is a common disorder. It has a variety of causes, including nutritional deficiencies, genetic disorders, inadequate RBC production, and loss of RBCs through bleeding or abnormal destruction. Too few RBCs or inadequate hemoglobin can lead to cellular hypoxia, causing weakness and fatigue.

- Polycythemia (too many RBCs) usually develops secondarily to chronic hypoxia, for example, in clients with chronic lung disease. Too many RBCs increase the viscosity or "stickiness" of the blood.

- The primary function of WBCs is to fight off infection, destroy foreign matter, and eliminate damaged or abnormal cells in the body; WBC disorders affect immune function.

- Leukemia is a malignancy in which abnormal WBCs multiply, gradually replacing normal bone marrow and impairing the ability to form normal blood cells and fight off infection. The risk factors, treatment, and prognosis for different types of leukemia vary.

- Multiple myeloma also is a WBC malignancy. It, however, affects B lymphocytes called plasma cells. These cells proliferate and invade bone marrow, lymph nodes, and other tissues. Clients with multiple myeloma have bone pain and a high risk for pathologic fractures.

- Platelets are vital to the process of blood clotting (coagulation) and control of bleeding. Clients with thrombocytopenia (low platelet count) are at significant risk for bleeding.

- Hemophilia is a clotting disorder that is genetically transmitted on the X chromosome from mothers to sons. In hemophilia, lack of a specific clotting factor interrupts the clotting cascade. Again, this leads to a significant risk for bleeding with minor injuries.

- The lymphatic system also is involved in the immune response. Lymph nodes often swell during infections. Painless swelling of a lymph node, however, may indicate a malignancy such as Hodgkin's disease, non-Hodgkin's lymphoma, or others.

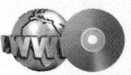 **EXPLORE MediaLink**

Additional interactive resources for this chapter can be found on the Companion Website at www.prenhall.com/burke. Click on Chapter 30 and "Begin" to select the activities for this chapter.

For chapter-related NCLEX-style review questions and an audio glossary, access the accompanying CD-ROM in this book.

FOR FURTHER Study

For more information about potassium, see Chapter 7.

Chapter 8 provides information about managing cancer pain.

For more information about corticosteroids and immunity, see Chapter 11.

For more information about malignancies, chemotherapy, and radiation therapy, see Chapter 12.

For more information about blood transfusions, see Chapter 13.

For more about loss and grieving, see Chapter 14.

For more information about proper foot care, see Chapter 28.

For more information about kidney damage and renal failure, see Chapter 32.

Critical Thinking Care Map

Caring for a Client with Acute Myelocytic Leukemia
NCLEX-PN® Focus Area: Safe, Effective Care Environment

Case Study: Catherine Cole is a 37-year-old secretary. About 2 months ago, she began to tire easily and experience night sweats and an intermittent fever. She also noticed that her skin was pale, she bruised easily, and she was having heavier menstrual periods. After seeing her primary care physician, Mrs. Cole is admitted to the hospital for a bone marrow biopsy.

Nursing Diagnosis: Ineffective Protection

COLLECT DATA

Subjective	Objective
_____	_____
_____	_____
_____	_____
_____	_____
_____	_____
_____	_____

Would you report this data? Yes/No

If yes, to: _____

Nursing Care

_____
_____
_____
_____
_____
_____
_____
_____

How would you document this? _____
_____
_____
_____

Data Collected
(use those that apply)

- States, "I'm so tired, and I have these bruises all over me. I'm so afraid of the results of the bone marrow test. I don't know what we will do if I have cancer."
- 5'4" inches (156 cm) tall, weighs 106 lbs (48.1 kg)
- Vital signs T 100°F; P 102; R 22; BP 130/82
- Night sweats and intermittent fever for past 2 months
- Numerous petechiae scattered over trunk and arms
- Ecchymoses lower right arm and right calf
- Relates menstrual periods heavier than normal
- Oral mucosa red, with several small ulcerations in buccal areas
- Low RBC count; low hemoglobin and hematocrit; low platelets; high WBC count; myeloblasts present

Nursing Interventions
(use those that apply; list in priority order)

- Place in a private room.
- Limit visitors to husband and daughter.
- Verbally and in writing remind staff, family, and client to practice good hand washing. Post a sign in the room as a reminder, and discuss the importance of hand washing with Mrs. Cole and her family.
- Take and record vital signs every 4 hours.
- Frequently assess for and report signs of bleeding such as increased bruising, joint pain, occult blood in body fluids, and menstrual pad count.
- Assist with oral hygiene every 2 to 4 hours, using a soft-bristle toothbrush or a sponge. Offer warm saline or dilute hydrogen peroxide mouth rinses.
- Encourage to alternate activity with rest.
- Teach about the bone marrow biopsy. Allow time for questions.
- Refer to oncology nurse specialist.

1   A 19-year-old client is admitted in sickle cell crisis. The FIRST nursing action would be to:

   A. administer pain medications.
   B. obtain blood samples for analysis.
   C. administer antibiotics.
   D. insert Foley catheter.

2   A client is admitted with a diagnosis of pernicious anemia. Priority nursing care would include:

   A. prevention of infection.
   B. increasing iron intake.
   C. providing rest periods.
   D. increasing fluid intake.

3   An LPN is assigned to a client with thrombocytopenia. A priority goal of nursing care is:

   A. prevention of infection.
   B. prevention of injury.
   C. prevention of dehydration.
   D. prevention of nutritional deficit.

4   A 19-year-old client with hemophilia A wants to join an athletic team in college. Which of the following would be most appropriate?

   A. hockey
   B. golf
   C. basketball
   D. baseball

5   The nurse establishes a nursing diagnosis of Impaired Oral Mucous Membrane for a client with leukemia who is experiencing stomatitis. Client teaching would include which of the following interventions? (Choose all that apply.)

   A. warm saline as a mouth rinse
   B. application of petroleum jelly to the lips
   C. increased intake of citrus fruit juice
   D. cool liquids for hydration
   E. use of viscous lidocaine to relieve discomfort

6   A client developed disseminated intravascular coagulation (DIC) following injuries sustained in an automobile collision. Which of the following, if observed, requires intervention by the nurse?

   A. The client has two pillows under her knees.
   B. The client is resting on her right side.
   C. The client has oxygen per nasal cannula at 5 L/min.
   D. The client has cool compresses to her knees.

7   The priority nursing care focus for a client diagnosed with multiple myeloma is:

   A. prevention of injury and pain control.
   B. balanced nutrition and prevention of injury.
   C. safety and preservation of mental status.
   D. control bleeding and preserve energy.

8   A client develops lymphedema of her left arm following a left radical mastectomy. Discharge teaching would include:

   A. removing antiembolic stockings or pressure devices daily.
   B. elevating extremity when seated or in bed.
   C. inspecting skin every other day.
   D. adding low-potassium foods to diet.

9   A client is evaluated for possible Hodgkin's disease. Which of the following assessment findings would be expected?

   A. enlarged cervical lymph node
   B. absent Reed–Sternberg cells
   C. negative Epstein–Barr virus
   D. immovable, painful inguinal lymph nodes

10   The nurse develops a nursing diagnosis of Risk for Infection for a client with leukemia. The BEST action by the nurse would be to:

   A. require visitors with colds or flu to wear masks.
   B. wash hands when leaving the room.
   C. document signs of infection in the medical record.
   D. maintain protective isolation protocols at all times.

Answers for Review Questions, as well as discussion of Care Plan and Critical Thinking Care Map questions, appear in Appendix V.

Thinking Strategically About...

Sheri Matthews is a 76-year-old widow who lives alone. She tells the clinic nurse, Lisa Apana, that she liked to cook when her husband was alive but that preparing an entire meal just for herself seems senseless. She relates she typically has nothing for breakfast, a bologna sandwich and cup of coffee for lunch, and a hot dog or two, a few cookies, and a glass of milk for dinner.

DATA COLLECTED

Mrs. Matthews has lost 20 lbs. (9 kg) since her husband died 8 months ago. She says she feels weak and sometimes has heart palpitations. Physical assessment data include: T 98.8°F (37.1°C); BP 90/52; P 110; R 22. Skin is warm, pale, and dry. Diagnostic tests indicate folic acid deficiency anemia. Mrs. Matthews is started on an oral folic acid supplement and is instructed to increase her intake of foods containing folic acid.

CRITICAL THINKING

1 Why was Mrs. Matthews placed on a folic acid supplement in addition to dietary modifications?

2 How was Mrs. Matthews's report of weakness related to her folic acid deficiency?

3 Why is the older adult at increased risk for developing folic acid deficiency anemia? Consider physiologic, economic, and social factors.

4 Design a three-day menu that includes foods high in folic acid that are easy and quick to prepare.

COORDINATION OF INTERDISCIPLINARY CARE

1 Suggest interventions that might assist Mrs. Matthews to have an improved nutritional intake.

MANAGEMENT OF CARE

1 What are nursing interventions that could help Mrs. Matthews regain her previous level of energy?

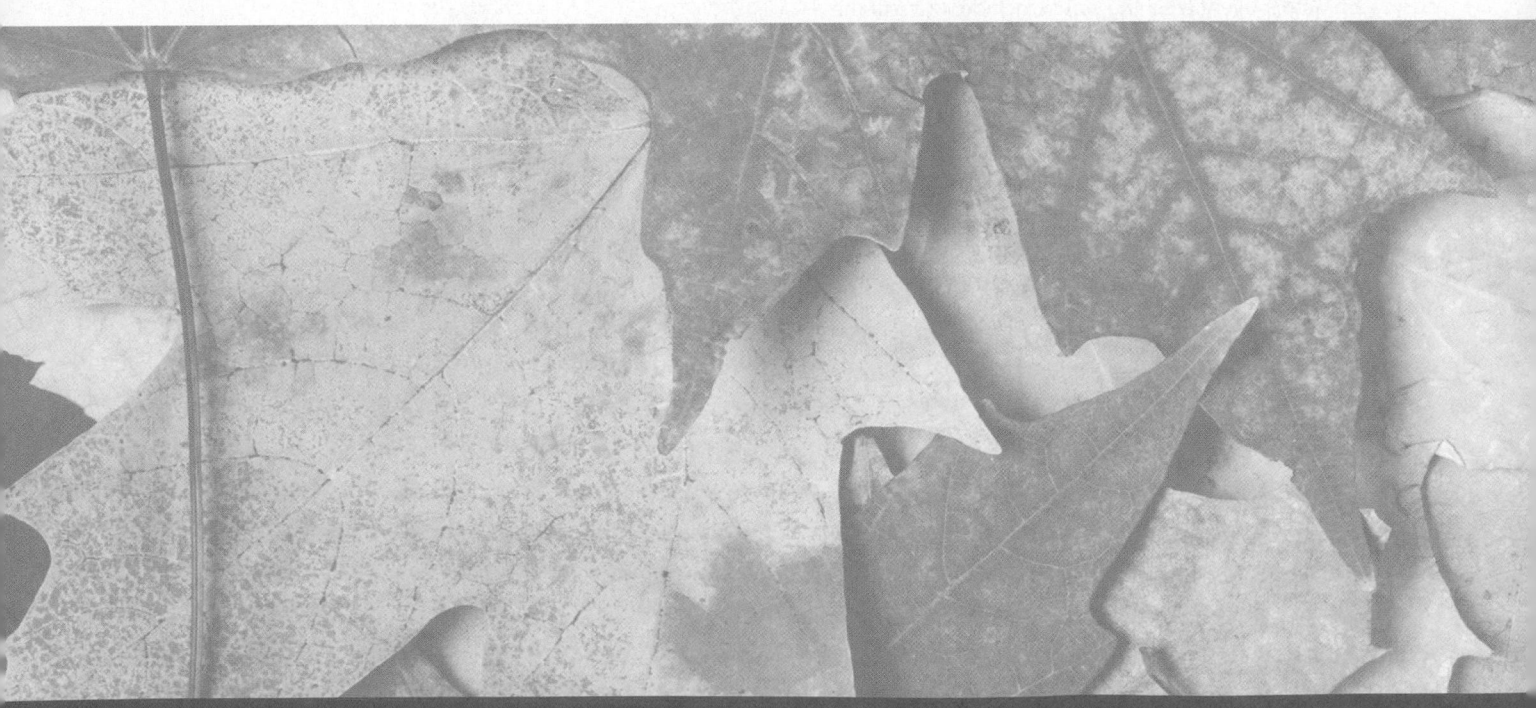

Disrupted Urinary Function

UNIT VIII

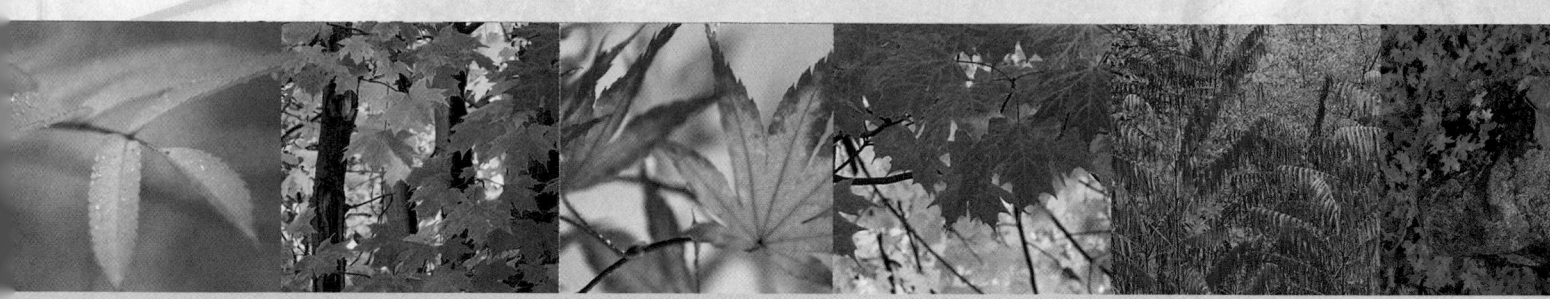

Chapter 31

The Urinary System and Assessment

BRIEF Outline

LEARNING Outcomes

After completing this chapter, you will be able to:

- Identify and describe the structures and functions of the renal and urinary system.
- Collect subjective information and physical assessment data related to the urinary system and kidney function.
- Provide appropriate nursing care for clients undergoing diagnostic tests to identify disorders of the urinary system or kidneys.

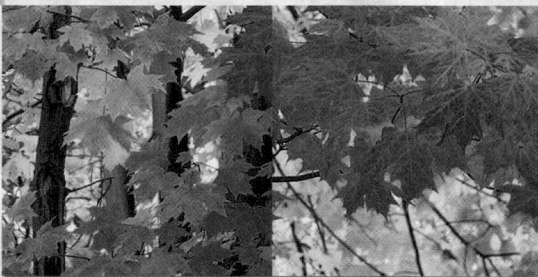

MediaLink

www.prenhall.com/burke
Use the address above to access the free, interactive Companion Website created for this textbook. Get hints, instant feedback, and textbook references to chapter-related NCLEX-style questions. Link to other interesting sites.

Audio Glossary:
Use the Companion Website, or the CD-ROM disk enclosed with your textbook, to hear the pronunciation of key terms in this chapter.

The urinary system plays a vital role in eliminating wastes and regulating fluid and electrolyte balance in the body. Changes in its structure or function can affect the entire body; likewise, it is affected by other body systems, particularly the cardiovascular and endocrine systems.

Structure and Function of the Urinary System

The urinary system includes the paired kidneys and ureters, the urinary bladder, and the urethra (Figure 31-1 ■). The urinary system is important in maintaining and regulating the body's internal environment. The urinary system excretes metabolic wastes. It also excretes or conserves water and solutes, as needed. The kidneys help regulate acid–base balance and blood pressure. Because these are vital functions, any disorder of the urinary system can affect the entire body.

KIDNEYS

The two kidneys sit behind the peritoneum (*retroperitoneal* space) on either side of the spine. They are partially protected by the rib cage. These highly vascular, bean-shaped organs are about the size of a closed fist. On the inner (*concave*) surface of each kidney is a notch known as the *hilum,* where the ureter, renal artery, renal vein, lymphatic vessels, and nerves enter or exit. The *renal fascia,* a layer of dense connective tissue, protects and anchors the kidney.

Each kidney has three distinct regions: the cortex, medulla, and pelvis (Figure 31-2 ■). The outer region, or *renal cortex,* contains the **glomeruli,** small clusters of capillaries. The glomeruli are part of the **nephrons,** the functional units of the kidney (Figure 31-3 ■). Each kidney contains approximately 1 million nephrons, which process the blood to make urine.

In the *renal medulla,* or inner portion of the kidney, nephrons form the *renal pyramids.* These pyramids channel

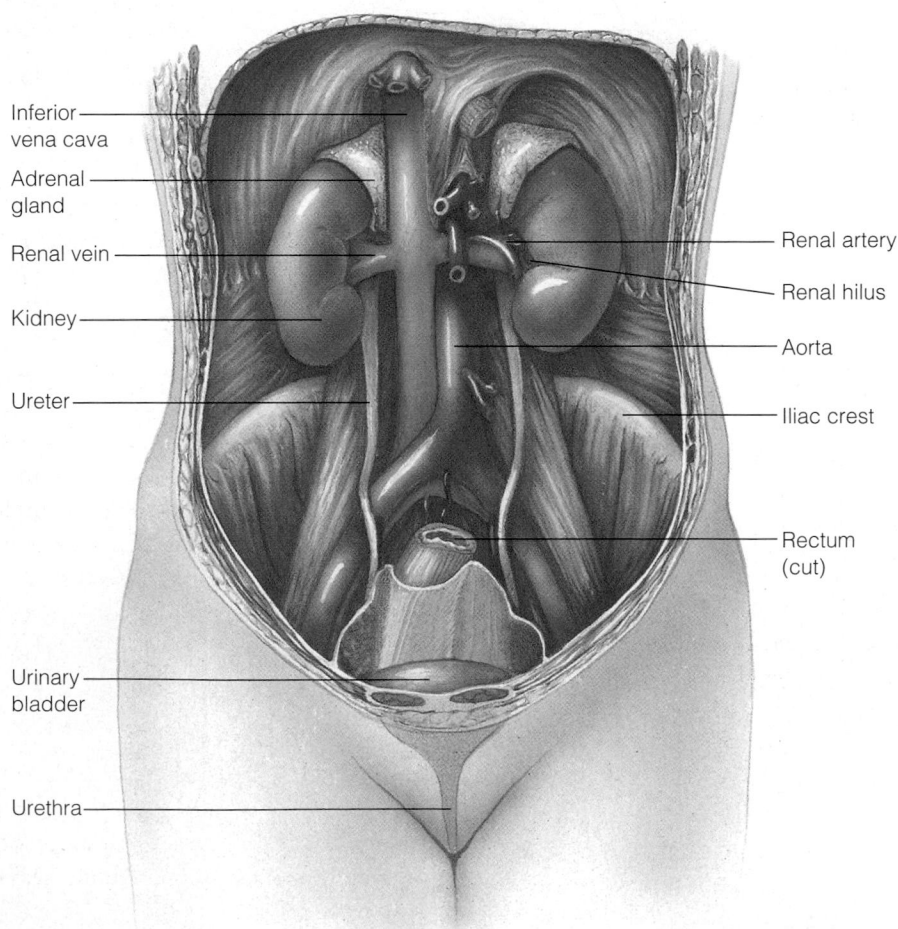

Inferior vena cava

Adrenal gland

Renal vein

Kidney

Ureter

Urinary bladder

Urethra

Renal artery

Renal hilus

Aorta

Iliac crest

Rectum (cut)

Figure 31-1. ■ Anterior view of the urinary system.

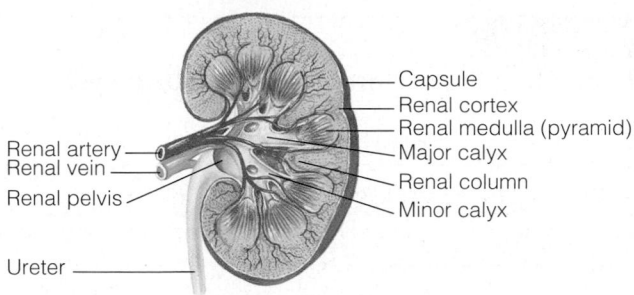

Figure 31-2. ■ Internal anatomy of the kidney.

urine into branches of the innermost region, the *renal pelvis*. These branches are known as *calyces* (singular, *calyx*). Urine is channeled from the pelvis through the ureter and into the bladder for storage.

URETERS

The *ureters* are bilateral tubes about 10 to 12 inches (25 to 30 cm) long. They move urine from the kidney to the bladder by peristaltic waves. The ureters contain smooth muscle and are innervated by the autonomic nervous system.

URINARY BLADDER

The urinary bladder is a hollow, muscular organ that lies behind the symphysis pubis. The ureters enter the bladder at its base, an area known as the *trigone* (Figure 31-4 ■). The

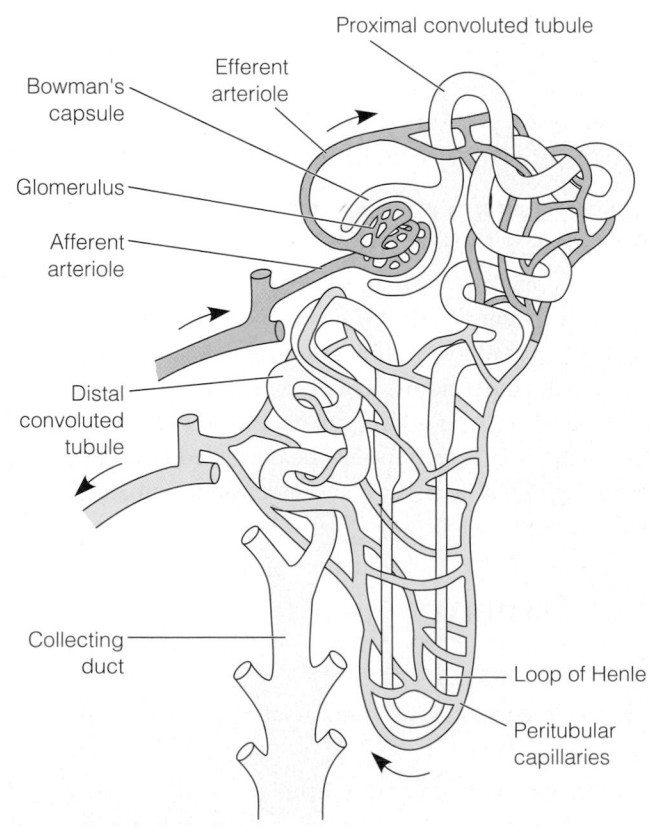

Figure 31-3. ■ Structure of a nephron.

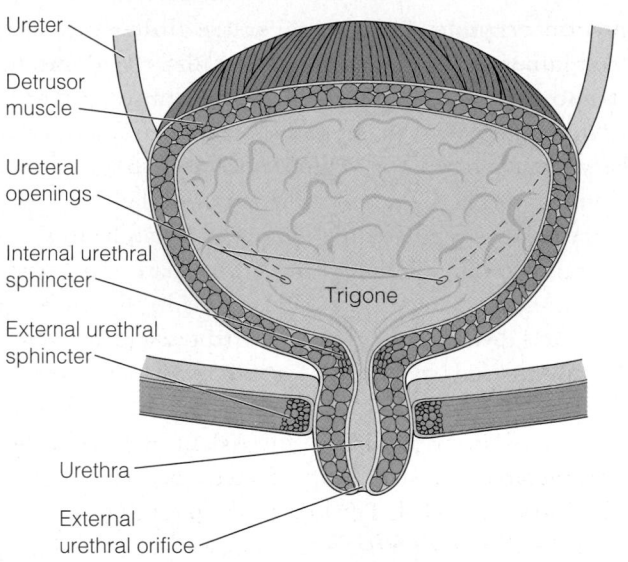

Figure 31-4. ■ Structure of the urinary bladder.

urethral opening is at the third point of this triangular region. Bladder muscle tone in this area prevents a backflow of urine from the bladder into the ureters.

The bladder is lined with epithelial mucosa. The muscle (*detrusor muscle*) is arranged in layers that allow the bladder to expand or contract. Healthy adults usually feel the urge to void when the bladder contains 300 to 500 mL of urine. However, the bladder can hold more than twice that amount if necessary. The *internal urethral sphincter* relaxes in response to a full bladder, signaling the need to urinate. A second *external urethral sphincter* formed by skeletal muscle is under voluntary control.

URETHRA

The *urethra* is a thin-walled muscular tube that channels urine out of the body. It extends from the base of the bladder to the *urinary meatus* (*opening*). In females, the urethra is approximately 1.5 inches (3 to 5 cm) long; the urinary meatus is anterior to the vagina. In males, the urethra is about 8 inches (20 cm) long; it serves as a channel for semen as well as urine. The prostate gland encircles the urethra at the base of the bladder in males. The male urinary meatus is at the end of the glans penis.

URINE FORMATION

The kidneys process about 180 liters (47 gallons) of filtrate each day. Of this, only 1% is excreted as urine; the rest is returned to the circulation. Urine is formed by the processes of glomerular filtration, tubular reabsorption, and tubular secretion.

Glomerular Filtration

Glomerular filtration is a passive process in which fluid and solutes move from the blood in the glomerulus into

Bowman's capsule. The amount of fluid filtered from the blood into the capsule per minute is called the **glomerular filtration rate (GFR)**. Normal GFR in adults is 120 to 125 mL/min. The blood pressure and volume are the primary factors controlling GFR. A drop in blood pressure or blood volume cause the GFR and urine output to fall.

The GFR is regulated by a number of mechanisms. Afferent (incoming) arterioles constrict or dilate in response to blood pressure changes. Specialized cells in the afferent arteriole and distal convoluted tubule (the *juxtaglomerular apparatus*) respond to changes in blood flow by releasing renin, an enzyme that affects systemic blood pressure. Glomerular filtration also is affected by the sympathetic nervous system.

Tubular Reabsorption

Tubular reabsorption begins as the filtrate enters the proximal tubules. In healthy kidneys, virtually all organic nutrients such as glucose and amino acids are reabsorbed. Water and electrolyte reabsorption is continuously regulated and adjusted to maintain homeostasis. Reabsorption occurs by both active and passive mechanisms.

Tubular Secretion

Through the process of *tubular secretion,* excess potassium and waste products such as hydrogen ion (H^+), creatinine, and ammonia are eliminated from the body. Both passive and active mechanisms work to eliminate waste products and regulate acid–base balance.

Urine Concentration

In the loop of Henle, urine is concentrated, and further wastes are excreted through reabsorption and secretion. In the distal tubule, antidiuretic hormone (ADH) determines the final dilution or concentration of urine (see Chapter 7). 〇⊃ When ADH is secreted, water is reabsorbed in the distal convoluted tubule and collecting duct, and urine is more concentrated. When ADH is not secreted, water cannot be reabsorbed and the urine is more dilute.

Urine is composed, by volume, of about 95% water and 5% solutes. Solutes normally excreted in the urine include urea, sodium, potassium, phosphate, sulfate, creatinine, uric acid, calcium, magnesium, and bicarbonate. The characteristics of normal urine are listed in Table 31-1 ■.

ENDOCRINE FUNCTION OF THE KIDNEYS

Besides producing urine, the kidneys produce renin and erythropoietin, and they activate vitamin D. The enzyme *renin,* produced by the juxtaglomerular apparatus, converts the plasma protein angiotensinogen to angiotensin I. Angiotensin I is converted in the lungs to angiotensin II. Angiotensin II, a potent vasoconstrictor, raises blood pressure. It also stimulates the adrenal cortex to release

TABLE 31-1	
Characteristics of Normal Urine on Urinalysis	
Color	Pale yellow to deep amber; clear
Odor	Aromatic
Specific gravity	1.005–1.030
pH	4.5–8.0
Protein	Negative to trace
Glucose	Negative
Ketones	Negative
RBC	0–5/high power field (HPF)
WBC	0–5/HPF
Casts	Negative to occasional
Bacteria	Negative

aldosterone, which promotes sodium and water retention. The net effect of the *renin–angiotensin–aldosterone* system is to raise the blood pressure and blood volume (see Chapter 7). 〇⊃

Erythropoietin is produced by the kidneys in response to hypoxia of renal cells. Erythropoietin stimulates the bone marrow to produce red blood cells.

Vitamin D is important for calcium regulation in the body. It is inactive when it enters the body either through the diet or by exposure to ultraviolet light (sunlight). It is activated in two steps by the liver and then the kidneys.

AGE-RELATED CHANGES IN KIDNEY FUNCTION

Nephrons are lost with aging, reducing kidney mass and the GFR. By age 80, the GFR may be less than half of what it was at age 30. The kidneys are less able to concentrate urine in the older adult. This fact, combined with diminished thirst in older adults, increases the risk for dehydration. Potassium excretion may be decreased in older adults, increasing the risk of fluid and electrolyte imbalances (see Table 31-2 ■).

Assessment

HEALTH HISTORY

Ask about current symptoms related to urinary function such as:

- Color, odor, and amount of urine
- Difficulty initiating urination or changes in the force of urine flow

TABLE 31-2

Nursing Implications of Age-Related Changes In Kidney Function

CHANGE	EFFECT	NURSING IMPLICATIONS
Decreased GFR	Decreased excretion of drugs primarily eliminated by the kidneys; increased risk of drug toxicity	Monitor clients carefully for signs of toxicity, especially when giving digoxin, certain antibiotics, cimetidine, and chlorpropamide.
Decreased number of nephrons; changes in aldosterone levels and response to ADH	Decreased ability to conserve water and sodium; increased risk of fluid, electrolyte, and acid–base imbalances	Monitor for fluid, electrolyte, and acid–base imbalances. Promote fluid intake of up to 2,500 mL/day unless contraindicated.
Decreased number of functional nephrons	Increased risk of kidney failure	Avoid nephrotoxic drugs if possible; monitor urine output and for signs of renal failure.

- Normal pattern of urination and recent changes from usual pattern
- Usual type and amount of fluid intake
- Painful urination (**dysuria**)
- **Nocturia,** urinating more than one time at night
- Blood in the urine (**hematuria**) or cloudy, foul-smelling urine (**pyuria**)
- Discharge from the penis or urinary meatus
- Abdominal, suprapubic, or flank pain.

Inquire about the onset, duration, and severity of symptoms, as well as associated symptoms such as nausea, general malaise, or fever. If pain is present, ask about the specific location and nature of the pain (sharp, burning, dull, constant, stabbing, intermittent), as well as its intensity.

Ask about previous urinary tract infections or surgeries. Determine what medications the client is taking (if any). Ask about chronic diseases such as diabetes, heart failure, or kidney failure. Ask women if pregnancy is a possibility and the type of birth control used. Determine family history of kidney disease or failure, kidney stones. Inquire about personal habits such as smoking or alcohol intake, and possible exposure to toxic chemicals (e.g., occupational exposure to dyes or chemicals).

PHYSICAL EXAMINATION

Assessment of the urinary system begins with obtaining a clean-catch urine specimen (Box 31-1 ■). Inspect the urine for color, odor, and clarity before sending it to the laboratory for analysis.

BOX 31-1   NURSING CARE CHECKLIST

Collecting a Midstream Clean-Catch Urine Specimen

- ☑ Explain the purpose of the procedure and specimen.
- ☑ If alert and ambulatory, provide instructions and supplies for the client to obtain the specimen:
  - ☑ Clean the genital and perineal area with soap and water.
  - ☑ Use each antiseptic towelette one time as follows:
    - ☑ Female clients: Cleanse front to back.
    - ☑ Male clients: Use a circular motion to clean the meatus. If uncircumcised, retract the foreskin before cleaning.
  - ☑ Start urine flow, then place the container into urine stream to collect the specimen.
  - ☑ Tightly cap the container, and, if necessary, rinse and dry the outside.

- ☑ If the client requires assistance:
  - ☑ Obtain all supplies; use Standard Precautions.
  - ☑ Provide perineal care.
  - ☑ Position on clean bedpan, commode, or toilet.
  - ☑ Cleanse perineal area with antiseptic towelettes as instructed above.
  - ☑ Ask to begin voiding. Place the specimen container into the stream of urine, taking care to avoid touching perineal tissues or hair. Collect 30 to 60 mL of urine.
  - ☑ Cap container, avoiding contamination of the inside of the cap.
- ☑ Label container and send with requisition to the laboratory.
- ☑ Document specimen collection and any pertinent information.

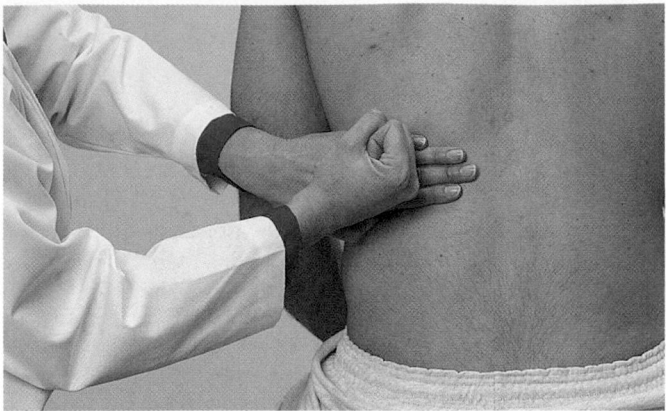

Figure 31-5. ■ Percussing the kidney.

Obtain vital signs. Assess skin color and condition, including looking for evidence of excessively dry skin or excoriations. Inspect the face (especially the periorbital area) and palpate the lower extremities for evidence of edema. Expose the abdomen, and assess its contour and symmetry. Auscultate bowel sounds. Lightly palpate the abdomen for tenderness, including the suprapubic region. With the client sitting and the back exposed, percuss the kidneys for tenderness (Figure 31-5 ■).

As indicated, inspect the genital area and urinary meatus for redness, swelling, discharge, or ulcerations. In the male, retract the foreskin if present with your gloved hands and gently compress the glans penis to expose the meatus (Figure 31-6 ■). Position the female client recumbent with the knees raised and spread apart. Spread the labia using gloved hands to expose the meatus.

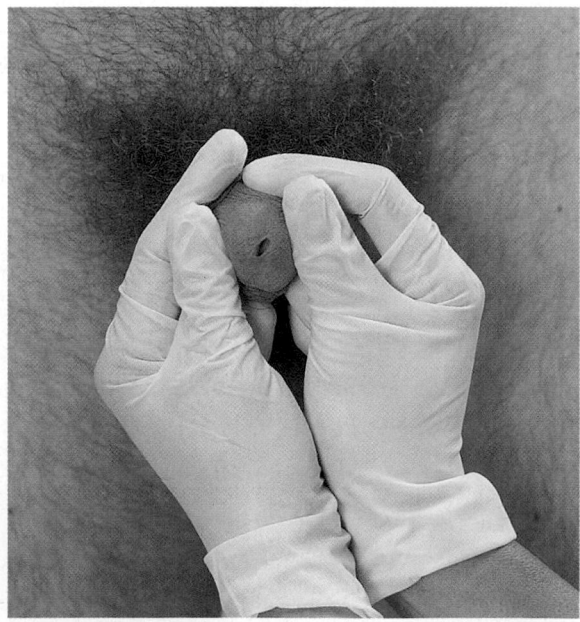

Figure 31-6. ■ Inspecting the urinary meatus of the male.

BOX 31-2

DOCUMENTATION OF URINARY SYSTEM ASSESSMENT

Client: Nguyen Trong, 26 y.o., presents with complaints of urinary frequency, urgency, and burning on urination that began the evening previously.

Assessment note: States she had to urinate 3 times during the night and says her urine is dark, cloudy, and "smells bad." Denies previous history of UTI or kidney problems. Is not sexually active, denies possibility of pregnancy. Does not use birth control. Has little information about family history as her family remains in Viet Nam. No known allergies or chronic diseases, not taking any medications currently.

BP 108/64, P 68, R 16, T 99.8 F PO. Skin pink, warm and dry. Good turgor. No edema noted. Abdomen flat, slightly tender to palpation in suprapubic region. No tenderness on percussion of kidneys. Clean-catch urine specimen obtained; urine dark brown, cloudy, malodorous. Sent to lab for urinalysis.

Box 31-2 ■ presents a sample documentation of the urinary system.

DIAGNOSTIC TESTS

Laboratory tests of blood and urine samples, ultrasound and x-ray studies, and direct visualization techniques are used to evaluate the urinary system.

Laboratory Tests

URINE STUDIES. The urinalysis is a key part of the diagnostic evaluation of the urinary system. Results of normal urinalysis are listed in Table 31-1. When abnormal results are obtained or a disorder of the kidneys or urinary tract is suspected, urine may be subjected to further analysis. Tests commonly performed on urine are outlined with their nursing responsibilities in Table 31-3 ■.

RENAL CLEARANCE. Two substances found in the blood are routinely used to evaluate renal function. *Urea* is formed in the metabolism of dietary and body proteins. *Creatinine* is produced in relatively constant quantities by muscle cell metabolism. Both of these substances are eliminated from the body by the kidneys by filtration and secretion; neither is reabsorbed. For this reason, *blood urea nitrogen (BUN)* and *serum creatinine* levels in the blood are effective indicators of renal function. The GFR can be evaluated by determining the amount of blood plasma cleared of creatinine during a specific period of time. This is known as the *creatinine clearance test*. The creatinine clearance test generally requires collection of a 24-hour urine sample, although shorter collection periods may be used. A blood sample is obtained at

TABLE 31-3			
Urine Studies			
TEST	**EXPECTED RESULTS**	**EXPLANATION**	**NURSING RESPONSIBILITIES**
Urinalysis	See Table 31-1	Urinalysis includes both chemical and microscopic analysis of the urine. Chemical analysis generally is performed by dipstick. Microscopic analysis is used to identify cells (blood cells or bacteria), casts (protein structures that develop in the tubules of the kidneys), or crystals.	Use midstream clean-catch technique to collect specimen in a sterile container. Provide appropriate teaching for the client to obtain the specimen. Use sterile technique to obtain a specimen from the drainage tubing if an indwelling catheter is in place.
Culture and sensitivity	No bacteria present	Urine is placed in or on an appropriate growth medium. If pathogens are present, they are microscopically identified. When combined in sensitivity testing, the specimen is grown in or on media containing disks of various antibiotics to identify those drugs that inhibit bacterial growth.	Obtain a specimen either by midstream clean-catch technique, straight catheterization, or from an indwelling catheter using sterile technique. Promptly send the specimen to the laboratory.
24-Hour urine tests			Obtain specimen container with appropriate preservative (if indicated) from the laboratory. Determine if specimen should be kept refrigerated or on ice during collection period. Follow procedures outlined in Box 31-1 for client teaching and specimen collection.
Electrolytes ■ Sodium ■ Chloride ■ Potassium ■ Calcium ■ Magnesium	 40–220 mEq/24 hr 110–250 mEq/24 hr (lower in >60 y.o.) 25–125 mEq/24 hr 100–300 mg/24 hr 7.3–12.2 mg/dL or 3–5 mmol/24 hr	The normal excretion of electrolytes in the urine depends on intake, serum levels, and fluid balance. Urine electrolytes are measured to help monitor kidney function, fluid and electrolyte balance, acid–base balance, and endocrine disorders.	
■ Protein ■ Creatinine	Resting: 50–80 mg/24 hr Ambulatory: <150–250 mg/24 hr Female: 600–1,800 mg/24 hr Male: 800–2,000 mg/24 hr	Urine creatinine and protein are used to help identify kidney disease. Protein molecules generally are too large to be filtered through the glomerular membrane; thus little protein is normally present in urine. Increased levels indicate kidney disease, urinary tract infection, or other serious conditions.	

some point during urine collection to measure serum creatinine. Nursing responsibilities for collecting a 24-hour urine specimen are outlined in Box 31-3 ■. Normal values of the BUN, serum creatinine, and creatinine clearance tests are in Table 31-4 ■. Serum albumin levels can be affected by kidney disease; Table 31-4 also includes normal values for the serum albumin.

Imaging Studies

X-rays, nuclear scans, and ultrasound examinations are used to assess the urinary system.

■ An abdominal x-ray known as the *KUB (kidney, ureter, bladder)* may be done to evaluate the size, shape, and position of organs in the urinary tract. This is a plain x-ray that requires no special preparation, although the client

may be asked to either empty the bladder or allow it to fill prior to the x-ray.

■ *Intravenous pyelography (IVP)* uses a contrast medium and x-rays to evaluate the urinary tract. The contrast medium is injected intravenously. It is filtered from the blood by the kidneys, allowing x-rays to show the contrast entering the kidney pelvis, flowing through the ureters, and into the bladder. This allows evaluation of renal function (by measuring the time required for filtration), and the position, size, shape, and structure of urinary tract organs. Box 31-4 ■ outlines nursing responsibilities related to IVP.

■ *Retrograde pyelography* may be done as an alternative to IVP, although it usually is done as part of cystoscopy or to evaluate placement of a stent or catheter. In this

BOX 31-3	NURSING CARE CHECKLIST

24-Hour Urine Specimen

☑ Note any diet or medication changes required during the collection period.

☑ Obtain specimen container with preservative (if indicated). Label with identifying data, the test, time started, and time of completion.

☑ Obtain a clean urine-collection device and place it in the room.

☑ Post notices—on chart, in Kardex, on the door, over the bed, and over the toilet—alerting all personnel that all urine is to be saved.

☑ At start time, have client empty bladder completely and *discard* urine.

☑ Save all urine for next 24 hours in the container, refrigerating as indicated. If any urine is missed, the collection must be restarted.

☑ At end of collection time, have client empty the bladder completely and save this urine in the container. Take entire specimen with requisition to the lab.

☑ Chart appropriately.

Teaching

☑ Save all your urine for the 24 hours.

☑ Urinate (and save) before moving bowels. Do not put any toilet tissue in the urine container.

BOX 31-4	NURSING CARE CHECKLIST

Intravenous Pyelography

Client Preparation

☑ Assess and clarify understanding of the procedure.

☑ Inquire about allergies to seafood, iodine, or x-ray contrast media. Notify the physician or radiologist of any known allergies.

☑ Verify signed consent for the procedure has been obtained.

☑ Instruct or administer preprocedure laxatives as ordered. Allow clear liquids only for 8 hours before the test.

☑ After IVP, monitor vital signs and urinary output. Report signs of reaction to contrast media such as dyspnea, tachycardia, itching, hives, or flushing. Check injection site for redness, pain, and warmth. Apply warm packs to the site if indicated.

Client and Family Teaching

☑ IVP uses x-rays to show the structures of the kidney, ureters, and bladder by injecting a dye that is rapidly excreted in the urine. The test takes about 30 minutes.

☑ As the dye is injected, you may experience transient flushing or burning, nausea, and a metallic taste.

☑ Immediately notify the physician if you develop a rash, difficulty breathing, rapid heart rate, or hives.

☑ Increase fluid intake after the test is completed.

exam, contrast media is instilled into the collecting system of the urinary tract (renal pelvis, ureters, and bladder) to outline their size, position, and structures.

■ *Computed tomography (CT) scan* or *magnetic resonance imaging (MRI)* also may be done to visualize structures of the

urinary tract. CT scan may be done with or without contrast media. If contrast is used, care of the client is similar to that provided for IVP (see Box 31-4).

■ *Renal scan (kidney scan)* is a nuclear medicine scan used to evaluate blood vessels and perfusion of the kidneys and the ureters. Renal scan can demonstrate blood flow obstructions to the kidneys as well as the functions of the nephron (filtration and tubular transport). It also can show obstructions of the ureters or backflow of urine from the bladder into the ureters (*reflux*). Nursing responsibilities for a renal scan are outlined in Box 31-5 ■.

■ *Ultrasound* examination of the bladder or kidneys may be performed to evaluate their size, shape, and position. This is a noninvasive examination that requires no preparation of the client other than explanation of the procedure. For this exam, the client may be instructed to either empty the bladder prior to the exam or to consume several glasses of water and come to the exam with a full bladder. Nurses may perform ultrasonic bladder scans to evaluate for urinary retention and to determine postvoiding residual volume (Box 31-6 ■).

TABLE 31-4	
Laboratory Tests Commonly Used to Evaluate Renal Function	

TEST	NORMAL VALUE
Blood urea nitrogen (BUN)	5–20 mg/dL; slightly higher in older adult
Serum creatinine	Female: 0.5–1.1 mg/dL Male: 0.6–1.2 mg/dL Slightly lower in older adult
Creatinine clearance	Female: 88–128 mL/min Male: 97–137 mL/min Values lower in older adult
Serum albumin	3.2–5 g/dL; 3.2–4.8 g/dL in older adult

Box 31-5	NURSING CARE CHECKLIST

Renal Scan

Client Preparation

☑ Informed consent is required. Clarify and reinforce teaching.

☑ Obtain weight.

☑ Provide 2 to 3 glasses of water before the procedure and encourage fluids after.

☑ Have client void prior to the procedure.

☑ Instruct to flush toilet immediately after voiding and to wash hands thoroughly to minimize exposure to radioactivity following the procedure.

☑ No pregnant personnel should care for client for 24 hours after the procedure.

Client and Family Teaching

☑ Increase fluid intake before and after the renal scan.

☑ No special diet or other preparation is required.

☑ A dilute radioactive substance will be injected to allow visualization of the kidneys.

☑ The test takes 1 to 4 hours.

☑ No anesthesia is required, and there will be no pain or discomfort other than that associated with remaining still for a period of time.

BOX 31-6	NURSING CARE CHECKLIST

Portable Ultrasonic Bladder Scan

☑ Explain the procedure and its purpose. This procedure is generally not done on pregnant clients.

☑ Perform the procedure within 15 minutes of voiding if it is being done to evaluate for residual urine.

☑ Obtain the portable ultrasonic bladder scan unit and warmed ultrasound gel.

☑ Position the client supine; expose the lower abdomen.

☑ Place the ultrasound probe just above the pubic bone to obtain the reading.

☑ The scanner shows an outline of the bladder and displays the volume of urine in milliliters (mL).

☑ Obtain several readings to ensure accuracy; the largest reading is the most accurate.

☑ Print the bladder outline, and place it in the client's chart. Document residual urine present.

☑ Remove ultrasound gel from the skin with a moist cloth, and reposition the client for comfort.

☑ Clean the portable scanner, following unit protocol, and return it to the appropriate location.

☑ Notify the charge nurse or physician if a significant amount of urine is present in the bladder.

■ *Cystoscopy,* direct visualization of the urethra and bladder using an endoscope, is used to diagnose conditions such as urethral strictures, bladder stones, tumors, and congenital abnormalities. This invasive examination is performed in an endoscopy laboratory or cystoscopy room of the surgical suite. Box 31-7 ■ outlines nursing care of the client undergoing cystoscopy.

BOX 31-7	NURSING CARE CHECKLIST

Cystoscopy

Client Preparation

☑ Assess and clarify understanding of the procedure and its purpose.

☑ Verify signed consent for the procedure has been obtained.

☑ Teach or assist with bowel preparation as ordered.

☑ Withhold food and fluids for 8 hours before the procedure as ordered.

☑ Administer sedation and other medications as ordered.

Client and Family Teaching

☑ The procedure takes about 30 to 45 minutes and is performed in a special cystoscopy room. Local or general anesthesia is used.

☑ You may feel pressure or an urge to urinate as the scope is inserted.

☑ Do not attempt to stand up without assistance after the procedure because you may feel dizzy or faint.

☑ Burning on urination for a day or two after the procedure is considered normal.

☑ Contact your physician immediately if your urine remains bloody or you experience bright red bleeding, low urine output, abdominal or flank pain, chills or fever.

☑ Warm sitz baths, analgesics, and antispasmodic medications help relieve discomfort.

☑ Increase fluid intake to decrease pain and difficulty voiding and reduce the risk of infection.

☑ Laxatives may be prescribed after the procedure to prevent constipation and straining.

Voiding Studies

Uroflowmetry is used to evaluate voiding and function of the lower urinary tract. It generally is used to evaluate urinary retention and incontinence. This is a noninvasive test that measures the volume and rate of urine flow. For this test, the client voids into a toilet equipped with a funnel and uroflowmeter. Prior to the test, the client is instructed to drink fluids and avoid urination for several hours. The client is placed in a specially equipped bathroom and advised to avoid discarding toilet tissue into the funnel or collection container. Privacy is provided, and the client voids into the urometer funnel without straining.

Note: The bibliography listings for this and all chapters have been compiled at the back of the book.

Chapter Review

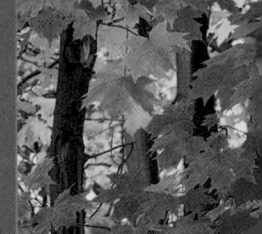

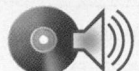 **KEY TERMS** by Topics

Use the audio glossary feature of either the CD-ROM or the Companion Website to hear the correct pronunciation of the following key terms.

Urinary system
glomeruli, nephrons, glomerular filtration rate (GFR)

Urinary and kidney function
dysuria, nocturia, hematuria, pyuria

KEY Points

- The urinary system includes the paired kidneys, which produce urine, and the urinary drainage system, including the ureters, urinary bladder, and urethra. Unimpaired urine flow through the system is vital to maintain normal fluid balance.

- The functional unit of the kidney is the nephron. The glomerulus of the nephron filters blood; this filtrate then is concentrated and refined in the tubule of the nephron to become urine. The urine flows from the collecting tubule into the renal pelvis and ureters to be stored in the bladder.

- Nursing assessment of urinary function generally is completed toward the end of the exam, to allow the client to develop trust and comfort with the nurse before discussing and examining potentially embarrassing topics or regions.

- Both blood tests and urine studies are used to evaluate the function of the urinary system. Imaging studies such as x-rays and ultrasound are important mechanisms for evaluating its structure.

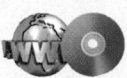 **EXPLORE Media**Link

Additional interactive resources for this chapter can be found on the Companion Website at www.prenhall.com/burke. Click on Chapter 31 and "Begin" to select the activities for this chapter.

For chapter-related NCLEX-style review questions and an audio glossary, access the accompanying CD-ROM in this book.

FOR FURTHER Study

For more information about antidiuretic hormone and the renin–angiotensin–aldosterone system, see Chapter 7.

For more information about the endocrine system, see Chapter 15.

For more information about the cardiovascular system, see Chapter 25.

NCLEX-PN® Exam Preparation

TEST-TAKING TIP Think about ways to manage stress and anxiety *before* you take the NCLEX-PN®. When you feel your muscles tensing, your heart rate increasing, and find you are having difficulty focusing on the question, use techniques such as visualization, meditation, or conscious relaxation to help you regain focus and composure.

1 A client is complaining of pain in the right flank region. The nurse recalls that the organs in this region of the abdomen include the:

   A. right kidney and ureter.
   B. spleen and pancreas.
   C. stomach and duodenum.
   D. bladder and uterus.

2 The nurse caring for a client with acute tubular necrosis knows that this is likely to affect:

   A. blood flow to the kidney pelvis.
   B. urine collection and voiding.
   C. the formation of urine in the nephron.
   D. the ability to maintain continence.

3 Digoxin 0.25 mg daily has been prescribed for an 80 y.o. client. The nurse observes closely for:

   A. evidence of drug excretion without the desired effect.
   B. Excretion of the drug unchanged in the urine.
   C. Impaired urination due to effects of the drug.
   D. Manifestations of drug toxicity due to impaired excretion.

4 In preparing a client who is scheduled for a creatinine clearance test, the nurse instructs the client to (select all that apply):

   A. note the time of the first saved urine sample as the start of the 24-hour collection.
   B. save a portion of each voiding for 24 hours.
   C. empty the bladder at the start time and discard this urine.
   D. avoid putting any toilet paper in the saved urine.
   E. prevent feces from contaminating the saved urine.

5 The nurse reviewing urinalysis (UA) results for a client notes that there is 2+ protein in the urine. The nurse correctly interprets this as:

   A. within normal limits for the UA.
   B. indicative of kidney failure.
   C. important to report to the physician.
   D. an indicator that the client has diabetes.

Answers for Review Questions appear in Appendix V.

Chapter 32

Caring for Clients with Renal and Urinary Tract Disorders

BRIEF Outline

Urinary Incontinence
Urinary Retention
Urinary Tract Infection
Glomerulonephritis
Nephrotic Syndrome
Urinary Calculi
Hydronephrosis
Polycystic Kidney Disease
Kidney Trauma
Bladder Cancer
Kidney Tumors
Acute Renal Failure
Chronic Renal Failure

LEARNING Outcomes

After completing this chapter, you will be able to:

- Describe the pathophysiology of common disorders of the kidneys and urinary tract.
- Compare and contrast the manifestations of common disorders of the kidneys and urinary tract.
- Discuss the nursing implications of medications prescribed for clients with these disorders.
- Provide appropriate nursing care for the client having surgery of the kidneys or urinary tract.
- Use the nursing process as a framework for providing individualized care to clients with disorders of the kidneys or urinary tract.

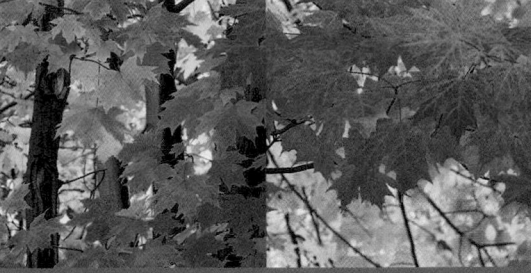

MediaLink

www.prenhall.com/burke
Use the address above to access the free, interactive Companion Website created for this textbook. Get hints, instant feedback, and textbook references to chapter-related NCLEX-style questions. Link to other interesting sites.

Audio Glossary:
Use the Companion Website, or the CD-ROM disk enclosed with your textbook, to hear the pronunciation of key terms in this chapter.

In this chapter, disorders of the kidneys and the urinary drainage system (kidney pelvis, ureters, urinary bladder, and urethra) are discussed. Review Chapter 31 ⊙⊙ for more information about structures of the urinary tract, their purpose, and urine formation. It is important to consider the client's modesty in voiding; possible reluctance to talk about the genitals; embarrassment about being exposed during examinations, tests, and procedures; and fear of potential changes in body function when caring for clients with kidney and urinary tract disorders. These issues can interfere with the client's willingness to seek help for problems.

VOIDING DISORDERS

Voiding disorders are common, although often unreported for reasons of modesty, embarrassment, difficulty discussing elimination, and the perception that the disorder is a normal part of the aging process.

Urinary Incontinence

Urinary incontinence, or involuntary urination, is a common problem, especially among older adults. Incontinence can cause physical problems (e.g., skin breakdown, infection, and rashes), as well as embarrassment, isolation and withdrawal, feelings of worthlessness and helplessness, and depression.

PATHOPHYSIOLOGY AND MANIFESTATIONS

Urinary continence requires a bladder that is able to expand and contract, and sphincters that can maintain a higher pressure in the urethra than that in the bladder. When bladder pressure is higher than urethral resistance, urine can escape. Any condition causing increased bladder pressures or lowered urethral resistance can cause incontinence. Pelvic muscle relaxation, impaired neural control, and bladder problems are common contributing factors.

Incontinence is commonly categorized as stress incontinence, urge incontinence, overflow incontinence, reflex incontinence, and functional incontinence (Table 32-1 ■).

Urinary Incontinence in Older Adults

Incontinence should *never* be considered a normal part of aging. However, age-related changes contribute to its development. Bladder capacity usually declines with age, and involuntary bladder muscle contractions are more common. In women, decreased estrogen levels and pelvic muscle relaxation cause urethral resistance to decrease, so stress

---

TABLE 32-1

Types of Urinary Incontinence

TYPE	DESCRIPTION	PATHOPHYSIOLOGY	CONTRIBUTING FACTORS
Stress	Loss of small amounts of urine when intra-abdominal pressure increases (sneezing, laughing, lifting)	Pelvic muscle relaxation; weakness of urethra and surrounding tissues decreases urethral resistance.	Multiple pregnancies Decreased estrogen levels (menopause) Prostate surgery
Urge	Inability to stop urine flow long enough to reach toilet after need to void is felt	Overactive detrusor muscle increases bladder pressure, causing inability to inhibit voiding.	Decreased bladder capacity Bladder irritation CNS disorders
Overflow	Urinary retention with bladder overdistention and frequent loss of small amounts of urine (25–50 mL)	Outlet obstruction or impaired detrusor muscle activity leads to overfilling and increased pressure.	Neurologic disorders or trauma Enlarged prostate Fecal impaction Anticholinergic drug effects
Reflex	Involuntary loss of moderate amount of urine occurring without warning	Altered spinal cord activity causes hyperreflexia of the detrusor muscle.	Neurologic disorders or trauma
Functional	Inability to get to toilet facilities to urinate	Self-care deficit interferes with ability to respond to urge to void.	Physical disability or impaired mobility, neurologic disorders Diuretic therapy or sedation Lack of facilities, privacy, or caregiver assistance

DATE ___4/15/06___

Please complete this chart prior to your visit. Choose a 24-hour period when it is convenient for you to measure and record the following: The amount of fluid you void (urinate), the amount of fluid you drink and type of beverage, the time, when leakage episodes occur, whether or not you have an urge to void just prior to leaking, and the activity you are doing when you leak or need to void.

VOIDING DIARY

DIARY.URO

Void Amount (oz.)	Fluid Intake Amount (oz.)	Time	Leak?	Urge prior to leak?	Activity
14 oz.		6:23 am	yes	yes	Awakening
8 oz.	14 oz. coffee	6:35			
		8:05	yes	yes	reading
	16 oz. coffee	8:30			
10 oz.		9:10	yes	yes	watch TV
10 oz.		9:30	"	"	"
12 oz.	8 oz. water	10:17	"	"	"
6 oz.		11:40	yes	yes	washing dishes
8 oz.	12 oz. coke	2:12 pm	yes	yes	Lunch
	16 oz. water	6:30			Dinner
10 oz.		8:00	yes	yes	Laundry
6 oz.		9:55	yes	yes	folding clothes
	8 oz. water	11:25			Bed time
6 oz.		1:30 am	—	yes	sleeping
8 oz.	—	5:05	—	yes	sleeping
5 oz.		6:30	—	yes	Awakening
		TOTAL			

Figure 32-1. ■ A sample voiding diary.

incontinence may occur. Decreased estrogen also may lead to dysuria and urgency. Other risk factors in older adults include immobility, chronic degenerative diseases or dementia, medications, diabetes, and stroke. Incontinence increases the risk for falls, fractures, pressure ulcers, urinary tract infection, and depression. It contributes to caregiver stress, and may be a major factor in institutionalizing the client.

INTERDISCIPLINARY CARE

The focus of interdisciplinary care is to identify and correct the cause if possible. If the underlying problem cannot be corrected, techniques may be taught to manage urine output.

Evaluation begins with a complete history, including the duration, frequency, volume, and associated circumstances of incontinence. A voiding diary (Figure 32-1 ■) is often used to provide detailed information. The history includes any chronic or acute illnesses, previous surgeries, and current medications (prescription and over the counter).

Physical assessment includes abdominal, rectal, and pelvic exams, as well as evaluation of mental and neurologic status, mobility, and dexterity. Women with incontinence often have weak abdominal and pelvic muscle tone, protrusion of the bladder or urethral wall into the vagina (cystocele or urethrocele), and thin vaginal tissues. In men, an enlarged prostate gland is commonly identified.

Diagnostic Tests

Diagnostic tests to identify the cause of urinary incontinence may include a *postvoid residual urine* measurement (Box 32-1 ■) or ultrasonic bladder scan (see Box 31-6) ∞ to determine how completely the bladder empties with voiding. Less than 50 mL of residual urine is expected; when 100 mL or more of residual urine is present, further tests are done. Additional studies may include *cystometrography* to evaluate bladder pressures and *uroflowmetry* to evaluate voiding patterns. See Chapter 31 ∞ for more information about uroflowmetry procedures.

Treatment

Urge incontinence may be treated with drugs to inhibit detrusor muscle contractions and increase bladder capacity. These may include tolterodine (Detrol) and oxybutynin

---

| BOX 32-1 | NURSING CARE CHECKLIST |

Postvoiding Residual Volume

Client Preparation

☑ Instruct to report when the urge to urinate is felt.

☑ Provide for privacy.

☑ Instruct to empty the bladder as completely as possible into a measuring device.

☑ Immediately after voiding, catheterize to drain the bladder completely. Measure amount obtained.

☑ Record and report: time; amount voided; amount obtained by catheterization; color, clarity, and odor of urine; and any other significant data.

Client and Family Teaching

☑ This test determines how completely the bladder empties with voiding.

☑ There is a slight risk of infection. Report frequency, urgency, pain on urination, nocturia, and cloudy, bloody, or malodorous urine.

(Ditropan). The anticholinergic effects of these drugs may cause dry mouth and eyes, constipation, confusion, and urinary retention.

When incontinence is associated with postmenopausal atrophic vaginitis, estrogen therapy may be effective. Both systemic estrogens and local creams are used.

When incontinence is associated with a cystocele or urethrocele, or is due to an enlarged prostate gland, surgery may be performed. *Bladder neck suspension* is used to treat urethrocele. Nursing care of the client having a bladder neck suspension is outlined in Box 32-2 ■.

Prostatectomy is indicated when an enlarged prostate gland obstructs urine outflow. (See care of the client with a prostatectomy in Chapter 34. ⊕)

NURSING CARE

ASSESSING

Collect subjective assessment data by asking about problems with urine loss, its frequency, and any contributing factors. Inquire about frequency, urgency, and burning on urination. Identify current medications and their timing. Assess patterns of fluid intake and output. Assess the abdomen for evidence of bladder distention or tenderness. Perform a mental status examination if indicated. Review any laboratory results, such as serum glucose and urinalysis for possible contributing factors such as diabetes or evidence of urinary tract infection.

| BOX 32-2 | NURSING CARE CHECKLIST |

Bladder Neck Suspension

Before Surgery

☑ Provide routine preoperative care and teaching as outlined in Chapter 9. ⊕

☑ Instruct to avoid straining and the Valsalva maneuver postoperatively.

After Surgery

☑ Provide routine postoperative care as outlined in Chapter 9. ⊕

☑ Frequently assess vaginal drainage or dressing. Notify the charge nurse or physician of bright red bleeding on dressing, from vagina, or in urine.

☑ Monitor and record quantity, color, and clarity of urine. Pink urine should gradually clear.

☑ Tape urinary catheters in position to prevent dislodging or pulling on incisions.

☑ Encourage activity and ambulation.

☑ Carefully monitor urine output following catheter removal.

☑ If a urethral or suprapubic catheter is in place at discharge, teach appropriate care.

☑ Stress importance of keeping scheduled appointments and contacting the physician if signs of a urinary tract infection or other complications develop.

DIAGNOSING, PLANNING, AND IMPLEMENTING

When planning care for clients with incontinence, consider mental and neurologic status, mobility, and motivation. Behavioral techniques require long-term commitment, as well as the physical and mental ability to implement them. Nursing interventions such as scheduled toileting, bladder training, and prompted voiding combined with praise can reduce the need for diapers, incontinence pads, and indwelling catheters in institutionalized clients.

Impaired Urinary Elimination

■ Monitor patterns of fluid intake and urination, including voluntary voiding and wetting accidents. *These data help identify the type and pattern of incontinence.*

■ Teach pelvic floor muscle exercises, called Kegel exercises (Box 32-3 ■). Instruct to consciously tighten pelvic muscles and relax the abdomen when the need to void is perceived. *Improved pelvic muscle strength helps prevent stress incontinence and decrease urge incontinence.*

■ Reduce delays in toileting. Ensure that the call light is within reach. Place a bedside commode in the room or provide clear access to the bathroom. Dress in

BOX 32-3	CLIENT TEACHING

Pelvic Floor (Kegel) Exercises

- Identify the pelvic muscles by:
  a. Attempting to stop the flow of urine during voiding and holding for a few seconds.
  b. Tightening the muscles of the vagina around a gloved finger or tampon.
  c. Tightening the muscles around the anus as though trying to avoid passing flatus.
- Perform exercises: Tighten pelvic muscles, hold for 10 seconds, and relax for 10 to 15 seconds. Continue the sequence (tighten, hold, relax) for 10 repetitions.
- Keep abdominal muscles and breathing relaxed while performing exercises.
- Initially, exercises should be performed twice per day, working up to four times a day.
- Exercise at a specific time each day or in conjunction with another daily activity (such as bathing or watching the news). Establish a routine, because these exercises should be continued for life.

loose-fitting clothing with elastic waistbands or Velcro closures. *These actions reduce the risk of wetting accidents.*

- After the evening meal, limit beverages, especially those that irritate the bladder, such as caffeine, Nutri-Sweet, and citrus juices. *Limiting evening fluid intake and bladder irritants reduces the risk of nighttime incontinence.*
- Administer diuretic drugs in the morning and midafternoon. *This timing allows the peak effect of the medication to occur while the client is awake and more able to respond to the urge to void.*

Toileting Self-Care Deficit

In institutions, functional incontinence (see Table 32-1) can be a significant problem in previously continent people. With functional incontinence, the primary problem is an outside factor that interferes with the ability to respond to the urge to void.

- Assess physical and mental capabilities and limitations, usual pattern of voiding, and ability to assist with toileting. *A thorough assessment helps address specific needs.*
- Provide assistive devices such as raised toilet seats, grab bars, a bedside commode, or night-lights. *Assistive devices help maintain independence.*
- Plan a toileting schedule to achieve approximately 300 mL of urine output with each voiding. *Allowing the bladder to fill until the urge to void is felt helps maintain normal bladder capacity.*
- Position for ease of voiding—sitting for females, standing for males—and provide for privacy. *Normal positioning and privacy enhance the ability to void.*

- Provide the majority of fluids during times of day when the client is most able to remain continent. *Unless restricted, maintain a fluid intake of at least 1.5 to 2 liters per day.*

Social Isolation

The client with any form of urinary incontinence is at risk for social isolation due to embarrassment, fear of not having ready access to a bathroom, body odor, or other factors.

- Refer for urologic examination and evaluation of incontinence. *Clients who assume that urinary incontinence is a normal part of aging may not be aware of treatment options.*
- Explore alternative coping strategies with client, significant others, staff, and other health team members. *Protective pads or shields, good perineal hygiene, scheduled voiding, and clothing that does not interfere with toileting can enhance continence.*

EVALUATING

To evaluate the effectiveness of nursing actions for the client with incontinence, keep a voiding diary of fluid intake, voidings, and wetting accidents. Identify wetting episodes that occur because of delayed toileting or difficulty manipulating clothing. Assess the client's willingness to participate in social activities.

Documenting. Document assessment data, teaching provided, and the client's ability and apparent willingness to continue with prescribed treatment measures, lifestyle changes, and exercises.

CONTINUING CARE

Appropriate home care and teaching can help keep the client in the home, reduce caregiver stress, and reduce the risk of institutionalization. Assess the home environment (whether in the community or a residential living facility) for possible barriers to urinary elimination such as:

- Inadequate lighting, particularly at night
- Narrow doorways that may interfere with access to the toilet
- Inadequate toilet facilities.

Teach the client with urinary incontinence to keep a voiding diary to help identify factors contributing to incontinent episodes. Instruct to maintain a generous fluid intake of 1.5 to 2 quarts of fluid per day. Advise restricting fluid intake after the evening meal. Discuss bladder irritants such as caffeine, citrus juices, and artificial sweeteners, and advise limiting their use. Teach Kegel exercises. Discuss the potential risks and benefits of hormone replacement therapy, surgery, and physical therapy with women. Encourage overweight clients to lose weight.

Discuss scheduled voiding and bladder training techniques with caregivers. Suggest taking the client to the toilet every 2 to 4 hours. To increase bladder capacity, the time between voidings may be gradually increased. Provide a list of resources for assistive devices such as a bedside commode, urinal, grab bars, or raised toilet seat.

Urinary Retention

Normal bladder emptying may be disrupted by an obstruction to urine flow or by a functional problem.

PATHOPHYSIOLOGY

When the bladder cannot empty, it becomes overstretched. This, in turn, affects detrusor muscle contraction and further impairs urination.

Benign prostatic hypertrophy (*BPH,* or enlargement of the prostate) is a common cause of *urinary retention.* Difficulty initiating and maintaining urine flow is often the presenting complaint in men with BPH. Acute inflammation associated with infection or trauma of the bladder, urethra, or perineal tissues may also interfere with the ability to urinate. Scarring caused by repeated urinary tract infections can narrow the urethra and obstruct output.

Surgery, particularly abdominal or pelvic surgery, can affect detrusor muscle function, leading to acute urinary retention. Medications also may affect bladder contraction. Drugs with anticholinergic effects may cause urinary retention. These include antianxiety drugs, antidepressant drugs, and many common over-the-counter cough, cold, allergy, and sleep-promoting drugs. Neurologic diseases or trauma may interfere with normal mechanisms of bladder emptying (*neurogenic bladder*). Voluntary urinary retention (particularly common among nurses) may lead to overfilling of the bladder and a loss of detrusor muscle tone.

MANIFESTATIONS AND COMPLICATIONS

The client with urinary retention is unable to empty the bladder completely. Overflow voiding or incontinence may occur (see Table 32-1). Assessment reveals a firm, distended bladder that may be displaced to one side of midline.

Acute or chronic urinary retention can lead to complications such as hydronephrosis (distention of the kidney with urine), acute renal failure, and urinary tract infection. These conditions are discussed in subsequent sections of this chapter.

INTERDISCIPLINARY CARE

A portable bladder scan (see Box 31-6) ⚭ or straight catheterization may be performed to determine the extent of urinary retention.

For the client with a mechanical obstruction to urine flow, retention is treated by removing or repairing the obstruction. The prostate gland may be resected in the client with BPH. Cholinergic medications such as bethanechol chloride (Urecholine) may be ordered to promote bladder emptying. Modifying the client's medication regimen may be necessary.

Techniques to stimulate reflex voiding and promote complete bladder emptying are used for neurogenic bladder. These include using trigger points, for example, stroking or pinching the abdomen, inner thigh, or glans penis. Pulling pubic hairs or tapping the suprapubic region can also stimulate urination.

The *Credé method* (applying pressure over the symphysis pubis with the fingers of one or both hands) may promote complete bladder emptying. Applying manual pressure to the abdomen and using the *Valsalva maneuver* (bearing down while holding one's breath) also promotes bladder emptying.

Intermittent straight catheterization following surgery can prevent overdistention of the bladder. Intermittent catheterization is less likely to cause a urinary tract infection than an indwelling catheter, and so is preferred. Clients with chronic urinary retention may perform intermittent self-catheterization every 3 to 4 hours (see Box 32-4 ■).

BOX 32-4	**CLIENT TEACHING**

Client Self-Catheterization Checklist

- Wash hands before and after the procedure, and clean the urinary meatus with soap and water.
- Attempt to void. If urine is not of sufficient quantity (at least 100 mL) or if you cannot void at all, do self-catheterization.

Female

- While sitting, locate the urethra by looking in a mirror, or feeling it with a fingertip.
- Lubricate the meatus with a water-soluble lubricant.
- Take a deep breath and insert the catheter tip 2 to 3 inches or until urine flows.

Male

- While sitting, hold the penis with slight upward tension and extend it to its full length.
- Lubricate the catheter from the tip to about 6 inches downward.
- Take a deep breath and insert the catheter 6 to 7 inches or until urine flows.

Both

- Hold the catheter securely and allow urine to drain until the flow stops.
- Withdraw the catheter and wash it with soap and water. Store in a clean container.

NURSING CARE

Careful nursing assessment can identify clients with problems of urinary retention. Note intake and output, paying close attention to voiding patterns as well as total output. Notify the charge nurse or physician if it has been 8 or more hours since the client has voided. Gently palpate the lower abdomen just above the symphysis pubis for tenderness and firm distention. Percussing the lower abdomen may be helpful; a full bladder has a dull percussion tone. If ordered or allowed by unit protocol, perform an ultrasonic bladder scan to measure the amount of urine present in the bladder.

Measures to promote urination can be helpful. Place the client in normal voiding position (sitting for females and standing for males) and provide privacy. Run water in the sink or shower, place the client's hands in warm water, pour warm water over the perineum, or provide a warm sitz bath as additional measures. Provide adequate time for voiding; allow up to 10 minutes.

When catheterization is necessary, use strict sterile technique. Nursing care related to catheterization is listed in Box 32-5 ■.

CONTINUING CARE

Assess the client's ability to provide self-care. Determine understanding of the problem, ability to recognize manifestations of urinary retention, and ability to perform maneuvers to stimulate voiding. If intermittent catheterization is required,

| BOX 32-5 | NURSING CARE CHECKLIST |

Urinary Catheterization

☑ Use Standard Precautions.

☑ Use sterile technique for catheter insertion.

☑ If possible, use intermittent catheterization instead of an indwelling catheter to reduce the risk of infection.

☑ Use an appropriate size catheter. A small catheter may leak; a large catheter may traumatize tissues.

☑ Provide perineal care before catheterization and for clients with an indwelling catheter. Use soap and water, rinsing carefully. Avoid pulling on an indwelling catheter.

☑ Do not drain more than 750 to 1,000 mL from the bladder at one time.

☑ Assess amount, color, clarity, and odor of urine. Collect a urine specimen as needed.

☑ Monitor intake and output.

☑ Secure tubing of an indwelling catheter to prevent trauma.

☑ Maintain gravity drainage; prevent loops of tubing or elevation of the drainage container higher than the bladder.

assess vision, ability to see the urinary meatus, and motor skills for inserting the catheter. Assess access to water and facilities for hand washing and for cleaning the catheter. Discuss the manifestations of acute urinary retention and urinary tract infection, and stress the importance of notifying a health care provider if these develop.

INFECTIOUS AND INFLAMMATORY DISORDERS

Urinary Tract Infections

Urinary tract infections (UTIs) affect up to 20% of adult women; they are much less common in men until age 50. Their incidence increases with aging in both sexes. Unfortunately, *nosocomial* (hospital-acquired) infections are among the most common UTIs.

UTIs can affect any portion of the urinary tract. They are broadly classified according to the region and primary site affected. *Lower urinary tract infections* include *urethritis* (inflammation of the urethra), *prostatitis* (inflammation of the prostate gland), and *cystitis* (inflammation of the bladder). The most common *upper urinary tract infection* is *pyelonephritis* (inflammation of the kidney and renal pelvis).

PATHOPHYSIOLOGY AND MANIFESTATIONS

The urinary tract is normally sterile above the urethra. The most important mechanisms to maintain its sterility are adequate urine volume, unimpeded urine flow, and complete bladder emptying. Other defenses include acid urine, ureteral peristalsis, bacteriostatic properties of the urinary tract, and a *ureterovesical junction* (where the ureters enter the bladder) that prevents backflow of urine toward the kidneys. In males, a long urethra and the antibacterial effect of zinc in prostatic fluid are also important.

Bacteria from the intestines (most commonly *Escherichia coli*) often infect the urinary tract by ascending from the perineal area into the lower urinary tract. Box 32-6 ■ lists risk factors for UTIs. Changes in the urinary tract associated with aging further increase the risk for UTIs in older adults. These changes are summarized in Box 32-7 ■.

Cystitis

Cystitis (inflammation of the urinary bladder) is the most common UTI. The bladder mucosa becomes inflamed and congested with blood. Pus may form, and the mucosa may

---

BOX 32-6

RISK FACTORS FOR UTIs

- Instrumentation of the urinary tract (e.g., catheterization, cystoscopy)
- Structural abnormalities, obstructions, or strictures
- Incomplete bladder emptying
- Chronic diseases such as diabetes

Females

- Short, straight urethra
- Proximity of urinary meatus to the vagina and anus
- Tissue trauma and possible contamination during sexual intercourse
- Use of a diaphragm for birth control
- Personal hygiene practices
- Voluntary urinary retention

Males

- An enlarged prostate gland

BOX 32-8

MANIFESTATIONS OF CYSTITIS

- **Dysuria**—difficult or painful urination
- Frequency
- Urgency—a sudden, compelling need to urinate
- **Nocturia**—voiding two or more times at night
- Pyuria—presence of pus in the urine (cloudy appearance, foul odor)
- **Hematuria**—blood in the urine
- Suprapubic discomfort

---

bleed. The inflammatory process causes the classic manifestations of cystitis (Box 32-8 ■). Older adults with UTIs may be asymptomatic, or may present with nocturia, incontinence, confusion, behavior change, lethargy, anorexia, or "just not feeling right."

Although cystitis is generally uncomplicated and often resolves spontaneously, the infection can ascend to involve the kidneys. In older adults or people with impaired immune responses, bacteremia, sepsis, and shock are possible serious complications.

Pyelonephritis

Pyelonephritis is an inflammatory disorder affecting the renal pelvis and *parenchyma* (the functional portion of the kidney tissue). It may be acute, caused by a bacterial infection; or chronic, associated with other disorders.

Bacteria usually enter the kidney from the lower urinary tract. Risk factors include pregnancy (because of slowed ureteral peristalsis), obstruction, and congenital malformation. *Vesicoureteral reflux* (a condition in which

---

BOX 32-7 | **FOCUS ON OLDER ADULTS**

Risk Factors for UTIs Associated with Aging

- Increased urine pH, promoting bacterial growth
- Higher incidence of diabetes leading to glucosuria (glucose in the urine provides a good culture medium for bacteria)
- Incomplete bladder emptying and urinary retention
- Changes in vaginal pH in women and decreased prostatic secretions in men

---

urine moves from the bladder back toward the kidney) is a common risk factor in children. It may occur in adults when bladder outflow is obstructed.

E. coli is responsible for most cases of acute pyelonephritis. The infection spreads from the renal pelvis to the cortex. The inflamed kidney becomes edematous. Localized abscesses may form, and kidney tissue can be destroyed by the inflammatory process.

The onset of acute pyelonephritis is typically rapid, with chills and fever, malaise, and vomiting, as well as localized manifestations of flank pain and costovertebral tenderness. The client also may have symptoms of cystitis. As with cystitis, older adults may present with a change in behavior, confusion, incontinence, or a general deterioration in condition.

Chronic pyelonephritis leads to fibrosis and scarring of the renal pelvis and calyces. The tubules are gradually destroyed. Chronic renal failure and end-stage renal disease are possible consequences.

INTERDISCIPLINARY CARE

Treatment of UTIs focuses on eliminating the cause, preventing relapse or reinfection, and identifying and correcting any contributing factors.

Diagnostic Tests

A *urinalysis* is ordered to identify blood cells and bacteria in the urine. A midstream, clean-catch urine specimen should be used (see Box 31-1). If necessary, urine may be obtained by a straight catheterization or "mini-cath," using aseptic technique. A urine *culture and sensitivity* also may be done to identify the causative organism. A *complete blood count (CBC) with differential* is done to assess for systemic responses to infection.

In men and in adult females with recurrent UTIs, more extensive diagnostic testing may be done. An *intravenous pyelogram (IVP)* is used to examine the kidneys, ureters, and bladder for abnormalities that may contribute to UTIs. *Voiding cystourethrography* allows assessment of bladder and urethral abnormalities. *Cystoscopy* is used to diagnose conditions that may contribute to UTIs such as an enlarged prostate, urethral strictures, bladder stones, tumors, and congenital abnormalities. See Chapter 31 ⚭ for nursing care related to diagnostic tests of urinary tract function.

Medications

An uncomplicated UTI is treated with a 3-day or a 7- to 10-day course of antibiotics. Drugs such as sulfonamides, trimethoprim–sulfamethoxazole (TMP-SMZ, Bactrim, Septra), and fluoroquinolones such as ciprofloxacin (Cipro) often are used. Treatment often is started before urine culture results are obtained, because these drugs are effective against the usual organisms. Compliance is better with a 3-day course of treatment; however, it is not used for clients with recurrent infections or acute pyelonephritis.

Acute pyelonephritis usually requires 10 to 21 days of antibiotic therapy. Intravenous antibiotics may be necessary if the infection is severe or nausea and vomiting are present. For resistant or recurrent UTIs, therapy with urinary anti-infectives may last from 2 weeks to 6 or 12 months (Table 32-2 ■).

NURSING CARE

ASSESSING

It is important to collect both subjective and objective assessment data from clients with a suspected or confirmed UTI. These data provide information that can be used to help the client recover fully from the infection and prevent future UTIs.

- *Subjective data:* symptoms, including onset and duration; associated symptoms (abdominal or back pain, fever, nausea, or vomiting); previous UTIs, including frequency, and treatment; current method of birth control; possibility of pregnancy; chronic diseases, medications, recent lifestyle changes (e.g., recent marriage or a new sexual relationship); hygiene practices (perineal cleansing after elimination, use of feminine hygiene sprays or bubble baths)

- *Objective data:* vital signs, including temperature; general appearance and apparent state of health; lower abdominal or costovertebral tenderness; obtain clean-catch midstream urine specimen
- *Laboratory studies:* WBC and differential; urinalysis and culture; serum glucose as indicated.

DIAGNOSING, PLANNING, AND IMPLEMENTING

Urinary tract infection interferes with comfort and with normal patterns of urination. If not effectively treated, the infection can ascend to the kidneys and lead to chronic kidney problems.

Priorities in Nursing Care. Ensuring effective urinary elimination and treatment of the infection are nursing care priorities.

Impaired Urinary Elimination

- Monitor urinary output and color, clarity, and character of urine, including odor. *The client with a UTI often experiences dysuria, frequency, urgency, and nocturia. Urine may appear rusty or blood tinged, cloudy, and malodorous. Urine normally returns to clear yellow within 48 hours. If it does not, report to the charge nurse or physician.*

- Provide for easy access to a bedpan, urinal, commode, or bathroom. Make sure lighting is adequate and pathways are clear. *Frequency, urgency, and nocturia increase the risk of urinary incontinence and injury due to falls.*

- Encourage fluid intake unless contraindicated. Tell the client to avoid caffeinated drinks. *Increased fluid dilutes urine, reducing irritation of the inflamed bladder and mucosa. Caffeine can increase bladder spasms and mucosal irritation.*

Noncompliance: Prescribed Antibiotic Regimen

- Work with the client to develop a plan for taking medications, such as taking them with meals (unless contraindicated) or setting out all doses for the day in the morning. *Missed doses of antibiotic can result in subtherapeutic blood levels and reduced effectiveness, and development of drug-resistant bacteria. Taking medication in association with a regular daily activity such as meals helps clients to remember doses.*

- Instruct to complete the full course of antibiotic therapy even though symptoms resolve rapidly. Explain that noncompliance can lead to recurrent infection and potential long-term problems. *Although symptoms may be relieved within 1 to 2 days, this may not be adequate time to eliminate bacteria from the urinary tract.*

- Instruct to keep appointments for follow-up and urine culture. *Follow-up urine culture, scheduled 1 to 3 days after*

TABLE 32-2

Nursing Implications for Pharmacology: UTI

AGENTS/DRUGS	PURPOSE	NURSING RESPONSIBILITIES	CLIENT TEACHING
Sulfonamides ■ Sulfisoxazole (Gantrisin) ■ Sulfamethoxazole (Gantanol) ■ Trimethoprim–sulfamethoxazole (TMP–SMZ, Bactrim, Septra)	Sulfonamides are effective and inexpensive for treating UTIs. They are the drug of choice for most UTIs. They may be given alone or in combination with another antibiotic or with a urinary analgesic.	Assess for allergies to sulfa drugs. Stop the drug and notify the physician if a rash develops. Administer on an empty stomach, 1 hour before or 2 hours after meals, with a full glass of water. Assess for bruising, bleeding, fever, and signs of systemic infection. Assess for other drugs that may interact with sulfonamides. Closely monitor diabetic clients receiving oral hypoglycemic agents for hypoglycemic reactions.	Take all of the medication as ordered. If you miss a dose, take it as soon as you can. Drink at least 8 full glasses of water per day. Avoid cranberry juice. Notify your doctor if you are taking any other medications. If you are diabetic, monitor blood glucose closely. Do not take if you are pregnant or breastfeeding. Use sunscreen to reduce the risk of sunburn. Your urine may turn orange. This is harmless.
Urinary Anti-Infectives ■ Methenamine, (Mandelamine, Hiprex) ■ Nalidixic acid (NegGram) ■ Nitrofurantoin (Furadantin, Macrodantin) ■ Trimethoprim (Proloprim, Trimpex)	Urinary anti-infectives are often used to prevent UTIs in clients with chronic infections. They also may be used if the client is allergic or sensitive to commonly used antibiotics.	Ensure fluid intake of 1,500 to 2,000 mL/day. Give drug with meals to minimize GI side effects. Monitor liver and renal function studies. Monitor closely for adverse effects. Do not administer to pregnant clients. These drugs interact with many other medications. Monitor closely for adverse effects.	Continue taking these drugs even after symptoms have cleared. Drink 6 to 8 glasses of water or fluid per day. Take with meals or food to minimize gastric upset. Do not take if you are pregnant or could become pregnant. Use sunscreen to prevent sunburn. Your urine may turn brown; this is not harmful.
Urinary Analgesic ■ Phenazopyridine (Pyridium)	Phenazopyridine is a urinary analgesic that may be used to relieve pain, burning, frequency, and urgency associated with UTIs. It does not treat the infection and must be used along with antibiotic therapy.	Phenazopyridine stains the urine reddish orange. Yellow-tinged sclera or skin may indicate toxicity. Stop the drug and notify the physician. Do not give to clients with impaired renal function; monitor liver and kidney function tests.	Protect your clothing to prevent staining. Do not use for more than 24 to 48 hours. If symptoms continue, contact your doctor. If your skin or eyes appear yellow, stop taking the drug and notify the physician. Take the drug after meals to minimize gastric upset.

single-dose therapy and 7 to 14 days after conventional therapy, is vital to ensure complete eradication of bacteria and to prevent relapse or recurrence.

CONTINUING CARE

Because both upper and lower urinary tract infections are usually managed in the community, teaching is the most important nursing intervention. Teach clients and their families about the risk factors that contribute to UTIs. Discuss measures to prevent future UTIs:

■ Empty bladder at least every 2 to 4 hours while awake. Avoid voluntary urinary retention.

■ Maintain intake of 2 to 2.5 quarts or 8 to 10 glasses of fluid per day.

BOX 32-9	COMPLEMENTARY THERAPIES

Preventing UTIs

Blueberries have been shown to contain a compound that prevents bacteria from attaching to the bladder wall to cause cystitis. Bilberry (a relative of the blueberry) also is recommended and is available as an herbal extract in capsules. Saw palmetto is another herbal urinary anti-infective used primarily by men with prostatic enlargement. Bromelain (an enzyme derived from pineapple) may increase the effectiveness of antibiotic therapy for treating UTIs. Vitamin C supplements can help treat and prevent UTIs. Dietary changes to prevent UTIs include reduced intake of sugar, alcohol, and fat.

- Complete the prescribed treatment and keep follow-up appointments. Failure to do so increases the risk of unresolved and recurrent infections.
- Unless contraindicated, maintain acidic urine (e.g., drink two glasses of cranberry juice per day; take vitamin C); avoid excess intake of milk products, other fruit juices, and sodium bicarbonate (baking soda). Box 32-9 ■ lists complementary health care practices to prevent UTIs.
- For women:
  - Cleanse perineal area front to back after voiding and defecating.
  - Void before and after sexual intercourse.
  - Avoid bubble baths, feminine hygiene sprays, and douches.
  - Wear cotton briefs; avoid nylon.

Like many infectious processes, urinary tract infection often occurs when immune defenses are low. Inform client that lack of adequate rest, poor nutrition, and high levels of emotional stress are often associated with UTIs. Discuss possible lifestyle changes to reduce future risk for UTIs. Teach clients to identify the early manifestations of UTIs, and stress the importance of seeking medical intervention promptly.

The client with an indwelling urinary catheter is at continued risk for UTIs. Provide information about alternatives such as scheduled toileting, incontinence pads or diapers, and external catheters. Teach the client with urinary retention or a family member to perform straight catheterization every 3 to 4 hours using clean technique (see Box 32-4). If no alternative to an indwelling catheter is feasible, teach clients and their families how to care for the catheter. This includes perineal care, managing and emptying the collection bag, maintaining a closed system, and bladder irrigation or flushing if ordered. Stress the importance of maintaining a generous fluid intake and supporting immune function to prevent upper urinary tract infection.

Glomerulonephritis

Disorders and diseases involving the glomerulus are the leading cause of chronic renal failure in the United States. **Glomerulonephritis** is an inflammatory condition that primarily affects the glomerulus. It may be an acute or a chronic disorder. Glomerulonephritis may be a primary kidney disorder or may develop secondarily to a systemic disease such as lupus erythematosus.

PATHOPHYSIOLOGY AND MANIFESTATIONS

Glomerulonephritis affects both the structure and function of the glomerulus. It damages the capillary membrane, allowing blood cells and proteins to escape from the vascular compartment into the filtrate. *Hematuria* (blood in the urine) may be either gross or microscopic. **Proteinuria** (protein in the urine) increases progressively with increased glomerular damage. Loss of plasma proteins in the urine causes *hypoalbuminemia* (low levels of albumin in the blood). Edema develops as a result, caused by reduced osmotic draw within blood vessels.

When glomerular filtration is disrupted, the GFR falls and **azotemia** (increased blood levels of nitrogenous wastes, including urea and creatinine) occurs. This activates the renin–angiotensin–aldosterone system, leading to salt and water retention and hypertension (Figure 32-2 ■).

Acute Glomerulonephritis

Acute glomerulonephritis usually follows an infection with group A beta-hemolytic *Streptococcus,* such as strep throat.

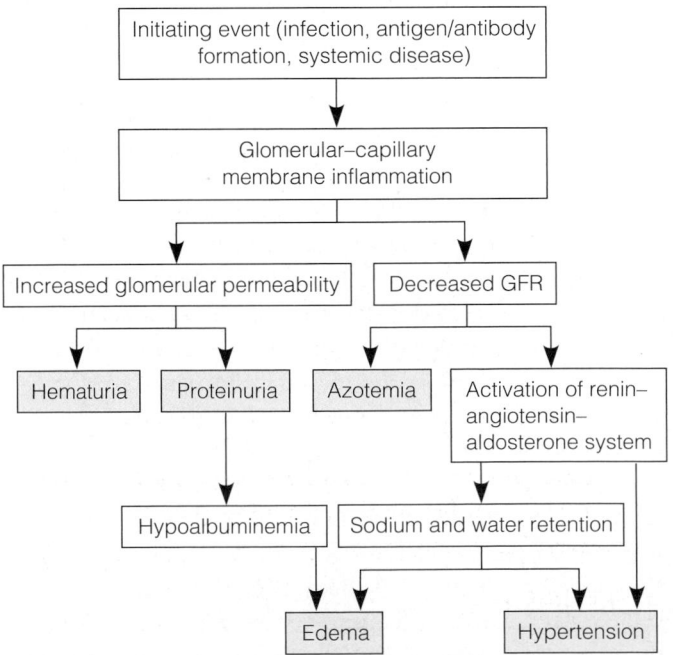

Figure 32-2. ■ The pathophysiology of glomerulonephritis.

BOX 32-10

MANIFESTATIONS OF ACUTE GLOMERULONEPHRITIS
- Hematuria; cola- or coffee-colored urine
- Proteinuria
- Edema: periorbital and facial; dependent (upper extremities in particular)
- Hypertension
- Fatigue
- Anorexia, nausea, vomiting
- Headache
- Elevated BUN and serum creatinine

Immune complexes become trapped in the glomerular membrane, causing an inflammatory response. Inflammation damages the glomerular capillary walls and makes them more porous. Plasma proteins and blood cells escape into the urine. Both kidneys are involved. This is primarily a disease of childhood, but it can affect adults.

Manifestations of acute glomerulonephritis typically develop abruptly, 10 to 14 days after the initial infection (Box 32-10 ■). Older adults may show less characteristic manifestations. Nausea, malaise, arthralgias, and proteinuria are common manifestations; hypertension and edema are seen less often in older adults.

The symptoms may subside spontaneously within 10 to 14 days. Most people recover completely, but some may develop chronic glomerulonephritis with persistent impaired renal function.

Chronic Glomerulonephritis

Chronic glomerulonephritis usually is the end stage of kidney damage by a systemic disease such as diabetes. In many cases, however, no previous kidney disease has been recognized. Chronic glomerulonephritis is characterized by slow, progressive destruction of the glomeruli and gradual loss of entire nephrons. The kidneys decrease in size and their surfaces become granular or rough as nephrons are destroyed.

Symptoms develop slowly, and the disease is often not recognized until signs of renal failure are evident. Renal failure may develop years to decades after the disease is diagnosed.

Diabetic nephropathy is common in the later stages of diabetes mellitus. Microproteinuria may be seen 10 to 15 years after the onset of diabetes. Overt proteinuria and nephropathy develop within 15 to 20 years of the initial diagnosis. The glomerular membrane becomes scarred and thickened, impairing glomerular filtration.

Systemic lupus erythematosus (SLE) is a disorder that affects the connective tissue of the body. Most people with SLE develop *lupus nephritis,* inflammatory lesions of the supportive tissues of the glomerulus. Both the glomerulus and the renal tubule may be affected. Clients with lupus nephritis

have hematuria and proteinuria. Renal failure ultimately may develop.

INTERDISCIPLINARY CARE

Care of the client with acute or chronic glomerulonephritis focuses on identifying and treating the underlying disease process and preserving kidney function. In most cases there is no specific treatment to achieve a cure.

Diagnostic Tests

Laboratory tests may help determine the cause of glomerulonephritis and evaluate its effects on kidney function. An *antistreptolysin-O (ASO) titer* identifies antibodies to group A beta-hemolytic streptococci. The *erythrocyte sedimentation rate (ESR)* is a general indicator of inflammation, and may be elevated in acute glomerulonephritis.

The *BUN* and *serum creatinine* levels increase in kidney disease. The *creatinine clearance,* a very specific indicator of renal function and the GFR, falls. Normal values for these tests are found in Table 31-4. ⬤⬤ *Serum electrolytes* show the effect of impaired kidney function on fluid and electrolyte balance.

A *urinalysis* is done to identify blood cells and protein in the urine. A 24-hour urine specimen may be ordered to measure protein and creatinine in the urine. (See Box 31-3 ⬤⬤ and Table 31-3 ⬤⬤ for nursing responsibilities for these tests.)

In addition, a *KUB (kidney, ureter, bladder) x-ray* may be done to evaluate kidney size. A *kidney scan* (see Box 31-5) or *biopsy* also may be ordered. The nursing implications for a kidney biopsy are outlined in Box 32-11 ■.

Medications

There is no specific drug treatment for glomerulonephritis. Glucocorticoids (such as prednisone) or other immunosuppressive drugs may be given for acute glomerulonephritis to reduce the risk of renal failure. Penicillin or other antibiotics may be ordered for the client with poststreptococcal glomerulonephritis to kill any remaining bacteria. Antihypertensives and diuretics may be prescribed to lower blood pressure and reduce edema.

Plasma Exchange Therapy

Plasma exchange therapy (plasmapheresis) removes harmful antibodies in the plasma by passing the blood through a blood cell separator and reinfusing the red blood cells (RBCs) with an equal amount of albumin or plasma. It may be used to treat acute glomerulonephritis. This procedure is usually done in a series, rather than a one-time-only treatment. Informed consent is required for this procedure.

Dietary Management

Sodium intake may be restricted. Dietary proteins may be increased when protein is being lost in the urine. However,

Renal Biopsy

Client Preparation

☑ Informed consent is required. Clarify and reinforce teaching.

☑ Withhold food and fluids for 8 hours before the procedure.

☑ After the procedure, apply pressure dressing and position supine to maintain pressure on the biopsy site.

☑ Monitor closely for bleeding during the first 24 hours after the procedure:

   a. Check vital signs frequently. Report tachycardia, hypotension, or other signs of shock.

   b. Monitor the biopsy site for bleeding.

   c. Check hemoglobin and hematocrit, comparing with preprocedure values.

   d. Report complaints of flank or back pain, shoulder pain, pallor, light-headedness.

   e. Monitor urine output. Initial hematuria should clear within 24 hours.

☑ Report manifestations of abdominal pain, guarding, and decreased bowel sounds.

☑ Encourage fluids.

Client and Family Teaching

☑ Local anesthesia is used. The procedure may be uncomfortable but should not be painful.

☑ When the needle is inserted, you will be instructed to hold your breath.

☑ The entire procedure takes about 10 minutes.

☑ Avoid coughing for 24 hours after the procedure. Avoid strenuous activity such as heavy lifting for about 2 weeks after the procedure.

☑ Report manifestations of complications to the physician.

if azotemia is present, dietary protein is restricted. When proteins are restricted, those included should be complete proteins such as meat, fish, eggs, soy, or poultry. These proteins supply all the essential amino acids required for growth and tissue maintenance.

NURSING CARE

ASSESSING

Assessment data provide valuable clues about the cause and effects of glomerulonephritis on the client. Subjective data to collect include the onset and duration of manifestations such as changes in urine output or color, weight gain or edema, and other symptoms such as nausea and vomiting. Ask about recent sore throat or other infection and its treat-

ment. Note any history of previous kidney disorders, UTIs, or chronic diseases such as diabetes or lupus. Inquire about current medications.

Obtain the vital signs and weight. Note any edema, particularly of the face, around the eyes, or of the upper extremities. Inspect the throat and skin for evidence of infection. Obtain a urine specimen, and note the color, clarity, and character of the urine. Review laboratory data such as the serum creatinine, BUN, and the creatinine clearance.

DIAGNOSING, PLANNING, AND IMPLEMENTING

Priorities in Nursing Care. Because there is no specific treatment for glomerulonephritis, nursing care focuses on the effects of the disorder on the client's comfort and ability to maintain ADLs.

Excess Fluid Volume

■ Monitor vital signs, including blood pressure, apical pulse, respirations, and breath sounds, at least every 4 hours. Report any significant changes. *Excess fluid volume increases the workload of the heart and the blood pressure. Tachycardia or dysrhythmias may be present. Tachypnea, dyspnea, and crackles may be noted.*

■ Record intake and output (I&O) every 4 to 8 hours, or more frequently as indicated. *Accurate I&O records help determine fluid volume status.*

■ Weigh daily under consistent conditions. *Daily weights are an accurate indicator of fluid volume status.*

■ Assess location and degree of edema. *Edema associated with glomerulonephritis often affects low-pressure tissues such as the face, around the eyes, and the upper extremities.*

■ Restrict fluids as ordered, offering ice chips (in limited and measured amounts) and frequent mouth care to relieve thirst. Develop a fluid intake schedule with the client. *Ice chips and frequent mouth care help relieve thirst while maintaining the integrity of oral tissues.*

■ Carefully monitor intravenous infusions. Include any fluid used to dilute medications as intake. *Significant "hidden" fluid intake can result from multiple intravenous medications.*

■ Arrange dietary consultation to plan the diet when sodium is restricted and when proteins are either restricted or increased. *Providing appealing foods can help maintain adequate nutrition despite anorexia and nausea.*

■ Provide frequent position changes and good skin care. *Tissue perfusion may be altered by edema, increasing the risk of skin breakdown.*

Fatigue

■ Provide for rest by scheduling procedures and activities. Assist with activities of daily living (ADLs) as needed.

Rest reduces fatigue and improves the client's ability to tolerate and cope with treatments and activities. The goal is to conserve limited energy reserves.

- Teach the client and family about the relationship between fatigue and the disease process. Limit visitors and visit length. *Understanding the cause of fatigue helps the client and family to cope with reduced energy and comply with prescribed rest.*

Ineffective Protection

- Monitor temperature, pulse, and mental status every 4 hours. *Fever, elevated pulse, increasing lethargy, or confusion may be early signs of infection.*
- Assess frequently for other signs of infection such as purulent wound drainage, productive cough, abnormal breath sounds, and red or inflamed lesions. Monitor for indications of UTIs such as dysuria, frequency and urgency, and cloudy, foul-smelling urine. *Infection may be masked by the prescribed drugs. Frequent assessment allows early identification.*
- Practice good hand washing. Provide a private room and restrict ill visitors. *Drugs used to treat acute glomerulonephritis may reduce the ability to resist infection.*

Ineffective Role Performance

Activity may be limited to minimize proteinuria. Fatigue and muscle weakness may limit physical and social activities. In addition, facial edema affects self-concept and may lead to isolation.

- Encourage self-care and participation in decision making. *Increased autonomy helps to restore self-confidence and reduce powerlessness.*
- Support coping measures, helping identify personal strengths. Whenever possible, enlist the support of family, other clients, and friends. *This support helps the client gain confidence and provide physical, psychologic, emotional, and social support.*
- Discuss the effect of the disease and treatments on roles and relationships. Help the client and family develop a plan to deal with potential changes and maintain usual roles to the extent possible. *Planning ahead reduces stress and helps the client and family maintain a sense of control.*
- Refer to social services and support groups as needed. *Groups can help the client and family cope with and adapt to the disease.*

EVALUATING

To evaluate the effectiveness of nursing care for the client with glomerulonephritis, collect data such as:

- Weight, presence of edema, and skin integrity; freedom from infection

- Ability to follow, prepare, and consume the prescribed diet
- Planning for additional rest and modification of usual roles and relationships.

Documenting. Document continuing assessment data and trends in symptoms, objective data, and laboratory results. Document all teaching and the client's and family's apparent understanding and acceptance of the information and treatment plan.

CONTINUING CARE

Glomerulonephritis may be self-limiting or progressive. Its course ranges from weeks to years. Self-management is essential, and the key to self-management is a good understanding of the disorder and treatment regimen.

Teach about the disease process and prognosis. Discuss the prescribed treatment, including activity and diet restrictions. Provide information about the use and potential effects, both beneficial and adverse, of all prescribed medications. Discuss the importance of contacting the physician prior to taking any other medications. It is vital to avoid drugs that are potentially toxic to the kidneys. Discuss the risks, manifestations, prevention, and management of complications such as edema and infection. Because the client and family may be monitoring kidney status to a certain extent themselves, teach the signs, symptoms, and implications of improving or declining renal function.

NURSING PROCESS CARE PLAN
Client with Acute Glomerulonephritis

Jung-Lin Chang is a 23-year-old graduate student who goes to the university health center when he notices that his urine is brown and foamy. The physician admits him to the infirmary and orders a throat culture, ASO titer, CBC, BUN, serum creatinine, and urinalysis.

Assessment. Connie King, the admitting nurse, notes that Mr. Chang's history is negative for past kidney or urinary problems. He states that he had a "pretty bad" sore throat a couple of weeks ago. He took a few antibiotics he had left from a previous bout of strep throat, increased his fluids, and did not see a doctor. The sore throat resolved, and he felt well until noticing the change in his urine. He thought the puffiness around his eyes was due to lack of sleep and fatigue. He has eaten little the past 2 days.

Assessment findings include BP 136/90, P 98, R 18, and T 98.8°F (37.1°C) PO; weight 165 pounds (75 kg), up from his normal of 160 lb (72.5 kg); and moderate periorbital edema and edema of his hands and fingers.

Lab results show a negative throat culture but high ASO titer. His CBC is normal, BUN 42 mg/dL, and serum creatinine 2.1 mg/dL. Urinalysis shows protein, red blood cells, and RBC casts. A subsequent 24-hour urine contains 1,025 mg of protein, compared to the normal of 30 to 150 mg/24 hours.

Mr. Chang is diagnosed with acute poststreptococcal glomerulonephritis. His orders include bed rest with bathroom privileges, fluid restriction (1,200 mL/day), and a low-sodium and low-protein diet.

Diagnosis

- *Excess Fluid Volume* related to plasma protein loss and sodium and water retention
- *Risk for Imbalanced Nutrition: Less than Body Requirements* related to anorexia
- *Anxiety* related to prescribed activity restriction
- *Deficient Knowledge: Glomerulonephritis* related to lack of information

Expected Outcomes. The expected outcomes for the plan of care are that Mr. Chang will:

- Maintain blood pressure within normal limits.
- Return to usual weight with no evidence of edema.
- Consume adequate calories following prescribed dietary limitations.
- Verbalize less anxiety regarding ability to continue with his program of study.
- Demonstrate an understanding of acute glomerulonephritis and his prescribed management regimen.

Planning and Implementation

- Monitor vital signs every 4 hours. Notify the physician of significant changes.
- Record intake and output every 8 hours.
- Schedule fluids: 650 mL day shift, 450 mL evening shift, and 100 mL night shift.
- Weigh daily.
- Arrange for dietary consultation.
- Provide small meals with high-carbohydrate snacks.
- Encourage Mr. Chang to talk about his condition and its potential effects.
- Enlist friends and family to listen and provide support.
- Teach about acute glomerulonephritis and prescribed management regimen.
- Instruct in the appropriate use of antibiotics.

Evaluation. Mr. Chang is released from the infirmary after 4 days. He decides to return to his parents' home for the 6 to 12 weeks of convalescence prescribed by his doctor. Mr. Chang's renal function gradually returns to normal with no further azotemia and minimal proteinuria after 4 months. Mr. Chang verbalizes an understanding of the relationship between the episode of strep throat, his inappropriate use of antibiotics, and the glomerulonephritis. He says, "I may not always remember to take every pill on time in the future, but I sure won't save them for the next time again!"

Critical Thinking in the Nursing Process

1. How did Mr. Chang's use of "a few" previously prescribed antibiotics to treat his sore throat affect his risk for developing poststreptococcal glomerulonephritis?
2. What additional risk factors did Mr. Chang have for developing glomerulonephritis?
3. What teaching should the nurse provide to reduce his risk for future episodes of acute glomerulonephritis?

Nephrotic Syndrome

Nephrotic syndrome is not a disease but a group of symptoms. It results from damage to glomerular membranes and severe protein loss in the urine. A number of disorders cause nephrotic syndrome. *Minimal change disease* is the most common cause in children. In adults, nephrotic syndrome may result from primary kidney disorders or from systemic diseases such as diabetes or lupus.

Clients with nephrotic syndrome have significant proteinuria, low serum albumin levels, high blood lipids, and edema. Edema may be severe, affecting the face and periorbital area as well as dependent tissues (Figure 32-3 ■). *Thromboemboli* (mobilized blood clots) are a relatively common complication of nephrotic syndrome. Peripheral veins and arteries, pulmonary arteries, and renal veins may be occluded.

Nephrotic syndrome usually resolves without long-term effects in children. Adults are less likely to recover completely. Many have persistent proteinuria and progressive renal impairment that may lead to renal failure.

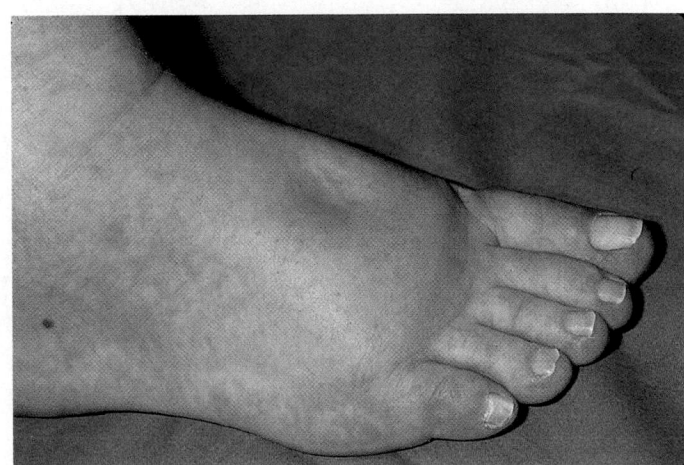

Figure 32-3. ■ Severe edema in a client with nephrotic syndrome. (*Source:* NMSB, Custom Medical Stock Photos, Inc.)

Clients with nephrotic syndrome are placed on a low-sodium diet, often with a moderate protein restriction. Diuretics and angiotensin-converting enzyme (ACE) inhibitors are prescribed to reduce the edema and protein loss. Drugs such as glucocorticoids (e.g., prednisone) may be given to induce remission. Nonsteroidal anti-inflammatory drugs (NSAIDs) also may be ordered.

Nursing care and teaching for clients with nephritic syndrome is similar to that provided for clients with glomerulonephritis.

OBSTRUCTIVE DISORDERS

Urinary Calculi

Urolithiasis (development of stones within the urinary tract) is the most common cause of obstructed urine flow. *Nephrolithiasis* indicates stone formation within the kidney. The stone (or *calculus*) may develop and cause obstruction at any point within the urinary tract (Figure 32-4 ■). In the United States, kidney stones are the most common. Males are affected more often than females by a 4:1 ratio. In other parts of the world, bladder stones are common.

PATHOPHYSIOLOGY

Calculi (stones) are masses of crystals formed from materials normally excreted in the urine. Most are made of calcium. Risk factors for kidney stones include personal or family history of urinary stones; dehydration; excess calcium, oxalate, or protein intake; gout; hyperparathyroidism; or urinary stasis. Stones form when a poorly soluble salt crystallizes. When the concentration of the salt in the urine is very high, very little stimulus is needed to start crystallization. A meal high in the mineral or decreased fluid intake, as occurs during sleep, may start stone formation. When fluid intake is adequate, no stone growth occurs. Lithiasis is also affected by the pH of the urine and compounds that inhibit stone development.

Calcium stones often are associated with hypercalcemia. Risk factors for calcium stones include hyperparathyroidism (see Chapters 7 and 16) ⚭ and immobility, as well as alkaline urine and dehydration.

MANIFESTATIONS AND COMPLICATIONS

Manifestations of urinary calculi are due to obstructed urine flow, distention, and tissue trauma from the rough-edged stone. They vary by stone location (Box 32-12 ■). Stones at any level may cause manifestations of UTI, including chills and fever, frequency, urgency, and dysuria.

Urinary tract obstruction by renal calculi may cause few symptoms if it develops slowly. Acute obstruction causes severe pain in the flank region, possibly radiating

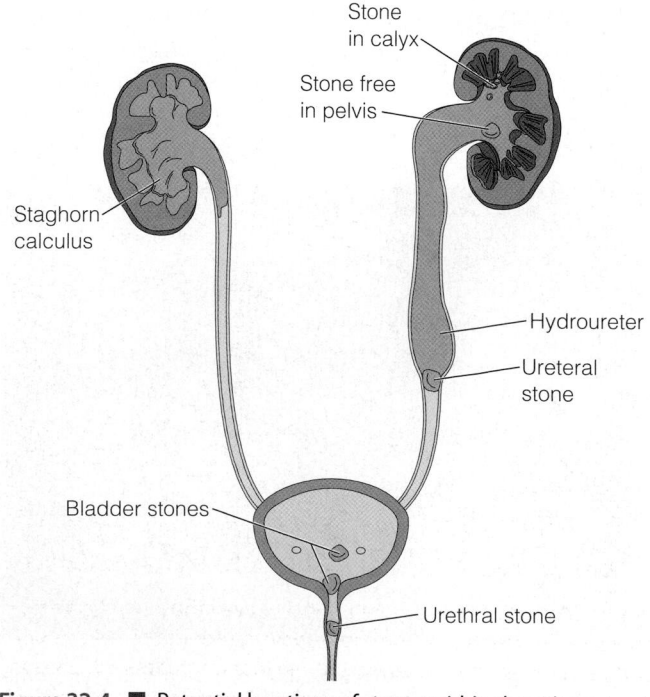

Figure 32-4. ■ Potential locations of stones within the urinary tract.

BOX 32-12

MANIFESTATIONS OF URINARY STONES

Kidney Pelvis
- May be asymptomatic
- Dull, aching flank pain

Ureter
- **Renal colic:** Acute, severe, intermittent flank pain on affected side
- Pain radiating to suprapubic region, groin, and scrotum or labia
- Nausea, vomiting
- Pallor; cool, clammy skin
- Microscopic hematuria

Bladder
- May be asymptomatic
- Dull suprapubic pain
- Microscopic or gross hematuria

to the genitals. If the obstruction is unrelieved, the kidney may be damaged. Urine production continues; however, the obstruction blocks its outflow. This leads to increased pressure and distention of the urinary tract behind the obstruction. *Hydronephrosis* (discussed in the next section of this chapter) and *hydroureter* (distention of the ureter with urine) may result. Urinary stasis increases the risk of infection as well.

INTERDISCIPLINARY CARE

Diagnostic Tests

Diagnostic tests are used to confirm the diagnosis and determine the type of stone. A *urinalysis* is done to detect hematuria. Any stones passed are analyzed to identify their composition. The nurse often is responsible for retrieving stones. All urine is strained and may be saved. Any visible stones or sediment are sent for analysis.

A *KUB x-ray* is done to identify the presence of calculi in the kidneys, ureters, and bladder. *IVP, renal ultrasound, CT scan,* or *MRI* may be used to locate calculi and identify hydroureter or hydronephrosis. *Cystoscopy* is used to visualize and possibly remove calculi from the urinary bladder and distal ureters. Review Chapter 31 ∞ for nursing implications for these studies.

Medications

Pain relief is vital for acute renal colic. Narcotic analgesics are used to provide analgesia and relieve ureteral spasms. Analgesics often are administered intravenously for rapid pain relief. Indomethacin (an NSAID) in suppository form can reduce the amount of narcotic analgesia required.

After stone analysis, medications may be prescribed to prevent further stone formation. Thiazide diuretics are frequently ordered for calcium stones. They reduce urinary calcium excretion and can prevent future stones.

Dietary Management

The diet may be modified to prevent further lithiasis. Fluid intake is increased to 2.5 to 3 liters per day to prevent concentration of stone-forming salts. Intake should be spaced throughout the day and evening. The client may be advised to drink one to two glasses of water at night to maintain dilute urine during sleep.

Foods that contributed to stone formation may be limited in the diet. For calcium stones, dietary calcium and vitamin D–enriched foods are restricted. Because calcium stones form more readily in alkaline urine, the diet is modified toward foods that lower the urinary pH (Table 32-3 ■).

Surgery

Stones that are too large to be passed spontaneously (>5 mm in diameter) may require removal. *Lithotripsy* (crushing of

TABLE 32-3	
Foods to Consume or Avoid to Prevent Urolithiasis	
Foods that acidify urine	Cheese, cranberries, eggs, grapes, meat and poultry, plums and prunes, tomatoes, whole grains
Foods that alkalinize urine	Green vegetables, fruit (except those noted above), legumes, milk and milk products, rhubarb
Foods high in calcium	Beans and lentils, chocolate and cocoa, dried fruits, canned or smoked fish except tuna, flour, milk and milk products
Foods high in oxalate	Asparagus, beer and colas, beets, cabbage, celery, chocolate and cocoa, fruits, green beans, nuts, tea, tomatoes
Foods high in purines	Goose, organ meats, sardines and herring, venison; moderate in beef, chicken, crab, pork, salmon, veal

renal calculi using sound or shock waves) is the preferred treatment. It may be done by laser or using an external lithotriptor device. In *extracorporeal shock-wave lithotripsy (ESWL),* shock waves generated outside the body are directed at the stone (Figure 32-5 ■). These shock waves travel harmlessly through soft tissue, but pulverize the stone into fragments that are small enough to be eliminated in the

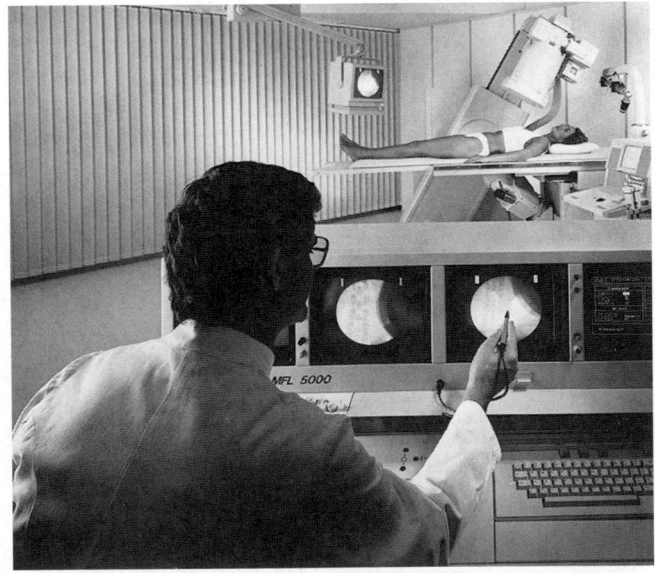

Figure 32-5. ■ Extracorporeal shock-wave lithotripsy. Acoustic shock waves created by the shock-wave generator travel through soft tissue to shatter the urinary stone into fragments, which are then eliminated in the urine. (Courtesy of Dormier Medical Products.)

BOX 32-13 NURSING CARE CHECKLIST

Lithotripsy

Before Surgery

☑ Clarify and reinforce teaching as needed.

☑ Provide routine preoperative care as outlined in Chapter 9. ⊚

After Surgery

☑ Frequently monitor vital signs. Report changes to the charge nurse or physician.

☑ Monitor amount, color, and clarity of urine output. Expect hematuria for 12 to 48 hours following surgery.

☑ Anchor ureteral catheters or nephrostomy tubes securely. Irrigate gently if ordered.

☑ Teach catheter and operative site care.

☑ Instruct client to report drainage of urine from incision for more than 4 days, symptoms of infection, pain, bright hematuria.

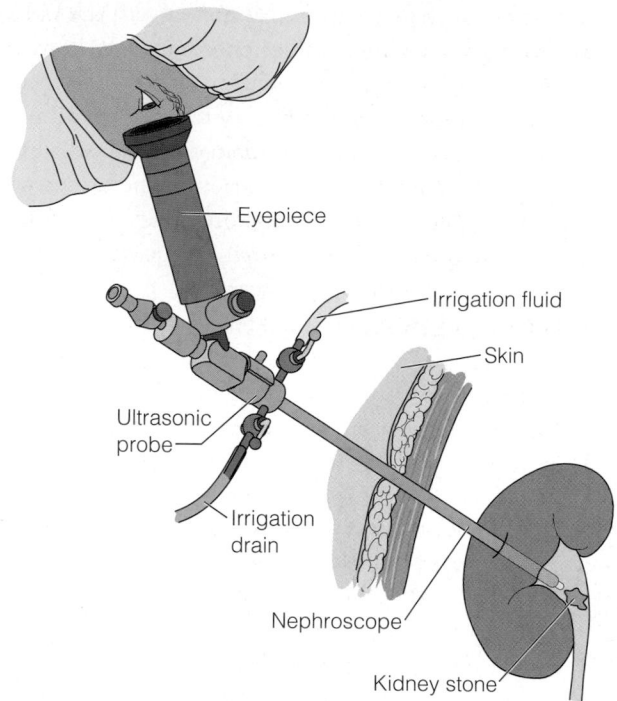

Figure 32-6. ■ Percutaneous lithotripsy. A nephroscope is inserted through the skin into the renal pelvis, and the stone is fragmented using ultrasonic waves or laser.

---

urine. Box 32-13 ■ outlines nursing care for clients having a lithotripsy.

Stones in the renal pelvis or calyces may require nephrostomy for removal. A small incision is made in the flank, and a nephroscope is inserted to visualize the renal pelvis. The stones may then be removed or crushed. With *percutaneous lithotripsy,* the stone is fragmented using a small ultrasonic transducer or a laser beam (Figure 32-6 ■). Fragments are removed by irrigation and suction.

Bladder stones may be crushed and removed by *cystoscopy.* Cystoscopy also may be used to advance a catheter or basket catheter into a ureter to remove a stone. A laser may be used to disintegrate a ureteral stone via a ureteroscope. Stone fragments are then flushed out with fluid.

Nephrolithotomy may be required to remove a *staghorn calculus,* which invades the calyces and renal parenchyma. If kidney damage has been severe, a partial or total *nephrectomy* (removal of the kidney) may be necessary. (See Box 32-18 later in this chapter for nursing care of clients having kidney surgery.)

NURSING CARE

ASSESSING

The client with a urinary stone often is in acute distress when seeking medical help. The nursing assessment is brief and focused. Ask about the onset, character, intensity, location, and radiation of pain, as well as associated symptoms such as nausea and vomiting. Inquire about previous episodes of pain

or a history of kidney stones. Ask about most recent food and fluid intake, and any factors that may have contributed to dehydration (such as physical labor on a hot day). Be sure to ask about known allergies to medications or foods (seafood in particular).

DIAGNOSING, PLANNING, AND IMPLEMENTING

Priorities in Nursing Care. Relieving the client's pain and retrieving stone fragments for analysis are the priorities for nursing care of the client with urinary stones.

Pain

■ Administer analgesia as ordered. *Pain control is vital to reduce anxiety and stress, and to facilitate healing after surgery.*

■ Unless contraindicated, increase fluid intake and encourage ambulation. *Increased fluids and ambulation increase urinary output, help to move the stone through the ureter, and decrease pain.*

■ Check urinary output, catheters, incision, and wound drainage. *Increased pain may indicate a blocked catheter, infection, or bleeding.*

Impaired Urinary Elimination

■ Measure urine output; document hematuria, dysuria, frequency, urgency, and pyuria. *Low urine output is a possible indicator of obstruction. Hematuria is often associated with calculi and with procedures for stone removal. A change in the degree of hematuria may indicate stone passage or a complication. Dysuria, frequency, urgency, and cloudy urine are symptoms of urinary tract infection, and may indicate the need for antibiotic treatment.*

■ Strain all urine for stones, saving recovered stones for laboratory analysis. *Analysis of recovered stones helps direct treatment to prevent further stone formation.*

■ Maintain patency of all catheters. Secure catheters well and label as indicated. Use sterile technique for all irrigations or other procedures. *A kinked or plugged catheter obstructs urine flow, increasing the risk of further urinary system damage. Labeling catheters prevents mistakes, such as inappropriate irrigation or clamping. Aseptic technique minimizes the risk of infection.*

EVALUATING

Collect data about pain level and urine output (amount, color, character) to evaluate the effectiveness of nursing care for the client with urinary stones.

Documenting. Document continuing pain assessment, relief measures provided, and their efficacy. Document urine output, including color and amount, and any fragments or stones retrieved and sent for analysis. Note all teaching provided and the client's understanding of measures to prevent future episodes of urinary stones.

CONTINUING CARE

Because a history of lithiasis increases the risk of future stone formation, teaching is essential. Assess level of understanding and previous learning. Clarify all diagnostic and therapeutic procedures. Clients whose pain can be managed with oral analgesics may be managed at home. Teach the client to:

■ Collect and strain all urine, saving any stones.

■ Report stone passage to the physician and bring the stone in for analysis.

■ Observe the amount and character of urine, reporting any changes to physician.

Discuss factors that increase the risk of urinary stones and how to minimize this risk. Emphasize the importance of drinking 2.5 to 3 quarts of fluid per day, following dietary recommendations, and taking medication as prescribed. Discuss the relationship between urolithiasis and urinary tract infection. Teach prevention, recognition, and management of UTIs.

When the client is discharged with dressings, a nephrostomy tube, or a catheter, teach dressing changes, tube care, and assessment of the wound and skin. Emphasize the need to keep tubes and catheters patent. Teach how to empty drainage bags, assess urine output, and when to contact the physician.

> **BOX 32-14**
>
> **MANIFESTATIONS OF HYDRONEPHROSIS**
>
> **Acute**
> - Colicky flank pain; may radiate into groin
> - Hematuria, pyuria
> - Fever
> - Nausea, vomiting, abdominal pain
>
> **Chronic**
> - Intermittent, dull flank pain
> - Hematuria, pyuria
> - Fever
> - Palpable mass

Hydronephrosis

Hydronephrosis (abnormal dilation of the renal pelvis and calyces) can result from urinary tract obstructions or from *vesicoureteral reflux* (backflow of urine from the bladder to the ureters). Pressure in the renal pelvis increases, and it dilates. The nephrons and collecting tubules may be damaged, affecting renal function. The manifestations of hydronephrosis depend on how rapidly it develops. (Box 32-14 ■). If both kidneys are affected, symptoms of acute renal failure may develop.

Hydronephrosis is diagnosed by *ultrasound* or *CT scan.* Other tests, such as *cystoscopy,* may be done to determine the cause. Prompt treatment is vital to preserve renal function. Immediate treatment involves reestablishing urine flow from the affected kidney. A nephrostomy tube, ureteral stent, or indwelling catheter may be required.

Ureteral stents (small, specialized catheters) are used to keep ureters open and promote healing. Stents can be positioned during surgery or cystoscopy. One or both ends of the stent may be pigtail or J-shaped to keep it in place (Figure 32-7 ■). A stent may be temporary, or it may be used for longer periods with ureteral obstruction due to tumors, strictures, or other causes. Box 32-15 ■ describes nursing care for a client with a ureteral stent.

Nursing care focuses on preventing hydronephrosis and ensuring urinary drainage. Monitoring intake, urine output, and bladder emptying helps identify impaired urine outflow. Monitoring urine output is vital for clients with risk factors such as pelvic or abdominal tumors, urinary calculi, adhesions and scarring from previous surgeries, or neurologic deficits. Ensuring urinary drainage is also vital in the client with a ureteral stent, nephrostomy, or surgical intervention for hydronephrosis. Label catheters and drainage tubes clearly, and measure outputs separately. Prevent kinking or obstruction. Irrigate tubes only as ordered by the physician.

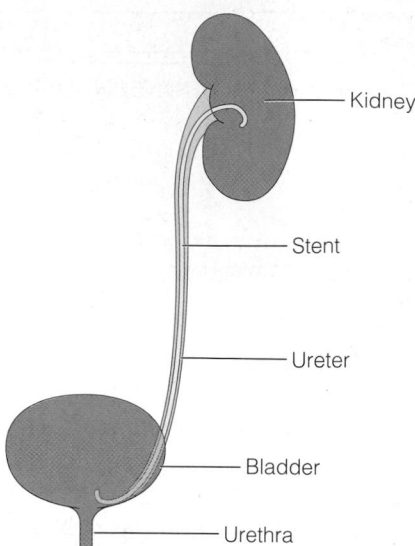

Figure 32-7. ■ A ureteral stent.

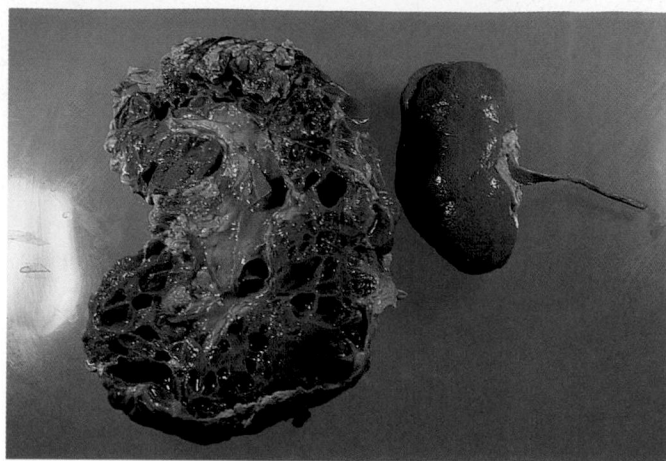

Figure 32-8. ■ A polycystic kidney and a normal kidney for comparison. (*Source:* NMSB, Custom Medical Stock Photos, Inc.)

Polycystic Kidney Disease

Polycystic kidney disease is a hereditary disease characterized by cyst formation and massive kidney enlargement. It is a relatively common disease that affects both children and adults.

PATHOPHYSIOLOGY AND MANIFESTATIONS

Renal cysts develop in the nephron. These fluid-filled sacs can range in size from microscopic to several centimeters in diameter. Both kidneys are affected. As the cysts fill, enlarge, and multiply, the kidneys also enlarge (Figure 32-8 ■). The cysts gradually destroy functional kidney tissue. Cysts also may develop elsewhere (e.g., liver, spleen, pancreas). Cardiac and vascular abnormalities also may be present.

Polycystic kidney disease is slowly progressive, with symptoms usually noticed in the 30s or 40s. Common manifestations include flank pain, microscopic or gross hematuria, proteinuria, and polyuria and nocturia. Urinary tract infections and stones are common. Most clients develop hypertension. The kidneys become enlarged, palpable, and knobby. Eventually, signs of renal failure develop.

INTERDISCIPLINARY CARE

Management of adult polycystic kidney disease is supportive. A *renal ultrasound* is done to diagnose polycystic kidney disease.

Care is taken to avoid further renal damage by nephrotoxins, urinary tract infection, obstruction, or hypertension. A fluid intake of 2,000 to 2,500 mL per day is encouraged to help prevent UTIs and lithiasis. ACE inhibitors or other antihypertensive agents are prescribed to manage hypertension. Ultimately, clients with polycystic kidney disease require hemodialysis or kidney transplantation. The section on chronic renal failure later in this chapter gives more information about dialysis and kidney transplants.

NURSING CARE

Although each client has individual nursing care needs, the following nursing diagnoses may be appropriate for the client with polycystic kidney disease:

- *Excess Fluid Volume* related to impaired renal function
- *Anticipatory Grieving* related to potential loss of kidney function
- *Deficient Knowledge* related to lack of information about how to maintain kidney function
- *Ineffective Coping* related to the potential for transmitting an inherited disorder to offspring.

CONTINUING CARE

Teach about polycystic kidney disease and how to maintain good kidney function. Instruct to drink about 2,500 mL of fluid per day. Include additional information about preventing

---

BOX 32-15 NURSING CARE CHECKLIST

Ureteral Stent

☑ Label all drainage tubes and stents for easy identification. Secure positions.

☑ Attach each catheter and stent to a separate closed drainage system.

☑ Monitor for infection or bleeding: fever, tachycardia, pain, hematuria, and cloudy or malodorous urine.

☑ Encourage fluids, especially those that acidify urine, such as apple and cranberry juice.

☑ For an indwelling stent, teach follow-up care and recognition and prevention of complications.

urinary tract infections, such as hygiene measures. Discuss early manifestations of UTIs, and stress the importance of seeking prompt treatment to prevent further kidney damage. Advise avoiding medications that are potentially toxic to the kidneys and checking with the primary care provider before taking any new drug.

Offspring of clients with adult polycystic kidney disease have a 50% chance of inheriting the disorder. Discuss genetic counseling and screening of family members, especially if renal transplantation is likely and family members are potential donors.

KIDNEY TRAUMA

The kidneys are relatively well protected by the rib cage and back muscles but may be injured by blunt force (most common) or penetrating injury. Falls, motor vehicle accidents, and sports injuries can all result in kidney damage. Renal contusion or a small hematoma may result or, more seriously, a laceration or other damage. Gunshot wounds, knife wounds, impalement injuries, and fractured ribs can cause penetrating damage. Because the kidney is a vascular organ, trauma can lead to hemorrhage and possible shock.

The primary manifestations of renal trauma are hematuria (gross or microscopic), flank or abdominal pain, and oliguria or **anuria** (absence of urine). There may be localized swelling, tenderness, or *ecchymoses* (bruising) in the flank region. Signs of shock may be present, including tachycardia, hypotension, tachypnea, cool and pale skin, and decreased level of consciousness.

Treatment of minor kidney injuries is generally conservative, including bed rest and observation. Bleeding is usually minor and self-limiting. Immediate treatment for major or critical trauma focuses on controlling hemorrhage and treating or preventing shock. Surgery may be required to stop the bleeding. (See Box 32-18 in the section on Kidney Tumors for nursing care of the client undergoing kidney surgery.)

TUMORS OF THE KIDNEY AND URINARY TRACT

Any part of the urinary tract can be affected by a tumor, but the most common site is the bladder. Tumors of the urinary tract may lead to obstruction, renal failure, hemorrhage, and invasion of surrounding tissues.

Bladder Cancer

Bladder cancer is the tenth leading cause of cancer deaths. People living in heavily industrialized states are more likely to be affected than those living in agricultural states. People in northern regions have a higher risk than people in southern regions.

Bladder cancer usually affects people over age 50. It is diagnosed in men two to four times more often than in women. Many clients with bladder cancer have more than one tumor at the time of diagnosis.

PATHOPHYSIOLOGY

The major risk factors for bladder cancer are carcinogens in the urine and chronic inflammation or infection of bladder mucosa. Chemicals from cigarette smoke and other chemicals such as those used in the plastics industry, by leather finishers, spray painters, and hairdressers are carcinogenic (cancer producing). They are excreted in the urine and stored in the bladder, increasing the risk of abnormal cell growth.

Bladder tumors begin as cell changes that develop into superficial or invasive lesions. Most are papillomas, with a polyp-like structure attached by a stalk to the bladder mucosa (Figure 32-9 ■). The prognosis for a full recovery is

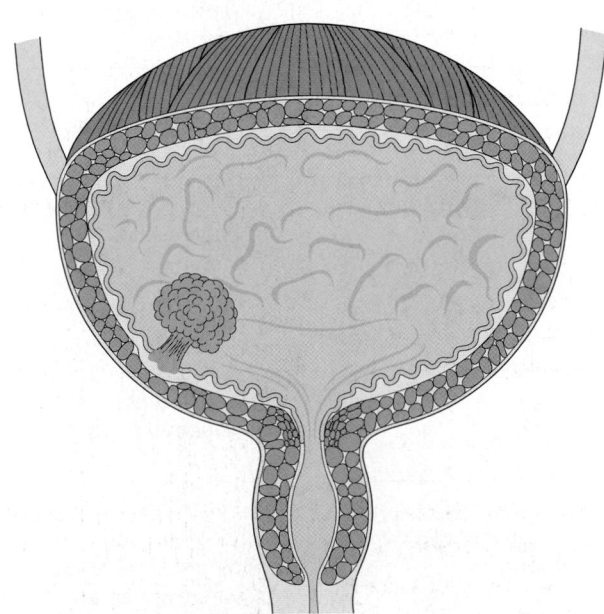

Figure 32-9. ■ A papillary lesion of the bladder wall.

good. When metastasis occurs, the pelvic lymph nodes, lungs, bones, and liver are most commonly involved.

MANIFESTATIONS

Painless hematuria is the most common initial manifestation of bladder cancer. Frequency, urgency, and dysuria are other manifestations of bladder cancer.

INTERDISCIPLINARY CARE

When *urinalysis* shows hematuria, a *urine cytology* may be done to assess for cancer cells. A *cystoscopy* is done to visualize and biopsy the lesion. Review Box 31-7 ⊘ for nursing implications of a cystoscopy.

Medications

Chemotherapeutic drugs may be instilled into the bladder as the primary treatment for bladder cancer or to prevent recurrence of the tumor after surgery. Bacillus Calmette–Guérin (BCG Live, TheraCys) causes a local inflammatory reaction that eliminates or reduces superficial tumors. Other chemotherapeutic drugs also may be used. Bladder irritation, frequency, dysuria, and contact dermatitis are possible adverse reactions to *intravesical* (within-bladder) chemotherapy.

Surgery

Surgery for bladder tumors ranges from simple resection of noninvasive tumors to removal of the bladder and surrounding structures (Table 32-4 ■). In a total or radical **cystectomy,** the bladder and adjacent muscles and tissues are removed. In men, the prostate and seminal vessels are also removed, resulting in impotence. In women, the uterus, fallopian tubes, and ovaries are removed, resulting in sterility. A *urinary diversion* is created for urine collection and drainage. The most common urinary diversion is the *ileal conduit;* a *continent urinary diversion* also may be created (Figure 32-10 ■). Box 32-16 ■ describes nursing care of the client undergoing a cystectomy and urinary diversion.

NURSING CARE

ASSESSING

Painless hematuria is the most common early manifestation of bladder cancer. Direct any client with blood in the urine to seek medical evaluation and care.

TABLE 32-4

Nursing Implications for Bladder Cancer Surgeries

PROCEDURE	DESCRIPTION	NURSING CONSIDERATIONS
Transurethral resection of bladder tumor (TURBT)	Tumor removal via cystoscope inserted through urethra	Maintain continuous bladder irrigation as ordered, ensure catheter patency. Monitor for excessive bleeding. Encourage fluids up to 2,500–3,000 mL/day. Give stool softeners to prevent straining.
Partial cystectomy	Resection of the tumor and a portion of the bladder wall	Maintain urethral and/or suprapubic catheter patency to reduce pressure on suture lines. Monitor for excessive bleeding.
Complete or radical cystectomy	Removal of the entire urinary bladder and surrounding tissues	Permanent urinary diversion required. Maintain stent position and patency. May have urethral catheter to drain pelvic cavity.
Cutaneous ureterostomy	One or both ureters brought to abdominal wall; urine drains via stoma	Requires urinary drainage appliance. Small stoma may make tight seal difficult. Risk of skin irritation from contact with urine. Increased risk of UTI due to direct access from skin to kidney.
Ileal conduit	Portion of ileum formed into pouch; ureters inserted into pouch and open end is brought to surface to form stoma	Continuous urine drainage requires appliance. Risk of infection is significant. Good skin care is vital due to constant contact with urine.
Continent internal ileal reservoir or continent ileal bladder conduit (Kock's pouch)	Pouch created from ileum; nipple valves formed by telescoping tissue where brought to skin and where ureters attach prevent urine leakage and reflux	Drainage-collection device is not necessary. Client must be willing and able to perform clean intermittent self-catheterization every 2 to 4 hours to drain pouch.

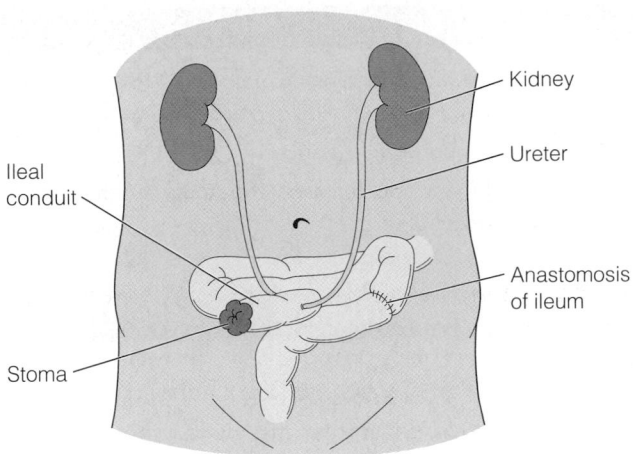

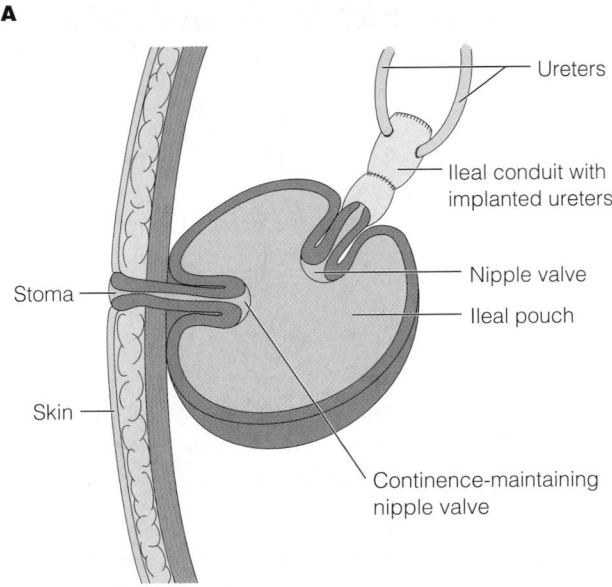

Figure 32-10. ■ Urinary diversion procedures. (**A**) Ileal conduit. (**B**) A continent urinary diversion.

DIAGNOSING, PLANNING, AND IMPLEMENTING

Priorities in Nursing Care. The client with bladder cancer faces an uncertain future. The priority focus for nursing care is ensuring effective urinary elimination.

Impaired Urinary Elimination

■ Monitor amount, color, and clarity of urine output from all catheters, stents, and tubes hourly for the first 24 hours postoperatively, then every 4 to 8 hours. *Output of less than 30 mL per hour may indicate low blood volume, impaired kidney function, or impaired drainage. A change in urine color or clarity may indicate infection or other complication.*

| BOX 32-16 | NURSING CARE CHECKLIST |

Bladder Tumor Surgery (Cystectomy)

Before Surgery

☑ Contact the enterostomal therapist to determine the stoma site(s).

☑ Provide routine preoperative care as ordered (see Chapter 9). ∞

After Surgery

☑ Monitor intake and output. Assess urine output hourly for the first 24 hours, then every 4 hours or as ordered. Notify the charge nurse or physician if less than 30 mL/hour.

☑ Assess urine color and consistency. Expect pink or bright red urine to clear by third postoperative day. Urine may be cloudy due to mucus produced by bowel mucosa, but excessive cloudiness or malodorous urine may indicate infection.

☑ Assess stoma and surrounding skin every 2 hours for the first 24 hours, then every 4 hours for 48 to 72 hours. Notify the charge nurse or physician if the stoma blanches when touched or is pale, gray, or cyanotic.

☑ Irrigate ileal diversion catheter with 30 to 60 mL sterile normal saline every 4 hours or as ordered.

☑ Teach stoma and urinary diversion care, including odor management, skin care, increased fluid intake, pouch application and leakage prevention, self-catheterization for clients with continent reservoirs, and signs of infection and other complications.

■ Label all catheters, stents, and their drainage containers. Maintain separate closed gravity drainage systems for each. *Clear labeling of tubes can prevent errors in irrigating and calculating outputs. Separate closed systems minimize the risk of infection.*

■ Secure catheters and stents with tape; prevent kinking or occlusion; maintain gravity flow by keeping drainage bags lower than the kidneys. *Impaired urine flow can lead to kidney damage or place pressure on suture lines.*

■ Encourage fluid intake of 3,000 mL/day. *Increased fluid intake reduces the risk of infection and dilutes urine, which is less irritating to the skin around the stoma site.*

■ After removal of any stents or ureteral catheters, monitor urine output closely for 24 hours. *Edema or stricture of ureters may impede output.*

■ Encourage activity. *Ambulation promotes urine drainage and helps prevent calcium loss from bones, which could lead to urinary calculi.*

Risk for Impaired Skin Integrity

■ Assess skin surrounding the stoma for redness, excoriation, or signs of breakdown. Assess for urine leakage

BOX 32-17   PROCEDURE CHECKLIST

Urinary Stoma Care

- ☑ Gather all supplies. Provide for privacy.
- ☑ Assess client's knowledge, ability, and willingness to assist; explain procedure as needed.
- ☑ Use Standard Precautions.
- ☑ Remove existing pouch, pulling gently away from skin. Warm water or adhesive solvent may be used to loosen the seal if necessary.
- ☑ Assess the stoma. Report a dark purple, black, or very pale stoma to the physician.
- ☑ Prevent urine flow during cleaning by placing a rolled gauze square or tampon over the stoma opening.
- ☑ Cleanse peristomal skin with soap and water, rinse, and pat or air dry.
- ☑ Use stoma guide to determine the correct size for the bag opening and/or protective ring seal. Trim the bag or seal as needed.
- ☑ Apply the skin barrier; allow to dry.

- ☑ Apply the bag with an opening no more than 1 to 2 mm wider than the stoma; prevent wrinkles or creases in the bag seal.
- ☑ Connect bag to urine-collection device.
- ☑ Chart, including the appearance of the stoma and the response of the client.

SAMPLE DOCUMENTATION

7/20/07 1400	Urinary stoma bag changed. Stoma bright pink and moist. Surrounding skin slightly pink but intact. Protective gel applied. Urine output yellow with mucous shreds noted, not malodorous. _____ _____Lynn Jones, LVN

Note: Refer to a nursing fundamentals or skills text for more detailed instruction. Check state guidelines and facility policy before performing any procedure.

---

from catheters, stents, or drains. Keep the skin clean and dry. *Urine irritates the skin, increasing the risk of breakdown. Meticulous skin care can prevent breakdown.*

- Ensure gravity drainage of urine-collection device or empty bag every 2 hours. Change urine-collection appliance as needed, removing any mucus from stoma. See the checklist in Box 32-17 ■ for care of a urostomy. *Overfilling may damage the seal, allowing leakage and urine contact with skin.*

Disturbed Body Image

- Use active listening and respond to concerns. *Surgical procedures and adjunctive cancer treatments can significantly affect the client's body image. Grieving is a normal response.*
- Encourage the client to look at, touch, and care for the stoma and appliance as soon as possible. Allow to proceed gradually, providing support and encouragement. *A willingness to provide self-care indicates adaptation to the changed body image.*
- Discuss concerns about resuming usual activities, perceived changes in relationships, and sexual relations. Refer to a support group or a person who has successfully adjusted to a urinary diversion. *If a radical cystectomy has been done, the client will no longer be able to bear children, and may experience erectile dysfunction. Clients and families may be reluctant to ask about sexual topics. Support groups allow open discussion of concerns and anxieties.*

EVALUATING

When evaluating the effectiveness of nursing care, collect data regarding urinary output, skin integrity, and the client's and family's acceptance of and ability to care for any urinary diversion or catheters.

Documenting. Document continuing assessments, including the amount, color, clarity, and odor of urine output from all catheters or stomas. Note the client's and family's response to the stoma and teaching about its care if one was created. Document all teaching provided and the understanding of the client and family.

CONTINUING CARE

For many clients, surgery for bladder cancer means a lifelong change in urinary elimination. Prior to discharge, assess the client's and family's knowledge and understanding of the cancer diagnosis and recommended treatment plan. When the tumor has been resected, stress the importance of regular follow-up care and monitoring for tumor recurrence.

Teach the client who has had a urinary diversion to care for the stoma and surrounding skin. Discuss strategies to prevent urine reflux and infection. Teach signs and symptoms of UTIs and renal calculi. If a continent urinary diversion has been created, teach self-catheterization using clean technique.

Stress the importance of follow-up care and of notifying the physician promptly if signs of a complication develop. Refer the client and family to a cancer support group, and, as appropriate, discuss hospice care.

NURSING PROCESS CARE PLAN
Client with Bladder Cancer

Ben Hussain is a 61-year-old man who became alarmed when his urine became bright red. Even though he had no other symptoms, he called his doctor. Urinalysis and cytology showed gross hematuria and abnormal cells. A cystoscopy and biopsy confirmed an invasive bladder tumor. He is admitted to the hospital for a radical cystectomy and ileal diversion.

Assessment. Mr. Hussain's admission history indicates that he has lost 10 to 15 pounds during the last few months. He has smoked two to three packs of cigarettes per day for 40 years, but he cut back to a pack a day about a year ago. Mr. Hussain says he is "a little nervous about surgery and what they're going to find." Ms. Mills, the admitting nurse, notes that he fidgets and talks rapidly throughout their interview. He is concerned about how he will handle the pain after surgery, because he has never been hospitalized before his cystoscopy. Physical assessment findings include BP 154/86; P 84; R 18; T 98.2°F (36.7°C) PO. He has scattered crackles throughout his lung fields. Mr. Hussain's urine is clear and bright pink. The remainder of his assessment is essentially normal.

Diagnosis. The following nursing diagnoses are identified for Mr. Hussain:

- *Anxiety* related to undetermined extent of disease and fear of pain
- *Deficient Knowledge* related to lack of information about ileal diversion
- *Impaired Urinary Elimination* related to cystectomy and ileal diversion
- *Risk for Impaired Gas Exchange* related to smoking history and effects of anesthesia

Expected Outcomes. The expected outcomes of the plan of care for Mr. Hussain are that he will:

- Verbalize a decrease in anxiety.
- Demonstrate ability to manage patient-controlled analgesia (PCA) for postoperative pain control.
- Report pain at a level of 3 or less on a scale of 1 to 10 postoperatively.
- Demonstrate care for his ileostomy stoma, surrounding skin, and collection appliance prior to discharge.

- Maintain urine output with acceptable color and clarity and no signs of infection.
- Maintain adequate gas exchange as evidenced by good skin color, O_2 saturation greater than 95%, and clear lung sounds upon auscultation.

Planning and Implementation. The following nursing interventions are planned and implemented for Mr. Hussain:

- Allow time to answer questions and verbalize fears pre- and postoperatively.
- Provide written as well as verbal explanations as needed.
- Maintain PCA or epidural infusion postoperatively. Monitor effectiveness of pain relief.
- Explain all procedures related to stoma and appliance care as they are being performed.
- Encourage Mr. and Mrs. Hussain to look at the stoma and touch it when ready.
- Teach stoma, skin, and appliance care, emphasizing techniques to prevent skin irritation and urinary tract infection.
- Monitor urine output, color, clarity, and consistency hourly for 24 hours, then every 4 hours for 24 hours, then every 8 hours. Report output less than 30 mL/hr, bright bleeding, and excessively cloudy or malodorous urine.
- Assist to use an incentive spirometer hourly while awake. Ambulate as soon as possible. Assess lung sounds every 4 hours, reporting increased crackles or diminished breath sounds.
- Refer to a local stoma group on discharge.

Evaluation. On discharge, Mr. Hussain has helped clean the stoma and surrounding skin several times. His wife is able to empty the drainage bag and change the appliance, cutting the opening to fit. His urine is pale yellow and slightly cloudy. Mr. Hussain is ambulating independently and using oxycodone (Percocet) twice a day for pain relief. His lungs are clear, and he is very proud of having "survived" 7 days without a cigarette. He says, "Now I'm going to shoot for 7 weeks, then 7 months, then 7 years without a smoke!" A home health referral is made to continue teaching Mr. Hussain to care for his diversion and appliance.

Critical Thinking in the Nursing Process

1. How does cigarette smoking contribute to the increased risk of urinary tract tumors?
2. The first time Mr. Hussain changes his urostomy appliance, he experiences a leak. What hints can you give Mr. Hussain to prevent leaks from occurring?
3. How would you respond if Mr. Hussain said "I'm not only giving up on cigarettes, I'm also giving up on sex from here on"?

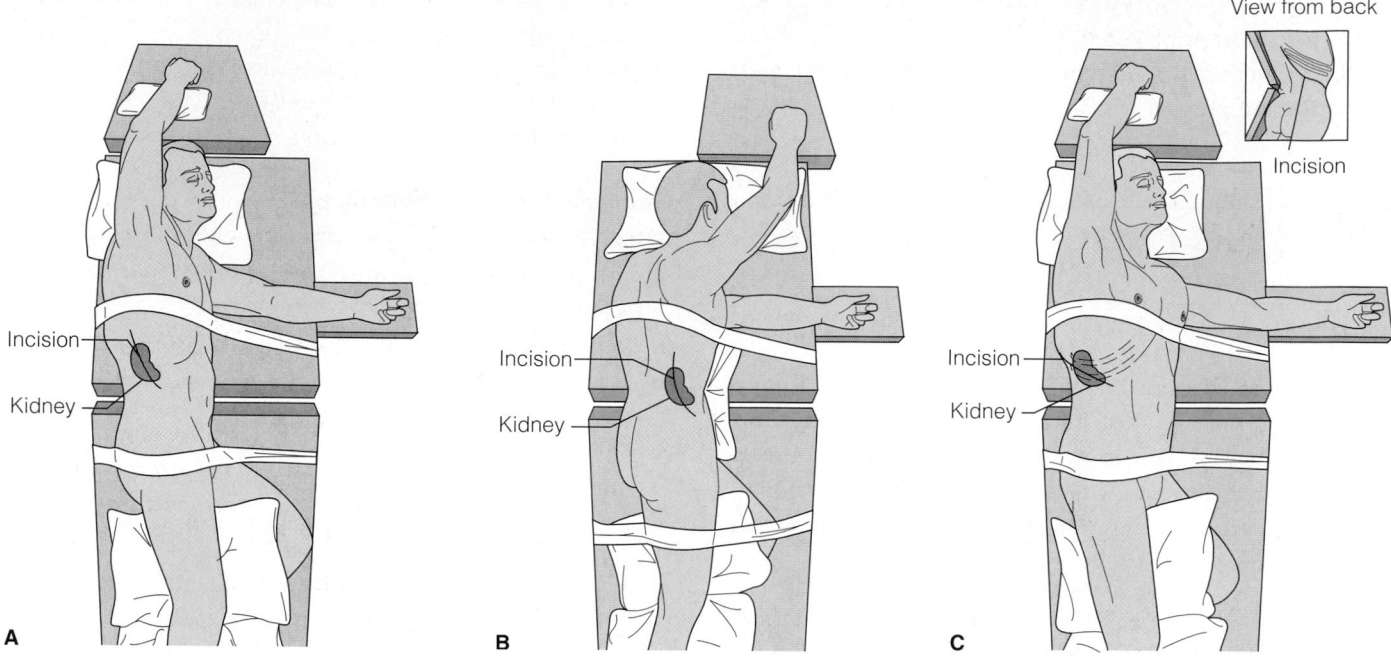

Figure 32-11. ■ Incisions used for kidney surgery. (**A**) flank, (**B**) lumbar, and (**C**) thoracoabdominal.

Kidney Tumors

Primary tumors of the kidney are uncommon. Renal cell carcinoma is the most common primary tumor. The highest incidence occurs in people over age 55. Men are affected twice as often as women. Smoking, obesity, and renal calculi are risk factors. Other primary cancers also may metastasize to the kidney.

PATHOPHYSIOLOGY AND MANIFESTATIONS

Most primary renal tumors arise from tubular epithelium. They can occur anywhere in the kidney, and tend to invade the renal vein. Renal tumors often have metastasized to other organs such as the lungs, bone, lymph nodes, liver, or brain at the time of diagnosis.

Renal cancer is often silent, with few signs or symptoms. Hematuria, often microscopic, is the most consistent manifestation. Other symptoms include flank pain, palpable abdominal mass, fever, fatigue, weight loss, and anemia or polycythemia (elevated RBCs). Renal tumors may produce hormones or other substances that can cause such manifestations as hypercalcemia, hypertension, and hyperglycemia.

INTERDISCIPLINARY CARE

Renal cancer is often diagnosed by a *renal ultrasound* or *computed tomography (CT) scan.* A *kidney biopsy* is done to identify the presence of cancer cells. (Review Box 32-11 for nursing care of the client undergoing a kidney biopsy.)

Radical nephrectomy (removal of the affected kidney and surrounding tissue) is performed if the cancer is limited to the kidney. Although the kidney itself can be removed using laparoscopic surgery, an open technique generally is used. (Figure 32-11 ■ shows common incisions used.) Box 32-18 ■ describes nursing care of a client having kidney surgery. If the cancer has spread beyond the kidney, chemotherapy or radiation therapy may be prescribed (see Chapter 12). ⚭

NURSING CARE

Priorities in Nursing Care. Nursing care priorities for the client with renal cancer include managing postoperative pain, preventing respiratory complications, and preserving renal function of the remaining kidney. Psychologically, the client may experience grieving due to the cancer diagnosis.

Pain

Pain management presents a challenge. Intercostal blocks, patient-controlled analgesia (PCA), or routine analgesic administration can effectively relieve discomfort. Nursing care focuses on assessing and managing pain, and preventing respiratory complications due to pain or fear of pain.

■ Assess frequently for adequate pain relief, using a pain scale and nonverbal signs such as grimacing, tense body position, increased pulse, blood pressure changes, or rapid, shallow respirations. Notify the physician of inadequate

BOX 32-18 NURSING CARE CHECKLIST

Partial or Total Nephrectomy

Before Surgery

☑ Assess understanding and reinforce teaching.

☑ Provide routine preoperative care and teaching as ordered (see Chapter 9). ∞

After Surgery

☑ Provide routine postoperative care as described in Chapter 9. ∞

☑ Assess urine output hourly for the first 24 hours then every 4 to 8 hours.

☑ Label and secure all catheters, stents, nephrostomy tubes, or drains. Irrigate only as ordered by the physician.

☑ Monitor for signs of hemorrhage or infection.

☑ Frequently monitor respiratory status and assist with respiratory care.

☑ Support grieving process and adjustment to the loss of a kidney.

☑ Teach home care:

    a. Maintain fluid intake of 2,000 to 2,500 mL/day.

    b. Gradually increase exercise to tolerance, avoiding heavy lifting for a year after surgery. Avoid contact sports to reduce the risk of injury to the remaining kidney.

    c. Care of the incision and any remaining drainage tubes, catheters, or stents.

    d. Prescribed medications, including their purpose, dose, scheduling, and potential side effects.

    e. Signs and symptoms of UTIs and other complications to report to the physician.

pain relief. *The client may assume that pain is to be expected or may fear becoming addicted to analgesics. Responses to analgesics vary, and the prescribed dose may need to be adjusted.*

■ Assess the incision for inflammation or swelling and drainage catheters and tubes for patency. *An obstructed catheter can lead to complications and increased pain.*

clinical ALERT

Assess for abdominal distention, tenderness, and bowel sounds. Intra-abdominal bleeding, infection, or paralytic ileus can cause pain that may be confused with incisional pain.

■ Use adjunctive pain relief measures such as positioning, diversion, and relaxation techniques. *These can enhance the effects of analgesia.*

Ineffective Breathing Pattern

■ Place in semi-Fowler's position and side-lying positions as allowed and tolerated. *Lung expansion is improved in semi-Fowler's and Fowler's positions.*

clinical ALERT

Assess respiratory status frequently, including rate and depth, cough, breath sounds, oxygen saturation, and temperature. Pneumothorax or atelectasis on the operative side are common.

■ Change position frequently, ambulate as soon as possible. *These measures promote ventilation and airway clearance.*

■ Encourage frequent (every 1 to 2 hours) deep breathing, spirometer use, and coughing. Assist to splint the incision. *These measures promote alveolar ventilation, gas exchange, and airway clearance.*

Risk for Impaired Urinary Elimination

■ Monitor vital signs, CVP, and urine output every 1 to 2 hours initially, then every 4 hours. *Hypovolemia and low blood pressure reduce blood flow to the kidney and increase the risk of acute renal failure.*

■ Frequently assess the amount and nature of drainage on surgical dressings and from drainage tubes, stents, and catheters. Measure and record output from each drain or catheter separately. *Frequent and accurate assessment of drainage helps to identify potential surgical complications.*

clinical ALERT

Prevent kinking, twisting, or tension on drains and tubes. Do not clamp. Irrigate carefully and only with a physician's order. Notify the physician or charge nurse immediately if any tube becomes obstructed or dislodged.

■ Maintain fluid intake of 2,000 to 2,500 mL/day. *A liberal fluid intake prevents dehydration and promotes good urinary output.*

■ Use strict aseptic technique in caring for all urinary catheters, tubes, stents, drains, and incisions. *Asepsis is vital to prevent infection of the remaining kidney.*

■ Following catheter removal, assess frequently for urinary retention. Notify the physician if the client is unable to void within 4 to 6 hours or if the client complains of a feeling of fullness or discomfort. *Maintenance of urine output is vital to prevent possible complications such as infection and hydronephrosis.*

■ Monitor laboratory results, including urinalysis, BUN, serum creatinine, and serum electrolytes. Report abnormal findings to the physician. *Abnormal values may indicate early acute renal failure; prompt intervention is necessary to preserve renal function.*

Anticipatory Grieving

- Listen actively, encouraging the client and family to express fears and concerns. *Expression of fears helps the client and family begin to deal more effectively with them.*
- Demonstrate respect for cultural, spiritual, and religious values and beliefs; encourage use of these resources to cope with losses. *Value and belief systems can provide a structure and form for dealing with the grieving process.*
- Refer to cancer support groups, social services, or counseling as appropriate. *Support groups and counseling services provide additional resources for coping.*

CONTINUING CARE

If renal cancer was detected at an early stage and cure is anticipated, teaching for home care focuses on protecting the remaining kidney. Emphasize the need to maintain a generous fluid intake of 2,000 to 2,500 mL/day, increasing fluid intake during hot weather and when exercising. Stress measures to prevent UTIs, such as urinating when the urge is perceived, hygiene, and voiding before and after sexual intercourse. Discuss manifestations of UTIs that should promptly be reported to the physician. With men, discuss the important of regular screening for an enlarged prostate after ages 45 to 50. Encourage the client to avoid contact sports such as football or hockey and use measures to prevent motor vehicle crashes and falls, which could damage the remaining kidney.

RENAL FAILURE

Renal failure is a condition in which the kidneys are unable to remove accumulated waste products from the blood. Renal failure may be acute or chronic. It is characterized by azotemia (a buildup of nitrogenous waste products in the blood), and leads to fluid, electrolyte, and acid–base imbalances.

Acute Renal Failure

Acute renal failure (ARF) is a rapid decline in renal function with an abrupt onset. It is often reversible with prompt treatment. It is relatively common, affecting at least 10,000 people in the United States every year. Major trauma or surgery, infection, hemorrhage, severe heart failure, and lower urinary tract obstruction are risk factors. *Iatrogenic* causes of ARF include nephrotoxic medications and contrast dye used in x-rays. Older adults are at particular risk.

PATHOPHYSIOLOGY

The most common causes of ARF are *ischemia* (poor perfusion) of the kidney and **nephrotoxins** (agents that damage

the kidney tissue). Causes of ARF can be classified as prerenal, intrarenal, and postrenal (Table 32-5 ■).

Hypovolemia is a common *prerenal* cause of ARF. It is readily reversible if promptly recognized and treated with measures to restore blood volume. If it is not, it can lead to acute tubular necrosis and intrarenal ARF. *Intrarenal* failure results from acute damage to the nephrons by inflammation (e.g., acute glomerulonephritis), by vascular disorders (such as severe hypertension), or by exposure to nephrotoxins (Figure 32-12 ■). The risk for *acute tubular necrosis (ATN)* is particularly high when ischemia and exposure to a nephrotoxin occur at the same time. Obstruction of urine outflow can lead to *postrenal* ARF.

MANIFESTATIONS

Acute renal failure is generally identified by *oliguria* (urine output < 400 mL/day) and rising BUN or serum creatinine levels. The GFR falls, tubular cells become necrotic and slough, and the nephron is unable to eliminate wastes

TABLE 32-5

Causes of Acute Renal Failure

CATEGORY	CAUSE	EXAMPLES
Prerenal failure	Impaired blood supply to kidney	Fluid volume deficit, hemorrhage, heart failure, shock
Intrarenal failure	Acute damage to renal tissue and nephrons or *acute tubular necrosis (ATN)*: abrupt decline in tubular and glomerular function due to either prolonged ischemia and/or exposure to nephrotoxins	Acute glomerulonephritis, malignant hypertension, ischemia; nephrotoxic drugs or substances; red blood cell destruction (e.g., hemolytic transfusion reaction); muscle tissue breakdown due to trauma, heatstroke
Postrenal failure	Obstruction of urine outflow	Urethral obstruction by enlarged prostate or tumor; ureteral or kidney pelvis obstruction by calculi

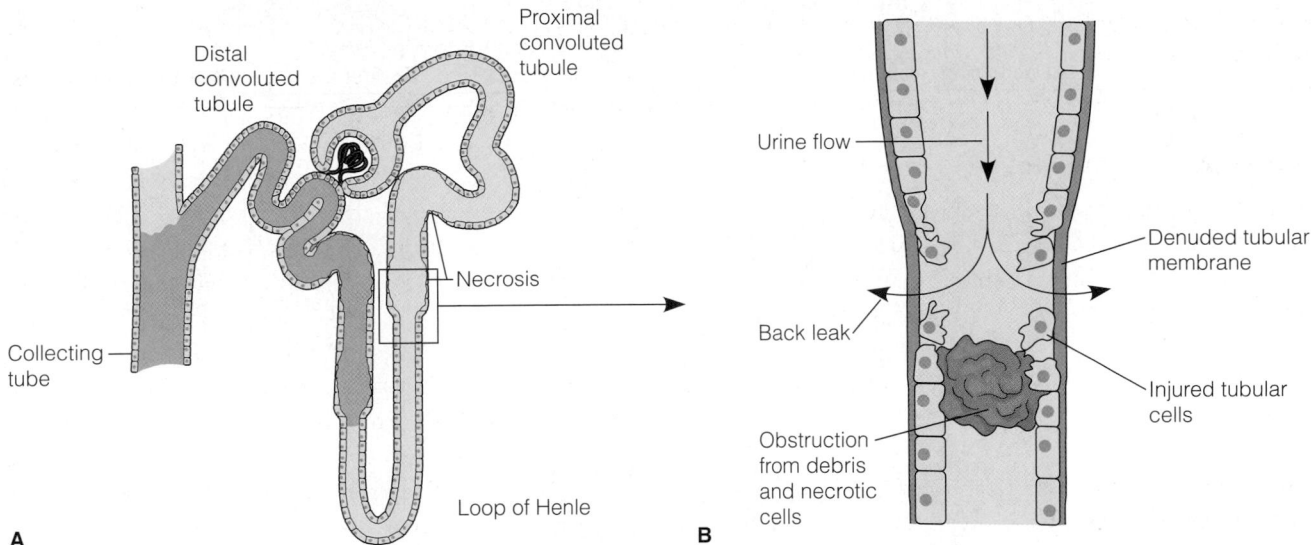

Figure 32-12. ■ **(A)** In acute tubular necrosis, tubular epithelium is damaged by hypotension and shock or by a toxin. **(B)** As a result, the flow of glomerular filtrate is blocked, and increased pressure in the tubule causes glomerular filtration to slow. The elimination of salt, water, and waste products is impaired.

effectively (Figure 32-12). The course of acute renal failure includes three phases: initiation, maintenance, and recovery.

1. The *initiation phase* begins with the initiating event and often is recognized only after the client has moved into the maintenance phase.
2. The *maintenance phase* of ARF begins within hours of the initiating event and typically lasts 1 to 2 weeks. Oliguria develops and the kidney cannot efficiently eliminate metabolic wastes, water, electrolytes, and acids. Azotemia can cause confusion and disorientation. Salt and water retention lead to fluid volume excess and edema. Hypertension and heart failure may develop. Hyperkalemia causes muscle weakness, nausea and diarrhea, and dysrhythmias. Metabolic acidosis results from inadequate elimination of hydrogen ions by the kidneys. In this phase, anemia may develop and immune function is impaired, increasing the risk for infections. Toward the end of the maintenance phase, urine output gradually increases, but the serum creatinine and BUN remain high.
3. The *recovery phase* of ARF is characterized by improving kidney function, urine output, and blood values. It lasts for up to 1 year.

Chronic Renal Failure

Chronic renal failure (CRF) is a slow, insidious process of kidney destruction. It may go unrecognized for years as nephrons are destroyed and renal mass is reduced. When the kidneys have too few nephrons to excrete metabolic wastes and regulate fluid and electrolyte balance adequately, the client is said to have *end-stage renal disease (ESRD)*, the final stage of CRF.

End-stage renal disease is increasing in incidence in all age groups, with a particularly sharp increase in people over age 70. The incidence of ESRD is highest in African Americans, followed by Native Americans, Asians, and European Americans. Diabetic nephropathy and hypertension are the leading causes of chronic renal failure in the United States. Among African Americans, hypertension is the leading cause.

PATHOPHYSIOLOGY

As nephrons are destroyed by the disease process, remaining nephrons hypertrophy to compensate for the lost renal mass. The increased demand on these nephrons increases their risk for destruction.

Chronic renal failure progresses over months to many years. In the early stage of *decreased renal reserve*, unaffected nephrons do the work of the lost nephrons, and the client remains free of symptoms. As kidney function is further reduced, BUN and serum creatinine levels begin to rise, and manifestations of *renal insufficiency* may be seen. Any further insult to the kidneys at this stage (infection, exposure to nephrotoxins) can precipitate *end-stage renal failure.* At this stage the GFR is less than 20% of normal, and serum creatinine and BUN levels rise sharply (Figure 32-13 ■). At this stage, **uremia** (which literally means "urine in the blood") develops.

MANIFESTATIONS

Chronic renal failure often is not identified until uremia develops. Early manifestations of uremia include nausea, apathy, weakness, and fatigue. As it progresses, the client may experience frequent vomiting, increasing weakness, lethargy, and confusion. The multisystem effects of uremia are illustrated in Figure 32-14 ■.

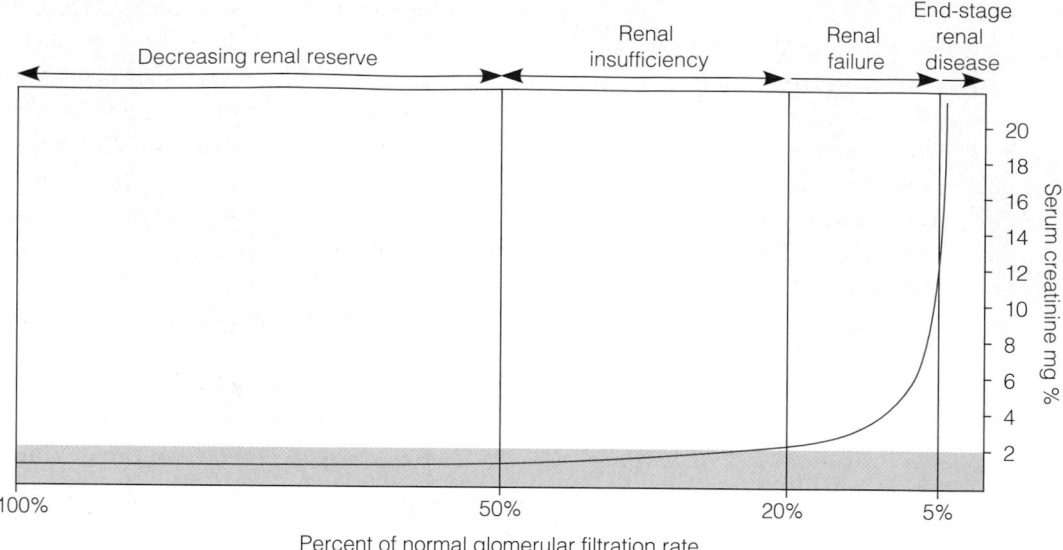

Figure 32-13. ■ The relationship of renal function to BUN and serum creatinine in the course of chronic renal failure.

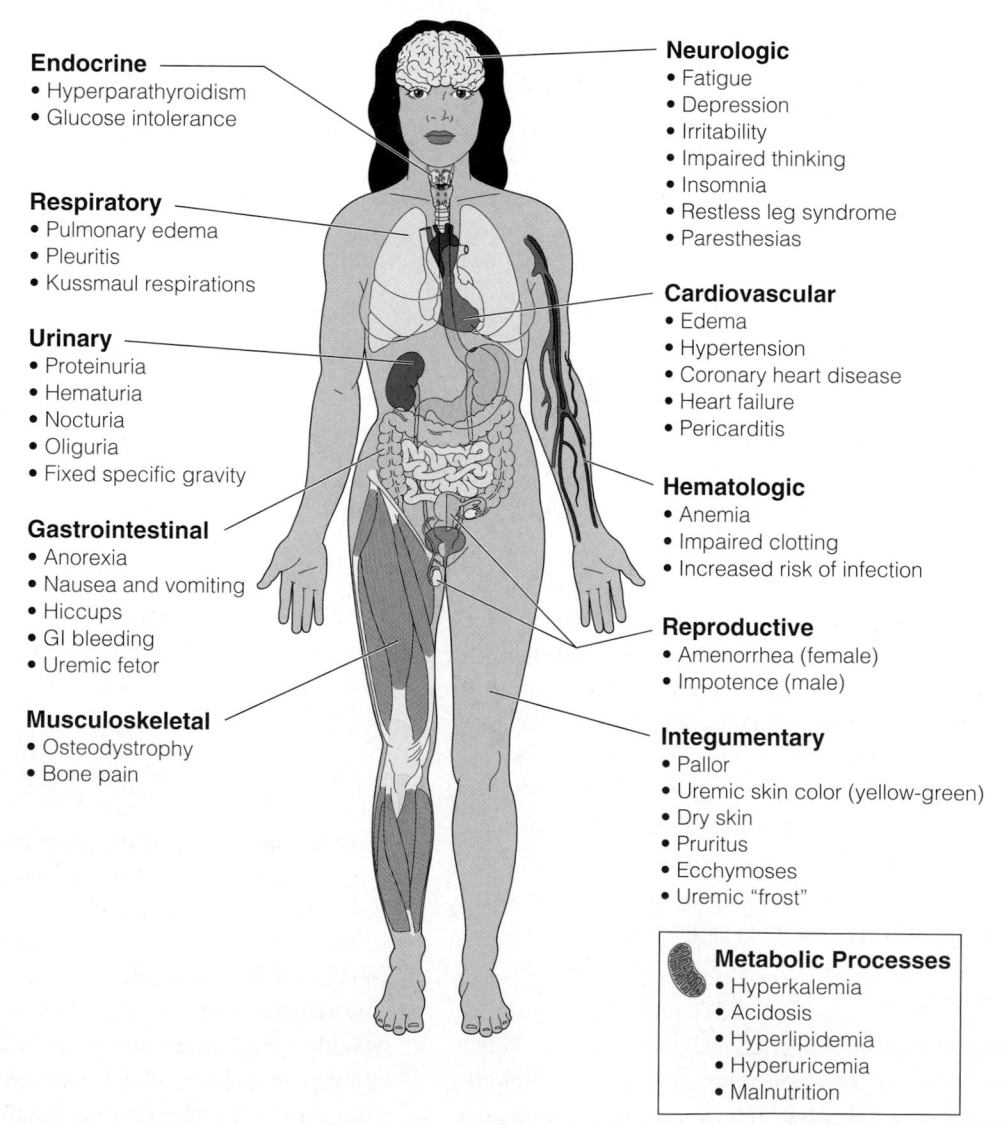

Figure 32-14. ■ The multisystem effects of uremia.

INTERDISCIPLINARY CARE

Preventing acute renal failure is a goal in the care of all clients, especially for those in high-risk groups. Maintaining blood volume, cardiac output, and blood pressure is vital to preserve kidney perfusion. Nephrotoxic drugs are avoided if possible. When a nephrotoxic drug must be used, keeping the client well hydrated and avoiding additional nephrotoxins help reduce the risk of renal failure. Care for the client with chronic renal failure focuses on eliminating factors that may further decrease renal function and on slowing the progress of the disease to ESRD.

Diagnostic Tests

- *Serum creatinine* and *BUN* are monitored to evaluate the disease progress and its treatment.
- *Creatinine clearance* is monitored to evaluate GFR and renal function. (See Table 31-4 ◯◐ for normal values.)
- *Serum electrolytes, arterial blood gases,* and *CBC* also are frequently monitored.
- *Urinalysis* may show a fixed specific gravity at 1.010, and abnormal substances such as protein, blood cells, and cell casts. *Casts* are protein and cellular debris molded in the shape of the tubular lumen.
- A *kidney biopsy* may be done to identify the underlying disease process (see Box 32-11).

Diet and Fluid Management

When the kidneys cannot effectively regulate fluid and electrolyte balance and eliminate metabolic waste products, intake of these substances must be regulated. Fluid and sodium intake are restricted. The daily fluid intake is calculated by allowing 500 mL for insensible losses (respiration, perspiration, bowel losses) and adding the amount of urine output (or lost in emesis or diarrhea) during the previous 24 hours. For example, if the client has 325 mL of urine output, intake for the next day is restricted to 825 mL, including both oral and intravenous fluids. Accurate weights and I&O records are essential. Clients with chronic renal failure should notify the physician of any weight gain of more than 5 pounds (2 to 2.5 kg) over a 2-day period. Sodium and potassium intake are regulated. Salt substitutes containing potassium are avoided.

The client with renal failure needs adequate nutrients and calories to prevent tissue breakdown. Proteins are limited to minimize azotemia and should be complete proteins (i.e., meat, fish, poultry, cheese, eggs, milk, or soy). Carbohydrates are increased to maintain adequate calorie intake. Total parenteral nutrition may be ordered if the client is unable to eat.

Medications

The fact that most medications are excreted by the kidney is a major consideration in treating clients with renal failure.

All nephrotoxic drugs (such as NSAIDs) are avoided or used with extreme caution. Drug dosages may be adjusted because excretion is slowed and half-life is prolonged.

Diuretics such as furosemide (Lasix) may be ordered to reduce fluid volume, lower blood pressure, and lower serum potassium levels. Other antihypertensive drugs such as ACE inhibitors are prescribed to maintain the blood pressure within normal levels.

Sodium bicarbonate or calcium carbonate may be used to manage the electrolyte imbalances and acidosis accompanying renal failure. When serum potassium levels are dangerously high, a potassium-binding exchange resin such as sodium polystyrene sulfonate (Kayexalate, SPS Suspension) may be ordered by oral or rectal route. Intravenous insulin and glucose also may be given to lower serum potassium levels.

Folic acid and iron supplements are used to combat anemia. A multiple-vitamin preparation is also often prescribed, because anorexia, nausea, and dietary restrictions may limit nutrient intake.

Renal Replacement Therapies

When conservative management is no longer effective to maintain fluid and electrolyte balance and prevent uremia, dialysis or kidney transplant is considered.

Dialysis is diffusion of solutes across a semipermeable membrane from an area of higher concentration to one of lower concentration. In dialysis, a semipermeable membrane separates the blood from an isotonic dialyzing solution. Water and solutes such as urea, creatinine, and electrolytes diffuse across this membrane, but proteins do not. Dialysis compensates for the kidneys' inability to eliminate excess water and solutes.

The decision to start dialysis is not an easy one. Like insulin therapy for a diabetic, dialysis manages symptoms but does not cure the disease. Dialysis requires a daily commitment. Clients on dialysis may have difficulty maintaining employment. Many families fall apart with the day-to-day stress. Even with dialysis, clients may have constant flulike symptoms and feel controlled by their illness. In the end, clients may choose to discontinue treatment, preferring death over continued dialysis.

HEMODIALYSIS. In *hemodialysis,* electrolytes, waste products, and excess water are removed from the body by diffusion and filtration (see Chapter 7). ◯◐ The client's blood is pumped to a dialyzing membrane unit (Figure 32-15 ■), where it moves past a semipermeable membrane. *Dialysate* (a solution similar to normal extracellular fluid) is warmed to body temperature and passed along the other side of the membrane. Solutes (electrolytes and waste products) diffuse through the membrane into the dialysate. Medications can be added to the dialysate to diffuse into the blood. Excess

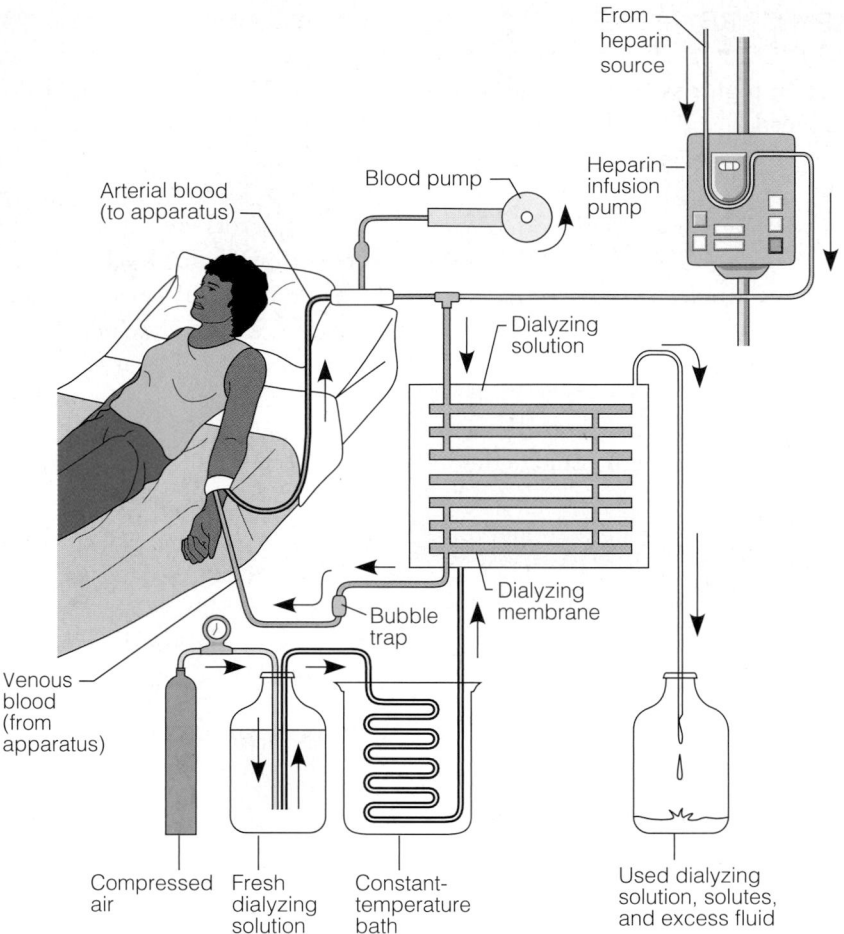

Figure 32-15. ■ A hemodialysis system.

water is removed from the blood by creating a higher fluid pressure on the blood side of the membrane. Clients typically undergo two or three sessions of hemodialysis per week for a total of 9 to 12 hours. Hemodialysis can be done at home but usually occurs in an outpatient dialysis center.

An arteriovenous (AV) fistula (Figure 32-16 ■) is commonly created for vascular access. Often the radial artery and

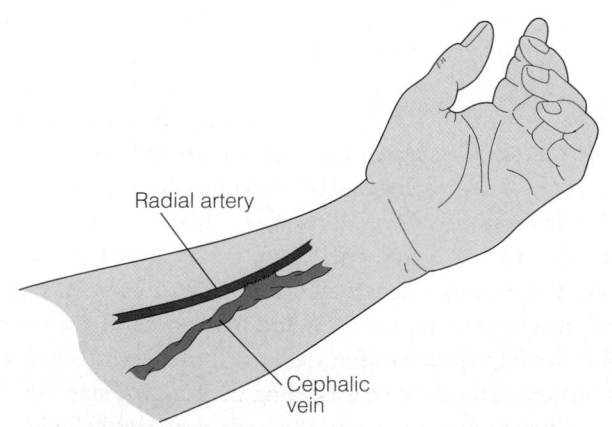

Figure 32-16. ■ An arteriovenous fistula.

cephalic vein are joined. A functional AV fistula has a palpable pulsation and a *bruit* (audible murmur) on auscultation. Some clients may have an arteriovenous graft for vascular access. Rarely, an arteriovenous shunt may be used. Box 32-19 ■ outlines nursing care for the client undergoing hemodialysis.

clinical ALERT

Do not take blood pressures or allow blood draws or IV starts on the nondominant arm of clients in renal failure, to avoid damaging blood vessels. If a fistula is in place, avoid taking blood pressures or doing venipunctures on the arm with the fistula.

Clients on hemodialysis may experience both systemic and fistula complications. Hypotension is the most frequent complication occurring during hemodialysis. Bleeding may occur due to altered clotting and the use of heparin during dialysis. Infection is a significant risk. Dialysis dementia is a progressive, potentially fatal neurologic complication that may affect clients on long-term hemodialysis.

BOX 32-19   NURSING CARE CHECKLIST

Hemodialysis

Before Dialysis

☑ Use Standard Precautions at all times.

☑ Document vital signs, including orthostatic blood pressures (lying and sitting), apical pulse, and respirations and also lung sounds and weight.

☑ Assess vascular access site for a palpable pulsation or vibration (*thrill*), an audible bruit, and signs of inflammation.

☑ Alert all personnel to avoid using the arm with the vascular access site (or the nondominant arm if a site has not yet been established) for blood pressure or venipuncture.

After Dialysis

☑ Document vital signs, weight, and vascular access site assessment. Monitor for orthostatic hypotension, tachycardia, and weight loss.

☑ Monitor BUN, serum creatinine, serum electrolytes, and hematocrit.

☑ Report possible adverse effects of dialysis such as muscle cramping, headache, nausea and vomiting, altered level of consciousness, seizures, or hypertension.

☑ Assess for bleeding at the access site or elsewhere.

☑ If a transfusion was given during dialysis, report manifestations of transfusion reaction, such as chills and fever; dyspnea; chest, back, or arm pain; and urticaria or itching.

☑ Provide psychologic support; listen actively for feelings of grief, hopelessness, or anger.

☑ Refer for social services and counseling as indicated.

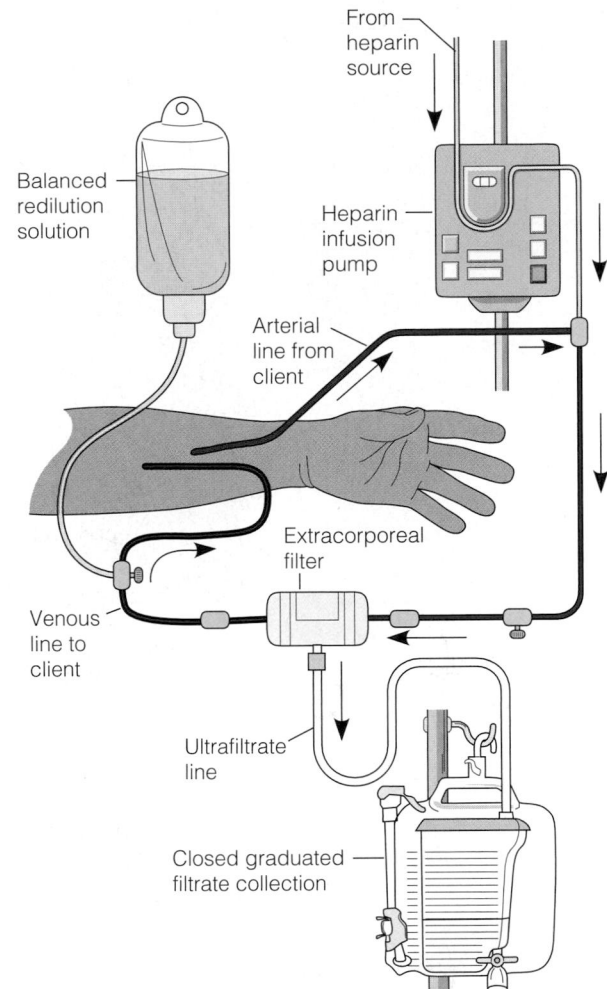

Figure 32-17. ■ Continuous renal replacement therapy (CRRT) from an artery to a vein.

AV fistula problems include infection and clotting or thrombosis. These complications may cause fistula failure and require development of a new site. AV fistula failure can have a psychologic impact, resulting in depression and an altered self-concept.

CONTINUOUS RENAL REPLACEMENT THERAPY. *Continuous renal replacement therapy (CRRT)* allows more gradual fluid and solute removal. CRRT may be used for clients whose condition is unstable. Blood is continuously circulated (artery to vein or vein to vein) and filtered, allowing excess water and solutes to drain into a collection device. Fluid may be replaced with a balanced electrolyte solution as needed during treatment (Figure 32-17 ■). The slower process of CRRT reduces the adverse effects associated with hemodialysis but may require prolonged immobilization.

PERITONEAL DIALYSIS. In *peritoneal dialysis,* the highly vascular peritoneum serves as the dialyzing membrane. Warmed dialysate is instilled into the peritoneal cavity through a peritoneal catheter (Figure 32-18 ■). Metabolic waste products and electrolytes diffuse into the dialysate while it remains in the abdomen. Excess water is drawn into the dialysate by osmosis. The fluid is then drained by gravity out of the peritoneal cavity into a sterile bag. Peritoneal dialysis is significantly less costly than hemodialysis, but is used by fewer people with renal failure in the United States.

Continuous ambulatory peritoneal dialysis (CAPD) is the most common form of peritoneal dialysis used today. Two liters of dialysate are instilled into the peritoneal cavity, and the catheter is sealed. The client can then continue normal daily activities, emptying the peritoneal cavity and replacing the dialysate every 4 to 6 hours. No special equipment is needed. A variation of CAPD is *continuous cyclic peritoneal dialysis (CCPD).* CCPD uses a delivery device during nighttime hours and a continuous dwell during the day. CAPD can be performed anywhere, and CCPD allows for home treatment at night, leaving the client free during the day. See Box 32-20 ■ for nursing care of the client having peritoneal dialysis.

Peritoneal dialysis is less likely to cause rapid fluid and electrolyte shifts than hemodialysis, but it is less efficient in

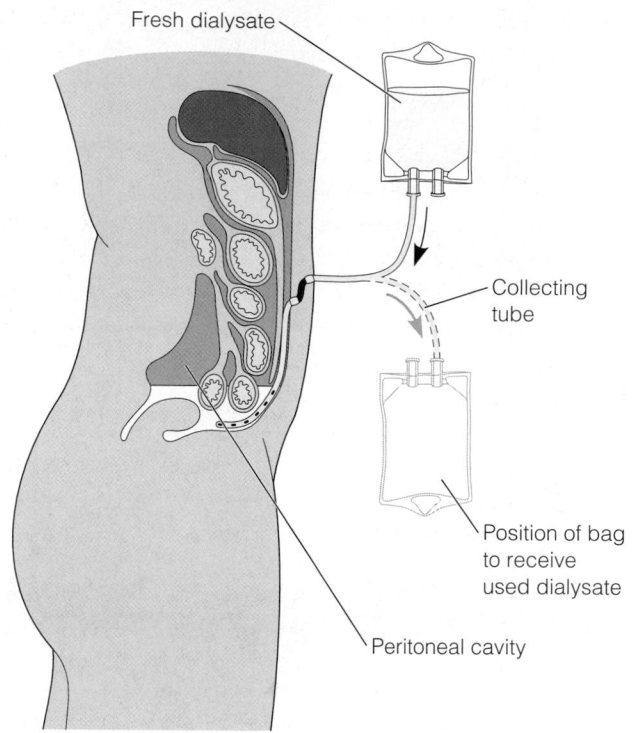

Figure 32-18. ■ Peritoneal dialysis.

Fresh dialysate

Collecting tube

Position of bag to receive used dialysate

Peritoneal cavity

removing waste products. It does not require vascular access, but it places the client at risk for developing peritonitis. The indwelling peritoneal catheter also may cause a body image disturbance.

Kidney Transplant

Kidney transplant, implanting a functioning kidney, is the treatment of choice for many clients with end-stage renal disease. The client is no longer tied to a dialysis catheter, machine, or center. Dietary and fluid restrictions are reduced, and the body image is one of increased "wholeness."

About 30% of transplanted kidneys in the United States are from living related donors. The rest are from cadavers. Living relatives with normal kidneys who are in good physical health and have the same ABO blood group as the recipient may serve as donors. Predonation counseling is essential because of the risks involved. Cadaver kidneys are obtained from people who meet the criteria for brain death, are less than 65 years old, and are free of systemic disease, malignancy, or infection, including HIV and hepatitis B or C. Kidneys are removed before or immediately after cardiac arrest and are preserved by hypothermia or continuous perfusion until they are implanted.

BOX 32-20   **NURSING CARE CHECKLIST**

Peritoneal Dialysis

Before Dialysis

☑ Use Standard Precautions at all times.

☑ Document vital signs, including temperature, orthostatic blood pressures (lying and standing), apical pulse, and respirations and also lung sounds.

☑ Weigh daily or between dialysis runs as indicated.

☑ Measure and record abdominal girth.

☑ Ask the client to urinate prior to peritoneal catheter insertion.

☑ Warm prescribed dialysate solution to body temperature (98.6°F or 37°C) using a warm water bath or heating pad on low setting.

☑ Explain all procedures and expected sensations.

During Dialysis

☑ Use aseptic technique during dialysis and when caring for the peritoneal catheter.

☑ Prime dialysis tubing with solution and connect it to the peritoneal catheter, avoiding kinks. Clamp drainage tubing.

☑ With the client sitting or in Fowler's position, instill dialysate into peritoneal cavity over approximately 10 minutes. Clamp tubing and allow the solution to remain in the abdomen for the prescribed dwell period.

☑ During instillation and the dwell time, observe for dyspnea, tachypnea, or other signs of respiratory distress.

☑ After the prescribed dwell time, open drainage tubing clamps and allow dialysate to drain by gravity into a sterile container. Observe solution for clarity and any evidence of blood, feces, odor, or cloudiness. Promptly report abnormal findings to the charge nurse or physician.

☑ Accurately record amount and type of solution instilled, including any added medications, the dwell time, and amount and character of the drainage.

☑ Monitor laboratory values, including BUN, serum creatinine, and serum electrolytes.

☑ Trouble-shoot for possible problems during dialysis:
   a. Slow instillation of dialysate: Raise the container and reposition the client. Check tubing and catheter for kinks. Check abdominal dressing for wetness, indicating leakage around the catheter.
   b. Excess dwell time.
   c. Poor dialysate drainage. Lower the bag; reposition the client, and check tubing for kinks.

After Dialysis

☑ Record vital signs, including temperature. Report significant changes from baseline.

☑ Time meals to correspond with solution drainage.

☑ Maintain fluid and dietary restrictions as ordered.

☑ Teach peritoneal dialysis procedure as indicated.

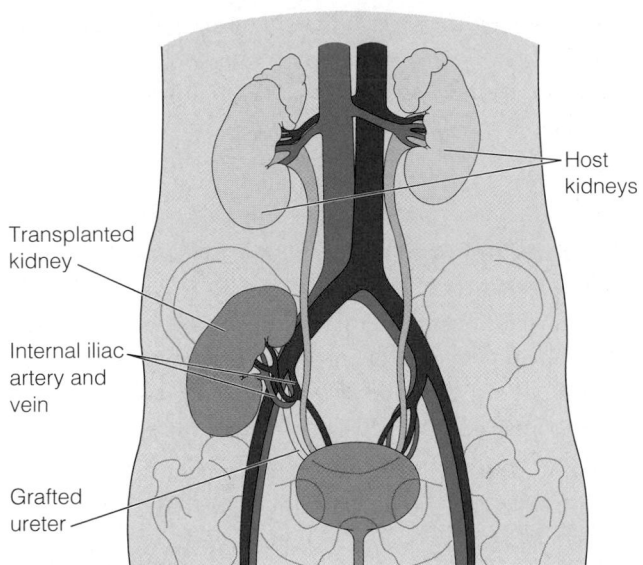

Host kidneys

Transplanted kidney

Internal iliac artery and vein

Grafted ureter

Figure 32-19. ■ Placement of a transplanted kidney.

The donor kidney is usually placed in the lower abdominal cavity of the recipient (Figure 32-19 ■). It is connected to arterial and venous blood supplies, and its ureter is connected to one of the recipient's ureters or directly to the bladder, using a tunnel technique to prevent reflux. Review Box 32-18 for nursing care for a living kidney donor. Box 32-21 ■ provides nursing care for the kidney recipient.

Unless the donor and recipient are identical twins, the transplanted organ stimulates a normal immune response to reject it. Drugs are given to suppress the immune system and the inflammatory response. Clients receiving immunosuppressive drugs have an increased risk of infections. Tumors may develop. Infants born to mothers undergoing immunosuppressive therapy have a higher risk of congenital defects. Corticosteroid use may lead to bone problems, peptic ulcer disease, and cataracts. (See nursing care of clients with altered immunity in Chapter 11. ∞) Even with immunosuppressive drugs, the transplanted kidney can be rejected at any time. Manifestations of rejection include a drop in urine output, increasing BUN and serum creatinine, and a fall in creatinine clearance. The client may develop a fever, swelling and tenderness at the graft site.

NURSING CARE

ASSESSING

Nurses caring for clients at risk for developing renal failure collect data related to the cardiovascular system and kidney perfusion, as well as data related to urinary function.

Subjective Data. Collect information about current symptoms, including urine output (color, quantity, any difficulty initiating urine flow or emptying the bladder completely).

BOX 32-21 **NURSING CARE CHECKLIST**

Kidney Transplant

Before Surgery

☑ Assess knowledge and reinforce teaching. Discuss concerns about surgery, the organ donor, and possible complications.

☑ Provide routine preoperative care as outlined in Chapter 9. ∞

After Surgery

☑ Provide routine postoperative care as outlined in Chapter 9. ∞

☑ Record urine output every 30 to 60 minutes initially. Maintain closed urinary drainage system.

☑ Closely monitor vital signs, arterial pressure, and hemodynamic pressures as ordered.

☑ Maintain intravenous fluids as ordered.

☑ Administer diuretics as ordered.

☑ Remove urinary catheter within 2 to 3 days or as ordered. Encourage voiding every 1 to 2 hours and assess frequently for urinary retention following catheter removal.

☑ Monitor serum electrolytes and renal function tests.

☑ Monitor for possible complications:
   a. Hemorrhage, as indicated by swelling at the operative site, increased abdominal girth, and changes in vital signs and level of consciousness.
   b. Urine leakage into the peritoneal cavity, as indicated by abdominal swelling and tenderness, and decreased urine output.
   c. Renal artery thrombosis, indicated by the abrupt onset of hypertension and a fall in GFR.
   d. Infection, indicated by possible fever, change in level of consciousness, cloudy or malodorous urine, or purulent drainage from the incision.
   e. Rejection, as indicated by fever, swelling and tenderness over the graft site, decreased urine output, and declining renal function.

☑ Reinforce teaching, including medications and potential side effects, vital sign and weight monitoring, signs of organ rejection, and any prescribed diet changes.

☑ Provide psychologic support; address concerns and provide information as needed.

Ask about recent weight changes and any noticeable swelling of the face, hands, legs, or ankles, as well as other symptoms such as nausea or vomiting. Obtain the client's medical history, including current or previous kidney problems, chronic diseases such as diabetes or lupus, recent surgery or diagnostic tests, and current or recent medications.

Objective Data. Vital signs, current weight, and intake and output (if known); level of consciousness and mental status; skin color, temperature, and moisture, and presence of any edema; auscultate heart, lung, and bowel sounds. Obtain a urine specimen for analysis, noting the color, clarity, character of the urine, and its specific gravity.

DIAGNOSING, PLANNING, AND IMPLEMENTING

Priorities in Nursing Care. The priority for nursing care is on preserving renal function to the extent possible and managing the effects of impaired output of fluids and waste products.

Excess Fluid Volume

■ Maintain accurate I&O records. *Accurate I&O records help determine treatment, especially fluid restriction. Hourly urine output measurements may be required in acute renal failure.*

■ Weigh daily or as ordered. Use consistent technique and timing to ensure accuracy. *Weight often provides a more accurate assessment of fluid volume than intake and output records, particularly in oliguric clients.*

■ Document vital signs at least every 4 hours. *Changes in vital signs may indicate either fluid volume excess or deficit. Hypertension can further damage the kidneys.*

■ Frequently assess heart and breath sounds. Assess the degree of peripheral edema and neck vein distention. *Excess fluid volume increases the risk for heart failure and pulmonary edema. An S_3 or S_4 gallop rhythm or crackles in the lungs may indicate heart failure and should be reported to the charge nurse or physician.*

■ Unless contraindicated, place in Fowler's position. *Fowler's position facilitates breathing and lung expansion and reduces the workload of the heart.*

■ Restrict fluids as ordered. Provide frequent mouth care and encourage using hard candies to decrease the thirst response. If ice chips are used to relieve thirst, include as intake (generally calculated as half of an equivalent volume of fluid; an 8-oz or 240-mL container of ice chips yields 120 mL of water). *Fluid restriction helps minimize fluid retention and the complications of fluid volume excess, especially in the client being managed without dialysis.*

■ Administer medications with meals. *This reduces total liquid consumed.*

■ Turn frequently and provide good skin care. *Edema can lead to skin breakdown, especially in the older or debilitated client.*

■ Administer diuretics as ordered and monitor response. *Diuretics may promote urination.*

■ Monitor serum electrolytes and for manifestations of imbalances. Report abnormal results. *Electrolyte imbalances may develop because of water retention and impaired renal function.*

Imbalanced Nutrition: Less than Body Requirements

The manifestations of uremia and dietary restrictions often affect food intake. The client may not eat enough to meet metabolic needs. *Catabolism* (breakdown of body proteins to meet energy needs) worsens azotemia and uremia.

■ Monitor and document food intake, including the amount and type of food consumed. *Food intake records help determine the adequacy of nutritional intake and identify the need for nutritional supplements.*

■ Administer antiemetic drugs 30 to 60 minutes before eating. *Anorexia, nausea, and vomiting are common. Antiemetics reduce nausea and the risk of vomiting with food intake.*

■ Provide mouth care just prior to meals. *The client may have a metallic taste and bad breath. Mouth care improves taste and stimulates the appetite.*

■ Provide frequent, small meals or between-meal snacks. *These measures promote food intake in the fatigued or anorectic client.*

■ Arrange for a dietary consultation. Provide preferred foods to the extent possible, and involve the client in planning menus. Allow family to prepare meals within dietary restrictions and encourage family members to eat with the client. *The client is more likely to eat favorite foods. Involving the client in planning promotes a sense of control and learning about dietary restrictions. Familiar foods and social interaction encourage eating and heighten the client's enjoyment of meals.*

■ Monitor serum electrolytes and albumin. *Changes in values may indicate either improving or declining nutritional status.*

■ Administer and monitor parenteral nutrition as ordered. *Parenteral nutrition may be necessary to prevent catabolism and increasing azotemia in the client with renal failure. Remember that intravenous lines and parenteral nutrition increase the risk for infection. Monitor sites carefully for signs of infection or inflammation.*

Risk for Infection

Renal failure affects immune function, increasing the risk for infection. Invasive treatments and catheters further increase this risk.

■ Use Standard Precautions and good hand washing at all times. *Hand washing and Standard Precautions help prevent spread of infection to and from the client. Clients on hemodialysis have an increased risk of hepatitis B, hepatitis C, and HIV infection.*

- Use strict aseptic technique when handling ports, catheters, and incisions. *Aseptic technique is vital to reduce the risk of introducing an infectious organism.*
- Monitor temperature and vital signs at least every 4 hours. *An elevated temperature or increased pulse rate may indicate infection.*
- Monitor WBC count and differential. *High or low WBC counts may indicate an infection. Increasing numbers of immature WBCs in circulation also may indicate infection.*
- Culture urine, peritoneal dialysis fluid, and other drainage as indicated. *Culture is used to determine the presence of pathogens.*
- Turn or ambulate frequently; encourage coughing and deep breathing. *These measures decrease the risk of respiratory infection.*
- Restrict visits from obviously ill family members. Teach the client and family how to reduce the spread of infection. *The client and family need to know and understand how to reduce the risk of infection at home and in the community.*

Disturbed Body Image

- Involve the client in decision making and encourage self-care. *Client involvement increases autonomy, improves acceptance, and promotes independence.*
- Encourage expression of feelings and concerns. Accept perceptions and feelings without criticism. *Self-expression enhances the client's self-worth and acceptance.*
- Work with the client to develop and achieve realistic goals. Provide positive reinforcement and feedback. Support positive gains. *Adapting to a change in body image and self-concept requires time and often occurs in a series of small steps. Realistic goals allow the client to see progress. Reinforcement helps develop positive coping strategies.*
- Encourage contact with a support group. Refer for counseling or social services as indicated. *Peer support and counseling can help the client and family develop effective coping and adaptation strategies.*

EVALUATING

When evaluating the effectiveness of nursing interventions for the client with renal failure, collect data related to fluid volume status, such as weight, intake and output, degree of edema, and cardiovascular status. Assess skin and mucous membrane integrity as well. Evaluate food and nutrient intake, and compliance with prescribed diet. Assess for freedom from infection. Look at coping strategies employed by the client, as well as active participation in care.

BOX 32-22	**ASSESSMENT**

Assessing for Discharge: Renal Failure

CLIENT

- Self-care: ability to independently perform ADLs; to prepare and eat prescribed diet; to manage peritoneal dialysis (CAPD or CCPD) or home hemodialysis
- Knowledge: disease process; fluid and diet restrictions; treatment options; strategies to preserve kidney function; prevention and recognition of infection; complications to report to physician; follow-up care and/or scheduled treatments
- Psychosocial: coping with diagnosis and treatments; support network and significant others; economic effects of treatments; acceptance of altered body image and roles
- Home environment: clean running water, hand washing and toilet facilities; clean area for home dialysis; transportation options

FAMILY AND CAREGIVERS

- Ability and willingness to assist with ADLs and to provide or assist with meal preparation and dialysis
- Financial and transportation resources; stability of family unit; effect of chronic illness on roles and relationships

---

Documenting. Document assessment data on a regular and continuing basis. Note the relationship between any changes in assessment findings and treatments provided. Document status of the AV fistula if present, or the clarity and amount of peritoneal dialysate returned. Document all teaching provided to the client and family, and their apparent understanding and acceptance of information.

CONTINUING CARE

Renal failure may be an acute disorder or a chronic disease. Even when manifestations of acute renal failure resolve before discharge, the healing process lasts for up to 1 year. Both acute and chronic renal failure can require long-term, day-to-day management. Box 32-22 ■ outlines assessment data to be collected before discharge.

Early teaching focuses on the nature of the renal failure. Teach clients with acute renal failure about the extended recovery period and the importance of avoiding exposure to nephrotoxins.

Educate all clients about prescribed dietary and fluid restrictions. Involve the client, a dietitian, and the family member usually responsible for cooking in teaching. Include strategies to improve flavor and to relieve thirst when fluid is restricted.

Teach the client on hemodialysis how to assess and protect the fistula or shunt. Refer home dialysis helpers for

---

BOX 32-23

RESOURCES FOR HOME CARE
The following resources may be useful for clients with kidney disease:

American Association of Kidney Patients
800-749-2257
www.aakp.org

National Kidney Foundation
800-622-9010
www.kidney.org

Kidney Foundation of Canada
514-369-4806
www.kidney.ca

---

formal training. Teach and demonstrate catheter care and the dialysis procedure to the client who will perform CAPD and a family member or significant other. When a kidney transplant has been done, teach about the prescribed medications, their adverse effects and management, infection prevention, and signs and symptoms of organ rejection.

Refer clients to local or state chapters of the National Kidney Foundation or the American Association of Kidney Patients (Box 32-23 ■).

Note: The bibliography listings for this and all chapters have been compiled at the back of the book.

Chapter Review

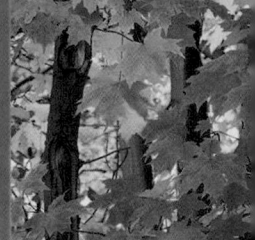

 **KEY TERMS** by Topics

Use the audio glossary feature of either the CD-ROM or the Companion Website to hear the correct pronunciation of the following key terms.

Voiding disorders
urinary incontinence

Infectious and inflammatory disorders
cystitis, dysuria, nocturia, hematuria, pyelonephritis, glomerulonephritis, proteinuria, azotemia

Obstructive disorders
urolithiasis, hydronephrosis, renal colic

Kidney trauma
anuria

Tumors
cystectomy

Renal failure
renal failure, nephrotoxins, uremia, dialysis

KEY Points

- Urinary incontinence, while often accepted as a normal part of aging in women, is not normal and can be treated.

- Lower urinary tract infections are common in women due to a short urethra and the proximity of the urethral meatus to the vagina and anus. Urinary tract infection in men, however, may indicate a structural, obstructive, or other problem of the urinary tract.

- A 3-day course of antibiotic therapy often is effective for treating uncomplicated UTIs. Added advantages of this shortened course are improved compliance and reduced adverse effects when compared to longer courses of treatment.

- Acute glomerulonephritis usually is due to an abnormal inflammatory response to beta-hemolytic streptococcal infection (strep throat). It usually resolves uneventfully in children and adults, but may lead to chronic glomerulonephritis and eventual kidney failure.

- Clients with a history of kidney or other urinary stones have a high risk of developing stones in the future. Emphasize the importance of maintaining a generous fluid intake, avoiding dehydration, and, for calcium stones, staying physically active and reducing calcium intake.

- Painless hematuria is a frequent initial manifestation of urinary tract cancer. Advise all clients with hematuria to see their physician for evaluation.

- Renal failure may be either acute or chronic:
  - Acute renal failure usually affects seriously ill older adults who experience hypovolemia or shock or who are exposed to a nephrotoxic drug or substance. Acute renal failure often resolves with treatment and kidney function is restored.
  - Chronic renal failure is the final stage of a long-term process of kidney destruction (due to diabetes, hypertension, lupus, or a primary kidney disease). Clients with chronic renal failure often require treatment to replace lost kidney function, such as dialysis or a kidney transplant.

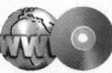 **EXPLORE Media**Link

Additional interactive resources for this chapter can be found on the Companion Website at www.prenhall.com/burke. Click on Chapter 32 and "Begin" to select the activities for this chapter.

For chapter-related NCLEX-style review questions and an audio glossary, access the accompanying CD-ROM in this book.

FOR FURTHER Study

For more information on calcium balance and the renin–angiotensin–aldosterone system, see Chapter 7.

Routine preoperative and postoperative care are covered in Chapter 9.

For further study about immunity, see Chapter 11.

For more about chemotherapy or radiation therapy, see Chapter 12.

For more information on hyperparathyroidism, see Chapter 16.

For more information about structures of the urinary tract and their purpose, urine formation, and normal values, see Chapter 31.

For more information about uroflowmetry procedures, see Chapter 31.

For more information about collecting a midstream, clean-catch urine specimen, see Box 31-1.

For more information about 24-hour urine specimens, see Box 31-3 and Table 31-3.

For discussion of prostatectomy, see Chapter 34.

Critical Thinking Care Map

Caring for a Client with Urinary Incontinence
NCLEX-PN® Focus Area: Health Promotion and Maintenance

Case Study: Anna Giovanni, a 76-year-old widow, lives alone. Her eldest daughter is concerned that her mother seems increasingly reluctant to leave the apartment to visit friends and family. She reports a strong odor of urine throughout her mother's apartment and that her mother's bed is often wet.

Nursing Diagnosis: Urinary Incontinence

COLLECT DATA

Subjective	Objective
_____	_____
_____	_____
_____	_____
_____	_____
_____	_____
_____	_____
_____	_____

Would you report this data? Yes/No

If yes, to: _____

Nursing Care

_____

_____

_____

_____

_____

_____

_____

_____

_____

How would you document this? _____

_____

_____

_____

Data Collected
(use those that apply)

- Relates urine leakage when laughing, coughing, and on hearing the sound of running water
- Often unable to reach bathroom in time at night
- Hysterectomy at age 52
- Estrogen-replacement therapy for approximately 10 years after hysterectomy
- Takes digoxin 0.125 mg qd, furosemide 40 mg bid, and KCl 20 mEq t.i.d.
- Moderate cystourethrocele
- Atrophy of vaginal tissues
- Pelvic floor strength weak
- Urinalysis within normal limits
- Postvoiding residual urine 5 mL
- Average of nine daytime voidings and four at night
- Urine leakage usually occurs in late afternoon and at night

Nursing Interventions
(use those that apply; list in priority order)

- Teach how to identify pelvic floor muscles and perform Kegel exercises.
- Suggest decaffeinated tea and noncitrus fruit juices (grape, apple, and cranberry).
- Encourage minimizing fluid intake after evening meal.
- Change afternoon dose of furosemide from 9:00 P.M. to 4:00 P.M.
- Encourage voiding by the clock, gradually increasing intervals from every 45 to 60 minutes to every 2 to 2.5 hours. Advise shorter intervals for 2 to 3 hours after furosemide doses.
- Suggest commercial products for protecting clothing and furniture.
- Provide bedside commode for nighttime use.
- Schedule follow-up visits and evaluations to reinforce teaching.

The LPN/LVN provides information to clients to prevent complications of disease or treatment. Be sure to study alterations in body systems and ways of teaching the client to manage his or her health after discharge from the health care facility.

1 A 79-year-old client with benign prostatic hypertrophy has not voided in the past 8 hours. The FIRST action by the LPN/LVN would be to:

A. provide 500 mL fluids orally.
B. perform a catheterization with a 14-Fr. straight catheter.
C. palpate the lower abdomen.
D. notify the physician.

2 A 50-year-old woman experiences stress incontinence. Which of the following assessment findings indicates a risk factor for this condition?

A. total abdominal hysterectomy 9 years ago
B. smokes one pack of cigarettes per day
C. exercises four times a week
D. history of two pregnancies

3 An LVN evaluates for residual urine on a client; 30 mL of clear yellow urine is returned. The appropriate action by the nurse would be to:

A. notify the physician.
B. document the finding in the medical record.
C. implement measures to assist the client to void.
D. increase client's fluid intake.

4 The nurse establishes a nursing diagnosis of Urinary Incontinence related to weak pelvic floor muscles for a 69-year-old client. Which of the following would be an appropriate nursing intervention?

A. Encourage client to drink orange juice and tea at each meal.
B. Schedule furosemide (Lasix) 40 mg at 8 P.M. daily.
C. Teach to perform Kegel exercises every 2 hours while awake.
D. Restrict fluid intake to 500 mL/day.

5 The nurse teaching a client to help prevent urinary tract infections includes which of the following instructions? (Select all that apply.)

A. Drink at least one 8-ounce glass of orange juice daily.
B. Increase your water intake to 6 or more glasses per day.
C. After voiding or defecating, wipe from back to front.
D. Wear cotton briefs under clothing.
E. Void before and after sexual intercourse.

6 A 19-year-old is admitted with acute glomerulonephritis. The nurse expects to obtain which of the following assessment findings?

A. "strep throat" 2 weeks ago
B. pneumonia 1 week ago
C. gastroenteritis
D. influenza 3 weeks ago

7 For a client with a ureteral calculus, a priority nursing action is to

A. wash hands.
B. restrict fluids.
C. strain all urine.
D. collect a sterile urine specimen.

8 A female client is discharged following a right nephrotomy to remove a urinary calculus. Discharge teaching should include:

A. maintaining oral fluid intake of 1,500 mL daily.
B. avoiding all sources of calcium.
C. signs and symptoms of urinary tract infection.
D. maintaining alkaline urine.

9 A client is diagnosed with chronic renal failure. The nurse explains that dietary management of a client with chronic renal failure includes:

A. a high-protein, low-carbohydrate diet.
B. a low-protein, high-carbohydrate diet.
C. a high-fat, moderate-sodium diet.
D. a low-fat, high-sodium diet.

10 A client has an arteriovenous (AV) fistula in his left arm for hemodialysis access. The nurse recognizes the need for further teaching if the client states:

A. "My wife gets the best blood pressure in my left arm."
B. "I check my fistula for pulsations."
C. "I remind the lab personnel to take blood from my right arm."
D. "I sleep on my left side with my left arm extended."

Answers for Review Questions, as well as discussion of Care Plan and Critical Thinking Care Map questions, appear in Appendix V.

CONSIDERING CULTURAL VARIATIONS RELATED TO TIME

Mrs. Torres, 42, a Puerto Rican American, arrived at the doctor's office a half-hour late for her Friday afternoon appointment. When the nurse at the desk asked her about this, she said, "I had a friend stop by who just arrived from Puerto Rico and we got busy talking. Is this a problem? The doctor is usually behind in his appointments." "Yes," the nurse said, "The doctor had an afternoon surgery scheduled and isn't here. He won't be back in the office until Monday. He waited as long as he could for you. You really needed to see him, because he needed to explain these test results for you, decide on a course of action, and give you prescriptions for medication. Now it will be two more days until you can see him and you will miss two days of medication that might have had you feeling better."

Time is an important but seldom recognized aspect of interpersonal communication. While the phenomenon of time varies among individuals, a person's concept of time is largely the result of experiences within his or her culture of origin (Giger & Davidhizar, 1999). Individuals learn the concept of time from persons and events in their environment, and it becomes integrated into every segment of their behavior and thought. Thus, it is essential for nurses to understand how perceptions of time vary, so culturally competent and sensitive care can be delivered. In the case of Mrs. Torres, the failure to arrive at her appointment on time will delay her recovery. If the nurse had emphasized the need to keep this appointment exactly as scheduled, Mrs. Torres might have made this a higher priority than visiting with her friend.

Temporal Orientation

Temporal orientation refers to the ordering of past, present, and future events. People who focus on the past have little motivation for formulating future goals that include primary prevention and health promotion activities. For example, Native Americans or the Old Order Amish may be viewed as past-oriented individuals. They hold strongly to traditions and values passed from generation to generation. This belief pattern directly reflects their social order and health care practices (Buccalo, 1997).

For people whose culture is oriented in the present, the present task is viewed as most important, such as visiting with a friend who has dropped by. These people are unlikely to adhere to rigid time schedules; instead, they focus on the current activity. Present-time orientation may also result in nonadherence to medication regimens, visiting hours at the hospital, and follow-up appointments. For example, a teenager may get caught up in an activity and miss an appointment that required arriving at a precise time (Davidhizar, Bechtel, & Giger, 1999).

People who have a future-time orientation organize and plan their activities to achieve future goals. Many middle-class Americans, regardless of ethnic or cultural origin, tend to be future oriented. They may delay starting a family, purchasing a house, or purchasing an expensive car until education is successfully completed and financial success has been attained. Future-oriented individuals may seem cold and detached and may focus more on tasks to accomplish future goals than on relationships.

Clock vs. Social Time

Most people in North America organize their activities around the clock, arriving at places or starting behaviors at a very specified time determined by hours and minutes. Some groups, however, initiate activities and behaviors on the basis of social time. For them, events such as weddings or church services may start when everyone arrives and stop when the event is completed. For these individuals, time is qualitative rather than quantitative (Giger & Davidhizar, 1999).

Nursing Implications

- *Assess **individuals for time orientation.*** The nurse needs to relate health care teaching to the client's perspective of time. For example, when a client is present rather than future oriented, the nurse needs to relate present actions to current health status, not to the future.
- *Care planning should be based on cultural orientation.* By acknowledging other time perceptions, the nurse can plan interventions to assist the client to adapt behavior to meet health needs. For example, stressing the importance of keeping appointments on time, of taking medication as ordered, and of complying with care regimens can increase the client's compliance.
- *Differences in behavior by health team members may be related to time perception.* Some team members who are social-time rather than clock-time oriented may have difficulty with punctuality and strict adherence to the time frames for treatments and medication administration.

Self-Reflection Questions

1. What is your predominant time orientation: past, present, or future?

2. Are you predominantly clock-time oriented or social-time oriented?

3. If your client or coworkers do not share your time orientation, what problems can occur?

Thinking Strategically About...

Walter Cohen, 45 years old, has been a type 1 diabetic since the age of 20. He was diagnosed with diabetic nephropathy 10 years ago, and has now progressed to end-stage renal disease. He enters the nephrology unit for temporary hemodialysis to treat uremia and to prepare for CAPD.

DATA COLLECTED

During the nursing assessment, Mr. Cohen states that he thought his lack of appetite, nausea, vomiting, and fatigue during the past month were caused by "a touch of the flu." His weight remained stable, so he didn't worry about not eating much. Objective data includes BP 178/100; P 96; R 20; T 97.8°F (36.5°C) PO. His skin is cool and dry, with minor excoriations on his forearms and lower legs. Mr. Cohen has a fetid breath odor. A few fine crackles are noted in lung bases bilaterally. Both lower extremities have 3+ pitting edema to just below the knees; his hands also appear edematous. Bowel sounds are hypoactive. Urinalysis shows gross proteinuria. CBC shows RBC 2.9 million/mm^3; hemoglobin 9.4 g/dL; hematocrit 28%. His BUN is 198 mg/dL; creatinine 18.5 mg/dL; sodium 125 mEq/L; potassium 5.7 mEq/L; calcium 7.1 mg/dL; and phosphate 6.8 mg/dL.

Mr. Cohen underwent four hemodialysis sessions to treat his uremia. An arteriovenous fistula was created in his left arm for possible future hemodialysis. A permanent catheter was surgically placed in the peritoneal cavity and he began peritoneal dialysis.

CRITICAL THINKING

1 How does diabetes mellitus damage the kidneys and lead to end-stage renal disease?

2 What are some advantages of CAPD?

3 What are some disadvantages of CAPD?

4 What is a likely cause of the excoriations on Mr. Cohen's extremities?

5 What are contraindications for CAPD?

MANAGEMENT OF CARE

1 What are the nursing implications when caring for a client with an arteriovenous fistula?

2 What nursing care would be implemented when caring for a client with a permanent peritoneal CAPD catheter?

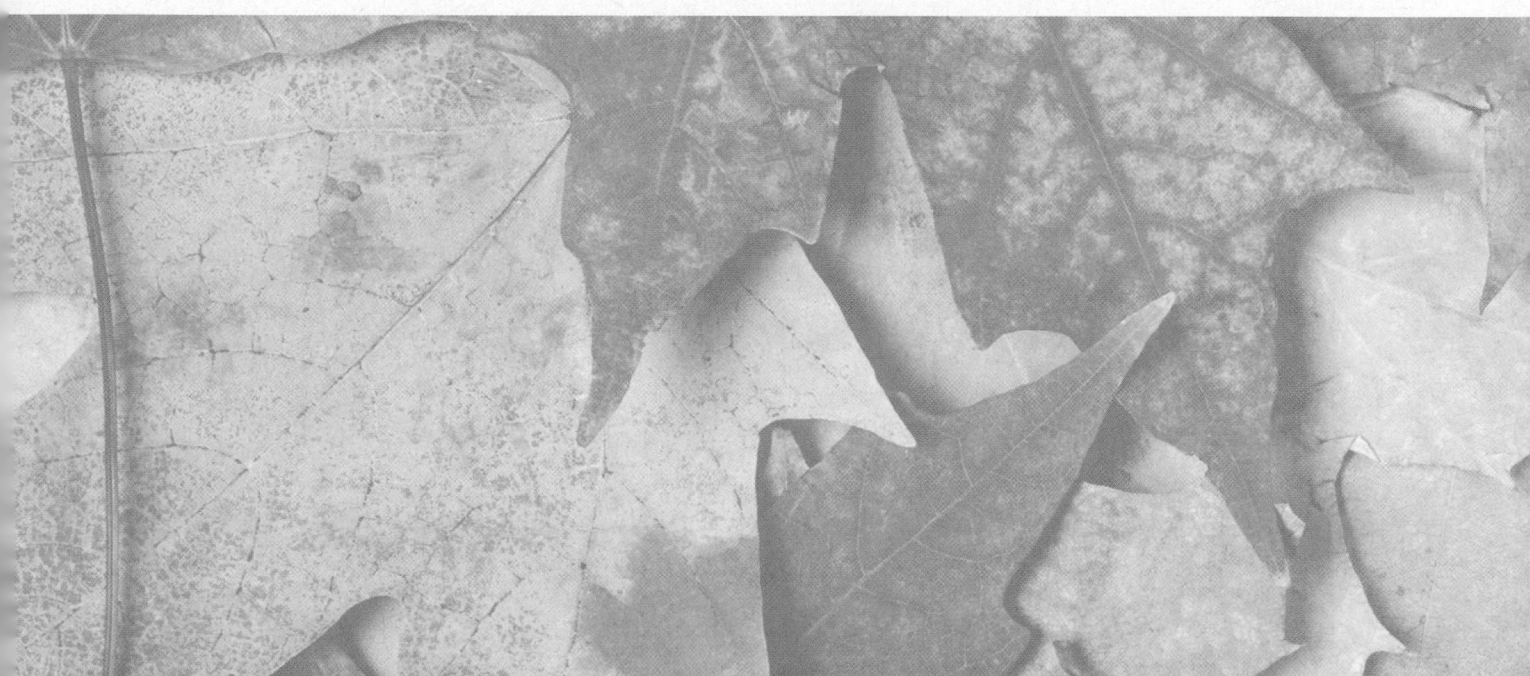

Disrupted Reproductive Function

UNIT IX

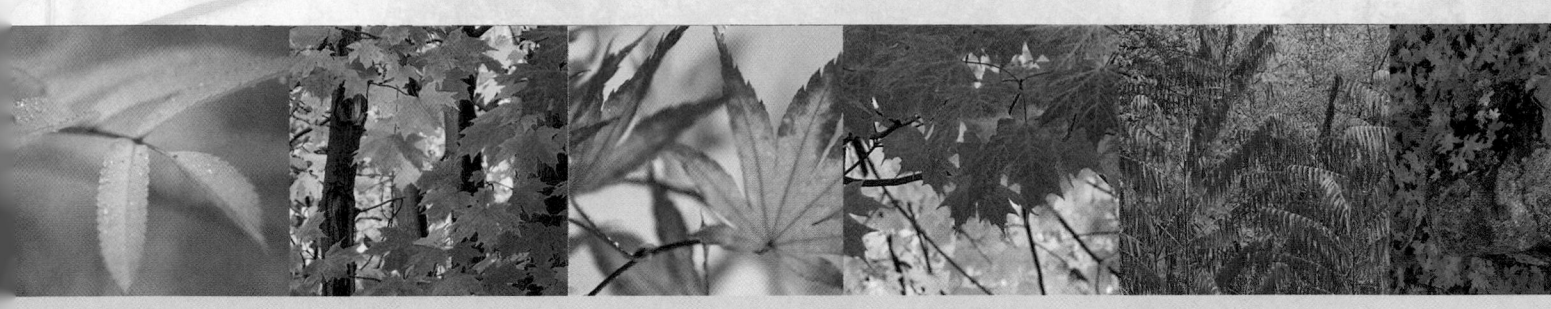

The Reproductive System and Assessment

LEARNING Outcomes

After completing this chapter, you will be able to:

- Identify the major structures and functions of the male reproductive system.
- Identify the major structures and functions of the female reproductive system.
- Identify and describe the functions of female sex hormones.
- Describe normal age-related changes in male and female reproductive system structure and function.
- Collect subjective and objective assessment data related to the reproductive system.
- Provide appropriate nursing care for clients undergoing diagnostic tests related to the reproductive system.

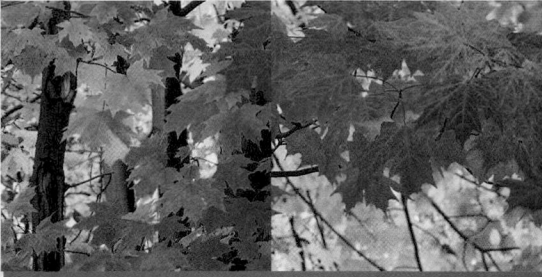

MediaLink

www.prenhall.com/burke

Use the address above to access the free, interactive Companion Website created for this textbook. Get hints, instant feedback, and textbook references to chapter-related NCLEX-style questions. Link to other interesting sites.

Audio Glossary:

Use the Companion Website, or the CD-ROM disk enclosed with your textbook, to hear the pronunciation of key terms in this chapter.

Although the reproductive organs in men and women are very different, they share common functions: providing sexual pleasure and producing children. The reproductive organs, in conjunction with the endocrine system, also produce hormones that are important in biologic development and sexual behavior.

Structure and Function of the Male Reproductive System

The reproductive system in men includes the paired testes, the scrotum, ducts, glands, and penis (Figure 33-1 ■).

TESTES AND SCROTUM

The *testes* produce sperm and testosterone. Sperm is produced in the *seminiferous tubules* of the testes. Leydig's cells within the testes produce testosterone.

The testes are suspended in the scrotum by the spermatic cord. The *scrotum* is a sac or pouch that regulates the temperature of the testes. The best temperature for producing sperm is about 2 to 3 degrees below body temperature. When the temperature is too low, the scrotum contracts to bring the testes up against the body. When the testes are too warm, the scrotum relaxes to allow the testes to lie further away from the body.

Spermatogenesis

Spermatogenesis is sperm production. This process begins with puberty and continues throughout a man's life, with several hundred million sperm produced daily. Spermatogenesis takes 64 to 72 days, and includes the following processes:

1. Sperm stem cells (*spermatogonia*) divide to produce daughter cells (*spermatocytes*) that have the same number of chromosomes (46) as the parent cell.

2. Spermatocytes further divide to produce *spermatids*, immature cells with half the number of chromosomes (23) as the spermatocyte.

3. Spermatids mature into sperm cells with a head and a tail. The head contains enzymes that allow the sperm to penetrate and fertilize the ova. The tail allows the sperm to move. When the sperm and ova fuse, the resulting cell has the normal number of chromosomes (46).

Male Sex Hormones

The male sex hormones are called **androgens.** Most are produced in the testes, although a small amount is produced by the adrenal glands. *Testosterone,* the primary male sex hormone, is essential to develop and maintain sexual function. It also promotes metabolism, muscle and bone growth, and **libido** (sexual desire).

DUCTS AND SEMEN

Sperm mature and are stored in the *epididymis,* a long coiled tube that lies over the outer surface of each testis. When a man is sexually excited, the epididymis contracts to push the sperm through the *vas deferens* to mix with seminal fluid.

Seminal fluid is made of secretions from the seminal vesicles, the epididymis, the prostate gland, and Cowper's glands. Seminal fluid nourishes the sperm, provides bulk, and increases its alkalinity. An alkaline pH is essential to mobilize the sperm and ensure fertilization of the ova. Sperm mixed with this fluid is called *semen.* During **ejaculation** (expulsion of seminal fluid) semen enters the urethra for expulsion.

The total amount of ejaculate is about 2 to 4 mL. The sperm count of ejaculate in a healthy male is from 100 million to 400 million.

PROSTATE GLAND

The *prostate gland* is about the size of a walnut. It encircles the urethra just below the urinary bladder (see Figure 33-1). Secretions of the prostate gland make up about one-third of the volume of the semen. These secretions enter the urethra through several ducts during ejaculation. For information about digital rectal examination of the prostate, see Chapter 34. ⬭

PENIS

The penis is composed of a *shaft* and a tip called the *glans,* which is covered in the uncircumcised man by the *foreskin* (or *prepuce*). The shaft contains three columns of erectile tissue: The two lateral columns are called the *corpora cavernosa,* and the central mass is called the *corpus spongiosum.*

Erection occurs when a reflex triggers the parasympathetic nervous system to stimulate arteriolar vasodilation, filling erectile tissue with blood. The erection reflex may be initiated by touch, pressure, sights, sounds, smells, or thoughts of a sexual encounter. After ejaculation, the arterioles constrict, and the penis becomes flaccid.

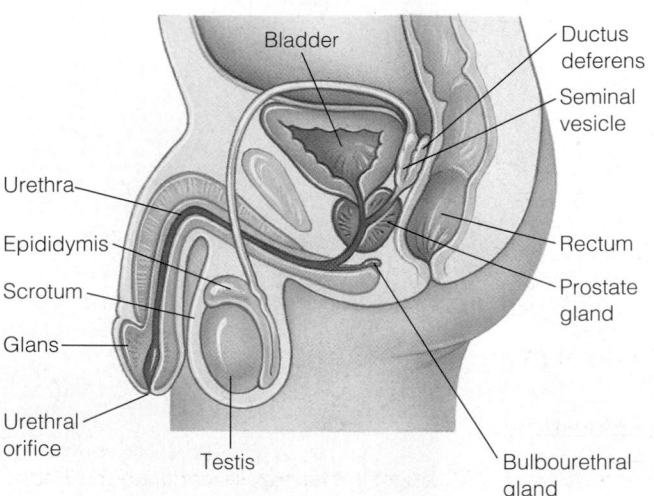

Figure 33-1. ■ The male reproductive system.

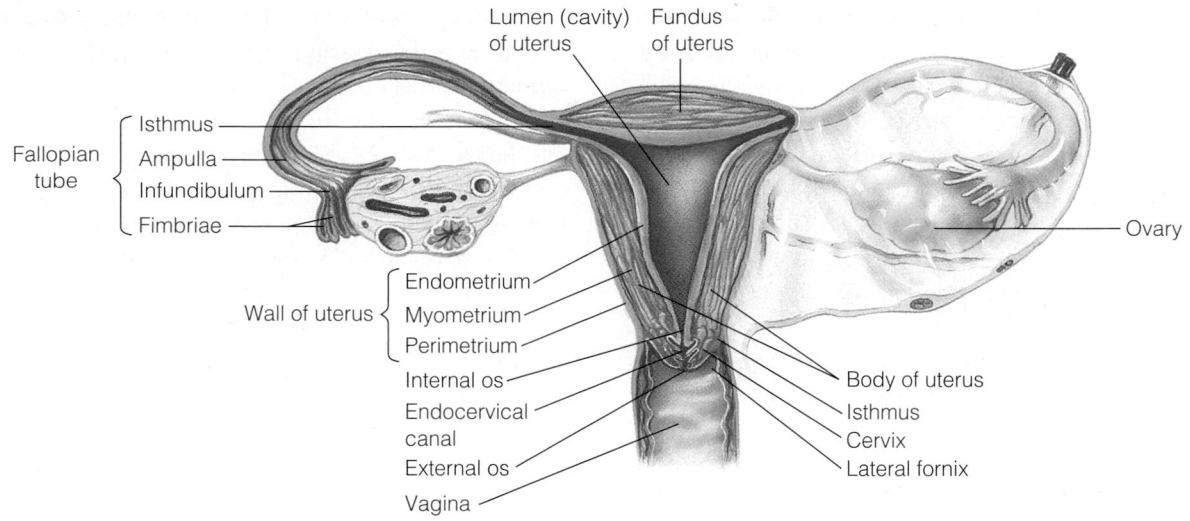

Figure 33-2. ■ The internal organs of the female reproductive system.

Structure and Function of the Female Reproductive System

The female reproductive system includes the paired ovaries and fallopian tubes, uterus, vagina, the external genitalia, and the breasts. In women, the urethra and urinary meatus are separated from the reproductive organs; however, they are in such close proximity that a health problem with one often affects the other.

INTERNAL STRUCTURES

The internal organs of the female reproductive system include the ovaries, fallopian tubes, uterus, and vagina (Figure 33-2 ■).

Ovaries and Ovulation

In adult women, the ovaries are flat, almond-shaped glands located below the ends of the fallopian tubes. The ovaries produce the female hormones estrogen and progesterone, and store immature ova called *oocytes*.

The ovaries produce estrogens, progesterone, and androgens in a cyclic pattern. **Estrogens** are steroid hormones essential to the development and maintenance of secondary sex characteristics. Along with other hormones, estrogens also help prepare the female reproductive organs for growth of a fetus. Estrogens help maintain skin, bone, and blood vessel structure; affect serum cholesterol and high-density lipoprotein (HDL) levels; enhance blood clotting; and affect sodium and water balance. Estrogen secretion varies with the menstrual cycle (see later discussion).

Progesterone primarily affects breast glandular tissue and the endometrium. During pregnancy, progesterone relaxes smooth muscle to decrease uterine contractions. It also increases body temperature. Androgens (produced in small amounts by the adrenal glands as well as the ovaries) are responsible for normal hair growth patterns at puberty and also have metabolic effects.

The *ovarian cycle* has three phases lasting about 28 days. The *follicular phase* lasts from the 1st to the 10th day of the cycle. The *ovulatory phase* lasts from the 11th to the 14th day, ending with ovulation. The *luteal phase* lasts from the 14th to the 28th day (Figure 33-3 ■).

Each ovary contains many small structures called *ovarian follicles*. Each follicle contains an immature ovum, called an *oocyte*. Each month, several follicles mature, stimulated by *follicle-stimulating hormone (FSH)* and *luteinizing hormone (LH)*. The mature follicles (*graafian follicles*) produce estrogen,

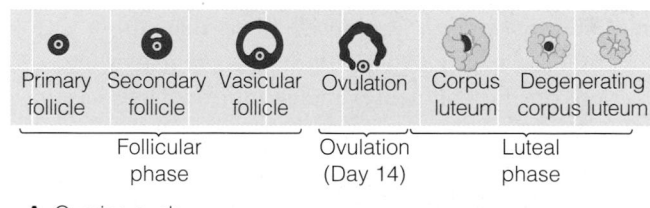

A Ovarian cycle

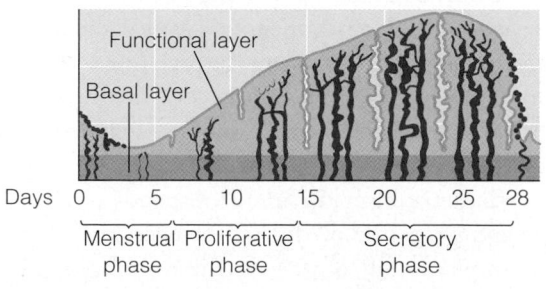

B Uterine cycle

Figure 33-3. ■ (A) Changes in ovarian follicles during the 28-day ovarian cycle. (B) Corresponding changes in the endometrium during the menstrual cycle.

which stimulates development of endometrium. When the estrogen level is high enough to stimulate the anterior pituitary gland, a surge of LH is produced. LH stimulates development of the oocyte into a mature ovum and causes the ovarian follicle to rupture, releasing the ovum. This is the process of *ovulation*. The ruptured follicle then becomes a *corpus luteum,* which produces estrogen and progesterone to support the endometrium until conception occurs or the cycle begins again. If pregnancy does not occur, the corpus luteum degenerates, and its hormone production ceases. Falling progesterone and estrogen levels allow LH and FSH levels to increase, and a new cycle begins.

Fallopian Tubes

The *fallopian tubes* (or uterine tubes) are thin tubes about 4 inches (10 cm) long and 1 cm in diameter. They are attached to the uterus on one end. The distal ends of the fallopian tubes are open, with projections called *fimbriae* that drape over the ovary. The fimbriae pick up the ovum after it is released from the ovary.

The fallopian tubes are made of smooth muscle and lined with cilia. Movement of the cilia and smooth muscle contractions move the ovum through the tubes toward the uterus. Fertilization of the ovum by sperm usually occurs in the outer portion of one of the fallopian tubes.

Uterus

The *uterus* is a thick-walled, pear-shaped muscular organ located between the bladder and rectum. Ligaments support it within the abdominal cavity. Its function is to receive the fertilized ovum and provide a site for growth and development of the fetus.

The uterine wall has three layers. The outer layer, the *perimetrium,* merges with the peritoneum. The middle layer, the *myometrium,* has muscle fibers that run in various directions, allowing expansion during pregnancy and contractions during the menses and childbirth. The *endometrium* lines the uterus. Its innermost layer is shed during menstruation.

The uterus is made up of three parts: the fundus, the body, and the cervix (see Figure 33-2). The cervix projects into the vagina. The uterine opening of the cervix is called the *internal os;* the vaginal opening is called the *external os.* The *endocervical canal* between the openings allows discharge of menstrual fluid and entrance of sperm. The cervix is a firm structure that softens in response to hormones during pregnancy.

The endometrium of the uterus responds to changes in estrogen and progesterone during the ovarian cycle to prepare for implantation of the fertilized embryo. The endometrium is receptive to embryo implantation for only about 7 days each month, during the time when the embryo would normally reach the uterus from the fallopian tube.

The menstrual cycle begins at the onset of menstruation (Figure 33-3B). During the *menstrual phase,* the inner endometrial layer detaches and is expelled as menstrual fluid. As the maturing follicle begins to produce estrogen, the *proliferative phase* begins. The inner endometrial layer is repaired and thickens, while spiral arteries proliferate and tubular glands form. Cervical mucus becomes thin, helping sperm move into the uterus. During the *secretory phase,* progesterone increases endometrial vascularity and prepares it to support the fertilized ovum. Cervical mucus thickens, blocking the internal os. If fertilization does not occur, hormone levels fall. Spasm of spiral arteries causes degeneration and sloughing of the inner endometrial layer, starting the process again.

Vagina

The vagina is a fibromuscular tube about 3 to 4 inches (8 to 10 cm) long located between the bladder and urethra and the rectum. The upper end contains the cervix in an area called the *fornix.* The mucous membrane walls of the vagina form folds, called *rugae.* Vaginal mucus is relatively acidic and bacteriostatic. Estrogen and normal vaginal flora help maintain its acid pH. The vagina is the birth canal, allows excretion of menstrual fluid, and is an organ of sexual response.

EXTERNAL GENITALIA

The external genitalia include the mons pubis, the labia, the clitoris, the vaginal and urethral openings, and glands (Figure 33-4 ■).

The *mons pubis* is a pad of adipose tissue anterior to the symphysis pubis. After puberty, the mons is covered with hair.

The labia are divided into two structures. The *labia majora* are folds of skin and adipose tissue covered with hair

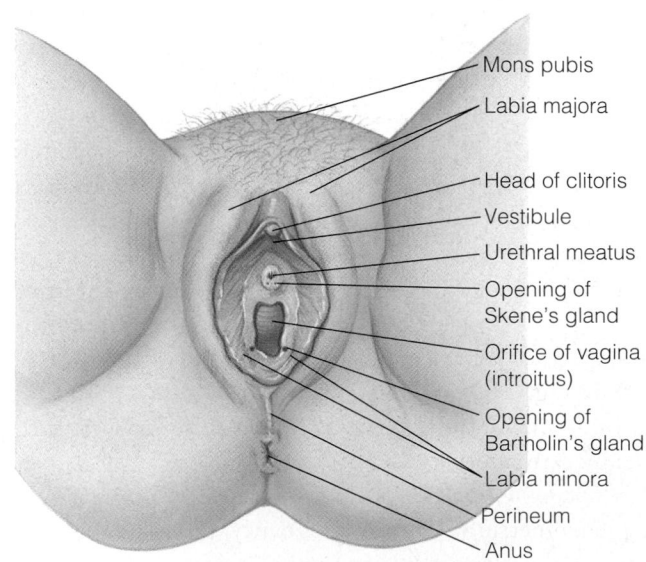

Mons pubis
Labia majora
Head of clitoris
Vestibule
Urethral meatus
Opening of Skene's gland
Orifice of vagina (introitus)
Opening of Bartholin's gland
Labia minora
Perineum
Anus

Figure 33-4. ■ The female external genitalia.

that enclose the labia minora. The *labia minora* are hairless and contain some erectile tissue. The area between the labia is called the *vestibule*. It contains the openings of the vagina and urethra, as well as *Bartholin's glands.* These glands secrete lubricating fluid during sexual activities. *Skene's glands,* which open onto the vestibule on each side of the urethra, produce fluid to moisten the vestibule.

The *clitoris* is an erectile organ, similar to the penis in the male. Like the penis, it is highly sensitive and distends during sexual arousal. The vaginal opening, called the *introitus,* is surrounded by a connective tissue membrane called the hymen, which determines the size and shape of the opening.

BREASTS

The *breasts* (or *mammary glands*) are supported by the pectoral muscles and are richly supplied with nerves, blood, and lymph (Figure 33-5 ■). The areola, a pigmented area near the center of the breast, contains sebaceous glands and a nipple. The *nipple* usually protrudes and becomes erect in response to cold and stimulation. The primary purpose of the breasts is to supply nourishment for the infant.

The breasts are made of adipose, connective, and glandular tissue. Cooper's ligaments, which support the breast, extend from the outer breast tissue to the nipple, dividing the breast into 15 to 25 lobes. Each lobe contains *mammary glands* connected by ducts that open to the nipple.

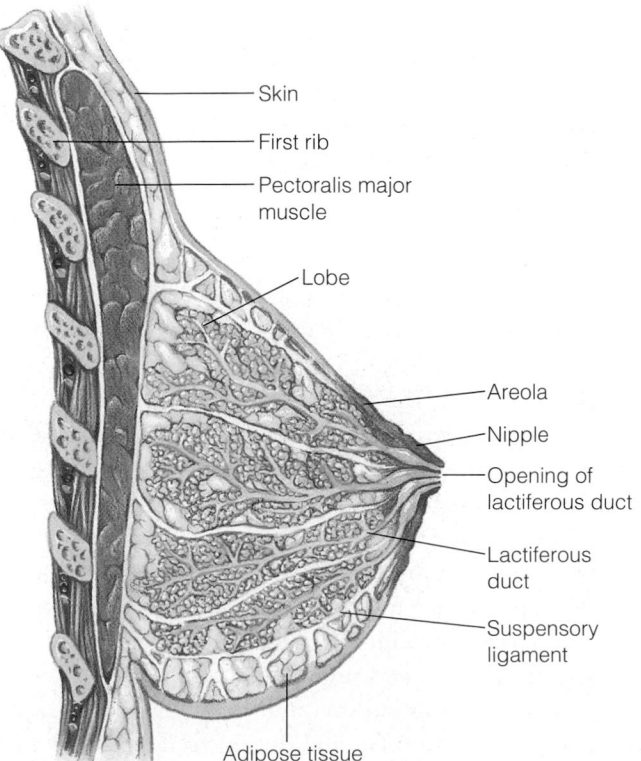

Figure 33-5. ■ Structure of the female breast.

Skin
First rib
Pectoralis major muscle
Lobe
Areola
Nipple
Opening of lactiferous duct
Lactiferous duct
Suspensory ligament
Adipose tissue

Age-Related Changes in the Reproductive System

With aging, the secretion of androgens, estrogens, and gonadotropic hormones declines. Reduced hormone levels lead to changes in secondary sex characteristics of both men and women.

In women, lower estrogen levels lead to atrophy of the ovaries, uterus, and vaginal tissue. Subcutaneous fat is lost from perineal tissues, and pelvic floor muscles weaken, increasing the risk for stress incontinence. The vagina becomes smooth and shiny as its elasticity is lost. Vaginal secretions diminish and become more alkaline. With loss of hormonal support, the breasts and nipples decrease in size. Fibrosis and calcification may develop in the ducts of the breasts.

The sperm count of older men is reduced, and the testes become firmer. Although the size of the penis may diminish, the ability to achieve erection is maintained. The prostate enlarges in most older men, and may interfere with urinary elimination.

Assessment

Assessment of reproductive function often is left until the latter part of an interview and examination to allow development of trust and comfort between the client and the nurse.

HEALTH HISTORY

It is important to use familiar terms and to ask questions in a nonthreatening manner and to avoid judging the client's responses. When interviewing, move from more general questions, for example, about previous pregnancies and a woman's menstrual cycle, to questions about problems such as sexually transmitted infections or difficulty maintaining an erection. For both male and female clients, first ask about the presenting problem. Identify its onset, manifestations, and effect on ADLs (such as difficulty urinating or dribbling, excessive menstrual flow). Inquire about possible contributing factors, such as a recent prescription for an antibiotic or using a different brand of condom. Also ask about associated symptoms such as fever or abdominal pain.

Because the urinary and reproductive systems are so closely linked in men, ask about problems such as difficulty urinating or dribbling when urinating. Ask about urethral discharge or any rash or sores on the penis.

In women, ask about the color, amount, and character of vaginal bleeding and its relationship to the menstrual cycle. Inquire about any vaginal discharge, including its onset, color, character, and odor, and any itching or rashes.

MediaLink Female Reproductive System

Obtain a history of any chronic diseases such as diabetes, heart disease, multiple sclerosis, or spinal cord problems. Ask about a family history of cancer; the risk for endometrial and breast cancer is higher in women with a family history of these cancers. Ask both men and women about possible intrauterine exposure to diethylstilbestrol (DES). This drug was used to prevent miscarriage during the 1940s and 1950s, and has been linked to an increased risk for urinary tract deformity and sterility in men, and cervical and vaginal cancer in women. Determine what medications the client is taking. Ask about physical or psychosocial stressors that may contribute to sexual problems.

Explore the client's lifestyle, specifically asking about use of alcohol, cigarettes, or street drugs. Inquire about sexual history (number and type of sexual partners), history of specific sexual problems (e.g., impotence or dyspareunia, painful intercourse) or sexual trauma, use of contraceptives, and current sexual satisfaction.

PHYSICAL ASSESSMENT

Men

Inspect and palpate the breasts, including the areola and nipple. Although breast problems are less common and easier to detect in men, it is important to not overlook this part of the examination.

Inspect and use a gloved hand to palpate the inguinal area and groin for bulges (Figure 33-6 ■). Inspect the penis; if the client is uncircumcised, retract the foreskin (or ask the client to do so). Inspect the urinary meatus (see Figure 31-6). ⊂⊃ Look specifically for skin irritation or sores, drainage from the meatus. Replace the foreskin. Inspect the skin around the base of the penis, and palpate the shaft of the penis. Inspect the scrotum; palpate each testes and epididymis.

Women

Inspect both breasts with the client seated. Inspect first with the arms at the sides, then overhead, follow by the hands pressed on hips, and then leaning forward. Observe

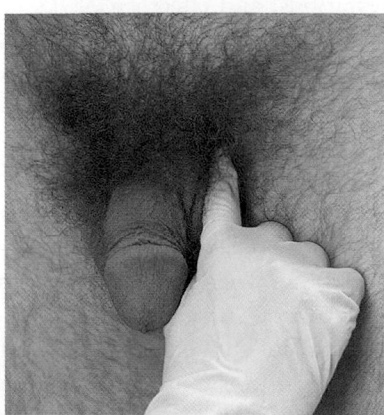

Figure 33-6. ■ Palpating the male inguinal area for bulges.

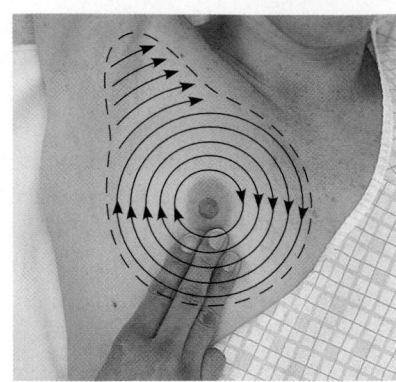

Figure 33-7. ■ A suggested pattern for palpating the breast.

size, symmetry, contour, skin color, texture, venous patterns, and any lesions. Inspect the areolae and nipples. Position the client supine, with a small pillow under the shoulder and the arm over the head. Palpate each breast, axilla, and supraclavicular area. Although various patterns of palpation can be used, it is important to palpate all areas of the breast including the axillary tail (Figure 33-7 ■). Note any tenderness, and describe any identified masses by location, size, shape, consistency, mobility, and borders. Palpate the nipple and compress it between the thumb and index finger. Note any discharge, and its color and consistency. See Chapter 35 for more information about clinical breast examination. ⊂⊃

With the client in *lithotomy position* (supine with the knees flexed and separated) and using a gloved hand, inspect and palpate the labia majora for excoriation, rashes, lesions, or bulging. Separate the labia minora; inspect and palpate the labia minora. Inspect the clitoris, vaginal opening, and perineum. Ask the client to strain or "bear down," looking for bulging of the vaginal wall, protrusion of the cervix or uterus, or urinary incontinence.

Documenting

Box 33-1 ■ presents two examples of documentation of assessment data collected related to the reproductive system.

DIAGNOSTIC TESTS

A variety of diagnostic tests may be used to identify disorders affecting the reproductive system, including diagnostic examinations, laboratory testing, imaging studies, and special procedures. Diagnostic examinations, such as digital prostate exam and clinical breast exam, are discussed in the chapters that follow. Diagnostic examinations and studies of the reproductive system often require use of invasive techniques and procedures such as a pelvic exam using a vaginal speculum and bimanual palpation of pelvic organs for women, and digital rectal exam in men. Box 33-2 ■ outlines nursing care of the woman undergoing a pelvic examination.

BOX 33-1

DOCUMENTING ASSESSMENT OF THE REPRODUCTIVE SYSTEM

Male client: George Jackson, a 68 y.o. black male, presents at his physician's office. Assessment note: Complains of increasing difficulty starting to urinate and dribbling on completion of urination. States he thinks the problem began about 6 months ago, but has recently become more noticeable. Also notes that it takes longer to fully empty his bladder, and he sometimes has to "bear down" to empty it completely. Denies other urinary symptoms, irritation of the urethra or penis, or difficulty maintaining an erection.

Healthy appearing black male who appears younger than his stated age. Color good. BP158/88, P 78, R 16, T 98.0 F PO. Pulses strong and equal ×4 extremities. Clean-catch urine specimen obtained. Urine clear, amber, no visible sediment. External genitalia appear normal; no inflammation or discharge noted. No tenderness or bulges noted on palpation of inguinal and groin regions.

Female client: Michelle Wu, a 55 y.o. Asian American woman, presents at her gynecologist's office. Assessment note: Complains of perineal and vaginal itching, burning, and discharge. States symptoms began about 24 hours ago, and have become so intense that she "can't stand it any longer." Denies previous history of vaginitis, recent antibiotic prescription, or other precipitating factors of which she is aware.

Appears healthy, but acutely uncomfortable. Skin warm and dry. BP 128/76, P 84, R 18, T 97.6 F PO. Pulses strong and equal. Clean-catch urine specimen obtained. Urine clear yellow, no sediment noted. External genitalia red and inflamed. No clear line of demarcation between inflamed and normal-appearing tissue. Creamy discharge with a slight "fishy" odor noted at vaginal os; no mucous tissue bleeding noted.

Laboratory Tests

Commonly used laboratory tests to evaluate the reproductive system are outlined, with normal values and their nursing implications, in Table 33-1 ■.

Imaging Studies

Radiologic studies, including x-rays and computed tomography (CT) scans, often are done as either screening tests to detect malignancy or to evaluate organs of the reproductive system.

Mammography is used to screen for breast cancer in women who have no symptoms. It can detect tumors that are too small to be detected by clinical breast exam or self-breast exam. Tumors as small as 5 mm in diameter can be identified on mammography. Mammography, which involves x-rays of each breast taken from different angles, also helps differentiate between benign breast changes and malignancy. Suggest that women who have tender breasts avoid coffee, colas, chocolate, and other products containing caffeine or methylxanthines for 5 to 7 days before mammography. Instruct the client to:

- Avoid using deodorants, creams, lotions, or powders on the day of the test.
- Remove all jewelry and clothing above the waist.
- Put on a hospital gown with the opening in front.

Plain x-ray films (abdominal x-ray) and abdominal CT scan may be ordered to evaluate for enlargement of reproductive organs or malignancy. Preparation and nursing care of the client vary; in many cases, no special preparation is required. If contrast media is used, ask the client about any

BOX 33-2 | NURSING CARE CHECKLIST

Pelvic Examination

Before the Procedure

☑ Obtain equipment: disposable exam gloves, light source, sterile cotton swabs, spatula, water-soluble lubricant, slides, fixative spray, vaginal specula of various sizes.

☑ Have the client empty the bladder; obtain a clean-catch urine specimen if indicated.

☑ Explain the procedure, answering any questions.

☑ If the physician is male, reassure the woman that a female nurse will remain in the room.

☑ Ask the client to remove all clothing and put on a gown. Provide a sheet for draping during the procedure.

During the Procedure

☑ Place the client in lithotomy position with the knees flexed and separated.

☑ Position the light source to illuminate the perineal area.

☑ Assist the physician, nurse practitioner, or other care provider as needed during the examination.

☑ Provide continuing support for the client.

After the Procedure

☑ Provide tissues and a towelette for cleansing lubricant from the perineal tissues.

☑ Provide a minipad to protect garments if any bleeding is expected (e.g., following a cervical biopsy). Allow privacy while the client dresses.

☑ Prepare requisitions and slides for laboratory testing as indicated.

☑ Provide information about when to expect test results, follow-up appointments, and answer any further questions.

TABLE 33-1			
Diagnostic Laboratory Tests			
TEST	NORMAL ADULT VALUES	EXPLANATION	NURSING IMPLICATIONS
Blood Tests Used to Evaluate Testicular and Ovarian Function, Infertility, and Sexual Dysfunction			
Progesterone	Male: 13–97 ng/dL (0.4–3.1 nmol/L) Female: 15–2,500 ng/dL (0.5–730 nmol/L), depending on menstrual phase	Progesterone (produced by the ovaries, adrenal glands, and the placenta) levels are used to identify ovulation and assess corpus luteum function.	Note sex, age, and day of last menstrual period or trimester of pregnancy on the requisition or lab slip. Schedule these tests either before or at least 7 days after any nuclear medicine scans because radioisotopes can interfere with results.
Serum estradiol	Male: 10–50 pg/mL (37–184 pmol/L) Female (menstruating): 30–400 pg/mL (110–1,470 pmol/L) Female (postmenopausal): 0–30 pg/mL (0–110 pmol/L)	Estradiol (an estrogen produced by the ovaries and the testes) decreases significantly after menopause. Levels are used to evaluate female infertility or amenorrhea.	
Follicle-stimulating hormone (FSH)	Male: 1.4–15.4 mLU/mL (1.4–15.4 IU/L) Female (menstruating): 1.1–9.9 mLU/ML (1.1–9.9 IU/L) Female (postmenopausal): 19–100 mLU/mL (19–100 IU/L)	FSH (produced by the anterior pituitary gland) levels are measured to evaluate menstrual disorders, amenorrhea, or infertility in women, and testicular dysfunction in men.	
Luteinizing hormone (LH)	Male: 1–8 mU/mL (1–8 U/L) Female (menstruating): 1–104 mU/mL (1–104 U/L), depending on phase Female (postmenopausal): 16–66 mU/mL (16–66 U/L)	LH (produced by the anterior pituitary gland) levels are used to evaluate delayed sexual development, amenorrhea, menstrual irregularity, and infertility.	
Serum testosterone	Male: 280–1,100 ng/dL (9.7–38 nmol/L) Female: 15–70 ng/dL (0.5–2.4 nmol/L)	Testosterone (produced by the testes, ovaries, and adrenal glands) levels are measured to evaluate function of the testes and ovaries, male infertility, and sexual dysfunction.	
Laboratory Tests Used to Detect and Evaluate Cancer of the Reproductive Organs			
Papanicolaou (PAP) smear	Within normal limits	The Pap smear is used to detect inflammation or infection, and cell changes characteristic of premalignancy or malignancy of the vagina and cervix.	Schedule the test when the client is not menstruating. Instruct to avoid sexual intercourse, douching, or vaginal medications for 48 hours prior to the exam. Have the client void before the exam. Place the client in lithotomy position. Support the client during and after the exam. Note age, date of last menstrual period, and source of specimen on the requisition.
Tumor markers: Human chorionic gonadotropin (hCG)	Male and nonpregnant female: <5 mLU/mL (<5 IU/L)	hCG is normally produced by the placenta; some malignant tumors (e.g., of the testes or ovaries) also produce hCG, causing serum levels to rise.	Schedule either before or at least 7 days after a nuclear scan because radioisotopes interfere with results. Note age, sex, and date of last menstrual period on requisition.

TABLE 33-1

Diagnostic Laboratory Tests (continued)

TEST	NORMAL ADULT VALUES	EXPLANATION	NURSING IMPLICATIONS
Alpha$_1$-fetoprotein (AFP)	<10 ng/mL (<10 µg/L)	AFP, normally present in maternal circulation during pregnancy, is used as a tumor marker for liver cancer, testicular cancer, and other malignancies.	
Prostate-specific antigen (PSA)	Male: 0–4 ng/mL (0–4 µg/L)	PSA is produced exclusively by the prostate gland. Levels rise in benign prostatic hypertrophy and malignancy of the prostate.	Schedule test before or at least 2 weeks after any manipulation of the prostate (DRE, biopsy, etc.) The specimen is obtained fasting; instruct the client to refrain from food intake for 8 hours prior to the exam.
Cancer antigen 125 (CA 125)	<35 U/mL (<35 kU/L)	CA 125 is produced by malignant cells; it is used to detect ovarian cancer and monitor its progression following removal of the tumor.	Schedule before or at least 7 days after any nuclear scan because radioisotopes interfere with test results.
Tests to Detect Genital Infections Syphilis serology: ■ VDRL (Venereal Disease Research Laboratory) ■ Rapid plasma regain (RPR) ■ Fluorescent treponemal antibody absorption (FTA-ABS)	Negative or nonreactive	These tests are used to detect antibodies produced in response to infection with *Treponema pallidum,* the spirochete that causes syphilis.	Instruct the patient to avoid alcohol intake for 24 hours prior to the test, and to avoid food intake for 8 hours prior to testing. Instruct to abstain from sexual contact until test results are known. Positive test results must be reported to the state health department. If positive, instruct client to abstain from sexual contact until effectively treated, and to notify all sexual partners of test results.
Genital culture (cervix, vagina, prostate fluid, urethral secretions)	Negative	Cultures of genital secretions are done to diagnose the cause of vaginitis, vulvovaginitis, urethritis, and urethral discharge. The infection may be sexually transmitted or result from causes unrelated to sexual contact. A number of different organisms can cause genital infections.	Men: Instruct to avoid urinating for at least an hour prior to the test because this will reduce the number of organisms present. Women: Instruct to avoid douching for 24 hours prior to the exam because this will reduce the number of organisms present. Obtain the specimen before antibiotic therapy is started. Position men supine; advise that temporary nausea, sweating, lightheadedness, or weakness may occur during specimen collection, but this is brief and temporary. Place women in lithotomy position; advise that discomfort may occur, but it should not be painful. Follow specific instructions for preparing slides such as a wet prep or saline prep.

TABLE 33-2

Diagnostic Ultrasound Studies

DIAGNOSTIC TEST	PURPOSE	NURSING IMPLICATIONS
Breast ultrasound	Primarily used to differentiate cystic from solid masses of the breast. Also may be used to guide a needle biopsy of a breast mass.	These exams are noninvasive and require no special preparation of the client. Provide support during the procedure. Assist the client to clean off ultrasound gel residue following the procedure.
Abdominal ultrasound	Used to demonstrate structures of the abdomen and pelvis, including size, position, and shape.	
Pelvic ultrasound (females)	Used to identify malignancy, benign or malignant uterine tumors, and to monitor ovulation in women. Both abdominal and vaginal approaches are used. For the vaginal approach, the transducer is covered with a condom and coated with transducer gel.	Place the client in lithotomy position when the transvaginal approach is used. Instruct to increase fluids and not void before the procedure to ensure a full bladder. Provide support during the procedure. Allow to empty the bladder as soon as possible.
Transrectal ultrasonography (TRUS) (males)	Used to assess the prostate gland, urethra, seminal vesicles, and vas deferens. May also be used to guide a needle biopsy of the prostate.	Instruct to use a disposable phosphate (Fleet) enema the evening or early morning before the procedure. Have the client void prior to the procedure. Place the client in lithotomy position. Administer sedation if ordered, and provide support during the procedure.

allergies to drugs, iodine, seafood, or previous reactions to contrast media.

A number of ultrasonography examinations may be used to detect reproductive system problems. While these exams do not expose the client to radiation and many are noninvasive, some specialized ultrasound exams are more invasive. Table 33-2 ■ outlines commonly used ultrasound procedures for evaluating the reproductive system.

Endoscopy

Several endoscopy procedures are used to evaluate the reproductive system. These procedures allow direct visualization of the organs of the abdominal and pelvic cavities. In addition, tissue can be obtained during procedures for biopsy.

Abdominal laparoscopy is done using local anesthesia and intravenous (conscious) sedation. During this procedure, the peritoneal cavity is filled with gas to allow better visualization of its organs (Figure 33-8 ■). It may be combined with laparoscopic ultrasound. The instruments are inserted through small abdominal incisions. Nursing care of the client undergoing abdominal laparoscopy is outlined in Box 33-3 ■.

In men, *cystoscopy* may be used to evaluate the size of the prostate gland and obtain tissue for biopsy. This procedure is discussed further in Chapter 31; ⊙⊙ nursing implications for cystoscopy are outlined in Box 31-7. ⊙⊙

Colposcopy is used to examine tissues of the vagina and cervix using a brightly lighted microscope. Colposcopy can

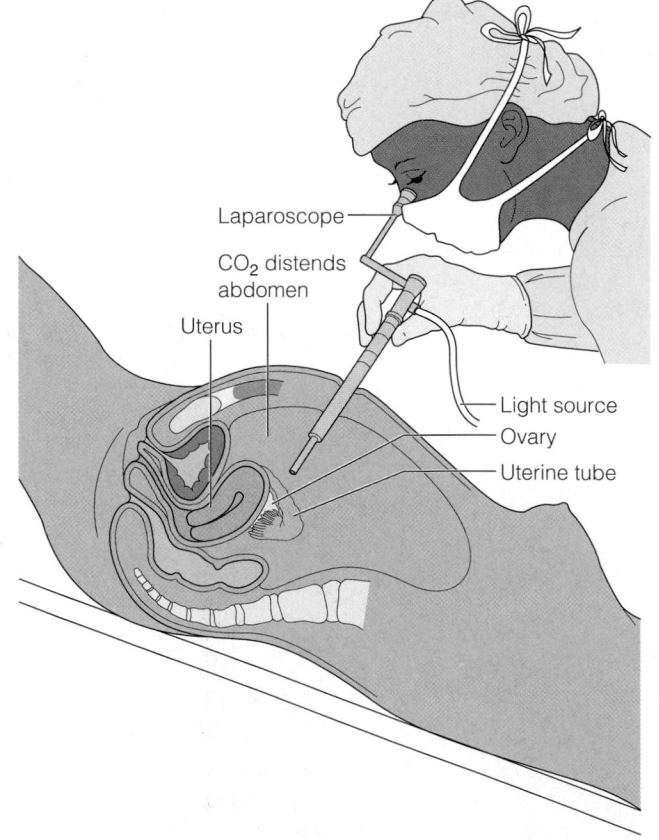

Laparoscope
CO_2 distends abdomen
Uterus
Light source
Ovary
Uterine tube

Figure 33-8. ■ Laparoscopy. A flexible, lighted instrument (laparoscope) is inserted through a small incision to visualize the abdominal and pelvic cavities.

BOX 33-3	NURSING CARE CHECKLIST

Laparoscopy

Before the Procedure

☑ Obtain informed consent.

☑ Reinforce teaching; clarify any questions the client or family members have.

☑ Instruct to douche (vaginal cleansing) and scrub around the umbilicus with povidone-iodine or other recommended antiseptic solution the night before the procedure.

☑ Ask to empty the bladder before the procedure.

☑ Obtain baseline vital signs and assessment data.

After the Procedure

☑ Monitor vital signs. Report data outside the established baseline or parameters. Report temperature greater than 101°F (38.3°C) PO.

☑ Apply a perineal pad. Instruct to change at least every 4 hours; keep a pad count.

☑ Observe dressings and surrounding tissue for drainage, bleeding, or hematoma formation.

☑ Monitor pain and provide analgesia as ordered. Instruct to report excessive pain at once.

☑ Explain that shoulder pain or release of gas through the vagina may occur.

☑ Maintain intravenous fluids until oral fluid intake is resumed.

☑ Provide discharge instructions, including potential problems about which the client should notify the physician: bleeding, intense abdominal pain, fever, fluid leakage, malaise, or difficulty breathing. Explain that hiccups may occur; a drug can be prescribed if they are disruptive.

---

identify early premalignant changes in cervical tissue, and is performed when Pap test results are abnormal. This procedure usually is accompanied by *endocervical curettage* to obtain cell samples for examination and biopsy. Colposcopy should be scheduled early in the client's menstrual cycle (between days 8 and 12). This invasive procedure requires informed consent. Instruct the client to avoid using any vaginal creams or medications prior to the procedure. The client is placed in lithotomy position during the procedure. Tell the client that she will feel a pinch or momentary cramping sensation when the specimen is obtained. Provide psychologic support, because this procedure often is performed when an abnormal Pap smear result has been obtained. Instruct the client to refrain from sexual intercourse or insertion of anything into the vagina (e.g., tampons) until the cervix has healed, approximately 7 to 10 days.

Note: The bibliography listings for this and all chapters have been compiled at the back of the book.

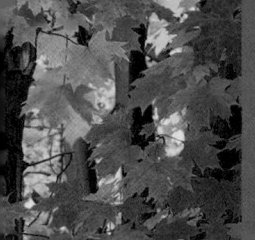

Chapter Review

 **KEY TERMS** by Topics

Use the audio glossary feature of either the CD-ROM or the Companion Website to hear the correct pronunciation of the following key terms.

Male reproductive structure and function
androgens, libido, ejaculation

Female reproductive structure and funcion
estrogens

Assessment
mammography

KEY Points

- Although the structures of the reproductive systems in men and women are very different, their functions are the same: reproduction, sexual pleasure, and development of secondary sexual characteristics.

- In men, the lower urinary and reproductive system are closely related, with the urethra and penis serving both as organs for urine elimination and ejaculation of semen. In women, the urinary and reproductive systems, although anatomically close to one another, are totally separated in structure and function.

- Modesty and fear may inhibit open discussion of reproductive system concerns and problems; establishing a trusting relationship with the client is vital.

- Although blood tests can be used to identify some reproductive system disorders, diagnostic tests frequently require direct examination of structures. These procedures vary from minimally invasive to very invasive (laparoscopy, cystoscopy).

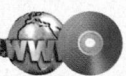 **EXPLORE Media**Link

Additional interactive resources for this chapter can be found on the Companion Website at www.prenhall.com/burke. Click on Chapter 33 and "Begin" to select the activities for this chapter.

For chapter-related NCLEX-style review questions and an audio glossary, access the accompanying CD-ROM in this book.

FOR FURTHER Study

For more information about the urinary system, urinary meatus, and cystoscopy, see Chapter 31.

For more information about digital rectal examination of the prostate, see Chapter 34.

For more information about clinical breast examination, see Chapter 35.

NCLEX-PN® Exam Preparation

TEST-TAKING TIP The practical nurse assists with many diagnostic procedures by collecting specimens, assisting with invasive procedures by setting up sterile fields and equipment and in other ways, and by caring for clients before and after procedures. Knowledge of these procedures and the nursing care associated with the procedures is vital.

1 A client asks the nurse how it is possible for the egg to make it all the way from the ovary to the uterus when it doesn't have a tail to propel it like the sperm. The nurse's response is based on the knowledge that movement of the egg to the uterus occurs

A. only when the egg has been fertilized by a sperm.
B. by smooth muscle contraction and ciliary movement.
C. by gravity.
D. through chemical messengers that attract the ovum.

2 Place the following structures in the order in which a sperm travels from its production through ejaculation:

A. vas deferens
B. testes
C. urethra
D. epididymis
E. seminal vesicle

3 A 45-year-old woman sees her gynecologist because she has stopped menstruating, and is concerned that it may be related to her exercise or signal a problem of the reproductive organs. Follow-up laboratory tests show the following: Serum estradiol 12 pg/mL, FSH 60 mLU/mL, LH 33 mU/mL. The nurse correctly interprets these results as

A. typical of a woman following menopause.
B. indicative of pregnancy.
C. significantly abnormal.
D. within normal limits for women of all ages.

4 A client scheduled for an abdominal laparoscopy asks the nurse if there will be much pain following the procedure. The most appropriate response by the nurse is

A. "No. You should have no pain or discomfort following this procedure because it is noninvasive."
B. "Yes. Because the abdominal muscles are disrupted during the procedure, you will have significant pain for about a week after the procedure."
C. "You will experience discomfort because the abdomen is inflated with gas during the procedure. Please notify us if you experience severe pain."
D. "Because local anesthesia and conscious sedation are used during the procedure, you will have no pain or discomfort afterward."

5 A male client tells the nurse that his doctor's office called and told him that he needs to come in for a DRE and PSA now that he is over age 50. He says he was too embarrassed to admit that he didn't know what that meant, and wonders if there is anything he needs to know ahead of time. The appropriate response by the nurse is

A. "No, no special preparation is required for a digital rectal exam and prostate-specific antigen test."
B. "Yes. The day surgery unit will call you a week before because informed consent is required for these invasive procedures."
C. "No. These tests are performed in the doctor's office. All required preparation will occur there under the doctor's direction."
D. "Yes. You should have the PSA (a blood test) drawn before the doctor does the digital rectal exam. Do not eat anything the morning of your blood test."

Answers for Review Questions appear in Appendix V.

Chapter 34

Caring for Male Clients with Reproductive System Disorders

BRIEF Outline

Benign Prostatic Hyperplasia
Cancer of the Prostate
Prostatitis
Structural and Inflammatory Disorders
Infertility
Scrotal Masses and Trauma
Testicular Cancer
Phimosis
Priapism
Cancer of the Penis
Erectile Dysfunction
Ejaculatory Dysfunction

LEARNING Outcomes

After completing this chapter, you will be able to:

- Describe the pathophysiology and manifestations of common disorders of the male reproductive system.
- Discuss nursing implications for medications used to treat disorders of the male reproductive system.
- Use the nursing process to provide care for clients with disorders of the male reproductive system.
- Contribute to the plan of care for male clients undergoing surgery for reproductive system disorders.

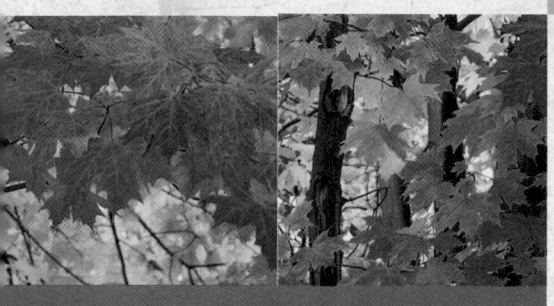

MediaLink

www.prenhall.com/burke
Use the address above to access the free, interactive Companion Website created for this textbook. Get hints, instant feedback, and textbook references to chapter-related NCLEX-style questions. Link to other interesting sites.

Audio Glossary:
Use the Companion Website, or the CD-ROM disk enclosed with your textbook, to hear the pronunciation of key terms in this chapter.

The male reproductive system may be affected by structural and functional disorders, infectious and inflammatory disorders, and malignancies. Many of these disorders and their treatments pose a risk to the client's fertility and sexuality, as well as urinary function.

PROSTATE DISORDERS

Benign Prostatic Hyperplasia

Enlargement of the prostate gland, **benign prostatic hyperplasia (BPH),** affects most men over the age of 50. The incidence of BPH increases with age: More than 90% of men over 70 years old have BPH. Its cause is unknown, but risk factors have been identified. These include age, family history, race, ethnicity, and hormonal factors. BPH tends to develop earlier in African Americans than in European Americans. Its incidence is lowest in native Japanese men.

PATHOPHYSIOLOGY

BPH only develops in men who have testes; it does not affect men who were castrated before puberty. *Testosterone,* the primary androgen produced primarily in the testes, is converted to dihydrotestosterone (DHT) in the prostate gland. DHT stimulates growth of the prostate. Although testosterone levels decrease in aging, estrogen (produced in small amounts in men) levels increase. Estrogen appears to make the prostate more responsive to DHT, promoting its growth. Increases in estrogen levels in relation to testosterone levels may contribute to BPH.

BPH develops as small nodules that form and grow in the central and transition zones of the prostate, next to the urethra. The expanding prostate compresses surrounding tissue, narrowing the urethra (Figure 34-1 ■).

MANIFESTATIONS AND COMPLICATIONS

Narrowing of the urethra partially or completely obstructs the urethra, impairing urine flow and bladder emptying. Obstruction causes the symptoms of BPH, including weak urinary stream, difficulty initiating urine flow, dribbling, and urinary retention. *Nocturia* (voiding more than once at night) is an early symptom. The manifestations of BPH are summarized in Box 34-1 ■.

If BPH is not treated, increased pressure in the bladder causes urine *reflux* (backflow) into the ureters. This can eventually lead to *hydronephrosis,* which can affect kidney function (see Chapter 32). ⊂⊃ Fortunately, these complications are rare, because the symptoms associated with BPH force most men to seek help before significant urinary retention and bladder distension develop.

INTERDISCIPLINARY CARE

Some men are diagnosed with BPH during a routine physical examination before symptoms develop. Others wait until the discomfort from dysuria, urgency, and urinary retention becomes almost unbearable before seeking care.

Diagnostic Tests

- A *digital rectal exam (DRE)* reveals an enlarged and asymmetrical prostate gland. To perform DRE, the primary care provider inserts a lubricated, gloved finger into the rectum to palpate the posterior surface of the prostate gland. This allows estimation of the size, shape, and consistency (firm but soft versus hard) of the gland.
- A routine *urinalysis* is done to detect signs of urinary tract infection.

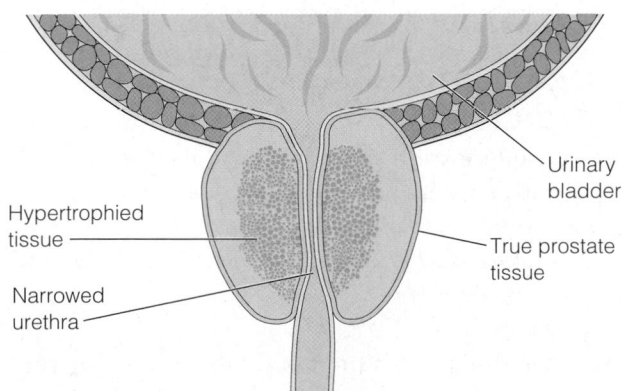

Figure 34-1. ■ Benign prostatic hyperplasia (BPH).

Hypertrophied tissue

Narrowed urethra

Urinary bladder

True prostate tissue

BOX 34-1	

MANIFESTATIONS OF BENIGN PROSTATIC HYPERPLASIA

- Nocturia (early symptom)
- Diminished force of urinary stream
- Hesitancy in starting voiding
- Dribbling after voiding
- Incomplete bladder emptying
- Frequency, urgency
- Urge incontinence
- Dysuria, hematuria

- *Prostate-specific antigen (PSA)* levels may be somewhat higher than normal in BPH (see Chapter 33), ⟨⟩ but are significantly elevated with prostate cancer.
- *Uroflowmetry* may be done to determine the degree of urethral obstruction.

Medications

Several drugs may be used to shrink the enlarged prostate and reduce the manifestations of BPH. Finasteride (Proscar) inhibits the conversion of testosterone to DHT in the prostate, causing the gland to shrink. It is most effective in men with significantly enlarged prostate glands. This drug affects libido and can cause impotence.

Alpha$_1$ blockers such as terazosin (Hytrin), doxazosin (Cardura), and tamsulosin (Flomax) relax smooth muscle in the prostate, the urethra, and the bladder neck. Smooth muscle relaxation reduces urethral obstruction and improves urinary flow and symptoms of BPH.

Complementary Therapies

Saw palmetto is an herbal therapy that reduces the symptoms of BPH. Its effects are similar to those of finasteride, although its mechanism of action is unknown. It causes few side effects and is considered to be a safe herbal remedy. Other plant extracts such as the bark of *Pygeum africanum,* the roots of *Echinacea purpurea,* pollen extract, and trembling poplar leaves are reported to have beneficial effects, although their safety and efficacy has not been established.

Surgery

Clients with BPH may need surgery to relieve urinary obstruction. Only the portion of the prostate gland surrounding the urethra is removed in BPH. *Transurethral incision of the prostate (TUIP)* and *transurethral resection of the prostate (TURP)* are the most common procedures used. In the TUIP procedure, small incisions are made in the prostate and the bladder neck to widen the urethra. No tissue is removed, and this procedure can be done on an outpatient basis.

In a TURP, obstructing prostate tissue is removed using the wire loop of a *resectoscope* inserted through the urethra (Figure 34-2 ■). Irrigating fluid carries resected tissue into the bladder to be flushed out on completion of the procedure. TURP is a relatively low-risk procedure with few complications. After surgery, *retrograde ejaculation* (discharge of seminal fluid into the bladder instead of through the urethra) is common. Fluid volume excess with hyponatremia, also known as *transurethral syndrome,* is a potential complication of TURP. Nursing care for the client having a TURP is outlined in Box 34-2 ■.

Balloon urethroplasty or destroying excess prostate tissue with lasers or microwaves also may be used to treat BPH. These minimally invasive procedures can be done on an outpatient basis.

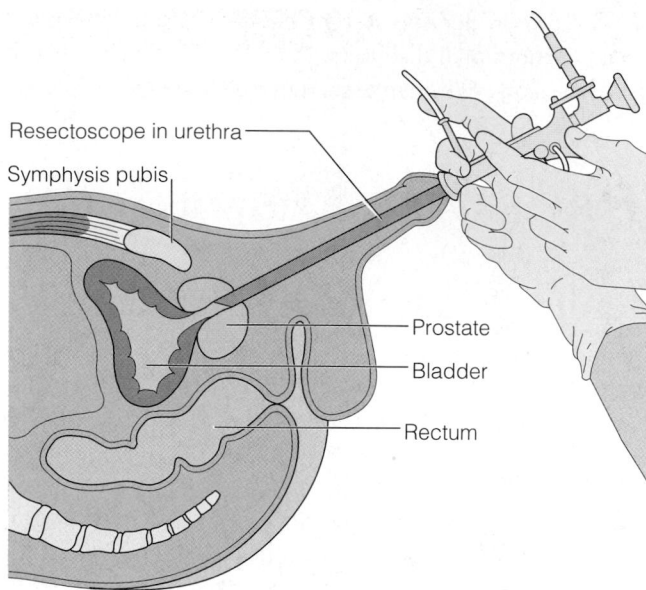

Figure 34-2. ■ Transurethral resection of the prostate (TURP). A resectoscope inserted through the urethra is used to remove excess prostate tissue.

NURSING CARE

ASSESSING

Ask older men about difficulty voiding, including difficulty starting and stopping the flow of urine, the size of the urinary stream, and any symptoms such as burning, frequency, urgency, or nocturia. Monitor urine output, including amount (total and per voiding), color, clarity, and odor.

DIAGNOSING, PLANNING, AND IMPLEMENTING

Although BPH itself is not a life-threatening condition, its consequences (urinary retention) can be.

Priorities in Nursing Care. Educating the client and monitoring for adverse effects of the disorder and its treatment are priority nursing responsibilities.

Ineffective Therapeutic Regimen Management

- Provide information about BPH and its treatment. Refer client to primary care provider or a urologist. *Most men are aware that BPH is very common, but are unsure of the function or exact location of the prostate gland. To make decisions, clients need to know about possible treatment options and their effects.*
- Advise to drink 2 to 3 liters of fluids daily, unless contraindicated by heart or kidney disease. *Fluids help prevent urinary tract infections and reduce dysuria.*

BOX 34-2	NURSING CARE CHECKLIST

Transurethral Resection of the Prostate (TURP)

Before Surgery

☑ Provide routine preoperative care and teaching (see Chapter 9). ⊂⊃

☑ Inform client that he will return from surgery with a urinary catheter in place.

After Surgery

☑ Provide routine postoperative care (see Chapter 9). ⊂⊃

☑ Assess and manage pain, which may include urethral discomfort, bladder spasms, and abdominal cramping due to gas.

☑ Use aseptic technique when managing urinary drainage and irrigation.

☑ Maintain accurate intake and output, accounting for amounts of irrigating solution used. Irrigant may be counted as intake, or, depending on hospital protocol, the amount of irrigant instilled may be subtracted from urinary output to accurately determine the amount of urine output.

☑ When allowed, encourage a liberal fluid intake.

☑ Frequently assess catheter patency; record color and character of urine. Light red to red urine with small clots is expected for up to 24 hours after surgery. The urine should gradually clear of clots and become light pink to yellow after 24 to 48 hours.

☑ For the first 24 to 48 hours, monitor for hemorrhage (frankly bloody urine, large blood clots, decreased urinary output, increasing bladder spasms, decreased hemoglobin and hematocrit, tachycardia, and hypotension). Notify physician if manifestations occur.

☑ Explain that catheter may cause a sensation of needing to void. Instruct to avoid straining to void or when having a bowel movement.

☑ If a continuous bladder irrigation (CBI) is present, maintain irrigating fluid flow rate to keep the output light pink or colorless.

☑ Report changes in vital signs, mental status, and laboratory results.

☑ If CBI is not used, follow agency procedure and physician orders for irrigating the indwelling catheter (usually when the urine is frankly bloody or has numerous larger blood clots, or when bladder spasms increase).

☑ After catheter removal, assess amount, color, and consistency of voided urine. Explain that burning, dribbling, and small clots in the urine are common after catheter removal.

☑ Teach Kegel exercises (see Chapter 32, Box 32-3) ⊂⊃ and to start and stop the urine stream several times during each voiding to reduce incontinence.

☑ Maintain antiembolic stockings and pneumatic compression devices as ordered. Assist with leg exercises and ambulation as ordered.

■ Advise to restrict alcohol intake, especially late at night, to minimize problems with nocturia. *Nocturia can pose a safety risk for older men who may have age-related changes in vision, muscle strength, and coordination.*

Excess Fluid Volume

■ Assess for manifestations of fluid volume excess and hyponatremia (see Chapter 7 ⊂⊃). *Irrigating fluid absorbed through disrupted tissues of the urethra and bladder can lead to fluid volume excess and hyponatremia.*

clinical ALERT

Transurethral syndrome, resulting from the large amounts of irrigating fluid used during and after surgery, can affect cardiovascular or pulmonary status, and lead to altered mental status.

■ Weigh daily. Monitor intake and output, including irrigating fluid used during and after surgery. Subtract the amount of irrigating solution used after surgery from the amount of output to determine the urine output. *Frequent assessments help identify fluid volume excess. Weight is an effective indicator of fluid volume status.*

■ Restrict fluids and administer diuretics as ordered. *Fluid restriction conserves sodium, and diuretics decrease total fluid load.*

Impaired Urinary Elimination

■ Change from leg drainage bag to a larger night drainage bag at bedtime. *A bag suspended from the bed frame at night permits gravity drainage of urine and prevents reflux of urine back into the bladder.*

■ Avoid strapping the leg bag on too tightly. *Tight straps can decrease venous return and increase risk for thrombophlebitis and complications such as pulmonary emboli.*

■ Place a soft cloth between the leg bag and thigh *to decrease friction and absorb dampness under the bag, reducing the risk of skin irritation.*

■ Empty the leg bag every 3 to 4 hours *to prevent overfilling.*

Promptly report any unexpected changes in urine color, consistency, or odor to the physician. Report continued hematuria, evidence of frank bleeding, or large blood clots, as well as a lack of or significant decrease in urine output because these may be manifestations of a complication such as hemorrhage or infection.

■ Obtain a bladder scan (see Chapter 31) 🔗 as ordered or as indicated to assess urinary retention following catheter removal. *Bladder scan is a noninvasive method of assessing bladder emptying that can be performed at the client's bedside.*

EVALUATING

Collect the following data to evaluate the effectiveness of nursing interventions for a client with BPH or who has had surgery to treat BPH:

■ Urine output, including amount, color, clarity, and odor
■ Ability to control urine flow without incontinence or dribbling

■ Knowledge and understanding of treatment options
■ Ability to manage home care, and understanding of when to contact the physician.

Documenting. Document continuing assessment data for clients treated medically in the community and for clients who undergo surgery. Include ability to initiate urine flow, amount and appearance of urine output, and residual urine remaining in bladder. If surgery is performed, document presence and degree of hematuria. Note level of pain, its location and type, as well as analgesia provided and its effectiveness. Document all teaching and recommendations for follow-up appointments or care.

CONTINUING CARE

Clients often are discharged within 2 days following a TURP. When TURP is done on an outpatient basis, the client may be discharged with an indwelling urinary catheter. Provide home care instructions as noted under Impaired Urinary Elimination above. Box 34-3 ■ outlines discharge instructions after prostate surgery. Address concerns about sexuality following prostate surgery, providing referral to counseling or support services as indicated.

BOX 34-3	CLIENT TEACHING

Prostate Surgery

Activity

Healing requires 4 to 8 weeks. Avoid strenuous activity and heavy lifting. Do not drive for 2 weeks. Take long walks, but take stairs slowly and carefully. Continue leg exercises (dorsiflexing the foot) to prevent blood clots in the legs. You can take showers, but avoid tub baths while the catheter is in place.

Bleeding

Bleeding may occur after a bowel movement, coughing, or increased exercise. If you notice blood in the urine, increase fluids and rest until urine is clear. If you have clots or are unable to urinate, call your doctor immediately. Avoid aspirin and nonsteroidal anti-inflammatory drugs (NSAIDs) for at least 2 weeks.

Bowel Movements

Keep bowel movements regular and soft to avoid pressure on the prostate area. Drink fruit juices and take stool softeners as ordered.

Diet

Resume your normal diet. Increase fluids to ten 8-ounce glasses daily. Avoid alcohol unless otherwise advised by your physician.

Sexual Intercourse

Do not have sex for 6 weeks after surgery to avoid bleeding. You may still have erections even with the catheter in place. When you resume sex, ejaculate may flow back into the bladder, so you express little or no semen.

Urination

After the catheter is removed, you may experience some burning, stinging, or leakage for several weeks, and you may pass small blood clots occasionally. These symptoms disappear as the area heals. Use pads to control leakage.

Work

If work is not strenuous, you may return in 4 weeks. Otherwise, wait 6 to 8 weeks.

Contact your doctor immediately if:
■ You are unable to urinate.
■ Bleeding is excessive or is not controlled by fluids and rest.
■ You have chills and fever or severe abdominal pain.
■ Your scrotum becomes swollen and tender.
■ You have pain in one calf, chest pain, or difficulty breathing.

Prostate Cancer

At all ages, African American men have a higher incidence of prostate cancer than European American men. African Americans also are more likely to die of prostate cancer, with a mortality rate more than double that of other racial and ethnic groups. Increasing awareness of the risk for prostate cancer and screening procedures is particularly important in populations of African American men. To improve care and reduce the risk for advanced prostate cancer, recommend that all African American men have a yearly DRE and serum PSA from age 45 on.

MANIFESTATIONS OF PROSTATE CANCER

Genitourinary
- Dysuria, hesitancy, reduced urinary stream
- Frequency, nocturia, hematuria
- Erectile dysfunction
- Hard, enlarged prostate on DRE

Musculoskeletal
- Bone or joint pain
- Back pain

Neurologic
- Lower extremity weakness
- Bowel or bladder dysfunction

Systemic
- Weight loss
- Anemia, fatigue

Cancer of the Prostate

Cancer of the prostate is the most common type of cancer in North American men and the second leading cause of cancer death, following lung cancer. It is primarily a disease of older men, increasing in incidence with age and rarely occurring before age 40. In addition to age, race is a significant risk factor for prostate cancer (Box 34-4 ■). Other risk factors include a family history of the disease. Occupational exposure to certain chemicals, a diet high in animal fat, and high serum testosterone levels also may contribute to the risk.

When diagnosed early, prostate cancer is curable. When the cancer is confined to the prostate at diagnosis, the 5-year survival rate is 100%. Prostate cancers may grow slowly or aggressively.

PATHOPHYSIOLOGY

Prostate cancer is usually an *adenocarcinoma,* arising from glandular epithelial cells. It usually begins in the peripheral, posterior tissue of the gland. As the tumor grows larger, it may compress the urethra, obstructing urine flow. The tumor may spread locally to involve the seminal vesicles or bladder. It rarely invades the bowel.

Tumor metastasis is common. The pelvic lymph nodes are the most frequently involved. Distant metastases usually affect bony tissue, especially the pelvic bones and spinal column. Prostate cancer may also spread to the liver and lungs.

MANIFESTATIONS AND COMPLICATIONS

In the early stages, prostate cancer usually causes no symptoms. As the tumor grows and spreads, manifestations of urinary obstruction, metastasis, and general symptoms of the disease develop, as described in Box 34-5 ■.

Compression fractures of the spine are common, potentially causing loss of mobility and bowel and bladder function. Tumors may eventually involve bone marrow, resulting in severe anemias and impaired immune function.

INTERDISCIPLINARY CARE

Because prostate cancer is curable when diagnosed early, screening measures for early detection help reduce mortality.

The American Cancer Society recommends offering an annual DRE and serum PSA check after age 50. Men at high risk, including African American males and men with a strong family history of prostate cancer, should receive annual screening exams including DRE and serum PSA beginning at age 45.

Many treatment options are available for prostate cancer. Watchful waiting may be the treatment of choice if the tumor is slow growing and the client is elderly or has a limited expected life span (less than 10 years).

Diagnostic Tests

- *DRE* is done as a screening measure and when an enlarged prostate is suspected. In prostate cancer, the gland is enlarged and hard to palpation.
- *Serum PSA levels* increase significantly in prostate cancer.
- *Transrectal ultrasonography (TRUS)* is used to help differentiate prostate cancer from BPH (see Chapter 33). ∞
- A *tissue biopsy* is done to establish the diagnosis of prostate cancer. Tissue is obtained by either needle biopsy or transrectal ultrasound-guided biopsy. See Box 34-6 ■ for nursing care of the client undergoing a transrectal ultrasound-guided biopsy.
- *Bone scan, magnetic resonance imaging (MRI),* or *computed tomography (CT) scans* may be done to identify possible tumor metastasis.

Hormone Therapy

Hormone therapy is used to treat advanced prostate cancer. Hormone therapy can be accomplished by removing the testes (**orchiectomy**) or by using drugs. Drugs that block the effects of testosterone and other androgens inhibit tumor growth but do not cure prostate cancer. In advanced prostate cancer, hormone therapy may improve length and

BOX 34-6	NURSING CARE CHECKLIST

Transrectal Ultrasound-Guided Biopsy of the Prostate

Before the Procedure

☑ Reinforce teaching. The client will remain awake; a local anesthetic will be used. The client will have a feeling of rectal fullness, which may be very uncomfortable. A sharp pain (a "pinch") may be felt as the biopsy is obtained.

☑ Instruct to avoid aspirin products and nonsteroidal anti-inflammatory agents for a week before the biopsy.

☑ An enema is usually given prior to the examination.

☑ This procedure requires a signed consent.

After the Procedure

☑ Monitor vital signs and urine output for an hour following the procedure.

☑ Instruct to avoid strenuous activity for the rest of the day.

☑ Hematuria and some bloody streaks in the stool are expected for 24 to 48 hours after the procedure. Ejaculate also may contain blood for up to 2 weeks.

☑ Report unusual bleeding, such as blood clots in urine, bloody stools, or signs of infection, such as rectal pain, dysuria, and urgency.

quality of life. The disadvantage of hormone therapy is side effects such as loss of libido, erectile dysfunction (ED) (*impotence*), hot flashes, and **gynecomastia** (breast enlargement). The client who has had an orchiectomy may have body image problems due to losing the testicles.

Radiation Therapy

Radiation therapy may be used to treat prostate cancer, avoiding many of the adverse effects of prostate surgery, such as impotence and urinary incontinence. Radiation may be delivered either by external beam or implants of radioactive seeds (*brachytherapy*). Radiation therapy also may be used to reduce the size of bone metastasis, control pain, and restore function in clients with advanced prostate cancer. (See Chapter 12 ⦿ for nursing care of the client receiving radiation therapy.)

Surgery

Prostatectomy, surgical removal of the prostate gland, may be done to treat prostate cancer. In a *simple prostatectomy,* only the prostate tissue is removed. A *radical prostatectomy* involves removal of the prostate, prostatic capsule, seminal vesicles, and a portion of the bladder neck. Prostatectomy may be done by several different approaches. Table 34-1 ■ outlines different types of prostatectomy procedures with their specific nursing implications.

Most clients have problems with urinary incontinence and erectile dysfunction following radical prostatectomy.

To prevent or treat urinary incontinence, an artificial urinary sphincter may be surgically implanted (Figure 34-3 ■). The client with an artificial urinary sphincter must be able to manipulate the pump in the scrotum and to recognize when a problem with the appliance occurs.

Cryosurgery is a possible treatment option. Guided by ultrasound, a cryoprobe is inserted into the tumor. Prostate tissue is destroyed by intermittent freezing and thawing. This surgical treatment is associated with a risk of bladder outlet injury, urinary incontinence, impotence, and rectal damage.

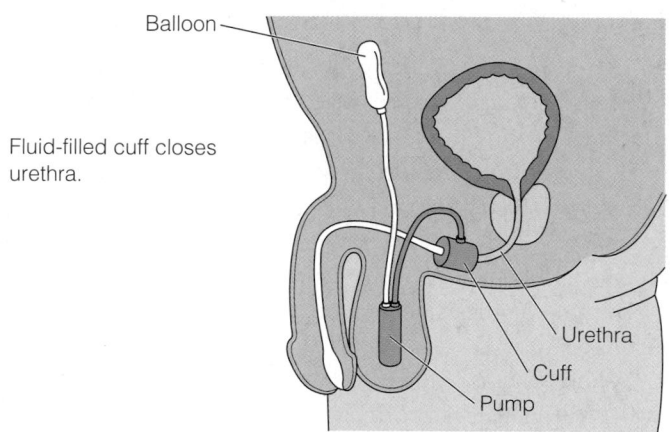

Fluid-filled cuff closes urethra.

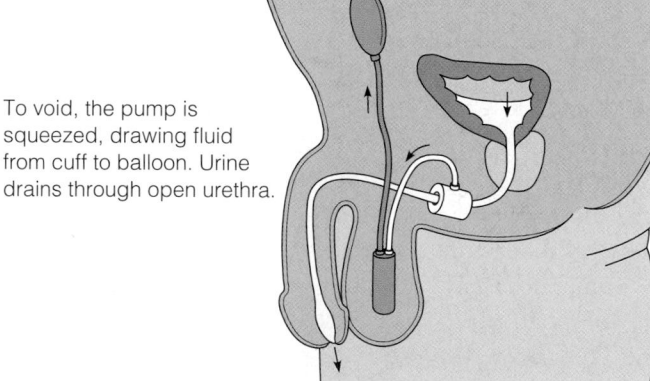

To void, the pump is squeezed, drawing fluid from cuff to balloon. Urine drains through open urethra.

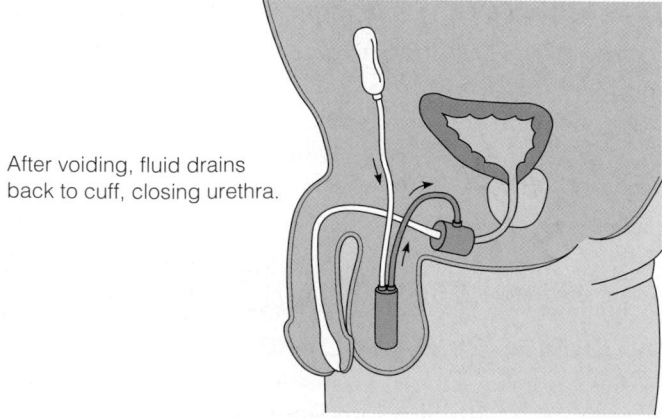

After voiding, fluid drains back to cuff, closing urethra.

Figure 34-3. ■ Operation of an artificial urinary sphincter.

TABLE 34-1

Approaches to Prostatectomy

ILLUSTRATION	DESCRIPTION	NURSING IMPLICATIONS
Retropubic prostatectomy 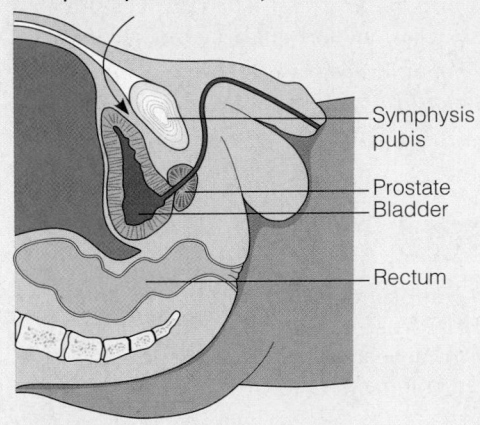 Symphysis pubis Prostate Bladder Rectum	The prostate gland is removed through an abdominal incision; the bladder is left intact.	Assess abdominal incision for urine drainage (none should be present) and signs of infection, such as redness, increased or purulent drainage, poor healing. Report to charge nurse or physician.
Suprapubic prostatectomy 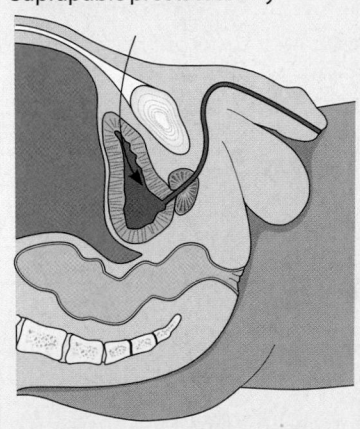	The prostate gland is removed through an abdominal incision into the bladder.	Assess urine output from suprapubic and urethral catheters. Assess abdominal dressing for urine drainage; change saturated dressings frequently. Consult with a skin care specialist if necessary. Following urethral catheter removal, clamp suprapubic catheter as ordered and encourage voiding. Assess residual urine by unclamping the catheter and measuring urine output after voiding.
Perineal prostatectomy 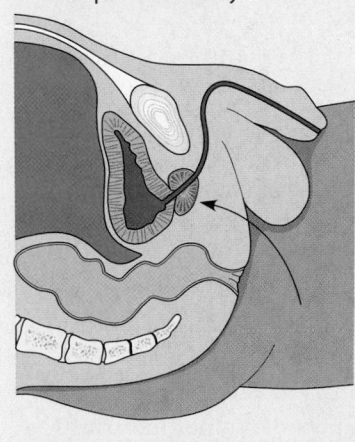	The prostate gland is removed through a perineal incision between the scrotum and anus.	Assess perineal incision for drainage and evidence of infection. Avoid rectal temperatures or enemas. Use a T-binder or padded scrotal support to hold dressing in place. Following dressing removal, heat lamps or sitz baths may be used to promote comfort and healing. Teach perineal irrigation as ordered and after bowel movements.

NURSING CARE

ASSESSING

In most cases, nursing assessment of a client with prostate cancer is done on admission to a facility for radiation ther-

apy or surgery. Refer to Chapter 12 ⦾ for assessment data to collect prior to radiation therapy. For the client undergoing prostate surgery, see Chapter 9 ⦾ for pre- and postoperative assessment data to collect. In addition, inquire about the client's understanding of his disease and the planned treatment.

DIAGNOSING, PLANNING, AND IMPLEMENTING

Priorities in Nursing Care. The effects of the enlarged prostate, the tumor, and treatment options on urinary elimination are the nursing care priority for clients undergoing treatment for prostate cancer. Because sexual dysfunction is a very real potential effect of treatment, it also is a nursing care priority.

Impaired Urinary Elimination (Risk for Incontinence)

- Assess the degree of incontinence and its impact on lifestyle. *Knowledge of the amount and type of incontinence and its effect on the client's life is used to plan appropriate nursing interventions.*
- Teach pelvic muscle exercises (Kegel exercises), and help plan a regular schedule to perform the exercises. *Pelvic muscle exercises can improve urine retention in the client with stress incontinence.*
- Refer to physical therapy or a continence specialist for additional measures. *Exercises, restricting some types of fluids, and other measures such as bladder training can often improve continence.*
- Teach methods to control dampness and odor.
  a. Advise maintaining a liberal fluid intake, only limiting fluids after dinner. *Restricting fluids does not prevent incontinence, although it may prevent nighttime episodes. Fluid restriction causes more concentrated urine, increasing odor problems.*
  b. Suggest using absorbent pads worn inside the underwear and changed as needed. *Most pads help control odor and dampness, increasing comfort.*
- Explore options such as an external collection device (external catheter or Texas catheter) for total incontinence. *This device, which collects urine as it leaves the urinary meatus, may improve self-esteem and allow resumption of social activities.*
- Encourage expression of feelings about the impact of incontinence on quality of life. *Listening to these concerns with sensitivity can help the client work through feelings and adapt to the inability to remain continent.*

Sexual Dysfunction

- Encourage discussion of sexual function between the client, his partner, and his physician. *Most older men are active sexually and fully capable of sustaining an erection. Some men may refuse therapy because they fear the effect of treatment on sexuality. Open discussion of concerns assists with decision making about treatment options.*
- Discuss various treatment options and their effects on sexual function. *The incidence of erectile dysfunction varies with different therapies for prostate cancer.*

- Encourage the client to discuss concerns about sexuality with a counselor or therapist. *A therapist or counselor may be able to suggest alternative ways for expressing sexuality.*

Pain

- Assess intensity, location, and quality of pain. *Because most clients with prostate cancer are over age 65, many have pain from other conditions such as osteoarthritis. Careful assessment helps identify its cause and direct treatment.*

> ### clinical ALERT
>
> Promptly report complaints of leg or chest pain. Pelvic surgery and pelvic tumors are risk factors for deep venous thrombosis, which can lead to pulmonary embolus, a potentially life-threatening emergency.

- Teach pain-control methods, including pharmacologic and nonpharmacologic measures. (See Chapters 8 ⚭ and 12 ⚭ for more information about pain control in the client with cancer.) *Adequate pain management enhances quality of life and allows the client to remain active.*

EVALUATING

To evaluate the effectiveness of nursing interventions for the client with prostate cancer, collect data such as the following:

- Ability to control urination and remain continent
- If incontinent, ability to control odor and dampness; maintain social activities
- Willingness to discuss sexuality and consider the effects of treatment on sexuality
- Pain level on a standard pain scale.

See the Critical Thinking Care Map at the end of this chapter on caring for a client with prostate cancer.

Documentation. Document all instruction provided about prostate cancer and its treatment, as well as responses of the client, spouse, and family to the information and treatment options. Document continuing assessment data, including effects of the tumor on urinary output, cancer manifestations, and any symptoms of possible tumor metastasis.

CONTINUING CARE

Clients with prostate cancer face both the diagnosis of cancer and a number of treatment options. The client and family must deal with often conflicting advice from the urologist, medical and radiation oncologists, friends, the media, and advocate groups. Provide accurate information about available treatments and their effects. Encourage discussion of concerns. Provide information about prostate cancer support groups (if available). Men struggling with treatment choices may learn about the options from men who have experience.

Emphasize the importance of keeping appointments for treatment and follow-up. Following treatment, yearly DRE and PSA levels are done. Discuss early warning signs of metastasis to the spinal column, such as intermittent back pain that is aggravated by activity. Other symptoms include leg weakness. Provide verbal and written instructions about prescribed medications, including their purpose, dose, timing, and expected and unintended effects.

If surgery has been done, provide postoperative instructions about catheter and dressing care, diet, activity resumption, and possible complications. Include family and significant others in teaching.

Provide information to all male clients about the importance of screening tests to detect prostate cancer early. The American Cancer Society has free pamphlets about early detection of prostate cancer.

Prostatitis

Prostatitis (inflammation of the prostate gland) is a relatively common problem in young and middle-aged men. While prostatitis may be caused by a bacterial infection, nonbacterial prostatitis is the most common type seen.

PATHOPHYSIOLOGY AND MANIFESTATIONS

Acute bacterial prostatitis is often associated with lower urinary tract infections. The infecting organism is usually *Escherichia coli,* but other pathogens may also invade the prostate. Infected urine may reflux into the prostatic ducts, or perhaps organisms may ascend the urinary tract. There is evidence that contamination of the urinary *meatus* (opening of the urethra) during vaginal or anal sexual intercourse may play a role in ascending infections.

Nonbacterial prostatitis may be caused by organisms such as chlamydiae, mycoplasmas, and viruses, but its exact

---

BOX 34-7

MANIFESTATIONS OF PROSTATITIS
- Pain, burning on urination
- Frequency, urgency
- Chills, fever
- Low back, perineal, or genital pain
- Pain following ejaculation
- Obstructed urine flow

---

cause is unknown. Nonbacterial prostatitis may be a type of sexually transmitted disease or an autoimmune disorder. Manifestations of prostatitis are listed in Box 34-7 ■.

INTERDISCIPLINARY CARE

It is often difficult to diagnose prostatitis. Urine and prostatic secretions are examined, and cultures are done to identify bacteria.

Bacterial prostatitis is treated with appropriate antibiotics. Extended antibiotic therapy may be necessary (up to 4 months) to eradicate the infection. Nonbacterial prostatitis is treated symptomatically. Nonsteroidal anti-inflammatory drugs (NSAIDs) are useful for pain, and anticholinergics may reduce voiding symptoms.

NURSING CARE

Instruct clients with prostatitis to increase fluid intake to about 3 liters daily and to void often. Advise them to maintain regular bowel habits. These measures help decrease pain with voiding and defecation. Local heat, such as sitz baths, may help relieve pain and irritation. Stress the importance of finishing the course of antibiotic therapy to effectively treat the infection. In nonbacterial prostatitis, frequent ejaculation may help decrease congestion of the gland.

Frank discussion with the client is important. It may help to explain nonbacterial prostatitis as a chronic inflammatory disorder, similar to arthritis. Address misconceptions about the disease with the client and his partner. Sexual intercourse is actually helpful, and men cannot "infect" their partners.

DISORDERS OF THE TESTES AND SCROTUM

Structural and Inflammatory Disorders

TESTICULAR TORSION

Testicular torsion, or twisting of the testes and spermatic cord, is a potential medical emergency. Boys and young

men up to age 20 are at greatest risk for testicular torsion. Its cause is unclear, although elevated hormone levels and abnormal attachment of the testicles to the scrotum may contribute. Trauma to the scrotum may precipitate the condition in clients who are already predisposed.

Testicular torsion causes acute scrotal pain with a sudden onset. Nausea and vomiting frequently occur. The *cremasteric reflex* (retraction of the testicles when the skin on the inside of the thigh is stroked) may be depressed or absent.

> ## clinical ALERT
>
> Advise men with symptoms of testicular torsion to seek immediate medical treatment because a delay in treatment can result in necrosis and loss of the affected testicle.

Diagnostic studies such as testicular scanning may be used to evaluate blood flow to the testicle. Emergency surgery is done to relieve testicular and spermatic cord twisting and to fix the testicle within the scrotum. Impaired blood flow to the testicle can lead to testicular ischemia and necrosis. If the testicle is necrotic or severely damaged, it will be removed.

An episode of torsion is frightening for the adolescent male. He is usually very embarrassed by the problem and may imagine that early sexual activity or even fantasies that result in erections are responsible. Because adolescents are not likely to volunteer these concerns, the nurse should provide information to relieve some of these anxieties. Postoperative nursing care is similar to that for clients with scrotal surgeries, as discussed later in the section on testicular cancer.

CRYPTORCHIDISM

Cryptorchidism is failure of one or both testes to descend through the inguinal ring into the scrotum. In most cases, the testes descend without intervention in the first year of life. Cryptorchidism is primarily a childhood problem, although on rare occasions it is missed and discovered later in adolescent or adult life. When the problem continues into adolescence and adulthood, cryptorchidism increases the risk for testicular cancer and problems of fertility. Men who have a history of cryptorchidism should be especially vigilant about testicular self-examination. Teach the client how to perform testicular self-examination (see Box 34-8 on page 828). Emphasize the importance of regular exams, and discuss findings that should be reported to the physician.

EPIDIDYMITIS

Epididymitis is inflammation of the epididymis. It is usually caused by an infection spread from the bladder, urethra, prostate gland, or seminal vesicles. In younger men, the cause is often a sexually transmitted organism such as *Chlamydia trachomatis* or *Neissena gonorrhoeae*. In older men, epididymitis usually is associated with a urinary tract infection or prostatitis. Early manifestations include pain and local swelling; the scrotum may swell to the extent that it interferes with walking. Fever and general malaise also may develop. Sterility is a potential complication of epididymitis. Antibiotics are prescribed to treat epididymitis. Nurs-

ing care focuses on relieving symptoms of the disorder. Ice packs may be applied to the scrotum to relieve pain. A scrotal support is usually applied. Discuss the possibility of infertility. The client may wish to seek evaluation for this problem at a later date.

ORCHITIS

Orchitis is inflammation of the testicle. It is commonly caused by an infection from other parts of the genitourinary tract. It also can occur as a complication of mumps; the mumps virus is excreted in the urine. Adult men with mumps are at highest risk for this complication. Trauma, including vasectomy and other scrotal surgeries, may cause inflammation of the testes. Manifestations of orchitis include severe testicular pain and swelling. Possible complications include hydrocele and abscess. These can lead to infertility or impotence. Bacterial orchitis is treated with antibiotics. Treatment for viral orchitis may be symptomatic. An abscess may require surgical drainage or orchiectomy. Nursing care is very similar to that of the client with epididymitis and other scrotal disorders.

Infertility

Infertility is the inability to conceive a child during a year or more of unprotected intercourse. *Sterility* is the absolute inability to conceive. When the sperm count drops below 20 million/mL, the client is likely to be infertile. Male infertility usually results from a testicular disorder, such as cryptorchidism or orchitis. Less often, it may be caused by a systemic disease, hormonal disorder, or obstructed outflow of sperm from the testes. In many cases, no specific cause can be found for the infertility.

A sperm count is obtained to evaluate infertility in men. If an identifiable cause such as an endocrine disorder or varicocele (see next section) can be identified and treated, this may restore fertility. In many cases of male infertility, it is appropriate to counsel the client about options such as using a sperm donor or adopting a child.

Nursing care for the infertile male client focuses on providing information and psychologic support for the man and his partner.

Scrotal Masses and Trauma

Scrotal masses such as hydroceles, spermatoceles, and varicoceles (Figure 34-4 ■) usually are benign and treatable.

SCROTAL MASSES

A *hydrocele* is a collection of fluid in the sac that encloses the testes. The cause is not always identifiable, but it may follow epididymitis, orchitis, injury, or a tumor. Scrotal enlargement may be the only manifestation of hydrocele, although it may cause pain or a tight sensation in the scrotum.

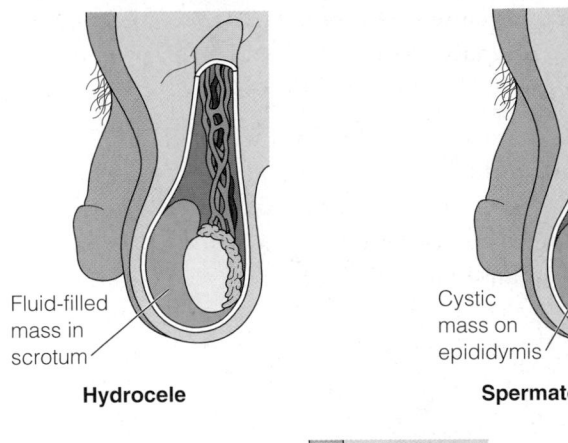

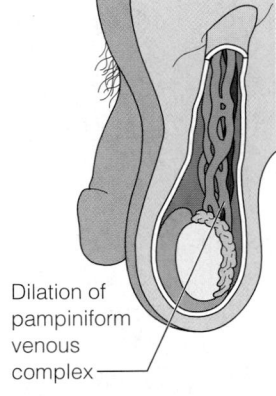

Figure 34-4. ■ Common scrotal masses.

Hydrocele is diagnosed by transillumination or ultrasound of the scrotum. Treatment is usually not necessary. If the hydrocele causes embarrassment or significant pain, a hydrocelectomy may be performed.

A *spermatocele* is a mobile, usually painless mass in the epididymis that contains dead sperm cells. The cause is thought to be leakage of sperm due to trauma or infection. Treatment is usually not necessary.

A *varicocele* is abnormal dilation of the spermatic veins above the testis. It is caused by incompetent or absent valves in the veins and almost always occurs on the left side. The dilated veins form a soft mass (often described as a "bag of worms") that can cause dull pain in the scrotum. This condition can decrease the sperm count and cause atrophy of the testicle, resulting in infertility. Varicoceles are usually treated, especially in younger clients.

SCROTAL TRAUMA

Scrotal trauma is usually minor, resulting in temporary hematomas caused by minor crushing or straddle-type injuries. More severe crush injuries can rupture the testicles. Occasionally, the client's clothing and scrotal skin can be trapped in moving machinery, resulting in avulsion injuries. Such an accident can tear the skin away from the penis and scrotum, sometimes releasing scrotal contents. Penetrating injuries of the scrotum due to knife or gunshot wounds also can occur. Treatment of scrotal trauma varies, depending on the extent of damage and the type of scrotal damage involved.

VASECTOMY-RELATED PROBLEMS

The most common surgery of the scrotum is **vasectomy,** a sterilization procedure in which a portion of the spermatic cord is removed. This surgery rarely causes long-term complications. However, some clients develop scar tissue that causes chronic pain. Other complications include chronic testicular pain and epididymal obstruction.

NURSING CARE

Obtain assessment data such as the following from clients who have a history of scrotal trauma, surgery, or who complain about scrotal swelling or pain:

- Ask about the onset, duration, and severity of symptoms.
- Inspect the scrotum for swelling, redness, and bruising or discoloration. Using a gloved hand, gently palpate each testis and epididymis for tenderness, warmth, or masses.

Teach the client with a scrotal disorder about the disorder and its treatment. If surgery is planned, discuss the client's fears about the surgery, pain management, and measures to reduce bleeding (see the section on testicular cancer that follows). Postoperatively, observe for swelling and discoloration of the scrotum. Report excessive swelling or discoloration to the physician, because this could indicate excessive bleeding. Discuss the possible effects of surgery on fertility, and actively listen to the client's concerns.

Testicular Cancer

Testicular cancer is the most common cancer in men between the ages of 15 and 35. Fortunately, it is one of the most treatable cancers, with a cure rate of greater than 90%.

Although its cause is unknown, risk factors for testicular cancer include the following:

- Age: Testicular cancer usually develops between ages 15 and 40, but may occur at any age.
- Cryptorchidism (undescended testicle)
- Family history
- Race and ethnicity: Men living in the United States, United Kingdom, and Scandinavia have a higher risk of developing testicular cancer than African and Asian men.

Unfortunately, most men who develop testicular cancer have no risk factors. Therefore, beginning at the age of 15, all men should perform monthly testicular self-examination (Box 34-8 ■).

BOX 34-8

TESTICULAR SELF-EXAMINATION

- Examine your testicles during or just after a warm shower or bath. Soap on your hands and scrotum allows easy manipulation of tissue.
- Gently roll each testicle between your thumb and fingers. The testicles normally feel smooth, rounded, walnut sized, and freely movable.

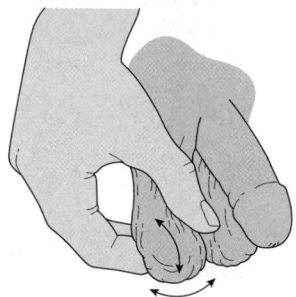

- If one testicle is significantly larger than the other, or if you feel any hard lumps, contact your health care provider immediately.
- Examine your testicles on the same day of each month (e.g., the first day of the month) to help you remember.

PATHOPHYSIOLOGY AND MANIFESTATIONS

Testicular cancer grows within the testicle, eventually replacing most of the normal tissue. Usually only one testicle is affected. Local spread is limited, but it often spreads rapidly through lymph and blood vessels to other organs. Spread by lymph vessels usually causes disease in retroperitoneal lymph nodes. Dissemination of the disease through the vascular system can lead to metastasis in the lungs, bone, or liver. The classic presenting symptom of testicular cancer is a painless hard nodule. Occasionally, the client may have a dull ache in the pelvis or scrotum. Acute pain related to the tumor is rare.

INTERDISCIPLINARY CARE

Care focuses on diagnosing and eliminating the cancer and preventing or treating metastasis. Treatment depends on the stage of the cancer at diagnosis: Stage I is confined to the testicle; stage II includes regional lymph node involvement; in stage III, distant metastases are present.

When testicular cancer is suspected, blood is drawn to identify tumor markers such as *alpha-fetoprotein (AFP)*, *human chorionic gonadotropin (HCG)*, *alkaline phosphatase*, and *lactic dehydrogenase (LDH)*. Elevated levels indicate probable testicular cancer. These markers are also measured after surgery to help monitor the effectiveness of treatment.

An *ultrasound of the testicle* is performed to rule out other causes of the mass. *CT scans* are done to detect possible metastasis to the lungs or abdominal organs. Biopsy is often done at the time of surgery.

Medications

Stage III testicular cancer is treated with a combination of surgery and chemotherapy. A combination of chemotherapy drugs is used. (See Chapter 12 for more information about chemotherapy for cancer and management of chemotherapy side effects.)

Surgery

Surgery to remove the affected testicle and spermatic cord (called a *radical orchiectomy*) is the primary treatment for early testicular cancer. This operation is performed through an incision in the inguinal area. Lymph nodes in the retroperitoneal area may also be removed, taking care to preserve the nerves necessary for ejaculation. Following removal of the testis, a saline-filled prosthesis may be inserted into the scrotum.

Radiation Therapy

Following surgery, radiation therapy is used to treat cancer in the retroperitoneal lymph nodes, the most frequent site of metastasis. The client may experience temporary diarrhea, nausea, or decreased bone marrow function. These problems are usually mild. (See Chapter 12 for more information about nursing care related to radiation therapy.)

NURSING CARE

ASSESSING

Nurses can be instrumental in identifying testicular cancer at an early, treatable stage. Ask men if they have noticed any change in the size of their testicles. In some cases, the client's partner may notice a change in the size or feel of one testicle compared to the other. Palpate the scrotum and testicles, noting any difference in size or changes from the normal. Promptly report to the physician a testicle that is hard, irregular in shape, or is fixed (not movable within the scrotum).

DIAGNOSING, PLANNING, AND IMPLEMENTING

Priorities in Nursing Care. The client with an orchiectomy often is discharged on the day of surgery. Nursing care focuses on teaching and psychologic support.

Deficient Knowledge

- Discuss using analgesics, ice bags, and a scrotal support to reduce postoperative pain. *Ice provides local analgesia and helps reduce scrotal swelling. A scrotal support is particularly helpful when the client ambulates. See Chapter 9 for routine pre- and postoperative care and teaching.*

- Instruct to contact the physician if complications develop: the incision gaps open, bleeding beyond slight oozing after 24 hours, or rapid scrotal swelling. *Because the client is usually discharged early, complications may not develop until after discharge.*

Risk for Sexual Dysfunction

- Assess current sexual function. To do this, establish an atmosphere of openness and permission to discuss sexual concerns. *After the initial shock of the diagnosis, clients often have intense concerns about sexual and reproductive issues, which can be relieved only by information.*
- Help the client express his concerns about altered sexual function and appearance. *The ability to express sexuality and father children is a basic human need. The client may fear the loss of this ability, and will grieve its loss if treatment affects it.*
- Reinforce teaching about the expected effect of surgery on sexuality. Reassure that erectile and climactic function is rarely affected by testicular cancer and treatment. *If the treatment involves only an orchiectomy, there should be no lasting effects on sexual or reproductive function.*
- Discuss the option of preserving sperm in a bank prior to treatment. *This option may help relieve fears about the ability to father children in the future. Sperm banking must be done prior to treatment with surgery, chemotherapy, or radiation therapy.*

EVALUATING

To evaluate the effectiveness of nursing care for clients with testicular cancer, collect data such as the following:

- Ability to demonstrate and relate the importance of regular testicular self-examination
- Understanding of ways to reduce pain and swelling after surgery

- Knowledge of manifestations of complications and when to contact the physician
- Willingness to discuss or ask questions about effect of treatment on sexuality and reproduction

Documenting. Document teaching provided, the client's and family's understanding of the information, and recommendations or appointments for follow-up care.

CONTINUING CARE

> **clinical ALERT**
>
> Teach all young men how to perform testicular self-examination and stress the importance of establishing a routine.

Shower cards that demonstrate testicular self-exam on one side and breast self-exam on the other are available through the American Cancer Society. These cards serve as useful reminders.

Include families in teaching for the client with testicular cancer. If the client is sexually active, his partner needs information about the effects of treatment on sexuality and reproduction. If the client is a teenager, his parents often are involved in postoperative care. The client facing cancer needs the support of knowledgeable loved ones.

Teach postoperative care, including incision care, use of ice and a scrotal support, and signs and symptoms of complications to report to the physician.

Discuss the need for continuing follow-up after treatment for testicular cancer. Surveillance includes periodic physical examinations, chest x-rays, tumor markers, and CT scans of retroperitoneal nodes for 5 to 10 years after orchiectomy.

DISORDERS OF THE PENIS

Phimosis

Phimosis is constriction of the foreskin so that it cannot be pushed back over the glans penis. It may be congenital or may follow infection or injury. Phimosis increases the risk of secondary infections, scarring, and perhaps cancer of the penis. Severe phimosis can interfere with urination. If the foreskin is forcibly retracted behind the glans, it may become trapped, impairing blood flow to the glans. Circumcision (removal of the foreskin) may be necessary to correct the condition. Teach clients and parents about the importance of hygiene measures to prevent infection and possible phimosis. Teach clients with phimosis to perform self-examination for cancer of the penis.

Priapism

Priapism is a sustained, painful erection that is not associated with sexual arousal. It is caused by impaired blood flow in the corpora cavernosa of the penis. Priapism may be idiopathic or be secondary to certain conditions or drugs (Box 34-9 ■). The sustained erection of priapism often is painful and harder than normal. If the condition continues, there is a risk of tissue damage and impotence.

Initial treatment of priapism includes analgesia, sedation, and fluids. In clients with sickle cell disease, transfusion and oxygen are provided. Ice packs to the perineum may provide relief. If other measures are ineffective, surgery may be done to temporarily drain blood out of the penis.

Inspect the penis for degree of erection and color; palpate its firmness and degree of rigidity. Monitor urine output. Report oliguria or signs of acute urinary retention. Provide analgesics as ordered to manage pain. Address the client's anxiety about the condition, pain, treatment, and the threat to sexual function. Reassure the client that potency usually is maintained after surgical shunting. The client may be acutely embarrassed by the erection; address his concerns and reassure him that the erection is not within his control.

Cancer of the Penis

Cancer of the penis is rare in North America. Older men are most often affected. Its cause is uncertain. Phimosis, tightening of the foreskin that prevents retraction over the glans, is a significant risk factor. Penile cancer also is linked to viral infections, human papillomavirus (HPV) in particular. Other risk factors include exposure to ultraviolet (UV) light, unprotected sex with multiple partners, and cigarette smoking.

PATHOPHYSIOLOGY AND MANIFESTATIONS

Squamous cell carcinoma accounts for 95% of all penile cancers. The tumor usually develops as a nodular or wartlike growth or a red velvety lesion on the glans or foreskin. The tumors tend to grow slowly. Penile cancer spreads to regional lymph nodes, and very late in the disease may spread to the bone, liver, or lungs. If the lesion is treated before nodes are involved, chances for a cure are good. Manifestations include a mass or persistent sore or ulcer at the distal end of the penis, involving the glans or foreskin. Most of these lesions are painless; however, they may ulcerate and bleed. Purulent, foul-smelling discharge may be noted under the foreskin.

INTERDISCIPLINARY CARE

Cancer of the penis is diagnosed by biopsy of the lesion and any suspicious lymph nodes. Small, localized lesions may be treated with a topical chemotherapy drug, external-beam radiation, laser, or surgical excision. The penis may be partially or totally amputated if the cancer has spread into deeper structures. If a total *penectomy* is done, a perineal urethrostomy is created to preserve urinary continence. Clients with distant metastases may be treated with chemotherapy.

NURSING CARE

When providing routine care, observe the penis for any visible lesions. If a lesion is noted, promptly report it to the physician. Following surgery, monitor the surgical site for healing and any signs of infection. Carefully monitor intake and output, and provide routine postoperative care. Inform the client that dribbling after voiding may occur for several weeks following surgery. Teach perineal care to reduce the risk of skin irritation and breakdown. Sitz baths may help relieve pain and promote healing. Carefully listen to concerns, being aware of the effect of a penectomy on body image, self-concept, and sexuality.

Documenting. Document assessment data, including any lesions. Note instructions provided and the client's and family's understanding of information.

CONTINUING CARE

To help prevent cancer of the penis, teach clients about the risks of unprotected sex, and encourage condom use. Inform clients about the possible link between UV rays and penile cancer, and encourage men to shield their genitals when sunbathing or using tanning salons. Discuss the importance of seeking prompt treatment for any lesion or abnormal drainage noted on the penis.

DISORDERS OF SEXUAL EXPRESSION

Erectile Dysfunction

Erectile dysfunction (ED) or **impotence** is the inability to attain and maintain an erection that allows satisfactory sexual intercourse. An estimated 10 million to 15 million men in the United States have ED. Most are older than 65. This problem may involve total inability to achieve erection, an inconsistent ability to achieve erection, or the ability to sustain only brief erections.

There are many possible causes of ED, including many chronic diseases such as diabetes and atherosclerosis, and many drugs. In most men, the cause of ED is primarily physiologic. Psychologic factors also contribute and are believed to cause 10% to 20% of cases of ED.

PATHOPHYSIOLOGY

A number of physiologic mechanisms work together to cause an erection. For an erection to occur, the blood supply to the penis must be adequate, normal nervous system and hormonal actions are necessary, and appropriate psychologic and social responses need to occur. Interruption of any of these factors and certain drugs can lead to impotence.

Atherosclerosis can interfere with the arterial blood supply to the penis. Surgeries such as radical prostatectomy or chronic diseases such as diabetes or multiple sclerosis can disrupt innervation. Decreased testosterone levels also can lead to erectile dysfunction. Many drugs, including antihypertensive medications, psychotropic drugs, hormones, and others, disrupt the normal mechanisms to achieve erection, leading to impotence.

INTERDISCIPLINARY CARE

ED often can be effectively managed using drugs, mechanical devices, or surgery.

Diagnostic Tests

Diagnostic tests are done to help identify the cause of the problem:

- *Blood tests,* such as a chemistry profile and testosterone, prolactin, thyroxine, and PSA levels, are done to identify systemic disorders that may be causing the dysfunction.
- *Nocturnal penile tumescence and rigidity (NPTR)* monitors erections that occur during rapid eye movement (REM) sleep. This test may be done in a sleep laboratory or at home with a portable device.
- *Cavernosometry* and *cavernosography* evaluate blood flow to and from the penis.

Medications

Erectile dysfunction can be treated with drugs that work in a variety of ways. Sildenafil (Viagra) for ED was approved for use in 1998. Sildenafil and related drugs do not directly cause an erection but enhance the natural response to sexual stimuli. At recommended doses, no effect occurs in the absence of sexual stimulation. Table 34-2 ■ discusses nursing implications for these drugs. The onset and duration of action of these drugs vary; review information specific to the prescribed drug before teaching.

> ### clinical ALERT
>
> Sildenafil and related drugs can cause a dangerous drop in blood pressure when used together with nitrates (including nitroglycerin to treat angina). Advise men who use nitrates to prevent or treat angina to talk to their cardiologist before taking ED drugs, and instruct all men using these drugs to avoid use of recreational nitrates.

Testosterone replacement also may be ordered for men with ED. Aldostadil (prostaglandin E_1) can be administered by inserting a semisolid pellet into the urethra or by direct injection into the penis. This drug stimulates an erection, but many men discontinue treatment because of the mode of delivery or dissatisfaction with lack of spontaneity. Transdermal nitroglycerin paste applied directly to the penis is another option to promote blood flow and erection.

Mechanical Devices

Men who cannot take sildenafil may use a *vacuum constriction device (VCD)* that draws blood into the penis with a vacuum, trapping it there with a constricting band at the base of the penis. This device, however, is cumbersome and may be an unacceptable option for many men.

TABLE 34-2

Nursing Implications for Pharmacology: Erectile Dysfunction

DRUG/CLASS	ACTION	NURSING IMPLICATIONS	CLIENT AND FAMILY TEACHING
Sildenafil (Viagra) Tadalafil (Cialis) Varderafil (Levitra)	These drugs are used to treat erectile dysfunction in men. They work together with nitric oxide and an enzyme released during sexual stimulation to increase the firmness and duration of an erection. The duration of effect varies among these drugs.	Contraindicated for men taking any form of nitrate drug (including recreational nitrates); combination can cause significant hypotension. Relatively contraindicated for men who have cardiovascular disease. May cause priapism, especially in men with other risk factors. Approved only for use in men.	Take the drug approximately 30 minutes to 1 hour before sexual activity. Drug effect may diminish after 2 to 36 hours; do not take more than once a day. If you have high blood pressure or cardiovascular disease, check with your doctor before taking. Promptly report erection that lasts more than 4 hours, chest pain, or shortness of breath.

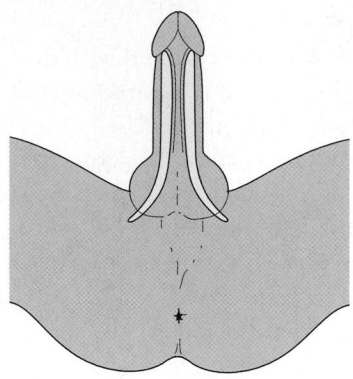

A Semirigid

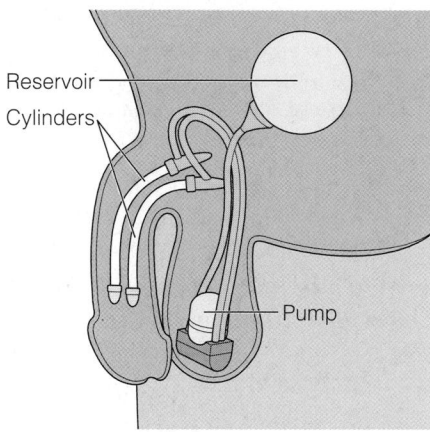

Reservoir
Cylinders
Pump

B Inflatable

Figure 34-5. ■ Types of penile implants. (**A**) Semirigid rods implanted in the corpora cavernosa keep the penis in a constant state of semierection. (**B**) With an inflatable penile implant, the client compresses a pump in the scrotum to fill cylinders in the corpora cavernosa and achieve an erection. Pressing a release valve returns the fluid to a reservoir.

Surgery

When ED does not respond to less invasive methods of treatment, a semirigid or inflatable prosthesis may be implanted (Figure 34-5 ■). Clients are generally satisfied with the results of a penile implant. Partners are also likely to report satisfaction, although the more firm erection can cause pain or prolong the duration of intercourse for an unacceptable period. Client and partner teaching is mandatory. Counseling by a sex therapist may be needed to facilitate adaptation to the implant.

NURSING CARE

ASSESSING

Problems with erectile dysfunction often are revealed in the course of a health assessment interview. Ask about chronic diseases such as diabetes and thyroid conditions,

hypertension and other cardiovascular disease, kidney failure, and neurologic conditions. Inquire about medications such as antihypertensive drugs (which often cause ED), antidepressants, tranquilizers, and sedatives. Explore psychosocial stressors that may contribute to ED. Discuss lifestyle and use of alcohol or street drugs. Finally, ask specific questions about sexual function, including a history of premature ejaculation, impotence, or other sexual problems.

DIAGNOSING, PLANNING, AND IMPLEMENTING

Willingness of the nurse to discuss the client's sexuality often is important to bring the subject of erectile dysfunction into the open and to inform the client (and partner) that treatment is available.

Sexual Dysfunction

- Assess for risk factors such as a new medication or recent surgery. *Although most older men have at least one risk factor for ED, identifying specific risk factors can help focus treatment strategies.*
- Ask specific questions about sexual function and current sexual practices. *Men with ED and their partners often live in isolation with the problem for many years. The partner may be unaware of the problem or may believe the client has lost his attraction to the partner. The client may keep his problem secret because of an intense feeling of shame. Many clients greet the information about the high incidence of ED with a sense of relief that they are not alone.*
- Discuss previous methods of coping with ED. *Current coping strategies provide insight into the problem and help guide teaching.*
- Provide information about treatment options. *Information provides hope for successful resolution of the problem and helps the client and his partner identify acceptable treatment options.*
- Refer the client and his partner for counseling. *Although ED is primarily a physiologic problem, many clients benefit from counseling to address psychologic issues of ED.*

EVALUATING

To evaluate the effectiveness of nursing care for a client with erectile dysfunction, collect data such as the following:

- Willingness to discuss sexual function with a health care professional
- Willingness to share concerns with partner
- Knowledge of medical and surgical treatment options, their risks and benefits.

Documenting. Document teaching provided, as well as the client's and partner's apparent understanding and acceptance of information. Note any referrals provided.

CONTINUING CARE

To reduce the risk of ED, advise clients to remain physically active, consume a low-fat diet, and avoid cigarette smoking and excess alcohol intake. Discuss the potential effects of high-risk medications on sexual function with clients during teaching. Provide information about various treatment options for ED, including their cost, intended benefit, and potential risks or drawbacks of each option. Stress the importance of contacting the primary care provider before taking any prescription or over-the-counter drug to treat ED. Encourage partners to be involved in the treatment plan.

NURSING PROCESS CARE PLAN
Client with Erectile Dysfunction

Donald Lawton, 68 years old, has been married for 40 years. At age 52, he was diagnosed with type 2 diabetes mellitus. He has had stable angina controlled with sublingual nitroglycerin for the past 5 years. Two years ago, he noticed that his erections were not as rigid as normal. Gradually, the problem has worsened until he can no longer attain an erection adequate for sexual intercourse. His libido remains unaffected. He relates shame and embarrassment, and is unable to discuss this problem with anyone, including his wife.

Assessment. Mr. Lawton talks to his doctor after his wife threatens to leave him, claiming neglect. He is referred to a urologist. Mr. Lawton says he values his relationship with his wife and that sexual intimacy has been important to them. He says their sexual activity has always been limited to foreplay and sexual intercourse, expressing mild distaste about other forms of sexual intimacy. He reports feeling as if he is no longer a man and that he is ashamed that he can no longer satisfy his wife. This has affected their entire relationship and communications.

Mr. Lawton's serum testosterone levels are normal. Nocturnal penile tumescence and rigidity monitoring in the sleep laboratory reveal an absence of erections during REM sleep. The urologist prescribes varderafil (Levitra) and suggests couples counseling.

Diagnosis. The following nursing diagnoses are identified for Mr. Lawton:

- *Sexual Dysfunction* related to diabetes
- *Ineffective Sexuality Patterns* related to lack of knowledge and poor communication patterns with wife
- *Disturbed Body Image* related to change in erectile function

Expected Outcomes. The expected outcomes for the plan of care are that Mr. Lawton will:

- Demonstrate the ability to discuss sexual concerns with his wife.
- State acceptance of the change in his erectile function.
- Verbalize understanding of the use and potential adverse effects of varderafil.

Planning and Implementation. The following interventions are planned and implemented for Mr. Lawton:

- With permission, include his wife in discussions and teaching sessions.
- Encourage couples counseling.
- Listen to concerns about ED, and encourage communication.
- Teach about varderafil, its use, precautions, and potential adverse effects.

Evaluation. Mr. Lawton begins to discuss his sexual and relationship problems more readily. He and Mrs. Lawton begin to attend counseling. Mrs. Lawton states that she was afraid her husband no longer found her attractive and that he had found another woman. She greets the knowledge of the true nature of the problem with relief and concern. Privately, Mr. Lawton tells the nurse that he feels his marriage is improving and that even though "things" will never be the same, he is beginning to look forward to some mutual exploration. Mr. Lawton is able to use varderafil without adverse effects, and 4 months later reports that he and his wife are "90% satisfied with the result."

Critical Thinking in the Nursing Process

1. Mr. Lawton's ED was directly related to his diabetes. Describe the pathophysiology of diabetes-induced ED (see Chapter 17). ∞
2. How does the nocturnal penile tumescence and rigidity test differentiate between physiologic and psychologic causes of ED?
3. Discuss the importance of Mr. and Mrs. Lawton's lack of communication on the development of their sexual problems. Include possible reasons for their difficulty in discussing sexual concerns.

Ejaculatory Dysfunction

There are many types of ejaculatory dysfunction. *Premature ejaculation* is often caused by psychologic factors; diabetes also can cause premature ejaculation. *Delayed ejaculation* may be related to aging changes, such as decreased penile sensation or decreased libido. Ejaculation also can be affected by drugs to treat hypertension, depression, anxiety, and narcotic medications. *Retrograde ejaculation* (semen discharged into the bladder rather than through the urethra) is usually related to treatment of prostate disorders or testicular cancer.

Medical and nursing care for clients with ejaculatory problems focus on assessing the problem and client teaching. Of these problems, premature ejaculation is most easily treated. Wearing a condom and techniques such as relaxation and guided imagery can delay sexual excitement and ejaculation. The client's partner can be taught how to avoid excessive stimulation until ejaculation. If the problem persists, referral to a specialist is appropriate.

Note: The bibliography listings for this and all chapters have been compiled at the back of the book.

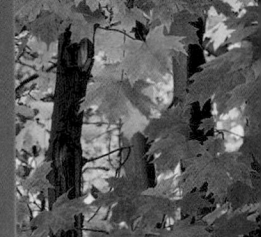

Chapter Review

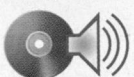 **KEY TERMS** by Topics

Use the audio glossary feature of either the CD-ROM or the Companion Website to hear the correct pronunciation of the following key terms.

Prostate disorders
benign prostatic hyperplasia (BPH), orchiectomy, gynecomastia, prostatectomy

Disorders of testes and scrotum
cryptorchidism, infertility, vasectomy

Disorders of sexual expression
erectile dysfunction (ED), impotence

KEY Points

- Prostate problems such as benign prostatic hyperplasia (BPH) and prostate cancer are the most common problems affecting the male reproductive system, especially in older adults.

- The manifestations of BPH and prostate cancer are similar: frequency, urgency, hesitancy, a reduced urine stream, and nocturia. Physical examination and diagnostic testing are necessary to differentiate these disorders.

- In both BPH and prostate cancer, medications or "watchful waiting" may be appropriate treatment; surgery, however, is often the treatment of choice. Minimally invasive procedures such as balloon dilation, laser prostatectomy, or transurethral incision of the prostate (TUIP) may be used to treat BPH. Prostate cancer, on the other hand, is treated with a prostatectomy.

- Following a prostatectomy, the client is at risk for deep venous thrombosis (DVT) and pulmonary embolism. Preventive measures such as leg exercises, elastic hose, pneumatic compression devices, and early ambulation are important to prevent these complications.

- Although testicular cancer is rare, its risk is highest in young men (15 to 35 years old). Teach all young men to perform testicular self-examination and stress the importance of doing it on a regular basis.

- Most clients with erectile dysfunction can be effectively treated with medication or an implanted prosthetic device.

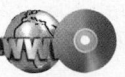 **EXPLORE Media**Link

Additional interactive resources for this chapter can be found on the Companion Website at www.prenhall.com/burke. Click on Chapter 34 and "Begin" to select the activities for this chapter.

For chapter-related NCLEX-style review questions and an audio glossary, access the accompanying CD-ROM in this book.

FOR FURTHER Study

See Chapter 7 for information about fluid volume excess and hyponatremia.

Chapter 8 discusses pain management.

Chapter 9 provides a discussion of routine preoperative and postoperative care.

For more information about radiation therapy and chemotherapy in the client with cancer, see Chapter 12.

For more information about the pathophysiology of diabetes-induced erectile dysfunction, see Chapter 17.

Chapter 31 gives more information about bladder scans.

For in-depth discussion of kidney function, see Chapter 32. For Kegel exercises, see Box 32-3.

For more information about prostate-specific antigen test and transrectal ultrasonography, see Chapter 33.

Critical Thinking Care Map

Caring for a Client with Prostate Cancer
NCLEX-PN® Focus Area: Safety and Infection Control

Case Study: William Turner is a 71-year-old African American man. He lives at home with his wife, who had a stroke 2 years ago. Mr. Turner has been in good health except for a "touch" of osteoarthritis in his hips and hands. He reports a gradual onset of urinary urgency during the past 2 years. During a routine physical examination, a hard nodule is palpated on his prostate gland, and his PSA level is found to be elevated. A radical retropubic prostatectomy is performed. He is discharged home several days later with an indwelling catheter in place. The home health nurse visits Mr. Turner 2 days after his discharge.

Nursing Diagnosis: Ineffective Health Maintenance

COLLECT DATA

Subjective	Objective
_____	_____
_____	_____
_____	_____
_____	_____
_____	_____
_____	_____
_____	_____

Would you report this data? Yes/No

If yes, to: _____

Nursing Care

_____
_____
_____
_____
_____
_____
_____
_____
_____
_____

How would you document this? _____
_____
_____
_____

Data Collected
(use those that apply)

- History of osteoarthritis in hands and hips
- Home clean and neat
- Fully dressed, carrying large night urinary drainage bag
- Relates difficulty getting out of house to buy groceries due to embarrassment of being seen with drainage bag
- Reports inability to change from large drainage bag to leg bag due to arthritis
- VS within normal limits
- Pelvic incision healing well with no evidence of infection
- Lung sounds clear
- Urine pale yellow, not malodorous
- Uncertain about whether to continue pelvic muscle and dorsiflexion exercises at home
- Questions need for follow-up visits now that his cancer is cured

Nursing Interventions
(use those that apply; list in priority order)

- Discuss the possibility of stress incontinence after the catheter is removed.
- Reinforce the need for perineal muscle exercises while the catheter is still in place.
- Explore available support systems to identify people to assist with catheter care.
- Provide teaching for Mr. Turner and care assistants as appropriate.
- Discuss potential postoperative complications.
- Reinforce the importance of follow-up care to monitor the disease and healing.

NCLEX-PN® Exam Preparation

1 Following a transurethral prostatectomy (TURP), a client confesses to the nurse that while he is able to maintain an erection, he "can't seem to produce anything" on orgasm. The nurse recognizes this as indicative of:

A. nocturia.
B. impotence.
C. decreased libido.
D. retrograde ejaculation.

2 Following TURP surgery, the nurse irrigates the bladder:

A. on an every-4-hours schedule.
B. as needed to clear blood clots and reduce spasms.
C. to reduce the sensation to void.
D. to prevent hyponatremia.

3 A client is about to be discharged following TURP. What statement indicates the need for additional instruction?

A. "I will continue taking one regular daily aspirin for my heart."
B. "I will not take a tub bath while the catheter is in place."
C. "I should not have sex for six weeks."
D. "I need to drink ten eight-ounce glasses of fluids a day."

4 Your client is 1 day postoperative from a TURP. In what order would you address the client's following complaints?

A. pain and bladder spasms
B. leakage around the irrigation catheter
C. blood clots in urinary catheter
D. dyspnea and chest pain
E. poor appetite and an "off" taste

5 Which of the following instructions should the nurse include when teaching a client with nonbacterial prostatitis?

A. Restrict fluids to avoid painful voiding.
B. Have frequent sex.
C. Wear a condom to avoid infecting their partner.
D. Finish the antibiotic therapy.

6 A 63-year-old client with no prior history of prostate problems has an elevated PSA level. He asks the nurse if this means that he has prostate cancer. The most appropriate response is:

A. "Yes. Prostate cancer increases the PSA level."
B. "No. The PSA increases when there is a prostate infection."
C. "Although the PSA increases with prostate cancer, it also increases in benign prostatic hypertrophy. Further tests are necessary."
D. "PSA levels increase with aging, so this test is ineffective to detect or diagnose prostate cancer."

7 A client with prostate cancer asks why the physician is planning to remove his testicles when the cancer is in his prostate gland, not his scrotum. The nurse responds based on the knowledge that

A. removing the testes reduces testosterone needed to support tumor growth.
B. prostate cancer frequently metastasizes to the testes.
C. this measure is important to prevent the client from engaging in sexual relations.
D. removing the testes is easier than administering hormones to treat prostate cancer.

8 Which of the following is an accurate statement regarding sildenafil (Viagra)?

A. Sildenafil is helpful in patients who have cardiovascular disease.
B. Sildenafil works better when combined with a nitrate drug.
C. Sildenafil may cause priapism.
D. Sildenafil is taken b.i.d. on an empty stomach.

9 A 19-year-old man presents at the walk-in clinic complaining of severe pain in his scrotum that began suddenly about an hour ago. The nurse should

A. obtain a complete medical history from the client.
B. advise the client to call his personal physician for an appointment.
C. provide a narcotic analgesic to relieve the pain.
D. notify the physician immediately.

10 A young woman tells the nurse that she has noticed that one of her husband's testicles is much harder than the other. She wonders if this is normal, because it isn't painful. The nurse responds that

A. this is a normal variation in many men.
B. if the testicle becomes painful, her husband should see his physician.
C. testicular cancer usually presents as a hard, painless nodule; he should see his physician.
D. this is a common manifestation of an infected testicle; her husband should see his physician for an antibiotic prescription.

Answers for Review Questions, as well as discussion of Care Plan and Critical Thinking Care Map questions, appear in Appendix V.

Chapter 35

Caring for Female Clients with Reproductive System Disorders

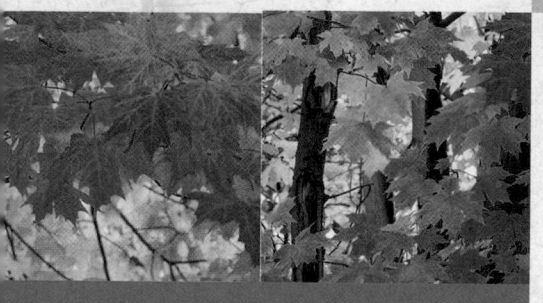

BRIEF Outline

Menopause
Premenstrual Syndrome and Dysmenorrhea
Dysfunctional Uterine Bleeding
Endometriosis
Ovarian Cysts
Vaginitis
Pelvic Inflammatory Disease
Toxic Shock Syndrome
Reproductive Organ Cancers
Structural Disorders
Breast Disorders
Breast Cancer

LEARNING Outcomes

After completing this chapter, you will be able to:

- Describe the pathophysiology of commonly occurring disorders of the breast and female reproductive system.
- Compare and contrast the manifestations of benign and malignant disorders of the breast and female reproductive system.
- Provide appropriate preoperative and postoperative nursing care for the client having gynecologic surgery.
- Use the nursing process when providing nursing care for female clients with disorders of the breast and reproductive system.

Disorders of the female reproductive system can occur at any point in a woman's adult life. They may affect her ability to bear children, her sexuality, and her sense of well-being as a woman. For many women, the ability to reproduce affects self-esteem, femininity, and general health. Women experiencing reproductive system problems may be asked to disclose personal, intimate information, which may be embarrassing and uncomfortable. Sensitivity on the part of the nurse is vital to establishing a caring, therapeutic relationship with the client.

PERIMENOPAUSE

Menopause

Menopause (or the *climacteric*) is the period during which menstruation permanently ceases. It marks the natural biologic end of reproduction. **Perimenopause** includes the 4 or 5 years surrounding menopause, during which estrogen production declines, and the menses permanently cease due to loss of ovarian function. It extends for 1 year after the final menstrual period. At this point, a woman is said to be postmenopausal.

Menopause is a normal physiologic process. However, the hormonal changes that occur can lead to unpleasant side effects. These side effects may vary from simply annoying to disruptive and difficult.

In the United States, menopause occurs usually between ages 45 and 55. *Surgical menopause* occurs when the ovaries are removed in premenopausal women. Certain health risks increase after menopause, including heart disease, osteoporosis, and breast cancer.

PHYSIOLOGY AND MANIFESTATIONS

During menopause, the number of ovarian follicles declines significantly, and the follicles that remain are less sensitive to FSH and LH. (Review the ovarian cycle in Chapter 33. ☮) As follicles cease to develop, ovarian estrogen production ceases. The ovaries continue to produce androgens, and small amounts of a less active form of estrogen are produced by the adrenal glands. This remaining estrogen is insufficient to maintain the female secondary sexual characteristics. This causes a loss of breast tissue, body hair, and subcutaneous fat. The ovaries and uterus shrink in size. The skin becomes less elastic, and vaginal and perineal tissues atrophy. Vaginal lubrication decreases.

An imbalance between estrogen and FSH from the pituitary gland causes *vasomotor instability*. This instability can lead to night sweats and hot flashes, palpitations, and headaches. The woman may have an increased incidence of vaginitis, as well as **dyspareunia** (pain during sexual intercourse). Menstrual cycles become irregular and eventually stop. Other common manifestations of menopause include possible irritability, anxiety, insomnia, difficulty concentrating, and depression.

INTERDISCIPLINARY CARE

Care related to menopause focuses on managing symptoms, teaching about menopause, and discussing postmenopausal health risks.

Medications

Hormone replacement therapy (HRT) is often used to relieve unpleasant manifestations of menopause and reduce some of the risks associated with estrogen deficiency. HRT relieves hot flashes and night sweats. It also decreases vaginal dryness and perineal tissue atrophy, which can lead to painful intercourse and urinary incontinence. Long-term benefits of HRT include reduced bone loss, with a lower risk for osteoporosis and resulting fractures, as well as a lower risk for colon cancer.

HRT, however, is not without risk. Nausea, vomiting, weight gain, breast tenderness and engorgement, and vaginal bleeding are common side effects of HRT. Fluid retention may be a problem. Long-term estrogen replacement increases the risk of endometrial cancer and ovarian cancer. A combination of estrogen with progestin reduces the risk of these cancers, but may contribute to bloating and irritability. HRT increases the risk of breast cancer and the formation of blood clots with resulting pulmonary emboli. Although initially thought to reduce the risk for coronary heart disease, HRT actually appears to increase this risk. Clients on HRT also may develop gallbladder disease. The decision to use HRT ultimately falls to the client, in consultation with her care provider. Table 35-1 ■ provides nursing implications and client teaching related to HRT.

Women for whom HRT is inappropriate or who choose not to use HRT may take drugs known as selective estrogen receptor modulators (SERMs), such as raloxifene (Evista), to prevent some of the long-term effects of menopause. SERMs act like estrogen in some tissues but not in others, and appear to reduce the risk of breast cancer and osteoporosis significantly in menopausal women. They do not prevent the manifestations of menopause.

Complementary Therapies

A number of complementary therapies may be used to help relieve the symptoms of menopause, although none are well supported in research. These include aromatherapy with

TABLE 35-1

Nursing Implications for Pharmacology: Hormone Replacement Therapy

DRUG CLASSIFICATION/DRUGS	ACTION	NURSING IMPLICATIONS	CLIENT AND FAMILY TEACHING
■ Conjugated estrogens/medroxyprogesterone acetate (Prempro, Premphase) ■ Estradiol/norethindrone acetate (CombiPatch)	These drugs replace lost estrogen to minimize the manifestations of menopause and potentially reduce some of the long-term risks of menopause. Progesterone is added to the estrogen to reduce the risk of endometrial cancer.	Notify physician of contraindications to HRT: pregnancy, breast cancer, undiagnosed vaginal bleeding, thrombophlebitis, or history of stroke. Women currently using any form of HRT should complete current cycle before changing products.	This replaces hormones lost during menopause. Do not use if you think you may be pregnant. You may have spotting or irregular menstrual bleeding while on HRT. Have yearly Pap smear and mammogram. Talk to your doctor about continuing HRT every 6 months; visit annually. Promptly report unusual bleeding, abdominal pain, or other adverse effects to your doctor.

geranium, rose, or fennel; herbs such as vitex, ginseng, and dong quai; meditation; and supplements such as vitamins D and E and soy protein.

NURSING CARE

ASSESSING

Collect subjective assessment data such as date of the last menstrual period, timing and regularity of the menstrual cycle, and duration and amount of menstrual flow. Ask the client if there is any risk that she could be pregnant. Inquire about menopausal symptoms such as night sweats, hot flashes, vaginal irritation or discomfort with intercourse, and measures that she has taken to relieve symptoms.

DIAGNOSING, PLANNING, AND IMPLEMENTING

Priorities in Nursing Care. Menopause is not a disorder, but a normal part of the life and reproductive cycle. The nursing role during menopause focuses on education.

Deficient Knowledge: Menopause

■ Discuss symptoms the client is experiencing, and suggest strategies for coping (see Continuing Care). *Appropriate information helps both understanding and decision making. Many effects of menopause can be managed with lifestyle and other nondrug strategies.*
■ Provide information about the benefits and risks of HRT. *Information helps the client decide whether HRT is right for her.*

clinical ALERT

Advise women who choose HRT to stop smoking and to consider limiting the number of years of therapy to 5 or less to reduce the short- and long-term risks associated with HRT.

■ Recommend a daily calcium intake of 1,500 mg for clients not on HRT and 1,000 mg for clients on HRT. *Adequate calcium is important to help reduce the risk of osteoporosis associated with menopause.*
■ Emphasize the importance of aerobic and weight-bearing exercise. *Exercise reduces the rate of bone loss, helps maintain optimal weight, and reduces cardiovascular risk.*

Sexual Dysfunction

■ Encourage the woman to express feelings and concerns about the effects of menopause on her sex life. *The client may not be comfortable expressing her feelings until the nurse shows comfort with the topic and encourages her.*
■ Suggest spending more time in foreplay and using water-soluble gels (e.g., Replens) for vaginal lubrication. *These measures can prevent vaginal pain and irritation and improve the quality of the sexual experience for the client and her partner.*

Risk for Situational Low Self-Esteem

■ Encourage expression of fears and concerns related to changes in interpersonal and family roles. *Some women associate aging with "uselessness" and unattractiveness.*
■ Encourage volunteer activities or employment for the woman who has extra time. *This promotes a sense of*

usefulness and contribution to society. Activities involving young people can help reduce anxiety about the loss of reproductive ability.

■ Discuss the importance of a healthy lifestyle in maintaining physical attractiveness. Identify risk factors and high-risk behaviors. *Lifestyle habits and behaviors (such as cigarette smoking and sun exposure) contribute to the aging process. Active women who exercise and eat a well-balanced diet look better and feel better.*

EVALUATING

To evaluate the effectiveness of nursing care and teaching, assess the client's level of understanding about the perimenopausal period and measures to reduce unpleasant effects. Openly discuss the effects of menopause on sexuality and self-esteem with the client to evaluate coping.

Documenting. Document teaching provided and the client's response to and apparent understanding of information. Note the client's decision regarding hormone replacement therapy or herbal preparations to deal with the manifestations of perimenopause.

CONTINUING CARE

Emphasize that menopause is a normal physiologic process, not a disease or an illness, and that symptoms are temporary and manageable. Discuss ways of coping with undesirable side effects (Box 35-1 ■). Explain that making healthy lifestyle changes and reducing risk behaviors may reduce the need for HRT. Health maintenance and self-care are

increasingly important: Encourage yearly mammograms, clinical breast examinations, Pap tests, and monthly breast self-examination and self-monitoring for vaginitis.

BOX 35-1	CLIENT TEACHING

Coping with Symptoms of Menopause
Vaginal Dryness
■ Use a water-soluble lubricant for comfort during intercourse.
■ Avoid vaginal douches or perineal powders.
■ Eat 6 to 8 oz. of yogurt with live cultures daily to help prevent vaginitis.

Hot Flashes
■ Let people know when you're having a hot flash—it's nothing to be ashamed of!
■ Use relaxation techniques such as meditation or guided imagery during hot flashes.
■ Stay active—activity relieves hot flashes and stress and improves sleep.
■ Avoid hot-flash triggers such as alcohol, caffeine, sugar, hot or spicy foods, and very large meals.
■ Dress in layers of natural fabrics.
■ Splash face and neck with cool water or put something cool on wrists and forehead.
■ Lower the thermostat, especially at night.

Irritability or Depression
■ Stay involved in work or meaningful volunteer activities.
■ Maintain balance—work, exercise, do something you enjoy, and get enough rest every day.

DISORDERS OF MENSTRUATION

Monthly menstruation often causes minor discomfort, such as breast tenderness, a feeling of heaviness and congestion in the pelvic area, cramping, and backache. Many women experience more serious effects, both physiologic and psychologic. This section discusses premenstrual syndrome, dysmenorrhea, and abnormal uterine bleeding.

Premenstrual Syndrome

Premenstrual syndrome (PMS) is a symptom complex of irritability, depression, edema, and breast tenderness preceding menses. It may affect more than half of all women during their reproductive years. Risk factors for PMS include major life stressors, age over 30, and depression. The actual cause of PMS is unknown, but it is thought to involve imbalances of estrogen and progesterone.

PATHOPHYSIOLOGY AND MANIFESTATIONS

The pathophysiology of PMS is not clearly understood. Hormonal changes such as altered estrogen–progesterone ratios, increased prolactin levels, and rising aldosterone levels during the luteal phase of the menstrual cycle (see Figure 33-3) ◯◯ are thought to contribute to the problem. Increased aldosterone levels cause salt and water retention and edema. Neurotransmitters such as monoamine oxidase and serotonin affect emotions and probably play a role in PMS.

Manifestations of PMS generally occur 7 to 10 days prior to the onset of the menstrual flow, and are relieved when the menstrual flow begins. The multisystem effects of PMS are shown in Figure 35-1 ■. The manifestations of PMS and their intensity vary remarkably for each client.

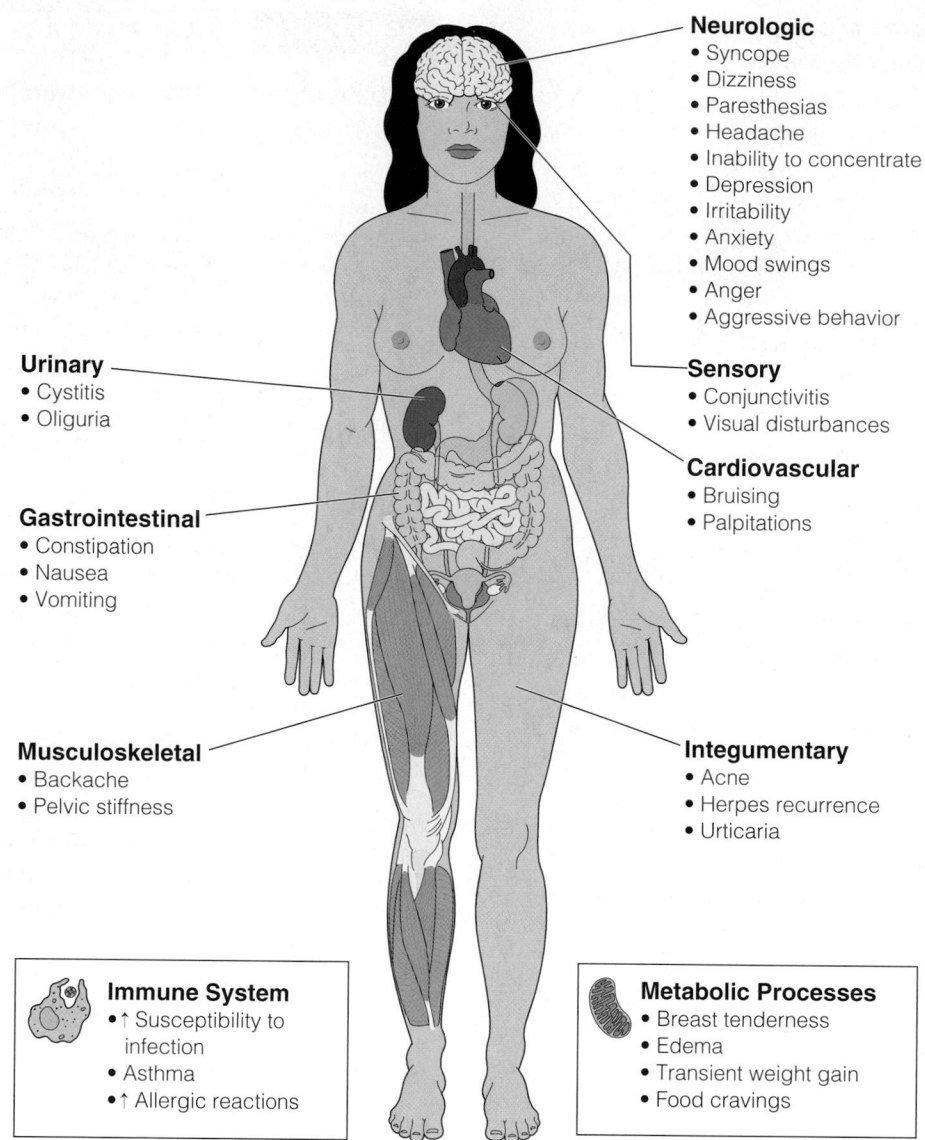

Neurologic
- Syncope
- Dizziness
- Paresthesias
- Headache
- Inability to concentrate
- Depression
- Irritability
- Anxiety
- Mood swings
- Anger
- Aggressive behavior

Sensory
- Conjunctivitis
- Visual disturbances

Cardiovascular
- Bruising
- Palpitations

Integumentary
- Acne
- Herpes recurrence
- Urticaria

Urinary
- Cystitis
- Oliguria

Gastrointestinal
- Constipation
- Nausea
- Vomiting

Musculoskeletal
- Backache
- Pelvic stiffness

Immune System
- ↑ Susceptibility to infection
- Asthma
- ↑ Allergic reactions

Metabolic Processes
- Breast tenderness
- Edema
- Transient weight gain
- Food cravings

Figure 35-1. ■ The multisystem effects of premenstrual syndrome.

INTERDISCIPLINARY CARE

The goals of care for PMS are to relieve manifestations and help the client develop self-care strategies for episodes of PMS. The client is advised to keep a daily diary of symptoms for several months to evaluate their timing and severity.

Management focuses on diet, exercise, relaxation, and stress management. A diet high in complex carbohydrates with limited simple sugars and alcohol is recommended. Reduced salt intake helps to minimize fluid retention. Caffeine is restricted to reduce irritability. Increased intake of calcium, magnesium, and vitamin B$_6$ may be helpful. Exercise is beneficial, but adequate rest also is necessary. The client needs to balance periods of activity and rest. Techniques for relaxation and stress management include deep abdominal breathing, meditation, muscle relaxation, and guided imagery.

If the manifestations of PMS are severe, drugs that affect hormone or neurotransmitter levels such as danazol (Danocrine), fluoxetine (Prozac), sertraline (Zoloft), or paroxetine (Paxil) may be prescribed.

Complementary therapies also may be used for PMS. These may include acupuncture, aromatherapy with various oils, herbs such as vitex or evening primrose oil, homeopathy, or reflexology.

NURSING CARE

Nursing care for the client with PMS focuses on teaching the client to manage manifestations of the disorder.

Effective Therapeutic Regimen Management

- Encourage keeping a journal of menstrual cycle, physical symptoms, and mood changes. *Recognizing the signs and timing of PMS is the first step in developing ways to cope with the problem.*
- Review symptoms, relating them to diet, activity, and stress levels. *Identifying relationships helps develop strategies to reduce and manage the symptoms of PMS.*
- Explore self-care measures that have helped the client cope with mood alterations in the past. Encourage coping strategies such as relaxation techniques and exercise. *Using some drugs or alcohol to relieve PMS may actually make symptoms worse.*
- Review daily activities and suggest ways to balance rest periods and activity. *Rest decreases energy and oxygen consumption, increasing the amount available to muscles.*
- Explore ways to rearrange or reschedule activities during PMS symptoms. *Planning ahead provides more control and promotes effective coping.*
- Teach self-care measures to relieve pain: heat application, relaxation techniques (such as breathing exercises, imagery techniques, or meditation), and exercise. *Heat relieves muscle spasms and dilates blood vessels, increasing blood supply to the pelvis and uterus. Relaxation and exercise promote release of naturally produced pain relievers (endorphins).*

EVALUATING

Assess the client's level of understanding about PMS and symptom management.

Documenting. Document information provided, as well as the client's apparent willingness to employ suggested measures to relieve symptoms.

CONTINUING CARE

Teach the client that PMS is not a disease, but a response to hormone changes of the menstrual cycle. Understanding the condition allows the client to assume control, manage anxiety, and use appropriate strategies to reduce symptoms. Discuss dietary measures, relaxation techniques and exercise, stress reduction techniques, and support systems in teaching about PMS management.

Dysmenorrhea

Dysmenorrhea, pain associated with menstruation, is experienced by up to 75% of menstruating women.

PATHOPHYSIOLOGY AND MANIFESTATIONS

In *primary dysmenorrhea,* no disease process is identified. Prostaglandins stimulate muscles in the uterus to contract. These contractions can cause mild cramping to severe muscle spasms. As the muscles contract, blood flow to the uterus is restricted, causing ischemia and pain. Abdominal pain begins with the onset of menses and lasts 12 to 48 hours. Pain may radiate to the lower back and thighs. Other manifestations may include headache, nausea, vomiting, diarrhea, fatigue, or breast tenderness. Psychologic factors, such as anxiety and tension, may contribute to dysmenorrhea. Childbirth tends to decrease the incidence and severity of symptoms.

Secondary dysmenorrhea is related to an underlying disorder that causes scarring or injury of reproductive organs. Endometriosis, fibroid tumors, pelvic inflammatory disease, or ovarian cancer may cause painful menses. These conditions are discussed later in this chapter.

INTERDISCIPLINARY CARE

Care of the client with menstrual pain focuses on identifying its cause, and on managing pain. Drugs such as mild analgesics, prostaglandin inhibitors such as nonsteroidal anti-inflammatory drugs (NSAIDs), or oral contraceptives may be recommended to relieve pain. Nonpharmacologic measures include dietary changes, exercise, relaxation, and stress management. Dietary measures such as reducing intake of sodium, sugar, caffeine, and alcohol; decreasing fluid consumption; and increasing intake of protein, calcium, magnesium, and vitamin B_6 may be helpful. A balance of rest and exercise is important. Techniques for relaxation and stress management include deep abdominal breathing, meditation, muscle relaxation, and guided imagery. Use of a heating pad also helps reduce pain. As with PMS, complementary therapies such as aromatherapy, herbal preparations, reflexology, acupressure, or massage may be helpful.

NURSING CARE

Nursing care focuses on helping the client develop effective coping strategies. Discuss using an NSAID such as ibuprofen on a regular basis during periods of menstrual pain. Teach nonpharmacologic pain relief measures, and encourage use of these as well for pain relief. Stress the benign nature of primary dysmenorrhea, being sure to validate the reality of the pain and discomfort. Discuss diet and exercise, as well as stress management techniques. Teach safe use of heat for pain relief. Provide information about engaging in sexual intercourse, explaining that orgasm may help relieve the client's symptoms.

Dysfunctional Uterine Bleeding

Dysfunctional uterine bleeding (DUB) is vaginal bleeding that is abnormal in amount, duration, or time of occurrence. Dysfunctional uterine bleeding is usually related to hormonal imbalances or pelvic tumors, either benign or malignant.

PATHOPHYSIOLOGY AND MANIFESTATIONS

Hormonal imbalance, especially progesterone deficiency with relative estrogen excess, causes endometrial tissue to proliferate. Unless this tissue is supported by adequate progesterone, sloughing occurs. Depending on ovarian function and the hormone imbalance, irregular, prolonged, or profuse vaginal bleeding may occur. *Anovulation,* absence of ovulation, is associated with both estrogen and progesterone deficiencies. Emotional upsets or stress also can cause hormonal imbalances and thus affect menstruation. Pelvic tumors can also cause abnormal bleeding. They are discussed in later sections of this chapter.

Amenorrhea is the absence of menstruation. It is usually caused by hormone imbalance. Because a certain percentage of body fat is required for menstruation to occur, anorexia nervosa or excessive athletic activity or training can also cause amenorrhea. Amenorrhea is a normal consequence of pregnancy, breastfeeding, and menopause, as well as removal of the uterus or ovaries.

Oligomenorrhea, scant menses, usually is related to hormonal imbalances. *Menorrhagia,* excessive or prolonged menstruation, may result from endocrine or reproductive system disorders. Clotting disorders and anticoagulant medications also can cause menorrhagia. Repetitive long or heavy cycles can lead to excessive blood loss, fatigue, anemia, hemorrhage, and sexual dysfunction.

Metrorrhagia, bleeding between menstrual periods, may be a sign of cervical or uterine cancer. For this reason, it is important to evaluate metrorrhagia promptly and thoroughly. *Mittleschmerz* (midcycle spotting associated with ovulation) occurs in many women and is not considered metrorrhagia.

Postmenopausal bleeding may be caused by endometrial polyps, endometrial hyperplasia, or uterine cancer. The possibility of cancer makes early evaluation and treatment essential.

INTERDISCIPLINARY CARE

The care of the client with DUB focuses on identifying and treating the underlying disease. A careful history and physical examination are obtained. Abdominal and pelvic exams are done to rule out abdominal masses. The client may need to keep a menstrual history and basal body temperature chart for several months to relate ovulation to bleeding.

Diagnostic Tests

- *Complete blood count (CBC)* to evaluate the effects of DUB.
- *Thyroid function tests* to rule out thyroid disorders such as hyper- or hypothyroidism as the cause of DUB.
- *Serum estradiol (estrogen)* and *progesterone* levels to evaluate ovarian function.
- *Serum hCG* and *LH* levels to evaluate pituitary function.
- *Pap smear* to rule out cervical cancer.
- *Pelvic ultrasound* to detect lesions such as fibroid or cancerous tumors. See Table 33-2 ⏺⏺ for nursing care related to pelvic ultrasound.
- *Laparoscopy* to visualize pelvic structures or hysteroscopy to detect abnormalities of the uterine cavity. Nursing care for the client undergoing a laparoscopy is outlined in Box 33-3. ⏺⏺
- *Endometrial biopsy* may be done to microscopically examine endometrial tissues.

Medications

For many clients, menstrual irregularities can be treated with hormones. Oral contraceptives or progesterone preparations may be ordered. Oral iron supplements may be prescribed to replace iron lost through menstrual bleeding.

Surgery

DUB is the leading cause of hysterectomy. However, the least invasive intervention that proves effective is preferred, beginning with a therapeutic dilation and curettage (D&C), then endometrial ablation, and, finally, hysterectomy.

In a *therapeutic D&C,* the cervical canal is dilated and the uterine wall is scraped. D&C is used to diagnose and treat DUB and certain other disorders. It is contraindicated for any woman who has been taking anticoagulant drugs. Nursing care of the client undergoing D&C is outlined in Box 35-2 ■.

Endometrial ablation permanently destroys the endometrial layer of the uterus by laser surgery or electrosurgical resection. It is done for women who do not respond to drug therapy or D&C. This procedure ends menstruation and reproduction.

In *uterine balloon heat therapy,* a specialized balloon is inserted through the cervix into the uterus, then inflated and heated. This outpatient procedure takes only 10 minutes and can be done using local anesthesia.

Hysterectomy, or removal of the uterus, may be done if other treatments are unsuccessful or malignancy is found, particularly if childbearing is no longer desired. In premenopausal women, the ovaries are usually left in place. In postmenopausal women, a total hysterectomy, or panhysterectomy, may be done, removing the uterus, fallopian tubes, and ovaries.

BOX 35-2	NURSING CARE CHECKLIST

Dilation and Curettage (D&C)

Before Surgery

☑ If ordered, ask to come in the day before surgery for insertion of a laminaria tent to absorb cervical secretions and slowly dilate the cervix.

☑ Provide routine preoperative care (see Chapter 9). ∞

After Surgery

☑ Provide routine postoperative care (see Chapter 9). ∞

☑ Monitor circulation and sensation in the legs; avoid placing a pillow under the knees.

☑ Instruct to use perineal pads and avoid tampons for 2 weeks.

☑ Explain that the next menstrual period may be delayed.

☑ Instruct to avoid intercourse until after follow-up visit and cessation of vaginal discharge.

☑ Advise to rest, avoid heavy lifting for several days, and report bright red or excessive bleeding (more than a normal menstrual period).

Hysterectomy may be done using an abdominal or a vaginal approach, or a vaginal approach with laparoscopic visualization of the pelvic cavity. Recovery is faster following vaginal or laparoscopic hysterectomy than with an abdominal hysterectomy. The abdominal approach, however, may be used when better access to and visualization of the pelvic cavity is needed. Nursing care of the client undergoing a hysterectomy is outlined in Box 35-3 ■.

clinical ALERT

Pelvic surgery, including hysterectomy, increases the risk of deep venous thrombosis and pulmonary embolism. Encourage leg exercises and early ambulation to promote venous return. Advise women who smoke to stop. Promptly report symptoms such as leg or calf pain, swelling of one leg, chest pain, or difficulty breathing.

NURSING CARE

ASSESSING

Nursing assessment focuses on subjective data related to the onset of symptoms, timing and amount of menstrual flow (in pads per day and duration of period), and associated symptoms such as pain or cramping, weakness, or excessive fatigue.

clinical ALERT

Advise women with complaints of bleeding between periods or after menopause to promptly seek medical attention because this can be a sign of endometrial or cervical cancer.

DIAGNOSING, PLANNING, AND IMPLEMENTING

Priorities in Nursing Care. Dysfunctional uterine bleeding often causes anxiety, and may threaten self-image, sexuality, or reproductive potential. In many cases, helping the client deal with the psychologic and emotional effects of DUB and

BOX 35-3	NURSING CARE CHECKLIST

Hysterectomy

Before Surgery

☑ Assess understanding and reinforce teaching as needed. Provide emotional support.

☑ Instruct to cleanse abdominal and perineal areas as ordered.

☑ If ordered, administer a small cleansing enema and have client empty bladder.

☑ Provide routine preoperative care as ordered (Chapter 9). ∞

After Surgery

☑ Provide routine postoperative care (see Chapter 9). ∞

☑ Report excess bleeding, especially following a vaginal hysterectomy.

☑ Monitor for potential complications, such as infection, ileus, venous thrombosis, and pulmonary embolus.

☑ Assess vaginal drainage; teach perineal care.

☑ Advise to restrict physical activity for 4 to 6 weeks, and avoid heavy lifting, stair climbing, douching, tampons, and sexual intercourse.

☑ Instruct to shower, avoiding tub baths, until bleeding has stopped.

☑ Instruct to report the following to the physician:
  a. Temperature greater than 100°F (37.7°C)
  b. Vaginal bleeding greater than a typical menstrual period or that is bright red
  c. Urinary incontinence, urgency, burning, or frequency
  d. Severe pain.

☑ Encourage expression of feelings and concerns.

☑ If appropriate, provide information about hormone replacement therapy.

☑ Reinforce the importance of regular gynecologic examinations even after hysterectomy.

its treatment (e.g., therapeutic D&C or hysterectomy) is the highest nursing care priority.

Ineffective Coping

- Discuss results of diagnostic tests and examinations with the client face to face. *This allows for open exchange of information.*
- Provide information about causes, treatment, risks, long-term effects, and prognosis for DUB. *This allows the client to assume responsibility for her own health and become involved in her own treatment plan.*
- Evaluate coping strategies and psychosocial support systems. Teach appropriate coping strategies if indicated. *The possibility of surgery or cancer may be a crisis for the client and her support system. Effective coping strategies help in dealing with this situational crisis.*

Sexual Dysfunction

- Discuss sexual intercourse during menstruation. Explain that orgasm may help relieve symptoms, but that it is necessary to use contraception to prevent pregnancy even during menstruation. *Orgasm frequently provides at least temporary relief of symptoms. Some women mistakenly believe that birth control measures are unnecessary during menstruation.*
- Provide an opportunity to express concerns related to effect of DUB on lifestyle and sexual functioning. *Some women abstain from sexual activity due to symptoms of DUB. Encouraging verbalization of concerns can assist to develop strategies to minimize the impact of DUB on sexuality and lifestyle.*
- Encourage frequent rest periods. *This conserves energy and may allow sexual function to resume.*
- Provide information about alternative methods of sexual expression. *Methods of sexual expression other than vaginal intercourse may satisfy the needs of both partners.*

EVALUATING

Collect data related to the following to evaluate the effectiveness of nursing interventions:

- Verbalizes ability to cope with symptoms and treatment of disorder.
- Discusses acceptable and satisfying sexual practices with partner.

Documenting. Document continuing assessment data. This is particularly important for the postoperative client who has undergone a D&C or hysterectomy. Document the number of perineal pads saturated as an estimate of bleeding. Document care and teaching, as well as the client's emotional responses to information and treatment options.

CONTINUING CARE

Provide support, reassurance, and information to help the client and her family understand her disorder and its treatment. Teach self-care measures to help minimize the effects of DUB on activities of daily living.

Discuss using ordered drugs, including oral contraceptives, iron supplements, or other agents, including dosage and side effects. Encourage to take an iron supplement with orange juice to improve absorption, and avoid taking it with foods high in calcium (such as milk), which interfere with its absorption. Provide information about maintaining a balanced diet, increasing iron-rich foods, such as eggs, beans, liver, beef, and shrimp. Encourage a fluid intake of 2,000 to 3,000 mL/day.

Emphasize the need to report recurring episodes of DUB (particularly in postmenopausal women) to the health care provider immediately.

DISORDERS OF FEMALE REPRODUCTIVE TISSUE

Disorders of female reproductive tissue include endometriosis, cysts and polyps, and benign tumors known as uterine leiomyomas (fibroids). Malignant tumors of reproductive tissue are discussed in the next section of this chapter.

Endometriosis

Endometriosis is a common condition in which endometrial tissue is found outside the uterus. Endometrial tissue may be found on the ovary and other pelvic organs or tissues, and rarely in other organs such as the lungs. Risk factors may include a family history of endometriosis; early menarche; and short, regular menstrual cycles with heavy flow.

PATHOPHYSIOLOGY

The cause of endometriosis is unknown. It may be caused by backflow of menstrual blood carrying endometrial cells through the fallopian tubes into the pelvis. Cells that can develop into endometrium may be implanted during embryonic development, or endometrial cells may spread through the blood or lymph to other sites. Inflammation or immune responses may contribute to endometriosis.

The **ectopic** (in an abnormal location) endometrial tissue responds to the ovarian cycle, and bleeding occurs during menses. The implants regress during pregnancy and atrophy at menopause. Bleeding of the ectopic tissue may cause cysts, scarring, inflammation, and adhesions. Scarring can lead to infertility and problems such as bowel obstruction.

MANIFESTATIONS

The manifestations of endometriosis occur just before and during the menses. They include dysmenorrhea with backache and cramps, painful defecation, dysuria, dyspareunia, and infertility. These manifestations may vary, depending on the site of ectopic tissue.

INTERDISCIPLINARY CARE

Endometriosis often is diagnosed by the history and physical exam. Firm, tender nodules are found in the pelvic cavity, and the uterus may be retroflexed. A *pelvic ultrasound* may be done, or a laparoscopy performed to visualize the implants. (Review Table 33-2 ⚭ and Box 33-3 ⚭ for nursing implications for these exams.)

Medications

Mild analgesics and NSAIDs are used to relieve pain associated with endometriosis. Hormones such as oral contraceptives, progesterone, or danazol (an androgen hormone) may be given to suppress ovarian function, at least temporarily. Suppressing ovarian function allows the ectopic tissue to shrink.

Surgery

Ectopic lesions may be treated by laser or electrocautery via laparoscopic surgery. When the disease is severe and childbearing is no longer desired, a bilateral **salpingo-oophorectomy** (BSO, removal of the fallopian tubes and ovaries) and hysterectomy may be performed. Nursing care for the client undergoing a hysterectomy is outlined in Box 35-3.

NURSING CARE

ASSESSING

When assessing the client with endometriosis, collect subjective data such as:

- Pain—timing in relation to menses; location, quality, and duration
- Other symptoms such as painful defecation, dysuria, painful intercourse, or other manifestations associated with menses
- Pregnancy history or desire for and attempts to conceive a child
- Affect of the condition on life, roles, and relationships.

DIAGNOSING, PLANNING, AND IMPLEMENTING

Pain often is the primary manifestation of endometriosis. Discomfort can be severe, impairing productivity and leading to lost work time.

Priorities in Nursing Care. Helping the client to deal with the manifestations and potential complications of endometriosis is the nursing care priority.

Pain

- Evaluate the severity and timing of the pain. *Although the severity of the pain may not directly relate to the severity of the disease, it will help guide the choice of treatment.*
- Discuss using drugs and nonpharmacologic measures for pain relief. *Heat to the abdomen or back, relaxation techniques (e.g., yoga and meditation), exercise, and biofeedback can help the client manage pain, particularly when used together with analgesics.*
- Suggest trying alternative positions for sexual intercourse. *Different positions may reduce discomfort during intercourse for the client with endometriosis.*

Anxiety

- Encourage discussion of concerns about infertility. Answer questions honestly. *Knowledge helps the client gain a sense of control and relieve anxiety and fear.*
- Discuss the advantages of having children soon and in rapid succession, and using oral contraceptives between pregnancies to minimize bleeding. *Ectopic endometrial tissue regresses during pregnancy and with oral contraceptives, reducing scarring.*
- Provide information about measures to promote conception, including measuring basal body temperature and other techniques to identify ovulation. *Using measures such as these helps optimize the chance of conception.*

EVALUATING

To evaluate the effectiveness of nursing interventions for the client with endometriosis, collect information about the client's ability to manage associated discomfort and cope with the effects of the disorder.

Documenting. Document care and teaching, as well as the client's understanding of the disorder and management options.

CONTINUING CARE

Teach the client and family about endometriosis and treatment options, including their side effects. Discuss the possible benefits of having children earlier in life, rather than delaying parenthood. If the client has undergone surgery, provide instructions for home care, including managing incisions, preventing infection, and follow-up care.

Ovarian Cysts

A cyst is a fluid-filled sac. Cysts can develop in the vulva, endometrium, or ovaries. This section focuses on ovarian cysts.

PATHOPHYSIOLOGY AND MANIFESTATIONS

Ovarian cysts may be either follicular cysts or corpus luteum cysts. Follicular cysts develop when a mature follicle does not rupture or when the fluid in an immature follicle does not reabsorb after ovulation. Corpus luteum cysts occur when the corpus luteum remains enlarged after ovulation. Most cysts regress spontaneously within two or three menstrual cycles. They often are asymptomatic, although the pain associated with cyst rupture may be confused with the pain of appendicitis.

Polycystic ovary syndrome (PCOS) is characterized by numerous follicular cysts. It is an endocrine disorder in which LH, estrogen, and androgen hormone levels are higher than normal, and FSH levels are low. This hormone imbalance causes irregular menstrual periods, *hirsutism* (excessive hair growth), acne, obesity, and infertility. Women with PCOS often have insulin resistance and may develop type 2 diabetes early in adulthood. PCOS also increases the risk of endometrial cancer, hypertension, and abnormal cholesterol levels.

INTERDISCIPLINARY CARE

Care focuses on identifying and correcting the disorder and preventing its recurrence.

Diagnostic Tests

Diagnostic tests may be used to diagnose and differentiate ovarian cysts:

- *LH, FSH,* and *serum testosterone* levels are measured. The FSH–LH ratio is reversed in PCOS, and serum testosterone levels are higher than normal.
- *Glucose tolerance tests* may be done to identify possible type 2 diabetes.
- *Laparoscopy* is done to visualize ovarian cysts. (See Box 33-3 ⚭ for nursing care of the client undergoing laparoscopy.)

Medications

Oral contraceptives often are ordered to regulate the menses in women with PCOS. If the client wishes to become pregnant, clomiphene (Clomid, Serophene) may be prescribed to stimulate ovulation. Other drugs such as progesterone or the corticosteroid dexamethasone can be given to control manifestations of hirsutism.

Surgery

Follicular cysts may be punctured through laser surgery, or a wedge resection of the ovary may be done to restore ovulation. Rarely, **oophorectomy** (removal of the ovary) is performed if the cysts are very large.

NURSING CARE

Unless surgery is performed, the focus of nursing care for clients with ovarian cysts is on education. Provide information about the disorder and prescribed treatment. Discuss the benign and temporary nature of most ovarian cysts other than PCOS. Discuss the risks and benefits of treatment options with the client. Encourage the client with PCOS to share concerns about potential risks and the effect of the disorder on the ability to conceive. Teach measures to reduce the risk of heart disease (control hypertension, exercise and diet management to control cholesterol levels, avoid smoking, manage stress) and type 2 diabetes (weight loss and diet management). Stress the importance of regular follow-up with a health care provider knowledgeable about PCOS. Teach the manifestations of endometrial cancer, and stress the importance of promptly notifying the health care provider if symptoms develop.

Uterine Fibroid Tumor

Fibroid tumors, or *uterine leiomyomas,* are benign tumors of the uterus or cervix. They are common among all women of childbearing age (see Box 35-4 ■), and are a leading reason for hysterectomy.

Fibroid tumors are classified by their location in the wall of the uterus (Figure 35-2 ■). *Intramural* tumors are within the uterine wall. *Subserous* fibroids are beneath the outer layer of the uterus, projecting into the peritoneal cavity. *Submuous* fibroid tumors are beneath the endometrial lining of the uterus.

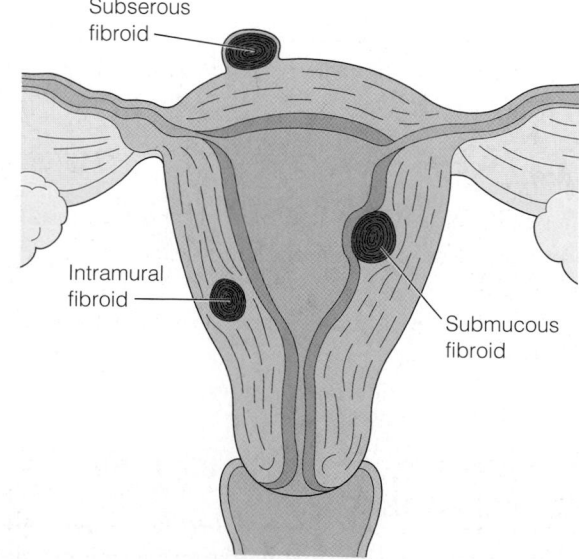

Figure 35-2. ■ Sites of uterine fibroid tumors.

Uterine Fibroid Tumors in African American Women

Uterine fibroid tumors are three to nine times more common in African American women than in white women: 40% to 50% of African American women between ages 30 and 60 develop fibroid tumors, whereas only 20% of Caucasian women in this age group develop them.

The cause of fibroid tumors is not clear, but they are probably related to estrogen secretion. Small tumors may be asymptomatic. Large fibroids can crowd other organs, causing pelvic pressure, pain, dysmenorrhea, menorrhagia, and fatigue. Depending on tumor location, constipation and urinary urgency and frequency are common.

The uterus is enlarged. Excessive bleeding often causes anemia.

In asymptomatic women who wish to bear children, fibroid tumors are monitored. Drugs may be given to reduce tumor size and slow their growth. *Laparoscopic myomectomy,* removal of the tumor without removing the entire uterus, may be performed in young women who wish to have a child. Hysterectomy is performed if tumors are large, and in women who are menopausal.

If surgery is deferred, client and family teaching emphasize the importance of regular follow-up appointments to monitor tumor growth. If surgery is chosen, teaching emphasizes pain control techniques and appropriate preoperative and postoperative teaching (see the previous discussion of the client undergoing a hysterectomy). Dietary modifications to increase iron intake, prevent constipation, and promote healing are important.

INFECTIONS OF THE FEMALE REPRODUCTIVE SYSTEM

Infections affecting the female reproductive tract may be local or systemic. Many are sexually transmitted infections (STIs), which are discussed in Chapter 36. ⬤ The most common local infections are vaginal, including simple vaginitis, candidiasis, and trichomoniasis. Systemic infections include pelvic inflammatory disease, toxic shock syndrome, and HIV/AIDS (see Chapter 11). ⬤

Vaginitis

Vaginitis, inflammation or infection of the vagina, is common. Vaginal infections are classified by cause, and may be fungal (candidiasis), protozoan (trichomoniasis), or bacterial (*Gardnerella*) infections.

Risk factors for vaginitis include unprotected sexual activity, multiple sexual partners, using a broad-spectrum antibiotic, obesity, diabetes, pregnancy, and poor personal hygiene. Sexual activity and swimming in contaminated water are risk factors for trichomoniasis.

PATHOPHYSIOLOGY AND MANIFESTATIONS

The low pH of vaginal secretions, normal vaginal flora, and estrogen normally protect against vaginal infections. An infection is more likely to develop when any or all of these factors are disrupted. When conditions are favorable, microorganisms invade the vulva and vagina. Simple vaginitis is the most common vaginal infection in women of reproductive age. *Gardnerella vaginalis* is the causative organism in many cases. Candidiasis (moniliasis or yeast infection) is caused by the organism *Candida albicans*. Candida organisms are part of the normal vaginal environment, causing problems only when they multiply rapidly. When increased estrogen levels, antibiotics, fecal contamination, or other factors alter the normal vaginal flora, *Candida* organisms multiply, causing a yeast infection.

Trichomoniasis, a protozoan infection, is a sexually transmitted infection. This organism frequently is carried asymptomatically by the male partner.

Most vaginal infections cause vaginal discharge, itching or burning, and dysuria. The specific manifestations of various vaginal infections are outlined in Table 35-2 ■.

INTERDISCIPLINARY CARE

Vaginitis is common and often is appropriate for self-care. Many topical agents are available over the counter.

clinical ALERT

Clients with persistent or recurrent episodes of vaginitis should be carefully evaluated. Repeated vaginal yeast infections may be a manifestation of diabetes or HIV infection.

TABLE 35-2

Vaginal Infections

INFECTION	TYPE OF DISCHARGE	OTHER MANIFESTATIONS	TREATMENT	NURSING CARE
Candidiasis (*Monilia*, yeast infection)	Thick white patches adhering to cervix and vaginal wall, resembling cottage cheese; little odor	Itching of vulva and vaginal area, redness, painful intercourse	Butoconazole, miconazole, clotrimazole, or terconazole creams, vaginal tablets, or suppositories	Teach perineal hygiene and use of vaginal applicators. Instruct to complete entire treatment.
Simple vaginitis (bacterial vaginosis, *Gardnerella* vaginosis)	Thin, white, "milklike," or gray with fishy odor, especially when mixed with potassium hydroxide	None to mild itching or burning in vulvar area; clue cells on microscopic examination	Oral metronidazole or metronidazole gel; clindamycin cream or oral clindamycin	Teach perineal hygiene. Instruct to complete treatment. Discuss relationship to PID.
Trichomoniasis	Frothy, yellow or white, foul odor	Burning and itching of vulva	Oral metronidazole for client and sexual partner	Teach perineal hygiene; avoid unprotected intercourse until treatment completed.
Atrophic vaginitis (senile vaginitis)	Thin, opaque discharge, may be blood tinged, odorless; pale, smooth, thin, dry vaginal walls	Painful intercourse, itching, vaginal dryness	Topical estrogen cream; water-soluble lubricant for intercourse; possible HRT	Discuss symptoms of menopause and sexual techniques to minimize trauma.

Diagnostic Tests

- Vaginal secretions are cultured and examined microscopically for the presence of "clue cells," a sign of bacterial vaginitis.
- *"Wet mount"* or *"wet prep"* with potassium hydroxide (KOH) reveals a fishy odor in bacterial vaginitis. The slide is examined microscopically to detect *hyphae* (filaments or threads) and *Candida* spores.
- *Normal saline wet prep* is used to detect the presence of protozoa if trichomoniasis is suspected.
- *Glucose tolerance tests* or *HIV screening* may be done at the time of the initial assessment.
- *Pregnancy tests* may be done because certain treatments are contraindicated during pregnancy.

Medications

Drugs used to treat vaginitis vary with the organism, as shown in Table 35-2. In many cases, the client's sexual partner must also be treated to prevent reinfection. Mild vinegar douches may be ordered, but should not be used routinely. Frequent douching washes away normal flora, affecting the natural defense mechanism against bacterial invasion.

NURSING CARE

ASSESSING

Collect subjective assessment data from the client with complaints of vaginal discharge or itching. Subjective data includes the onset, duration, and severity of the symptoms, as well as any associated manifestations (such as dysuria, frequency, and urgency, or abdominal pain) and circumstances (such as antibiotic therapy). Ask to describe the amount, color, odor, and consistency of vaginal discharge. Inquire about perineal care (use of bubble baths, perineal powders or sprays, and douching) and usual dressing habits (underwear of synthetic materials, tight jeans or pants). Ask if the client could be pregnant and about menstrual history. Inquire about any chronic diseases such as diabetes or HIV infection, and current medications. Finally, ask what self-care measures she has used to treat her symptoms.

DIAGNOSING, PLANNING, AND IMPLEMENTING

Priorities in Nursing Care. Nursing care focuses on teaching the client and, if necessary, her sexual partner to comply with the treatment regimen, use safer sex practices, and prevent future transmission of the infection.

Deficient Knowledge: Prevention of Vaginitis

- Explain how the infection is transmitted. *The infection may be acquired through sexual activity, from inappropriate perineal hygiene measures, or overgrowth of certain organisms that normally reside on perineal and vaginal tissues. A clear understanding of how the infection developed allows the client to use measures to prevent future infections.*
- If advised, emphasize the need for both the client and her partner to complete the course of treatment. *Many*

infections are asymptomatic in one partner. Incomplete treatment allows the infection to recur and reinfect the partner.

- Teach hygiene measures such as the following:
  - Avoid bubble baths, douches, feminine hygiene sprays, synthetic underwear, and tight pants.
  - Cleanse the perineum from front to back after voiding and defecating.
  - Cleanse genitals before and after sexual intercourse. *These measures help maintain the normal vaginal environment and prevent irritation and contamination of perineal tissues that can increase the risk of infection.*

clinical ALERT

Advise women taking an antibiotic prescription to consume at least 6 to 8 ounces of yogurt containing live bacterial cultures daily to help prevent vaginitis.

Pain

- Suggest using cool compresses and mild vinegar douches. *Cool compresses relieve itching. Vinegar has a fungicidal and bactericidal effect.*
- Recommend sitz baths to alleviate discomfort. *Sitz baths cleanse the perineal area and wash away irritating discharge.*

EVALUATING

To evaluate the effectiveness of nursing interventions, collect data related to the client's and her partner's understanding of the treatment and prevention of vaginitis, as well as the client's level of comfort.

Documenting. Document subjective and objective assessment data, including the duration and circumstances of the infection, appearance of perineal tissues, and the character of any vaginal discharge, including its odor. Document teaching provided, as well as the client's understanding of the information and willingness to comply with recommended treatment measures.

CONTINUING CARE

To prevent vaginitis, teach all women about personal hygiene and safer sex practices. Teach women to avoid douching and wearing nylon underwear and/or tight pants. Unprotected sexual activity, particularly with multiple partners, greatly increases the risk of vaginal infections and STIs. Unless contraindicated, encourage the client with repeated mild candidiasis infections to consume 8 oz. of yogurt containing live active cultures daily to help restore normal vaginal flora.

Many postmenopausal women experience atrophic vaginitis due to the thinning and drying of the vaginal mucosa that result from lack of estrogen. Teach these clients about using topical estrogen creams, water-soluble lubricants for intercourse, and other methods to minimize the undesirable effects of menopause.

Pelvic Inflammatory Disease

Pelvic inflammatory disease (PID) is an infection of the pelvic organs (fallopian tubes, ovaries, uterus, and cervix). PID is usually caused by infection with *Neisseria gonorrhoeae* and/or *Chlamydia trachomatis*. Clients with PID often are infected with more than one organism. PID is a major cause of female infertility.

PID usually affects young, sexually active women who have multiple partners. Other risk factors include use of an intrauterine device (IUD) for birth control. Oral contraceptives and barrier contraceptives such as condoms reduce the risk of PID.

PATHOPHYSIOLOGY

Infectious organisms enter the vagina and travel to the uterus during intercourse or other sexual activity. They can also enter during childbirth, abortion, or reproductive tract surgery. The infection then spreads through the fallopian tubes, leading to inflammation and obstruction due to scar tissue. It settles on the ovary and also may enter the lymphatic system or bloodstream, leading to systemic infection.

MANIFESTATIONS

The manifestations of PID include high fever, vaginal discharge, severe lower abdominal pain, nausea, malaise, and dysuria. Scarring of the fallopian tubes can lead to infertility and an increased risk of ectopic pregnancy. The client also may experience pain during intercourse and dysmenorrhea.

INTERDISCIPLINARY CARE

The diagnosis of PID often is based on the history and physical examination.

Diagnostic Tests

Endocervical secretions are cultured to identify the infecting organism. The *WBC* often is markedly elevated, a sign of infection. *Ultrasonography* is performed to rule out ectopic pregnancy. *Laparoscopy* may show inflammation, edema, and possible abscess of pelvic structures.

Medications

Treatment usually is started with antibiotics that are effective to treat gonorrhea and chlamydia. If PID is not acute, outpatient antibiotic treatment is prescribed. In acute cases, however, the client is hospitalized. Analgesics are given, and antibiotics and fluids are administered intravenously. In either case, the woman's sexual partner is treated at the same time. Nursing implications for antibiotic use are discussed in Chapter 10. 🔗

Surgery

The surgeon may insert a drain into an abscess, if present, and remove any adhesions. If the infection is overwhelming or chronic, a hysterectomy with bilateral salpingo-oophorectomy may be necessary.

NURSING CARE

ASSESSING

Ask about abdominal pain, including its location, intensity, character, timing, and duration. Inquire about associated symptoms such as nausea, vomiting, and vaginal drainage. Ask if the client could be pregnant. Inquire about risk factors such as multiple sexual partners, unprotected sexual activity, and recent STIs.

Objective data include vital signs and temperature, shape and contour of the abdomen, bowel sounds, and abdominal tenderness. Note the color, odor, and amount of any vomitus or vaginal drainage.

DIAGNOSING, PLANNING, AND IMPLEMENTING

PID can have severe, even life-threatening complications. Scarring of the fallopian tubes can lead to ectopic pregnancy or pelvic abscess. Adhesions (bands of scar tissue) within the pelvis can obstruct the bowel.

Priorities in Nursing Care. Promoting prompt and effective treatment of PID and compliance with the prescribed treatment is the priority for nursing care.

Risk for Injury

- Maintain bed rest in semi-Fowler's position. *This promotes drainage and helps localize the infection in the pelvic cavity.*
- Maintain Standard Precautions and meticulous hand washing. Wear gloves when handling perineal pads and linens. Disinfect bedpans and toilet seats. *These measures help prevent spread of the infection to others.*
- Administer antibiotics as ordered, monitoring closely for adverse effects. *Antibiotics used in acute PID are potent agents; some can have life-threatening side effects.*
- Teach to recognize and report potential complications such as ectopic pregnancy, abscess, or bowel obstruction. *Reporting early manifestations of these potential complications reduces the risk of delayed treatment.*

Deficient Knowledge: STI Prevention

- Explain how infection is spread and how to prevent future infections. *Knowledge of the spread of infections allows control in preventing exposure to future infections.*

- Stress the importance of completing the treatment regimen and of follow-up visits. *Incomplete treatment can lead to chronic infection and bacteria that are resistant to antibiotics. Noncompliance and recurrence are common.*
- Teach perineal care, especially wiping from front to back. *This reduces transmission of fecal organisms to reproductive tissues and reduces the incidence of urinary tract infections.*
- Instruct to avoid using tampons until the infection has completely cleared. Advise changing tampons or pads at least every 4 hours. *Menstrual flow provides a favorable environment for microorganisms to multiply.*
- Discuss safer sex practices and family planning. Instruct to remove diaphragms within 6 hours after use. IUDs are contraindicated. Latex condoms offer the most effective protection against infection. *These measures help prevent recurrence of infection.*
- Teach to report any unusual vaginal discharge or odor to the health care provider. Emphasize the importance of seeking treatment if her partner develops an STI. *Treatment is most effective early in the disease process. STIs such as gonorrhea and* Chlamydia *often are asymptomatic in women.*

EVALUATING

To evaluate the effectiveness of nursing care for the client with PID, collect data related to manifestations of the disease and its complications, as well as the client's and her partner's understanding of and willingness to use measures to prevent future infections.

Documenting. Document continuing assessment data and the client's response to treatment measures (e.g., reduced fever and abdominal pain). Document all teaching provided and the client's and partner's apparent understanding and acceptance of measures to prevent future episodes of PID.

CONTINUING CARE

Emphasize the importance of completing the prescribed treatment and keeping follow-up appointments as directed to ensure eradication of the infection. Discuss safer sex practices, and measures to prevent recurrence of PID. Address the manifestations of potential complications of PID.

clinical ALERT

Stress the importance of seeking care promptly if manifestations of ectopic pregnancy (intermittent colicky abdominal pain, sharp abdominal or shoulder pain, symptoms of hypovolemic shock) or bowel obstruction (abdominal pain and distention, nausea and vomiting, high-pitched or absent bowel sounds) develop.

Inform the client that the patency of the fallopian tubes can be evaluated after several menstrual cycles, to allow for complete resolution of the inflammatory process.

Toxic Shock Syndrome

Toxic shock syndrome (TSS) is a rare but acute illness caused by *Staphylococcus aureus* infection. Although it may be related to using tampons during menstruation, TSS also has been associated with the use of vaginal barrier contraceptives such as the sponge, the diaphragm, and the cervical cap. About half of all cases of TSS are related to other factors such as childbirth, abdominal surgery, septic abortion, burns, and skin lesions.

PATHOPHYSIOLOGY

TSS is caused by virulent strains of *Staphylococcus aureus* that enter the bloodstream through open blood vessels during the menses, the placental site after childbirth, or other open wound. Once inside the body, the organism produces toxins that cause vasodilation, hemodynamic instability, and shock. The clinical manifestations of TSS are presented in Box 35-5 ■.

INTERDISCIPLINARY CARE

The goals of care for a client with TSS are to identify the source of the infection, eradicate the infection, and restore stability of the cardiovascular and other body systems. The diagnosis is based on the history and physical examination. Wounds and vaginal secretions are cultured for *Staphylococcus aureus*. Treatment includes administering intravenous fluids to restore blood volume and blood pressure. Antibiotics are given to eliminate the infection. Drugs to restore the blood pressure and perfusion of vital organs also may be given.

BOX 35-5

MANIFESTATIONS OF TOXIC SHOCK SYNDROME

- High fever
- Nausea, vomiting, abdominal pain, diarrhea
- Muscle pain
- Sore throat
- Headache
- Dizziness, low blood pressure
- Diffuse red rash, conjunctivitis
- Peeling skin on palms and soles
- Altered mental status

NURSING CARE

ASSESSING

Ask about the onset and duration of symptoms. Inquire about use of tampons, diaphragm, or vaginal barrier contraceptive devices. Ask about other risk factors such as recent surgery or abortion, or disruption of the skin by an infection or wound.

Obtain complete head-to-toe physical assessment data, including vital signs.

DIAGNOSING, PLANNING, AND IMPLEMENTING

Clients with TSS may be critically ill, requiring intensive nursing care.

Ineffective Tissue Perfusion

- Administer intravenous fluids and blood expanders as ordered. *Vascular dilation causes blood pooling and impaired organ and tissue perfusion. Increasing intravascular volume improves venous return, cardiac output, and tissue perfusion.*
- Administer oxygen as ordered. Monitor oxygen saturation, reporting levels less than 95% to the charge nurse or physician. *Increasing the oxygen content of blood increases oxygen reaching peripheral tissues.*

Decreased Cardiac Output

In the client with TSS, low circulating blood volume may decrease cardiac output.

- Monitor vital signs hourly or more often, as indicated. *An increase in pulse and respiratory rates often is the earliest sign of shock. The blood pressure may remain within normal limits, even though tissues are not receiving adequate blood flow.*
- Monitor urine output hourly; notify the physician if urinary output falls below 30 mL per hour. *Urine output falls when the kidneys do not receive adequate blood flow. This indicates compromised perfusion to other tissues as well, and an increased risk for renal and other organ system failure.*
- Monitor respiratory status, including rate, depth, and breath sounds. *Rapid fluid administration increases the risk of pulmonary edema, which increases the work of breathing and interferes with gas exchange.*

EVALUATING

To evaluate the effectiveness of nursing care for the client with TSS, collect continuing assessment data, comparing it to objective data collected on admission.

Documenting. Document continuing assessment data and the client's response to treatment measures. Note all teaching provided, referrals made for continuing care, and follow-up appointments.

CONTINUING CARE

Teach the client and family about the causes of TSS and self-care measures to prevent future infection (Box 35-6 ■).

Emphasize the importance of completing the prescribed course of antibiotics, even after manifestations have subsided. Stress the need to keep follow-up appointments. Advise women who have had TSS to avoid using tampons and vaginal barrier contraceptives. Stress the importance of reporting manifestations of the disorder to primary care provider, because women who have had TSS have a high risk for recurrence.

BOX 35-6	CLIENT TEACHING

Preventing Toxic Shock Syndrome

- Use the lowest absorbency tampon possible to contain menstrual flow.
- Change tampons at least every 4 hours, and use sanitary pads at night.
- Wash hands with soap before inserting a tampon, diaphragm, or vaginal medication.
- Remove diaphragms when recommended following intercourse. Do not use during menses.
- Do not use tampons during the first 12 weeks after childbirth.
- If you have had TSS, avoid using tampons or a diaphragm.

MALIGNANT TUMORS

Cervical Cancer

Cervical cancer is common. Early detection and intervention have substantially reduced the incidence of invasive cervical cancer and deaths due to cervical cancer.

Most cervical cancers are related to infection of the cervix with human papillomavirus (HPV). The other risk factors for cervical cancer include early sexual experience, multiple sex partners, HIV infection, unprotected sex, smoking, and a poor diet.

PATHOPHYSIOLOGY

Most cervical cancers begin as changes in squamous cells of the cervix. These changes are called *cervical intraepithelial neoplasia (CIN).* Over a number of years, these cells become more abnormal and the number of affected cells increases, developing into carcinoma *in situ.* Carcinoma *in situ* is localized, but if it is not treated, it becomes invasive, spreading into the underlying connective tissue. Cervical cancers spread by direct invasion of surrounding tissues such as the vagina, bladder, and rectum, as well as by metastasizing to the pelvis and other organs.

MANIFESTATIONS

Early cancer causes no symptoms. Invasive cancer produces bleeding and leukorrhea (whitish discharge from the vagina), which increase as the cancer progresses. Other manifestations include pain in the back or thighs, hematuria, bloody stools, anemia, and weight loss.

INTERDISCIPLINARY CARE

Screening

A *Papanicolaou (Pap) smear* is used to screen for cervical cancer. Cells and secretions from the cervix are collected and spread on a glass slide for examination. Infectious or abnormal cell changes can be identified. Abnormal cells may be described as atypical, mild dysplasia, or moderate to severe dysplasia (carcinoma *in situ*). See Box 33-2 ⚭ and Table 33-1 ⚭ for nursing responsibilities related to a Pap smear. Abnormal Pap smear results are reported by the type and severity of cellular changes (Table 35-3 ■).

Diagnostic Tests

- If the initial *Pap smear* shows abnormal cells, it is repeated.
- The *Digene Hybrid Capture II HPV test* may be done to identify the presence of high-risk strains of HPV.
- *Colposcopy* and *biopsy* of the suspicious area may be done if the second Pap smear shows abnormal cells. Box 35-7 ■ describes nursing implications for cervical biopsy.
- *MRI* or *CT* of the pelvis, abdomen, or bones may be done to evaluate for tumor spread.

Treatment

When the tumor is limited to cervical tissue (not invasive), it may be excised by laser, heated or cooled probes, or cauterization. *Conization,* removal of a cone-shaped wedge of cervical tissue (Figure 35-3 ■), may be done if the lesion extends into the endocervical canal.

Radioactive implants of needles, tubes, or seeds into the uterine cavity (brachytherapy) are used to treat locally invasive tumors. For invasive lesions, hysterectomy or radical hysterectomy (removal of the uterus, fallopian tubes, lymph nodes, and ovaries) is performed. A *pelvic exenteration*—removal of all pelvic contents, including the bowel, vagina, and bladder—may be done for locally invasive cancer. A colostomy is created for bowel elimination and a urinary diversion for urine elimination. See Chapter 20 ⚭ for more

TABLE 35-3

Abnormal Pap Smear Result Classifications

DYSPLASIA	CERVICAL INTRAEPITHELIAL NEOPLASIA (CIN)	BETHESDA SYSTEM
Benign	Benign	Normal
Benign with inflammation	Benign with inflammation	Normal, atypical squamous cells of undetermined significance (ASC-US)
Mild dysplasia	CIN I	Low-grade squamous intrapithelial lesion (SIL)
Moderate dysplasia	CIN II	High-grade SIL
Severe dysplasia	CIN III	
Carcinoma *in situ* (CIS)		
Invasive cancer	Invasive cancer	Invasive cancer

information about colostomy, and Chapter 32 ∞ for more information about urinary diversion. Radiation therapy also is used to treat invasive cervical cancer. External radiation beam therapy may be used before surgery to decrease the size of the tumor. Chemotherapy may be used when surgery or radiation therapy cannot be used or if the cancer has metastasized (see Chapter 12). ∞

NURSING CARE

ASSESSING

Because the client with cervical cancer rarely has symptoms until the cancer is advanced, nursing assessment focuses on collecting data related to risk factors for cervical cancer. Ask:

BOX 35-7   **NURSING CARE CHECKLIST**

Cervical Biopsy

Before the Procedure

☑ Explain the procedure. Discomfort is minimal, although cramping may be felt during cervical dilation.

☑ Have client empty her bladder.

After the Procedure

☑ Cleanse the area, apply a perineal pad, and assist to a comfortable position.

☑ Explain that minor bleeding and vaginal discharge are expected; use perineal pads and avoid tampons for at least 1 week.

☑ Caution to avoid sexual intercourse until discharge has stopped.

☑ Instruct to notify physician of heavy bleeding, pain, foul-smelling discharge, fever, or malaise.

- The age at which the client began having sexual intercourse
- Number of partners
- Use of barrier protection (male or female condoms)
- History of sexually transmitted diseases
- Smoking history.

DIAGNOSING, PLANNING, AND IMPLEMENTING

Priorities in Nursing Care. Nursing care priorities include helping the client deal with the physical and psychologic effects of cervical cancer, providing information needed to make informed decisions, and minimizing the adverse effects of treatment.

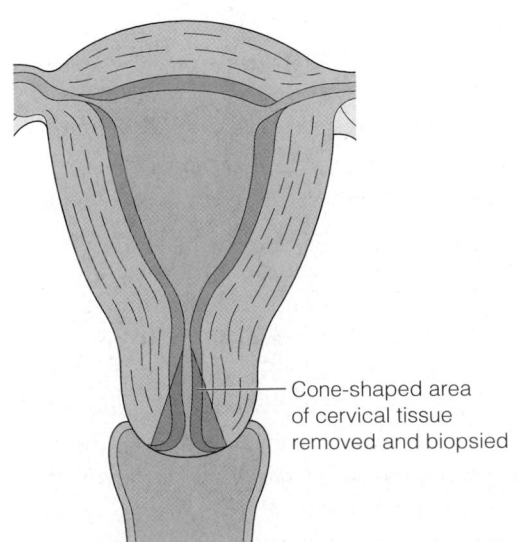

Cone-shaped area of cervical tissue removed and biopsied

Figure 35-3. ■ Conization, removal of a cone-shaped section of the cervix.

Impaired Tissue Integrity

- Teach wound and skin care specific to needs. *Open and damaged tissue increases the risk for infection. Meticulous skin and wound care helps prevent infection and further tissue destruction.*
- Apply non–oil-based lotions to skin to reduce itching and help maintain integrity. *Oil-based lotions are not recommended for tissue undergoing radiation.*
- Instruct to preserve markings used to localize the radiation beam to the target area. *Markings are used in future radiation treatments.*
- Observe for manifestations of fistula, and teach the client to do the same. *Fistulas may form as a complication of radiation to the pelvic or abdominal cavities.*

Fear

- Explain that most women with cervical cancer survive for 5 years or more, and that the earlier the cancer is detected, the better the prognosis. *The cure rate for early cervical cancer is 90%. This fact can provide hope, an essential ingredient in recovery.*
- Allow time to express concerns and to ask questions. *Unexpressed feelings and fears and lack of understanding may cause the client to view the situation as worse than it is.*
- Refer to counselor or support group for additional information. *Cancer survivors provide proof that people can survive the diagnosis and treatment of cancer and lead normal, productive lives.*

Disturbed Body Image

- Actively listen and acknowledge concerns about effect of the disease and its treatment on self-concept, attractiveness, and sexuality. *Hysterectomy represents loss of a significant body part, significantly changing body image. If surgery is extensive, the client may also need to adjust to the presence of a colostomy and urinary diversion.*
- Encourage the client and family to share their feelings and concerns with one another. *Family members provide support for each other, and can be instrumental in helping the client adjust to the change in body image and function.*
- Allow the client and family to grieve for not only lost body image and function, but also for the potential loss of life. *Cervical cancer presents a threat to overall life span, as well as a threat to reproductive function.*
- Assist the client and family to identify and use coping mechanisms that have been successful in the past. *Coping mechanisms help the client and family deal with stressors during diagnosis and treatment of the disease.*
- Help the client select clothing, wigs, and cosmetics, as appropriate, to project a positive body image. *Appearance to the outside world is a significant contributor to body image.*

EVALUATING

To evaluate the effectiveness of nursing interventions, collect data related to skin integrity and absence of infection. Ask the client and family members about coping with the diagnosis and treatment, and provide additional information and support as needed.

Documenting. Document all information and teaching provided, and the client's and family's apparent understanding of treatment options. Document continuing assessments, postoperative care, and the client's response to other treatments such as radiation therapy.

CONTINUING CARE

Teach all clients and the public how to control risk factors for cervical cancer. Stress the importance of regular pelvic exams and Pap smears throughout the life span. Teach young women about the relationship between early sexual activity, multiple partners, and risk for sexually transmitted diseases and cervical cancer. Discuss safer sex alternatives and using condoms for protection. Emphasize the importance of continued screening exams for the older client who may not see a gynecologic specialist on a regular basis.

Client and family teaching vary according to the stage of the cancer and the treatment selected. Provide information concerning radiation, chemotherapy, or surgery, as indicated. Refer the client to home health services and/or a cancer support group.

NURSING PROCESS CARE PLAN
Client with Cervical Cancer

Anna Eliza Gillam is a 45-year-old divorced woman with four children ranging in age from 16 to 23. She was married at age 18 and had several sexual partners prior to marriage. She has had three sexual partners since her marriage ended. Her Pap smear 2 weeks ago showed atypical cells. A repeat Pap smear and biopsy of a cervical lesion is positive for squamous cell carcinoma of the cervix.

Assessment. The nursing assessment reveals: BP 130/80; P 72; R 18; T 99.2°F (37.3°C). Weight 142 lbs (64.5 kg), approximately 15% over ideal for height. Smokes about one-half pack of cigarettes per day, and does not drink alcohol.

Ms. Gillam is very fearful and has told no one about her abnormal Pap smear. She says that she has had back pain radiating down her thighs for several months and a foul vaginal discharge that increases after intercourse. Until 2 weeks ago, she had not had a Pap smear for 5 years.

Laparoscopy shows the disease to be widespread in the pelvic cavity. A CT scan is scheduled.

Diagnosis. The nursing diagnoses for Ms. Gillam include the following:

- *Decisional Conflict* related to treatment options
- *Pain* related to metastasis and surgery
- *Risk for Impaired Skin Integrity* related to radiation
- *Anticipatory Grieving* related to cancer diagnosis and potential loss of life

Expected Outcomes. The expected outcomes for the plan of care specify that Ms. Gillam will:

- Gain knowledge to make informed decisions about treatment options.
- Develop strategies for pain control.
- Maintain skin and tissue integrity during radiation therapy.
- Develop effective coping strategies for dealing with life-threatening illness and pain.

Planning and Implementation. The following interventions are planned and implemented for Ms. Gillam:

- Explore treatment alternatives, including the prognosis with each option.
- Administer pain medications as ordered.
- Inspect skin surfaces daily before and after radiation therapy.
- Provide information about additional strategies for pain control.
- Refer to a local cancer support group.
- Refer to clinical social worker for discharge and home care planning.
- Assess response to treatment and understanding of her disease.
- Recommend a high-protein, high-carbohydrate diet.

Evaluation. Ms. Gillam has begun radiation therapy following pelvic exenteration. She controls her pain with relaxation and imagery techniques, requiring only occasional analgesics. Her skin is reddened but intact in the area of radiation. Ms. Gillam seems optimistic and has quit smoking. She and her family are continuing to attend the cancer support group meetings.

Critical Thinking in the Nursing Process

1. Develop a teaching outline to use with groups about reducing modifiable risks for cervical cancer.
2. Following an abnormal Pap smear, a second smear reveals inflammatory changes consistent with HPV but no cell changes. What advice will you provide to the client?
3. Explain the terms *noninvasive* and *invasive* in relation to cervical cancer and its methods of treatment.

Endometrial Cancer

Endometrial cancer is common. It usually affects older women between ages 50 and 70. In addition to age, risk factors for endometrial cancer include early menarche, late menopause, history of infertility, extended use of tamoxifen or estrogen therapy (without progestins), obesity, and diabetes. Endometrial cancer is curable. With early diagnosis and treatment, the 5-year survival rate exceeds 90%.

PATHOPHYSIOLOGY

Most endometrial malignancies are slow to grow and metastasize. These tumors tend to be associated with estrogen excess, and begin with endometrial hyperplasia. This type of endometrial cancer occurs more commonly in perimenopausal white women. Endometrial cancers seen in postmenopausal Asian and African American women may be more aggressive and are not associated with known risk factors.

The tumor usually begins in the fundus of the uterus, invades the muscle of the uterus, and spreads throughout the female reproductive tract. Metastasis occurs by the lymphatic system and bloodstream, as well as through the fallopian tubes to the peritoneal cavity. Target areas for metastasis include the lungs, liver, and bone.

MANIFESTATIONS

Abnormal uterine bleeding after menopause is the most common manifestation of endometrial cancer. This bleeding is usually painless but may be moderate to large in amount. Vaginal discharge is another sign of endometrial cancer. On pelvic examination, the uterus often is enlarged.

INTERDISCIPLINARY CARE

The preliminary diagnosis of endometrial cancer is made based on the history and physical examination. An endometrial biopsy or D&C is performed to obtain cells for examination. (Review Box 35-2 for nursing responsibilities related to a D&C.)

Treatment

The treatment of choice for primary endometrial carcinoma is a total abdominal hysterectomy and bilateral salpingo-oophorectomy (removal of the uterus, fallopian tubes, and both ovaries). Pelvic lymph nodes also may be resected during surgery. Radiation therapy may be done before surgery to shrink the tumor or after surgery to eliminate cancer cells in lymph nodes. Progesterone is ordered to treat recurrent disease. Chemotherapy is less effective than other forms of therapy, although it may be used to treat disseminated disease.

NURSING CARE

Nursing care involves helping the client deal with the physical and psychologic effects of endometrial cancer, make informed decisions, and minimize the adverse effects of therapy. The client who has had a hysterectomy requires pre- and postoperative nursing care (review Box 35-3). Encourage the client to perform self-care and resume normal activities of daily living.

Disturbed Body Image

- Review the side effects of treatment (hair loss, nausea, vomiting, fatigue, diarrhea, stomatitis, and surgical scarring), and help develop a plan to deal with these effects. *This promotes a sense of control.*
- Provide information about measures to alleviate adverse effects of chemotherapy, such as premedicating with antiemetic drugs, using viscous lidocaine for stomatitis, and obtaining a wig or using hats and scarves to cover the head. *Knowledge helps reduce the sense of helplessness clients often feel in dealing with these effects.*

CONTINUING CARE

Provide information about the disease and proposed specific treatments. To clients receiving radiation therapy, emphasize the importance of keeping appointments. If necessary, help them arrange transportation to and from the facility. Teach appropriate skin care. Explain the expected side effects of radiation implant therapy (see Chapter 12). ∞ Pain control measures are also an essential part of the teaching plan (see Chapter 8). ∞ Emphasize the importance of follow-up care as recommended.

Ovarian Cancer

Ovarian cancer is the most lethal of the gynecologic cancers, because it is often asymptomatic. In most cases, the disease has spread beyond the ovaries at the time of diagnosis. Ovarian cancer is more common in European American women than in African American women. However, the mortality rate is higher in African American women.

Risk factors for ovarian cancer include older age, early menarche and late menopause, history of infertility, treatment for infertility with clomiphene (Clomid), and a personal or family history of breast or ovarian cancer.

PATHOPHYSIOLOGY

Because the ovaries contain several different tissue types, there are different types of ovarian cancers. These cancers grow and spread at different rates. The most common type of ovarian cancer is an epithelial tumor. Malignant tumors usually present as solid masses with areas of necrosis and hemorrhage.

Ovarian cancer spreads by shedding cancer cells into the peritoneal cavity and by direct invasion of the bowel and bladder. Tumor cells also spread through the lymph system and blood to lymph nodes and such organs as the liver and the lungs.

MANIFESTATIONS

Early ovarian cancer generally has no symptoms. When manifestations do develop, they are often vague and mild, such as indigestion, urinary frequency, abdominal bloating, and constipation. Pelvic pain sometimes occurs. An enlarged abdomen with ascites (a collection of fluid in the abdomen) is a late manifestation of ovarian cancer.

INTERDISCIPLINARY CARE

While an enlarged ovary may be palpated on physical examination, diagnostic tests usually are required to detect ovarian cancer. These tests may include:

- *CA125,* a tumor marker, may not be elevated in early ovarian cancer and is not specific for ovarian cancer.
- *Transvaginal ultrasonography* may be done to detect ovarian masses.
- *Laparoscopy* is performed to obtain tissue for biopsy and determine organ involvement.

Surgery is the treatment of choice for ovarian cancer. In most cases, a total hysterectomy with bilateral salpingo-oophorectomy is performed, and other organs and tissues in the abdomen are inspected for spread of the cancer. Following surgery, chemotherapy may be used to eliminate cancer cells in other tissues. Paclitaxel (Taxol), a chemotherapy drug, may help achieve and maintain remission. See Chapter 12 ∞ for more information about nursing care of the client receiving chemotherapy.

NURSING CARE

Nursing care for the client with ovarian cancer is similar to the nursing care for clients with other gynecologic cancers. The side effects of treatment and generally poor prognosis affect the quality of life and have major psychosocial implications. Anticipatory grieving may begin at the time of diagnosis.

Educate women who have significant risk factors for ovarian cancer, such as a positive family history of the disease or previous breast cancer, about the importance of having regular pelvic examinations. Suggest regular screening with transvaginal ultrasound and CA125 measurements for this high-risk group. Teach clients not to ignore symptoms such as indigestion, nausea, or urinary frequency, because these may be early manifestations of ovarian tumors. Emphasize, however, that ovarian cancer usually has no symptoms in early stages. Instruct any woman with a palpable abdominal mass to see her primary care provider.

Discuss recommended treatment with women who have ovarian cancer. Suggest ways to minimize or manage side effects. Provide emotional and psychologic support throughout the course of the disease, and refer the client to hospice services when appropriate.

Cancer of the Vulva

Cancer of the vulva usually affects older women between the ages of 60 and 70. In younger women, it is strongly associated with sexually transmitted infections, particularly HPV. Herpes simplex type 2 (HSV-2) infection also is a risk factor for vulvar cancer.

The prognosis of vulvar carcinoma generally is good, with an 85% to 90% five-year survival rate when there is no lymph node involvement.

PATHOPHYSIOLOGY AND MANIFESTATIONS

Cancer of the vulva usually arises in epithelial cells. The primary site is usually the labia majora, but it also may be found on the labia minora, clitoris, vestibule, and other perineal tissues. It spreads by direct extension into surrounding tissues, as well as through the lymph system to regional and pelvic lymph nodes.

Cancer of the vulva often causes no symptoms, and lesions are discovered on routine examination or self-examination. The lesion may appear as a white macular patch, a small raised lump, an ulceration, or a red painless sore.

Persistent pruritus (itching) and irritation of the vulva is the most common symptom. Perineal pain and bleeding occur with advanced disease.

INTERDISCIPLINARY CARE

Visible lesions are carefully examined, excised, and biopsied. Early, noninvasive lesions are excised using laser surgery, cryosurgery, or electrocautery. For more advanced disease, vulvectomy may be performed (Figure 35-4 ■).

In a simple *vulvectomy,* the vulva, labia majora and minora, clitoris, and prepuce are removed. In a radical vulvectomy, subcutaneous tissue and regional lymph nodes are removed as well. If surgery is contraindicated, lesions may be treated with locally applied chemotherapy or by laser.

NURSING CARE

Priorities in Nursing Care. Disruption of perineal tissues is a priority nursing problem for clients being treated for cancer of the vulva. Sexuality also is significantly affected, and

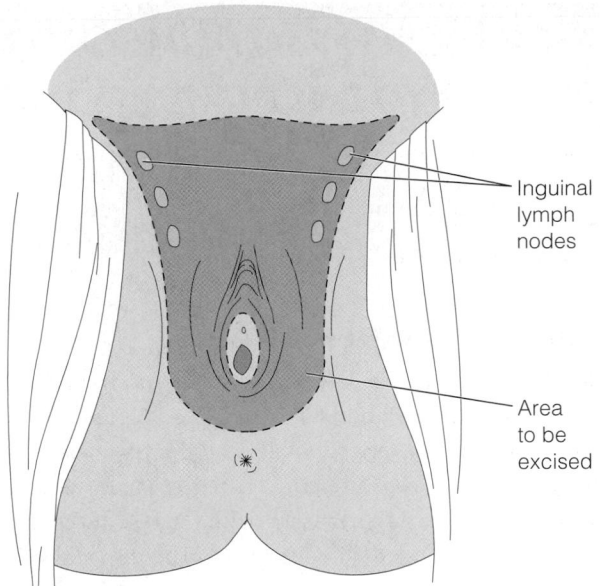

Figure 35-4. ■ Vulvectomy for cancer of the vulva.

Inguinal lymph nodes

Area to be excised

must be considered as a nursing care problem. Body image also is affected; see also the nursing interventions for Disturbed Body Image under the section on cervical cancer.

Impaired Tissue Integrity

- Teach the client and/or her partner or other family member how to irrigate perineal tissues. *Irrigation helps prevent skin breakdown and infection.*
- After irrigation, apply dry heat using a heat lamp positioned about 18 inches from the area; emphasize safety precautions, including use of a low-wattage bulb (40 to 60 watts). *Dry heat helps promote healing and comfort.*
- Discuss dietary measures (high protein, iron, and vitamin C) to promote healing. *These nutrients promote collagen formation and wound healing.*

CONTINUING CARE

Because many clients who undergo treatment for cancer of the vulva are older, consider referral to home health services for wound management. Discuss early manifestations of infection or impaired healing, and stress the importance of contacting the physician if these develop. Instruct the client to cleanse the perineum by pouring warm water over it after voiding and using a sitz bath after defecation. If lymph nodes have been removed, the client may experience lower extremity edema. Teach the client to elevate the feet and legs when sitting, and to wear antiembolic elastic hose when out of bed.

STRUCTURAL DISORDERS OF THE FEMALE REPRODUCTIVE SYSTEM

Structural disorders of the female reproductive system include displacement of the uterus from its normal position within the pelvis, prolapse of pelvic organs, and vaginal fistulas.

Uterine Displacement

The uterus is not fixed within the pelvis. It normally is positioned with the body and fundus facing anteriorly and the cervix more posterior, but its position may vary among women. An *anteverted* uterus is tilted toward the bladder, whereas a *retroverted* uterus is tilted toward the rectum (Figures 35-5A and B ■). Changes in the upper portion of the uterus in relation to the cervix also can occur (Figures 35-5C and D). An *anteflexed* uterus is flexed forward on itself. Backward flexion of the uterus is called *retroflexion*.

Uterine displacement can be congenital or acquired. Childbirth or inflammation and scarring within the pelvic cavity can lead to displacement of the uterus. Clients with uterine displacement may experience manifestations such as painful menses (dysmenorrhea), discomfort during intercourse, and backache. The client also may have difficulty conceiving a child.

The diagnosis of uterine displacement is made by physical examination. A history of infections or difficulty conceiving

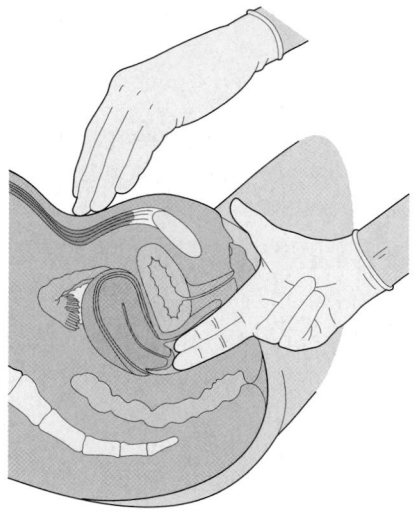

A Anteversion

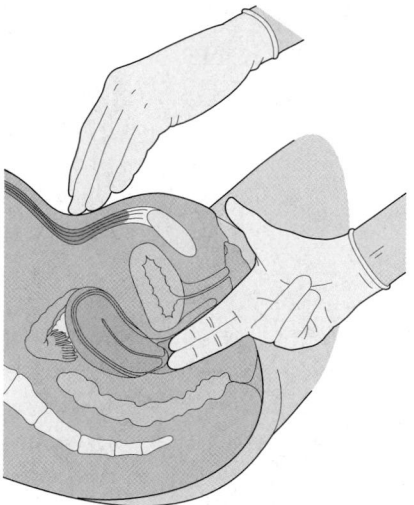

B Retroversion

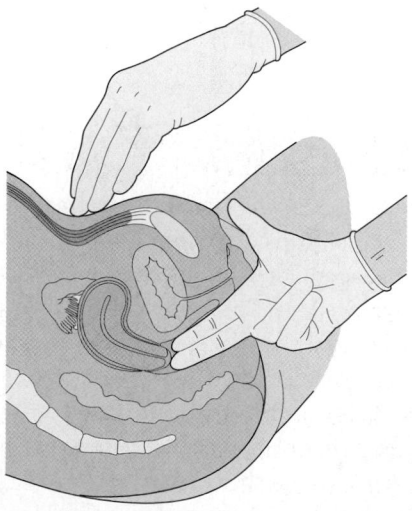

C Anteflexion

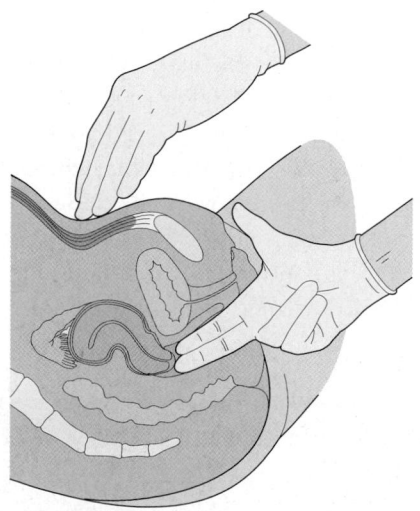

D Retroflexion

Figure 35-5. ■ Common uterine displacements.

support this diagnosis. In most cases, no treatment is necessary. Surgical suspension of the uterus may be done to treat associated infertility.

Nursing care focuses on teaching about the disorder. Many women have a poor understanding of their reproductive anatomy. This lack of knowledge may cause anxiety about the cause and seriousness of the disorder. Use drawings and models to explain the nature of the displacement disorder and its effects. Encourage the client and her partner to ask questions. Suggest trying alternate positions during sexual intercourse to relieve any discomfort. Reassure the client that the ability to have an orgasm is not affected.

Pelvic Organ Prolapse

Relaxation or damage of the pelvic floor muscles puts additional tension on the ligaments and structures that support the bladder, uterus, and rectum within the pelvis. When this occurs, these organs may prolapse, or drop down.

PATHOPHYSIOLOGY AND MANIFESTATIONS

Cystocele

A **cystocele** is prolapse of the urinary bladder into the vagina. It develops as the ligaments that support the bladder are stretched. Thinning of the vaginal wall commonly occurs during menopause, increasing the risk of cystocele. Cystocele often is accompanied by a urethrocele, or prolapse of the urethra into the vagina. The client with a cystocele often develops stress incontinence (see Chapter 32). ⚭ Other manifestations include urinary frequency and urgency, and difficulty emptying the bladder. Frequent bladder infections may develop due to urinary retention.

Rectocele

Rectocele, protrusion of the anterior rectal wall into the vagina, may be caused by trauma during childbirth or chronic constipation with straining to defecate. The client may have a sense of pelvic pressure and difficulty defecating.

Uterine Prolapse

Prolapse of the uterus into the vagina can vary from mild to complete prolapse outside the body (Figure 35-6 ■). **Uterine prolapse** is caused by stretching of the ligaments that normally support the uterus within the pelvis. Increased pressure within the abdomen also can lead to uterine prolapse. The client experiences a heavy or dragging sensation in the groin and lower back that is relieved by lying flat. She may notice a mass protruding from the vagina, especially after bearing down or with heavy lifting. Constipation, urinary incontinence, and painful intercourse are common.

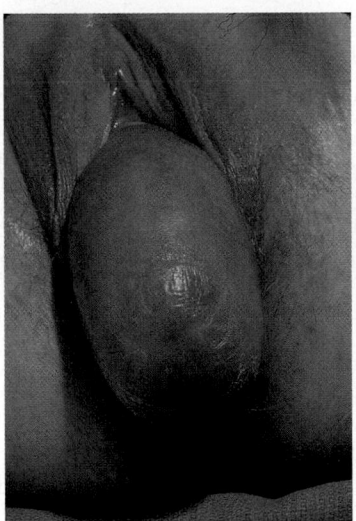

Figure 35-6. ■ Complete uterine prolapse with inversion of the vagina. (*Source:* Custom Medical Stock Photos, Inc.)

INTERDISCIPLINARY CARE

If pelvic organ prolapse is suspected, the client is asked to bear down or cough during pelvic examination to help identify the problem.

Kegel exercises or physical therapy may be ordered to strengthen weakened pelvic muscles. (See Kegel exercises as outlined in Box 32-3. ⚭) Pelvic organ prolapse often is treated surgically with procedures to repair the vaginal wall, shorten pelvic muscles, and resuspend pelvic organs. In postmenopausal clients, hysterectomy is the preferred treatment for significant uterine prolapse.

When surgery is contraindicated or refused by the client, a pessary may be inserted into the vagina to provide temporary support for the uterus or bladder. At regular intervals, the pessary is removed, cleaned, and reinserted.

NURSING CARE

Stress incontinence is a common problem in clients with pelvic organ prolapse. Teach the client how to perform Kegel exercises. These exercises strengthen perineal muscle tone, minimize urinary leakage, and minimize descent of the bladder and rectum into the vagina. Discuss hormone replacement therapy with postmenopausal women. It helps maintain pelvic tissue, reducing the risk for prolapse. Suggest using perineal pads to absorb urine leakage, and teach appropriate perineal care measures:

- Cleanse the perineum from front to back.
- Change perineal or incontinence pads frequently.
- Avoid using perineal sprays or powders.

Suggest reducing or eliminating caffeine intake and minimizing consumption of diet sodas. Both caffeine and artificial sweeteners can aggravate urinary incontinence.

Teach the client for whom a pessary is ordered how to insert, remove, and care for the device.

Because obesity is a risk factor for pelvic organ prolapse, diet counseling may be indicated. Suggest self-help diet organizations such as Weight Watchers or TOPS.

Vaginal Fistula

A *fistula* is an abnormal opening or passage between two organs or spaces that are normally separated. A vaginal fistula may develop between the vagina and the urinary bladder or between the vagina and the rectum. The fistula may be a complication of childbirth, surgery, or radiation therapy. Bladder cancer also may lead to vaginal fistula. Urine or stool and flatus enter the vagina through this abnormal opening, causing complaints of involuntary leakage of urine or gas. A small vaginal fistula may resolve without treatment. Larger fistulas may require surgical repair.

Nursing care is similar to that provided for any client undergoing pelvic surgery (see Chapter 9). Teaching is important. Stress the importance of careful perineal cleansing to reduce irritation and prevent further tissue breakdown. Suggest perineal irrigation or sitz baths for cleansing. Perineal pads may be used to absorb urine or fecal drainage. Provide information about avoiding gas-forming foods to minimize embarrassment from odor.

BREAST DISORDERS

Breast disorders are common. Women are primarily affected, but men also can develop them. Breast tissue changes in response to hormones, nutrition, and physical and environmental factors. Most women notice increased tenderness and lumpiness prior to menses. More than half of all women who menstruate regularly find a lump in the breast; 80% of these lumps are not cancerous. When a woman discovers a breast lump, her first response is often fear: of breast cancer, of losing her breast, and perhaps of losing her life. Because American society views the breast as a significant part of feminine beauty, breast problems often threaten a woman's self-image.

Nurses play a critical role in teaching about normal breast tissue, common disorders, screening and risk factors for breast cancer, and breast self-examination.

Fibrocystic Breast Changes

Fibrocystic breast changes are noncancerous changes in breast tissue, causing swelling, pain, tenderness, and lumpiness. They are thought to be caused by an excessive response to cyclic hormone changes. Fibrocystic changes are common in women 30 to 50 years old and rare in postmenopausal women.

PATHOPHYSIOLOGY

Fibrocystic changes are classified as nonproliferative or proliferative changes. *Nonproliferative* fibrocystic changes involve fibrosis of connective tissue, cyst formation, and inflammation (Figure 35-7 ■). These changes do not increase the risk for breast cancer. *Proliferative* fibrocystic changes involve cell growth, with an increase in cell numbers, especially of epithelial gland cells. The risk for cancer is higher in clients with proliferative breast changes. Both forms of fibrocystic changes may be present.

MANIFESTATIONS

Fibrocystic breast changes cause bilateral or unilateral breast pain or tenderness and a sense of fullness that increases just prior to menstruation. Lumps may be felt in the breasts, and discharge from the nipple may be noted. Multiple, mobile cysts can form, usually in both breasts. Fluid may be aspirated from these cysts.

INTERDISCIPLINARY CARE

Diagnosis of fibrocystic breast changes is based on the history, physical exam, and mammography. A needle biopsy may be done to rule out malignancy.

Aspiration of a large cyst may relieve pain. A well-fitting supportive brassiere worn day and night helps relieve discomfort. Some women report that avoiding caffeine and chocolate relieves symptoms; both contain methylxanthines,

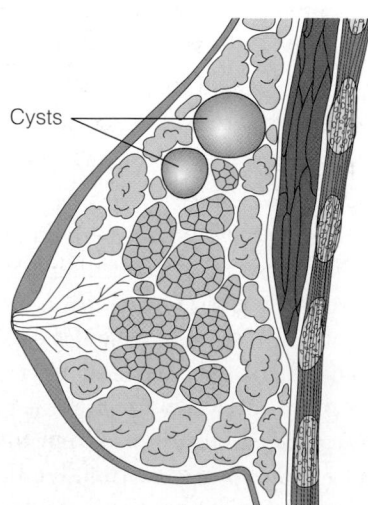

Cysts

Figure 35-7. ■ Fibrocystic breast changes.

believed to contribute to fibrocystic changes. Women who smoke report a reduction in breast lumps when they quit smoking. Mild analgesics and local heat or cold also are recommended. Vitamin E also may help relieve breast pain.

NURSING CARE

The nursing role for women with fibrocystic breast changes is primarily educational. Provide preoperative teaching and psychologic support before breast biopsy. After the procedure, discuss home care and possible complications that should be reported to the physician. Reinforce teaching about measures to promote comfort. Suggest that although research has not confirmed the role of abstaining from caffeine or taking vitamin E to relieve discomfort, many women find these measures beneficial.

Mastitis

Mastitis is inflammation that causes tenderness, swelling, and redness of the breast. Mastitis usually affects lactating women, caused by organisms from the infant's nose and throat.

Mastitis is treated with antibiotics. Increasing fluid intake, wearing a supportive bra, and taking mild analgesics, such as aspirin or ibuprofen, help relieve symptoms. If lactating, the woman should continue to breast feed from the unaffected breast and express milk from the affected breast.

Nursing care of the woman with mastitis includes teaching about the importance of hand washing, breast and nipple care, and, in lactating women, regular, thorough emptying of the breasts to prevent engorgement.

Disorders Related to Breast Augmentation

An estimated 4 million American women have undergone breast augmentation or reconstruction following mastectomy. Several problems are associated with breast implants:

- Scarring may occur around the implant, causing excessive firmness and distortion of the breast.
- The implant may rupture or bleed silicone gel through the capsule, causing local inflammation.
- While implants do not appear to increase the risk of breast cancer, they make early detection more difficult.

Other disorders such as connective tissue disease and chronic fatigue syndrome have been linked with silicone breast implants, although a connection has not been proved. Most current implants are saline filled.

Nurses should reassure clients with implants that removing the implant is not recommended unless it has ruptured or the client has symptoms of an autoimmune disorder. Inform clients who have reconstructive breast surgery following

BOX 35-8	POPULATION FOCUS

Breast Cancer

The incidence of breast cancer is decreasing, with the largest declines occurring in younger women. Although the incidence of breast cancer is lower in African American women than in Caucasian women, the mortality rate is higher. It often is detected at a later stage, and survival rates for African American women are lower at all stages.

mastectomy for cancer that local cancer recurrence usually is superficial and easily detected by palpation. Recurrent cancer is treated the same for clients with implants as for those without them.

Breast Cancer

Breast cancer is second only to lung cancer as a cause of cancer-related deaths among women. Breast cancer also strikes men, although rarely. While the incidence of breast cancer remains stable, mortality rates are decreasing (see Box 35-8 ■).

Breast cancer is not one disease, but many, depending on the affected breast tissue, the effect of estrogen on the tumor, and the age of the person at onset. The two most significant risk factors for breast cancer are female gender and age over 50. Other risk factors for breast cancer are listed in Table 35-4 ■.

TABLE 35-4	
Breast Cancer Risk Factors	
Gender	Female
Race	White
Age	Over 50
Family history	Breast cancer in mother or sister
Medical history	Cancer of other breast; endometrial cancer; proliferative fibrocystic breast changes
Menstrual history	Early menarche (before age 12); late menopause (after age 50)
Reproductive history	First birth after age 30; prolonged use of estrogen replacement therapy
Radiation exposure	Multiple chest x-rays or fluoroscopic exams, particularly before age 30
Lifestyle	More than two alcoholic drinks daily Obesity; smoking High economic status Breast trauma

PATHOPHYSIOLOGY

Breast cancer is unregulated growth of abnormal cells in breast tissue. It begins as a single transformed cell, which then multiplies. Breast cancer is hormone dependent: It does not develop in women without functioning ovaries who have never received estrogen replacement therapy. Most tumors occur in the ductal areas of the breast. Breast cancers are classified as noninvasive (*in situ*) or invasive. Invasiveness refers to penetration of the tumor into surrounding tissue. Two atypical types of breast cancer are inflammatory carcinoma and Paget's disease.

Noninvasive (*in Situ*) Carcinoma

In *noninvasive* breast cancer, malignant cells proliferate within the ducts or lobules of the breast without invading surrounding tissue. The nipple and the subareolar region are usually involved. Noninvasive cancers are typically diagnosed when the mass is seen on mammography rather than by a palpable breast mass or nipple discharge. Noninvasive cancers appear to increase the risk for invasive breast cancer.

Invasive Carcinoma

Most breast cancers are *invasive*, arising from the intermediate ducts of the breast. These tumors can be differentiated by cell type. However, the prognosis and treatment of the disease depend on the stage of the disease (see later section on staging), rather than on cell type. Invasive breast cancers spread to involve surrounding breast tissue, lymph, and blood vessels. The cancer can metastasize to distant sites through the bloodstream or lymphatic system. The common sites of metastasis of breast cancer are regional lymph nodes, bone, brain, lung, liver, and skin.

Inflammatory Carcinoma

Although rare, inflammatory breast cancer is the most malignant form of breast cancer. The client presents with a diffuse redness, warmth, and edema of the breast. A discrete mass may not be palpable. Metastases develop early and widely in clients with inflammatory carcinoma. The prognosis for this type of breast cancer is poor.

Paget's Disease

Paget's disease is a rare breast cancer that involves the nipple ducts. Initial symptoms are itching or burning of the nipple with superficial erosion, crusting, or ulceration.

MANIFESTATIONS

Most breast tumors are discovered by the client as small, hard, and painless lumps or masses. The mass is usually found in the upper outer quadrant of the breast. Other symptoms are listed in Box 35-9 ■. Skin changes such as dimpling, peau d'orange skin (Figure 35-8 ■), and engorged vessels on the affected breast may occur.

BOX 35-9

MANIFESTATIONS OF BREAST CANCER
- Small, hard, painless lump in breast
- Change in size or shape of breast
- Nipple discharge
- Breast pain
- Dimpling, pulling, or retraction in an area of the breast
- Persistent skin rash near the nipple area
- Flaking or eruption near the nipple
- Unusual lump in the underarm or above the collarbone

Clients with bone metastasis may have pathologic fractures, chronic pain, and hypercalcemia. Clients with lung metastasis may have difficulty breathing, and brain metastasis can affect mental processes.

INTERDISCIPLINARY CARE

Diagnosis of breast cancer begins with detection. The earlier breast cancer is detected, the more likely it is that treatment will be effective in curing the disease or extending survival.

Breast Cancer Screening

Breast cancer screening includes breast self-exam, clinical breast examination, and mammography. These are usually used in combination.

Recommendations for breast cancer screening are:
- BSE monthly starting at age 20
- Clinical breast examination every 3 years from ages 20 through 39 and annually after age 40
- Baseline mammogram between age 40 and 49; annual mammogram after age 50.

BREAST SELF-EXAMINATION (BSE). All women should be familiar with their own breasts so they can identify changes if they develop. BSE is an option for detecting breast cancer: Most breast cancers are found by the women themselves. Women should be taught how to perform BSE

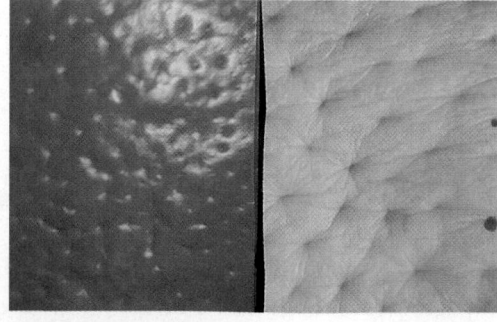

Figure 35-8. ■ Left, orange peel; right, peau d'orange skin. (*Source:* CNRI/Phototake.)

Step 1. Teach the client to observe her breasts in front of a mirror and in good lighting. Tell her to observe her breasts in four positions:

  With her arms relaxed and at her sides
  With her arms lifted over her head
  With her hands pressed against her hips
  With her hands pressed together at her waist, leaning forward

Instruct her to look at each breast individually, and then to compare them. She should observe for any visible abnormalities, such as lumps, dimpling, deviation, recent nipple retraction, irregular shape, edema, discharge, or asymmetry.

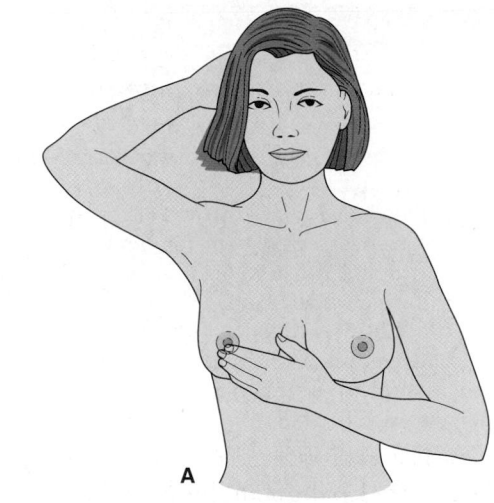

A

Step 2. Teach the client to palpate both breasts while standing or sitting, with one hand behind her head (Figure A). Tell her that many women palpate their breasts in the shower because water and soap make the skin slippery and easier to palpate. Show the woman how to use the pads of her fingers to palpate all areas of her breast, using the concentric circles technique (Figure B). Tell her to press the breast tissue gently against the chest wall, and to be sure to palpate the axillary tail.

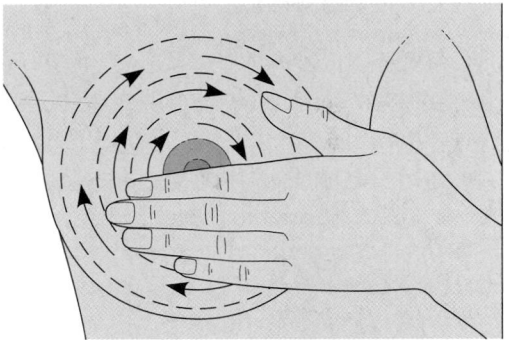

Step 3. Instruct the client to palpate her breasts again while lying down, as described in Step 2. Suggest that she place a folded towel under the shoulder and back on the side to be palpated. The arm on the examining side should be over the head, with the hand under the head (Figure C).

B

Step 4. Teach the client to palpate the areola and nipples next. Show her how to compress the nipple to check for discharge (Figure D).

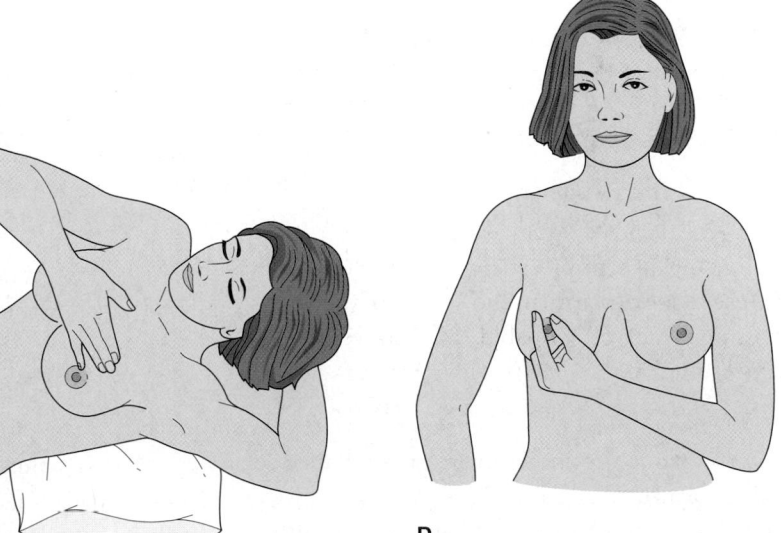

Step 5. Remind the client to use a calendar to keep a record of when she performs BSE. Teach her to perform BSE at the same time each month, usually 5 days after the onset of menses, when there is less hormonal influence on tissues.

C

D

Figure 35-9. ■ Teaching breast self-examination (BSE).

(Figure 35-9 ■). Premenopausal women should perform BSE after their menstrual period, because hormonal changes increase breast tenderness and lumpiness prior to menses. Suggest that postmenopausal women perform BSE on the first day of each month.

clinical ALERT

Emphasize the importance of continuing regular breast examinations after menopause because the risk for breast cancer increases with increasing age.

Breast Cancer in Older Women

Breast cancer is primarily a disease of older women: More than 60% of all breast cancers are diagnosed in women age 50 and older.

Women between ages 50 and 65 are the most likely to benefit from annual screening mammography, yet many women in this age group have never had a mammogram. Failure of physicians to refer older women for mammography is the usual reason. Nurse practitioners and female physicians are more likely to refer women for mammography.

Breast-conserving surgery is offered to older women less often than modified radical mastectomy. Yet the choice of surgical treatment, particularly for older women, is highly individual. Many older women wish to preserve their breasts.

CLINICAL BREAST EXAMINATION. In clinical breast examination, a trained health professional inspects and palpates the breasts and axillae, and checks for nipple discharge.

SCREENING MAMMOGRAPHY. Mammography is a low-dose x-ray of the breast used to detect breast lesions before they can be felt. Although mammography can detect breast tumors 2 years before they are palpable, most of these tumors have been present for 8 to 10 years. Mammography compresses breast tissue. It is uncomfortable to painful, depending on breast size and tenderness, and pain tolerance.

Box 35-10 ■ discusses concerns about screening and treatment for older women.

Diagnostic Tests

- *Diagnostic mammography* is done to visualize a palpable breast mass or identify a possible tumor in a client with other symptoms of breast cancer but no palpable mass.
- *Ultrasonography* is done to localize and distinguish between solid and cystic masses.
- *Computed tomography (CT) scans, magnetic resonance imaging (MRI),* and *positron emission tomography (PET)* scans may be done to locate and evaluate possible metastasis of breast cancer.
- *Cytologic examination* of fluid from nipple discharge may reveal the presence of cancer cells.
- *Tissue biopsy,* or examination of tissue from the lesion for cancer cells, is vital to diagnose breast cancer. Tissue for biopsy can be obtained in several ways:
  a. Fine-needle aspiration biopsy uses a fine needle to remove fluid and cells from the breast lesion (Figure 35-10A ■). Aspiration biopsy may be done using a stereotactic biopsy device; mammography and a computer are used to guide the needle.

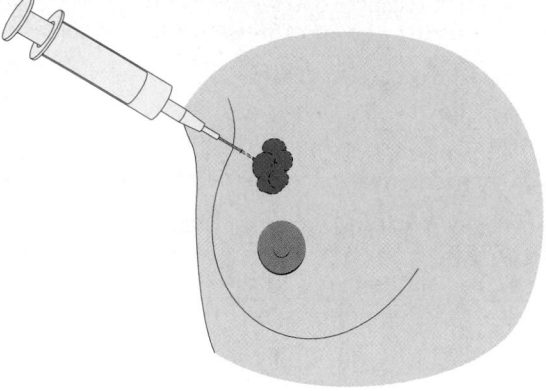

A Aspiration biopsy

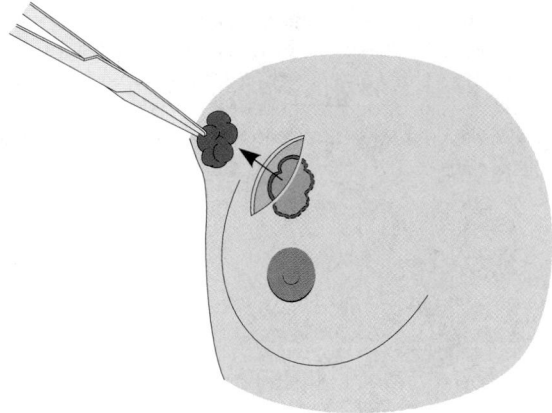

B Excisional biopsy

Figure 35-10. ■ Types of breast biopsy. (**A**) In an aspiration biopsy, a needle is used to aspirate fluid or tissue from the breast. (**B**) In an excisional biopsy, the breast lesion is removed surgically, and its tissue is examined.

  b. Core-needle biopsy uses a large, hollow-core needle to remove one or more cores of tissue from the breast lesion.
  c. Excisional biopsy is an open technique, in which the lesion is surgically removed and the tissue examined (Figure 35-10B).

Box 35-11 ■ outlines nursing care for a client undergoing a breast biopsy.
- In some centers, a *breast cancer risk profile* may be done to identify women who might benefit from aggressive therapy. This study subjects tumor cells to tests to determine their response to hormones, aggressiveness, and likelihood of recurring.

Staging of Breast Cancer

Staging (classifying the tumor by size, lymph involvement, and metastasis) provides important information for deciding on treatment options. The choice of treatment also

BOX 35-11   NURSING CARE CHECKLIST

Breast Biopsy

Before the Procedure

☑ Provide routine preoperative care as ordered (see Chapter 9). ∞

☑ Provide psychologic support.

Client and Family Teaching

☑ You will be notified of the results within a few days.

☑ Use a mild analgesic to relieve discomfort.

Fine-Needle Aspiration Biopsy

☑ Tissue and fluid are withdrawn from the lesion using a fine needle.

☑ This procedure takes only a few minutes and may be done in the physician's office.

Core-Needle Biopsy

☑ You will lie on a special table with your breast protruding through a hole.

☑ Local anesthesia will be used.

☑ Tissue from the lesion will be removed with a needle.

Excisional Biopsy

☑ The biopsy is done in ambulatory surgery with local anesthesia.

☑ The entire lesion and a small amount of surrounding tissue are removed.

☑ A nurse will explain what's happening, answer questions, and offer support during the biopsy.

☑ Tell the doctor if you have pain during the procedure.

☑ The incision is closed with sutures or tape and covered with a small dressing.

☑ Wear a well-fitting bra and apply ice packs to relieve discomfort and bruising after the procedure.

---

depends on age and the woman's preferences. Breast cancer tends to be more aggressive in premenopausal women (probably because of hormonal factors), requiring more aggressive treatment.

Medications

Systemic therapy (tamoxifen, chemotherapy, or biologic therapy) is used to prevent breast cancer or to delay the recurrence of cancer in all client groups.

Tamoxifen (Nolvadex) interferes with estrogen activity. It is used to treat existing breast cancer and to reduce the

risk for developing breast cancer in women who are at high risk (see Table 35-5 ■).

clinical ALERT

Although tamoxifen reduces the risk for developing breast cancer, it increases the risk of endometrial cancer, deep venous thrombosis, and pulmonary embolism. Teach women taking tamoxifen the early warning signs of endometrial cancer. Stress the importance of yearly pelvic examinations. Emphasize the need to stop smoking.

TABLE 35-5

Nursing Implications for Pharmacology: Tamoxifen

DRUG CLASSIFICATION/ DRUGS	ACTION	NURSING IMPLICATIONS	CLIENT AND FAMILY TEACHING
Estrogen Blocker/Antineoplastic Agent			
■ Tamoxifen (Nolvadex)	Tamoxifen inhibits tumor growth by blocking estrogen receptor sites of cancer cells. It is used to reduce the risk of breast cancer in high-risk women, prevent cancer recurrence after treatment, and as adjunctive therapy for advanced breast cancer. Tamoxifen increases the risk for endometrial cancer, deep venous thrombosis (DVT), and pulmonary embolism.	Assess for increased bone or tumor pain; provide analgesics as ordered. Monitor CBC, serum electrolytes, liver function tests, and thyroid hormone levels during treatment. Report abnormal results to the charge nurse or physician.	Use a diaphragm, condom, or other barrier contraception while taking this drug and for 1 month following. Weigh yourself weekly. Promptly report bone pain, weight gain, swelling, shortness of breath, nausea or vomiting, changes in mental status, headache, blurred vision, menstrual irregularities, or vaginal bleeding. This drug may cause hot flashes. Do not smoke while you are taking this drug.

When tamoxifen is ineffective or poorly tolerated, other hormone therapies may be used. In premenopausal women, the ovaries may be removed to reduce estrogen levels. Drugs such as diethylstilbestrol (DES), megestrol acetate (Megace), or aminoglutethimide (Cytadren) may be prescribed. However, these drugs have more side effects than tamoxifen.

Chemotherapy is commonly used to treat breast cancer when lymph nodes in the axilla are involved. It also is used to prolong life in late metastatic disease. (See Chapter 12 ⊂⊃ for more information about chemotherapy and its nursing implications.)

Radiation Therapy

Radiation therapy is typically used following breast cancer surgery to destroy any remaining cancer cells that could cause recurrence or metastasis. It is usually used in combination with lumpectomy for early-stage breast cancer. If a tumor is unusually large, radiation shrinks the tumor prior to surgery. Palliative radiation therapy is also used to treat chest wall recurrences and to help control pain and prevent fractures with bone metastases. Radiation is delivered by external beam or tissue implants.

Surgery

When breast cancer has not metastasized, the treatment of choice is surgery to remove the primary tumor combined with radiation therapy to reduce the risk of tumor recurrence or spread.

BREAST-CONSERVING SURGERY. Breast-conserving surgery involves removing the tumor and a disease-free margin surrounding the tumor (Figure 35-11A ■). Lymph nodes under the arm (axillary nodes) are removed as well. Surgery is followed by whole-breast radiation to destroy remaining cancer cells. This treatment is as effective as total mastectomy in treating breast cancer.

MASTECTOMY. Mastectomy (removal of the breast) is often done to treat breast cancer. *Radical mastectomy* is removal of the entire affected breast, underlying chest muscles, and lymph nodes under the arms. *Modified radical mastectomy* is removal of the breast tissue and lymph nodes under the arm, leaving the chest wall muscles intact (Figure 35-11B). Box 35-12 ■ outlines nursing care and teaching for the client undergoing a mastectomy.

Axillary node dissection usually accompanies breast cancer surgeries. Dissection may be limited to a single node to check for cancer cells or may involve removal of all axillary lymph nodes. This surgery can lead to long-term complications, such as lymphedema, nerve damage, and adhesions. Exercises to promote optimal use of the affected arm are discussed in the Continuing Care section that follows.

BREAST RECONSTRUCTION SURGERY. Breast reconstruction is common following mastectomy. It may be done at the time of surgery or at a later date, depending on factors such as physical condition, need for additional therapy, and preference. An implant may be used under the muscle if sufficient tissue to cover the implant is available (Figure 35-12A ■). Following radical surgery, muscle from the back or abdomen may be transplanted and used with or without an implant to reconstruct the breast (Figure 35-12B). A new nipple may be created by using tissue from the opposite nipple or other sites.

Metastatic Breast Cancer Treatment

If breast cancer has metastasized to other sites, the focus of treatment is *palliation* (symptom relief), extending life, and ensuring the comfort of the client. Therapies such as radiation therapy, hormone therapy, chemotherapy, or surgery may be used for palliative treatment, depending on the sites of metastases. Quality of life may take precedence over quantity of life.

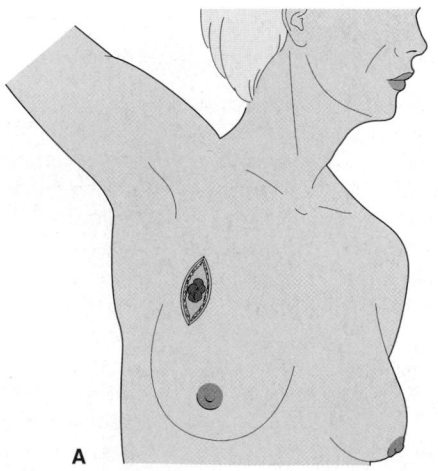 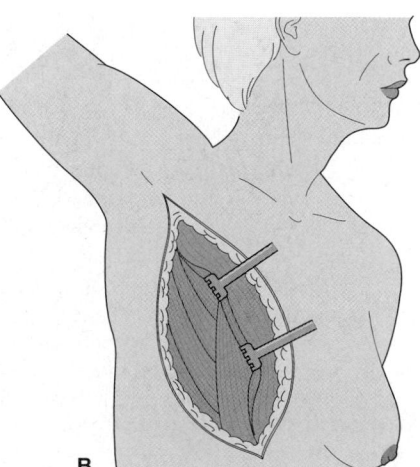

Figure 35-11. ■ Surgery for breast cancer. (**A**) In a lumpectomy, the tumor and a small margin of surrounding tissue are removed. (**B**) In a modified radical mastectomy, the entire breast and axillary lymph nodes are removed.

BOX 35-12	**NURSING CARE CHECKLIST**

Mastectomy

Before Surgery

☑ Provide routine preoperative care as outlined in Chapter 9. ⓒⓓ

☑ Reinforce teaching as needed.

☑ Allow access to support persons (significant others, religious or spiritual, or counselors).

☑ Offer emotional support.

After Surgery

☑ Provide routine postoperative care as outlined in Chapter 9. ⓒⓓ

☑ Reinforce teaching about postoperative care and exercises (discharge may occur within hours or the day after surgery).

Client and Family Teaching

☑ Empty the drain and replace the dressing daily.

☑ Return for drain removal in 2 to 4 days or as ordered.

☑ Take the prescribed analgesic before pain becomes severe and before performing exercises.

☑ Report excessive bleeding to your doctor.

☑ Numbness and tingling in the axillary area are common.

☑ Begin arm and shoulder exercises to restore full mobility as recommended by your doctor.

☑ You may drive within 7 to 10 days and return to work within 4 to 6 weeks.

☑ Do not lift heavy objects with the arm on the operated side.

☑ Protect the affected arm from injury and infection: Wear rubber gloves when washing dishes, garden gloves when working outside; avoid having blood pressures taken or blood drawn on the operative side.

NURSING CARE

ASSESSING

Obtain subjective information from all women about their risk factors for breast cancer, such as a history of the disease in a close female relative (mother, grandmother, sibling), early menarche or late menopause, and childbearing. Ask about breast self-exam, including how they do it, how often, and their knowledge of abnormal findings and what to do if a lump is discovered. Ask about breast pain, nipple discharge, change in breast size, or a change in the appearance or skin of the breast.

With the client disrobed to the waist, inspect the breasts and nipples for size, symmetry, contour, skin color and texture, venous patterns, and lesions. With the client supine and the arm behind the head, palpate each breast. Be sure to include the nipple and the axillary tail of breast tissue. Figure 33-7B ⓒⓓ shows one possible pattern for breast palpation. Note any palpable masses by location, size, shape, consistency, tenderness, mobility, and borders (sharp or poorly defined). Palpate each axilla for enlarged lymph nodes (Figure 35-13 ■).

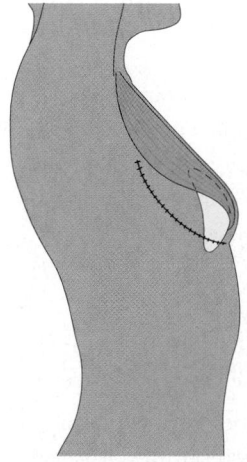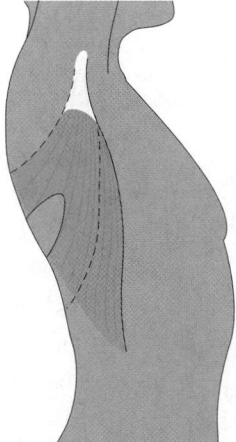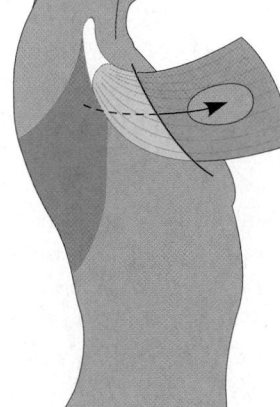

A Implant   **B** Latissimus dorsi myocutaneous flap

Figure 35-12. ■ Breast reconstruction surgeries. (**A**) An implant is inserted under the pectoris muscle. (**B**) A latissimus dorsi flap is used to reconstruct the breast.

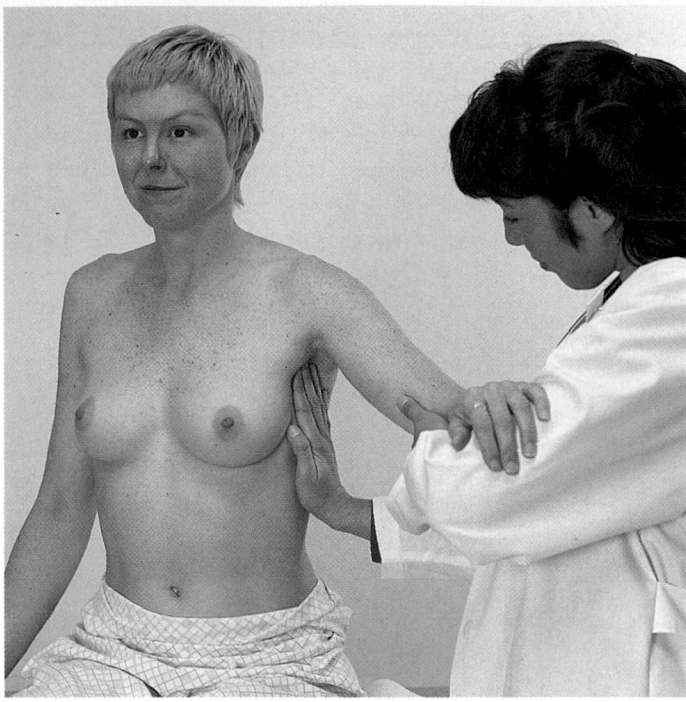

Figure 35-13. ■ Palpating the axillary lymph nodes. (Photographer: Richard Tauber.)

DIAGNOSING, PLANNING, AND IMPLEMENTING

Priorities in Nursing Care. Nursing care priorities for the client with breast cancer focus on supporting the client's decision making and grieving processes, as well as promoting rehabilitation following treatment.

Decisional Conflict: Treatment Options

■ Discuss the disease process and treatment options. Provide an opportunity for questions. Answer as simply and directly as possible. Make eye contact with the client and pay attention to body language. *Providing factual information and an opportunity to ask questions helps the client make an informed decision during a highly stressful time.*

■ Focus on immediate concerns, and provide up-to-date written material for review. *Stress and anxiety interfere with the ability to process information. Written materials can be reviewed later.*

■ Listen in a nonjudgmental manner during the decision-making process. *Nonjudgmental, empathic listening helps the client process information and make informed decisions.*

■ Provide opportunities to meet with other women who have had breast cancer surgery. *Breast cancer survivors often can answer questions the client is unable or unwilling to ask of care providers. They also can be a resource after surgery.*

Anticipatory Grieving

■ Listen attentively to expressions of loss and observe for nonverbal cues (failure to make eye contact, crying, silence). *Breast surgery, even lumpectomy, alters the appearance*

of the breast. This loss is expressed through grief. Not all women grieve openly. Attending to nonverbal cues helps open discussion of feelings of loss and grieving.

■ Spend time with the client. Do not rush interactions. *Taking time to be with the client communicates caring.*

■ Explain that periods of depression, anger, and denial after breast surgery are normal. *They are expected responses to loss and grieving.*

■ Enlist support from significant others to help the woman cope with her grief. *The client's family and friends can provide support during the grieving process.*

Risk for Infection

■ Assess dressings for bleeding, drainage, color, and odor every 4 hours for 24 hours. Circle any visible bleeding and drainage on the dressing as a baseline for subsequent assessment. *Excessive bleeding or drainage may indicate a postoperative complication that requires intervention.*

■ Observe incision and IV sites for pain, redness, swelling, and drainage. Assess the wound drainage system for patency; note the color and amount of drainage. *A local inflammatory response or wound drainage that is cloudy or malodorous may indicate an infection.*

■ Use aseptic technique when changing dressings, emptying wound drainage, and caring for intravenous tubing and sites. *Aseptic technique minimizes the risk of contamination with pathogens.*

■ Encourage a well-balanced diet. Refer to a dietitian as indicated. *Adequate nutrition promotes healing and immune function.*

■ Teach how to care for the incision and drainage system (cleansing, securing, and emptying). *The client is often discharged before the drainage system is removed, and needs teaching to provide self-care.*

■ Instruct to report fever, redness or hardness at the surgical site, or purulent drainage to the surgeon. *Early identification and treatment of infection can prevent more serious or long-term consequences.*

■ Instruct to avoid deodorants and talcum powder on the affected side until the incision is completely healed. *These substances may irritate the skin and impede healing.*

■ Discuss skin care during radiation therapy to reduce the risk of infection. *Radiation can cause dryness, itching, rash, or scaling of skin, increasing the risk of infection.*

Risk for Injury

Removing axillary lymph nodes increases the risk for problems such as lymphedema and infection.

■ Use the arm on the nonsurgical side for taking blood pressures and blood samples. *Compression of the arm on the surgical side may cause lymphedema.*

■ Elevate the affected arm on a pillow. *Elevating the arm permits drainage, prevents swelling, and promotes circulation.*

■ Encourage range-of-motion (ROM) exercises of the affected arm. *Exercise helps develop new drainage channels.*

- Teach protective measures: Avoid constricting sleeves, avoid lifting heavy objects, use a heavy oven mitt or potholder when cooking, and promptly apply antibiotic ointment to any cut or burn. Wear gloves when working in the yard or garden to prevent skin injury. *These measures help prevent infection and lymphedema.*

Risk for Disturbed Body Image

- Encourage verbalization of feelings. *Breast surgery can change body image. Talking about feelings of loss and change helps the client cope with the changes her body is experiencing due to surgery and treatment.*
- Explain that redness and swelling will fade with time. *Surgical changes may be compounded by side effects of chemotherapy or hormone therapy. Knowing that the scar will fade may help develop a more realistic view of the changes.*
- Include the partner (as desired) in discussions about physical changes caused by surgery and treatment. *The client may fear her partner's response to surgery. Open discussions facilitate adaptation of both partners to the changes.*
- Provide resources (pamphlets, books, referral to counselors or support groups) as appropriate. *Information and resources can assist with coping and adaptation to the changed body image.*
- Encourage the client to look at the incision when she feels ready. *Often, the reality is not as frightening as was imagined.*
- Reassure her that the decision about a prosthesis or reconstruction can be made at a later time. *Physical and emotional healing help the client make a better decision for long-term body image.*
- If the client is interested, provide written material about breast reconstruction and encourage meeting with a plastic surgeon and with women who have had reconstruction. *These steps allow the client to make a fully informed decision about available options.*

EVALUATING

To determine the effectiveness of nursing interventions, collect data such as the following:

- Makes an informed choice of treatment options based on extent of disease and personal preferences.
- Expresses feelings of anger or sorrow related to potential consequences of breast cancer.
- Looks at and touches incision; cares for incision and drainage system.
- Remains free of infection or injury.

Documenting. Document teaching and discussions about treatment options. Following surgery and during radiation or chemotherapy, document continuing assessment data, including healing, skin condition, adverse effects, and the client's and family's emotional and psychologic responses to treatment. Note all teaching provided and the client's understanding and acceptance of information presented.

CONTINUING CARE

Limited postoperative exercises are started within 24 hours after surgery, beginning with ROM of the elbow, wrist, and hand. Encourage performance of activities of daily living (ADLs), such as eating, combing her hair, and washing her face. If wound drains are present, tell to avoid abducting the arm or raising the elbow above shoulder height until drains are removed.

When wound healing is complete, abduction and external rotation of the upper arm may begin. Activities that require complete ROM include vacuuming and dusting. Forward and lateral elevation of the arms also increases function. Postmastectomy exercises such as wall climbing, overhead pulley, rope turning, and arm swings (Figure 35-14 ■) should be discussed with the physical therapist.

Advise that adequate rest and emotional support are important to promote healing and recovery. Both radiation and chemotherapy can cause fatigue and other symptoms. Use measures (outlined in Chapter 12) 🔗 to manage these symptoms.

Encourage participation in a breast cancer support group to share thoughts, feelings, experiences, and information about treatments, side effects, insurance problems, and other practical aspects of living with breast cancer. Discuss using online information services and bulletin boards for additional information and support.

Discuss manifestations of breast cancer recurrence, either as a second primary tumor or as metastasis from the original site. Advise to report signs and symptoms promptly (new breast lumps, a persistent cough or shortness of breath, jaundice or pain in the upper right quadrant of the abdomen, bone pain, or lumps around the collarbone or under the arm).

Advise a wholesome, balanced diet for healing and to deal with the effects of treatment, particularly chemotherapy. Maintaining body weight during chemotherapy can be difficult because of nausea and vomiting. Discuss potential solutions such as eating cold foods, which may be better tolerated than hot foods. Suggest complementary therapies such as guided imagery and meditation to help cope with the adverse effects of treatment. Discuss the potential benefits of vitamin supplements (vitamins A, C, and E) to help promote healing and recovery.

Advise women who choose a prosthesis that a temporary lightweight prosthesis can be worn immediately after the drains and sutures have been removed. Because prostheses are expensive, advise not purchasing a permanent prosthesis until the wound has healed completely. Prostheses are available at medical suppliers and many larger department stores. Most private and government insurance policies pay for the first prosthesis.

Note: The bibliography listings for this and all chapters have been compiled at the back of the book.

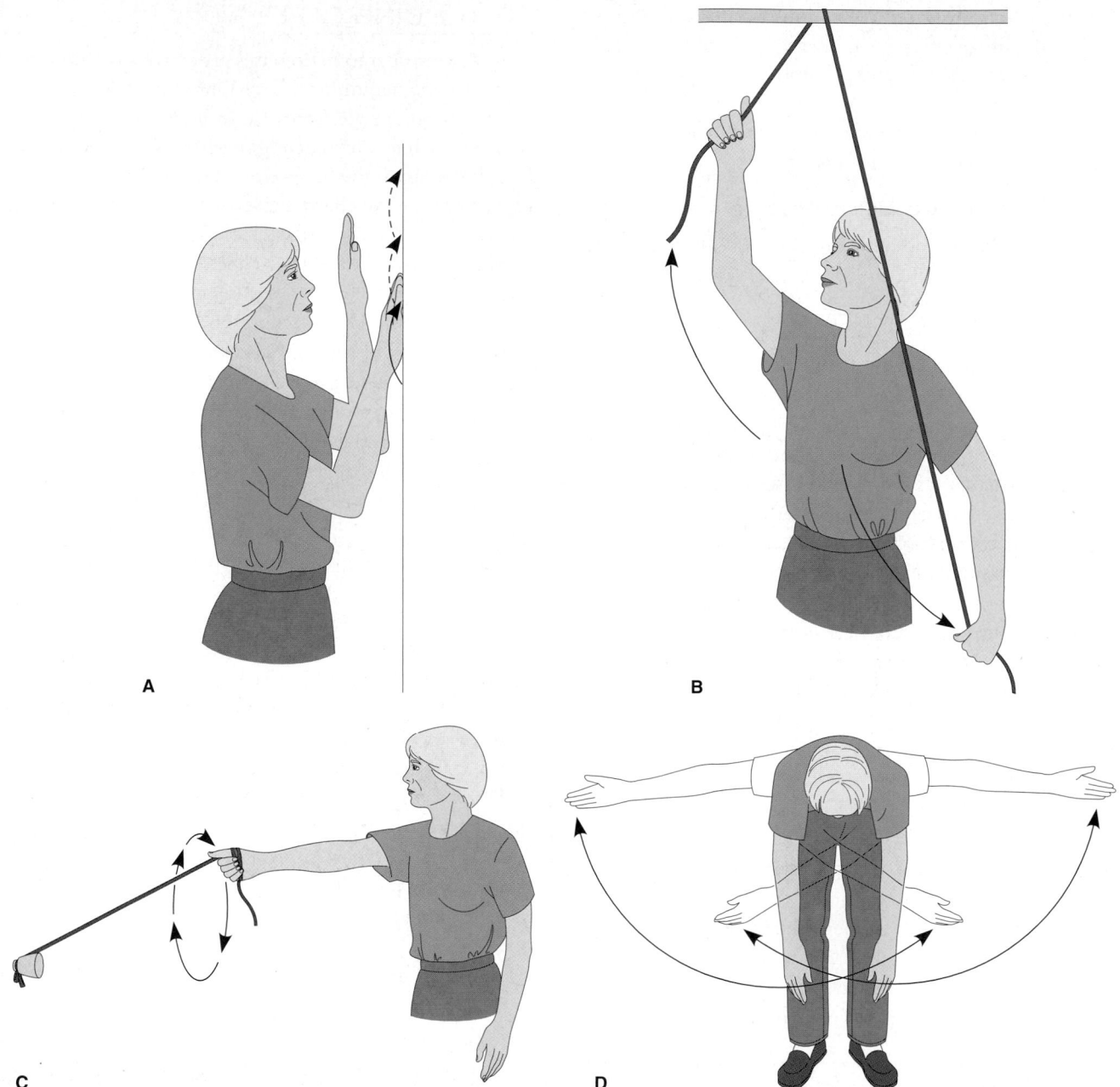

A

B

C

D

Figure 35-14. ■ Postmastectomy exercises. (**A**) Wall climbing: Stand facing wall with toes 6 to 12 inches from wall. Bend elbows and place palms against wall at shoulder level. Gradually move both hands up the wall parallel to each other until incisional pulling or pain occurs. (Mark that spot on wall to measure progress.) Work hands down to shoulder level. Move closer to wall as height of reach improves. (**B**) Overhead pulley: Using operated arm, toss 6-foot rope over shower curtain rod (or over top of a door that has a nail in the top to hold the rope in place for the exercise). Grasp one end of rope in each hand. Slowly raise operated arm as far as comfortable by pulling down on the rope on opposite side. Keep raised arm close to your head. Reverse to raise unoperated arm by lowering the operated arm. Repeat. (**C**) Rope turning: Tie rope to door handle. Hold rope in hand of operated side. Back away from door until arm is extended away from body, parallel to floor. Swing rope in as wide a circle as possible. Increase size of circle as mobility returns. (**D**) Arm swings: Stand with feet 8 inches apart. Bend forward from waist, allowing arms to hang toward floor. Swing both arms up to sides to reach shoulder level. Swing back to center, then cross arms at center. Do not bend elbows. If possible, do this and other exercises in front of mirror to ensure even posture and correct motion.

Chapter Review

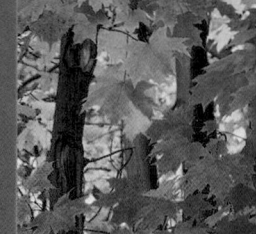

 KEY TERMS by Topics

Use the audio glossary feature of either the CD-ROM or the Companion Website to hear the correct pronunciation of the following key terms.

Perimenopause
menopause, perimenopause, dyspareunia

Disorders of menstruation
premenstrual syndrome (PMS), dysmenorrhea, dysfunctional uterine bleeding (DUB), amenorrhea, metrorrhagia, hysterectomy

Female reproductive tissue disorders
ectopic, salpingo-oophorectomy, oophorectomy

Female reproductive system infections
vaginitis, pelvic inflammatory disease (PID)

Structural disorders
cystocele, rectocele, uterine prolapse

Breast disorders
staging, mastectomy

KEY Points

- Disorders affecting the female reproductive system often affect the client's sexuality and body image in addition to their physical effects.

- Many disorders of the female reproductive system, including structural disorders, endometriosis, ovarian cysts, uterine fibroid tumors, and pelvic inflammatory disease, increase the risk of infertility.

- A number of tumors of the female reproductive system, including some breast, cervical, and endometrial cancers, are estrogen dependent. Women who have a history of early menarche, late menopause, few or no pregnancies or late childbearing, and estrogen replacement therapy have an increased risk for these cancers.

- Current technology has resulted in alternatives to hysterectomy as the primary treatment for many female reproductive disorders.

- Although specific genes have been identified that increase the risk of breast and ovarian cancer, the majority of these cancers occur in women who do not have the identified gene or genes.

- Screening measures such as breast self-examination, mammography, and Pap smears allow early detection and treatment of breast and cervical cancer, significantly reducing their mortality rates.

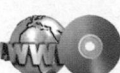 EXPLORE MediaLink

Additional interactive resources for this chapter can be found on the Companion Website at www.prenhall.com/burke. Click on Chapter 35 and "Begin" to select the activities for this chapter.

For chapter-related NCLEX-style review questions and an audio glossary, access the accompanying CD-ROM in this book.

⊙ FOR FURTHER Study

See Chapter 8 for discussions of pain control measures.

For more information about caring for the client undergoing surgery, see Chapter 9.

Nursing implications for antibiotic use are discussed in Chapter 10.

For nursing care of clients with HIV and AIDS, see Chapter 11.

For more discussion of symptoms related to radiation and chemotherapy, see Chapter 12.

See Chapter 20 for more information about colostomy, and Chapter 32 for more information about urinary diversion.

For Kegel exercises, see Box 32-3.

For more information about hormonal changes during the menstrual cycle, see Chapter 33.

For more information about pelvic ultrasound, laparoscopy, Pap smear, and clinical breast examination, see Chapter 33.

For further study of sexually transmitted infections, see Chapter 36.

Caring for a Client Experiencing Menopause

NCLEX-PN® Focus Area: Health Promotion and Maintenance: Growth and Development Through the Life Span

Case Study: Maria Villagrana, age 49, is having her annual checkup. She is concerned about recent symptoms, including palpitations, hot flashes, night sweats, and periods of anxiety and insomnia. During the past year, her menstrual periods have become short and erratic, and she has not menstruated for the past 3 months. Her most recent period lasted only 1 day.

Nursing Diagnosis: Anticipatory Grieving

COLLECT DATA

Subjective	Objective
_____	_____
_____	_____
_____	_____
_____	_____
_____	_____
_____	_____

Would you report this data? Yes/No

If yes, to: _____

Nursing Care

_____
_____
_____
_____
_____
_____
_____
_____
_____
_____

How would you document this? _____
_____
_____
_____

Data Collected (use those that apply)

- Often feels as though her "heart is running away with her"
- Hates thought of growing older
- Thinks her husband is losing interest in sex
- Wonders about decision not to have children
- Breaks down in tears for no reason
- Reports absentmindedness and difficulty concentrating
- BP 140/70; P 74; R 18; T 98.2°F (36.7°C)
- Smokes one pack of cigarettes daily
- Weighs 152 lbs (69 kg) (approximately 25% over ideal body weight)
- No history of uterine or breast cancer
- High-fat, high-carbohydrate, low-protein and low-fiber diet
- Calcium intake is less than 30% of recommended level
- Thyroid hormone levels normal
- FSH level elevated
- All other laboratory findings within normal ranges

Nursing Interventions (use those that apply; list in priority order)

- Teach coronary heart disease risk factors.
- Refer to smoking cessation program.
- Arrange consultation with a registered dietitian.
- Explain risks and benefits of hormone replacement therapy.
- Refer to midlife women's support group at the local community center.
- Arrange sexual counseling for Mr. and Mrs. Villagrana regarding techniques, positions, and modifications to accommodate midlife changes.

NCLEX-PN® Exam Preparation

TEST-TAKING TIP Nurses use a variety of tubes when caring for clients: feeding tubes, suction tubes, drainage tubes, chest tubes, tracheostomy tubes. Know the purpose of each, how to care for each, and what the necessary infection control measures are for each.

1 A woman experiencing frequent hot flashes and night sweats associated with perimenopause asks the nurse whether she should take hormones. The nurse's response is based on the knowledge that hormone replacement therapy (select all that apply)

  A. is recommended for all women during the 5 to 6 perimenopausal years.

  B. is associated with a higher risk of breast cancer.

  C. can reduce the risk of fractures associated with osteoporosis.

  D. does little to relieve menopausal symptoms such as hot flashes and night sweats.

  E. reduces the risk of developing coronary heart disease following menopause.

2 A client with nonproliferative fibrocystic breast changes complains of monthly breast pain. She is likely to be advised to do all of the following (select all that apply):

  A. Consider prophylactic mastectomy to reduce her risk for breast cancer.

  B. Use NSAIDs such as acetaminophen or ibuprofen for discomfort.

  C. Try local heat or cold applications.

  D. Eliminate caffeine and chocolate from her diet.

  E. Wear a supportive brassiere to reduce discomfort.

3 A 23-year-old woman being seen for a pelvic exam and Pap smear confesses to the nurse that she is terrified of cervical cancer because her mother died of the disease at age 35. The nurse recommends measures to reduce her risk, including

  A. practicing monogamy and using barrier protection during sexual activity.

  B. taking prophylactic tamoxifen until menopause.

  C. having a pelvic examination and Pap smear every 6 months.

  D. using oral contraceptives to regulate hormone secretion.

4 All of the following are good advice; which are especially important for the woman taking tamoxifen?

  A. Eat a low-fat, low-cholesterol diet.

  B. Stop smoking.

  C. Get regular aerobic exercise.

  D. Get regular dental care.

5 A 52-year-old woman tells the clinic nurse that her husband felt a lump in the area between her breast and axilla. She wonders if this is anything to worry about, given that it really isn't in her breast. The nurse's response is based on the knowledge that the most frequent location for breast cancer is:

  A. upper outer quadrant.

  B. peri-areolar area.

  C. lower outer quadrant.

  D. upper inner quadrant.

6 A client has had a simple mastectomy with dissection of the lymph nodes. She has a Jackson–Pratt drain in place. Your discharge instructions would include:

  A. getting a permanent prosthesis as soon as possible.

  B. how to empty the drain and clean around the insertion site.

  C. keeping her arm elevated with the elbow above shoulder height as much as possible.

  D. wrapping the chest and arm with elastic bandage to reduce scarring.

7 A client, age 22, has primary dysmenorrhea. Which of the following statements indicates that she may need more instruction regarding self-care?

  A. "It is okay to have sexual relations during my periods."

  B. "A heating pad may help relieve symptoms."

  C. "I should take an analgesic like ibuprofen right before and regularly during my period."

  D. "I will need another form of birth control, since this means I can't continue taking the pill."

8 Your 65-year-old neighbor asks you about some vaginal bleeding she has been having. She is postmenopausal and not on hormone replacement therapy. You advise her:

  A. that she still has some hormones present, simulating a period.

  B. to see her doctor immediately.

  C. to increase her use of soy products.

  D. that hormone replacement therapy would relieve this.

9 A client relates a history of periods that last up to 2 weeks, with heavy bleeding for the first 5 days. The nurse appropriately charts this as

  A. amenorrhea.

  B. metrorrhagia.

  C. Mittleschmerz.

  D. menorrhagia.

10 A client has a history of PID. She is at increased risk for:

  A. cervical cancer.

  B. passing this tendency on to her daughter.

  C. infertility and ectopic pregnancy.

  D. toxic shock syndrome.

Answers for Review Questions, as well as discussion of Care Plan and Critical Thinking Care Map questions, appear in Appendix V.

Chapter 36

Caring for Clients with Sexually Transmitted Infections

BRIEF Outline

Overview of STIs
Chlamydia
Genital Herpes
Genital Warts
Gonorrhea
Syphilis

LEARNING Outcomes

After completing this chapter, you will be able to:

- Describe the pathophysiology of the most common sexually transmitted infections (STIs).
- Identify laboratory and diagnostic tests used for STIs.
- Identify general measures to prevent and treat common STIs.
- List the signs and symptoms of the most common STIs.
- Discuss nursing implications for medications prescribed for clients with STIs.
- Use the nursing process to provide individualized care for clients with STIs.

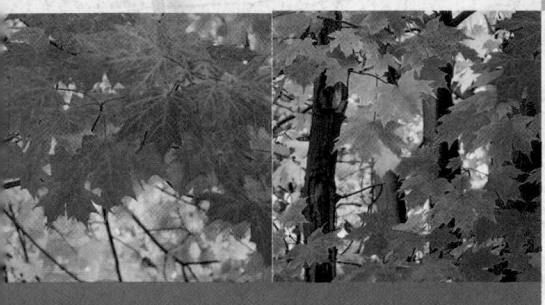

MediaLink

www.prenhall.com/burke
Use the address above to access the free, interactive Companion Website created for this textbook. Get hints, instant feedback, and textbook references to chapter-related NCLEX-style questions. Link to other interesting sites.

Audio Glossary:
Use the Companion Website, or the CD-ROM disk enclosed with your textbook, to hear the pronunciation of key terms in this chapter.

Any infection transmitted by sexual contact, including vaginal, oral, and anal intercourse, is referred to as a **sexually transmitted infection (STI),** also known as a *sexually transmitted disease (STD)*. Every sexually active person is at risk for STIs. STIs affect the client's general and reproductive health; some, such as HIV and hepatitis B, can be life threatening.

Every year, an estimated 15 million people in the United States acquire an STI. Because of tissue trauma that occurs during sexual intercourse, many STIs are more easily transmitted from a man to a woman than from a woman to a man. Women often experience few early manifestations of the infection and have a greater risk for complications of STIs such as pelvic inflammatory disease and genital cancers.

The incidence of STIs is highest among young people: Two-thirds of all STIs occur in people under age 25. However, people of all ages are at risk. Anyone who is sexually active can be infected with STIs, and infants can be infected by their mothers *in utero* or during delivery. Children can be infected through incest or sexual abuse. Victims of sexual assault are also at risk.

People with multiple sexual partners have the highest risk of acquiring an STI. The incidence also is high in people of color in urban settings with lower socioeconomic status and less education (Box 36-1 ■). Drug abuse, unprotected sexual activity, and sexual activity with multiple partners also are risk factors for STIs (Box 36-2 ■).

clinical ALERT

All states require reporting of syphilis, gonorrhea, and AIDS to state and federal agencies. Chlamydia is reportable in most states; requirements for reporting other STIs vary by state. For this reason, the exact incidence of many STIs is unknown.

Overview of STIs

Although STIs are caused by many different organisms, including bacteria, viruses, and parasites, they have several characteristics in common:

1. Most can be prevented by the use of latex condoms.

BOX 36-1   POPULATION FOCUS

Sexually Transmitted Infections

The incidence of STIs differs among racial and ethnic groups. African American adolescents are 25 times more likely to have gonorrhea than European American teens. The rate of primary and secondary syphilis is 50 times greater in African Americans than in European Americans. Hispanics have a rate of syphilis infection that is three times that of European Americans. The overall incidence of congenital syphilis is decreasing. However, 90% of reported cases occur in infants born to African American or Hispanic mothers.

BOX 36-2

RISK FACTORS FOR STIs

- Personal or partner history of STI
- Adolescent sexual activity
- Use of oral contraceptives
- Unprotected sexual activity
- Multiple sexual partners
- Pregnancy

---

2. They can be transmitted during both heterosexual and homosexual activities.
3. For treatment to be effective, sexual partners of the infected person must also be treated.
4. Two or more STIs frequently coexist in the same client.

Some STIs can be cured with appropriate antibiotic treatment. Others, such as genital herpes and genital warts, are chronic conditions caused by viruses. These infections may be managed but not cured. Some, such as HIV and hepatitis B, are potentially fatal. (HIV is discussed in Chapter 11; hepatitis B in Chapter 21. ⚭) Common STIs, their manifestations, treatment, and possible complications are outlined in Table 36-1 ■. The five most common STIs in the United States are discussed next in greater detail.

Chlamydia

Chlamydial infections are thought to be the most common STIs in the United States and the leading cause of pelvic inflammatory disease (PID) (see Chapter 35). ⚭ Because the infection often is asymptomatic, the incidence of the disease is thought to be nearly 10 times what is reported. Incidence is highest among sexually active teenagers. The risk factors for chlamydia are those for nearly all STIs (see Box 36-2).

PATHOPHYSIOLOGY

Chlamydia trachomatis is a bacterium that behaves like a virus, reproducing only within the host cell. It is spread by any sexual contact and to the neonate by passage through the birth canal of an infected mother. The incubation period is from 1 to 3 weeks. The bacteria typically invade the cervix in women and the urethra in men. In addition to causing genital infections, *C. trachomatis* causes *trachoma,* a chronic, contagious type of conjunctivitis prevalent in Asia and Africa.

MANIFESTATIONS AND COMPLICATIONS

Chlamydial infections are asymptomatic in most women until they have invaded the uterus and uterine tubes. Early manifestations, when present, include dysuria, urinary frequency, and vaginal discharge. Nearly a third of men with chlamydia are also asymptomatic. Manifestations of the infection in men include dysuria, urethral discharge, and possible testicular pain. Although clients may be asymptomatic, they are still potentially infectious.

If untreated, chlamydial infection in women ascends into the upper reproductive tract, causing such complications as PID, which includes endometritis, salpingitis, and chronic pelvic pain. These infections are a major cause

---

TABLE 36-1

Selected Sexually Transmitted Infections

DISEASE/ORGANISM	MANIFESTATIONS	TREATMENT	COMPLICATIONS
Chancroid[a] (rare in United States) *Haemophilus ducreyi*	**Females:** Frequently asymptomatic **Males:** Painful penile ulcers and *lymphadenopathy* (tender, enlarged lymph nodes)	Azithromycin PO once *or* ceftriaxone IM once *or* ciprofloxacin PO for 3 days *or* erythromycin PO for 7 days	Secondary infection of lesions, fistulas, chronic ulcers
Chlamydia *Chlamydia trachomatis*	**Females:** Asymptomatic; may have dysuria, vaginal or cervical discharge, vaginal bleeding or pelvic pain **Males:** May be asymptomatic or have dysuria, white or clear urethral discharge, testicular pain (epididymitis)	Doxycycline PO for 7 days *or* azithromycin PO once	**Females:** Pelvic inflammatory disease (PID), infertility, pelvic abscesses, spontaneous abortion, stillbirth, postpartum endometritis **Neonates:** Ophthalmia neonatorum or pneumonia **Males:** Urethritis, epididymitis, prostatitis
Genital herpes Herpes simplex virus, usually type 2	Single or multiple vesicles on the genitals with associated pruritus, followed by painful ulcers	No cure; acyclovir PO *or* famciclovir PO *or* valacyclovir PO for 7–10 days or until symptoms resolve	Herpes keratitis, a severe eye infection **Females:** Cervical cancer **Neonates:** Herpes affecting the eye, skin, mucous membranes, and CNS **Males:** Neuralgia, meningitis, urethral strictures, pus forming in lymph nodes
Genital warts (condyloma acuminatum) Human papillomavirus (HPV)	Single or multiple painless warts on genitals or perianal area	No cure, usually recur. Cryotherapy, *or* podophyllin 10–25% in tincture of benzoin compound applied to wart, *or* client-applied podofilox topical solution or gel *or* imiquimod cream	Urinary obstruction and bleeding **Females:** Enlargement during pregnancy; increased risk of cancer of the cervix, vagina, vulva, and anus **Neonates:** Respiratory papillomatosis, a chronic condition
Gonorrhea[a] *Neisseria gonorrhoeae*	**Females:** Often asymptomatic; may have vaginal discharge, abnormal menses, dysuria **Males:** Dysuria, increased urinary frequency, purulent urethral discharge	Cefixime PO *or* ciprofloxacin PO *or* ceftriaxone IM in a single injection *plus* azithromycin PO in a single dose *or* doxycycline PO for 7 days to treat possible coexisting chlamydia	**Females:** Pelvic inflammatory disease (PID), sterility, ectopic pregnancy, abdominal adhesions **Males:** Prostatitis, urethritis, nephritis, epididymitis, sterility
Granuloma inguinale[a] (rare in United States) *Calymmatobacterium granulomatis*	Single or multiple subcutaneous nodules that erode to form painless, bleeding, enlarging ulcers	Trimethoprim–sulfamethoxazole PO for 21 days *or* doxycycline PO for 21 days	Secondary infection of lesions, *keloid* (excess scar tissue) on genitals, tissue necrosis, fever, malaise, secondary anemia, cachexia, and death
Lymphogranuloma venereum[a] (rare in United States) *Chlamydia trachomatis*	Painless vesicle or ulcer, followed by regional lymphadenopathy, inguinal abscess	Doxycycline PO for 21 days *or* erythromycin PO for 21 days	Ruptured abscesses with draining sinuses or fistulas, nephropathy, hepatomegaly, or phlebitis
Pelvic inflammatory disease (PID) *Chlamydia trachomatis, Neisseria gonorrhoeae, Mycoplasma hominis,* and others	Pain and tenderness in lower abdomen, uterus and surrounding tissues; possible fever, chills, and elevated WBC and sedimentation rate	Combined drug therapy such as cefotetan IV *plus* doxycycline IV or PO *or* clindamycin IV *plus* gentamicin IV or IM; may require hospitalization	Ectopic pregnancy, pelvic abscess; infertility, recurrent or chronic PID, chronic abdominal pain, pelvic adhesions, depression

TABLE 36-1			
Selected Sexually Transmitted Infections (continued)			
DISEASE/ORGANISM	MANIFESTATIONS	TREATMENT	COMPLICATIONS
Syphilis[a] *Treponema pallidum*	**Primary:** Painless chancre at site of exposure; regional lymphadenopathy **Secondary:** Skin rash; oral mucous patches; generalized lymphadenopathy; mucous patch on vulva or anus; fever; malaise; patchy alopecia **Tertiary** (late): Tumors of skin, bone, liver; inflammation of aorta, aneurysms; central nervous system degeneration	Penicillin G IM in a single injection *or* doxycycline PO for 14 days Syphilis of unclear or more than 1 year's duration: penicillin G IM weekly for 3 weeks *or* doxycycline PO for 28 days	**Primary and secondary:** Disease progression **Tertiary:** Heart failure, blindness, paralysis, skin ulcers, liver failure, mental illness
Trichomoniasis *Trichomonas vaginalis*	**Females:** Asymptomatic or may have frothy, excessive vaginal discharge, erythema, edema and pruritus **Males:** Usually asymptomatic; may have urethritis, penile lesions, or inflammation	Metronidazole PO in a single dose or for 7 days	**Females:** Recurrent infections, salpingitis, low-birth-weight infants, prematurity

[a] Reporting to state and federal agencies required by law.

of infertility and ectopic pregnancy, a potentially life-threatening condition. Complications in men include epididymitis, prostatitis, sterility, and Reiter's syndrome (an autoimmune disorder). In the newborn, chlamydia can lead to blindness or pneumonia.

INTERDISCIPLINARY CARE

Because chlamydial infections are often asymptomatic, treatment is often begun on a presumptive basis. The Centers for Disease Control and Prevention (CDC) recommends screening asymptomatic women who are at high risk for chlamydia.

Diagnostic Tests

Chlamydial infection can be diagnosed in several ways. Infected tissue can be cultured to identify the presence of the bacteria. This test is expensive and not readily available in all areas, however. More often, the diagnosis is made based on detection of chlamydial antigens or nucleic acid, or by detecting antibodies to *Chlamydia* in the blood or local secretions. These tests are particularly effective in diagnosing chlamydial infection in high-risk populations.

Medications

The drug of choice for chlamydial infections in men and non-pregnant women is a single oral dose of azithromycin (Zithromax) or a 7-day course of oral doxycycline (Vibramycin). For pregnant women, erythromycin is the alternative therapy. Ofloxacin (Floxin) for 7 days is another alternative treatment. Nursing implications for these antibiotics are discussed in Chapter 10. 🔗

NURSING CARE

Nursing care of the client with chlamydia focuses on identifying the infection, eradicating it, preventing future infections, and managing any complications.

ASSESSING

Box 36-3 ■ outlines nursing assessment as it relates to clients with an STI.

DIAGNOSING, PLANNING, AND IMPLEMENTING

Consider the following nursing diagnoses and interventions when planning and delivering care for a client with an STI.

Priorities in Nursing Care. Teaching about the infection, its treatment, and potential effects on reproductive health for the client and his or her partners is the priority for nursing care.

Ineffective Health Maintenance

- Teach about the disease, its transmission, treatment, and measures to prevent its spread or reinfection. *Understanding the disease and how it is spread helps the client gain a sense of control and prevent future STIs.*
- Discuss safer sex practices outlined in Box 36-4. *Clients can prevent future STIs by making lifestyle changes and conscious decisions about safer sex practices.*
- Emphasize the importance of referring all sex partners for testing and treatment as needed. *Unless both partners in a relationship are effectively treated, reinfection is likely.*

BOX 36-3	ASSESSMENT

Assessing Clients with an STI

SUBJECTIVE DATA

- Current symptoms: pain or itching; onset, duration, relieving and aggravating factors; dysuria, frequency, urgency, or other urinary symptoms; vaginal or urethral drainage, color, amount, odor; visible lesions.
- General health, including any chronic diseases or conditions.
- Past medical history, particularly any previous history of STIs or reproductive system problems and their treatment.
- Sexual activity and measures used to prevent pregnancy or infection.
- Possibility of pregnancy; last menstrual period (date, characteristics).
- Social habits such as tobacco, alcohol, or other drug use; frequency and amount.

OBJECTIVE DATA

- Vital signs, including temperature.
- Inspect skin, including palms of hands and soles of feet; mucous membranes of mouth and oropharynx; abdomen for contour, visible peristalsis; genitalia, including penis, external urinary meatus, scrotum, and anus in men; perineum, labia majora, labia minora, vaginal opening, and anus in women. Note any redness, rash, ulcers, or lesions, swelling or drainage. Obtain sterile swab of drainage for culture or Gram stain.
- Auscultate bowel sounds.
- Palpate abdomen and suprapubic region for tenderness; inguinal lymph nodes for swelling or tenderness (lymphadenopathy); perineal tissues for tenderness or swelling.

- Stress the importance of completing the prescribed treatment plan and returning for follow-up visits as recommended. *Incomplete treatment may result in continued infection and organisms that are resistant to antibiotic therapy.*

Impaired Skin Integrity

- Teach the client to keep perineal tissues clean and dry. Advise cleansing front to back after urinating and defecating, using soap and water as needed to clean the area, and a blow drier on cool setting to dry. *Keeping tissues clean and dry promotes healing and reduces the risk of secondary infection of lesions.*
- Instruct to avoid perineal powders or sprays, as well as bubble baths. *Feminine hygiene sprays and bubble baths can excessively dry perineal tissues, increasing the risk of infection.*
- Advise client to wear cotton underwear, avoiding tight-fitting jeans and pantyhose. *These measures allow moisture to evaporate, rather than keeping it against the skin.*

Risk for Injury

- Stress the importance of taking all prescribed medication. *Completing the prescribed course of antibiotic helps ensure elimination of the infecting organism.*
- Instruct to abstain from sexual contact until client and partners are cured, and to use condoms to prevent future infections. *Abstinence prevents reinfection and spread of the STI. Condoms provide barrier protection, reducing the risk of infection during sexual activity.*
- Provide information about signs and symptoms of reinfection and other STIs. Stress the importance of prompt diagnosis and treatment of all STIs. *Successful treatment of the disease does not prevent possible subsequent infections.*

Anxiety

- Emphasize that most STIs can be effectively treated, preventing serious complications and transmission to the infant. *This information provides a sense of control and helps decrease anxiety.*
- Discuss with women of childbearing age that cesarean delivery can prevent transmission of infection to the neonate. *Understanding that infection of the neonate can be prevented helps relieve anxiety.*

Situational Low Self-Esteem

- Create an environment in which the client feels respected and safe to discuss concerns about the disease and its effect on the client's life. *Being treated with respect and privacy helps the client realize that the disease does not change his or her worth as a person.*
- Provide privacy and confidentiality. *Clients are often embarrassed to discuss intimate details of their sex lives.*
- Communicate caring for the client. *Unfortunately, many people affected by STIs lack family and other social support networks. The nurse's concern can enhance self-esteem.*

Sexual Dysfunction

- Provide a supportive, nonjudgmental environment to discuss feelings and questions about the effect of the STI on future sexual relationships. *Feelings of guilt, shame, and anger are natural responses to the diagnosis of an STI and can lead to a total avoidance of sexual intimacy.*
- Offer information about support groups and other resources for people with specific STIs. *Information can offset feelings of shame and hopelessness. Many people have learned to live with and manage these disorders without infecting their partners or their children.*

Impaired Social Interaction

- Help the client understand that an STI is a consequence of sexual behavior, not a "punishment," and that it can be avoided in the future. *This knowledge enhances the client's ability to relate to others.*

EVALUATING

To evaluate the effectiveness of nursing care, collect data such as the following:

- Completed prescribed medication regimen as ordered?
- Kept all recommended follow-up appointments?
- Able to identify measures to prevent future STIs?
- Engaging in safer sex practices with an uninfected partner?
- Resumed social activities?
- If pregnant, can state measures to prevent disease transmission to unborn child?

Documenting. Document subjective and objective assessment data, including the circumstances under which the infection was obtained (if known) and the number of recent sexual partners. Document all teaching provided and the client's understanding and apparent willingness to comply with prescribed treatment. Note information provided about safer sex practices and the receptiveness of the client and partner to safer sex practices.

CONTINUING CARE

Nurses have a critical role in preventing STIs by teaching clients about these diseases, their prevention, treatment, and potential complications (Box 36-4 ■).

Stress the importance of complying with the prescribed treatment and referring partners for examination and treatment as needed. Discuss safer sex practices and using condoms to avoid reinfection. Teach about the complications of chlamydia, such as PID, and their manifestations. Instruct the client to seek medical attention promptly if symptoms of PID develop. If the infection has progressed to PID, provide additional information about PID and its treatment (see Chapter 35). ∞

Genital Herpes

Genital herpes (*Herpes genitalis*) is a chronic and often asymptomatic STI. Currently, no cure is available for genital herpes. As many as 45 million people in the United States are infected with the herpes simplex virus type 2 (HSV-2), the usual cause of genital herpes. Most of these people, however, have unrecognized infections. Like other STIs, the incidence of genital herpes is highest among adolescents and young adults.

PATHOPHYSIOLOGY AND MANIFESTATIONS

HSV-2 is closely related to HSV-1, which commonly causes fever blisters or cold sores. HSV-1 also can infect the genitalia; likewise, HSV-2 can infect other parts of the body. Genital herpes is spread by vaginal, anal, or oral–genital contact. Its incubation period is 3 to 7 days. Within a week

BOX 36-4	CLIENT TEACHING

Preventing STIs: A Checklist for Clients

- You can eliminate your risk entirely by not having sex with anyone (**abstinence**) or by having sex only with an uninfected partner who has sex only with you (*mutual monogamy*).
- The more sexual partners you have, the greater your risk of contracting an STI.
- Latex condoms, used consistently and correctly, can prevent many STIs, including HIV infection. Use a new condom each time, lubricating the condom with a water-based lubricant.
- When a male condom cannot be used appropriately, the female condom, a lubricated polyurethane sheath inserted into the vagina, reduces the risk of STIs, including HIV.
- Vaginal spermicides reduce the risk for gonorrhea and chlamydia but do not prevent HIV infection.
- If you suspect you've been exposed to an STI, see a doctor or clinic right away. Encourage your partner to seek treatment, too.
- Follow the doctor's instructions carefully and take all the medicine prescribed for you. Continue the medication even when the symptoms go away. (The infection sometimes remains active after symptoms go away.)
- Go back to your doctor for a follow-up exam according to his or her instructions.
- Don't have sex until you *and* your partner are completely cured.
- If you use drugs by injection, enroll in or continue a drug-treatment program. Do not use injection supplies that have been used by another person under any circumstances. Thoroughly and consistently clean injection equipment with bleach between uses.

after exposure, painful red papules appear in the genital area. In men, the lesions usually occur on the glans or shaft of the penis. In women, the lesions often occur on the labia, vagina, and cervix. Anal intercourse may result in lesions in and around the anus.

Soon after the papules appear, they form small painful blisters filled with clear fluid containing virus particles (Figure 36-1 ■). The blisters break, shedding the virus and creating painful ulcers that last 6 weeks or longer. Touching these blisters and then rubbing or scratching in another place can spread the infection to other areas of the body.

The first outbreak of herpes lesions is called the *first episode infection.* Subsequent episodes, or *recurrent infections,* are usually less severe. The period between episodes is called *latency.* Even though no symptoms are present, the person remains infectious. During latency, the virus withdraws into the nerve fibers that lead from the infected site to the

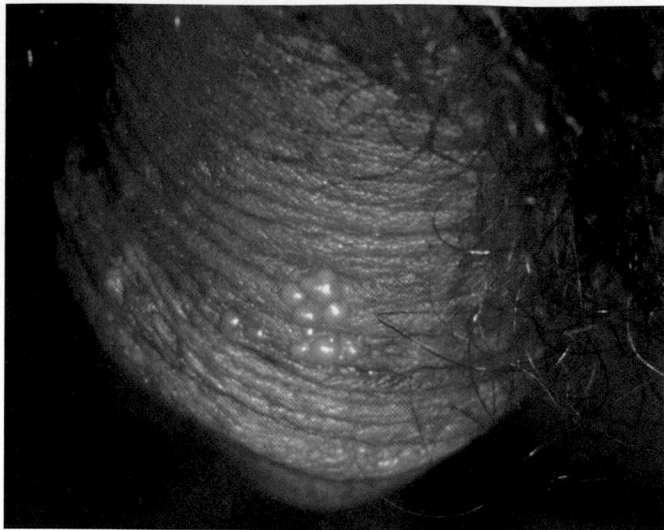

Figure 36-1. ■ Genital herpes blisters as they appear on the penis. (*Source:* Camera M. D. Studios, Carroll H. Weiss, Director, 8290 N.W. 26th Place, Sunrise, FL 33322.)

lower spine, remaining dormant until recurrence, at which time it retraces its path to the genital area.

Prodromal symptoms (warning signals or clues) of herpes outbreaks include burning, itching, tingling, or throbbing at the sites where lesions commonly appear. There may be pain radiating to the legs, thighs, groin, or buttocks. The infection may be more infectious during the prodromal period, so sexual contact should be avoided.

Recurrent infections have symptoms of herpetic lesions, general malaise or headache, fever, dysuria and urinary retention, and vaginal or urethral discharge.

Men are not likely to experience serious complications of genital herpes. Women, however, face more serious concerns. Neonatal infection from a mother with herpes can range from asymptomatic to widely disseminated, fatal disease. Transmission occurs during passage through the birth canal. The risk is highest during the first episode of infection. Women also face an increased risk of cervical cancer. In rare cases, the herpes virus can spread to the brain, causing herpes encephalitis, a life-threatening complication.

INTERDISCIPLINARY CARE

Because there is no cure for genital herpes, treatment focuses on relieving symptoms and preventing spread of the infection. Teaching is an essential component of care.

Genital herpes is usually diagnosed by the history (including lesion characteristics and patterns of recurrence) and physical exam. Antiviral drugs such as acyclovir (Zovirax) or famciclovir (Famvir) help reduce the length and severity of the first episode and decrease the frequency of recurrent episodes. These drugs usually are given orally; for severe episodes, acyclovir also can be given intravenously.

NURSING CARE

In addition to the nursing care as outlined for chlamydia, the nursing diagnoses of Pain and Impaired Health Maintenance should be considered for the client with genital herpes.

Pain

- Teach the client to keep herpes blisters clean and dry. A solution of warm water, soap, and hydrogen peroxide can be used to cleanse the lesions two or three times daily. Burow's solution (an aluminum acetate solution) can also be used. Lesions should be dried using a hair dryer on the cool setting. Instruct to wear loose cotton clothing that will not trap moisture; pantyhose and tight jeans should be avoided. *Keeping the lesions clean and dry reduces the risk of secondary infection and promotes healing.*
- For dysuria, suggest pouring water over the genitals while urinating. Encourage increased fluid intake. Fluids that increase urine acidity, such as cranberry juice, should be avoided. *These measures help relieve dysuria by diluting or reducing the acidity of the urine.*

Ineffective Health Maintenance

- Discuss cesarean delivery to prevent transmission of infection to the neonate. In women without manifestations of recurrence, vaginal delivery is possible. *Understanding that infection of the neonate can be prevented helps relieve anxiety.*
- Discuss the need for annual Papanicolaou (Pap) smears; Pap smears every 6 months may be recommended for women with genital herpes. *Careful monitoring will identify early changes in cervical tissues, allowing effective treatment.*

clinical ALERT

Instruct the client to use barrier protection for all sexual intercourse because the infection can be transmitted from the onset of prodromal symptoms until all symptoms are cleared.

CONTINUING CARE

With teaching, clients with genital herpes can learn to manage this chronic disease with the least possible disruption in lifestyle and relationships. Teach the client to recognize prodromal symptoms of recurrence, and discuss factors that seem to trigger recurrences (such as emotional stress, acidic food, sun exposure). Explain the need for abstinence from sexual contact from the time prodromal symptoms appear until 10 days after all lesions have healed.

Encourage the client to use oral antiviral drugs to reduce the frequency and duration of outbreaks. Painful lesions can be protected with sterile Vaseline or aloe vera gel. Because viral shedding can occur at any time, emphasize the importance of using latex condoms and careful hygiene practices (such as not sharing towels or other personal items) even during latency periods.

Genital Warts

Genital and anal warts, also known as *condyloma acuminatum* or venereal warts, are caused by human papillomavirus (HPV). HPV is one of the most common STIs in the United States. Most HPV infections are asymptomatic or unrecognized. Like most STIs, genital warts are usually found in young, sexually active adults and are associated with early onset of sexual activity and multiple sexual partners.

PATHOPHYSIOLOGY AND MANIFESTATIONS

HPV is transmitted by all types of sexual contact. The incubation period for genital warts is about 3 months. Many different types of HPV cause chronic genital infections.

Although most people who carry HPV have no symptoms, others develop single or multiple painless, cauliflower-like growths on the vulvovaginal area, perineum, penis, urethra, or anus (Figure 36-2 ■). In women, the growths may appear in the vagina or on the cervix and be apparent only during a pelvic examination.

Several subtypes of HPV are strongly associated with cervical dysplasia and an increased risk of cervical cancer. HPV also is associated with a higher risk of vaginal, vulvar, penile, and anal cancers.

Potential complications of genital warts include destruction of normal tissue or obstruction of the urethra. The virus also can be transmitted to the fetus during pregnancy

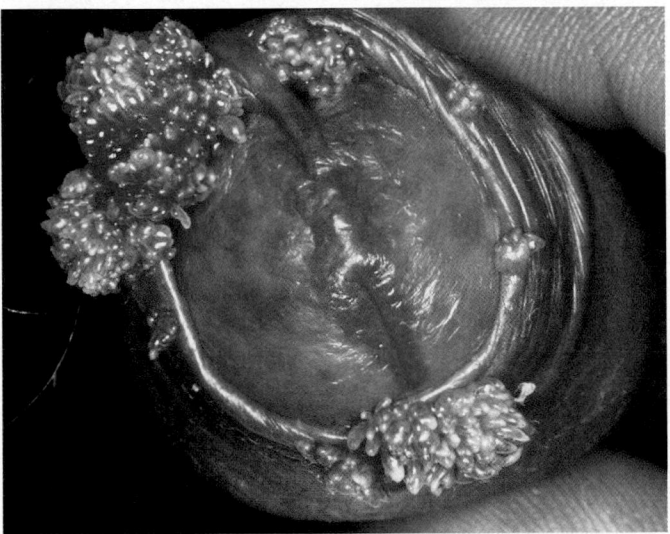

Figure 36-2. ■ Genital warts (condyloma acuminatum) on the penis. (*Source:* Photo Researchers, Inc.)

or delivery. The lesions enlarge during pregnancy and may obstruct the birth canal, necessitating cesarean delivery. Infants infected with HPV can develop respiratory papillomatosis, a chronic respiratory condition.

INTERDISCIPLINARY CARE

Genital and anal warts are diagnosed primarily by their clinical appearance; HPV also may be diagnosed by examination of cervical cells taken during a Pap smear or cervical biopsy.

Genital warts on the vulva, perineum, or penis can be treated with a topical agent (podophyllin resin) applied directly to the warts. This treatment is done in the physician's office, with the client returning weekly until the warts are gone.

Genital warts may be removed by cryotherapy, electrocautery, or surgical excision. Carbon dioxide laser surgery is increasingly used to remove extensive warts.

NURSING CARE

In addition to the general nursing care for clients with an STI (see the section on chlamydia), the client with genital warts needs pretreatment teaching if the warts are to be removed.

Emphasize the need for the client and infected partners to return for regular treatment and abstain from sexual relations until lesions have resolved, and to use condoms to prevent reinfection.

clinical ALERT

Stress the importance of annual Pap smears for female clients because of the increased risk for cervical cancer.

Genital warts can enlarge and destroy normal tissue or block the urethra. Instruct the client to report difficulty urinating or symptoms of urinary retention or infection. Discuss the risk of transmitting the disease to the fetus or neonate and the need for cesarean delivery. Stress the importance of telling the women's health care provider about the infection.

Gonorrhea

Gonorrhea, also known as *GC* or *clap*, is the most common reportable communicable disease in the United States. The rate of gonorrhea infection among African Americans is significantly higher than in non-Hispanic whites. Among women, 15- to 19-year-olds have the highest rate of infection, while among men, 20- to 24-year-olds have the highest rate.

PATHOPHYSIOLOGY AND MANIFESTATIONS

Gonorrhea is caused by *Neisseria gonorrhoeae*, a gram-negative diplococcus. Its incubation period is 2 to 8 days. Gonorrhea is transmitted by direct sexual contact and during delivery as the neonate passes through the birth canal.

The organism initially targets the cervix and the male urethra. Without treatment, the disease spreads to other organs. In men, gonorrhea can cause acute, painful inflammation of the prostate, epididymis, and periurethral glands and can lead to sterility. In women, it can cause PID, endometritis, salpingitis, and pelvic peritonitis. In the neonate, gonorrhea can infect the eyes, nose, or anorectal region.

Manifestations of gonorrhea in men include dysuria and serous, milky, or purulent urethral discharge. Some men also develop regional lymphadenopathy. Some men and most women have no symptoms until the disease is advanced. When manifestations of gonorrhea are present in women, they include dysuria, urinary frequency, or abnormal vaginal discharge.

INTERDISCIPLINARY CARE

Treatment of gonorrhea is directed toward eradicating the organism and any coexisting disease (see later section), preventing reinfection, and preventing spread of the disease.

Diagnostic Tests

In men, the diagnosis of gonorrhea can usually be confirmed by obtaining a smear of urethral discharge. Cultures are not necessary unless Gram stains of smears are negative despite typical clinical symptoms of gonorrhea. In women, cultures of cervical discharge are necessary to confirm the diagnosis of gonorrhea. Because cultures require 24 to 48 hours for confirmation, treatment is usually begun on a presumptive diagnosis.

People with gonorrhea often are infected with another STI. For this reason, the client and his or her partners are tested for other STIs such as syphilis, chlamydia, and possibly HIV.

Medications

Because many strains of *N. gonorrhoeae* are resistant to penicillin, an alternative antibiotic, such as a single dose of cefixime (Suprax), ceftriaxone (Rocephin), ciprofloxacin (Cipro), or ofloxacin (Floxin), is used to treat gonorrhea infection of the urethra, cervix, or rectum. The same antibiotics are used to treat pharyngeal gonorrhea infection. However, a longer course of treatment may be required.

NURSING CARE

Review Box 36-3 for areas to assess with clients who have STIs. Also review nursing care as described under chlamydia at the beginning of this chapter, and the Nursing Process Care Plan provided here.

If single-dose antibiotic therapy has not been ordered, emphasize the importance of taking all of the prescribed medication as directed. Encourage referral of sexual partners for evaluation and treatment. Stress the need to abstain from all sexual contact until the client and partners are cured of the disease, and instruct to use a condom to avoid transmitting or contracting infections in the future. Emphasize the need for a follow-up visit 4 to 7 days after treatment is completed to ensure that the infection has been cured.

NURSING PROCESS CARE PLAN
Client with Gonorrhea

Janet Cirit, a 33-year-old legal secretary, is unmarried but dating a man named Jim Adkins. Ms. Cirit visits her gynecologist because her periods have become irregular and she is having pelvic pain and abnormal vaginal discharge. Recently, she developed a sore throat, and the pelvic pain is keeping her awake at night.

Assessment. In the gynecologist's office, the nurse obtains a complete history, including questions about menstrual periods, pain associated with urination or sexual intercourse, urinary frequency, most recent Pap smear, birth control method, history of STI and drug use, and types of sexual activity. Ms. Cirit reports her symptoms and indicates that she is taking oral contraceptives for birth control so she and Mr. Adkins do not use a condom during sexual relations.

Physical examination reveals both pharyngeal and cervical inflammation, and lower abdominal tenderness. Ms. Cirit's temperature is 98.5°F (37.0°C). She is not pregnant. Diagnostic tests are positive for gonorrhea and negative for *Chlamydia*. The white blood count (WBC) is slightly elevated, indicating possible salpingitis. Because Mr. Adkins has been Ms. Cirit's only sexual partner, it is clear that he needs to be treated as well.

Diagnosis. The following nursing diagnoses are identified for Ms. Cirit:

- *Pain* related to the infectious process
- *Situational Low Self-Esteem* related to shame and guilt of having an STI
- *Ineffective Sexuality Patterns* related to impaired relationship and fear of reinfection

Expected Outcomes. The expected outcomes are that Ms. Cirit will:

- Report relief of pelvic pain.
- Verbalize an understanding of the cause and transmission of gonorrhea.
- Verbalize that she will insist her partner use condoms during future sexual activity.

Planning and Implementation. The following interventions are planned and implemented during care of Ms. Cirit:

- Administer ceftriaxone IM as ordered and document.
- Discuss feelings and concerns about the diagnosis of gonorrhea.
- Emphasize relationship of STI to behavior, not cleanliness or self-worth.
- Help identify ways to talk with a future sexual partner about condom use.

Evaluation. During her follow-up visit, Ms. Cirit states that she is feeling much better and sleeping well at night since the pain has ended. She has ended her relationship with Mr. Adkins and is considering joining a health club in the hope of increasing her level of fitness and perhaps meeting someone new.

Critical Thinking in the Nursing Process

1. What signs might have caused Ms. Cirit to suspect that Mr. Adkins had gonorrhea?
2. How are Ms. Cirit's signs and symptoms related to the infectious process of gonorrhea?
3. How might Ms. Cirit convince a future sexual partner to use condoms during sexual activity without spoiling the romantic aspect?

Syphilis

Syphilis is a complex systemic STI that, if not treated appropriately, can lead to blindness, paralysis, mental illness, cardiovascular damage, and death. Penicillin has significantly reduced the incidence of syphilis. The current rate of infection is low and falling among most racial and ethnic groups. It is higher among African Americans, American Indians, and Alaska Natives. Syphilis infection rates also remain high in the South and in many urban centers.

Syphilis often occurs with one or more other STIs, such as HIV or chlamydia.

PATHOPHYSIOLOGY AND MANIFESTATIONS

Syphilis is caused by a spirochete, *Treponema pallidum,* which may infect almost any body tissue or organ. It is transmitted from open lesions during any sexual contact (genital, oral–genital, or anal–genital). The organism can survive for days in fluids. It may also be transmitted by infected blood or other body fluids such as saliva. The average incubation period is 20 to 30 days. Once it has entered the system, *T. pallidum* spreads through the blood and lymphatic system. Congenital syphilis is transferred to the fetus through the placental circulation.

Syphilis is characterized by three clinical stages: primary, secondary, and tertiary, with an extended period of latency

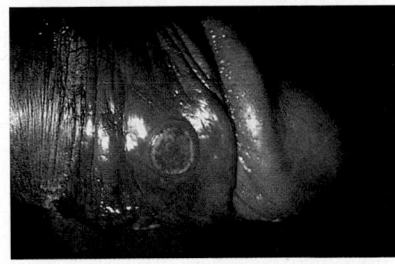

Figure 36-3. ■ Chancre of primary syphilis on the penis.
(*Source: Custom Medical Stock Photos, Inc.*)

between the last two stages. Each stage has characteristic clinical manifestations.

Primary Syphilis

The primary stage of syphilis is characterized by the appearance of a painless ulcer called a **chancre** (Figure 36-3 ■) at the site of inoculation (genitals, anus, mouth, breast, finger). Regional lymph nodes (e.g., inguinal nodes) also may be swollen. The chancre appears 3 to 4 weeks after the infectious contact. In women, a genital chancre may go unnoticed, disappearing within 4 to 6 weeks. In both primary and secondary stages, syphilis is highly infectious, even if no symptoms are evident.

Secondary Syphilis

Manifestations of secondary syphilis may appear any time from 2 weeks to 6 months after the initial chancre disappears. These symptoms can include a skin rash, especially on the palms of the hands (Figure 36-4 ■) or soles of the

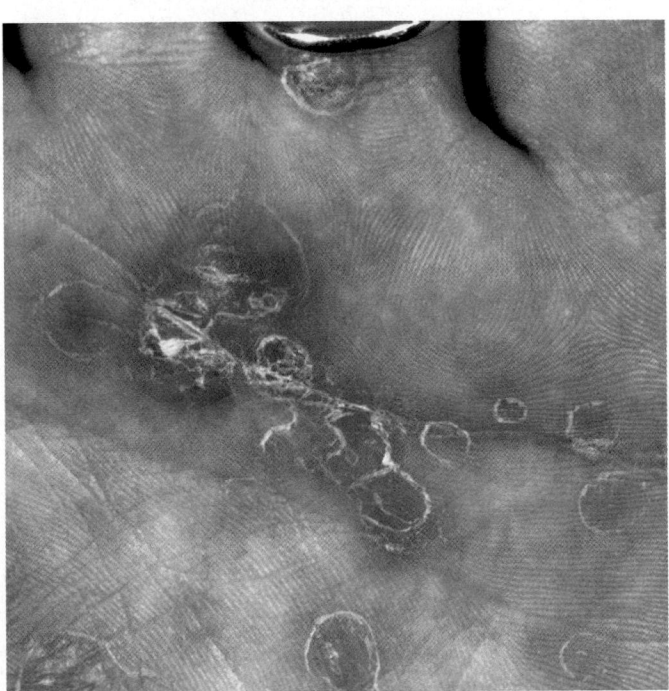

Figure 36-4. ■ Palmar rash of secondary syphilis. (*Source:* Photo Researchers, Inc.)

feet; mucous patches in the oral cavity; sore throat; generalized lymphadenopathy; condyloma lata (flat, broad-based papules, unlike the pedunculated structure of genital warts) on the labia, anus, or corner of the mouth; flulike symptoms; and alopecia. These manifestations generally disappear within 2 to 6 weeks.

Latent-Stage Syphilis

The latent stage of syphilis can last up to 50 years. During this stage, no symptoms of syphilis are apparent, and the disease is not transmissible by sexual contact. It can be transmitted by infected blood, however. All prospective blood donors are screened for syphilis. In two-thirds of all cases, the latent stage persists without further complications. Unless treated, the remaining one-third of infected people progress to late-stage or tertiary syphilis. The latent stage is shortened in people with HIV disease.

Tertiary Syphilis

Tertiary syphilis can be manifested in two different ways. *Benign late syphilis* is characterized by localized infiltrating tumors (*gummas*) in skin, bones, and liver. This form of tertiary syphilis generally responds promptly to treatment. A *diffuse inflammatory response* that involves the central nervous system and the cardiovascular system has a more insidious onset. Although the disease can still be treated at this stage, much of the cardiovascular and central nervous system damage is irreversible.

INTERDISCIPLINARY CARE

As with other STIs, the goals of treatment for syphilis are to inactivate the spirochete and educate the client about how to prevent reinfection or further transmission. In addition, clients should be screened for chlamydial infection and advised to have an HIV test.

Diagnostic Tests

The following tests are widely used to diagnose syphilis:

- The *VDRL (Venereal Disease Research Laboratory)* and *RPR (rapid plasma reagin)* become positive about 4 to 6 weeks after infection. Because these tests are not specific, additional tests may be necessary.
- The *FTA-ABS (fluorescent treponemal antibody absorption)* test is specific for *T. pallidum* and can be used to confirm VDRL and RPR findings.

- *Immunofluorescent staining* or *dark-field microscopy* can be used to identify the presence of *T. pallidum* in a specimen obtained from a chancre or by aspirating a lymph node.

Medications

A single intramuscular (IM) dose of penicillin G is the treatment of choice for primary and secondary syphilis. If the duration of the disease is unknown or more than 1 year, the total dosage is increased and given in three weekly injections. Clients allergic to penicillin are given oral doxycycline (Vibramycin). The nursing implications of antibiotic therapy are discussed in Chapter 10.

NURSING CARE

The nursing assessment, diagnoses, interventions, and evaluation for a client with syphilis are similar to that for a client with chlamydia discussed earlier in this chapter. In addition, see the Critical Thinking Care Map at the end of the chapter for an opportunity to plan care for a client with syphilis.

CONTINUING CARE

Early symptoms of syphilis resolve with or without treatment. Teach clients that syphilis is a chronic disease that can be spread to others even when no symptoms are evident. Stress the importance of (1) taking all prescribed medications, (2) referring all sexual partners for evaluation and treatment, (3) abstaining from all sexual contact for a minimum of 1 month after treatment, and (4) using a condom to avoid transmitting or contracting infections in the future. Emphasize the need for follow-up testing at 3 and 6 months for clients with primary or secondary syphilis, and at 6 and 12 months for those with late-stage disease. Discuss integrating safer sex practices into the client's lifestyle to prevent future episodes of STIs.

Note: The bibliography listings for this and all chapters have been compiled at the back of the book.

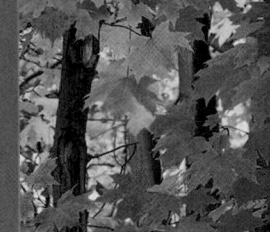

Chapter Review

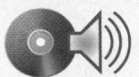 **KEY TERMS** by Topics

Use the audio glossary feature of either the CD-ROM or the Companion Website to hear the correct pronunciation of the following key terms.

Sexually transmitted infections
sexually transmitted infection (STI), abstinence, chancre

KEY Points

- The risk for contracting a sexually transmitted infection is directly related to lifestyle. Teach all clients to use safer sex practices such as abstinence, mutual monogamy with an uninfected partner, and barrier protection during sexual relations.

- Many STIs such as chlamydia, gonorrhea, and syphilis can be effectively treated with single-dose antibiotic therapy. Others, such as genital herpes and genital warts, are chronic viral infections that can be managed but not cured.

- Human papillomavirus (HPV) infection significantly increases a woman's risk for cervical cancer. Recommend that all women with HPV have annual Pap tests for early detection of cervical cancer.

- Many STIs such as syphilis, gonorrhea, and other less common diseases must be reported to state and federal agencies.

- Screening and treatment of the client's partner is necessary to prevent reinfection during or after treatment for an STI.

- Complications of STIs can include pelvic inflammatory disease and problems of fertility, as well as systemic responses (e.g., cardiovascular and neurologic manifestations of tertiary syphilis).

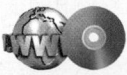 **EXPLORE MediaLink**

Additional interactive resources for this chapter can be found on the Companion Website at www.prenhall.com/burke. Click on Chapter 36 and "Begin" to select the activities for this chapter.

For chapter-related NCLEX-style review questions and an audio glossary, access the accompanying CD-ROM in this book.

FOR FURTHER Study

For review of nursing implications for antibiotics, see Chapter 10.

For discussion of human immunodeficiency virus (HIV) and AIDS, see Chapter 11.

For more about hepatitis B, see Chapter 21.

For further study about pelvic inflammatory disease (PID), see Chapter 35.

Critical Thinking Care Map

Caring for a Client with Syphilis
NCLEX-PN® Focus Area: Reduction of Risk Potential

Case Study: Eddie Kratz, a 22-year-old man, shares a small apartment with Marla Jones, who is 7 months pregnant with his child. Although he intends to marry Ms. Jones before the baby is born, he has continued a previous relationship with a woman named Justine Simpson. His sexual activities with Ms. Simpson have increased in frequency as Ms. Jones's pregnancy has advanced. Recently, Mr. Kratz has noticed a swelling in his groin and a sore on his penis.

Nursing Diagnosis: Risk for Injury

COLLECT DATA

Subjective	Objective
_____	_____
_____	_____
_____	_____
_____	_____
_____	_____
_____	_____

Would you report this data? Yes/No

If yes, to: _____

Nursing Care

_____

_____

_____

_____

_____

_____

_____

_____

_____

_____

How would you document this? _____

_____

_____

_____

Data Collected
(use those that apply)

- Regional lymphadenopathy
- Having unprotected sex with Ms. Jones and Ms. Simpson
- Syphilitic chancre on the shaft of the penis
- Believes that Ms. Jones is not having sex with anyone else, but is not sure
- ELISA results negative for HIV
- Dark-field analysis of chancre exudate confirms syphilis

Nursing Interventions
(use those that apply; list in priority order)

- Administer and document IM injection of benzathine penicillin G as ordered.
- Teach the importance of treatment to the health of their infant.
- Discuss importance of abstaining from sexual activity until client and partners are cured, and using condoms to prevent reinfection.
- Explain the need for follow-up testing in 3 and 6 months.
- Notify Ms. Jones and Ms. Simpson of need for testing.
- Send reminders for follow-up at 3- and 6-month intervals.
- Refer Mr. Kratz and Ms. Jones for counseling about the impact of the disease on their relationship.
- Provide a copy of STI prevention checklist.

1 A woman has been diagnosed with a chlamydia infection. As you explain her prescription to her, she states, "I don't need any medicine. I feel fine." Your response is based on the knowledge that:

A. the body often clears chlamydia by itself.
B. fever and dysuria usually accompany chlamydia in women.
C. clients with STIs often deny symptoms.
D. if untreated, chlamydia can progress to PID.

2 Using azithromycin (Zithromax) instead of doxycycline (Vibramycin) can improve compliance primarily because:

A. Zithromax has fewer side effects.
B. Zithromax is taken in a single oral dose.
C. Zithromax costs less.
D. Zithromax tastes better.

3 An 18-year-old college student has just been diagnosed with a first episode infection of herpes simplex type 2. She says, " I can't believe this. I'm so embarrassed. How could he? I trusted him." Your initial response is:

A. "You can't believe this has happened to you."
B. "You need to use barrier protection so you do not pass this on."
C. "You can't trust what these college guys tell you."
D. "We will provide you with prescriptions that will make you more comfortable."

4 Teaching the client with genital warts (HPV) should include:

A. measures to relieve pain.
B. how to take acyclovir.
C. avoiding acidic foods.
D. importance of regular Pap testing.

5 A client with newly diagnosed gonorrhea also undergoes testing for HIV infection. She asks why this is necessary. The nurse's response is based on the knowledge that

A. it is likely the client has been using injection drugs, increasing her risk for HIV.
B. gonorrhea is an opportunistic infection that usually doesn't occur in clients with intact immune systems.
C. other STIs including HIV often coexist in clients with gonorrhea.
D. both gonorrhea and HIV occur more frequently in women who have sex with other women.

6 A client with syphilis is reluctant to take the prescribed antibiotic. The nurse stresses which of the following as the most important reason for treating this disease?

A. To prevent transmission of the disease to others.

B. To promote healing of the initial chancre without secondary infection.
C. To ensure that the disease will not progress to tertiary syphilis.
D. To prevent reinfection of the client.

7 Your client has been diagnosed with syphilis. Which allergy would necessitate a change in the usual treatment?

A. penicillin
B. eggs
C. acyclovir
D. sulfa

8 A male client diagnosed with genital herpes says that he does not want to use condoms because they are uncomfortable. He asks if there is another way to prevent spreading this infection to his partners. The nurse responds that:

A. it is only necessary to use condoms when lesions are visible.
B. condoms should be used for all sexual relations, especially from the onset of prodromal symptoms until all lesions are healed.
C. it isn't necessary to use condoms if sexual relations are limited to oral sex during outbreaks of the infection.
D. practicing mutual monogamy will prevent spreading this infection to others even if a condom is not used.

9 Which comment by a 20-year-old indicates the client needs additional teaching about STIs?

A. "My boyfriend needs to see his doctor for treatment also."
B. "If we only engage in oral sex, we cannot transmit STIs."
C. "Use of latex condoms can prevent most STIs."
D. "Some STIs cannot be cured, but symptoms can be treated."

10 Important nursing responsibilities related to the sexually transmitted infections of syphilis and gonorrhea are (select all that apply):

A. reporting cases of the infection to state agencies.
B. discussing the need for cesarean delivery with infected women.
C. emphasizing the need to identify and treat infected partners.
D. teaching safer sex practices to infected clients and their partners.
E. stressing the importance of abstinence until the infection is cleared.

Answers for Review Questions, as well as discussion of Care Plan and Critical Thinking Care Map questions, appear in Appendix V.

Assessing Communication Variables from a Cultural Perspective

Mrs. Kin-Lee, a 25-year-old Vietnamese woman, arrived in the emergency room in transition with very strong and closely spaced contractions. Despite her imminent delivery she did not initiate conversation or communicate urgency about getting attention from the staff. She answered questions politely, nodding and smiling respectfully at the staff between occasional grimaces during the contractions. The only other sign of pain was her white knuckles as she grasped the armrests on the wheelchair in which she was placed. Many Vietnamese, as most Asians, believe that a woman must experience pain as part of childbirth, and that expressing these feelings will bring on shame.

Verbal and nonverbal methods of communication vary among persons in different cultures. Communication presents the most significant challenge in working with clients from diverse cultural backgrounds, since the meaning of communication may vary by culture. The nurse who is aware of communication variables can be more attentive to nuances and different meanings of communication across cultures.

Communication

Communication embraces the entire world of human interaction and behavior. Communication provides the means by which people connect, and it is also the means by which culture is transmitted and preserved. Regardless of culture, individuals learn to think, feel, believe, and strive for what their culture considers proper. Both verbal and nonverbal communications are learned within one's culture (Giger & Davidhizar, 1999). The nurse should be aware of these communication variables:

Dialect	Dialect largely depends on geographic location. For example, clients from Appalachia, Australia, and England speak English quite differently from one another.
Language style	Words may have *different meanings* in different cultures. For example, the word "bad" may have a positive meaning to a teenager and have a more typical, negative meaning to an adult (Giger & Davidhizar, 1999).
Volume of speech	Volume of speech may be culturally determined. Irish people, for example, frequently raise their voices. In contrast, others (such as the Japanese) tend to keep their voices low.
Touch	Use of touch varies widely among cultures. Because nurses use touch to reassure, provide affirmation, and decrease loneliness, we must be aware of how it is perceived. Depending on the situation and the culture of the person, touch can also be perceived as threatening, intrusive, or seductive.
Context of speech or emotional tone	Context of speech refers to the use *of emotion* when communicating. The Black American, Jewish,

or German client is less likely to use an emotional tone than one who is Italian, Irish, or Mexican (Giger & Davidhizar, 1999). Arabs may express their emotions openly through nonverbal cues and voice, but may withhold some feelings from strangers. Arabs may express agreement in front of strangers that does not reflect their true meanings (Meleis, 1996). An Arab may tend to protect others from disagreements or indicate disagreement by simply raising an eyebrow rather than responding verbally.

Kinesics

Kinesics refers to the use of stances, gestures, and eye behavior when communicating with others. Vietnamese individuals typically nod and smile to indicate respect when interacting with a health care professional (Giger & Davidhizar, 1999). However, they may or may not be agreeing with what is being said.

Nursing Implications

- **Assess verbal and nonverbal communication for cultural variations in meaning.** The nurse should be attentive to variations between and within cultures in relation to dialect, language style, volume of speech, touch, context of speech, and kinesics. A misinterpretation of communication due to cultural differences can create misunderstanding and deficits in meeting a client's needs.

- **Determine how respect can be communicated within a particular culture.** In some cultures a client will not confide information until a relationship with the caregiver has developed. Thus, use of "small talk" may be essential to develop a therapeutic relationship. In other cases, calling clients by their last names or greeting them by name is important. It may be helpful to greet an individual by title and first name, to approach and shake hands or to smile with direct eye contact. In every case, it is important to assess the response of the individual, to determine the client's comfort level, and to adapt communication strategies depending on the response of the individual.

Self-Reflection Questions

1. What personal communication techniques do you use when approaching individuals for the first time?

2. What communication techniques do you observe among other cultures during your initial greeting?

3. What generally accepted communication techniques can you use to communicate respect to persons from another culture?

Thinking Strategically About...

Rachel Clemments is a 44-year-old divorced mother of two teenage girls. Because of a strong family history of breast cancer, she has been closely monitored (annual mammograms and clinical breast examination, monthly BSE) for the past 4 years. In spite of careful monitoring, however, 2 weeks ago she discovered a thickened area in her left breast. An incisional biopsy revealed invasive lobular carcinoma.

DATA COLLECTED

Ms. Clemments's history reveals that her mother, two aunts, and one sister were diagnosed with breast cancer. Her mother and one of the aunts died before age 45. Physical assessment findings on admission include T 98.5°F (37.0°C); BP 110/62; P 65; R 14. Her weight is 120 lbs. (54 kg); she is 5′6″ (168 cm) tall.

Based on biopsy findings and her fear of future tumors, Ms. Clemments chooses to have a modified radical mastectomy and axillary node dissection. She is debating whether to have reconstructive breast surgery. Her oncologist has recommended a 6-month course of adjuvant chemotherapy, and she is concerned about side effects. One of her greatest concerns is how her illness will affect her ability to support and care for her daughters. She is afraid that treatment will limit her ability to keep her job and continue to meet her daughters' needs. Since breast cancer seems part of the family legacy, she worries that it will happen to her girls.

CRITICAL THINKING

1 What knowledge deficits does the nurse need to address with Ms. Clemments?

2 What are some of the common side effects of chemotherapy and what are some of the medications that help minimize them?

MANAGEMENT OF CARE

1 Most chemotherapeutic agents cause myelosuppression (depression of bone marrow function). This means the client has decreased WBC (leukopenia), decreased RBC (anemia) and decreased platelets (thrombocytopenia). What are the nursing implications when caring for a client with neutropenia?

2 What client education would be important for a client with thrombocytopenia?

COORDINATION OF INTERDISCIPLINARY CARE

1 What resources might be available to assist Ms. Clemments in coping with her diagnosis and treatment?

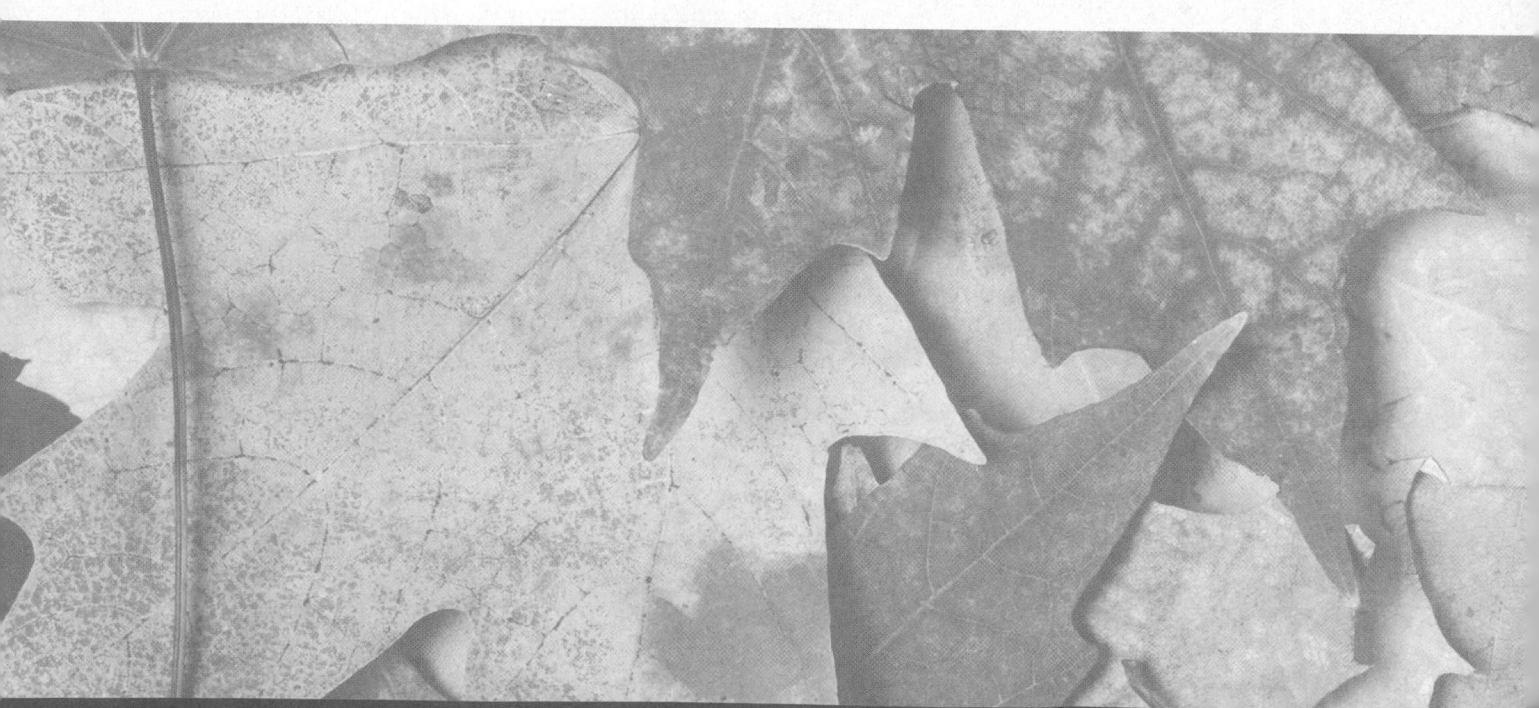

Disrupted Neurologic Function

UNIT X

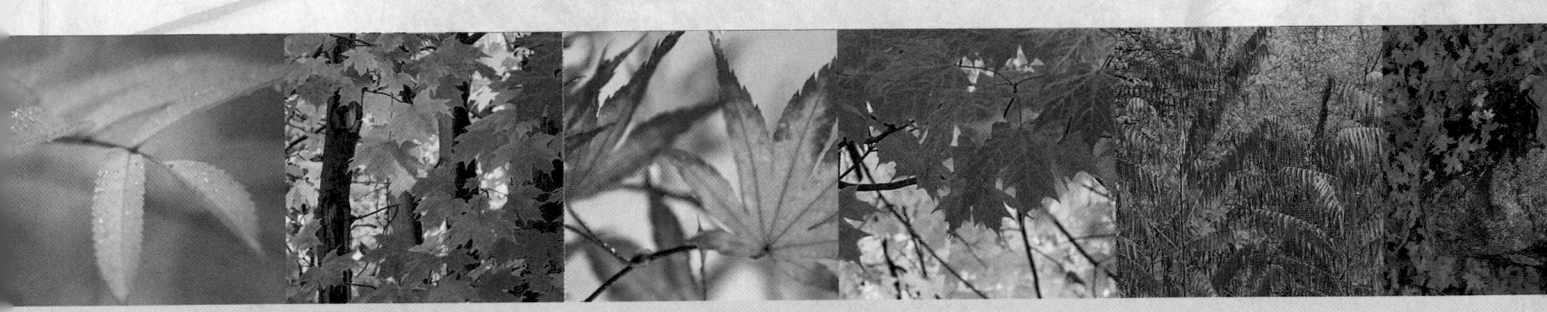

Chapter 37

The Nervous System and Assessment

BRIEF Outline

LEARNING Outcomes

After completing this chapter, you will be able to:

- Describe the structure and functions of the central and peripheral nervous systems.
- Identify subjective and objective assessment data to collect for clients with neurologic or sensory disorders.
- Identify nursing responsibilities for common diagnostic tests and monitors for clients with neurologic or sensory disorders.
- Identify the major structures and functions of the eye and the ear.
- Describe changes in neurologic function, vision, and hearing that occur with aging.

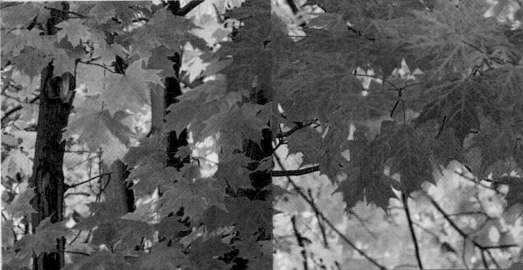

MediaLink

www.prenhall.com/burke
Use the address above to access the free, interactive Companion Website created for this textbook. Get hints, instant feedback, and textbook references to chapter-related NCLEX-style questions. Link to other interesting sites.

Audio Glossary:
Use the Companion Website, or the CD-ROM disk enclosed with your textbook, to hear the pronunciation of key terms in this chapter.

The nervous system consists of the brain, spinal cord, and peripheral nerves. It is a very complex system that controls all motor, sensory, and autonomic activities of the body. It responds to changes within the body and to environmental stimuli. When the nervous system malfunctions, the person may experience acute or chronic disorders.

The visual system includes internal and external structures, which are important for visual function. The auditory system functions to receive and perceive sounds as well as maintain position sense and balance. The major sensory organs, including the eyes and ears, are vital in providing input to the nervous system.

The Nervous System

The nervous system is divided into the central nervous system (CNS) and the peripheral nervous system (PNS). The brain and spinal cord make up the CNS. The PNS consists of the cranial nerves, the spinal nerves, and the autonomic nervous system.

A **neuron** (basic cell of the nervous system) is made up of a dendrite, a cell body, and an axon (Figure 37-1 ■). Dendrites are short, branch-like extensions on the cell body. They carry impulses to the cell body from other cells. The cell body controls the function of the neuron. At the other end of the neuron is a single, long projection known as the

axon. It carries impulses away from the cell body. Many axons are protected and insulated by a white fatty substance called **myelin sheath.** Nerves covered with a myelin sheath are known as *myelinated* or white nerve fibers. Axons without myelin are unmyelinated or gray nerve fibers.

Neurons are responsible for neurotransmission. Nerve impulses move from one neuron to another neuron across a **synapse.** A chemical **neurotransmitter** (see Figure 37-1) such as acetylcholine either helps the impulse cross the synapse or stops it. *Sensory* (or afferent) neurons carry impulses from the skin and muscles to the CNS. *Motor* (or efferent) neurons carry impulses from the CNS to the muscles for contraction and to glands in order to release secretions.

THE CENTRAL NERVOUS SYSTEM

The Brain

The brain is the control center of the nervous system. A rigid, bony skull protects the brain from external injury. Beneath the skull are three protective membranes or **meninges:** (1) dura mater, the outer layer; (2) arachnoid, the middle layer; and (3) pia mater, the inner layer directly attached to the brain (Figure 37-2 ■ *inset*). Arterial blood vessels are located in the *epidural space* between the skull and dura mater. Cerebrospinal fluid (CSF) is found in the *subarachnoid space* between the arachnoid and the pia mater.

There are four major regions of the brain: cerebrum, diencephalon, brainstem, and cerebellum (see Figure 37-2).

CEREBRUM. The cerebrum is the largest area of the brain and is divided into a right and left hemisphere. Deep grooves called **fissures** separate the hemispheres and separate the cerebrum from the cerebellum. The cerebral hemispheres are connected by a thick band of nerve fibers called *corpus callosum,* which lies deep in the brain. It allows communication between the two hemispheres. Each hemisphere receives sensory and motor impulses from the opposite side of the body. The right hemisphere controls sensation and movement on the left side of the body, whereas the left hemisphere controls sensation and movement on the right side of the body. In every individual one hemisphere is more dominant than the other. The left hemisphere is responsible for speech, problem solving, reasoning, and calculations. The right hemisphere controls visual-spatial information such as art, music, and the surrounding physical environment.

The cerebrum consists of gray matter and white matter. The outer layer or *cerebral cortex* contains the gray matter, which is made up of neurons. The rest of the cerebrum is made up of myelinated nerve fibers called white matter. Each cerebral hemisphere is divided into four lobes: frontal, parietal, temporal, and occipital (Figure 37-3 ■). They are separated by fissures.

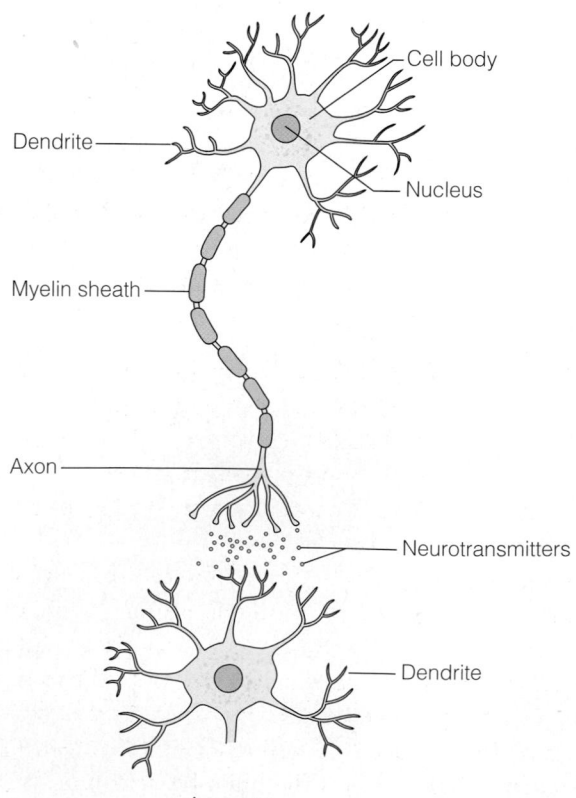

A neuron

Figure 37-1. ■ A neuron.

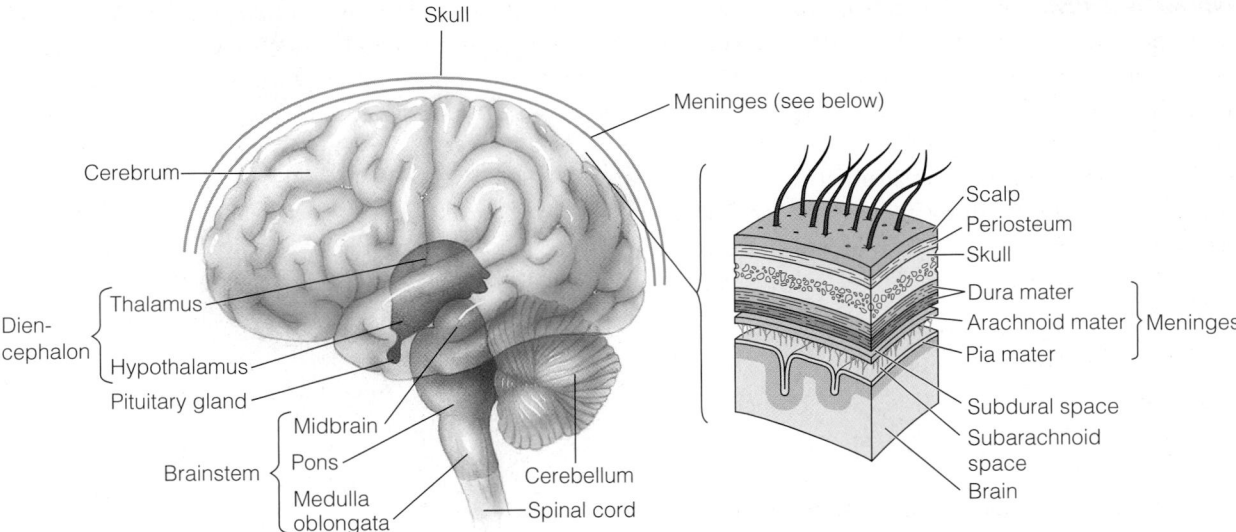

Figure 37-2. ■ The four major regions of the brain with an illustration of the meninges.

DIENCEPHALON. The diencephalon contains the thalamus and hypothalamus. The thalamus relays all sensory information to the cortex. The hypothalamus regulates temperature, fluid balance, thirst, appetite, emotions, and the sleep/wake cycle.

BRAINSTEM. The brainstem consists of the midbrain, pons, and medulla oblongata. The midbrain is the center for

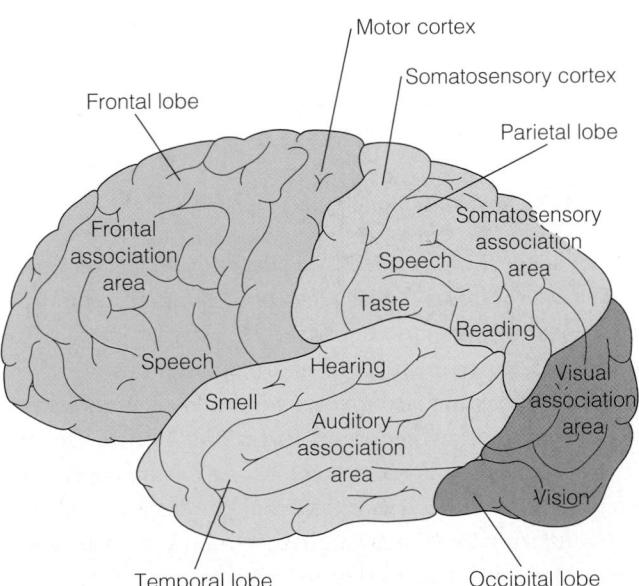

Figure 37-3. ■ Cerebral lobes with their functions. The *frontal lobe* controls voluntary motor control on the opposite side of the body and determines emotions, motivation, complex thinking, judgment, and personality. Broca's area promotes speaking ability. The *parietal lobe* interprets sensations and determines right from left and where the body is in relation to the environment. The *temporal lobe* processes taste, smell, and hearing stimuli; it is also important in long-term memory. Wernicke's area promotes understanding of the spoken and written word. The *occipital lobe* processes visual stimuli.

auditory and visual reflexes. It serves as a nerve pathway between the cerebral hemispheres and lower brain. The pons controls respiration. The medulla oblongata is located at the base of the brainstem. It controls heart rate, blood pressure, respirations, coughing, swallowing, and vomiting.

CEREBELLUM. The cerebellum is connected to the midbrain, pons, and medulla. Like the cerebrum, it has two hemispheres. It coordinates involuntary muscle activity and fine motor movements as well as balance and posture.

CEREBROSPINAL FLUID. Four ventricles within the brain make and circulate CSF in the subarachnoid space of the brain and spinal cord. CSF is a clear, colorless liquid that protects the brain and spinal cord from trauma. It also provides a place for nutrient exchange and waste removal. The daily production of CSF is about 125 to 150 mL. CSF has a high glucose content with very few white blood cells and no red blood cells.

BLOOD SUPPLY TO THE BRAIN. The brain receives about 750 mL of blood each minute and uses approximately 20% of the body's cardiac output. This large oxygen demand is necessary for glucose metabolism, which is the brain's only source of energy. The brain cannot store oxygen or glucose so it needs a constant supply of both.

Two arterial systems supply blood to the brain: (1) internal carotid arteries and (2) vertebral arteries. Most of the cerebrum is supplied blood by the internal carotid arteries. The brainstem and cerebellum receive their blood supply from the vertebral arteries. These major arteries are connected by smaller arteries forming a ring called the *circle of Willis*. This circle protects the brain by providing alternative blood flow routes when an artery is blocked. Cerebral veins drain venous blood into the jugular veins.

BLOOD–BRAIN BARRIER. The *blood–brain barrier* is composed of astrocytes that are joined by tight junctions. This decreases permeability so that harmful substances in the blood cannot enter the brain. It allows only the passage of glucose, some amino acids, respiratory gases, and water. Substances such as urea, some toxins, and most antibiotics cannot pass this barrier. However, brain injury may cause a local breakdown of the barrier.

The Spinal Cord

The spinal cord exits the skull through the foramen magnum and extends to the first or second lumbar vertebra, where it ends in the cauda equina. It is about 17 inches long and 3/4 inch thick. The spinal cord is surrounded and protected by the vertebral column. The column consists of 7 cervical, 12 thoracic, 5 lumbar, 5 sacral, and 4 fused vertebrae, which form the coccyx.

The inside of the spinal cord is H shaped and consists of gray matter surrounded by white matter. The gray matter contains three specialized areas called horns: (1) the ventral horn (motor neurons), (2) dorsal horn (sensory neurons), and (3) lateral horn (sympathetic neurons). The white matter forms ascending and descending pathways known as *spinal tracts*. These tracts carry messages to and from the brain: ascending sensory pathways and descending motor pathways. On exiting the brain, motor and sensory nerve fibers cross to the opposite side of the spinal cord. This is why a stroke in the left hemisphere affects motor and sensory function on the right side of the body.

THE PERIPHERAL NERVOUS SYSTEM

The peripheral nervous system links the CNS with the rest of the body. It receives and conducts information from the external environment, and transmits signals to muscles and organs of the body. Spinal nerves, cranial nerves, and ganglia make up the PNS. The PNS is divided into the somatic and autonomic nervous systems. The somatic system connects the skin and muscles to the CNS. The autonomic nervous system controls visceral organs and some glands.

Spinal Nerves

There are 31 pairs of spinal nerves (Figure 37-4 ■). These nerves are named in reference to the corresponding vertebrae of the spine:

- Cervical: 8 pairs (C_1 to C_8)
- Thoracic: 12 pairs (T_1 to T_{12})
- Lumbar: 5 pairs (L_1 to L_5)
- Sacral: 5 pairs (S_1 to S_5).

Each spinal nerve contains sensory and motor fibers. The dorsal and ventral root of each spinal nerve attaches it to the spinal cord. Sensory fibers are in the dorsal root with motor fibers in the ventral root. Damage to the dorsal root causes loss of sensation, whereas damage to the ventral root results in flaccid paralysis.

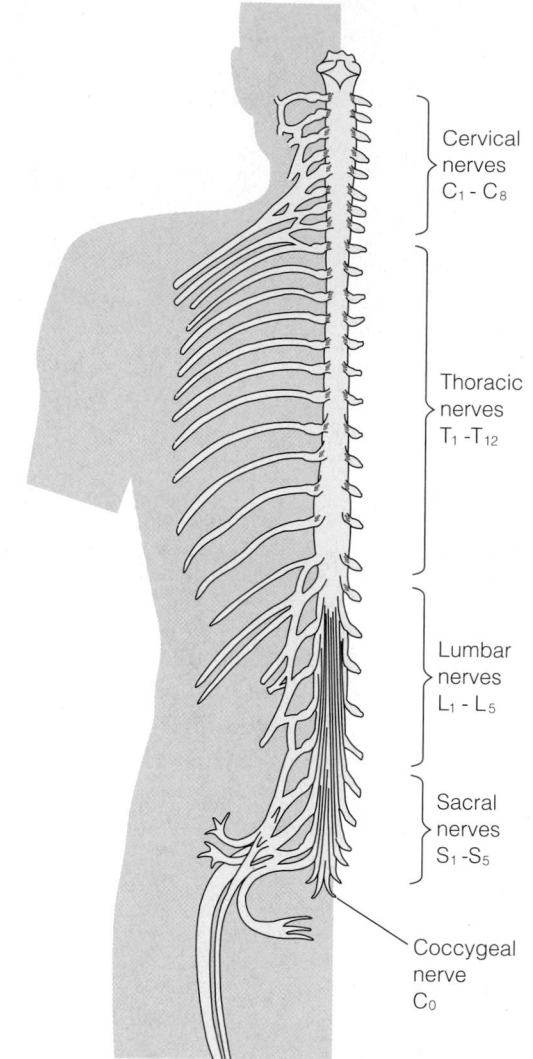

Cervical nerves C_1 - C_8

Thoracic nerves T_1 - T_{12}

Lumbar nerves L_1 - L_5

Sacral nerves S_1 - S_5

Coccygeal nerve C_0

Figure 37-4. ■ Distribution of spinal nerves.

An area of skin supplied by a single spinal nerve is called a **dermatome.** The dorsal roots of the spinal nerves carry sensations from specific dermatomes. Dermatomes are useful for locating pain sites and neurologic lesions.

Spinal nerves are also involved in reflexes. A **reflex** is an involuntary motor response to a stimulus. Reflexes follow a pathway known as a **reflex arc.** The reflex arc consists of a receptor, an afferent sensory neuron, the response center in the spinal cord or brain, an efferent motor neuron, and an effector muscle or gland (Figure 37-5 ■).

Common reflexes include stretch, deep tendon, withdrawal, and superficial. *Stretch reflexes* control muscle tone and help maintain posture. *Deep tendon reflexes (DTRs)* are assessed at the wrists, elbows, knees, and Achilles tendon with a reflex hammer. *Withdrawal reflexes* occur when a person expects pain and automatically withdraws the threatened body part. *Superficial reflexes* result from gently stimulating the skin. For example, the plantar reflex is elicited by stroking the sole of the foot. The normal response is to curl the toes downward.

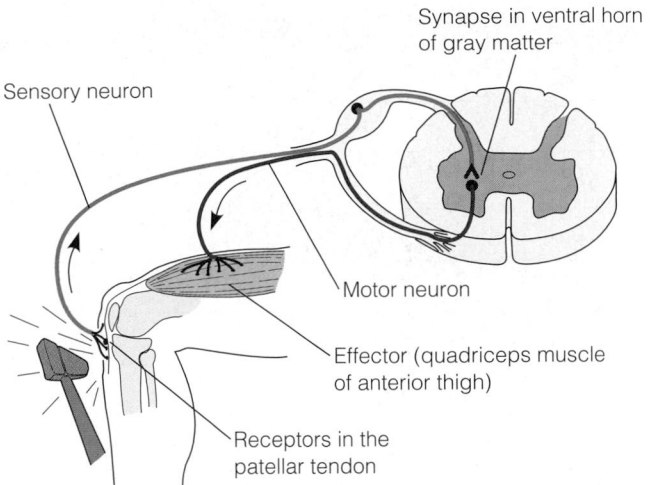

Figure 37-5. ■ A typical reflex arc of the spinal nerve. The stimulus is transferred from the sensory neuron directly to the motor neuron at the point of synapse in the spinal cord.

Cranial Nerves

Twelve pairs of cranial nerves begin in the brain or brainstem (Table 37-1 ■). They have sensory or motor functions or both. The vagus nerve extends into the thoracic and abdominal areas, but the other 11 cranial nerves innervate only head and neck regions. Cranial nerves I (olfactory), II (optic), and VIII (vestibulocochlear) control sensory function only.

THE AUTONOMIC NERVOUS SYSTEM

The autonomic nervous system (ANS) is part of the peripheral nervous system. It is responsible for maintaining the body's internal homeostasis. The ANS regulates respiration, heart rate, digestion, urinary excretion, body temperature, and sexual function.

There are two divisions: (1) the sympathetic nervous system (SNS) and (2) the parasympathetic nervous system (PNS). Fibers from both systems can affect the same structures. Generally when one system increases an action, the other system decreases the action. This process keeps the body in balance so that one action does not dominate.

The SNS prepares the body to handle stress. It plays a key role in the body's "fight-or-flight" response. The parasympathetic nervous system operates during nonstressful situations. It conserves the body's energy by regulating digestion, elimination, and other activities. The actions of the SNS and PNS are shown in Figure 37-6 ■.

Structure and Function of the Eye

The eyes are complex structures. The primary function of the eye is to convert patterns of light from the environment into a message that is transmitted via the optic nerve to the

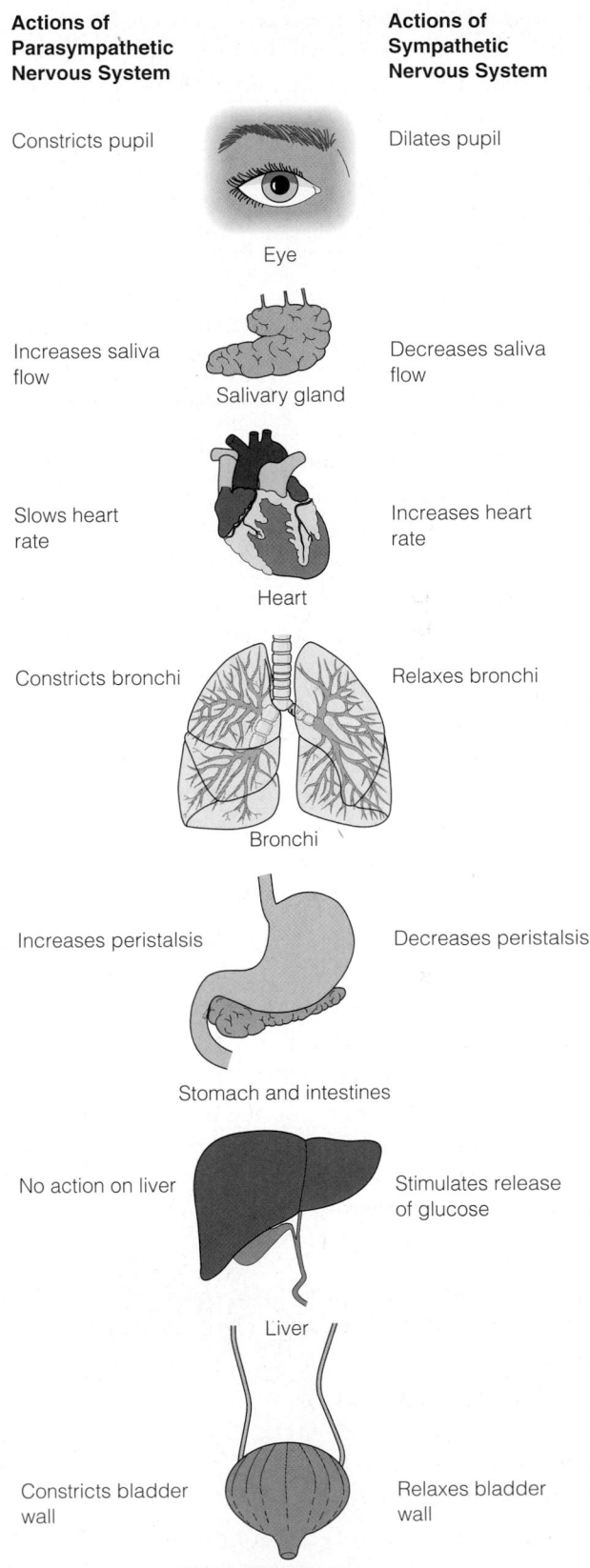

Actions of Parasympathetic Nervous System		Actions of Sympathetic Nervous System
Constricts pupil	Eye	Dilates pupil
Increases saliva flow	Salivary gland	Decreases saliva flow
Slows heart rate	Heart	Increases heart rate
Constricts bronchi	Bronchi	Relaxes bronchi
Increases peristalsis	Stomach and intestines	Decreases peristalsis
No action on liver	Liver	Stimulates release of glucose
Constricts bladder wall	Bladder	Relaxes bladder wall

Figure 37-6. ■ Autonomic nervous system and the organs it affects. The right side shows the actions of the sympathetic nervous system. The left side shows the actions of the parasympathetic nervous system.

TABLE 37-1

The Cranial Nerves

CRANIAL NERVE	FUNCTION
I Olfactory	Smell
II Optic	Vision
III Oculomotor	Pupil constriction Eyeball movement Raising of upper eyelid
IV Trochlear	Eyeball movement
V Trigeminal	Sensation of the scalp, nose, mouth, and cornea Chewing
VI Abducens	Lateral movement of the eyeball
VII Facial	Movement of facial muscles Secretions from lacrimal and salivary glands Taste in anterior two-thirds of tongue
VIII Vestibulocochlear	Sense of hearing and equilibrium
IX Glossopharyngeal	Taste in posterior one-third of tongue Sensation of pharynx and tongue Gag reflex Swallowing Secretions of parotid gland
X Vagus	Swallowing Controls parasympathetic nervous system activities (e.g., heart and respiratory rates, digestion) Sensation in pharynx and larynx
XI Accessory	Neck and shoulder movement
XII Hypoglossal	Tongue movement

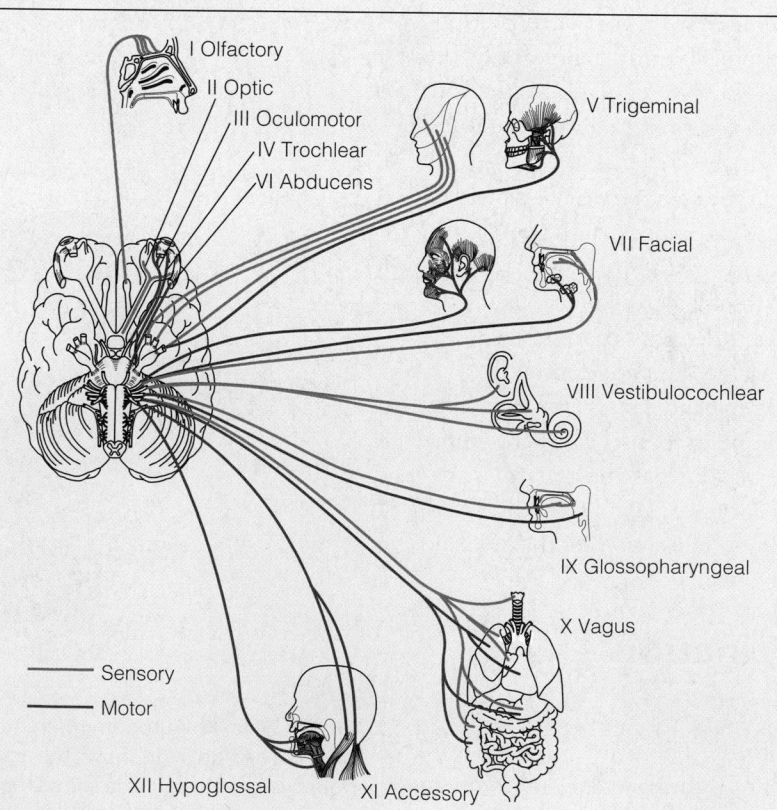

I Olfactory
II Optic
III Oculomotor
IV Trochlear
VI Abducens
V Trigeminal
VII Facial
VIII Vestibulocochlear
IX Glossopharyngeal
X Vagus
Sensory
Motor
XII Hypoglossal
XI Accessory

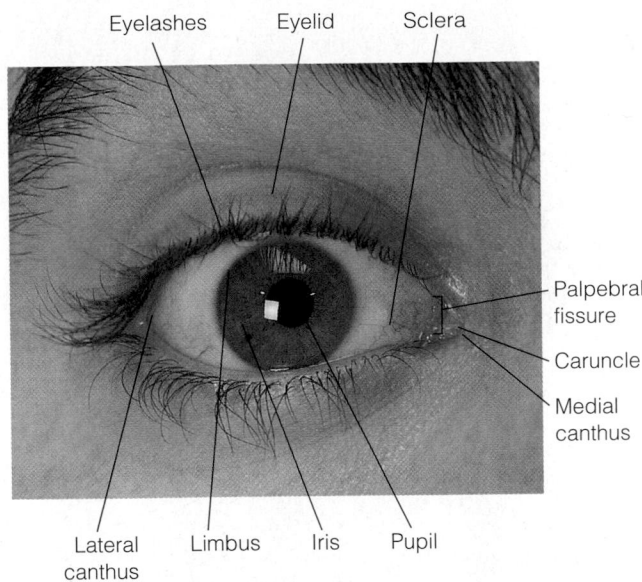

Figure 37-7. ■ The external and accessory structures of the eye.

brain. The brain gives meaning to the message, allowing us to make sense of what we see.

The eye is protected and supported by the *accessory structures.* They include (Figure 37-7 ■):

■ The *eyelids* and *eyelashes,* which protect the eye, trap dirt and debris, regulate the amount of light entering the eye, and spread tears.

■ The *conjunctiva,* a thin mucous membrane that covers the anterior surface of the eye and lines the inner surfaces of the eyelids.

■ The *lacrimal apparatus,* which secretes and drains tears to cleanse and moisten the eye's surface. Tears are produced by the *lacrimal gland.* They contain an antibacterial enzyme that protects the eye from infections. Tears drain into the *lacrimal ducts* and from there into the nose.

■ The *eye muscles* control eye movement and help maintain the shape of the eyeball.

Each eye is a hollow sphere about 1 in. (2.5 cm) in diameter, surrounded and protected by bone and cushions of fat. The wall of the eyeball has three layers. The outermost layer consists of the white, fibrous *sclera* and the transparent *cornea* (Figure 37-8 ■). The sclera protects and gives shape to the eyeball. The border between the sclera and the cornea is called the *limbus* (see Figure 37-7). The cornea is a transparent window that allows light to enter the eye. It contains no blood vessels and is very sensitive to touch. When the cornea is touched, the eyelids blink (the *corneal reflex*) and tears are secreted.

The middle layer of the eyeball, the *uvea,* is very vascular. It includes the iris, the ciliary body, and the choroid. The *iris,* the colored part of the eye, regulates light entering the eye by controlling the size of the pupil. The *pupil* is the dark center of the eye through which light enters. The pupil constricts in bright light and dilates in dim light or darkness. The *ciliary body*

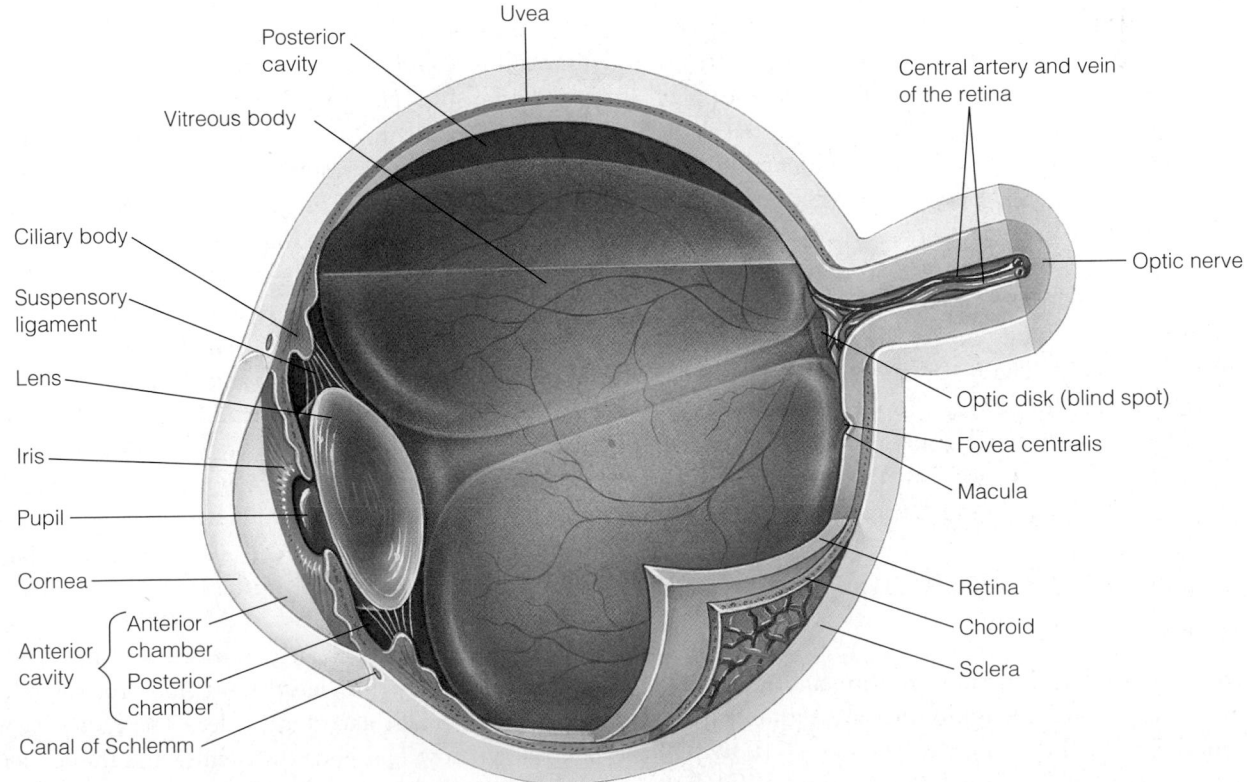

Figure 37-8. ■ The internal structures of the eye.

encircles the lens. It controls the shape of the lens to focus light on the retina. The *lens* is a transparent structure behind the pupil that can change shape to focus light onto the retina. Like the cornea, the lens contains no blood vessels. The vascular *choroid* nourishes the other layers of the eyeball and absorbs light, preventing it from scattering within the eyeball.

The *retina* is the innermost lining of the eyeball. It contains millions of light receptors called rods and cones. *Rods* are very light sensitive and allow us to see in dim light. *Cones* allow us to see in color and provide a sharper image than rods. Most cones are located in the *macula,* the area where light passing through the pupil and lens focuses on the retina. The macula provides our central vision. In the center of the macula, the *fovea centralis* allows detailed color vision. The optic nerve enters the eye at the *optic disk.*

The hollow eyeball is divided into two interior cavities. The larger *posterior cavity* behind the lens contains the clear gelatinous *vitreous body.* The vitreous body shapes and supports the eye.

The *anterior cavity* is further divided into the *anterior chamber* (the space between the cornea and the iris) and the *posterior chamber* (the space between the iris and the lens). Aqueous humor, a clear fluid, circulates through the anterior cavity, nourishing the lens and cornea. Aqueous humor is constantly formed and drained to maintain a relatively constant pressure within the eye. The *canal of Schlemm* at the junction of the sclera and the cornea allows aqueous humor to flow between the anterior and posterior chambers.

As light enters the eye, it is bent (**refraction**) to focus on the retina. The cornea, aqueous humor, lens, and vitreous body bend light rays to focus the image. To change the point of focus from far to near, the lens changes shape, the pupil constricts, and the eyes converge. This is called *accommodation.*

The *optic nerves* are cranial nerves that meet at the *optic chiasma.* Here nerve fibers from the medial half of each retina cross to the opposite side to join nerve fibers from the lateral half of the other eye (Figure 37-9 ■). The impulses generated in the retina travel to the *visual cortex* in the occipital lobe of the brain. The brain translates the impulses into the image we see, our *vision.*

The visual fields of each eye overlap considerably, and each eye sees a slightly different view. This allows *depth perception,* the ability to identify differences in distance between objects.

Structure and Function of the Ear

The ear has two primary functions: hearing and maintaining balance. The ear is divided into three areas, the external ear, the middle ear, and the inner ear (Figure 37-10 ■). All three areas are needed for hearing. The inner ear also helps maintain balance.

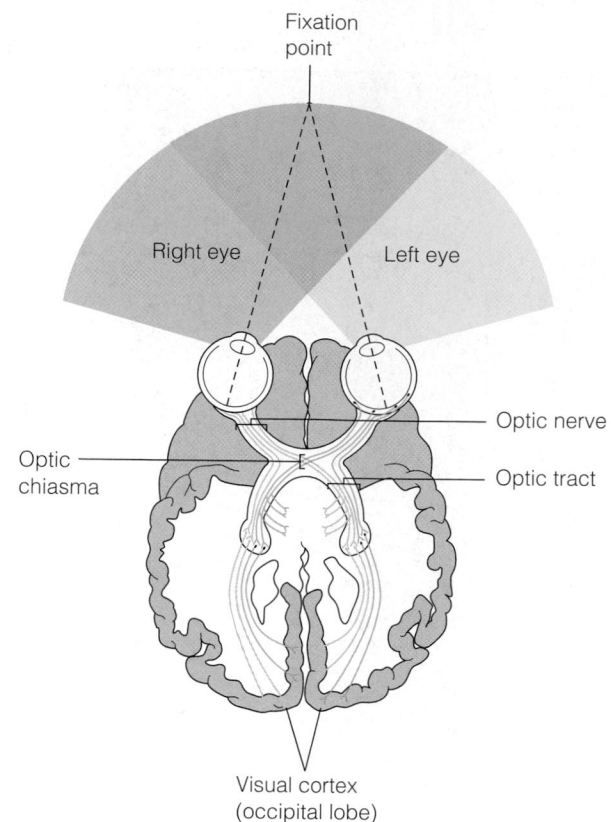

Figure 37-9. ■ The visual fields of the eyes and the optic pathways.

The *external ear* includes the auricle (or pinna), the auditory canal, and the tympanic membrane (eardrum). The *auricles* direct sound waves into the ear. The *auditory canal* is about 1 in. (2.5 cm) long. It focuses sound waves on the eardrum. Glands in the canal secrete **cerumen** (earwax), a yellow to brown waxy substance. Cerumen traps dirt and debris, protecting the tympanic membrane and middle ear from infection. The **tympanic membrane** (eardrum) separates the external ear and the middle ear.

The *middle ear* contains the auditory ossicles (bones): the malleus, the incus, and the stapes. These bones transmit vibrations from the tympanic membrane to the oval window of the inner ear. The middle ear is filled with air. It opens into the *eustachian tube,* which connects it with the nasopharynx. This proximity to the nasopharynx increases the likelihood for middle ear infections associated with upper respiratory infections. The eustachian tube helps equalize the pressure in the middle ear with atmospheric pressure.

The inner ear (*labyrinth*) is a maze of bony, fluid-filled chambers. The labyrinth has three regions: the vestibule, the semicircular canals, and the cochlea. The *vestibule* contains the oval window, and joins the cochlea and the semicircular canals. Receptors in the vestibule respond to changes in gravity and head position, helping maintain balance. The

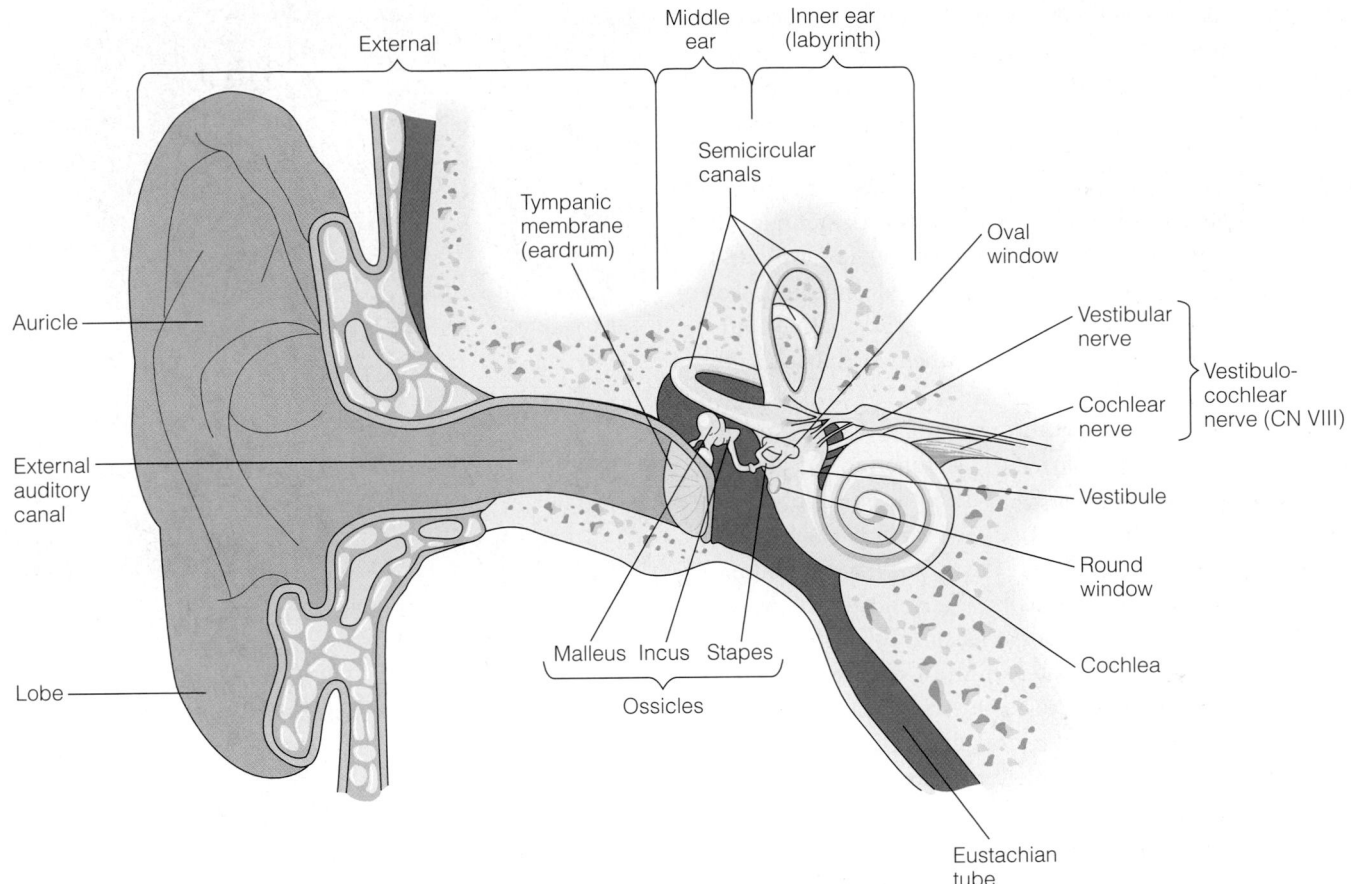

Figure 37-10. ■ Structures of the external, middle, and inner ear.

three *semicircular canals* also contain receptors that respond to head movements. The *cochlea* contains the *organ of Corti,* the receptor for hearing. The organ of Corti is sensory hair cells innervated by cranial nerve (CN) VIII, the vestibulocochlear nerve.

Hearing is the perception and interpretation of sound. Sound waves entering the external auditory canal cause the eardrum to vibrate. The ossicles transmit this vibration to the oval window, setting fluid within the vestibule into motion. The fluid movement stimulates receptors in the organ of Corti, which then send signals to the brain via CN VIII. Nerve fibers from each ear cross, so the auditory centers on each side of the brain receive impulses from both ears. The brain can receive and interpret a wide variety of sounds, as well as localize the source of the sound.

The inner ear also provides information to the brain about head position. This information is used to coordinate body movements so that *equilibrium* and *balance* are maintained. Changing head position sends different patterns of nerve impulses to the brain from the inner ear. The brain interprets these messages, stimulating motor centers to coordinate body movements.

Assessment

HEALTH HISTORY

Focused assessment of the client with a neurologic disorder begins with identifying the client's level of consciousness (LOC). When the client's LOC is altered, the nurse may need to ask the family for information.

Ask about numbness, tingling, sensations, tremors, problems with coordination or balance, loss of movement in any part of the body, or difficulty walking or using the hands. Determine when symptoms first began and whether they are constant or intermittent. If the client is experiencing pain, ask if coughing, sneezing, or walking increases the pain.

Determine whether the client has difficulty with speaking, seeing, hearing, tasting, or detecting odors. Inquire about memory, feelings of anxiety or depression, recent changes in sleep patterns, ability to perform activities of daily living, sexual activity, and weight. If the patient is taking any medications (prescription, over-the-counter, and natural or herbal preparations), ask about the purpose, frequency and duration of use, and any side effects.

Obtain the client's past medical history and family health history, focusing on previous incidents of seizures, fainting, dizziness, headaches, and any trauma, surgery, or tumors of the brain, spinal cord, or nerves. Ask about the presence or a family history of diabetes, high blood pressure, stroke, seizures, or mental health problems. Ask about recent and remote memory.

Question about occupational exposure to toxic chemicals or materials, use of protective headgear, and the amount of time doing repetitive motion tasks such as data entry and assembly work. Determine diet and use of alcohol, tobacco, or recreational drugs. Ask if the client wears a helmet during bicycle or motorcycle riding or when participating in contact sports.

Observe the client for squinting or abnormal eye movements that indicate problems with eye function. Ask about watery, irritated eyes or changes in vision. Inquire about the use of eye medications, corrective eyewear, and care of eyeglasses or contact lenses. Identify any history of eye trauma, surgery, or infections as well as the date and results of the last eye examination. Ask about a personal or family history of glaucoma, cataracts, diabetes, high blood pressure, thyroid disorders, and eye infections. Question whether there is a history of nearsightedness or farsightedness, cancer of the retina, or color blindness. Collect information about work exposure to chemicals or participation in sports that increase the risk of eye injury.

Explore changes in hearing such as difficulty hearing high-pitched or low-pitched sounds, ringing in the ears (*tinnitus*), ear pain, drainage from the ears, or use of hearing aids. Ask about trauma, surgery, or infections of the ear as well as infections such as meningitis or mumps. Determine the use of medications that may affect hearing such as aminoglycoside antibiotics. Obtain the client's family history of hearing loss or ear problems.

PHYSICAL EXAMINATION

The focused physical examination for the client with a neurologic problem begins by assessing the client's posture, movement, and appearance, and identifying orientation, mental, and emotional state. Identify if the client can see, hear, and feel your touch.

Assess dress, hygiene, and grooming as well as gait and posture. Observe the client's actions and affect. Note the LOC, content and quality of speech, mood swings, personality changes, and orientation to time, place, and person. Assess for memory or perceptual deficits.

Obtain blood pressure in both arms (unless contraindicated), pulse, respiratory rate, and temperature. Note any abnormal breathing patterns such as **Cheyne–Stokes** (periods of apnea for 10 to 60 seconds followed by gradual increased rate and depth of breathing). Check pupil response to light by using a penlight. Normal response should be PERRLA (pupils equally round and reactive to light and accommodation). Observe for **ptosis** (eyelids dropping) and **nystagmus**

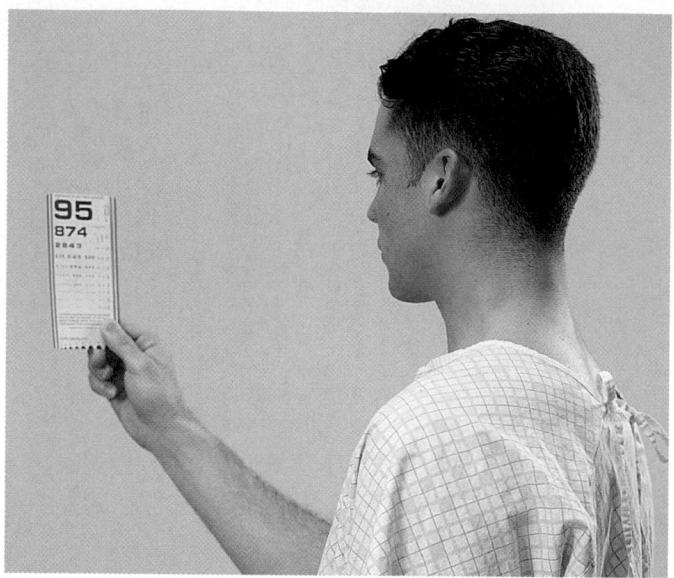

Figure 37-11. ■ Testing vision using a Rossenbaum eye chart. (Photographer: Richard Tauber.)

(involuntary eye movement). Assess ability to swallow a small drink of water, noting presence of **dysphagia** (difficulty swallowing).

Determine the client's ability to shrug the shoulders and to stick out the tongue. Note that the tongue should be midline. Assess for facial droop. Have client turn head side to side against resistance. Assess Romberg.

Assess upper and lower extremities for weakness, atrophy, and tremors as well as identifying decreased muscle tone (**flaccidity**) or increased muscle tone (**spasticity**). Ask the client to squeeze your hands, push feet against the resistance of your hands, and raise both legs off the bed. Note any difference between left or right side. Assess gait and ability to stand on one foot and walk heel to toe. Assess deep tendon reflexes (DTRs). Abnormal DTRs require further medical evaluation.

Assess distant vision by using the Snellen chart and asking the client to cover one eye at a time to read the chart; then repeat the test for the other eye. Assess near vision in the same manner, using a Rosenbaum chart (Figure 37-11 ■). To test extraocular movements, ask the client to follow a pen or your finger while keeping the head stationary. Inspect the eyelids for unusual redness or discharge. Note abnormal wideness of the lids, which may be due to *exophthalmos*. Inspect the cornea and iris for cloudiness or irregularities and the sclera for redness or yellow discoloration.

Assess for hearing loss by performing the whisper test and the Rinne and Weber tests (see Box 40-9). ◑ Inspect the auricle for redness, drainage, scales, or skin lesions. Palpate the auricles and over the mastoid process for tenderness, swelling, or nodules.

For more information about assessment techniques, see Chapter 5. ◑ See Box 37-1 ■ for an example of a neurologic assessment.

DOCUMENTATION OF NEUROLOGIC ASSESSMENT

Client: A 50-year-old male arrives on the neurologic unit at 5:00 P.M. following a motor vehicle accident. He is diagnosed with a concussion. He has no significant other medical problems.

Assessment note: Alert and oriented × 3. PERRLA. Able to move all extremities and resist pressure equally. Denies numbness or tingling in all extremities. Hand grasps strong and equal.

At 8:00 P.M. difficult to arouse. Oriented to person only. Pupils unequal with right greater than left, sluggish reaction. Speech slightly slurred. Left hand grasp weak. States numbness in left hand. Has difficulty raising left leg and has decreased ability to push against resistance. Charge nurse notified and physician paged.

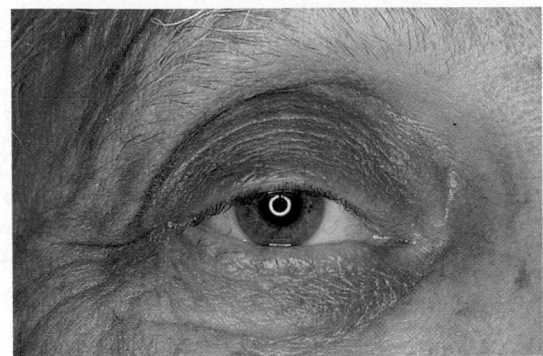

Figure 37-12. ■ Ptosis. (Photographer: Elena Dorfman.)

The Older Adult

In the older adult the brain atrophies, causing slower movement and reflexes as well as a degree of forgetfulness. However, significant short- and long-term memory loss, mental status changes, altered coordination, loss of motor skills, and altered speech signal a need for further assessment. The client may have difficulty changing position or standing up without assistance. This may be accompanied by dizziness, which is the result of anemia, ear infection, eye problems, stroke, or drug toxicity. These changes are often related to common chronic diseases that develop in older adults.

Often older adults experience sleep disorders and reduced pain perception. This may result from other chronic diseases and medication use or more serious neurologic dysfunction. Depression, delirium, and dementia develop in many older adults, which usually signals underlying disease. Confusion, memory loss, and depression are not associated with normal aging. Further information on assessing psychologic status may be found in Chapter 47. ◐◑

A number of changes in the eye and vision occur with aging. The lens becomes less elastic, affecting near vision. This is known as **presbyopia.** Clients with presbyopia may feel that their arms have become too short to read the newspaper comfortably.

Eyelid muscles may lose tone, causing the lower lid to turn out (*ectropion*) or the upper lid to droop (*ptosis,* Figure 37-12 ■). The lid margin may turn inward (*entropion*), causing the lashes to irritate the eye. Tears are decreased, so the eyes may feel dry and scratchy. Other eye and vision changes commonly seen with aging are summarized in Table 37-2 ■.

Hearing difficulties may be mechanical or natural. Inability to hear high-frequency sounds may develop from degeneration in the cochlea or the loss of small hairs in the ears. Increased accumulation of cerumen or earwax can also reduce hearing ability.

DIAGNOSTIC TESTS

Laboratory Tests

Several nonspecific laboratory tests are done to rule out other causes of neurologic dysfunction. A blood glucose level is done to identify the presence of hypoglycemia. Serum sodium and osmolarity are measured because low sodium levels, or increased or decreased osmolarity, may cause a coma. Arterial blood gases are used to rule out low oxygen or high carbon dioxide levels, another cause of altered LOC. To identify infectious diseases such as meningitis or encephalitis, a complete blood count (CBC) with differential and cultures from blood, urine, throat, and nose are done.

Elevated serum creatinine and BUN, which reflect decreased kidney function, can decrease LOC. Liver studies

TABLE 37-2

Age-Related Changes in the Eye and Vision

CHANGE	EFFECT ON VISION
Decreased corneal sensation and tear secretion	Increased risk of damage due to foreign body or trauma; increased risk of infection
Constriction of the pupil	Reduced light entering the eye; difficulty with night vision
Decreased elasticity and increased density of the lens	Difficulty focusing, especially for near vision Increased problems with glare Decreased color perception (especially blues, greens, and violet)
Loss of rods at periphery of retina	Decreased peripheral vision
Loss of fat and subcutaneous tissue around the eyes	Eyes appear sunken; decreased peripheral vision

TABLE 37-3

Imaging Techniques

DIAGNOSTIC STUDY	EXPLANATION AND PURPOSE	NURSING IMPLICATIONS
Radiography	Used to identify neurologic abnormalities such as lesions and tumors; when combined with use of an injected contrast medium, used to study blood flow through vessels.	If contrast media used, ask about allergies to iodine and seafood before the exam; ensure good hydration before and after the exam to reduce the risk of kidney damage. Although noninvasive, they expose the client to potentially damaging radiation. Ask women of childbearing age about possible pregnancy before the exam.
Skull and spine x-rays	Used to identify fractures, bone erosion, and calcifications.	Noninvasive test. Explain if different positions are needed.
Computed tomography (CT) scans	Specialized radiographic procedures that produce computer-generated images with significantly more detail than standard x-rays allow. May be done with or without contrast media. Detects problems such as hemorrhage, edema, hematoma, infarction, tumor, brain abscess, aneurysm, as well as size and location of CVA.	See Box 38-9 🔗 for nursing care checklist of a client undergoing a CT scan of the head.
Magnetic resonance imaging (MRI)	MRI uses a super magnet and radio-frequency signals to elicit a response from hydrogen nuclei. Used to identify stroke, tumor, trauma, multiple sclerosis, and seizures.	The client is not exposed to radiation during an MRI. Ask about implanted devices such as pacemakers or defibrillators. Provide teaching as the experience can be frightening.
Cerebral angiography	Invasive procedure that combines x-ray and fluoroscopy (a radiographic image displayed on a screen) with injection of contrast media into the vessel to illuminate blood flow through the vessel and evaluate its patency. Used to detect an aneurysm, brain tumor, and stroke.	Withhold meal prior to test. Explain that client will have hot flush of head and neck when contrast media is injected. **clinical ALERT** Closely monitor neurologic and VS; maintain pressure dressing and ice to injection site. Immediately report bleeding or swelling to the charge nurse and physician.
Myelography	X-ray of spinal cord and canal after injection of contrast media. Identifies spinal cord tumors, herniated intervertebral disks, and arthritic bone spurs.	See Box 39-11 for nursing care of a client undergoing myelography. **clinical ALERT** Closely monitor neurologic and VS. Immediately report leakage or bleeding from lumbar puncture site to charge nurse and physician.
Positive emission tomography (PET)	A radioactive agent is injected and computed tomography measures metabolic activity of the brain. Used to detect brain cancer, Alzheimer's disease, epilepsy, and Parkinson's disease.	Withhold food and fluids 4 hours before the exam. Explain that an IV line will be inserted. Instruct client to drink extra fluids to aid removal of radioisotope.
Ultrasound	Echoes from high-frequency sound waves are used to study blood flow within a vessel.	
Carotid duplex study	Sound waves identify blood flow velocity to determine the presence of occlusive vascular disease.	Explain study to client.

TABLE 37-4

Electrographic Studies

ELECTROGRAPHIC STUDY	EXPLANATION AND PURPOSE	NURSING IMPLICATIONS
Electroencephalography (EEG)	Electrodes are placed on the scalp to record brain electrical activity. Done to diagnose epilepsy, brain disorders such as tumor, abscess, or hematoma, and brain death.	Noninvasive procedure that does not cause electric shock. Assist client to wash electrode paste out of hair.
Electromyography (EMG)	Needles are inserted into muscles to record electrical activity. Used to diagnose such disorders as multiple sclerosis, myasthenia gravis, and spinal cord injury or disease.	Explain that there is slight discomfort when the needles are inserted.
Evoked potentials	Either a visual or auditory stimulus evokes electrical activity related to nerve conduction along the sensory pathway. This activity is recorded with electrodes placed on the scalp and skin. Done to diagnose multiple sclerosis, acoustic neuroma, Parkinson's disease, spinal cord disease, or blindness.	Instruct client to wash hair before the exam.

TABLE 37-5

Diagnostic Tests for Visual and Auditory Systems

DIAGNOSTIC TEST	EXPLANATION AND PURPOSE	NURSING IMPLICATIONS
Fluorescein stain	Fluorescein dye is injected onto the cornea and the cornea is viewed with a slit lamp. The green staining allows identification of corneal ulceration or abrasion.	Explain that the dye may sting slightly when inserted, and the staining will wash away with tears.
Visual field testing	A semicircular bowl-like instrument that shows light in different parts of the bowl to map field of vision. Used to evaluate the progression of glaucoma.	Procedure does not cause pain but can tire the client.
Facial x-rays and CT scan	X-rays and CT scan used to identify orbital fractures or the presence of foreign bodies in the eye.	Explain procedure to client.
Ultrasonography	A probe is placed against the cornea to measure for lens implant after cataract removal and to diagnose retinal detachment.	Explain to client that cornea is anesthetized before the procedure is done.
Audiometry	Client wears earphones through which sounds are presented to determine the hearing range. Used to diagnose conductive hearing loss.	Explain that test is done by an audiologist.
X-ray and CT scan	X-rays and CT scan used to evaluate the auditory canal for diagnosing Ménière's disease.	Explain procedure to client.
Electronystagmography	In electronystagmography, cold or warm water is injected into the semicircular canals. Client observed for nystagmus, nausea, vomiting, falling, or vertigo, indicating labyrinth disease.	Ensure client safety by observing for vomiting and assisting as necessary to prevent aspiration.

such as ALT, AST, and serum ammonia are elevated in liver failure, which also affect LOC. Blood and urine toxicology screenings are useful in identifying drug or alcohol toxicity.

Normal CSF is clear, colorless, contains no RBCs, a few WBCs, very little protein, and glucose of 50 to 70 mg/dL. A lumbar puncture is done to obtain cerebrospinal fluid, which is sent for a culture and sensitivity and Gram stain, in order to identify intracranial infections. The nursing care before and after a lumbar puncture as well as client teaching is summarized in Chapter 38 (see Box 38-3). 🔗

Imaging Techniques

Imaging techniques used to identify neurologic function may be invasive and noninvasive. Table 37-3 ■ summarizes these diagnostic procedures and their nursing implications.

Electrographic Studies

Electrographic studies are used to evaluate electrical activity of the brain, nerve and skeletal muscles, and sensory pathways. These diagnostic procedures with their nursing implications are presented in Table 37-4 ■.

Diagnostic Tests for Visual and Auditory Systems

Specific studies are used for evaluating the visual and auditory systems. These tests and appropriate nursing implications are summarized in Table 37-5 ■.

Note: The bibliography listings for this and all chapters have been compiled at the back of the book.

Chapter Review

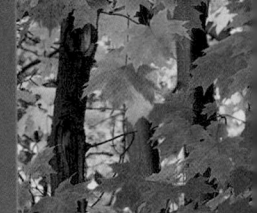

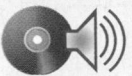 **KEY TERMS** by Topics

Use the audio glossary feature of either the CD-ROM or the Companion Website to hear the correct pronunciation of the following key terms.

Structure and function of the nervous system

neuron, myelin sheath, synapse, neurotransmitter, meninges, fissures, dermatome, reflex, reflex arc

The eye
refraction

The ear
cerumen, tympanic membrane

Assessment
Cheyne–Stokes, ptosis, nystagmus, dysphagia, flaccidity, spasticity, presbyopia

KEY Points

- The brain and spinal cord comprise the central nervous system (CNS). The peripheral nervous system (PNS) includes the cranial and spinal nerves along with the autonomic nervous system (ANS).

- The ANS consists of two divisions: sympathetic and parasympathetic. Both regulate visceral functions such as respiration, heart rate, digestion, urinary excretion, body temperature, and sexual function.

- The eyes and ears provide the major proportion of the body's sensory functions. Without vision or hearing, significant changes in lifestyle occur.

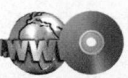 **EXPLORE MediaLink**

Additional interactive resources for this chapter can be found on the Companion Website at www.prenhall.com/burke. Click on Chapter 37 and "Begin" to select the activities for this chapter.

For chapter-related NCLEX-style review questions and an audio glossary, access the accompanying CD-ROM in this book.

FOR FURTHER Study

For more information about assessment techniques, see Chapter 5.

The nursing care and client teaching for a lumbar puncture are summarized in Box 38-3.

The Rinne and Weber hearing tests are explained in Box 40-9.

Chapter 47 provides further information about assessing psychologic status.

NCLEX-PN® Exam Preparation

1 Which of the following visual changes should the nurse expect the older adult client to report?

A. increased tear secretion
B. reduced ability to differentiate blue and green colors
C. reduced vision during daylight hours
D. difficulty focusing on objects in the distance

2 Following electroencephalography (EEG), what nursing action should the nurse implement?

A. Monitor for signs of bleeding at insertion site.
B. Encourage client to increase fluid intake.
C. Monitor for nausea and vomiting.
D. Assist client to shampoo hair.

3 Stimulation of the sympathetic nervous system would cause which of these actions? Select all that apply.

A. decreased peristalsis
B. slower heart rate
C. dilation of skin blood vessels
D. increased blood glucose levels
E. dilation of the pupils
F. constriction of the bronchi

4 When the client has difficulty maintaining balance, what cranial nerve is involved?

A. cranial nerve III
B. cranial nerve V
C. cranial nerve VIII
D. cranial nerve XI

5 A client arrives in the emergency department after a bicycle accident. Which of the following assessment questions is most important for the nurse to ask?

A. "Were you wearing a helmet?"
B. "Have you had difficulty sleeping at night?"
C. "Do you have a family history of diabetes?"
D. "Do you take any herbal preparations?"

Answers for Review Questions appear in Appendix V.

Chapter 38

Caring for Clients with Intracranial Disorders

BRIEF Outline

Head Injuries
Altered Level of Consciousness
Brain Tumor
Cerebrovascular Accident
Cerebral Aneurysm
Seizure Disorder
Intracranial Infections
Headaches

LEARNING Outcomes

After completing this chapter, you will be able to:

- Identify common manifestations and neurologic effects of head injuries, increased intracranial pressure, tumors, cerebrovascular accident, seizures, brain infections, and headaches.
- Identify laboratory and diagnostic tests used to diagnose intracranial disorders.
- Describe the interdisciplinary care required for managing clients with increased intracranial pressure.
- Discuss the nursing implications for medications ordered for clients with intracranial disorders.
- Identify the preoperative and postoperative care for clients undergoing a craniotomy.
- Use the nursing process to collect data, establish outcomes, provide individualized care, and evaluate nursing responses for the client with an intracranial disorder.

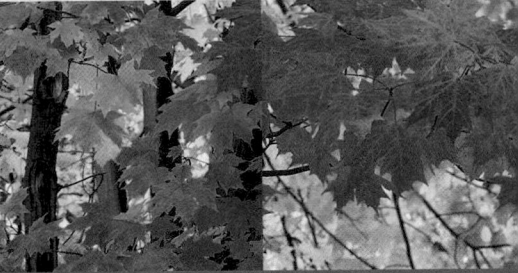

MediaLink

www.prenhall.com/burke
Use the address above to access the free, interactive Companion Website created for this textbook. Get hints, instant feedback, and textbook references to chapter-related NCLEX-style questions. Link to other interesting sites.

Audio Glossary:
Use the Companion Website, or the CD-ROM disk enclosed with your textbook, to hear the pronunciation of key terms in this chapter.

Intracranial disorders can be acute and life threatening or occur over a long period of time. These disorders often result in long-term problems that affect the client's and family's quality of life.

This chapter presents common head injuries followed by a discussion on increased intracranial pressure and altered level of consciousness. Additional topics include brain tumors, cerebrovascular accidents, aneurysms, seizures, brain infections, and headaches. Basic nursing care for the client having neurosurgery is described.

Head Injuries

Head injuries can cause minor damage such as that seen in scalp lacerations or cause major damage to the skull or brain. The most serious form of head injury is traumatic brain injury. Traumatic brain injury (TBI) is a leading cause of death and disability in the United States. Males ages 15 to 24, children ages 5 and younger, and elderly clients (75 years or older) are at an increased risk for TBI injuries. The Centers for Disease Control and Prevention (CDC) estimates that at least 1.4 million people in the United States sustain head injuries each year. Of these, 235,000 are hospitalized and 50,000 die. Motor vehicle accidents (MVAs) are a major cause of head injuries, followed by falls, violent assaults, and sports injuries. Elevated blood alcohol levels often increase the risk of an MVA.

PATHOPHYSIOLOGY AND MANIFESTATIONS

Head injuries include scalp lacerations, skull fractures, concussion, contusion, and hematomas. Scalp lacerations are classified as a minor head injury and often look worse than they are because they bleed profusely. A *skull fracture* is a break in the skull. It is usually caused by extreme force and can possibly result in brain damage. Skull fractures are either open (from a tear in the dura) or closed. There are four types of skull fractures:

1. *Linear*—a simple, clean break in the skull.
2. *Comminuted*—the skull is crushed into small, fragmented pieces.
3. *Depressed*—bone fragments may be pushed into the brain; usually caused by a powerful blow to the skull.
4. *Basilar*—occurs at the base of the skull and may extend to the paranasal sinus of the frontal bone or the middle ear found in the temporal bone. This can cause blood or cerebrospinal fluid (CSF) to leak from the nose (**rhinorrhea**) or the ears (**otorrhea**). Other manifestations include *Battle's sign* (bruising over the mastoid process) and *periorbital ecchymosis,* sometimes called "raccoon eyes." If CSF leakage is present, the risk of infection is high.

In any head injury, it is important to determine whether the brain has sustained damage. Brain damage may result

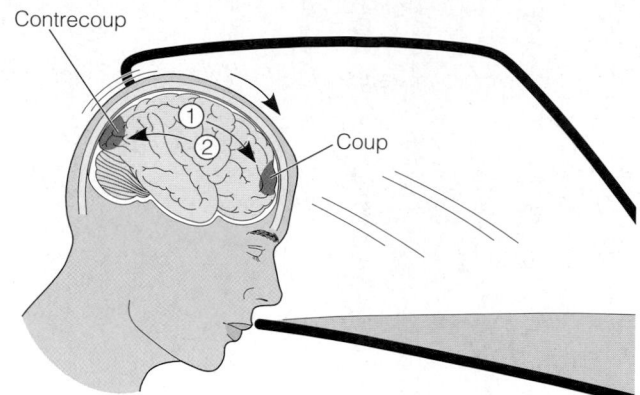

Figure 38-1. ■ Coup–contrecoup head injury. Following the initial injury (coup), the brain rebounds within the skull and sustains additional injury (contrecoup) in the opposite part of the brain.

from open or closed head injuries. O*pen head injuries* occur in two ways. Severe blunt trauma can create an opening through the scalp, skull, and dura to expose the brain as seen in a depressed skull fracture. An object such as a bullet or knife can penetrate the skull and damage the brain. Clients with open injuries have a higher risk for meningitis.

Closed head injuries usually result from an acceleration–deceleration injury, also called the coup–contrecoup phenomenon (Figure 38-1 ■). For instance, when the head hits an object (e.g., dashboard), the brain bounces forward (acceleration) and then rapidly rebounds and hits the back of the skull (deceleration). Thus, the brain sustains bruising at two points, resulting in extensive brain damage. **Concussion** or **contusion** are other types of closed head injuries. The amount of damage from a head injury relates to how the injury occurred, the type of injury, and its location. Brain damage develops from either direct trauma to the tissue or increased **intracranial pressure (ICP)** and cerebral edema. Table 38-1 ■ lists common brain injuries.

Intracranial hemorrhage is defined as bleeding within the skull and is the most serious type of brain injury. Intracranial hemorrhage may result from the tearing of cerebral arteries or veins or from direct trauma. This bleeding leads to formation of a **hematoma** (an accumulation of blood). Blood accumulates in the epidural, subdural, or subarachnoid spaces, or within the cerebral lobes. Pressure on surrounding tissues leads to increased intracranial pressure. If the pressure is unrelieved, neurologic changes occur. Hematomas are classified by their location: epidural, subdural, or intracerebral (Figure 38-2 ■ and Table 38-1).

COMPLICATIONS

Increased Intracranial Pressure

The cranium has three compartments: (1) the brain (80%), (2) blood (10%), and (3) cerebrospinal fluid (10%). Intracranial pressure is the pressure exerted within the cranium by

TABLE 38-1

Common Brain Injuries with Pathophysiology and Manifestations

BRAIN INJURY	PATHOPHYSIOLOGY	MANIFESTATIONS
Concussion	Brain injury is caused by violent shaking of the brain.	Immediate loss of consciousness for <5 minutes. Drowsiness, confusion, dizziness. Headache, blurred or double vision.
Contusion	Bruising of the brain tissue caused by blunt trauma. More severe than a concussion because brain swelling occurs.	Varies with the size and location of the injury. Initial loss of consciousness; if LOC remains altered, the client may become combative. During unconsciousness, lies motionless; has pale, clammy skin; faint pulse; hypotension; shallow respirations; and altered motor responses.
Epidural hematoma	Severe blow to brain causes arterial bleeding that collects between the skull and dura mater. May be caused by skull fractures or contusion.	Brief loss of consciousness followed by a short period of alertness. Then the client rapidly progresses into a coma with decorticate or decerebrate posturing, *ipsilateral* (same-side) pupil dilation, and seizures.
Subdural hematoma	Closed head injury causes venous blood to collect between dura mater and the subarachnoid layer.	There are three types of subdural hematomas: *Acute:* Rapid deterioration from drowsiness and confusion to coma, ipsilateral pupil dilation and contralateral hemiparesis.
	Subacute occurs from less severe head injury.	*Subacute:* Manifestations appear 48 hours to 2 weeks later; alert period followed by slow progression to coma.
	Chronic occurs most often in elderly, alcoholics, and those on long-term anticoagulant therapy.	*Chronic:* Manifestations develop weeks to months after initial injury. Slowed thinking, confusion, drowsiness; may progress to pupil changes and motor deficits.
Intracerebral hematoma	Bleeding into the brain tissue; may be caused by gunshot wound or a depressed skull fracture.	Decreasing level of consciousness; pupil changes and motor deficits.

these contents. This pressure normally ranges from 5 to 15 mm Hg. If the volume of one component increases, the volume of the other components must decrease to keep the pressure within its normal range. When this does not occur, increased intracranial pressure (IICP) develops. Normal

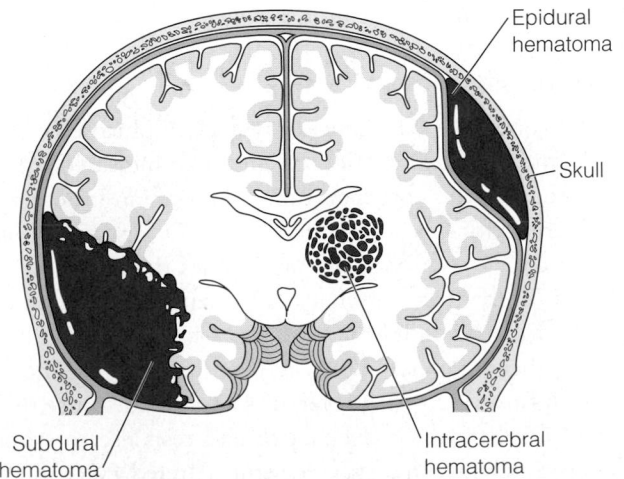

Figure 38-2. ■ Three types of hematomas: epidural, subdural, and intracerebral.

activities such as coughing, sneezing, straining, or bending forward can briefly increase ICP. Brief pressure increases are not harmful; however, prolonged increases can damage delicate brain tissue. IICP can develop with a head injury, brain surgery, or meningitis.

Cerebral blood flow is vital to deliver the required oxygen and glucose. For the brain to function properly, an adequate blood supply must travel to the brain. When ICP increases, cerebral vasoconstriction occurs, which reduces cerebral blood flow and causes ischemia. If ischemia lasts longer than 5 minutes, the result is irreversible brain damage. Cerebral blood flow is also affected by the amount of carbon dioxide and oxygen in the blood. Increased carbon dioxide levels ($PaCO_2$) and/or decreased oxygen levels (PaO_2) cause vasodilation of the cerebral arteries. Either one of these conditions will increase intracranial pressure.

Any increase in ICP causes changes in the client's level of consciousness (LOC), pupil response, speech, motor function, and vital signs. The changes become more dramatic as ICP increases. Manifestations may be labeled as early or late (Box 38-1 ■) and develop slowly or rapidly. Not all manifestations occur in all clients. The location and cause of IICP will determine the symptoms. Because the

BOX 38-1

MANIFESTATIONS OF INCREASED INTRACRANIAL PRESSURE

	Early	Late
Level of consciousness	Irritability; personality changes; restlessness; short-term memory changes; disorientation to time, then to place and person; confusion	Decreasing LOC that progresses to coma. No response to painful stimuli.
Pupils	Pupils equal, round, and reactive to light	Sluggish response to light progressing to fixed (no response to light). First, pupils may be dilated on one side (ipsilateral), then progress to bilateral dilation.
Vision	Decreased visual acuity, blurred vision, diplopia	Cannot assess due to decreasing LOC or coma.
Motor function	Weakness in one extremity or side; hemiplegia on the opposite side of the brain injury	Decorticate or decerebrate positioning.
Speech	Difficulty speaking	Cannot assess due to decreasing LOC or coma.
Blood pressure	Elevated blood pressure	*Cushing's triad:* increased systolic blood pressure, widening pulse pressure, bradycardia.
Pulse	Slightly elevated pulse	
Respiration	Rate may increase	Decreased respiratory rate with altered respiratory patterns (e.g., Cheyne–Stokes).
Temperature	May be increased or decreased	Significantly elevated.
Other symptoms	Headache worse on rising in the morning and with position changes	Continual headache. Projectile vomiting. Loss of pupil, corneal, gag, and swallowing reflexes.

symptoms may be subtle, the nurse must closely observe the client for any changes. Two later symptoms, decorticate and decerebrate posturing, indicate increasing ICP in the client and must be treated immediately. Cushing's triad occurs late in the development of IICP. This is an ominous sign of impending death.

clinical ALERT

The earliest sign of increasing ICP is a change in the level of consciousness.

Cerebral Edema

Cerebral edema, an abnormal accumulation of fluid, increases the amount of extracellular or intracellular brain tissue volume. As the brain swells within the rigid skull, intracranial pressure increases. Brain injury, intracranial surgery, tumors, hemorrhage, and infections can cause cerebral edema. Edema rises to its highest level within 48 to 72 hours after an insult to the brain, then gradually subsides. Without early recognition and treatment, the client's condition can deteriorate rapidly.

Head injuries severe enough to cause IICP can lead to altered LOC, brain herniation, and brain death. The following information shows how these additional complications affect the client.

ALTERED LEVEL OF CONSCIOUSNESS. *Consciousness* means that the client is oriented to time, place, and person, and responds appropriately to external stimuli. To maintain normal consciousness, the brain must receive its constant supply of oxygen and glucose. It also requires an intact reticular activating system (RAS), located in the brainstem. The RAS keeps a person alert and responsive to the environment.

Many neurologic conditions can affect the client's level of consciousness. Usually LOC is altered by IICP and cerebral edema because the increased pressure in the cranium reduces the blood supply to the brain. The following disorders will likely increase ICP and affect the person's ability to remain alert and oriented:

- Head injury
- Hematoma
- Cerebrovascular accident or stroke
- Tumors
- Infections.

Any condition that reduces oxygen and glucose levels in the brain may decrease LOC. Clients at an increased risk include those with poorly controlled diabetes and those with long-term cardiac or respiratory disease. Drugs such as alcohol, narcotics, sedatives, and anesthetics depress the CNS, which in turn alters consciousness. Seizures and toxins produced by liver or kidney failure may also alter LOC.

The client's altered LOC may be described using the terms in Box 38-2 ■. However, it is best for the nurse to describe the client's actual behavior and response to stimuli instead of relying on a specific term. Altered LOC and behavior are early changes associated with IICP (see Box 38-1). As brain function deteriorates, more stimuli are needed to

BOX 38-2

ALTERED LEVELS OF CONSCIOUSNESS

Full Consciousness: alert; oriented to time, place, and person; fully understands written and spoken words

Confusion: disoriented to time, place, and person; unable to think clearly; short attention span; poor memory

Delirium: motor restlessness; agitated and irritable; may have hallucinations; may be combative

Obtundation: appears drowsy and lethargic; responds to verbal and tactile stimuli but quickly drifts back to sleep

Stupor: generally unresponsive; may withdraw purposefully with vigorous or painful stimuli

Coma: does not respond to stimuli

elicit a response from the client. Eventually, no response is obtained.

The Glasgow Coma Scale (Table 38-2 ■) provides a quick guide for assessing LOC. It measures how well the client responds with eye opening and verbal and motor responses. The lower the score, the worse the client's condition. To prevent permanent brain damage, the nurse must act quickly. The physician must be notified and measures started to lower IICP.

BRAIN HERNIATION. Brain herniation occurs late in the course of IICP. In an attempt to save brain tissue, the brain shifts from an area of high pressure to low pressure. One common site of herniation is the foramen magnum (the hole at the base of the brain where the spinal cord exits). As pressure rises, the brain is pushed through the foramen magnum. This compresses the brainstem so that vital functions such as respiration cease. Without prompt recognition, the client eventually dies.

BRAIN DEATH. Brain death occurs when cerebral blood flow stops, resulting in irreversible loss of brain function. (The criteria for determining brain death can be found in Chapter 13, Box 13-11. ○○) If organ donation is planned, the appropriate agencies are contacted.

INTERDISCIPLINARY CARE

It is most important to identify and prevent IICP in any client with a neurologic problem. Medications are given immediately to lower ICP. Clients with severe brain injuries need their ICP monitored. Uncontrolled intracranial bleeding requires immediate surgery.

Diagnostic Tests

The type and extent of neurologic deficits are often discovered during the history and physical examination. The following laboratory tests are ordered to determine the cause of the client's altered LOC:

- *Blood glucose* is measured when hypoglycemia is suspected.
- *Arterial blood gases* monitor pH and levels of oxygen and carbon dioxide. They can identify hypoxia and increased carbon dioxide levels. See Chapter 7 ○○ for more information about arterial blood gases.
- *Toxicology screening* of blood and urine is done to identify alcohol or drug toxicity.
- *Serum creatinine and BUN* are measured when renal failure is suspected (see Chapter 31 for normal levels). ○○
- *Liver function tests* (alanine transaminase [ALT], aspartate transaminase [AST]) can evaluate liver function (Chapter 18). ○○
- *Complete blood count with differential* is used to assess for anemia or infectious disease.

The following diagnostic tests are ordered to determine the cause of IICP:

- *Computed tomography (CT) scan* or *magnetic resonance imaging (MRI)* detects hemorrhage, edema, hematoma, or tumor.
- *Cerebral angiography* provides x-ray views of cerebral blood flow and is used when a stroke is suspected.
- *Lumbar puncture* provides a sample of CSF to analyze for possible meningitis. It is performed only when there is danger of IICP. Removal of CSF during IICP greatly increases the risk of brain herniation. Nursing interventions for the client having a lumbar puncture are described in Box 38-3 ■.

TABLE 38-2

Glasgow Coma Scale

BEHAVIOR	RESPONSE	SCORE
Eye opening response	Spontaneously	4
	To speech	3
	To pain	2
	No response	1
Best verbal response	Oriented to time, place, and person	5
	Confused	4
	Inappropriate words	3
	Incomprehensible sounds	2
	No response	1
Best motor response	Obeys commands	6
	Moves to localized pain	5
	Flexion withdrawal from pain	4
	Abnormal flexion (decorticate)	3
	Abnormal extension (decerebrate)	2
	No response	1
Total score:	*Best response*	15
	Comatose client	8 or less
	Totally unresponsive	3

BOX 38-3	NURSING CARE CHECKLIST

Lumbar Puncture

Before the Procedure

☑ Obtain a signed consent form.

☑ Obtain lumbar puncture tray and additional equipment requested by the physician.

☑ Have client empty the bowel and bladder before the procedure begins.

☑ Position the client in a lateral recumbent position on the side of the bed with the back toward the physician (see figure).

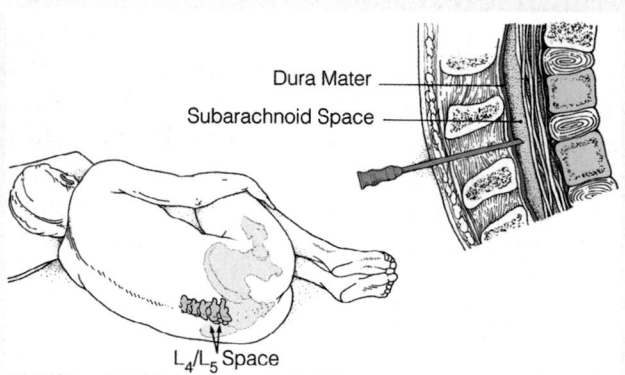

Dura Mater

Subarachnoid Space

L₄/L₅ Space

☑ Assist client to take slow, deep breaths and maintain position during the procedure.

After the Procedure

☑ Monitor vital signs and neurologic signs following facility policy.

☑ Monitor the puncture site for leakage of cerebrospinal fluid or hematoma formation.

☑ Encourage fluid intake to replace fluids lost (up to 3,000 mL in 24 hours) if cardiac disease not present.

☑ Give analgesics as prescribed for pain.

Client and Family Teaching

☑ Reinforce and clarify information about the procedure.

☑ Explain the importance of not moving during the procedure.

☑ A Band-Aid will cover the place where the needle was inserted.

☑ After the procedure, remain flat in bed for 4 to 24 hours as ordered by the physician.

☑ If you have a headache or backache, ask for medications for pain.

Medications

Medications play an important role in managing clients with IICP. The most frequently ordered drugs include (1) osmotic diuretics, (2) loop diuretics, (3) corticosteroids, (4) anticonvulsants, (5) antipyretics, and (6) histamine antagonists.

Intravenous *fluids* are used to maintain the client's fluid and electrolyte balance and to prevent hypotension. Only 0.9% normal saline and lactated Ringer's solution are given because they do not cross the blood–brain barrier and increase cerebral edema. They are infused at low rates such as 50 to 75 mL/hr. All IV solutions should be given using an intravenous pump to prevent volume overload.

Osmotic diuretics (e.g., mannitol [Osmitrol]) draw water out of the edematous brain tissue to be excreted by the kidneys. Large or frequent doses of mannitol cause dehydration and electrolyte losses. Loop diuretics decrease cerebral edema but cause less fluid and electrolyte losses.

clinical ALERT

Closely monitor the client who is receiving diuretics for dehydration and electrolyte losses especially sodium and potassium.

Dexamethasone (Decadron), a *corticosteroid,* reduces inflammation, which in turn decreases cerebral edema but causes GI irritation and possibly gastric ulcers. A histamine H_2-receptor antagonist like ranitidine (Zantac), a proton pump inhibitor such as pantoprazole (Protonix), or antacids are given to prevent gastric irritation. Antiemetics are used to prevent vomiting and the risk for aspiration.

Anticonvulsants may treat or prevent seizure activity associated with a head injury. One of three anticonvulsants may be ordered: (1) phenytoin (Dilantin), (2) diazepam (Valium), or (3) phenobarbital. Acetaminophen, an antipyretic, is used alone or in combination with a hypothermia blanket to treat hyperthermia. Hyperthermia raises cerebral metabolism and increases ICP.

Clients with severe TBI and continually elevated ICP may be given *barbiturates.* Barbiturate therapy places the client in a coma, reducing metabolism of the injured brain. Lowering metabolism allows the brain time to heal without permanent damage. During this therapy, the client is closely monitored in the critical care unit.

ICP Monitoring

An ICP monitoring device is inserted into the skull to assess for IICP. This device is used only for clients in the critical care unit. Intracranial pressures are constantly monitored so that immediate treatment can be started before brain

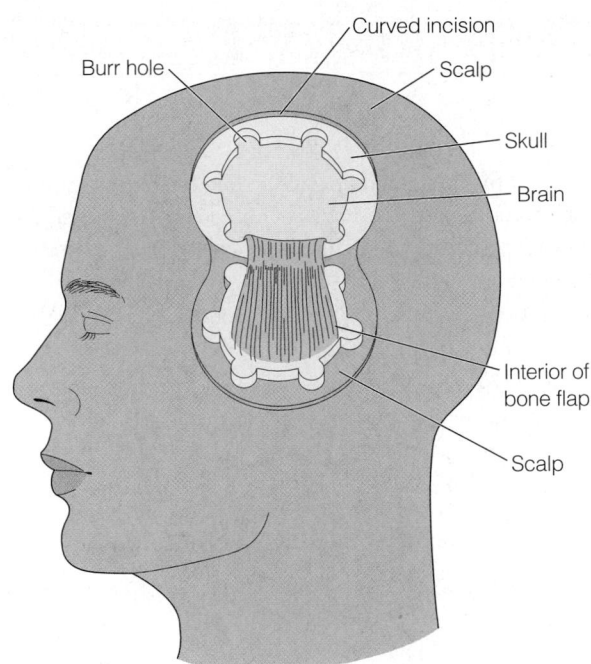

Figure 38-3. ■ Burr holes are made in the skull to create a bone flap or to remove a blood clot or evaluate a hematoma.

damage occurs. Because bacteria could enter the brain via the monitoring device, the client is assessed for symptoms of meningitis.

Surgery

Different cranial surgical procedures are done to reduce the client's ICP. A bone flap may be removed from the skull to allow room for the brain to expand (Figure 38-3 ■). *Burr holes* are holes drilled into the skull to remove a blood clot or evacuate a hematoma. A craniotomy can relieve the pressure of a brain tumor. Care of the client following a craniotomy is presented under the section on brain tumor.

NURSING CARE

ASSESSING

Clients with IICP need frequent nursing assessments. The nurse observes and reports immediately to the physician any sudden change in neurologic function. Subjective and objective findings help to identify the type of nursing interventions the client will need (Box 38-4 ■).

DIAGNOSING, PLANNING, AND IMPLEMENTING

Priorities in Nursing Care. The client with a head injury has multiple nursing needs. Besides preventing IICP, it is important to avoid its potential complications. If the client is

unconscious, care is directed at maintaining the airway, nutrition, and skin integrity, as well as preventing problems that can arise due to immobility and the risk of infection. Unconscious clients are usually cared for in the critical care unit. Persons with mild neurologic deficits may be treated in the emergency department, then monitored at home.

Ineffective Tissue Perfusion: Cerebral

- Elevate the head of the bed 30 degrees and keep the head in a midline position. *These measures promote venous drainage from the head so that pressure does not build up.*
- Give oxygen as ordered. Use pulse oximetry to measure oxygen levels. Keep PaO_2 levels above 94% and $PaCO_2$ levels between 35 and 45. *The brain needs a constant supply of oxygen to prevent brain damage. Increased carbon dioxide levels can cause cerebral vasodilation, leading to cerebral edema.*
- Avoid hip flexion and abdominal distention. Give stool softeners as ordered. Monitor patency of nasogastric tube. *Hip flexion, gastric distention, and constipation can increase ICP. Stool softeners and a nasogastric tube may prevent IICP.*

> **clinical ALERT**
>
> Avoid Valsalva maneuver (e.g., coughing, straining during bowel movements) to prevent IICP.

- Monitor temperature every 2 hours for hyperthermia. If possible, avoid taking rectal temperatures. *Temperature is monitored to prevent brain damage from an increased metabolic rate. Taking a rectal temperature can increase ICP.*
- Keep the client quiet; reduce noise and lights in the room; and space nursing activities over the shift. Speak softly and calmly. *Loud noises and bright lights plus constant nursing care activities can increase ICP.*
- Turn client slowly and gently with a turn sheet. *Sudden movement can increase ICP.*
- Limit fluid over a 24-hour period. *Fluid restrictions may prevent and decrease cerebral edema.*

> **clinical ALERT**
>
> Monitor urine output every 1 to 2 hours for signs of diabetes insipidus or syndrome of inappropriate antidiuretic hormone (SIADH).

- If client is combative, avoid using restraints. Have nursing staff or family sit quietly with the client. *Restraining the client increases ICP. Family may provide a soothing atmosphere.*
- Monitor for seizure activity and maintain seizure precautions:
  - Keep oral airway and suction equipment at bedside.

| BOX 38-4 | ASSESSMENT |

Assessing Clients with Increased Intracranial Pressure

SUBJECTIVE DATA

- When did change in LOC or memory occur first; onset slow or rapid?
- Presence of headache, nausea, or vomiting.
- Visual changes such as double vision or blurring.
- Ringing in the ears; dizziness or feeling faint.
- Any numbness or tingling in extremities.
- History of trauma, infection, cranial surgery, seizures, or loss of consciousness.
- Medication and alcohol use.

OBJECTIVE DATA

- Blood pressure, pulse, respirations, temperature.
- Observe for memory lapses or altered thought processes.
- Assess LOC and orientation to time, place, and person. If client is unconscious or his or her condition is unstable, use the Glasgow Coma Scale (Table 38-2).
- Check pupil response to light.
- Assess strength of hand grip and movement of extremities.
- Note nausea or vomiting.
- Note color and amount of drainage from ears and nose. Assess for halo sign: Collect fluid on gauze, noting presence of a yellowish ring which indicates CSF.
- Note presence of raccoon eyes or Battle's sign.

ADDITIONAL DATA FOR UNCONSCIOUS CLIENTS

- Note any change in breathing pattern.

- Assess for the Babinski reflex by stroking the bottom of the foot. An abnormal or positive response in adults is when the big toe flexes upward and the other toes fan out. This indicates upper motor neuron disease.
- Assess corneal reflex by touching the corneal surface with a wisp of cotton. Normally, the client blinks.
- Assess the gag reflex by touching the back of the client's throat gently with a tongue blade. Normally, the client will show a gag reflex.
- Assess for abnormal posturing (decorticate or decerebrate posturing).

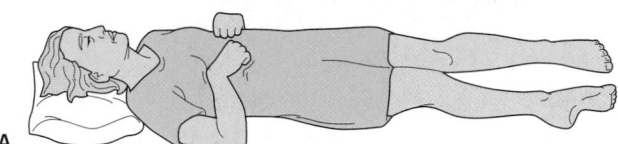

A

Decorticate Posturing

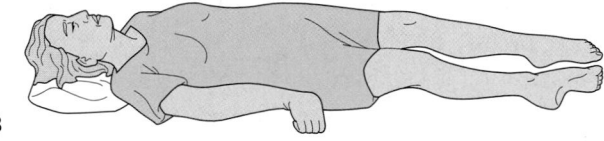

B

Decerebrate Posturing

- Monitor and report diagnostic test results beyond expected range.

- Pad side rails with blankets or seizure pads.
- Keep bed in low position with side rails up.

Clients with neurologic injuries are prone to developing seizures and are at risk for injury.

Ineffective Breathing Pattern

- Monitor respiratory rate, depth, and rhythm for changes. *As ICP increases, the risk of respiratory distress rises. IICP is known to cause respiratory arrest. Unconscious clients may lose their cough reflex. Head injuries will decrease respiratory function.*
- Assess the client's ability to clear secretions. If unconscious or the client has a poor cough, suction the airway for less than 10 seconds. *Suctioning longer reduces oxygen levels and increases carbon dioxide levels, which can increase ICP.*

clinical ALERT

Never suction nasally the client with a basilar skull fracture who is draining CSF from the nose or ears.

- Insert an oral airway as needed. *This prevents the tongue from obstructing the airway.*
- Turn the client from side to side every 2 hours; keep in a side-lying position with head of bed elevated. *Turning prevents pooling of secretions in one area of the lungs. Side positioning prevents the tongue from obstructing the airway.*
- If client is unconscious, keep NPO and provide oral hygiene. *Oral hygiene removes secretions that could dry and be aspirated.*

clinical ALERT

Never give oral food or fluids to the unconscious client to prevent aspiration.

Risk for Imbalanced Nutrition: Less than Body Requirements

- Give tube feeding through a nasogastric or gastrostomy tube or administer total parenteral nutrition (TPN) as ordered. *Head injuries increase the client's metabolic rate and risk for malnutrition. Tube feedings or TPN are ordered to prevent malnutrition.*

■ Before each tube feeding, check gastric residual. *Excess gastric residual means that the tube feeding is not being absorbed. This places the client at risk for malnutrition and aspiration.*

■ Monitor daily weights. *Daily weights help determine the client's nutritional and fluid status.*

Risk for Impaired Skin Integrity

■ Turn the client every 2 hours. Use a special mattress or bed as available. Lift rather than drag the client across the sheet. *Turning relieves pressure over bony prominences. Special mattresses (e.g., egg crate cushion or beds) distribute the client's weight more evenly. Dragging can cause skin tears.*

■ Prevent skin breakdown by:
  ■ Keeping bed linens clean, dry, and wrinkle free
  ■ Bathing the client daily with mild soap
  ■ Cleansing the skin following urine and fecal soiling with a mild cleansing agent
  ■ Providing adequate hydration.

Keeping linens clean, dry, and wrinkle free decreases the risk of skin injuries. Daily hygiene keeps the skin soft and supple. Adequate hydration prevents the skin from drying out and cracking.

■ Provide oral care and lubricate the lips every 2 to 4 hours. *This removes dried crusts and prevents drying and cracking of oral mucous membranes.*

■ Keep the cornea moist by instilling methyl cellulose solution (0.5% to 1%). Apply protective eye shields if the corneal reflex is absent. *Proper eye care prevents corneal abrasion and irritation.*

Impaired Physical Mobility

■ Maintain extremities in position of function with support devices. Remove support devices every 4 hours for skin care. Place a pillow in the axilla area; use hand splints; use foam boots or high-top tennis shoes on the feet. *Pillows in the axilla area prevent abduction of the shoulder. Hand splints may prevent flexion contractures of the hands. Foam boots or high-top tennis shoes are used to prevent footdrop.*

■ Perform passive range-of-motion (ROM) exercises at least four times per day. *Passive ROM exercises done routinely maintain muscle tone and function, prevent contractures, and restore impaired motor function in unconscious clients.*

clinical ALERT

Do not perform passive ROM on the client with IICP.

Risk for Infection

■ Assess for a CSF leak and monitor for signs of infection. *Open head wounds such as a depressed skull fracture increase the risk for infection. They can be contaminated with dirt, hair, or other debris.*

■ Test clear drainage from ear and nose for glucose by using a glucose reagent strip. *Clear drainage that tests positive for glucose indicates the presence of CSF.*

■ Keep the nasopharynx and external ear clean. Place a sterile piece of cotton in the ear and loosely tape a 4 × 4 gauze under the nose to collect any drainage. Change the dressings when they become wet. *Bacteria can enter through these openings when wet dressings are present.*

■ Remind client not to blow the nose, cough, or stop a sneeze. *Blowing the nose or coughing increases ICP. Stopping a sneeze can force bacteria up into the brain.*

■ Use strict aseptic technique when changing head dressings or handling the ICP monitoring device. *Aseptic technique decreases the risk of introducing bacteria.*

EVALUATING

To evaluate the effectiveness of nursing care for a client with IICP, collect and record data such as level of alertness and orientation; strong hand grip, extremity movement, and steady gait; and absence of diplopia, tinnitus, dizziness, nausea, vomiting, or abnormal pupil response.

Documenting. Documentation also includes client and family teaching about home care such as skin care, ROM exercises, medication administration and side effects, and symptoms to report.

CONTINUING CARE

The nurse assesses clients to determine whether they can manage their care at home or if they need to be transferred to a long-term care facility. Clients with a mild head injury should be observed for at least 24 hours. If they are not hospitalized, they must be closely monitored at home. For example, with a linear skull fracture, the family is taught to wake and observe the client every 2 hours during the first 8 hours after the accident. The client and family should return to the emergency department if the client develops any of the following manifestations:

■ Increasing drowsiness, confusion, or slurred speech
■ Difficulty waking the client
■ Vomiting
■ Blurred vision; one or both pupils dilated
■ Prolonged headache
■ Blood or clear fluid leaking from the nose or ears
■ Weakness in arm or leg
■ Seizures.

Clients and their families should receive a copy of the home care instructions that were reviewed in the emergency department. The nurse must document all teaching done for observation after a head injury.

Clients with a concussion may develop postconcussion syndrome. They may experience headache, poor concentration, dizziness, personality changes, and fatigue for weeks to months. Family support is important during this phase of recovery.

Clients with severe head injuries usually require extensive rehabilitation either as inpatients or outpatients. Rehabilitation may include physical, speech, and occupational therapy. The client and family need teaching about medications, exercises and positioning, skin care, diet, use of assistive devices, and potential complications. Families providing long-term home care may need respite care.

Unconscious clients need placement in a long-term care facility. A social services department can help the family find a suitable facility and also assist with financial concerns. Because the prognosis of the client is uncertain, the family may need support services from counselors and the clergy.

NURSING PROCESS CARE PLAN
Client with Increased Intracranial Pressure and Altered Level of Consciousness

---

Martin Straton, 52 years old, fell during his daily run in the park. He hit his head on the right side and was knocked unconscious. A bystander called an ambulance, which arrived in 10 minutes to transport him to the local hospital.

Assessment. BP 150/90, P 60, R 14. He responds to verbal and tactile stimuli but quickly falls back asleep. His right pupil is dilated and does not react to light. He is unable to move his extremities on the left side. Oxygen is given by a face mask. CT scan shows an epidural hematoma on the right side with edema. The neurologist discusses the need for immediate surgery with Mr. Straton's wife. He was taken to surgery in the evening for burr holes to evacuate the hematoma. His surgery is successful, and he is transferred to the critical care unit.

Diagnosis. After surgery, the following diagnoses are made for Mr. Straton:

- *Risk for Ineffective Tissue Perfusion: Cerebral* related to increased intracranial pressure and edema
- *Risk for Aspiration* related to altered level of consciousness
- *Risk for Impaired Skin Integrity* related to immobility
- *Risk for Imbalanced Nutrition: Less than Body Requirements* related to inability to eat

Expected Outcomes. The expected outcomes for the plan of care are that Mr. Straton will:

- Maintain adequate cerebral tissue perfusion as evidenced by stable vital signs and neurologic status, and no decrease in LOC.
- No aspiration as evidenced by clear lung sounds.
- Maintain intact skin.
- Maintain normal body weight.

Planning and Implementation. The following interventions are planned and implemented for Mr. Straton:

- Perform neurologic and respiratory assessment with vital signs every 2 hours or as needed. Monitor pulse oximetry.
- Use measures to reduce cerebral edema such as:
  - Elevate head of bed 30 degrees; keep head in neutral alignment; avoid flexion of head and hips.
  - Provide calm environment and allow for rest periods.
- Assess ability to clear secretions; check gag reflex every shift; and suction posterior pharynx as needed.
- Turn side to side every 2 hours, and maintain side-lying position. Turn slowly with a turn sheet.
- Maintain NPO status and provide frequent oral hygiene.
- Assess skin over bony prominences every shift.
- Assess fluid status and document intake and output.

Evaluation. Twenty-four hours after surgery, Mr. Straton slowly starts to regain consciousness. His right pupil slowly reacts to light, and he moves his left extremities slightly. Mr. Straton continues to improve and is discharged to his home a week later.

Critical Thinking in the Nursing Process

1. Mr. Straton was found unconscious. What assessments would you make and how could you maintain an open airway at the scene?
2. During the immediate postoperative period, Mr. Straton becomes confused and tries to pull out his ICP monitoring device. You know you cannot restrain him. What other nursing interventions could you try?
3. Describe oral hygiene measures for clients who are unconscious.

Brain Tumor

Brain tumors are abnormal growths within the cranium. Their cause is unknown, but prolonged exposure to certain chemicals and radiation increases the incidence. Brain tumors occur at any age. The incidence is highest among young children and adults between the ages of 50 and 70.

Intracranial tumors are classified as either benign or malignant, based on tissue type and cell characteristics. The term *benign* can be misleading, because the tumor may be

TABLE 38-3

Classification of Brain Tumors

TUMOR	CHARACTERISTICS
Glioma	
■ Astrocytoma	Most common glioma
	Graded I to IV according to degree of cell differentiation
■ Glioblastoma multiforme	Highly malignant
	Fast growing and highly invasive of other tissues
Meningioma	Slow-growing tumor developing in the meninges
Acoustic neuroma	Benign, slow-growing tumor of the acoustic nerve
Metastatic brain tumor	Slow growing and malignant
	Develops from primary sites in the lung and breast

BOX 38-5

MANIFESTATIONS OF BRAIN TUMORS

Frontal Lobe Tumors
- Personality changes, inappropriate behavior, impaired judgment, inability to concentrate
- Recent memory loss
- Motor deficits
- Expressive aphasia
- Seizures

Parietal Lobe Tumors
- Sensory–perceptual deficits
- Seizures

Temporal Lobe Tumors
- Psychomotor seizures
- Receptive aphasia

Occipital Lobe Tumors
- Visual deficits
- Headache

inaccessible by surgery, and as it grows, it presses on vital centers. If the compression increases, it leads to disability and death. Malignant tumors invade other areas of the brain and eventually cause death unless effectively treated.

Brain tumors are also categorized as primary or secondary. Primary tumors develop from cells and structures within the brain. Secondary brain tumors develop in areas outside of the brain and metastasize to the brain. The most common brain tumors are listed in Table 38-3 ■.

PATHOPHYSIOLOGY AND MANIFESTATIONS

Brain tumors invade, displace, and destroy brain tissue. As the tumor grows, it disrupts the normal balance of brain tissue, blood, and CSF within the skull. When the brain fails to compensate for the increase in volume, increased intracranial pressure develops. This will lead to the typical manifestations of IICP discussed earlier in the chapter. If untreated, the final result is brain herniation and death.

Manifestations are either local or generalized. Local manifestations relate to the location and function of that specific site, for example, frontal lobe or temporal lobe (Box 38-5 ■). Knowing the tumor site helps the nurse plan the client's care. Tumors can press on cerebral blood vessels, decreasing their blood supply. This leads to complaints of dizziness. Generalized manifestations include headache that is usually worse in the morning, nausea, vomiting, changes in mental functioning, and seizures.

INTERDISCIPLINARY CARE

A brain tumor is treated with chemotherapy, radiation therapy, surgery, or any combination of these. The choice of treatment is based on the size and location of the tumor, the type of tumor, and the client's physical condition. The following tests aid in diagnosing a brain tumor:

- A *CT scan* or *MRI* is ordered to locate and define the size of the tumor.
- An *electroencephalogram (EEG)* is ordered if seizures are present.
- A *cerebral angiogram* is used to measure blood flow through the cerebral blood vessels.
- A *stereotactic needle biopsy* may be performed for some tumors.

Medications

Chemotherapy may be used to treat a brain tumor. One way to administer the chemotherapy is by an Ommaya reservoir. This device is surgically implanted into the lateral ventricle of the brain (Figure 38-4 ■). It allows the chemotherapy to be absorbed along with CSF. New timed-release chemotherapy wafers can be placed directly into the tumor cavity after the tumor is removed by surgery.

Intracranial Surgery

Surgery can remove a tumor, reduce its size (also known as **debulking**), or relieve symptoms. Some of the common intracranial surgeries are:

- *Burr Hole:* A hole is drilled into the skull to remove a clot or to relieve pressure.
- *Craniotomy:* A surgical opening is made into the cranial cavity (Figure 38-5 ■). A craniotomy is done by making a series of burr holes. The bone between the holes (bone flap)

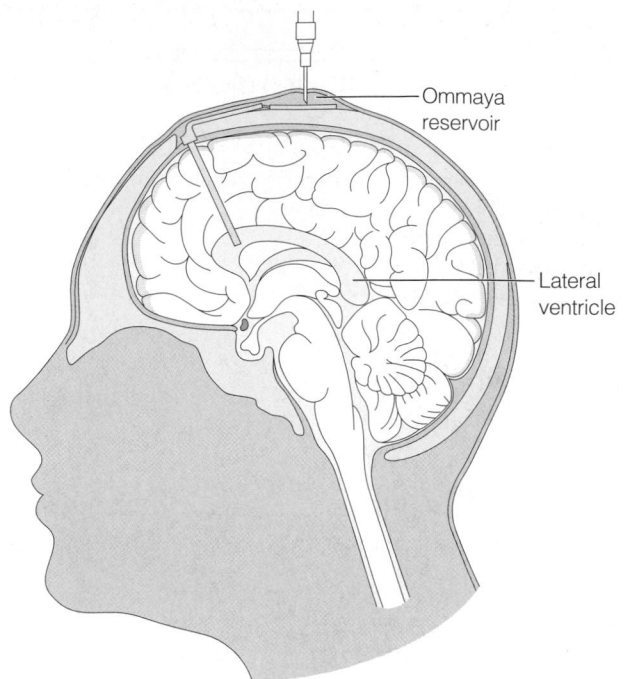

Figure 38-4. ■ Ommaya reservoir for medication administration.

is cut with a saw and then turned down. After the tumor is removed, the bone flap is sutured in place. A craniotomy is also used to repair defects following a head injury.

- *Supratentorial craniotomy* (above the tentorium) allows access to the frontal, temporal, occipital, and parietal lobes.
- *Infratentorial craniotomy* (below the tentorium) provides access to the cerebellum and brain stem.
- *Craniectomy:* Complete removal of a bone flap decreases cerebral edema.
- *Cranioplasty:* Synthetic material, a metal plate, or wire mesh is inserted where the skull was removed.

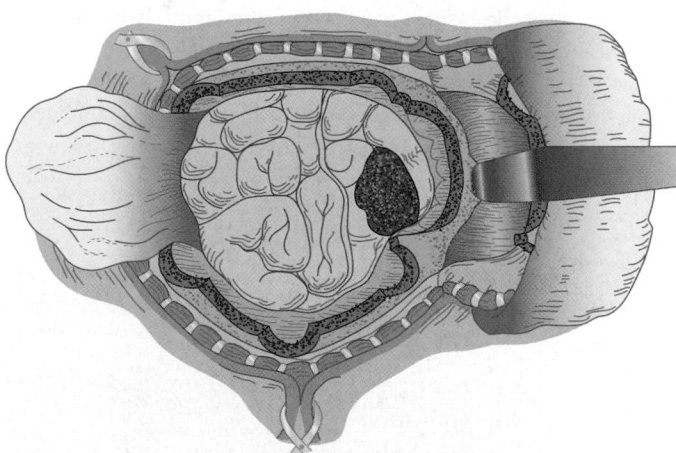

Figure 38-5. ■ In a craniotomy, a portion of the skull is surgically opened to allow access to the brain.

Radiation Therapy

Radiation therapy may be given to slow tumor growth or following surgery. The purpose is to destroy abnormal tumor cells that are sensitive to radiation. Conventional external radiation may be given daily, five times per week for 6 weeks. A procedure called *stereotaxic radiation* or "gamma knife" is used for deep tumors. A stereotaxic frame is attached to the client's head, allowing a large, single dose of radiation to be directed at a small specific site so that normal cells are not harmed.

NURSING CARE

The nursing care of a client with a brain tumor requires support during diagnosis and specific interventions as determined by the treatment used. The diagnosis of a brain tumor is frightening. Both the client and family need ongoing emotional support throughout all phases of care.

ASSESSING

Before delivering care, the nurse gathers information about the client's history and performs a basic neurologic examination. If the client is confused or has difficulty answering questions, the family should be included in the interview. Assessment data can identify how the brain tumor is interfering with the client's life (Box 38-6 ■).

BOX 38-6	ASSESSMENT

Assessing Clients with Brain Tumors

SUBJECTIVE DATA

- Change in memory, ability to concentrate, personality, or behavior.
- Describe frequency and location of headache.
- Difficulty speaking; double or blurred vision; ringing in the ears.
- Dizziness or changes in coordination or balance.
- Any numbness, tingling, or weakness in extremities.
- History of seizures or brain tumors.

OBJECTIVE DATA

- Blood pressure, pulse, respirations, temperature.
- Observe for orientation to time, place, and person, and memory lapses.
- Assess strength of hand grip and movement of extremities.
- Assess gait by asking the client to walk normally, then in a heel-to-toe fashion.
- Assess coordination.
- Monitor and report diagnostic test results.

DIAGNOSING, PLANNING, AND IMPLEMENTING

Priorities in Nursing Care. The client with a brain tumor has many nursing care needs. Both clients and their families face an uncertain future. The client may experience side effects from chemotherapy, radiation, or surgery. Following surgery, the client may develop an altered LOC, IICP, and seizures. The client will require intensive care in the immediate postoperative period. Nursing care following a craniotomy is found in Box 38-7 ■. The client may also experience anxiety and an altered body image.

Anxiety

■ Explain diagnostic procedures and treatment methods to the client and family. Repeat information as needed. *The client and family need time to adjust to the diagnosis and its implications. If urgent treatment is necessary, they will not have time to adjust. Explaining the procedures and treatments may decrease anxiety.*

■ Encourage client and family to express their feelings. *Talking about their feelings and fears can reduce anxiety.*

■ Provide emotional support by listening and staying with the client. If the client prefers, arrange for a member of the clergy to visit. *Provide a calm environment. Listening and the nurse's physical presence may make the client feel calmer.*

Disturbed Body Image

■ Assess for signs and symptoms of a negative body image (e.g., refusal to look in the mirror, denial, and withdrawal from family and friends). *Physical changes; dependence on others for basic needs; and long-term speech, vision, and motor deficits can cause low self-esteem.*

■ Provide or arrange for a client to have surgical cap, scarf, or turban. Assist the client to obtain a wig or hairpiece. Reinforce the fact that the hair will grow back. *These interventions can decrease the client's embarrassment about hair loss.*

EVALUATING

The nurse collects and documents the following data to evaluate the effectiveness of nursing interventions for the client following a craniotomy: absence of neurologic deficits and signs of infection, level of anxiety, and knowledge of follow-up care at home.

Documenting. Documentation about client and family teaching includes wound care, medications, symptoms of complications, and safety precautions.

BOX 38-7	NURSING CARE CHECKLIST

Clients Having a Craniotomy

Before Surgery

☑ Provide routine preoperative care (see Chapter 9). ⚭

☑ Assess understanding and level of anxiety of the planned surgery.

☑ Prepare the family for how the client will appear after surgery: a large dressing covering the head; possible swollen, bruised eyelids; and an endotracheal tube.

After Surgery

☑ Provide routine postoperative care (see Chapter 9). ⚭

☑ Review nursing care intervention for IICP.

☑ Monitor respiratory status every 1 to 2 hours and assess airway patency.

☑ Monitor oxygen saturation levels as needed.

☑ Position on the nonoperative side if a bone flap or large mass was removed, to decrease venous collection and pressure on the surgical incision.

☑ Apply cool cloth over client's eyes. Reduce noise and bright lights in the room.

☑ For pain, use acetaminophen with codeine.

☑ Assess and report CSF leak from ears, nose, or wound; a leak might indicate an opening in the dura that could allow bacteria into the brain.

☑ Provide interventions to prevent infection:

  ☑ Use strict aseptic technique when changing dressings and caring for wound drains and ICP monitor lines. Monitor for any purulent drainage.

  ☑ Administer prescribed antibiotics.

  ☑ Assess for manifestations of meningitis (see later discussion in this chapter).

  ☑ After the head dressing is removed (usually 3 days postsurgery), clean the incision with half-strength hydrogen peroxide to remove dried blood.

☑ If CSF leak is present, place a sterile dressing over the drainage area and change when damp.

  ☑ If CSF leaks from the nose, elevate head of bed 20 degrees unless contraindicated. Do not suction nasally; do not clean the nose; tell client not to put fingers in the nose.

  ☑ If CSF leaks from the ear, position client on side of leakage unless contraindicated. Do not clean the ear; tell client not to put fingers in the ear.

☑ Monitor for seizures and maintain seizure precautions.

CONTINUING CARE

Clients diagnosed with a brain tumor have short- and long-term needs. They may require chemotherapy or radiation treatments. If surgery is planned, the client and family need to discuss their fears about the potential side effects. Assess the client's and family's capabilities and resources to provide care after discharge.

If chemotherapy or radiation therapy is ordered, the following information should be given to the client and family:

- Importance of keeping appointments for chemotherapy or radiation therapy
- Adverse effects of chemotherapy or radiation
- Skin care with radiation therapy
- How to manage nausea or vomiting; nutritional support.

Following a craniotomy, the client and family require emotional support. The recovery process is lengthy. It involves adapting to body image changes and managing motor and sensory deficits. Encourage the family to be involved in the client's care. For example, they can assist the client with personal hygiene and meals. As clients are able, they should be encouraged to take an active role in their own care.

The client and family may need information about support groups and community resources. Clients with neurologic deficits are referred for physical, occupational, and speech therapy and those with inoperable brain tumors are referred to hospice. Before the client is discharged home, the nurse should provide verbal and written information on the following topics:

- The use and side effects of anticonvulsant and anti-inflammatory medications
- Wound care:
  - Do not shampoo hair until the incision is healed, then pat the incision dry after shampooing. Avoid a curling iron or hair dryer on hot setting until hair has grown back.
  - When outside, wear a hat to prevent sunburn.
  - Protect the head until the wound is healed.
- Signs and symptoms to report:
  - Swelling at incision site; bloody, yellow, or clear drainage from ears, nose, or incision
  - Increased drowsiness
  - Changes in behavior
  - Stiff neck, severe headache, and elevated temperature
  - New sensory or motor deficits, vision changes, or seizures
- Safety precautions for motor deficits, sensory deficits, lack of coordination, seizures, and cognitive deficits
- Importance of follow-up appointments.

Cerebrovascular Accident

A **cerebrovascular accident (CVA)** is also called a brain attack or stroke. It leads to neurologic deficits from decreased blood supply to a local area of the brain. Approximately 700,000 people suffer a CVA each year in the United States. CVAs are the third leading cause of death in the United States and frequently leave clients with some type of physical disability. They occur most often in people over 65 years of age. Males have an increased incidence as do those people with a family history of CVA. African Americans have twice the risk of Caucasians.

Other risk factors include hypertension, diabetes mellitus, obesity, atrial fibrillation, and atherosclerosis. Lifestyle habits such as smoking, high cholesterol diet, excessive use of alcohol, and cocaine and heroin use increase the risk. Women who take oral contraceptives are at a higher risk.

PATHOPHYSIOLOGY AND MANIFESTATIONS

A **transient ischemic attack (TIA)**, a brief episode of reversible neurologic deficits, lasts from a few minutes to less than 24 hours. It results from a temporary reduction of blood flow to a specific area of the brain. Usually TIA is caused by atherosclerosis or a small embolus, which obstructs a small cerebral blood vessel. TIA is often a warning signal of a future CVA. The client may experience several TIAs before a CVA. The time between the TIA and a CVA ranges from hours to months. Manifestations include dizziness, visual loss in one eye, one-sided numbness or weakness of the fingers, arms, or legs or aphasia.

A CVA is the sudden loss of neurologic function. There are three causes of CVAs: (1) thrombus, (2) embolus, and (3) hemorrhage (Table 38-4 ■). CVAs caused by thrombus occur most often in older adults who are resting or sleeping. Any one of these causes can partially or completely reduce blood flow to cerebral tissues. This decreases oxygen to the area of the brain supplied by the involved blood vessels. Initially, the brain cells are ischemic but quickly die, resulting in a cerebral infarction. If the brain experiences **anoxia** (lack of oxygen to the brain) for more than 10 minutes, irreversible brain damage occurs. Adequate collateral blood supply can decrease the amount of damage. Collateral circulation occurs when areas of the brain have decreased blood flow over a long period of time. Smaller blood vessels develop to supply blood to areas with reduced blood supply. Large areas of infarction usually result in severe disability or death.

When cerebral blood supply is altered, there is temporary or permanent loss of neurologic function. The signs and symptoms of a CVA vary, depending on the area of the brain involved, the size of the area, and collateral blood flow. Typical manifestations alter movement, sensation,

TABLE 38-4

Comparison of the Types of CVA (Stroke)

TYPE	CAUSE	ONSET	PATHOPHYSIOLOGY
Thrombotic CVA	Atherosclerosis of large cerebral arteries	During or after sleep	Atherosclerosis causes plaque to build up in cerebral arteries. If plaque is not removed or treated, a thrombus or clot develops. This leads to ischemia in the brain tissue supplied by the vessel.
Embolic CVA	Atrial fibrillation, congestive heart failure (CHF), rheumatic heart disease Mitral valve disease Endocarditis	Sudden onset with immediate deficits	Embolus travels to a cerebral artery from a distant site, especially the heart. It usually lodges in a narrow portion of a cerebral artery causing necrosis.
Hemorrhagic CVA	Hypertension	Occurs suddenly, often during some activity	Hypertension weakens a cerebral blood vessel causing it to rupture. This leads to bleeding into the brain tissue or subarachnoid space.

thought, memory, behavior, or speech (Table 38-5 ■). However, the effects of a CVA are not limited to the nervous system. Complications of a CVA can affect respiration, elimination, and muscle function.

TABLE 38-5

Manifestations and Complications of Cerebrovascular Accident

MANIFESTATIONS	POTENTIAL COMPLICATIONS
Motor Deficits ■ Hemiparesis ■ Hemiplegia ■ Facial droop	**Respiratory Problems** ■ Airway obstruction ■ Decreased ability to cough ■ Pneumonia
Speech Deficits ■ Expressive aphasia ■ Receptive aphasia ■ Global aphasia ■ Dysarthria	**Gastrointestinal Problems** ■ Dysphagia ■ Constipation
Visual Deficits ■ Diplopia ■ Homonymous hemianopia	**Genitourinary Problems** ■ Incontinence ■ Frequency ■ Urinary retention
Sensory-Perceptual Deficits ■ Agnosia ■ Apraxia ■ Neglect syndrome	**Musculoskeletal Problems** ■ Contractures ■ Muscle atrophy ■ Footdrop ■ Shoulder adduction
Cognitive and Behavior Changes ■ Memory loss ■ Short attention span ■ Poor judgment ■ Poor problem-solving ability ■ Emotional lability ■ Depression	**Integumentary Problems** ■ Decubitus ulcers

Right and Left Hemisphere Problems

Strokes usually occur in one hemisphere. Recent studies have shown that people who are left hemisphere dominant (right-handed) show certain symptoms. A comparison of right and left hemisphere strokes is given in Box 38-8 ■.

Motor Deficits

Motor deficits commonly follow a CVA. Depending on the area of the brain involved, CVAs may cause weakness, paralysis, or spasticity. Because the sensory and motor nerves cross at the neck, sensory and motor deficits develop on the opposite side of the damage. For example, a CVA in the right hemisphere causes deficits in the left side of the body and vice versa. This is known as **contralateral** (opposite side) deficit. The deficits include:

■ *Hemiparesis:* weakness of the left or right half of the body.
■ **Hemiplegia:** paralysis of the left or right half of the body (Figure 38-6 ■). Initially, the affected arm and leg are flaccid; they become spastic within 6 to 8 weeks. Spasticity can lead to adduction of the shoulder; flexion of the

BOX 38-8

RIGHT-HEMISPHERE VERSUS LEFT-HEMISPHERE CVA

Right-Hemisphere CVA	Left-Hemisphere CVA
Left hemiplegia	Right hemiplegia
Left visual field deficits	Right visual field deficits
Spatial-perceptual deficits	Aphasia
Denies or unaware of deficits	Aware of deficits
Easily distracted	Impaired intellectual ability
Poor judgment	Slow, cautious behavior
Impulsive	High level of frustration over losses

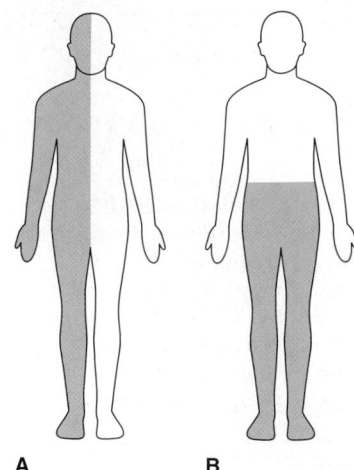

Figure 38-6. ■ Types of paralysis. (**A**) Hemiplegia is paralysis of one-half of the body. (**B**) Paraplegia is paralysis of the lower part of the body.

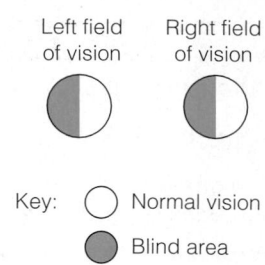

Figure 38-7. ■ Homonymous hemianopia. Loss of vision in the nasal field of the right eye and temporal field of the left eye.

fingers, wrist, elbow, and knee; and external rotation of the hip. These problems limit the client's mobility and increase risk for immobility complications including thrombophlebitis, orthostatic hypotension, aspiration and pneumonia, contractures, and decubitus ulcers.

Speech Deficits

Speech deficits usually result from a CVA affecting the dominant hemisphere. The left hemisphere is dominant in all right-handed people and most left-handed people. Strokes cause many speech and language problems. Among these problems are:

■ *Expressive aphasia:* an inability to speak or write due to damage of Broca's area. The client usually can understand what is being said.
■ *Receptive aphasia:* an inability to understand the spoken word due to damage of Wernicke's area. The client can speak but the words do not make sense.
■ *Global aphasia:* a combination of expressive and receptive aphasia.
■ *Dysarthria:* difficulty in speech caused by paralysis of the muscles that control speech.

Visual Deficits

When a CVA damages the parietal and temporal lobes, vision is impaired. The client may experience diplopia or **homonymous hemianopia** (the loss of vision in half of the eye). The visual loss is opposite to the side affected by the stroke. The client sees only one-half of the normal vision and must turn the head to see the environment (Figure 38-7 ■).

Sensory–Perceptual Deficits

A CVA may alter sensation and perception of temperature, vibration, pain, pressure, and *proprioception* (awareness of the body's position). The loss of these sensory abilities increases the client's potential for injury. Common sensory–perceptual deficits include:

■ *Agnosia:* the inability to recognize a familiar object such as a toothbrush
■ *Apraxia:* the inability to carry out a familiar routine, e.g., brushing teeth or combing hair, even when paralysis is not present
■ *Neglect syndrome* (or unilateral neglect): client ignores the affected side of the body; tends to bump into walls, walk to one side, or fail to dress the affected side.

Cognitive and Behavioral Changes

Clients who have had a CVA may have cognition changes. For example, damage to the right-hemisphere frontal lobe can cause memory loss, decreased attention span, poor judgment, and an inability to solve problems. Behavioral changes include **emotional lability** (the client may laugh or cry inappropriately) or loss of self-control such as swearing or refusing to wear clothes. Depression is common, especially when there are functional and speech losses. Stress is poorly tolerated and is seen as uncontrolled anger.

Urinary and Gastrointestinal Problems

When the stroke damages only one hemisphere, bladder and bowel problems are usually short term. Initially, the client may experience urinary frequency, urgency, or incontinence. These problems last longer when there are cognitive deficits. Constipation develops as a complication of immobility. A stroke can impair the ability to swallow. Factors such as attention deficits and weakness or lack of coordination of the tongue often contribute to this problem. *Dysphagia* may result in choking, drooling, aspiration, or regurgitation. Nursing care focuses on preventing aspiration and promoting adequate nutrition.

INTERDISCIPLINARY CARE

The client with a TIA receives medications or has surgery to prevent a stroke. Once a CVA has occurred, immediate medical attention is needed. At first, the medical team concentrates on diagnosing the type of CVA and preserving life. Drugs are ordered to reduce IICP and prevent neurologic

BOX 38-9	NURSING CARE CHECKLIST

Clients Having CT Scan of the Head

Preparation of Client

☑ Obtain a signed consent form.

☑ Check facility policy on withholding food and fluids. For A.M. test: NPO 8 hours before test. For P.M. test: May have a liquid breakfast.

☑ Give medications up to 2 hours before test.

☑ Identify for allergy to iodine dye (by asking about allergy to seafood).

☑ Remove hairpins, clips, and earrings.

Client and Family Teaching

☑ Follow the guidelines for not drinking or eating before the test.

☑ If contrast dye is injected, a warm sensation may be felt in the face or body.

☑ The exam lasts from 30 to 90 minutes.

☑ The CT scanner is a narrow circular enclosure with a round opening. You are strapped to a special table while the scanner revolves around your head. This test is painless, but the scanner makes a loud clicking noise.

☑ Someone is always immediately available during the test.

deficits. Following the acute phase, care focuses on the client's rehabilitation.

Diagnostic Tests

The following diagnostic tests are used to detect the potential for a stroke or to identify physiologic changes once the CVA has occurred:

- *CT scan* identifies the size and location of the CVA. It is useful to differentiate between an infarction and hemorrhage. Nursing interventions for the client having a CT scan of the head are described in Box 38-9 ■.
- *MRI* detects areas of infarction earlier than a CT scan.
- *Cerebral arteriography* identifies vessel abnormalities such as an aneurysm.
- *Doppler ultrasound* studies evaluate the flow of blood through the carotid arteries and identify if a vessel is partially or completely occluded.
- *Positron emission tomography (PET)* identifies the amount of tissue damage following a CVA.
- *Lumbar puncture* is used to obtain cerebrospinal fluid for examination. Blood in the CSF indicates a hemorrhagic CVA (see Box 38-3).

Medications

Medications are given to prevent a CVA in clients with TIAs or a previous CVA. Antiplatelet medications are most frequently ordered. Platelets can collect in the cerebral arteries and potentially block a vessel. Daily use of low-dose aspirin effectively reduces clot formation. Other antiplatelet medications include dipyridamole (Persantine), ticlopidine (Ticlid), and clopidogrel (Plavix).

CVAs are now referred to as "brain attack" so that everyone realizes the urgency of seeking immediate medical help. If a thrombotic or embolic stroke is suspected, the client is given a thrombolytic drug, alteplase (Activase r-tpa). This drug dissolves blood clots, increases blood flow, and prevents damage to the brain cells. To be effective, it must be started within the first 3 hours after symptoms appear. It is not given when intracerebral bleeding is present.

Thrombotic strokes are treated with anticoagulant therapy. They do not dissolve an existing clot but prevent new clots from forming. Anticoagulants are never given to a client who is bleeding within the brain. The most common anticoagulants are heparin and warfarin (Coumadin). Newer low-molecular-weight heparin such as Lovenox may be ordered. Antiplatelet medications or heparin are started 24 hours after thrombolytic therapy. See Chapter 28 ∞ for more information about anticoagulant therapy.

During the acute phase, the client may receive antihypertensive drugs to control blood pressure. Hypertension can increase the area of infarction. If the client has IICP, mannitol (an osmotic diuretic) or furosemide (a loop diuretic) is used to decrease cerebral edema. An anticonvulsant such as phenytoin is given to prevent or control seizures.

Surgery

Surgery may be performed to prevent a stroke. Persons with a history of TIAs or in danger of having another CVA may undergo a **carotid endarterectomy.** Surgery removes atherosclerotic plaque or a thrombus (Figure 38-8 ■). Nursing care for the client following a carotid endarterectomy is

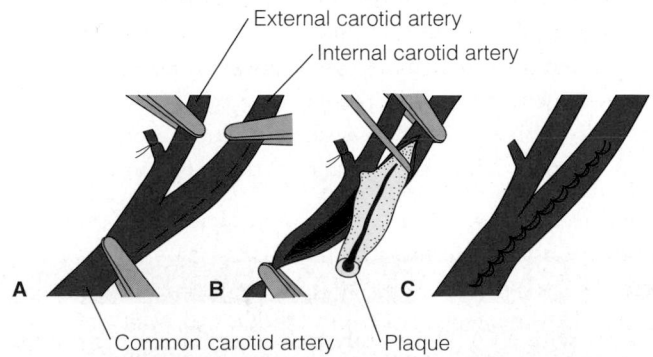

Figure 38-8. ■ Carotid endarterectomy. (**A**) The occluded area is clamped off and an incision is made in the artery. (**B**) Plaque is removed from the inner layer of the artery. (**C**) To restore blood flow through the artery, the artery is sutured or a graft is inserted.

BOX 38-10	NURSING CARE CHECKLIST

Post Carotid Endarterectomy

☑ Place in a supine position with head and neck in midline alignment. Elevate the head of the bed 30 degrees unless contraindicated.

☑ Teach client to support the head with the hands when changing position.

☑ Maintain patency of wound drains.

☑ Monitor for *hemorrhage:* Assess for hematoma or bleeding at incision site. Assess neck size and check for drainage under the client's neck and shoulders.

☑ Monitor for *respiratory distress:* Assess respiratory rate, rhythm, depth, and effort. Assess for difficulty swallowing, tracheal deviation from the midline, and restlessness. Keep a tracheostomy set at the bedside.

☑ Monitor for *cranial nerve impairment:* Assess for facial drooping, hoarseness, dysphagia, tongue deviation, speech difficulty, or shoulder sag on one side.

☑ Monitor for *carotid artery occlusion* or *CVA:* Assess for confusion, dizziness, slurred speech, or hemiparesis. Check for carotid bruit.

☑ Monitor for *hypertension* or *hypotension:* Monitor blood pressure at least hourly. Report hypertension immediately because of the risk of CVA, artery rupture, or hypotension that could lead to myocardial ischemia.

BOX 38-11	ASSESSMENT

Assessing Clients with CVA

SUBJECTIVE DATA

- Change in memory or confusion.
- Any sudden severe headache.
- Difficulty speaking or understanding speech.
- Visual changes such as double vision or blurring.
- Any dizziness, loss of coordination or balance.
- Any numbness, tingling, or weakness of the face, arm, or leg.
- History of hypertension, previous TIA or CVA, diabetes, dysrhythmias, or cardiac disease.
- History of alcohol abuse, smoking.
- Use of antihypertensive, anticoagulant, or oral contraceptive medication.

OBJECTIVE DATA

- Blood pressure, pulse, respirations, temperature.
- Monitor for manifestations of IICP (see Box 38-1).
- Assess orientation; observe for memory lapses.
- Assess for slurred speech, expressive or receptive aphasia.
- Test facial sensation by stroking face with cotton ball.
- Assess strength of hand grip, movement of extremities, gait, and bilateral foot strength.
- Assess ability to swallow.
- Note presence of bowel and/or bladder incontinence. Palpate bladder for distention.

described in Box 38-10 ■. For the first 24 hours after surgery, the client is cared for in the critical care unit. Transluminal angioplasty, a nonsurgical procedure, compresses plaque against the arterial wall, increasing blood flow to the cerebrum. Once the vessel is opened, a stent may be placed to maintain arterial patency.

Complementary Therapy

Clients taking antihypertensive medications should not use black cohosh because it increases the antihypertensive drugs' hypotensive effects. Feverfew, garlic, ginger root, and ginkgo can suppress platelet aggregation and increase the risk of bleeding for those clients taking aspirin and anticoagulants such as heparin and warfarin (Coumadin).

NURSING CARE

Clients with a CVA may fully recover or have some residual effects from the stroke. They may experience problems with mobility, speech, and swallowing and an inability to perform ADLs. As clients progress from the acute to the recovery phase, they are cared for in a long-term care facility, rehabilitation center, and the home.

ASSESSING

Subjective and objective information is obtained from the client with a suspected TIA or CVA. On admission to the hospital, the client is assessed for any neurologic deficits. If the client's condition is unstable, respiratory and cardiac status are closely monitored. Box 38-11 ■ suggests additional data to collect.

DIAGNOSING, PLANNING, AND IMPLEMENTING

Priorities in Nursing Care. Many nursing diagnoses are appropriate for the client with a CVA. Each person is affected differently, depending on the amount of brain damage and the area involved. The priority of care during the initial period is preserving functional brain cells and preventing acute complications. Once the client's condition is stable, problems of physical mobility, communication, sensory-perceptual deficits, bowel and urine elimination, and swallowing present the major nursing challenges.

Ineffective Tissue Perfusion: Cerebral

The acute phase of a CVA is 24 to 72 hours after admission. If the CVA is extensive, the client is cared for in the critical care unit. ICP is monitored closely. See the section on IICP earlier in this chapter.

Risk for Ineffective Airway Clearance

■ Monitor respiratory status and airway patency. Suction the airway as necessary. Place the client in a side-lying position to prevent aspiration. Monitor respiratory status and give oxygen as ordered. *Breathing may be affected by the CVA. If the client is unconscious, suctioning is important to prevent airway obstruction. The client is at risk for developing atelectasis and pneumonia.*

Impaired Physical Mobility

■ Turn the client from side to side every 2 hours around the clock. Keep the body aligned and place extremities in proper position with pillows (Figure 38-9 ■). *Mobility can be impaired by weak extremities, muscle wasting, or hemiplegia. Proper positioning and turning maintain joint function*

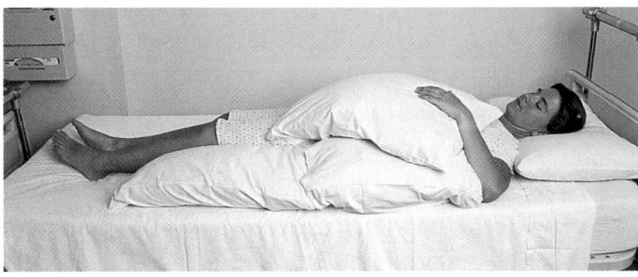

A

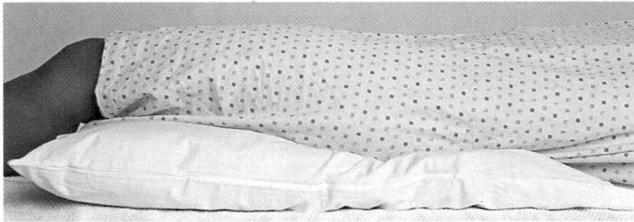

B

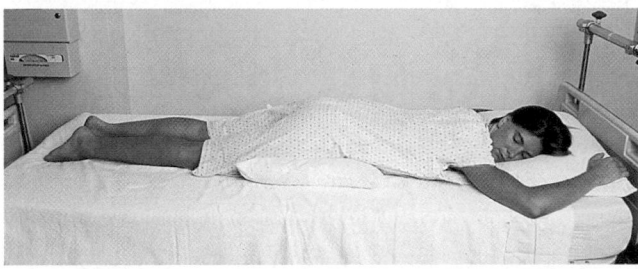

C

Figure 38-9. ■ Positioning the client with hemiplegia is important to prevent deformity of the affected extremities. **(A)** With the client in a supine position, place a pillow in the axilla (to prevent adduction) and under the hand and arm, with the hand higher than the elbow (to prevent flexion and edema). **(B)** When the client is lying supine, use a pillow from the iliac crest to the middle of the thigh to prevent external rotation of the hip. **(C)** When the client is in the prone position, place a pillow under the pelvis to promote hip hyperextension.

and decrease skin breakdown and dependent edema in the hands and feet. These actions also reduce the risk of other complications resulting from immobility.

■ Monitor calves each shift for symptoms of thrombophlebitis: redness, warmth, and tenderness. *Clients on bed rest can develop thrombophlebitis.*

■ Do not use a footboard. Use hand splints as directed by the physical therapist. *Footboards are no longer recommended. Hand splints may prevent contractures of the fingers and wrist.*

■ Perform active ROM exercises on unaffected extremities and passive ROM exercises on affected exercises every 4 hours. *Active ROM exercises can improve muscle strength. Passive ROM exercises improve joint mobility.*

clinical ALERT

Active and passive ROM exercises increase venous return and decrease risk of thrombophlebitis.

■ Collaborate with the physical therapist to teach the client transfer and ambulation. *The physical therapist knows the correct transfer and ambulation techniques for the CVA client.*

Impaired Verbal Communication

■ Use the following guidelines when communicating with the client:
  ■ Speak to the client as an adult. Do not raise your voice when speaking to the client.
  ■ Allow adequate time for the client to answer.
  ■ Face the client and speak slowly.
  ■ When you do not understand the client's speech, be honest and say so.
  ■ Use short, simple statements and "yes" and "no" questions.
  ■ If clients cannot speak, ask them to nod the head or blink their eyes.
  Communication may be altered by expressive or receptive aphasia. All of these techniques can decrease the client's frustration and may motivate the client to communicate.

■ Provide pad and pencil, magic slate, flash cards, computerized talking board, and/or picture board. *Other techniques may help the client communicate.*

Disturbed Sensory Perception

■ Keep the environment free of clutter and well lit. Keep the bed in the low position with side rails elevated. *Clients with a CVA are at risk for injury.*

■ Place items on the unaffected side. *Clients with a visual field deficit may ignore items on the affected side of the body.*

■ Teach the client to turn the head and move the eyes toward the affected side of the body. *Clients with homonymous hemianopia cannot see half of their environment; turning the head and moving the eyes in one direction increases mobility and decreases the risk of injury.*

- Approach the client from the unaffected side and speak before touching. *These actions prevent startling the client.*
- If unilateral neglect is present, encourage client to handle affected extremities. *This increases the client's awareness of the affected side.*

Impaired Urinary Elimination and Constipation

- Offer the bedpan or urinal, or assist client to bedside commode every 2 to 4 hours. *This reduces the risk of urinary incontinence and helps establish a regular voiding pattern.*
- Promote daily intake of 2,000 mL, but limit oral intake at night. *Adequate fluid intake may prevent urinary tract infection (UTI). Limiting intake may prevent incontinence at night.*
- Keep the skin dry and monitor for signs of redness. *Clients who are incontinent are at risk for skin breakdown.*
- Reinforce the client's pre-CVA bowel habits:
  - Drink 2,000 mL/day and eat a high-fiber diet.
  - Increase physical activity as tolerated.
  - Offer the bedpan or bedside commode at the same time each day; ensure privacy; and have the client sit in an upright position.
  - Give stool softeners as ordered.

  Increased fluids, fiber, and activity stimulate bowel activity. A regular daily time for bowel movements in the upright position and privacy promotes normal bowel elimination. Stool softeners help prevent hard stool that is more difficult to expel.

Impaired Swallowing

- Place the client in an upright position for meals and 30 minutes afterward. Tilt the head slightly forward. *The client's swallowing reflex or ability to concentrate may be affected by a CVA. Upright position and tilting head forward prevent aspiration.*

clinical ALERT

Do not feed a client who does not have a functioning gag reflex.

- Provide oral care before meals. *Oral care stimulates saliva and eases swallowing.*
- Serve thickened liquids and pureed or soft food such as custard and canned fruits and vegetables. *Thickened liquids and pureed and soft foods are easier to swallow and may prevent aspiration.*
- Encourage client to eat small bites of food and place food on the unaffected side of the mouth. *Small bites and using the unaffected side prevents food from collecting in the mouth and makes swallowing safer.*

clinical ALERT

After eating, check the client's mouth for "pocketing" of food especially on the affected side.

- Limit distractions during mealtime. *Distractions increase the risk of aspiration.*
- Have suction equipment available during mealtime. *Suction will be needed if the client starts to choke or aspirate.*

Self-Care Deficit

- Encourage the client to use the unaffected arm to bathe, brush teeth, comb hair, dress, and eat. *Self-care to the extent the client is able reduces their frustration, increases independence, and improves self-esteem. Using the unaffected arm will promote the client's feeling of independence.*
- Teach the client and family to put clothing on the affected extremity first and then dress the unaffected extremities. *This technique increases awareness of the affected extremity and promotes independence.*
- Consult with an occupational therapist to teach the client how to use assistive devices for eating, hygiene, and dressing. *An occupational therapist's role is to teach clients how to use their upper extremities and appropriate assistive devices.*

EVALUATING

Evaluate the effectiveness of nursing care of the client with a CVA by collecting data on the following:

- Airway remains patent
- Provides self-care or with assistance
- Communicates care needs effectively
- Copes with illness
- Demonstrates willingness to participate in rehabilitation
- Knowledge of medications.

Documenting. Documentation includes VS, assessment of speech, ability to move extremities, strength of hand grip, swallowing, bowel and breath sounds, intake and output. Client teaching about self-care, complications, medications, diet, assistive devices, ROM exercises, and safety measures are recorded.

CONTINUING CARE

After a CVA, the client and family face many changes. The middle-aged adult family member may become the caretaker for an older parent. An older adult may be unable to care for a spouse who has had a stroke. They may have to accept placement of the spouse in a long-term care facility.

Discharge planning includes assessing the client's and family's ability to care for the client. The client and family need teaching before the client can be sent home. The following topics should be included:

- Prevention of CVA; symptoms of TIA and CVA
- When to seek medical care (provide physician's name and emergency numbers)
- Complications such as aspiration, pneumonia, UTI, blood clots, and skin breakdown
- Medications: use, dose, and side effects
- Equipment modifications in the home; for example, a raised toilet seat, grab bars in the bathroom, a bath chair, a vise-type jar lid opener, a long-handled shoehorn
- Safety measures to prevent falls
- Demonstration of feeding techniques and use of assistive devices
- Demonstration of ROM exercises and the use of any splints
- Physical care (ADLs, transfer techniques, skin care)
- Psychologic support for client and family; respite care for the caregiver
- Community resources such as home health agency, Meals-on-Wheels, elder care (day care for adults); sources for special equipment (e.g., walker); support groups and stroke clubs.

Rehabilitation is a lengthy process. The family will need to be patient as the client relearns ADLs. Emphasize that physical function may continue to improve for up to 3 months, and speech may continue to improve even longer.

Cerebral Aneurysm

A cerebral **aneurysm** is an abnormal outpouching or dilation of a cerebral artery. It occurs at the point where the arterial wall is the weakest. The weakness is related to atherosclerosis, hypertension, or a congenital defect. Cerebral aneurysms usually develop in the circle of Willis. There are several types

of aneurysms: (1) berry, (2) saccular, (3) fusiform, and (4) dissecting (Figure 38-10 ■). A ruptured cerebral aneurysm is the most common cause of a hemorrhagic CVA.

PATHOPHYSIOLOGY AND MANIFESTATIONS

At first, the weakened portion of the artery enlarges and presses on nearby cranial nerves. Unless it affects cranial nerve function, the person is asymptomatic. As the aneurysm enlarges, it may periodically leak blood into the brain. The person complains of headache, nausea, vomiting, and pain in the neck and back. If the leak can spontaneously seal itself with a clot, the client again becomes asymptomatic. If the aneurysm keeps expanding, it is likely to rupture, forcing blood into the subarachnoid space at the base of the brain. This is known as a **subarachnoid hemorrhage.** Bleeding into the subarachnoid space causes meningeal irritation.

Manifestations of a subarachnoid hemorrhage include (1) sudden, explosive headache; (2) stiff neck (*nuchal rigidity*); (3) change in consciousness; (4) photophobia; (5) nausea and vomiting; and (6) cranial nerve deficits. The major complications are rebleeding and vasospasm. Rebleeding can occur within the first 48 hours and later in 7 to 10 days. The later rebleeding occurs when the initial clot breaks down as part of the body's normal process. A *cerebral vasospasm* occurs when one or more cerebral arteries narrow, leading to ischemia and infarction. Both complications have a high mortality rate.

INTERDISCIPLINARY CARE

Diagnosis is made by a CT scan, angiography, and lumbar puncture. A *CT scan* of the brain shows the location and size of the aneurysm. *Cerebral angiography* is done to view the cerebral arteries, locate the aneurysm, and identify a vasospasm. The presence of blood in the cerebrospinal fluid during a *lumbar puncture* confirms a subarachnoid hemorrhage.

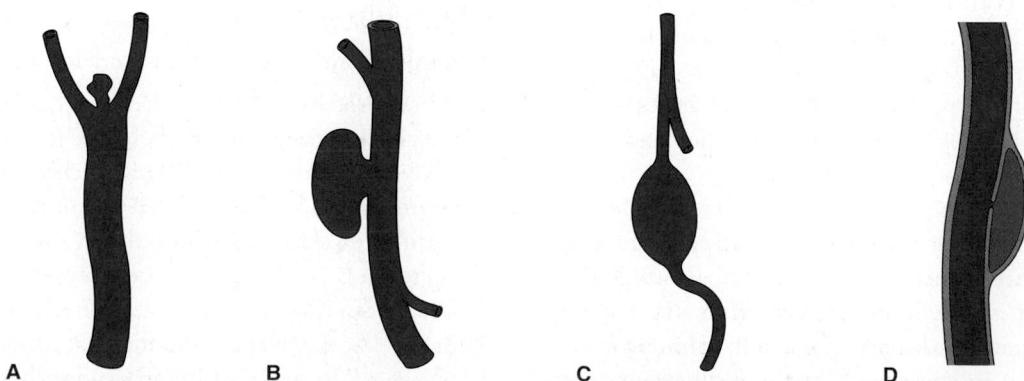

Figure 38-10. ■ Types of aneurysms. (**A**) A berry aneurysm is a small sac on a stem or stalk. (**B**) A saccular aneurysm is formed from a distended small portion of the vessel wall. (**C**) A fusiform aneurysm is an enlarged area of the entire blood vessel. (**D**) A dissecting aneurysm is formed when blood fills the area between the tunica media and the tunica intima.

Several medications are given to avoid rebleeding and vasospasm until surgery is possible. Aminocaproic acid (Amicar) prevents the clot from being destroyed. A calcium channel blocker, such as nimodipine (Nimotop), decreases vasospasm. The client is given anticonvulsants to prevent seizures. Stool softeners prevent unnecessary straining that can increase intracranial pressure. Acetaminophen or codeine is used for pain control.

Surgery is the treatment of choice to prevent additional bleeding. It is preferred as soon as the client's condition is stable. The skull is opened and either a metal clip is placed at the neck of the aneurysm or the aneurysm is wrapped with synthetic material.

If the size or location of the aneurysm prohibits surgery, the client is managed conservatively. The nurse monitors the client for signs of deterioration by doing neurologic checks, and taking blood pressure, pulse, and respirations hourly (more frequently if the client's condition worsens). The following aneurysm precautions are instituted to prevent an increase in ICP and the risk of rebleeding:

■ Place the client in a private, quiet, darkened room.
■ Limit visitors to two family members at any one time.
■ Elevate the head of the bed 15 to 30 degrees.
■ Keep on complete bed rest. Feeding and bathing may be allowed.
■ Avoid activities that increase ICP such as coughing, sneezing, straining, blowing the nose, moving self up in bed, or smoking.

Discharge teaching following a subarachnoid hemorrhage is similar to that for a CVA, as discussed earlier in this chapter. Clients with significant neurologic deficits are referred for rehabilitation services. The client and family need to follow postop craniotomy guidelines (see Box 38-7).

Seizure Disorder

A **seizure** is a brief disruption of brain function caused by abnormal electrical activity in the nerve cells of the brain. This electrical activity may involve all or part of the brain and may cause sensory, motor, or autonomic manifestations. A **convulsion** is involuntary muscle contraction and relaxation, which involves the entire body.

Seizures can occur as an isolated event. For example, it is not uncommon for a client to have a few seizures following a severe head injury. When seizures occur in a chronic pattern, the disorder is called **epilepsy** or *seizure disorder*. The cause of most seizure disorders is unknown. However, seizures beginning in adulthood usually result from other conditions such as a brain infection, CVA, or brain tumor. Approximately 2.4 million people in the United States are affected by epilepsy and seizures.

PATHOPHYSIOLOGY AND MANIFESTATIONS

Neurons carry messages by electrical impulses from the body to the cerebral cortex. If a few unstable neurons continue sending electrical impulses, a seizure occurs. A group of abnormally firing neurons that start a seizure is called an **epileptogenic focus.** The part of the body controlled by these neurons performs abnormally. Certain conditions such as hypoglycemia, high fever, and hypoxia can trigger seizure activity. When seizures occur, they greatly increase metabolism and therefore consumption of oxygen and glucose to the brain. Seizures are classified as partial or generalized.

Partial Seizures

Partial (or focal) seizures start in one area of the cerebral cortex. There are two types of partial seizures:

1. *Simple partial seizures* cause uncontrolled jerking movements of a finger, hand, foot, leg, or the face. This motor activity may spread to other body areas and is known as the **jacksonian march.** Sometimes simple partial seizures involve the sensory part of the brain. Symptoms include flashing lights, tingling sensations, or hallucinations. The seizure activity usually lasts 20 to 30 seconds, and the client does not lose consciousness.

2. *Complex partial seizures* are also known as psychomotor seizures. Manifestations include repetitive, nonpurposeful actions: lip smacking, aimless walking, or picking at clothing. These behaviors are called **automatisms** and last less than 1 minute. During the seizure, the person has an altered level of consciousness. Afterward, the client may be confused or not remember the seizure. The seizure can be preceded by an **aura** (a warning sign that something is going to happen). The aura may be an unusual smell, a sense of déjà vu, or a sudden intense emotion.

Generalized Seizures

Generalized seizures involve both hemispheres of the brain and result in loss of consciousness. There are two common forms of generalized seizures:

1. *Absence seizures* occur more frequently in children. They are characterized by a brief change in consciousness such as a blank stare, blinking of the eyes, eyelid fluttering, and lip smacking. All motor activity is stopped during the seizure. Because the seizure lasts only 5 to 10 seconds, the client may be unaware of it. Some clients can experience many seizures per day.

2. *Tonic-clonic seizures* are the most common seizure disorder in adults and children. Because these seizures can develop suddenly, the client risks potential injury such as head trauma, fractures, burns, or motor vehicle accidents. Tonic-clonic seizures follow a typical pattern:

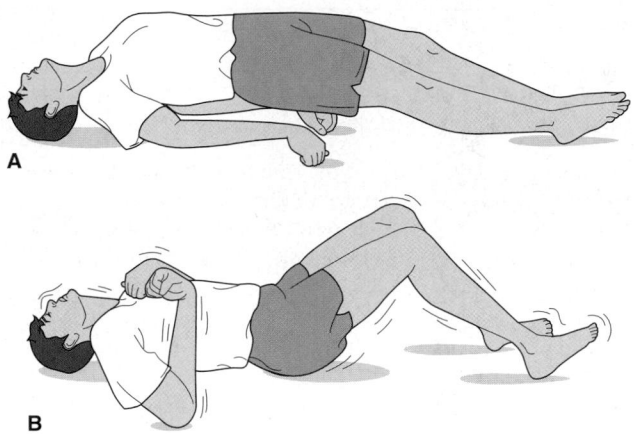

Figure 38-11. ■ Tonic-clonic contractions in generalized seizures. (**A**) Tonic phase. (**B**) Clonic phase.

(1) aura, (2) tonic phase, (3) clonic phase, and (4) post-ictal phase.

The client experiences an aura such as a bright light, an odd taste in the mouth, or an unusual sound. A loud cry may be heard when air is forced out of the lungs. The client falls to the ground, loses consciousness, and has tonic contractions followed by clonic contractions (Figure 38-11 ■). In **tonic contractions,** muscles are rigid with the arms and legs extended and jaws clenched. Pupils become fixed and dilated. Breathing stops briefly and cyanosis develops. During **clonic contractions,** movements are jerky as the muscles alternately contract and relax. The eyes roll back; tongue and cheek biting, as well as frothing from the mouth, may occur. Urinary and bowel incontinence are common. The entire seizure generally lasts about 1 to 2 minutes.

In the postictal phase, the client is unconscious for up to 30 minutes. The client regains consciousness slowly and may be confused and disoriented on waking. Individuals often experience headache, muscle aches, and fatigue following the seizure. Many people sleep for several hours afterward. Amnesia of the events prior to the seizure is normal.

Status Epilepticus

Status epilepticus is a continuous period of tonic-clonic seizures in which the client does not regain consciousness. Constant seizure activity can harm the brain's nerve cells due to depletion of oxygen and glucose and impaired ventilation and perfusion. It also causes physical exhaustion and respiratory distress. Status epilepticus is considered a life-threatening medical emergency to prevent permanent brain damage. It can be triggered by abrupt discontinuation of anticonvulsant medication, acute head injury, or hypoxia.

INTERDISCIPLINARY CARE

Initial treatment focuses on controlling the seizure. Long-term management involves identifying the cause and pre-

Electroencephalogram (EEG)

Preparation of the Client

☑ Explain the procedure to the client.

☑ Withhold tranquilizer and depressant medications 24 to 48 hours before and caffeine-containing foods (e.g., coffee, tea, cola, and chocolate).

☑ Shampoo hair the night before.

Client and Family Teaching

☑ The test lasts from 1 to 2 hours.

☑ The test is painless. It is done while you lie on a stretcher or sit in a reclining chair.

☑ Electrodes are applied to the scalp with a thick paste.

☑ After the test, the nurse will help you remove the paste from your hair.

venting future seizures. Collaborative care includes diagnostic testing, medications, and, in some cases, surgery.

Diagnostic Tests

A complete neurologic exam is done to identify the site of the seizures. The following diagnostic tests may be ordered:

■ *EEG* can determine the type of seizure and locate the seizure focus. See Box 38-12 ■ for nursing implications with an EEG.
■ *Skull x-rays* may identify possible skull fractures.
■ *CT scan* or *MRI* may detect a tumor, CVA, or hemorrhage.
■ *Blood studies* are done to assess CBC, electrolytes, blood urea nitrogen (BUN), blood glucose, and to test for syphilis.

Medications

Most seizure activity can be decreased or controlled with anticonvulsant medication. The goal is to use the lowest possible dose of medication with the fewest side effects. It takes several weeks to adjust the dose. Routine serum drug levels are drawn to determine effective doses and the potential for toxicity, as well as to identify clients who are not taking their medications. Each medication has a therapeutic and toxic level. Consult a drug handbook for the appropriate levels. If the client's seizures are not well controlled, a second medication is added. Many clients often need these drugs for their entire life. Anticonvulsant drugs may interact adversely with other drugs. Nursing implications are discussed in Table 38-6 ■.

Status epilepticus must be treated immediately. First, an airway is established. This is followed by intravenous

TABLE 38-6			
Nursing Implications for Pharmacology: Anticonvulsant Drugs			
DRUGS	**ACTIONS**	**NURSING IMPLICATIONS**	**CLIENT TEACHING**
Clonazepam (Klonopin) Carbamazepine (Tegretol) Ethosuximide (Zarontin) Gabapentin (Neurontin) Lamotrigine (Lamictal) Phenobarbital Phenytoin (Dilantin) Fosphenytoin (Cerebyx) Primidone (Mysoline) Valproic acid (Depakene)	Anticonvulsant agents act in the motor cortex of the brain to prevent abnormal electrical discharges from the epileptic foci in this area. They control chronic seizures but do not cure seizure disorders. Also, they raise the seizure threshold so that a seizure cannot begin.	Give at the same time each day with meals to prevent gastric upset. Monitor for side effects (e.g., drowsiness, sedation, ataxia, diplopia, rash, or nystagmus). Check clients taking phenytoin for gingival hyperplasia. Monitor CBC, platelet count, and liver tests for adverse reactions. Monitor serum drug levels for therapeutic range.	Take at the same time each day with meals to prevent gastric upset. If omit a dose, call MD immediately. Do not drive a car or operate machinery when drowsy. If taking Dilantin, brush and floss daily. Report rash, bleeding, unsteady gait, or yellow eyes. Keep follow-up appointments with physician and lab for drug levels. Carry ID card identifying the type of seizures and the medications you are taking.

administration of diazepam (Valium) or lorazepam (Ativan) to stop seizure activity. Because these drugs are short acting, the dose may need to be repeated. For longer control, phenytoin and phenobarbital are given.

Surgery

When medications do not control a client's seizures, surgery may be an option. New techniques allow the client to be awake during the surgery. While the client is awake, the surgeon can map the area of abnormal electrical discharges and remove it. It is important to identify the abnormal area of epileptogenic tissue clearly, so that normal brain tissue is not removed.

Complementary Therapy

Ginkgo decreases the effectiveness of phenytoin (Dilantin). Clients taking anticonvulsants should avoid drinking grapefruit juice because it reduces metabolism of these drugs, raising plasma levels.

NURSING CARE

Nursing assessments and interventions focus on care during and immediately after a seizure. Once the client's condition is stable, client and family teaching are emphasized for discharge.

ASSESSING

The nurse collects subjective assessment data to determine the extent to which the seizure activity is interfering with the client's life and the type of medical intervention needed. Objective observations are made before, during, and after a seizure (Box 38-13 ■).

DIAGNOSING, PLANNING, AND IMPLEMENTING

Priorities in Nursing Care. Nursing care for clients with a seizure disorder focuses on providing care during and immediately after a seizure. Priorities of care for these clients include Risk for Ineffective Airway Clearance, Risk for Injury, and Anxiety.

BOX 38-13   **ASSESSMENT**

Assessing Clients with Seizure Disorders

SUBJECTIVE DATA

- Describe where seizures begin in your body. What are you told happens during a seizure? How do you feel after the seizure? Do you have a warning sign (aura)?
- History of birth or head injuries, brain tumor or infections, CVA, liver or renal disease, alcohol or drug addiction.
- Anticonvulsant medications.

OBJECTIVE DATA

- Observe before, during, and after a seizure:
  - Precipitating factors; sudden onset or warning aura; length of seizure; urine or bowel incontinence; clenched teeth; foaming or bleeding from the mouth.
  - Where did the seizure begin; did it involve both sides? Were there tonic to clonic movements?
  - Loss of consciousness during and after seizure? How long?
  - Presence of automatisms, e.g., lip smacking, eyelid fluttering.
  - Rate, quality, or absence of respirations; presence of cyanosis.
  - Amnesia about the seizure and events before it.

Risk for Ineffective Airway Clearance

- Loosen clothing around the neck. *Loosening clothing can maintain a patent airway.*
- Turn the client on the side. *During a seizure, the tongue may fall back and obstruct the airway. Secretions may pool at the back of the mouth. Turning the client on the side allows secretions to drain from the mouth.*

clinical ALERT

Do not force anything into the client's mouth because it could obstruct the airway.

- Give oxygen by mask as needed. *Seizures can cause hypoxia, so the client may need supplemental oxygen.*
- Provide suction at the bedside. *Suction is used to prevent aspiration.*

Risk for Injury

- Maintain the bed in a low position and keep side rails up. *A low bed position helps the client avoid falls and injuries. Side rails prevent the client from falling out of bed during a seizure.*
- Place blankets or protective pads over the side rails. *Padding decreases the risk of injury.*
- If the client is sitting or standing when the seizure begins, gently lower the client to the floor. *Loss of consciousness during a seizure would cause the client to fall.*
- If on the floor, place a folded towel or pillow under the client's head. *The head is protected to prevent injury.*
- Never restrain the client during a seizure. *Physically restraining the client could cause fractures of the arms or legs.*
- Clear the area of objects that could cause harm. *This provides an environment free of potential harm.*

Anxiety

- Clients with a seizure disorder worry about having a seizure in public and fear rejection by others. Encourage the client to identify potential concerns and misconceptions. *The client needs time to accept the diagnosis and its effect on family, work, and future lifestyle. Misconceptions cause unnecessary worry and anxiety.*
- Provide information about community support groups. *Sharing information with other people with similar health problems may decrease the client's anxiety.*
- Refer the client to any local and state agencies for information about driving or operating dangerous machinery. *Accurate information decreases anxiety. The client needs to know there are legal limitations on driving until a person is proven free of seizures. A driver's license may be reinstated after a seizure-free period and a letter from a physician.*

EVALUATING

Collect the following data to evaluate the effectiveness of nursing care for the client with a seizure disorder:

- Seizures are controlled
- Free from injury
- Knowledge of medications.

Documenting. Documentation includes describing any seizure activity; for example, precipitating factors, length and number of seizures, involvement of one or both sides of the body, tonic-clonic movements, automatisms, urine or bowel incontinence, apnea or cyanosis, and foaming from mouth. Client teaching about safety measures, medications and side effects, and importance of wearing an ID bracelet should be recorded.

CONTINUING CARE

Seizure disorders require lifelong management. Teach the client and family to understand the disorder, medications, and injury prevention.

Discuss the care and observations necessary before, during, and after a seizure. Stress the importance of safety and keeping the airway patent. Teach the client and family ways to prevent injury at home by (1) not smoking in bed or alone, (2) installing grab bars in the shower and tub area, (3) taking a shower rather than a tub bath to prevent drowning, and (4) keeping the bedroom and bathroom doors unlocked in case of an emergency.

The following points should be emphasized:

- Teach about medication use, side effects, and the need to take at prescribed intervals.
- Record any seizure activity and medications taken daily.
- Avoid activities that require alertness and coordination until medication levels are stable.
- Stress importance of follow-up care and keeping appointments with physician and laboratory.
- Instruct to wear ID bracelet identifying seizure condition and medications.
- Limit intake of coffee; avoid alcohol.
- Avoid factors that may trigger a seizure: fatigue, fasting, excessive stress, flashing or blinking lights.
- Provide information on the Epilepsy Foundation of America.

Intracranial Infections

The most common inflammatory conditions of the brain are meningitis, encephalitis, and brain abscesses. They are caused by bacteria and viruses (Table 38-7 ■). If untreated, these conditions may lead to long-term neurologic deficits or death.

TABLE 38-7		
Comparison of Intracranial Infections		
INFECTION	**CAUSATIVE ORGANISM**	**SUSCEPTIBLE CLIENTS**
Bacterial meningitis ■ Pneumococcal meningitis	*Streptococcus pneumoniae*	Children under 2; adults over 65
■ *Haemophilus influenzae* meningitis	*Haemophilus influenzae*	Children under 5
■ Meningococcal meningitis	*Neisseria meningitidis*	Children under 5, adolescents, college students living in dormitories
Viral (aseptic) meningitis	Herpes simplex and zoster; mumps, Epstein–Barr virus; cytomegalovirus (CMV)	All ages
Encephalitis	St. Louis encephalitis virus, Eastern and Western equine virus transmitted by ticks and mosquitoes; herpes simplex; rabies; after vaccination with measles, mumps, or rubella	All ages
Brain abscess	Secondary infection from streptococci, staphylococci, pneumococci	30 to 40 years old; higher incidence in men

MENINGITIS

Meningitis is an inflammation of the meninges of the brain and spinal cord. Bacterial meningitis may result from *Neisseria meningitidis* (meningococcal meningitis), *Streptococcus pneumoniae,* or *Haemophilus influenzae.* Organisms enter the brain by way of (1) the bloodstream, (2) the respiratory tract, or (3) penetrating wounds of the skull or cranial surgery. Most often, meningitis is secondary to another infection such as otitis media, an upper respiratory infection, or pneumonia. Viral meningitis, also called aseptic meningitis, is a less severe disease than bacterial meningitis. It is caused by several common viruses (see Table 38-7).

Once the bacteria or virus enters the central nervous system, it begins an inflammatory response in the meninges, CSF, and ventricles. The inflammatory process increases production of CSF. This can lead to cerebral edema and increased ICP. Although viral infection also triggers the inflammatory response, the course of the disease is shorter. Recovery is usually uneventful.

Manifestations show an irritation of the meninges, as outlined in Box 38-14 ■. Two positive signs of meningeal irritation are Brudzinski's sign and Kernig's sign. In Brudzinski's sign, when the client's neck is flexed, the knees and hips flex. Kernig's sign is an inability to extend the leg when the hip is flexed at a 90-degree angle. The client may also show signs of IICP, including decreased LOC, seizures, and changes in vital signs and respiratory pattern.

Complications of meningitis may include seizures, hydrocephalus, cerebral infarction, coma, and death. Meningitis may leave residual effects such as visual deficits, deafness, cranial nerve palsies, or hemiplegia.

Meningococcal meningitis can progress to the devastating complication of meningococcemia. This form of meningitis is spread by airborne droplets and is highly contagious. It can cause death within 10 to 12 hours after the client develops a high fever and petechial rash. Death results from an overwhelming septicemia, vascular collapse, and adrenal hemorrhage.

ENCEPHALITIS

Encephalitis is an acute inflammation of the white and gray matter of the brain and spinal cord. It is almost always caused by a virus, but it may also be caused by bacteria or fungi (see Table 38-7). Many of the viruses are associated with certain seasons of the year or particular geographic regions. The virus may be transmitted by ticks or mosquitoes.

Encephalitis ranges from a mild infection to a serious disease that could be fatal. There is widespread inflammation of the white and gray matter of the brain and spinal cord. Nerve cells may be extensively damaged. Edema and areas of necrosis may lead to localized hemorrhage. IICP develops, progressing to brain herniation, unless treated. Certain viruses tend to affect specific areas of the brain. For example, herpes simplex virus involves the frontal and temporal lobes. Manifestations are similar

BOX 38-14

MANIFESTATIONS OF MENINGITIS

- Headache
- High fever
- Photophobia
- Nausea, vomiting
- Nuchal rigidity (stiff neck)
- Positive Brudzinski's sign
- Positive Kernig's sign
- Restlessness and irritability
- Confusion, altered LOC
- Signs of IICP (elevated blood pressure, bradycardia, change in respiratory pattern, decreased LOC)
- Seizures
- Petechial rash (in meningococcal meningitis)

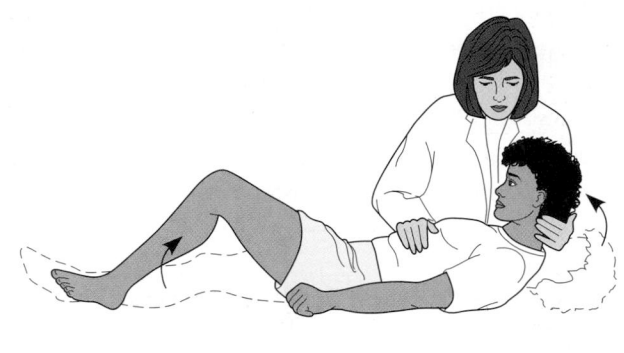

A   Brudzinski's Sign

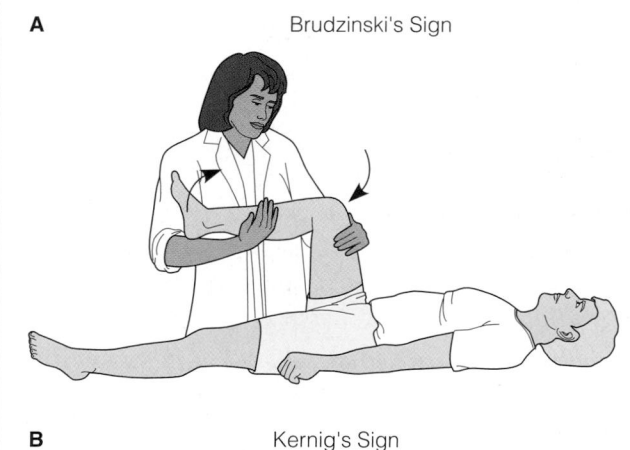

B   Kernig's Sign

The microorganisms in the brain tissue cause local inflammation. As the white blood cells destroy the organisms, pus forms. The body tries to protect the rest of the brain by forming a capsule around the pus. Unless the abscess is treated, the capsule enlarges and compresses nerves and brain tissue. Chronic inflammation can lead to edema and IICP.

Initially, the client complains of a headache, fever, chills, and malaise. As the abscess expands, nausea, vomiting, drowsiness, confusion, weakness on one side, and seizures develop.

INTERDISCIPLINARY CARE

Bacterial meningitis is a medical emergency that could be fatal within days. Treatment focuses on a rapid diagnosis and starting antibiotic therapy immediately. Depending on hospital policy, the client may be placed in Airborne Precautions isolation. Management of viral meningitis focuses on relieving client symptoms with antipyretics and analgesics. Antibiotic therapy and specific isolation precautions are not indicated for viral meningitis

The treatment for encephalitis is similar to that for meningitis, with the exception that antiviral medications are used. Isolation is not necessary, because encephalitis is not transmitted from person to person.

Treatment of the client with a brain abscess focuses on prompt beginning of antibiotic therapy. Other manifestations are treated symptomatically. When antibiotics are unsuccessful, the abscess may be surgically drained or, if encapsulated, removed during a craniotomy.

Diagnostic Tests

The diagnosis of bacterial or viral meningitis or encephalitis is based on clinical manifestations. Diagnosis of a brain abscess is more difficult because there are unclear symptoms. The following diagnostic tests may be ordered:

- *Lumbar puncture* is done to collect samples of CSF. The following findings indicate a positive diagnosis of bacterial meningitis: (1) CSF appears cloudy, (2) an elevated protein level and white blood cell count, (3) a decreased glucose level, and (4) elevated CSF pressure.
- *Culture and sensitivity* and *Gram stain* of the CSF can identify the bacteria or virus causing meningitis or encephalitis.
- *Cultures from the blood, urine, throat, and nose* are performed to identify the bacterial source of infection.
- *CT scan, MRI,* or *skull x-rays* may identify the infection source causing a brain abscess.

Medications

In cases of bacterial meningitis, high doses of intravenous penicillin or third-generation cephalosporins are started immediately. The specific antibiotic is chosen after the

to those of meningitis, including high fever, headache, stiff neck, seizures, confusion, and disorientation. As the disease progresses, the LOC deteriorates, and the client becomes comatose.

BRAIN ABSCESS

A **brain abscess** is a collection of purulent material within the brain. Many brain abscesses occur from an infection in the middle ear or nasal sinuses. They may develop after a head injury or intracranial surgery. Other sources include bacterial endocarditis; osteomyelitis; and lung, pelvic, or skin infections. Streptococci, staphylococci, and pneumococci are often the underlying causes.

culture and sensitivity report identifies the causative organism. Antibiotic therapy is given in high doses so that it will cross the blood–brain barrier and reach the CSF. (For an in-depth discussion of antibiotic therapy, see Chapter 10. 🔗) Drug therapy is continued from 7 to 21 days. The CDC recommends that isolation be continued for 24 hours after antibiotic therapy started. Antibiotics are also used to treat brain abscesses.

Anyone exposed to meningococcal meningitis is started on prophylactic antibiotic therapy immediately. The drugs of choice are rifampin (Rifadin) and ciprofloxacin (Cipro). All cases of meningitis must be reported to the local public health department.

Treatment for encephalitis consists of antiviral drugs such as vidarabine (Vira-A) and acyclovir (Zovirax). If started early in the disease course, they may decrease mortality. They are most effective if used before the client becomes comatose.

Additional medications are given to relieve symptoms and to prevent complications from any one of the intracranial infections. Anticonvulsant medications prevent or control seizures. Antipyretics are used to reduce fever. Analgesics such as acetaminophen are given to relieve headache and neck pain. Osmotic diuretics and corticosteroids may decrease cerebral edema. The client initially may require antiemetics to control nausea and vomiting. Intravenous fluids may be necessary to prevent dehydration until the client is able to take oral fluids.

NURSING CARE

Clients with an intracranial infection are acutely ill. Depending on the extent of their illness, they may be cared for in the critical care unit or on a medical unit. If neurologic deficits are present, long-term nursing may be needed. The combination of fever, dehydration, and cerebral edema predisposes the client to seizures.

ASSESSING

An important aspect of care is to obtain a careful history and identify subjective and objective data. Box 38-15 ■ outlines data to collect on the client with an intracranial infection.

DIAGNOSING, PLANNING, AND IMPLEMENTING

Priorities in Nursing Care. When caring for clients with intracranial infections, the priority nursing diagnoses are Risk for Ineffective Tissue Perfusion: Cerebral, and Hyperthermia. Nursing care also focuses on reducing the client's headache and photophobia caused by meningeal irritation.

BOX 38-15	ASSESSMENT

Assessing Clients with Intracranial Infections

SUBJECTIVE DATA

- Presence of nausea, vomiting, photophobia, or stiff neck.
- Confusion or headache.
- Exposure to mosquitoes or ticks.
- History of head injury, brain surgery, otitis media, or bacterial endocarditis.

OBJECTIVE DATA

- Blood pressure, pulse, and temperature.
- Assess orientation, LOC, memory, and response to stimuli.
- Assess for dizziness, diplopia, drooping eyelids, pupil changes, and hearing difficulty due to cranial nerve damage.
- Assess for Brudzinski's or Kernig's signs (see Box 38-14, Figures A and B).
- Observe for any seizure activity, restlessness, and/or agitation.
- Inspect skin for presence of petechial rash over the body.

Risk for Ineffective Tissue Perfusion: Cerebral

- Monitor for altered neurologic function. See interventions for IICP discussed earlier in this chapter. *Inflammation from intracranial infections increases the client's risk for developing altered levels of consciousness, seizures, increased IICP, and cranial nerve dysfunction.*

Hyperthermia

- Monitor body temperature at least every 4 hours. *Clients with intracranial infections can spike high fevers, which could lead to seizures.*
- Remove unnecessary clothing and bed linen. Give antipyretic medications, tepid sponge baths, or use a cooling blanket as ordered. *Antipyretic drugs, tepid sponge baths, and a cooling blanket can reduce a fever. Removing unnecessary clothing and bed linen promotes cooling. The temperature is decreased slowly to prevent shivering, which can raise the temperature higher.*
- Monitor for signs and symptoms of dehydration noting skin turgor, mucous membranes, and daily body weight. Measure and compare intake and output every 2 to 4 hours. Note urine concentration. *Fluids are restricted in clients with intracranial disorders to prevent cerebral edema. When a high fever exists, fluids are quickly lost, increasing risk for dehydration.*

Acute Pain

- Reduce environmental stimuli; keep room quiet and dim bright lights. *Environmental stimuli can increase the client's headache. Low lighting may decrease hallucinations and photophobia.*

- Provide gentle ROM exercises. *ROM exercises reduce joint stiffness and promote circulation.*
- Place client in position of comfort. *Positioning may decrease the client's muscle and joint aches.*
- Place a cool cloth over the client's eyes. *This may decrease the client's headache and the discomfort of photophobia.*
- Give a mild analgesic such as acetaminophen or codeine. *Meperidine and morphine sulfate are avoided because they can alter the size and reaction of the client's pupils.*

EVALUATING

Evaluate the effectiveness of the nursing care for a client with an intracranial infection by collecting the following data:

- Temperature within normal range
- Absence of headache and neurologic irritation
- No signs of IICP
- Knowledge of anti-infective therapy.

Documenting. Documentation focuses on VS; LOC; neurologic deficits such as dizziness, diplopia, hearing loss, and seizures; and presence of headache, photophobia, and petechial rash. The nurse records client teaching related to medications, symptoms to report, diet, and rest.

CONTINUING CARE

Following the acute phase of an intracranial infection, the client requires several weeks of convalescence. The client and family need to understand home management. The nurse assesses the client's and family's abilities and resources to provide care after discharge.

Include the following topics in the teaching session:

- Medications: use, dose, and side effects. Emphasize the importance of taking all antibiotic or antiviral medica-

tion until completely gone to prevent new organisms from growing.
- Emphasize the importance of reporting fever, headache, or neck stiffness in people who had close contact with the client with meningitis.
- Encourage adequate rest and sleep as well as a well-balanced diet.
- Advise to increase physical activity gradually.
- Stress the importance of reporting any signs or symptoms of ear infection, sore throat, or upper respiratory infection.

The client with permanent neurologic deficits resulting from encephalitis is usually discharged to a rehabilitation setting or a long-term care facility. For infections transmitted by mosquitoes, the client and family need to know how to destroy breeding sites of insect larvae. They are also taught to avoid mosquito and tick bites by wearing protective clothing and insect repellents.

Headaches

Headache is one of the most common symptoms people experience at all ages. They may result from brain tumors, meningitis, head injuries, stress, muscle tension, or a combination of these factors. Most headaches are mild and are relieved by a mild analgesic. Other headaches are chronic, intense, and recurring. Clinical manifestations vary according to the cause and type of the headache.

The cranium has many pain-sensitive structures. These include the skin, muscles, and periosteum of the skull; the nasal cavities and sinuses; parts of the meninges; cerebral blood vessels; and cranial nerves with sensory function. Stretching, inflammation, pressure, and dilation of the pain-sensitive structures can produce a headache. The most common types of headaches are migraine, cluster, and tension headaches (Table 38-8 ■).

TABLE 38-8			
Types of Headaches			
TYPE	RISK FACTORS	DESCRIPTION	MANIFESTATIONS
Migraine	More common in women. Family history of migraine headaches	May be triggered by stress or crisis; foods such as alcohol, chocolate, caffeine, or nuts. Often correlates with menstrual cycle. May last hours to days. Migraine with aura usually lasts less than an hour.	*No aura:* pulsating or throbbing headache on one side of the head. Accompanied by nausea, vomiting, and sensitivity to light and sound. *Aura:* Preceded by aura, then same symptoms as above.
Cluster	More common in men	Series of headaches over a 2- to 3-month period, then disappear for a long period of time.	Unilateral pain located around or behind the eye that can wake the client; also nasal congestion, tearing, facial flushing.
Tension	More common in women	May be triggered by stress, eyestrain, or poor posture. These triggers can cause muscle contraction in neck, face, and scalp.	Bilateral pain, tightness, pressure, or viselike feeling; pain is most common on awakening.

MIGRAINE HEADACHE

Migraine headaches are the most common type of vascular headache. The exact causes are uncertain. It is believed that they result from abnormal cerebral blood flow, increased release of serotonin, or abnormal genes that control the activities of certain brain cells. Migraines differ in intensity, duration, and frequency from client to client, and episodes may be different in the same person (see Table 38-8).

CLUSTER HEADACHE

The cluster headache is a form of vascular headache. It typically begins 2 to 3 hours after the person falls asleep. The attacks usually occur in clusters of 1 to 8 daily for weeks or a few months; then they disappear for an extended period. Usually, the same side of the head is involved in each cluster of attacks. Cluster headaches can be triggered by alcohol consumption.

TENSION HEADACHE

Tension headaches often result from prolonged muscle contraction of the head and neck. They are poorly localized with a gradual onset. Occupations that require a prolonged period of abnormal posture such as bending over a desk often precipitate tension headache. Slouching while reading or watching television can lead to muscle contraction. Most headaches are tension headaches.

INTERDISCIPLINARY CARE

The first priority of care is to identify the underlying cause of the headache. If the cause is treatable, the headache symptoms should decrease or disappear. Migraine headaches are managed by drug therapy, client teaching, and controlling of triggers. Eliminating alcohol may reduce the incidence of cluster headaches. Improving poor posture and initiating comfort measures such as gentle massage or heat may help reduce tension headaches.

A thorough history and physical examination are part of the diagnosis and treatment. A brain scan, MRI, x-ray studies of the skull and cervical spine, EEG, and lumbar puncture for CSF are used to rule out other neurologic problems. Serum metabolic screens and hypersensitivity testing also may be performed if systemic problems are suspected.

Medications

The choice of medications for managing headaches depends on the specific type of headache. The goals are to reduce the frequency and severity of headaches and to limit or stop a headache when it occurs.

To reduce the frequency and severity of migraines, several prophylactic medications are ordered. Propranolol (Inderal) prevents dilation of cerebral blood vessels, and verapamil (Isoptin) controls cerebral vasospasms. Amitriptyline (Elavil) blocks the uptake of serotonin and catecholamines.

Methysergide maleate (Sansert) decreases serotonin action; however, it can produce severe side effects and must be used cautiously.

Before a migraine becomes severe, ergotamine (Ergomar) or ergotamine with caffeine (Cafergot) is given by oral, sublingual, rectal, or intranasal route. When given at the first sign of an attack, ergotamine is effective in controlling up to 70% of acute attacks. Two serotonin agonists, sumatriptan (Imitrex) and zolmitriptan (Zomig), act rapidly to stop migraines. Sumatriptan (Imitrex) is available for oral, subcutaneous, or intranasal use.

Once a migraine attack is in progress, narcotic analgesics such as codeine or meperidine (Demerol) may be needed. Antiemetics such as promethazine (Phenergan) or metoclopramide (Reglan) are given to control nausea and vomiting.

Many of the same medications used for migraines may treat cluster headaches. Some clients gain relief from a cluster headache by inhaling 100% oxygen at 7 to 9 L/min for 15 minutes. Ergotamine tartrate may be given in suppository form at bedtime to prevent cluster headaches.

Nonnarcotic analgesics such as aspirin or acetaminophen may be effective in relieving tension headaches. For prophylaxis, amitriptyline (Elavil) may be given at bedtime.

Complementary Therapy

Biofeedback and meditation are used to reduce stress and possible tension headaches. Kava relaxes skeletal muscles, relieving tension that may lead to a tension headache. Some clients with migraines have received relief from acupuncture, exercise, biofeedback, and the herbal supplement feverfew. Other complementary therapies for headaches include riboflavin, vitamin D, and magnesium.

NURSING CARE

Nursing care begins by obtaining a history and description of the headache. It is important to identify the effects of recurring headaches on the client's daily life. Box 38-16 ■ lists assessment data to collect. Nursing interventions focus on controlling the pain and discomfort of the headache.

Pain

- Ask the client to rate the pain on a scale of 0 to 10 (10 = the worst pain) or provide a visual analog of faces that show different levels of discomfort. *Rating scales provide objective data about the client's subjective pain or discomfort. They can also evaluate the effectiveness of pain relief measures.*

- Minimize light, noise, and activity. Provide rest in a quiet, nonstimulating environment when the headache is present. *Reducing environmental stimuli may decrease pain.*

BOX 38-16 ASSESSMENT

Assessing Clients with Headaches

SUBJECTIVE DATA

- Describe headaches: type of pain, frequency, duration, location, radiation, precipitating factors, time of day it occurs, relieving factors.
- Any light flashes or bright spots before the headache begins?
- Does nausea, vomiting, or numbness accompany headache?
- Interference with daily activities or associated with stress.
- Exposure to toxic chemicals at work.
- Family history of migraines.
- Medication and alcohol use.

OBJECTIVE DATA

- Observe for facial flushing and tearing (present with cluster headaches).
- Observe for pallor, diaphoresis, and one-sided weakness (present with migraines).
- Note presence of nausea, vomiting, or diarrhea.
- Palpate neck and shoulder muscles for tightness (present with tension headaches).

- Encourage the client to use deep breathing or relaxation techniques. *These strategies reduce tension and may help the client gain a sense of control over the pain.*
- Apply cold or warm cloth to the head and neck as ordered. *Cold causes vasoconstriction, which may reduce pain in vascular headaches. Heat reduces muscle tension and improves circulation.*

- Offer a back massage. *Massage promotes muscle relaxation, which is especially useful for tension headaches.*

Collect the following information to evaluate the effectiveness of providing care to the client with headaches:

- Decreased or absence of pain
- Understands medications
- Modifies lifestyle to reduce headaches.

CONTINUING CARE

Because headaches are managed at home, client education is the main focus. Teach the client how to limit attacks and to reduce the effects of headaches. Clients with long-term or migraine headaches may be referred for stress reduction or biofeedback classes. The teaching session should include the following points:

- Teach about medication use, dosage, and side effects.
- Report ergotamine side effects (e.g., numbness and tingling in fingers and toes, leg weakness, and aching muscles)
- Eliminate caffeine, cured meats, monosodium glutamate (MSG), and foods containing tyramine (chocolate, red wine, aged cheese); avoiding smoking.
- Participate in regular moderate exercise.
- Avoid fasting, fatigue, and irregular sleep patterns.
- Keep a headache diary.
- Identify comfort measures during a headache: darkened, quiet room and applying a cool cloth to the forehead.

Note: The bibliography listings for this and all chapters have been compiled at the back of the book.

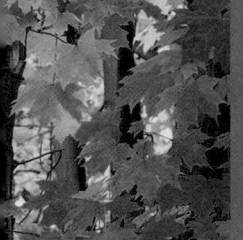

Chapter Review

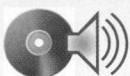 KEY TERMS by Topics

Use the audio glossary feature of either the CD-ROM or the Companion Website to hear the correct pronunciation of the following key terms.

Head Injuries
rhinorrhea, otorrhea, concussion, contusion, intracranial pressure (ICP), hematoma

Brain Tumor
brain tumors, debulking

Cerebrovascular Accident
cerebrovascular accident (CVA), transient ischemic attack (TIA), anoxia, contralateral, hemiplegia, aphasia (expressive, receptive, or global), homonymous hemianopia, emotional lability, carotid endarterectomy

Aneurysm
aneurysm, subarachnoid hemorrhage

Seizure Disorder
seizure, convulsion, epilepsy, epileptogenic focus, jacksonian march, automatisms, aura, tonic contractions, clonic contractions, status epilepticus

Intracranial Infections
meningitis, encephalitis, brain abscess

KEY Points

- The highest incidence for traumatic brain injuries is for people between the ages of 1 and 35 and the older adult. In the elderly, falls are a frequent cause of brain trauma.

- Increasing ICP is a medical emergency and must be treated immediately to prevent permanent brain damage or death.

- Subtle changes such as restlessness and drowsiness indicate a change in neurologic function and must be reported promptly.

- Intracranial surgery increases the risk of meningitis. It is extremely important to use aseptic technique when changing any wound dressing.

- Older adults often ignore the symptoms of a TIA, mistakenly thinking it is part of the normal aging process because the symptoms disappear after a short time.

- The primary risk factors for a stroke are hypertension, atherosclerosis, cardiac disease, smoking, and age. Discuss potential lifestyle changes with high-risk clients.

- Clients with seizure disorders must understand their anticonvulsant medications and the importance of not discontinuing them without medical supervision.

- Meningococcemia, a complication of meningococcal meningitis, can cause death in 10 to 12 hours. Any client with a high fever and petechial rash must be seen by a physician immediately.

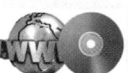 EXPLORE MediaLink

Additional interactive resources for this chapter can be found on the Companion Website at www.prenhall.com/burke. Click on Chapter 38 and "Begin" to select the activities for this chapter.

For chapter-related NCLEX-style review questions and an audio glossary, access the accompanying CD-ROM in this book.

FOR FURTHER Study

See Chapter 7 for more information about arterial blood gases.

See Chapter 9 for a discussion of routine preoperative and postoperative care.

For an in-depth discussion of antibiotic therapy, see Chapter 10.

For brain death criteria, see Box 13-11 in Chapter 13.

For more information on liver function tests, see Chapter 18.

See Chapter 28 for more information about anticoagulant therapy.

See Chapter 31 for normal levels for serum creatinine and BUN tests.

Critical Thinking Care Map

Caring for a Client after a Cerebrovascular Accident
NCLEX-PN® Focus Area: Physiologic Integrity; Reduction of Risk Potential

Case Study: Mr. Boren, a 68-year-old African American male, had a CVA this morning. He is drowsy but responds to verbal stimuli by nodding his head to indicate "yes" when asked questions. He has flaccid paralysis in his left arm and left leg (he is left-handed). He shows visual field deficits that indicate homonymous hemianopia. A CT scan confirms the diagnosis of a right-brain CVA due to a thrombus of the middle cerebral artery. Mr. Boren is started on a continuous IV heparin infusion.

Nursing Diagnosis: Impaired Verbal Communication

COLLECT DATA

Subjective	Objective
_____	_____
_____	_____
_____	_____
_____	_____
_____	_____

Would you report this data? Yes/No

If yes, to: _____

Nursing Care

_____

_____

_____

_____

_____

_____

_____

_____

_____

_____

How would you document this? _____

_____

_____

_____

Data Collected
(use those that apply)

- Lack of eye contact
- Left arm and leg flaccid
- Nods off while people speak to him
- Nods head to answer questions
- Makes a clenched fist of right hand when trying to speak
- Eyes look pleading

Nursing Interventions
(use those that apply; list in priority order)

- Provide a large marker and tablet.
- Place objects, call bell, and tissues on Mr. Boren's unaffected side.
- Use short, simple sentences when talking to Mr. Boren.
- Provide adaptive devices (silverware with thick handles and nonslip plates) for Mr. Boren to use.
- Contact speech therapy for consultation.
- Encourage Mrs. Boren to visit at mealtimes.
- Explain all health care procedures.
- Maintain a calm, unhurried manner.

NCLEX-PN® Exam Preparation

1 A client was accidentally struck in the head by a baseball bat. Which condition should the nurse anticipate as a serious complication?

A. clear fluid draining from the ears
B. large hematoma at the impact site
C. headache
D. complaints of dizziness

2 Which of the following risk factors in the client's history is most likely to increase the potential in developing a CVA?

A. age 50 or older
B. use of oral contraceptives for the past 10 years
C. presence of atherosclerosis
D. consumption of one beer per day
E. overweight by 50 pounds
F. Caucasian race

3 Following a lumbar puncture, which nursing action should the nurse implement?

A. Remind the client to not move legs after the procedure.
B. Monitor the puncture site for CSF leakage.
C. Have the patient empty his bladder.
D. Limit the client's fluid intake.

4 What teaching point should the nurse emphasize to a client taking phenytoin (Dilantin) on a daily basis?

A. Check urine for brownish color.
B. Report fatigue and weakness.
C. Do not take with food.
D. Brush and floss daily.

5 A client experienced a blow to the right frontal region of the head. If the client begins to develop increased intracranial pressure, which manifestation should the nurse see first?

A. decreased heart rate
B. sluggish response by pupils to light
C. irritability
D. projectile vomiting

6 What manifestation is most often seen in a client with brain tumor located in the occipital lobe?

A. diplopia
B. psychomotor seizures
C. contralateral hemiparesis
D. expressive aphasia

7 Which nursing diagnosis has the highest priority for a client with status epilepticus?

A. Anxiety
B. Risk for Injury
C. Risk for Ineffective Airway Clearance
D. Risk for Ineffective Tissue Perfusion: Cerebral

8 A client is being discharged from the emergency department with a diagnosis of migraine headaches. It is most important to include which of the following teaching points?

A. Keep a headache diary.
B. Identify comfort measures during a headache.
C. Refer client to stress reduction classes.
D. Teach client how to reduce frequency of attacks.

9 The physician notes the following findings: positive Brudzinski's and Kernig's signs, increased ICP, sputum cultures positive for *Streptococcus pneumoniae*. Based on this information, the nurse can anticipate that the physician will diagnose this client with:

A. encephalitis.
B. brain abscess.
C. bacterial meningitis.
D. subdural hematoma.

10 A client begins to seize during your assessment. Place these actions in the sequence that the nurse should do them.

A. Clear area of objects that could cause injury.
B. Loosen the gown.
C. Turn the client on his side.
D. Pad the side rails as soon as possible.
E. Provide supplemental oxygen.
F. Place pillow under the client's head.

Answers for Review Questions, as well as discussion of Care Plan and Critical Thinking Care Map questions, appear in Appendix V.

Chapter 39

Caring for Clients with Degenerative Neurologic and Spinal Cord Disorders

BRIEF Outline

Alzheimer's Disease
Multiple Sclerosis
Parkinson's Disease
Myasthenia Gravis
Huntington's Disease
Amyotropic Lateral Sclerosis
Guillain–Barré Syndrome
Spinal Cord Injury
Herniated Intervertebral Disk

LEARNING Outcomes

After completing this chapter, you will be able to:

• Describe the causes, pathophysiology, and manifestations of common degenerative neurologic disorders and spinal cord injuries.

• Discuss the nursing implications for medications and treatments ordered for clients experiencing degenerative neurologic disorders.

• Describe the client's functional ability according to the level of damage to the spinal cord.

• Describe the interdisciplinary care required for clients with quadriplegia and other spinal cord disorders.

• Reinforce teaching to clients with a degenerative neurologic disorder.

• Use the nursing process to assess, plan, and implement individualized care for the client with degenerative neurologic and spinal cord disorders.

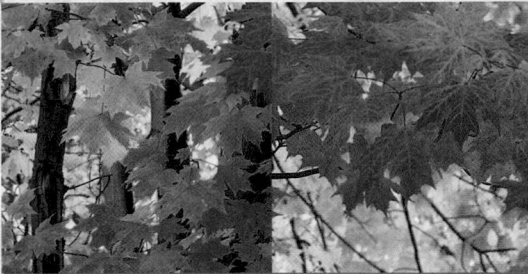

MediaLink

www.prenhall.com/burke
Use the address above to access the free, interactive Companion Website created for this textbook. Get hints, instant feedback, and textbook references to chapter-related NCLEX-style questions. Link to other interesting sites.

Audio Glossary:
Use the Companion Website, or the CD-ROM disk enclosed with your textbook, to hear the pronunciation of key terms in this chapter.

Degenerative neurologic disorders disrupt the central nervous system (CNS) and the peripheral nerves. They can cause devastating physical and emotional changes. The client and family often face lifestyle and role changes and may even experience financial difficulties. The exact cause of these disorders is uncertain. Some may have a genetic or autoimmune cause.

Spinal cord injuries and herniated disk problems are also discussed in this chapter. Permanent damage to the spinal cord can also present physical and psychologic challenges to the client and caregiver.

DEGENERATIVE NEUROLOGIC DISORDERS

Common degenerative disorders of the CNS include Alzheimer's disease, multiple sclerosis, Parkinson's disease, myasthenia gravis, Huntington's disease, and amyotrophic lateral sclerosis. Guillain–Barré syndrome is an example of a disorder affecting the peripheral nerves.

Cranial nerve disorders may be caused by trauma or inflammation. The pairs of cranial nerves are described in Chapter 37. ⚭ The most common cranial nerve disorders affect the trigeminal (cranial nerve V) and the facial (cranial nerve VII) nerves.

A variety of nervous system disorders may have toxic or infectious causes. These disorders are rare but require significant nursing care when they occur. Rabies, tetanus, and Creutzfeldt–Jakob disease are presented in the last part of this section.

Alzheimer's Disease

Alzheimer's disease (AD) is a progressive, irreversible deterioration of the brain. It is characterized by a gradual loss of intellectual functioning. An estimated 4 million adults in the United States have Alzheimer's disease, the most common type of dementia. It affects adults in middle to late life. As one ages, the risk of developing AD increases. Genetic defects on chromosomes 1, 14, 19, and 21 are associated with Alzheimer's disease.

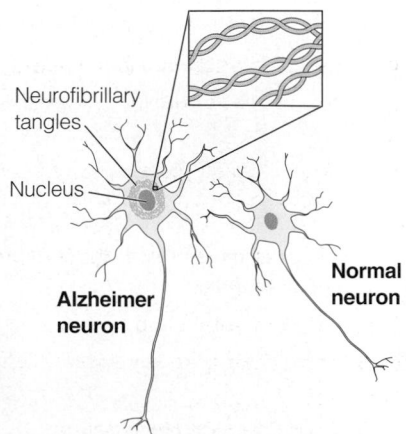

Figure 39-1. ■ Neuron with neurofibrillary tangles seen in Alzheimer's disease.

PATHOPHYSIOLOGY AND MANIFESTATIONS

Four pathologic changes are seen in the brains of AD clients: (1) loss of nerve cells, (2) reduced brain size, (3) presence of neurofibrillary tangles (Figure 39-1 ■), and (4) neuritic plaques. A protein substance called amyloid causes the plaque formation. The neurofibrillary tangles and plaque lead to altered nerve impulse transmission. This results in loss of memory and cognition. There is also a decrease in acetylcholine, a neurotransmitter that is essential for memory. AD affects the frontal lobe first and then involves the entire brain.

Alzheimer's disease is staged according to the client's symptoms and abilities (Box 39-1 ■). It develops slowly over a long period of time, with the first sign being memory loss.

BOX 39-1

MANIFESTATIONS OF ALZHEIMER'S DISEASE

Stage 1 (Approximately 2 to 4 Years)
- Short-term memory loss; forgets location and names of objects
- Attempts to cover up memory loss
- Has difficulty learning new information or making decisions
- Decreased attention span
- Can be angry or depressed

Stage 2 (Approximately 2 to 12 Years)
- Unable to remember names of family members and gets lost in familiar locations
- Easily agitated and irritable
- Has difficulty using objects, reading, writing, and speaking
- Cannot follow a conversation
- Personal hygiene declines
- Unable to make decisions (e.g., choose clothing)
- Walks with unsteady gait, head down, shoulders bent, shuffles
- Exhibits "sundowning" and wandering behavior

Stage 3 (Approximately 1 to 4 Years)
- Cannot recognize self or others
- Inability to communicate
- Has delusions and hallucinations
- Bowel and bladder incontinence

Memory deficits are subtle so that family and friends may not suspect a problem or deny that a problem exists. There is a progressive decline in cognition and judgment. The client exhibits **sundowning syndrome** (behavior characterized by increased agitation, disorientation to time, and wandering during afternoon and evening hours). In the last stage, the caregiver must meet the client's activities of daily living (ADLs). Common complications include pneumonia, dehydration, malnutrition, and falls. Prognosis is poor, and death frequently occurs from pneumonia secondary to aspiration.

INTERDISCIPLINARY CARE

Without the hope of a cure, the client and family face a long, devastating illness. They will need long-term followup and support.

Diagnostic Tests

Diagnosing AD begins by ruling out other causes for the client's symptoms. A complete blood count (CBC), thyroid studies, and electrolyte levels are used to exclude the following conditions: urinary tract infection (UTI) or pneumonia, hypothyroidism, and malnutrition and fluid or electrolyte imbalances. The only definitive method of diagnosis is postmortem examination of brain tissue. The following diagnostic tests are performed:

- *Electroencephalogram (EEG)* may show a slowed brain wave pattern in the late stages.
- *Magnetic resonance imaging (MRI)* and *computed tomography (CT) scan* of the brain may show decreased brain size in the late stages.
- *Positron emission tomography (PET) scan* can show reduced glucose levels in the affected areas of the brain.
- *Mini-Mental Status Examination (MMSE)* shows the loss of memory and other cognitive skills over time.

Medications

Cholinesterase inhibitor drugs, such as tacrine hydrochloride (Cognex), donepezil (Aricept), and rivastigmine (Exelon) block the breakdown of acetylcholine. They seem to slow cognitive decline and in some clients improve reasoning and memory. Because they cause liver toxicity, liver function is monitored frequently. Memantine (Ebixa), a new drug that blocks glutamate to protect the brain cells, is being used in late-stage AD. Selective serotonin reuptake inhibitors such as fluoxetine (Prozac) are given to treat depression. To control behavioral symptoms, risperidone (Risperdal) is used because it has fewer side effects than haloperidol (Haldol).

Complementary Therapy

Ginkgo biloba seems to improve memory but does not cure AD. It must be used cautiously in clients taking anticoagulants because it increases bleeding. Antioxidants such as vitamin C, vitamin E, and coenzyme 10 may slow the progression of AD. Huperzine A, a traditional Chinese medicine, acts as an acetylcholinesterase inhibitor. Massage, art, and music therapy can help reduce agitation.

NURSING CARE

Clients with AD require supportive nursing interventions to help them cope with their physical and psychological needs. The nurse assumes an important role in reinforcing teaching of the client and family as well as assisting with referrals to community services.

ASSESSING

The nurse collects subjective and objective data to guide the type of care the client will need (Box 39-2 ■).

DIAGNOSING, PLANNING, AND IMPLEMENTING

Priorities in Nursing Care. Nursing care focuses on assisting the client and caregiver to maintain the highest quality of life. Care can be as simple as altering the client's environment to full nursing assistance as the client declines.

Disturbed Thought Processes

- Orient the client to person, place, and time frequently; place large, easy-to-read calendars and clocks within

---

BOX 39-2	ASSESSMENT

Assessing Clients with Alzheimer's Disease

SUBJECTIVE DATA

- Change in memory or concentration.
- Difficulty making everyday decisions.
- Easily irritated or restless; frequency of nighttime wakening.
- Has difficulty using the correct word for an object.
- Past medical history of head trauma, CNS infection, or exposure to metals.
- Family history of Alzheimer's disease.

OBJECTIVE DATA

- Observe client for lapses in memory or thought processes and ability to recognize family.
- Assess orientation to time, place, and person.
- Observe for unkempt physical appearance in client's clothing and grooming.
- Note affect and ability to follow conversation.
- Note any deficits in speaking or reading.

client's line of vision. *Orientation promotes reality and reduces confusion.*

- Keep the daily routine the same. Assign the same caregivers. *Daily routines and familiar staff decrease confusion and help the client cope.*
- Place client in a quiet environment with soft music. *A quiet environment is less distracting to a confused client and reduces agitation. Soft music may be soothing.*
- Schedule rest periods or quiet times throughout the day. *Fatigue contributes to confusion.*
- Keep familiar objects in the same place. *This will help them remember where objects are and decreases confusion.*
- Set boundaries by placing red or yellow tape on the floor. *Boundaries help the client stay within safe areas.*

clinical ALERT

Older adults see red or yellow more easily.

Self-Care Deficits

- Encourage as much self-care as possible. *This promotes independence and activates the client's memory.*
- Demonstrate use of equipment (e.g., comb, toothbrush, eating utensils). *Visual cues help client remember prior tasks.*
- Perform daily bathing and hygiene measures as needed. *Clients in stages 2 and 3 often forget ADLs or fight bathing. Pressure ulcers may go unnoticed unless daily bathing is done.*
- Modify clothing with Velcro and lay out daily clothing. *Velcro closures are easier for client to use. Preselected clothing decreases frustration.*
- Encourage fluids during the day. *AD clients forget to drink fluids and may become dehydrated.*
- If hyperactive, provide a high-calorie diet. Encourage "finger foods" such as sandwiches and fruit. *Hyperactivity increases metabolism and the risk for malnutrition.*
- Limit the number of foods placed in front of the client at one time. Cut food into bite-size pieces. *Too many foods at one time can be confusing.*

Caregiver Role Strain

- Discuss the physical and emotional demands of caregiving with the caregiver and family. *Discussion allows the caregiver and family an opportunity to think about their future needs.*
- Teach the caregivers to take rest periods and avoid fatigue. *Caregivers feel overwhelmed by their responsibilities. They become physically and mentally exhausted and socially isolated.*
- Refer client and family to local AD support groups, national AD association, and home health. *Support groups and home health can assist in coping with the diagnosis.*

- Provide financial or social service referrals. *Referrals assist families in planning for long-term care.*

EVALUATING

Evaluate the effectiveness of nursing care by collecting data on the client's level of altered thought processes and self-care deficits. Also, evaluate the caregiver's physical and emotional endurance to care for the client.

Documenting. Documentation includes description of memory, cognitive, and thought deficits, ability to provide self-care, and client and caregiver teaching.

CONTINUING CARE

The nurse assesses the client's ability to stay in his or her home and the caregiver's ability to provide care. Review the disease process and help identify potential support systems within the family and community. If the client will be cared for at home, address safety concerns (Box 39-3 ■). Also, suggest the following strategies for helping the client:

- Make a schedule of the client's daily activities.
- Label drawers containing client's clothes and label rooms.
- Use communication techniques to the client's level of ability.
- When the client is agitated, divert his or her attention by walking or rocking in a rocking chair.
- If the client wanders, have him or her wear a Medic-Alert bracelet or pendant.

Refer clients to social services for help with such legal matters as wills, advanced directives, and powers of attorney. Caregivers often feel alone as friends and family drift away. They become depressed and exhausted. When appropriate, recommend respite care. The need for a skilled nursing facility will cause the family many conflicting emotions. They need time to adjust to the idea but are often relieved to hand over the physical care to someone with more experience.

NURSING PROCESS CARE PLAN
Client with Alzheimer's Disease

Arthur and Ruth Joste have been married for 47 years; both are 73 years old. Their two children live in the same town. For the past 9 months, Arthur has not been able to remember friends' names and phone numbers. He miscalculates the checkbook balance and neglects his hygiene needs.

Assessment. In the neurologist's office, Mr. Joste scores 20 out of a possible 30 points on the Mini-Mental Status

BOX 39-3	CLIENT TEACHING

Safety Concerns for Client with Alzheimer's Disease

Safety Interventions

- Keep furniture in the same place and keep traffic areas free from clutter.
- Apply skidproof surface on stairs, install handrails, and mark stairs to show depth.
- Make sure that the client's shoes fit properly.
- Omit alcohol use, and limit medications that affect balance (e.g., antihypertensives).
- Use night-lights; provide ample lighting in hallways and on stairs.
- Lock cleaning solutions, pesticides, medications, and nonedible food in a cabinet.
- Protect the client from fire hazards; make matches, lighters, and cigarettes inaccessible. Modify the controls on the oven and stove.
- Install protective covers over electrical sockets, fans, and motors.
- Adjust the water heater to a safe temperature.

- Provide double lock systems to outside doors and fence the yard with a locked gate to prevent the client from wandering. Install alarms and bells on doors to sound when client attempts to exit.
- Lock up client's car keys.
- Have family or neighbor check on client at the same time every day.

Communication Techniques

- Face the client and talk directly to him or her; call the client by name.
- When first approaching the client, identify yourself.
- Use simple sentences and words with few syllables; repeat explanations as needed.
- Speak in a calm, low voice; have a relaxed approach.
- Ask one question at a time. Use questions that require only a "yes" or "no" response.
- Allow the client time to process what you are trying to say.

Examination. His wife says that she covers up mistakes for her husband and that he wanders the house for several hours at night. After an evaluation, Mr. Joste is diagnosed with Alzheimer's disease. Both have feared this diagnosis and are overwhelmed.

Diagnosis. Nursing diagnoses for Mr. Joste and his family include the following:

- *Self-Care Deficit* related to forgetfulness and declining physical abilities
- *Risk for Injury* related to decreased orientation
- *Disturbed Sleep Pattern* related to time disorientation and daytime sleeping

Expected Outcomes. The Jostes are referred to Mr. Dixon Montane, a home health nurse. The expected outcomes of care specify that Mr. Joste will:

- Participate in grooming and hygiene activities as able.
- Remain free of injury.
- Obtain a minimum of 7 uninterrupted hours of sleep a night.

Planning and Implementation. Mr. Montane makes a home visit to assess for potential hazards and to meet the Jostes' children. After touring the home, Mr. Montane recommends that Mrs. Joste remove throw rugs from hallways, and provide extra lighting in dark areas. He suggests that Mrs. Joste add a night-light in the bathroom and modify the doors with a safety lock system. He also suggests that Mr. Joste walk everyday and do simple chores to decrease daylight

sleep time and stimulate memory. He recommends labeling drawers with their contents. He reviews new communication techniques with the family.

A part-time homemaker will help Mrs. Joste with housekeeping chores. Mr. Montane also suggests hiring a home health aide to provide daily hygiene care. Mr. and Mrs. Joste will attend the weekly support group meetings for Alzheimer's disease for about 3 months.

Evaluation. Six months later, Mr. Montane's follow-up visit finds that Mr. Joste has become increasingly confused. It seems unlikely that Mr. Joste will be able to remain at home and will need placement in a long-term care facility.

Critical Thinking in the Nursing Process

1. Identify several safety interventions to teach Mr. and Mrs. Joste.
2. List five interventions to decrease agitation in clients with AD.
3. A client with stage 2 Alzheimer's disease cannot focus on eating and is easily agitated. What strategies could you use to ensure that she eats enough to meet her needs?

Multiple Sclerosis

Multiple sclerosis (MS) is a chronic, degenerative disease that damages the myelin sheath surrounding the axons of the CNS. This disorder is marked by periods of exacerbation (symptoms appear) followed by periods of remission. In the end the person is chronically disabled and may become wheelchair bound.

MS affects Caucasian females more frequently between the ages of 20 and 40. A family history and living in the cold, damp, northern part of the United States increase the risk. The exact cause is unknown, but viral infections seem to trigger an autoimmune response. Emotional stress, fatigue, pregnancy, and acute respiratory infections tend to occur before the onset of MS.

PATHOPHYSIOLOGY AND MANIFESTATIONS

Myelin sheaths make up what is known as white matter in the CNS. Multiple sclerosis destroys the myelin sheath of the spinal cord, brain, and optic nerve and replaces it with *plaque.* The plaque can develop throughout the white matter of the CNS. This process is called **demyelination.** When the myelin is destroyed, nerve impulse conduction slows.

Manifestations vary according to the area of the nervous system affected (Figure 39-2 ■). They may appear suddenly and last for days to months. As the disease progresses, exacerbations last longer and occur more often. When the nerve cells are finally destroyed, the manifestations become permanent. Fatigue is a common but often ignored symptom. Medical care is sought when the client develops diplopia, weakness, and tingling and numbness in the extremities.

An unusual characteristic of MS is the worsening of motor symptoms after a hot shower or exercise.

As the disease progresses, the client is prone to UTIs, pressure ulcers, joint contractures, injuries from falls, pneumonia, and depression. Death often results from pneumonia and a debilitated condition.

INTERDISCIPLINARY CARE

The treatment goal is to keep the client functioning for as long as possible. As the client becomes more disabled, speech, physical, and occupational therapists are consulted.

Diagnostic Tests

Manifestations are vague or mild, making an early diagnosis difficult. A positive diagnosis is based on the client's history, physical examination, and symptoms. Periodic diagnostic testing is done to follow the course of the disease. The following laboratory and diagnostic tests may be ordered:

- *Cerebrospinal fluid (CSF) analysis* reveals increased T lymphocytes, protein, and immunoglobulin G (IgG). IgG indicates increased immune system activity.
- *MRI* studies detect the plaque lesions in the white matter.
- *EEG* may show slowed brain activity during the acute stage of MS.

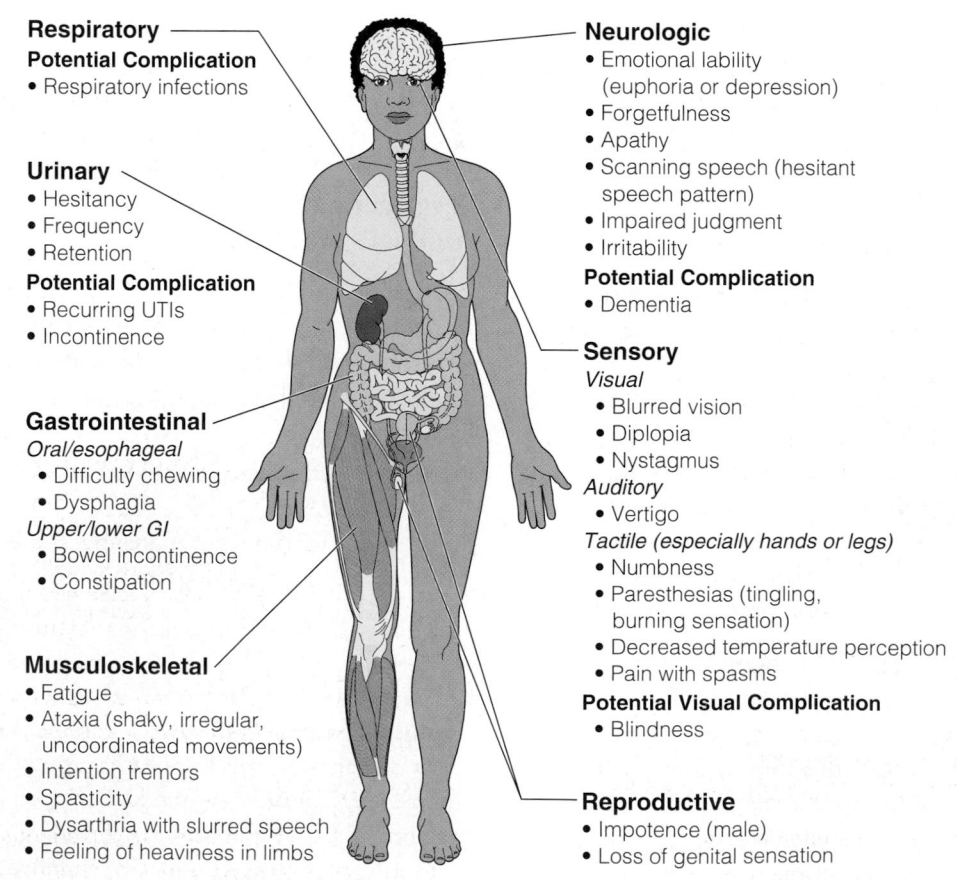

Respiratory
Potential Complication
- Respiratory infections

Urinary
- Hesitancy
- Frequency
- Retention
Potential Complication
- Recurring UTIs
- Incontinence

Gastrointestinal
Oral/esophageal
- Difficulty chewing
- Dysphagia
Upper/lower GI
- Bowel incontinence
- Constipation

Musculoskeletal
- Fatigue
- Ataxia (shaky, irregular, uncoordinated movements)
- Intention tremors
- Spasticity
- Dysarthria with slurred speech
- Feeling of heaviness in limbs

Neurologic
- Emotional lability (euphoria or depression)
- Forgetfulness
- Apathy
- Scanning speech (hesitant speech pattern)
- Impaired judgment
- Irritability
Potential Complication
- Dementia

Sensory
Visual
- Blurred vision
- Diplopia
- Nystagmus
Auditory
- Vertigo
Tactile (especially hands or legs)
- Numbness
- Paresthesias (tingling, burning sensation)
- Decreased temperature perception
- Pain with spasms
Potential Visual Complication
- Blindness

Reproductive
- Impotence (male)
- Loss of genital sensation

Figure 39-2. ■ Multisystem effects of multiple sclerosis.

Medications

A class of drugs known as immunomodulators seems to slow MS progression and reduce the number of attacks. They include beta-interferon (Avonex) and glatiramer (Copaxone). Clients with advanced MS are being treated with mitoxantrone (Novantrone), but use is limited because of its cardiotoxicity. Newer treatments include using a monoclonal antibody, natalizumab (Antegren), to alter the immune response.

Steroids are given to decrease inflammation and increase periods of remission. Muscle spasms along with pain develop in the client's extremities, which may be reduced with baclofen (Lioresal) and dantrolene (Dantrium). Fatigue is controlled with amantadine (Symmetrel). Clients with urinary retention and frequency are given bethanecol (Urecholine) and propantheline (Pro-Banthine).

Other Therapies

Physical therapists teach the client ways to maintain balance. For example, the client should stand with the feet slightly apart to give a wider base of support. The client with ataxia is taught to use a walker or cane. Spasticity is managed with stretching exercises, gait training, and the use of braces or splints. Severe spasticity and uncontrolled pain may be treated with surgical procedures such as a neurectomy (cutting a nerve), *rhizotomy* (cutting a nerve root), or cordotomy (cutting of lateral pathways in the spinal cord).

Plasmapheresis, or plasma exchange, is a procedure that removes plasma from whole blood. Its purpose is to remove T lymphocytes that cause inflammation. There has been some success with plasmapheresis causing a remission for clients with MS.

Nutrition

Diet therapy does not treat MS, but a well-balanced diet provides energy and strengthens the immune system. Reduced physical activity tends to cause weight gain and bone loss. Consult a dietitian about a diet low in calories but high in calcium and vitamin D. To prevent additional bone loss, encourage the client to perform weight-bearing activities (e.g., walking).

If the client has dysphagia, change the diet to make chewing and swallowing easier. For example, thickened drinks and small bites of food can prevent choking and fatigue. Avoid serving crackers, dry toast, or chips because they may cause choking.

NURSING CARE

MS is a lifelong illness that the client and family can manage at home. When acute infections threaten the client's life, admission to a hospital may be necessary. As the disease

| BOX 39-4 | **ASSESSMENT** |

Assessing Clients with Multiple Sclerosis

SUBJECTIVE DATA
- Extreme fatigue; diplopia or blurred vision.
- Mood swings: depression to euphoria.
- Muscle weakness or ataxia; numbness and tingling in extremities.
- Urinary frequency, retention, or incontinence; constipation.
- Difficulty chewing or swallowing; weight loss.
- Past history of viral infections, living in northern United States, physical or emotional stress, or pregnancy.
- Use of steroid or immunosuppressant medications.
- Family history of multiple sclerosis.

OBJECTIVE DATA
- Observe client for inattentiveness, difficulty finding the right word, poor coordination, muscle weakness, ataxia, and tremors.
- Note disheveled appearance or signs of incontinence.
- As the client speaks, listen for slurred speech or hesitating speech pattern.
- Auscultate for bowel tones; decreased bowel tones indicate slowed peristalsis.

advances, weakened muscle strength and spasticity increase the potential for complications from immobility. If the client becomes totally disabled and the family cannot provide care, a long-term care facility will be necessary.

ASSESSING

Assessment data collected by the nurse can help identify the diagnosis, can determine the extent to which the disease is interfering with the client's life, and can indicate the type of treatment required at this stage of the disease (Box 39-4 ■).

DIAGNOSING, PLANNING, AND IMPLEMENTING

Priorities in Nursing Care. The client experiences fatigue, decreased mobility, urinary and bowel incontinence, and altered respiratory status. In addition, the client may be unable to perform ADLs. Coping with changes in lifestyle may cause depression. Priorities of care for clients with MS include focusing on Fatigue, Self-Care Deficits, and Ineffective Coping.

Fatigue

- Observe how fatigue affects the client's ability to perform ADLs. *Knowing how fatigue affects the client will assist in planning care.*

- Plan daily activities to include rest periods. *Rest is essential to manage feelings of fatigue; relaxation periods can restore energy reserves.*

clinical ALERT

Fatigue in clients with MS is different from being "tired," so rest and sleep may not cause an improvement.

- Encourage the client to perform tasks in the morning hours. *Fatigue usually worsens in the afternoon.*

Self-Care Deficits

- Encourage the client perform as much self-care as possible. *This promotes independence and decreases feelings of helplessness.*
- Allow adequate time to perform tasks. *Weak muscles and spasticity slow the client's ability to perform all tasks.*
- Provide adaptive devices such as arm or wrist braces, long-handled combs, or modified clothing. Provide shower chair or raised toilet seat. *Adaptive devices encourage the client to perform ADLs and may reduce fatigue.*

Ineffective Coping

- Encourage the client to state his or her feelings. Consult with a counselor or psychiatrist as needed. *Clients with MS feel helpless and isolated. They often believe they cannot effectively manage the symptoms of MS.*
- Refer to a support group and provide information about the National MS Society. *Support groups and the National MS Society can offer suggestions for coping with MS.*
- Refer to state vocational rehabilitation agency as needed. *Vocational rehabilitation agencies can assist the client with job retraining.*

EVALUATING

The nurse collects data to evaluate the effectiveness of care by assessing the client's ability to perform ADLs; ability to cope with a chronic illness; and knowledge of medications, diet, and ways to prevent complications.

Documenting. Documentation includes presence of neurologic deficits, coping strategies, and teaching content related to medications, diet, potential complications, and stressors.

CONTINUING CARE

The newly diagnosed client needs a realistic explanation of MS. Early in the course of the disease refer clients to a support group. Encourage clients to keep a diary about symptoms and activities in order to identify stressors. Teaching is best done when the client is in a period of remission. Discuss the following topics with the client and family:

- Avoiding stress, extremes of heat or cold, high humidity, physical overexertion, and infections
- Preventing fatigue and acute exacerbations
- Medications, side effects, and interactions with prescription or other drugs
- Adequate fluid intake, regular bowel and bladder elimination schedule, well-balanced meals, daily physical exercise, and weight control
- Ways to prevent complications such as pressure ulcers, respiratory and urinary tract infections
- Ways to cope with pain, dysphagia, spasticity, and vision changes
- Importance of follow-up care with physician, nurses, and rehabilitation team
- Need for counseling if client is planning a future pregnancy.

If the client is employed, discuss the availability of sick leave during periods of exacerbation. As the disease progresses, the client will require assistance from many community agencies including home health nursing.

Parkinson's Disease

Parkinson's disease (PD) is a chronic, progressive, degenerative neurologic disease that alters motor coordination. It is one of the most common neurologic disorders, affecting approximately 1.5 million people in the United States. Most people are diagnosed after the age of 40. It seems to affect Caucasian men more often than women.

The cause of primary Parkinson's disease is unknown. *Secondary parkinsonism* may be caused by repeated head trauma, encephalitis, or exposure to carbon monoxide or cyanide poisoning. Drugs such as phenothiazines, haloperidol (Haldol), and methyldopa (Aldomet) may induce parkinsonism. The symptoms disappear when the drug is stopped.

PATHOPHYSIOLOGY AND MANIFESTATIONS

Parkinson's disease results from a deficiency of **dopamine**, which is produced in the substantia nigra of the midbrain. In PD, neurons in the cerebral cortex atrophy and the number of dopamine receptors decreases. This results in a decrease in dopamine (a neurotransmitter responsible for voluntary motor function). The balance of dopamine (an inhibitory neurotransmitter) and acetylcholine (an excitatory neurotransmitter) is upset. When dopamine levels drop, acetylcholine is no longer inhibited. This means

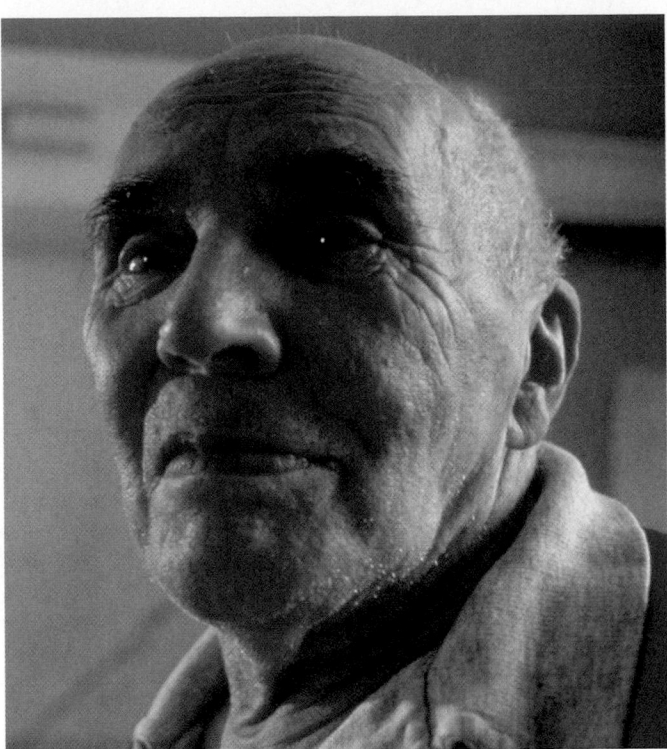

Figure 39-3. ■ In Parkinson's disease, the client's face lacks expression. (*Source:* Phototake NYC.)

that acetylcholine causes constant excitement of the motor neurons, which is the basis for the manifestations of PD.

Manifestations are subtle and may be mistaken as signs of normal aging (Figure 39-3 ■). The onset is gradual and the disease progresses slowly. There are three cardinal signs: (1) tremor, (2) rigidity, and (3) **bradykinesia** (slowed voluntary movements and speech). The classic "pill-rolling" tremor occurs when the thumb and fingers move like they are rolling a pill. Tremors disappear during sleep and movement. Other manifestations are noted in Box 39-5 ■.

BOX 39-5

MANIFESTATIONS OF PARKINSON'S DISEASE

- Tremor that moves from one arm to both arms and may involve lips, jaw, head, and lower extremities
- Rigidity of neck, shoulders, and trunk
- Bradykinesia:
  - Inability to initiate voluntary movements
  - Slurred speech, low amplitude
  - Decreased blinking
  - Masklike, expressionless face
- Drooling
- Excess sweating on face and neck
- Excessively oily skin
- Depression or memory loss

INTERDISCIPLINARY CARE

There are no specific tests to diagnose PD. Diagnosis is based on the client's history and the presence of two of the three cardinal symptoms. A PET scan may show decreased levels of levodopa (a precursor of dopamine).

Interventions vary with the extent of the client's manifestations and disability. The client may be treated with medication, surgery, and rehabilitation. The goal is to retain the highest level of function for as long as possible.

Medications

Drug therapy does not cure Parkinson's disease, but rather is used to control symptoms. Four different classes of drugs are used: *dopaminergics, dopamine agonists, anticholinergics,* and *monoamine oxidase inhibitors (MAOIs)* (Table 39-1 ■). Drugs are chosen based on the client's symptoms, individual response, and the length of effectiveness. For example, over time levodopa, a dopaminergic, loses its effectiveness, and side effects increase. Dopamine agonists are added to increase the effectiveness of levodopa. Eventually, drugs no longer control the symptoms, and the client's condition declines. Catechol-*O*-methyltransferase (COMT) inhibitors, such as tolcapone (Tasmar), are a newer class of drugs that reduce symptoms caused by the "wearing-off" of Sinemet.

Surgery

Two primary surgeries, pallidotomy and stereotaxic thalamotomy, are used to relieve symptoms. Both procedures are done under local anesthesia. In the *pallidotomy,* part of the globus pallidus (basal ganglia located in cerebral cortex that is responsible for skilled movement) is destroyed to control rigidity and tremors. *Stereotaxic thalamotomy* destroys part of the thalamus to reduce tremors; it is reserved for younger people with extreme unilateral tremor.

Electrical Stimulation

Deep brain stimulation (DBS) involves surgically implanting a battery-operated neurostimulator device. An insulated wire is placed in the thalamus and connected to a pulse generator, which is placed under the skin near the clavicle. Once in place, the device sends mild electrical impulses into the brain. The impulses block the signals that cause PD tremors.

Complementary Therapy

Yoga and t'ai chi are well-established therapies to improve strength, balance, and flexibility in clients with PD along with traditional medicines. Massage therapy and acupuncture seem to decrease the muscle stiffness and aching that accompanies PD. No specific herbal supplements are recommended and should only be used with the guidance of a physician.

TABLE 39-1

Nursing Implications for Pharmacology: Parkinson's Disease

DRUG CLASS/DRUGS	ACTION	NURSING IMPLICATIONS	CLIENT TEACHING
Dopaminergics ■ Levodopa (Larodopa) ■ Carbidopa–levodopa (Sinemet) ■ Amantadine (Symmetrel)	Levodopa is converted to dopamine in the brain and carbidopa prevents levodopa from being destroyed. Levodopa is the most effective drug for Parkinson's disease. Amantadine, an antiviral drug, raises dopamine levels.	Check for drug interactions before giving. Do not give to clients with angle-closure glaucoma. Monitor for nausea, hypotension, confusion, and dyskinesia. Assess for "on–off" effect—symptoms may appear or improve suddenly. Hold levodopa for 8 hours prior to giving Sinemet to avoid toxicity.	Take medication as directed. Do not alter dosages. Inform physician of other drugs you are taking. Change position slowly to avoid hypotension. Increase fluid intake and exercise regularly. Report the "on–off" effect, decreased motor movements, insomnia, and rapid heartbeat to your physician.
Dopamine Agonists ■ Bromocriptine (Parlodel) ■ Pergolide (Permax) ■ Pramipexole (Mirapex) ■ Ropinirole (Requip)	They are given to decrease tremor, rigidity, and bradykinesia.	Monitor for adverse reactions: nausea, orthostatic hypotension, and psychosis. See nursing implications under the dopaminergics.	Client teaching information is similar to that found under the dopaminergics.
Anticholinergics ■ Trihexyphenidyl (Artane) ■ Benztropine (Cogentin) ■ Biperiden (Akineton) ■ Procyclidine (Kemadrin)	They are given during the early stages of the disease or when the client can no longer take levodopa. These medications ease drooling, tremors, and rigidity.	Do not give to clients with glaucoma, cardiac dysfunction, and prostatic hypertrophy. Check for drug interactions. Monitor for side effects of dry mouth, blurred vision, constipation, urinary retention, and confusion. Taper off slowly to avoid parkinsonism.	Take the medication as prescribed. Check with physician before taking with other medications. Do not suddenly stop taking anticholinergics. Report blurred vision, constipation, difficulty urinating, or increased temperature. Drink adequate amounts of fluid to prevent dehydration.
Monoamine Oxidase Inhibitor (MAOI) ■ Selegiline (Eldepryl)	It reduces tremor, rigidity, and bradykinesia.	Monitor for ataxia, insomnia, dizziness, or postural hypotension.	Take the medication as directed. Report signs of insomnia, difficulty moving, or dizziness.

NURSING CARE

Clients with PD have complex needs. In the early stages, most clients remain at home with limited family assistance. As the client deteriorates and care increases, the family may want to consider placement in a long-term care facility. Throughout this illness, the client and family need continued support and counseling.

ASSESSING

Assessment should identify the client's symptoms and the extent to which the disease is affecting the client's daily life

(Box 39-6 ■). It is important to note the client's ability to function safely.

DIAGNOSING, PLANNING, AND IMPLEMENTING

Priorities in Nursing Care. Clients with PD develop problems similar to other degenerative neurologic disorders. Refer to previous nursing care sections in this chapter for discussions on fatigue, self-care deficits, and ineffective coping. This section focuses on mobility, communication, and nutrition. In later stages, the client may develop airway management problems.

BOX 39-6	ASSESSMENT

Assessing Clients with Parkinson's Disease

SUBJECTIVE DATA

- Difficulty making decisions.
- Mood swings; depression; insomnia.
- Drooling or difficulty swallowing; weight loss.
- Arm or leg stiffness; frequent falls.
- Loss of dexterity or ability to write.
- Urinary incontinence; constipation.
- Past medical history of head trauma, exposure to metals, or carbon monoxide.
- Use of major tranquilizers.

OBJECTIVE DATA

- Height and weight.
- Observe client for infrequent blinking, expressionless face, slow slurred speech, stooped posture, shuffling gait, or depression.
- Assess for muscles that move in small jerky movements.
- Assess for tremors at rest that disappear with movement, or "pill-rolling" tremor.
- Palpate skin for excessive sweating or oiliness; inspect for injury from falls.

Impaired Physical Mobility

- Perform ROM exercises at least twice a day, emphasizing the trunk, neck, arms, hips, and legs. *ROM exercises promote joint function, strengthen muscles, and prevent contractures.*
- Assist with ambulation at least four times a day. *Exercise fosters independence and self-esteem.*
- Use assistive devices such as canes, splints, or braces as needed. *Assistive devices improve balance and help the client maintain the correct position.*
- Consult with a physical therapist. *Physical therapy can help to improve coordination, balance, gait, and transfers. Exercise is also important in preventing contractures.*

Impaired Verbal Communication

- Teach the client to face the listener and speak in short sentences. Allow extra time for self-expression. *These strategies reduce the client's frustration in communicating.*
- Provide a write-on, wipe-off slate; flash cards with common phrases; or ask client to point to objects. *Individualizing communication decreases anxiety and isolation.*
- Suggest possible referral to a speech therapist. *Speech therapists can teach breathing patterns to improve voice tone and pitch.*
- Try to anticipate the client's needs. *This reduces the client's frustration.*

Imbalanced Nutrition: Less than Body Requirements

- Place in upright position for all meals and keep suction equipment at the bedside *to decrease the risk for aspiration.* Massage the throat as the client swallows *to help swallowing.*
- Cut food into small pieces *for easier swallowing.*

clinical ALERT

Serve semisolid or thickened liquid foods to prevent aspiration.

- Reduce distractions during mealtime. *This allows the client to focus on eating, chewing, and swallowing.*
- Obtain utensils that are easier for the client to grasp. *Modified utensils help the client eat and maintain a sense of self-esteem.*
- Increase daily fluid intake and fiber. *Fluids and fiber prevent constipation caused by several of the anti-Parkinson medications.*

EVALUATING

Evaluate the effectiveness of nursing care by collecting data related to ability to ambulate, chew, swallow, and communicate. In addition, evaluate for the absence of complications and knowledge of disease process and medications.

Documenting. Documentation includes noting the client's tremors, gait, speech pattern, skin integrity, and swallowing. Referrals to speech, occupational, and speech therapy and dietitian are recorded. Client and family teaching about safety measures, diet, medications, and exercise are also noted.

CONTINUING CARE

Persons with PD face such complications as skin breakdown from incontinence or immobility; falls; and joint contractures. As their condition progresses, they may develop malnutrition, constipation, or infection. Provide information about the disease, its management, and strategies for coping with tremors, dysphagia, and speech problems. Explain the purpose, side effects, and directions for taking each medication. Reinforce gait training, ROM exercises, and proper posture. Explain the importance of follow-up meetings with speech therapy, physical therapy, and occupational therapy.

Refer the client to home health services so that the nurse can assess the home for potential hazards. Poor vision, stooped posture, and confusion increase the client's risk for injury. Discuss safety measures such as removing loose rugs and excess furniture, installing a raised toilet seat and handrails in the bathroom, and providing adequate lighting throughout the home and in outside areas. Refer to local support groups and the American Parkinson's Disease Association.

Myasthenia Gravis

Myasthenia gravis is a chronic, autoimmune disorder affecting women most often between the ages of 20 and 30. Clients experience periods of exacerbations and remissions. Stress, pregnancy, and secondary infections may trigger an acute onset.

PATHOPHYSIOLOGY AND MANIFESTATIONS

For an unknown reason, the thymus gland produces antibodies that block or reduce the number acetylcholine receptors at each neuromuscular junction. Nerve impulses cannot be sent to the cranial nerves that control muscles of the face, lips, tongue, neck, and throat. This causes weakness of the facial, speech, and chewing muscles. Characteristic manifestations include eyelid ptosis, diplopia, slurred speech, nasal voice, difficulty chewing and swallowing, and fatigue. A smile appears as a snarl or grimace. There is progressive difficulty in performing fine motor tasks such as writing and progressive weakness of the respiratory muscles. The client faces the risk of aspiration and respiratory insufficiency. Onset is gradual, and manifestations may vary each day.

Two life-threatening emergencies are possible:

1. *Myasthenic crisis* is due to missed doses of medication or an infection. Clients suddenly develop increased muscle weakness, an inability to speak or swallow, and respiratory distress.
2. *Cholinergic crisis* is caused by overmedication with anticholinesterase (cholinergic) medications. The symptoms are similar to myasthenic crisis: severe muscle weakness plus nausea, vomiting, abdominal cramps, increased salivation, sweating, and bradycardia.

Either crisis requires immediate treatment and the possible need for mechanical ventilation.

INTERDISCIPLINARY CARE

A physical examination of the facial, oculomotor, laryngeal, and respiratory muscles is done. Diagnosis is confirmed by injecting edrophonium chloride (Tensilon), a short-acting anticholinesterase. Clients with myasthenia gravis show dramatic improvement in muscle strength, but the improvement lasts only about 5 minutes. *Electromyographic (EMG) studies* show increased muscle fatigue. *CT scan* of the chest may show a tumor of the thymus gland.

Pyridostigmine (Mestinon), an anticholinesterase medication, is the treatment of choice for myasthenia gravis. Dosage is adjusted until the client's symptoms decrease. It is difficult to balance the correct dose without causing myasthenic or cholinergic crisis. The client is taught to record all signs and symptoms carefully so that medication doses can be adjusted (Table 39-2 ■). Prednisone and cytotoxic agents, such as cyclosporine or azathioprine (Imuran), are added to block antibody production or decrease circulating antibodies.

---

clinical ALERT

Administer anticholinesterase drugs on a strict time schedule. Clients with dysphagia may not be able to swallow the medication unless it is taken exactly on time. Doses taken too late may cause myasthenic crisis. Taking doses early may result in cholinergic crisis.

TABLE 39-2

Nursing Implications for Pharmacology: Myasthenia Gravis

DRUG GROUP/DRUGS	ACTION	NURSING IMPLICATIONS	CLIENT TEACHING
Anticholinesterase Drugs ■ Neostigmine (Prostigmin) ■ Ambenonium (Mytelase) ■ Pyridostigmine (Mestinon, Regonol) ■ *For diagnosis*: Edrophonium (Tensilon)	Anticholinesterase drugs prolong the action of acetylcholine to improve muscle contraction. Dose is adjusted to obtain maximum benefit with the fewest side effects. They are contraindicated in clients with urinary or GI tract obstruction, asthma, or hyperthyroidism.	Identify client's ability to swallow. Give the medication on a regular schedule at the exact time. Monitor for *myasthenic crisis*: severe muscle weakness, difficulty breathing, swallowing, or speaking. Notify physician immediately. Monitor for *cholinergic crisis*: excess salivation and sweating, bradycardia, nausea and vomiting.	Take drug as directed on a regular schedule at the exact time. Report symptoms of *myasthenic crisis* immediately: severe muscle weakness, fast heartbeat, difficulty breathing, swallowing, or speaking. Report symptoms of *cholinergic crisis* immediately: slow heartbeat, increased salivation or sweating, decreased blood pressure. Wear Medic-Alert ID. Be sure a family member is trained in CPR.

Along with drug therapy, a **thymectomy** (surgical removal of the thymus gland) may be performed to remove the source of the antibodies. A short-term treatment option involves plasmapheresis. This procedure removes the anti-acetylcholine receptor antibodies so that muscle weakness and fatigue decrease.

NURSING CARE

The nurse collects data about the client's muscle weakness; speech, chewing, or swallowing difficulties; and changes in vision. Nursing care focuses on decreasing or preventing respiratory and swallowing problems as well as reducing fatigue. The nursing diagnoses and interventions are similar to those presented earlier in caring for the client with MS or PD.

Once the client and family understand the disease and ways to cope with the physical and psychosocial problems, the client can be managed at home. Review home care assessment and strategies found in the MS and PD sections. In addition, be sure the family knows cardiopulmonary resuscitation (CPR), and demonstrate how to insert an airway, suction, and use an Ambu bag.

Teaching should emphasize medication actions, side effects, scheduling, and symptoms of myasthenic and cholinergic crisis. Stress the importance of taking medications on an exact schedule. Advise the client to wear a Medic-Alert bracelet.

Refer the client and family to local support groups and provide information about the Myasthenia Gravis Foundation. Pregnancy should be discussed with the physician because it may cause manifestations to worsen. Also, medications such as neostigmine (Prostigmin) cross the placenta.

OTHER NEUROLOGIC DISORDERS

Huntington's Disease

Huntington's disease (HD) is a progressive, inherited neurologic disease. Men and women are affected equally between the ages of 40 and 50. It is transmitted as an autosomal-dominant genetic trait. Each child of a parent with HD has a 50% chance of inheriting the disease. There is no cure for this disease.

HD involves a lack of a neurotransmitter, gamma-aminobutyric acid (GABA). This causes acetylcholine levels to drop and dopamine levels to rise. Unlike PD in which a dopamine deficit slows movement, in HD the excess dopamine causes uncontrolled movement. Without GABA, there is premature death of basal ganglia and cerebral cortex cells. All of these changes develop slowly, affecting (1) personality, (2) intellectual function, and (3) movement. Emotional lability ranges from irritability and anger to depression. Delusions and hallucinations are not unusual. Memory and intellectual function decline to the point of dementia.

Chorea (constant, jerky, uncontrolled movements of the body) is a characteristic manifestation. The client exhibits mild fidgeting or writhing and twisting of the entire body. Motor symptoms are worse with emotional stress but decrease during sleep. Facial grimaces and tics affect speech, chewing, and swallowing, leading to choking and malnutrition. Bowel and bladder control are lost. As the chorea increases, the client is confined to bed. Prognosis is poor, with inevitable total dependence. Death is usually from aspiration pneumonia.

There is no specific test for this disease. Diagnosis is based on symptoms and family history. A PET scan shows changes in the brain. Offspring concerned about their chances of developing HD should have genetic testing.

Medications are given to control the symptoms of HD. The chorea movements may be modified by haloperidol (Haldol) or diazepam (Valium). Antidepressants and antipsychotics are prescribed in the early stage of the disease.

At first, the client and family can manage care at home. Many families are overwhelmed with the future physical and psychologic debilitation that the disease brings. Refer them to local support groups or a psychologist. As the client declines, care is similar to care for other deteriorating neurologic disorders. Eventually, skilled long-term care is needed.

Amyotrophic Lateral Sclerosis

Amyotrophic lateral sclerosis (ALS), also called *Lou Gehrig's disease* after the famous baseball player who suffered from it, is a rapidly progressive, fatal neurologic disease. The exact cause is unknown. More men are affected between the ages of 40 and 70.

ALS involves loss of motor neurons in the spinal cord and brainstem. When electrical impulses cannot be sent from the brain to the voluntary muscles, they lose strength and atrophy. Although body function decreases, the person remains mentally alert.

This disorder is characterized by muscle weakness, **fasciculations** (involuntary contractions of the voluntary muscles, or twitching), and muscle wasting of the arms, legs, and trunk. Brainstem involvement causes speech and swallowing difficulties. Toward the end, clients develop breathing problems, and death is from aspiration pneumonia or respiratory failure. About 50% of clients die within 2 to 5 years of diagnosis.

Diagnosis is based on the client's symptoms. A series of different tests are done to rule out other conditions that mimic ALS. An EMG confirms muscle weakness. Muscle biopsies show loss of muscle fiber.

There is no cure for ALS. Only one medication, riluzole (Rilutek), seems to slow the destruction of motor neurons. Other medications include baclofen and diazepam to relieve muscle spasms. Psychologic support is important for the client and family as the disease progresses.

For as long as possible, promote the client's independence in performing daily ADLs. The client and family should be referred to an ALS support group. Nursing care is similar to that for the client with MS, discussed earlier in this chapter. Before speech is lost, develop communication signals such as blinking for yes and no answers. When swallowing or breathing problems develop, anticipate enteral feedings and mechanical ventilation. To manage the client at home, the family is taught (1) suctioning techniques and the Heimlich maneuver, (2) bowel and urinary catheter care, (3) enteral feedings, (4) skin care, and (5) turning and positioning the client.

Guillain–Barré Syndrome

Guillain–Barré syndrome (GBS) is an acute, progressive inflammation of the peripheral nervous system (PNS). The cause is unknown but most often follows a recent respiratory or gastrointestinal (GI) infection, viral vaccination, or surgery. Infection with *Campylobacter jejuni* causes about 60% of Guillain–Barré cases.

PATHOPHYSIOLOGY AND MANIFESTATIONS

A cell-mediated immune system reaction destroys the myelin sheath covering the peripheral nerves. Without myelin, impulses are poorly conducted to the sensory and motor nerves. This causes rapid, muscle weakness, loss of reflexes, and paralysis.

Manifestations of GBS start in the lower extremities and move upward. The first symptoms are bilateral weakness and numbness and tingling in the legs. Within 24 to 72 hours, weakness extends to the arms and respiratory muscles and then progresses to paralysis. Cranial nerve involvement causes chewing, swallowing, and talking problems. If the autonomic nervous system is affected, blood pressure and pulse changes develop. Throughout this process, the person remains alert and oriented.

The most serious complication is respiratory failure. If this develops, a tracheostomy and mechanical ventilation are used for 2 to 3 weeks, but the time frame can vary. (See nursing care for the client with a tracheostomy in Box 23-10, 🔗 and mechanical ventilation in Chapter 24. 🔗) Other complications, such as skin breakdown and deep venous thrombosis (DVT), relate to the length of time the client is paralyzed.

INTERDISCIPLINARY CARE

Most clients with GBS recover with few or no residual effects. Recovery time depends on how fast the myelin sheath can rebuild itself. Average rehabilitation is about 6 months but may take as long as 1 year. As the nerves recover, the client's symptoms improve in reverse order.

Diagnosis of GBS is based on clinical symptoms and a recent viral infection. A lumbar puncture shows elevated CSF protein levels. The results of EMG studies show a definite slowing of nerve conduction.

Medical management consists of plasmapheresis and intravenous immune globulin. Plasmapheresis removes the antibodies that caused GBS. It is beneficial when used within the first 2 weeks. Clients typically have five exchanges over 8 to 10 days. The action of intravenous immune globulin is unclear, but the effects are similar to plasmapheresis. Antibiotics are prescribed for urinary tract or respiratory infections. Anticoagulants are given to prevent DVT and pulmonary embolism.

NURSING CARE

Clients are acutely ill and are managed in a critical care unit. Nursing assessments are done every 1 to 2 hours. Nursing interventions focus on preventing immobility problems; promoting adequate hydration, nutrition, and respiratory function; and providing psychosocial support. It is important to anticipate the needs of the client and family. They are stunned by the rapid deterioration of function and fear permanent paralysis.

After the acute phase, the client is transferred to a skilled nursing facility or home. Those with extensive paralysis need inpatient or outpatient physical, occupational, and speech therapy. The caregiver may need help from a homemaker or home health aide. When recovery is long, the caregiver will need respite care.

Trigeminal Neuralgia

Trigeminal neuralgia (*tic douloureux*) involves two sensory branches of the trigeminal nerve: the maxillary and mandibular (Figure 39-4 ■). Pain occurs along one or both

Sensory distribution

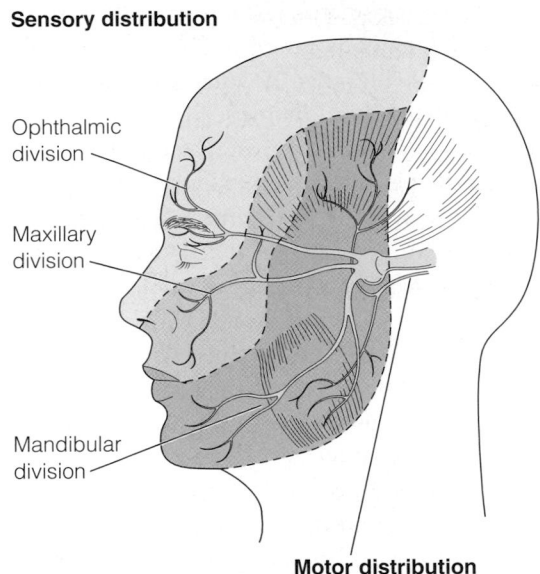

Ophthalmic division

Maxillary division

Mandibular division

Motor distribution

Figure 39-4. ■ Sensory and motor branches of the trigeminal nerve. There are three sensory branches: ophthalmic, maxillary, and mandibular.

of these branches. It usually affects women between the ages of 50 and 60. The actual cause is unknown but may be from dental or surgical procedures, facial trauma, infection, or pressure on the nerve by a tumor.

Trigeminal neuralgia is characterized by severe, one-sided facial pain lasting a few seconds to a few minutes. The pain is described as stabbing or burning in the forehead, along the nose, lips, or cheek. Attacks occur for several weeks and then suddenly disappear. The client may remain pain free for days to years. With age, remissions become shorter.

Trigger zones on the face initiate an attack when they are stimulated. Simple actions such as shaving, chewing, brushing the teeth, or washing the face, or wind or a change in temperature can set off an attack. An attack may cause wincing, grimacing, or tearing of the eye. To control pain, clients may refuse to wash, shave, eat, or talk.

Diagnosis is based on the characteristic location and type of pain. The drug most useful in controlling the pain is the anticonvulsant carbamazepine (Tegretol). When ineffective, other medications such as phenytoin (Dilantin) and baclofen (Lioresal) are added. If drug therapy fails, biofeedback and nerve blocks with local anesthetics are tried. Another option is a **rhizotomy** (the surgical severing of a nerve root to control pain). Only the sensory nerve root is destroyed. Motor function is preserved so that eating is unaffected. If the ophthalmic branch is damaged, the corneal reflex is lost.

Nursing care focuses on teaching self-care strategies including medications and potential side effects. Because

this is a chronic condition, long-term use of narcotics is avoided. Discuss ways to avoid trigger points, such as using room temperature water and soft cotton pads to wash the face. If the client refuses to eat during periods of pain attacks, encourage a soft high-protein and high-calorie diet.

After surgery, the client may lose sensation and corneal reflex on the involved side. Teach the client to chew on the unaffected side, to avoid hot foods or liquids, and to brush the teeth and check for food pockets between gums and cheek after every meal. Men should use an electric razor to shave. Clients should also protect the face from very cold or windy conditions, and, if necessary, wear a protective eye shield.

Bell's Palsy

Bell's palsy (facial paralysis) is associated with the herpes simplex virus. Inflammation causes edema and pressure on the facial nerve, resulting in necrosis. This leads to sudden weakness and paralysis on one side of the face. Paralysis distorts the affected side, causing ptosis of the eyelid, tearing, mouth drooping, drooling, an inability to smile, and difficulty chewing (Figure 39-5 ■). There is also pain around or behind the ear. Most clients improve within a few weeks to months, although some are left with residual paralysis.

Diagnosis is based on the client's facial appearance. Treatment is a short-term course of steroids. Because it is linked to the herpes virus, clients are given antiviral drugs. Mild analgesics may reduce the facial pain. Nursing and home care is similar to that for the client with trigeminal neuralgia. (Review the strategies listed after surgery.) In addition, teach the client to apply warm, moist heat such as gel packs, which increases circulation and relieves pain. A facial sling may be applied during meals to prevent muscle stretching.

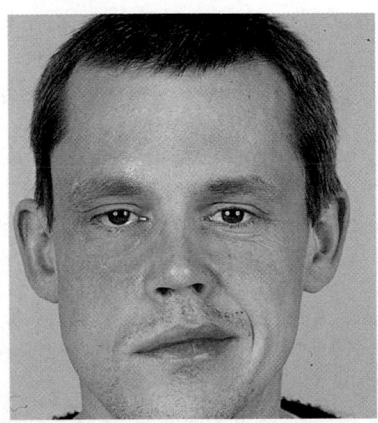

Figure 39-5. ■ The client with Bell's palsy shows the typical drooping of one side of the face. (*Source:* Phototake NYC.)

The loss of blinking increases the risk for corneal drying. Demonstrate how to instill artificial tears four times a day and how to apply an eye patch at night. Be sure the client understands how to inspect the eye each day and to report eye pain, redness, swelling, or discharge. Recommend wearing dark glasses or goggles when outside or working in dusty conditions.

Rabies

Rabies is a viral infection of the CNS caused by an animal bite. The rabies virus is carried by wild and domestic animals, including bats, skunks, foxes, raccoons, cats, and dogs. The virus spreads from the wound to the peripheral nerves and eventually travels to the CNS. Incubation varies from 14 days to 3 months. Any animal that has bitten someone is observed for 1 to 2 weeks to detect rabies symptoms. Sick animals are euthanized and their brains examined for the rabies virus.

Clinical manifestations occur in three stages. In *stage 1,* the wound is painful, with a tingling sensation. The client experiences malaise, fever, headache, and sensitivity to light and loud noises. *Stage 2* develops within 24 to 72 hours. Any attempt at swallowing causes forceful spasms of the larynx. The person refuses to drink (*hydrophobia*). Swallowing problems lead to frothy drooling. Eventually, the sight or sound of water triggers the muscle spasms and excessive salivation. *Stage 3:* Without treatment, death occurs in about 7 days from cardiopulmonary arrest.

To prevent rabies, it is recommended that all household dogs and cats be immunized. Any animal bite or scratch is thoroughly cleaned with soap and water to remove the saliva and dilute the virus. The person is taken immediately to the emergency department to receive rabies immune globulin (RIg) as soon as possible after the bite if the bite is from a wild animal or a domestic animal that has not been immunized. This is followed by five doses of inactivated human diploid cell rabies vaccine (HDCV) intramuscularly on the day of exposure and on days 3, 7, 14, and 28 after exposure.

Clients who show signs of rabies are cared for in the critical care unit with the room dark and quiet to decrease stimulation. Nursing care focuses on airway maintenance and seizure control. Standard Precautions are essential, because the rabies virus is present in the saliva of the client. If an open wound of a health care provider is contaminated with infected saliva, the provider must receive postexposure immunizations.

Tetanus

Tetanus, or *lockjaw,* is a disorder of the nervous system caused by *Clostridium tetani.* This anaerobic bacillus produces spores that live in the soil and enter the body through open wounds contaminated with dirt, street dust, or feces. Most cases of tetanus occur in adults over age 50 whose tetanus booster is older than 10 years. Incubation period averages 24 hours to several months.

When the spores enter an open wound, two exotoxins are absorbed by the peripheral nerves and carried to the spinal cord. They interfere with the transmission of neuromuscular impulses leading to uncontrolled muscle spasms. Initially, the client exhibits pain at the wound site, stiffness of the jaw and neck, mild spasms, and difficulty swallowing. As it advances, the person has difficulty opening the jaw (**trismus**). Spasms of the facial muscles give the person a grinning expression. Painful seizures cause the back to arch. Despite these physical effects, the client remains alert and oriented. The mortality rate is high and usually due to asphyxia from spasms of the glottis and respiratory muscles.

There are no specific laboratory tests for tetanus. The diagnosis is based on the clinical manifestations. Active immunization can prevent tetanus. Children should receive tetanus toxoid as part of the diphtheria–tetanus–pertussis (DPT) immunization series. Adults should be given two doses of tetanus toxoid 4 to 6 weeks apart, with a third dose in 6 to 12 months. The Centers for Disease Control and Prevention (CDC) recommends a booster dose every 10 years.

If a wound is extensive or heavily contaminated or if the person's immunization status is unknown, give tetanus immune globulin (TIG) to destroy the tetanus toxins. This is followed by injections of tetanus toxoid according to the schedule mentioned before. All wounds, no matter how small, are thoroughly cleaned with soap and water. Foreign material is carefully flushed out or removed from a wound. Only hydrogen peroxide and iodine kill the tetanus organism.

Clients who develop tetanus are cared for in a critical care unit with minimal stimulation. They are given antibiotics to destroy the organism and anticonvulsants to stop any seizures. When muscle spasms and seizures are severe, paralytic agents are used. Airway obstruction is managed by mechanical ventilation. The recovery periods varies from 2 to 5 weeks.

Creutzfeldt–Jakob Disease

Creutzfeldt–Jakob disease (CJD) is a rare, progressive neurologic disease causing brain degeneration. The disease is transmissible and fatal within 6 to 12 months after diagnosis. It primarily affects adults over 60, with more cases in England, Chile, and Italy.

CJD destroys the brain's gray matter. On autopsy, the brain has numerous tiny holes resembling a sponge (called spongiform encephalopathy). The underlying cause seems to be an infective protein pathogen called a *prion.* It is resistant to normal chemical and physical sterilization methods. A few cases have been transmitted through corneal transplants and human growth hormone from cadavers.

Early manifestations include memory loss and personality and visual changes. Then the person rapidly develops dementia, muscle contractions, speech problems, and ataxia. Clients in the terminal stage are comatose until death.

Diagnosis is difficult because CJD mimics other degenerative neurologic diseases such as Alzheimer's disease. A thorough neurologic examination, EEG changes, and CT scan help confirm a diagnosis. However, the final diagnosis of CJD is made only by an autopsy.

No specific treatment exists for CJD. Medical and nursing care focus on providing support and comfort. Standard Precautions are followed when handling all blood and body fluids. A 5% bleach solution seems to be most effective in disinfecting contaminated surfaces and equipment. It is not necessary to place the client in isolation.

A new disease, *new variant CJD,* seems to be linked to eating meat from animals infected with bovine spongiform encephalopathy (BSE), or "mad cow disease." It is a rare, degenerative, fatal brain disease that appears in younger clients. To date, no cases of variant CJD have occurred in the United States.

SPINAL CORD DISORDERS

The spinal cord, vertebrae, intervertebral disks, and spinal nerves are anatomically close to each other. Because of this, damage to the vertebrae or an intervertebral disk can affect the spinal cord and nerve impulse transmission through it. For example, if the client suffers a thoracic vertebrae injury, pressure is applied to the spinal cord. Unless the pressure is relieved, the client could be paralyzed.

Spinal Cord Injury

A spinal cord injury (SCI) is usually due to trauma. Adolescent and adult males experience most spinal cord injuries. Motor vehicle crashes cause most of the injuries, followed by falls, violent acts, and sports injuries.

The spinal cord provides a two-way path to conduct impulses between the brain and body. Nerves in the spinal cord connect to the body through nerve roots that exit the spinal column. These nerves provide motor and sensory information to the entire body below the head. Just like the spinal column, the spinal cord is divided into cervical, thoracic, and lumbar regions. The cervical region carries sensations from the head, neck, diaphragm, shoulders, and arms. The thoracic region supplies nerves to the chest that help in breathing and nerves of the sympathetic nervous system. The lumbar region supplies the legs, pelvis, and bowel and bladder.

PATHOPHYSIOLOGY AND MANIFESTATIONS

A number of factors cause spinal cord injuries. The neck can be forcibly bent forward or backward, compressing the vertebrae. Diving into shallow water also compresses the vertebrae and spinal cord (Figure 39-6 ■). A bullet may penetrate the cord, or a fall may cause a fracture of the neck or back. Most injuries occur in the lumbar and cervical regions, where the vertebrae are not protected by other parts of the skeleton such as the rib cage or pelvis.

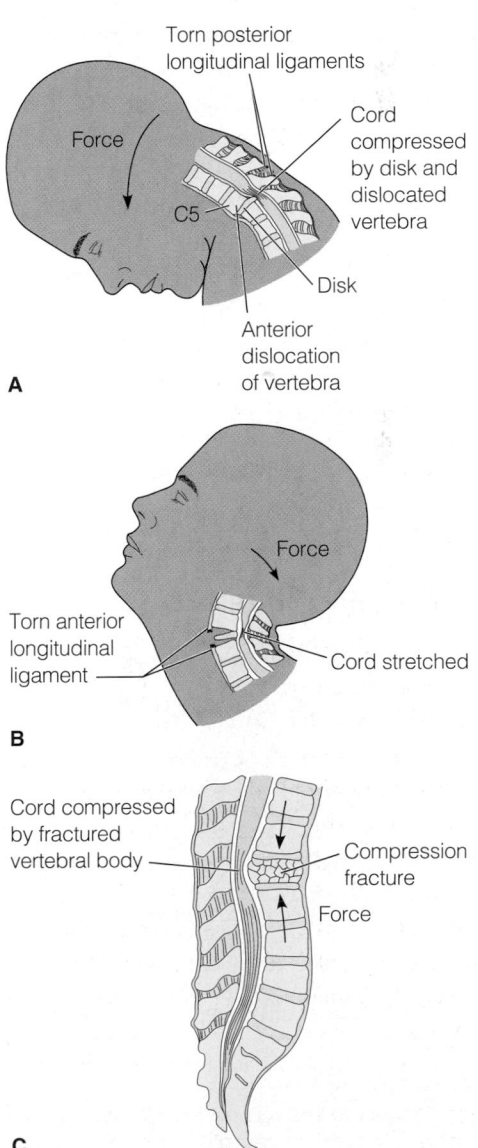

Figure 39-6. ■ Spinal cord injury mechanisms. **(A)** Hyperflexion. **(B)** Hyperextension. **(C)** Cord compression.

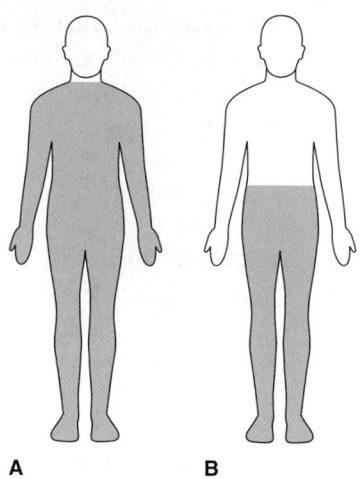

Figure 39-7. ■ Types of paralysis. **(A)** Tetraplegia. **(B)** Paraplegia.

Spinal cord injuries are classified according to the level of injury and the amount of cord damage. For example, an injury at the sixth cervical vertebra is called a C_6 SCI. Cord damage is described as complete or incomplete. A *complete SCI* results in total loss of motor and sensory function below the level of injury. *Incomplete injury* causes varying degrees of function below the level of injury. The level of the injury determines whether the client develops paraplegia or tetraplegia (Figure 39-7 ■). Damage at the thoracic level causes **paraplegia** (paralysis of the lower part of the body). High cervical injuries result in **tetraplegia,** formerly called quadriplegia, which is paralysis of the arms, trunk, legs, and pelvic organs.

As soon as bruising or compression occurs to the spinal cord, there is bleeding into the gray matter. At this point the damage may be reversible. However, the body's inflammatory response causes edema, hypoxia, and ischemia of the spinal cord. This process actually expands the injury area and may cause more damage than the original injury. If the cord has not suffered irreversible damage, corticosteroids given within the first 4 to 6 hours after injury may stop the inflammation. Tissue repair occurs over a period of 3 to 4 weeks, but the spinal cord does not regenerate.

The client may have deficits in movement, sensation, and reflex activity. The level of the injury determines the client's deficits and potential for rehabilitation (Table 39-3 ■). Complications occur either immediately after an injury or later (Box 39-7 ■). Clients with tetraplegia are prone to more complications than those with paraplegia.

SPINAL SHOCK

Spinal shock is a temporary loss of reflex activity below the level of spinal cord injury. It typically occurs 30 to 60 minutes after a complete SCI. There is loss of motor function, sensation, spinal reflexes, and autonomic function. Other manifestations include (1) bradycardia, (2) hypotension, (3) loss of sweating and temperature control below the level of injury, (4) bowel and bladder dysfunction, (5) flaccid paralysis, and (6) loss of ability to perspire. Spinal shock usually lasts from days to weeks, and then reflex activity returns. Until it resolves, the client needs medical support, such as intravenous (IV) fluids.

TABLE 39-3

Functional Abilities by Level of Spinal Cord Injury

LEVEL	FUNCTION	ADL	ELIMINATION	MOBILITY
C_1–C_3	No movement or sensation below the neck; Ventilator-dependent	D	D	Voice or sip-n-puff controlled electric WC
C_4	Movement and sensation of head and neck; some partial function of the diaphragm	D	D	Chin-operated electric WC
C_5	Controls head, neck, and shoulders; flexes elbows	WA	D	Electric WC
C_6	Uses shoulder, extends wrist	I or WA	WA	WC, self-transfer
C_7 and C_8	Extends elbow, flexes wrist, some use of fingers	I	I	Manual WC
T_1–T_5	Has full hand and finger control, full use of thoracic muscles	I	I	Manual WC
T_6–T_{10}	Controls abdominal muscles, has good balance	I	I	Manual WC
T_{11}–L_5	Flexes and abducts the hips; flexes and extends the knees	I	I	Ambulates with leg braces, short braces, or canes
S_1–S_5	Full control of legs; progressive bowel, bladder, and sexual function	I	I	

D = dependent, I = independent, WA = with assistance, WC = wheelchair.

COMPLICATIONS OF SPINAL CORD INJURY

- *Integument:* decubitus (pressure) ulcers
- *Neurologic:* pain, hypotonia, autonomic dysreflexia
- *Cardiovascular and peripheral vascular:* spinal shock, orthostatic hypotension, bradycardia, DVT
- *Respiratory:* limited chest expansion, pneumonia
- *Gastrointestinal:* stress ulcers, paralytic ileus, stool impaction, stool incontinence
- *Genitourinary:* urinary retention, urinary incontinence, neurogenic bladder, UTIs, impotence, decreased vaginal lubrication
- *Musculoskeletal:* joint contractures, muscle spasms, muscle atrophy, pathologic fractures, hypercalcemia

Autonomic Dysreflexia

Autonomic dysreflexia is an exaggerated sympathetic response in clients with SCIs at or above the T_6 level. This occurs because impulses from the autonomic nervous system are blocked by the SCI. Stimuli such as a full bladder or fecal impaction trigger a hypertensive crisis. The client develops pounding headache; flushed, diaphoretic skin above the lesion and pale, cold, and dry skin below it; goosebumps; and anxiety. If untreated, autonomic dysreflexia can cause seizures, a cerebrovascular accident (CVA), or death.

clinical ALERT

Blood pressure readings may reach a systolic up to 300 mm Hg.

This is a medical emergency. Elevate the head of the bed 45 degrees to lower the blood pressure. If this does not lower it, give antihypertensive medications as ordered. Monitor blood pressure every 2 to 3 minutes while at the same time assessing for the cause. If the client has a Foley catheter, check the tubing for kinks or irrigate the catheter to check for patency. When the client does not have a catheter, insert a straight catheter. If a fecal impaction is present, insert Nupercaine cream into the anus, wait 10 minutes, and manually remove the impaction.

INTERDISCIPLINARY CARE

Immediate Care

Care of the client with an SCI begins at the accident scene. Moving a client at the scene can further damage the spinal cord. If the client is moved incorrectly, pieces from a fractured vertebrae could penetrate the cord and cause permanent damage. Clients are not moved unless there is a life-threatening danger, such as being burned, crushed, or drowned.

clinical ALERT

Manage all accident victims as if they have a SCI.

At the accident scene, assess the client's airway, breathing, and circulation immediately. Next, assess the client for complaints of neck pain or changes in movement or sensation. Then immobilize the neck until emergency personnel arrive. They will apply a rigid cervical collar and place the client on a spinal backboard in a neutral position.

In the emergency department, the client is assessed for other injuries, respiratory distress, and neurologic deficits. The neck and spine remain immobilized throughout assessment and diagnostic testing. Oxygen is given to clients with cervical or thoracic injuries. An intravenous line and fluids are started to prevent shock. Until the client's condition is stable, closely monitor for respiratory, cardiac, urinary, and GI complications. High-dose methylprednisolone (Solu-Medrol), a corticosteroid, is started immediately to prevent secondary spinal cord damage from edema and ischemia.

Diagnostic Tests

The following diagnostic studies are used to diagnose SCIs:

- *Cervical spine x-rays* show fracture or displacement of the vertebrae.
- *CT scan* or *MRI* shows damage to the vertebrae, spinal cord, and tissues around the cord.

Medications

Corticosteroids are given for 1 to 2 weeks to decrease or control edema of the cord. Muscle spasms are treated with antispasmodics (Table 39-4 ■). *Histamine H_2-receptor antagonists* (e.g., ranitidine [Zantac]) are used to prevent stress-related gastric ulcers. Thrombophlebitis is prevented with *anticoagulants* (see Chapter 28 🔗 for more information). Stool softeners may be given as part of a bowel-training program.

Stabilization and Immobilization

Early management includes stabilizing and immobilizing the spinal cord. Thoracic and lumbar injuries are immobilized with braces or body casts. Cervical injuries are treated with cervical tongs (see Gardner–Wells tongs, Figure 39-8 ■) or a halo vest. The tongs are inserted into the skull and attached to weights to keep the spine in correct alignment. The disadvantage is that the client must be monitored closely for displacement of the tongs. If traction is interrupted, the client

TABLE 39-4			
Nursing Implications for Pharmacology: Antispasmodics in Spinal Cord Injury			
DRUG GROUP/DRUGS	**ACTION**	**NURSING IMPLICATIONS**	**CLIENT TEACHING**
Baclofen (Lioresal) Diazepam (Valium) Dantrolene (Dantrium)	They are used to control muscle spasm and pain associated with acute or chronic musculoskeletal conditions. They are not always effective in controlling spasticity resulting from cerebral or spinal cord conditions.	Assess the client's spasticity and involuntary movements. Give with food to decrease gastrointestinal symptoms. Monitor for drowsiness and dizziness. Monitor for therapeutic effect.	Take with meals to decrease gastric irritation. These drugs may cause drowsiness or dizziness. If drowsy, avoid activities that require mental alertness or coordination. Check with physician before taking with other drugs. Do not stop the drug abruptly without discussing with your physician.

faces additional spinal cord damage. Tongs are less frequently used today.

The halo vest (Figure 39-9 ■) is used for stable cervical or thoracic fractures without cord damage. It allows greater mobility, self-care, and participation in a rehabilitation program. This device is secured through four pins inserted into the skull, two in the frontal bone and two in the occipital bone. The halo ring is then attached to a rigid plastic vest lined with sheepskin. Nursing care is described in Box 39-8 ■.

Clients with cervical tongs and traction are placed on a kinetic bed, which provides a continuous side-to-side slow rotation. It helps to prevent immobility problems yet keep the spine aligned. Those with the halo vest can be placed in a regular bed.

Surgery

Surgery is necessary when bone fragments or a hematoma compresses the spine. It is also done to stabilize and support the spine. Different spinal surgeries may be performed such as a spinal fusion, decompression laminectomy, or insertion of metal rods. These surgeries are discussed later in the chapter.

NURSING CARE

Clients with an SCI need acute care in the hospital followed by rehabilitation. The care plan focuses on preventing complications of immobility, promoting self-care, and teaching the client and family.

ASSESSING

On arrival at the hospital the client is assessed from head to toe. Box 39-9 ■ presents subjective and objective data to collect. During the acute phase, perform assessments at frequent intervals.

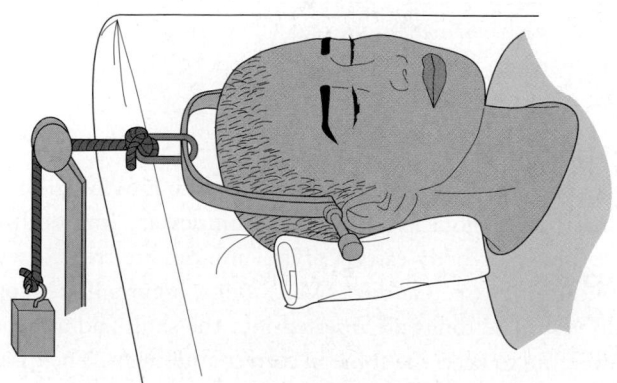

Figure 39-8. ■ Cervical traction with Gardner–Wells tongs.

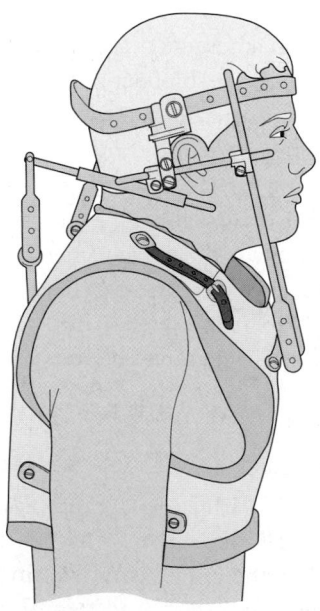

Figure 39-9. ■ Halo vest.

BOX 39-8	NURSING CARE CHECKLIST

Clients in Halo Vests

☑ Inspect pins and traction bars for tightness; report loose pins to physician.

☑ Check for access to the front of the vest for emergency intervention.

☑ Never use the halo ring to lift or reposition the client.

☑ Assess the pin sites for redness, edema, and drainage.

☑ Clean pin sites daily.

☑ Inspect the skin under the vest for pressure areas.

☑ To provide skin care, loosen the sides of the vest. Wash and thoroughly dry the skin. Prevent the lining from becoming wet.

☑ Change the sheepskin lining when it is soiled or at least once each week.

☑ Turn the client every 2 hours.

☑ Provide mild analgesic for headache.

DIAGNOSING, PLANNING, AND IMPLEMENTING

Priorities in Nursing Care. Spinal cord injuries can affect all body systems. The nurse monitors for and plans interventions to prevent problems with breathing, physical immobility,

BOX 39-9	ASSESSMENT

Assessing Clients with Spinal Cord Injury

SUBJECTIVE DATA

■ Breathing difficulty.

■ Loss of strength, movement, or sensation below level of injury.

■ Numbness or tingling in extremities.

■ Presence of fear, anger, or depression.

■ Past history of traumatic injury (circumstances of the accident/injury).

OBJECTIVE DATA

■ Blood pressure, pulse, and temperature.

■ Respiratory rate, depth, and breath sounds; ability to cough; use of accessory muscles.

■ Test motor strength.

■ Assess sensation, noting areas where the client cannot feel the touch.

■ Palpate the bladder for fullness.

■ Auscultate bowel sounds.

■ Monitor and report diagnostic test results.

bowel and bladder elimination, skin integrity, nutrition, and self-esteem. The highest priority nursing diagnoses focus on promoting respiratory function and preventing complications of immobility such as UTI, paralytic ileus, and pressure ulcers.

Ineffective Breathing Pattern

■ Monitor pulse oximetry levels. *It is important to measure oxygen levels in order to prevent respiratory problems.*

clinical ALERT

Monitor for difficulty swallowing or coughing, respiratory stridor, and increased motor and sensory loss. Injuries above the C_4 level alter respiratory function from edema of the cord or paralysis of the respiratory, chest, and abdominal muscles.

■ Turn, cough, and deep breathe at least every 2 hours. Suction PRN. *These measures decrease the risk for pneumonia and atelectasis.*

■ Increase fluids to 2,000 mL/day. *Increased fluids thin secretions, making them easier to expel and expectorate.*

Impaired Physical Mobility

■ Perform passive ROM exercises to all extremities twice a day. *ROM exercises help prevent contractures and improve circulation.*

■ Use splints, trochanter rolls, and high-top tennis shoes *to prevent wrist drop, footdrop, and external rotation of the hips.*

■ Inspect skin daily for pressure ulcers. Use a special bed if necessary. Turn client every 2 hours. *The lack of sensation along with immobility increases the risk for pressure ulcers.*

■ Provide diet high in protein, carbohydrate, and calories. *Stress from an SCI increases metabolism and the risk for malnutrition.*

■ Assess the lower extremities each shift for thrombophlebitis. Apply thromboembolytic disease (TED) hose and remove for 30 to 60 minutes each shift. *Immobile clients are at risk for DVT. TED hose prevents blood from pooling in the lower extremities and reduces the risk for DVT.*

clinical ALERT

Removing TED hose each shift promotes healthy skin and allows the nurse to assess skin integrity.

Impaired Urinary Elimination and Constipation

■ During spinal shock, insert a Foley catheter or perform intermittent catheterization. After spinal shock, reinforce the bladder training program. *A catheter prevents urinary retention and possible bladder rupture. Clients have a high risk for UTIs; the use of catheters is limited.*

■ Teach the client to use trigger voiding techniques such as stroking inner thigh, pulling the pubic hair, tapping on the suprapubic area or abdomen. *These trigger voiding techniques cause reflex activity that may initiate voiding.*

clinical ALERT

Palpate the bladder for fullness because clients with cervical injuries cannot feel a full bladder.

■ Place the client on a bedside commode if possible. *Upright position facilitates complete bladder and bowel emptying.*
■ Monitor for cloudy, foul-smelling urine and increase fluid intake. *These clients have a high potential for UTIs.*

clinical ALERT

Monitor for decreased or absent bowel tones that could indicate paralytic ileus.

■ Begin a bowel retraining program using stool softeners, rectal suppositories, and digital stimulation as needed. *These measures stimulate peristalsis and initiate bowel movements.*

Situational Low Self-Esteem

■ Allow the client time to grieve or to express denial, depression, and anger over the changes in social, financial, and personal roles. *The client needs time to adjust to the lifestyle changes.*
■ Provide accurate information based on the physician's prognosis. *Accurate information helps the client understand his or her present and future needs.*
■ Include family and significant others to treat the client as normally as possible. *These strategies can make the client feel worthy and of value.*
■ Refer the client and family to support groups. *Support groups can help the client and family adjust to the changes.*

EVALUATING

To evaluate the effectiveness of care for a client with an SCI, collect data on bowel and bladder elimination, ability to manage ADLs, and absence of complications such as contractures, pressure ulcers, DVT, and infection.

Documenting. Documentation includes vital signs, motor and sensory deficits, respiratory depth and presence of crackles and wheezes, skin integrity, and bowel and bladder function. Client and family teaching about skin care, bowel and bladder training, exercises, nutrition, medications, and potential complications are also recorded.

CONTINUING CARE

The nurse assesses the client's ability to live independently and, if necessary, the family's ability to provide care. This assessment provides information about whether the client can live at home or will need care in a rehabilitation center.

The client's physical and emotional needs determine the type of rehabilitation program. Rehabilitation centers can offer specialized assistance but may not be near the client's home. These centers teach the client to function at the highest level possible.

Discharge responsibilities include teaching the client and family how to provide medications, ADLs, exercises, bowel and bladder programs such as urinary catheterization, and skin care. Discuss ways to prevent potential complications such as constipation, urinary retention, pressure ulcers, contractures, DVT, autonomic dysreflexia, and infections. Emphasize indications for notifying the physician. A physical therapist will demonstrate the use of any assistive devices such as wheelchair or crutches, and the need for position changes. Social services can arrange referral to a home health agency, transfer to a rehabilitation center, or a job retraining program. A home health nurse can evaluate the suitability of the living area in the home.

Herniated Intervertebral Disk

A **herniated intervertebral disk**, also called *ruptured* or *slipped disk*, usually occurs in men between the ages of 30 and 50. Disk injury can develop from trauma, lifting incorrectly, sudden twisting of the spine, or degenerative changes due to arthritis. The majority of herniated disks occur in the lumbar (L_4 or L_5 to S_1) or cervical regions. Herniated disks are a common cause of chronic back pain.

PATHOPHYSIOLOGY AND MANIFESTATIONS

The intervertebral disks are located between the vertebrae of the spinal column. They are made of an inner *nucleus pulposus* and an outer fibrous ring, the *annulus fibrosus*. The disks allow the spine to absorb compression by acting as shock absorbers. A herniated intervertebral disk occurs when the nucleus pulposus protrudes through a weakened or torn annulus fibrosus (Figure 39-10 ■). When the disk herniates or "slips," it compresses the nearby spinal nerve root and causes motor and sensory changes, pain, and altered reflexes (Box 39-10 ■).

The herniation may be abrupt or gradual. Sudden straining of the back may cause immediate intense pain and muscle spasms. Gradual herniation resulting from degenerative changes and osteoarthritis has a slow onset of pain. The classic manifestation of a ruptured lumbar disk is recurrent low back pain. **Sciatica** describes pain that follows along the sciatic nerve. The pain ranges from mild to excruciating. It

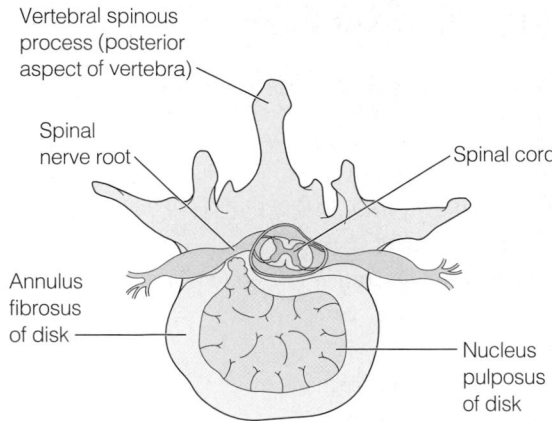

Vertebral spinous process (posterior aspect of vertebra)

Spinal nerve root

Spinal cord

Annulus fibrosus of disk

Nucleus pulposus of disk

Figure 39-10. ■ A herniated intervertebral disk. The herniated nucleus pulposus is applying pressure against the nerve root.

is increased by sitting, straining, coughing, sneezing, and walking. Sciatica is usually elicited when the client performs straight-leg raises.

INTERDISCIPLINARY CARE

Medical care focuses on identifying the location of herniation and determining the type of treatment. Nursing care is directed toward preparing clients for diagnostic tests. The nurse also cares for the client following surgery and provides teaching for discharge.

Diagnostic Tests

A complete neurologic examination is part of diagnosing a herniated disk. Spinal *x-rays* can identify skeletal deformities and narrowing of the disk spaces. *CT scan* and *MRI* show the site of the herniation. *Myelography* is used both to rule out tumors and locate the herniation. Nursing implications for myelography are found in Box 39-11 ■. *EMG* identifies specific spinal nerves that are affected by the pressure.

BOX 39-10

MANIFESTATIONS OF HERNIATED INTERVERTEBRAL DISK

Lumbar–Sacral Area (L$_4$ to L$_5$ and S$_1$)
- Pain that radiates from hip down the leg, usually unilateral
- Muscle spasms
- Numbness and tingling of the leg and foot
- Decreased or absent knee and/or ankle reflexes

Cervical Area (C$_5$ to C$_7$)
- Neck stiffness
- Pain radiating from shoulder down arm to hand
- Numbness and tingling of neck, shoulder, arm, and possibly hand
- Decreased arm strength
- Decreased triceps reflex

BOX 39-11   **NURSING CARE CHECKLIST**

Myelography
☑ Check facility policy for client preparation.

Pretest Teaching
☑ Do not eat or drink for several hours before the test.
☑ You will be placed on a table that tilts so the dye can circulate in the spinal column.
☑ Dye is injected through a lumbar puncture. You may feel warmth or a burning sensation. Tell the physician if you feel pain.
☑ Stay in bed and follow the doctor's orders for position.
☑ Immediately report fever, stiff neck, or seizures.

Post-Test Nursing Care
☑ Monitor vital signs and assess neurologic status every 1 to 4 hours for 24 hours.
☑ Monitor lumbar puncture site for leakage of CSF or bleeding every 4 hours. Notify the physician of leakage or bleeding.
☑ Increase fluids to 2,400 to 3,000 mL in 24 hours. (This may reduce the headache.)
☑ Make sure that the client voids within 8 hours after the examination.
☑ Give analgesics and antiemetics as needed for pain, headache, or nausea.
☑ If oil- or water-based dye is used, elevate the client's head 30 to 45 degrees for 8 to 12 hours.

Medications

Pain is managed with *nonsteroidal anti-inflammatory drugs (NSAIDs)* such as aspirin, ibuprofen (Motrin), and naproxen (Naprosyn). Narcotics are avoided in clients with chronic pain because of the risk of dependency. Muscle spasms are treated with *muscle relaxants. Transcutaneous electrical stimulation (TENS)* may relieve uncontrolled pain.

Medical Management

Besides medication, the client with disk herniation is managed with bed rest for 1 to 2 days. This is followed by a physical therapy program. It may include proper body mechanics and positioning and exercises to strengthen the back. Clients should sleep on a firm mattress. Those with cervical injuries may need to wear a cervical collar or brace. Hot, moist compresses to the neck are useful to relieve muscle spasms. Most clients respond well to these conservative treatments.

Surgery

Surgery is necessary when conservative measures fail or there are serious neurologic deficits. The following surgical procedures may be used:

- *Diskectomy:* removal of the herniated disk or disk fragments

BOX 39-12	NURSING CARE CHECKLIST

Laminectomy

Before the Procedure

☑ Provide routine preoperative care (see Chapter 9). ⊙⊙

☑ Teach client logrolling technique.

After the Procedure

☑ Provide routine postoperative care (see Chapter 9). ⊙⊙

☑ After a cervical laminectomy:

☑ Place small pillow under the neck.

☑ Keep cervical collar in place.

☑ After a lumbar laminectomy:

☑ Keep the bed flat or elevate the head of the bed slightly.

☑ Place a small pillow under the head and a pillow under the knees.

☑ Logroll the client every 2 hours.

☑ Assess sensation and movement of arms and hands (cervical) and lower extremities and feet (lumbar). Report motor or sensory impairment immediately.

☑ Inspect dressing for drainage with halo sign; test for glucose.

☑ Palpate operative site for a hematoma. Maintain wound suction and patency of drains.

☑ For cervical laminectomy, assess for difficulty swallowing, hoarseness, increased swelling at neck, or labored breathing.

- *Laminectomy:* removal of the vertebral lamina to relieve pressure on the nerves. This is the most common surgical procedure. Nursing care is discussed in Box 39-12 ■.
- *Spinal Fusion:* insertion of bone graft (from iliac crest) between the vertebrae, which fuses the vertebra so they are more stable
- *Chemonucleolysis:* injection of the enzyme chymopapain into the nucleus pulposus to shrink or dissolve the protruding herniation

The surgical approach depends on the location and size of the ruptured disk. The posterior approach is used for lumbar surgery. An anterior or posterior approach is used for cervical disks.

After a successful surgery, the majority of clients are able to return to their jobs in about 6 weeks. They may experience a few small areas of permanent numbness in the involved leg.

NURSING CARE

Clients with a herniated disk experience pain and possibly reduced mobility. These problems can affect everyday life. Nursing care focuses on managing pain and preventing any further injury.

BOX 39-13	ASSESSMENT

Assessing Clients with Herniated Intervertebral Disk

SUBJECTIVE DATA

- Pain radiating from hip to foot or neck to hand.
- Muscle weakness or spasms.
- Numbness and tingling of the leg, foot, or neck, shoulder, arm, or hand.
- Neck stiffness.
- Difficulty sleeping at night.
- Past medical history of falls, sudden straining of back, heavy lifting, osteoarthritis, or having a myelogram.

OBJECTIVE DATA

- Observe for abnormalities of the posture when standing.
- Assess ROM of affected extremity.
- Assess level of muscle weakness in arm or leg.
- Assess location and type of pain and aggravating and relieving factors.
- Test patellar, Achilles, or triceps reflexes.
- Note changes in gait, for example, walking with a limp.
- Monitor and report diagnostic test results.

ASSESSING

The client is assessed for the degree to which a herniated intervertebral disk affects the client's daily life. Data can determine possible treatment options (Box 39-13 ■).

DIAGNOSING, PLANNING, AND IMPLEMENTING

Priorities in Nursing Care. Nursing care for the client with a herniated intervertebral disk focuses on pain management during medical management or after surgery.

Acute Pain

- Maintain bed rest as prescribed. Teach to logroll when changing positions. *Restricting activity and proper positioning may prevent muscle spasms.*
- Use a firm mattress or place a board under the mattress. *A firm bed supports the spinal column and muscles.*
- Elevate the client's head and place a small pillow under the knees (for herniated lumbar disk) or under the neck (for herniated cervical disk). *Correct body positions can decrease intervertebral disk pressure.*
- Give muscle relaxant and analgesic medications on a regular basis around the clock. *Giving the medications around the clock lessens periods of severe pain.*

- Apply moist heat as ordered. *Moist heat increases blood flow and relaxes muscles.*
- Do not refer to the client as an addict. *Clients with chronic pain develop a tolerance to pain medications and may require higher dosages.*

clinical ALERT

Clients with chronic pain often develop tolerance to their pain medications, which does not mean addiction.

- When chronic pain is unrelieved, refer client to a pain management clinic. *These clinics offer specialists in pain management techniques.*

EVALUATING

To evaluate the effectiveness of nursing care for a client with a herniated disk, collect and record data related to absence of pain, muscle spasms, numbness, tingling, and neurologic deficits.

Documenting. Documentation about client teaching includes proper body mechanics, pain control, and, if applicable, follow-up after surgery.

CONTINUING CARE

Preparing the client for care at home may involve teaching about pain control or follow-up after surgery. Review medications and potential side effects. Teach the client and family about relaxation techniques. Listening to the client is important to determine the best methods for pain management. If needed, discuss referral to a pain management center with the physician.

The client is taught to maintain proper body positioning and body mechanics. The following are some of the guidelines to reinforce:

- Sleep on a firm mattress or use a bedboard. Use a small pillow under the neck and sleep on the side with the knees flexed.
- Sit in straight-backed chairs.
- Avoid activities that flex the spine, such as bending or lifting, and do not twist the back.
- Follow the prescribed exercise program.
- Wear flat-heeled shoes that provide good support.
- Use proper body mechanics.

Following surgery, discuss incision site care and the symptoms of wound infection and healing. The client and family also need to understand the client's limitations. For example, driving is prohibited for the first 6 weeks. All activities that involve bending, twisting, and lifting are avoided. Clients should not lift more than 10 pounds. Review the use of a cervical collar, back brace, or corset. Reinforce indications for when to seek medical care.

Spinal Cord Tumor

Spinal cord tumors may be benign or malignant, primary or secondary. Primary tumors develop from a part of the cord. Secondary tumors start from lung, breast, or other cancer sites, then spread to the spinal cord. Spinal cord tumors are also classified as *intramedullary* (within the spinal cord) or *extramedullary* (outside the spinal cord). Most tumors occur in the thoracic and cervical areas.

Spinal cord tumors compress the cord, spinal nerve roots, and surrounding blood vessels. Manifestations relate to how fast or slow the tumor grows, the tumor site, and spinal nerve involvement. Slow-growing tumors allow the cord to adapt to the compression. Symptoms do not appear until the tumor is quite involved. Metastatic tumors usually grow quickly, causing symptoms to appear sooner.

Pain is often the first sign and is described as localized or radiating. Localized pain accompanies metastatic tumors involving the vertebrae. Radiating pain follows a path along the spinal nerve root. There are also motor and sensory deficits on one side of the body. Motor deficits include weakness and clumsiness; sensory deficits consist of numbness, tingling, and coldness in an extremity. Bladder involvement causes urinary frequency, urgency, and difficulty voiding.

The diagnosis of a spinal cord tumor begins with a history and neurologic exam. This is followed by a CT scan or MRI study to visualize the tumor. A lumbar puncture can identify the presence of tumor cells in the cerebrospinal fluid.

Spinal cord tumors are treated by surgical excision and radiation therapy. Surgery is most successful for extramedullary tumors. Intramedullary and metastatic tumors may be only partially removed due to their location or invasiveness of surrounding tissues. Surgery is followed with radiation therapy. Severe pain is managed by inserting an epidural catheter for continuous narcotic analgesic administration. Corticosteroids are given to control edema of the cord.

Assessments and nursing interventions are similar to those described for clients with an SCI or surgery for a herniated intervertebral disk. Care is different depending on whether the client has a benign or metastatic tumor. Discharge teaching includes how the family can provide physical care and manage pain (See Chapter 12 ⚭ for cancer pain control methods.)

Note: The bibliography listings for this and all chapters have been compiled at the back of the book.

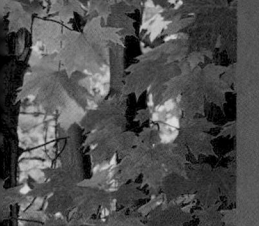

Chapter Review

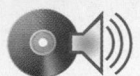 **KEY TERMS** by Topics

Use the audio glossary feature of either the CD-ROM or the Companion Website to hear the correct pronunciation of the following key terms.

Degenerative Neurologic Disorders
Alzheimer's disease (AD), sundowning syndrome, multiple sclerosis (MS), demyelination, plasmapheresis, Parkinson's disease (PD), dopamine, bradykinesia, myasthenia gravis, thymectomy, Huntington's disease (HD), chorea, amyotrophic lateral sclerosis (ALS), fasciculations, Guillain–Barré syndrome (GBS), trigeminal neuralgia, rhizotomy, Bell's palsy, rabies, tetanus, trismus, Creutzfeldt–Jakob disease (CJD)

Spinal Cord Disorders
paraplegia, tetraplegia, spinal shock, autonomic dysreflexia, herniated intervertebral disk, sciatica, spinal cord tumors

KEY Points

- Clients with advanced Alzheimer's disease must be monitored closely for disorientation and wandering to prevent injury.

- Multiple sclerosis is characterized by periods of exacerbation and remission, with remissions occurring less often as the disease progresses.

- Early manifestations of Parkinson's disease are managed with the administration of levodopa medications.

- The client with myasthenia gravis and family are taught to identify the two life-threatening emergencies: myasthenic or cholinergic crisis.

- Clients with trigeminal neuralgia experience severe facial pain when their trigger zones are stimulated.

- Spinal cord injury at C_4 or higher threatens the client's respiratory function. Report any symptoms of respiratory distress immediately to the physician.

- Clients with tetraplegia are at an increased risk for urinary tract infections and pneumonia. Any manifestation of these disorders should be treated immediately.

- Nursing care following a lumbar laminectomy focuses on logrolling the client every 2 hours until mobile. Immediately report any motor or sensory impairment.

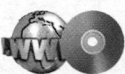 **EXPLORE MediaLink**

Additional interactive resources for this chapter can be found on the Companion Website at www.prenhall.com/burke. Click on Chapter 39 and "Begin" to select the activities for this chapter.

For chapter-related NCLEX-style review questions and an audio glossary, access the accompanying CD-ROM in this book.

FOR FURTHER Study

See Chapter 9 for a discussion of routine preoperative and postoperative care.

For more about control of cancer pain, see Chapter 12.

For care of a client with a tracheostomy, see Chapter 23.

For more information about mechanical ventilation, see Chapter 24.

For more information on anticoagulants, see Chapter 28.

For the paired cranial nerves, see Chapter 37.

Caring for a Client with Herniated Intervertebral Disk

NCLEX-PN® Focus Area: Physiologic Integrity

Case Study: A 50-year-old woman is thrown over the handlebars of her bicycle and sustains an intervertebral injury at C_5 and C_6. At the hospital a CT scan shows damaged ligaments and herniation of the C_7 disk. She is sent home with a cervical collar to stabilize the area. Two weeks later she complains of insomnia, acute pain in her neck and shoulders, and numbness and tingling in her left hand. She is concerned about when she can return to work.

Nursing Diagnosis: Impaired Physical Mobility

COLLECT DATA

Subjective	Objective
_____	_____
_____	_____
_____	_____
_____	_____
_____	_____
_____	_____

Would you report this data? Yes/No

If yes, to: _____

Nursing Care

_____

_____

_____

_____

_____

_____

_____

_____

_____

_____

_____

How would you document this? _____

_____

_____

_____

Data Collected (use those that apply)

- Insomnia
- Decreased ability to use left hand
- Pain in the neck and shoulders
- Concern about returning to work
- BP 110/78, P 68
- Complains of muscle weakness in left arm
- Unable to ride her bicycle at home
- Decreased reflexes in left arm

Nursing Interventions (use those that apply; list in priority order)

- Consult with physical therapist for mobility plan.
- Increase fiber in the diet.
- Instruct her to sleep on a firm mattress.
- Instruct her to keep the cervical collar on at all times.
- Give analgesics around the clock.
- Encourage six to eight glasses of water per day.
- Teach her to not lift objects or twist neck.

NCLEX-PN® Exam Preparation

TEST-TAKING TIP Be familiar with the relationship of functional abilities as they relate to specific levels of spinal cord injuries.

1 A client is being evaluated for a possible diagnosis of Alzheimer's disease. The client's symptoms include forgetfulness, difficulty making decisions, decreased ability to concentrate, and depression. The nurse knows that these are symptoms of:

A. stage 1.
B. stage 2.
C. stage 3.
D. pre-Alzheimer's.

2 The nurse is caring for a client with multiple sclerosis. Which one of these medications should the nurse expect to give if the client develops urinary frequency?

A. amantadine (Symmetrel)
B. dexamethasone (Decadron)
C. dantrolene (Dantrium)
D. propantheline (Pro-Banthine)

3 The client with Parkinson's disease is being taught about taking carbidopa-levodopa (Sinemet). What teaching points should the nurse emphasize? Select all that apply.

A. Report the "on–off" effect.
B. Change position slowly.
C. Report blurred vision or a rash.
D. Avoid taking medication with meals.
E. Monitor the color of your urine.
F. Increase fluid intake.

4 The nurse is caring for a client who has sustained a spinal cord injury above the sixth cervical vertebrae. Which of the following stimuli could trigger autonomic dysreflexia?

A. bladder distention
B. a headache
C. sneezing
D. cold feet

5 If a client is developing Guillian–Barré syndrome, what manifestation should the nurse expect to find first?

A. weakness in the arms
B. hypotension
C. dysphagia
D. numbness in the lower extremities

6 What functional ability should the nurse expect a client with a spinal cord injury at the fifth cervical vertebrae to achieve?

A. Use a voice-controlled wheelchair.
B. Can self-transfer.
C. Operate an electric wheelchair.
D. Operate a manual wheelchair.

7 When caring for the client with a herniated lumbar disk, the nurse should:

A. encourage the client to sit in a comfortable chair.
B. elevate the client's head and place a small pillow under the knees.
C. encourage the client to move as little as possible.
D. turn the client once a shift.

8 The nurse is caring for a client with myasthenia gravis. When planning the client's care, the nurse knows that it is critical to:

A. note any complaints by the client of changes in vision.
B. administer medications on a strict time schedule.
C. do the client's care quickly because she tires easily.
D. turn the client every 2 hours.

9 Which one of the following self-care strategies should the nurse teach to the client with trigeminal neuralgia?

A. Increase fluid intake.
B. Chew on the affected side.
C. Monitor calorie intake.
D. Ways to avoid trigger points.

10 The nurse is caring for a client who has just had a myelogram (water-soluble dye was used). It is important for the nurse to encourage the client to:

A. avoid coughing or sneezing.
B. stay flat in bed for 8 to 12 hours.
C. drink plenty of fluids.
D. not eat for several hours.

Answers for Review Questions, as well as discussion of Care Plan and Critical Thinking Care Map questions, appear in Appendix V.

Chapter 40

Caring for Clients with Eye and Ear Disorders

BRIEF Outline

Infectious or Inflammatory Eye Disorders
Eye Trauma
Refractive Errors
Cataracts
Glaucoma
Detached Retina
Macular Degeneration
Diabetic Retinopathy
Enucleation
Blindness
External Otitis
Impacted Cerumen and Foreign Bodies
Otitis Media
Otosclerosis
Inner Ear Disorders
Hearing Loss

LEARNING Outcomes

After completing this chapter, you will be able to:

- Describe the pathophysiology and manifestations of common eye and ear disorders.
- Describe nursing implications for drugs prescribed for clients with eye and ear disorders.
- Provide appropriate nursing care for a client having eye or ear surgery.
- Use the nursing process to provide individualized care for clients with problems that affect vision or hearing.

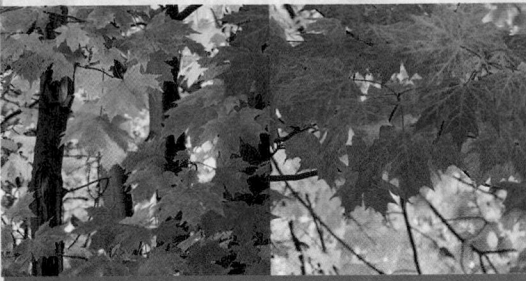

MediaLink

www.prenhall.com/burke
Use the address above to access the free, interactive Companion Website created for this textbook. Get hints, instant feedback, and textbook references to chapter-related NCLEX-style questions. Link to other interesting sites.

Audio Glossary:
Use the Companion Website, or the CD-ROM disk enclosed with your textbook, to hear the pronunciation of key terms in this chapter.

Vision and hearing are special senses that allow us to experience the world in which we live. The eyes allow us to see by providing a pathway for light, color, and images to reach the brain. The ears allow us to hear by providing a pathway for sounds to reach the brain. The special senses warn us of danger and protect us from injury. In addition, specialized structures within the ear help maintain position sense and balance. Deficits in the special senses may limit self-care, mobility, independence, communication, and relationships with others.

EYE DISORDERS

Infectious or Inflammatory Eye Disorders

The normally protective structures of the eye—the eyelids, eyelashes, and conjunctiva—may become inflamed or infected because they are constantly exposed to the environment.

DISORDERS AFFECTING THE EYELID

Blepharitis, inflammation of the eyelid, may be caused by an infection or by dermatitis. The eyelid is irritated and itchy. The eyelid margins are red, crusted, and scaly. A *hordeolum (sty)* is an infection of the sebaceous glands of the eyelid, usually caused by *Staphylococcus aureus* (Figure 40-1A ■). A sty is red and painful. It may affect either the external or internal lid margin. *Chalazion* is a painless cyst or nodule of the eyelid (Figure 40-1B).

CONJUNCTIVITIS

Conjunctivitis (inflammation of the conjunctiva) is a common eye disease. It is usually caused by a bacterial or viral infection spread by direct contact, for example, from hands, tissues, or towels. Acute conjunctivitis, also known as "pink eye," is usually mild, with redness, itching, tearing, and discharge of the eye (Figure 40-2 ■).

Some conjunctival infections, such as gonorrhea and trachoma, can damage the cornea, threatening vision. *Trachoma* is a major cause of blindness in parts of Africa, the Middle East, and Asia.

DISORDERS AFFECTING THE CORNEA

The clear cornea transmits and helps focus light and images onto the retina. It also protects the internal eye. The cornea has no blood supply. Scarring or ulceration of the cornea can lead to blindness.

Keratitis is inflammation of the cornea, usually caused by infection, lack of tears, or trauma. **Corneal ulcers** (Figure 40-3 ■) may be caused by infection, trauma, or contact lens overuse. Herpes viruses such as herpes zoster (shingles) can cause corneal ulcers. Corneal ulcers may be superficial or deep. Scarring may occur, clouding the cornea. If the cornea is perforated, infection of the internal eye and vision loss may result.

Inflammation of the cornea causes discomfort, tearing, discharge, and **photophobia** (extreme sensitivity to light). *Blepharospasm* (spasm of the eyelid and inability to open the

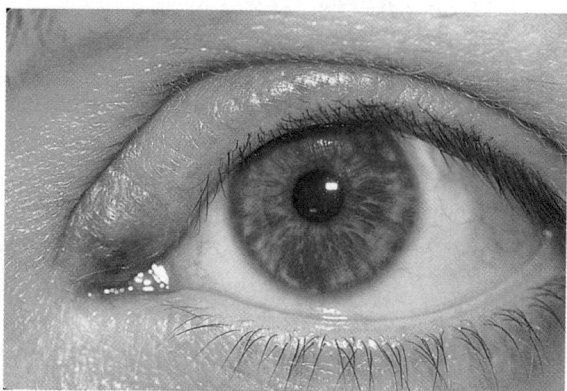

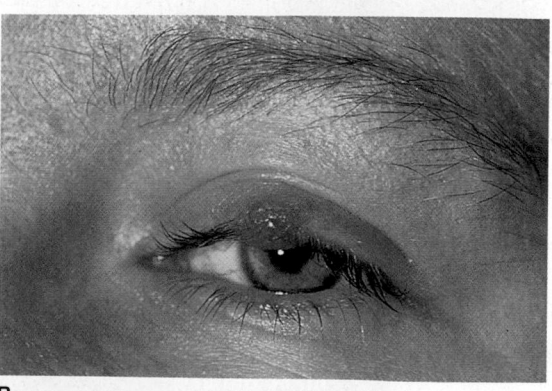

Figure 40-1. ■ **(A)** Hordeolum (sty); (*Source:* Sph Photo Researchers) **(B)** Chalazion (*Source:* Custom Medical Stock Photos, Inc.)

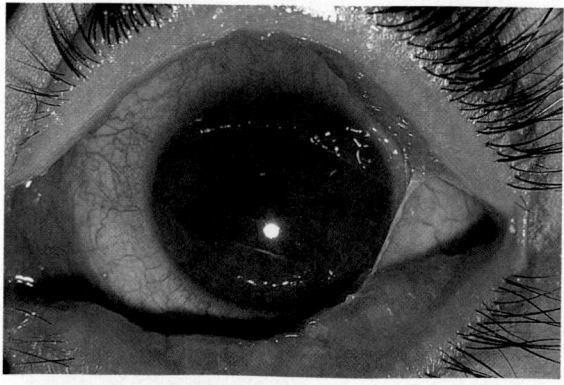

Figure 40-2. ■ An eye with acute conjunctivitis. (*Source:* Buddy Crofton/Medical Images, Inc.)

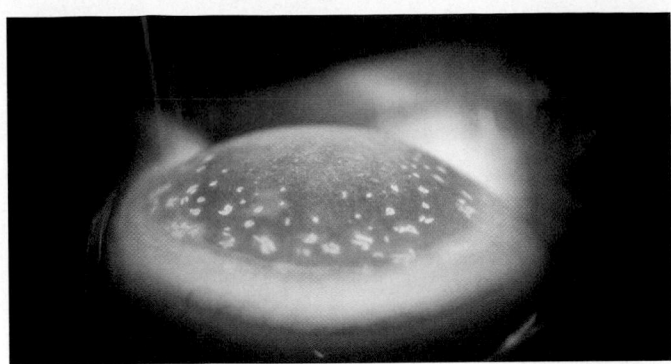

Figure 40-3. ■ Corneal ulcers. (*Source:* Custom Medical Stock Photos, Inc.)

eye) may develop. Sudden, severe eye pain may indicate corneal perforation.

UVEITIS AND IRITIS

Uveitis is inflammation of the middle vascular layer of the eye. *Iritis* (inflammation of the iris only) is more common. The client complains of severe eye pain, photophobia, and blurred vision. The pupil is constricted, and the limbus (where the cornea meets the conjunctiva) is red.

INTERDISCIPLINARY CARE

Prompt treatment of infectious or inflammatory eye disorders is important to preserve vision. Corneal ulcers are medical emergencies that must be referred to an ophthalmologist promptly for treatment.

Most of these disorders can be diagnosed by the history and examination of the eye. Usually, no diagnostic tests are required, although the following tests may be ordered:

- *Fluorescein stain with slit lamp examination* will show corneal ulcers or abrasions, which appear green with staining.
- *Conjunctival or ulcer scrapings* may be examined or cultured.

Medications

Topical anti-infectives applied as eyedrops or ointment often are ordered to treat eye infections. Antihistamines or corticosteroids may be prescribed when the eye is inflamed but no infection is present. Clients with uveitis may be given eyedrops to keep the pupil dilated and reduce discomfort.

Corneal Transplant

When the cornea is scarred and opaque (see Figure 40-3), a corneal transplant can restore vision. Corneas may be taken from people who died as a result of acute trauma or a noninfectious illness. Transplant rejection is low because the cornea has a limited blood supply, which limits the client's exposure to rejection antibodies. The client's scarred cornea is removed, and the graft is sutured in place. The sutures remain in place for up to a year. The eye is patched for 24 hours after surgery. The client must avoid activities that can increase intraocular pressure, such as straining to have a bowel movement, bending over, and lifting or pushing heavy objects. Eyedrops are ordered to reduce inflammation and prevent infection. Nursing care of the client undergoing eye surgery is discussed later in this chapter (see Box 40-2).

Complementary Therapies

Careful cleansing of the lid margins using a "no-tears" baby shampoo is often recommended for marginal blepharitis. Soaking the lids with warm saline compresses before cleansing may ease removal of the crusts and exudates seen in blepharitis and conjunctivitis. Eye irrigation may be ordered to remove the purulent discharge associated with conjunctivitis. Local heat applications may be used to treat hordeolum or chalazion.

NURSING CARE

The nursing care for clients with infections and inflammatory eye disorders may involve direct care. More often care focuses on prevention and client teaching. Nurses working in outpatient surgical centers provide care to clients undergoing corneal transplant.

ASSESSING

Ask the client to describe the symptoms, their onset, and any relationship between the symptoms and an injury or exposure to an infection or allergen. Inquire about the effect on vision and any associated symptoms, such as chills or fever. Identify the date of the client's most recent eye examination. Ask about corrective lens use, including type of lenses. Obtain past medical history, especially any chronic diseases, previous eye problems, and current medication use.

Test vision (with client wearing corrective lenses if normally worn) using a Snellen chart (see Chapter 5, Figure 5-5) ⬭⬭ or Rosenbaum chart. The Rosenbaum chart (see Chapter 37, Figure 37-11) ⬭⬭ is held 12 to 14 inches from the eyes, with vision assessed in the same manner as with the Snellen chart. Inspect the eye, including the conjunctiva, lids, and surrounding tissues. Check pupil size and response to light and accommodation.

DIAGNOSING, PLANNING, AND IMPLEMENTING

Priorities in Nursing Care. The priority nursing diagnoses for clients with infectious and inflammatory eye disorders focus on the risk for impaired vision, pain, and risk for injury.

Risk for Disturbed Sensory Perception: Visual

- Instruct to wash the hands thoroughly before inserting or removing contact lenses or instilling any eye medications. Teach to avoid touching or rubbing the eyes. *Hand washing is the single most important measure to prevent transmission of infection to the eye.*
- Emphasize the importance of proper contact lens care, including periodic lens removal and cleaning. *Improper cleaning and wearing contact lenses longer than recommended are major risk factors for infection and corneal damage.*
- If the cornea perforates, place the client in the supine position, close the eye, and cover it with a dry, sterile dressing. Notify the physician immediately. *Corneal perforation can lead to loss of eye contents.*

clinical ALERT

Suspect corneal perforation with complaints of sudden, severe eye pain and photophobia.

Pain

- Administer analgesics routinely in the first 12 to 24 hours after corneal surgery. *The outer portion of the eye, the cornea in particular, is extremely sensitive. Giving analgesics on a schedule prevents pain from becoming severe.*
- Patch both eyes if necessary. *Patching both eyes reduces eye movement and irritation of the affected eye.*
- Teach the client to apply warm compresses for 15 minutes, three to four times a day. *Warm compresses reduce inflammation and promote comfort.*
- Instruct to use dark sunglasses with ultraviolet (UV) protection when out of doors, even on cloudy days. *Bright light can cause eye pain in clients with an inflammation or infection.*
- Advise to avoid excessive reading or other close tasks. *Eye rest also promotes comfort.*

Risk for Injury

- Discuss the effect of an eye patch on depth perception and peripheral vision. Teach the client to scan from side to side and to be careful when judging distances or speed. *Patching one eye affects depth perception, increasing the risk for falling, traffic accidents, or other trauma.*
- Instruct not to rub or scratch the eye. *Rubbing or scratching may spread infection or damage a corneal graft.*
- Teach how to apply an eye shield at night. *An eye shield helps prevent inadvertent rubbing or trauma of the eye during sleep.*
- Teach clients to use eye protection during activities that can damage the eye. *Trauma increases the risk of infection and scarring of the cornea.*

EVALUATING

Collect and record the following data to evaluate the effectiveness of nursing care:

- Appearance of the eye
- Vision (using a chart to measure visual acuity)
- Demonstrates proper contact lens care
- Demonstrates instillation of eye drops using appropriate technique.

Documenting. Documentation includes the appearance of the eye, visual deficits, and ability to instill eye drops.

CONTINUING CARE

Teach all clients about hand washing and proper eye care. Instruct clients to use a new, clean cotton-tipped swab or cotton ball for each eye when cleansing eyelids. Teach how to instill eyedrops and ointments. If an eye patch is ordered, be sure the client or a family member knows how to apply it and where to obtain necessary supplies.

Teach contact lens users how to care for and clean the lenses. Stress the importance of periodically removing lenses, even extended-wear lenses. In general, lenses should be removed at night. Advise the client who has a corneal abrasion or keratitis to avoid wearing contact lenses until the cornea has healed completely.

Stress the importance of follow-up appointments after a corneal transplant. Reinforce teaching about how to prevent increased intraocular pressure (e.g., avoiding straining, vomiting, coughing, and lifting). Instruct the client and family to promptly report inflammation, graft cloudiness, or increased pain to the physician.

Eye Trauma

Any part of the eye, especially the exposed parts, can be affected by trauma. Foreign bodies, abrasions, and lacerations are the most common types of eye injury.

A *corneal abrasion* is a "scratch" of the cornea. Contact lenses, eyelashes, small foreign bodies, and fingernails often cause corneal abrasions. Corneal abrasions are extremely painful, causing photophobia and tearing. They usually heal rapidly without scarring.

Burns can affect the outer portion of the eye. Chemicals such as ammonia, oven and drain cleaners, and acids from car batteries commonly burn the eye. Thermal burns often occur in an explosion. UV light burns may be called other names depending on the source such as snowblindness or welder's-arc burn. A burn causes pain and affects vision. Eyelids are swollen and the conjunctiva is red and edematous; it may slough. The cornea often appears cloudy or hazy.

The eye may be *perforated* by metal flakes produced by high-speed drilling or grinding, glass shards, or weapons such as gunshots (including BBs), arrows, and knives. The layers of the eye can close after being penetrated by a small or sharp object. In these cases, the injury may not be apparent. Eye perforations cause pain, partial or complete loss of vision, and possibly bleeding or loss of eye contents.

Blunt eye trauma is often caused by sports injuries. The injury may be minor, such as lid *ecchymosis* (black eye) or *subconjunctival hemorrhage* (bleeding into the conjunctiva). These minor injuries typically do not need to be treated. *Hyphema,* bleeding into the anterior chamber of the eye, causes a reddish tint to the client's vision and visible blood in the anterior chamber. The eye orbit may be fractured by blunt trauma. The client experiences **diplopia** (double vision) and pain with eye movement. The eye appears sunken (*enophthalmos*).

INTERDISCIPLINARY CARE

The extent of injury caused by trauma is determined by eye exam. Unless immediate treatment is required, as with a chemical burn, vision is evaluated with corrective lenses if normally worn. Eye movement is evaluated unless a penetrating object is present (Box 40-1 ▪). The lid and conjunctiva are inspected for foreign objects and lacerations. A topical anesthetic may be used to relieve eye pain and photophobia prior to inspection. *Fluorescein staining* can help identify the presence of foreign bodies and abrasions. *Ophthalmoscopic examination* is done to detect bleeding or trauma to the interior chamber. Facial x-rays and computed tomography (CT) scans are used to identify orbital fractures or the presence of foreign bodies within the globe.

The eye is irrigated with sterile saline to remove small foreign bodies. Copious amounts of fluid are used to flush the eye when a chemical burn occurs. A special contact lens irrigating unit or a bottle of irrigant with intravenous tubing held to flush all eye surfaces may be used. During irrigation, fluid is directed from the inner canthus of the eye to the outer. The client's head is tipped slightly to the affected side to prevent contamination of the other eye. A sterile, moistened, cotton-tipped applicator or other instrument may be used to remove a foreign body. After the procedure, a topical antibiotic ointment is applied. An eye patch may be applied to keep the eye closed for approximately 24 hours.

Penetrating wounds usually require surgery. Narcotic analgesics, sedatives, and antiemetic drugs are given to relieve pain and anxiety and prevent vomiting, which increases intraocular pressure.

NURSING CARE

Nursing care for clients with eye trauma focuses on protecting the eye and preserving vision.

Impaired Tissue Integrity: Ocular

- Assess and record vision in each eye and both eyes, with and without corrective lenses. *The initial assessment provides a baseline and data about the effect of the injury on the client's vision.*
- Assess eye(s) and surrounding tissues for foreign bodies, burns, penetrating injury, or blunt trauma. *Eye trauma may be hidden by other injuries.*
- Immediately irrigate the eye if a chemical burn is suspected. *Irrigation to remove the chemical is of higher priority than assessment of the eye.*
- Remove loose foreign bodies using a moist, sterile, cotton-tipped applicator. *Prompt removal of foreign bodies may prevent corneal abrasion.*
- For a severe or penetrating injury, place the client on bed rest and stabilize the injured eye by applying an eye pad or gauze dressing loosely over both eyes. Stabilize any penetrating object if possible. *These measures reduce eye movement and can help preserve vision.*
- Following treatment, apply eyedrops or ointment and an eye pad or shield as ordered. *An eye pad is often applied to the affected eye to reduce pain and photophobia and to promote healing.*

BOX 40-1 | **ASSESSMENT**

Assessing Clients: The Cardinal Fields of Vision

Eye movement is assessed using the *six cardinal fields of vision.* Ask the client to follow a pen or your finger while keeping the head still. Move the pen or your finger through the six fields one at a time, returning to the central starting point and pausing before proceeding to the next field (see figure). The eyes should move through each field without involuntary movements.

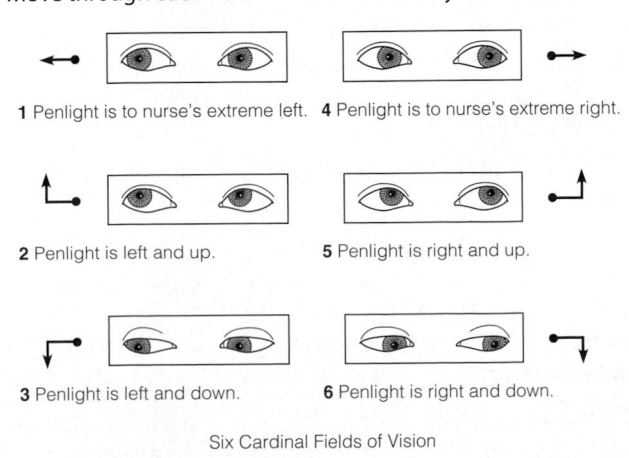

1 Penlight is to nurse's extreme left. **4** Penlight is to nurse's extreme right.

2 Penlight is left and up. **5** Penlight is right and up.

3 Penlight is left and down. **6** Penlight is right and down.

Six Cardinal Fields of Vision

CONTINUING CARE

Teaching people how to prevent eye injuries is an important nursing responsibility. Teach employees and people participating in high-risk sports and activities how and when to use eye protectors. Stress the importance of using seat belts and air bags to prevent eye injury in car crashes. Teach clients to immediately flush the eye with copious amounts of water if a chemical splash occurs. Loose, visible foreign bodies can be removed using a clean, moistened, cotton-tipped swab. If an abrasion or penetrating or blunt injury is suspected, loosely cover the eye with sterile gauze and immediately seek medical attention. Instruct clients not to remove objects that penetrate the eye. Both eyes should be patched to prevent movement until medial help is obtained.

Following an injury, reinforce teaching about follow-up treatment. Discuss the ordered medications, including how to instill eyedrops and ointments. Stress the need to avoid rubbing or scratching the eye. Teach the client or family how to apply the eye pad or shield if ordered. If ordered, instruct the client to avoid activities that increase intraocular pressure, such as lifting, straining, or bending over, to prevent further eye damage.

Refractive Errors

Changes in the shape of the cornea, lens, or the eyeball affect the focus of light on the retina. The result is blurred or indistinct vision. These *refractive errors* or defects are the most common cause of impaired vision. Common refractive errors include *myopia* (nearsightedness), *hyperopia* (farsightedness), and *astigmatism.* The causes and effects of these errors are summarized in Table 40-1 ■. Refractive errors often are detected through routine vision screening.

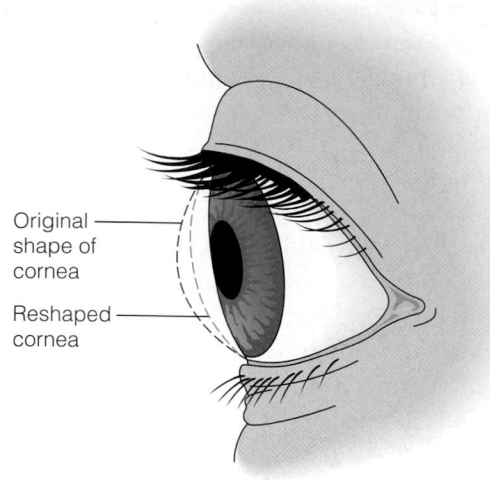

Figure 40-4. ■ LASIK surgery corrects refractive error by flattening the cornea of the eye.

The refractive error can usually be corrected with eyeglasses or contact lenses.

Several surgical procedures have been developed to correct refractive errors. *Radial keratotomy* uses a series of shallow radial incisions in the cornea to flatten it. In a *photorefractive keratectomy (PRK),* a very thin layer of corneal tissue is shaved to reshape the cornea. *Laser in situ keratomileusis (LASIK)* is similar. A thin flap of the cornea is lifted, then the center of the cornea is shaved to flatten it (Figure 40-4 ■). The flap is then replaced; it is held in place by the eye's natural stickiness. These surgeries require only minutes to complete and are done on an outpatient basis.

Nurses can help identify clients with refractive disorders and encourage them to seek treatment. Check the vision of clients who have difficulty reading printed material,

TABLE 40-1			
Common Refractive Errors			
PROBLEM	**CAUSE**	**EFFECT**	**CORRECTION**
Myopia (nearsightedness)	Abnormally long eyeball	Light rays focus in front of the retina. Distant objects are unclear. Focus improves as object is closer to the eye.	Concave corrective lenses Radial keratotomy Photoreceptive keratectomy (PRK) Laser *in situ* keratomileusis (LASIK)
Hyperopia (farsightedness)	Abnormally short eyeball	Light rays focus behind the retina. Close objects are unclear. Able to focus on distant objects through accommodation.	Convex corrective lenses Laser thermokeratoplasty
Presbyopia	Impaired accommodation of the lens caused by aging		
Astigmatism	Irregularities in the curvature of the cornea and lens	Light rays are imperfectly focused on the retina.	Requires correction only when refractive error affects vision

identifying objects, or following visual directions using a standard eye chart. First test each eye, then test vision using both eyes (see Chapter 5). ⚭ Refer clients whose vision is poorer than 20/40 in either or both eyes to an optometrist or ophthalmologist for further evaluation. In addition to the obvious nursing diagnosis of Disturbed Sensory Perception, the following nursing diagnoses may be appropriate:

- Risk for Injury related to inability to clearly see traffic signs and directions
- Risk for Noncompliance related to financial or cosmetic concerns.

Discuss the effect of eyeglasses on depth perception, and advise the client to be careful on stairs until he or she is used to the lenses. If contact lenses have been prescribed, teach and have the client demonstrate how to insert, remove, and care for them. Emphasize the importance of proper care to prevent eye infections or corneal abrasion. For clients who have had surgical correction of their vision, provide verbal and written instructions about postoperative care and follow-up. Teach the client and significant other how to instill prescribed eyedrops.

Cataracts

A **cataract** is clouding of the lens of the eye that impairs vision. Cataracts are common. Most people over age 65 have some cataracts. The cataract affects vision in only a few of these people, however. Cataracts usually affect both eyes, but tend to develop at different rates. Risk factors for cataracts include exposure to sunlight (UV-B rays), cigarette smoking, heavy alcohol consumption, congenital conditions, eye trauma, diabetes mellitus, and drugs such as corticosteroids and chlorpromazine (Thorazine).

PATHOPHYSIOLOGY AND MANIFESTATIONS

Most cataracts are *senile cataracts,* caused by aging. As the lens ages, its cells become less clear. First, this usually affects the edges of the lens, gradually spreading toward the center. Eventually, the entire lens may be clouded. When only a portion of the lens is affected, the cataract is called *immature.* A *mature cataract* involves the entire lens.

As a cataract matures, both near and distance vision are affected. Details become obscured (Figure 40-5 ■). The clouded lens scatters light rays, causing problems with glare and difficulty adjusting between light and dark environments. With a mature cataract, the pupil appears cloudy gray or white rather than black.

INTERDISCIPLINARY CARE

The diagnosis of a cataract is made based on the history and eye examination. As the cataract matures, the **red reflex** is lost. The location and extent of a cataract can be seen with

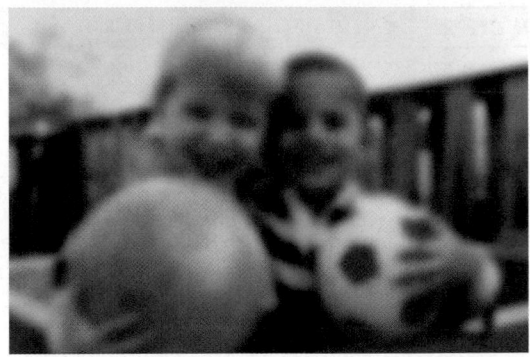

Figure 40-5. ■ Blurring of near and distant vision with a cataract. *(Courtesy National Eye Institute, National Institutes of Health.)*

ophthalmoscopic examination. No special diagnostic or laboratory procedures are required.

Cataracts are treated by surgical removal. This is an elective surgery, usually delayed until the cataract interferes with the client's activities of daily living and enjoyment of life. Cataract surgery is usually done on an outpatient basis, using local anesthesia. The clouded lens is removed through a small incision in the cornea (Figure 40-6 ■). An **intraocular lens** is implanted during the surgery to focus light and restore clear vision.

NURSING CARE

Nursing care for clients with cataracts focuses on teaching/ learning needs in both the pre- and postoperative periods. Cataract surgery is usually done as an outpatient procedure, and the client is often discharged within 1 hour

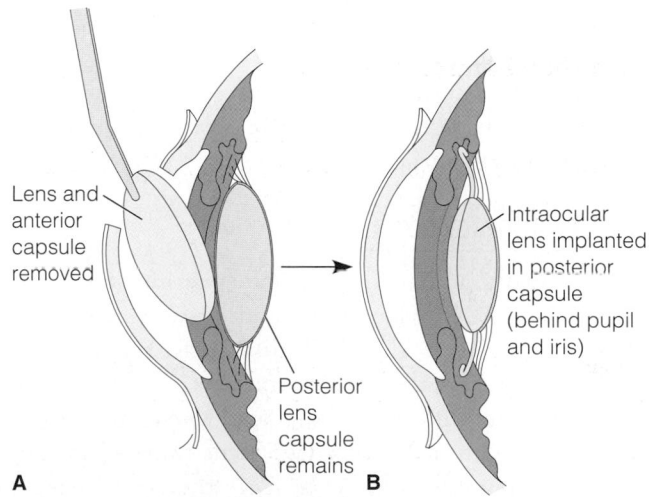

Figure 40-6. ■ Cataract removal with intraocular lens implant. (**A**) The lens and anterior capsule are removed. (**B**) The intraocular lens is implanted within the posterior capsule behind the pupil.

BOX 40-2	NURSING CARE CHECKLIST

Eye Surgery

Before Surgery

☑ Provide routine preoperative care as indicated (see Chapter 9). ⚭

☑ Assess understanding of the procedure. Clarify information as needed.

☑ Orient to the environment.

☑ Assess vision in the unaffected eye before surgery.

☑ Reinforce teaching about postoperative restrictions to prevent increased intraocular pressure: Avoid vomiting, straining at stool, coughing, sneezing, lifting more than 5 lbs, and bending over at the waist.

☑ Remove all eye makeup and contact lenses or glasses. Store them in a safe place.

☑ Administer preoperative medications and eyedrops or ointments as ordered.

After Surgery

☑ Assess and document vital signs, level of consciousness, comfort, and status of the eye dressing.

☑ Maintain the eye patch and shield as ordered.

☑ Place in semi-Fowler's or Fowler's position or as ordered.

☑ Approach client on unaffected side.

☑ Intervene as necessary to prevent vomiting, coughing, sneezing, or straining.

☑ Immediately report sudden, sharp eye pain to the physician.

☑ Place all personal articles and call bell within easy reach.

☑ Assist with ambulation when allowed.

☑ Administer eyedrops and other medications as ordered.

☑ Teach the client and family:

   a. How to instill eyedrops and about ordered medications
   b. How and when to apply eye patch and eye shield
   c. To avoid scratching, rubbing, touching, or squeezing the affected eye
   d. How to prevent constipation and straining, and about activity limitations
   e. Symptoms that should be reported to the physician, including eye pain or pressure, redness or cloudiness, drainage, decreased vision, floaters or flashes of light, or halos around bright objects
   f. To wear sunglasses with side shields when outdoors
   g. To make and keep recommended follow-up appointments.

☑ Arrange or refer the client for assistance with other health care needs (such as insulin injections) as needed following discharge.

after surgery. Box 40-2 ■ outlines nursing care of the client having eye surgery.

Deficient Knowledge: Cataracts

■ Provide information about cataracts and their surgical removal. Explain that cataracts usually are removed only when they interfere with vision and activities of daily living (ADLs). *This helps the client decide about surgery.*

■ Demonstrate a caring, understanding attitude toward concerns about vision. *Accepting the client's fears promotes trust and reduces anxiety.*

CONTINUING CARE

Clients usually are discharged home within hours after cataract surgery. Provide verbal and written instructions about postoperative care and directions for follow-up appointments. Include a family member in the teaching. Teach the client and family how and when to instill the prescribed eyedrops. Instruct the client to avoid reading, lifting, or strenuous activity; to leave the eye dressing in place; and to take prescribed medications during the initial 24-hour period. During the return visit, reinforce teaching about activity limitations to prevent increased intraocular pressure, protecting the operative eye, and symptoms of complications. Instruct to report eye pain, worsening of vision, headache, nausea, or itching and redness of the affected eye to the physician.

Glaucoma

Glaucoma is characterized by increased intraocular pressure and gradual loss of vision. It is a "silent" thief of vision: Peripheral vision is lost so slowly that it often is not noticed until late in the disease. This vision loss is permanent. Glaucoma is a leading cause of blindness worldwide and affects certain populations (Box 40-3 ■).

BOX 40-3	POPULATION FOCUS

Glaucoma

■ Open-angle glaucoma occurs more frequently and at an earlier age in African Americans. African Americans and people with a family history of glaucoma should be screened every 2 years over the age of 40.

■ Angle-closure glaucoma occurs more frequently in older adults and in people of Asian ancestry.

PATHOPHYSIOLOGY AND MANIFESTATIONS

Aqueous humor fills the space between the lens and the cornea. It is produced by the ciliary body and flows through the pupil into the anterior chamber. From there, it drains through the trabecular mesh into the canal of Schlemm. The normal intraocular pressure of 12 to 20 mm Hg is maintained by a balance between aqueous humor production and drainage. When this balance is disrupted, intraocular pressure increases.

In *open-angle glaucoma,* aqueous humor drainage through the trabecular meshwork into the canal of Schlemm is obstructed (Figure 40-7A ■). The amount of fluid in the eye increases. As a result, intraocular pressure increases. The increased pressure damages retinal neurons and the optic nerve. Peripheral vision is gradually lost and the visual field narrows (Figure 40-8 ■). Both eyes are usually affected. Untreated glaucoma eventually leads to blindness.

In *angle-closure glaucoma,* the angle between the cornea and iris closes, completely blocking drainage of aqueous

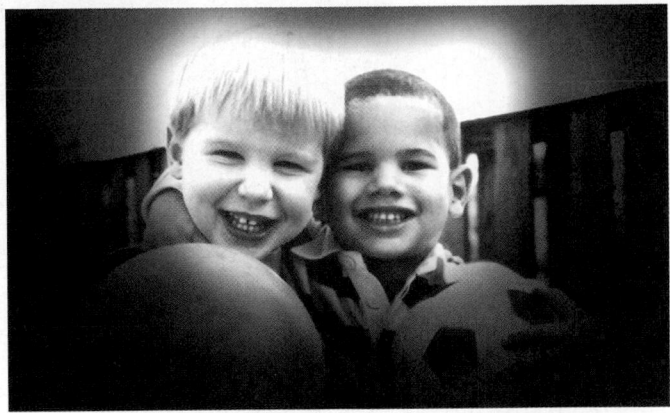

Figure 40-8. ■ Narrowing of the visual field with glaucoma. *(Courtesy National Eye Institute, National Institutes of Health.)*

humor from the eye (see Figure 40-7B). Intraocular pressure rises abruptly, damaging the retina and the optic nerve. Box 40-4 ■ lists the manifestations of chronic open-angle and angle-closure glaucoma.

clinical ALERT

Angle-closure glaucoma is a medical emergency. Without prompt treatment, the affected eye will become blind. Immediately report manifestations of acute angle-closure glaucoma to the charge nurse or physician.

Angle-closure glaucoma usually affects one eye. Episodes often occur when the pupil dilates (in darkness or with emotional upset), closing the angle. Angle-closure glaucoma can recur, therefore it is *vital* to avoid medications that can dilate the pupil. A client who has experienced an

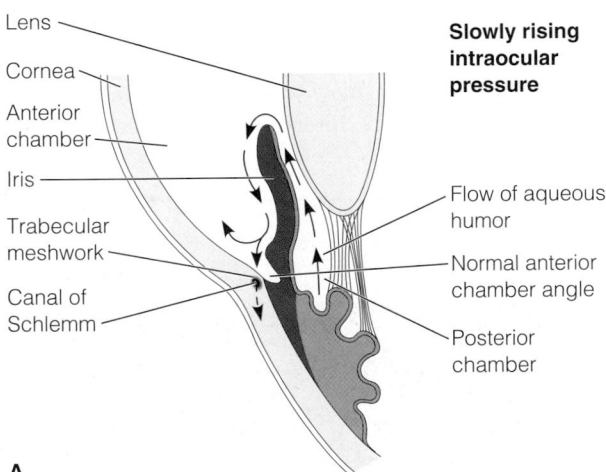

Slowly rising intraocular pressure

Lens
Cornea
Anterior chamber
Iris
Trabecular meshwork
Canal of Schlemm

Flow of aqueous humor
Normal anterior chamber angle
Posterior chamber

A

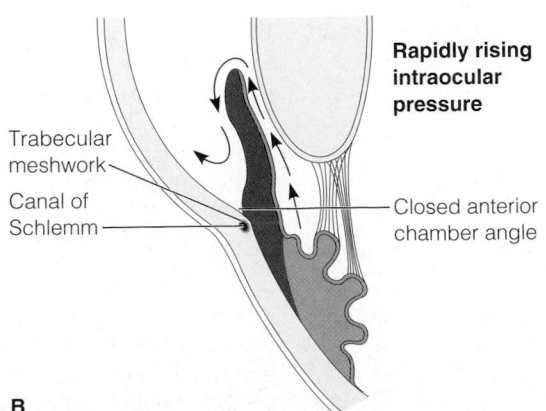

Rapidly rising intraocular pressure

Trabecular meshwork
Canal of Schlemm

Closed anterior chamber angle

B

Figure 40-7. ■ Types of glaucoma. **(A)** Chronic open-angle glaucoma. Drainage of aqueous humor through the trabecular meshwork is impaired. **(B)** Angle-closure glaucoma. The angle between the cornea and iris closes, completely blocking aqueous humor drainage.

BOX 40-4

MANIFESTATIONS OF GLAUCOMA

Open-Angle Glaucoma
- Painless
- Gradual loss of peripheral vision
- Difficulty adapting from light to dark
- Blurred vision
- Halos around lights
- Difficulty focusing on near objects

Angle-Closure Glaucoma
- Acute severe eye pain
- Blurred or cloudy vision
- Nausea and vomiting
- Halos around lights
- Affected eye red, cornea clouded
- Fixed (nonreactive) pupil

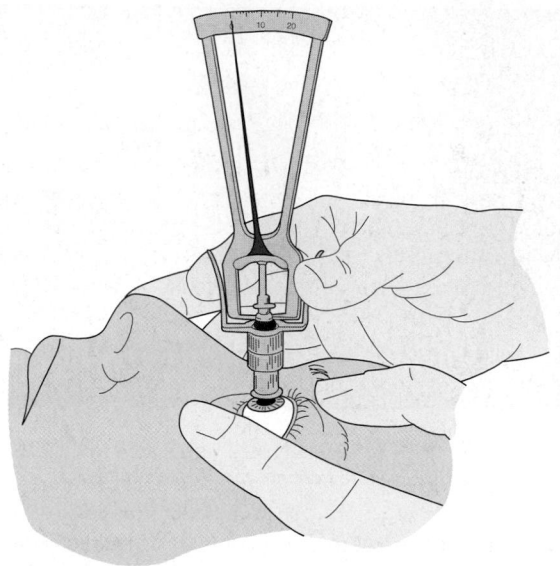

Figure 40-9. ■ The Schiötz tonometer for measuring intraocular pressure.

episode of angle-closure glaucoma in one eye is at risk for developing it in the other eye.

INTERDISCIPLINARY CARE

Although glaucoma cannot be cured, it can be controlled and vision preserved if it is diagnosed and treated early.

Routine eye examinations are recommended for early detection.

Diagnostic Tests

- *Tonometry* is done to measure the intraocular pressure. Tonometry screening is recommended for all people over the age of 60. The intraocular pressure is measured using a Schiötz tonometer (Figure 40-9 ■) or other tonometry instrument.
- The angle of the anterior chamber of the eye is assessed with *gonioscopy*. The gonioscope measures the depth of the anterior chamber, and helps differentiate between open-angle and angle-closure glaucoma.
- *Visual field testing* is used to identify loss of peripheral vision. The visual field is the entire area seen by the eye when focused on a central point.

Medications

Drugs often are used to reduce intraocular pressure and preserve vision. They usually are administered as eyedrops. Several classes or groups of drugs are used, including drugs that affect pupil size or the production of aqueous humor. Table 40-2 ■ outlines commonly used drugs and their nursing implications.

Acute angle-closure glaucoma is an ocular emergency that requires immediate intervention. Diuretics are given

TABLE 40-2

Nursing Implications for Pharmacology: Glaucoma

DRUG/CLASS	DESCRIPTION	NURSING RESPONSIBILITIES	CLIENT AND FAMILY TEACHING
Miotic Pilocarpine (Isopto Carpine, Ocusert-Pilo)	Miotic drugs constrict the pupil and contract the ciliary muscle. This stretches and opens the trabecular meshwork, promoting aqueous humor drainage and reducing intraocular pressure.	Report contraindications such as asthma, peptic ulcer disease, or urinary retention. After instilling drops, gently squeeze bridge of nose for 1 minute to increase local effect and reduce systemic absorption. Follow directions for using Ocusert-Pilo system.	To administer eyedrops: a. Wash your hands. b. Do not touch dropper. c. Squeeze bridge of nose and keep eye closed for 1 minute after using drops. Follow directions for using the Ocusert system. Drug causes blurred vision at first; this will clear. Avoid night driving and use night-lights in halls. Report abdominal cramps, difficulty breathing, or sweating, to your doctor.
Sympathomimetic ■ Epinephrine (Epifrin) ■ Dipivefrin (Propine) ■ Apraclonidine (Iopidine) ■ Brimonidine (Alphagan)	Sympathomimetic drugs reduce intraocular pressure by reducing aqueous humor production and increasing its absorption.	Report adverse reactions such as acute angle-closure glaucoma, hypertension, or an irregular pulse. Report itching, lid edema, and discharge from the eyes.	Report any change in vision or eye pain, which may indicate acute angle-closure glaucoma; contact your doctor immediately. Avoid over-the-counter sinus and cold medications that may increase the risk of angle-closure glaucoma.

TABLE 40-2			
Nursing Implications for Pharmacology: Glaucoma (continued)			
DRUG/CLASS	DESCRIPTION	NURSING RESPONSIBILITIES	CLIENT AND FAMILY TEACHING
Beta Blockers ■ Betaxolol (Betoptic) ■ Carteolol (Cartrol, Ocupress) ■ Levobunolol (Betagan) ■ Metipranolol (Opti-Pranolol) ■ Timolol (Timoptic)	Beta blockers decrease intraocular pressure by reducing the production of aqueous humor in the ciliary body. They do not affect vision like miotics and sympathomimetic drugs do, and they have a longer duration of action.	Report contraindications such as asthma, chronic obstructive pulmonary disease (COPD), heart block, and heart failure. Hold pressure over bridge of nose after instilling drops to prevent systemic absorption. Report side effects such as bradycardia, hypotension, and difficulty breathing.	Press on bridge of nose for 1 minute after instilling drops to keep the drug from entering your blood. Vision may be blurry at first but will improve. Report worsening vision, difficulty breathing, and reduced exercise tolerance to your doctor.
Prostaglandin Analog ■ Latanoprost (Xalatan)	Latanoprost reduces intraocular pressure by improving the outflow of aqueous humor.	Administer once daily at bedtime. Report side effects such as burning, stinging, or redness of the eye.	Instill drops at bedtime, as vision blurs after using the drops. The iris of the eye darkens while using this drug. This is not harmful. Report eye discomfort or redness to your doctor.
Carbonic Anhydrase Inhibitors ■ Acetazolamide (Diamox), PO, IV ■ Dorzolamide (Trusopt) eyedrops	Carbonic anhydrase inhibitors reduce aqueous humor production, lowering intraocular pressure. Intravenous acetazolamide rapidly reduces intraocular pressure in acute angle-closure glaucoma.	*Topical* ■ Squeeze the bridge of nose for 1–2 minutes after instilling the drug. ■ Report adverse or allergic effects, such as conjunctivitis or redness and itching of the lid. *Systemic* ■ Monitor daily weight, intake and output. ■ Report laboratory value changes for electrolytes, renal and liver function tests to the physician	*Topical* ■ May cause eye stinging and a bitter taste in your mouth immediately after using the drops. ■ If eye or lid become red or itchy, stop using the drug and notify your physician. *Systemic* ■ Drink 2–3 quarts of fluid daily. ■ Change positions slowly to prevent dizziness on standing.

intravenously to lower intraocular pressure rapidly. Acetazolamide, a carbonic anhydrase inhibitor, and osmotic diuretics, such as mannitol, are used. Fast-acting miotic drops are also used to constrict the pupil and help open the angle.

Surgery

Surgery is indicated when chronic open-angle glaucoma cannot be controlled by medication or for treating acute angle-closure glaucoma. The main purpose of surgery is to lower intraocular pressure. The most common surgeries used to manage clients with chronic open-angle glaucoma are *laser trabeculoplasty* and *cyclocryotherapy*. In laser trabeculoplasty, a laser is used to open drainage into the canal of Schlemm by burning holes into the trabecular meshwork. During cyclocryotherapy, a cryoprobe freezes and destroys a portion of the ciliary body, reducing aqueous humor production. For angle-closure glaucoma, a noninvasive procedure called *laser iridotomy* is done. The laser makes multiple small perforations in the iris, allowing aqueous humor to drain from the posterior chamber into the canal of Schlemm.

Complementary Therapy

Kava-kava must be used cautiously in clients with glaucoma because it causes pupil dilation, which can increase intraocular pressure.

NURSING CARE

Glaucoma is a chronic disease that requires lifelong management. The nurse must help the client and family understand the nature of the disease and its potential to cause blindness.

ASSESSING

Nursing assessment related to glaucoma focuses on identifying clients at risk. Ask about vision, including recent changes, difficulty seeing at night, and halos around lights. Inquire about a family history of glaucoma or any previous episodes of angle-closure glaucoma and the date of the most recent eye examination.

Inspect the eye for possible redness or clouding of the cornea. Assess vision (with corrective lenses if worn) using a standard eye chart. Assess pupil response to light (see Chapter 5). ∞ Evaluate peripheral vision (Box 40-5 ∎).

DIAGNOSING, PLANNING, AND IMPLEMENTING

Priorities in Nursing Care. Reduced vision caused by the glaucoma can affect the client's ability to provide self-care as well as manage other conditions, such as diabetes. Glaucoma also increases the client's risk for injury due to altered peripheral vision. The psychologic effects of a chronic disease can increase anxiety.

BOX 40-5	ASSESSMENT

Assessing Visual Fields by Confrontation

- Face the client, seated about 2 feet apart.
- Instruct the client to cover the right eye and focus on your face.
- Cover your left eye, and focus on the client's face.
- Midway between the client and yourself, bring a light-colored object into the field of vision from the side (see figure).

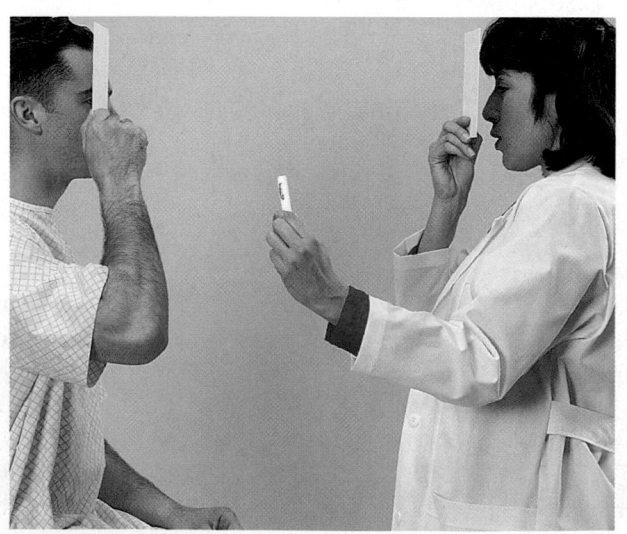

- Ask the client to indicate when the object is seen.
- Check all visual fields of both eyes in this manner.

Ineffective Health Maintenance

- Provide detailed verbal and written instructions about the ordered drugs. *Written instructions reinforce teaching and are a resource for the client.*
- Teach how to instill eyedrops, and have the client show you that he or she can do so. *Impaired vision, manual dexterity, or mobility may interfere with the ability to get drops into the eye. In some cases, a family member may need to do this for the client.*
- If taking other medications, ensure that the client can identify each and can take the appropriate dose if the drug is in injectable or liquid form. *Impaired vision and coexisting chronic diseases may make it difficult for the client to read medication labels or to draw up or pour an accurate dose.*
- Emphasize the importance of keeping all follow-up appointments to monitor intraocular pressure and vision. *Inadequate treatment can allow vision loss to continue.*

Risk for Injury

- Assess ability to provide self-care. Provide assistance as needed. *Clients may be reluctant to ask for help, believing that they should be able to perform these familiar tasks.*

> **clinical ALERT**
>
> Keep traffic area free of clutter to reduce the risk of injury in clients with visual impairments.

- Alert caregivers and housekeepers not to move items in the client's room. *Unexpected changes in the environment increase the risk for falls.*
- With the client's permission, raise the side rails on the bed. *Raised rails help remind the client to ask for help until the environment is familiar.*

Anxiety

- Assess for evidence of anxiety. Repeated expressions of concern or denial that altered vision will affect the client's life are indicators of anxiety. *Identifying and acknowledging anxiety helps the client recognize and deal with it.*
- Discuss the effects of glaucoma and possible vision loss on lifestyle and roles. *This allows the client to express concerns and fears. It also provides an opportunity to suggest alternative activities and assistive devices.*

EVALUATING

Look at the following data to evaluate the effectiveness of nursing care for the client with glaucoma:

- Able to state the purpose, dose, time, and side effects of medications.

- Can instill eyedrops as ordered.
- Able to safely perform ADLs.
- Relates the importance of follow-up care and can state the date of next vision exam.

Documenting. Documentation includes level of visual deficits and ability to perform ADLs and instill eyedrops. Client teaching is recorded about medications, warning signs of acute angle-closure glaucoma, and importance of regular eye examinations.

CONTINUING CARE

Discuss the prescribed drugs, including the name, dose, timing, and possible adverse effects. Teach the client how to instill eyedrops. Stress the importance of continuing treatment and periodic eye examinations with intraocular pressure measurements.

Discuss the risks, warning signs, and management of future attacks with the client who has had an episode of acute angle-closure glaucoma. If a permanent vision loss has resulted, discuss the effect of loss of vision on depth perception and safety.

If a significant amount of vision in both eyes has been lost, help identify changes in the home that can help the client remain safe and independent. Suggest removing scatter rugs and small items of furniture to allow the client to navigate safely in this already familiar environment. Refer to local and national resources that can help with assistive devices and modifications of the home.

NURSING PROCESS CARE PLAN
Client with Glaucoma and Cataracts

Lila Rainey is an 80-year-old widow who lives alone in the family home. She has worn glasses for myopia since she was a young girl. Four years ago she was diagnosed with chronic open-angle glaucoma, for which she takes timolol maleate (Timoptic) 0.5%. Recently, she has had increasing difficulty reading and watching television. She no longer drives at night because the glare of oncoming headlights makes it very difficult for her to see. Mrs. Rainey is now being admitted to the day surgery unit for a cataract removal and intraocular lens implant in her right eye.

Assessment. Mrs. Rainey is alert and oriented, though apprehensive about surgery. Vital signs are BP 134/72; P 86; R 18. Assessments of other body systems are essentially normal. Mrs. Rainey's pupils are round, equal, and react briskly to light and accommodation. Her conjunctivae are pink; sclera and corneas clear. The red reflex in the right eye

is diminished. Her visual acuity is 20/150 OD (right eye) and 20/50 OS (left eye) with corrective lenses. Her intraocular pressures are 16 mm Hg OD and 12 mm Hg OS. The nurse reviews the operative procedure with Mrs. Rainey, answering her questions and telling her what to expect after surgery.

Diagnosis. The following nursing diagnoses are identified for Mrs. Rainey:

- *Disturbed Sensory Perception: Visual* related to myopia and lens extraction
- *Anxiety* related to anticipated surgery
- *Deficient Knowledge* related to a lack of information about postoperative care

Expected Outcomes. The expected outcomes for the plan of care are that Mrs. Rainey will:

- Regain sufficient vision to maintain ADLs, including reading and watching television for enjoyment.
- Demonstrate a reduced level of anxiety.
- Demonstrate eyedrop instillation postoperatively.
- Verbalize postoperative care including signs of complications to be reported.

Planning and Implementation. The following interventions are implemented for Mrs. Rainey:

- Place call light and personal care items within easy reach.
- Encourage expression of fears about surgery and its potential effect on vision.
- Explain all procedures related to surgery and recovery.
- Instruct her to avoid shutting eyelids tightly, sneezing, coughing, laughing, bending over, lifting, or straining to have a bowel movement.
- Instruct to wear glasses during the day and an eye shield at night to prevent injury to the surgical site.
- Explain and demonstrate the procedure for administering eyedrops.
- Provide verbal and written instructions about postoperative care, including follow-up examinations, potential complications, and actions to take in response.

Evaluation. Mrs. Rainey is discharged 3 hours after surgery. She is visibly relieved the following morning when the eye patch is removed and her vision is better than before surgery, even without her glasses. Mrs. Rainey instills her own eyedrops before discharge and relates an understanding of the postoperative care and safety precautions. Mrs. Rainey's daughter plans to visit her mother several times a week to help with household chores. Mrs. Rainey understands the chronic nature of her glaucoma and says that her vision is too important for her to neglect her timolol drops and routine eye exams.

Critical Thinking in the Nursing Process

1. Mrs. Rainey was taught to hold pressure over the bridge of her nose for several minutes after instilling her timolol eyedrops. Why?
2. Timolol drops are not appropriate for all clients. Which common chronic conditions would contraindicate the use of timolol drops and why?
3. What community resources would you suggest to Mrs. Rainey if she did not have a close family member to assist with housework?

Detached Retina

The retina contains neurons that allow us to see light and images. A *detached retina* is separation of the retina from the choroid, the vascular layer of the eye. **Retinal detachments** can occur spontaneously or result from trauma. The vitreous humor shrinks with aging, increasing the risk for detached retina.

PATHOPHYSIOLOGY AND MANIFESTATIONS

The retina can remain intact but separate from the choroid, or tear and fold back on itself (Figure 40-10 ■). A break or tear in the retina allows fluid to seep between the retina and choroid, separating these layers. If the layers remain separated, the neurons of the retina become ischemic and die, causing permanent vision loss. For this reason, retinal detachment is a medical emergency that requires prompt treatment.

A detached retina is painless. The client may sense that a curtain or veil is being drawn across the vision. The affected area of vision relates to the area of detachment. Because light rays cross as they pass through the lens, a detachment in the upper part of the eye affects vision in the lower part of the visual field. Other common manifestations of a

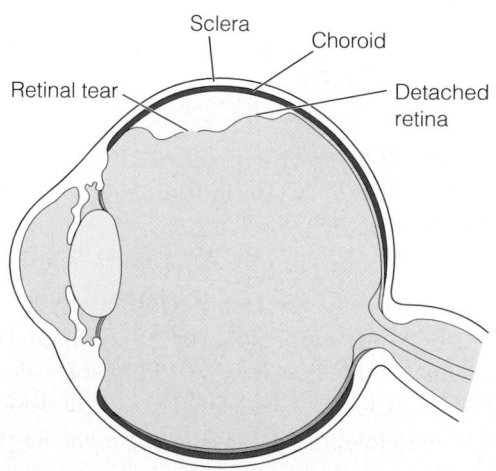

Figure 40-10. ■ Detached retina.

Sclera

Choroid

Retinal tear

Detached retina

detached retina include floaters (irregular, dark lines or spots in vision) and flashes of light.

INTERDISCIPLINARY CARE

A detached retina is diagnosed by the client's symptoms and examination of the eye. Until definitive treatment is available, the client's head is positioned so that the detached portion of the retina is lower than the rest of the eye.

Retinal detachment is often treated in an ophthalmologist's office. Several procedures may be used to reestablish contact between the retina and choroid. Air may be injected into the vitreous cavity, and the client positioned so that the air bubble pushes the detached portion of the retina against the choroid. Either laser therapy or cryotherapy, which uses a supercooled probe, may be used to initiate scarring that will "weld" the layers together. A surgical procedure, *scleral buckling,* creates an indentation or fold in the sclera, bringing the choroid into contact with the retina.

NURSING CARE

Early identification and treatment of a detached retina are vital to preserve sight. Most eye disorders cause a gradual loss of vision.

clinical ALERT

Carefully assess the client who complains of a sudden change in vision because these are often medical emergencies.

Promptly report rapid changes in vision to the charge nurse or physician. Remember that retinal detachment is painless; clients may seem to be more confused than concerned about what they are seeing. Review Box 40-2 for nursing care of the client undergoing eye surgery for a detached retina.

Ineffective Tissue Perfusion: Retinal

■ Position client with area of detachment dependent. For instance, if vision is lost in the upper outer portion of the left eye, indicating an inferior medial retinal detachment of the left eye, place the client on the right side with the head of the bed elevated. *Correct positioning allows the vitreous humor to press on the detached area, bringing the retina closer to blood vessels in the choroid and preserving retinal perfusion until treatment is available.*

Anxiety

■ Maintain a calm, confident attitude while providing priority care. *Maintaining a calm but urgent manner helps reassure the client.*

- Reassure the client that a detached retina is treatable, usually on an outpatient basis. *Reassurance helps relieve the fear of permanent vision loss.*
- Explain all procedures fully, including the reason for positioning. *Complete explanations help relieve anxiety and promote understanding.*
- Allow supportive family members or friends to remain with the client as much as possible. *Additional support helps reduce anxiety.*

To evaluate the effectiveness of nursing care, collect the following data:

- Did vision remain stable until treatment was provided?
- Was vision fully or partially restored by treatment?
- Did anxiety remain within acceptable limits?

CONTINUING CARE

Following treatment for a detached retina, stress the importance of positioning as ordered. The client may be instructed to maintain a position with the affected area of the eye inferior to maintain contact between the retina and choroid.

The client who has had a spontaneous retinal detachment has an increased risk of future detachments. Discuss early symptoms, and emphasize the importance of seeking immediate treatment if they occur. Emphasize the need to maintain follow-up treatment with the ophthalmologist. If the retina remains detached, discuss safety measures to accommodate the loss of vision and changes in depth perception.

Macular Degeneration

Macular degeneration is a common cause of blindness in older adults. With aging, the neurons of the macula (the area of central vision) may atrophy or separate from the choroid.

When the macula is damaged, central vision becomes blurred and distorted, but peripheral vision remains intact (Figure 40-11 ■). Distortion of vision in one eye is a common early symptom; straight lines appear wavy or distorted. Macular degeneration particularly affects activities that require close central vision, such as reading and sewing.

Laser treatment may slow macular degeneration, but often no effective treatment is available. Large-print books and magazines, the use of a magnifying glass, and high-intensity lighting can help the client to cope with reduced vision.

Promptly report new or rapid loss of central vision because early treatment may help preserve vision and slow the disease. Help clients with slowly progressive vision loss to adapt by recommending visual aids and other coping strategies.

Diabetic Retinopathy

Approximately 85% of diabetics develop *diabetic retinopathy,* a disorder affecting the capillaries of the retina. The capillaries are no longer able to transport blood and oxygen to the retina. Retinopathy affects clients with both type 1 and type 2 diabetes. Its extent seems to mostly relate to how long the client has had diabetes.

Initially, the venous capillaries dilate and develop microscopic aneurysms that may leak or rupture. These cause edema and small hemorrhages into the retina. As the disease progresses, large areas of the retina become ischemic, and new blood vessels form, spreading over the surface of the retina and into the vitreous body. These vessels are fine and fragile. They may leak or rupture, causing bleeding into the vitreous body. The vessels also increase the risk for a detached retina.

A yearly eye examination is recommended for all adults with diabetes. Laser treatment may be done to seal microaneurysms and destroy new, fragile blood vessels. Treatment slows the disease progress but does not cure it.

The nursing care focus for diabetic retinopathy is on education. Stress the importance of regular eye examinations for all clients with diabetes. Teach the client to report promptly any change in vision, including blurring; black spots (floaters), cobwebs, or flashing lights in the visual field; or a sudden loss of vision in one or both eyes. Emphasize that controlling blood glucose levels and maintaining blood pressure within normal limits will help limit diabetic retinopathy or slow its progress.

Enucleation

Occasionally, an eye must be removed. This procedure is known as *enucleation.* After the eye is removed, the conjunctiva and eye muscles are sutured to a round implant inserted into the orbit to maintain its shape. A permanent prosthesis is individually designed to closely resemble the client's other eye. The prosthesis can be fitted 1 to 2 months after surgery.

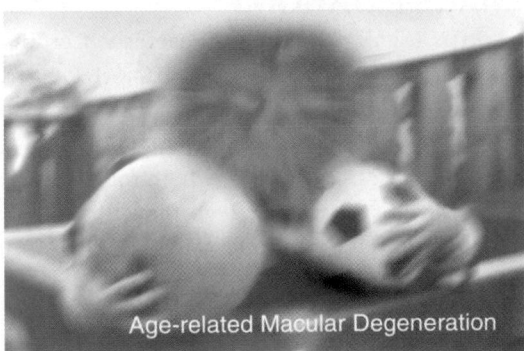

Age-related Macular Degeneration

Figure 40-11. ■ Blurred central vision occurs in age-related macular degeneration. *(Courtesy National Eye Institute, National Institutes of Health.)*

Often, it is difficult to discern which eye is functional and which is the prosthesis.

clinical ALERT

Don't make the mistake of charting, "Pupils equal, round, and react to light and accommodation (PERRLA)" on a client with an eye prosthesis!

Postoperative nursing care includes teaching, psychologic support, and observing for potential complications. The client may be instructed to apply warm compresses and instill antibiotic ointment or drops postoperatively.

Blindness

Visual impairment ranges from blindness to decreased visual acuity that can be corrected with refractive lenses. *Blindness* is defined as severely limited vision that cannot be corrected. Total blindness usually means the client cannot see light at all. In practical terms, a person who needs assistive devices or help from others for normal activities of daily living due to impaired vision is considered blind. Most blindness is preventable with early recognition and treatment of common eye disorders such as cataract and glaucoma.

Nurses can foster independence in the hospitalized client who is blind by doing the following:

- Orient to the environment verbally and physically. Describe the client's room using a central point such as the bed. Lead the client around the room, identifying chairs, sink, bathroom, and other landmarks. Be sure that objects such as chairs, personal items, and clothing are not moved within the room unless the client moves them. Leave doors either fully open or closed as the client wishes, but, to preserve safety, do not leave doors partially open. Keep the room and hallways free of clutter where the client will be ambulating.
- Use verbal communication freely. Describe activities going on around the client. Introduce yourself as you enter the room and let the client know when you are leaving.
- Provide other sensory stimuli such as radio and television as desired by the client.
- Orient to food trays, describing the position of food items on the plate and tray using the face of a clock as a reference (unless the client has always been blind and cannot visualize a clock face).
- When assisting with ambulation, allow the client to hold your arm as you walk slightly ahead. Do not hold the client's arm. Verbally describe the environment, such as "There will be two steps up five feet ahead."
- Do not be afraid to ask what assistance the client desires.
- For the client with a new loss of sight, refer for services as appropriate. Persons who are blind can receive mobility training, assistance with relearning of self-care activities, education about communication tools, and vocational and other forms of rehabilitation. State, local, and national agencies help coordinate services for the blind. Many assistive devices are available, including guide or pilot dogs, computer services, talking books and tape players, and low-vision aids.

EAR DISORDERS

Disorders of the external ear can alter sound wave conduction and hearing. The most common disorders of the external ear include infection or inflammation, trauma, and obstruction of the ear canal with *cerumen* (wax).

Middle ear disorders may be either acute or chronic. They require immediate treatment to prevent damage and scarring of the middle ear structures, which could result in conductive hearing loss. Otitis media and mastoiditis are the common conditions affecting the middle ear.

Common inner ear disorders include labyrinthitis and Ménière's disease. They are less common than external and middle ear disorders.

External Otitis

Disorders of the external ear—such as external otitis and impacted cerumen—can affect sound conduction and hearing. **External otitis**, or **swimmer's ear**, is inflammation of the ear canal. Swimmers, divers, and surfers are particularly prone to external otitis. Wearing a hearing aid or earplugs, which hold moisture in the ear canal, also is a risk factor.

PATHOPHYSIOLOGY AND MANIFESTATIONS

External otitis usually is caused by bacteria. Cerumen (earwax) is water repellent and has an antibacterial effect. Moisture, cleaning, or drying of the ear canal can remove earwax, increasing the risk of infection.

External otitis causes ear pain, which may be severe, and a feeling of fullness in the ear. Manipulating the outer ear increases the pain. Drainage may be present. The ear canal appears inflamed and swollen.

INTERDISCIPLINARY CARE

Treatment of otitis externa usually includes:

- Thorough cleaning of the ear canal, particularly if drainage or debris is present
- Treating the infection with a topical antibiotic

BOX 40-6	CLIENT TEACHING

Tips to Prevent External Otitis

- Stay out of the water for 7 to 10 days or until completely healed.
- When you resume water activities, use earplugs, a tight-fitting swim cap, or a wetsuit hood to keep water out of the ears or protect the ear from cold water temperatures.
- Use a hair dryer on the lowest setting to dry ear canals after swimming.
- Do not insert cotton swabs or any other object into the ear canals.

- Topical corticosteroid drops (often combined with the antibiotic) to relieve the pain, itching, and swelling
- Teaching to prevent future episodes of swimmer's ear (see Box 40-6 ■).

NURSING CARE

External otitis can cause severe pain and discomfort, but rarely requires hospitalization. The nurse teaches the client about the disorder, comfort measures, and strategies to prevent future episodes.

ASSESSING

When assessing a client with external otitis, ask about ear cleaning practices and participation in water sports or activities. Have the client describe ear pain, including its character, timing, aggravating factors (e.g., pulling or moving the auricle of the ear), and relieving factors. Assess hearing in both ears, using the whisper test (see Chapter 5) ⚭ or an audiometer. Inspect the external ear for drainage, redness, or evidence of trauma. Using an otoscope, insert the speculum just inside (no more than 1 cm) the canal to inspect for redness, swelling, drainage, or trauma.

DIAGNOSING, PLANNING, AND IMPLEMENTING

Priorities in Nursing Care. The priority of care of clients with external otitis is Impaired Tissue Integrity. In addition, the nurse focuses on teaching the client to manage external otitis at home.

Impaired Tissue Integrity

- Teach clients not to clean the ear canal with a toothpick, cotton-tipped applicator, or other tool. *This damages the skin and disrupts the protective cerumen, allowing infection to develop.*

BOX 40-7	NURSING CARE CHECKLIST

Instilling Eardrops

- ☑ Wash hands.
- ☑ Warm the drops by holding the bottle or putting it in a pocket for about 5 minutes before instilling.
- ☑ Place the client on the unaffected side or tilt the head toward the unaffected side.
- ☑ Partially fill the ear dropper with medication.
- ☑ Using the nondominant hand, straighten the ear canal by pulling the pinna of the ear up and back.
- ☑ Instill the prescribed number of drops into the ear canal.
- ☑ Keep the client on the side for about 5 minutes after putting in the drops.
- ☑ Loosely place a small piece of cotton in the opening to the ear canal for 15 to 20 minutes.

- Teach how to instill prescribed eardrops (Box 40-7 ■). *The medication is more effective when it is allowed to reach the inner portion of the ear canal.*
- Instruct to avoid getting water in the affected ear until it is fully healed. Cotton balls may be used while showering to prevent water from entering the ear canal. Instruct to avoid water sports and activities until allowed by the primary care provider. *Moisture in the ear canal can interfere with healing.*

EVALUATING

To evaluate the effectiveness of teaching related to external otitis, have the client demonstrate instilling eardrops. Review knowledge and willingness to avoid water sports until healing is complete. Ask to describe measures for preventing future episodes of external otitis.

Documenting. Documentation includes any hearing deficits, ability to instill eardrops, and knowledge about preventative strategies.

CONTINUING CARE

The client is ultimately responsible for following the prescribed treatment and preventing future episodes of external otitis. Provide verbal and written instructions for the prescribed medications. Teach the client how to prevent recurrent episodes. Inform all clients that ear canals rarely need cleaning beyond washing the external opening with soap and water. Teach clients of all ages not to clean ear canals with any implement.

Instruct the client to report any increase in pain, swelling, or redness around the ear, fever, malaise, or increased fatigue to the primary care provider.

Impacted Cerumen and Foreign Bodies

The ear canal is narrow and curved. It can become obstructed by earwax or foreign objects such as insects.

As earwax dries, it moves out of the ear canal. In some people, however, it accumulates. Older adults in particular are at risk for *impacted* (tightly wedged) cerumen. With aging, earwax becomes harder and drier. Attempting to remove earwax with cotton-tipped swabs often packs it more deeply into the ear canal.

Ear canal obstruction interferes with sound conduction and hearing. The client reports a sensation of fullness and **tinnitus** (ringing) in the ear. A foreign body or impacted cerumen can be seen using an otoscope.

Treatment focuses on clearing the canal. The canal may be irrigated to clear the obstruction. Impacted wax, objects, or insects may need to be removed using an ear curet, forceps, or other implement. Mineral oil or topical lidocaine drops are used to immobilize or kill insects before they are removed.

clinical ALERT

If a foreign body such as a bean or an insect occludes the canal, do not irrigate with water. Water may cause the object to swell, making it more difficult to remove.

Teaching is important to prevent obstruction of the ear canal with earwax. Advise the client with impacted cerumen to use mineral oil or commercial products to soften wax and remove it by irrigating the canal with water. Stress the risk of impacting cerumen against the eardrum if cotton-tipped swabs are used to clean the ear canal. The swab also may break and lodge in the canal. If eardrops have been prescribed, teach the client and a family member how to instill them.

Otitis Media

Middle ear disorders can lead to permanent hearing loss without effective treatment. **Otitis media,** inflammation or infection of the middle ear, is the most common middle ear disorder. It usually affects infants and young children but can occur in adults. While the eardrum protects the middle ear from the environment, the eustachian tube connects it with the nasopharynx. Organisms can enter the middle ear from the nose and throat through the eustachian tube.

PATHOPHYSIOLOGY AND MANIFESTATIONS

Upper respiratory infection (URI) and eustachian tube dysfunction are risk factors for otitis media. The tube is narrow and flat, normally opening only during yawning and swallowing. Allergies or URI can cause it to swell, impairing its function.

Serous otitis media occurs when the eustachian tube is obstructed. Air in the middle ear is gradually absorbed, causing negative pressure in the middle ear. The negative pressure draws serous fluid from the capillaries into the space.

Manifestations of serous otitis media include decreased hearing and a "snapping" or "popping" sensation in the affected ear. The eardrum moves less freely and may appear retracted ("sucked in") or bulging. Fluid or air bubbles may be seen behind the drum. Changes in atmospheric pressure (e.g., flying or underwater diving) can cause acute pain, bleeding into the middle ear, or rupture of the eardrum.

Acute otitis media usually follows URI. Drainage through the eustachian tube is impaired. Mucus and serous fluid collect in the middle ear. Bacteria enter from the nasopharynx, growing and multiplying in this fluid. The infection causes an immune response, and pus forms in the middle ear. The pus increases pressure in the middle ear and can rupture the eardrum.

Acute otitis media causes pain, often severe, in the affected ear. The client may have a fever, and complain of hearing loss, dizziness, vertigo (a sensation of whirling or rotation), and tinnitus. The eardrum is red and inflamed or dull and bulging (Figure 40-12 ■). It does not move normally and may rupture, causing purulent drainage.

COMPLICATIONS

Acute mastoiditis may develop when acute otitis media is not effectively treated. Pus fills the air cells of the mastoid process of the temporal bone, which is next to the middle ear. Acute mastoiditis destroys these air cells, causing recurrent earache and hearing loss on the affected side. The mastoid process (behind the ear) is tender and may be swollen, red, and inflamed. The client may complain of tinnitus, headache, and fever. Acute mastoiditis may lead to meningitis, although this condition occurs rarely.

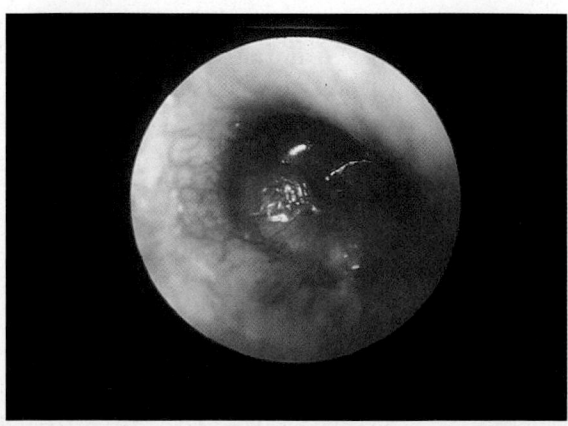

Figure 40-12. ■ A red, bulging tympanic membrane of otitis media. (*Source:* Medical Images, Inc.)

Chronic otitis media is a permanent perforation of the eardrum. Middle ear infections are recurrent, and structures of the middle ear are destroyed. Severe conductive hearing loss may result.

INTERDISCIPLINARY CARE

Otitis media is usually diagnosed by the client's history and the physical examination. A *pneumatic otoscope* is used to examine the eardrum. A puff of air is blown into the ear canal; this normally causes slight movement of the eardrum. In otitis media, the drum moves less freely. A diagnostic test called *impedance audiometry* may also be done to assess movement of the eardrum and middle ear structures.

Medications

Decongestants are used to improve eustachian tube function and treat serous otitis media. (See Chapter 23 ⊂⊃ for more information about and the nursing implications of decongestants.) Acute otitis media is treated with antibiotics, often in combination with decongestants. Antibiotic treatment may be continued for 5 to 10 days. (See Chapter 10 ⊂⊃ for more information about antibiotic treatment.) Mild analgesics such as acetaminophen are recommended to relieve pain and reduce fever. Acute mastoiditis needs aggressive treatment with intravenous antibiotics.

Autoinflation

The client with eustachian tube dysfunction may learn to open the tube by performing the Valsalva maneuver, or by forcefully exhaling through the nose against closed nostrils.

Surgery

Surgery may be done to relieve pressure in the middle ear and prevent spontaneous eardrum rupture. In a *tympanocentesis,* a needle is inserted through the eardrum to draw fluid and pus out of the middle ear. *Myringotomy,* surgical drainage of the middle ear, may be done. Clients who do not respond to antibiotics may need *ventilation (tympanostomy) tubes* inserted during myringotomy. This procedure allows ventilation and drainage of the middle ear during healing. The tube eventually comes out of the ear, and the eardrum heals. While the tube is in place, it is important to avoid getting any water in the ear canal. A *mastoidectomy,* removal of infected air cells, bone, and pus, may be done on a client with mastoiditis.

Complementary Therapies

Complementary therapies may help promote comfort in the client with otitis media. A drop of lavender oil on cotton in the ear canal helps relieve discomfort. A warm cloth or a chamomile tea bag steeped in warm water can be used to apply heat to the side of the face or ear, reducing pain. A

naturopathic practitioner may prescribe remedies such as pulsatilla, belladonna, or aconite.

NURSING CARE

Clients with otitis media are commonly seen and treated in community settings. The nursing role focuses on prevention and teaching.

ASSESSING

Collect data about the onset and duration of symptoms, including pain, popping or snapping sensations in the ear, and any drainage from the ear. Ask about any recent URIs. Move the auricle of the ear, asking how movement affects the pain. The pain of otitis media usually does not change with manipulation of the external ear. Inspect the client's throat for redness, swelling, or drainage. Obtain the client's temperature. Assess hearing in both ears, using the whisper test or an audiometer. If trained, use an otoscope to inspect the ear canal and eardrum. Inspect and palpate the mastoid process for tenderness.

DIAGNOSING, PLANNING, AND IMPLEMENTING

Priorities in Nursing Care. Pain and the risk of damage to the middle ear are priority nursing care problems for the client with otitis media. Box 40-8 ■ outlines nursing care of the client having ear surgery.

Pain

- Advise using mild analgesics every 4 hours as needed to relieve pain and fever. *Nonprescription drugs help relieve pain and reduce fever.*
- Advise the client to apply heat to the affected side of the face and head unless contraindicated. *Heat dilates blood vessels, promoting fluid reabsorption and reducing swelling.*
- Instruct to promptly report abrupt pain relief to the physician. *Abrupt pain relief may mean the eardrum has ruptured, releasing pressure from the middle ear.*

Deficient Knowledge: Antibiotic Therapy

- Stress the importance of completing the full course of antibiotic therapy. *Taking all of the ordered antibiotic is important to eliminate the infection and prevent antibiotic-resistant bacteria from developing.*
- Discuss the desired and potential adverse effects of the prescribed antibiotic. Tell the client to report any adverse effects to the physician. *If the medication is ineffective or the client has an adverse reaction to it, a different antibiotic may be ordered.*

| **BOX 40-8** | **NURSING CARE CHECKLIST** |

Ear Surgery

Before Surgery

☑ Provide routine preoperative care as ordered (see Chapter 9). ⚭

☑ Assess hearing or verify that hearing has been assessed before surgery.

☑ Discuss postoperative communication strategies.

☑ Explain postoperative restrictions such as avoiding blowing the nose, coughing, and sneezing. Instruct to leave the mouth open if coughing or sneezing is necessary.

After Surgery

☑ Provide routine postoperative care as ordered (see Chapter 9).

☑ Assess for bleeding or drainage from the affected ear. Note color, character, and amount of any drainage.

☑ Assess for nausea; administer antiemetics as ordered to prevent vomiting.

☑ Elevate the head of bed and position on the unaffected side.

☑ Assess for vertigo or dizziness, especially with movement. Avoid unnecessary movements such as turning. Ensure safety during ambulation.

☑ Assess hearing.

☑ Stand on the client's unaffected side to communicate. Use alternate strategies, such as writing, when needed.

☑ Remind to avoid coughing, sneezing, or blowing the nose.

☑ Provide instructions for home care.

  a. Avoid showers, shampooing, and immersing the head until approved by the physician.

  b. Keep the outer earplug clean and dry, changing it as needed. Do not remove inner ear dressing until ordered by the physician.

  c. Avoid blowing the nose; if you need to cough or sneeze, keep mouth open.

  d. Do not swim, dive, or travel by air until allowed by the physician.

  e. You may need to take an antiemetic/antihistamine drug for up to 1 month after surgery.

  f. Notify the physician if you develop a fever, bleeding, increased drainage, increased dizziness, or decreased hearing.

■ Inform the client that the antibiotic may cause diarrhea, vaginitis, or thrush. Unless contraindicated, instruct the client to eat 8 oz of yogurt with live bacterial cultures daily during antibiotic therapy. *Antibiotics destroy normal body flora as well as infectious organisms. Live yogurt cultures help restore these beneficial microbes, preventing superinfection.*

■ Stress the importance of keeping follow-up appointments. *Follow-up is important to confirm cure of the infection and prevent complications.*

Impaired Tissue Integrity

■ Instruct the client with ventilation tubes to avoid swimming, diving, or submerging the head while bathing. *Water can enter the middle ear through the ventilation tubes.*

■ Instruct the client to avoid air travel, rapid changes in elevation, or diving. *A rapid change in pressure can damage the inflamed middle ear.*

■ Encourage to rest, increase fluid intake, and eat a nutritious diet. *These general health measures improve immune function and promote healing.*

EVALUATING

Collect the following data to evaluate the effectiveness of care:

■ Knowledge of the treatment plan

■ Understanding of symptoms to report to the primary care provider

■ On follow-up visits, relief of symptoms, compliance with prescribed treatment, and hearing in both ears.

Documenting. Documentation includes improvement of symptoms, hearing ability, and teaching about antibiotics, preventive measures, and postoperative care if surgery was done.

CONTINUING CARE

Teach about otitis media, its causes and prevention, and any specific treatment. Provide verbal and written instructions about the ordered antibiotic, its effects, recommended timing (with or without food, doses evenly spaced throughout the day), and possible side effects. Discuss the symptoms of allergic or adverse reactions that should be reported to the physician. Stress the importance of completing the full course of therapy.

If surgery has been performed, teach the client and family members about postoperative care. Discuss postoperative precautions, such as avoiding water in the ear canals and sudden changes in air pressure.

Otosclerosis

Otosclerosis is a hereditary disorder that usually affects white females. Abnormal bone forms, immobilizing the stapes and causing a conductive hearing loss.

Hearing loss usually begins in adolescence or early adulthood. Both ears are affected. Air conduction of sound is lost. However, sound is conducted through bone. As a result, the client may be able to use a telephone but have difficulty conversing in person. The client also may experience tinnitus. Otosclerosis may be treated with surgical reconstruction of the middle ear.

Education and referral of the client to appropriate community agencies are important nursing care priorities for the client with otosclerosis. For the client who has surgery, nursing care is similar to that for other clients undergoing ear surgery (see Box 40-8).

Inner Ear Disorders

Inner ear disorders occur less frequently than other ear disorders. Labyrinthitis and Ménière's disease are the most common diseases of the inner ear.

PATHOPHYSIOLOGY AND MANIFESTATIONS

The inner ear (or labyrinth) contains the semicircular canals that help maintain balance, and the neural receptors for hearing. Inner ear disorders affect balance and may cause permanent hearing loss. **Vertigo,** a sensation of whirling or movement when there is none, is the key symptom of inner ear disorders.

clinical ALERT

Vertigo is a disorder of equilibrium (balance). It can be disabling, causing falls, injury, and difficulty walking. *Dizziness,* on the other hand, is a feeling of unsteadiness, lack of balance, light-headedness, or movement within the head. It is not as severe as vertigo.

Labyrinthitis

Labyrinthitis is inflammation of the inner ear. It may be caused by bacteria or viruses. Labyrinthitis is uncommon. It causes severe vertigo, hearing loss, and *nystagmus* (rapid involuntary eye movements). Nausea and vomiting often accompany the vertigo. Falling is a significant risk if the client attempts to stand.

Ménière's Disease

Ménière's disease is a chronic inner ear disorder caused by excess fluid and pressure in the labyrinth of the inner ear. Its onset may be gradual or sudden. Clients with Ménière's disease have recurring attacks of vertigo with tinnitus and gradual hearing loss. The hearing loss usually affects one ear, although the other ear also may be affected. Attacks of severe vertigo occur abruptly and are unpredictable, lasting from minutes to hours.

INTERDISCIPLINARY CARE

There is no cure for inner ear disorders. Treatment focuses on managing symptoms and preventing permanent hearing loss.

Several diagnostic tests may be done to identify inner ear disorders.

- *Electronystagmography* is used to assess involuntary eye movements (nystagmus) in response to the stimuli of warm and cool water instilled into the ear canal.
- *X-rays* and *CT scans* of the inner ear structures may be done.
- *Glycerol test* is done by giving the client oral glycerol to decrease pressure in the inner ear.

Hearing improves temporarily in clients with Ménière's disease. Clients with labyrinthitis or an acute attack of Ménière's disease may need hospitalization to manage the vertigo and its effects. Drugs such as meclizine (Antivert), prochlorperazine (Compazine), or hydroxyzine (Vistaril) are given to relieve vertigo and nausea. If nausea and vomiting are severe, intravenous fluids may be used to maintain fluid and electrolyte balance. Bed rest in a quiet, darkened room with minimal sensory stimuli and minimal movement provides the most comfort for the client.

The client with Ménière's disease may be placed on a low-salt diet and a diuretic to reduce the frequency of attacks. Tobacco, which can precipitate an attack, is avoided, along with alcohol and caffeine.

Surgery may be necessary to relieve excess pressure in the inner ear or to block transmission of stimuli related to balance and vertigo. There is a risk of hearing loss when surgery is required. Following surgery, the client is positioned to minimize ear pressure and vertigo. Movement is restricted, and the client is assisted during ambulation. Antiemetics and antivertigo drugs are used to manage the nausea and vertigo after surgery. Complications include infection and leakage of cerebrospinal fluid.

NURSING CARE

The client with inner ear disorders has multiple nursing care needs related to the manifestations of the disease. Persistent episodes of dizziness, tinnitus, balance problems, or hearing loss should be reported to a health care provider. Clients diagnosed and treated early may have a lower risk for injury.

ASSESSING

Assess the effects of the disorder on balance and the ability to safely ambulate. Assess hearing, using the whisper test (see Chapter 5). ⊕ Ask about tinnitus, including pitch, tone, quality, and duration. Refer for a complete hearing and ear examination if this has not been done. Assess for nystagmus by having the client follow an object through the six cardinal fields of vision (see Box 40-1). Nausea and vomiting may interfere with nutrition. Ask about usual food and fluid intake, and assess height and weight, skin color and condition, and for other signs of nutritional status. Discuss the effect of the disorder on the client's life. Unpredictable attacks of vertigo, tinnitus, and hearing loss can affect lifestyle, employment, sleep, rest, and ability to cope.

DIAGNOSING, PLANNING, AND IMPLEMENTING

Priorities in Nursing Care. The highest priority nursing diagnoses are risk for trauma and disturbed sleep pattern. Attacks of vertigo may occur without warning. They can be so severe that the client cannot remain upright.

Risk for Trauma

- Ask the client not to get up without assistance during acute attacks of vertigo. *During attacks of vertigo, assistance reduces the risk of falling.*

> ### clinical ALERT
>
> During an acute attack of vertigo, keep the client on bed rest with side rails raised and the call light within easy reach.

- Teach the client to avoid sudden head movements or position changes. *Sudden movement may precipitate an attack of vertigo.*
- Administer drugs as ordered, including antiemetics, diuretics, and sedatives. *These medications may reduce the frequency, severity, and duration of attacks.*
- Teach the client who senses an oncoming attack to take the prescribed medication and lie down in a quiet, darkened room. *This decreases the risk of injury, and may reduce the duration and severity of the attack.*
- Instruct the client to pull to the side of the road and wait for the symptoms to subside if an attack occurs while driving. *This is vital to protect the safety of the client and others.*
- Discuss the importance of wearing a Medic-Alert bracelet or necklace. *A Medic-Alert bracelet or tag helps ensure appropriate treatment if the client is unable to answer questions or respond in an emergency.*
- Discuss the effect of one-sided hearing loss on the ability to identify sound direction. Encourage the client to use

other senses as well, for example, when crossing the street. *Sound perception and the ability to identify its direction change when hearing is lost in one ear.*

Disturbed Sleep Pattern

Tinnitus can interfere with concentration, relaxation, and sleep.

- Discuss options for masking tinnitus:
  a. Ambient noise from a radio or sound system
  b. A masking device or white-noise machine
  c. A hearing aid that produces a tone to mask the tinnitus
  d. A hearing aid that amplifies ambient sound.
  Masking the perception of tinnitus may allow the client to focus on something other than the sound.
- Suggest that the client discuss possible medications to treat tinnitus with the physician. *Drugs, including antidepressants such as nortriptyline (Aventyl, Pamelor), taken at bedtime may relieve tinnitus and promote rest.*

EVALUATING

To evaluate the effectiveness of nursing care, assess the safety measures. Discuss the client's and family's understanding of the disease and measures to reduce the frequency and severity of attacks. Discuss coping strategies the client will use to manage the effects of the disorder on his or her lifestyle.

Documenting. Documentation includes noting manifestations of dizziness, tinnitus, balance problems, or hearing loss. Effectiveness of interventions to relieve these symptoms is noted. Record client and family teaching about strategies to reduce and cope with the attacks, safety, medications, and possible community resources.

CONTINUING CARE

Safety is a primary focus of teaching for home care. Teach the client to change positions slowly, especially when ambulating. Turning the whole body rather than just the head helps to prevent vertigo. Because attacks can be unpredictable, the client should not ambulate alone unless in a safe environment. Instruct to sit down immediately when vertigo occurs and lie down if possible. Teach about prescribed medications, providing both verbal and written instructions about their use, desired effects, and possible adverse effects and precautions.

If the client has had surgery, provide information about postoperative care and follow-up. Teach techniques to minimize postoperative vertigo and associated nausea. Surgery may cause permanent hearing loss in the affected ear; discuss safety and communication strategies.

Hearing Loss

Hearing loss impairs the ability to communicate in a world filled with sound and hearing individuals. Approximately 10 million adults in the United States are hearing impaired. Hearing loss is more common in older adults, affecting a quarter to a third of older adults. Up to 70% of long-term care residents have impaired hearing.

PATHOPHYSIOLOGY AND MANIFESTATIONS

Hearing loss is classified as conductive, sensorineural, or mixed, depending on what portion of the auditory system is affected. A hearing deficit can be partial or total, congenital or acquired. It may affect one or both ears. Some types of hearing loss affect the ability to hear specific frequencies of sound.

Conductive Hearing Loss

Anything that affects sound transmission from the external opening of the ear to the inner ear causes a *conductive hearing loss*. Obstruction of the ear canal, for example, by impacted cerumen, is the most common cause. Other causes of conductive loss include perforated eardrum, damage to the ossicles of the middle ear, fluid, scarring, or tumors of the middle ear. The client with a conductive hearing loss benefits from sound amplification by a hearing aid.

Sensorineural Hearing Loss

Disorders that affect the inner ear or the auditory pathways of the brain may cause a *sensorineural hearing loss*. Trauma, infection, diseases such as Ménière's disease, and ototoxic medications can lead to sensory hearing loss. In the United States, noise exposure is the major cause. Exposure to a high level of noise, for example, standing close to the stage or speakers at a rock concert, damages the hair cells of the organ of Corti. Ototoxic drugs such as aspirin, furosemide (Lasix), vancomycin, and aminoglycoside antibiotics also damage the hair cells.

Sensory hearing losses usually affect the ability to hear high-frequency sounds more than low-frequency sounds. This affects speech discrimination and communication, especially in a noisy environment. Hearing aids may not help.

Presbycusis

With aging, the hair cells of the cochlea degenerate, causing progressive hearing loss. Hearing begins to decline in early adulthood and progresses with time. **Presbycusis** is a type of sensorineural loss. Because hearing loss is gradual, the client and family may not realize the extent of the deficit. Hearing aids and other amplification devices are useful for most clients with presbycusis.

INTERDISCIPLINARY CARE

Hearing evaluation includes gross tests of hearing (such as the whisper test), the Rinne and Weber tests, and audiometry.

- The *Rinne and Weber tests* (Box 40-9 ■) compare sound conduction by air and through bone. Bone conduction of sound is better than air conduction with a conductive hearing loss. With a sensory hearing loss, both air and bone sound conduction are affected.
- *Audiometry* is used to quantify hearing deficits. Specific sound frequencies are presented to each ear by either air or bone conduction to identify the type and pattern of hearing loss.

Amplification

A hearing aid or other amplification device can help many clients with hearing loss. These devices amplify sound, increasing the sound level so it can be heard by the client. This improves the perception and interpretation of the sound. Hearing aids must be individually prescribed by an audiologist. To be effective, proper design and fit as well as regular maintenance are necessary.

The least noticeable style of hearing aid fits entirely in the ear canal. It allows telephone use and can be worn during exercise. Because it is small, good manual dexterity is needed to insert it, clean it, and change the batteries. An in-ear hearing aid fits into the external ear (Figure 40-13A ■). It is easier to handle and provides greater amplification than the in-canal style of hearing aid. With both the in-canal and in-ear style, cleaning is important. Small openings may become plugged with wax, interfering with sound transmission.

The behind-the-ear hearing aid is easier to manipulate (Figure 40-13B). For the client who wears glasses, it can be integrated into the earpiece of the eyeglasses.

Clients with profound hearing loss may require a body hearing aid. The microphone and amplifier of this aid are contained in a pocket-sized case that the client clips onto clothing, slips into a pocket, or carries in a harness. The receiver is attached by a cord to the case and clips onto the ear mold, which delivers the sound to the ear canal.

For the client who does not have a hearing aid, an assistive listening device, or "pocket talker," with a microphone and "Walkman"-type earpieces, is useful. Pocket talkers are available over the counter and are relatively inexpensive. The earpiece requires no special fitting, and the external microphone allows the client to focus on the desired sound rather than simply amplifying all sounds.

Surgery

Surgery may be done to correct damage to the middle ear. The client with a sensory hearing loss may require a cochlear implant to allow sound perception. Cochlear

| BOX 40-9 | **ASSESSMENT** |

Assessing Clients: The Rinne and Weber Tests

The Rinne and Weber tests are used to help determine if hearing loss is conductive or sensory.

- *The Rinne test:* Strike the tines of a tuning fork on the heal of your hand to start it vibrating (see figure A). Place the base of the tuning fork behind the ear, on the mastoid bone. Ask the client to tell you when the sound is no longer heard, then quickly move the tuning fork in front of the ear canal. Ask if

the client can hear the sound. If the client says yes, air conduction of sound is better than bone conduction, the normal finding.

- *The Weber test:* Place the base of a vibrating tuning fork on the middle of the top of the client's head (see figure B). Ask where the client best hears the sound. Sound is normally heard equally in both ears.

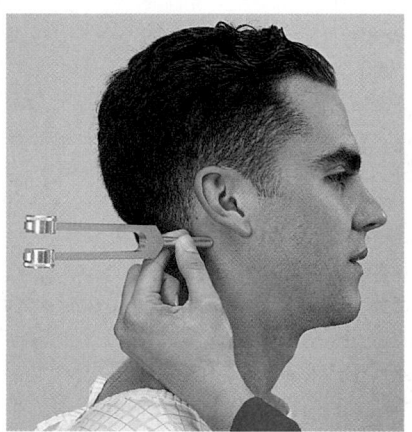 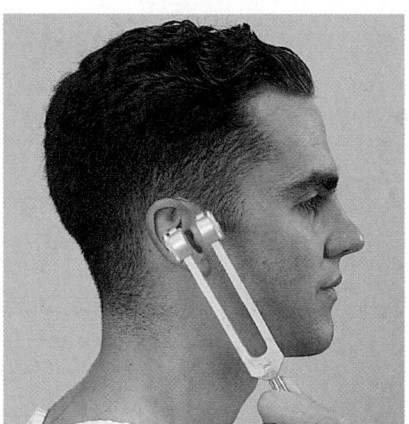

A Rinne Test

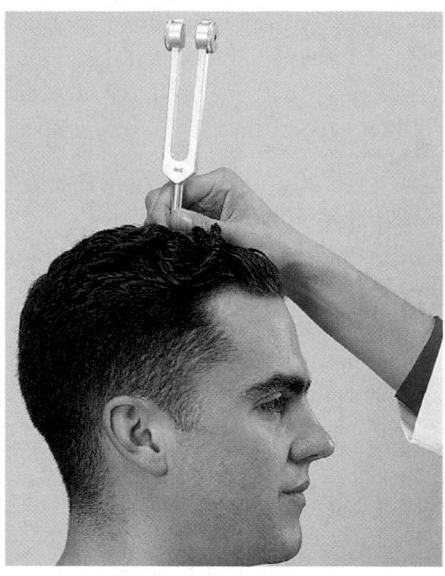

B Weber Test

implants provide sound perception but do not restore normal hearing. The client can recognize warning sounds such as automobiles, sirens, telephones, and doors opening or closing. They also are alerted to speech so they can focus on the person speaking. Many clients can learn to interpret the perceived sounds as words, especially with newer implant devices.

NURSING CARE

Planning and implementing nursing care for the client with a hearing deficit focuses on the type and extent of hearing loss and on how well the client has adapted to the loss. It also considers the availability of hearing aids and the client's ability and willingness to use them.

ASSESSING

Clients with a hearing loss often display signs that caregivers can recognize. Voice volume frequently increases, and the client positions the head with the better ear

toward the speaker. Be alert for signs of impaired hearing such as cupping an ear, difficulty understanding verbal communication when the person cannot see the speaker's face, difficulty following conversation in a large group, and withdrawal from social activities. The client may appear unsociable or paranoid.

Inspect the external ear canal and eardrum, using an otoscope. Perform the whisper test and Rinne and Weber tests to evaluate hearing. Document findings, and recommend an audiologist for further evaluation if indicated.

DIAGNOSING, PLANNING, AND IMPLEMENTING

Priorities in Nursing Care. Priority nursing care problems for a client with a hearing loss include loss of a sensory function, impaired communication, and social isolation.

Disturbed Sensory Perception: Auditory

- Encourage the client to talk about the hearing loss and its effect on activities of daily living. *Listening to and providing support encourage the client to develop coping strategies.*

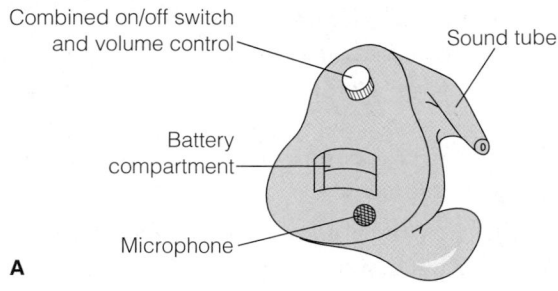

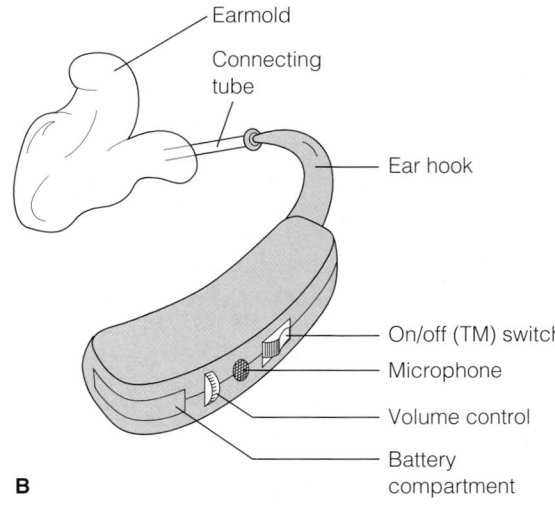

Figure 40-13. ■ Types of hearing aids. **(A)** An in-ear hearing aid. **(B)** A behind-the-ear hearing aid.

■ Provide information about hearing loss and available services to the client and family. *Information about hearing aids, amplification devices, and other services helps the client plan ways to compensate for the loss.*

■ Replace batteries in hearing aids on a regular and as-needed basis. *Hearing aid batteries last approximately 1 week.*

■ If the hearing aid has a toggle switch for microphone/telephone, be sure it is in the appropriate position. *This ensures proper amplification with the hearing aid.*

clinical **ALERT**

Check hearing aids for patency, cleaning out earwax as needed.

Impaired Verbal Communication

■ Get the client's attention before beginning to speak. Use a wave of the hand or tap on the shoulder. *This allows the client to focus on the person speaking.*

■ When speaking, face the client and keep the hands away from the face. Avoid making the client look into glare or

standing so that your face is in shadow. Trim mustaches so the lips are visible. *People with a hearing loss often use lip-reading consciously or unconsciously to help understand spoken words.*

■ When speaking, use a low voice pitch with normal loudness. The voice tends to become higher in pitch when loudness increases. *The ability to hear higher pitch tones often is lost; lowering the voice pitch allows the client to hear it more clearly.*

■ Speak at a normal rate, and do not overarticulate. Use shorter sentences and pause at the end of each sentence. *Changing the pace of speech may make conversation more difficult to follow and to lip-read. Using short sentences and pausing gives the client time to interpret the message.*

clinical **ALERT**

Reduce the noise in the environment before speaking with the client

■ Use nonverbal and written communication as needed. *Nonverbal cues and written messages may improve understanding.*

■ Rephrase sentences as necessary. *Some words are more difficult to perceive than others; rephrasing often clarifies the message for the client.*

■ Ask the client to repeat important information. *This helps ensure that the client understood the information.*

■ Share information about the client's hearing loss and effective communication strategies with other staff. *Consistent use of effective communication strategies decreases the client's frustration.*

Social Isolation

■ Help the client identify the extent and cause of social isolation. *Identifying the hearing deficit as a contributing factor to a sense of isolation may prompt the client to seek ways to improve hearing.*

■ Encourage interaction with friends and family on a one-to-one basis in quiet settings. *Conversations in small groups and quiet settings are easier for the client to follow and participate in.*

■ Treat the client with dignity. Remind friends and family that hearing loss does not mean loss of mental faculties. *Inappropriate responses to questions and comments can lead others to think of the client as "stupid" or demented.*

■ Involve the client in activities that do not require acute hearing, such as checkers and chess. *Activities such as these allow social interactions without the stress of straining to hear.*

■ Obtain a pocket talker or encourage the client and family to do so.

- Refer to an audiologist for evaluation and possible hearing-aid fitting.
- Refer to resources such as support groups and senior citizen centers. *These groups provide new social outlets.*

EVALUATING

Listen to the client's responses, and observe behavior, interactions with others, and signs of anxiety or stress to help determine the effectiveness of nursing interventions for the client with hearing loss.

Documenting. Documentation includes noting behaviors such as increased voice volume, cupping an ear, positioning the head with the better ear toward the nurse. Also note the client's withdrawal from social situations. Record client and family teaching about caring for a hearing aid, strategies to cope with a hearing loss, and possible community resources.

CONTINUING CARE

Teaching is vital to help prevent hearing loss. Teach all clients:

- How to safely clean ear canals
- The importance of preventing and treating ear infections

- To use earplugs when swimming or diving
- To use ear protectors when operating loud equipment, shooting, or when exposed to constant high-pitched sound
- To avoid frequent exposure to loud noise such as extremely loud music.

Help the client learn to manage and cope with hearing loss. Discuss evaluation by an audiologist to determine the usefulness of a hearing aid. Teach the client how to use, care for, and maintain a hearing aid. Encourage the client to acknowledge the deficit and ask people to speak clearly and repeat statements as needed. Voicing a preference for individual visits and small group interactions rather than large social functions can help the client to remain connected to friends and family.

Refer the client and family to national, state, and local agencies that provide education and assistance. Local and regional agencies are often listed in the telephone book. An audiology center may also have a list of local resources.

Note: The bibliography listings for this and all chapters have been compiled at the back of the book.

Chapter Review

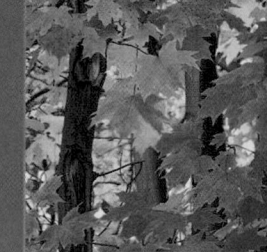

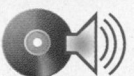 **KEY TERMS** by Topics

Use the audio glossary feature of either the CD-ROM or the Companion Website to hear the correct pronunciation of the following key terms.

Eye disorders
conjunctivitis, keratitis, corneal ulcers, photophobia, diplopia, cataract, red reflex, intraocular lens, glaucoma, retinal detachment, macular degeneration

Ear disorders
external otitis (swimmer's ear), tinnitus, otitis media, vertigo, presbycusis

KEY Points

- Glaucoma and cataracts, both very treatable conditions, are leading causes of blindness.

- Collect complete subjective and objective assessment data on clients who complain of changes in vision or a red, painful eye. While the cause may be minor and treatable, such as conjunctivitis, some conditions such as acute glaucoma may have similar symptoms and lead to permanent vision loss if not promptly treated.

- Teaching and maintaining client safety are primary nursing roles when caring for clients with eye or ear conditions.

- Most outer and middle ear conditions are minor and treatable, but can lead to conductive hearing loss if ignored.

- Vertigo, a sensation of movement, is a common manifestation of inner ear disorders. Clients with vertigo are at risk for falls, and often experience nausea and vomiting with the vertigo.

- Inspect the ear canal of clients who complain about recent hearing loss, especially if the client is older or wears a hearing aid or earplugs. Impacted cerumen can interfere with sound conduction and hearing.

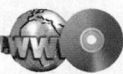 **EXPLORE Media**Link

Additional interactive resources for this chapter can be found on the Companion Website at www.prenhall.com/burke. Click on Chapter 40 and "Begin" to select the activities for this chapter.

For chapter-related NCLEX-style review questions and an audio glossary, access the accompanying CD-ROM in this book.

FOR FURTHER Study

For vision testing using the Snellen chart, assessment of pupil reflex, and more on hearing assessment, see Chapter 5.
For in-depth discussion of the client having surgery, see Chapter 9.
For nursing implications for antibiotics, see Chapter 10.
For more information about decongestants, see Chapter 23.
For vision testing using the Rosenbaum chart, see Figure 37-11.

Critical Thinking Care Map

Caring for a Client with Age-Related Hearing Loss
NCLEX-PN® Focus Area: Coping and Adaptation

Case Study: Carl Aaron is an 85-year-old retired logger who has been caring for his disabled wife in their home for the past 3 years. Mr. Aaron has osteoarthritis, which now makes it difficult for him to continue providing all the care his wife requires. They move into a care center where his wife can receive nursing care while he resides in the assisted living wing.

Nursing Diagnosis: Disturbed Sensory Perception: Auditory

COLLECT DATA

Subjective	Objective
_____	_____
_____	_____
_____	_____
_____	_____
_____	_____
_____	_____

Would you report this data? Yes/No

If yes, to: _____

Nursing Care

_____
_____
_____
_____
_____
_____
_____
_____
_____
_____
_____

How would you document this? _____
_____
_____
_____

Data Collected
(use those that apply)

- Proximal interphalangeal (PIP) and distal interphalangeal (DIP) joints swollen, cool, and hard bilaterally
- Weber test, no lateralization
- Answers not always appropriate to the question
- Rinne test AC>BC
- Appears depressed
- Mental status exam is normal
- Frequently asks nurse to repeat questions
- Ear canals clean, no redness, small amount of dark earwax noted
- C/O hip pain when ambulating
- Audiometric testing reveals significant hearing loss consistent with presbycusis
- BP 144/86, P 78, R 18
- Expresses concerns about wife's care
- Ignores conversation at his table during meals about wife's care

Nursing Interventions
(use those that apply; list in priority order)

- Teach Mr. Aaron how to use and care for hearing aids.
- Provide a schedule of small group activities for Mr. Aaron.
- Supplement verbal with nonverbal communication strategies.
- Obtain a temperature-controlled heating pad to promote comfort.
- Use a pocket talker as needed until hearing aids are available.
- Ask Mr. Aaron's family to obtain headphones for radio and television use.
- Administer ordered nonsteroidal anti-inflammatory drug (NSAID) every 6 hours.
- Use effective communication techniques.
- Encourage Mr. Aaron to shower on arising to relieve morning stiffness.
- Face Mr. Aaron when speaking with him.
- Facilitate one-on-one interactions between Mr. Aaron and other residents.
- Speak distinctly in a low voice.

NCLEX-PN® Exam Preparation

1 A client arrives in the outpatient clinic with a possible corneal abrasion. What diagnostic test would confirm this diagnosis?
- A. tonometry
- B. visual field testing
- C. facial x-rays
- D. fluorescein staining

2 The nurse is caring for an elderly male client who wears eyeglasses to correct myopia. When planning the client's care, the nurse understands that the client's lenses are used to correct:
- A. nearsightedness.
- B. farsightedness.
- C. astigmatism.
- D. nystagmus.

3 The nurse is teaching a client the correct method for administering eardrops. Place the steps in the correct order that the client should do them.
- A. Tilt the head toward the unaffected side.
- B. Instill the ordered number of drops.
- C. Pull the pinna (auricle) upward and backward.
- D. Place a loose cotton ball in the ear canal for 15 to 20 minutes.
- E. Partially fill the ear dropper with medication.
- F. Warm the drops by holding the bottle.

4 The nurse is caring for an older client who has a severe hearing impairment. An appropriate nursing intervention would be to:
- A. encourage the client to learn sign language.
- B. write out questions and responses.
- C. reduce environment noise before speaking with the client.
- D. raise the voice to a higher pitch.

5 A client is being taught about taking pilocarpine (Isopto Carpine). Which of the following side effects should the client report to a health care provider?
- A. darkening of the iris
- B. stinging in the eyes
- C. bitter taste in your mouth
- D. increased sweating

6 The nurse is irrigating a client's eye with a sterile normal saline solution. The nurse should direct the flow of the solution from the:
- A. center of both eyes to the lower conjunctiva.
- B. inner to the outer canthus.
- C. lower to the upper conjunctiva.
- D. outer to the inner canthus.

7 When educating a client about acute angle-closure glaucoma, what point should the nurse emphasize to the client about this condition?
- A. Immediately report symptoms to your physician.
- B. Do not use medications that cause pupil constriction.
- C. Wear sunglasses when outdoors.
- D. Lie down for 30 minutes until symptoms disappear.

8 Immediately following eye surgery, it is important for the nurse to place the client in what position?
- A. flat in bed
- B. turned on affective side
- C. high Fowler's position
- D. semi-Fowler's position

9 During the nurse's initial assessment of an elderly woman with open-angle glaucoma, what symptoms might the history reveal?
- A. light flashes in both eyes
- B. difficulty focusing on near objects
- C. acute severe eye pain
- D. watery drainage from both eyes

10 When teaching the client about Ménière's disease, which of the following diet changes should the nurse emphasize?
- A. Avoid foods high in sodium.
- B. Increase the amount of green leafy vegetables.
- C. Reduce the intake of milk and milk products.
- D. Increase fluid intake before meals.

Answers for Review Questions, as well as discussion of Care Plan and Critical Thinking Care Map questions, appear in Appendix V.

Thinking Strategically About...

Wong Lee is a 50-year-old tug boat mechanic who is married with three sons. He has been through rehabilitation twice for alcoholism, but continues to drink. Mr. Lee takes an anticoagulant for chronic atrial fibrillation. While attending a family reunion, Mr. Lee joins a game of softball. During the end of the second inning, the batter hits a ball that strikes Mr. Lee in the head. He stumbles and drops to the ground, but eventually gets up on his own and insists that he feels fine.

Two weeks later, after an evening of socializing and drinking, Mr. Lee develops a headache. He attributes it to a hangover, but the headache becomes steadily worse the next day. He becomes confused and disoriented. His wife takes him to the local emergency department where a CT scan is performed. The diagnosis of subdural hematoma is made and Mr. Lee is transferred to the neurosurgical unit.

DATA COLLECTED

Physical assessment findings on admission include T 98.5°F (37.0°C), BP 160/72, P 62, and R 14. Mr. Lee continues to be disoriented, but does complain of a worsening headache. Over the next few hours, Mr. Lee becomes drowsy. He suddenly vomits without any complaints of nausea. The nurse reports a Glasgow Coma Scale score of 11. An ICP monitor is inserted and reveals increased intracranial pressure. Mr. Lee is scheduled to have burr holes with hematoma evacuation that afternoon.

CRITICAL THINKING

1 Mr. Lee's hematoma is classified as subacute. How does this compare with other types of intracranial hematomas?

2 What are factors in Mr. Lee's history that make an intracranial bleed more likely following a minor head injury?

3 What manifestations of increased ICP did Mr. Lee display on admission to the neurosurgical unit?

4 Why is an anticoagulant necessary for a client with chronic atrial fibrillation?

5 What is a factor in Mr. Lee's history that makes him at higher risk for atrial fibrillation?

PRIORITIES IN NURSING CARE

1 You are caring for Mr. Lee 2 days postoperatively. You also are caring for Mrs. Smith, a 62-year-old client recovering from a mild stroke; Mr. Hines, a 28-year-old with a traumatic sports-induced head injury; and Mr. Mullins, a 58-year-old with a spinal cord injury that occurred 10 years ago, who is admitted for upper body strengthening. As you leave the report room at 0730, the night nurse tells you that Mr. Mullins is upset with the care that the night CNA provided and wants to speak to the charge nurse. She adds that Mr. Lee has complained of constipation and is sitting on the commode trying to have a bowel movement. The unit secretary tells you that the doctor is asking for a set of vital signs on Mr. Hines and that Mrs. Smith would like something for back pain. In what order would you address these needs and why?

MANAGEMENT OF CARE

1 Mr. Lee keeps trying to pull out his ICP line postoperatively. Knowing he is at risk for elevated ICP, what are the nursing implications indicated for Mr. Lee and in general for any client with an increased ICP?

COMMUNICATION

1 Describe what communication and education need to be provided for Mr. Lee's wife and sons to assist in coping with this event.

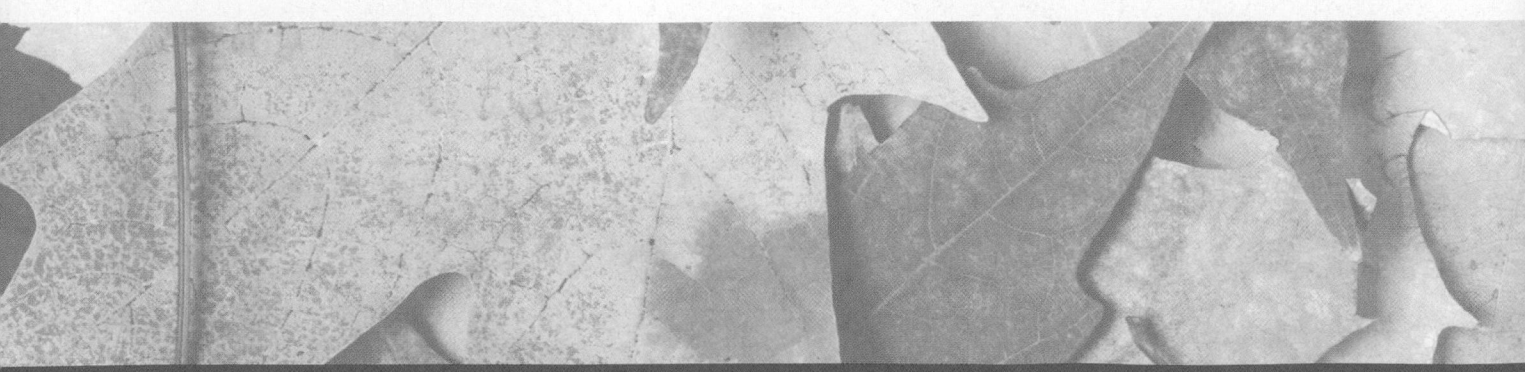

Disrupted Musculoskeletal Function

UNIT XI

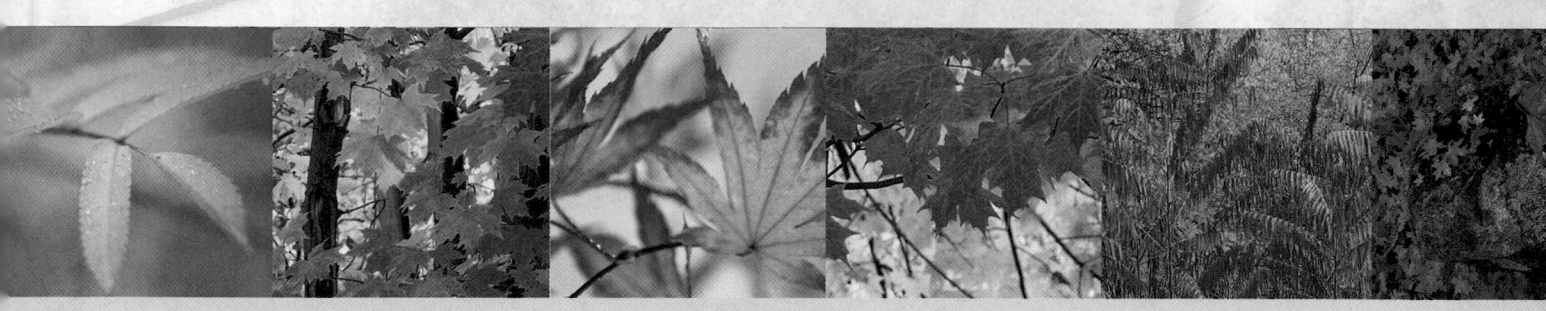

Chapter 41

The Musculoskeletal System and Assessment

BRIEF Outline

Structure and Function of the Musculoskeletal System
- Bones
- Joints, Ligaments, and Tendons
- Muscles
- Changes in the Older Adult

Assessment
- Health History
- Physical Examination
- Diagnostic Studies

LEARNING Outcomes

After completing this chapter, you will be able to:

- Describe the structure and function of bones, joints, muscles, ligaments, and tendons.
- Identify age-related changes in the musculoskeletal system.
- Collect appropriate subjective and objective assessment data related to the musculoskeletal system and its function.
- Provide nursing care for clients undergoing diagnostic tests for musculoskeletal system disorders.

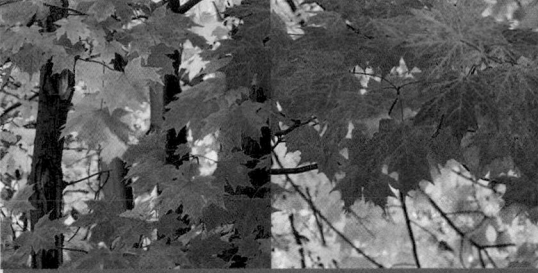

MediaLink

www.prenhall.com/burke
Use the address above to access the free, interactive Companion Website created for this textbook. Get hints, instant feedback, and textbook references to chapter-related NCLEX-style questions. Link to other interesting sites.

Audio Glossary:
Use the Companion Website, or the CD-ROM disk enclosed with your textbook, to hear the pronunciation of key terms in this chapter.

Structure and Function of the Musculoskeletal System

The musculoskeletal system includes bones and joints of the skeleton, connective tissues such as tendons and ligaments, and the skeletal muscles. The musculoskeletal system allows us to remain upright and to move and protects our vital organs.

BONES

The human skeleton has 206 bones (Figure 41-1 ■). Bones provide structure and support soft tissues. They protect vital organs from injury. Bones are classified by shape (Figure 41-2 ■):

- *Long bones,* such as those in the arms and legs, have a shaft, called a *diaphysis,* and two broad ends, called *epiphyses.*
- *Short bones* include those of the wrist and ankle.
- *Flat bones,* including skull bones, the sternum, and ribs, are thin and flat; most are curved.
- *Irregular bones* vary in size and shape. They include the vertebrae, the scapulae, and the bones of the pelvis.

Bone cells include *osteoblasts* (cells that form bone), *osteocytes* (cells that maintain bone), and *osteoclasts* (cells that resorb bone). Bones also contain collagen (a type of connective tissue) and minerals (primarily calcium and phosphate). Bones are covered with *periosteum,* a double-layered connective tissue that contains blood vessels and nerves.

There are two types of bone: *Compact bone* is smooth and dense, whereas *spongy bone* contains spaces. Both types are found in almost all bones of the body. Compact bone forms the shaft of long bones and the outside layer in other types of bones. The spongy sections of bones contain bone marrow. *Red bone marrow,* found mostly in flat bones such as the sternum, ribs, and ileum, makes blood cells and hemoglobin. *Yellow bone marrow,* found in the shaft of long bones, primarily contains fat and connective tissue.

Bones that are being used and subjected to stress (such as weight-bearing activity) are constantly remodeled. In this process, bone is resorbed and new bone is deposited. Bone remodeling is regulated by hormones, the effects of gravity, and mechanical stress from the pull of muscles. Without activity and stress on the bones, more bone is resorbed and less new bone is formed.

JOINTS, LIGAMENTS, AND TENDONS

Joints, also called *articulations,* are where two or more bones meet. Joints hold the skeleton together while allowing the body to move. The three primary types of joints are:

1. *Synarthrosis*—immovable joints (e.g., such as skull sutures)
2. *Amphiarthrosis*—slightly movable joints (e.g., vertebral joints)

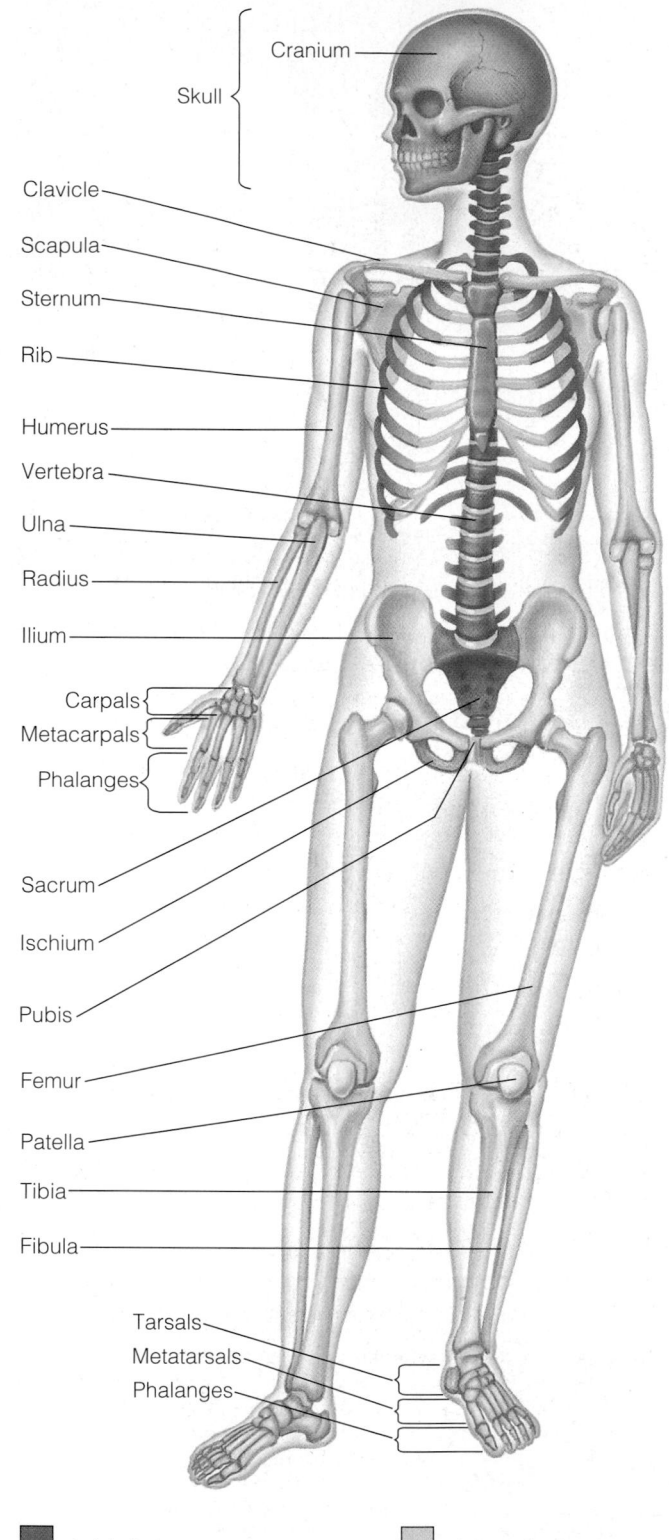

Figure 41-1. ■ Bones of the human skeleton.

3. *Diarthrosis or synovial*—freely movable joints (e.g., shoulders, hips)

Synovial joints are found at all limb articulations. The surfaces of synovial joints are covered by cartilage, and the

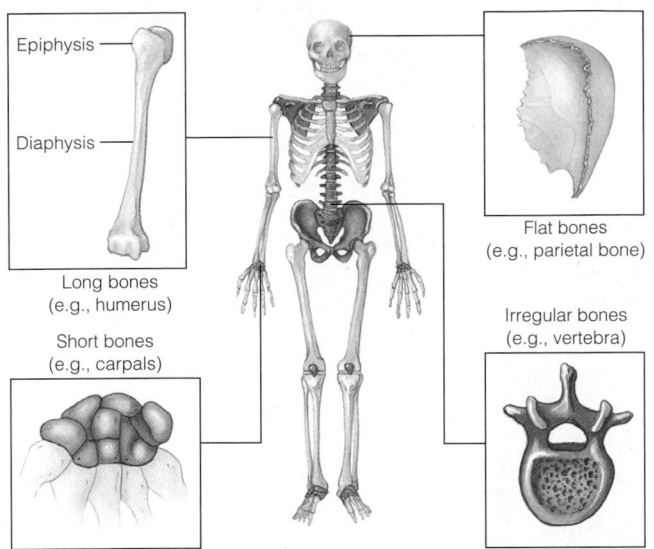

Figure 41-2. ■ Classification of bones by shape.

Epiphysis

Diaphysis

Long bones
(e.g., humerus)

Short bones
(e.g., carpals)

Flat bones
(e.g., parietal bone)

Irregular bones
(e.g., vertebra)

joint cavity is enclosed by a tough, fibrous capsule. This cavity is lined with synovial membrane and filled with synovial fluid. Synovial fluid lubricates the joint, facilitating smooth movement of the articulating bones. Synovial joints allow many different kinds of movements (Table 41-1 ■).

Ligaments are bands of connective tissue that connect bones to bones. Ligaments either limit or enhance movement, provide joint stability, and enhance joint strength.

TABLE 41-1	
Movement of Synovial Joints	
MOVEMENT	**DESCRIPTION**
Abduction	Move away from the midline of the body
Adduction	Move toward the midline of the body
Extension	Straighten limb at a joint
Flexion	Bend limb at a joint
Dorsiflexion	Bend ankle to bring top of foot toward shin
Plantar flexion	Straighten ankle to point toes down
Pronation	Turn forearm to place palm down
Supination	Turn forearm to place palm up
Eversion	Turn out
Inversion	Turn in
Circumduction	Move in a circle
Internal rotation	Move inward on a central axis
External rotation	Move outward on a central axis

Tendons are fibrous connective tissue bands that connect muscles to bones and enable the bones to move when skeletal muscles contract. *Bursae* are small sacs of synovial fluid that cushion and protect bony areas that are at high risk for friction, such as the knee and the shoulder.

MUSCLES

There are three types of muscle tissue: skeletal muscle, smooth muscle, and cardiac muscle. *Skeletal muscle,* also known as *voluntary muscle,* allows voluntary movement. Both *smooth muscle* and *cardiac muscle* are involuntary; their movement is controlled by internal mechanisms. The muscles of the bladder wall, gastrointestinal system, and bronchi are smooth muscle. Cardiac muscle is in the heart.

Skeletal muscles are thick bundles of parallel fibers. Each muscle fiber is a bundle of smaller structures called *myofibrils.* Myofibrils are strands of smaller repeating units called *sarcomeres,* which allow the muscle to contract. Skeletal muscle contracts when motor neurons release acetylcholine, a neurotransmitter. This produces an action potential (electrical impulse) that spreads through the muscle fiber, causing it to contract. The more fibers that contract, the stronger the muscle contraction. Skeletal muscles can be moved through conscious, voluntary control or be reflex activity. There are approximately 600 skeletal muscles in the body (Figures 41-3A and B ■).

Nerve impulses maintain muscle tone. Lack of use causes muscle atrophy, whereas regular exercise increases the size and strength of muscles. Prolonged strenuous activity can cause a buildup of lactic acid and muscle fatigue.

CHANGES IN THE OLDER ADULT

Aging commonly affects the musculoskeletal system. Although some musculoskeletal system changes appear to relate to the aging process itself, others result from decreased activity, lifestyle factors, or pathophysiologic processes.

Older adults, women in particular, tend to lose bone mass with aging. Joint and disk cartilage dehydrates and loses its flexibility as well. Together, these changes contribute to a loss of height (an average of about 1.5 to 2 inches) and a stooped posture. The hips and knees are somewhat flexed, and the head tilted slightly backward to maintain eye contact. This posture changes the older adult's center of gravity, increasing the risk for falls. Dehydration of joint cartilage contributes to degenerative joint disease (osteoarthritis) in older adults. Affected joints tend to stiffen and lose range of motion. Cartilage deteriorates, and pieces of cartilage may be loose in the joint space, contributing to joint pain and stiffness. Ligaments and tendons lose flexibility with aging, increasing the risk of tears and joint instability.

Reduced activity levels, decreased muscle cell innervation, and endocrine changes associated with aging contribute to skeletal muscle atrophy in the older adult. Muscle

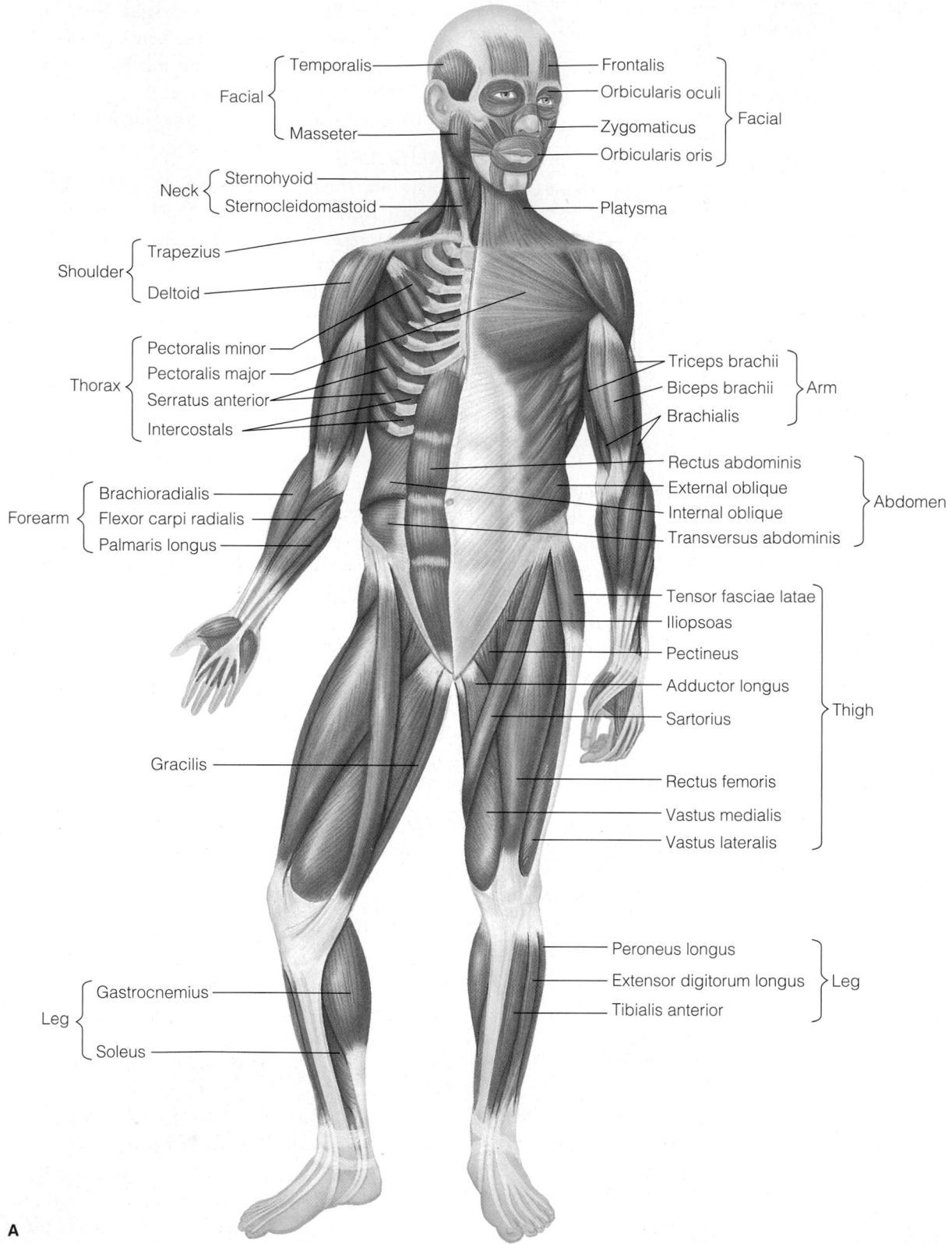

Figure 41-3. ■ **(A)** Muscles of the anterior body.

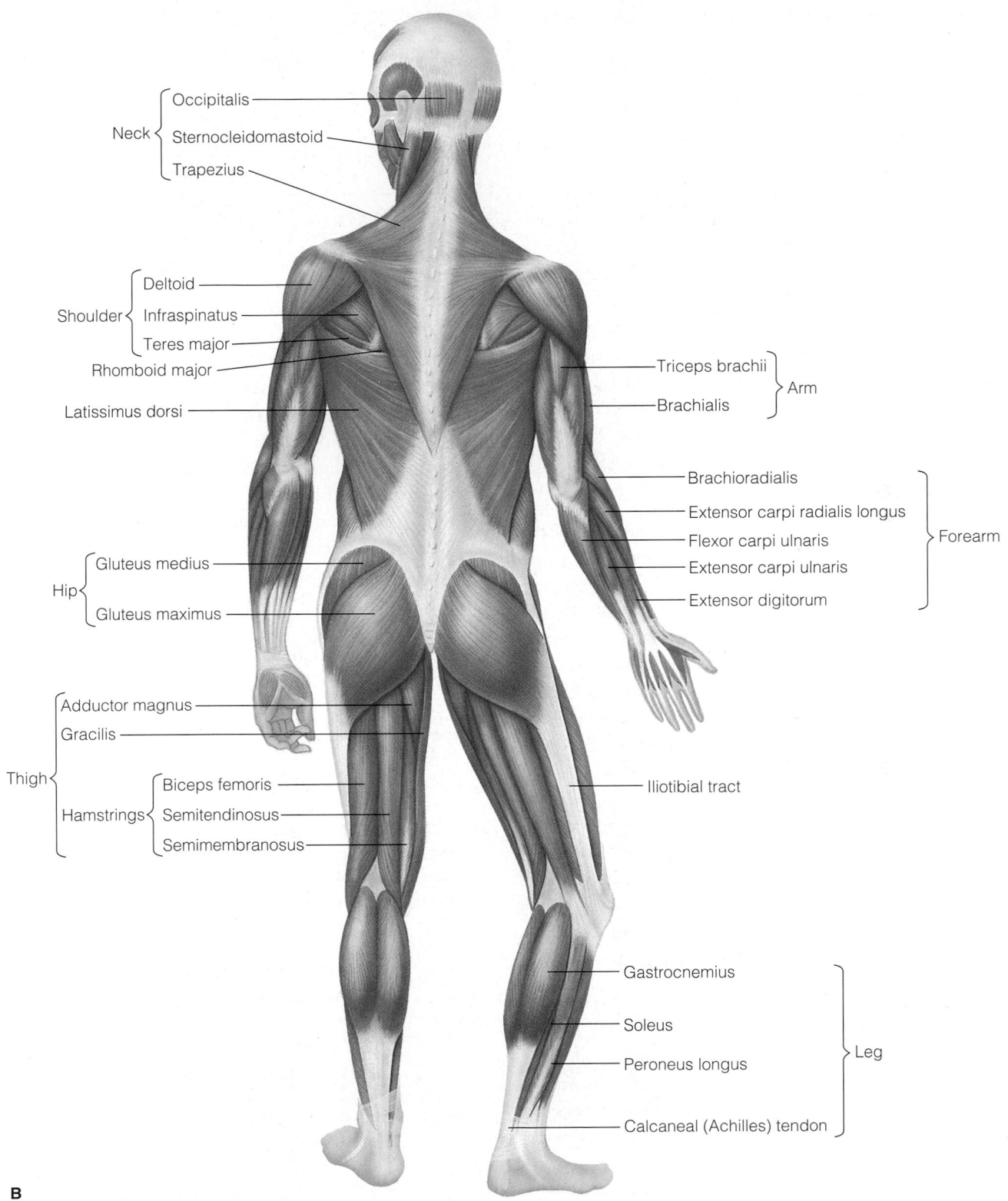

B

Figure 41-3. ■ *(continued)* **(B)** Muscles of the posterior body.

tone decreases, as does muscle strength and stamina. Maintaining an active lifestyle and specific exercises such as weight training help counteract these changes, maintain muscle mass, and prevent osteoporosis.

Assessment

This section focuses on assessment data that relates to the musculoskeletal system. This data may be collected as part of the total health assessment of the client, or may be collected from a client with a complaint or disorder related to musculoskeletal function.

Pain and limited mobility are the primary manifestations of musculoskeletal trauma and disorders. Because the neurologic and musculoskeletal systems are closely interrelated, a neurologic disorder may have musculoskeletal effects (e.g., a stroke or multiple sclerosis). Assessment of neurologic function is presented in Chapter 37. ⚭

HEALTH HISTORY

Explore the client's chief complaint (for example, wrist pain), inquiring about the onset of the problem, its duration and specific manifestations, and the effect of the problem on function and ability to maintain activities of daily living (ADLs). Ask about any precipitating events such as trauma (e.g., a fall, motor vehicle crash, hyperextension of a joint), significantly increased life stressors, or other associated events. Explore complaints of pain, determining the location and any radiation of the pain, its character (sharp, dull, aching, constant or intermittent), duration and timing, aggravating and alleviating factors, and the effect of the pain on function (e.g., resulting limitations in joint range of motion, ability to complete ADLs, and occupation and other life roles). Inquire about associated complaints such as fever, fatigue, weight changes, rash, or swelling. Explore past injuries or related or similar problems and treatment measures (prescribed or self-care) and their effectiveness.

PHYSICAL EXAMINATION

Depending on the circumstances, physical assessment of the musculoskeletal system may be very focused or may include overall assessment of musculoskeletal structure and function. In most cases, the practical/vocational nurse focuses on collecting assessment data related to the client's primary problem/complaint.

Begin by assessing the client's posture, gait, ability to walk and change directions with or without assistive devices, and ability to sit and to rise from a chair. Additional functional assessment data, collected as indicated, includes the client's ability to manipulate clothing for toileting and complete other hygiene activities (e.g., bathing) and ADLs.

Inspect general muscle mass and symmetry of muscle development, as well as equality of limb length. Assess and

document muscle strength, grading muscle strength from 0 to 5, with 0 being no muscle contraction or paralysis, and 5 begin full range of motion (ROM) against resistance (Table 41-2 ■). Table 41-3 ■ provides suggested instructions for clients to evaluate various muscle groups. The nurse provides resistance to muscle movement by pushing in the opposite direction.

Inspect and palpate bones and joints for obvious deformity, tenderness or pain, swelling, warmth, and ROM. Joint ROM often is assessed only when a musculoskeletal problem is present. When ROM is assessed, it is important to assess and compare corresponding joints on both sides of the body. Palpate joints such as the shoulders and knees for **crepitus,** a grating sound or sensation, during ROM. Table 41-4 ■ identifies the normal movements for the major joints.

TABLE 41-2

Grading Muscle Strength

GRADE	DESCRIPTION
0	No contraction; paralysis
1	Contraction felt, but no limb movement
2	Passive ROM
3	Full ROM against gravity
4	Full ROM against some resistance
5	Full ROM against full resistance

TABLE 41-3

Instructions to Evaluate Muscle Strength

MUSCLE GROUP	INSTRUCTIONS
Eyes and lids	Close eyes tightly.
Facial muscles	Blow out cheeks, stick out tongue.
Neck	Put chin on chest, look up at ceiling, touch ear to the shoulder.
Deltoid	Hold arms up.
Biceps, triceps	Bend arm, straighten arm.
Wrist	Bend hand forward and backward.
Fingers	Shake hands, make a fist, squeeze nurse's fingers, spread fingers.
Gluteal and leg	Alternately cross legs while sitting, straighten leg.
Ankle and foot	Bend foot up and down.

TABLE 41-4

Assessing Joint Range of Motion

JOINT(S)	MOTION	CLIENT INSTRUCTIONS
Temporomandibular (TM)	Extension, flexion	Open mouth wide, then close it.
Cervical spine	Flexion	Put your chin to your chest.
	Extension	Look at the ceiling.
	Lateral flexion	Touch your ear to your shoulder.
	Rotation	Touch your chin to your shoulder.
Lumbar spine	Flexion	Touch your toes with your fingers.
	Extension	Slowly bend backward.
	Lateral flexion	Bend right and left.
	Rotation	Twist your shoulders right and left.
Shoulders	Flexion	Raise your arms straight up and out.
	Extension	Reach back with your straight arm.
	Internal rotation	Touch your left shoulder with your right hand, repeat with other side.
	Abduction	Raise your arm straight out to the side.
	Adduction	Move your straight arm across your chest.
Elbows	Flexion	Touch your hands to your shoulders.
	Pronation	With elbows bent, turn your hand palm down.
	Supination	With elbows bent, turn your hand palm up.
Fingers	Flexion	Make a fist.
	Extension	Open your hand.
	Abduction	Spread your fingers.
	Adduction	Close your fingers.
Hips	Flexion	Bring your knee to your chest.
	Extension	Reach behind you with your foot.
	Abduction	With your leg straight, move it out to the side.
	Internal rotation	Bend your knee and swing it toward your other leg.
	External rotation	Bend your knee and swing it out to the side.
Knees	Flexion	Bend your knee.
	Extension	Straighten your leg.
Ankles	Dorsiflexion	Pull your toes up toward your head.
	Plantar flexion	Point your toes toward the floor.
	Inversion	Turn the sole of your foot inward.
	Eversion	Turn the sole of your foot outward.
Toes	Flexion	Curl your toes.
	Extension, abduction	Spread your toes.

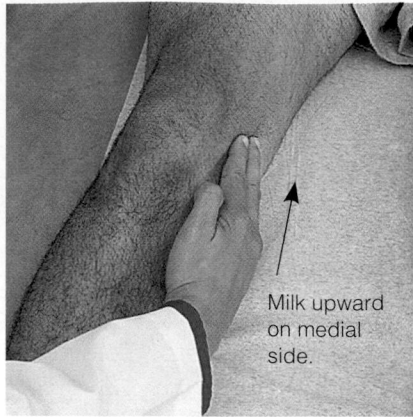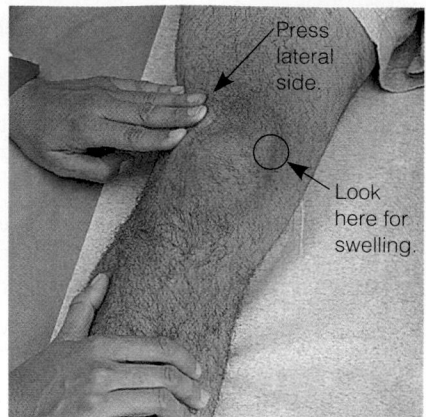

Figure 41-4. ■ Checking for the bulge sign.

clinical ALERT

Never attempt to move a joint past its normal range of motion for the client or past the point at which pain is experienced.

Several special physical assessment maneuvers may be performed with additional training and as indicated. The "*bulge sign*" and *ballottement* are used to assess for fluid in the knee joint.

- *Bulge Sign:* With the client supine, milk upward on the medial side of the knee, then tap the lateral side of the patella while observing for a fluid bulge (Figure 41-4 ■).
- *Ballottement:* Apply downward pressure with one hand placed just above the knee. With the other hand, tap the

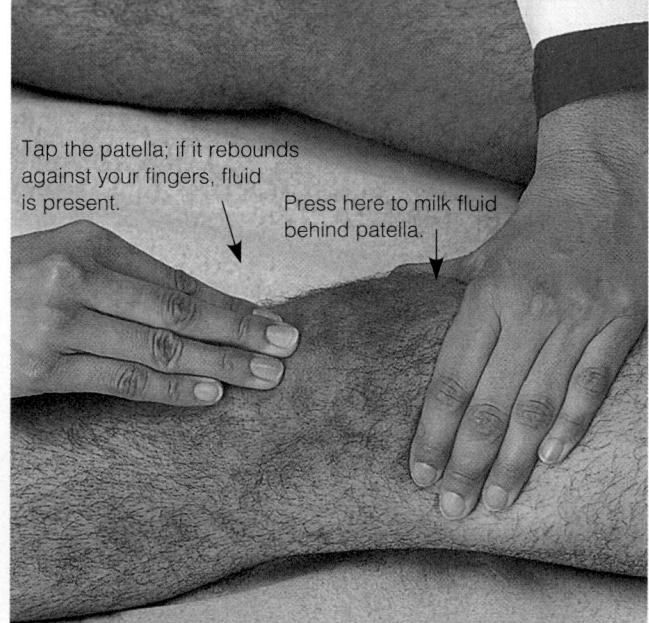

Figure 41-5. ■ Checking for ballottement.

patella (knee cap); fluid in the knee causes the patella to rebound against the fingers (Figure 41-5 ■).

The *Thomas test* may be performed when a hip flexion contracture is suspected. The reclining client is asked to bring one knee up to the chest while keeping the other leg straight. With a hip flexion contracture, the extended leg rises off the examining table.

Box 41-1 ■ presents an example of a documented focused musculoskeletal assessment.

DIAGNOSTIC STUDIES

Diagnostic imaging studies (e.g., x-rays) are extensively used to evaluate bones and joints. Laboratory testing may be indicated to evaluate some musculoskeletal disorders and systemic diseases (such as rheumatoid arthritis) with musculoskeletal effects.

Laboratory Tests

Blood tests used in diagnosing musculoskeletal disorders include measures of inflammation, selected serum electrolytes

---

BOX 41-1

DOCUMENTING MUSCULOSKELETAL ASSESSMENT

Client: Mary Simmons presents at her primary care practitioner's office complaining of right elbow pain.

Assessment note: Sharp, intermittent R elbow pain began approximately 6 days ago. No known injury; does relate that she has been taking tennis and golf lessons for the past 3 months, and is playing both sports several times a week. Pain aggravated by movement and lifting. No previous known injuries or history of similar problems. Describes self as healthy and physically active. Denies history of joint swelling, pain, or arthritis symptoms. No known chronic diseases or medications. No known allergies. Appears healthy, weight appropriate for height. No joint swelling, warmth, or erythema noted, proximal R elbow tender to palpation. Arm strength 5/5 bilaterally, pain experienced on flexion and extension against resistance. Full ROM all upper extremity joints, no crepitus noted.

and enzymes, and indicators of autoimmune disorders. Table 41-5 ■ identifies commonly used laboratory studies for diagnosing musculoskeletal disorders with their nursing implications.

Synovial fluid may be analyzed to diagnose joint disorders. Normally, joints contain very small amounts of fluid. Inflammatory processes and trauma can increase this fluid volume, and affect the composition of synovial fluid. *Arthrocentesis* is the procedure used to obtain fluid from a joint. It often is performed in a physician's office or at the client's bedside.

Box 41-2 ■ outlines nursing care for the client undergoing arthrocentesis.

Imaging Techniques

Radiologic studies, x-rays in particular, are commonly used to diagnose musculoskeletal trauma and bone and joint disorders. Although the x-ray table may be uncomfortable, these procedures generally are noninvasive. Plain x-ray films require no special client preparation, but do expose the client to radiation. Ask female clients of childbearing age if there is any

TABLE 41-5

Laboratory Tests to Evaluate Musculoskeletal Disorders

TEST	NORMAL VALUE	EXPLANATION	NURSING IMPLICATIONS
Erythrocyte sedimentation rate (ESR)	0–20 mm/hr	A nonspecific measure of inflammation, the ESR measures the rate at which RBCs settle out of blood. The rate increases in inflammation.	No special client preparation is required for this blood test.
C-reactive protein (CRP)	<0.5 mg/dL (0–5 mg/L)	CRP is an abnormal protein that is a sensitive indicator of inflammation.	No special client preparation is required for this blood test.
Calcium (Ca^{2+})	8.5–10.0 mg/dL (2.15–2.5 mmol/L)	Most of the body's calcium is in the bones and teeth. Adequate total body calcium is vital to maintain bone mass. Blood levels increase when calcium is released from the bone.	Instruct the client to withhold all calcium preparations for 8–12 hours prior to the test; the client may be advised to fast for 8 hours prior to the test.
Phosphate (Ph)	2.5–4.5 mg/dL (1.0–1.5 mmol/L)	Phosphate is primarily combined with calcium in bones and teeth in the body. Calcium and phosphorus have an inverse relationship; when blood levels of one increase, the other decreases.	Fasting may be recommended for this blood test.
Alkaline phosphatase (ALP)	Women: 81–234 U/L Men: 98–251 U/L	ALP is an enzyme found in bone, liver, and other cells of the body. ALP levels rise during bone healing and with bone tumors.	Instruct the client to fast for 12 hours prior to the test.
Uric acid	Women: 2.6–6.6 mg/dL (137–393 μmol/L) Men: 3.5–7.6 mg/dL (210–452 μmol/L)	Uric acid is the end product of protein metabolism, excreted by the kidneys and in feces. Elevated levels are found in gout, a metabolic disorder in which urate crystals are deposited in joints and other tissues.	Fasting for 8 hours prior to the test may be recommended.
Rheumatoid factor (RF)	Negative	RF is a group of antibodies directed against normal antibodies. Presence of RF is strongly associated with rheumatoid arthritis and other connective tissue diseases.	No special client preparation is required for this blood test.
Antinuclear antibodies (ANA)	Negative at a 1:20 dilution	Antinuclear and anti-DNA antibodies attack antigens in cell nuclei, and are found in autoimmune disorders such as systemic lupus erythematosus (SLE).	No special client preparation is required for these blood tests.
Anti-DNA antibodies	Negative		
Lupus erythematosus test (LE prep)	Negative	The LE prep is an indirect measure of the presence of antinuclear antibodies used to diagnose SLE.	Do not schedule within 2 days of heparin administration. List client medications on requisition.

BOX 41-2	NURSING CARE CHECKLIST

Arthrocentesis

☑ Reinforce teaching, clarifying information as needed. Instruct the client that local anesthesia will be used. Fasting for 6 to 8 hours prior to the procedure may be recommended.

☑ Obtain informed consent for this invasive procedure.

☑ Assist with positioning of the extremity.

☑ Assist with cleaning and draping of the site as directed.

☑ Assist with anesthetic preparation and specimen collection as directed.

☑ Apply a pressure dressing to the site following aspiration to prevent bleeding into the tissues.

☑ Instruct to apply a cold pack, maintain the pressure dressing (elastic binding), and elevate the extremity for 8 to 24 hours as indicated.

☑ Instruct to rest the affected joint for 2 to 3 days following the procedure.

chance they could be pregnant before the x-ray is performed and alert the physician and radiologic technician if there is.

Bone density scans (bone densitometry) are used to diagnose osteoporosis by measuring bone mineral density. These procedures use special x-ray imaging techniques that expose the client to very low amounts of radiation. Bone density scans help predict fracture risk by comparing the individual's bone mass to that of a healthy 25- to 35-year-old person.

Computed tomography (CT) scans and other imaging techniques may be used in diagnosing musculoskeletal disorders.

- *CT scans* are specialized radiographic procedures that produce computer-generated images with significantly more detail than standard x-rays allow. CT scan may be done to detect small fractures and bone erosions and to evaluate bone density. They also may be used to evaluate the spinal column and spinal curvatures and to detect tumors.
- *Magnetic resonance imaging (MRI)* uses a super magnet and radio-frequency signals to elicit a response from hydrogen nuclei. The client is not exposed to radiation during an MRI. MRI is useful in evaluating soft tissue injuries, degenerative disk changes in the spine, and joint inflammation and injuries.

clinical ALERT

Always ask clients scheduled for MRI about the presence of a pacemaker, prosthetic device (such as a hip joint prosthesis), or other metallic objects. Pacemakers and other implanted devices can be damaged by MRI; metallic objects such as surgical clips and joint prostheses can overheat or become dislodged during MRI.

BOX 41-3	NURSING CARE CHECKLIST

Bone Scan

Before the Procedure

☑ Verify the presence of a signed consent for the procedure.

☑ Assess knowledge and reinforce teaching.

☑ Notify physician and nuclear medicine technician if the client is or might be pregnant.

☑ Client may eat, drink, and ambulate.

☑ Remove all clothing and jewelry.

☑ Empty bladder.

During the Procedure

☑ Radioactive material is injected intravenously.

☑ Instruct to drink four to six glasses of water after the injection and before scanning.

☑ Scanning takes 30 to 60 minutes to complete.

After the Procedure

☑ Apply warm compresses to injection site if red or swollen.

☑ Increase fluid intake and activity to promote excretion of the radioactive material.

☑ No radioactive substance precautions are necessary.

- *Ultrasound* procedures use echoes from high-frequency sound waves to evaluate tissues. These tests are noninvasive. Ultrasound devices may be used to evaluate overall bone density by estimating bone density over the heel or kneecap.
- *Bone scan* is a nuclear medicine procedure in which the amount of an injected radioactive isotope taken up by bones is evaluated. Abnormal bone scans may reveal "hot spots" where uptake of the material is increased (e.g., a malignant tumor or infected area), or "cold spots" where its uptake is diminished (e.g., an area of bone that is ischemic, or has decreased blood flow). Box 41-3 ■ describes nursing care of the client undergoing a bone scan.

Arthroscopy

Arthroscopy uses a flexible fiberoptic endoscope to view joint structures and tissues. This procedure is used to identify torn tendons or ligaments, an injured meniscus, inflammatory joint changes, and damaged cartilage. Box 41-4 ■ outlines nursing care of the client undergoing diagnostic arthroscopy.

Note: The bibliography listings for this and all chapters have been compiled at the back of the book.

BOX 41-4	NURSING CARE CHECKLIST

Diagnostic Arthroscopy

Before the Procedure

☑ Reinforce teaching about the purpose of the procedure and what to expect during and after the procedure.

☑ Mild postoperative pain is expected, but will be controlled with analgesics.

☑ Instruct the client to fast for 8 hours before the procedure.

☑ Obtain informed consent or ensure that it has been obtained.

☑ Obtain baseline vital signs and assessment data.

☑ Provide routine preoperative care as indicated (see Chapter 9). ⦾⦿

After the Procedure

☑ Provide routine postoperative care as indicated (see Chapter 9). ⦾⦿

☑ Assess neurovascular status (color, temperature, pulses, movement, and sensation) of the distal extremity every 15 minutes; compare with the unaffected side.

☑ Monitor pain and provide analgesics as ordered.

☑ Observe elastic compression dressing for evidence of bleeding, excessive swelling, or constriction of the extremity.

☑ Instruct to keep the extremity elevated for 24 to 48 hours, applying ice to the affected area for the first 24 hours.

☑ Knee arthroscopy: Teach the client how to use crutches to avoid weight bearing on the joint for 24 hours following the procedure.

☑ Shoulder arthroscopy: Place the affected arm in a sling and provide instructions as directed by the physician.

☑ Provide instructions for ROM exercises or referral to physical therapy as directed.

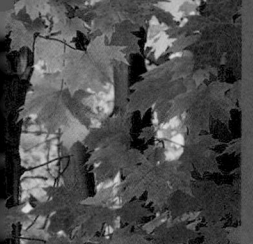

Chapter Review

 **KEY TERMS** by Topics

Use the audio glossary feature of either the CD-ROM or the Companion Website to hear the correct pronunciation of the following key terms.

Structure and function
synovial joints
Assessment
crepitus, arthroscopy

KEY Points

- Bones and muscles and the structures that connect them (tendons, ligaments, and joints) provide structure to the body, allow people to remain upright, and allow movement.

- The musculoskeletal and neurologic systems are closely related in function. Neurologic disorders may have musculoskeletal manifestations.

- Aging affects both the structure and function of the musculoskeletal system, increasing the risk for traumatic injury due to falls.

- Imaging studies such as x-rays, CT scans, and arthroscopy are widely used to diagnose musculoskeletal trauma and disorders.

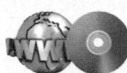 **EXPLORE MediaLink**

Additional interactive resources for this chapter can be found on the Companion Website at www.prenhall.com/burke. Click on Chapter 41 and "Begin" to select the activities for this chapter.

For chapter-related NCLEX-style questions and an audio glossary, access the accompanying CD-ROM in this book.

FOR FURTHER Study

See Chapter 9 for a discussion of routine preoperative and postoperative care.

Assessment of neurologic function is presented in Chapter 37.

NCLEX-PN® Exam Preparation

Although the majority of NCLEX-PN® test items are multiple choice, with one *best* response out of four choices, some items are in alternative formats. These formats include multiple response questions in which you will be asked to "select all that apply" of five or six choices. For these questions, you must choose all the appropriate responses to get the question correct. Read all the possible responses carefully, and look at each, keeping the stem of the question in mind. Some responses may be appropriate nursing care activities or assessments, but may not apply to the question. Use your best judgment and clinical decision-making skills to respond to these questions.

1 In reviewing an x-ray report that states "distal epiphyseal fracture of the radius," the nurse correctly interprets this as meaning a fracture:

A. close to the elbow.
B. of the shaft of the radius.
C. at the wrist end of the bone.
D. that has broken the skin.

2 The physician's orders for a client following hip replacement surgery are to maintain the operative leg in a position of abduction. The nurse positions the client:

A. with the legs together and bent at a 60° angle.
B. on the side, with the knees bent.
C. supine, with the knees crossed.
D. with the leg positioned away from the center of the body.

3 The nurse assessing hand strength asks the client to (select all that apply):

A. shake hands.
B. move the hand up (extended).
C. spread the fingers against resistance.
D. make a fist.
E. flex the hand against resistance.

4 When assessing range of motion of the client's knee, the nurse notes a grating sound. This is appropriately charted as:

A. crepitus.
B. synovitis.
C. erythema.
D. inflammation.

5 The nurse preparing a client for a bone scan provides which of the following instructions?

A. You should have nothing to eat for 8 to 12 hours before the procedure.
B. When the injection is given, you will be instructed to drink four to six glasses of water.
C. Following the procedure, it is important to avoid close contact with others for 4 hours to avoid exposing them to radiation.
D. This test is noninvasive; no special preparation is required.

Answers for Review Questions appear in Appendix V.

Chapter 42

Caring for Clients with Musculoskeletal Trauma

BRIEF Outline

Soft Tissue Trauma
Fractures
Hip Fracture
Joint Trauma and Injury
Repetitive Use Injuries
Amputation

LEARNING Outcomes

After completing this chapter, you will be able to:

- Discuss risk factors for and mechanisms of musculoskeletal trauma.
- Safely and appropriately assess clients with musculoskeletal trauma.
- State how fractures are classified.
- Discuss interdisciplinary care for clients who have experienced musculoskeletal trauma.
- Discuss common complications of fractures, their manifestations, and nursing strategies to prevent them.
- Discuss psychologic effects unique to amputation.
- Describe the difference between skin and skeletal traction.
- Provide individualized care for clients who have experienced musculoskeletal trauma.

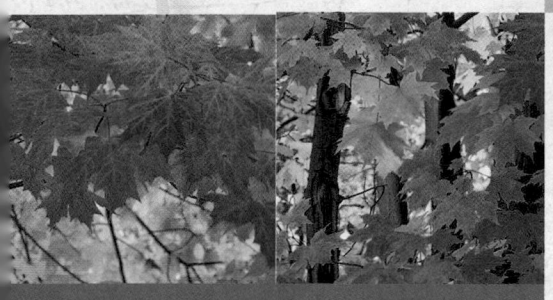

MediaLink

www.prenhall.com/burke
Use the address above to access the free, interactive Companion Website created for this textbook. Get hints, instant feedback, and textbook references to chapter-related NCLEX-style questions. Link to other interesting sites.

Audio Glossary:
Use the Companion Website, or the CD-ROM disk enclosed with your textbook, to hear the pronunciation of key terms in this chapter.

MUSCULOSKELETAL TRAUMA

Musculoskeletal **trauma** occurs when tissues are subjected to more force than they are able to absorb. The severity of trauma depends on both the amount of force and the location of impact, because different parts of the body can withstand different amounts of force. For example, small bones in the hand cannot absorb as much energy as the femur. Many external sources can cause trauma, and the force can vary in severity. A step off the curb, a fall, being tackled in a football game, and a motor vehicle crash are a few examples.

Musculoskeletal trauma ranges from mild to severe, for example, soft tissue injury, fracture, or complete amputation. Musculoskeletal trauma often affects surrounding tissues. A bone fracture can affect the function of muscles, tendons, and ligaments that attach to it.

Nurses can play a major role in trauma prevention. Teach children and young adults the importance of using safety equipment—such as automobile seat belts, bicycle helmets, football pads, proper footwear, protective eyewear, and hard hats—to prevent or decrease the severity of injury from trauma.

Older clients are at higher risk for musculoskeletal trauma due to falls. Assess the home for potential hazards such as poorly lighted stairs or no hand railings. Encourage removing throw rugs and clutter from travel areas. Discuss using bath mats and installing grab bars in bathrooms. Advise wearing shoes with good treads to decrease the risk of slipping.

Soft Tissue Trauma

Sprains, strains, and other soft tissue injuries are common injuries. The lower back and cervical spine are the most common sites for muscle strains. The ankle is the most commonly sprained joint, usually caused by inversion of the foot.

PATHOPHYSIOLOGY AND MANIFESTATIONS

A **contusion,** the simplest musculoskeletal injury, is bleeding into soft tissue resulting from blunt force. With significant bleeding, a **hematoma** forms. A contusion causes swelling and discoloration (a bruise), which initially appears purple or blue ("black-and-blue"). As blood cells break down and are reabsorbed, the mark becomes brown, then yellow, and finally disappears.

A **sprain** is a ligament injury. Sprains are caused by a twisting motion that overstretches or tears the ligament. Sprains are graded by the extent of damage:

- *Grade I*—overstretching with mild bleeding and inflammation
- *Grade II*—severe stretching and some tearing with inflammation and hematoma
- *Grade III*—complete tearing of the ligament
- *Grade IV*—the bony attachment of the ligament is broken away.

A **strain** is a microscopic tear in the muscle that causes bleeding into the tissues. A strain (or "pulled muscle") occurs when a muscle is forced to extend past its elasticity. Strains may be caused by inappropriate lifting or by a sudden acceleration–deceleration injury, such as a motor vehicle crash. The characteristics of sprains and strains are compared in Box 42-1 ■.

INTERDISCIPLINARY CARE

An x-ray may be done to rule out fracture. If further evaluation is necessary, an MRI may be done.

Soft tissue trauma is treated with measures to decrease swelling, alleviate pain, and encourage rest. The client is instructed to avoid using the injured area. A splint may be applied. Ice is applied for the first 48 hours, after which heat can be applied. A compression dressing, such as an Ace bandage, may be applied. The injured extremity should be elevated to the level of the heart to increase venous return and decrease swelling. If the lower extremity is injured, crutches are provided. A knee injury also requires a knee immobilizer. If the upper extremity is injured, a sling is provided.

Nonsteroidal anti-inflammatory drugs (NSAIDs) and analgesics, including narcotics, may be ordered to manage pain and reduce the inflammatory response.

BOX 42-1

CHARACTERISTICS OF SPRAINS AND STRAINS

Sprain
- Ligament injury
- Joint instability
- Pain, swelling, discoloration
- Increased pain with joint use

Strain
- Muscle tear
- Swelling, local tenderness
- Sharp or dull pain
- Increased pain with muscle contraction

NURSING CARE

ASSESSING

To assess soft tissue injury, collect both subjective and objective data. Ask about the mechanism of injury and when it occurred. Ask about any protective devices that were being used at the time of injury (e.g., seat belt or air bag). Obtain specific information about pain, including location, character, intensity, and aggravating and relieving factors. Ask about the effect of the injury or pain on use of the extremity and ability to bear weight. Ask about movement and sensation distal to the injury, especially numbness, tingling, or inability to move. Also inquire about previous injuries and self-care measures that have been used for this injury (e.g., analgesics, ice or heat, wrapping, or rest).

Inspect the injured area for redness, swelling, or deformity. Assess active range of motion of affected joints.

clinical ALERT

Do not attempt to move an injured joint beyond the point of comfort. If fracture is suspected, immobilize the joint and do not assess range of motion until the fracture has been ruled out. This is especially important when there is a risk of cervical spine fracture.

Palpate for swelling, warmth, tenderness, deformity, and crepitus (a grating sensation or sound). Check movement and sensation distal to the injury.

DIAGNOSING, PLANNING, AND IMPLEMENTING

Priorities in Nursing Care. Teaching measures to promote comfort, prevent further injury, and allow healing are the priorities for nursing care for the client with soft tissue trauma.

Pain

The pain of soft tissue injuries is caused by tissue damage and edema.

- Instruct to rest the injured extremity. *Rest allows the injured muscle or ligament to heal.*
- Apply ice to the injury. *Ice causes vasoconstriction and decreases swelling in the injured area. Ice may also numb the tender area.*
- Maintain compression dressing, such as an Ace bandage. *A compression dressing decreases swelling, edema, and pain.*
- Elevate the extremity 2 inches above the heart. *Elevating the extremity promotes venous return and decreases swelling.*

- Teach the acronym RICE to remember acute injury care: rest, ice, compression, elevation. *Acronyms help memory. Knowing the treatment plan decreases anxiety and pain.*
- If pain continues after several days, instruct to apply heat. *Heat increases blood flow and venous return, decreasing edema and pain.*
- Advise to take aspirin or NSAIDs on a regular basis (around the clock as recommended) with food. *When a therapeutic blood level is maintained, these drugs reduce inflammation, relieving pain. Taking the drug with food reduces gastrointestinal upset.*
- Instruct to use analgesics (over the counter or prescribed) to maintain comfort, preventing pain from becoming severe. *Severe pain increases muscle tension and can make it more difficult to relieve pain with medications.*

Impaired Physical Mobility

- Teach correct use of crutches, canes, or slings if prescribed. *Using correct technique increases the safety and effectiveness of these devices.*
- Remind to rest injured extremity. *Using the extremity can delay healing and increase the risk of further injury.*
- Encourage follow-up with primary care provider. *Severe sprains may require further treatment such as a brace or surgical intervention.*

EVALUATING

To evaluate the effectiveness of nursing care, assess pain, safety when ambulating, and knowledge of home care.

Documenting. Document assessment data and emergent care provided. Document teaching, including the client's apparent understanding of instructions and willingness to comply with self-care measures.

CONTINUING CARE

Teach about ordered medications, splints, dressings, and assistive devices. Always observe use of assistive devices. If the device is inappropriate, the risk of falling can be increased. Older adults often have less muscle mass in the upper extremities; a walker may be safer than crutches. Specify when to schedule a follow-up appointment with the physician. Explain that activity limitations will be evaluated at the follow-up appointment. Reinforce the RICE acronym (rest, ice, compression, elevation). Emphasize the importance of rest to allow complete healing. Instruct to report any complications, such as numbness, coolness of the limb, or severe pain, to the physician immediately. Warn that severe swelling can lead to compartment syndrome, discussed in the next section of this chapter.

Fractures

A **fracture** is a break in the continuity of a bone. Fractures vary in severity according to the location and the type of fracture.

PATHOPHYSIOLOGY

A fracture occurs when bone is subjected to more force than it can absorb. Fractures may result from a direct blow, a crushing force (*compression*), a sudden twisting motion (*torsion*), a severe muscle contraction, or disease that has weakened the bone (*pathologic fracture*).

Types of Fractures

Fractures are classified in a number of different ways (Table 42-1 ■). A *closed* or *simple fracture* is the most common. *Open* or *compound fractures* disrupt the skin over the fracture, allowing bacteria to enter the wound. This increases the risk of complications such as infection or nerve damage. *Complete fractures* involve the entire width of the bone, whereas *incomplete fractures* do not. In a *stable (nondisplaced) fracture,* the pieces of bone remain in alignment. In an *unstable (displaced) fracture,* the bones move out of correct alignment.

The direction of the fracture line is also used to classify fractures. The fracture line may be *oblique,* at a 45-degree angle to the bone, *spiral,* or along the lengthwise plane of the bone (*greenstick fracture*).

Fracture Healing

Fracture healing is affected by age, physical condition, and the type of fracture. When a bone fractures, blood vessels tear and a *hematoma* forms between the fractured bone ends and around bone surfaces (Figure 42-1A ■). Bone and tissue damage cause a local inflammatory response. Clotting factors within the hematoma form a fibrin meshwork (Figure 42-1B). Within 48 hours, fibroblasts and new capillaries growing into the fracture form *granulation tissue* that gradually replaces the hematoma. Phagocytes remove cell debris. Bone-forming cells called *osteoblasts* migrate to the fracture site, where they build a web of collagen fibers from both sides of the fractured bone. Chondroblasts lay down patches of cartilage as a base for bone growth. This *fibrocartilaginous callus* connects bone fragments, splinting the fracture (Figure 42-1C). Osteoblasts continue to form collagen fibers and bone matrix, which are gradually mineralized with calcium and mineral salts to form *bony callus* (Figure 42-1D). Osteoblasts promote new bone formation. *Osteoclasts* migrate to the repair site to remove damaged and excess bone in the callus (Figure 42-1E). This process usually continues for 2 to 3 months. In the final phase of healing, excess callus is removed and new bone is laid down along the fracture line. As the bone heals and again is subjected to the mechanical stress of everyday use, osteoblasts and osteoclasts remodel the repair site along the lines of force.

Healing time varies with the individual. An uncomplicated fracture of the arm or foot can heal in 6 to 8 weeks. A fractured vertebra takes at least 12 weeks to heal. A fractured hip may require 12 to 16 weeks.

TABLE 42-1 **Types of Fractures**	
FRACTURE TYPE	**DESCRIPTION**
Closed (simple)	Skin over fracture remains intact.
Open (compound)	Broken bone protrudes through skin.
Comminuted	Bone fragments into many pieces.
Compression	Bone is crushed.
Impacted	Broken ends of bone are forced together.
Depressed	Broken bone is pressed inward (e.g., the skull).
Spiral	Jagged break occurs due to twisting force.
Greenstick	Incomplete break occurs along the length of the bone.

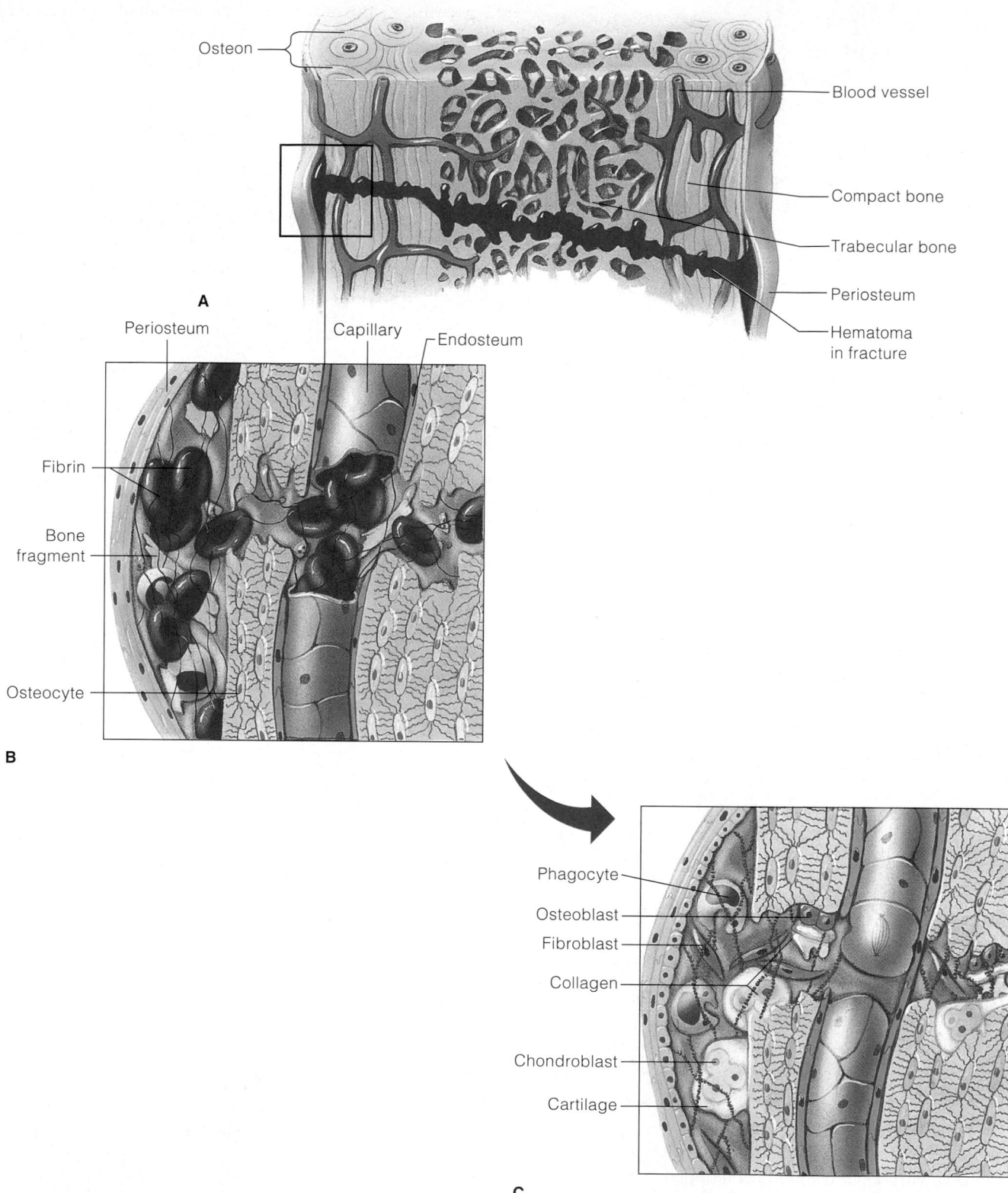

Figure 42-1. ■ Fracture healing.

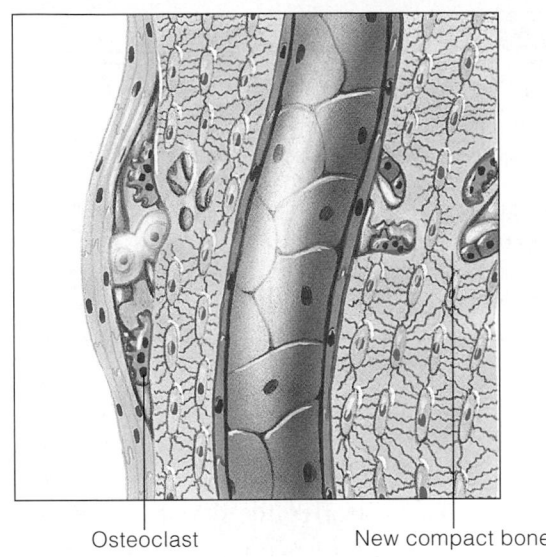

Osteoclast   New compact bone

E

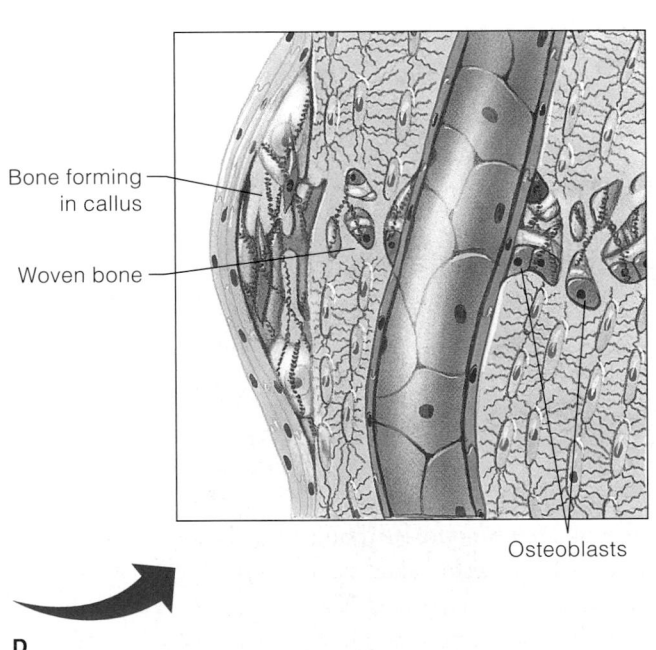

Bone forming
in callus

Woven bone

Osteoblasts

D

MANIFESTATIONS AND COMPLICATIONS

Common manifestations of fractures are listed in Box 42-2 ■. Fractures are frequently accompanied by soft tissue injuries that involve muscles, arteries, veins, nerves, or skin. The extent of soft tissue injury depends on the amount of energy or force transmitted to the area.

While most fractures are uncomplicated, serious complications can develop. A fractured pelvis or femur may cause significant bleeding and hypovolemic shock. Up to 4.5 liters of blood can be lost with a pelvic fracture, for example. Open fractures may be complicated by infection. Significant tissue trauma may accompany open fractures. The fractured bone may damage peripheral nerves,

---

BOX 42-2

MANIFESTATIONS OF FRACTURES

- Deformity
- Swelling, ecchymosis (bruising)
- Pain
- Tenderness, guarding, immobility
- Numbness
- Crepitus
- Muscle spasms

---

affecting movement and/or sensation distal to the fracture. Blood flow to a portion of fractured bone may be disrupted, causing necrosis. Blood vessel damage and immobility increase the risk for developing deep venous thrombosis (DVT) (see Chapter 28). ⦻ Other serious complications such as compartment syndrome, fat embolism, and delayed union are discussed next.

Compartment Syndrome

A *compartment* is a space enclosed by a fibrous membrane or fascia. Compartments within the limbs may enclose and support bones, nerves, and blood vessels. **Compartment syndrome** occurs when excess pressure restricts blood vessels and nerves within a compartment. It may be caused by bleeding or edema within the compartment, or by external compression of the limb by a too-tight cast. Nerve damage occurs within 30 minutes. Impaired tissue perfusion may lead to necrosis. Unless promptly relieved, compartment syndrome may lead to loss of the limb and sepsis. Compartment syndrome usually develops within the first 48 hours of injury, when edema is at its peak. Manifestations of compartment syndrome are shown in Box 42-3 ■. Use the "5 Ps" to help remember these manifestations.

---

clinical ALERT

Closely monitor for manifestations of compartment syndrome with forearm and tibia fractures. Notify the physician promptly if symptoms develop. Immediate intervention is necessary to preserve limb function.

BOX 42-3

MANIFESTATIONS OF COMPARTMENT SYNDROME

- **P**ain unrelieved by narcotic analgesics
- **P**allor and decreased capillary refill
- **P**aresthesias (numbness and tingling)
- **P**aresis (weakness) or paralysis
- **P**ulselessness (pulse may be normal early)

If compartment syndrome develops, pressure is relieved by removing the tightly fitting cast or performing a *fasciotomy*, a surgical procedure to relieve pressure within the compartment.

Fat Embolism

Fat emboli occur when fat globules lodge in a pulmonary vessel or the peripheral circulation. When a bone breaks, fat globules can leave the bone marrow and enter the bloodstream. In the bloodstream, fat globules combine with platelets and travel to the brain, lungs, kidneys, and other organs, blocking small vessels and causing tissue ischemia. Fracture of a long bone, the femur in particular, is the primary risk factor for fat emboli.

Manifestations of fat emboli usually develop within a few hours to a week after injury. The symptoms result from occluded blood flow to the tissues and from fatty acids in the circulation. Altered cerebral perfusion causes confusion and changes in level of consciousness. If pulmonary circulation is affected, chest pain and acute shortness of breath develop. Manifestations of pulmonary edema and acute respiratory distress syndrome (ARDS) may occur (see Chapter 24). ⦻ Normal clotting is disrupted, and petechiae develop on the skin and mucous membranes.

Delayed Union

Delayed union is prolonged healing of bones beyond the usual time period. Bone healing may be impaired by factors such as delayed fracture reduction, inadequate immobilization, infection, and age. Delayed union may lead to *nonunion* with persistent pain and movement at the fracture site.

INTERDISCIPLINARY CARE

A fracture requires prompt treatment. The fracture is *reduced* (the normal alignment of bone restored) and immobilized as soon as possible.

Emergency Care and Diagnosis

When fracture is suspected, the extremity or affected body part is immobilized before the client is moved. The neck and back are immobilized using a rigid cervical collar and backboard if a vertebral fracture is suspected. The joints above and below a suspected extremity fracture are immobilized. Pulses, color, movement, and sensation of the extremity are checked both before and after splinting. Open wounds and fractures are covered with a sterile dressing.

On arrival in the health care setting, x-rays of the affected body part are usually obtained to confirm the diagnosis of a fracture.

Fracture Reduction

Before the fractured bone is stabilized for healing, **reduction** (restoration of normal alignment) must be done. In *closed*

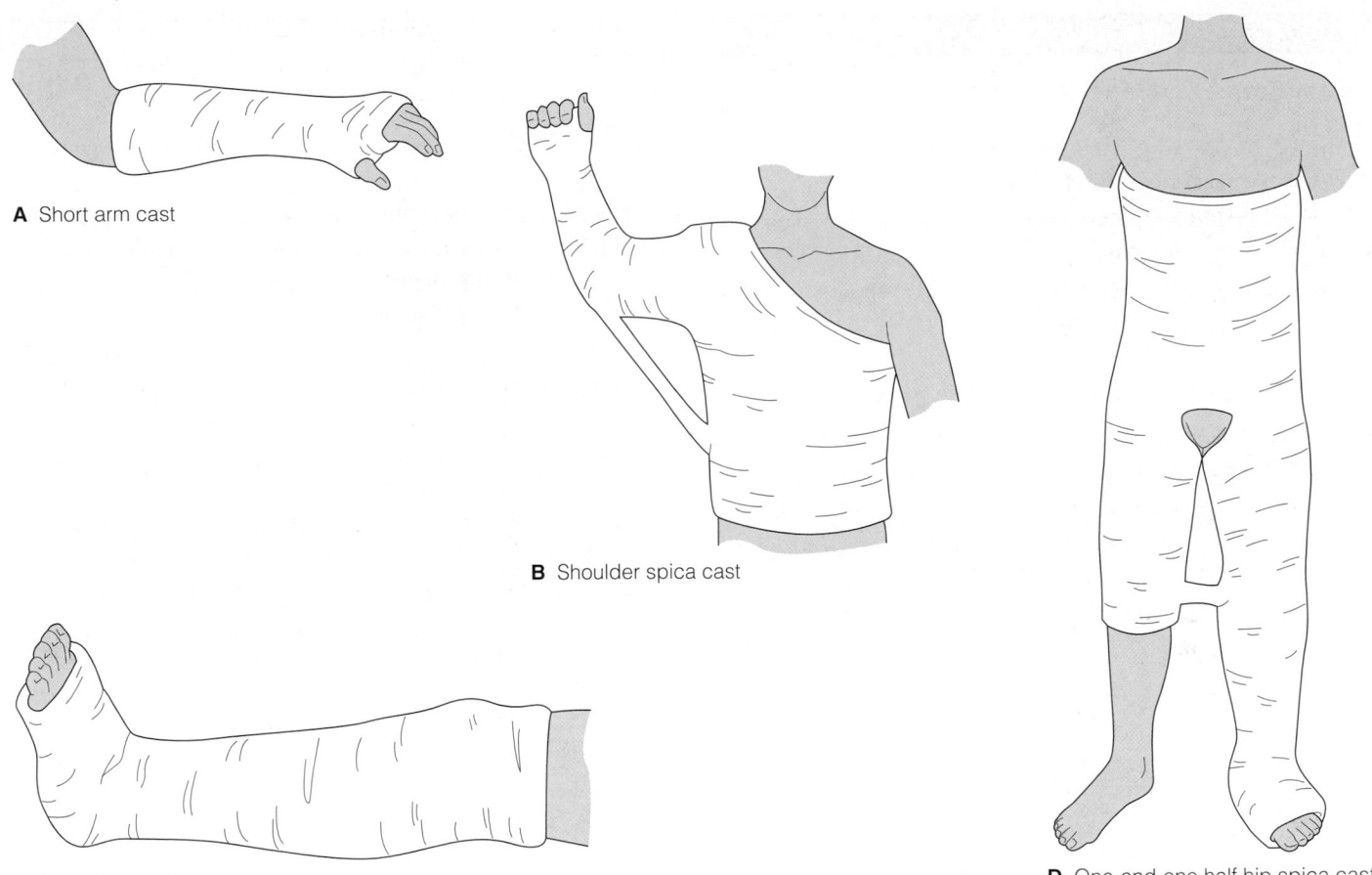

A Short arm cast

B Shoulder spica cast

C Long leg cast

D One-and-one half hip spica cast

Figure 42-2. ■ Common types of casts.

reduction, external manipulation is used to reposition the bone. Local or regional anesthesia or conscious sedation usually is given prior to closed reduction. (See Chapter 9 ⚭ for more information about anesthesia and conscious sedation.) The fracture is then immobilized with a splint, cast, or traction. An x-ray may be done to verify proper position, and neurologic and circulatory status are assessed distal to the fracture. An *open reduction* is done in surgery. The bone is exposed and realigned; nails or screws may be used to maintain its position.

Casts

A *cast* is a rigid device used to immobilize broken bones and promote healing. Casts may be made of plaster or fiberglass. The joints above and below the fracture are immobilized by the cast so the bone will not move during healing. The cast is applied over a thin cushion of padding and molded to the normal contour of the body. Until the cast is completely dry, care is taken to avoid placing pressure on it; simply palpating a wet cast with the fingertips can leave dents that may cause pressure sores. A plaster

cast may need up to 48 hours to dry, whereas a fiberglass cast dries in less than 1 hour. The type of cast applied depends on the location of the fracture (Figure 42-2 ■). Nursing care and teaching for clients with casts is outlined in Box 42-4 ■.

Significant swelling under the cast can impair blood flow and damage nerves and tissues of the extremity. If this occurs, the cast may be *bivalved,* or split down both sides, to relieve the pressure (Figure 42-3 ■). The two halves of the cast are then held in place with Velcro straps to keep the fracture immobilized.

clinical ALERT

Assess and document color, pulses, movement, and sensation distal to the fracture before the fracture is reduced and a cast is applied, as well as after the procedure and prior to discharge. Document all teaching provided, as well as the client's and family's apparent understanding of instructions.

BOX 42-4	NURSING CARE CHECKLIST

Cast Care

☑ Support drying cast on pillows; do not cover.

☑ Use the palms of the hands to handle a drying cast.

☑ Frequently assess pulses, color, movement, and sensation of the affected extremity.

☑ Promptly report increased or severe pain; changes in pulses, color, movement, or sensation distal to the cast; or a "hot spot" or drainage on the cast.

☑ Pad or tape rough cast edges to reduce skin irritation.

☑ Use plastic wrap as needed to keep the cast clean and dry.

Client and Family Teaching

☑ The cast dries from the inside out; do not use a blow dryer to speed drying; do not cover the cast while it is drying.

☑ A sensation of warmth during drying is normal.

☑ Keep the cast clean and dry.

☑ If a fiberglass cast gets wet, dry it with a blow dryer on cool setting.

☑ Notify your doctor immediately if you develop increased pain, coolness, color changes, increased swelling, or loss of sensation in the injured limb.

☑ Do not put anything into the cast.

☑ Relieve itching by blowing cool air into the cast with a blow dryer on a cool setting.

☑ A sling may help distribute the weight of the cast evenly around the neck; do not roll the sling because this may impair circulation.

☑ Use crutches as taught to prevent weight bearing on the affected leg.

☑ The cast will be removed with a cast saw. You will feel its vibration, but the saw will not cut the skin.

Traction

Muscle spasms can pull bones out of alignment after a fracture. **Traction** uses a straightening or pulling force to return or maintain the fractured bones in normal position. Various types of traction may be used:

1. *Manual traction* is applied by physically pulling on the extremity. Manual traction often is used to reduce a fracture or dislocation. Other types of traction use ropes, pulleys, and weights to maintain alignment of the bones.

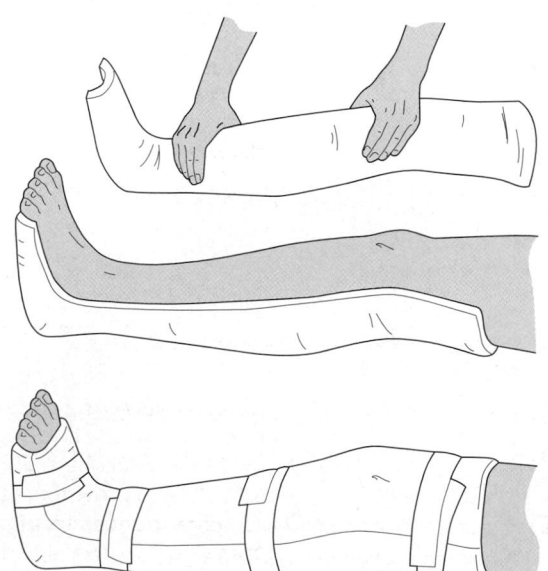

Figure 42-3. ■ Bivalving a cast.

2. *Skin traction* applies the pulling force through the client's skin. Skin traction is noninvasive and is relatively comfortable for the client.

3. In *skeletal traction,* the pulling force is applied directly through pins inserted into the bone. Skeletal traction allows use of more weight to maintain bone alignment. The risk of infection is greater, however, and it may cause more discomfort.

4. *Straight traction* applies a pulling force in a straight line to the injured body part. The body provides a counterweight or opposing force to the traction. The most common type of straight traction is *Buck's traction* (Figure 42-4A ■), in which the pulling force is applied to the skin of the affected leg.

5. *Balanced suspension traction* uses more than one force of pull to raise and support the injured extremity off the bed and maintain its alignment (Figures 42-4B and C). Balanced suspension traction increases mobility while maintaining bone position. It also makes it easier to change linen and perform back care. Box 42-5 ■ outlines nursing care for clients in traction.

Surgery

Surgery may be required to align and stabilize a fractured bone. In the simplest form of surgery, an external fixator device is applied to immobilize the fracture. An *external fixator* uses a frame connected to pins inserted into the bone (Figure 42-5 ■). The pins require care similar to that of skeletal traction pins. The client is monitored for infection, and frequent neurovascular assessment is performed.

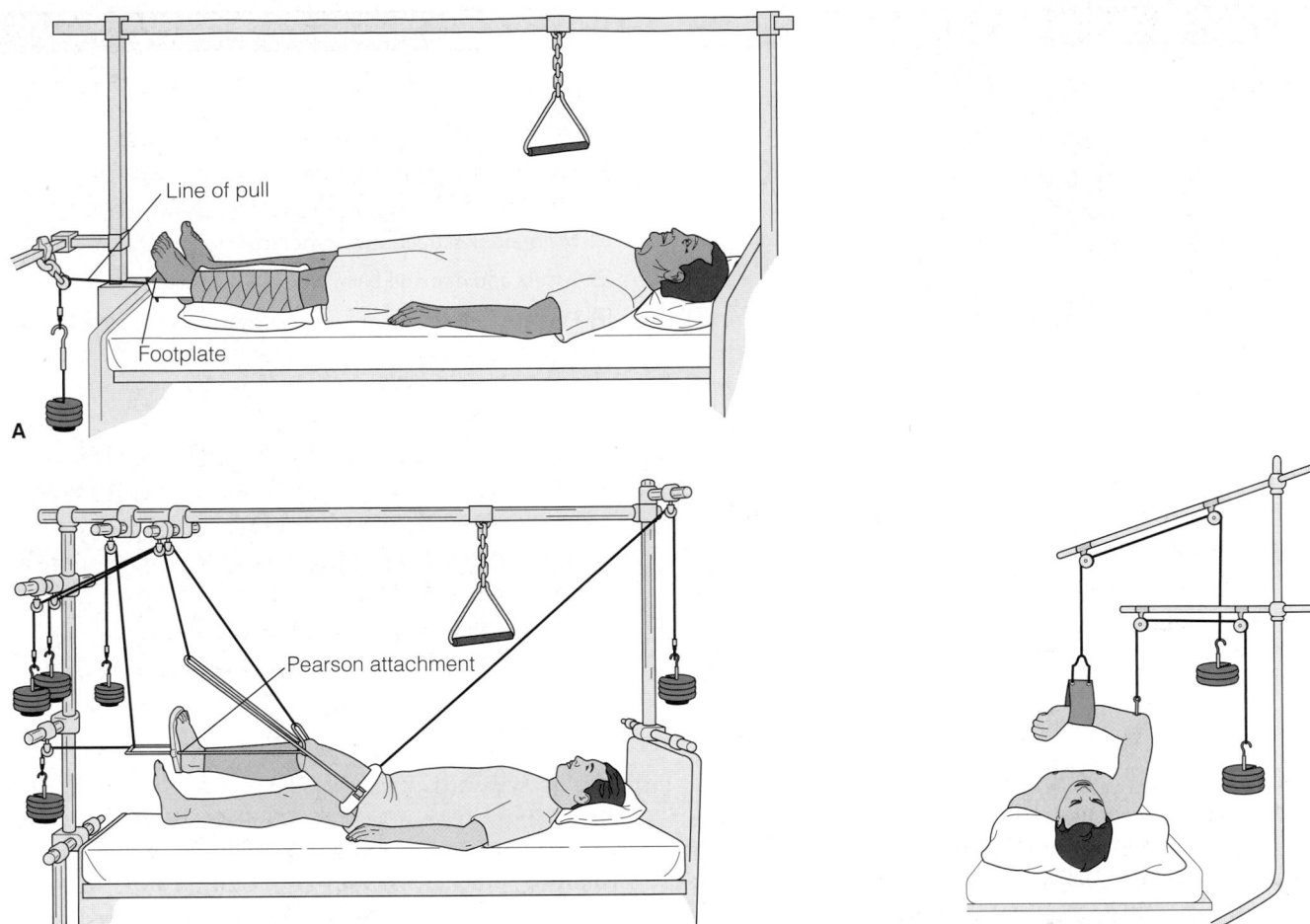

Figure 42-4. ■ Examples of traction. (**A**) Buck's traction, a straight, skin traction. (**B**) Balanced suspension traction for a femur fracture. (**C**) Skeletal traction to stabilize a fractured humerus.

BOX 42-5	NURSING CARE CHECKLIST

Traction

☑ Maintain the pulling force and direction:

   ☑ Center client on the bed; maintain body alignment with the direction of pull.

   ☑ Ensure that nothing is lying on or obstructing the ropes.

   ☑ Tape knots; do not allow knots to come in contact with the pulley.

   ☑ Ensure that weights hang freely and do not touch the floor.

☑ *For skin traction:*

   ☑ Frequently assess pulses, color, sensation, and movement distal to wrappings; notify physician or rewrap (if ordered) as necessary.

   ☑ Remove weights only if intermittent traction has been ordered and to rewrap bandages.

☑ Frequently assess skin, bony prominences, and pressure points for irritation or breakdown.

☑ Protect pressure sites with padding and protective dressings.

☑ *For skeletal traction:*

   ☑ Never remove weights.

   ☑ Frequently assess neurovascular status, skin, and pin insertion sites.

   ☑ Provide pin site care as ordered (or per protocol).

   ☑ Report signs of infection, such as redness, drainage, and increased tenderness.

   ☑ Report manifestations of complications of immobility, including pressure ulcers, DVT, atelectasis or pneumonia, paralytic ileus, and constipation.

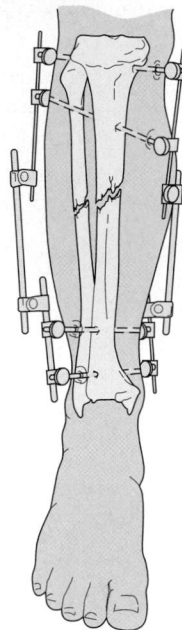

Figure 42-5. ■ An external fixator device used to stabilize a fractured tibia and fibula.

Internal fixation is usually done in a surgical procedure called an *open reduction and internal fixation (ORIF)*. In this procedure, the fracture is directly reduced, and a nail, screws, plates and screws, or pins are inserted to hold the bones in place (Figure 42-6 ■). Open fractures and hip fractures are frequently repaired with ORIF. Nursing considerations for a client undergoing ORIF are outlined in Box 42-6 ■.

Other Interventions

Analgesics and NSAIDs are ordered to relieve pain following a fracture. Parenteral analgesics or patient-controlled analgesia (PCA) may be used for the first 24 to 48 hours. (See discussion of PCA in Chapter 8. 🔗)

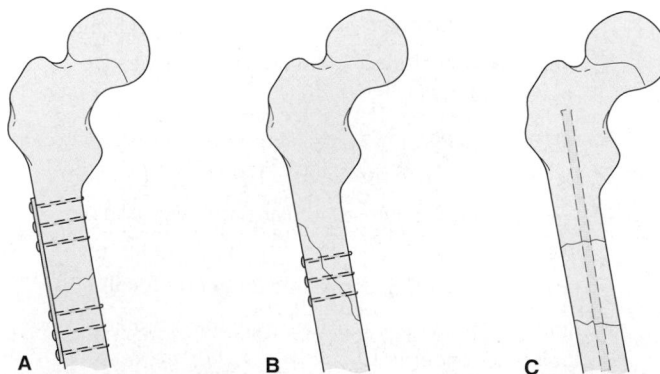

Figure 42-6. ■ Internal fixation devices. (**A**) A plate and screws used to stabilize an oblique fracture. (**B**) Screws inserted through the fracture. (**C**) A medullary nail inserted into the bone to stabilize a segmental fracture.

| BOX 42-6 | NURSING CARE CHECKLIST |

ORIF

Before Surgery

☑ Provide routine preoperative care as outlined in Chapter 9. 🔗

☑ Maintain skin traction as ordered.

☑ Assess and manage pain.

☑ Frequently assess neurovascular status of affected extremity.

☑ Reinforce teaching.

After Surgery

☑ Provide routine postoperative care (Chapter 9). 🔗

☑ Frequently assess neurovascular status; promptly report changes to charge nurse or physician.

☑ Assess wound drainage (on dressing and in surgical drain such as Hemovac).

☑ Maintain alignment of affected extremity as ordered.

☑ Encourage and assist with mobility as soon as allowed.

Stool softeners may be given and dietary fiber increased to decrease the risk of constipation secondary to narcotics and immobility. An antiulcer drug such as a histamine blocker, proton pump inhibitor, or antacid may be ordered to prevent gastrointestinal bleeding. Antibiotics may be given, particularly with open or complex fractures.

Electrical bone stimulation may be used to treat fractures that are not healing appropriately. An electrical current is used to increase the migration of osteoblasts and osteoclasts to the fracture site. Mineral deposition increases, promoting bone healing.

NURSING CARE

ASSESSING

Assess pain in the injured extremity using a standard pain scale. Assess the effectiveness of analgesia in relieving pain. Remember also that pain may be an early symptom of compartment syndrome. Assess distal pulses beginning with the unaffected extremity. Then compare the quality of pulses in the affected limb to those of the unaffected limb. Assess sensation proximal and distal to the fracture. Ask about changes in sensation (paresthesias). Check skin color and temperature in the extremity. Coolness may indicate arterial compromise, whereas warmth and a bluish tinge may indicate venous blood pooling. Assess motion distal to the fracture site. Limited range of motion (ROM) may indicate such problems as nerve damage and paralysis.

clinical ALERT

Spiral fractures often are associated with abuse (e.g., someone deliberately twisting the client's arm). Be alert for other evidence of abuse, such as bruises of various color and age, a record of frequent emergency care for traumatic injuries, and x-ray reports of multiple healed fractures. Notify the charge nurse and physician if abuse is suspected.

DIAGNOSING, PLANNING, AND IMPLEMENTING

Priorities in Nursing Care. The priorities for nursing care of the client with a fracture include managing pain and impaired mobility, and preventing complications. Nursing implications for fractures of specific bones are listed in Table 42-2 ■.

Pain

- Administer analgesics as ordered on a regular basis to prevent intense pain. *Pain is more effectively relieved if analgesics are given before pain becomes severe.*

TABLE 42-2

Nursing Implications of Specific Fractures

FRACTURE	USUAL TREATMENT	NURSING IMPLICATIONS	CLIENT TEACHING
Clavicle	Figure-8 or clavicular strap (see Figure 42-7 ■)	Frequently assess neurovascular status of injured arm.	Applying a figure-8 splint or strap; skin care Wrist and elbow ROM exercises
Humerus	Hanging arm cast, traction, or ORIF, depending on location and severity	Frequently assess neurovascular status of injured arm.	Cast care, sling application Finger and shoulder ROM exercises as indicated
Wrist and hand	Posterior plaster splint and sling; short arm cast; or finger splint	Frequently assess neurovascular status of injured hand. Compartment syndrome is a risk.	Manifestations of complications to report Elevate arm Finger exercises
Femur	Skeletal traction followed by external fixator, ORIF, or cast brace that allows limited weight bearing	Frequently assess vital signs and neurovascular status of affected leg. Bleeding may lead to shock. Assess respiratory status; fat embolism is a risk.	Analgesic use Reporting signs of complications ROM exercises of lower legs, feet, and toes Pin site or incision care
Tibia and fibula	Long leg cast for 3–4 weeks, followed by short leg cast. External fixation device or ORIF may be used.	Frequently assess neurovascular status; blood vessels or nerves may be damaged. Compartment syndrome is a risk. Assess knee; bleeding into joint may occur.	Weight-bearing restrictions as ordered Pin or incision site care Crutch walking
Ankle and foot	Closed reduction and short leg cast	Assess neurovascular status of distal foot and toes.	Cast care, crutch walking
Skull	Observation for simple fracture; surgical elevation of depressed skull fracture	Frequently assess neurologic status: LOC; mental status; pupil response to light; extremity movement and strength; vital signs. Promptly report changes. See Chapter 38. ⚭	Observations for altered mental or neurologic status Prescribed activity restrictions Preventing future head injuries
Face	Monitoring; ORIF if severely displaced	Monitor airway and breathing. Monitor neurologic status as noted above. Promptly report changes.	Analgesic use Effect of swelling on appearance and expected changes Indications or options for plastic surgery

(continued)

TABLE 42-2

Nursing Implications of Specific Fractures (continued)

FRACTURE	USUAL TREATMENT	NURSING IMPLICATIONS	CLIENT TEACHING
Spine	Immediate immobilization. For nondisplaced fractures, cervical collar, halo immobilizer, thoracic brace, or body cast. For displaced fractures, surgical stabilization and/or skeletal traction	Frequently assess extremity movement and sensation. Promptly report changes to the physician. Maintain spinal immobilization and alignment. Provide good skin care. See Chapter 39. ⚭	Skin care under the brace Pin site care Length of immobilization Preventing complications of immobility See Chapter 39. ⚭
Rib	Analgesia and respiratory care to prevent atelectasis or pneumonia. Fracture of two or more adjacent ribs in two or more places causes *flail* chest (see Chapter 24). ⚭	Frequently assess respiratory status (rate, depth and equality of chest movement, breath sounds). Provide adequate pain relief to encourage deep breathing. Encourage use of incentive spirometer.	Analgesic use Avoid rib belt or tape unless ordered by physician Splint chest with hand or pillow to cough and deep breathe Use of incentive spirometer Contact doctor if fever or shortness of breath develops
Pelvis	Bed rest on firm mattress; if unstable or displaced, pelvic sling followed by surgery	Closely monitor for bleeding and shock. Monitor neurovascular status of lower extremities. Report hematuria, rectal bleeding, or blood in feces. Logroll for comfort.	Analgesic use Activity restrictions Contact doctor for blood in urine or feces, difficulty voiding or defecating Report numbness, tingling, or weakness of lower extremities to doctor

- Splint and support the injured area. *Splinting helps relieve pain by immobilizing the fracture.*
- Elevate the injured extremity above the heart. *Pain is caused by the fracture itself as well as muscle spasms and swelling. Elevating the extremity promotes venous return and decreases edema, which decreases pain.*
- Apply ice. *Ice causes vasoconstriction, decreasing swelling. It may also numb the area.*
- Move gently and slowly. *Gentle movement reduces the risk of muscle spasms.*
- Encourage distraction and other adjunctive pain relief measures such as meditation and visualization. *These measures promote relaxation and reduce the intensity of pain.*

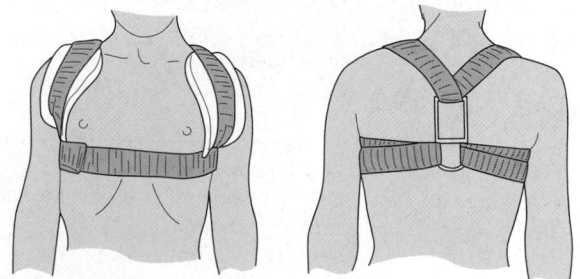

Figure 42-7. ■ A clavicular strap to immobilize a fractured clavicle.

Impaired Physical Mobility

- Assist with active ROM exercises of the unaffected limbs. *ROM helps prevent muscle atrophy and maintain strength and joint function.*
- Teach isometric exercises, and encourage them every 4 hours. *Isometric exercises help prevent muscle atrophy.*
- Encourage ambulation when able; provide assistance as needed. *Ambulation maintains and improves circulation and helps prevent muscle atrophy and bone loss.*
- Reinforce teaching and observe use of assistive devices (canes, crutches, walkers, slings, etc.). *Proper use of devices maintains safety and helps prevent falls and complications of immobility.*
- Encourage flexion and extension exercises of the lower extremities. *Flexion and extension exercises promote venous return, helping prevent DVT.*
- Turn the client on bed rest every 2 hours. If in traction, teach client to shift weight hourly. *Turning and weight shifts increase circulation and help prevent skin breakdown.*
- Encourage frequent use of incentive spirometer, deep breathing, and coughing. *Immobilized clients have an increased risk for developing atelectasis and pneumonia due to retained respiratory secretions.*

Risk for Ineffective Tissue Perfusion: Peripheral

Tissue perfusion can be affected by bleeding, edema, compartment syndrome, and immobility.

- Assess the 5 Ps (pain, pallor, pulse, paresthesias, and paresis) every 1 to 2 hours. *Unrelenting pain, pallor, diminished distal pulses, paresthesias, and paresis are indicators of compartment syndrome. Notify the physician immediately. (Note that pulses may not change with compartment syndrome.)*

- Assess cast for tightness. *Edema can cause the cast to become too tight; a tightly fitting cast affects distal circulation.*

- If the cast is too tight, prepare to assist with bivalving (see Figure 42-3). *Bivalving (splitting the cast) relieves pressure caused by a too-tight cast.*

- Elevate the injured extremity above the heart. *Elevating the extremity increases venous return and decreases edema.*

- Administer anticoagulants as ordered. *Anticoagulants may be ordered to reduce the risk for DVT.*

- Apply antiembolism stockings or pneumatic compression boots. *These devices increase venous return, decrease blood pooling, and the risk of DVT.*

EVALUATING

To evaluate the effectiveness of nursing care, collect data related to pain and the effectiveness of analgesia, safety and mobility, and tissue perfusion.

Documenting. Document assessment findings, including neurovascular status, before and after fracture reduction. Document level of pain before and after interventions, as well as analgesia provided. If traction is used, note type of traction and amount of weight applied. Record any drainage noted on cast, from incision, or from pin sites. Document skin care and measures to prevent complications. Document all teaching and discharge instructions, and the client's understanding of information. Note client's ability to demonstrate techniques such as crutch walking.

CONTINUING CARE

The needs for teaching and home care vary, depending on the type and severity of the fracture and its location. For example, a client with a simple fracture of the tibia may need only teaching about cast care and crutch walking. An older client who has surgery to repair a hip fracture has more teaching needs, including using an abduction pillow and restrictions on weight bearing and hip flexion. Referrals to visiting nurses and community services are more likely in older clients. Teach measures to reduce the risk of falls and fractures (see Box 42-7 ■).

BOX 42-7	FOCUS ON OLDER ADULTS

Decreasing Fractures in Older Adults

Falls are the most common cause of fractures in older adults. Hip fractures are the leading cause of hospitalization for injuries in older adults. The clavicles and wrists are also commonly fractured. Fractures in older adults can lead to loss of functional ability or death. Fall-related deaths are usually related to complications from prolonged immobility, not the act of falling.

A number of measures can reduce the risk of falling and fracture:

- Encourage children, adolescents, and younger adults to maintain an adequate calcium intake to prevent osteoporosis (see Chapter 43). ∞
- Remove scatter rugs and obstacles in traffic areas of the home.
- Paint a contrast stripe on the edge of stairsteps.
- Provide night-lights and transition lighting between bedroom and bath.
- Install grab bars in the bath and railings on stairs.
- Teach to turn using a series of small steps.
- Instruct to wear well-fitting shoes or hard-soled slippers when ambulating.
- Encourage regular aerobic and strength-training exercises.
- Review medication regimen with the physician.
- Teach safe use of assistive devices such as canes and walkers.

Teach about ordered activity restrictions. If a cast has been applied, discuss cast care and dealing with irritants such as itching. Instruct about slings, crutches, or a walker as appropriate. Instruct to elevate the extremity to reduce swelling. Ice may be applied initially to reduce both pain and edema. Instruct to perform range-of-motion exercises of affected extremity as allowed. Teach the importance of eating well-balanced meals to promote healing. Stress the importance of follow-up care, and provide information about manifestations of complications to report to the physician.

Suggest resources for clients who need an extended period of immobilization or limited activities:

- Home care agencies for wound care and monitoring healing
- Physical therapy to evaluate home safety and suggest modifications as needed, and to teach crutch walking, limited weight bearing, transferring, and other activities
- Local medical suppliers for equipment and supplies such as slings or braces, crutches, walkers, wheelchairs, overhead trapeze units, shower chairs, elevated toilet seats, grab bars, and bedside commodes
- Local pharmacies for dressing supplies
- Fitness equipment suppliers for rehabilitation needs such as hand or ankle weights for strengthening exercises

Hip Fracture

Hip fractures are a significant problem, especially in older adults. Decreased bone mass and muscle strength, slowed reflexes, and medications that can affect cognition or balance all contribute to the increased risk for hip fracture in older adults. Osteoporosis and loss of bone mass can lead to spontaneous hip fracture or one resulting from minor trauma such as stepping off a curb. Hip fracture often leads to loss of independence and restricted activity, even after healing is complete.

PATHOPHYSIOLOGY AND MANIFESTATIONS

A hip fracture is a break of the femur at the head, neck, or trochanteric regions (Figure 42-8 ■). Fractures of the head or neck of the femur are called *intracapsular fractures; extracapsular fractures* are fractures of the trochanteric region. Most hip fractures occur in the neck or trochanteric regions. When the head or neck of the femur is involved, impaired blood supply to the bone increases the risk of poor healing and *avascular necrosis.*

Manifestations of a hip fracture include pain, and shortening and external rotation of the affected lower extremity.

INTERDISCIPLINARY CARE

A hip fracture usually is diagnosed by the history, physical examination, and an x-ray of the affected hip. Buck's traction may be applied to reduce muscle spasm until surgery can be done.

An ORIF procedure is performed to promote mobility, decrease pain, and prevent complications. Fixation is accomplished by securing the femur with pins, screws, nails, or plates (Figure 42-9A ■). ORIF works well for fractures in the trochanteric area. If the femoral head or neck is fractured, a prosthesis is inserted to replace the femoral head

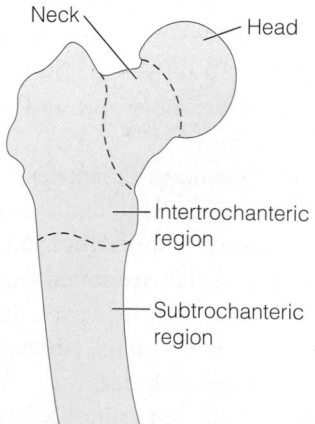

Figure 42-8. ■ The *head* of the femur fits into the socket of the pelvis. The *neck* is the narrower area below the head. The *trochanteric* region is below the neck.

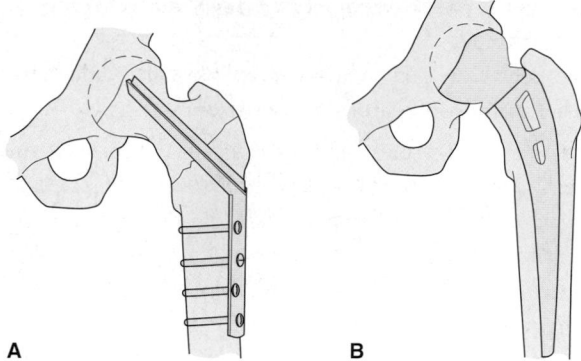

Figure 42-9. ■ (A) A surgical nail or screw is used to stabilize an intertrochanteric hip fracture. (B) A hip prosthesis is used if the femoral head is damaged.

(Figure 42-9B). This procedure is called an *arthroplasty.* If both the femoral head and the hip socket (the acetabulum) must be replaced, a *total hip replacement* or *arthroplasty* is performed. (See Chapter 43 ◯◯ for more information about total joint replacement.)

NURSING CARE

ASSESSING

Careful assessment is vital both before and after surgery. Monitor vital signs frequently, and report changes from baseline. Monitor temperature, reporting any elevation. Increased temperature may indicate wound infection, respiratory infection, or sepsis. Assess color, temperature, capillary refill, pulses, and movement and sensation of affected leg, comparing findings with the unaffected leg. Report changes to the charge nurse or physician. If surgery has been performed, assess the wound for healing, drainage, and signs of infection or inflammation. Promptly report shortening and internal rotation of the affected leg, which could indicate dislocation of the affected hip.

DIAGNOSING, PLANNING, AND IMPLEMENTING

Nursing care of a client with a hip fracture is challenging. After age 50, the risk of hip fracture increases every year. Many clients with a hip fracture are older and have several underlying health problems.

Priorities in Nursing Care. Nursing care priorities include relieving pain, maintaining circulation to the injured extremity, and increasing mobility.

Pain

■ Ask about location and nature of pain. *It is important to differentiate pain caused by the fracture or surgery from pain of other causes such as angina, a respiratory infection, or intestinal ileus.*

- Ask to rate pain using a standardized pain scale before and after any intervention. *The pain scale provides a means of evaluating the effectiveness of pain relief measures.*
- Apply Buck's traction as ordered. *Buck's traction immobilizes the fracture before surgery, reducing pain and additional trauma.*
- Administer analgesia as ordered. A PCA pump may be ordered. *Analgesics relieve pain and reduce muscle tension and spasm. PCA pumps allow more effective pain control with lower total doses of analgesia.*
- Move gently and slowly. *Gentle turning prevents severe muscle spasms.*
- Encourage distraction, deep breathing, relaxation, and other adjunctive pain relief measures. *Adjunctive measures improve the effectiveness of analgesics.*

Impaired Physical Mobility

Maintaining mobility is important to prevent complications of immobility (such as atelectasis, pressure sores, and DVT), especially in older adults.

- Turn clients on bed rest at least every 2 hours. Encourage hourly weight shifts when in traction. *Turning and weight shifting increase circulation and help prevent skin breakdown.*
- Place a pillow or abductor splint between the legs when in bed and during turning. *A pillow or splint prevents adduction of the affected hip, which could lead to dislocation.*
- Encourage isometric exercises and flexion and extension exercises of the feet, ankles, elbows, shoulders, and knees every 4 hours. *These exercises help maintain muscle tone and promote venous return from the extremities.*
- Work with physical therapy to promote activities as allowed. *The physical therapist can help mobilize the client when weight bearing is limited, and can provide assistive devices and teaching about their appropriate use.*
- Assist to a hip chair (reclining wheelchair) at the bedside. *A hip chair, which allows the client to sit with no more than 60 degrees of hip flexion, prevents excess hip flexion and reduces the risk of dislocating the hip joint while muscles heal. Sitting at the bedside several times per day improves circulation and lung expansion.*
- Assist and encourage ambulation per physician's orders. *Ambulation helps prevent muscle atrophy and other complications of immobility.*
- Apply antiembolism (TED) hose or pneumatic compression devices (PCDs) as ordered. Remove hose or the PCD at least every 8 hours to inspect the skin. *TED hose and PCDs promote venous return from the lower extremities, reducing the risk of DVT.*

- Administer anticoagulants as ordered and monitor for adverse effects (bleeding). *Anticoagulants may be ordered to reduce the risk of DVT. While the risk for bleeding is low, it is important to monitor for abnormal bleeding of the wound, gums, GI tract, or other sites.*

Impaired Skin Integrity

- Use sterile technique for dressing changes. *Sterile technique reduces contamination of the wound by infectious organisms.*
- Assess wound color, healing, and the presence of any drainage. *Redness, swelling, and purulent drainage may indicate infection.*
- Administer antibiotics as ordered. *Prophylactic antibiotics may be ordered to prevent wound infection.*
- Promptly report any temperature elevation, tachycardia, or signs of wound infection to the physician. *Prompt identification and treatment of a wound infection promote healing and may prevent the development of osteomyelitis (see Chapter 43).* ∞

EVALUATING

Collect data regarding level of pain and pain relief, ability to resume physical mobility, wound healing, and skin integrity to evaluate the effectiveness of nursing care for the client with a fractured hip.

Documenting. Document pre- and postoperative assessment data, including neurovascular assessments of the affected leg and indicators of complications such as lung sounds, incisional drainage, and skin condition. Document pain level and the effectiveness of measures to relieve pain. Record activity and teaching.

CONTINUING CARE

Hip fracture in the older adult can lead to loss of independence and long-term disability. Box 42-7 outlines teaching to help prevent hip fractures. Helping the client regain independence in activities of daily living (ADLs) is a priority in planning for discharge. Box 42-8 ∎ outlines assessment data to help determine an older adult's ability to return to his or her previous living situation after a hip fracture.

Explain activity restrictions. Teach how to limit the amount of weight placed on the affected extremity. Discuss the importance of sitting in a high, firm chair to minimize hip flexion; a high toilet seat can be added to a regular toilet seat. Encourage equipping a shower with a rail to aid stability and prevent falls. If a walker is needed, teach how to use it. Explain that the walker should not be carried. Instruct client to lift it, advance it, and then take two steps. If a cane is needed, teach how to use it to reduce weight

BOX 42-8 **ASSESSMENT**

Assessing for Discharge: Hip Fracture

CLIENT

- Self-care: ability to independently perform ADLs, and to use assistive devices such as a walker, elevated toilet seat, grab bars, shower seat
- Knowledge: cognitive function; understanding of activity and weight-bearing limitations; understanding of complications to report to physician
- Psychosocial: acceptance of help from others
- Home environment: adequate lighting, grab bars in bathroom, level floors; barriers to independence (stairs, small bathrooms, or deep tubs for bathing)

FAMILY AND CAREGIVERS

- Cognitive status of primary caregiver; ability and willingness to assist with ADLs and household chores; understanding of activity restrictions
- Resources for medications and treatments, in-home caregivers, or long-term care if necessary
- Availability of home health services and long-term care facilities as needed

bearing on the affected side. Stress the importance of well-balanced meals, and explain all ordered medications.

The client who is cognitively impaired does not learn as effectively and is less able to independently perform ADLs following hip fracture. The stress of the injury and surgery also may worsen manifestations of dementia. Teaching needs to be very focused, presented in brief sessions, and repeatedly reinforced. Temporary or permanent placement in a long-term care facility may be necessary following a hip fracture. This also may be the case if the primary caregiver is cognitively impaired. Discharge planning needs to begin on admission to the hospital. Provide information and referrals for home care services or long-term care facilities as appropriate. Recommend facilities that provide physical therapy and structured activities to promote independence and recovery.

NURSING PROCESS CARE PLAN
Client with Hip Fracture

Stella Carbolito, 74 years old, lives alone. She depends on a pension check and Social Security for her income. While walking to the market, Mrs. Carbolito falls and breaks her left hip. She is transported by ambulance to the nearest hospital.

Assessment. On admission, Mrs. Carbolito's left leg appears shorter than her right, and it is externally rotated. Distal pulses are present and strong bilaterally; both legs are warm.

Mrs. Carbolito complains of severe pain but denies any numbness or burning. She can wiggle the toes on her left leg and has full movement of her right leg. Her vital signs are T 98.0°F (36.6°C); P 100; R 18; BP 120/58. X-ray shows a fracture of the left femoral neck. Mrs. Carbolito is admitted with an order for 10 lbs of straight leg traction. An ORIF is planned for the following day.

Diagnosis. Mrs. Carbolito's nurse, Maria Davis, identifies the following nursing diagnoses:

- *Pain* related to fracture and muscle spasms
- *Impaired Physical Mobility* related to bed rest and left hip fracture
- *Risk for Ineffective Tissue Perfusion: Peripheral* related to fracture and swelling
- *Risk for Disturbed Sensory Perception: Tactile* related to risk of nerve impairment

Expected Outcomes. The expected outcomes for Mrs. Carbolito's care specify that she will:

- Verbalize adequate pain control.
- Relate an understanding of the purpose of traction and surgery.
- Demonstrate exercises as taught.
- Report increased pain, numbness, tingling, or weakness to the nurse.

Planning and Implementation. The following nursing interventions are planned and implemented:

- Assess pain using a standard scale before and after giving analgesics.
- Give analgesics on a regular basis as ordered to control pain.
- Document color, pulses, temperature, movement, and sensation in left leg every 2 to 4 hours.
- Apply straight leg (Buck's) traction as ordered.
- Teach deep breathing and relaxation techniques, as well as isometric and flexion/extension exercises.
- Discuss the purpose of traction and surgery to repair the hip fracture.

Evaluation. Two days after surgery, Mrs. Carbolito is out of bed and in a hip chair. Her pain is effectively managed with the ordered analgesic and relaxation exercises. She does isometric and flexion/extension exercises when reminded. Plans are being made for Mrs. Carbolito's discharge to her daughter's home. A community nurse and physical therapist will visit, and the hospital social worker has ordered a trapeze for her bed, an elevated toilet seat and cushion for her chair, and a walker.

Critical Thinking in the Nursing Process

1. What preoperative teaching does Mrs. Carbolito need before the planned ORIF of her left hip?

2. Explain why Mrs. Carbolito was placed in traction when she was going to the operating room anyway.

3. List all the departments in the hospital that will be involved in Mrs. Carbolito's care. Describe their roles.

JOINT TRAUMA AND INJURY

Joint dislocations and subluxations usually result from trauma, although they also may occur spontaneously.

PATHOPHYSIOLOGY AND MANIFESTATIONS

A **dislocation** is separation of contact between two bones of a joint. Traumatic dislocations result from sudden force; joint disease can cause a spontaneous dislocation. A *subluxation* is partial separation of the bones of a joint. While any joint may be affected, shoulder and hip dislocations are the most common. Joint dislocations often are recurring injuries for clients actively participating in contact sports and other vigorous physical activities.

The manifestations of a dislocation include pain, change in shape of the joint, change in length of the extremity, immobility, and change in the axis of the bone.

INTERDISCIPLINARY CARE

Manual traction is used to reduce the dislocation (reduction restores the usual relationship of the bones). Narcotic analgesics, muscle relaxants, or conscious sedation may be given before the dislocation is reduced. (See Chapter 9 ⟳ for more information about conscious sedation.)

When the shoulder is dislocated, it is placed back in the joint by manual traction and then immobilized in a sling for 3 weeks. A rehabilitation program is then initiated.

A dislocated hip requires immediate reduction. If a displaced hip is not reduced within 6 hours of injury, necrosis of the femoral head may result. The dislocated hip also threatens the sciatic and femoral nerves. Movement, sensation, pallor, and pulses must be assessed frequently. After reduction, the hip is immobilized with bed rest and a cast or traction. Immobilization allows the tendons and ligaments to heal.

NURSING CARE

When joint dislocation or subluxation is suspected, carefully assess for manifestations of the disorder and possible complications such as neurovascular trauma. Assess pain, including location, severity, character, timing, and factors that aggravate or relieve it. Assess color, warmth, pulses and capillary refill, sensation, and movement of the affected extremity. Compare the affected extremity with the corresponding unaffected extremity. Promptly report any changes or abnormal findings to the charge nurse or physician.

If traction is required, maintain the alignment of the affected extremity. Carefully assess for and implement nursing care to prevent complications of immobility (such as impaired skin integrity or atelectasis).

CONTINUING CARE

Stress the importance of following recommendations for immobilization. Discuss skin care and suggest ways to prevent skin-to-skin contact, particularly in the axillary area. Advise rehabilitation exercises to strengthen muscles and other supportive structures in the shoulder, decreasing the risk of future dislocations. Discuss activities that may precipitate recurrent dislocations and suggest alternatives.

When a hip dislocation has occurred, weight bearing may be limited for up to 6 months. Provide instructions or refer to physical therapy for teaching about crutch walking or using a walker. Discuss cast and skin care if a cast is applied after reduction (see the fracture section of this chapter). Suggest lining the edges of the cast in the groin area with plastic to avoid soiling. Teach the client in traction or a spica cast about possible complications of immobility and measures to reduce their risk. Provide referrals to physical and occupational therapy and home health services as needed.

Repetitive Use Injuries

Repetitive use injuries can result from repeated twisting and turning of the wrist, pronating and supinating of the forearm, kneeling, or raising the arms over the head. Common repetitive use injuries include carpal tunnel syndrome, bursitis, and epicondylitis. These injuries can result in significant disability and lost work time.

PATHOPHYSIOLOGY AND MANIFESTATIONS

Carpal Tunnel Syndrome

The carpal tunnel is a canal through which tendons and the median nerve pass from the wrist to the hand. *Carpal tunnel syndrome* is one of the most common work-related injuries. It occurs more commonly in women. It develops when the tunnel narrows, compressing and irritating the median nerve. This usually results from inflammation and swelling of structures in the wrist joint. Numbness and tingling of the thumb, index finger, and middle finger of the affected hand develop. The affected hand is weak, and "falls asleep" at night, with pain that is relieved by shaking or massaging the hand and fingers. The client may have difficulty holding utensils or performing precise activities with the affected hand.

Bursitis

Bursitis is inflammation of a bursa. A *bursa* is a closed, fluid-filled sac found in areas where there is friction, for example, where a tendon passes over a bony prominence. Bursae in the shoulder, hip, leg, and elbow often become inflamed due to friction between the bursa and surrounding tissue. Manifestations of bursitis include local tenderness and pain with joint movement. The client guards the joint to decrease pain.

Epicondylitis

Epicondylitis is inflammation of a tendon where it inserts into the bone. Epicondylitis is also called *tennis elbow* or *golfer's elbow*. Repeated trauma that causes tears, bleeding, and inflammation of the tendon can lead to epicondylitis. Its manifestations include point tenderness, pain radiating down the forearm, and a history of repetitive use.

INTERDISCIPLINARY CARE

Repetitive use injuries are diagnosed by history and physical examination. History may reveal an occupation that involves computer work, jackhammer operation, mechanical work, gymnastics, or percussive devices. Leisure activities or participating in sports such as tennis, golf, softball, or baseball also increase the risk for these disorders. Fractures of the arm or wrist, or diseases such as rheumatoid arthritis, increase the risk of carpal tunnel syndrome. When carpal tunnel syndrome is suspected, *Phalen's test* (see Figure 42-10 ■) may be done to help make the diagnosis.

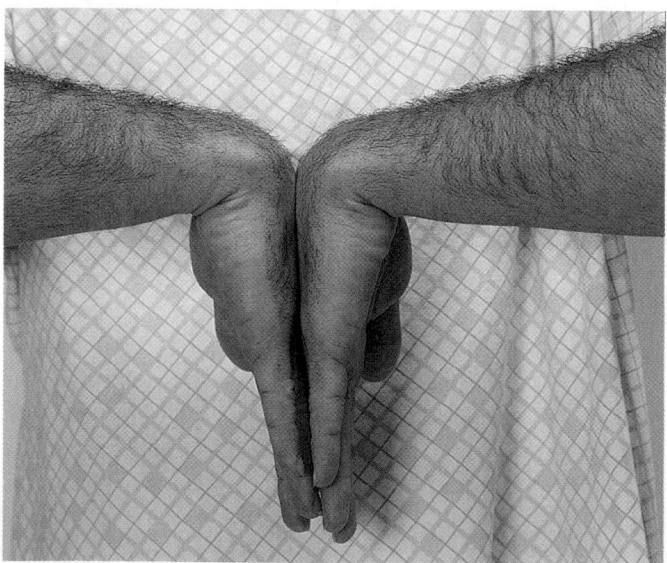

Figure 42-10. ■ Phalen's test. The wrist is flexed 90 degrees with the fingers extended. Finger numbness during the test may indicate carpal tunnel syndrome.

Initial treatment for repetitive use injuries is rest and immobilization of the involved joint. The joint may be splinted, and ice applied in the first 24 to 48 hours to decrease pain and inflammation. After this period, heat may be applied every 4 hours.

NSAIDs are usually given to reduce inflammation. In some cases, corticosteroids may be injected into the joint.

For carpal tunnel syndrome, surgery may be necessary. In carpal tunnel surgery, the carpal ligament is resected to enlarge the tunnel and relieve pressure on the nerve.

NURSING CARE

Nursing care for repetitive use injuries usually occurs in a community-based care setting. Teaching is a primary focus of nursing care.

Pain

- Encourage use of an appropriate splint or joint immobilizer. *Splinting maintains joint alignment and reduces pain and inflammation.*
- Teach safe application of ice or heat to the affected joint as indicated. *Ice causes vasoconstriction and numbs the tender area; heat decreases swelling by increasing venous return. Inappropriately applied, both ice and heat can damage tissues.*
- Instruct about using NSAIDs as ordered. *Taken on a regular basis (not as needed for pain), NSAIDs decrease swelling and inflammation, reducing pain.*
- Instruct not to discontinue treatment abruptly. *Stopping treatment abruptly may cause the injured joint to become reinflamed.*

Impaired Physical Mobility

- Refer to physical therapy for appropriate exercises. *The physical therapist can teach exercises to maintain joint mobility.*
- Suggest occupational therapy. *Occupational therapy can help the client learn new ways to perform tasks to prevent recurring symptoms.*

EVALUATING

To evaluate the effectiveness of nursing care, assess the client's knowledge and understanding of the disorder and its treatment.

Documenting. Document assessment data and teaching provided for the client to promote self-care.

CONTINUING CARE

Teach about repetitive use injury and its causes and treatments. Rehabilitation may be necessary to restore independence. Help identify ways to avoid activities that increase risk of injury. Suggest that an environmental risk manager or ergonomic specialist evaluate the client's workstation and recommend measures to reduce the risk of repetitive use injuries. Wrist supports or an ergonomic keyboard may be useful for the client who uses a computer extensively. Appropriate desk and chair height also are important in maintaining correct anatomic position while working. Provide information about sources for braces or other assistive devices.

Amputation

Amputation is partial or total removal of a body part. Amputation may be done to treat bone cancer, may be the result of a chronic condition (such as peripheral vascular disease or diabetes), or it may occur due to trauma. Regardless of the cause, amputation is devastating to the client. The loss of a limb has significant physical and psychosocial effects on the client and family. Adapting to amputation may take a long time and significant effort.

Peripheral vascular disease (PVD) is the major cause of lower extremity amputation (see Chapter 28). ⚮ Peripheral neuropathy in clients with diabetes also increases the risk for amputation.

Trauma is the major cause of upper extremity amputation. Most traumatic amputations result from motor vehicle crashes or accidents involving machinery at work.

PATHOPHYSIOLOGY AND MANIFESTATIONS

Impaired blood flow and untreated infection that causes **gangrene** (tissue death) can lead to amputation. In PVD, circulation to the extremities is impaired. This leads to edema and tissue damage. Healing also is impaired. Minor injuries and stasis ulcers can become infected because altered immune function can allow bacteria to invade and proliferate. In peripheral neuropathy, loss of sensation frequently leads to unrecognized injury and infection. Untreated infection can lead to gangrene and amputation.

A limb may be partially or completely severed by acute trauma. In some cases the severed limb may be reattached. Extensive tissue damage, however, may make reattachment impossible.

Level of Amputation

The level of amputation is determined by the extent of tissue damage and remaining healthy tissue. When possible, joints are preserved for better function of the extremity. Figure 42-11 ■ illustrates common sites of amputation.

COMPLICATIONS

Potential complications of amputation include infection, delayed healing, and contracture.

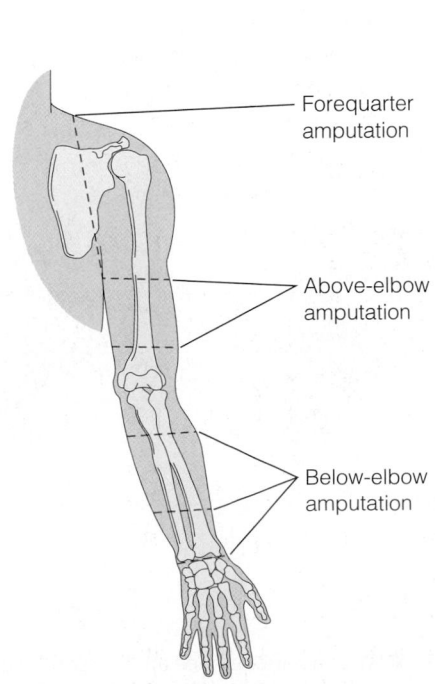

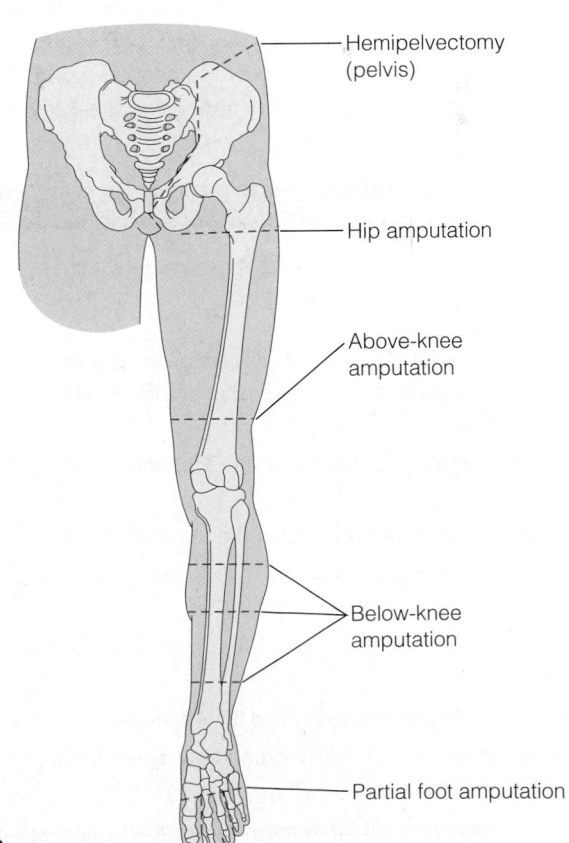

Figure 42-11. ■ Common sites of amputation. (**A**) The upper extremities and (**B**) the lower extremities.

Infection

As with all surgeries, infection is a risk following amputation. The client who is older, has diabetes, or has PVD is at a particularly high risk for infection. Local manifestations of infection include drainage, odor, redness, positive wound cultures, and increased discomfort at the suture line. Systemic manifestations include chills and fever, tachycardia, and possibly a fall in blood pressure. If any of these manifestations develop, immediately notify the charge nurse or physician. Pneumonia may develop, with a productive cough, pain on deep inspiration, and malaise. Provide good skin care, maintain aseptic technique during dressing changes, and encourage coughing and deep breathing to prevent infection.

Delayed Healing

Delayed healing is healing that occurs at a slower rate than expected. Infection or impaired circulation can lead to delayed healing. It is a particular risk in older clients who are more likely to have chronic diseases such as diabetes or PVD. Poor nutrition and smoking also are risk factors for delayed healing. Notify the physician if the wound is not healing appropriately or if the stump is cool to the touch.

Contractures

A **contracture** is abnormal flexion and fixation of a joint caused by muscle atrophy and shortening. Contracture of the joint above the amputation is a common complication. Measures to prevent contractures are outlined in Box 42-9 ∎.

BOX 42-9	NURSING CARE CHECKLIST

Preventing Contractures after Amputation

☑ Encourage joint extension.

☑ With above-knee amputation, place in prone position several times daily; do not elevate stump on pillows after the first 24 hours.

☑ For below-knee amputation, elevate foot of bed, keeping knee extended.

☑ Position upper extremities using the same principles.

☑ Provide active or passive ROM exercises every 2 to 4 hours for all joints.

☑ Use trapeze on bed frame to encourage frequent position changes.

☑ Teach importance of moving and ROM exercises.

☑ For a thigh or above-knee amputation, avoid sitting for prolonged periods.

☑ Teach postural exercises to compensate for loss of weight on affected side.

Phantom Pain

Phantom pain is felt along nerves of the body part that has been amputated. Although its exact cause is unknown, it may be caused by trauma to the nerves serving the amputated part. The missing extremity feels numb, crushed, trapped, twisted, or burning. Management of phantom pain is challenging, often requiring referral to a pain clinic and a comprehensive pain management program.

INTERDISCIPLINARY CARE

Following amputation, the wound may be open (*guillotine*) or closed (*flap*). Open amputations are done when an infection is present. The end of the stump (remaining portion of the limb) is left open to drain. Continuous skin traction is applied to the limb. When the infection has cleared, the wound is closed.

In a closed amputation, a flap of skin is formed to cover the end of the wound. A rigid plaster shell or a soft compression dressing is applied to the stump after amputation to reduce edema, prevent infection, and promote healing. The rigid dressing helps mold the stump to fit a prosthesis. A soft compression dressing (gauze covered by an elastic wrap) is used when frequent wound checks are necessary. The elastic wrap helps prevent edema and forms a conical shape on the stump. The bandage is applied from distal to proximal (Figure 42-12 ∎). After the wound is dressed, the client is encouraged to toughen the stump skin by pushing it into first soft and then harder surfaces.

The client with a closed amputation may return from surgery with a temporary prosthesis. Limited weight bearing may be allowed within 24 to 48 hours after surgery. Once the stump is completely healed, a *prosthetist* (a professional who makes and fits artificial limbs) discusses available prosthetic options with the client. The prosthesis is custom made and fitted to the client. Some clients may have several prostheses

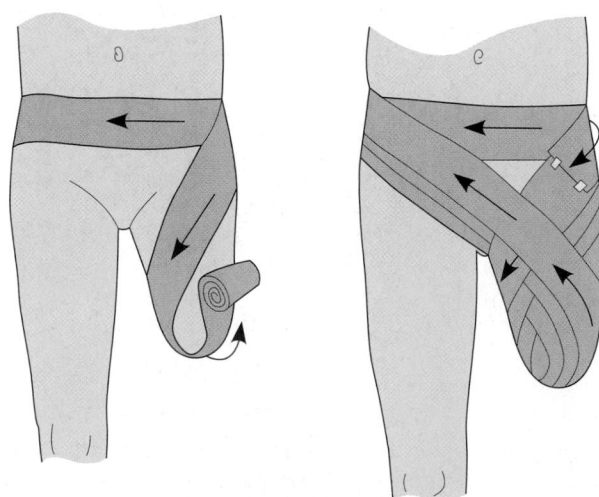

Figure 42-12. ∎ With an above-knee amputation, a figure-8 bandage is wrapped around the waist, then brought down over the stump and back up around the hips.

made for different functions, depending on their age, occupation, and activity level. Options available for arm amputees include:

- A shoulder harness with cables attached to a hook. The hook functions as a hand and fingers, activated by chest and shoulder muscle contraction.
- A cosmetic hand, also activated by shoulder and chest muscle contractions.
- A myoelectric arm operated by battery-powered motors. The motors are activated by electrodes, which transmit neuromuscular impulses.

Physical and occupational therapy are provided to help regain optimal function. The client with a leg amputation is taught how to use crutches or a walker for ambulation. The client with an arm amputation may need to relearn how to perform many ADLs such as bathing, dressing, and eating.

A member of the clergy, psychologist, or social worker may help the client cope with the loss of a limb and the grieving process.

NURSING CARE

ASSESSING

Initial assessment focuses on responses to surgery and identifying potential complications. Frequently assess vital signs and pain. Report significant changes in vital signs (such as a fall in blood pressure, tachycardia, or difficulty breathing) to the charge nurse or physician. Monitor temperature every 4 hours, reporting an elevation. Monitor urine output, reporting an output of less than 30 mL/hr.

Have client describe location and character of pain, and rate the pain using a pain scale. Report pain unrelieved by analgesics or that changes in location or character.

Assess wound and dressing, reporting excessive or bright red drainage that could indicate hemorrhage. Monitor wound healing, assessing for redness, swelling, purulent drainage, or evidence of a hematoma.

Observe the client's responses to the wound and amputated limb. The client may initially refuse to look at the affected limb, but should gradually begin taking interest in the limb and wound care.

DIAGNOSING, PLANNING, AND IMPLEMENTING

Priorities in Nursing Care. Nursing care priorities are to relieve pain, promote healing, prevent complications such as infection, promote mobility, and support the client and family as they grieve and adapt to the loss of a limb. Box 42-10 ■ describes special considerations for the older adult with an amputation.

BOX 42-10	**FOCUS ON OLDER ADULTS**

The Older Adult with an Amputation

Holistic nursing care is especially important for the older client with an amputation.

- Renal and liver function decline with aging, increasing the risk of adverse and toxic drug effects. Closely monitor response to medications.
- Altered circulation prolongs wound healing, and immune function often declines with aging, increasing the risk for infection. Monitor for local and systemic signs of infection.
- Slowed reflexes and gait alterations may disrupt balance. Introduce assistive devices in stages.
- A walker may be more appropriate than crutches, because older clients have less upper body strength. Address safety issues, such as the risk for falling.
- Assess the need for in-home assistance and make appropriate referrals to visiting nurses and home health aides.

Pain

- Administer analgesics as ordered. A PCA pump may be used initially. *Postoperative pain can be compounded by muscle spasms, swelling, and phantom pain. PCA pumps increase client control over and allow early relief of pain before it intensifies.*
- Splint and support injured area. *Splinting reduces muscle spasm and decreases edema, relieving pressure and pain.*
- Unless contraindicated, elevate the stump for 24 hours. *Elevating the stump promotes venous return and decreases edema, which will decrease pain.*
- Frequently reposition, turning slowly and gently. *Repositioning relieves pressure on tissues. Slow, gentle turning helps prevent severe muscle spasms.*
- Encourage distraction, meditation, deep breathing, and relaxation exercises. *These adjunctive measures help the client refocus, reducing the intensity of pain, including phantom pain.*

Risk for Infection

- Change wound dressing as ordered, using aseptic technique. *Aseptic technique prevents contamination of the wound with bacteria.*
- Protect wound and dressing from contamination by urine or feces. *A high above-knee (AK) or hip amputation wound can be contaminated during toileting, increasing the risk for infection.*
- Administer antibiotics as ordered. *Antibiotics inhibit bacterial growth and help prevent or eliminate infection.*
- Teach stump-wrapping techniques. *Correctly wrapping the stump improves circulation, reducing the chance of infection.*
- Report elevated WBC count. *The WBC count rises as the body tries to rid itself of infection.*

Risk for Dysfunctional Grieving

- Encourage verbalization of feelings, asking open-ended questions. *Open-ended questions allow discussion of feelings and communicate a willingness to listen.*
- Maintain eye contact and actively listen. *Eye contact and active listening communicate respect for the client and his or her feelings.*
- Reflect on the client's feelings. *Reflection statements, such as "You seem angry," allow the client to recognize feelings and validate their presence.*
- Allow unlimited visiting hours, if possible. *Unlimited visiting hours promote increased social supports.*

Disturbed Body Image

- Encourage verbalization of feelings, and validate that feelings are real and appropriate. *This allows communication of fears and lets the client know the nurse is willing to listen.*
- Allow to wear clothing from home. *Familiar clothing provides emotional comfort and helps the client retain a sense of identity.*
- Encourage looking at the stump. *Looking at and touching the stump helps the client face fear of the unknown and move from denial to acceptance.*
- Encourage participation in stump care. *Active participation in care increases self-esteem and independence.*
- Offer visitation by another amputee. *A support person who has experienced the same change provides hope for regaining independence.*
- Encourage active participation in rehabilitation. *Active participation in rehabilitation increases independence and mobility.*

Impaired Physical Mobility

- Perform ROM exercises on all joints. *ROM exercises help prevent contractures that limit mobility.*
- Maintain postoperative dressing (rigid or compression). *Postoperative dressings help mold the stump and promote healing.*
- Frequently turn and reposition. Place the client with a lower extremity amputation in the prone position every 4 hours. *Repositioning increases blood flow to muscles. The prone position helps prevent hip contracture.*
- Teach crutch walking or the use of assistive devices. *These devices allow more rapid resumption of activity.*
- Encourage active participation in physical therapy. *Physical therapy may initially be fatiguing; continuing participation increases energy level and activity tolerance.*

EVALUATING

To evaluate the effectiveness of nursing care for the client with an amputation, assess pain and the effectiveness of relief measures. Note the presence or absence of wound infection or a complication such as pneumonia. Note the client's and family's response to the wound and the loss of a body part. Assess physical mobility and participation in physical therapy.

Documenting. Document continuing assessment data, including condition of the incision and the stump. Document nature and amount of pain and the effectiveness of analgesia. Record the client's and family's responses to the amputation, to teaching, and to the prospect of a prosthesis.

CONTINUING CARE

Assess knowledge of care needs, activity restrictions or special needs, and resources for home care. Discuss home management—who is responsible for household activities such as cleaning and cooking. Inquire about arrangements that have been made for home care activities and ADLs. Evaluate use of prescription and nonprescription medications, paying particular attention to interactions and drugs that may affect balance, mental alertness, or appetite. Ask about social habits, such as cigarette smoking, alcohol use, or other drug use, that may affect healing or the ability to provide self-care.

Assess the home environment for potential safety hazards and access to care needs, such as:

- Scatter rugs
- Stairs between living areas of the house
- Grab bars to facilitate toileting and bathing
- Clean water and other needs for wound care.

Teach stump bandaging to prepare for fitting the prosthesis. Discuss positioning to prevent contractures. Teach stump exercises to maintain joint mobility and muscle tone of the affected limb. Encourage resumption of physical activities as soon as possible. Discuss household modifications to promote independence, such as grab bars in the bathroom, faucets with single-handle controls for water flow and temperature, and handheld shower heads and shower chairs for bathing. Encourage to contact local and national agencies and support groups such as these:

American Amputee Foundation
P.O. Box 250218 Hillcrest Station
Little Rock, AR 72225
501-666-2523

National Rehabilitation Information Center
8455 Colesville Road, Suite 935
Silver Spring, MD 20919-3319
800-346-2742

Note: The bibliography listings for this and all chapters have been compiled at the back of the book.

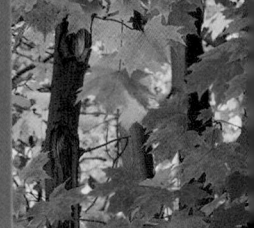

Chapter Review

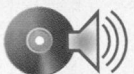 **KEY TERMS** by Topics

Use the audio glossary feature of either the CD-ROM or the Companion Website to hear the correct pronunciation of the following key terms.

Musculoskeletal trauma
trauma, contusion, hematoma, sprain, strain, fracture, compartment syndrome, reduction, traction

Joint trauma and injury
dislocation, amputation, gangrene, contracture, phantom pain

KEY Points

- Musculoskeletal injury, from minor strains to amputation, affects comfort and interferes with mobility and maintenance of ADLs. An extended period of recovery and rehabilitation may be required to recover previous function.

- Common complications of immobility, such as pneumonia and DVT, are a risk for clients with musculoskeletal injuries.

- With all musculoskeletal injuries, assessment of circulation, movement, and sensation distal to the injury is important both initially and as part of continuing care.

- Fractures may be stabilized for healing with a cast, surgical insertion of pins or plates, or using traction. Skin and wound care are important to prevent infection and complications of immobility.

- Compartment syndrome is a serious complication of fracture that requires immediate attention. Remember the 5 Ps: pain, pallor, paresthesias, paresis, and possible pulselessness. Do not assume, however, that compartment syndrome is not developing if the client has a strong pulse distal to the injury.

- Hip fractures are a significant risk in older adults and can lead to loss of independence. Provide meticulous nursing care focusing on rehabilitation from the time of hospital admission to full recovery.

- Carpal tunnel syndrome is a common repetitive use injury that can impair fine motor function of the hands. Prevention is the best treatment.

- Amputation due to trauma or disease is traumatic both physically and psychologically. Loss of a body part causes grieving and disturbs body image. Many ADLs need to be relearned following amputation.

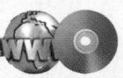 **EXPLORE Media**Link

Additional interactive resources for this chapter can be found on the Companion Website at www.prenhall.com/burke. Click on Chapter 42 and "Begin" to select the activities for this chapter.

For chapter-related NCLEX-style review questions and an audio glossary, access the accompanying CD-ROM in this book.

FOR FURTHER Study

For discussion of patient-controlled analgesia (PCA), see Chapter 8.

For more information about anesthesia, conscious sedation, and routine preoperative and postoperative care, see Chapter 9.

For more about manifestations of pulmonary edema and acute respiratory distress syndrome, see Chapter 24.

For more information on deep venous thrombosis, see Chapter 28.

For discussion of peripheral vascular disease (PVD), see Chapter 28.

For further study about prevention of osteomyelitis, see Chapter 43.

For information about total joint replacement, see Chapter 43.

For more information about intracranial disorders, see Chapter 38.

For more information about spinal disorders, see Chapter 39.

Critical Thinking Care Map

Caring for a Client with a Below-Knee Amputation
NCLEX-PN® Test Focus Area: Psychosocial Integrity: Coping and Adaptation

Case Study: John Rocke is a 45-year-old divorced man with a history of poorly controlled diabetes mellitus. He lives alone in a second-floor apartment. Two days ago, Mr. Rocke underwent a left below-knee amputation as a result of gangrene of his left foot, a consequence of his diabetes.

Nursing Diagnosis: Ineffective Individual Coping

COLLECT DATA

Subjective

_____
_____
_____
_____
_____
_____

Objective

_____
_____
_____
_____
_____

Would you report this data? Yes/No

If yes, to: _____

Nursing Care

_____
_____
_____
_____
_____
_____
_____
_____
_____
_____
_____

How would you document this? _____
_____
_____
_____

Data Collected
(use those that apply)

- Vital signs stable
- Stump splinted; covered by soft dressing
- Wound healing without signs of infection
- Refuses ROM exercises and turning
- Complaining of severe pain
- Yells "Get out! I don't want anyone to see me like this" when anyone enters room
- Tolerating 1,800-calorie American Diabetes Association (ADA) diet

Nursing Interventions
(use those that apply; list in priority order)

- Encourage verbalization of feelings.
- Contact the physician for a referral to a psychologist or social worker.
- Request a change from prn analgesia to a PCA pump.
- Teach the importance of moving and ROM exercises to prevent contractures.
- Encourage turning and lying prone.

NCLEX-PN® Exam Preparation

1 The nurse is caring for a client who has a new cast. Which of the following are appropriate nursing care measures? (Select all that apply.)

A. Use a blow dryer to apply heat to dry the cast.
B. Cover the extremity and cast with a blanket to prevent chilling.
C. Elevate the extremity on a pillow to reduce swelling.
D. Handle the cast with the palms of the hands only.
E. Pad rough edges of the cast to prevent skin excoriation.

2 When caring for a client with an above-knee amputation (AKA), it is important for the nurse to encourage the client to spend time in:

A. the prone position.
B. the supine position.
C. a flexed position.
D. a position of comfort.

3 The nurse is caring for a client who has just had an ORIF of the right hip. It is important for the nurse to keep the hip in a position of:

A. comfort.
B. adduction.
C. flexion.
D. abduction.

4 The nurse is caring for a client who has just had surgery to repair a fracture of the tibia. The client's leg is in a cast and he is receiving PCA morphine for pain. He continues to complain of severe pain and paresthesias in his foot. The nurse should:

A. elevate the leg above the heart.
B. bivalve the cast.
C. immediately notify the physician.
D. request an increase in the dose of morphine.

5 When educating the client with a sprained ankle about home care, the nurse should teach the client the acronym:

A. BRAT.
B. RICE.
C. RACE.
D. ROSE.

6 The nurse is caring for a client who earlier in the day had surgery to repair a fractured femur. The client's temperature has been elevated since the previous shift. Current assessment findings include a temperature of 101.5°F, facial petechiae, and confusion. The nurse recognizes these as possible manifestations of:

A. hemorrhage.
B. infection.
C. compartment syndrome.
D. fat embolism.

7 The nurse is caring for a client who has recently had a below-knee amputation (BKA) of the left leg. The nurse knows that the most common cause for amputation of the lower extremities is:

A. motor vehicle accidents.
B. accidents involving machinery at work.
C. bone cancer.
D. peripheral vascular disease (PVD).

8 Which of the following nursing care activities are appropriate for the client in skeletal traction? (Select all that apply.)

A. Position to maintain alignment of the body with the direction of pull.
B. Cleanse pin sites per unit protocol.
C. Assist the client to the bedside commode for toileting.
D. Release the weights when repositioning the client in bed.
E. Slide, do not lift, the client when repositioning.

9 The nurse evaluates teaching as effective when the client with a sprained ankle states the need to

A. begin exercising the ankle immediately.
B. apply ice to the ankle for the first 24 hours.
C. soak the injured extremity in warm water.
D. avoid taking analgesics to avoid masking signs of complications.

10 Which of the following types of traction increases the client's mobility while maintaining appropriate bone position?

A. balanced suspension
B. straight traction
C. skin traction
D. skeletal traction

Answers for Review Questions, as well as discussion of Care Plan and Critical Thinking Care Map questions, appear in Appendix V.

CONSIDERING CULTURAL VARIATIONS RELATED TO SPACE

A 25-year-old male Cuban American client says to the nurse, "Everybody in this culture is so cold. When I talk up to them they are always backing away. I think the nurses think I'm going to attack them sexually or something. They keep backing away from me. It's especially noticeable if I'm in line waiting for something. I may be standing close to the person in front of me, and they turn around and glare."

All verbal communication occurs in the context of space (Giger & Davidhizar, 1999). *Personal space* is the area needed by an individual to maintain intimacy and safety in relationships. Because health care providers frequently invade a person's space when providing direct care, understanding the cultural perceptions of space is important. For example, among Americans and most Europeans, personal space is highly valued, and an unannounced invasion will often result in the client's becoming suspicious and tense (Bechtel & Davidhizar, 1988).

Proximity to Others

Hall (1966) established three different dimensions of personal space: *intimate zone* (0–18 inches), *personal zone* (18 inches to 3 feet), and the *social zone* (3 to 6 feet). The intimate zone is used for close, personal encounters like comforting, counseling, and direct care activities. Invading this area without the client's acknowledgment may lead to suspicion and hostile feelings.

For most interactions not involving direct care or intimate conversation, the personal zone is considered most appropriate. In presenting client education and information, a distance of 18 inches to 3 feet is close enough for privacy yet far enough away to avoid intimate touch. Health care providers who have the respect of their clients and families are often able to interact well in this zone.

Individuals are frequently not conscious of their personal space requirements, although they react to invasion of their territory. The nurse should always be aware of clients' and families' body language during interactions. Signs that suggest the client's personal space is being invaded include stepping back, looking uncomfortable and tense, and not facing the nurse during communication.

Objects in the Environment

Objects in the environment can have great meaning for clients of different cultures, and the client may feel uncomfortable when the nurse discards or moves these objects. Objects can also affect client care and teaching. For example, when the nurse sits behind a desk, a position of authority is assumed. This may be appropriate in some cases, but usually communication is improved by sitting across from or at a 90-degree angle to the client.

Removal of a client's personal items can create distrust. For example, it may be necessary to remove a wedding ring prior to treatment, but the client may feel this takes away a strong sense of support. Likewise, placing a Roman Catholic person's rosary on a table out of reach can cause anxiety.

Items that may seem worthless to the caregiver can be of great significance to the client. For example, some clients collect plastic medicine cups to symbolize the adversities overcome in the treatment plan. If the nurse discards the medicine cups, the client may lose track of how much success has taken place and may not be as motivated to comply with treatment.

Nursing Implications

- *Provide information about the need to invade a client's space.* When it is necessary to invade a client's space, the nurse should provide information about what will be done and how long it will take. This information will enhance compliance and increase the client's comfort.

- *Assess the client for degree of comfort when invading personal space.* Personal space boundaries vary from individual to individual. While most individuals are comfortable in a conversational space of 3 to 6 feet, some individuals need more space. It is important to be alert for reactions of clients during close physical contact.

- *Provide privacy for clients during close physical care.* Use of privacy curtains, keeping the client covered whenever possible, exposing only the necessary body part, and asking other persons to leave the room during close physical care can increase feelings of security.

Self-Reflection Questions

1. How much space do you need to feel comfortable during interactions with strangers?

2. How much space do you prefer when you are with friends?

3. What do you do when your personal space is invaded?

4. How can you assist clients to accept your care when you must invade their personal space?

Chapter 43

Caring for Clients with Musculoskeletal Disorders

BRIEF Outline

Scoliosis and Kyphosis
Osteoporosis
Osteomalacia and Paget's Disease
Osteomyelitis
Bone Tumors
Common Foot Disorders
Osteoarthritis
Rheumatoid Arthritis
Systemic Lupus Erythematosus
Gout
Lyme Disease
Ankylosing Spondylitis
Fibromyalgia
Low Back Pain
Muscular Dystrophy

LEARNING Outcomes

After completing this chapter, you will be able to:

• Relate the effects of common musculoskeletal disorders to the normal structure and function of the musculoskeletal system.
• Identify manifestations of impaired musculoskeletal function.
• Describe the pathophysiology of common musculoskeletal disorders.
• Discuss interdisciplinary care measures to diagnose and manage musculoskeletal disorders.
• Provide individualized nursing care for clients with musculoskeletal disorders.
• Care for clients undergoing musculoskeletal surgery.
• Provide teaching and home care for clients with musculoskeletal disorders.

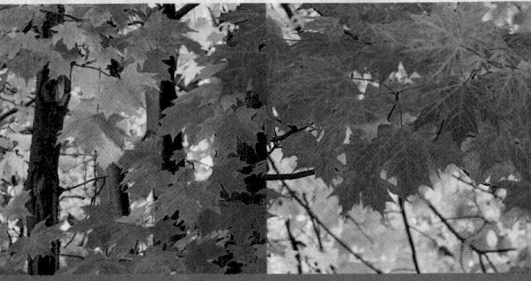

MediaLink

www.prenhall.com/burke
Use the address above to access the free, interactive Companion Website created for this textbook. Get hints, instant feedback, and textbook references to chapter-related NCLEX-style questions. Link to other interesting sites.

Audio Glossary:
Use the Companion Website, or the CD-ROM disk enclosed with your textbook, to hear the pronunciation of key terms in this chapter.

The tissues and structures of the musculoskeletal system may be affected by a variety of disorders. When these problems occur, clients may experience impaired physical mobility, altered body image, discomfort or pain, and difficulty completing self-care activities. Many musculoskeletal conditions are chronic. Nursing care focuses not only on physical care needs, but also on teaching and providing psychosocial support for the client and family.

STRUCTURAL AND BONE DISORDERS

Scoliosis and Kyphosis

Scoliosis and kyphosis are the two most common deformities of the spinal column. **Scoliosis** is a lateral curvature of the spine. **Kyphosis** is exaggeration of the normal posterior curve of the thoracic spine (Figure 43-1 ■).

PATHOPHYSIOLOGY AND MANIFESTATIONS

Scoliosis

Scoliosis is usually diagnosed in adolescence. It affects girls much more often than boys. In most cases it is *idiopathic* (has no identified cause). The lateral curve of scoliosis is usually seen in the thoracic, lumbar, or thoracolumbar regions of the spine. As it develops, muscles and ligaments on the concave side of the curvature shorten. In scoliosis, the shoulders and hips are not level, and the creases of the waist are asymmetric. A lateral curvature and rotation of the spine are seen on x-ray. Severe scoliosis causes back pain and possible dyspnea, anorexia, and nausea because internal organs are crowded.

Kyphosis

Kyphosis often is caused by structural changes in the spine from congenital disorders, Paget's disease, osteoporosis, or osteomalacia. The manifestations of kyphosis include moderate back pain and increased curvature of the thoracic spine as viewed from the side ("hunchback"). Impaired mobility and respiratory problems may occur in cases of severe curvature.

INTERDISCIPLINARY CARE

Diagnosis of scoliosis and kyphosis is made by inspection and x-rays of the spine. The client stands with the arms relaxed and hanging freely at the sides while the examiner evaluates the client from both the back and the front for symmetry of the shoulders, scapulae, waist creases, and the length of the arms. The client then bends forward, and the examiner observes for prominence of the scapula or hip. The client is then viewed from the side while the screener looks for increased thoracic rounding or lumbar swayback. Using x-rays, the degree of curvature and rotation can be measured.

Conservative treatment of scoliosis and kyphosis may include weight loss, active and passive exercises, and braces

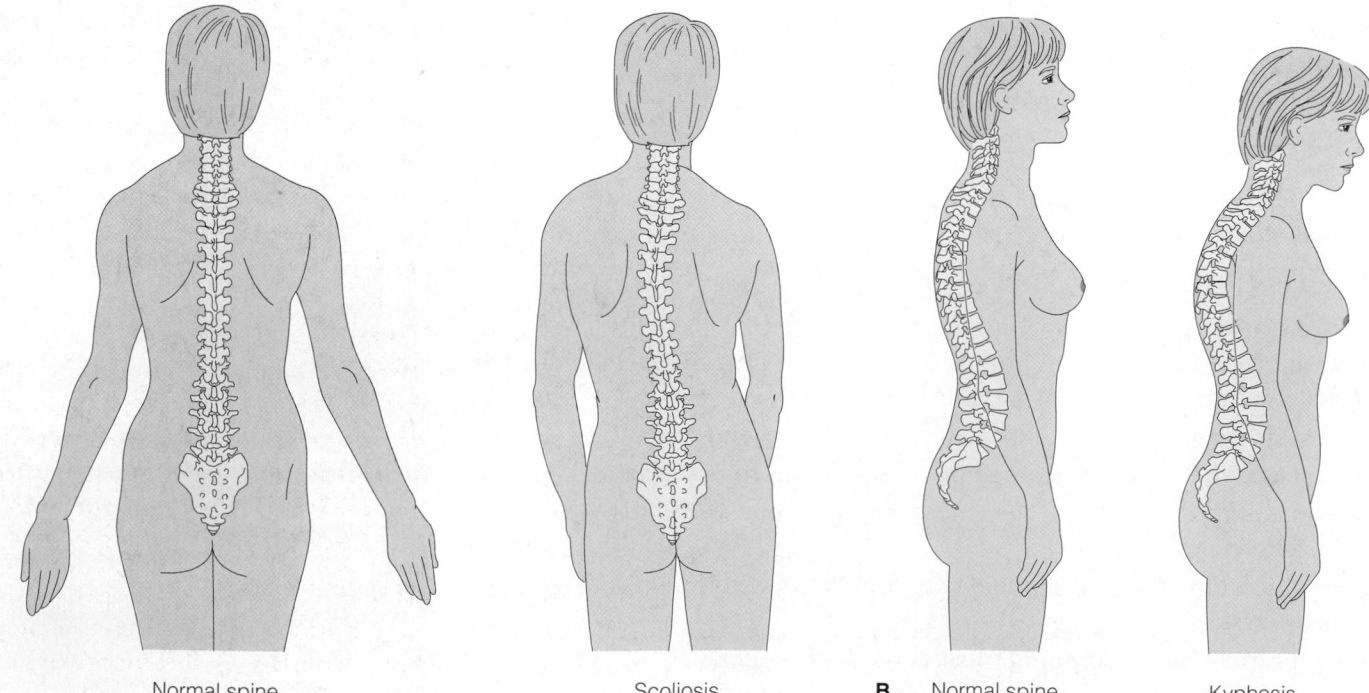

| A | Normal spine | | Scoliosis | **B** | Normal spine | | Kyphosis |

Figure 43-1. ■ (A) Scoliosis, a lateral curvature of the spine. (B) Kyphosis, exaggerated posterior curvature of the thoracic spine.

for support. Clients with severe scoliosis or kyphosis may require surgery to reduce the degree of curvature.

NURSING CARE

Scoliosis and kyphosis can change the client's center of gravity, increasing the risk for falls. Braces can pose a risk for skin irritation. Teaching and reducing the risk for injuries are the priorities for nursing care.

Risk for Injury

- Assess the environment for safety hazards. *Some braces may not allow bending or twisting of the spine.*
- Advise to use the handrail on stairways and take precautions when walking on slippery surfaces, throw rugs, and so on. *A brace may increase the risk of falling and impair the ability to prevent falls.*
- Instruct to wear a smooth cotton T-shirt or cotton tube under the brace, change undergarments at least daily, and wash them with a mild soap. Avoid lotion and body powders. *The brace can irritate the skin and increase the risk of skin breakdown.*
- Advise to loosen brace during meals and for the first 30 minutes after each meal. *Loosening the brace promotes food intake and comfort while eating.*
- Teach how to apply the brace, and explain any activity restrictions. *Prolonged sitting may be restricted. The brace is worn when ambulating.*

CONTINUING CARE

Reassure clients with scoliosis or kyphosis that the condition was not caused by poor posture. If a brace is ordered, provide verbal and written instructions for wearing the brace, such as the number of hours per day it is to be worn and activity restrictions to follow when wearing or not wearing the brace. Teach how to protect and care for skin under the brace.

If scoliosis or kyphosis restricts lung expansion, discuss the importance of not smoking and of avoiding respiratory infections. Encourage these clients to obtain pneumococcal and influenza immunizations.

Osteoporosis

Osteoporosis, literally defined as "porous bones," is a bone disorder in which bone mass is lost. Bones become more fragile, increasing the risk of fractures. Osteoporosis usually is associated with aging. Eighty percent of those affected are women, and most are over the age of 60.

Although the cause of osteoporosis remains unclear, several risk factors have been identified. Some risk factors cannot be changed; others can be changed. Box 43-1 ■ lists the risk factors for osteoporosis.

BOX 43-1

RISK FACTORS FOR OSTEOPOROSIS

Risk Factors that Cannot Be Changed
- Age, female gender
- Race (Caucasian or Asian)
- Family history
- Endocrine disorders

Risk Factors that Can Be Changed
- Calcium deficiency
- Estrogen deficiency
- Smoking, excess alcohol intake
- Sedentary lifestyle
- Medications

PATHOPHYSIOLOGY

The reduced bone mass of osteoporosis is caused by an imbalance of the processes that influence bone growth and maintenance. Peak bone mass is achieved at about age 35. After that time, bone formation does not keep pace with resorption, and bone mass is lost.

Two types of osteoporosis have been identified. *Type I osteoporosis* occurs in postmenopausal women between ages 51 and 75 and is caused by estrogen deficiency. *Type II osteoporosis,* or *senile osteoporosis,* affects both men and women over age 70. It develops more slowly and is associated with calcium deficiency.

MANIFESTATIONS AND COMPLICATIONS

The usual manifestations of osteoporosis are loss of height, progressive curvature of the spine, low back pain, and fractures.

Height is lost as vertebral bodies collapse. Characteristic dorsal kyphosis and cervical lordosis develop, causing the "dowager's hump" often associated with aging. The abdomen tends to protrude and knees and hips flex as the body attempts to maintain its center of gravity (Figure 43-2 ■).

A fracture may be the first obvious sign of osteoporosis. Some fractures are spontaneous. Others may result from everyday activities (twisting, bending, lifting, rising from bed). These are known as **pathologic fractures**, fractures that occur with minimal or no trauma. Wrist and vertebral fractures are common. Hip fractures associated with osteoporosis often interfere with the ability to maintain normal activity and live independently.

INTERDISCIPLINARY CARE

The care of the client with osteoporosis focuses on stopping or slowing the process, relieving the symptoms, and preventing complications. Proper nutrition and exercise are important components of treatment.

MediaLink

Video: Osteoporosis

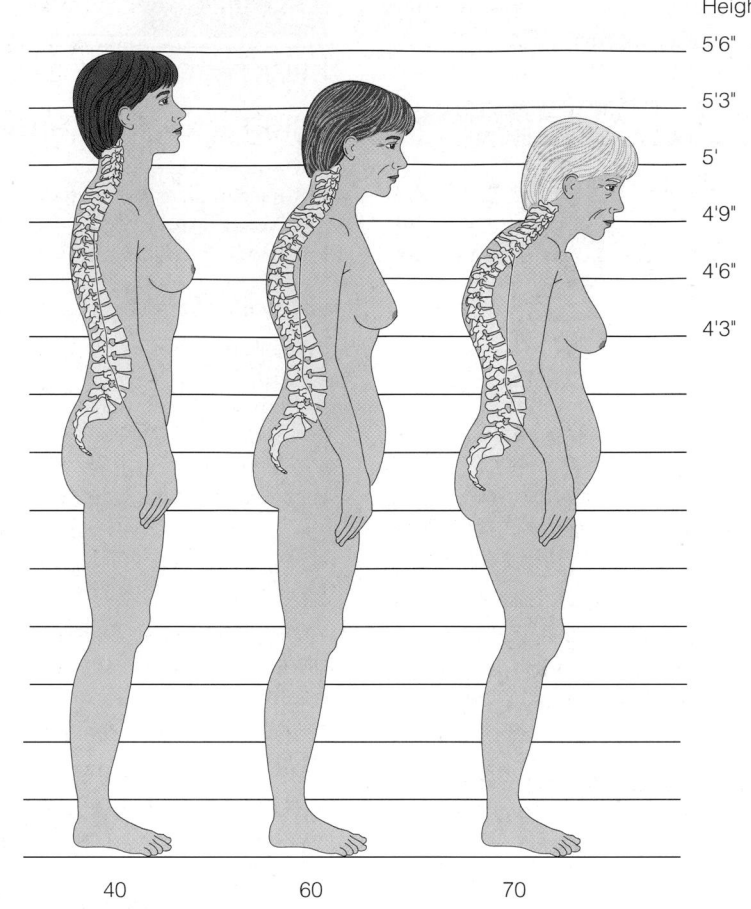

Height
5'6"
5'3"
5'
4'9"
4'6"
4'3"

Age   40   60   70

Figure 43-2. ■ Changes in height, posture, and spinal curves caused by osteoporosis.

Bone density measurements can help predict the risk for fracture; x-rays may not show osteoporotic changes until more than 30% of the bone mass has been lost. A baseline bone density exam is now recommended for premenopausal women in their 40s.

Calcium

Calcium is vital to preventing osteoporosis. Adequate calcium intake in the older adult may slow bone loss. Adequate calcium intake before age 30 to 35 increases peak bone mass and reduces the risk of osteoporosis later in life. Calcium needs change over the lifetime. See Table 43-1 ■ for National Institutes of Health (NIH) calcium intake recommendations. Box 43-2 ■ lists foods high in calcium.

Calcium supplements are available in many forms. A combination of calcium with vitamin D is recommended, particularly for older adults who may have limited sun exposure.

Medications

Estrogen or hormone replacement therapy (HRT) or selective estrogen receptor modulators (SERMs) may be ordered

TABLE 43-1	
NIH Recommended Daily Calcium Intake	
AGES	**MILLIGRAMS OF CALCIUM**
0–6 months	400
6 months–1 year	600
1–5 years	800
6–10 years	800–1,200
11–24 years	1,200–1,500
25–50 years	1,000
Pregnant or lactating	1,200–1,500
51–64 years: Women on HRT and men	1,000
51 years: Women not on HRT	1,500
65 and older	1,500

BOX 43-2

FOODS HIGH IN CALCIUM

- Dairy products (best source):
  - Milk, yogurt
  - Cheese
- Tofu
- Sardines, with bones
- Clams, oysters
- Canned salmon
- Spinach, greens
- Broccoli, cauliflower, bok choy
- Green beans
- Dark molasses

to prevent or treat bone loss in postmenopausal women. These drugs are discussed in Chapter 35. 🔗 Other drugs that may be used to prevent or treat osteoporosis include:

- Alendronate (Fosamax) and risedronate (Actonel) to inhibit bone resorption
- Calcitonin, a hormone

- Sodium fluoride, a mineral.

Table 43-2 ■ outlines the nursing implications of these drugs.

NURSING CARE

Priorities in Nursing Care. Nursing care focuses on preventing osteoporosis itself, and preventing injuries in clients who have osteoporosis.

Risk for Injury

- Keep bed in low position. Use side rails if indicated to prevent client from getting up alone. Provide nighttime lighting to toilet facilities. *Most falls are preventable, particularly in hospitals and long-term care facilities.*
- Avoid using restraints if at all possible. *Restraints may increase the risk of falling and the risk of injury due to a fall. Clients also may fracture osteoporotic bones when pulling against restraints.*
- Encourage weight-bearing exercises for 30 to 40 minutes at least three times a week. *Weight-bearing exercises*

TABLE 43-2

Nursing Implications for Pharmacology: Osteoporosis

DRUG/CLASSIFICATION	DESCRIPTION	NURSING RESPONSIBILITIES	CLIENT TEACHING
Bisphosphonates ■ Alendronate (Fosamax) ■ Risedronate (Actonel)	The bisphosphonates inhibit bone resorption, increasing the bone density and reducing the risk of fractures. They are used to prevent and treat osteoporosis.	Give with water on arising, 30 minutes before food or other medications. Hold calcium supplements and foods high in calcium for 2 hours after giving the drug. Instruct to avoid lying down for 30 minutes after taking the drug. Report changes in renal function studies (BUN and creatinine) and serum electrolytes to physician.	Take with clear water only; avoid eating or drinking for 30 minutes. Do not lie down until after you have eaten breakfast. Report heartburn or difficult or painful swallowing to your health care provider. Report tingling around the mouth or numbness and tingling of fingers or toes. Take calcium and vitamin D supplements as instructed.
Calcitonin ■ Calcitonin-salmon injection, synthetic ■ Calcimar ■ Miacalcin (injection or nasal spray)	Calcitonin prevents further bone loss and increases bone mass in osteoporosis if adequate calcium and vitamin D are consumed. Calcitonin may be used by postmenopausal women who cannot or will not take estrogen.	Observe for possible anaphylactic reaction for 20 minutes after giving; have resuscitation equipment available. Alternate nostrils daily when giving by nasal spray. Report nausea and vomiting, anorexia, mild flushing of the hands or feet, and urinary frequency. Teach how to handle and inject the drug at home.	Take in the evening to reduce side effects. Warm nasal spray to room temperature before using. Rhinitis (runny nose) is common with calcitonin nasal spray. Nasal sores or itching may occur. Report nosebleed to your health care provider. Nausea and vomiting will improve as treatment continues. Be sure to consume adequate calcium and vitamin D.
Fluoride ■ Slow-release sodium fluoride (Slow Fluoride)	Fluoride stimulates bone growth by stimulating the proliferation of osteoblasts.	Give with crackers or bread to reduce nausea. Monitor serum fluoride levels and report levels outside the normal range (95–185 ng/mL) to the health care provider.	Take with crackers or bread to minimize nausea. Maintain adequate calcium intake. Keep follow-up appointments as directed.

such as walking or low-impact aerobics promote bone growth. Swimming (including walking on the bottom of the pool) is not a weight-bearing activity.

- Encourage older adults to use assistive devices as needed to remain active and independent. *Walking sticks, canes, and other tools help the client engage in activities that promote bone growth.*
- Teach older clients about safety and fall precautions. *Helping identify and correct safety hazards in the home can reduce the risk of falls, fractures, and potential disability.*
- Evaluate medication regimen for drugs that may increase the risk of falling (some antihypertensives, antianxiety agents, antihistamines, or sedatives). *Many drugs may cause orthostatic hypotension or sedation, increasing the risk for falling.*

Imbalanced Nutrition: Less than Body Requirements

- Teach all clients recommended calcium intake for their age (see Table 43-1). *An adequate calcium intake is vital to prevent and treat osteoporosis.*
- Provide a list of foods high in calcium (see Box 43-2), and help identify ways to include these foods in the diet. *Calcium obtained through the diet is an effective way to maintain adequate calcium levels in the body.*
- Teach clients using calcium supplements to take calcium carbonate supplement (e.g., Tums) 30 to 60 minutes before meals. Calcium citrate supplements should be taken with meals to prevent gastrointestinal (GI) distress. All supplements should be taken in divided doses (two to three times daily). *Taking calcium supplements at the appropriate time and in divided doses increases their absorption and effectiveness.*

Pain

- Assess acute or new complaints of pain. *Acute pain usually results from a fracture, such as compression fracture of the vertebrae.*
- Give acetaminophen or anti-inflammatory drugs as indicated for pain. *Acetaminophen often is well tolerated by older adults. Regular doses of nonsteroidal anti-inflammatory drugs (NSAIDs) can help manage chronic pain.*
- Apply heat to the painful area, being careful to avoid burning the client. *A controlled heating pad (e.g., Aqua-K) may offer temporary pain relief. To avoid the "rebound effect," remove the heating pad every 20 to 30 minutes.*
- Assist physical therapy to plan an exercise regime. *Exercise is vital to maintain bone mass, but modifications may be necessary to promote comfort.*

CONTINUING CARE

Teaching about osteoporosis is important to prevent the disease and its consequences. Stress the importance of maintaining the recommended daily calcium intake. This is particularly important for adolescent girls and young adult women, who may avoid eating many high-calcium foods such as dairy products because of concerns about weight. Emphasize that low-fat (or nonfat) dairy products also contain calcium. For clients who avoid dairy products because of lactose intolerance or a vegetarian diet, suggest alternate sources such as sardines, salmon, broccoli, and dark-green, leafy vegetables. Refer to a dietitian for further teaching and diet planning.

Teach the importance of physical activity and weight-bearing exercise to prevent bone loss. Suggest regular exercise such as walking for at least 20 minutes four or more times a week. Inform that swimming and pool aerobic exercises are not as helpful to maintain bone density because of the lack of weight bearing.

Teach postmenopausal women about hormone replacement therapy (HRT) to prevent bone loss. Refer to primary care provider for more information about the risks and benefits of HRT.

Stress the importance of not smoking. Provide information about smoking cessation programs and support groups. Discuss the effect of heavy alcohol use on bone mass, and suggest it be used moderately, if at all.

Discuss safety and fall prevention with the client who has osteoporosis. Advise to remove scatter rugs and clutter from walkways in the house. Instruct to use a night-light or graduated lighting from the bedroom to the bathroom to reduce the risk of nighttime falls. Discuss placing grab bars in strategic locations such as the shower and next to the toilet to reduce the risk of falling.

Provide a list of local and national resources, such as medical equipment supply retailers and osteoporosis support groups and foundations. The National Osteoporosis Foundation and the Osteoporosis and Related Bone Diseases National Resource Center have many client information pamphlets and resources. Refer to a health care provider, social services, or occupational therapy as indicated for bone density testing, home care services, or rehabilitation.

Osteomalacia and Paget's Disease

Osteomalacia and Paget's disease also affect the structure and integrity of bone.

PATHOPHYSIOLOGY AND MANIFESTATIONS

Osteomalacia, also known as *adult rickets,* results from inadequate mineralization of bone. When insufficient amounts of calcium or phosphate are available, the bone matrix is not mineralized and the bone is unable to bear weight. This causes deformities of weight-bearing bone and pathologic fractures. Osteomalacia is commonly caused by a lack of

MANIFESTATIONS OF OSTEOMALACIA AND PAGET'S DISEASE

Osteomalacia

- Bone pain
- Difficulty changing positions (lying to sitting; sitting to standing)
- Muscle weakness
- Waddling gait
- Dorsal kyphosis
- Pathologic fractures

Paget's Disease

- Bone pain
- Deformity
- Pathologic fractures
- Chalk-stick fractures of lower extremities
- Compression fractures
- Kyphosis, loss of height
- Muscle weakness

RISK FACTORS FOR OSTEOMYELITIS

- Open fracture
- Gunshot or deep puncture wound
- Orthopedic surgery
- Soft tissue infection
- Pressure ulcers
- Impaired immune function
- Venous stasis or arterial ulcers of the legs
- Diabetes mellitus

Box 43-4 ■ lists risk factors for osteomyelitis. The older adult is at risk for several reasons: reduced immune function, chronic diseases, impaired circulation, and a higher risk of pressure ulcers.

PATHOPHYSIOLOGY AND MANIFESTATIONS

Pathogens usually enter the bone through an open wound, such as an open fracture or a gunshot or puncture wound. Bacteria also may spread to the bone from a local tissue infection. After entry, bacteria lodge and multiply in the bone, causing an inflammatory and immune system response. Phagocytes attempt to contain the infection. In the process, they release enzymes that destroy bone tissue. Pus forms, followed by edema and vascular congestion. Canals in the marrow cavity of the bone allow the infection to spread to other parts of the bone. If the infection reaches the outer margin of the bone (Figure 43-3 ■), it raises the periosteum of the bone and spreads along the surface. Blood supply to the bone is disrupted, leading to ischemia and, eventually, necrosis of the bone. Blood and antibiotics cannot reach the bone tissue, making it difficult to treat the infection.

vitamin D. Vitamin D, obtained from certain foods and ultraviolet (UV) radiation from the sun, is necessary to maintain calcium and phosphate levels in the body. Osteomalacia can be corrected with treatment. For more information about the relationship of vitamin D, calcium, and phosphorus in the body, see Chapter 7. ⬭

In Paget's disease of the bone, the activity of *osteoclasts* (which break down and resorb bone) increases. This stimulates activity in *osteoblasts* (cells that form new bone) to replace lost bone. However, the new bone formed is soft and poorly mineralized, so it is prone to fractures. The cause of this disease is unknown. The manifestations of osteomalacia and Paget's disease are listed in Box 43-3 ■.

INTERDISCIPLINARY CARE

Clients with osteomalacia often are placed on vitamin D supplements. Calcium and phosphate supplements also may be ordered. Drugs such as the bisphosphonates and calcitonin are used along with calcium supplements for clients with Paget's disease. Review Table 43-2 for the nursing implications of these drugs.

Nursing care for clients with osteomalacia or Paget's disease is similar to that provided for clients with osteoporosis.

Osteomyelitis

Osteomyelitis is an infection of the bone. It is usually caused by *Staphylococcus aureus* bacteria, although other pathogens also can infect the bone. Osteomyelitis can occur at any age, but usually affects children under age 12 and adults over age 50.

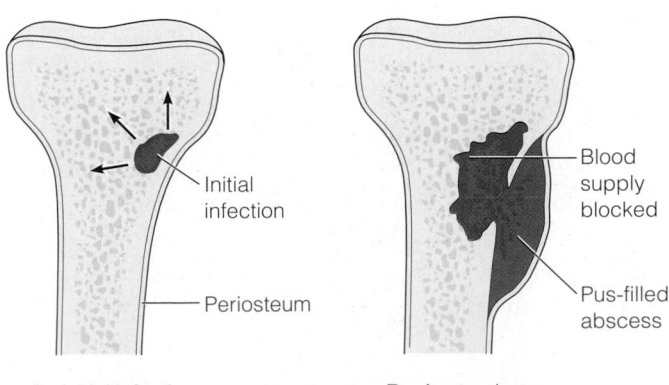

Figure 43-3. ■ Osteomyelitis. (**A**) Bacteria enter and multiply in the bone. (**B**) The infection spreads to other parts of the bone. If the infection reaches the outer part of the bone, the periosteum separates from the surface of the bone.

BOX 43-5

MANIFESTATIONS OF OSTEOMYELITIS
- Chills and fever
- General malaise, fatigue
- Pain in the affected limb
- Limited weight bearing in extremity
- Redness, swelling, heat, tenderness over site
- Purulent wound drainage, slowed healing

The diagnosis of osteomyelitis often is not made until the infection has become chronic. A surgical wound or fracture that does not heal may be the initial sign of infection. Box 43-5 ■ lists the manifestations of osteomyelitis.

INTERDISCIPLINARY CARE

Early diagnosis and treatment of osteomyelitis with antibiotic therapy is important to prevent bone necrosis.

Diagnostic Tests

- The *white blood cell count (WBC)* and *erythrocyte sedimentation rate (ESR)* are elevated, nonspecific signs of infection.
- *Blood* and *tissue cultures* are obtained to identify the infecting organism.
- *Magnetic resonance imaging (MRI), computed tomography (CT) scan,* or *ultrasound* are performed to identify the infection site.
- A *bone scan* may be ordered to help identify active infection (see Box 41-3 ⊚ for nursing care of a client having a bone scan).

Medications

Antibiotics initially are given intravenously. This may be continued after discharge from the hospital, or an oral antibiotic may be used. Treatment is continued for 4 to 6 weeks.

Surgery

Surgery may be done to obtain a specimen for culture. It may also be done to **debride** the area (remove foreign material and dead or damaged tissue). In surgical debridement, the periosteum is excised and the *cortex* (outer portion of the bone) is drilled to release the pressure from accumulated pus. Following irrigation, drainage tubes connected to an irrigation system may be inserted to keep the cavity clean. After surgery, the nurse is responsible for instilling and removing dilute antibiotic solutions through the drainage tubes.

clinical ALERT

Use strict sterile technique when caring for a wound irrigation to prevent additional contamination of the infected bone.

NURSING CARE

ASSESSING

The nurse can be instrumental in identifying early manifestations of osteomyelitis. Frequently and carefully assess at-risk clients for manifestations (see Box 43-5). The older adult may have less specific symptoms, presenting instead with confusion and vague complaints.

DIAGNOSING, PLANNING, AND IMPLEMENTING

Priorities in Nursing Care. Priority nursing diagnoses for the client with osteomyelitis focus on comfort and limited mobility. Because osteomyelitis can be difficult to treat, it also is important to address emotional responses to the disease.

Pain

- Provide analgesics on a scheduled basis over 24 hours rather than as needed. *Scheduled analgesic doses allow maintenance of constant blood levels.*
- Offer analgesic 20 to 30 minutes prior to tests, procedures, or exercises. *Premedicating allows time for the medication to take effect prior to a procedure.*
- Splint or immobilize the affected extremity. *Splinting or immobilizing the involved extremity provides support and reduces pain caused by movement.*
- Use adjunctive strategies (e.g., distraction, relaxation) for pain management. *Muscle or joint pain may be relieved with measures that promote relaxation and vasodilation, such as warm, moist packs; warm baths; or heating pads to the involved extremity.*
- Provide assistive devices (such as a splint, walker, or crutches) for ambulation. *Assistive devices help support the involved extremity and reduce weight bearing when ambulating.*
- Handle the affected area gently. *Gentle handling and minimal manipulation help reduce pain.*

Hyperthermia

- Monitor temperature every 4 hours and during periods of chilling. Report fever to the charge nurse or physician. *A sudden rise in temperature or continued elevation may indicate a lack of response to treatment. Blood cultures may be ordered when an acute temperature elevation occurs.*
- Keep environment cool and provide light clothing and bedding during fever. *A cool environment and light clothing promote comfort when the temperature is elevated.*
- Promote fluid intake of 2,000 to 3,000 mL/day. *The client with an elevated temperature needs additional fluid to replace losses through perspiration.*

Impaired Physical Mobility

- Keep the affected limb in functional position when immobilized. *Keeping the affected extremity in functional position reduces the risk of contractures.*

- Maintain rest. Avoid weight bearing on the affected extremity. *Stress on the weakened bone can lead to pathologic fractures.*
- Assist with active or passive range-of-motion (ROM) exercises every 4 hours. *ROM exercises help maintain normal joint mobility.*

EVALUATING

Collect assessment data related to pain, fever, and fluid balance (urine output, skin turgor, and temperature) to evaluate the effectiveness of nursing care. Also assess physical mobility, strength, and skin condition when evaluating nursing care.

Documenting. Document continuing assessment data, including temperature and other vital signs, appearance of the affected extremity, and general appearance of the client. Record the amount, color, odor, and other characteristics of any wound drainage. Document all teaching provided, as well as the client's and family's understanding of the disease and prescribed care, including wound care and medications.

CONTINUING CARE

Reinforce teaching about medications and wound management at home. Emphasize the importance of taking all antibiotics as prescribed. Instruct to use pain medications as needed to prevent pain from becoming severe. Discuss possible drug side effects, and provide information about managing these effects. For example, increase fluid and fiber intake to prevent constipation caused by many analgesics, and consume 8 ounces of live-culture yogurt to help prevent diarrhea and yeast infections (mouth or vagina) often associated with prolonged antibiotic therapy.

Teach wound care as needed. Refer for home health services as appropriate. Provide a list of resources for wound care supplies such as local medical suppliers. Teach general principles of infection control, including the importance of good hand washing, especially after toileting or contact with wound drainage.

Rest or limited weight bearing generally is ordered for the affected limb. Bed rest is recommended for vertebral osteomyelitis until back pain has eased enough to allow ambulation. Teach how to avoid complications of immobility. Suggest frequent position changes, keeping skin and linens clean and dry, and active ROM exercises for unaffected joints.

Emphasize the importance of good nutrition. An adequate supply of calories, protein, and other nutrients is necessary for immune function and healing. Suggest frequent small meals and the use of supplements such as Ensure.

Stress the need to keep all follow-up appointments to ensure complete eradication of the infection.

Bone Tumors

Bone tumors (or *neoplasms*) may be either benign or malignant, primary or secondary. Benign tumors are more common than malignant. *Primary* bone tumors are rare in adults, occurring more frequently in adolescents. *Metastatic* bone tumors (that is, seeded from a tumor elsewhere in the body) are more common in adults, often originating from tumors of the prostate, breast, kidney, thyroid, and lung.

PATHOPHYSIOLOGY AND MANIFESTATIONS

Primary bone tumors are classified by the tissue from which they arise: bone (*osteogenic*), cartilage (*chondrogenic*), collagen (*collagenic*), and bone marrow (*myelogenic*) (Table 43-3 ■).

TABLE 43-3

Common Primary Bone Tumors

TUMOR ORIGIN	BENIGN TUMORS	MALIGNANT TUMORS	SITE
Bone (osteogenic)	Osteoma	Osteosarcoma—most common malignant tumor of bone tissue	Long bones (femur, tibia), knee
Cartilage (chondrogenic)	Osteochondroma—most common benign tumor		Pelvis, scapula, ribs
		Chondrosarcoma	Femur, pelvis, ribs, head of long bones
Collagen (collagenic)		Fibrosarcoma	Femur, tibia
Bone marrow (myelogenic)		Multiple myeloma—most common primary malignancy of the bone	Vertebrae, ribs, skull, pelvis
Unknown		Ewing's sarcoma—usually occurs in adolescence	Long bones; pelvis, ribs, scapula, sternum

---

BOX 43-6

MANIFESTATIONS OF BONE TUMORS

- Deep bone pain; worse at night and at rest
- Redness, warmth, swelling over the affected bone
- Enlarging mass over affected bone
- Muscle weakness or atrophy
- Fever

Primary tumors cause bone breakdown (*osteolysis*), which weakens the bone, resulting in fractures. Malignant bone tumors invade and destroy adjacent bone tissue by producing substances that promote bone resorption or by interfering with a bone's blood supply. Benign bone tumors, unlike malignant ones, have a symmetric, controlled growth pattern. As they grow, they push against neighboring bone tissue. This weakens the bone's structure until it is unable to withstand the stress of ordinary use and frequently causes pathologic fracture.

Bone tumors are usually identified when an injury brings the mass to the client's attention. Box 43-6 ■ lists the common manifestations of bone tumors.

INTERDISCIPLINARY CARE

Because symptoms are usually vague, tumor diagnosis may be delayed.

Diagnostic Tests

- Conventional *x-rays* show the location of the tumor and the extent of bone involvement.
- *CT scan* and *MRI* are used to identify the extent of tumor invasion into surrounding tissue.
- A *biopsy* is done to identify the type of tumor.
- The *serum alkaline phosphatase, red blood cell (RBC) count,* and *serum calcium* levels are elevated.

Chemotherapy

Chemotherapeutic drugs are given to shrink the tumor before surgery, to prevent recurrence after surgery, or to treat tumor metastasis. See Chapter 12 ◯◯ for further discussion of chemotherapy and its nursing implications.

Radiation Therapy

Radiation therapy may be used in combination with chemotherapy. Radiation therapy is frequently applied to metastatic bone lesions to control pain. It is also used to eliminate bony tumors or to eliminate any remaining tumor after surgery. Radiation therapy is discussed in Chapter 12. ◯◯

Surgery

Surgery is performed to remove the tumor. The tumor itself may be excised, or the affected limb amputated. To avoid amputation, a bone graft from a cadaver or metal prostheses often is used to replace missing bone. Care of the client undergoing amputation is presented in Chapter 42. ◯◯

NURSING CARE

Nursing care needs for the client with a bone tumor focus on both the physical aspects of care as well as the psychosocial effects of the diagnosis and its treatment.

Priorities in Nursing Care. Pain related to the tumor is a priority for nursing interventions.

Pain

- Assess pain, including location, intensity (ask the client to rate the pain on a standard pain scale), quality or type, aggravating and relieving factors, and duration. *An accurate assessment of pain is necessary to help determine its cause and to evaluate the effectiveness of interventions.*
- Develop strategies for controlling both acute pain (from surgery, fracture, or inflammation) and chronic pain (from tumor growth and spread). *Effective pain management is based on the acuity and intensity of the pain. See Chapter 8 ◯◯ for more information about pain management.*
- Encourage use of both pharmacologic and nonpharmacologic methods to prevent pain from becoming intense. *Pain relief measures are more effective when used to control pain before it becomes intense.*
- Provide assistive devices (e.g., canes, walkers, crutches) when ambulating. *Assistive devices reduce pain by supporting weight bearing during ambulation.*
- Provide regular rest periods between scheduled treatments. *Rest reduces muscle tension and pain.*

Impaired Physical Mobility

- Teach correct use of trapeze. *Using the trapeze helps strengthen the biceps of the arm and allows clients to reposition themselves, get out of bed, and perform other activities.*
- Begin muscle-strengthening and active and passive ROM exercises immediately after surgery. A continuous passive motion (CPM) machine may be used after surgery on an extremity. *Muscle-strengthening and ROM exercises maintain joint function and prevent muscle wasting.*
- Assist the client who has leg surgery or amputation with exercises to strengthen the triceps muscles of the arms and with quadriceps and gluteal setting exercises and leg raises. *Muscle-strengthening exercises prepare the client for using assistive devices (e.g., crutches) for ambulation and other activities until a prosthesis is fitted.*
- Refer to physical or occupational therapy for fitting of and teaching about assistive devices such as a cane,

crutches, or a walker. *Assistive devices promote mobility and reduce the risk of falling.*

Disturbed Body Image

- Listen to and support the client who is grieving loss of a limb or other changes such as hair loss associated with treatment. *The client who has lost a body part or experienced a change in body image will go through a grieving process.*

- Allow time for open discussions of feelings about changes in body image and potential changes in social and personal life. *Open and accepting discussion helps the client work through grieving and begin coping with the changes.*

Anticipatory Grieving

- Listen actively and encourage verbalization of feelings and concerns about the diagnosis and treatment. *Active listening promotes trust and provides an opportunity for the client and family to work through accepting the diagnosis.*

- Present information in a matter-of-fact manner, taking time to listen to and address concerns. Discuss expected effects and potential side effects of surgery, chemotherapy, and radiation therapy. *Accurate and appropriate information empowers the client and family to make decisions about treatment.*

- Refer to a counselor, the clergy, or, as appropriate, hospice services. *The client with a malignant bone tumor faces the very real possibility of dying as a result of the disease, particularly when the tumor is metastatic from another site. Trained professionals can help the client and family identify and express their feelings, and work through the grieving process.*

CONTINUING CARE

Teach about the disease, its potential consequences, and treatment options. Provide information about how to minimize side effects. Depending on the location of the tumor and planned treatment, modifications of the home environment may be necessary. Discuss potential barriers to mobility, such as stairs or lack of access to transportation. Help identify a network of support people who can assist with coping, care, and treatment as needed. If surgery has been performed, teach wound care, demonstrating dressing changes and stump care (if amputation has occurred). Provide a list of local resources for obtaining supplies. Discuss activity and weight-bearing restrictions. Refer to physical therapy for teaching about ambulation and appropriate muscle-group strengthening exercises. Ensure that the client who has experienced an amputation is working with or has a referral to a prosthetic specialist. For the client with metastatic disease, discuss hospice services and support groups for clients with cancer.

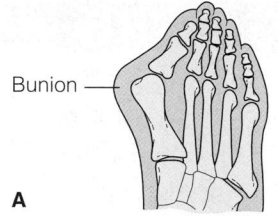

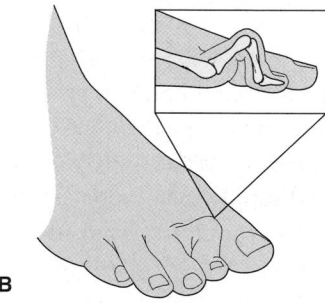

Figure 43-4. ■ **(A)** Hallux valgus (bunion). **(B)** Hammertoe.

Common Foot Disorders

Hallux valgus and hammertoe are common foot disorders that cause pain or difficulty in walking. Wearing poorly fitting or confining shoes may contribute to these disorders.

HALLUX VALGUS

Hallux valgus, or *bunion,* is enlargement and lateral displacement of the great toe (Figure 43-4A ■). They develop due to chronic pressure against the great toe. Heredity and joint disorders contribute, as does wearing pointed, narrow-toed shoes or high heels. The toe bends away from the midline of the body, and the metatarsophalangeal (MTP) joint becomes enlarged. Calluses develop over the joint. Hallux valgus is obvious on physical examination of the foot. The client may complain of pain and difficulty fitting into shoes.

HAMMERTOE

Hammertoe (claw toe) is a deformity of the toe characterized by flexion of the proximal interphalangeal (PIP) joint with hyperextension of the MTP and distal interphalangeal (DIP) joints. It may affect any toe, but the second toe is usually affected. The flexed PIP joint rubs against the shoe, causing painful corns to develop (Figure 43-4B).

INTERDISCIPLINARY CARE

Corrective shoes often are ordered for clients with foot disorders. Orthotic devices that cushion and stretch the affected joints may be placed within shoes or between the toes. Analgesics may be ordered, or corticosteroid drugs injected into the affected joints to relieve acute inflammation. A bunionectomy may be done to treat hallux valgus. Surgery also may be done to correct hammertoe.

NURSING CARE

Priorities in Nursing Care. The focus and priority for nursing care of the client with a foot disorder is managing discomfort associated with the disorder and teaching measures to maintain mobility and prevent injury.

Pain

- Instruct to wear appropriate or corrective footwear. *Shoes that fit well and provide enough foot space laterally and dorsally, such as running shoes, are recommended. In some cases, the client may need special shoes or orthotics.*
- Provide information about resources for obtaining a proper shoe fit. *Shoe stores and repair shops often can stretch a shoe at the pressure area. Fabric shoes are more comfortable for people with bunions because fabric stretches more readily than leather or synthetic materials.*
- Suggest protective pads to wear over bunions, calluses/corns, and the ball of the foot. *Protective pads help reduce pain and irritation when shoes are worn.*
- Instruct to remove pads and inspect skin every other day. Clients who have difficulty reaching or observing the foot should ask another person to do the inspection for them. *Skin inspection is particularly important if sensation has been lost in the feet due to diabetes or chronic peripheral vascular disease.*

Risk for Infection

Risk for infection following foot surgery may be increased because of impaired peripheral circulation and exposure of the feet to the environment.

- Teach proper care and cleaning of incision and exposed pins implanted during surgery. *Pins may be inserted to maintain the position of the bones and joints.*
- Instruct to wear a plastic bag over the cast or pins when bathing or walking in rain or snow. *When casts or pins are exposed in water, infection may result.*

CONTINUING CARE

Teach clients in all age groups the importance of well-fitting footwear. Discuss with women in particular the long-term effects of wearing high-heeled shoes with constricting toes. Suggest alternatives for stylish footwear, and encourage clients to wear supportive and nonrestrictive footwear at all times. Discuss the possible effects of bunions on balance, and talk about safety measures to prevent falls and injury. Teach techniques to relieve pressure on affected joints as discussed in the nursing care section.

JOINT AND CONNECTIVE TISSUE DISORDERS

The term **arthritis,** which literally means inflammation of a joint, is often used for any disorder that causes pain and stiffness of the musculoskeletal system. *Rheumatism* is another term used to describe pain in the joints and related tissues. Some arthritic disorders are limited to the joint and surrounding tissues; others are more widespread systemic diseases. Several, such as rheumatoid arthritis and systemic lupus erythematosus, are *connective tissue disorders.*

Connective tissue is the most abundant and widely distributed body tissue. It connects body parts; provides support; forms bones, cartilage, and the walls of blood vessels; and attaches muscles to bones. Connective tissue diseases have diverse manifestations. Arthritic disorders, regardless of their cause, can create problems of mobility, deformity, and disability.

Osteoarthritis

Osteoarthritis (OA) is a degenerative joint disease characterized by progressive loss of joint cartilage in synovial joints. Osteoarthritis is the most common type of arthritis and is a leading cause of disability in older adults. It affects men and women equally. Risk factors for OA include age, repetitive joint use or trauma, heredity, obesity, and congenital or acquired defects.

PATHOPHYSIOLOGY

Osteoarthritis affects the entire joint: the cartilage, bone, synovial membrane, and the ligaments, muscles, and tendons that surround the joint. The joint cartilage loses its strength and elasticity and is gradually destroyed. As the cartilage erodes and ulcerates, the underlying bone is exposed. The bone thickens in exposed areas, and cysts develop. Cartilage-coated *osteophytes* (bony outgrowths) change the anatomy of the joint. As these spurs or projections enlarge, small pieces may break off, leading to mild inflammation of the joint.

The hips, knees, lumbar and cervical vertebrae, proximal and distal interphalangeal (PIP and DIP) joints of the fingers, wrist, and big toe joint of the foot are affected most frequently by osteoarthritis.

MANIFESTATIONS AND COMPLICATIONS

The onset of OA is usually gradual and insidious, and the course slowly progressive. Localized joint pain (**arthralgia**) is the most common symptom of OA. Following periods of immobility (e.g., on awakening in the morning or after an automobile ride), involved joints may stiffen. Range of motion of the joint decreases as the disease progresses, and grating or crepitus may be noted during movement. Bony overgrowth may cause joint

BOX 43-7

MANIFESTATIONS OF OSTEOARTHRITIS

- Deep, aching pain in affected joints
- Pain aggravated by use, relieved by rest
- Stiffness following immobility
- Limited ROM
- Crepitus with movement
- *Heberden's nodes* on DIP joints
- *Bouchard's nodes* on PIP joints

BOX 43-8 **COMPLEMENTARY THERAPIES**

Osteoarthritis

Many complementary therapies may help relieve the discomfort of osteoarthritis and maintain mobility. Refer the client to a trained practitioner or naturopathic physician. Selected complementary therapies for OA include:

- Aromatherapy: massage or compress of cypress or rosemary to affected joints
- Herbs: glucosamine and chondroitin; natural anti-inflammatories such as willowbark
- Magnets over affected joints
- Reflexology
- Therapeutic touch
- Yoga

enlargement. Enlarged joints are characteristically bony-hard and cool on palpation. The manifestations of OA are listed in Box 43-7 ■.

Osteoarthritis of the spine may cause degeneration of disks between the vertebrae and narrowing of the joint spaces. Degenerative disk disease may be complicated by a *herniated disk,* the protrusion of the nucleus pulposus of the disk. Herniation can compress nerve roots, causing severe pain and muscle weakness. See Chapter 39 🔗 for further discussion of disk disorders. Loss of cartilage between the processes of the vertebrae causes localized pain, stiffness, muscle spasm, and limited range of motion. Osteophytes may form on these processes, increasing pain and muscle spasm.

INTERDISCIPLINARY CARE

The diagnosis of OA is based on the history and on physical and x-ray examination of affected joints. Initially, the joint space narrows. As the disease progresses, bone density increases, osteophytes are seen at the joint periphery, and bone cysts may be noted.

Clients with OA are encouraged to lose weight if obese and to remain physically active. Exercise helps maintain muscle tone and joint support, and promotes weight loss. Exercise in water (non–weight bearing) may help clients with OA of the knees or hips. Heat applied locally to affected joints can relieve discomfort. Box 43-8 ■ provides selected complementary therapies that may be beneficial for clients with OA.

Medications

The pain of OA often can be managed with mild analgesics such as aspirin or acetaminophen. Acetaminophen is preferred for use in older clients because it has fewer toxic side effects. Nonsteroidal anti-inflammatory drugs (NSAIDs) may also be ordered. These medications are discussed in more detail in the section of this chapter on rheumatoid arthritis. Capsaicin cream can reduce joint pain and tenderness when applied topically to affected joints such as the knees or hands. In some cases, a long-acting corticosteroid mixed with a local anesthetic may be injected directly into the affected joint. Although this procedure relieves pain, it can increase cartilage breakdown if done frequently.

Surgery

Surgery may be done when pain and limited joint motion interfere with ADLs. *Arthroscopy* may be done for osteoarthritis of the knee. Using an arthroscope, the joint is inspected, and damaged cartilage and osteophytes can be removed. Nursing care of the client undergoing arthroscopy is outlined in Box 41-4. 🔗

Arthroplasty, reconstruction or replacement of a joint, is often done when the client has severely restricted mobility and pain at rest. In most cases, both surfaces of the affected joint are replaced with prosthetic parts in a procedure known as a *total joint replacement.* Joints that may be replaced include the hip, knee, shoulder, elbow, ankle, wrist, and joints of the fingers and toes.

In a *total hip replacement,* the joint surfaces of the acetabulum and femoral head are replaced (Figure 43-5A ■). The entire head of the femur and part of the femoral neck are removed and replaced with a prosthesis. In a *total knee replacement* (Figure 43-5B), the femoral side of the joint is replaced with a metallic surface, and the tibial side with polyethylene.

Infection is the major complication of total joint replacement surgery. Infection impairs healing and can lead to failure and removal of the prosthesis. Box 43-9 ■ outlines nursing care for the client undergoing total joint replacement. See Chapter 9 🔗 for more information about caring for the client undergoing surgery.

NURSING CARE

OA frequently complicates pain management and interferes with mobility in both home and institutional settings. It rarely is the primary nursing care problem unless the client is having joint surgery for the effects of OA.

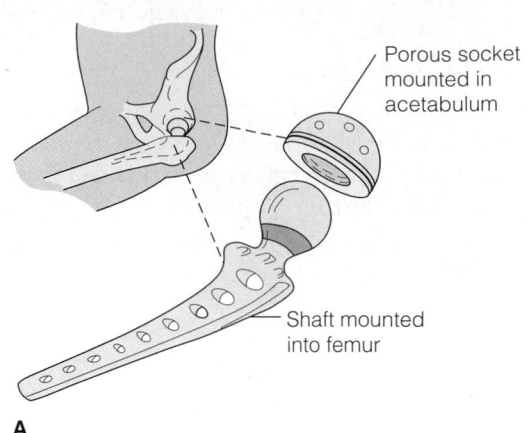

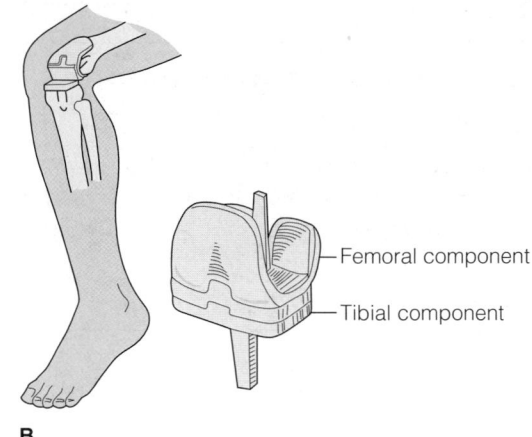

Porous socket mounted in acetabulum

Shaft mounted into femur

A

Femoral component

Tibial component

B

Figure 43-5. ■ (**A**) Total hip replacement. (**B**) Total knee replacement.

BOX 43-9	NURSING CARE CHECKLIST

Total Joint Replacement

Before Surgery

☑ Provide routine preoperative care and teaching. See Chapter 9. ⚭

☑ Reinforce teaching as indicated.

☑ Teach use of overhead trapeze for changing positions.

☑ Teach or provide ordered skin preparation such as shower, shampoo, and skin scrub with antibacterial solution.

☑ Administer intravenous antibiotic as ordered.

After Surgery

☑ Provide routine postoperative care (see Chapter 9). ⚭

☑ Assess neurovascular status (color, temperature, pulses and capillary refill, movement, and sensation) of the affected limb hourly for the first 12 to 24 hours, then every 2 to 4 hours. Report abnormal findings immediately.

☑ Empty and record wound suction drainage every 4 hours.

☑ Frequently assess for bleeding. Reinforce the dressing as needed. Report significant bleeding to the charge nurse or physician.

☑ Maintain extremity position using sling, abduction splint, brace, immobilizer, or other ordered device.

☑ Help shift position at least every 2 hours while on bed rest.

☑ Encourage frequent use of incentive spirometer, deep breathing, and coughing.

☑ Assist out of bed as soon as allowed (usually 24 to 48 hours postoperatively). Reinforce teaching about avoiding weight bearing on affected extremity; use overhead trapeze, pivot turning, and toe-touch.

☑ Initiate physical therapy and exercises as prescribed.

☑ Use sequential compression devices or antiembolism stockings as ordered.

☑ For total hip replacement, prevent hip flexion greater than 90 degrees and adduction of the affected leg. Provide a seat riser for toilet or commode.

☑ Report signs of hip prosthesis dislocation, including pain or shortening and internal rotation of the affected leg.

☑ For total knee replacement, use a continuous passive range-of-motion (CPM) device or range-of-motion exercises as prescribed.

☑ When CPM is ordered, set prescribed degree of flexion and extension and speed of movement per manufacturer's instructions.

☑ With the machine in extension, pad the CPM with sheepskin before placing the extremity in the CPM. Adjust frame length and foot plate to the extremity; align joints with frame joints.

☑ Disable electric bed controls as indicated to maintain alignment of the extremity with the CPM. Elevate the head of the bed up to 20 degrees if allowed.

☑ Start CPM, observing rate, degree of flexion, and client responses. Maintain CPM as ordered, frequently assessing comfort, incision, skin condition, and neurovascular status.

☑ Reinforce teaching about postdischarge exercises and activity restrictions. Emphasize the importance of scheduled follow-up physician visits.

☑ Make referrals as needed to home health agencies and physical therapy.

BOX 43-10   **ASSESSMENT**

Assessing Clients with Osteoarthritis

SUBJECTIVE DATA

- Pain: location and characteristics; effect on ADLs (occupation, household tasks, activities, self-care, sleep/rest); relief measures used (analgesics, heat or cold, splinting or wrapping, rest)
- Changes in mobility; usual activities and any limitations
- Patterns of sleep/rest
- Coping with effects of joint pain, stiffness, and limited mobility

OBJECTIVE DATA

- Mobility: gait, ability to sit and rise from sitting, ability to step into and out of tub or shower, negotiate stairs
- Ability to perform ADLs: manipulate clothing for toileting, perform hygiene and grooming activities, feed self
- Joint swelling, redness, tenderness, warmth; range of motion
- Effect on function; observe ability to:
  - Comb hair, pick up and hold a utensil with each hand, write
  - With each leg, run heel of one foot down shin of opposite leg; stand from sitting position and walk
  - In sitting position, bend down to tie shoes

ASSESSING

Nursing assessment of the client with OA focuses on the effects of the disease on ADLs (functional assessment). Assessment data to collect for a client with OA are outlined in Box 43-10 ■.

DIAGNOSING, PLANNING, AND IMPLEMENTING

Priorities in Nursing Care. Teaching and assisting the client with osteoarthritis to manage discomfort and maintain mobility are the priorities for nursing care.

Chronic Pain

- Administer analgesic or anti-inflammatory medication as needed. *Analgesics reduce the perception of pain; anti-inflammatory drugs reduce local inflammation, swelling, and pain in affected joints.*
- Teach use of splints or other devices on affected joints as needed. *The pain of OA is often relieved by joint rest.*
- Apply heat to painful joints using the shower, a tub or sitz bath, warm packs, hot wax dips, heated gloves, or *diathermy,* which uses high-frequency electrical currents to generate heat. *Heat reduces muscle spasm, relieving pain. Moist heat penetrates deeper than dry heat; diathermy delivers heat to deeper body tissues.*

- Emphasize the importance of proper posture and good body mechanics for walking, sitting, lifting, and moving. *Good body mechanics and posture reduce stress on affected joints.*
- Encourage the overweight client to lose weight. *Excess weight places abnormal stress on joints, particularly the knees.*
- Encourage use of nonpharmacologic measures such as progressive relaxation, meditation, visualization, and distraction. *These adjunctive pain-relief measures can reduce muscle tension and spasm, promoting comfort.*

Impaired Physical Mobility

- Teach active and passive ROM exercises as well as isometric, progressive resistance exercises. *These exercises help maintain muscle tone and strength and mobility of affected joints and prevent contractures.*
- Encourage participation in low-impact aerobic exercises such as water aerobics. *Aerobic exercise improves endurance and cardiovascular fitness.*
- Provide analgesics or other pain-relief measures prior to exercise or ambulation. *With decreased pain, exercise tolerance improves.*
- Teach good body mechanics and encourage to avoid heavy lifting. *Good body mechanics reduce the stress on joints.*
- Encourage planned rest periods during the day. *Rest reduces fatigue, pain, and joint stress.*
- Teach use of ambulatory aids such as a cane or walker as ordered. *These devices help relieve some weight bearing and stress on affected joints.*

Self-Care Deficit

- Assist with ADLs as needed. *OA can significantly interfere with ADLs such as cooking, brushing hair, bathing, and toileting. Minimal assistance can promote self-esteem and as much independence as possible.*
- Refer to an occupational therapist for exercises and assistive devices. *The occupational therapist can identify measures that will help the client remain independent.*
- Help obtain assistive devices such as long-handled shoehorns, zipper grabbers, long-handled tongs or grippers for retrieving items from the floor, jar openers, and special eating utensils. *These devices can promote independence in performing ADLs.*

EVALUATING

To evaluate the effectiveness of nursing care, collect data regarding ability to manage pain, maintain mobility, and perform ADLs.

Documenting. Document assessment data and any changes from baseline assessment. Record level of pain and the effectiveness of anti-inflammatory medications to reduce pain. Note mobility and any restrictions or needed accommodations to maintain mobility.

CONTINUING CARE

With environmental modifications and assistive devices, the client with OA often can remain home and independent. Assess the home for hazards to mobility, such as scatter rugs. Identify the need for assistive devices such as handrails, grab bars, walk-in shower stall, or shower chair and handheld shower head. Help obtain and install assistive devices as indicated.

Teach ways to help maintain joint function and mobility:

- Exercise helps maintain joint mobility, and develops supportive muscles and tendons. Walking is an effective low-impact, aerobic exercise.
- Do not overuse or stress affected joints.
- Balance exercise with rest of affected joints.
- If obese, lose weight to decrease stress on weight-bearing joints.
- Sit in a straight chair without slumping; avoid soft chairs or recliners.
- Sleep on a firm mattress or use a bed board.

Teach about prescribed or over-the-counter medications for OA. Discuss their use, side effects, and any particular precautions specific to the medication. Discuss nonpharmacologic pain-relief measures such as heat, rest, massage, relaxation, and meditation.

If arthroplasty has been done, reinforce teaching about activity and weight bearing. Teach use of splints, braces, slings, or other devices to maintain the desired limb position during healing. Discuss assistive devices such as overhead trapeze for getting out of bed, elevated toilet seats, and chairs to use and avoid when sitting. Encourage practice of prescribed exercises. Observe and reinforce teaching as needed for using crutches or a walker.

Discuss possible complications, including signs of infection or dislocation, and instruct to notify the physician promptly if these occur. Refer for home care, physical or occupational therapy, or other community resources as indicated. See the Critical Thinking Care Map at the end of this chapter for an opportunity to use the nursing process to plan care for a client with osteoarthritis and total hip replacement.

Rheumatoid Arthritis

Rheumatoid arthritis (RA) is a chronic, systemic inflammatory disorder that primarily affects the joints. It is a connective tissue disorder that affects more women than men, and usually develops between the ages of 30 and 50 years. Usually, multiple joints are affected. The disease has periods of remission and exacerbation. RA is an autoimmune disorder of unknown cause. See Chapter 11 ⨀ for more information about autoimmune disorders.

PATHOPHYSIOLOGY AND MANIFESTATIONS

In rheumatoid arthritis, T lymphocytes (T cells) migrate to the joint and infiltrate the synovial membrane. An immune response is initiated, and IgG, an immunoglobulin, is produced. The body sees this as a foreign substance, and produces autoantibodies to the IgG. These autoantibodies, known as *rheumatoid factors,* bind with the IgG to form immune complexes. Complement is activated, and a variety of white blood cells are attracted to the area. These cells phagocytize immune complexes. In the process, they release enzymes that destroy joint tissue.

The resulting inflammation affects the joint and surrounding tissues. Affected joints are swollen, red, and painful. Joint tissue is destroyed by an extensive network of new blood vessels (vascular granulation tissue known as *pannus*) in the synovial membrane. Pannus erodes the cartilage and bone of affected joints and invades surrounding tissues, including ligaments and tendons (Figure 43-6 ■).

Rheumatoid arthritis is a systemic disease that affects other tissues as well as joints. Symptoms such as fatigue, anorexia, weight loss, and nonspecific aching and stiffness often occur before typical joint changes are evident. Joint manifestations of rheumatoid arthritis often develop slowly and insidiously. Joint swelling with stiffness, warmth, tenderness, and pain are typical. The pattern of joint involvement is usually *polyarticular* (involving multiple joints) and *symmetric.* The joint and systemic manifestations of RA are listed in Box 43-11 ■. Clinical features of RA and OA are compared in Table 43-4 ■.

The course of rheumatoid arthritis is variable and fluctuating. Early disease progression is more rapid than later in the disease. Destruction of affected joints and

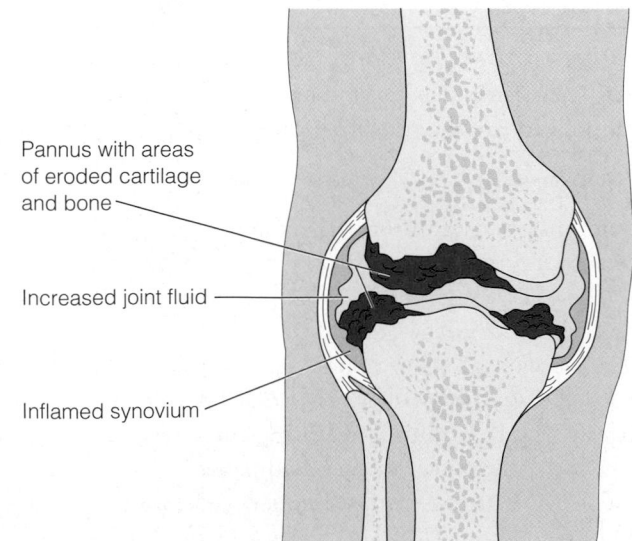

Pannus with areas of eroded cartilage and bone

Increased joint fluid

Inflamed synovium

Figure 43-6. ■ Joint inflammation and destruction in rheumatoid arthritis.

BOX 43-11

MANIFESTATIONS OF RHEUMATOID ARTHRITIS

Joint

- Swelling, warmth, tenderness, and pain; usually affects PIP and metacarpophalangeal (MCP) joints of fingers, wrists, knees, ankles, and toes
- Limited range of motion
- Morning stiffness lasting more than 1 hour
- Joint destruction and deformity (see Figure 43-7):
  - *Swan-neck deformity:* flexion of DIP joint with hyperextension of PIP joint
  - *Boutonnière deformity:* hyperextension of DIP joint with flexion of PIP joint
  - *Ulnar deviation* and *subluxation* of MCP joints
  - Carpal tunnel syndrome
  - Hallux valgus and hammertoe deformities of the foot

Systemic

- Fatigue, weakness
- Anorexia, weight loss
- Low-grade fever
- Anemia
- *Rheumatoid nodules:* firm subcutaneous tissue nodules over elbow, MCP joints, toes

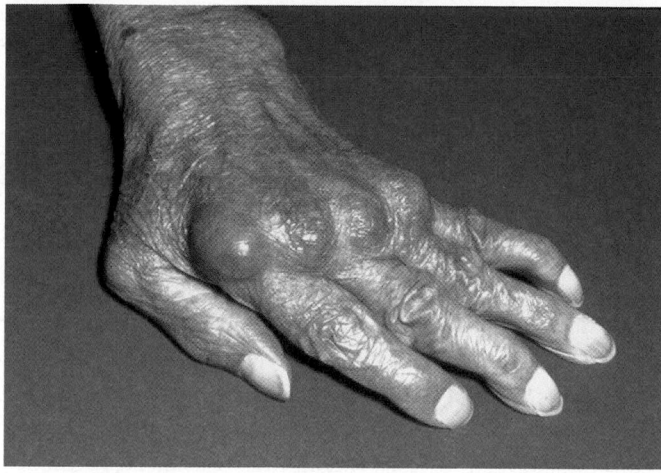

Figure 43-7. ■ Typical hand deformities associated with rheumatoid arthritis. (*Source:* Custom Medical Stock Photos, Inc.)

reduce joint destruction, and maintain function. A multidisciplinary approach is used, with a balance of rest, exercise, physical therapy, and treatments to modify the disease process. For the older adult, less emphasis may be placed on preventing joint deformity and more emphasis on maintaining function.

Diagnostic Tests

- *Rheumatoid factors (RF)* are present in most people with RA.
- *ESR* is typically elevated, often markedly.
- *Synovial fluid* aspirated from inflamed joints is analyzed.
- *X-ray* of affected joints shows characteristic joint changes as the disease progresses.

Rest and Exercise

During an acute disease flare, both joint and total body rest are ordered. Regular rest periods during the day are recommended. Inflamed joints may be splinted to provide local joint rest. Rest is balanced with physical therapy and

problems of immobility are the primary complications of RA (Figure 43-7 ■). Clients with severe RA may develop vasculitis (blood vessel inflammation), pleuritis (inflammation of the pleura covering the lungs), or pericarditis (inflammation of the pericardial covering of the heart).

INTERDISCIPLINARY CARE

The diagnosis of rheumatoid arthritis is based on the history, physical exam, and diagnostic tests. There currently is no cure for RA. Treatment goals are to relieve symptoms, stop or

TABLE 43-4

Characteristics of Rheumatoid Arthritis and Osteoarthritis

FEATURE	RHEUMATOID ARTHRITIS	OSTEOARTHRITIS
Onset	Usually insidious, may be abrupt	Insidious
Course	Often progressive, with remissions and exacerbations	Slowly progressive
Pain and stiffness	On arising, lasting > 1 hour; following prolonged immobility	Following activity or periods of immobility; short duration
Affected joints	Red, hot, swollen; tender to palpation; decreased ROM Multiple joints affected	May be swollen; cool and bony hard to palpation; decreased ROM One or several joints affected
Systemic manifestations	Fatigue, weakness, anorexia, weight loss, fever, anemia	Fatigue

exercise to maintain muscle strength and joint mobility. Range-of-motion exercises are ordered to maintain joint function and prevent contractures. Isometric, isotonic, and low-impact aerobic exercises such as swimming and walking also may be ordered.

Medications

A variety of drugs and drug groups are used to manage RA. Aspirin and other NSAIDs and mild analgesics are used to reduce inflammation and manage the signs and symptoms of the disease (see Table 43-5 ■). Because some NSAIDs have been associated with an increased risk for heart attack, they are used with caution. The class of NSAIDs known as COX-2 inhibitors appears to carry the highest risk for heart disease;

they may, however, be prescribed when other NSAIDs have been ineffective or the client is unable to tolerate the gastrointestinal effects of other NSAIDs. Corticosteroids may also be used to reduce acute pain and inflammation. A diverse group of drugs called disease-modifying or slow-acting antirheumatic drugs appears to alter the disease course and reduce joint destruction. Drugs such as leflunomide (Arava) and etanercept (Enbrel) modify the autoimmune and inflammatory responses to RA. Gold salts can cause remission of the disease. Other disease-modifying drugs used to treat RA include hydroxychloroquine (Plaquenil), an antimalarial agent, sulfasalazine, and penicillamine. Immunosuppressive or cytotoxic drugs may be used to manage RA when the disease is aggressive or unresponsive to other medications.

TABLE 43-5

Nursing Implications for Pharmacology: Rheumatoid Arthritis

DRUG/CLASSIFICATION	DESCRIPTION	NURSING RESPONSIBILITIES	CLIENT TEACHING
Aspirin ■ Acetylsalicylic acid, aspirin, Ecotrin, Empirin, others	Aspirin inhibits prostaglandin synthesis and activity, reducing inflammation. It also has an analgesic and antipyretic effect. It inhibits platelet aggregation and normal blood clotting. Doses of up to 3.6 to 4.8 g/day are required for the best anti-inflammatory effect.	Assess for contraindications such as allergy or bleeding disorders. Give crushed or whole with food or milk to prevent gastric irritation. Do not crush enteric-coated or sustained-release forms. Stop the drug and notify the doctor if rash, hives, or signs of gastrointestinal bleeding develop.	Always take with food or milk. If gastric upset or nausea develops, try enteric-coated aspirin. Do not substitute acetaminophen for aspirin because it does not have anti-inflammatory effects. Report dark stools, vomiting of blood, abnormal bleeding, blurred vision, ringing in the ears, rashes, or difficulty breathing to your doctor. Check labels of other over-the-counter drugs carefully; many contain aspirin. Do not use alcohol while taking aspirin; it greatly increases the risk of gastrointestinal bleeding.
Other Nonsteroidal Anti-Inflammatory Drugs (NSAIDs) ■ Ibuprofen (Motrin, others) ■ Indomethacin (Indocin) ■ Ketoprofen (Orudis) ■ Naproxen (Anaprox, Naprosyn) ■ Piroxicam (Feldene) ■ Sulindac (Clinoril) ■ Tolmetin (Tolectin) ■ Others	NSAIDs are used to manage arthritis and other causes of inflammation. Although each is different, all inhibit prostaglandin synthesis, reducing inflammation. More costly than aspirin, they may allow fewer daily doses to be effective. For most, adverse effects are similar to aspirin. All NSAIDs may increase the risk of heart attack or stroke when used in large doses for a long time.	Obtain baseline weight and vital signs. Carefully monitor clients who are elderly or have reduced kidney function for toxicity. Give with food or milk to minimize gastric effects. Report possible adverse effects such as GI bleeding; impaired renal function; and CNS effects.	Take as ordered to maintain a constant blood level for the best effect. It may take several weeks for the full effect to occur. Take with food or milk. Weigh weekly; report sudden weight gain of more than 3 to 5 pounds to your doctor. Report changes in vision, hearing, mood, urination; or bloody urine, bloody vomit; or blood in stool to your doctor. Avoid alcohol and aspirin while taking NSAIDs. Use acetaminophen as needed for pain relief.
Second-Generation NSAIDs: COX-2 Inhibitors ■ Celecoxib (Celebrex) ■ Rofecoxib (Vioxx)	COX-2 inhibitors are NSAIDs that suppress inflammation and pain. They are associated with an increased risk for heart attack and stroke when used long term.	Assess for contraindications such as allergy to aspirin or other NSAIDs or advanced kidney disease Administer by mouth without regard to meals.	Take with a full glass of water; stay upright for 15–30 minutes after taking. Promptly notify your doctor if you develop abdominal pain, tarry stools, rash, edema, or unexplained weight gain. Notify your doctor if you are or plan to become pregnant.

Methotrexate is the most commonly used immunosuppressive drug; others include cyclosporine, azathioprine, and monoclonal antibodies. Treatment with immunosuppressive drugs increases the risk for infection and certain cancers.

Surgery

Surgery may be done to relieve pain and repair or replace joints damaged by RA. *Arthrodesis* (joint fusion) may be used to stabilize joints such as cervical vertebrae, wrists, and ankles. Arthroplasty, or total joint replacement, may be necessary in cases of gross deformity and joint destruction. Total joint replacement and nursing care needs of clients undergoing this surgery were discussed in the previous section on osteoarthritis.

Other Therapies

Several newer treatments may be used to treat progressive RA. *Plasmapheresis* may be used to remove circulating antibodies, moderating the autoimmune response. *Total lymphoid irradiation,* another option, decreases total lymphocyte levels.

For most clients with rheumatoid arthritis, an ordinary, well-balanced diet is recommended. Some clients may benefit from substituting usual dietary fat with omega-3 fatty acids found in certain fish oils.

NURSING CARE

Clients with rheumatoid arthritis have multiple nursing care needs involving all functional health patterns. In addition to its physical manifestations, the disease also has many psychosocial effects. It is an incurable chronic disease that may lead to severe crippling. Pain and fatigue can interfere with the ability to perform expected roles, such as home maintenance or job responsibilities. Other people may not understand the systemic nature of the RA or realize the difference between rheumatoid arthritis and osteoarthritis.

ASSESSING

Assessment of the client with RA focuses on the progress of the disease and on its effect on functional abilities (see Box 43-12 in the continuing care section that follows). To assess the status of the disease, collect data such as the following:

- Pain level; number of affected joints
- Duration of morning stiffness
- Redness, heat, and swelling of affected joints
- Other symptoms such as fatigue, weakness, anorexia, fever.

DIAGNOSING, PLANNING, AND IMPLEMENTING

Priorities in Nursing Care. Rheumatoid arthritis is a chronic, systemic disease. Nursing care priorities are on relieving pain and discomfort, managing fatigue, and teaching the client how to live with the disease.

Pain

The pain of active RA is constant. It affects self-care, ADLs, and contributes to fatigue.

- Encourage to adjust activities according to pain level. *Pain is an indicator of stress on inflamed joints. Increasing pain indicates a need to decrease activity.*
- Teach use of heat or cold for pain relief. A warm shower, tub bath, warm compresses, or paraffin dips can be used to apply heat. If heat increases pain and swelling during periods of acute inflammation, cold packs may be more effective. *Both heat and cold have analgesic effects and can help relieve associated muscle spasms.*
- Discuss the importance of taking anti-inflammatory medications as ordered, and the relationship between inflammation and pain. *Anti-inflammatory agents reduce chemical mediators of inflammation and swelling, relieving pain.*
- Encourage use of other nonpharmacologic pain-relief measures such as visualization, distraction, meditation, and progressive relaxation techniques. *These techniques can reduce muscle tension and help the client focus away from the pain, decreasing the intensity of the pain experience. See Chapter 8 ∞ for further discussion of adjunctive pain-relief measures.*

Fatigue

- Encourage a balance of activity with periods of rest. Stress the importance of planned rest periods during the day. *Both joint and whole-body rest are important to reduce the inflammatory response.*
- Assist to prioritize activities, scheduling the most important ones early in the day. *Prioritizing allows the client to maintain activities that are meaningful and important.*
- Encourage to engage in regular physical activity in addition to ordered ROM exercises. *Aerobic exercise promotes a sense of well-being and restful sleep.*
- Help identify tasks that can be delegated to others. *Enlisting the help of family and friends can help the client maintain those activities that are important.*

Ineffective Role Performance

- Discuss effects of the disease on career and other life roles. *Discussion helps the client accept changes and begin to identify strategies for coping with them.*
- Encourage discussion of feelings about the disease and its effect on client and family roles. *Open discussion helps family members identify and accept feelings about losses and changes.*
- Listen actively to concerns, acknowledging their validity. *Demonstrating acceptance of these feelings and concerns promotes trust.*
- Help identify strengths to use in coping with role changes. *Past coping strategies and family strengths can be used to deal with necessary role changes.*
- Encourage client to make decisions and assume personal responsibility for disease management. *Clients who assume*

an active role in managing their disease maintain a greater sense of self-control and self-esteem.

- Encourage to maintain life roles to the extent possible. *Maintaining roles helps the client cope with this chronic and potentially crippling disease.*
- Refer to counseling or support groups. *Counseling and support groups can help the client and family develop effective coping strategies.*

Disturbed Body Image

- Demonstrate a caring, accepting attitude. *This helps the client accept physical changes caused by RA and avoid feelings of hopelessness or powerlessness.*
- Encourage discussion about the effects of RA, both physical and psychosocial. *Verbalization helps the client identify feelings and provides an opportunity to validate these feelings.*
- Involve client in decision making and provide choices whenever possible. *Autonomy enhances the sense of control.*
- Discuss clothing and adaptive devices that promote independence. *Independence enhances self-esteem.*
- Provide positive feedback for self-care activities and adaptive strategies. *Positive reinforcement encourages the client to continue adaptive measures and maintain independence.*
- Refer to self-help groups, support groups, the Arthritis Foundation, and other agencies for assistive devices and literature. *These groups can help the client develop strategies to cope with the effects of RA, enhancing self-concept, body image, and independence.*

EVALUATING

To evaluate the effectiveness of nursing care for a client with RA, collect data such as quality and quantity of rest; effective use of NSAIDs and analgesics; ability to maintain ADLs and usual roles; statements about body image and coping with disease effects.

Documenting. Document continuing assessment data, including the appearance, swelling, and movement of inflamed joints. Record fatigue level and the ability of the client to perform ADLs. Document all teaching provided, and the client's and family's understanding and acceptance of information. Note specific instructions for medication use, recommended activity, and measures to rest inflamed joints.

CONTINUING CARE

The client has the primary responsibility for managing rheumatoid arthritis. Assessment and teaching are vital to prepare for this responsibility. Box 43-12 ■ outlines assessment data to collect related to home care.

Teach about the disease and its systemic effects. Stress the importance of following all aspects of the treatment plan. Encourage active involvement in planning care.

BOX 43-12 **ASSESSMENT**

Assessing for Discharge: Rheumatoid Arthritis

CLIENT
- Ability to perform ADLs; need for help or assistive devices; ability to cope with activity limitations and economic effects; acceptance of assistance from others
- Understanding of rheumatoid arthritis and its effects; prescribed medications; activity and rest recommendations; long-term prognosis
- Home environment: stairs, environmental barriers that limit independence (e.g., small bathrooms, deep tubs for bathing); energy-saving features (such as easily loaded clothes washer and dryer, easy-to-clean floors)

FAMILY AND CAREGIVERS
- Ability and willingness to assist with ADLs and household tasks; acceptance of rest needs and altered roles and relationships
- Financial resources for prescribed drugs and treatments

COMMUNITY
- Availability of home health services; access to public transportation, medical services, pharmacies
- Support groups and other resources

Help identify strategies to balance rest and exercise. Instruct to reduce exercise and increase rest if pain and stiffness increase. Teach to use heat and cold to promote comfort and activity.

Teach about prescribed medications. Emphasize the need to take NSAIDs as ordered, not on an as-needed basis for pain. Review Table 43-5 for additional client and family teaching about NSAIDs. Emphasize the importance of keeping regular follow-up appointments to monitor the disease and treatment.

Suggest assistive devices to maintain independence. Include ambulatory aids, such as canes and walkers, and self-care aids, such as handheld showers, long-handled brushes and shoe horns, and eating utensils with oversized or special handles. Discuss clothing options to help maintain independence, such as elastic waist pants without zippers, Velcro closures, zippers with large pull tabs, and slip-on shoes. Refer to local and community agencies as indicated.

clinical ALERT

Remember that the client with rheumatoid arthritis is vulnerable to quackery and unproven alternative treatment strategies. Maintain open lines of communication to encourage discussion of these options and possible experimental therapies with the treatment team.

NURSING PROCESS CARE PLAN
Client with Rheumatoid Arthritis

Janice James, 42 years old, first noticed vague joint pain, fatigue, poor appetite, and general malaise about 6 weeks ago. Her symptoms have continued, and she reports feeling very stiff in the mornings, often lasting until 10:00 or 11:00 A.M. She sees her nurse practitioner (NP) when she notices that her knuckles and finger joints are not just achy but also swollen and hot. The NP tentatively diagnoses rheumatoid arthritis and refers Mrs. James to a rheumatology clinic.

Assessment. Mrs. James's past medical history reveals only the usual childhood diseases and three uncomplicated pregnancies and deliveries. Mrs. James states that she is allergic to penicillin.

Objective assessment data reveals swelling of PIP and MCP joints of both hands. The second and third PIP and second MCP joints on the right hand appear red and shiny, and are hot, spongy, and tender to palpation. Mrs. James can extend her fingers to 180 degrees but cannot make a complete fist with either hand. Her grip strength is weak bilaterally. Wrist ROM is limited in all directions. Mrs. James's knees also appear swollen, and flexion is slightly limited.

Blood work shows ESR 52 mm/hr and hematocrit 30%. She has a positive rheumatoid factor.

Diagnosis. The following nursing diagnoses are identified for Mrs. James:

- *Pain* related to joint inflammation
- *Impaired Home Maintenance* related to fatigue
- *Activity Intolerance* related to the effects of inflammation
- *Risk for Noncompliance* with therapeutic regimen related to lack of information and understanding

Expected Outcomes. The expected outcomes are that Mrs. James will:

- Verbalize effective pain-management strategies.
- Verbalize a plan to reduce her responsibilities for home maintenance.
- Express a willingness to plan rest breaks during the day.
- Demonstrate understanding of the prescribed treatment and the importance of compliance for both short- and long-term benefit.

Planning and Implementation. The following nursing interventions are implemented over the first 6 weeks of Mrs. James's care at the rheumatology clinic:

- Teach ways to relieve pain and morning stiffness, including:
  a. Take NSAIDs at equal intervals throughout the day.
  b. Take morning NSAID dose with milk and crackers about 30 minutes before arising.
  c. Perform ROM exercises in shower or bathtub.
- Teach ways to minimize joint stress while performing ADLs.
- Discuss delegation of household tasks to other family members.
- Explore ways to incorporate 30-minute rest breaks into work schedule.
- Reinforce teaching about disease process, prescribed drugs and their effects, and the importance of balanced rest and exercise.

Evaluation. After 6 months, Mrs. James's "morning sickness" now lasts about 45 minutes, and her hand and wrist ROM have improved. She has had difficulty scheduling rest periods at work and has had to struggle to delegate household tasks. "I don't look sick to the kids, and they seem to think housecleaning is a terrible imposition on their time. It's often easier to just do it myself than to fight about it. Besides, that way it gets done right." Mrs. James has faithfully followed her treatment plan, keeping her scheduled appointments and maintaining contact with the treatment team.

Critical Thinking in the Nursing Process

1. Explain the normal inflammatory process and relate this to the inflammatory joint changes Mrs. James experienced. Discuss the systemic effects of inflammation on Mrs. James as well.
2. When Mrs. James experiences an acute exacerbation of her disease 1 year later, the rheumatologist orders prednisone, 40 mg daily. The effect is dramatic in relieving Mrs. James's pain and stiffness. She asks why the physician did not prescribe this drug in the first place. How will you respond?
3. Following Mrs. James's acute exacerbation, the rheumatologist prescribes methotrexate. What short- and long-term adverse effects of this drug will you teach Mrs. James about?

Systemic Lupus Erythematosus

Systemic lupus erythematosus (SLE) is a chronic inflammatory connective tissue disease. SLE affects multiple body systems. It can range in severity from mild and episodic to a rapidly fatal disease.

SLE is much more common in women than in men and in Asians and Hispanics. It is more common and severe in people of African ancestry. Its cause is unknown, but genetic, environmental, and hormonal factors play a role in its development.

PATHOPHYSIOLOGY

In SLE, autoantibodies are produced that target normal body cells and cell components such as DNA, blood cells, and proteins involved in normal coagulation. These autoantibodies react with their corresponding antigen to

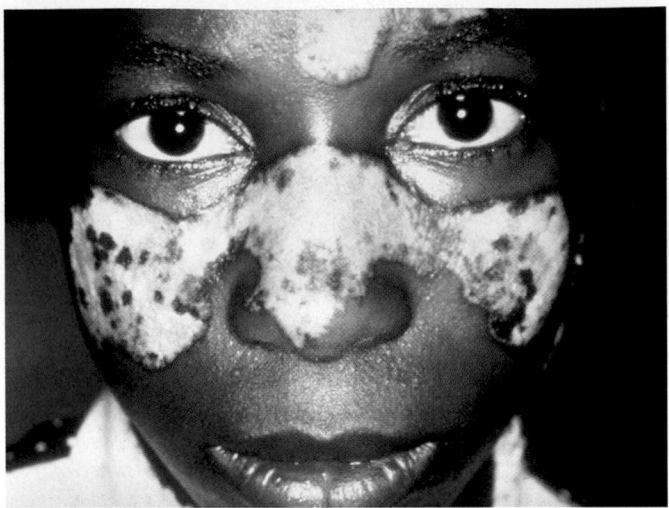

Figure 43-8. ■ The butterfly rash of systemic lupus erythematosus. (*Source:* Photo Researchers, Inc.)

form immune complexes, which are then deposited in the connective tissue of blood vessels, lymphatic vessels, and other tissues. This causes an inflammatory response that damages the tissues. Immune complexes frequently are de-

posited in and damage the kidneys. Other affected tissues include the musculoskeletal system, brain, heart, spleen, lung, GI tract, skin, and peritoneum.

MANIFESTATIONS AND COMPLICATIONS

Early in the disease, the manifestations of SLE mimic those of rheumatoid arthritis, including fever, anorexia, malaise, weight loss, and joint pain, inflammation, and stiffness. Skin manifestations are common. SLE was named for its characteristic red *butterfly rash* across the cheeks and bridge of the nose (Figure 43-8 ■). This rash was thought to resemble the bite of a wolf, hence *lupus* (wolf) *erythematosus* (red). Many clients with SLE are photosensitive. A diffuse rash on skin exposed to the sun is common. Because SLE affects many body systems, its manifestations can be diverse (Figure 43-9 ■).

The course of SLE is mild and chronic in most clients, with periods of remission and exacerbation. The number and severity of exacerbations tend to decrease with time.

Clients with SLE often have difficulty carrying a pregnancy to term. They also have an increased risk for infections, which may be severe. Infections such as pneumonia and septicemia are the leading cause of death in clients with SLE, followed by the effects of kidney or central nervous system involvement.

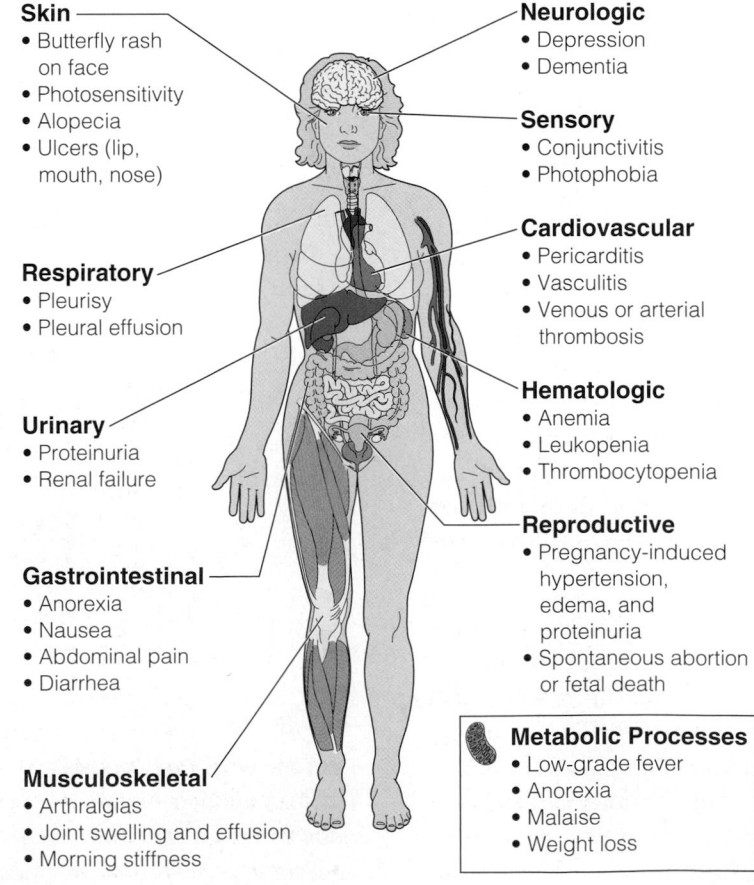

Skin
• Butterfly rash on face
• Photosensitivity
• Alopecia
• Ulcers (lip, mouth, nose)

Respiratory
• Pleurisy
• Pleural effusion

Urinary
• Proteinuria
• Renal failure

Gastrointestinal
• Anorexia
• Nausea
• Abdominal pain
• Diarrhea

Musculoskeletal
• Arthralgias
• Joint swelling and effusion
• Morning stiffness

Neurologic
• Depression
• Dementia

Sensory
• Conjunctivitis
• Photophobia

Cardiovascular
• Pericarditis
• Vasculitis
• Venous or arterial thrombosis

Hematologic
• Anemia
• Leukopenia
• Thrombocytopenia

Reproductive
• Pregnancy-induced hypertension, edema, and proteinuria
• Spontaneous abortion or fetal death

Metabolic Processes
• Low-grade fever
• Anorexia
• Malaise
• Weight loss

Figure 43-9. ■ The multisystem effects of systemic lupus erythematosus.

INTERDISCIPLINARY CARE

The diagnosis of SLE is based on the history and physical exam, along with diagnostic tests. As with RA, effective management requires teamwork, with active participation by the client and the health care team.

Diagnostic Tests

- *Antinuclear antibodies (ANA)* are identified. While virtually all clients with SLE have positive ANA tests, so do many clients who do not have SLE.
- *Anti-DNA antibody testing* is a more specific indicator of SLE.
- *C-reactive protein (CRP)* levels are elevated during acute exacerbations.
- The *erythrocyte sedimentation rate (ESR)* often is elevated, and the CBC shows anemia and low RBC, WBC, and platelet counts.
- *Urinalysis* and renal function studies such as the *serum creatinine* and *blood urea nitrogen (BUN)* may be ordered to assess for kidney damage.

Medications

Aspirin and NSAIDs often are used to manage joint pain and inflammation, fever, and fatigue. Table 43-5 outlined nursing responsibilities for aspirin and NSAIDs. The antiplatelet actions of aspirin make it particularly useful for clients with SLE, because it also helps prevent thrombosis. Antimalarial drugs such as hydroxychloroquine (Plaquenil) may be ordered. Hydroxychloroquine can damage the retina of the eye; for this reason, an ophthalmologic exam is done every 6 months during treatment.

Corticosteroid drugs are used to treat severe and life-threatening manifestations of SLE. Some clients require long-term corticosteroid therapy to manage symptoms and prevent major organ damage. These clients have a high risk for corticosteroid side effects, such as cushingoid effects, weight gain, hypertension, infection, accelerated osteoporosis, and hypokalemia. See Chapter 11 ∞ for more information about corticosteroid therapy and its nursing implications. Immunosuppressive agents may be used alone or in combination with corticosteroids. These drugs increase the risk for infection and malignancy, and have other toxic effects.

Other Therapies

Because of the photosensitivity associated with SLE, sun exposure should be avoided. Sunscreens with a sun protection factor (SPF) rating of 15 or higher are recommended when out of doors. Some physicians recommend avoiding oral contraceptives, because estrogen can trigger an acute episode of SLE.

Clients with lupus nephritis who develop end-stage renal disease are treated with dialysis (hemodialysis or peritoneal dialysis) and kidney transplantation. These treatment strategies are discussed in Chapter 32. ∞

NURSING CARE

Many of the nursing care needs and priorities for the client with SLE are similar to those for clients with rheumatoid arthritis. This section focuses on the needs related to dermatologic symptoms of lupus, the increased risk for infection, and health maintenance problems.

Impaired Skin Integrity

Skin lesions are a common manifestation of SLE. They disrupt skin integrity and can be disfiguring.

- Discuss the relationship between sun exposure and disease activity, both dermatologic and systemic. *It is important for the client to understand that sun exposure can worsen both skin and systemic manifestations of SLE.*
- Help identify strategies to limit sun exposure:
  a. Avoid being outside when sun is most intense (10:00 A.M. to 3:00 P.M.).
  b. Use sunscreen with an SPF of 15 or higher.
  c. Reapply sunscreen after swimming, exercising, or bathing.
  d. Wear loose clothing with long sleeves and wide-brimmed hats when outside.
  These strategies can help the client maintain a normal lifestyle while helping to prevent acute episodes.
- Keep skin clean and dry; apply therapeutic creams or ointments to lesions as ordered. *These measures promote healing and reduce the risk of infection.*

Ineffective Protection

- Wash hands on entering room and before providing direct care. *Hand washing is the best defense against transmitting infection.*
- Use strict sterile technique in caring for intravenous lines and indwelling urinary catheters or performing any wound care. *Aseptic technique reduces the risk of contamination by microorganisms.*
- Monitor temperature and vital signs every 4 hours. Report signs of infection, including tenderness, redness, swelling, and warmth. *Prompt identification of an infection allows early initiation of appropriate treatment.*
- Report abnormal laboratory values. *Increased WBCs may indicate infection; changes in liver or renal function studies, myocardial enzymes, or other laboratory values may indicate organ system involvement.*
- If necessary, use protective isolation. *Treatment with corticosteroids or immunosuppressive agents impairs the ability to fight infection. Protective isolation may be necessary to prevent infection.*
- Instruct family members and visitors to avoid direct contact with the client when they are ill. *A "minor" upper respiratory infection can be a significant illness for the client with SLE.*

- Help ensure adequate food intake, offering supplementary feedings as indicated or maintaining parenteral nutrition if necessary. *Adequate nutrition is important for healing and immune system function.*
- Teach the importance of good hand washing after using the bathroom and before eating. *Hand washing reduces the risk of infection with endogenous organisms.*
- Provide good mouth care. *Good oral hygiene reduces the risk of infection from oral bacteria.*

CONTINUING CARE

Teach about SLE and its potential effects. Both physical manifestations of SLE and psychosocial issues can affect the ability to effectively manage the disease. Encourage discussion about the impact of the disease. Refer the client and family to counseling as needed. Provide information about community and social service agencies, and local support groups.

Discuss the importance of skin care. Instruct to avoid irritating soaps, shampoos, or chemicals (e.g., hair dyes and permanent wave solution) to prevent excessive drying of the skin. Encourage use of hypoallergenic products. Stress the importance of limiting sun exposure, particularly between 10:00 A.M. and 3:00 P.M. Encourage use of appropriate sunscreen and the wearing of long sleeves and wide-brimmed hats. For clients with hair loss, discuss using wigs, turbans, or other head coverings. Remind that the hair will regrow during remission.

Stress the importance of avoiding exposure to infection. Encourage to avoid crowds and infectious people. Teach the importance of adequate rest and nutrition and avoiding stress to increase resistance to infection.

Teach about treatment plan, including rest and exercise, medications, and follow-up appointments. Stress the importance of contacting the physician promptly if symptoms of an exacerbation develop. Encourage to wear a Medic-Alert bracelet or tag with their condition and therapy such as corticosteroids or immunosuppressives.

Discuss family planning. Oral contraceptives may be contraindicated; provide information about alternative means of birth control. Pregnancy is not contraindicated; however, the client should tell her women's health care practitioner about her SLE and notify her primary care physician of her pregnancy.

Gout

Gout is a metabolic disorder that leads to accumulation of urate crystals in joints and surrounding tissues. It affects more men than women, and its incidence increases with age.

Gout may be primary or secondary. *Primary gout* is a genetic disorder characterized by elevated serum uric acid levels. It is the most common form of gout. In *secondary gout*, uric acid levels increase due to another disorder or treatment with certain drugs. Disorders such as leukemia, chronic renal disease, and diabetic ketoacidosis can raise uric acid levels, as can drugs such as some diuretics and antituberculosis drugs. Alcohol ingestion also increases serum uric acid levels.

PATHOPHYSIOLOGY AND MANIFESTATIONS

Uric acid is the breakdown product of purine metabolism. Normally, a balance exists between the production and excretion of uric acid, with most of what is produced each day excreted via the kidneys and the rest in the feces. The serum uric acid level is normally between 3.4 and 7.0 mg/dL in men and 2.4 and 6.0 mg/dL in women. At levels greater than 7.0 mg/dL, urate crystals may form. Crystals tend to form in peripheral tissues of the body, where lower temperatures reduce the solubility of the uric acid.

Unless treated, gout may progress from *asymptomatic hyperuricemia,* with high serum uric acid levels but no symptoms, to *acute gouty arthritis.* The acute attack, usually affecting a single joint, occurs unexpectedly, often beginning at night. About half of initial attacks are in the joint of the great toe. The affected joint becomes red, hot, swollen, and exquisitely painful and tender. The client also may have fever, chills, and general malaise.

Acute attacks last from days up to several weeks and typically subside spontaneously. The interval between acute attacks is called the *intercritical period.* It may last years, although most people have another acute attack within 1 year. In *chronic tophaceous gout,* deposits of urate crystals known as tophi develop in cartilage, synovial membranes, tendons, and soft tissues. Tophi may be seen in the helix of the ear and on the extremities. The skin over tophi may ulcerate. Tophi can also develop in the tissues of the heart and spinal epidura. In some cases, uric acid stones may form in the kidney.

INTERDISCIPLINARY CARE

The classic presentation of acute gout is so distinctive that the diagnosis often is based on the history and physical exam. *Serum uric acid* is nearly always elevated, usually above 7.5 mg/dL. Fluid aspirated from the inflamed joint shows typical needle-shaped urate crystals.

Treatment focuses on relieving an acute attack and preventing recurrent attacks.

Medications

NSAIDs are used to treat an acute attack of gout. Indomethacin (Indocin) is the most frequently used NSAID for gout. Aspirin is avoided because it may interfere with uric acid excretion. Review Table 43-5 for nursing implications for NSAIDs.

Colchicine, a drug that inhibits the deposition of urate crystals in tissues, also may be ordered to stop an acute attack. The use of colchicine, however, is limited by side effects such as abdominal cramping, diarrhea, nausea, or vomiting. Colchicine

TABLE 43-6

Nursing Implications for Pharmacology: Gout

DRUG/CLASSIFICATION	DESCRIPTION	NURSING RESPONSIBILITIES	CLIENT TEACHING
Colchicine	Colchicine prevents urate crystals from being deposited in tissues. It does not lower serum uric acid levels. It is available in combination with a uricosuric agent, probenecid. Plain colchicine is used to treat an acute attack of gout; combination therapy is used to prevent further attacks.	Assess for contraindications, such as serious GI, kidney, liver, or heart disease. Administer by mouth on an empty stomach. Report nausea, vomiting, or diarrhea to the physician; these side effects may require stopping the drug.	Drink 3–4 quarts of liquid per day. Report reactions such as GI distress, fatigue, bleeding, easy bruising, or recurrent infections to your doctor. Avoid using alcohol while you are taking this drug.
Uricosuric Drugs ■ Probenecid (Benemid)	Probenecid inhibits the tubular reabsorption of urate, increasing the excretion of uric acid and decreasing serum uric acid levels.	Give after meals or with milk. Monitor intake and output. Increase fluid intake to at least 3 L/day. Report adverse effects such as headache, dizziness, nausea and vomiting, flank pain, fever, hives, pruritus, and abnormal lab values.	Do not take aspirin or products containing aspirin while taking probenecid. Use acetaminophen for relief of mild pain. Drink at least 3 quarts of fluids per day.
■ Sulfinpyrazone (Anturane)	Sulfinpyrazone improves uric acid excretion, reducing serum uric acid levels. It is used to prevent recurrent attacks of acute gout and treat chronic gout.	Give with meals or antacid. Monitor diabetic clients for hypoglycemia. Monitor for bleeding in clients receiving warfarin. Encourage fluid intake of at least 3 L/day. Do not give concurrently with aspirin. Report signs of peptic ulcer disease to the physician promptly.	Drink at least 3 quarts of fluid per day. Take with meals to minimize gastric distress. Do not take aspirin; use acetaminophen for relief of mild pain. Report epigastric pain, nausea, or black stools to the physician promptly. Discontinue the drug immediately.
Allopurinol (Zyloprim)	Allopurinol reduces uric acid production, lowering serum uric acid levels. It is used for clients with manifestations of primary or secondary gout.	Monitor intake and output. Increase fluids to 3 L/day. Report adverse effects such as nausea, diarrhea, and rash. Give with meals. Report abnormal kidney and liver function tests, CBC, and prothrombin time or INR to the physician. Discontinue drug and notify the physician immediately if a rash develops.	Stop the drug and report skin rash, painful urination, bloody urine, eye irritation, or swelling of lips or mouth to your doctor. Take after meals. Drink 3–4 liters of fluid daily. Report abnormal bleeding, bruising, fatigue, pallor, sore throat, or frequent infections to your doctor. Acute gout may occur when you start this drug; continue drug as ordered. Do not take a double dose if you miss a dose. Use caution when driving, operating machinery, or performing other activities that require alertness; may cause drowsiness.

may be used in smaller doses (with fewer side effects) to prevent attacks of gout.

Drugs to promote uric acid excretion or block its production may be ordered to prevent attacks. *Uricosuric* drugs block reabsorption of uric acid in the kidney tubules, promoting its excretion and reducing serum levels. Allopurinol affects purine metabolism, decreasing the production of uric acid (see Table 43-6 ■).

Other Therapies

During an acute attack of gout, bed rest is ordered. It is continued for about 24 hours after the attack has subsided.

The affected joint may be elevated, and hot or cold compresses may be applied for comfort.

A liberal fluid intake (3 or more liters per day) is ordered. Sodium bicarbonate or potassium citrate may be ordered to minimize the risk of uric acid renal stones.

clinical ALERT

Carefully monitor clients receiving sodium bicarbonate or potassium citrate for fluid and electrolyte or acid–base imbalances (see Chapter 7). ⚭

Often, no specific diet is recommended. The obese client is advised to lose weight, but fasting is contraindicated. Alcohol intake and specific foods that tend to precipitate attacks are avoided.

NURSING CARE

Priorities in Nursing Care. Pain is a primary focus for nursing assessment and interventions during an acute attack of gout.

Acute Pain

- Ask client to rate pain using a standard pain scale. Note the location and quality of the pain. *Acute gout causes exquisite tenderness of the affected joint. Accurate assessment of pain facilitates evaluation of treatment measures.*
- Position for comfort. Elevate the joint or extremity (usually the great toe) on a pillow, maintaining alignment. *Elevating the joint improves blood return, relieving some of the edema.*
- Protect the affected joint from pressure, using a foot cradle to keep covers off the foot. *Affected joints are so tender that even the weight of a sheet can be unbearable.*
- Administer prescribed anti-inflammatory and antigout medications as ordered. In the initial period, colchicine may be given hourly. *These medications reduce the acute inflammatory response, gradually relieving discomfort.*
- Administer analgesics as prescribed. *Analgesics often are ordered until the acute inflammation is relieved.*
- Monitor for desired and adverse effects of medications. Report adverse effects to the physician. *Anti-inflammatory and antigout medications can have significant side effects that may require a change of therapy.*
- Maintain bed rest. *Rest and immobilizing the affected joint help reduce joint inflammation.*

CONTINUING CARE

Without appropriate treatment between episodes of acute gout, recurrences are likely. Teaching is a vital nursing responsibility for the client with gout.

Teach about the disease and its manifestations. Advise that initial attacks cause no permanent damage but recurrent attacks can lead to permanent damage and joint destruction. Discuss other potential effects of continued hyperuricemia, including tophaceous deposits in subcutaneous and other connective tissues. Discuss the risk for kidney damage and stones.

Teach about prescribed medications. Stress the need to continue medications until discontinued by the physician, even if there are no symptoms. Discuss potential side effects of the drugs, and their management. Instruct to drink about 3 quarts of fluid per day and to avoid using alcohol. Instruct to avoid over-the-counter medications without talking to the physician. Encourage to keep scheduled follow-up appointments.

Lyme Disease

Lyme disease is an inflammatory disorder caused by a spirochete, *Borrelia burgdorferi,* which is usually spread by ticks. It is the most commonly reported tick-borne illness in the United States. Although Lyme disease is usually seen in children, adults also can be affected. Geographically, Lyme disease is more common in the Northeast, upper Midwest, and along the Pacific Coast. Ticks that act as vectors for Lyme disease are usually carried by mice or deer. The usual time of onset is the summer months.

PATHOPHYSIOLOGY AND MANIFESTATIONS

Borrelia burgdorferi enters the skin at the site of the tick bite. After an incubation period of up to 30 days, it migrates outward in the skin, forming a characteristic lesion called *erythema migrans.* It may spread via lymph or blood to other skin sites, nodes, or organs.

Erythema migrans is the initial manifestation of Lyme disease. This flat or slightly raised red lesion at the site of the tick bite expands over several days (up to a diameter of 50 cm), with the central area clearing as it expands. Systemic symptoms such as fatigue, malaise, fever, chills, and muscle pain often accompany the initial lesion. As the disease spreads, secondary skin lesions develop, as do migratory musculoskeletal symptoms, including muscle and joint pain, and tendonitis. Headache and stiff neck are common. If untreated, the client may develop chronic arthritis, myocarditis, meningitis, encephalitis, and other neurologic manifestations.

INTERDISCIPLINARY CARE

A number of antibiotics may be used to treat Lyme disease. Treatment may be continued for up to 1 month to ensure that the organism has been eradicated. Aspirin or another NSAID may be prescribed to relieve arthritic symptoms. The affected joint may be splinted to rest the joint. When the knee is involved, weight bearing may be restricted and the client instructed to use crutches.

NURSING CARE

Priorities in Nursing Care. The nursing role in treating Lyme disease is primarily educational. Teach about the disease and its transmission. Emphasize the importance of completing the full course of antibiotic therapy. Discuss possible adverse effects of treatment and their appropriate management. Teach the client with arthritic manifestations about using NSAIDs, including the importance of maintaining a consistent schedule of doses rather than taking the medication only as needed for pain.

Nurses can take a major role in educating the public about Lyme disease and its prevention. Box 43-13 ■ provides important information about preventing Lyme disease.

Ankylosing Spondylitis

Ankylosing spondylitis is a chronic inflammatory arthritis that primarily affects the spine, causing pain and progressive stiffening. The cause of ankylosing spondylitis is unknown. Heredity plays a role in its development. It affects men more often than women.

BOX 43-13	CLIENT TEACHING

Preventing Lyme Disease

- Avoid tick-infested areas, particularly tall grasses and dense brush.
- When walking or working in potentially infested areas, wear clothing that completely covers the extremities (e.g., long pants tucked into boot tops or long socks, and long-sleeved shirts tucked into pants).
- Use an insect repellent such as diethyltoluamide (DEET) or permethrin on skin and clothing.
- Inspect skin and clothing for ticks after you have been outside.
- Protect pets with tick collars and inspect them frequently for ticks.
- Remove any ticks found on the body or pets immediately. Grasp the mouth portion of the tick with fine tweezers where it enters the skin, and pull steadily and firmly until the tick releases. Do not twist or jerk.
- Put the tick in alcohol and save it for future examination in case you develop symptoms. Do not crush the tick.
- Wash the affected area thoroughly with soap and water; apply an antiseptic.
- If you develop flulike symptoms or a "bull's-eye" rash around the tick bite, notify a physician immediately.

PATHOPHYSIOLOGY AND MANIFESTATIONS

The onset of ankylosing spondylitis is usually insidious. Clients may complain of persistent or intermittent bouts of low back pain. The pain is worse at night, followed by morning stiffness that is relieved by activity. Pain may radiate to the buttocks, hips, or down the legs. As the disease progresses, back motion is limited, the lumbar curve is lost, and the thoracic curvature is accentuated. In severe cases, the entire spine is fused, preventing any motion. Clients with ankylosing spondylitis may also develop arthritis in other joints, primarily the hip, shoulders, and knees. Systemic manifestations include anorexia, weight loss, fever, and fatigue. Many clients develop uveitis, inflammation of the iris and the middle, vascular layer of the eye.

INTERDISCIPLINARY CARE

Physical therapy and daily exercises are important to maintain posture and joint range of motion. NSAIDs relieve pain and stiffness and allow the client to perform necessary exercises.

As with other chronic arthritic disorders, the primary nursing role in ankylosing spondylitis is providing supportive care and education. Encourage to maintain a fluid intake of 2,500 mL or more per day. Suggest performing exercises in the shower because warm, moist heat promotes mobility.

Uveitis may cause photophobia and blurred vision in the affected eye. Provide indirect lighting and a darkened room for photophobia. If vision is significantly impaired, use appropriate measures such as:

- Orient to surroundings; do not move furniture or place objects in usual pathways.
- Introduce yourself verbally when entering the room. Tell client what you are doing during procedures.
- Assist during ambulation by allowing client to hold your elbow.

Fibromyalgia

Fibromyalgia, also known as *fibrositis,* is a common rheumatic syndrome of musculoskeletal pain, stiffness, and tenderness. Fibromyalgia usually affects women over the age of 50. It may be precipitated or aggravated by stress, sleep disorders, trauma, or depression.

The cause of fibromyalgia is unknown, and its pathophysiology is unclear. A gradual onset of chronic, achy muscle pain is typical. The pain may be localized or involve the entire body. The neck, shoulders, lower back, and hips are often affected. Tenderness is present, usually in small, localized trigger points. Local tightness or muscle spasm may also occur. Systemic manifestations of fibromyalgia include fatigue, sleep disruptions, headaches, and an irritable bowel. Pain and fatigue are aggravated by exertion.

This disorder may resolve spontaneously or become chronic and recurrent. The client with fibromyalgia needs reassurance of the benign nature of the disorder along with validation of its reality. Other therapeutic measures include local heat, massage, stretching and low-impact aerobic exercises, and sleep improvement. Amitriptyline, a tricyclic antidepressant, has been found to promote better sleep and relieve symptoms of fibromyalgia.

Nursing care for clients with fibromyalgia is supportive and educational, provided in community settings such as clinics and other primary care settings. It is important to validate concerns and reassure clients that their symptoms are not "all in the head." This syndrome is recognizable and manageable; its course is not progressive. Teach about the disorder. Provide verbal and written instructions about management strategies. Instruct to take prescribed medications at bedtime, because they may cause drowsiness. Caution about driving while taking the medication.

Low Back Pain

Acute or chronic low back pain usually is due to strains in the muscles and tendons of the back caused by abnormal stress or overuse. It involves the lumbar, lumbosacral, or sacroiliac areas of the back. Low back pain caused by degenerative disk disease and herniated vertebral disks is covered in Chapter 39. 🔗

PATHOPHYSIOLOGY AND MANIFESTATIONS

In general, there are five types of back pain:

- *Local pain,* often caused by fractures, strains, or sprains. Tumors also may press on pain-sensitive structures, causing local pain.
- *Referred pain* is caused by disorders of organs in the abdomen or pelvis, such as gastrointestinal or genitourinary disorders or an abdominal aortic aneurysm.
- *Pain of spinal origin* is associated with pathology of the spine such as disk disease or arthritis.
- *Radicular back pain* radiates from the back to the leg along a nerve root. It is sharp pain that may be aggravated by movement, such as coughing, sneezing, or sitting.
- *Muscle spasm pain* is associated with many spine disorders. This type of back pain is dull and may be accompanied by abnormal posture and taut spinal muscles.

Low back pain may range from mild discomfort lasting a few hours to chronic, debilitating pain. Acute pain is usually caused by an activity such as lifting and bending or twisting.

INTERDISCIPLINARY CARE

Low back pain usually is diagnosed by the history and physical exam. X-rays, CT scan, and MRI are ordered only when a potentially serious underlying condition is suspected.

Most clients with acute low back pain need only short-term treatment. Ice packs or ice massage can be applied or rubbed over the painful area for 15 minutes every hour or more. Moist, warm towels or a heating pad can be used as an alternative to ice therapy.

Prolonged rest is not recommended. In fact, increased activity helps to restore function and may increase endorphin levels. Exercise is initiated and increased gradually. Physical therapy frequently is used in combination with exercise. Diathermy (deep heat therapy), ultrasonography, hydrotherapy, and transcutaneous electrical nerve stimulation (TENS) units may be used to reduce the muscle spasms and relieve pain.

Other treatments include chiropractic manipulation of the spine to reduce spasms and pain. *Back school* is a rehabilitation program that teaches about the anatomy of the spine and ways to decrease the risk of recurring back injury.

Low back pain often can be managed with NSAIDs and analgesics. Muscle relaxants also may be ordered. For intense, intractable pain, a steroid solution may be injected into the epidural space. This helps decrease the swelling and inflammation of the spinal nerves.

NURSING CARE

Priorities in Nursing Care. Because low back pain often is chronic in nature, teaching the client measures to reduce the risk of injury and manage the discomfort are priorities for nursing care.

Ineffective Health Maintenance

- Teach appropriate body mechanics in lifting and reaching. Instruct to plan the lift, keep the object being lifted close to the body, and avoid twisting when lifting. Encourage to obtain help when lifting. *Using good body mechanics can prevent many back injuries.*
- Encourage to avoid prolonged standing or sitting, lying prone, and wearing high heels. *These activities exacerbate back pain.*
- Encourage an exercise program to strengthen abdominal and back muscles. Teach or refer for teaching about exercises such as partial sit-ups with the knees bent and knee–chest exercises to stretch hamstrings and spinal muscles. Instruct to do each exercise five times, gradually increasing to ten repetitions. Advise to stop any exercise that increases pain, and seek professional advice before continuing. *Prescribed back exercises, such as the pelvic tilt, partial sit-ups, and back rolls, strengthen back and abdominal muscles, reducing the risk of back injury and pain.*
- Suggest workplace or environmental modifications to minimize stress on the lower back. *Lumbar supports in*

chairs, adjustments to chair or table height, and rubber floor mats help prevent back strain or injury.

- Encourage obese clients to lose weight. *Obesity changes the center of gravity, and increases the risk of injury when lifting.*
- Encourage to stop smoking. *Smoking contributes to disk degeneration and the risk of injury.*

Pain

- Assess the quality, severity, and location of pain, as well as factors that tend to aggravate or relieve it. *Accurate assessment data can help identify the cause and type of pain.*
- Instruct to take NSAIDs or analgesics on a routine schedule rather than as needed. *Maintaining a constant blood level of NSAIDs or analgesics reduces inflammation and improves pain relief.*
- Instruct the client on bed rest to assume a side-lying position with the hips and knees flexed. Keep a pillow under or between the knees. Instruct to use a footstool when seated to support the weight of the feet. *These measures decrease pressure on intervertebral disks and spinal nerves.*
- Teach about the "rebound phenomenon" of prolonged heat or ice therapy. *Ice remaining on the skin longer than 15 minutes or heat longer than 30 minutes causes a reverse effect known as the rebound phenomenon, and can increase inflammation and pain.*

CONTINUING CARE

Back pain is a common problem. Nurses can make an impact on this significant problem by teaching health practices to prevent back pain. Teach safe lifting, bending, and turning during physical activity. Stress the importance of using large muscle groups of the legs to lift rather than bending and lifting with the smaller muscles of the back. Teach other aspects of good body mechanics, including posture, sleeping on a firm mattress, and sitting in chairs that provide good support. Discuss the positive effect of maintaining optimal body weight and good physical fitness.

In industrial and work settings, nurses should be alert for situations that increase the risk of back pain and injury. Office workers should have chairs with appropriate seat height

and length and back support. Modifications of work space or machinery may be necessary for industrial workers to avoid excess stresses on back muscles. Finally, it is important to remember that back pain is a leading cause of lost work time for nurses themselves. Remind coworkers to use good body mechanics and to seek help when lifting or moving clients.

Muscular Dystrophy

Muscular dystrophy (MD) is a group of inherited muscular diseases that cause progressive muscle degeneration and wasting. The most common form of MD, *Duchenne's muscular dystrophy,* is inherited as a sex-linked recessive disorder, and is therefore transmitted from the mother to male children. This disorder affects males exclusively and occurs in 1 out of 3,500 live male births.

Muscle fiber atrophy, necrosis, regeneration, and fibrosis lead to progressive weakness of voluntary muscles in MD. The pattern of muscle weakness and the rate at which it progresses vary, depending on the type of MD. As the disease progresses, the person develops difficulty ambulating and eventually becomes wheelchair bound and finally bed bound.

There is no cure or specific treatment for MD. Care focuses on preserving and promoting mobility. A multidisciplinary approach, involving many members of the health care team, is necessary to meet the physical and psychologic needs of these clients and their families.

Nursing care focuses on promoting independence and mobility and providing psychologic support. Teach about prescribed exercises such as stretching and counterposturing exercises. Discuss skin care and ways to prevent irritation under braces. Because the muscles of respiration may be affected, discuss ways to prevent respiratory infections, such as avoiding crowds during flu season and being immunized against pneumococcal pneumonia and influenza. Provide information about support services and organizations such as the Muscular Dystrophy Association.

Note: The bibliography listings for this and all chapters have been compiled at the back of the book.

MediaLink · Video: MD

MediaLink · Video: Muscle Atrophy

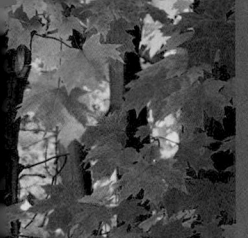

Chapter Review

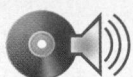 **KEY TERMS** by Topics

Use the audio glossary feature of either the CD-ROM or the Companion Website to hear the correct pronunciation of the following key terms.

Structural and bone disorders
scoliosis, kyphosis, osteoporosis, pathologic fractures, osteomyelitis, debride

Joint and connective tissue disorders
arthritis, osteoarthritis (OA), arthralgia, arthroplasty, rheumatoid arthritis (RA), systemic lupus erythematosus (SLE), gout, muscular dystrophy (MD)

KEY Points

- Musculoskeletal system disorders affect comfort, mobility, ADLs, and safety. Education is a primary nursing role in all of these disorders.

- Prevention is a key strategy for osteoporosis. Stress the importance of adequate calcium intake throughout the life span, and encourage menopausal clients to discuss preventive measures with their health care provider.

- Osteomyelitis, infection of the bone, is difficult to treat; prevention and early identification are vital. Promptly report general signs of infection, as well as redness, heat, wound drainage, continued pain, and refusal to use or bear weight on an extremity.

- Benign bone tumors and metastasis of tumors from other locations are more common than primary malignancy of the bone.

- Most people develop osteoarthritis as they age. The pain and joint effects of osteoarthritis are localized and are managed symptomatically with balanced rest and activity.

- Rheumatoid arthritis, on the other hand, is a systemic inflammatory disease. Its management is directed toward reducing inflammation and preventing joint destruction. Rheumatoid arthritis can have crippling effects. Stress the importance of a multidisciplinary treatment regimen to maintain function and mobility.

- Systemic lupus erythematosus also is a systemic connective tissue disease with symptoms similar to RA. It is less likely to cause joint crippling, but has more widespread effects than RA in many people. Reducing inflammation is a priority in both disorders.

- The arthritis of gout is caused by a disorder of purine metabolism and excess uric acid buildup in the body. It is not caused by eating too much rich food.

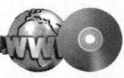 **EXPLORE Media**Link

Additional interactive resources for this chapter can be found on the Companion Website at www.prenhall.com/burke. Click on Chapter 43 and "Begin" to select the activities for this chapter.

For chapter-related NCLEX-style review questions and an audio glossary, access the accompanying CD-ROM in this book.

FOR FURTHER Study

For more information about the relationship of vitamin D, calcium, and phosphorus in the body, see Chapter 7.

See Chapter 8 for more information about pain management.

For in-depth discussion of care of the surgical client, see Chapter 9.

See Chapter 11 for more information about autoimmune disorders.

For radiation therapy and chemotherapy related to bone cancer, see Chapter 12.

Dialysis and kidney transplantation are discussed in Chapter 32.

For further study about selective estrogen receptor modulators (SERMs), see Chapter 35.

See Chapter 39 for further discussion of disk disorders.

See Box 41-3 for information about bone scans and Box 41-4 for information about arthroscopy.

For more about care of the client undergoing amputation, see Chapter 42.

Caring for a Client with Osteoarthritis and Total Hip Replacement

NCLEX-PN® Focus Area: Physiologic Integrity: Physiologic Adaptation

Case Study: Robert Cerulli is a 72-year-old retired commercial fisherman who has significant degenerative changes in both hip joints. He is admitted for a right total hip replacement; a left total hip replacement is planned to follow in 6 to 12 months.

Nursing Diagnosis: Impaired Physical Mobility

COLLECT DATA

Subjective	Objective
_____	_____
_____	_____
_____	_____
_____	_____
_____	_____
_____	_____

Would you report this data? Yes/No

If yes, to: _____

Nursing Care

_____
_____
_____
_____
_____
_____
_____
_____
_____
_____
_____

How would you document this? _____
_____
_____
_____

Data Collected (use those that apply)

- Takes carbidopa/levodopa (Sinemet 25-100) 4 times a day for Parkinson's disease
- No other chronic medical conditions
- No known medication allergies
- Does not smoke; consumes only small amounts of alcohol
- Alert and oriented
- Speech is soft but clear
- Vital signs: BP 116/64; P 68 regular; R 18; T 97.4°F (36.3°C) PO
- Color good, skin warm and moist
- Peripheral pulses strong and equal in upper extremities; slightly weaker but equal in lower extremities
- Feet cool to touch, good capillary refill
- Walks with a limp; shuffling gait noted

Nursing Interventions (use those that apply; list in priority order)

- Assess pain hourly first 24 to 48 hours post-operatively, and as needed thereafter.
- Teach to use patient-controlled analgesia (PCA) and monitor effectiveness.
- Help change position every 2 hours; encourage use of overhead trapeze to shift positions.
- Maintain sequential compression device and antiembolic stocking as ordered.
- Remind to use incentive spirometer hourly for first 24 hours, then every 2 hours while awake.
- Assist out of bed three times a day after the first 24 hours.
- Maintain right hip abduction with abduction pillow.
- Perform passive ROM exercises of unaffected extremities every shift.
- Encourage frequent quadriceps-setting exercises and plantar and dorsiflexion of feet.
- Assess the surgical site frequently; report signs of excess bleeding or inflammation.
- Monitor temperature every 4 hours.
- Assess pulses, color, movement, and sensation of right foot hourly for the first 24 hours, then every 2 hours for 24 hours, then every 4 hours.

NCLEX-PN® Exam Preparation

1 When caring for a client who sustained a gunshot wound to the femur 4 days ago, which of these assessments requires immediate nursing intervention?

A. soiled dressing
B. tenderness, swelling, redness over incision site
C. increased capillary refill
D. pain scale of 6

2 A client diagnosed with osteoporosis and a right hip replacement is preparing for discharge. All of the following are important discharge instructions; place them in order of priority.

A. use of walker and elevated toilet
B. pain medication
C. list of calcium-enriched foods
D. smoking cessation programs and tools
E. schedule for increasing activity

3 A nurse teaches the mother of a 4-year-old child how to prevent Lyme disease. Which of these statements indicates that further teaching is necessary?

A. "We are going camping, but I'll make sure she stays out of the brush."
B. "Even though it's warm, I'll make her wear long pants."
C. "If a tick gets on my child, I'll pull it off immediately and squash it."
D. "I'll buy some insect repellant before we leave on our vacation."

4 When assessing a client who has osteoarthritis, the nurse should expect to observe which of these findings?

A. superficial, sharp pain
B. stiffness following joint use
C. full ROM
D. crepitus with movement

5 Which of the following is an appropriate goal for teaching of a client with SLE?

A. Experiences no joint pain or inflammation.
B. States rationale for maintaining vegetarian diet.
C. Uses SPF 15 or higher sunscreen when outside.
D. Relates importance of splints to prevent joint damage.

6 The nurse is teaching a client who is recovering from an acute gout attack about his prescription for sulfinpyrazone (Anturane). Which statement by the client would indicate an understanding of the instructions?

A. "I'm going to drink less water so I won't swell up."
B. "I'll take the colchicine every day."
C. "I'll let my doctor know if my stomach begins to hurt."
D. "I will take my medicine on an empty stomach."

7 A client is diagnosed with chronic low back pain. The physician has asked the nurse to provide information related to this condition. Which of the following nursing diagnoses would the nurse be expected to address?

A. Disturbed Body Image
B. Ineffective Health Maintenance
C. Hopelessness
D. Acute Pain

8 The nurse is teaching a client with rheumatoid arthritis about the prescribed drug, celecoxib (Celebrex). Which of the following does the nurse include? (Select all that apply.)

A. Always take this drug with food or milk to avoid gastric upset.
B. Take the drug as needed to manage pain and stiffness.
C. Contact your doctor if you develop stomach or abdominal pain.
D. You may use acetaminophen as needed for pain.
E. Like aspirin, this drug reduces your risk for heart attack.

9 An x-ray done on a client admitted to the emergency department with an injury to the right tibia shows a mass in the tibia. The client asks the nurse if this means his leg will need to be amputated. The appropriate response by the nurse is:

A. "The prospect of amputation must be frightening to you."
B. "Do you have other symptoms of bone cancer?"
C. "Most bone tumors are benign. I'm sure you won't need anything that drastic."
D. "Bone masses usually occur secondarily to cancer elsewhere. Treatment will focus on the primary tumor."

10 The student nurse is assisting with basic assessments at a local middle school. A young girl is noted to have a lateral curvature of the spine and asymmetry of the shoulders. The nurse recognizes this as a manifestation of:

A. scoliosis.
B. kyphosis.
C. Paget's disease.
D. osteomalacia.

Answers for Review Questions, as well as discussion of Care Plan and Critical Thinking Care Map questions, appear in Appendix V.

Thinking Strategically About...

Nancy Bauer is a 53-year-old schoolteacher. She comes into the clinic with complaints of low back pain.

DATA COLLECTED

Mrs. Bauer has smoked a pack of cigarettes a day for 30 years and drinks one to two glasses of wine with dinner each evening. She does not routinely exercise. Mrs. Bauer has had symptoms of menopause for 8 years, but she has never been on estrogen therapy. Both Mrs. Bauer's mother and her 60-year-old sister have osteoporosis.

Mrs. Bauer is having continuous low back pain unrelieved by mild analgesics. She frequently wakes up during the night because of the pain. She states, "I don't know what can be causing this pain."

Mrs. Bauer's vital signs are all within normal limits. She has full range of motion of all extremities. She reports discomfort when bending over and returning to an upright position. She has a noticeable "hump" on her upper back and is 1 inch shorter than her stated height. When asked about her diet, she reports that she has never been a "milk drinker" even as a child. She indicates that on a typical day, she takes in only one-half to one dairy serving.

CRITICAL THINKING

1 What knowledge deficits can the nurse identify for Mrs. Bauer?

2 Why is Mrs. Bauer shorter than she was as a younger adult?

3 What physical activities should the nurse encourage for Mrs. Bauer and why?

4 What education about lifestyle changes should the nurse include in the teaching plan for Mrs. Bauer and why?

5 Is Mrs. Bauer typical of the usual osteoporosis client and why?

MANAGEMENT OF CARE

1 Discuss the management of dietary needs and exercise therapy for Mrs. Bauer.

COORDINATION OF INTERDISCIPLINARY CARE

1 What resources might be available to assist Mrs. Bauer in implementing changes to her lifestyle that could decrease the risk of more bone loss?

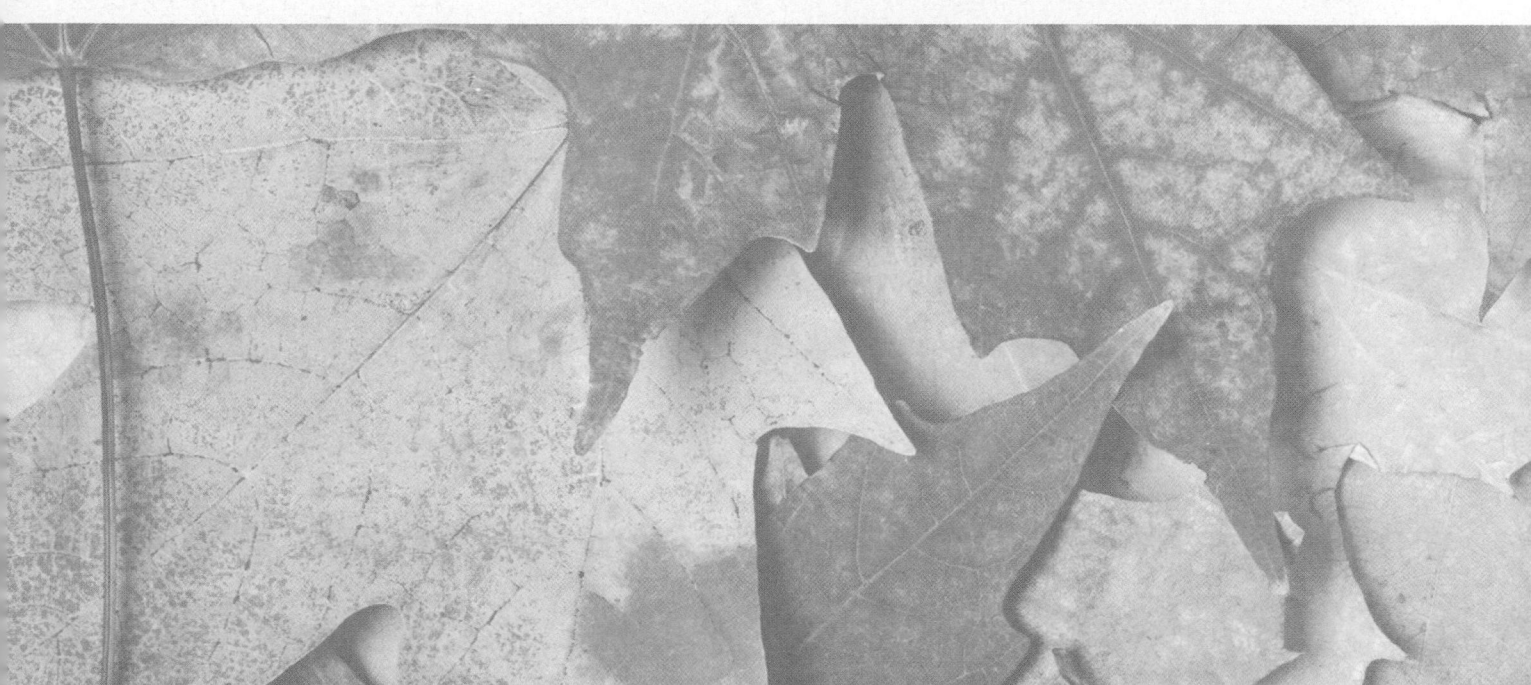

Disrupted Integumentary Function

UNIT XII

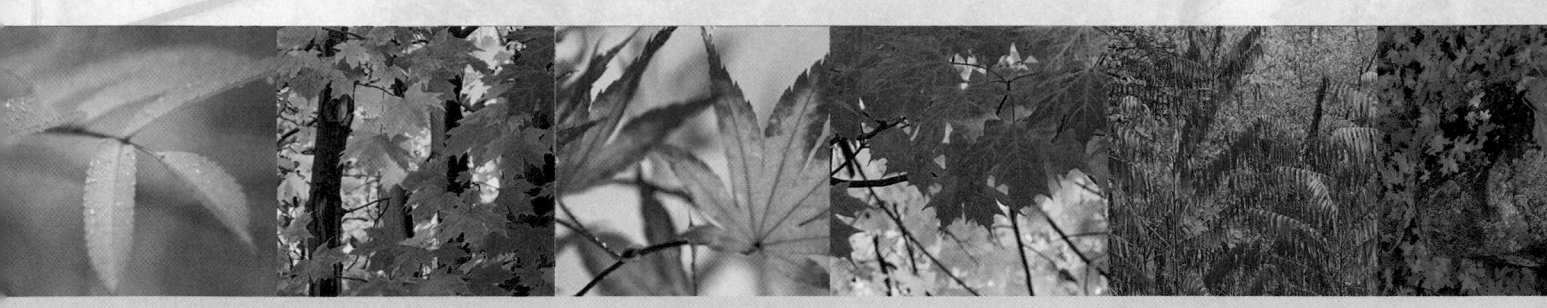

Chapter 44

The Integumentary System and Assessment

BRIEF Outline

Structure and Function of the Integumentary System
- The Skin
- The Hair and Nails

Assessment
- Health History
- Physical Examination
- The Older Adult
- Diagnostic Tests

LEARNING Outcomes

After completing this chapter, you will be able to:

- Identify the structure and functions of the skin and its appendages.
- Describe factors that influence skin color.
- Describe skin changes in the older adult.
- Identify subjective and objective assessment data to collect for clients with integumentary disorders.
- Identify nursing responsibilities for common diagnostic tests and monitors for clients with integumentary disorders.

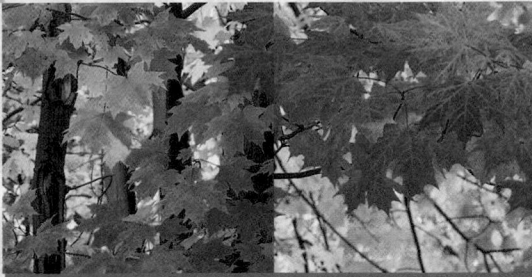

MediaLink

www.prenhall.com/burke
Use the address above to access the free, interactive Companion Website created for this textbook. Get hints, instant feedback, and textbook references to chapter-related NCLEX-style questions. Link to other interesting sites.

Audio Glossary:
Use the Companion Website, or the CD-ROM disk enclosed with your textbook, to hear the pronunciation of key terms in this chapter.

Structure and Function of the Integumentary System

The skin, glands, hair, and nails make up the integumentary system. The skin provides an external covering for the body, separating the body's organs and tissues from the external environment. The skin contains receptors for touch and sensation, helps regulate body temperature, and assists in fluid and electrolyte balance. It provides cues to racial and ethnic background, conveys emotional responses, and helps determine self-concept, roles, and relationships. Functions of the skin, glands, hair, and nails are described in Table 44-1 ■.

THE SKIN

The skin has a surface area of 15 to 20 square feet and weighs about 9 pounds. It has been estimated that each square inch of skin contains 15 feet of blood vessels, 4 yards of nerves, 650 sweat glands, 100 oil glands, 1,500 sensory receptors, and more than 3 million cells that are constantly dying and being replaced.

The skin is composed of two regions: the epidermis and the dermis (Figure 44-1 ■). The **epidermis,** the surface or outermost part of the skin, is made up of several layers of epithelial cells. The deepest layer of the epidermis contains cells that produce melanin and keratin. *Melanin* forms a shield to protect nerve endings in the dermis from the damaging effects of ultraviolet light. *Keratin* is a fibrous, water-repellent protein that makes the epidermis tough and protective. The outermost layer of the epidermis makes up about 75% of the epidermis's total thickness. It consists of about 20 to 30 sheets of dead cells filled with keratin fragments arranged in "shingles" that flake off as dry skin. The **dermis,** the second, deeper layer of skin, is made up of a flexible connective tissue. This layer is richly supplied with blood cells, nerve fibers, and lymphatic vessels. Most of the hair follicles, sebaceous glands, and sweat glands are located in the dermis.

The color of the skin is the result of varying levels of pigmentation. *Melanin,* a yellow-to-brown pigment, is darker and is produced in greater amounts in persons with dark skin color than in those with light skin. Exposure to the sun causes a buildup of melanin and a darkening of the skin in people with light skin. *Carotene* (a yellow-to-orange pigment) is more abundant in the skins of persons of Asian ancestry, and together with melanin accounts for their golden skin tone. The epidermis in Caucasian skin has very little melanin and is almost transparent. The color of their red blood cells shows through, lending Caucasians a pinkish skin tone.

Skin color is influenced by emotions and illnesses. **Erythema** (a reddening of the skin) may occur with embarrassment such as blushing, fever, hypertension, or inflammation. It may also result from a drug reaction, sunburn, or other

---

TABLE 44-1

Functions of the Skin and Its Appendages

STRUCTURE	FUNCTIONS
Epidermis	Protects tissues from physical, chemical, and biologic damage. Prevents water loss and serves as a water-repellent layer. Stores melanin, which protects tissues from harmful effects of the ultraviolet radiation in sunlight. Converts cholesterol molecules to vitamin D when exposed to sunlight. Contains phagocytes, which prevent bacteria from penetrating the skin.
Dermis	Regulates body temperature by dilating and constricting capillaries. Transmits messages via nerve endings to the central nervous system.
Sebaceous (oil) glands	Secrete sebum, which lubricates skin and hair and plays a role in killing bacteria.
Eccrine sweat glands	Regulate body heat by excretion of perspiration.
Apocrine and ceruminous sweat glands	Unknown.
Hair	Cushions the scalp. Eyelashes and cilia protect the body from foreign particles. Provides insulation in cold weather.
Nails	Protect the fingers and toes, aid in grasping, and allow for various other activities, such as scratching the skin, picking up small items, peeling an orange, and so on.

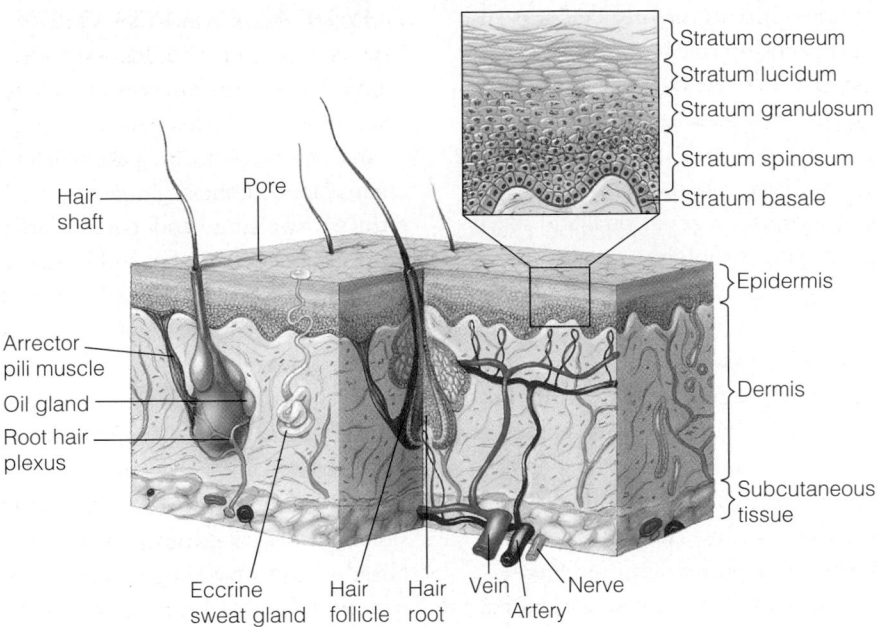

Figure 44-1. ■ Anatomy of the skin.

factors. **Cyanosis** (bluish discoloration of the skin and mucous membranes) results from poor oxygenation of hemoglobin or lack of adequate hemoglobin or RBCs. **Pallor,** or paleness of skin, may occur with shock, fear, or anger, or in anemia and hypoxia. **Jaundice** is a yellow-to-orange color visible in the skin and mucous membranes; it most often results from a liver disorder.

Glands of the Skin

The skin has three types of glands: sebaceous (oil) glands, sweat glands, and ceruminous glands. Each of these glands has a different function (see Table 44-1).

Sebaceous glands are found all over the body except the palms and soles. These glands secrete an oily substance (*sebum*) that softens and lubricates the skin and hair. Sebum also protects the body from infection by killing bacteria. The secretion of sebum is stimulated by hormones, especially androgens.

There are two types of sweat glands: eccrine and apocrine. The production of sweat is regulated by the sympathetic nervous system and serves to maintain normal body temperature. The secretions from apocrine glands are similar to those of sweat glands. Ceruminous glands are modified apocrine sweat glands that secrete yellow-brown waxy cerumen. This substance provides a sticky trap for foreign materials.

THE HAIR AND NAILS

Hair is distributed and scattered all over the body, except the lips, nipples, parts of the external genitals, the palms of the hands, and the soles of the feet. Hair is produced by a hair bulb, and its root is enclosed in a hair follicle. The visible hair is composed of dead cells. Many factors, including nutrition and hormones, influence hair growth. Hair in various parts of the body has protective functions. A nail is a modified scalelike epidermal structure. Like hair, nails consist mainly of dead cells. Review Table 44-1 for hair and nail functions.

Assessment

HEALTH HISTORY

The health history may be part of a health screening, total health assessment, or focused on the client's chief complaint such as a rash or itching. Ask about any change in health, skin color changes, dryness or oiliness, growth of or changes in warts or moles, the presence of lesions, and delayed wound healing. Determine whether the client takes hormones, vitamins, steroids, or antibiotics, which may cause skin side effects. For obese clients, inquire about any chafing in areas where moisture accumulates such as overlapping skin folds.

When the client complains about itching, ask the client to describe the type of itching. Inquire about precipitating causes such as medications, soaps, shampoos, cosmetics, skin care products, pets, travel, stress, or diet changes. Ask about skin reactions to insect bites and stings.

In assessing the hair, ask about problems with thinning or baldness, excessive hair loss, change in distribution of hair, use of hair-care products, diet, and dieting. When assessing nail problems, ask about nail splitting or breakage, discoloration, infection, diet, and exposure to chemicals.

Obtain the client's past medical history, focusing on previous problems, allergies, surgery, and lesions. Skin problems may be symptoms of other health disorders, such as cardiovascular, diabetes mellitus, thyroid disease, liver disease, and hematologic disorders. Occupational and social history may provide cues to skin problems; ask the client about exposure to chemicals at work, travel, use of alcohol, and responses to stress.

Assess the presence of risk factors for skin cancer carefully. These include male gender; age over 50; family history of skin cancer; light-colored hair and eyes; extended exposure to sunlight; tendency to sunburn; history of sunburn or other skin trauma; live in high altitudes or near equator; exposure to radiation, x-rays, coal, tar, or petroleum products; and the use of sun-protection products.

Also explore the risk factors for malignant melanoma. These include a large number of moles, the presence of atypical moles, a family history of melanoma, prior melanoma, repeat severe sunburns, ease of freckling and sunburning, or inability to tan.

PHYSICAL EXAMINATION

The examination should be conducted in a warm, private room. The client removes all clothing and puts on a gown that allows access to all skin areas.

Inspect the skin for pallor or cyanosis. In dark-skinned clients, look at the sclera of the eyes for jaundice. Assess for redness, swelling, and pain related to various rashes, inflammation, infections, and burns. First-degree burns cause painful erythema and swelling. Red, painful blisters occur in second-degree burns and white or blackened areas appear in third-degree burns. Check for *vitiligo*, an abnormal, patchy loss of melanin, over the face, hands, and groin. Assess for *petechiae*, small, reddish-purple pinpoint spots, over the abdomen and buttocks.

Inspect the skin for lesions. Primary and secondary lesions are described and shown in Table 44-2 ■. Look for raised bluish or yellowish bruises. Note bruises that are in varying stages of healing. Assess for lesions that appear in circles, groups, or along the sensory nerves.

Palpate skin temperature, texture, moisture, and turgor. Note warmth and redness associated with inflammation and coolness related to decreased blood flow. Observe

---

TABLE 44-2

Primary and Secondary Skin Lesions

Macule, Patch 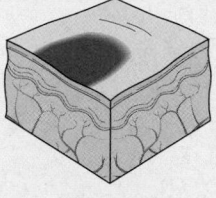	Flat, nonpalpable change in skin color. Macules are smaller than 1 cm, with a circumscribed border, and patches are larger than 1 cm and may have an irregular border. **Examples** Macules: freckles, measles, and petechiae. Patches: mongolian spots, port-wine stains, vitiligo, and chloasma.	**Vesicle, Bulla** 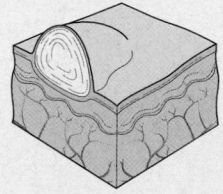	Elevated, fluid-filled, round or oval-shaped, palpable mass with thin, translucent walls and circumscribed borders. Vesicles are smaller than 0.5 cm, bullae are larger than 0.5 cm. **Examples** Vesicles: herpes simplex/zoster, early chickenpox, poison ivy, and small burn blisters. Bullae: contact dermatitis, friction blisters, and large burn blisters.
Papule, Plaque 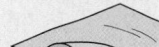 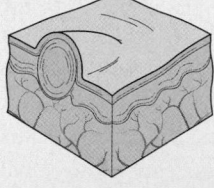	Elevated, solid, palpable mass with circumscribed border. Papules are smaller than 0.5 cm; plaques are groups of papules that form lesions larger than 0.5 cm. **Examples** Papules: elevated moles, warts, and lichen planus. Plaques: psoriasis, actinic keratosis, and also lichen planus.	**Wheal** 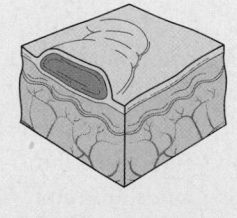	Elevated, often reddish area with irregular border caused by diffuse fluid in tissues rather than free fluid in a cavity, as in vesicles. Size varies. **Examples** Insect bites and hives (extensive wheals).
Nodule, Tumor 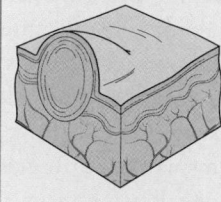	Elevated, solid, hard or soft palpable mass extending deeper into the dermis than a papule. Nodules have circumscribed borders and are 0.5 to 2 cm; tumors may have irregular borders and are larger than 2 cm. **Examples** Nodules: small lipoma, squamous cell carcinoma, fibroma, and intradermal nevi. Tumors: large lipoma, carcinoma, and hemangioma.	**Pustule** 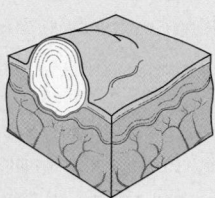	Elevated, pus-filled vesicle or bulla with circumscribed border. Size varies. **Examples** Acne, impetigo, and carbuncles (large boils).

TABLE 44-2

Primary and Secondary Skin Lesions (continued)

Cyst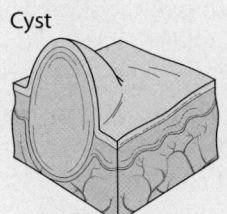

Elevated, encapsulated, fluid-filled or semisolid mass originating in the subcutaneous tissue or dermis, usually 1 cm or larger.

Examples Varieties include sebaceous cysts and epidermoid cysts.

Atrophy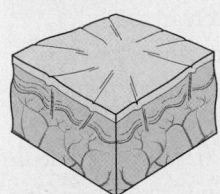

A translucent, dry, paper-like, sometimes wrinkled skin surface resulting from thinning or wasting of the skin due to loss of collagen and elastin.

Examples Striae, aged skin.

Erosion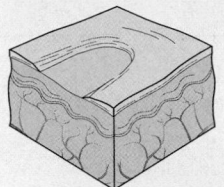

Wearing away of the superficial epidermis causing a moist, shallow depression. Because erosions do not extend into the dermis, they heal without scarring.

Examples Scratch marks, ruptured vesicles.

Lichenification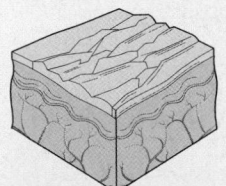

Rough, thickened, hardened area of epidermis resulting from chronic irritation such as scratching or rubbing.

Example Chronic dermatitis.

Scales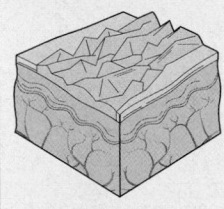

Shedding flakes of greasy, keratinized skin tissue. Color may be white, gray, or silver. Texture may vary from fine to thick.

Examples Dry skin, dandruff, psoriasis, and eczema.

Crust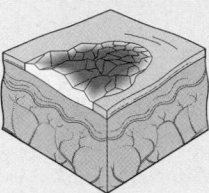

Dry blood, serum, or pus left on the skin surface when vesicles or pustules burst. Can be red-brown, orange, or yellow. Large crusts that adhere to the skin surface are called scabs.

Examples Eczema, impetigo, herpes, or scabs following abrasion.

Ulcer

Deep, irregularly shaped area of skin loss extending into the dermis or subcutaneous tissue. May bleed. May leave scar.

Examples Decubitus ulcers (pressure sores), stasis ulcers, chancres.

Fissure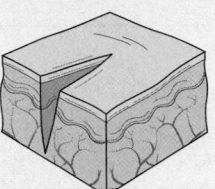

Linear crack with sharp edges, extending into the dermis.

Examples Cracks at the corners of the mouth or in the hands, athlete's foot.

Scar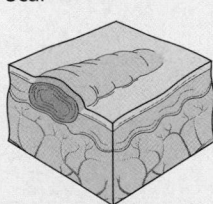

Flat, irregular area of connective tissue left after a lesion or wound has healed. New scars may be red or purple; older scars may be silvery or white.

Examples Healed surgical wound or injury, healed acne.

Keloid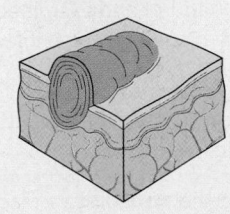

Elevated, irregular, darkened area of excess scar tissue caused by excessive collagen formation during healing. Extends beyond the site of the original injury. Higher incidence in people of African descent.

Examples Keloid from ear piercing or surgery.

---

for rough, dry or smooth, oily skin as well excessive perspiration. Inspect for *tenting* (Figure 44-2 ■). Tenting is the term used when the skin is pinched gently over the collarbone or back of the hand and remains pinched for a few moments before returning to its normal position. This is a common finding in the elderly. Note decreased skin turgor as seen in dehydration. Assess for **edema** (accumulation of fluid in the body's tissues) by depressing the client's skin over the ankle.

Inspect the distribution and quality of hair. Look for *hirsutism* (excessive hair) or **alopecia** (hair loss). Palpate the hair for coarseness or fineness. Inspect the scalp for lesions such as pustules or scales. Look for nits (eggs) seen with head lice adhering to the base of the hair shaft. Note excessive greasy flakes rather than mild dandruff.

Inspect nails for **clubbing** (angle of nail base is greater than 180 degrees). Observe nail surface for inflammation, separation from the nail bed, grooves, pitting, or spoon-shape.

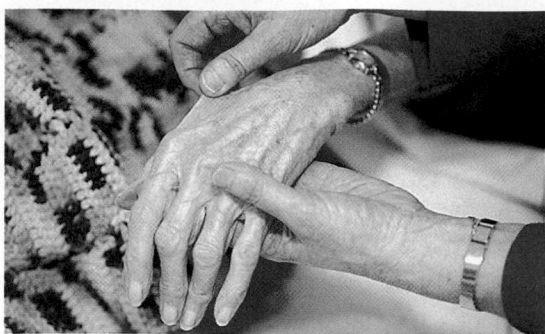

Figure 44-2. ■ Tenting in an elderly client.

Inspect for yellowish-colored, bluish-green, or dark nails. Look at the nails for red splinter hemorrhages and pigmented bands, which are normal in 90% of African Americans.

For additional information about assessment techniques, see Chapter 5. ◍ See Box 44-1 ■ for an example of how to document an integumentary assessment.

THE OLDER ADULT

A variety of normal skin changes are seen in the older adult. Loss of subcutaneous tissue, dermal thinning, and decreased elasticity may cause wrinkles and sagging of the skin. The skin is thinner, and turgor is decreased. Older adults are unable to respond to heat or cold quickly, increasing their risk for heat stroke and hypothermia. (For more information about older adults, see Chapter 3. ◍)

Other age-related changes include the following:

■ Dry, itchy skin may result from the reduced number of sweat and oil glands.
■ Overall production of melanocytes decreases, while abnormal localized proliferations of melanocytes may occur in specific areas. This localized hyperpigmentation may lead to the development of senile lentigines, commonly called "liver spots." These flat, brown macules commonly appear on the arms and hands in areas of sun exposure. Keratoses also result from hyperpigmentation.

TABLE 44-3

Common Diagnostic Tests for Integumentary Disorders

TEST	EXPLANATION AND PURPOSE	NURSING IMPLICATIONS
Biopsy	A special biopsy instrument is used to obtain a skin sample of a nodule to rule out malignancy.	Verify that consent form has been signed. Assist with obtaining supplies that physician will need. Apply dressing and give follow-up instructions. Send specimen to laboratory.
Cutaneous immuno-fluorescence biopsy	A skin biopsy is obtained and a fluorochrome dye applied. Under a microscope antibodies become fluorescent. Done to diagnose immune-mediated dermatitis.	Verify that consent form has been signed. Assist with obtaining supplies that physician will need. Apply dressing and give follow-up instructions. Send specimen to laboratory.
Potassium hydroxide (KOH)	Hair, nail, or scale specimen collected, placed on a glass slide with KOH added, and examined under the microscope. Used to diagnose fungal infections.	Teach client about purpose of test. Send specimen to laboratory.
Culture and sensitivity	Fluid obtained from intact bullae, pustules, or abscesses to identify bacterial or viral infections and the appropriate medication for treatment.	Explain the purpose and send specimen to laboratory.
Tzanck test	Fluid and cells collected from blisters, placed on slide, stained, and examined microscopically. Used to identify herpes infections.	Explain the purpose and send specimen to laboratory.
Skin scraping	Tissue sample scraped from lesion with a scalpel moistened with oil so skin sticks to blade, transferred to slide, and examined to diagnose fungal infections or scabies.	Explain the purpose and send specimen to laboratory.
Patch test	Suspected allergens applied to normal skin under patches. Reaction ranges from weak with redness or itching, to strong with pain and blisters.	Explain purpose and instruct client to return in 48 hours for removal of patches and evaluation.
Wood's light examination	A special lamp with ultraviolet rays is shown on areas of skin to differentiate hyperpigmented from hypopigmented lesions.	Explain the purpose of the examination and that ultraviolet is not harmful to eyes or skin.

BOX 44-1

DOCUMENTATION OF INTEGUMENTARY ASSESSMENT

Client: A 60-year-old male is seen in an outpatient clinic for psoriasis. States, "This episode is worse than before. I just returned from vacation and this happened." Has a family history of psoriasis.

Assessment note: Raised, red, round plaques noted on anterior part of both arms, back of hands, and scalp. Thick gray scales found between the toes. Toenails yellow with pitting. States, "I just can't seem to stop scratching."

Seborrheic keratoses are dark, raised lesions. Actinic keratoses are reddish, raised plaques on areas of high sun exposure. They may become malignant.

■ Skin tags, small flaps of excess skin, are normal in aging skin.

■ Both hair and nail growth decrease with aging. Older men may develop coarse hair in the ears and nose and over the eyebrows. Decreased estrogen levels may cause postmenopausal women to develop dark facial hair over the upper lip and under the chin.

■ Hair becomes gray due to a reduction of melanocytes.

■ Nails may thicken, yellow, and peel.

DIAGNOSTIC TESTS

Laboratory Tests

Diagnosis of skin problems relies on the client's history and inspection of the lesion. When diagnosis remains uncertain, other diagnostic procedures are used. The most common test is the skin biopsy. Other tests include stains and cultures to identify bacterial, fungal, and viral infections. Photographs may be taken to document wound healing or to record wounds in suspected abuse cases. Table 44-3 ■ lists the diagnostic tests, purpose, and nursing implications.

Note: The bibliography listings for this and all chapters have been compiled at the back of the book.

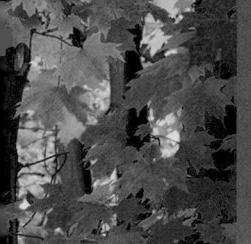

Chapter Review

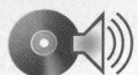 **KEY TERMS** by Topics

Use the audio glossary feature of either the CD-ROM or the Companion Website to hear the correct pronunciation of the following key terms.

Structure and function
epidermis, dermis, erythema, cyanosis, pallor, jaundice

Assessment
edema, alopecia, clubbing

KEY Points

- The skin and its appendages provide an external covering for the internal tissues and organs, help regulate body temperature, assist in fluid and electrolyte balance, protect tissues, and convey emotions.

- Two layers compose the skin: the epidermis and dermis. Epidermis contains cells that produce melanin and keratin. The dermal layer includes blood cells, nerve fibers, lymph vessels, hair follicles, and sebaceous and sweat glands.

- Older adults experience loss of subcutaneous tissue, dermal thinning, and decreased elasticity, which increases fragility of skin.

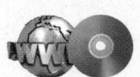 **EXPLORE Media**Link

Additional interactive resources for this chapter can be found on the Companion Website at www.prenhall.com/burke. Click on Chapter 44 and "Begin" to select the activities for this chapter.

For chapter-related NCLEX-style review questions and an audio glossary, access the accompanying CD-ROM in this book.

⊘ **FOR FURTHER** Study

For more about the older adult client, see Chapter 3.

For further study about assessing the integumentary system, see Chapter 5.

NCLEX-PN® Exam Preparation

1 Which of the following age-related changes occur in the skin? Select all that apply.

A. increased blood supply
B. decreased skin elasticity
C. development of liver spots
D. appearance of petechiae
E. increased response to heat
F. thick yellow nails

2 When inspecting the skin for tenting, the nurse should:

A. pinch the skin gently over the collarbone.
B. depress the client's skin over the ankle.
C. palpate the client's skin for moisture.
D. assess the client's skin for lesions appearing in a group.

3 Which one of the following risk factors should the nurse ask the client in regards to the potential for skin cancer?

A. female under 50
B. dark-colored hair and eyes
C. living near a lake or river
D. exposure to radiation

4 A skin lesion that is described as elevated, fluid-filled with thin translucent walls is known as a:

A. macule
B. wheal
C. vesicle
D. pustule

5 What diagnostic test would be ordered to identify a fungal infection?

A. skin biopsy
B. skin scraping
C. patch testing
D. Wood's light examination

Answers for Review Questions in Appendix V.

Chapter 45

Caring for Clients with Skin Disorders

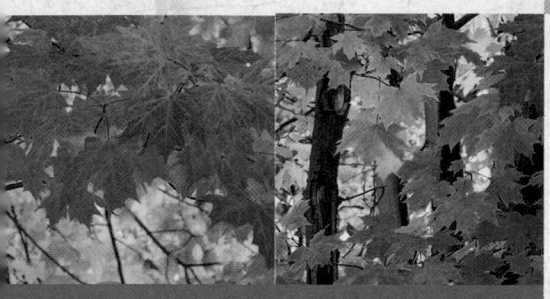

BRIEF Outline

Common Skin Disorders
    Pruritus
    Psoriasis
    Dermatitis
    Acne

Infections and Infestations of the Skin
    Bacterial Infections
    Fungal Infections
    Viral Infections
    Parasitic Infestations

Malignant Skin Disorders
    Pressure Ulcers

LEARNING Outcomes

After completing this chapter, you will be able to:

- Relate skin changes in the older adult to an increased risk for dry skin, pruritus, skin cancer, and pressure ulcers.
- Compare and contrast the pathophysiology, manifestations, and interdisciplinary care of clients with common skin disorders, infections and infestations of the skin, malignant skin disorders, and pressure ulcers.
- Use the nursing process to collect data and provide interventions for clients with common skin disorders, infections and infestations of the skin, malignant skin disorders, and pressure ulcers.
- Provide client and family teaching appropriate for prevention and self-care of disorders of the skin.

MediaLink

www.prenhall.com/burke
Use the address above to access the free, interactive Companion Website created for this textbook. Get hints, instant feedback, and textbook references to chapter-related NCLEX-style questions. Link to other interesting sites.

Audio Glossary:
Use the Companion Website, or the CD-ROM disk enclosed with your textbook, to hear the pronunciation of key terms in this chapter.

There are many different disorders of the skin. The client with a minor or benign disorder is often treated in a physician's office or outpatient setting. The client with a disorder that involves large areas of the body, is chronic, or is malignant may require inpatient care. The nurse collects data about client needs and implements interventions to meet a wide variety of physical, emotional, and social responses.

Refer to Chapter 44 for the common primary and secondary skin lesions (Table 44-2). ⊘ These terms are used throughout this chapter and in Chapter 46. This chapter discusses common disorders of the skin. Chapter 46 ⊘ discusses burns.

Common Skin Disorders

PRURITUS

Pruritus is a subjective itching sensation that produces an urge to scratch. Pruritus may occur in a small, circumscribed area, or it may involve a widespread area; it may or may not be associated with a rash. Pruritus is not a disorder itself but is rather a manifestation of an underlying irritation or condition. Itching is triggered by heat and prostaglandins and is increased by release of histamine and other chemical mediators. Almost anything in the internal or external environment can cause pruritus. Insects, animals, plants, fabrics, metals, medications, allergies, and emotional distress are among the most common causes. Pruritus also may occur as a secondary manifestation of systemic disorders, such as certain types of cancer, diabetes mellitus, liver disease, and kidney failure.

Pruritus is initiated by a stimulation or irritation of receptors in the junction between the epidermis and dermis. The response by the person is to scratch or rub the affected area. This may irritate the skin and cause further inflammation, setting off a cycle of increasingly intense itching and scratching, called the *itch–scratch–itch* cycle.

The secondary effects of pruritus include skin excoriation, erythema, wheals, changes in pigmentation, and infections. Pruritus that persists may interrupt sleep patterns, because the itching sensation is often more intense at night. Long-term pruritus may be debilitating; broken skin also increases the risk of infection.

DRY SKIN

Dry skin (*xerosis*) is most often a problem in the older adult (see Chapter 44). ⊘ In older adults, decreased activity of sebaceous and sweat glands reduces the skin's lubrication and moisture retention. However, dry skin may occur at any age as a result of exposure to environmental heat and low humidity, sunlight, excessive bathing, and a decreased intake of liquids.

The primary manifestation of dry skin is pruritus. Other manifestations include visible flaking of surface skin and

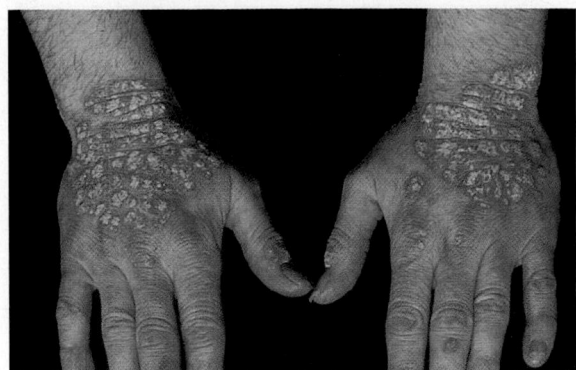

Figure 45-1. ■ The characteristic lesions of psoriasis are raised, red, round plaques covered with thick, silvery scales. (*Source:* NMSB, Custom Medical Stock Photos, Inc.)

an observable pattern of fine lines over the area. If the skin has been excessively dry and pruritic for a long period, the client may have secondary skin lesions and *lichenification* (thickening).

PSORIASIS

Psoriasis is a chronic, noninfectious skin disorder. It is characterized by raised, reddened, round circumscribed plaques of varied size, covered by silvery white scales (Figure 45-1 ■). The plaques shed thick gray scales. The lesions may appear anywhere on the body. However, they are most commonly found on the scalp, extensor surfaces of the arms and legs, elbows, knees, sacrum, and around the nails. As with any chronic illness, the skin manifestations may disappear and recur throughout life.

The actual cause of psoriasis is unknown, but some evidence suggests it may be an autoimmune disorder. Sunlight, stress, seasonal changes, hormone fluctuations, steroid withdrawal, and certain drugs (such as alcohol, corticosteroids, lithium, and chloroquine) appear to make the disorder worse. About one-third of clients have a family history of psoriasis. Trauma to the skin from surgery, sunburn, or excoriation may also precipitate it.

Pruritus is common over the lesions. If the lesions are located in an *intertriginous zone* (between toes, under breasts, or in the perianal region), the psoriatic scales may soften, allowing painful fissures to form. When psoriasis affects the nails, pitting and a yellow or brown discoloration results. The nail may separate from the nail bed, thicken, and crumble, increasing the risk for infection.

DERMATITIS

Dermatitis is an acute or chronic inflammation of the skin characterized by erythema and pain or pruritus. Various agents or illnesses cause the inflammatory response of the skin. Initial skin responses include erythema, formation of vesicles and scales, and pruritus. Later, irritation from

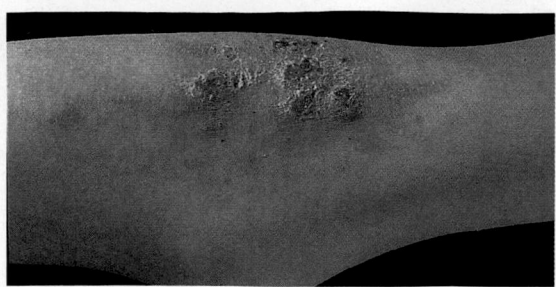

Figure 45-2. ■ Atopic dermatitis or eczema. (*Source:* NMSB, Custom Medical Stock Photos, Inc.)

scratching promotes edema, a serous discharge, and crusting. Long-term irritation in chronic dermatitis causes the skin to become thickened, leathery, and darker in color.

Contact (allergic) dermatitis is caused by a hypersensitivity response or chemical irritation. The major sources known to cause contact dermatitis are dyes, perfumes, poison plants (ivy, oak, sumac), chemicals, and metals. Latex dermatitis is a contact dermatitis that is common in the health care field.

Atopic dermatitis is also called *eczema*. The exact cause is unknown, but related factors include depressed cell-mediated immunity, elevated immunoglobulin E (IgE) levels, and increased histamine sensitivity. Clients with atopic dermatitis have a family history of hypersensitivity reactions, such as eczema, asthma, and allergic rhinitis. Characteristic lesions include chronic lichenification, erythema, and scaling, the result of pruritus and scratching. The lesions are usually found on the hands, feet, or flexor surfaces of the arms and legs (Figure 45-2 ■). Scratching and excoriation increase the risk of secondary infections, as well as invasion of the skin by viruses such as herpes simplex.

Seborrheic dermatitis is a chronic inflammatory disorder that involves the scalp, eyebrows, eyelids, ear canals, nasolabial folds, axillae, and trunk. The cause is unknown. This disorder is seen in all ages, from the very young (called "cradle cap") to the very old. Clients taking methyldopa for hypertension occasionally develop this disorder, and it is a component of Parkinson's disease. Seborrheic dermatitis is also frequently seen in clients with AIDS. The lesions are yellow or white plaques with scales and crusts. The scales are often yellow or orange and have a greasy appearance. Mild pruritus is also present.

Exfoliative dermatitis is an inflammatory skin disorder characterized by excessive peeling or shedding of skin. A preexisting skin disorder such as psoriasis, atopic dermatitis, contact dermatitis, or seborrheic dermatitis may be present. Exfoliative dermatitis is also associated with leukemia and lymphoma. Systemic manifestations include weakness, malaise, fever, chills, and weight loss. Scaling, erythema, and pruritus may be localized or involve the entire body. In addition to peeling of skin, the client may lose the hair and nails.

ACNE

Acne is a disorder of the sebaceous glands. These glands empty into the hair follicles and are open to the skin surface through a pore. They produce sebum in response to direct hormonal stimulation by testicular androgens in men and to adrenal and ovarian androgens in women. Most sebaceous glands are on the face, scalp, and scrotum.

Acne lesions are primarily *comedones* (pimples, whiteheads, and blackheads). Whiteheads are pale, slightly elevated papules. Blackheads are plugs of material that accumulate in the sebaceous glands. Inflammatory acne lesions include comedones, erythematous pustules, and cysts (Figure 45-3 ■). The lesions may itch. The common types of acne are as follows:

- *Acne vulgaris* is common in adolescents and young to middle-aged adults. Many factors once thought to cause acne vulgaris, including high-fat diets, chocolate, infections, and cosmetics, have been disproved (Porth, 2005).
- *Acne rosacea,* a chronic facial acne, occurs more often in middle and older adults. The lesions begin with erythema over the cheeks and nose. Over years of time, the skin color changes to dark red, and the pores over the area become enlarged.

INTERDISCIPLINARY CARE

Pruritus, dry skin, psoriasis, dermatitis, and acne are most often treated by self-care at home. Treatment focuses on identifying and eliminating or modifying any precipitating factors, providing relief from itching and pain, and reducing the risk of further damage to the skin.

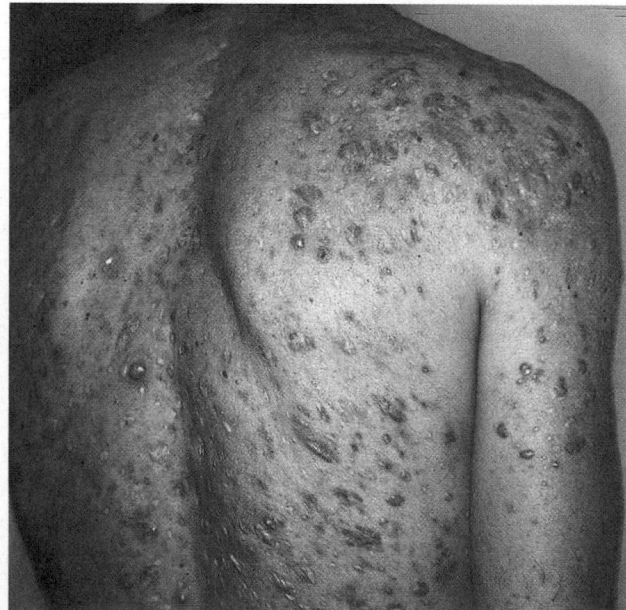

Figure 45-3. ■ Inflammatory acne lesions include comedones, erythematous pustules, and cysts. These lesions often leave scars when they heal. (*Source:* Camera M.D. Studios, Carroll H. Weiss, Director, 8290 N.W. 26th Place, Sunrise, FL 33322.)

Diagnostic Tests

Culture and sensitivity of skin scrapings and studies for fungal infections are conducted by microscopic examination to distinguish pruritus from psoriasis, dermatitis, and other disorders. Cutaneous scratch or patch testing may be performed if allergic reactions are the suspected cause.

If the client has atypical manifestations, or to differentiate psoriasis from inflammatory or infectious dermatitis, a skin biopsy may be done. Ultrasound tests may be performed to measure skin thickness. Results reveal typical psoriatic changes in the stratum corneum layer (see Figure 44-1) 🔗 of the epidermis and dermal inflammation.

Medications

PRURITUS. If possible, the client discontinues all medications to determine whether the pruritus is due to a drug reaction. Oral medications include antihistamines, tranquilizers, and antibiotics. Antihistamines provide relief from pruritus in some clients. Tranquilizers provide sedation, which may relieve the emotional stress associated with pruritus. Systemic antibiotics are used to treat infection resulting from the scratching and excoriation.

Topical medications that contain corticosteroids are often used to relieve pruritus and inflammation. Topical medications may also be administered through therapeutic baths or soaks with agents that relieve pruritus, such as cornstarch, baking soda, or coal tar concentrates (see Box 45-1 ■).

PSORIASIS. Topical corticosteroids, tar preparations, and retinoids decrease inflammation and suppress mitotic activity of psoriatic cells. The most effective topical corticosteroids are potent preparations. They are well absorbed through the skin and are used under an occlusive dressing. Corticosteroids may also be taken systemically or injected directly into the lesions. Tar preparations, applied topically or in a bath, are effective in some cases. They do have the undesirable side effect of staining. A topical retinoid (Tazarotene [Tazorac]) gel results in longer lasting remissions, but may cause skin irritation and pruritus. Calcipotriene (Dovonex), a vitamin D analogue, has been shown to be effective and safe in both short- and long-term treatment of psoriasis.

Photochemotherapy, using methoxsalen, is a treatment for severe psoriasis. This drug is an antimetabolite that inhibits deoxyribonucleic acid (DNA) synthesis. Exposure to ultraviolet-A (UVA) rays activates methoxsalen. It is administered orally, and the client is exposed to UVA 2 hours later. Treatments are administered 2 to 3 times a week. Usually, 10 to 20 total treatments are given over 1 to 2 months. The eyes are covered by dark glasses during the treatment. Treatment causes tanning, and direct sunlight

---

BOX 45-1

THERAPEUTIC BATHS

Agents Used in Therapeutic Baths

- Saline or tap water
- Antibacterial agents: potassium permanganate, acetic acid, hexachlorophene
- Colloid substances: oatmeal (Aveeno), cornstarch, sodium bicarbonate
- Potassium permanganate
- Emollients: Alpha-Keri, Lubath, mineral oil

Therapeutic baths have a variety of uses in treating skin disorders. Depending on the agent used, therapeutic baths soothe the skin, lower the skin bacteria count, clean and hydrate the skin, loosen scales, and relieve itching.

Nursing Responsibilities

- Ensure that the bathwater is at a comfortable temperature that is neither too hot nor too cool (usually 110 to 115°F [43 to 46°C]).
- Fill the tub one-third to one-half full.
- Mix the agent well with the water.
- Assist the client into and out of the tub to prevent falls.
- Dry the client by blotting with the towel.

Client and Family Teaching

- Use a bath mat in the tub: The medications may cause the tub to become slippery.
- Keep the bathroom warm but adequately ventilated.
- Follow directions carefully for the amount of medication to use in the bath.
- Fill the bath one-third to one-half full of water that is at a comfortable temperature.
- Stay in the bath for 20 to 30 minutes, and immerse the areas to be treated.
- Do not get the bathwater in your eyes.
- Dry by blotting (not rubbing) with the towel.
- If the medications cause staining, use old towels or linens.
- If the itching is not relieved or the skin becomes excessively dry, call your health care provider.

---

must be avoided for 8 to 12 hours thereafter. If the client has erythema, the treatments are stopped until the redness and swelling resolve. Photochemotherapy can accelerate aging of exposed skin, induce cataract development, alter immune function, and increase the risk of melanoma.

Ultraviolet-B (UVB) light is often used to treat psoriasis. UVB light decreases the growth rate of epidermal cells. Mercury vapor lights or fluorescent UV tubes provide the UVB light. Fluorescent tubes are often arranged in a cabinet so the client can stand and expose psoriatic lesions more easily. These units may be purchased or constructed to be used in the client's home. The light therapy is administered in gradually increasing exposure times, until the client experiences a mild erythema, like a mild sunburn. Treatments

TABLE 45-1

Nursing Implications for Pharmacology: Acne

DRUG GROUP/DRUGS	ACTION/USES	NURSING IMPLICATIONS	CLIENT TEACHING
Antiacne Retinoids ■ Isotretinoin (Accutane) ■ Tretinoin (Retin-A)	These agents are vitamin A metabolites that, depending on the drug, either act as an irritant to decrease comedone formation or decrease sebum production. Baseline lipid levels are measured at the onset of treatment, at 2 weeks, and then monthly during treatment (lipids > 500–800 mg/dL indicates a need to stop the drug to prevent acute pancreatitis). Liver function tests are performed at 2- to 3-week intervals for 6 months and then once a month during treatment.	Do not administer to clients with eczema or who are sensitive to the sun. Do not administer to pregnant women. Assess for side effects of redness, scaling, severe erythema with topical use.	Cleanse affected skin areas well with a bland soap and dry completely before applying drug. Expect redness and peeling of skin. Use only nonmedicated cosmetics, lotions, or shaving lotions and wash them off before applying drug. Use sunscreen and protective clothing when outside. Do not take vitamin A supplements or drink alcohol while using the drugs. Use a reliable contraceptive from 1 month before beginning treatment to 1 month following the end of treatment. A pregnancy test should be conducted within 2 weeks of beginning treatment to rule out pregnancy. Report jaundice, pruritus, and/or dark urine immediately. If visual disturbances, nausea, vomiting, and headache occur, stop the drug at once and report manifestations to the physician.

are given daily and are measured in seconds of exposure. The eyes are shielded during the treatment. The erythema response occurs in about 8 hours. Careful assessment is necessary to prevent more severe burning, which could exacerbate the psoriasis.

ACNE. Treatment for acne is based on the type and severity of the lesions. For acne with comedones, tretinoin (retinoic acid, Retin-A) or benzoyl peroxide preparations are prescribed. Azelaic acid (Azelex) may also be used. Benzoyl peroxide preparations are found in over-the-counter medications such as Fostex, Acne-Dome, Desquam-X, Benzagel, Clear By Design, and Xerac BP. These products loosen the comedones. Inflammatory acne is treated with oral or topical antibiotics, such as tetracycline, erythromycin, and minocycline. Severe forms of inflammatory acne are treated with isotretinoin (Accutane), which is effective but has serious side effects. Nursing responsibilities for these medications are discussed in Table 45-1 ■. The treatment for acne lasts months, and in some cases for the rest of one's life.

Surgery

Dermabrasion of inactive acne lesions can improve the client's appearance, especially if the scars are flat. The skin is first frozen (and anesthetized) with Freon or ethyl chloride. The lesions are carefully abraded with fine sandpaper or abrasive brushes.

Complementary Therapy

Topical aloe therapy may be used for managing psoriasis, acne, and eczema. Overuse of aloe may result in atopic dermatitis. Goldenseal can be applied topically to treat eczema, acne, and itching. Peppermint oil is applied to the skin to decrease pruritus but use cautiously because skin irritation and contact dermatitis may develop.

NURSING CARE

Nursing care for the client with common skin problems focuses on promoting comfort and decreasing the risk of infection. Because clients care for themselves at home, nursing interventions are primarily educational. Teaching focuses on methods of relieving itching and dry skin and preventing infection. Clients with psoriasis require information about medications and light treatments.

ASSESSING

Assessment data are collected by the nurse to determine the degree of discomfort, the extent to which the skin condition is interfering with the client's activities of daily living and usual lifestyle, and the risk factors for complications. Box 45-2 ■ suggests subjective and objective data to collect.

BOX 45-2   **ASSESSMENT**

Assessing Clients with Common Skin Problems

SUBJECTIVE DATA

- Location, duration, and type of itching or skin lesion present.
- Ability to sleep at night.
- Skin oily or dry, amount of sweating.
- Medications used to treat dry skin, itching, or skin lesions.
- History of allergies.
- History of exposure to environmental substances.
- Chronic illness, such as thyroid disorders, diabetes mellitus, or liver disease.

OBJECTIVE DATA

- Inspect the entire skin for color and lesions:
  - Redness, swelling, and pain may indicate a secondary infection from itching, or may follow phototherapy treatments for psoriasis.
  - Dry, rough skin with visible flaking indicates severe xerosis.
- Palpate the skin for temperature, texture, moisture, and turgor:
  - Increased warmth may indicate infection. Dry skin is rough.
  - Pinch the skin gently over the collarbone or top of the hand; tenting (in which the skin remains in a fold for a few moments) is common in older adults.

DIAGNOSING, PLANNING, AND IMPLEMENTING

Priorities in Nursing Care. Although pruritus, dry skin, psoriasis, dermatitis, and acne are not life threatening, they may result in physical and emotional distress. The highest priority nursing diagnosis is impaired skin integrity due to the high risk for infection. Clients with chronic skin disorders experience disturbed body image and have deficient knowledge about medication administration.

Impaired Skin Integrity

- Recommend that the nails be trimmed short, the environmental temperatures be slightly cool, and loose clothing be worn. *These measures relieve pruritus and decrease the risk of infection.*
- Suggest the following strategies to relieve itching:
  - Rub the pruritic area with the surface of the hand rather than scratching with the nails, briefly apply pressure or cold to help relieve pruritus, and wear cotton gloves at night.
  - Use distraction or relaxation techniques.
  - Wash clothing in a mild detergent and rinse twice. Do not use fabric softeners.
  - Avoid using perfumes and lotions containing alcohol, and apply skin lubricants after a bath to help retain moisture.

  These strategies relieve itching and prevent excoriation.
- Demonstrate methods of taking therapeutic baths or treatments. Gently rub lesions with a soft washcloth, using a circular motion. *Gentle rubbing reduces the risk of injury to the skin.*

---

clinical ALERT

Use warm—not hot—water because hot water dries the skin and increases itching.

- Dry the skin with a soft towel, using a blotting or patting motion. *Washing or drying the skin with rough linens may excoriate the skin over lesions.*
- Teach the client and family to watch for and report to the health care provider any complications of treatment, such as excoriation, increased redness, increased skin peeling, or blister formation. *The medications and treatments may cause damage to skin cells through chemical burns or exposure to ultraviolet light. Times and methods of treatment need to be adjusted if these occur.*

Disturbed Body Image

- Establish a trusting nurse–client relationship by verbally and nonverbally expressing acceptance. For example, touching the client on the shoulder demonstrates that the lesions and the client's appearance are not offensive. *One's body image is affected not only by self-perception but also by the responses of others. The skin eruptions and lesions, especially chronic ones, often cause clients to isolate themselves from social contacts, withdraw from normal roles and responsibilities, and feel helpless or powerless.*
- Encourage talking about self-perception and questions about the disease and the treatment. *The client adapts to a changed body image through a process of recognition, acceptance, and resolution. Each person responds individually to changes in body image and loss.*
- Encourage interaction with others through family involvement in care, referral to support groups, and referral to organizations such as the National Psoriasis Foundation. *Acceptance of others is critical to acceptance of self. By becoming involved in care, the family demonstrates love and acceptance. Sharing experiences with others who have the same health problem is a source of strength in adjusting to a visible health problem. Local, state, and national organizations can provide resources and information.*

Deficient Knowledge: Medication Administration

Teach the client the following general guidelines for applying topical medications:

- Each time a medication is applied, the skin surface must be clean and dry. Remove creams by washing with tap water. Remove ointments by first washing the skin with mineral oil, and then with mild soap and water.
- To apply *gels, creams,* and *pastes:* Squeeze about 1/2 to 1 inch of the medication into the palm of the hand and rub the hands together. Apply with the hands to the affected areas using long strokes until the skin is thinly covered. Exceptions:
  - *Corticosteroids* are usually applied two or three times a day in small amounts and rubbed directly into the skin. If prescribed, cover with a dressing.
  - Medications containing *tar* are applied in the direction of the hair growth. Do not apply these medications to the face, the genitals, or in skin folds. These medications will stain clothing.
- To apply *lotions:* Shake the bottle well. Pour a small amount into the palm of the hand and pat the medication on the skin. If the lotion is thin, use a gauze pad.
- To apply *sprays:* Hold the container about 6 inches from the skin and apply the medication in a short spray.
- To apply *medicated shampoo:* Rinse the hair. Apply the shampoo, massage into the hair and scalp. Allow it to remain for the prescribed time. Rinse.
- To apply *pastes:* Use enough paste on an applicator (such as a wooden tongue depressor) to cover the lesion thinly. *Teaching guidelines ensure accurate administration.*

EVALUATING

Collect data to determine the client's understanding of medications and their use, the client's degree of comfort, and any changes in the level of skin integrity or involvement.

Documenting. Document appearance of lesions, effectiveness of pruritic-relief measures, and client teaching about medications and therapeutic baths.

CONTINUING CARE

In addition to teaching the client how to administer topical medications, the nurse should provide the following information for self-care:

- Medications and treatments do not cure the disease. They only relieve the symptoms.
- Dry skin increases pruritus, which stimulates scratching. Scratching may in turn cause excoriation, and excoriation increases the risk of infection.
- It may be necessary to change the diet or environment to avoid contact with allergens.

clinical ALERT

Teach clients using oral corticosteroids to never stop taking the medication abruptly.

Infections and Infestations of the Skin

The skin's resistance to infections and infestations is provided by normal skin flora, sebum, and the immune response. Disorders may occur from a break in the skin surface, a virulent agent, or decreased resistance due to a compromised immune system.

BACTERIAL INFECTIONS

Bacterial infections of the skin arise from the hair follicle, where bacteria can accumulate and grow and cause a localized infection. If the bacteria invade deeper tissues, they can cause a systemic infection, a potentially life-threatening disorder. Most bacterial infections are treated by a primary care provider, and the client remains at home for care. Nosocomial (occurs in the hospital) infections of wounds or open lesions in hospitalized clients are often the result of bacterial infections, especially by methicillin-resistant *Staphylococcus aureus* (MRSA). (See Chapter 10. ⊂⊃)

Folliculitis

Folliculitis is most often caused by *Staphylococcus aureus.* The infection begins at the skin surface and extends down into the hair follicle. The bacteria release enzymes and chemical agents that cause an inflammation. The lesions appear as pustules surrounded by an area of erythema on the surface of the skin. Folliculitis is found most often on the scalp and extremities, on the face of bearded men, on the legs of women who shave, and on the eyelids (called a *stye*). Although folliculitis may appear without any apparent cause, contributing factors include poor hygiene, poor nutrition, prolonged skin moisture, and trauma to the skin.

Furuncles

A **furuncle** ("boil") is also an infection of the hair follicle. A group of infected hair follicles is called a *carbuncle*. It often begins as folliculitis, but the infection spreads down the hair shaft, through the wall of the follicle, and into the dermis. The causative organism is commonly *Staphylococcus aureus*. Contributing factors include poor hygiene, trauma to the skin, areas of excessive moisture including perspiration, and systemic diseases, such as diabetes mellitus.

A furuncle is initially a deep, firm, red, painful nodule from 1 to 5 cm in diameter. After a few days, the nodule changes into a large, tender cystic nodule. The cysts may contain purulent drainage. Carbuncles have multiple openings onto the skin and may cause fever, chills, and malaise.

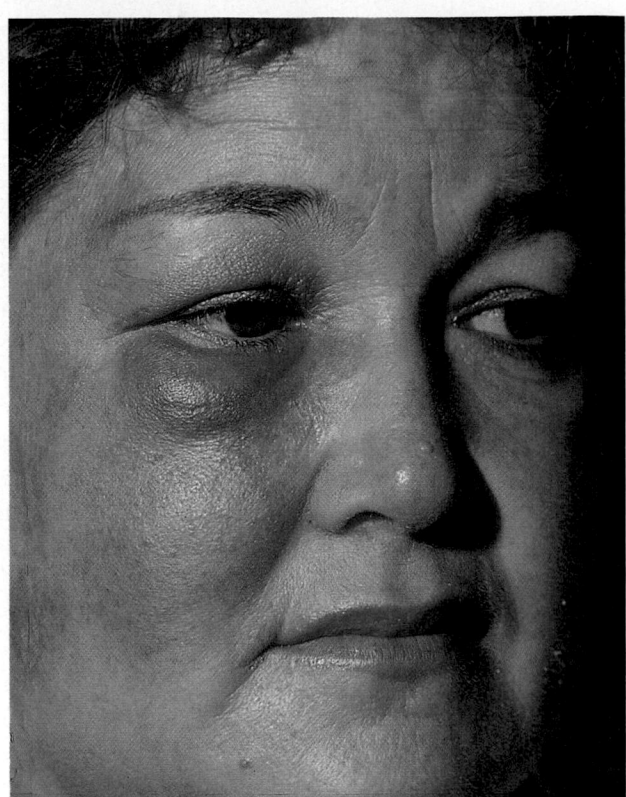

Figure 45-4. ■ Cellulitis is a bacterial infection localized in the dermis and subcutaneous tissue. The involved area is red, swollen, and painful. (*Source: Camera M.D. Studios, Carroll H. Weiss, Director, 8290 N.W. 26th Place, Sunrise, FL 33322.*)

Cellulitis

Cellulitis is a localized infection of the dermis and subcutaneous tissue. Cellulitis can occur following a wound or skin ulcer or as an extension of furuncles or carbuncles. The infection spreads as a result of a substance called *spreading factor,* or *hyaluronidase,* which is produced by the causative organism. Hyaluronidase breaks down the fibrin network and other barriers that normally localize the infection in the skin.

The area of cellulitis is red, swollen, and painful (Figure 45-4 ■). In some cases, vesicles may form over the area of cellulitis. The client may also experience fever, chills, malaise, headache, and swollen lymph glands.

FUNGAL INFECTIONS

Fungi are plantlike organisms that live in the soil, on animals, and on humans. The fungi that cause superficial skin infections are called **dermatophytes.** In humans, the dermatophytes live on keratin in the stratum corneum, hair, and nails. Superficial fungal infections of the skin are often referred to as *ringworm* or *tinea.* Fungal disorders are also called *mycoses.*

The organism may be transmitted by direct contact with animals or other infected persons or by inanimate objects such as combs, pillowcases, towels, and hats. The onset and spread of the fungal infection is greatest in moist areas, such

as in skin folds, between the toes, and in the mouth. Other factors that increase the risk of a fungal infection include the use of broad-spectrum antibiotics that kill off normal flora and allow the fungi to grow, the presence of diabetes mellitus, immunodeficiencies, nutritional deficiencies, pregnancy, increasing age, and iron deficiency.

Dermatophyte (Tinea) Infections

The dermatophyte (*tinea*) infections are named by the body part affected. Those most common in adults are as follows:

- *Tinea pedis (athlete's foot)* affects the soles of the feet, the space between the toes, and the toenail. The lesions vary from mild scaliness to painful fissures with drainage, and they are usually accompanied by pruritus and a foul odor.
- *Tinea cruris* is an infection of the groin that may extend to the inner thighs and buttocks. Also called "jock itch," it is often associated with tinea pedis and is more common in people who are physically active, are obese, and/or wear tight underclothing.

Candidiasis Infections

Candidiasis infections are caused by *Candida albicans,* a yeastlike fungus. This fungus is normally found on mucous membranes, on the skin, in the vagina, and in the gastrointestinal tract. The fungus becomes a pathogen when certain conditions encourage its growth: an environment of moisture, warmth, or altered skin integrity; systemic antibiotics; pregnancy; birth control pills; poor nutrition; immunosuppression; or diabetes mellitus, Cushing's disease, or other chronic debilitating illnesses.

Candidiasis affects only the outer layers of the skin and mucous membranes. It occurs in the mouth, vagina, uncircumcised penis, nails, and deep skin folds. The first sign of infection is a pustule that often burns and itches. As the infection spreads, a white to yellow curdlike substance covers the infected area.

VIRAL INFECTIONS

Viruses are pathogens that consist of a ribonucleic acid (RNA) or DNA core surrounded by a protein coat. They depend on live cells for reproduction. The viruses that cause skin lesions either increase cellular growth or cause cellular death. An increase in the incidence of viral skin disorders has been attributed to a variety of causes, including some commonly used drugs such as birth control medications, corticosteroids, and antibiotics.

Warts

Warts (*verrucae*) are lesions caused by the human papillomavirus (HPV). Warts may be found on skin and mucous membranes. Nongenital warts are benign lesions; genital warts may be precancerous. Warts are transmitted through skin contact. Warts may be flat, fusiform (tapered at both ends), or round, but most are round and raised and have a rough, gray surface. Warts resolve spontaneously when immunity to the virus develops. This response may take up to 5 years. There are many different types of HPV. Those most common are described here:

- A *common wart* may occur anywhere on the skin or mucous membranes. It grows above the skin surface and may be dome shaped with ragged borders. A flat wart is a small flat lesion, usually seen on the forehead or dorsum of the hand.
- *Plantar warts* occur at pressure points on the soles of the feet. The pressure of shoes and walking prevents these warts from growing outward. They tend to extend deeper beneath the skin surface than common warts, and they are often painful.
- *Condylomata acuminata (venereal warts)* occur in moist areas, along the glans of the penis, in the anal region, and on the vulva. They are usually cauliflower-like in appearance and have a pink or purple color.

Herpes Simplex

Herpes simplex ("fever blister," "cold sore") infections are caused by two types of herpesvirus: HSV I and HSV II. Most infections above the waist, most commonly on lips, face, and mouth, are caused by HSV I. (Genital herpes infections, which result from either HSV I or HSV II, are classified as sexually transmitted infections and are discussed in Chapter 36. ⊙) The virus may be transmitted by physical contact, oral sex, or kissing. The virus lives in nerve ganglia and may cause recurrent lesions in response to sunlight, menstruation, injury, or stress.

The infection begins with a burning or tingling sensation, followed by the development of erythema, vesicle formation, and pain. The vesicles progress through pustules, ulcers, and crusting until healing occurs in 10 to 14 days. The initial infection is often severe and accompanied by systemic manifestations, such as fever and sore throat. Recurrences are more localized and less severe.

Herpes Zoster

Herpes zoster ("shingles") is a viral infection of the skin caused by varicella zoster, the same herpesvirus that causes chickenpox. The varicella virus remains dormant in the sensory dorsal ganglia. Years after the initial chickenpox infection, the virus becomes reactivated. This most often occurs when the client is immunosuppressed. Once the virus is reactivated, inflammation and painful vesicles develop in the skin area connected to the same sensory dorsal ganglia.

Clients with Hodgkin's disease, certain types of leukemia, and lymphomas are more susceptible to an outbreak of herpes zoster. Herpes zoster is more prevalent in people who are immunocompromised (e.g., by HIV), those who are receiving radiation therapy or chemotherapy, and those who have had major organ transplants. In people with HIV infections, the appearance of the lesions may be one of the first manifestations of immune compromise.

The lesions are vesicles with an erythematous base. The lesions usually appear unilaterally on the face, trunk, and/or thorax; continue to erupt for 3 to 5 days; then crust and dry. Recovery occurs in 4 to 6 weeks. The client experiences severe pain before and during eruption of the lesions. The older adult is especially sensitive to the pain and often experiences more severe outbreaks of herpes zoster lesions. In most cases, the disease is benign and localized. Complications of herpes zoster include *postherpetic neuralgia* (a sharp, spasmodic pain along the course of one or more nerves) and vision loss. The neuralgia, described as burning or stabbing, results from inflammation of the root ganglia. Permanent loss of vision may follow occurrence of lesions that arise from the ophthalmic division of the trigeminal nerve.

PARASITIC INFESTATIONS

The skin may be invaded by parasites or insects. Infestations affect people of all social classes but are associated with crowded or unsanitary living conditions. Two of the more common parasites are mites and lice.

Pediculosis

Pediculosis is often found in overcrowded living conditions or in people who do not have access to bathing and clothes-washing facilities. Children tend to contract head lice while attending day care or school. Infestation occurs through contact with an infected person, or contact with clothing and linen infested with the parasites.

Pediculosis is an infestation with lice. Lice are parasites that ingest the blood of an animal or human host. One louse (a 2- to 4-mm oval organism) is capable of laying hundreds of eggs. All species of lice have a similar life cycle. The first stage is an unhatched egg (a *nit*) laid by the female louse on a hair shaft. The nit is a small pearl-gray or brown egg visible to the naked eye. Three types of lice live on human hosts:

- *Pediculosis corporis* is an infestation with body lice. The lice live in clothing fibers and are transmitted primarily by contact with infested clothes and bed linens. The louse bites cause a macule, followed by wheals and papules. Itching is common.
- *Pediculosis capitis* is an infestation with head lice. The lice are most often found behind the ears and nape of the neck, but may spread to other hairy areas of the body. Transmission is by contact with an infected person or object such as a comb. The infestation causes itching, scratching, and erythema.
- *Pediculosis pubis* is an infestation with pubic lice ("crabs"). The lice are spread through sexual activity or

contact with infested clothing or linens. The infestation causes skin irritation and intense itching.

Scabies

Scabies infestation affects people of all races, ages, and socioeconomic classes. Outbreaks of scabies occur frequently in shelters, college dormitories, and long-term care facilities. It is spread from skin-to-skin contact but the mite can live for 2 days on clothing and bedding.

Scabies is caused by the female mite. The infestation is found between the fingers, the inner surfaces of the wrist and elbow, the axillae, the female nipple, the penis, the belt line, and the gluteal crease. Lesions appear about 4 weeks after contact with an infected individual. The lesions are small red-brown burrows, about 2 mm in length, sometimes covered with vesicles that appear as a rash. Pruritus is common, especially at night. Excoriations from scratching predispose the person to secondary bacterial infections.

INTERDISCIPLINARY CARE

Clients with infections and infestations of the skin and mucous membranes are usually diagnosed and treated by their primary health care provider, and then provide self-care at home. Treatment is focused on identifying the causative agent and administering medications to kill the bacteria or eradicate the organism, and preventing secondary infections. Environments such as day care centers, schools, hospitals, and long-term care facilities that are infested with lice or scabies must be vacuumed and cleaned thoroughly.

Diagnostic Tests

Bacterial infections are diagnosed by a culture and sensitivity of the drainage from a lesion to identify organisms and to target the most effective antibiotic. If the infection is systemic, a blood culture may be conducted to identify the causative organism.

Fungal infections are diagnosed by various methods. Cultures of skin scrapings, nail scrapings, or hairs are done. Microscopic examination of scrapings may be done to visualize spores and filaments. The affected skin may be inspected under ultraviolet light (called a Wood's lamp); fungal spores fluoresce blue-green.

Laboratory tests may be necessary to differentiate herpes zoster from impetigo, contact dermatitis, or herpes simplex. Cultures of fluids from vesicles and antibody tests are used to identify the herpesvirus types.

When a client has pediculosis, the hair shaft and clothing are inspected, with microscopic examination used for a positive diagnosis. Scabies is diagnosed by skin scrapings and microscopic examination of the mites or their feces.

Medications

BACTERIAL INFECTIONS. The primary treatment for bacterial infections is an antibiotic specific to the organism. The antibiotic is usually administered systemically, but may also be applied topically. Multiple furuncles and carbuncles may be treated with cloxacillin, a penicillinase-resistant penicillin; the cephalosporins also are often effective. Antibiotic therapy is discussed in Chapter 10. 🔗

FUNGAL INFECTIONS. Fungal infections are treated by topical or systemic antifungal medications. Nursing implications for antifungal medications are discussed in Table 45-2 ■. Dermatophyte infections are usually treated with topical antifungals. Candidiasis infections are treated with nystatin (Mycostatin) in powder, tablet, or vaginal suppository form. Other medications that may be used include ketoconazole and fluconazole, administered orally.

TABLE 45-2			
Nursing Implications for Pharmacology: Fungal Infections			
DRUG GROUP/DRUGS	ACTION/USES	NURSING IMPLICATIONS	CLIENT TEACHING
Antifungal Agents ■ Amphotericin B (Fungizone) ■ Clotrimazole (Mycelex) ■ Fluconazole (Diflucan) ■ Griseofulvin Microsize (Fulvicin-U/F) ■ Ketoconazole (Nizoral) ■ Miconazole (Monistat) ■ Nystatin (Mycostatin)	Some drugs interfere with the fungal cell membrane permeability; others interfere with DNA synthesis. They are prepared in many forms: powders, shampoos, suspensions, troches, oral tablets, and vaginal tablets.	Assess for known hypersensitivity to these agents. Assess for side effects: skin rash, gastrointestinal symptoms, and mental status. Administer ketoconazole with food. Shake suspensions well before administering, and ask clients to swish them around in the mouth before swallowing. Tell clients to let oral tablets dissolve in the mouth.	Treatment continues for a long time, but it is important to complete the full prescription. Take griseofulvin with meals. Avoid alcohol and exposure to sunlight. Continue vaginal applications through the menses, and either refrain from sexual intercourse or have partner wear a condom. Your sexual partner must be treated at the same time or the infection will be passed back and forth.

VIRAL INFECTIONS. Most viral skin infections are treated with antiviral medications, and other medications are used to relieve pruritus and pain in clients with herpes zoster. A common method of wart removal is acid therapy, using a colloidal solution of 16% salicylic acid and 16% lactic acid. The solution is applied to the wart every 12 to 24 hours, and the wart disappears in 2 or 3 weeks. Other methods of eradicating warts are cryosurgery, freezing with liquid nitrogen, and electrodesiccation with an electric cautery. Herpes lesions are treated with acyclovir (Zovirax), an antiviral agent that may be administered topically, orally, or parenterally.

PARASITIC INFESTATIONS. Lice are eradicated with topical agents that kill the parasite, such as medications that contain gamma benzene hexachloride, malathion (Prioderm lotion), or permethrin (NIX). Scabies may be eradicated with a single treatment of lindane lotion or Kwell, applied to the entire skin surface.

Complementary Therapy

Tea-tree oil, taken from the Australian tea tree (*Melaleuca alternifolia*), has been used to relieve discomfort and speed healing of boils and carbuncles. Most natural food stores carry tea-tree oil products. If these products cause allergic reactions, they should be stopped immediately.

NURSING CARE

Nursing care of the client with a skin infection or infestation focuses on preventing the spread of infection and restoring normal skin integrity. Most clients provide self-care at home. If the hospitalized client develops a secondary bacterial infection, isolation procedures should be implemented to limit the spread of infection to others.

One of the most effective methods of reducing the spread of infection in any setting is careful hand washing. Health care providers must wash their hands with soap and water before and after every client contact, even if gloves are worn. All clients, family members, and visitors should be taught how to wash their hands effectively, and the importance of this procedure should be stressed.

ASSESSING

The nurse collects subjective and objective assessment data to identify the manifestations of an infection or infestation, and to determine the degree to which the client is at risk for complications. Ask the client about personal and intimate contact with others who may have been infected or infested, manifestations of increased infection (increased erythema, fever, purulent drainage), and living conditions. Include questions about any chronic illnesses, such as diabetes

mellitus, immune disorders, and previous viral infections (including having chickenpox as a child). Inspect the skin, hair, and mucous membranes. Note the location, appearance, and size of lesions; type and color of lesions; and nits. Take and record vital signs. Report abnormal findings.

DIAGNOSING, PLANNING, AND IMPLEMENTING

Priorities in Nursing Care. Nursing interventions for most infections and infestations of the skin focus on providing information so the client can perform self-care at home (see Continuing Care). However, the client with herpes zoster may have increased nursing care needs, with such priority nursing diagnoses as Pain, Disturbed Sleep Pattern, and Risk for Infection.

Acute Pain

- Assess and monitor the location, duration, and intensity of the pain. *Each person experiences and expresses pain differently. Pain tolerance is individualized.*
- Administer prescribed medications regularly and evaluate their effectiveness. *Regular administration prevents the pain from reaching an intensity at which the medication would be less effective.*
- Use measures to relieve pruritus. Administer prescribed antipruritic medications. Apply calamine lotion or cool compresses, if prescribed. Keep the room temperature cool. *Pruritus is a common problem for these clients, and it may intensify pain. Lotions and cool compresses are often effective in decreasing the itch–scratch–itch cycle.*

clinical ALERT

Scratching increases the risk of secondary infection.

- Encourage the use of distraction such as music or a specific relaxation technique such as progressive muscle relaxation or deep breathing. *Noninvasive methods help the client manage the pain and also increase the effectiveness of pain medications.*

Disturbed Sleep Pattern

- Provide appropriate interventions (above) to relieve pain and pruritus. *The pain and pruritus of herpes zoster are often more intense at night, probably as a result of decreased distraction. Analgesics and noninvasive methods of relief may be necessary before bedtime.*
- Maintain a cool environment and avoid heavy bed covers. Use a bed cradle if necessary to keep bed linens off the client. *Heat and touch intensify pruritus. Pruritus stimulates scratching, which awakens the client. Pain may then be perceived as being more acute. A cycle is established that interferes with sleep.*

Risk for Infection

- Take and record vital signs every 4 hours. Report increased body temperature. Assess skin lesions for increased erythema, formation of pustules, or purulent drainage. Monitor white blood cell (WBC) count. Palpate lymph nodes for enlargement. *Secondary bacterial infections may occur, manifested by fever, changes in lesions or drainage, an increased WBC, or enlarged lymph nodes.*

- Use interventions to decrease the itch–scratch–itch cycle. *Clients with herpes zoster have increased risk for infection because of pruritus, scratching, and skin excoriation. Excoriations from scratching provide a portal for bacterial infection.*

- Institute infection control procedures. Maintain strict isolation for immunocompromised clients. Wear gloves and gown if contact with lesions is likely. Instruct pregnant women (visitors and health care providers) to avoid exposure until lesions have crusted over. *Isolation procedures are instituted for the immunocompromised client to protect the client from infection. The client is also contagious to others who did not have chickenpox or varicella vaccine as a child. The nurse wears gloves and a gown to prevent spreading the infection to self and others. Pregnant women must avoid exposure because the herpesvirus can cross the placental barrier.*

EVALUATING

To evaluate the effectiveness of nursing care for clients with a skin infection or infestation, collect assessment data, evaluating for changes in skin integrity and the need for additional measures to protect skin and underlying tissues from injury. Determine the client's understanding of medications and their use, and of how to prevent transmission of the infection or infestation.

Documenting. Documentation includes the location, appearance, and size of lesions as well as the presence of nits. Record measures to protect the skin and client teaching including medications and ways to prevent transmission of infection or infestation.

CONTINUING CARE

Planning and teaching for home care are important nursing responsibilities when caring for the client with a skin infection or infestation. Specific teaching for each type of illness follows.

Bacterial Infections

Teaching focuses on facilitating tissue healing and eliminating the infection. Stress the importance of bathing daily with antibacterial soap, gently washing off crusts during the bath. Warm compresses may be applied to the lesions two or three times a day to increase comfort and decrease swelling. Teach the client to cover draining lesions with a sterile dressing, to handle soiled dressings or linens according to Standard Precautions, and to wear disposable rubber gloves when changing dressings. Other instructions should be given:

- Maintain good nutrition.
- Carefully wash hands before and after dressing changes.
- Do not share linens and towels. Wash all linens and towels in hot water.
- Never squeeze or try to open a lesion. Clean the skin and keep it dry, especially in hot weather. Do not pluck nasal hair or pick the nose.
- Take the full course of prescribed medications until the supply is finished.

Fungal Infections

Many people treat themselves with over-the-counter antifungal medications. It is recommended that the person be diagnosed at the first occurrence. The nurse should provide the following information:

- Fungal infections are contagious. Do not share linens or personal items with others. Use a clean towel and washcloth each day.
- Carefully dry all skin folds, including those under the breasts, under the arms, and between the toes. Do not wear the same pair of shoes every day. Wear cotton socks or hose with cotton feet. Do not wear rubber or plastic-soled shoes. Use talcum powder or an antifungal powder twice a day.
- For vaginal yeast infections: Avoid tight jeans and pantyhose. Wear cotton or cotton-crotch panties. Bathe more frequently, and dry the genital area well. Have your sexual partner treated at the same time you are so you don't pass the infection back and forth.

Viral Infections

The nurse provides the following information:

- The diseases are usually self-limiting and heal completely.
- Do not have contact with children or pregnant women until crusts have formed over the blistered areas in clients with herpes zoster.

Parasitic Infestations

Client and family teaching is necessary to facilitate treatment at home, to prevent the spread of the infestation, and to dispel the myth that only dirty people have lice. Teach this specific information:

- Wash clothing and linens in soap and hot water, or have them dry-cleaned.
- Iron clothing to kill lice eggs.
- Boil personal care items, such as combs and brushes, to kill parasites.

- Treat all family members and sexual partners.
- Do not use combs, brushes, or hats of others.

See Critical Thinking Care Map on herpes zoster at the end of this chapter.

Malignant Skin Disorders

The skin is a common site for malignancy. Many of these lesions are found on skin surfaces that have had long-term exposure to the sun or the environment. Skin cancer is the most common of all cancers. This section of the chapter discusses the various types of malignant skin disorders.

NONMELANOMA SKIN CANCER

The skin is a fragile organ and is subject to damage from ultraviolet radiation and chemicals. Over time, this damage results in alterations in cellular structure and function, and malignancies may occur. The two types of **nonmelanoma skin cancers** (named because they do not arise from melanin-producing cells) are basal cell carcinoma and squamous cell carcinoma.

The American Cancer Society estimates that more than 1 million new cases of nonmelanoma skin cancer are diagnosed each year. If diagnosed and treated early, 95% to 99% can be cured. Nonmelanoma skin cancer is the most common malignant growth found in fair-skinned people. Of the two types of nonmelanoma skin cancer, basal cell carcinoma is the most common, outnumbering squamous cell carcinoma three to one. Men develop nonmelanoma skin cancer more often than do women, probably because of occupational exposures. Adults between the ages of 30 and 60 have the majority of these cancers. The factors involved in the development of nonmelanoma skin cancer include ultraviolet radiation, chemicals, skin pigmentation, and preexisting pigmented skin lesions.

Ultraviolet radiation (UVR) from the sun is believed to be the cause of most nonmelanoma skin cancers. Sun rays are believed to either alter DNA or suppress T-cell and B-cell immunity. People who live in higher altitudes receive greater ultraviolet radiation exposure. The amount of clothing worn, the time of day, and the amount of time in the sun also determine the amount of exposure. Exposure to ultraviolet radiation in tanning booths also has been implicated in nonmelanoma skin cancer development.

Certain chemicals have also been associated with nonmelanoma skin cancer. Hydrocarbons, found in mixtures of coal, tar, asphalt, soot, and mineral oils have been linked with skin cancer. Other factors associated with nonmelanoma skin cancer are the use of ionizing radiation, viruses, and physical trauma. Human papillomavirus is implicated in the development of squamous cell carcinoma, as is damage to the skin from burns.

Skin pigmentation affects the development of nonmelanoma skin cancer. The more melanin a person has, the more the skin is protected from damaging ultraviolet rays. Thus, African Americans, Asian Americans, and people of Mediterranean descent have a much lower incidence of nonmelanoma skin cancer than do people who have red hair and fair complexions and who tend to freckle or sunburn easily.

Most people have many pigmented moles or other lesions on their body, of which most are normal. However, a major risk factor in the development of nonmelanoma skin cancer is a change in an existing lesion or the presence of a premalignant lesion, such as actinic keratosis.

BASAL CELL CARCINOMA

Basal cell carcinoma begins in the basal cell layer of the epidermis, usually on sun-exposed areas of the body, especially the head and neck. Basal cell carcinomas are the most common and the least deadly. They are slow-growing and rarely metastasize, but they can invade nearby areas. They can recur in the same location after treatment.

Nodular basal cell carcinoma appears as a smooth, itchy pimple but as they grow, the skin becomes shiny, and either pearly white, pink or skin-colored. Superficial basal cell carcinoma is a flat papule, often red, and may ulcerate.

SQUAMOUS CELL CARCINOMA

Squamous cell carcinoma is a malignant tumor of the squamous epithelium of the skin or mucous membranes. It occurs most often on areas of skin that are exposed to ultraviolet rays and weather, such as the forehead, helix of the ear, top of the nose, lower lip, and back of the hands. Squamous cell carcinoma may also arise on skin that has been burned or has chronic inflammation. This is a much more aggressive cancer than basal cell cancer, with a faster growth rate and a much greater potential for metastasis if untreated.

Pathophsyiology and Manifestations

Squamous cell carcinoma begins as a firm, flesh-colored or erythematous papule. The tumor may be crusted. As it grows, it may ulcerate, bleed, and become painful. As the tumor extends into the surrounding tissue and becomes a nodule, the area around the nodule becomes *indurated* (hardened) (Figure 45-5 ■). Recurrent squamous cell carcinoma can be invasive, increasing the person's risk of metastasis.

MELANOMA

Melanoma, also called *cutaneous* or *malignant melanoma,* is a skin cancer that arises from melanocytes, the cells that produce melanin. The incidence of this serious skin cancer is

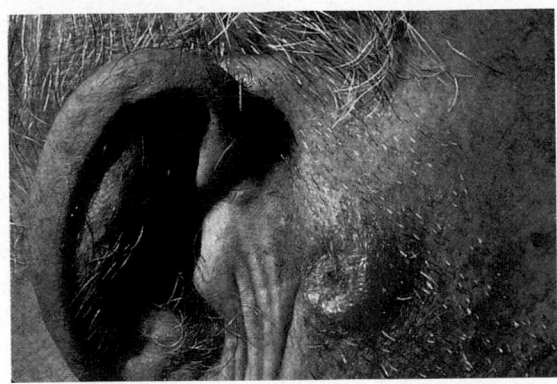

Figure 45-5. ■ As a squamous cell cancer grows, it tends to invade surrounding tissue. It also ulcerates, may bleed, and is painful. (Reprinted with permission from the American Academy of Dermatology. All rights reserved.)

increasing annually; its incidence doubled in the past three decades. Melanoma is the cause of 4% of all skin cancer cases, but contributes to a large number of skin cancer deaths. The American Cancer Society estimates that more than 60,000 new melanoma cases will be diagnosed in the United States in 2005.

Pathophysiology and Manifestations

The incidence is highest in Caucasians, people who had severe, blistering sunburns during childhood, and in people who live in sunny climates, burn easily, and visit tanning parlors. However, melanoma may arise from lesions that are already present or from skin that is normally covered with clothing. While they are still confined to the epidermis, the lesions are flat and relatively benign. However, when they penetrate the dermis, they mingle with blood and lymph vessels and are capable of metastasizing. At this latter stage, the tumors develop a raised or nodular appearance and often have smaller nodules, called satellite lesions, around the periphery.

The prognosis for survival for people diagnosed with malignant melanoma is determined by several variables, including tumor thickness, ulceration, metastasis, site, age, and gender. Younger clients and women have a somewhat better chance of survival. Tumors on the hands, feet, and scalp have a poorer prognosis. Tumors of the feet and scalp may not be noticed and diagnosed until they grow into the dermis.

Precursor lesions for the development of melanoma are dysplastic **nevi** (moles), congenital nevi, and lentigo maligna. *Dysplastic nevi* (also called atypical moles) appear during childhood and become dysplastic (have abnormal development) after puberty. They most often appear on the face, trunk, and arms but also are seen on the scalp, female breast, groin, and buttocks. They have irregular borders and pigmentation colors. A client with classic dysplastic nevi has more than 100 nevi, at least one of which is larger than

8 mm in diameter, and at least one has the characteristics of melanoma. *Congenital nevi* are present at birth. They are often slightly raised, with an irregular surface and a fairly regular border. *Lentigo maligna* is a tan or black patch on the skin that looks like a freckle. It grows slowly, becoming mottled, dark, thick, and nodular. It is usually seen on one side of the face of an older adult who has had a large amount of sun exposure.

A change in the color or size of a nevus is reported in 70% of people diagnosed with a melanoma. The ABCD rule (American Cancer Society, 2005) is used to assess suspicious lesions:

A = asymmetry; one-half of the nevus does not match the other half

B = border irregularity (edges are ragged, blurred, or notched)

C = color variation or dark black color

D = diameter greater than 5 mm (size of a pencil eraser)

During the initial radial phase, which may last from 1 to 25 years (depending on the type), the melanoma grows parallel to the skin surface. During this phase, the tumor rarely metastasizes and is often curable by surgical excision. However, during the next vertical growth phase, atypical melanocytes penetrate into the dermis and subcutaneous tissue, greatly increasing the risk for metastasis and death. When the lesion enters the vertical growth phase, it grows rapidly, and its color changes from a mixture of tan, brown, and black to a characteristic red, white, and blue color. The lesion also develops irregular borders and often has raised nodules and ulcerations (Figure 45-6 ■).

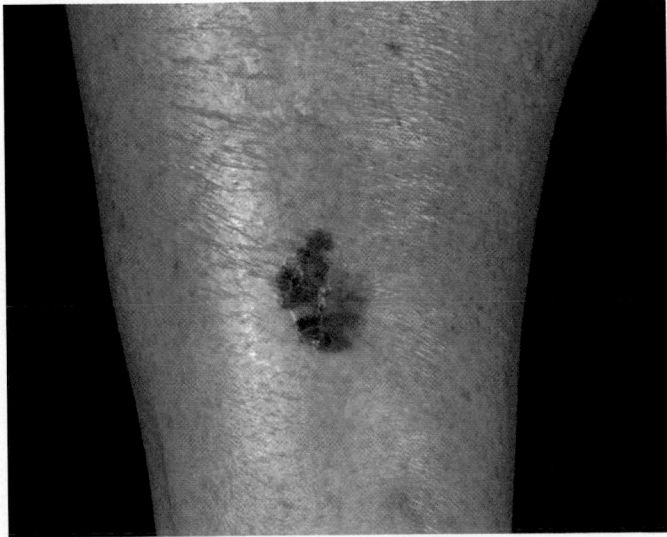

Figure 45-6. ■ Malignant melanoma is a serious skin cancer that arises from melanocytes. (*Source:* Caliendo/Custom Medical Stock Photo, Inc.)

INTERDISCIPLINARY CARE

Treatment of all skin cancers focuses on removal of malignant tissue using such methods as surgery, curettage and electrodesiccation, cryotherapy, or radiotherapy. These treatments offer a greater than 90% cure rate. The management of melanoma begins with identification, diagnosis, and tumor staging. Besides surgical excision, melanoma is also treated with chemotherapy, immunotherapy, radiation therapy, and biological therapies (interleukin-2 and interferon, or therapeutic vaccines containing melanoma antigens).

Diagnostic Tests

Skin cancer is diagnosed by microscopic examination of tissue biopsied from any suspicious lesion. The biopsies are usually done as office procedures under local anesthesia. Laboratory and diagnostic tests are also conducted to determine whether a melanoma has metastasized.

Liver function tests are done. The combination of an elevated lactic dehydrogenase (LDH), alkaline phosphatase, and aspartate aminotransferase (AST) suggests metastasis to the liver. If liver enzymes are abnormal, a computed tomography (CT) scan of the liver is conducted. A complete blood count is done to determine hematologic abnormalities. Serum blood chemistry tests are conducted to identify electrolyte and mineral abnormalities.

Chest x-rays for possible lung metastasis are taken if the client has respiratory difficulty or hemoptysis. If there is undetermined bone pain, a bone scan is performed. If the client has headaches, seizures, or neurologic deficits, a CT scan or magnetic resonance imaging (MRI) of the brain is conducted.

The systems used to describe the level of invasion of a melanoma and the maximum tumor thickness are called *microstaging* systems. In the Clark system of microstaging, the vertical growth of the lesion is measured from the epidermis to the subcutaneous tissue. In the Breslow system, the vertical thickness is measured from the granular level of the epidermis to the deepest level of tumor invasion. This determination is important, because as the thickness of the melanoma increases, survival rate decreases. Staging of malignant tumors is discussed in Chapter 12. ⬭

Surgery

Nonmelanoma skin cancers may be removed through Mohs' micrographic surgery or surgical excision. In Mohs' micrographic surgery, thin layers of the tumor are shaved off horizontally. A frozen section of the tissue is stained at each level to determine tumor margins. This is the most accurate method of assessing the extent of nonmelanoma skin cancer, and it conserves the most normal tissue. Cure rates with Mohs' microscopic surgery are at 99% for primary basal cell

cancer and 94% for squamous cell carcinoma. For melanoma, surgical excision is the preferred treatment. A wide excision is used that includes the full thickness of the skin and the subcutaneous tissue.

Curettage and Electrodesiccation or Cryosurgery

Small basal cell cancers may be removed with curettage and electrodesiccation. This procedure provides good cosmetic results and preserves normal tissue. However, healing time is longer, and it is difficult to ensure that all tumor margins have been removed. Cryosurgery is noninvasive; liquid nitrogen is used to freeze and destroy the tumor tissue. The area of the tumor is locally anesthetized. Then, liquid nitrogen is applied to the lesion by either a spray or cryoprobes. Cryosurgery is used for some primary basal cell cancers and for low-risk squamous cell cancers.

Radiation

Radiation is used for lesions that are inoperable because of their location (e.g., on the eyelid, the canthus, or the lip) or their size (between 1 and 8 cm). Radiation is also used for clients who are older and of poor surgical risk. The treatment is given over a 3- to 4-week period in a clinical facility. It does not allow control of tumor margins, and may itself cause skin cancer.

Immunotherapy

Immunotherapy is a relatively new treatment for melanoma. The immunologic response was explored because the number of spontaneous remissions in clients with melanoma was higher than with any other adult tumor. Tumor-specific antigen–antibodies have also recently been identified. Agents such as interferons, interleukins, monoclonal antibodies, bacille Calmette–Guérin (BCG), levamisole, transfer factors, and tumor vaccines have all shown activity in melanoma, with varying response rates. The effectiveness of these agents alone, in combination with chemotherapy, or in combination with each other is under investigation.

NURSING CARE

Surgical excision is the most common form of treatment for skin cancer. Nursing care depends on the treatment employed and on the extent of the procedure.

ASSESSING

The nurse assesses the skin of clients who seek care for many different health problems and may be the first to identify suspicious lesions. Assessment data is collected by the nurse to determine factors in the client's history that

ASSESSMENT

Assessing Clients with Skin Cancer

SUBJECTIVE DATA

- Any change in the size, shape, or color of a mole, wart, birthmark, or scar.
- Bleeding, crusting, itching, or pain of a mole, wart, birthmark, or scar.
- Exposure to hazardous chemicals.
- Use of sunscreen.
- Use of tanning salons.
- Knowledge about and frequency of skin examinations.
- Previous removal of skin cancer.
- Family history of treatment for skin cancer.
- Geographic area of residence during lifetime.
- Previous serious sunburn.

OBJECTIVE DATA

- Inspect and palpate the entire skin for lesions. Use a good light and stretch the skin as tightly as necessary to better view lesions. Pay special attention to areas covered with hair, skin folds (such as under the breasts), the axilla, webs between the fingers and toes, soles of the feet, the area between the buttocks, oral cavity, ear canals, and mucous membranes. Assess for:
  - Obvious lesions
  - Visible swelling
  - Contour, size, and color of moles, warts, birthmarks, and scars
  - Enlarged lymph nodes
  - Discoloring of the skin
  - Areas of ulceration, scaling, crusting, or erosion.
- Measure and document all skin lesions on an anatomic chart. If possible take photographs of any suspicious lesions to use in future comparison.
- Monitor and report results above expected range for liver function tests.

may have increased the risk for skin cancer and to identify any skin lesions. Box 45-3 ■ lists subjective and objective data to collect.

DIAGNOSING, PLANNING, AND IMPLEMENTING

Priorities in Nursing Care. The increasing incidence of skin cancer requires that nurses be involved in early detection and in teaching preventive behaviors in all settings. Information about skin self-examination, sunscreens, and skin cancer prevention are discussed in the Continuing Care section.

Wide excision and the high risk of metastasis from melanoma usually require inpatient surgical treatment. The nurse provides care and teaching. The most common nursing diagnoses are Anxiety, Impaired Skin Integrity, and Hopelessness.

Anxiety

- Provide reassurance by sitting quietly with the client, speaking slowly and calmly, and conveying empathetic understanding by touch. Support the client's coping mechanisms, such as crying and talking. Use short, simple sentences; focus on the here and now, and provide concise information. *Higher levels of anxiety result in a focus on the present, inability to concentrate, and difficulty understanding verbal communications.*
- Provide accurate information to the client and family about the illness, treatment, and expected length of recovery. *Accurate information enables a person to make informed decisions.*
- Encourage discussion of expected physical changes and ways to minimize disfigurement through cosmetics and clothing. Provide the client with strategies for participating in the recovery process. *Coping behaviors differ from person to person and from situation to situation. Surgical incisions to remove melanoma may cause disfigurement. Active participation in care provides the client with some control over the future and is often an effective means of coping with anxiety.*

Impaired Skin Integrity

- Monitor the client every 4 hours for fever, tachycardia, and malaise, as well as for incisional erythema, swelling, pain, or drainage that increases or becomes purulent. *These manifestations may indicate infection. Skin cancers not only destroy skin layers but also can invade body structures. Both open lesions (from tumors that ulcerate before diagnosis) and incisions (from biopsy and surgery) increase the risk for secondary infection.*
- Keep the incision line clean and dry by changing dressings as necessary. *Moisture increases the risk of infection.*
- Follow principles of medical and surgical asepsis when caring for a client's incision. Teach family members and visitors the importance of careful hand washing. Maintain standard precautions if drainage is present. *Aseptic techniques are necessary when caring for any surgical incision to prevent infection. Careful hand washing helps prevent the spread of infection. Nurses must use precautions with blood and body fluids to protect themselves from exposure to HIV.*
- Encourage and maintain adequate calories and protein intake in the diet. Suggest a consultation with the dietitian if client does not want to eat. *The client with cancer has increased metabolic needs. If these are not met, healing may be impaired.*

Hopelessness

- Use active listening, ask open-ended questions, and reflect on the client's statements. Acknowledge and respect the client's feelings of apathy or anger as expressions of distress. Convey an empathetic understanding of the client's fears and concerns. *Hopelessness is a common response to the diagnosis of cancer. Clients who experience hopelessness are often withdrawn, passive, and apathetic. An empathetic listener can help them face their concerns.*

- Provide opportunities for the client to express hope, faith, a sense of purpose, and the will to live. *The client with melanoma faces the possibility or reality of metastasis; the possibility that the cancer may recur and cause death; and alterations in self-concept, roles, and relationships. Inspiring hope in clients during this health crisis is a legitimate nursing action.*

- Explore the client's perceptions. Provide information, and correct misconceptions if necessary. *Verbalizing feelings, concerns, and goals allows others to validate or correct them, promotes a therapeutic nurse–client relationship, and fosters feelings of self-worth.*

- Encourage the client to identify support systems and past sources of strength and coping. *Identifying support systems and effective coping strategies from past crises helps the person resolve the current crisis and develop hope.*

- Encourage the client to participate in self-care, mutual decision making, and goal setting. *Meeting self-care needs and making decisions about one's own care build self-confidence.*

- Encourage focusing not only on the present but also on the future: Review past occasions for hope, discuss personal meaning of hope, establish and evaluate short-term goals with the client and family, and encourage them to express hope for the future. *Mobilizing the client's resources strengthens motivation, hope, and the will to live.*

EVALUATING

Evaluating the effectiveness of nursing care for the client with skin cancer requires ongoing assessment. Collect data about effectiveness of treatment measures, client's understanding of and compliance with treatments, and effectiveness of medications.

Documenting. Documentation includes effectiveness of treatment measures, medications and side effects. Record teaching provided to the client and family about wound care, regular checkups with a health care provider, and skin self-examination.

CONTINUING CARE

Nurses provide client and family education for prevention and early detection of skin cancer (Box 45-4 ■). Numerous

---

BOX 45-4	CLIENT TEACHING

Preventing Skin Cancer

It is well known that cumulative sun exposure positively correlates with nonmelanoma skin cancers. Many skin cancers can be prevented by limiting exposure to risk factors. Primary prevention behaviors recommended by the American Cancer Society and the Skin Cancer Foundation follow:

- Minimize exposure to the sun between the hours of 10 A.M. and 4 P.M., when ultraviolet rays are the strongest.
- Cover up with a wide-brimmed hat, sunglasses, long-sleeved shirt, and long pants made of tightly woven material when you are in the sun.
- Use a waterproof or water-resistant sunscreen with a sun protective factor (SPF) of 15 or more before every exposure to the sun. Apply sunscreen not only on sunny but also on cloudy days, when ultraviolet rays can penetrate 70% to 80% of the cloud cover.
- Reapply the sunscreen before the protection time is up. If you are at risk for skin cancer, apply sunscreen daily.
- Use sunscreen and protective clothing when you are on or near sand, snow, concrete, or water, which can reflect more than half of the ultraviolet rays onto the skin.
- Avoid tanning booths; UVA radiation emitted by tanning booths damages the deep skin layers.

---

brochures are also available from the American Cancer Society, health education and support agencies, and pharmaceutical companies that manufacture sunscreen. Most of this literature is provided free of charge.

Teach the client or family who is at risk for, or has been diagnosed with, skin cancer how to conduct a self-examination of the skin. Stress that it should be conducted on the same day of each month. Family members can help with areas that are hard to examine (ears, scalp, back, extremities), or the client can use a mirror. Showing photographs of both normal and cancerous skin lesions may help teach the client and family what to watch for when doing self-examination. Teach about the following changes:

- Color, especially any lesion that becomes darker or variegated in shades of tan, brown, black, red, white, or blue
- Size, especially any lesion that becomes larger or spreads out
- Shape, especially any lesion that protrudes more from the skin or begins to have an irregular outline
- Appearance, especially bleeding, drainage, oozing, ulceration, crusting, scaliness, or development of a mushrooming outward growth
- Consistency, especially any lesion that becomes softer or is more easily irritated

- Surrounding skin—redness, swelling, or leaking of color from a lesion into the surrounding skin
- Sensation—itching or pain.

If any of these changes occurs, the client should immediately contact the health care provider for further assessment. If treatment is conducted in an outpatient setting, teach the client and family specific measures for self-care, including how and when to change dressings, the use of aseptic technique and careful hand washing when caring for the wound, symptoms to report (such as bleeding, fever, or signs of wound infection), and how to protect the operative site against trauma and irritations. The client who undergoes extensive surgery will require preoperative and postoperative care (see Chapter 9). ⚭

Encourage clients with melanoma to schedule regular medical checkups every 3 months for the first 2 years, every 6 months for the next 5 years, and yearly thereafter. Emphasize that proper self-care combined with regular medical care can help the client lead a fairly normal life. If assistance for home care is necessary, provide referrals to a community health or home care agency. Refer the client to a local cancer support group if the client believes this will be helpful.

Pressure Ulcers

Pressure ulcers (bedsores, decubitus ulcers) are ischemic lesions of the skin and underlying tissue caused by external pressure that impairs the flow of blood and lymph (Porth, 2005). The ischemia causes tissue necrosis and eventual ulceration. Pressure ulcers tend to develop over a bony prominence (e.g., heels, greater trochanter, sacrum, and ischia), but they may appear on any part of the body that is subjected to external pressure, friction, or shearing forces. Pressure causes more damage when it is applied to a small area than when it is distributed over a large surface.

PATHOPHYSIOLOGY AND MANIFESTATIONS

When a person lies or sits in one position for an extended length of time without moving, pressure on the tissue between a bony prominence and the external surface of the body distorts capillaries and interferes with normal blood flow. If the pressure is relieved, blood flow to the area increases, a brief period of reactive hyperemia occurs, and no permanent damage occurs. However, if the pressure continues, platelets clump in the endothelial cells surrounding the capillaries and form *microthrombi* (very small blood clots). These microthrombi impede blood flow, resulting in ischemia and hypoxia of tissues. Eventually, the cells and tissues of the immediate area and of the surrounding area die and become necrotic.

Alterations in the involved tissue depend on the depth of the injury. Injury to superficial layers of skin results in blister formation. Injury to deeper structures causes the pressure ulcer area to appear dark reddish-blue. As the issues die, the ulcer becomes an open wound that may be deep enough to expose the bone. The necrotic tissue elicits an inflammatory response. The client experiences fever and pain and has an increased white blood cell count. Secondary bacterial invasion is common. Enzymes from bacteria as well as macrophages dissolve necrotic tissue, resulting in a foul-smelling drainage.

Shearing forces result when one tissue layer slides over another. The stretching and bending of blood vessels cause injury and thrombosis. Clients in hospital beds are subject to shearing forces when the head of the bed is elevated and the torso slides down toward the foot of the bed. Pulling the client up in bed also subjects the client to shearing forces. For this reason, clients are always lifted up in bed. In both cases, friction and moisture cause the skin and superficial fascia to remain fixed to the bed sheet, while the deep fascia and bony skeleton slide in the direction of body movement.

Although pressure ulcers may occur in an adult with impaired mobility, those most at risk are older adults with limited mobility, people with quadriplegia, and clients in the critical care setting. Others at risk are clients with fractures of large bones (e.g., hip or femur), and those who have undergone orthopedic surgery or sustained spinal cord injury. Incontinence, nutritional deficit, chronic illnesses (like renal failure and anemia), edema, and infection also create increased risk.

Because of age-related skin changes, the older adult is at increased risk for the development of pressure ulcers. The skin of the older adult has a thicker epidermis, a thinner dermis with decreased vascularity, decreased sebaceous gland activity, and decreased strength and elasticity. The more fragile and less nourished dermal layer is more prone to shear and friction problems. The skin of the older adult responds more slowly to inflammation, and wounds heal more slowly. When pressure ulcers occur, they are more difficult to reverse.

Pressure ulcers are graded or staged to classify the degree of damage. The stages, defined by the Panel for the Prediction and Prevention of Pressure Ulcers in Adults as part of the U.S. Department of Health and Human Services are listed in Box 45-5 ■.

INTERDISCIPLINARY CARE

If a client is at risk for pressure ulcers, the goal is prevention. Ulcers that are already present require collaborative treatment to promote healing and restore skin integrity.

Laboratory tests are conducted to determine the presence of a secondary infection and to differentiate the cause of

MediaLink

Pressure Ulcers

BOX 45-5

PRESSURE ULCER STAGING

Stage I

Nonblanchable erythema of intact skin; the heralding lesion of skin ulceration. Identification of stage I pressure ulcers may be difficult in clients with darkly pigmented skin. *Note:* Reactive hyperemia can normally be expected to be present for one-half to three-fourths as long as the time the pressure occluded blood flow to the area. This should not be confused with stage I pressure ulcer.

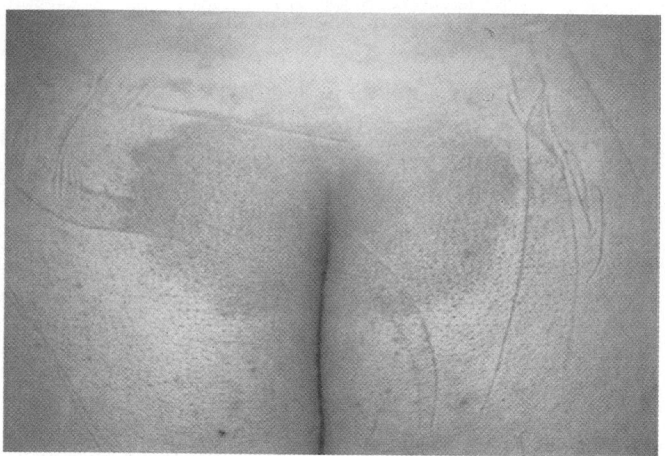

Stage II

Partial-thickness skin loss involving epidermis and/or dermis. The ulcer is superficial and presents clinically as an abrasion, blister, or shallow crater.

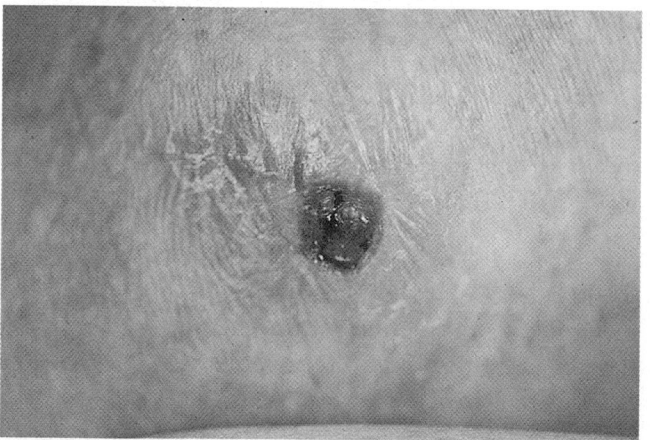

Stage III

Full-thickness skin loss involving damage or necrosis of subcutaneous tissue that may extend down to, but not through, underlying fascia. The ulcer presents clinically as a deep crater with or without undermining of adjacent tissue.

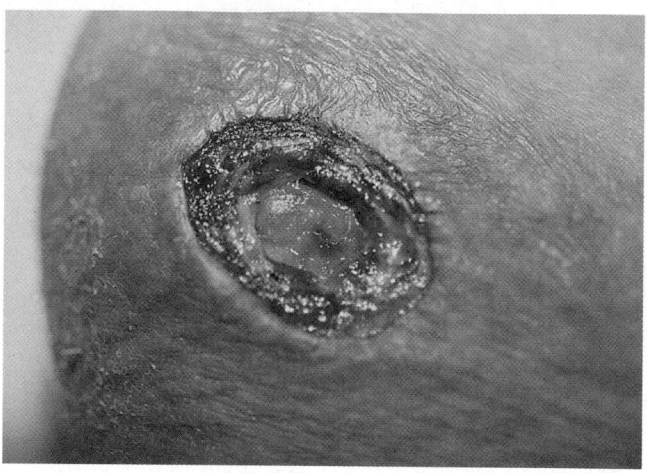

Stage IV

Full-thickness skin loss with extensive destruction; tissue necrosis; or damage to muscle, bone, or supporting structures (e.g., tendon or joint capsule). Sinus tracts may also be associated with stage IV ulcers.

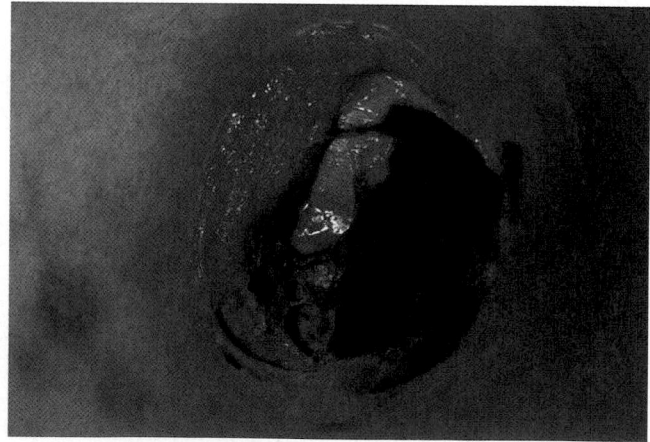

Note: When eschar is present, accurate staging of the pressure ulcer is not possible until the eschar has sloughed or the wound has been debrided.

Text is from Agency for Health Care Policy and Research. (1992). *Pressure Ulcers in Adults: Prediction and Prevention.* Rockville, MD: U.S. Department of Health and Human Services. Photos courtesy of Karen Kennedy, RN, FPN.

the ulcer. If the ulcer is deep or appears infected, drainage or biopsied tissue is cultured to determine the causative organism.

Topical and systemic antibiotics specific to the infectious organism are used to eradicate any infection present and to promote healing. Special wound care products and dressings may be used to manage the care of pressure ulcers (Table 45-3 ■). Surgical debridement may be necessary if the pressure ulcer is deep; if subcutaneous tissues are involved; or if an *eschar* (a scab or dry crust) has formed over

TABLE 45-3

Products Used to Treat Pressure Ulcers

STAGE	PRODUCT	PURPOSE
I	Skin Prep	Toughens intact skin and preserves skin integrity.
	Granulex	Prevents skin breakdown, increases blood supply, adds moisture; contains trypsin to aid in removal of necrotic tissue.
	Hydrocolloid dressing (e.g., DuoDERM)	Prevents skin breakdown and promotes healing without the formation of a crust over the ulcer. Is permeable to air and water vapor; prevents the growth of anaerobic organisms.
	Transparent dressing (e.g., Tegaderm)	Prevents skin breakdown; prevents entrance of moisture and bacteria but allows oxygen and moisture vapor permeability.
II	Transparent dressing	Enhances healing.
	Hydrocolloid dressing	*Note:* If infection is present, these types of dressings are contraindicated. A sterile dressing should be applied instead.
III	Wet-to-dry gauze dressing with sterile normal saline	Allows necrotic material to soften and adhere to the gauze, so that the wound is debrided.
	Hydrocolloid dressing	Enhances healing.
	Proteolytic enzymes (such as Elase)	Proteolytic enzymes serve as a debriding agent in inflamed and infected lesions.
IV	Wet-to-dry gauze dressing with sterile normal saline	Enhances healing. *Note:* Transparent or hydrocolloid dressings or skin barriers are contraindicated.
	Vacuum-assisted closure (VAC)	Creates a negative pressure to help reduce edema, increase blood supply and oxygenation, and decrease bacterial colonization. Also helps promote moist wound healing and the formation of granulation tissue.

the ulcer, preventing healing by granulation. Large wounds may require skin grafting for complete closure.

NURSING CARE

The client with one or more pressure ulcers not only has impaired skin integrity but also is at increased risk for infection, pain, and decreased mobility; prolonged treatment for other conditions; increased health care costs; and diminished quality of life.

Risk for Impaired Skin Integrity and Impaired Skin Integrity

The interventions and rationales below are adapted from the clinical guidelines of the Agency for Health Care Policy and Research (1992) (now the Agency for Healthcare Research and Quality) for identifying adults at risk and treating those with stage I pressure ulcers.

- Identify at-risk individuals and the specific factors that place them at risk.
  - Assess bed- and chair-bound clients, as well as those who cannot reposition themselves, for immobility, incontinence, nutritional status, and altered level of consciousness.

- Assess clients on admission to acute care and rehabilitation hospitals, nursing homes, home care programs, and other health care facilities, using a validated risk assessment tool.
- Document all assessments of risk.

Identifying individuals at risk for pressure ulcers allows reduction of risk factors. Clients who cannot reposition themselves or whose activity is limited to bed or a chair should be assessed. Using a validated assessment tool ensures systematic evaluation and allows reassessment over time. Accurate and complete documentation ensures continuity of care.

- Conduct a systematic skin inspection at least once a day, paying particular attention to the bony prominences. *Systematic, comprehensive, and routine skin care decreases incidence. Data from skin inspection are used to design interventions to reduce risk and evaluate outcomes.*

- Clean the skin at the time of soiling and at routine intervals, as frequently as the client's need or preference dictates. Avoid hot water, use a mild cleansing agent, and clean the skin gently, applying as little force and friction as possible. *Metabolic wastes and environmental contaminants accumulate on the skin and should be removed regularly. Feces and urine cause chemical irritation. Hot water may cause skin injury. Mild cleansing agents are less likely to remove the skin's natural resistance to injury.*

■ Minimize environmental factors leading to skin drying, such as low humidity and exposure to cold. Treat dry skin with moisturizers. *Well-hydrated skin resists mechanical trauma. Low humidity dries the skin, making it less pliable. Severe dryness is associated with fissures and cracks in the stratum corneum. Moisturizers help reduce dryness of skin.*

clinical ALERT

Do not massage over bony prominences. Evidence suggests that massage may lead to deep tissue trauma in at-risk clients.

■ Minimize skin exposure to moisture from incontinence, perspiration, or wound drainage. Use materials that absorb moisture and present a quick-drying surface to the skin. Change underpads and briefs frequently. Do not place plastic directly against the skin. *Factors in urine, perspiration, or wound drainage may irritate the skin. Moisture alone can increase the skin's susceptibility to injury.*

■ Minimize friction and shearing forces. Use proper positioning, transferring, and turning techniques. Lubricants such as cornstarch or creams, protective films such as transparent dressings and skin sealants, protective dressings such as hydrocolloids, and protective padding may also reduce friction injuries. *Proper positioning can eliminate most shear injury. Friction injuries to the skin occur from moving across a rough surface (e.g., bed linens). Any agent that eliminates contact or decreases friction reduces this risk.*

■ For inadequate dietary intake of protein or calories, offer nutritional supplements and support the client during mealtimes. If dietary intake remains inadequate, enteral or parenteral feedings may be needed. *Poor dietary intake of protein, calories, and iron has been associated with pressure ulcer development.*

■ Maintain the client's current level of activity, mobility, and range of motion. *Frequent turning, repositioning, and movement are essential in reducing risk.*

■ Teach clients who can do so to shift their weight every 15 minutes. *Data support that spontaneous movements by older, bedridden clients lower the incidence of pressure ulcers.*

clinical ALERT

Reposition all at-risk clients at least every 2 hours, using a written schedule for systematic turning and repositioning. Avoid leaving clients sitting in a chair or wheelchair. Fewer pressure ulcers develop in clients who are turned every 2 to 3 hours.

■ For clients on bed rest, use positioning devices, such as pillows or foam wedges, to protect bony prominences. For clients who are completely immobile, use devices that relieve pressure on the heels. The most common method is to raise the heels off the bed. Place any at-risk client on a pressure-reducing device, such as foam, static air, alternating air, gel, or water mattress. Do not use donut-type devices. *Suspending the heels is the best way to redistribute pressure to those areas. Pressure-reducing devices and beds can reduce the incidence of pressure ulcers. Donut cushions may actually contribute to pressure ulcer development.*

clinical ALERT

Avoid placing clients in the side-lying position directly on the trochanter.

■ Maintain the head of the bed at the lowest degree of elevation consistent with the client's medical condition and other restrictions. Limit the amount of time the head of the bed is elevated. *Proper positioning can reduce pressure on body prominences.*

■ Use assistive devices, such as a trapeze or bed linen, to move clients in bed who cannot assist during transfers and position changes. *Lifting, rather than dragging, clients up in bed is less likely to cause friction injury.*

CONTINUING CARE

Client and family teaching focus on prevention of pressure ulcers as discussed. Because many clients at risk for pressure ulcers are older or have other serious illnesses, the nurse may need to teach a caregiver about the following topics:

■ Definition, description, and common locations of pressure ulcers
■ Risk factors for the development of pressure ulcers
■ Skin care
■ Ways to avoid injury
■ Diet.

Depending on the stage of the pressure ulcer, teach the client or caregiver how to care for ulcers that are already present: how to change wet-to-dry dressings, apply skin barriers, and avoid injury and infection. Referrals to a home health agency or community health department can help the family through the lengthy healing process.

Note: The bibliography listings for this and all chapters have been compiled at the back of the book.

Chapter Review

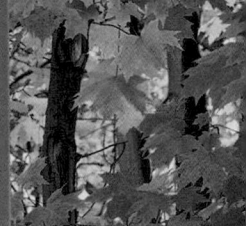

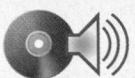 **KEY TERMS** by Topics

Use the audio glossary feature of either the CD-ROM or the Companion Website to hear the correct pronunciation of the following key terms.

Skin disorders
pruritus, psoriasis, dermatitis, acne

Skin infections and infestations
folliculitis, furuncle, cellulitis, dermatophytes, candidiasis, warts, herpes simplex, herpes zoster, pediculosis, scabies

Skin malignancy
nonmelanoma skin cancers, basal cell carcinoma, squamous cell carcinoma, melanoma, nevi

Pressure ulcers
pressure ulcers

KEY Points

- Common skin disorders include pruritus (itching), dry skin, psoriasis, dermatitis, and acne. The goals of client care are to identify and eliminate precipitating factors, provide relief from itching and pain, and reduce the risk of further damage to the skin.

- The skin may be infected or infested with various agents, including bacteria, fungi, viruses, and parasites. Treatment is provided to identify the causative agent, administer medications to kill or eradicate the organism, and prevent secondary infections.

- Nonmelanoma skin cancers (basal cell carcinoma and squamous cell carcinoma) are the most commonly occurring of all cancers. They are believed to be primarily due to damage from ultraviolet radiation from sun exposure. They do not tend to metastasize and are treated by excision.

- Melanoma skin cancers are serious malignancies that do metastasize. Any change in the shape, border, color, size, consistency, or sensation of a nevus (mole) should be immediately evaluated for transformation into a malignant melanoma.

- Pressure ulcers are ischemic lesions of the skin and underlying tissue. They are caused by external pressure or shearing forces that cause ischemia. The most common sites of development are over bony prominences. Older adults, as well as clients who are immobile, are most at risk for pressure ulcers. Nursing interventions are implemented to reduce risk factors and maintain intact skin.

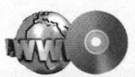 **EXPLORE Media**Link

Additional interactive resources for this chapter can be found on the Companion Website at www.prenhall.com/burke. Click on Chapter 45 and "Begin" to select the activities for this chapter.

For chapter-related NCLEX-style review questions and an audio glossary, access the accompanying CD-ROM in this book.

⊘ FOR FURTHER Study

For more about surgery in the care of a client with cancer, see Chapter 9.

For more about treatment of infections, see the discussion of antibiotic therapy in Chapter 10.

For further study of the staging of malignant tumors, see Chapter 12.

Sexually transmitted infections are discussed in Chapter 36.

See Chapter 44 for information about common primary and secondary skin lesions, and skin changes in older adults.

For discussion of the nursing care of burns, see Chapter 46.

Critical Thinking Care Map

Caring for a Client with Herpes Zoster
NCLEX-PN® Focus Area: Prevention and Health Maintenance

Case Study: Jesus Rivera is a 34-year-old migrant farm worker living in temporary housing in a rural area of southwestern America. He visits a free clinic and reports that he has not felt well for a week, and has had chills and fever. He has painful oozing blisters in a line on his left thorax. His vital signs are T 99°F (37.2°C), P 74, R 22, BP 148/88. He does remember having chickenpox as a child. He is afraid that exposure to pesticides has caused his blisters. The primary health care provider diagnoses Mr. Rivera with herpes zoster and prescribes a topical antiviral medication and an oral pain medication.

Nursing Diagnosis: Risk for Infection

COLLECT DATA

Subjective

_____
_____
_____
_____
_____
_____

Objective

_____
_____
_____
_____
_____
_____

Would you report this data? Yes/No

If yes, to: _____

Nursing Care

_____
_____
_____
_____
_____
_____
_____
_____
_____

How would you document this? _____
_____
_____
_____

Data Collected
(use those that apply)

- Age 34
- Migrant farm worker
- Reports chills and fever
- T 99°F
- BP 148/88
- Open blisters on thorax
- Exposure to pesticides

Nursing Interventions
(use those that apply; list in priority order)

- Provide chickenpox immunization.
- Teach how to apply topical medications.
- Stress importance of avoiding intimate contact with family members.
- Report migrant status to local authorities.
- Discuss need for careful hand washing.
- Teach effects of pain medications.

NCLEX-PN® Exam Preparation

1 A client diagnosed with psoriasis is preparing for bed. Which nursing intervention should be given the highest priority at this time?

A. Prepare the ordered therapeutic bath.
B. Administer a pain medication.
C. Teach the client to scratch the lesions to decrease discomfort.
D. Decrease the temperature in the client's room.

2 The nurse recognizes that which factors in a client's history are most likely to be related to a diagnosis of herpes zoster? (Select all that apply.)

A. cervical cancer
B. kidney transplant
C. childhood infection of chickenpox
D. measles at the age of 20
E. client receiving chemotherapy
F. menstruating female

3 A client has been receiving antibiotics for 3 days. The nurse should observe for the development of which side effect?

A. furuncles.
B. candidiasis.
C. tinea pedis.
D. folliculitis.

4 Topical acyclovir has been ordered for a client with genital herpes. The nurse should teach the client to:

A. use bare hands when applying the medication.
B. avoid taking hot baths.
C. use the medication once a week.
D. abstain from sexual intercourse.

5 A client diagnosed with pediculosis corporis returns to the clinic on two separate occasions with complaints of itching. The client states that all of the medicine given to treat the condition was taken as directed. The most important question to ask the client at this time is:

A. "Are other family members affected by the itching?"
B. "Are you having difficulty sleeping at night?"
C. "Do you have any pets living in your home?"
D. "Did you wash all of your bed linen after taking the medicine?"

6 Which factor relates directly to a diagnosis of nonmelanoma skin cancer?

A. exposure to ultraviolet radiation
B. client who is African American
C. decreased estrogen levels
D. appearance of liver spots

7 A client has developed a small basal cell cancer on the forearm and has been scheduled for cryosurgery. The client tells you that life is not worth living now that cancer has been found. An appropriate nursing diagnosis for this client might be:

A. Anxiety.
B. Fear.
C. Hopelessness.
D. Impaired Skin Integrity.

8 The most important instruction given to clients who are at risk for the development of skin cancer should be:

A. self-examination of skin.
B. the major risk factors for developing skin cancer.
C. treatments for the various types of skin cancer.
D. prognosis for skin cancer.

9 Which of these observations would be most significant when assessing the condition of a client who is at risk for a pressure ulcer?

A. diminished lung sounds
B. decreased appetite
C. permanent redness over the sacrum
D. contracture of the lower extremities

10 Nursing interventions that should be included on the care plan for a client diagnosed with impaired skin integrity are:

A. massage over the bony prominences.
B. reposition the client every 4 hours.
C. use hot water for bathing.
D. diet high in proteins and calories.

Answers for Review Questions, as well as discussion of Care Plan and Critical Thinking Care Map questions, appear in Appendix V.

Chapter 46

Caring for Clients with Burns

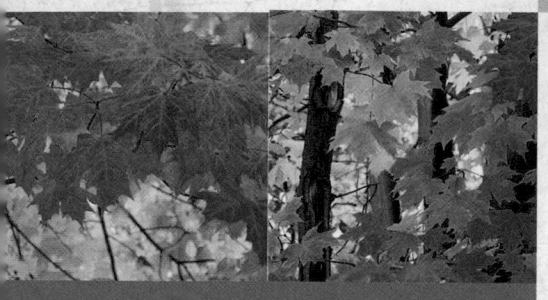

BRIEF Outline

Types of Burn Injury
  Classification of Burn Depth
Major Burns

LEARNING Outcomes

After completing this chapter, you will be able to:

- Discuss types, classification, extent estimation, and stages of treatment for burns.
- Describe the pathophysiology of a major burn.
- Identify the interdisciplinary care necessary for the client with a major burn, including diagnostic tests; medications; fluid resuscitation; respiratory management; nutritional support; wound management; surgery; biologic and biosynthetic dressings; scar, keloid, and contracture prevention; and wound dressings.
- Use the nursing process to collect data and provide interventions for clients with major burns.
- Provide client and family teaching for care of the burn after discharge.

MediaLink

www.prenhall.com/burke
Use the address above to access the free, interactive Companion Website created for this textbook. Get hints, instant feedback, and textbook references to chapter-related NCLEX-style questions. Link to other interesting sites.

Audio Glossary:
Use the Companion Website, or the CD-ROM disk enclosed with your textbook, to hear the pronunciation of key terms in this chapter.

It is estimated that more than 2.5 million burns occur each year in the United States, resulting in more than 100,000 hospitalizations and 4,500 deaths. The home is the most common site for fire-related burns. Home fires cause 80% of all fire-related deaths, with about 8 people dying in home fires each day. Factors associated with deaths from burns are age (especially children under 4 and adults 65 and older), careless smoking, alcohol or drug intoxication, and physical and mental disabilities.

Burns range from minor loss of the outermost layer of the skin to a complex injury involving all body systems. Treatments vary from simple application of a topical antiseptic agent in an outpatient clinic to an invasive, multisystem, interdisciplinary health team approach in the sterile environment of a burn center.

Types of Burn Injury

A **burn** is an injury in which a transfer of energy from a heat source to the human body results in tissue loss, damage, or irreversible destruction. Burns may be the result of thermal, chemical, electrical, or radiation damage. Although all four types can lead to generalized tissue damage and multisystem involvement, the causative agents and priority treatment measures are unique to each.

- *Thermal burns* result from exposure to dry heat (flames) or moist heat (steam and hot liquids). They are the most common burns and occur mostly in children and older adults.

- *Chemical burns* are caused by direct skin contact with either acid or alkaline agents. More than 25,000 products found in the home or workplace can cause chemical burns.
- The severity of *electrical burns* depends on the type and duration of current and amount of voltage. Electricity follows the path of least resistance, which in the human body tends to lie along muscles, blood vessels, nerves, and bone. Necrosis of the tissue results from impaired blood flow secondary to blood coagulation at the site of the electrical injury.
- *Radiation burns* are usually associated with sunburn or radiation treatment for cancer. These kinds of burns tend to be superficial, involving only the outermost layers of the epidermis.

CLASSIFICATION OF BURN DEPTH

After a burn, tissue damage is determined primarily by the extent of the burn (the percentage of body surface area involved) and the depth of the burn (affected layers of underlying tissue). The American Burn Association uses both the extent and depth of burn to classify burns as minor, moderate, or major. Characteristics of burns within each classification are summarized in Table 46-1 ■ and illustrated in Figure 46-1 ■.

A **superficial burn** (first-degree burn) involves only the epidermal layer. This type of burn most often results from sunburn, ultraviolet light, minor flash injury from a sudden ignition or explosion, or mild radiation burn associated with cancer treatment. Because the skin remains intact, this

---

TABLE 46-1

Characteristics of Burns By Depth

CHARACTERISTIC	SUPERFICIAL (FIRST DEGREE)	PARTIAL THICKNESS (SECOND DEGREE)	FULL THICKNESS (THIRD DEGREE)
Skin layers lost	Epidermis	Epidermis and dermis	Epidermis, dermis, and underlying tissues
Skin appearance over burn	Red; may have local edema	Fluid-filled blisters; bright pink; may appear waxy white with deep partial-thickness burns	Waxy white; dry, leathery, charred
Skin function	Present	Absent	Absent
Pain sensation	Present	Present	Absent
Manifestations at the burn site	Pain; local edema	Severe pain; edema; weeping of fluid	Little pain; edema
Treatment	Regular cleaning Topical agent of choice Mild analgesics	Regular cleaning Topical agent of choice May require skin grafting	Regular cleaning Topical agent of choice Skin substitutes Excision of eschar Skin grafting
Scarring	None; outer layer peels	May occur in deep burns	Occurs in grafted area
Time to heal	3 to 6 days	14 to > 21 days	Requires skin grafting to heal

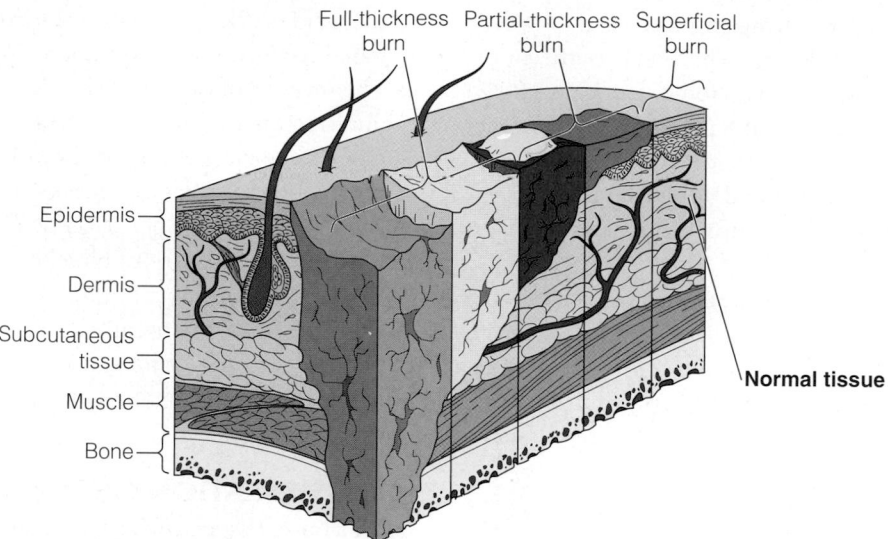

Figure 46-1. ■ Burn injury classification according to the depth of the burn.

degree of burn is not calculated into the estimates of burn injury. Clients with superficial burns involving large body surface areas may have chills, headache, nausea, and vomiting. Extensive superficial burns, especially in older adults, may require intravenous fluid treatment.

Partial-thickness burns (second-degree burns) may be subdivided into superficial or deep, depending on the depth of the burn.

A *superficial partial-thickness burn* involves the entire dermis. Causes may include a brief exposure to flash flame or dilute chemical agents, or contact with a hot surface. This burn is often bright red, and has a moist, glistening appearance with blister formation. The burned area blanches on pressure. Pain in response to temperature and air is usually severe. Pigment changes are common.

A *deep partial-thickness burn* involves the entire dermis plus hair follicles, but sebaceous glands and epidermal

sweat glands remain intact. This level of burn may be caused by hot liquids or solids, flash flame, direct flame, intense radiant energy, or chemical agents (Figure 46-2 ■). The surface of the burned skin appears pale and waxy and may be moist or dry. Large, easily ruptured blisters may be present. Capillary refill is decreased, but sensation to deep pressure is present. The wound is less painful than a superficial partial-thickness burn, but areas of both pain and decreased sensation may be present. Healing often requires more than 21 days. Necrosis may extend the depth of the wound. Contractures are possible, as are hypertrophic scarring and functional impairment.

A **full-thickness burn** (third-degree burn) involves all layers of skin (Figure 46-3 ■). The wound may extend into the subcutaneous fat, connective tissue, muscle, and bone. Full-thickness burns are caused by prolonged contact with flames, steam, chemicals, or high-voltage electric current.

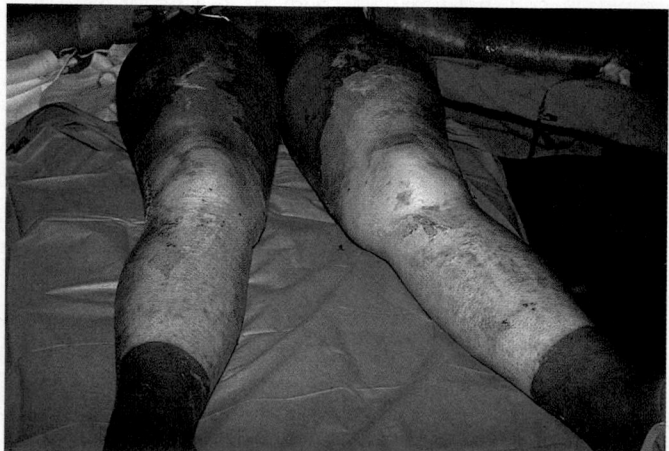

Figure 46-2. ■ Partial-thickness burn injury. (Courtesy of Dr. William Dominic, Valley Medical Center.)

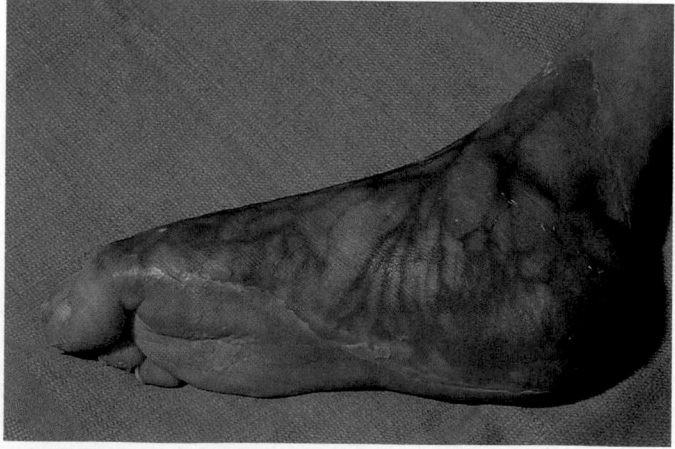

Figure 46-3. ■ Full-thickness burn injury. (Courtesy of Dr. William Dominic, Valley Medical Center.)

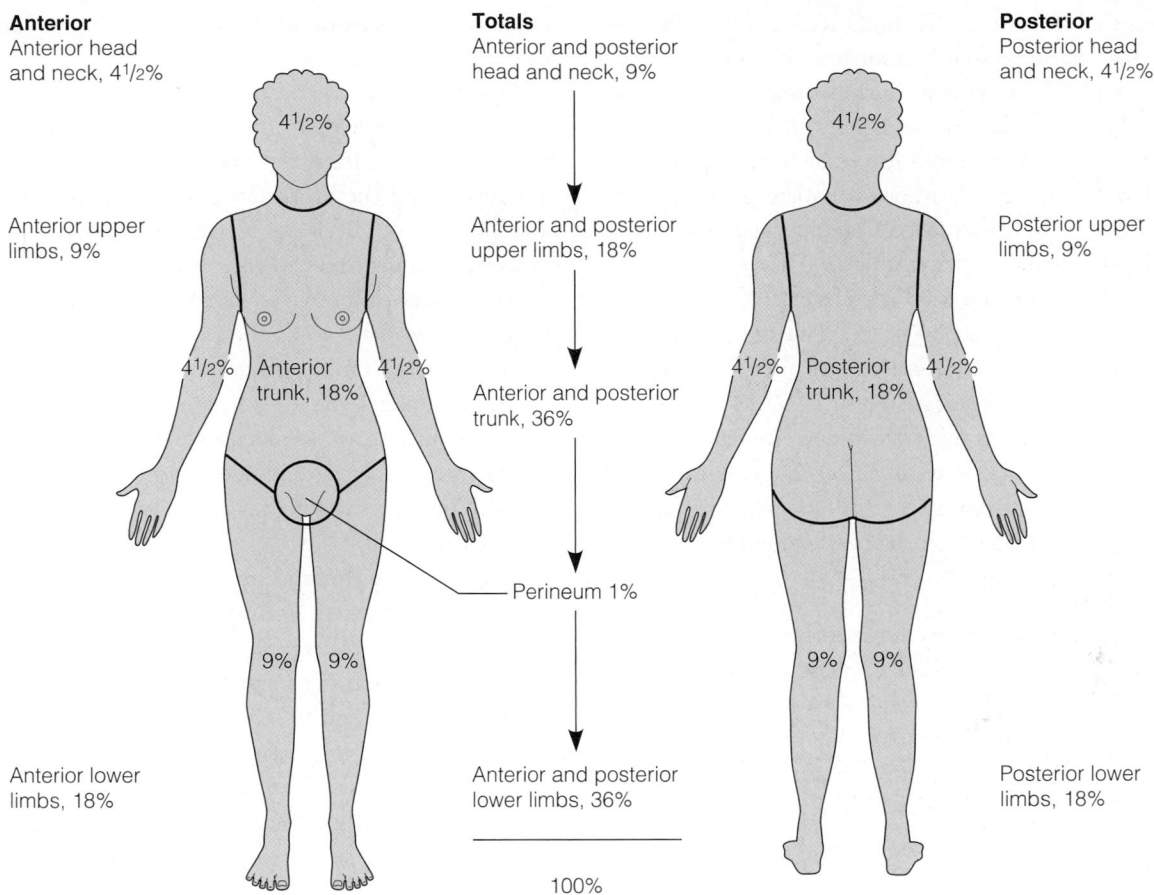

Figure 46-4. ■ The "rule of nines" is a way to estimate the percentage of TBSA affected by a burn injury. This quick method is useful in emergency situations, but it is not accurate for adults who are short, obese, or very thin.

Depending on its cause, the burn may appear pale, waxy, yellow, brown, mottled, charred, or nonblanching red. The wound surface is dry, leathery, and firm to the touch. Pain and touch receptors are destroyed.

Estimating the Extent of a Burn

The **"rule of nines"** is a rapid method of estimating the extent of partial- and full-thickness burns. It is used during prehospital and emergency care phases (Figure 46-4 ■). The head, trunk, arms, legs, and perineum are assigned percentages. For example, a client with burns of the face, anterior right arm, and anterior trunk has burn injury involving 27% of total body surface area (TBSA). On the client's admission to a facility, more accurate methods for estimating the extent of injury are employed.

Major Burns

PATHOPHYSIOLOGY AND MANIFESTATIONS

The pathophysiologic changes associated with major burns involve all body systems.

Cardiovascular System

Within minutes of the burn, there is loss of cell wall integrity at the injury site and in the capillary bed. This causes a massive amount of fluid to shift from the intracellular space into the interstitial space. The capillary walls also become more permeable so that fluid leaks from the capillaries at the burn wound site and throughout the body, decreasing intravascular fluid volume. Without adequate fluids in the intracellular and intravascular spaces, the client becomes hypovolemic. Plasma proteins and sodium escape, further increasing edema formation. Blood pressure falls as cardiac output diminishes. The net result is hypovolemic shock, which is called **burn shock.**

Vasoconstriction occurs as the vascular system attempts to compensate for fluid loss (see Chapter 13). ⚭ Abnormal platelet aggregation and white blood cell (WBC) accumulation result in ischemia and eventual thrombosis (clotting) in the deeper tissue below the burn. Red blood cells (RBCs) are hemolyzed due to direct damage from the burn. Because plasma fluid is lost rather than RBCs, hemoconcentration develops, which is seen as an elevated hematocrit. Neutrophils accumulate at the burn site, producing an elevated leukocyte count.

The leakage of fluid into the interstitial spaces compromises the lymphatic system, resulting in intravascular hypovolemia and edema at the burn wound site. Edema impairs peripheral circulation and results in necrosis of the underlying tissue. Potassium ions leave the cells due to burn injury and RBC hemolysis. Without adequate potassium to maintain normal cardiac rhythms, the client is at an increased risk of developing cardiac dysrhythmias.

Burn shock reverses when fluid is reabsorbed from the interstitium into the intravascular space. The blood pressure rises as cardiac output increases, and urinary output improves. Diuresis continues from several days to 2 weeks postburn. During this phase, the extra cardiac workload may predispose the older client or the client with cardiovascular disease to fluid volume overload. Even after capillary integrity is restored, fluid losses continue until the burn wound is closed.

Immune System

The capillary leakage that occurs in the early stages of a burn continues throughout the burn shock phase and impairs the active components of both the cell-mediated and humoral immune systems. Serum levels of all immunoglobulins are significantly diminished. Serum protein levels remain persistently low until the wound closure is closed. These changes in the immune system create a state of acquired immunodeficiency, which places the burn client at risk for infection for up to 4 weeks following the injury. During this time, infections can develop and cause death despite aggressive antimicrobial therapy.

Integumentary System

The burn injury impairs the normal physiologic functions of the skin (see Chapter 44). ⚭ If the microcirculation of the skin remains intact during burning, it cools and protects the deeper portions of the skin and cools the outer surface once the heat source is removed. With extensive burn injury, however, the microcirculation is lost, and the burning process continues even after the heat source is removed.

The thickness of the dermis and epidermis varies considerably from one area of the body to another. A temperature that damages the medial aspect of the forearm may not cause damage to the skin covering the same person's back.

Respiratory System

Inhalation injury is a complication that may range from mild respiratory inflammation to massive pulmonary failure. Exposure to toxic chemicals that can cause asphyxia, smoke, and heat initiates the pathophysiologic processes.

Carbon monoxide, produced by incomplete burning of materials, is a colorless, tasteless, odorless gas. It displaces oxygen and binds with hemoglobin, causing carboxyhemoglobinemia. Without oxygen, tissue hypoxia and eventually death occur. The manifestations of carbon monoxide

poisoning range from mild visual impairment and headache to coma and death.

Smoke inhalation and poisoning result when toxic gases and soot are deposited on the pulmonary mucosa. Inflammation occurs at localized sites within the airways, cells are destroyed, and the bronchial cilia that help clear the lungs are inactivated. Because of this, the client may develop bronchial congestion and infection.

Interstitial pulmonary edema develops secondary to the movement of fluid from the pulmonary blood vessels into the interstitial compartment of the lung tissue. Smoke inhalation damages the alveoli, which inactivates surfactant. Without surfactant the alveoli collapse, leading to atelectasis. Sloughing of the damaged and dead lung tissue occasionally produces debris that may lead to complete airway obstruction.

Upper airway thermal injury results from the inhalation of heated air. Physical findings include the presence of soot, charring, edema, blisters, and ulcerations along the mucosal lining of the oropharynx and larynx. The resulting edema in the airway peaks within the first 24 to 48 hours of injury. Because laryngeal reflexes protect the lower airway, thermal injury below the vocal cords is seldom seen. When it does occur, it is typically associated with the inhalation of steam or explosive gases or the aspiration of hot liquids.

Gastrointestinal System

Curling's ulcer is an acute ulceration of the stomach or duodenum that may form following a burn injury. Abdominal pain, acidic gastric pH levels, hematemesis (vomiting blood), and occult blood in the stool may indicate the presence of gastric ulcer formation.

Paralytic ileus may occur secondary to burn trauma. Lack of intestinal motility leads to gastric distention, nausea, vomiting, and hematemesis.

Urinary System

During the early stages of the burn injury, massive fluid losses occur. These losses lead to dehydration, hemoconcentration, and decreased urinary output. Dark brown concentrated urine may indicate hemoglobinuria, which is the result of the release of large amounts of dead or damaged erythrocytes after a major burn. The pigments can occlude the renal tubules and cause renal failure, especially when dehydration, acidosis, or shock is also present.

Metabolism

Two distinct metabolic phases occur as the body responds to the burn injury. The ebb phase, lasting during the first 3 days of the injury, is manifested by decreased oxygen consumption, fluid imbalance, shock, and inadequate circulating volume. These responses protect the body from the initial impact of the injury.

A second phase, the flow phase, occurs when adequate burn resuscitation has been accomplished. This phase is characterized by increased cellular activity and protein catabolism, lipolysis, and gluconeogenesis. The basal metabolic rate (BMR) reaches twice the normal rate. Body weight and heat drop dramatically. Hypermetabolism persists until after wound closure and may reappear if complications occur.

INTERDISCIPLINARY CARE

After stabilization in the emergency department, the client is transferred to the critical care unit or a specialized burn center. In both settings, continuous monitoring of laboratory tests, administration of fluids and pharmaceutical agents, pain control, wound management, and nutrition support therapies are the focus of care.

Diagnostic Tests

Laboratory and diagnostic tests are conducted to assess and monitor the client's response to the burn injury as well as to the treatment prescribed. Cultures of sputum, blood, urine, and wound tissue are done to indicate the presence of infection. Blood is typed and crossmatched upon the client's arrival to the unit, in case transfusions are required.

- *Urinalysis* is done to evaluate renal perfusion and nutritional status. In catabolic states, nitrogen is excreted in large amounts into the urine. Nitrogen loss is measured through 24-hour urine collections for total nitrogen, urea nitrogen, and amino acid nitrogen. Loss of plasma protein and dehydration lead to proteinuria and elevated urine specific gravity.
- The *complete blood count* is checked regularly. Hematocrit is elevated secondary to hemoconcentration and fluid shifts from the intravascular compartment during the emergent phase. Hemoglobin is decreased secondary to hemolysis. White blood cells are elevated in the presence of infection.
- *Serum electrolytes* are monitored frequently. Sodium levels are decreased secondary to massive fluid shifts into the interstitium. Potassium levels initially are increased, but decrease after burn shock resolves, as fluid shifts back to intracellular and intravascular compartments.
- *Total protein* and *albumin* indicate nutritional status during the rehabilitative stage.
- *Arterial blood gases* are used to monitor oxygen status and acid–base disturbances. The burn-injured client may demonstrate elevated or lowered pH, decreased P_{CO_2}, decreased P_{O_2}, and low-normal bicarbonate levels.
- *Pulse oximetry* allows continuous assessment of oxygen saturation levels. The burn-injured client may have saturation levels below 95%.
- *Chest x-ray* studies document changes within the first 24 to 48 hours that may reflect the presence of atelectasis,

pulmonary edema, or acute respiratory disease. If an upper airway injury is manifested, a *flexible bronchoscopy* permits direct visualization.
- *Electrocardiograms* (ECGs) are necessary to monitor the development of dysrhythmias, especially those associated with hypokalemia and hyperkalemia.

Stages of Burn Injury Care

The treatment for the burn client is divided into three, sometimes overlapping, stages. At each stage, different groups of nurses, physicians, and allied health care specialists collaborate to manage the client's recovery.

EMERGENT OR RESUSCITATIVE STAGE. This stage lasts from the onset of injury through successful fluid resuscitation. It includes estimating the extent of the burn, instituting initial first-aid measures, and implementing fluid resuscitation therapies. The client is assessed for shock and respiratory distress. Health care workers determine whether the client is to be transported to a burn center.

ACUTE STAGE. The acute stage begins with the start of diuresis and ends with closure of the burn wound. Hydrotherapy and excision and grafting of full-thickness wounds are performed as soon as possible. Enteral and parenteral nutritional interventions are started early to address caloric needs. Topical and systemic antimicrobial agents are administered to combat infection. Narcotic agents must be administered before all invasive procedures to maximize client comfort and to reduce the anxieties associated with wound debridement and intensive physical therapy.

REHABILITATIVE STAGE. This stage begins with wound closure and ends when the client returns to the highest level of health, which may take years. The primary focus is biopsychosocial adjustment: the prevention of contractures and scars, and the client's successful resumption of work, family, and social roles through physical, vocational, occupational, and psychosocial rehabilitation.

MEDICATIONS

Burns often cause excruciating pain. In the early stages of care, intravenously administered narcotics such as morphine, hydromorphone, or fentanyl are the best means of managing pain. Once the client has been stabilized, it is appropriate to administer narcotic agents prior to wound care or intensive exercising routines.

To eliminate infection on the surface of the burn wound, topical antimicrobial therapy is used, depending on protocol. Many antimicrobial agents are available. The three most widely used are mafenide acetate (Sulfamylon), silver sulfadiazine (Silvadene), and 0.5% silver nitrate soaks. The first two agents are broad-spectrum antibiotics that are supplied in a cream form. The choice of antibiotic is based on the burn

TABLE 46-2

Nursing Implications for Pharmacology: Topical Antimicrobial Agents

DRUGS	ACTION/USES	NURSING RESPONSIBILITIES	CLIENT TEACHING
Mafenide acetate (Sulfamylon)	A synthetic antibiotic that appears to interfere with the metabolism of bacterial cells. Effective against many gram-positive and gram-negative organisms. Used to prevent burn wound infections.	Use with caution in clients with renal or pulmonary disease. Assess for itching, swelling, or blisters on unburned areas, which indicate an allergy to the drug.	When applied, the drug causes pain or burning. Apply one to two times a day until the burn is healed. If symptoms of an allergy develop, stop using the drug and notify your health care provider.
Silver nitrate	A bacteriostatic agent that inhibits many different gram-positive and gram-negative organisms. Used as a 0.5% solution in distilled water to prevent burn wound infections.	Apply the solution to gauze dressings every 2 hours and change dressings completely two times a day. Monitor the client for decreased blood sodium and chloride levels because large amounts of water are absorbed from the dressing site.	Silver nitrate causes the skin and dressings to turn black. Saturate the dressings with the solution every 2 hours, and change all dressings two times a day. Report symptoms of infection, swelling, weight gain, or breathing difficulty to your health care provider.
Silver sulfadiazine (Silvadene)	Acts on bacterial cell membranes as a bactericidal. Effective against many gram-negative and gram-positive organisms. Used to prevent burn wound infections.	Monitor for WBC because client can develop leukopenia.	Apply the drug one to two times a day, completely covering the burn wound.

depth, wound location, the presence and type of identified bacteria, and whether the wound is treated with an open method (exposing the wound to air) or closed method (covered with bulky dressings). See Table 46-2 ■.

Other medications that may be used include histamine receptor antagonists and antacids to reduce gastric acidity, and medications to decrease respiratory mucous production. If unsure about immunization status, tetanus toxoid is given intramuscularly to prevent *Clostridium tetani* infection.

Fluid Resuscitation

To counteract the effects of burn shock, fluid resuscitation guidelines are used to replace the extensive fluid and electrolyte losses associated with major burn injuries. Fluid replacement is necessary in all burn wounds that involve more than 20% of the TBSA. Colloids, crystalloids, blood, and blood products are used for fluid resuscitation and maintenance. Crystalloid fluids are administered through two large-bore peripheral or central lines at rates sufficient to maintain urine output at 30 to 50 mL/hr. Lactated Ringer's solution is the intravenous fluid of choice, because it most closely approximates the body's extracellular fluid composition.

Fluid resuscitation rates are adjusted periodically throughout the emergent stage of care. During the fluid resuscitation stage, the client may require invasive hemodynamic monitoring (see Chapter 26 ⌬). A pulmonary artery catheter monitors cardiac output, cardiac index, and pulmonary artery wedge pressures. All measurements must be maintained within normal limits to attain adequate fluid resuscitation.

RESPIRATORY MANAGEMENT

The client's head is elevated to 30 degrees or more to maximize respiratory efforts. Airways may need frequent suctioning. If airway obstruction occurs, the client will require intubation. Oxygen flow rate is based on arterial blood gas results. The client may be placed on a face mask, steam collar, T-piece, mechanical ventilation with positive end-expiratory pressure (PEEP), pressure support ventilation, or high-frequency jet ventilation. The goal of all therapies is to maintain adequate tissue oxygenation with the least amount of inspired oxygen flow necessary.

NUTRITION

Oral intake can seldom meet the caloric requirements necessary to reverse the excessive protein breakdown and to begin the healing process. Caloric needs may be as great as 4,000 to 6,000 kcal/day. Enteral feedings are started within 24 to 48 hours of the burn injury to offset hypermetabolism, improve nitrogen balance, and decrease length of hospital stay.

A gastrointestinal feeding tube is inserted, with the tip extending past the pylorus to prevent reflux and aspiration. Enteral feeding is contraindicated in Curling's ulcer, bowel obstruction, feeding intolerance, pancreatitis, or septic ileus. When the enteral route cannot be used, a central venous catheter is inserted via the subclavian or jugular vein for the administration of total parenteral nutrition (TPN). (See Chapter 19 ⟳ for nursing care of the client receiving enteral feedings or TPN.)

WOUND MANAGEMENT

Burn wounds must be cleaned and debrided of necrotic tissue and blisters to promote healing and prevent prolonged inflammation. **Debridement** is the process of removing dead tissue from the wound.

The wound is cleaned with an antimicrobial soap, such as chlorhexidine gluconate (Hibiclens, Hibistat). However, Dial soap or Shur-Clens is used for facial burns, because chlorhexidine gluconate is toxic to eyes and ears. The area is shaved close to the burn wound before debridement to decrease the risk of infection, and intravenous narcotics are administered during debridement to control pain.

Mechanical debridement is performed during hydrotherapy. In this procedure, loose necrotic tissue is gently washed with a washcloth or gauze pad to remove dead skin and **eschar** (a hard crust that forms over the burn wound). Blistered skin is grasped with a dry gauze and gently removed. The edges of blisters or eschar are trimmed with blunt scissors. Wounds should be rubbed hard enough to remove debris yet not cause bleeding. Hydrotherapy measures include showering, using a spray table, or immersion in a tub of water. Although tubbing has traditionally been the method of choice, it is currently used less often because of the increased risk of wound infection.

Enzymatic debridement involves the use of a topical agent to dissolve and remove necrotic tissue. Following hydrotherapy, an enzyme of choice is applied in a thin layer directly to the wound and covered with one layer of fine mesh gauze. A topical antimicrobial agent is applied, covered with a bulky wet dressing, and the wound is immobilized with expandable mesh gauze.

Surgery

Various surgical procedures are performed to treat the burn wound:

- *Surgical debridement* is the process of excising tissue from the burn wound to the level of viable tissue. The most common technique is electrocautery. Debridement may also be performed by using a dermatome to slice off thin layers of damaged skin.
- *Escharotomy* is performed by the physician with a scalpel or by electrocautery. A sterile surgical incision is made

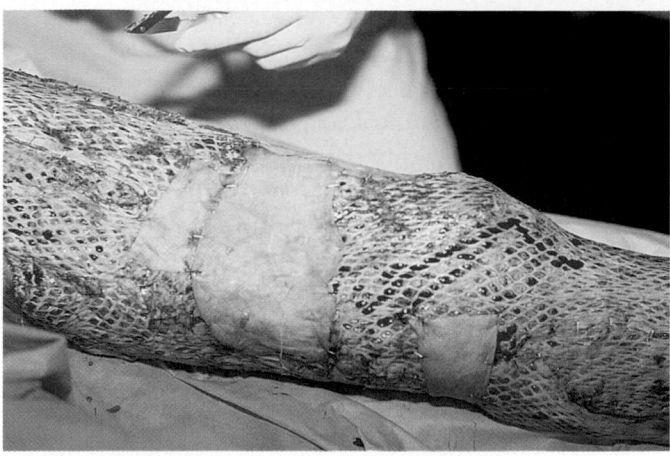

Figure 46-5. ■ Skin graft for burn injury (autograft). (Courtesy of Dr. William Dominic, Valley Medical Center.)

longitudinally along the extremity or the trunk to prevent constriction, impaired circulation, and possible gangrene.
- *Autografting* is used to effect permanent skin coverage of the wound. Early burn wound excision and skin grafting decrease the hospital stay and enhance rehabilitation. Skin is removed from healthy tissue (donor site) of the burn-injured client and applied to the burn wound (Figure 46-5 ■). After the autograft is applied, the grafted area is immobilized.
- *Cultured epithelial autografting* is a technique in which skin cells are removed from unburned sites on the client's body, minced, and placed in a culture medium for growth. With this technique, enough skin can be grown over a period of 3 to 4 weeks to cover an entire human body. The cells are prepared in sheets and attached to petroleum jelly gauze backing, which is applied to the burn wound site.

Biologic and Biosynthetic Dressings

Biologic dressing and biosynthetic dressing refer to any temporary material that rapidly adheres to the wound bed, promotes healing, or prepares the burn wound for permanent autograft coverage. Ideally, these kinds of dressings should be easy to apply and remove, inexpensive, elastic, able to reduce pain, able to serve as a bacterial barrier, and able to enhance the natural healing process. The dressings are applied to the burn wound as soon as possible. They help eliminate the loss of water through evaporation, reduce infection, and promote wound healing. Biologic and biosynthetic dressings that are currently in use include Biobrane, Dermagraft, Integra, AlloDerm, and TransCyte.

Scar, Keloid, and Contractures

Following a minor burn, the newly formed skin closely resembles its neighboring tissue. The epidermis does not thicken or heighten as a scar. However, when a burn extends into the dermal layer of skin, the skin is repaired through scar formation. Two types of excessive scar may develop. A **hypertrophic scar** is an overgrowth of dermal tissue that remains within the boundaries of the wound. A **keloid** is a scar that extends beyond the boundaries of the original wound. People with dark skin are at greater risk for the formation of hypertrophic scars and keloids. During the healing process, the burn scar shrinks and becomes fixed and inelastic, resulting in **contracture** of the wound (permanent shortening of connective tissue). Once a contracture forms, the tissue resists being stretched, and its inelasticity limits body movement. Positioning, splinting, exercise, and constant pressure application help prevent contractures from forming.

Wound Dressings

After the wound has been cleaned and debrided, it may be dressed by the open or closed method. In the open method, the burn wound remains open to air, covered only by a topical antimicrobial agent. This method allows easy wound assessment. However, it can be used only where strict isolation precautions are followed. Topical agents must be reapplied frequently because they tend to rub off onto the bedding.

In the closed method, a topical antimicrobial agent is applied to the wound site, which is covered with gauze or a nonadherent dressing and then gently wrapped with a gauze roll bandage. With the closed method, burn wounds are usually dressed twice daily and as needed. Dressings are applied circumferentially in a distal-to-proximal manner. All fingers and toes are wrapped separately. For wet-to-dry dressings, a thick gauze is applied to maintain moisture and is soaked every 2 hours with the ordered solution.

Splints are used to immobilize body parts and prevent contractures of the joints. They are applied and removed according to schedules established by the physical therapist. Early in the acute phase of care, the physical therapist also prescribes active and passive ROM exercises, which are performed during hydrotherapy and every 2 hours at the bedside. Early ambulation is also part of the plan of care once the client's condition becomes stable.

Applying uniform pressure can prevent or reduce hypertrophic scarring. Tubular support bandages are applied 5 to 7 days postgraft. They maintain a tension ranging from 10 to 20 mm Hg to control scarring. The client wears custom-made elastic pressure garments for 6 months to a year postgraft.

COMPLEMENTARY THERAPY

Clients with minor burns may apply aloe gel, a clear gel-like substance, three to five times per day. Occasionally,

local rashes may develop but will disappear when the gel is discontinued.

NURSING CARE

The client with a burn injury may require care ranging from education for self-care at home to complex care planning involving the multidisciplinary team. The client and family will experience a wide range of psychologic and emotional responses. Part of the nurse's role is to support them and to address their concerns.

ASSESSING

The nurse initially assesses all body systems of the client with a major burn to identify not only actual abnormal findings but also potential problems that may occur as a result of the injury. Chapter 5 ⊙⊙ discusses the assessment of each body system; Box 46-1 ■ summarizes data to collect when the client is admitted to an emergency department or burn center. This information is necessary to determine fluid resuscitation, causative agent, any on-the-scene treatment, health history, and age. Body weight on admission is necessary to monitor nutritional status during treatment.

DIAGNOSING, PLANNING, AND IMPLEMENTING

Priorities in Nursing Care. The priority nursing diagnoses for the client with a major burn are Impaired Skin Integrity, Deficient Fluid Volume, Risk for Infection, Impaired Physical Mobility, Imbalanced Nutrition: Less than Body Requirements, Acute Pain, and Powerlessness.

Impaired Skin Integrity

Nursing care for burn injuries focuses on assessing and cleaning the wound and controlling infection.

■ Monitor appearance of burn wound, amount and type of drainage, body temperature, and white blood cell count.

BOX 46-1	ASSESSMENT

Initial Focused Assessment of the Client with a Major Burn

- Time of the injury
- Cause of the injury
- First-aid treatment
- Past medical history
- Age
- Medications
- Body weight

Report changes from usual condition. *Early signs of infection include increased redness and swelling, increased or purulent drainage, fever and increased WBC.*

- Assist with hydrotherapy. Explain the procedure. Administer medications to control pain as prescribed. Keep environment warm. *Hydrotherapy is used to remove topical agents and debride the wound. The procedure is often painful and the client is likely to be easily chilled.*
- Apply topical antimicrobial agents as prescribed. Reapply as necessary. *Controlling infection is an essential component in restoring skin integrity for burn wounds.*
  - Provide special skin care to sensitive body areas.
  - Clean burns involving the eyes with normal saline or sterile water. If contracture of the eyelid develops, apply drops or ointment to the eye to prevent corneal abrasion.
  - Gently wipe burns of the lips with saline-soaked pads. Apply an antibiotic ointment as ordered. Assess the mouth frequently, and perform mouth care routinely. If an oral endotracheal tube is in place, reposition it often to prevent pressure sore formation.
  - Position nasogastric and nasotracheal tubes to prevent excessive pressure.
  - Do not cover ears with dressings. Do not use pillows.
  - Clean burns of the perineum during hydrotherapy. Assess the area for evidence of infection, and rinse thoroughly after toileting.
  The eyes, mouth, nose, ears, perineum, and exposed deeper tissues require special interventions.
- Change dressings as prescribed. When the open method is used, follow strict isolation procedures. If the closed method is used, apply in a distal-to-proximal manner. Wrap all fingers and toes separately. *These guidelines are necessary to prevent infection, maintain circulation, and cover all burned areas with dressings.*

Deficient Fluid Volume

Massive fluid losses occur immediately following the injury and continue throughout the first 2 to 5 days. During this period, nursing care focuses on restoring fluid losses and continuously assessing hemodynamic parameters.

- Assess vital signs frequently. Note increased and weak pulse, decreasing blood pressure, and increased respiratory rate. Document and report changes. *Vital signs change rapidly when fluid resuscitation is inadequate. Those listed indicate decreased fluid volume.*
- Monitor intake and output hourly. Report urine outputs of less than 50 mL/hr. *Urine output less than 50 mL/hr indicates decreased circulatory volume and renal perfusion.*
- Weigh daily. *Body weight is used to calculate fluid requirements.*

Risk for Infection

From the onset of the burn injury, the client is at risk for infection.

- Monitor and record body temperature every 1 to 2 hours. Document and report increased body temperature. Monitor WBC counts. *Body temperature increase and increased WBC counts indicate infection.*
- Determine tetanus immunization status. *Clients with burns are at risk for infection caused by* Clostridium tetani.
- Maintain an aseptic environment. *Isolation techniques decrease the risk of secondary infections.*
- Monitor for the presence of urgency, frequency, dysuria, bacteria in urine, and fever. *These are manifestations of urinary tract infections.*

Impaired Physical Mobility

- Perform active or passive range-of-motion (ROM) exercises to all joints every 2 hours. Ambulate when stable. *Physical therapy begins in the early stages of treatment. As the burn wound heals and new skin tissue forms, the involved area tends to shrink. Contractures significantly limit mobility, especially at joints. Regular exercise prevents further loss of mobility, restores movement, and improves functional status.*
- Apply splints as prescribed. Maintain antideformity positions, and reposition hourly. *Splinting and positioning help prevent contractures.*

- Maintain limbs in functional alignment. *This helps preserve joint mobility.*

Imbalanced Nutrition: Less than Body Requirements

Daily calorie requirements are determined by the dietitian. As soon as possible, enteral feedings are started. Parenteral nutrition is reserved for instances in which enteral feedings are contraindicated.

- Maintain nasogastric/nasointestinal tube placement. *This ensures appropriate absorption of nutrients and prevents aspiration.*
- Maintain enteral/parenteral nutritional support as prescribed. Observe and report any evidence of feeding intolerance. *Diarrhea, vomiting, excessive gastric residue, abdominal distention, absent bowel sounds, and constipation indicate intolerance to the strength or amount of tube feedings.*
- Weigh daily. *The client's weight is used to measure the adequacy of the nutritional support.*

Acute Pain

- Assess level of pain. *With extensive superficial and all partial-thickness burns, the client experiences excruciating pain. Pain tolerance is highly individual.* (Pain and pain management are discussed in detail in Chapter 8.) ⚭
- Anticipate the need for prophylactic analgesia. Determine whether patient-controlled analgesia (PCA) is appropriate. Administer narcotic analgesics as ordered. *Narcotic analgesics are administered regularly to minimize discomfort and also before any painful procedure. An inability to manage pain results in client feelings of despair and frustration. Invasive procedures and exposed nerve endings increase the client's pain.*
- Explain all procedures and expected levels of discomfort. *Clients who are prepared for painful procedures experience less stress and are better able to manage pain.*
- Explore noninvasive methods of pain control. *As the client progresses to the rehabilitative stage, non-narcotic analgesia and relaxation techniques are implemented. Methods such as relaxation, distraction, and massage can enhance the therapeutic effects of pain medications.*

Powerlessness

- Allow as much control over the surroundings and daily routine as possible, such as choosing times for dressing changes. *The client with a major burn injury usually endures a lengthy hospital stay. The burn unit is a strange environment, with hospital personnel and even family wearing sterile masks and gowns at client's bedside; everyone appears different. Feelings of powerlessness during the emergent and acute stages of burn care often pose a challenge to the nurse. Powerlessness results from the belief that one is unable to influence the outcome of a situation.*
- Keep needed items within reach, such as call light, urinal, water pitcher, and tissues. *These items reinforce the client's feelings of control.*
- Encourage expression of feelings. *Careful listening, a caring presence, and positive reinforcement can help the client cope.*
- Help set short-term, realistic goals, such as walking from the bedside to the chair twice daily. *Small gains are easier to achieve and allow for ongoing positive reinforcement.*
- Help access support systems, such as spiritual/cultural healing, support group consultation, and psychologic intervention. *Support systems help the client cope more effectively.*

EVALUATING

Evaluate the effectiveness of nursing care by collecting data about wound healing, fluid status, absence of infection, adequate nutrition, pain relief, and client's perceptions of ability to control the outcomes of treatment and care. As the burn heals, evaluate effectiveness of exercises and splinting in preventing contractures.

Documenting. Documentation includes VS, appearance of wounds, intake and output, breath and bowel sounds, nutrition intake, CMS of any involved extremity, and effectiveness of pain relief measures. Record client teaching related to wound care including skin graft and donor sites, diet, prevention of infection, hydration, pain management, and physical activity.

CONTINUING CARE

Client and family teaching are an important component of all phases of burn care. As treatment progresses, encourage family members to assume more responsibility in providing care. From admission to discharge, teach them to assess all findings, implement therapies, and evaluate progress.

Early in the plan of care, explain to the client and family the long-term goals of rehabilitation care: to prevent soft tissue deformity, protect skin grafts, maintain physiologic function, manage scars, and return the client to his or her optimal level of independence. The teaching plan focuses on helping the client and family prevent dehydration, infection, and pain; maintain adequate nutrition and skin integrity; and restore mobility and psychosocial well-being.

Teach the client and family how to assess for evidence of fluid volume deficit. Explain the rationale supporting all fluid therapies and emphasize the need to report immediately all signs and symptoms of fluid imbalance: weight loss, scanty urine output, dry mucous membranes.

Explain the rationale about asepsis. Instruct caregivers to protect the client from exposure to people with colds or infections and to follow aseptic technique meticulously when caring for the wound. Ensure that the client and family are able to recognize all signs and symptoms of infection: fever, poor wound healing, purulent drainage, malaise.

Consultation with physical therapy begins early in the treatment plan and continues throughout the long-term rehabilitative process. Explain to the client and family the need for progressive physical activity, and help them establish realistic goals. Explain the rationale supporting the use of splints, pressure support garments, and other assistive devices, and demonstrate how to apply them. Ensure that the client and family understand the importance of reporting any evidence of lack of progress.

Identify and answer all questions related to the client's nutritional therapies and maintaining adequate daily caloric intake. Consult with a dietician early in the treatment plan and throughout rehabilitation.

Encourage the client and family to express concerns related to pain management. Explain the causes of pain and discomfort and the rationale supporting the use of analgesia. Instruct them to report inadequate pain control. Teach the client and family alternative pain-control therapies.

Instruct the client and family in the care of the graft and donor sites. Provide the rationale for use of all pressure support garments. Emphasize the need to report any evidence of inadequate wound healing: altered skin integrity, drainage, swelling, redness.

Encourage the client and family to express their fears and concerns, and provide referrals to appropriate community resources. The circumstances surrounding the burn injury are often emotionally charged and challenge the nurse to consider all psychosocial implications. Powerlessness, anger, guilt, anxiety, and feelings of loss are common reactions to burn injury. The goal of psychosocial nursing care is to promote functional adaptation, encourage coping mechanisms and facilitate psychologic adjustment. The burn injury can create dramatic changes in the client's self-concept, role function, value system, and interpersonal relationships. Direct the client and family to occupational therapy, social services, clergy, or psychiatric services as appropriate.

NURSING PROCESS CARE PLAN
Client with a Major Burn

Craig Howard, a 39-year-old truck driver, is admitted to the hospital following an accident in which the cab of his truck caught on fire. He was freed from the truck by a passing motorist, who stayed with him until the rescue team arrived and transported him to a local ED. Mr. Howard's wife, Mary, and twin daughters, Jessica and Jane, age 10, have been notified.

Assessment. On his admission to the ED, Mr. Howard is diagnosed with deep partial-thickness and full-thickness burns of the anterior chest, arms, and hands. A quick assessment based on the rule of nines estimates the extent of his burn injury at 36% of TBSA. His vital signs are as follows: T, 96.2°F (35.6°C); P, 140; R, 40; BP, 98/60. In the field, the paramedics had inserted a large-bore central line into Mr. Howard's right subclavian vein and started a rapid infusion of lactated Ringer's solution. Mr. Howard is receiving 40% humidified oxygen via face mask. Initial ABGs are as follows: pH, 7.49; Po_2, 60 mm Hg; Pco_2, 32 mm Hg; bicarbonate, 22 mEq/L. Lung sounds indicate inspiratory and expiratory wheezing, and a persistent cough reveals sooty sputum production. A Foley catheter is inserted and initially drains a moderate amount of dark, concentrated urine. A nasogastric tube is inserted and connected to low-intermittent suction. Mr. Howard is alert and oriented and complains of severe pain associated with the burn injuries. The burn unit is notified, and Mr. Howard is prepared for transfer.

Diagnosis. On Mr. Howard's arrival to the burn unit, Ana Salazar, LVN, assesses Mr. Howard and assists in establishing the following prioritized nursing diagnoses:

- *Risk for Ineffective Airway Clearance* related to increasing lung congestion secondary to smoke inhalation
- *Deficient Volume Deficit* related to abnormal fluid loss secondary to burn injury
- *Risk for Ineffective Tissue Perfusion* related to peripheral constriction secondary to circumferential burn wounds of the arms

Expected Outcomes. The expected outcomes established in Ms. Salazar's plan of care specify that during the emergent phase of care, Mr. Howard will:

- Demonstrate a patent airway, as evidenced by clear breath sounds; absence of cyanosis; and vital signs, chest x-ray findings, and arterial blood gases (ABGs) within normal limits.
- Demonstrate adequate fluid volume and electrolyte balance, as evidenced by urine output, vital signs, mental status, and laboratory findings within normal limits.
- Demonstrate adequate tissue perfusion, as evidenced by palpable pulses, warm extremities, and normal capillary refill (fingernails).

Planning and Implementation. Ms. Salazar plans and implements the following interventions for Mr. Howard during the emergent phase of care:

- Prepare Mr. Howard for prophylactic nasotracheal intubation to maintain airway patency.

■ Initiate fluid resuscitation therapy using the prescribed formula to calculate intravenous fluid rate for the first 24 hours postburn.

■ Assist the physician to perform escharotomies of both upper extremities.

Evaluation. The nurse anesthetist has inserted a nasotracheal tube and connected Mr. Howard to a T-piece delivering 40% oxygen. His ABGs have significantly improved. Bronchodilators have been parenterally administered and mucolytic agents added to his respiratory treatments. His tracheal secretions have begun to show evidence of clearing. Hourly urine outputs are 60 to 90 mL, and color and concentration have improved. Blood pressure has increased to 100/64 and the pulse rate has decreased to 100. To improve tissue perfusion of both arms, the physician has performed bilateral escharotomies and Ms. Salazar has dressed the wounds using sterile procedure. The extremities have demonstrated improved circulation.

Critical Thinking in the Nursing Process

1. Explain the rationale for the immediate insertion of a Foley catheter and nasogastric tube.
2. What is the rationale supporting the intravenous administration of narcotics to control Mr. Howard's pain?
3. Explain why Mr. Howard would need escharotomies of his upper arms.

Note: The bibliography listings for this and all chapters have been compiled at the back of the book.

Chapter Review

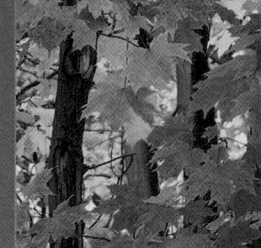

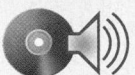 **KEY TERMS** by Topics

Use the audio glossary feature of either the CD-ROM or the Companion Website to hear the correct pronunciation of the following key terms.

Types of burn injury
burn, superficial burn, partial-thickness burn, full-thickness burn, "rule of nines"

Major burns
burn shock, debridement, eschar, hypertrophic scar, keloid, contracture

KEY Points

- A burn is an injury resulting from a heat source that results in tissue loss, damage, or irreversible destruction. The heat source may be thermal, chemical, electrical, or radiation.

- Burns are classified as superficial, partial thickness, or full thickness. The classification is made based on the depth of the burn.

- The "rule of nines" is often used to estimate the extent of a burn by assigning percentages to different parts of the body.

- The pathophysiology of a burn involves all body systems. One of the most critical is the shift of fluid into the extravascular space, resulting in a type of hypovolemic shock called burn shock. Other pathologic processes include an impaired immune system, disturbed functions of the skin, inhalation injury, gastrointestinal ulcerations and ileus, renal failure, and hypermetabolism.

- The treatment of a major burn includes fluid resuscitation, wound management, respiratory management, and nutritional support.

- Nursing care of the client with a burn is provided from initial emergency assessment and treatment through convalescence and rehabilitation. Priority nursing diagnoses focus on skin integrity, fluid volume, infection, physical mobility, nutrition, pain, and powerlessness.

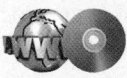 **EXPLORE MediaLink**

Additional interactive resources for this chapter can be found on the Companion Website at www.prenhall.com/burke. Click on Chapter 46 and "Begin" to select the activities for this chapter.

For chapter-related NCLEX-style review questions and an audio glossary, access the accompanying CD-ROM in this book.

FOR FURTHER Study

For further study about assessing each body system, see Chapter 5.

For more about nursing care of pain, see Chapter 8.

For more information on fluid loss in clients experiencing trauma, see Chapter 13.

See Chapter 19 for more information about enteral and TPN feedings.

For information on fluid resuscitation and hemodynamic monitoring, see Chapter 26.

For more about normal physiologic functions of the skin, see Chapter 44.

Critical Thinking Care Map

Caring for a Client with Major Burns
NCLEX-PN® Focus Area: Physiologic Integrity: Reduction of Risk Potential

Case Study: Akisha Moore, age 78, was burned over 40% TBSA when her nightgown caught on fire as she was heating coffee in a saucepan. The burns are both partial thickness and full thickness. The partial-thickness burns are covered with large blisters. On admission to the ED, Mrs. Moore is confused. Her blood pressure is 92/62, and her pulse (right wrist is not burned) is 110 and weak. A Foley catheter is inserted, and hourly urine outputs are averaging less than 20 mL per hour. Mrs. Moore is moaning with pain. Her respiratory rate is 36 and shallow and her temperature is 98°F.

Nursing Diagnosis: Risk for Deficient Fluid Volume

COLLECT DATA

Subjective	Objective
_____	_____
_____	_____
_____	_____
_____	_____
_____	_____
_____	_____

Would you report this data? Yes/No

If yes, to: _____

Nursing Care

_____
_____
_____
_____
_____
_____
_____
_____
_____
_____
_____

How would you document this? _____
_____
_____
_____

Data Collected (use those that apply)

- Age 78
- 40% TBSA burns
- T 98°F
- BP 92/62
- P 110, weak
- R 36, shallow
- Output averages <20 mL/hr
- Moans in pain
- Confused

Nursing Interventions (use those that apply; list in priority order)

- Report and continue to monitor vital signs.
- Report and continue to monitor urine output.
- Report and continue to monitor confusion.
- Report and continue to monitor body temperature.
- Administer morphine intravenously as prescribed.
- Determine body weight.
- Monitor IV fluid flow rate.
- Prepare to debride burned areas.
- Cover with a warm blanket.

1 During a soccer game, a young student was injured due to a lightning strike. The student began to jerk and speak incoherently. Based on this observation, which body system would be the most affected by the electrical current?

A. cardiac
B. pulmonary
C. urinary
D. nervous

2 A client was admitted to the intensive care unit with severe burns to the face and chest. The injured skin is dry and leathery, with no pain sensations present. The nurse recognizes that this burn is classified as:

A. full thickness.
B. partial thickness.
C. superficial.
D. deep partial thickness.

3 A client arrives in the emergency room suffering from burns received in a house fire. What assessment data should be obtained first?

A. pain
B. respiratory
C. mobility
D. urinary

4 An 85-year-old client, diagnosed with third-degree burns to the lower extremities, is complaining of dyspnea. Crackles are heard in all lung fields. The nurse is justifiable in determining that this client may have:

A. excess intercellular fluid.
B. early stages of heart failure.
C. portal hypertension.
D. increased circulatory volume.

5 A client suffered burns to the anterior trunk and left arm anterior and posterior. Using the "rule of nines," what percent of total body surface area (TBSA) was burned?

A. 27%
B. 30%
C. 35%
D. 42%

6 A client with extensive second- and third-degree burns is experiencing severe pain. Which method of administering narcotics is the most effective for this client?

A. PO
B. IM
C. IV
D. rectal

7 A burn client has developed a Curling's ulcer related to the trauma from his injuries. The nurse anticipates that the physician will order which nutrition therapy?

A. enteral feeding via gastrointestinal tube
B. high-calorie, high-protein diet
C. central venous total parenteral nutrition
D. peripheral venous total parenteral nutrition

8 Which of these measures should be included in the nursing care plan for a client with burns to the lower extremities?

A. meticulous wound care
B. vital signs every 8 hours
C. daily weights
D. range-of-motion exercises
E. assess peripheral pulses
F. apply aloe to the burn area

9 A burn client complains of chills and headache. Which nursing intervention should be the highest priority at this time?

A. Remove the dressings to examine the wound.
B. Obtain a set of vital signs.
C. Notify the physician.
D. Touch the skin to determine temperature.

10 The doctor has ordered silver sulfadiazine (Silvadene) for a client with a second-degree burn. The nurse is knowledgeable that the medication may cause:

A. dehydration.
B. pain.
C. bleeding.
D. leukopenia.

Answers for Review Questions, as well as discussion of Care Plan and Critical Thinking Care Map questions, appear in Appendix V.

ASSESSING THE CLIENT FROM ANOTHER CULTURE IN A SOCIAL CONTEXT

Mr. Ararnak, 27, a Saudi man, refused to allow a male lab technician to enter his wife's room to draw blood. She had just had a radical mastectomy. The nurse finally convinced the husband of the need for the blood sample and he reluctantly allowed the technician in the room. However, he made sure his wife was completely covered. Only her arm stuck out from beneath the covers. The nurse was careful to accommodate this request. The nurse knew that for Arab families, honor is one of the highest values. Since family honor is dependent on female purity, many Arabs feel that sexual segregation and extreme modesty must be maintained at all times.

Most clients are part of one or more social organizations, which play an important role in their lives. Thus, the social organizations of which the client is a part and their effect on the client need to be assessed, so culturally appropriate and effective care can be delivered to the client and family.

Family

For many individuals the most significant social organization influencing behavior is the family. However, the primary responsibility for decision making varies among cultural groups (Giger & Davidhizar, 1999). Some individuals, such as those from Appalachia or Mexico, rely heavily on family members for decision making. Some religious groups, such as the Amish, may also want to have the church fellowship involved. On the other hand, many mainstream Americans make decisions for themselves without consulting anyone.

The family structure may be male or female dominated. For example, in some Hispanic families the father is the primary decision maker and controller of the family. The Hispanic female is usually submissive and frequently puts the needs and wants of others above her own. In contrast, in many black American families the female is dominant and has a greater role in decision making.

The family should be viewed in two separate ways (Friedman, 1986). On the one hand, the family is the environment that supports the client and provides values and practices. On the other hand, the family itself should be treated as a client. When an individual is ill, the whole family unit is affected, and care should be delivered to everyone who is part of the family unit.

For some clients, the most important single organization is the nuclear family or the extended family. For others, the family unit may not be composed of blood relatives. The nurse should recognize those individuals who assume the functions customarily provided by blood relatives (Murray, Meili, & Zentner, 1993).

Church or Religious Affiliations

In the United States there are many church types and many major denominations. This is very different from countries such as Mexico or Spain, where most people belong to one faith and one church. In the United States some churches are identified with an ethnic group. For example, in the Amish church, religious beliefs are synonymous with the Amish life experience.

Nursing Implications

- **Assess the client–family relationship.** Nurses need to assess the client–family relationship in order to learn their values, the flow of authority, and how decisions are made.
- **Be aware that unrelated persons may provide the functions of a family.** Rules related to "family members" may need to be interpreted flexibly.
- **Involve the family as needed to achieve optimal outcomes.** The person with the decision-making power needs to be included in discussions about treatment options. When client education is done, the individual with the decision-making power should usually be involved. This improves compliance.
- **Respect religious customs.** Personal articles such as statues, shrines, rosaries, amulets, or pictures may have special religious meaning and should be treated with respect.
- **Communicate with health team members if they are unfamiliar with the family's decision-making structure.** The nurse may need to provide insight for team members regarding which family members the client feels need to be included in health care decisions.

Self-Reflection Questions

1. Who made the decisions about health care in your family of origin?

2. When making decisions, do you need or not need input from your family?

3. Do your religious values influence the way you feel about some clients?

4. What conflicts might you have in caring for a client whose religious values differ from your own?

5. What conflicts might you have in dealing with a male physician who is accustomed to male-dominated relationships with women?

Thinking Strategically About...

Geoff Sanders, age 69, is retired from the postal service. He has always been an avid participant in outdoor sports. When he was younger he played baseball and tennis, and for the last 10 years he has played golf at least twice a week. He now lives in Connecticut, but as a younger man he lived in Florida for almost 15 years. Mr. Sanders has a variety of warts and moles scattered over his body and has rarely paid attention to them. After taking a shower one day he noticed that a mole on his left lower leg looked bigger and darker. Mr. Sanders had just seen a public announcement on television about the dangers of changes in moles. He immediately called his primary care physician for an appointment at the dermatology clinic.

DATA COLLECTED

On arriving at the clinic for his appointment, Mr. Sanders is interviewed and assessed by nurse Tom Hall. Mr. Sanders reports a family history of skin cancer. His father had several squamous cell carcinomas removed from his face. Mr. Sanders has numerous nevi on his body. The one causing concern is located on the medial anterior left leg, 2 inches below the patella. The lesion has been present for years, but Mr. Sanders only noticed yesterday that it has become larger and darker. On further questioning, he states that the mole itches sometimes but has never hurt or bled. Mr. Sanders experiences a sunburn early each summer before he tans. The sunburn involves the lower legs because he always wears shorts during his twice-weekly golf game.

A complete assessment reveals various freckles, warts, and nevi. With the exception of the nevus that prompted Mr. Sanders to come to the clinic, all lesions appear normal. The nevus in question is raised, 3 cm in diameter, has an uneven shape with irregular borders and a nodular surface.

It is variegated in color, with various shades from brown to black. The skin surrounding the nevus is slightly erythematous. Mr. Sanders's inguinal lymph nodes are not enlarged or tender. With Mr. Sanders's permission, a photograph of the lesion is taken.

After discussing the lesion with a surgeon, Mr. Sanders is scheduled for a biopsy under a local anesthetic the following morning. Following the biopsy, the histologic examination reveals lentigo maligna melanoma. Staging of the tumor reveals no metastasis to regional lymph nodes. Mr. Sanders enters the hospital and undergoes a wide excision of the lesion the following morning and goes home the day after.

CRITICAL THINKING

1. Compare the description of Mr. Sanders's lesion with the ABCD skin cancer rule from the American Cancer Society, which outlines warning signs of skin lesions.

2. What nursing diagnoses could be identified for Mr. Sanders?

3. The worldwide incidence of malignant melanoma is increasing rapidly. What is the probable cause of this rapid increase?

4. Consider reasons why people who notice a change in a skin lesion put off seeking health care. What can nurses do to effect change?

COMMUNICATION

1. What guidelines should be included when teaching any client about prevention of skin cancer?

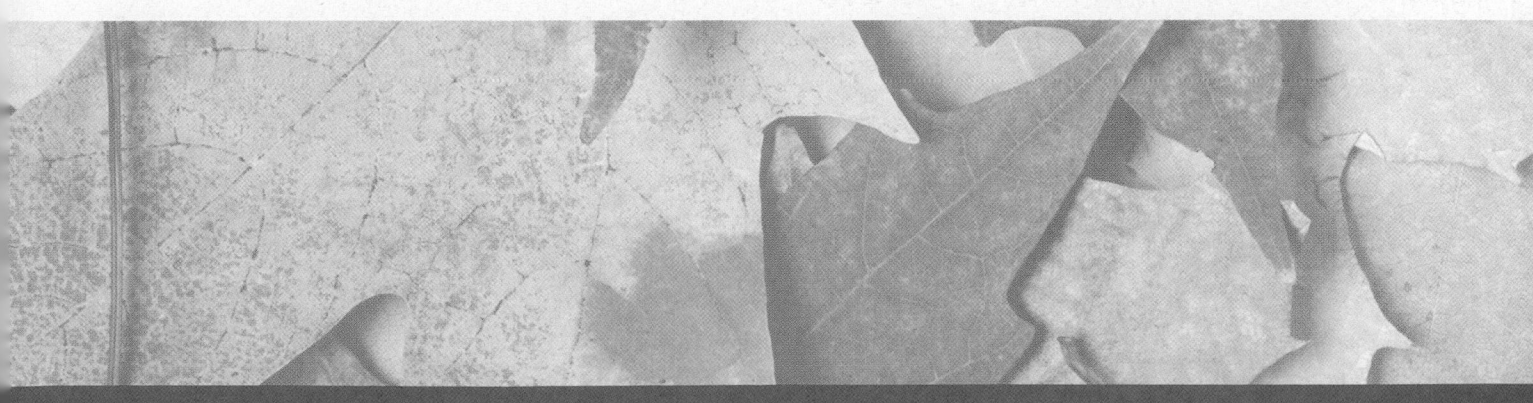

Disrupted Mental Health Function

UNIT XIII

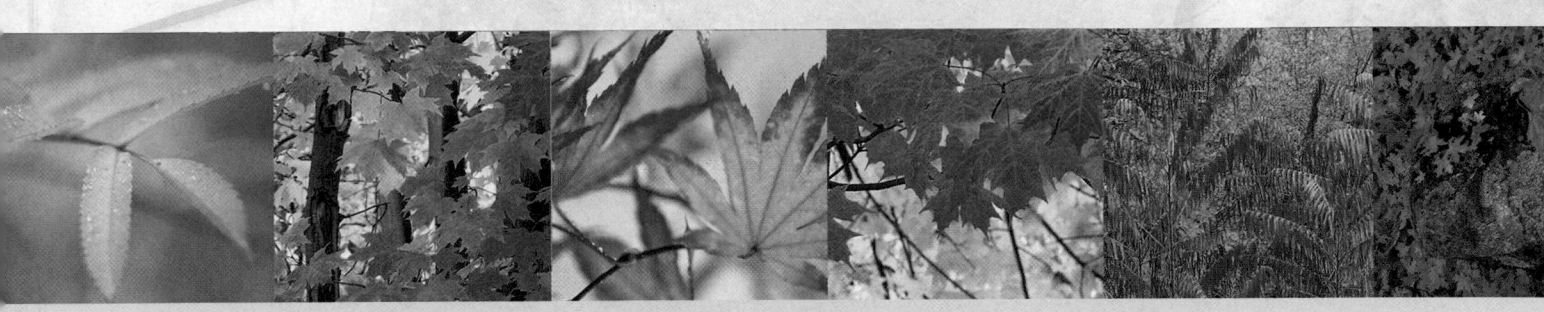

Mental Health and Assessment

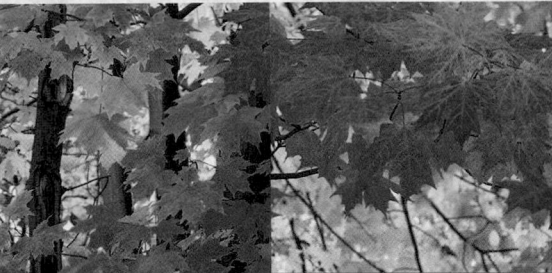

LEARNING Outcomes

After completing this chapter, you will be able to:

- Compare and contrast mental health and mental illness.
- Describe neurotransmission in the brain.
- Explain why psychosocial assessment is important.
- Identify risk factors for mental illness.
- Identify factors that promote mental health.
- Identify subjective and objective psychosocial assessment data.

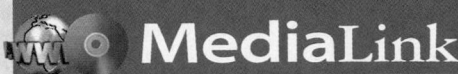

MediaLink

www.prenhall.com/burke
Use the address above to access the free, interactive Companion Website created for this textbook. Get hints, instant feedback, and textbook references to chapter-related NCLEX-style questions. Link to other interesting sites.

Audio Glossary:
Use the Companion Website, or the CD-ROM disk enclosed with your textbook, to hear the pronunciation of key terms in this chapter.

Nursing is holistic, which means that nurses treat clients as whole people. Nurses see clients as people who have diseases or disorders, but who are people first. Nurses do not define clients by their medical diagnoses or treatments, such as: "the asthmatic" or "schizophrenic" or "total hip in room 237." The body, mind, and spirit are each integral parts of the whole person (see Figure 47-1 ■). Nurses diagnose and treat problems affecting all aspects of the client: body, mind, and spirit. Refer to the list of nursing diagnoses in Appendix II to find diagnoses in each category. Because mental health is an important aspect of the health of each person, assessment of the mental health status of clients is an essential part of nursing practice.

Nurses encounter clients with psychosocial problems in all areas of nursing practice. Clients in the hospital or long-term care settings are likely to have mental health care needs as well as physical needs.

Mental Health

In general, there are seven important aspects of a mentally healthy person:

- Accurate assessment of reality
- Healthy self-concept
- Ability to relate to others
- Sense of meaning in life
- Creativity/productivity
- Control over one's own behavior
- Adaptability to change and conflict.

The ability to accurately determine reality is a basic part of mental health. It includes the abilities to differentiate between what really is and what might be, and to reasonably

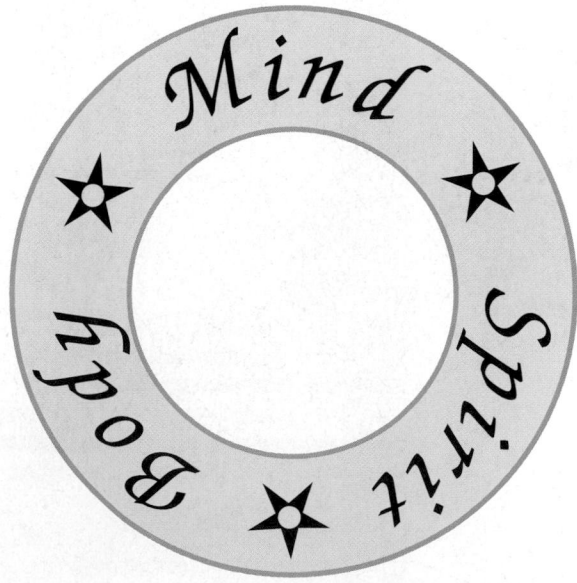

Figure 47-1. ■ Dimensions of a person. All are included in holistic nursing care.

predict the consequences of one's behavior (for example, knowing that the stove will be hot).

A healthy self-concept includes a realistic appraisal of the self (abilities, function, appearance) and a positive acceptance of the self as it is. **Insight,** or self-understanding, is important because it allows people to see their own motivations or reasons behind their feelings and behavior. A person lacking insight might refuse to take a medication because it causes his mouth to be dry. With insight a person could decide that he does not like to take the medication, but because it helps his mental illness he will take it. Insight is critical for problem solving. Without it people often do not realize that they have a mental illness.

Human beings are creatures that thrive best when they are with others. Love is the most important human emotion. Normal human development is not possible in isolation. People must be able to interact with and relate to others in order to flourish. Without the ability to relate to others in a satisfying way, a person cannot be fully healthy.

Humans seek reasons and meaning in life. Many people find a sense of meaning in the world through religion. Many others find meaning in nature, philosophy, ethics, or service to others. Spirituality is an important part of what it means to be a person. A fully mentally healthy person will have a sense of what is important in life and what gives life meaning.

A person does not have to be an artist to be creative. Healthy people can solve problems creatively. They can interpret experiences abstractly. Some people think *concretely,* meaning literally or without creativity. For example, a person who uses **concrete thinking** may say that the proverb "A rolling stone gathers no moss" means that if a stone rolls it will not collect moss. A more abstract thinker might say it means that a person who keeps moving around will not accumulate responsibilities, or that someone who keeps working will be able to function smoothly. Another aspect of healthy creativity is a sense of productivity or contribution. Healthy people want to feel like they are doing something to make a difference to others or a contribution to the world in their own way.

Control of behavior means that mentally healthy people can balance conflicts with their instincts, conscience, and reality before they act. Healthy people do not act out violently just because they are frustrated in the moment, nor would they steal something just because they want to have it. Mentally healthy people can delay gratification. They can act in a way that helps someone else, even if it is difficult for them. The healthiest people have the integrity to act on their values, even when this is difficult.

Adaptability is critical to success as a person. The one consistent thing around us is that the world is changing. Healthy people can compromise, plan, and be flexible. They can manage conflict successfully. Learning to change is not easy, but if people are healthy they will manage it.

Mental health is really a range of behaviors, a relative state instead of an absolute thing. Nobody is at the ultimate level of health in each of the above areas all the time. A person can have anywhere from minimal to maximal mentally healthy behavior, whether he or she has a mental disorder or not. Just as all people are developing throughout their lives, all people have the potential for growth toward greater mental health. Because nurses treat clients holistically, an important aspect of nursing is to promote the mental health of clients. Figure 47-2 ■ depicts the risks for mental illness and factors that promote mental health.

Brain Structure and Function of Brain Neurotransmitters

The brain is divided into the cerebrum, the limbic system, the brainstem, and the cerebellum. Figure 47-3 ■ illustrates brain anatomy. (Also see Chapter 38 ⬤⬤ for more information about brain structure and function.)

The work of the human brain is performed by approximately 100 billion neurons. The neurons are all interconnected, with an average neuron receiving input from 1,000 to 10,000 neighboring neurons. The complexities of the interrelatedness of the human brain are currently incomprehensible (Torrey, 2001). Research is seeking the answers to questions

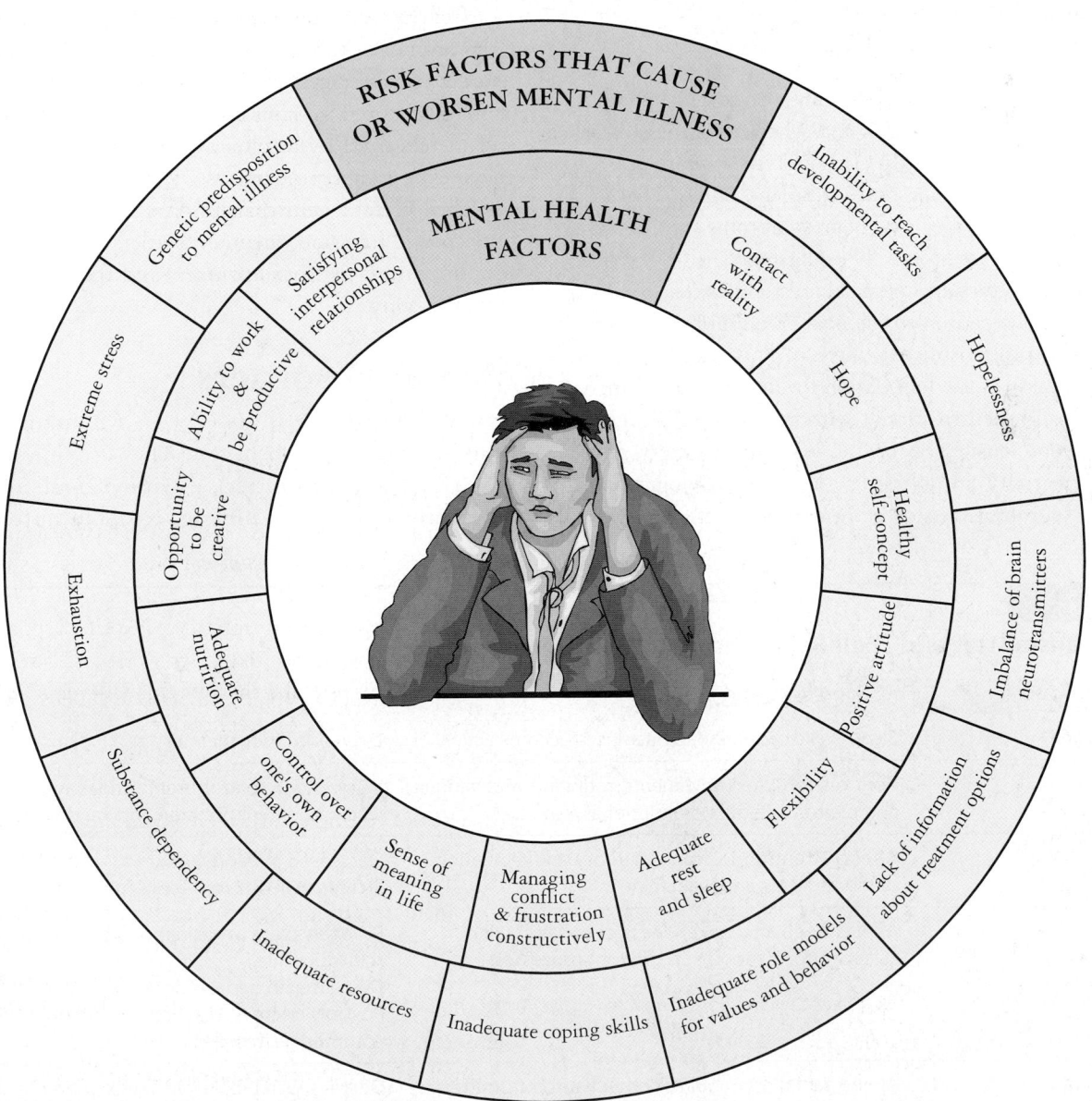

Figure 47-2. ■ Risk factors for mental illness and factors that promote mental health.

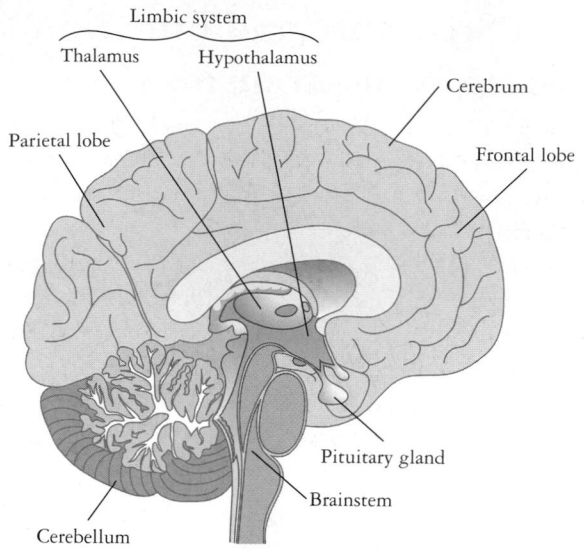

Figure 47-3. ■ Brain anatomy.

about the exact causes of brain disorders such as schizophrenia, depression, and bipolar disorder, and what treats these disorders specifically and efficiently. Although new information is rapidly becoming available, some treatments are used because they are effective at relieving client symptoms, not because their mechanism of action is fully understood.

Neurotransmitters are chemical messengers that conduct impulses from one neuron to the next. See Figure 47-4 ■ for a drawing of neurotransmitter function. This is an important concept because it is the foundation for understanding mental disorders and their treatment with psychotropic drugs.

Human consciousness, behavior, learning, memory, emotion, and creativity are all the result of physiologic brain functions. Neurotransmission is the communication between neurons conducted by neurotransmitter chemicals. Neurotransmission must occur for the brain to perform normally.

Neurotransmitters are manufactured in the **neuron** (nerve cell), and are released from the axon (the part of the nerve cell conveying an impulse away from the cell body) into the **synapse** (space between the axon and its target cell's dendrite). The neurotransmitter chemical stimulates the dendrite (the part of the neuron that conveys impulses toward the cell body) of the cell after the synapse.

The neurotransmitter must fit into a specific receptor site on the surface of the dendrite. The receptor site that is stimulated by the appropriate transmitter opens the ion channel into the dendrite. The ion channel allows for interchange of ions (sodium, potassium, and calcium), which changes the electrical charge of the cell (depolarization). Thus, the electrical impulse passes from one neuron to the next.

After the neurotransmitter is released into the synapse, it either excites or inhibits the next neuron (depending on the neurotransmitter). Then it is either taken back into the axon to be stored for later use (reuptake), or it is inactivated and metabolized by enzymes. The most common of these enzymes is monoamine oxidase.

When certain neurotransmitters have abnormally high or decreased function, mental disorders result. Table 47-1 ■ lists important neurotransmitters and their relationship to mental disorders.

Mental Disorders

Mental disorders are illnesses with symptoms related to thinking, feeling, or behavior. They are due to genetic, biologic (neurotransmitter), environmental, or psychologic influences. These illnesses result in impairment of

TABLE 47-1		
Neurotransmitters and Their Relationship to Mental Disorders		
NEUROTRANSMITTER	**PHYSIOLOGIC EFFECTS**	**RELATIONSHIP TO MENTAL DISORDERS**
Acetylcholine	Sleep/wake cycle. Signals muscles to become active.	Decreased in Alzheimer's and Parkinson's diseases.
Dopamine	Controls complex movements, cognition, motivation, and pleasure. Regulates emotional responses.	Increased in schizophrenia and mania. Decreased in depression and Parkinson's.
Norepinephrine	Affects attention, learning, memory, and regulation of mood, sleep, and wakefulness.	Decreased in depression. Increased in schizophrenia, mania, and anxiety.
Serotonin	Affects sleep and wakefulness, especially falling asleep. Affects mood and thought processes.	Probably plays a role in thought disorders of schizophrenia. Decreased in depression. Possibly decreased in anxiety and obsessive-compulsive disorder.
Gamma-aminobutyric acid (GABA)	Amino acid that modulates other neurotransmitters.	Decreased in anxiety and schizophrenia.

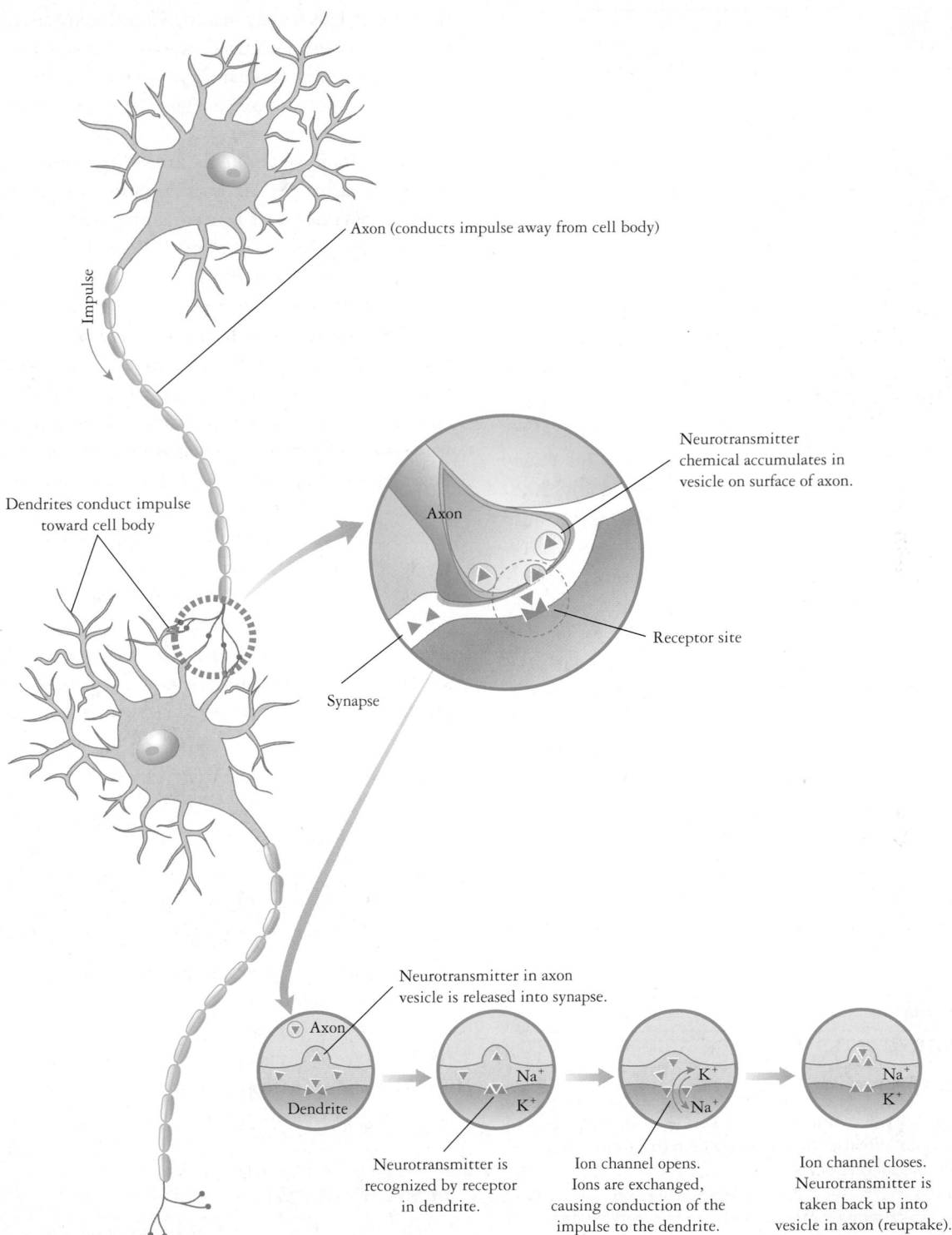

Figure 47-4. ■ Neurotransmission. First inset shows axon-dendrite interface. Second inset illustrates step-by-step neurotransmission.

functioning and other symptoms. Mental disorders are diagnosed according to the diagnostic criteria published in the *Diagnostic and Statistical Manual of Mental Disorders* (American Psychiatric Association, 2000). Specific mental disorders are covered in Chapters 48 through 51. ⬤

Physicians look at mental disorders in terms of disease processes and medical management. Nurses are more interested in how people are affected by these disorders. Nurses diagnose and treat clients' responses to illness, both physical and mental.

Mental disorders are a major problem for people all over the world. The incidence of mental disorders is often underestimated. One reason for this is that the severe impact of mental disorders is not always recognized. In 1996 the enormous Global Burden of Disease Study was done. The study showed that mental illnesses make up 5 of the 15 leading causes of disability in developed countries. Box 47-1 ■ lists the most common mental illnesses in the world. By 2020 major depressive disorder is projected to be the leading cause of disability in developed countries (Murray & Lopez, 1996). See Box 47-2 ■ for more details about the incidence of mental illness in the United States (National Institute of Mental Health, 2001).

There is currently no laboratory test to diagnose mental disorders. Research has been done to document brain changes in clients with major mental disorders. See Table 47-2 ■ for a summary of these tests, which are used for research, not individual client management.

THE STIGMA OF MENTAL ILLNESS

Try to list all the popular terms you have heard used to refer to people with mental illness: *crazy, nuts, bonkers, one-fry-short-of-a-happy-meal, wacko, goofy, psycho,* and *mental* are a few. Can you list others? What do all these terms have in common?

BOX 47-2

FACTS ABOUT MENTAL ILLNESS IN THE UNITED STATES
- One out of every five American adults suffers from a diagnosable mental disorder in any given year. This represents more than 44 million people.
- Depression is the most common mental disorder.
- Nearly twice as many women as men are affected by a depressive disorder each year.
- In 2000, 29,350 people died by suicide in the United States.
- More than 90% of people who kill themselves have a diagnosable mental disorder (commonly depressive or substance abuse disorders).
- 1.1% of the adult population has schizophrenia.
- Nineteen million Americans ages 18–54 have anxiety disorders.
- About 25% of jail inmates have major mental disorders.
- At least two-thirds of the elderly in nursing homes suffer from a mental disorder, such as major depressive illness.

They are all negative, insulting, and demeaning. When we talk about physical illnesses, we would not use such insulting terms. We would never call a person with diabetes an "insulin junkie" or a "sugar fool." These labels are inaccurate, inappropriate, and ignorant.

Simply talking about mental illness often causes people to laugh nervously. This is because mental illness has a **stigma** (negative attitude marking people with certain conditions as less valuable) in our culture.

It can feel so shameful to have a mental illness that people often refuse to seek treatment, even when that treatment can save their lives. Even physicians sometimes hesitate to give their clients the diagnosis of a mental disorder for fear that the clients will be "labeled" and treated badly as a result.

It is true that people with mental disorders have symptoms and impairment in their functioning (the specifics depend on which disorder they have). However, these disorders are treatable. Affected people can be and often are successful at being productive members of society such as politicians (including heads of state), artists, teachers, and nursing students. The stigma against the mentally ill is certainly not warranted. As client advocates, nurses should stop using the negative labels about people who have mental illnesses, and should educate the public that mental illnesses should be treated in the same way as physical illnesses.

There is a human tendency to want to be able to explain the things around us. This may be what makes people who do not truly understand mental illness fill in the blanks in their knowledge with fears and guesses. Nurses must base their practice on evidence, not guesses or stereotypes.

The stigma against mental illness makes nursing assessment of mental symptoms more challenging. Clients may be embarrassed or hesitant to talk about their feelings, ideas, or behavior. Nurses can make it easier for clients to cooperate by taking a confident and competent approach. When a nurse is giggling or hesitant, the client is more likely to be embarrassed. This is also true when the nurse is asking about other topics that are not appropriate in social conversation, such as bowel movements and urinary output.

Assessment

Nurses assess how clients' psychosocial functioning is affected by physical and mental disorders. Both subjective and objective data are important. Nurses, physicians, social workers, therapists, and other members of the health care team are involved in promoting the psychosocial health of clients. Psychosocial assessment at a general level is appropriate for all clients. A more specific assessment called a *mental status examination* or *mental status assessment* is appropriate for clients with mental disorders. Both assessments are included in this chapter.

TABLE 47-2

Diagnostic Tests for Mental Disorders

TEST	NORMAL VALUES	SIGNIFICANCE IN MENTAL HEALTH
Brain imaging ■ Computerized tomography (CT) scan ■ Magnetic resonance imaging (MRI) scan	CT and MRI studies show the structure of the brain.	Decrease in size of hippocampus in depression. Amygdala is enlarged in mania. MRI studies in schizophrenia have shown enlarged lateral and third brain ventricles, decreased volume of temporal lobe, and a worsening of several brain structural abnormalities over time.
Positron emission tomography (PET)	PET scan shows brain metabolism.	Mood disorders cause decreased frontal lobe metabolism. Increased blood flow to amygdala is seen in depression. PET shows functional abnormalities in brain glucose metabolism in the prefrontal cortex in schizophrenia.

PSYCHOSOCIAL ASSESSMENT

Psychosocial is a broad term that refers to things that affect psychologic and social functioning. Psychologic functions include:

■ Thinking
■ Feelings
■ Behavior
■ Responses to current stressors.

Social functions include:

■ Relationships with self and others
■ Community support.

When a client is admitted to a health care facility, the nurse may do an initial psychosocial assessment in addition to the physical assessment. Each facility will have its own format. Each aspect of the psychosocial assessment is described in the following paragraphs.

Culture and Family

Information about a client's family and culture are important parts of the psychosocial assessment, because they affect each person's health attitudes and behaviors related to health and illness. **Culture** is the attitudes, beliefs, customs, and behaviors that are passed from one generation to the next. Culture influences how we dress, what we eat, what work we do, our religion, language, customs, family roles, parenting behavior, the way we relate to other people, how we educate our children, our values, attitudes about right and wrong, and the priorities we set for our lives.

For the purposes of the nurse and the health care system, a client's **family** can be defined as a group of people who live together or in close contact, who take care of each other and provide assistance for their dependent members (Patterson, 1995). A more recent definition of family is an institution where individuals related through biology or enduring commitments participate in roles involving mutual socialization,

nurturance, and emotional commitment (Hockenberry, 2005). There are many different concepts of family, but the best definition of any client's family is what the client says it is. The psychosocial assessment includes the client's marital status and the members of the client's household because this information helps the health care team understand what family roles and responsibilities the client has and the kind of support the client might receive at home.

The client decides who may visit and who may receive information about the client's condition. The release of information is noted on a legal document in the client's medical record.

The languages spoken in the client's home are an aspect of psychosocial assessment because language affects the client's ability to relate and communicate with others. The nurse's ability to communicate with the client will affect the quality of nursing assessments, some interventions, and teaching. It is important for nurses to know that it requires different skills to understand technical or medical language than it does to conduct social conversation. Some clients will be independent for everyday communication, but will require an interpreter for informed consent or discharge teaching situations. When clients speak English as a nonnative language, even if they speak English well enough to have a social conversation, the nurse should ask whether they need an interpreter for health teaching. When a facility does not have an interpreter on staff, an interpreting agency can be accessed on the telephone.

Religious affiliation is an important psychosocial issue. Clients may have special religious-oriented dietary needs (such as Jewish clients who adhere to kosher dietary laws, Hindus or Seventh-Day Adventists who are vegetarians, Mormons who cannot consume caffeine, and many religious traditions that require special foods or restrict foods for certain holy days).

Religion can be very important to people when they are ill. Catholics and other Christians may want to be visited by their religious leaders when they are sick. The nurse may be able to help clients by asking if they have any religious needs while they are hospitalized. Some people will want to wear items of religious significance (a garment, symbol, amulet, or jewelry). Others may have traditions that require prayer at specified times or certain hygiene practices. Nurses cannot be expected to know about all potential religious or cultural needs, but can discover these issues during the psychosocial assessment.

Reason for Admission

The nurse can find out why the physician has admitted a client to a health care facility by reading the chart. It is still valuable to ask the client why he or she was admitted. The question "What happened that caused you to come to the hospital?" can give the nurse information about the client's perception of his or her situation.

Current Medical Problems

Assessing the client's medical problems might seem misplaced under psychosocial issues. However, medical history is helpful in psychosocial assessment because the client's health status certainly affects psychosocial functioning. Chronic illnesses provide significant stressors that will challenge clients' ability to cope when they are discharged. The client's behavior and relationships with self and others can be affected by health problems. Nurses should consider the client's whole health status, not only the specific issue for which she or he was admitted, when planning for discharge.

Substance Use

The use of alcohol or drugs as a way to cope with stress is an unhealthy coping mechanism, even if a client does not have alcohol dependency. (See Chapter 52 ⊂⊃ to learn more about substance abuse.) The crisis of hospitalization can be an opportunity for a client to change behavior and to begin new ways of coping. The nurse should ask every client about alcohol and drug use. Many will underestimate their use. Some will lie and say that they "never touch a drop." But occasionally when the nurse asks these questions a client will be ready to talk. This is a great opportunity to help clients. If nurses do not ask about alcohol and drug use, the opportunity will be lost.

Another reason to ask about recent alcohol and drug use when clients are admitted is to find out if the client is currently under the influence of intoxicants. Many prescribed medications interact in potentially dangerous ways with alcohol and other drugs. The physician must be notified immediately if the client is currently under the influence of alcohol or other intoxicants.

The final reason for assessing alcohol use history is to predict the likelihood of alcohol withdrawal syndrome. People who consume large amounts of alcohol regularly are likely to experience elevated vital signs and other symptoms of CNS stimulation if they stop drinking abruptly. Chapter 52 ⊂⊃ describes alcohol withdrawal in more detail.

When asking about alcohol or drug use, the nurse must avoid being judgmental. Clients are often embarrassed about these issues and are more likely to speak honestly with a nurse who is accepting of the client as a person. Ask how often clients drink rather than if they drink at all. Be careful not to suggest that the "correct" answer is that the client does not drink. Many people want to give the answer that the nurse wants to hear.

Assess smoking history to determine risk of respiratory illness and nicotine withdrawal symptoms, such as anxiety, insomnia, and irritability. The surgeon and anesthesiologist should be notified if a surgical client smokes, due to increased risk of respiratory complications in these clients. A smoking history gives the nurse another opportunity for health teaching.

Clients who drink large amounts of coffee or other caffeinated beverages regularly are at risk for caffeine withdrawal when they are hospitalized. Symptoms of caffeine withdrawal include headache, decreased energy, and constipation.

Support Systems

When people are mentally and psychosocially healthy, they usually have a network of people in their lives. Support systems include people who might be able to help a client with anything from ADLs to shopping, refilling prescriptions, going to see a movie, walking the dog, or checking books out of the library. Information about a client's social support system is helpful in discharge planning. Social support may come from family, friends, members of religious groups, fellow club members, charitable organizations, neighbors, coworkers, and so forth. When clients do not have an adequate social support system of their own, the nurse should contact a social worker who may need to arrange for help through a public agency.

Self-Concept

Our self-concept affects how we relate to ourselves and to others. Self-concept includes:

- Body image
- Role performance
- Identity
- Self-esteem.

See Table 47-3 ■ for some questions that can be used to assess a client's self-concept.

Coping Skills

Coping skills are the behaviors people use to relieve (cope with) their stress. Some coping skills are healthy and others are not. Knowledge of the client's usual coping behaviors will help the nurse promote healthy coping behavior, or plan for teaching to promote the client's health. For example, if a client who has just been diagnosed with cancer usually cries

TABLE 47-3

Assessing Self-Concept

COMPONENT OF SELF-CONCEPT	QUESTIONS TO ASK THE CLIENT
Body image	"How do you feel about your body?" "How has the surgery changed the way you feel about yourself?" "What do you like or not like about your body?"
Role performance	"Are you able to do all the things that are important to you?" "What were you able to do before that you cannot do now?" Ask about the client's ability to do something that is expected during the client's developmental stage (school, independent adult living, maintaining a relationship, parenting, work, teaching the younger generation).
Identity	"Of all the things you currently do, which ones define who you are the most?" "What are the most important things to you?" "Tell me five words that describe who you are."
Self-esteem	"Would you describe yourself in twenty-five words or less?" "How do you feel about yourself?" "What would you change about yourself if you could?"

alone in her room when she experiences stress, the nurse may be able to help this client talk about her fears and concerns. Learning to talk with others to express feelings and start problem solving might help the client begin to develop a new healthy way of coping. Table 47-4 ■ includes some questions to help the nurse assess clients' coping skills.

MENTAL STATUS ASSESSMENT

When asked, "What is the client's mental status?" the nurse will often reply: "Alert and oriented" or "Oriented times three." Many of the signs and symptoms of mental disorders such as schizophrenia and mood disorders are not covered

TABLE 47-4

Assessing Coping Skills

COPING ASSESSMENT	QUESTIONS TO ASK THE CLIENT
Past coping behaviors	"What have you done in situations like this in the past?" "How do you usually handle problems like this?" "How do you manage this at home?" "When the stress gets really bad, what do you do?" "Do you ever drink when the stress gets too high?"
Plans for coping	"What will you do when this happens again?" "What can you do differently the next time that will give you a different result?" "Now that we have talked, how will you manage when you go home?" "What might work better for you?"

by the "alert and oriented" assessment. A client could say, "I am Linda Eby. I am in the hospital. It is Tuesday at 8:00 P.M.," which sounds pretty good, but does this statement show if the client is experiencing hallucinations, if she feels like killing herself, or if her thinking is disorganized? The major clinical findings of the mental disorders are not covered in a simple assessment of orientation, so a more thorough assessment tool is needed.

Nurses and others on the health care team use mental status assessment to provide a clearer picture of the client's thinking processes. Because nurses do not read minds, thought processes are best assessed through systematic observation of the client's speech and behavior. A complete mental status assessment includes:

- Appearance (dress, grooming, posture, activity)
- Orientation (to person, place, time, situation)
- Mood and affect (depressed, elated, flat, anxious, changeable, angry)
- Speech characteristics (rate, content logical, pressured, loose associations)
- Thought disorder (delusions, obsessions, phobias)
- Hallucinations (auditory, visual, kinesthetic, olfactory)
- Behavior (aggressive, withdrawn, suicidal, homicidal, manipulative, intimidating, confused, intrusive, impulsive)
- Memory (short term and long term)
- Judgment/insight (understands illness, understands need for treatment, able to maintain own safety, able to maintain safety of others)

Note: The bibliography listings for this and all chapters have been compiled at the back of the book.

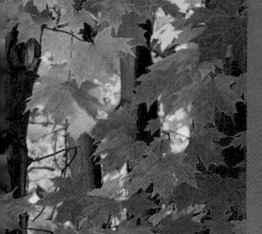

Chapter Review

 **KEY TERMS** by Topics

Use the audio glossary feature of either the CD-ROM or the Companion Website to hear the correct pronunciation of the following key terms.

Mental health
insight, concrete thinking

Neurotransmitters
neurotransmitters, neuron, synapse

Mental disorders
stigma

Assessment
psychosocial, culture, family

KEY Points

- Aspects of mental health are accurate assessment of reality, healthy self-concept, ability to relate to others, achieving a sense of meaning in life, creativity/productivity, control over one's own behavior, and adaptability to change and conflict.

- Psychosocial assessment is important because nurses treat the whole client: body, mind, and spirit. Each aspect of the person affects the others.

- Psychosocial assessment includes client's thinking, feelings, behavior, coping skills, relationships with self and others, and community support. The nurse should assess some psychosocial issues for every client.

- Mental disorders are brain diseases that affect clients' thoughts, feelings, and behavior.

- Mental status assessment is used to gain information about the symptoms of mental disorders.

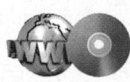 **EXPLORE Media**Link

Additional interactive resources for this chapter can be found on the Companion Website at www.prenhall.com/burke. Click on Chapter 47 and "Begin" to select the activities for this chapter.

For chapter-related NCLEX-style review questions and an audio glossary, access the accompanying CD-ROM in this book.

FOR FURTHER Study

See Chapter 38 for more information about brain structure and function.

See also Chapters 48 through 51 for information on specific mental disorders.

Chapter 52 provides information about substance abuse.

See Appendix II for the 2005–2006 NANDA-approved nursing diagnoses.

NCLEX-PN® Exam Preparation

1 A postsurgical client who speaks English as a nonnative language will be discharged this afternoon. She is able to have social conversations with the nurse in English. How should the nurse ensure the best communication of discharge instructions for this client?

A. Bring in an interpreter to translate discharge instructions.
B. Ask the client if she needs an interpreter.
C. Give the client the instructions, since she speaks English.
D. Ask the interpreter if the client needs his services.

2 What happens when the brain has too much or too little function of neurotransmitter chemicals?

A. The client will lose consciousness.
B. The client will lose control of his behavior.
C. This can cause mental disorders.
D. The brain is completely unable to function when neurotransmitters are not within a normal range.

3 Select the data that are part of a psychosocial assessment. (Select all that apply.)

A. the client's attitudes about his surgeon, and the intensity of his surgical pain
B. client's coping skills, self-concept, and social support
C. the expected length of a client's stay in the nursing home, client's daughter's hobbies, and the ages of her grandchildren
D. the age at which the client began sexual activity, how many steps the client has to climb to get to her apartment
E. the client's role in the family, and the members of the client's household

4 Which question by the nurse is most likely to obtain information about the client's skills for coping with stress?

A. "What would you usually do in a situation like this?"
B. "How many children do you have?"
C. "How do you feel about yourself after the surgery?"
D. "What are your coping strategies?"

5 How will the nurse find out if a client is experiencing suicidal thoughts?

A. Read the psychiatrist's progress notes.
B. Assess the client's behavior.
C. Assess for a sense of hopelessness in the client's verbalizations.
D. Ask the client directly.

Answers for Review Questions appear in Appendix V.

Chapter 48

Caring for Clients with Psychotic Disorders

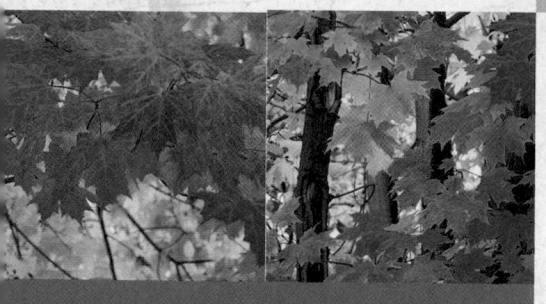

BRIEF Outline

Schizophrenia

LEARNING Outcomes

After completing this chapter, you will be able to:

- Explain the role of brain neurotransmitters in causing schizophrenia.
- Describe the actions and side effects of antipsychotic drugs.
- Identify subjective and objective data to collect for clients with schizophrenia.
- Identify nursing responsibilities for clients with schizophrenia.
- Identify appropriate nursing interventions for clients experiencing psychosis.

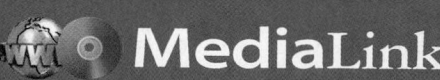

MediaLink

www.prenhall.com/burke

Use the address above to access the free, interactive Companion Website created for this textbook. Get hints, instant feedback, and textbook references to chapter-related NCLEX-style questions. Link to other interesting sites.

Audio Glossary:

Use the Companion Website, or the CD-ROM disk enclosed with your textbook, to hear the pronunciation of key terms in this chapter.

Psychosis refers to a thought disorder that causes the following symptoms: delusions, hallucinations, disorganized speech, and/or disorganized behavior (American Psychiatric Association [APA], 2000). See Table 48-1 ■ for definitions of these psychiatric terms. Psychosis is a major feature of schizophrenia, which is the most common thought disorder. There are other disorders that cause psychosis, including schizoaffective disorder, bipolar mania, and depression with psychotic features. Psychosis may also be a symptom of some general medical conditions or drug effects, but this chapter will focus on schizophrenia as the prototype for nursing care of people with psychotic disorders.

Schizophrenia

Schizophrenia is a complex disorder of the brain. Schizophrenia affects a person's thinking, mood, and behavior. Affected people experience psychosis; personality disorganization; and an impaired ability to interpret reality, to relate to self and others, and to function in daily life.

Approximately 2.2 million people in the United States have schizophrenia (Torrey, 2001). The disorder affects approximately 1% of the adult population. It affects women, men, people of all races and nationalities, and people of all socioeconomic classes. The age of onset is usually between the late teens and the early 30s. Diagnosis prior to adolescence is rare. See Box 48-1 ■ for information about late onset of schizophrenia in older adults.

Late-Onset Schizophrenia

The onset of schizophrenia is usually in young people, but it can begin in later life. Those who have a late onset of the disease are more likely to be women. It causes social isolation and all the positive symptoms of usual onset schizophrenia. Affected people tend to have delusions of persecution and hallucinations. It is a chronic long-term illness, but in elderly people, as in young people, antipsychotic medications can be very effective. Older adult clients tend to respond to lower doses of antipsychotic medications, whether they have the usual or late-onset form.

PATHOPHYSIOLOGY

E. Fuller Torrey, M.D., describes 10 findings relating to the cause of the disorder, accumulated in years of research and experience by scientists all over the world (Torrey, 2001):

1. *Neurochemical changes.* Neurotransmitters and their receptors, especially dopamine, norepinephrine, serotonin, GABA (gamma-aminobutyric acid), and glutamate, are altered in schizophrenia (Goff & Coyle, 2001). Antipsychotic drugs are effective because they affect the function and availability of neurotransmitters. Medical treatment of schizophrenia focuses largely on this area.

2. *Genetic component.* Schizophrenia is more likely to recur in a family that already has a family member with schizophrenia. There is a genetic component, but

TABLE 48-1		
Terms Related to Schizophrenia		
TERM	**DEFINITION**	**EXAMPLE**
Delusion	A false belief that is inconsistent with reality. It is not consistent with what the person's culture or religion accepts as real. It does not respond to reasoning or evidence that it is false.	One client believes that he is the supreme commander of all the world military. Another believes that the CIA is monitoring her conversations through a filling in her tooth.
Disorganized thinking	Thoughts are not related to each other or to the present situation. The normal flow of thought is disrupted. Thoughts may not form properly. Disorganized thoughts lead to disorganized speech and behavior.	Nurse says, "Would you like some breakfast?" Client says, "I would like something. I like dogs. I know the rules of fifty-two card games."
Hallucination	A sensory experience that seems real to the client but is not related to external stimuli. Most common are auditory, then visual. Can involve any of the senses.	The client hears voices commenting on everything he is doing. They tell him that he is bad, stupid, and worthless. Others cannot hear them.
Negative symptoms	These symptoms represent a reduction in normal functions such as reduced movement, thinking, motivation, and expression of emotion. In contrast, the delusions, hallucinations, and disorganized thinking are called *positive symptoms*.	The client spends most of his time lying in bed or sitting in a chair. He does not want to go outside. He does not read or listen to music or talk to others. Even when he hears something funny or sad, he shows very little emotion.

genetics is not the whole story. If it were purely genetic, both identical twins would always have it or not have it. Siblings of a person with the disorder are nine times more likely to have schizophrenia than the general population. Recent research implicates several genes that code for susceptibility to schizophrenia (Harrison & Owen, 2003). People with one or more of these susceptibility genes may manifest the disease only after they experience some stressor.

3. *Changes in brain structure and function.* Structural changes have been repeatedly found by imaging studies of the brains of people with schizophrenia. The structural abnormalities include enlargement of the brain ventricles, decrease in the size of the limbic system, and changes in the cell structure in the hippocampus, amygdala, parahippocampal gyrus, entorhinal cortex, and cingulate, which are located in the inferior part of the cerebrum.

4. *Cognitive impairments.* Four types of **cognitive** (thinking) function are affected by schizophrenia:
   - Attention
   - Executive function (abstract thinking and problem solving)
   - Awareness of the illness (insight)
   - Short-term memory.

   These thinking impairments affect people who have never taken medication, so they are not due to medication side effects. While the disease affects some aspects of thinking, other aspects remain intact, such as language skills, knowledge of information, and visual spatial abilities.

5. *Neurologic abnormalities.* The disease can cause abnormal reflexes (such as the grasp reflex found normally only in infants) and other less obvious neurologic abnormalities such as inability to perceive two simultaneous touches on the body and confusion between right and left. Abnormal eye movements (rapid eye movement and blinking too frequently or not often enough) have been associated with the disease. Abnormal body movements can be caused by the disease itself, as well as by medications used to treat it. (For more about the neurologic system, see Chapter 37. ∞)

6. *Brain electrical abnormalities.* Electroencephalograms (EEGs) have shown that people with schizophrenia are more likely to have abnormal electrical activity in the brain.

7. *Immunologic and inflammatory abnormalities.* Reduced immune function (leukocyte and immunoglobin abnormalities) has been documented in people with schizophrenia. Antipsychotic medications can also affect immune function, so it is difficult to determine what the disease causes and what the medication causes.

8. *Season of birth.* People with schizophrenia are born more frequently in the winter and spring. Numerous studies in 34 countries have shown a 5% to 8% increase in the birth rate of people with schizophrenia during the months of December through April. The reason for this seasonality is not known, although a maternal virus infection, especially during the second trimester of pregnancy, may be a causative factor. The increased frequency of influenza infection in the winter and in crowded areas supports this theory (Battle et al., 1999).

9. *Urban living.* People born or raised in an urban area have a greater risk for having schizophrenia. One reason for the increased number of people with the disorder in cities is that people move to the city for better mental health services. However, the birth rate of affected people in the city is twice that of the rate in rural areas (the suburbs have a rate between the two).

10. *Other.* Pregnancy and birth complications, minor physical anomalies, and an absence of rheumatoid arthritis are associated with schizophrenia.

In summary, schizophrenia is caused by abnormalities in brain structure and function. Genetic factors and environmental influences contribute to its development. Schizophrenia is probably more than one distinct disorder. People may have similar symptoms with different causes.

The pathophysiology most pertinent to nursing care involves the excess of the neurotransmitters dopamine and norepinephrine in the brain. Treatment of psychosis with antipsychotic medications is based on reducing the function of these neurotransmitters. Table 47-1 ∞ shows the various brain neurotransmitters and their relationship to mental disorders.

MANIFESTATIONS

The standard for diagnosis of mental disorders is the *Diagnostic and Statistical Manual of Mental Disorders,* fourth edition, text revision (APA, 2000), known as the DSM. The DSM diagnostic criteria for schizophrenia include:

- Characteristic symptoms: The client must have two or more of the following:
  Delusions
  Hallucinations
  Disorganized speech
  Grossly disorganized or catatonic behavior
  Negative symptoms.
- Seriously impaired social or occupational function
- Duration of symptoms must be at least 6 months.

The symptoms associated with schizophrenia may be placed into three major categories: positive, disorganized, and negative symptoms.

Positive (or *psychotic*) *symptoms* seem to be an excess or distortion of normal functions (APA, 2000). They include hallucinations and delusions.

■ **Hallucinations** are sensory perceptions that seem real but occur without external stimuli. The client may or may not have the insight that these are not real sensory experiences. Auditory hallucinations are the most common in schizophrenia, often experienced by the client as voices. Approximately 75% of people with schizophrenia hear voices at some time during their illness (Torrey, 2001). Visual hallucinations are the next most common. Hallucinations can also be tactile, gustatory (taste), olfactory (smell), or somatic (involving body sensations, such as electricity).

■ **Delusions** are fixed false beliefs. These beliefs persist despite evidence that they are not true. A delusional belief is one not ordinarily accepted by the members of the person's culture or religion. See Table 48-2 ■ for a list of types of delusions, which are categorized by their content.

Disorganized symptoms include disorganized thinking and disorganized behavior.

■ *Disorganized thinking* is a major feature of schizophrenia. Schizophrenia causes an inability to sort and interpret incoming sensory information and, as a result, an inability to respond appropriately. Because the observable demonstration of a person's thinking is speech, speech is the way thinking is assessed. Disorganized speech suggests disorganized thinking. Clients may have incoherent speech (in which subjects change every few words). At its worst, this becomes "word salad" in which words

are thrown together without relationship to each other, such as "Dogs, hat, fight, door, happening, machine, quickly." An example of a loose association is "You know I live in the zoo, I like animals, I plan to wear my new shoes when I go on the walk, are you coming?"

■ *Disorganized behavior* lacks goal orientation. The lack of goal orientation makes activities of daily living, such as personal hygiene or preparing meals, difficult. The client may have odd, unusual, or purposeless behavior such as walking in circles or pacing. Affected people sometimes dress in unusual ways, perhaps wearing several coats and hats on a hot day. Schizophrenia causes an altered sense of the self and affects movement and behavior. Disorganized behavior may also include unpredictable agitation (pacing, shouting, profanity) or inappropriate personal behavior, such as public masturbation (APA, 2000). It may also include catatonic behavior (a marked decrease in response to the environment). Clients with catatonia may have a rigid posture, resisting efforts to be moved. They may have excessive purposeless movement, or take on bizarre positions.

Negative symptoms of schizophrenia, in contrast to the positive ones, involve a deficit or decrease of normal functions. Negative symptoms include:

■ *Flat affect.* **Affect** is the nonverbal expression of emotion. The person with schizophrenia may have a decrease (blunting) or absence of nonverbal emotional expression, or *flattening* of affect. The person would not show facial expressions or other body language indicating feelings.

TABLE 48-2		
Types of Delusions		
TYPE OF DELUSION	**CONTENT**	**EXAMPLES**
Grandiose	The affected person has beliefs of inflated powers, knowledge, identity, or relationship to a deity or famous person.	"I am Spiderman."
Delusion of reference	Events, objects, or other people in the immediate environment have a particular and unusual significance.	"The TV newsman is talking to me."
Persecutory	The central belief is that the affected person is being conspired against, harassed, cheated, or persecuted.	"The food here is poisoned."
Somatic	The content of the delusion relates to the structure or function of the patient's body.	"There is a machine inside my body."
Bizarre	Believes clearly improbable ideas that are not derived from real-life experiences.	"My neighbor planted a fish inside my brain that tells me when to drink water."
Thought broadcasting	One's thoughts are being transmitted out loud so other people can hear them.	"I don't want to go to the store. Maybe I'll hurt somebody's feelings if I think they are fat or something."
Thought insertion	One's thoughts are not one's own, but are inserted into one's mind.	"You think I'm bad, but it's not me. The devil puts those ideas there."

BOX 48-2

REALITY CHECK ON SCHIZOPHRENIA

"At first it just sounds like wind in the leaves, rustling and soft. Then it becomes voices, whispering then talking louder. If I concentrate I can hear them more clearly."

"I am just here [psychiatric hospital] because I had a fight with my brother. There is nothing wrong with me. You are the one who is crazy!"

"I talk to the animals, you know, through their bellies. I am a vegetarian. I could never hurt them. I know what it is like to be eaten alive."

"The voices are talking to me all the time. They comment on everything, like 'You want that but it's too good for you, or you are so bad, or that man is going to kill you.'"

"Sometimes I wonder: Did I really see that, or was it in my imagination? Is that a real memory, or not? Is that person trying to kill me? My mother killed herself. I know why."

- *Alogia.* Alogia is decreased amount and richness of speech. It is thought that this reflects a reduction in thinking. A person with alogia has brief verbal responses, with little emotional expression. The speech may also be very concrete, lacking abstract ideas.
- *Avolition.* Avolition is a lack of motivation. Clients with avolition have difficulty initiating and persisting in goal-directed activities. This symptom can make it difficult for affected people to work or care for themselves.
- **Anhedonia.** Anhedonia is the lack of ability to feel pleasure.

Nursing practice is concerned with the client's response to illness, so the client's signs and symptoms are of interest to nurses. See Box 48-2 ■ for a description of the experience of schizophrenia by the real experts (people who have it and their families).

Course of the Disease

In addition to the thought and neurologic symptoms, schizophrenia affects the person's abilities to relate to self and others, and to function in society. Most people with schizophrenia do not marry, and are more likely than their parents to be unemployed (APA, 2000).

Like many chronic illnesses, schizophrenia is characterized by *exacerbations* when the client has psychotic and other symptoms, and then periods in which the symptoms subside (*remissions*). Many clients experience a **prodromal phase** with early symptoms before a full psychotic episode. If individuals recognize the symptoms of their prodromal phase, treatment with medication may prevent or lessen the psychotic episode to follow. For many individuals, the prodromal phase starts with negative symptoms. Often family members can look back and remember that the client spent a lot of time in bed, or became more distant or isolated before a psychotic episode (APA, 2000).

In the acute phase of the disorder, the affected person may experience hallucinations, delusions, disorganized speech or behavior, and the negative symptoms (alogia, flattened affect, social isolation, loss of motivation, and anhedonia). The affected person is usually unable to maintain employment, participate in school, contribute to household maintenance, or even do activities of daily living such as personal hygiene and cooking while in an acute episode.

Schizophrenia is associated with a shortened life expectancy. Females have a 5.6 times greater risk of early death than the general population. Males have a 5.1 times greater risk of early death. Suicide is the largest contributor to this excess mortality. Untreated people with schizophrenia who are experiencing depression and psychosis are at risk for suicide. Other risks associated with schizophrenia are accidents, diseases (heart disease, infections, and breast cancer), and homelessness. Homelessness probably contributes to the incidence of accidents and diseases (Torrey, 2001).

The brain disorder in schizophrenia renders many affected people unable to understand that they are mentally ill. As a result, effective treatments for schizophrenia often are avoided because clients lack the **insight** (self-understanding) to use them. Some health care providers blame the failure of many people with schizophrenia to take their disease seriously on denial. Denial is not the problem. In fact, lack of insight is one of the cognitive deficits in schizophrenia (Amador, 2001). At any given time 40% of people with schizophrenia are not receiving treatment (Torrey, 2001).

Early diagnosis and treatment of schizophrenia is important to prevent frequent relapses and rehospitalizations. Early intervention may prevent the worst long-term outcomes (homelessness and death) of this devastating brain disorder (Torrey, 2001).

Clients with schizophrenia often have a dual diagnosis, coexisting problems of mental illness and substance abuse. In combination, these problems lead to even more homelessness, disease, violence, incarceration, and death. Chapter 52 ⚭ covers this problem in more depth.

INTERDISCIPLINARY CARE

Continuum of Care

Because schizophrenia is a chronic illness that affects all aspects of life, the best approach to care is on a continuum. A continuum, or range, of services provides assistance for people who have different needs and for individuals as their needs change. A community should provide a continuum of services such as these:

- Hospitalization for acute episodes
- Case management to ensure that the client receives services
- Resources such as housing, food, medical care, transportation, clothing, employment, and socialization opportunities

- A range of housing and care options, such as subacute care, day hospitalization, supervised/assisted living, group homes, and foster care homes
- Outpatient treatment (including mental health clinics, and mandatory medication supervision as indicated)
- Support for families, including respite care, education, support groups, and referral services. Local affiliates of the National Alliance for the Mentally Ill are excellent resources for families.

People with schizophrenia have better outcomes if they receive appropriate services throughout their lives, and yet the resources do not exist in many communities. There may be many reasons for this lack: Our society values independence so highly that we reject the idea of treating people against their will; schizophrenia has such a stigma that people do not value spending tax money on people who suffer from it; and because of their disease, people with schizophrenia are not able to speak for themselves.

Milieu Therapy

For psychiatric inpatients, the environment or **milieu** can be used as part of therapy. Consider the needs of people with psychosis who are having hallucinations, poor judgment about safety, difficulty relating to others, and delusional thinking. The environment should be pleasant, simple, and safe. There should be minimal stimulation: no background music, loud television, loud talking, or flashing lights.

Consistent nursing staff helps promote development of trust. Nurses also serve as role models for normal behavior. Nurses demonstrate how to interact with other people, how to dress, how to ask someone to change their behavior, and how to participate in unit activities. Clients have the opportunity to practice and receive feedback on their behavior in the milieu.

Clients may need reminders to bathe, comb their hair, or attend group activities. Group activities often include recreation, simple exercise, arts and crafts, music, medication management, substance abuse treatment, relaxation techniques, or watching movies. To encourage independence, the nurse may allow clients to do unit activities independently first (for example, to comb hair before breakfast). If clients do not comb their hair, the nurse will prompt them to do so.

Milieu therapy also provides structure for clients' daily living. Meals and group activities are scheduled. Unit policies are followed consistently. Structure offers a predictable environment that is less stressful for a client with impaired thinking.

Psychosocial Rehabilitation

The goal of psychosocial rehabilitation is for individuals with mental illness to adjust to living in the community. Psychosocial rehabilitation begins during hospitalization, and continues in a community mental health program.

People with mental illnesses learn social skills, including ways to deal with other people in a variety of settings. Behavioral techniques are often used: People practice the skills they are learning. Skills training may include money management, using public transportation, recreation skills, personal hygiene, food preparation, and job skills.

Psychopharmacology

Medication is not the only treatment, but it is a cornerstone in the treatment of schizophrenia. Antipsychotic medications help relieve the hallucinations, delusions, and disordered thinking associated with the disorder.

Antipsychotic Agents

Antipsychotic medications (also called neuroleptics) are used to treat disorders such as schizophrenia that are characterized by psychosis. They are also used to treat the thought disorders sometimes associated with dementia, mania, or major depression with psychotic features. See Box 48-3 ■ for a list of antipsychotic medications.

Because schizophrenia affects people differently, a client may need to try several different antipsychotics before finding the one that works well. This trial process can be demoralizing. The nurse should explain that the health care provider will work with the client until the right one is found, and that no one will give up hope.

Medication compliance is a major problem for clients with schizophrenia. It can also create problems for nurses, especially when clients do not believe that they are sick. Approximately 80% of those who stop taking their medication after an acute episode have a relapse of psychosis within a year. Even people who continue to take their medications

---

BOX 48-3

ANTIPSYCHOTIC MEDICATIONS

Traditional or Typical Antipsychotics
- Chlorpromazine (Thorazine)
- Fluphenazine (Prolixin)
- Haloperidol (Haldol)
- Loxapine (Loxitane)
- Mesoridazine (Serentil)
- Molindone (Moban)
- Perphenazine (Trilafon)
- Thioridazine (Mellaril)
- Thiothixene (Navane)
- Trifluoperazine (Stelazine)

Atypical Antipsychotics
- Clozapine (Clozaril)
- Olanzapine (Zyprexa)
- Quetiapine (Seroquel)
- Ziprasidone (Geodon)

experience relapse at the rate of approximately 30% in a year (Torrey, 2001). Medication clearly improves the quality and quantity of life for people with severe mental illnesses such as schizophrenia. Unfortunately, the people who need medications the most often do not realize this. Also, certain medications cause side effects that combine with lack of insight to further decrease client compliance.

The antipsychotics are grouped as either typical (first-generation), atypical (second-generation), or new generation antipsychotic drugs.

The goals of treatment with antipsychotic agents are to:

- Relieve symptoms of psychosis
- Provide for safety
- Improve clients' function and quality of life.

TYPICAL (FIRST-GENERATION) ANTIPSYCHOTICS. The typical antipsychotics tend to be effective in treating psychosis or the positive symptoms of schizophrenia. The typical antipsychotics are especially effective in the treatment of acute psychosis with agitation. The negative symptoms are not very responsive to the typical antipsychotic medications.

It may take 2 days to 2 weeks for the onset of effects of the typical antipsychotic drugs. Full effect (*efficacy*) may take 4 weeks or longer. Clients and families need to be aware of this, so they do not give up hope and stop taking the medication too soon (Stuart & Laraia, 2001).

After approximately 12–24 months of stable maintenance on antipsychotic medication, clients can be slowly tapered from the drug to assess the need to continue this treatment. Some people with schizophrenia require a lifetime of continuous medication therapy (Stuart & Laraia, 2001).

Mechanism of Action. Psychotic symptoms are thought to be related to excess dopamine activity. Typical antipsychotic medications target the dopamine-2 (D_2) receptors, acting as antagonists to reduce dopamine activity in the brain.

Side Effects. Side effects are common and often cause clients to stop taking their medications when they are at home. Management of side effects is a critical part of the care of clients taking these medications.

Extrapyramidal Side Effects. While antagonism of D_2 receptors reduces psychosis, it causes extrapyramidal symptoms (EPS). Box 48-4 ■ lists extrapyramidal side effects. EPS result from the effects of antipsychotic drugs on the extrapyramidal tracts of the central nervous system, which control involuntary movement.

In the normal nervous system, the neurotransmitters dopamine and acetylcholine must be balanced to maintain normal muscle function. The client with untreated psychosis has increased dopaminergic activity. The balancing mechanism responds by increasing cholinergic activity. When an antipsychotic medication is given, dopaminergic activity is

---

BOX 48-4

EXTRAPYRAMIDAL SIDE EFFECTS FROM ANTIPSYCHOTIC DRUGS

- *Dystonia:* muscle rigidity
- *Dyskinesia (pseudoparkinsonism):* stiffness, tremors, shuffling gait
- *Akathisia:* restlessness, inability to sit still
- *Tardive dyskinesia:* late-onset permanent movement disorder with involuntary movements of face and tongue, or less commonly limbs and trunk

---

decreased, but the cholinergic activity is still high, leading to an imbalance. An anticholinergic drug can restore this balance and relieve the EPS. See Figure 48-1 ■ for a diagram of the process of EPS and its treatment. EPS include:

- **Dystonia:** muscular rigidity, abnormal muscle contraction. It can be mild, such as jaw muscle tightening, or as severe as oculogyric crisis (eyes uncontrollably rolled back), torticollis (neck twists head to side and back), and opisthotonos (generalized muscle spasms that result in arching of the back and neck). If the tongue or larynx are involved, choking can result. Dystonia occurs in approximately 20% of clients taking typical antipsychotics.
- Pseudoparkinsonism or **dyskinesia** (abnormal movement): stiff, stooped posture; shuffling gait; tremor; slow movements; cogwheel rigidity (jerky, ratchet-like movements of the joints); masklike facies (loss of facial expression). These symptoms are caused by the imbalance between dopamine and acetylcholine. Dystonia affects 20% of clients taking typical antipsychotics.
- **Akathisia:** restlessness, intense need to move. The client may report a sense of "jumping out of my skin" or an inability to sit still. Akathisia may cause clients to pace (walk back and forth continuously), fidget with fingers, or move arms and legs while sitting. Akathisia can make rest or sleep impossible for days. It is the most common EPS, affecting 25% of clients. It responds poorly to treatment (Keltner et al., 2003).
- **Tardive dyskinesia** (late onset of abnormal movement) is an extrapyramidal effect that develops after extended antipsychotic drug therapy. The symptoms of tardive dyskinesia (TD) include involuntary movements such as lip smacking, facial grimacing, tongue protrusion, tongue writhing, blinking, or other involuntary movements of the limbs and trunk. The most common TD symptoms involve abnormal involuntary movements of the face and tongue. The symptoms disappear during sleep. Sometimes clients can voluntarily suppress the abnormal movements briefly, but they recur when the client concentrates on something else.

A. Balance occurs in schizophrenic client's steady state of high dopamine.

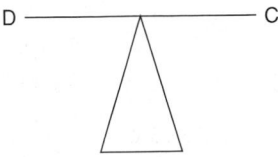

B. Antipsychotic med, decreases dopamine activity, putting dopamine, D, and acetylcholine, C, out of balance, Client has EPS.

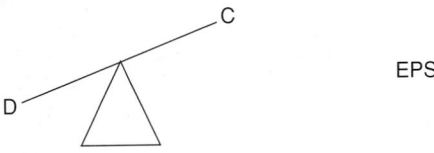

EPS

C. Anticholinergic med, is given to bring cholinergic activity down, restoring balance and treating EPS.

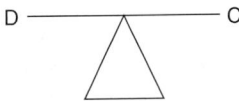

Figure 48-1. ■ Mechanism of extrapyramidal side effects (EPS).

TD may be due to development of hypersensitivity to dopamine. It is not caused by the same dopamine-acetylcholine imbalance as the other EPS. It does not respond to anticholinergic medications (Keltner et al., 2003).

It is important to assess clients on antipsychotic therapy for abnormal involuntary movement with a scale such as the AIMS (Abnormal Involuntary Movement Scale) to identify TD early. There is no effective treatment for TD, but it can be prevented by the use of the lowest effective dose of antipsychotic medication. Changing to another antipsychotic may be able to arrest the progression of TD. TD is irreversible; therefore, early recognition of the signs of TD is a critical nursing function.

EPS are very uncomfortable for clients. When they occur, the antipsychotic dose may be reduced, a different antipsychotic medication prescribed, or an anticholinergic or other medication may be used to treat the symptoms. Anticholinergic medications are usually given orally, but may be given intramuscularly in emergent situations. It is the responsibility of the nurse to ask whether the client is uncomfortable and to advocate for the client to obtain relief. See Table 48-3 ■ for a list of drugs used to treat EPS.

Neuroleptic Malignant Syndrome. Neuroleptic malignant syndrome (NMS) is a potentially fatal side effect of antipsychotic drugs. The major symptoms are high fever, muscle rigidity, autonomic instability (unstable blood pressure, diaphoresis, pale skin), delirium, inability to speak, tremors, and elevated levels of enzymes that indicate muscle damage (CPK). Temperatures may rise as high as 108°F (42.2°C). It is important for nurses to monitor vital signs on clients receiving antipsychotic medications.

Less than 1% of people who take antipsychotic drugs develop NMS, but for these it can be fatal. Early diagnosis and treatment are the keys to client survival.

Clients are at higher risk for developing NMS if they have dehydration, poor nutrition, or concurrent medical illness. Treatment involves discontinuing antipsychotic drugs

TABLE 48-3

Anticholinergic Drugs Used to Treat Extrapyramidal Side Effects

GENERIC (TRADE) NAME	DRUG CLASSIFICATION	AVAILABLE IN INJECTABLE FORM?
Benztropine (Cogentin)	Anticholinergic	Yes
Biperiden (Akineton)	Anticholinergic	Yes
Diphenhydramine (Benadryl)	Antihistamine (has strong anticholinergic side effects)	Yes
Procyclidine (Kemadrin)	Anticholinergic	No
Trihexyphenidyl (Artane)	Anticholinergic	Yes

and providing supportive treatment for dehydration and other symptoms (Videbeck, 2004).

NMS is an idiosyncratic reaction to antipsychotic (neuroleptic) drugs. It usually, but not always occurs early in therapy. It is not a toxic or allergic effect. High-potency typical antipsychotics are most frequently involved.

clinical ALERT

Neuroleptic malignant syndrome is a potentially fatal side effect of antipsychotic drugs. It usually occurs early in therapy. Nurses should assess for high fever, muscle pain, and unstable vital signs, and report these to the physician immediately.

Endocrine Side Effects. Dopamine inhibits the hormone prolactin, which promotes breast enlargement and milk production. Typical antipsychotics elevate levels of prolactin because they inhibit dopamine. Chronic prolactin elevation can cause decreased libido (sexual drive), breast enlargement (gynecomastia), and galactorrhea (leakage of milk) in women or men. It can also cause menstrual dysfunction in women.

The incidence of type 2 diabetes is increased in people with schizophrenia, even in those who are not obese. This increase may be in part due to adverse effects on the endocrine system caused by antipsychotic medications. Nurses should be alert for the development of signs and symptoms of hyperglycemia in clients taking antipsychotics.

Anticholinergic Side Effects. Anticholinergic side effects often result from the use of antipsychotics. See Box 48-5 ■ for a list of anticholinergic symptoms. Clients taking anticholinergic medications for EPS have an increased risk for these side effects.

Weight Gain. Most of the antipsychotics can cause weight gain. Weight gain with antipsychotics is associated with increased appetite, binge eating, carbohydrate craving, decreased

satiety, and change in food preferences in some clients. Increased insulin may also contribute to weight gain in people taking antipsychotic drugs.

Obesity is common in people with schizophrenia. They are less likely than the general population to exercise or eat a healthy low-fat diet. Appetite changes, sedentary lifestyle, and unhealthy food choices all add up to an increased risk for obesity and therefore type 2 diabetes and cardiovascular diseases.

Medical opinion is that the therapeutic effects of these drugs outweigh the importance of weight gain. However, weight gain can be a very important body image, self-esteem, and general health issue for clients.

The best approach to the risk of weight gain is prevention. Nurses can teach clients and their families about this risk and about how to reduce the likelihood of obesity with healthy nutrition and exercise.

Orthostatic Hypotension. The hypotension caused by antipsychotics is an antiadrenergic effect. Normally the blood vessels can respond to changes in body position by constricting, ensuring adequate blood flow to the brain. When sympathetic alpha-1 receptors are blocked, the vessels are prevented from responding automatically to body position changes.

BOX 48-5

ANTICHOLINERGIC SIDE EFFECTS

- Dry mouth
- Orthostatic hypotension
- Constipation
- Urinary hesitancy or retention
- Pupil dilation (*mydriasis*)
- Blurred near vision
- Dry eyes
- Photosensitivity
- Increased heart rate

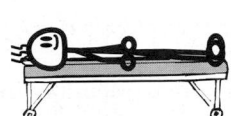 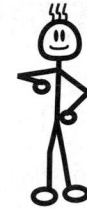

Figure 48-2. ■ Orthostatic blood pressure measurement. Take BP and pulse while client is supine. Repeat one minute after client stands up. A drop of 15–20 mmHg in systolic BP with increased P indicates orthostatic hypotension.

Orthostatic (position-related) hypotension happens when the individual stands up or changes position quickly. It is also called postural hypotension. Orthostatic hypotension is more likely to occur in older adults. It can create a safety hazard for the client who becomes dizzy or falls when the blood pressure drops (Keltner et al., 2003). See Figure 48-2 ■ for a reminder on how to measure for orthostatic hypotension.

Cardiac Side Effects. Antipsychotics may cause increased heart rate as an anticholinergic side effect. They may also cause prolonged conduction time through the heart's electrical system. On EKG a prolonged QT interval indicates prolonged conduction.

Seizures. The antipsychotics tend to decrease the seizure threshold; that is a smaller stimulus is required to cause a seizure in a client taking these medications. Epilepsy or a history of seizures is not a contraindication for the use of antipsychotic drugs, but the physician should be notified of any such history.

Photosensitivity. Some clients taking antipsychotics experience photosensitivity, which is an increased sensitivity to the effects of the sun. Photosensitive clients experience severe sunburn with minimal sun exposure. Dark-skinned as well as light-skinned clients can experience photosensitivity. They should be counseled to avoid prolonged exposure to sunlight or to wear long sleeves, a hat, or sunscreen on their skin whenever they are outdoors.

ATYPICAL ANTIPSYCHOTICS. The atypical antipsychotics have been used since the 1990s to treat schizophrenia and other psychotic disorders. Their mechanism of action differs from that of the typical agents. The typical agents act largely on dopamine-2 receptors, whereas the atypical agents influence a variety of dopamine receptor sites, serotonin receptors, muscarinic receptors, alpha-receptors, and histamine receptors.

Atypical agents differ from typical antipsychotic agents in several important ways. The atypical agents (Rankin, 2000):

1. Are effective in treating the negative symptoms of schizophrenia.
2. Cause fewer extrapyramidal side effects.

3. Are effective against the symptoms of schizophrenia for some people who do not respond to typical agents.

Side Effects. EPS are the side effects most commonly cited by clients as their reason for noncompliance with antipsychotic medications at home. As a group, the atypical agents cause fewer EPS, less prolactin increase, and less tardive dyskinesia. The atypicals treat psychosis effectively in some people who are resistant to the typical antipsychotics. Because of their efficacy and more favorable side effect profile, the atypical antipsychotics are currently prescribed more frequently than typical agents.

Individually, the atypical antipsychotics have some of the same side effects as the typical agents. Examples are the increased risk of weight gain with olanzapine, increased prolactin with risperidone, and the risk of increased heart conduction time with ziprasidone.

Diabetes. Clients receiving atypical antipsychotics are 9% more likely to have diabetes than people taking typical agents. In one study, the likelihood was significantly increased for clients taking clozapine, olanzapine, or quetiapine. The mechanism may be an increase in insulin resistance in body cells. Clients taking these drugs should be monitored regularly for development of diabetes. Other risk factors, such as African American, Native American, or Latino ethnicity, obesity, female gender, and family history of type 2 diabetes increase the client's risk (Keltner et al., 2003).

Agranulocytosis. Even though their side effect profile is favorable, the atypical agents still have side effects. The most notable is that clozapine can cause agranulocytosis, a life-threatening decrease in white blood cell production. This effect happens to 1% of clients who take clozapine. Therefore, clozapine is only used for clients who are resistant to treatment with other antipsychotics. Treatment resistance is established by failure to respond to at least two different antipsychotic agents. Clozapine is effective in treating 25% to 50% of clients whose symptoms do not respond to typical agents (Keltner et al., 2003).

clinical ALERT

All clients receiving clozapine should have their WBC measured once per week during the first 6 months of therapy, and every other week after that, to assess whether their white blood cell count is stable. If a client's WBC drops (indicating bone marrow suppression), clozapine should be permanently discontinued.

NEW GENERATION ANTIPSYCHOTICS. Unlike the other antipsychotic agents, aripiprazole (Abilify, Abilitat), a dopamine system stabilizer, has a stabilizing and modulating effect on brain dopamine. This drug is intended to reduce dopamine transmission when it is too high and to preserve it when it is too low, thus maintaining the dopaminergic-cholinergic balance. It therefore does not cause abnormal involuntary movements (EPS).

Depot Injection and Other Drug Forms

Several antipsychotic agents are currently available in long-acting decanoate (depot injection) form. The depot form of the drug is injected intramuscularly and lasts for several weeks. Haloperidol (Haldol) and fluphenazine (Prolixin) are the typical agents available in depot form. They are supplied in a sesame oil solution. Haloperidol is repeated every 4 weeks, and fluphenazine every 1 to 4 weeks. Risperidone is the only atypical antipsychotic agent currently in depot form. It is administered every 2 weeks and is supplied in a saline solution.

The advantages of the long-acting form of antipsychotic drugs relate to compliance with drug therapy. Clients may be able to comply with a clinic visit once every few weeks more consistently than they can take daily oral medications.

Several antipsychotic agents are available in liquid oral concentrate forms. The liquid form can be used to prevent situations in which clients move pills to their cheeks instead of swallowing them to spit them out later. It is also helpful when the client has difficulty swallowing or prefers the liquid to the pill form. The liquid concentrates must be mixed with a small amount of juice or other liquid to improve the taste.

Drug Interactions

All antipsychotic agents potentially interact with other CNS agents. There is an additive CNS depressant effect when they are combined with sedatives, narcotics, or alcohol. Antacids can decrease gastrointestinal absorption of the antipsychotics, reducing their effectiveness. Anticholinergic drugs can add to the anticholinergic side effects, and decrease the effectiveness of the antipsychotic. Tricyclic antidepressants add to the anticholinergic side effects (Rankin, 2000).

Abuse Potential

The antipsychotic medications do not cause euphoria, so there is virtually no abuse potential from these drugs. They also do not cause addiction or dependency. This lack of abuse potential is an important teaching point, because many consumers believe that any drug that affects the mind is addictive.

clinical ALERT

Nurses often hesitate to give prn medications, perhaps from fear of responsibility for making the decision to give them. If your client has EPS, do not hesitate to give these anticholinergics when they are ordered prn. EPS are very uncomfortable for clients, and are a major reason for non-compliance with antipsychotic medications.

NURSING CARE

ASSESSING

In psychiatric nursing the client's potential for violence is assessed first because it is a safety issue. Mentally ill people in general are no more violent than the general public, but there are groups of mentally ill people with increased risk for violence toward others (Torrey, 1997). The risk factors for violence are:

- Previous violent acts at home or in treatment
- History of substance abuse, especially if currently under the influence of substances
- Paranoid delusions
- Command hallucinations (commanding the client to hurt someone)
- History of being a victim of violence (violence is a learned behavior).

Certain behaviors may suggest that a client is becoming increasingly agitated and more likely to act out violently. These behaviors are clenched fists, loud talking or yelling, threatening, increasing motor activity (was sitting, then walking, then pacing back and forth quickly), hitting walls or furniture, wincing or looking afraid.

Mental Status Assessment

Nurses regularly assess and document the client's behavior, mood, and thought content (which is reflected in what the client says). See Chapter 47 ⬭ for information about mental status assessment.

Cultural Issues

Interpreting the meaning of client behaviors can be difficult if the client is from a different culture from the nurse. Box 48-6 ■ describes cultural sensitivity issues in psychiatric care. The nurse's goal is to see the client's behavior from the client's point of view.

BOX 48-6	POPULATION FOCUS

Cultural Care in Psychiatric Nursing

It is especially challenging to offer culturally sensitive psychiatric nursing. When the nurse and client are from different cultures, the nurse may misinterpret behavior that would be considered normal in the client's culture. For example, in some Latino cultures, people talk to the spirits of their dead relatives. What is really meant to be thinking about what the loved one would have wanted might appear to be hallucinating to a nurse. Some African and Caribbean cultures recognize witches and sorcerers, which might seem like delusional thinking to an outsider. The nurse should always try to interpret client behavior relative to the client's cultural background, rather than through the cultural standards of the nurse. When available, a cultural facilitator who can translate the client's language and culture-oriented behaviors can be very helpful.

Physical Assessment in the Psychiatric Setting

Although physical assessment plays an important role in nursing in every setting, the psychiatric nurse must be creative when assessing mental and physical health. When clients are hallucinating, they may not be sure what is real and what is not. Physical touching may be perceived as part of a threatening hallucination. Delusional thinking may make even the well-intentioned nurse seem menacing. Physical assessment may be very stressful for the client. Some clients mistake physical touch for sexual advances. Therefore, only priority physical assessments should be done in the acute psychiatric situation. A physician or nurse practitioner will perform an initial physical assessment as part of the psychiatric client's admission process. A trusting nurse–client relationship will make it easier for the nurse to gain client cooperation for necessary assessments.

Nurses must understand the desired effects and potential side effects of all medications and treatments received by their clients and assess for these. In addition, psychiatric clients may not be able to clearly articulate what is wrong with them. Careful listening is another important nursing skill. When a client with psychosis says, "The snake is squeezing my chest!" it is possible that this client is experiencing a heart attack.

The Client's Family

The client's family is a critical aspect of psychiatric care. It is important to obtain written permission from clients to communicate with anyone about them, including their family members. Families can make a big difference as allies in treatment for psychiatric clients, yet health care providers often overlook them, out of a mistaken sense of protecting the client's confidentiality. They are important members of the treatment team.

DIAGNOSING, PLANNING, AND IMPLEMENTING

Data about the client's mental status, observation of the client's behavior and interactions with others, physical assessment findings, and information from family all contribute data for establishing nursing diagnoses.

Priorities in Nursing Care. In the acute phase of psychosis, treatment should focus on the client's basic needs. Safety, nutrition, and rest are the priorities. Acute symptom management is also important.

Priority nursing diagnoses that often apply to clients with schizophrenia include Risk for Violence, Self-Directed or Other-Directed, Disturbed Thought Processes, Ineffective Coping, Impaired Social Interaction.

Desired outcomes for a client with schizophrenia include the following (Mills, 2000). The client will:

- Cause no harm to self or others.
- Have reality-based thinking.
- Use healthy coping skills.
- Take medications regularly.
- Continue to be active (employment, hobbies, exercise).
- Have a routine daily and weekly schedule.
- Include enjoyable activities in schedule.
- Perform activities of daily living independently.
- Keep in touch with family and important friends.

Risk for Violence, Self-Directed or Other-Directed

- Avoid touching an actively hallucinating client. *Touch may be perceived as part of a threatening hallucination, and client may hit in self-defense.*
- Intervene early as soon as you have identified increased agitation. Reassure clients that they are safe in the hospital. *Agitation can escalate quickly. Early intervention can prevent the situation from getting worse. Fear may motivate agitation. Clients often benefit from reassurance that they are safe.*
- Avoid confronting clients aggressively about their behavior. When inappropriate behavior arises, tell the client simply and calmly that the behavior is not acceptable and redirect the client to another activity. *Clients may not realize that their behavior is inappropriate. Aggressive behavior by the nurse may make clients feel defensive. The nurse's nonverbal behavior should be open and nonthreatening. Hold your hands at your sides. Keep your voice quiet and controlled. Your self-control can be "contagious" to the client.*
- Start with less restrictive interventions when clients have inappropriate behavior: Try to talk first then redirect, offer meds, isolate/medicate, restrain last. *Clients have the ethical and legal right to the least restrictive alternative treatment that is effective.*
- Maintain a low stimulation environment. *Clients with schizophrenia may have difficulty processing multiple stimuli, and extra stimuli may lead to agitation.*
- Talk with client about signs and symptoms of anxiety and agitation and the triggers that start these feelings. Discuss options for appropriate behavior and anxiety management techniques. *If client can recognize anxiety and agitation early, client can notify staff who can help identify coping mechanisms to prevent violent acting out. Clients with schizophrenia often have short attention spans and inadequate coping skills and may have impulsive behavior. Cognitive approaches to planning for future episodes help clients try appropriate new behavior.*
- Observe people experiencing paranoia or command hallucinations closely. *Even a person who has a nonviolent personality may act out violently when confronted with an apparently life-threatening hallucination, or when terrorized by a paranoid*

BOX 48-7	NURSING CARE CHECKLIST

Interacting with a Person Who Is Hallucinating

☑ Only one person should interact with the client at a time. *The client is having difficulty interpreting stimuli, so it will be easier for the client to respond to one person.*

☑ Keep environmental noise to a minimum. Do not speak loudly. *The client is having difficulty filtering sensory stimuli. A low stimulation environment will make it easier for the client to differentiate real stimuli from the voices.*

☑ Initially specifically ask the client about the hallucinations (usually voices) and what they are saying or telling the client to do. *It is helpful to know if clients are experiencing voices commanding them to hurt themselves or others.*

☑ Focus on reality. Do not continually ask clients to describe the hallucinations. Do not react to clients' report of hallucinations as if they are real. *Often hallucinations are transitory experiences for clients. Describing the hallucination can form it more clearly in the client's mind, and reinforce it. The nurse's role is to help clients recognize reality, not to further confuse them about their hallucinations or delusions. When the nurse keeps the conversation in reality, reality is reinforced and the hallucinations may be minimized.*

☑ Do not argue with the client's experience. Share your own perceptions. Reassure the clients that they are safe. *The client is truly hearing the voices. The goal is to present reality, not to convince the clients that they are wrong. Respectful disagreement can help the client understand what is real. For example, "I know you hear voices, but I don't hear them." Reassurance may help clients see that they are not in danger and do not need to defend themselves.*

☑ Avoid touching a person who is actively hallucinating. *During a hallucination, any touch may be perceived by the client as part of the hallucination. If the hallucination is threatening, the client may strike out in self-defense.*

■ Reinforce reality. Talk about what is really happening. *Even conversations about the simple realities of daily life (the weather, doing laundry, meals, etc.) focus the client's attention away from disordered thoughts and into the here and now. The nurse's role is to help the client recognize what is real.*

■ Do not argue with the client about delusional thoughts. *Clients do not recognize that they are delusions, and arguments can force the client to focus on defending the false ideas. Change the subject to reality-based topics.*

■ Encourage or assist the client to express feelings of fear or anxiety. Provide validation for the client's feelings. *The sense of losing contact with reality can be frightening. Expressing feelings to the nurse who accepts them without judgment and validates how difficult the situation must be can be affirming and helpful to clients.*

Ineffective Coping

■ Establish a trusting relationship in which the client is safe to express true feelings, especially negative ones. *The client may feel that only positive feelings are appropriate and not know an appropriate way to express negative feelings. A nonthreatening relationship provides the opportunity to express unresolved feelings. A strong reaction to client's feelings may indicate rejection.*

■ Offer medications in a confident way, expecting the client to take them. *The nurse's confident attitude promotes client trust.*

■ Teach clients stress management techniques such as going to their rooms and doing relaxation exercises. *Practicing new coping behavior teaches adaptive coping skills.*

Impaired Social Interaction

■ Approach client with an accepting attitude. Be honest and sincere. *Acceptance, honesty, and sincerity promote trust.*

■ Interact with the client individually and model appropriate social behavior (body language, topics of conversation). *People with schizophrenia often lack social skills and benefit from role modeling as a way to learn them.*

■ Give positive reinforcement for client's voluntary interactions with others. *Positive reinforcement is an effective behavioral approach to behavior change.*

■ Encourage client to attend group activities in the hospital. Accompany client at first if necessary. *Client may respond positively to encouragement from a trusted nurse.*

delusion that threatens the person's life. Many people will never be violent unless they are in a life-threatening situation. When people with schizophrenia are violent, usually the violent act is a matter of self-defense from their point of view.

See Box 48-7 ■ for help on interacting with clients who are actively hallucinating.

Disturbed Thought Processes

■ Provide antipsychotic medications as ordered and monitor effects. *It is the responsibility of nurses to assess the client's response to medications for the purpose of evaluating their effectiveness.*

■ Look for the client's strengths and abilities when providing nursing care. *When a person has a severe mental illness such as schizophrenia, it is easy to see the pathology. It is important to look for the person's strengths and to acknowledge the normal parts of the person. Even the psychotic client has coping or survival skills that the nurse can draw on for the client's benefit.*

EVALUATING

When evaluating the effectiveness of nursing care for clients with schizophrenia, the nurse looks to the desired outcomes. The nurse will determine whether the client:

■ Demonstrates reality-based thinking.
■ Performs ADLs independently.
■ Demonstrates an understanding of medication management.
■ Interacts effectively with others.

Documenting. The nurse should document data that describe clients' mental status and response to medications. Describing client statements and behaviors is preferable to writing conclusions, because the goal of documentation is to give the reader specific, concise, objective information about clients' responses to their disorders and treatments. For example, charting "The client states that he is Spiderman and plans to jump from roof to roof" illustrates his condition better than "Client has delusional thinking." Charting "Client has EPS" is not as clear as "Client states that his 'jaws feel tight' and he has been pacing the halls for 3 hours."

CONTINUING CARE

As the client recovers from psychosis and moves into the rehabilitation phase, the intervention focus changes to teaching and psychosocial rehabilitation issues. Medication teaching, group therapies, self-care skills, and social skills become more important. Clients can learn strategies to decrease the likelihood of relapse of schizophrenia. See Box 48-8 ■ for client teaching strategies to prevent relapse. Learning these strategies can give clients more control over their lives and disease processes.

Some people with schizophrenia will continue to have auditory hallucinations after they are discharged. Strategies for stopping these voices include *distraction,* which is listening to music, reading aloud, counting backwards from 100, watching television, and describing an object in detail. Some clients report that listening to music through headphones is most effective for overriding voices. *Interacting* is another strategy, and includes telling the voices to stop, talking to the voices while pretending to use a mobile phone, and agreeing to listen to the voices at certain times. The *activity* strategy includes walking, doing housework, taking a relaxing bath, playing the guitar, singing, and going to the gym. The *social* strategy involves talking to a trusted person, phoning a help line, avoiding people, going to a drop-in center, and going to a favorite place (Mills, 2000). The *stop technique* involves clients wearing a rubber band on one wrist. When they hear the voices, the clients snap the rubber band while telling the voices to stop.

Socialization

Relating to others is difficult for people with schizophrenia. In the community the nurse can refer the client to community socialization programs at mental health clinics or encourage the client to try recreational activities.

People with schizophrenia need a network of social contacts. Nurses foster relationships and group participation in all settings.

BOX 48-8	CLIENT TEACHING

Strategies for Preventing Relapse of Mental Illness

Discuss the following suggestions for reducing the chance of relapse of mental illness with the client:

- Learn from your experience. In the past how did you feel in the weeks before you needed to be hospitalized? What feelings or symptoms did you experience? These are the **predictors of relapse** for you. Tell your family about them, and watch for these symptoms. When they happen, get help from your psychiatrist who can change your treatment to help prevent or reduce the severity of the relapse.
- How do you feel about your **medication?** (Look for some positive aspect of client's attitude and repeat it.) What are your goals for the long term? Whatever you want to accomplish (becoming the president, going to Disneyland) will not happen if you do not take your medication. If medication is part of your treatment, take it. It is what keeps you out of the hospital. Tell your prescriber about side effects. Most can be treated.
- Do what you can to decrease the **stress** in your life. Keep your surroundings quiet. Go to a room alone or with one person if you want to. When someone argues with you, go to a quiet place. Know what is most stressful for you. If you know something is really stressful for you, avoid it.

- Know your **resources** and have a plan. Make a list of people who can give help when you need it. For example: Adam can take me to the pharmacy to refill my prescription. Betty can talk when I am lonely or scared. Carlos can take care of my fish if I am too tired. Dad can call the doctor or the hospital if I need to go. Write down all their phone numbers.
- Think of some **things that make you feel better.** Write them on a list. Take it out and do them when you start to feel bad. Maybe you feel better when you take a walk, do relaxation techniques, have a snack, paint, draw, take a nap, look at pictures, listen to music, talk to a trusted person, or pet a dog. The list has to be things you would really do.
- **Avoid risky situations.** Stay away from people who want you to use drugs or alcohol with them. It is too hard to say no. Stay away from negative people who criticize you or make you feel bad about yourself. Avoid situations that increase the voices or your stress.
- **Keep healthy.** Eat right. Sleep regularly. Stay active with hobbies, work, and exercise.
- **Keep hope alive.** Remember how life is always changing. Do you agree that some days you feel bad and some days you feel better?

Advocating for Clients

The treatments and knowledge needed to treat schizophrenia already exist. Financial commitment by the government and insurance companies, and community priorities must change to bring the resources to the people who need them. The role of nursing in this process is in client advocacy.

Nurses are experts on the subject of how people are affected by diseases and disorders. Nurses can influence their legislators to prioritize funding for mental illness treatment. Nurses can act collectively through their unions, employers, and professional organizations to influence insurance companies to cover mental illness equally with physical illness (called mental health parity). They can advocate in their communities for improved housing and other social services for mentally ill people. They can raise the consciousness of the people in their communities by writing to local newspaper editors about the issue of mental illness treatment. We can work to make the invisible people with mental illness visible so our society can see who truly needs help.

NURSING PROCESS CARE PLAN
Client with Schizophrenia

Anya Daeva is a 30-year-old woman who was diagnosed with schizophrenia 8 years ago. She has been hospitalized several times both for psychiatric admissions and general medical admissions. When she does not take her Risperdal (risperidone) she has a relapse of psychosis within 2 months. At this time she is experiencing psychosis again and suffered a compound fracture of the humerus and multiple ecchymoses when she ran into traffic. She has been hospitalized on the medical surgical unit since yesterday.

Assessment. The client's pain is managed by her ordered medications. The circulation, movement, and sensation in her fingers distal to the full arm cast are within normal limits. The capillary refill is 2 to 3 seconds. She states, "I was running away from the demons!" She appears to be afraid. She is seen talking when no other people are present, sometimes yelling at unseen others. She has been compliant with taking medications since admission. She told the nurse that when her prescription ran out at home, she felt like she didn't need the medicine any more.

Diagnosis. The following nursing diagnoses are identified for Ms. Daeva:

- Disturbed Thought Processes R/T disorganized thinking secondary to schizophrenia

- Disturbed Sensory Perception (auditory) R/T hallucinations secondary to schizophrenia
- Ineffective Coping R/T inadequate coping skills

Expected Outcomes. The client will:

- Maintain reality orientation.
- Have brief reality-based conversations with staff.
- State that she has a decrease in frequency and severity of "voices."
- Cooperate by taking all ordered medications during hospitalization.
- Engage in a trusting relationship with the nurse.
- Verbalize her willingness to participate in supervised medication management as an outpatient.

Planning and Implementation. The nurse caring for Ms. Daeva will:

- Establish a trusting relationship with the client.
- Reassure her that she is safe in the hospital, while not arguing with the delusional thinking.
- Reinforce reality.
- Monitor the client's mental status for improvement in psychotic symptoms (auditory hallucinations and delusional thinking).
- Reinforce the importance of taking antipsychotic medications consistently.
- Ask the hospital social worker to be involved in discharge planning.

Evaluation. After 2 days on the medical surgical unit, Ms. Daeva was still experiencing auditory hallucinations, but they were much less frequent. She complied with all her ordered medications. She was transferred to the inpatient psychiatric unit for 1 week, during which her thinking continued to be intermittently reality based and delusional. The social worker made arrangements for her to be discharged to a supervised apartment living situation, where a staff member would administer her medications.

Critical Thinking in the Nursing Process

1. Why was the social worker asked to participate in this client's discharge planning?
2. What factors led to this client's frequent hospitalizations?
3. Why is the nurse planning to have brief conversations with this client while she is experiencing psychosis?

Note: The bibliography listings for this and all chapters have been compiled at the back of the book.

Chapter Review

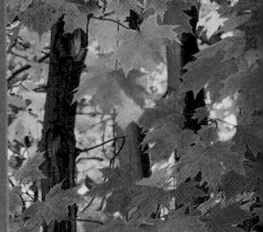

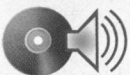 **KEY TERMS** by Topics

Use the audio glossary feature of either the CD-ROM or the Companion Website to hear the correct pronunciation of the following key terms.

Psychotic Disorders
psychosis

Schizophrenia
cognitive, hallucination, delusion, affect, anhedonia, prodromal phase, insight, dual diagnosis, milieu, dystonia, dyskinesia, akathisia, tardive dyskinesia

KEY Points

- Schizophrenia affects approximately 1% of all people in the United States.
- Schizophrenia is a complex disorder caused by functional and structural abnormalities of the brain.
- The disorder is characterized by positive, disorganized, and negative symptoms.
- People with schizophrenia have disordered thinking, decreased motivation, difficulty relating to other people and to themselves, and an increased risk of suicide.
- It usually starts in young adulthood and has periods of acute psychosis alternating with periods of reduced or absent symptoms.
- Most people with schizophrenia require a range of services throughout their lives.
- Families are important members of the treatment team.
- Antipsychotic medications work by reducing the function of neurotransmitters such as dopamine in the brain.
- Antipsychotic medications improve the symptoms of the majority of people with schizophrenia.
- Antipsychotic medications have side effects. Some (NMS and TD) are life threatening or long lasting, others (EPS) cause clients discomfort and may discourage compliance with medication therapy.
- There is hope for people with schizophrenia. Most people respond well to treatment. Research is promising new medications.

EXPLORE MediaLink

Additional interactive resources for this chapter can be found on the Companion Website at www.prenhall.com/burke. Click on Chapter 48 and "Begin" to select the activities for this chapter.

For chapter-related NCLEX-style review questions and an audio glossary, access the accompanying CD-ROM in this book.

FOR FURTHER Study

For more about the neurologic system, see Chapter 37.

See Chapter 47 for more about assessment of clients with mental disorders.

Table 47-1 shows the various brain neurotransmitters and their relationship to mental disorders.

For more about substance abuse and dependency, see Chapter 52.

Caring for a Client with Schizophrenia

NCLEX-PN® Focus Area: Physiologic Adaptation

Case Study: Craig Koda, age 21, was diagnosed with schizophrenia 6 months ago. He has tried two different antipsychotic medications during this time without full remission of his symptoms. He was admitted to the psychiatric unit through the emergency department today with an exacerbation of psychosis with agitation. His mother states that he resists taking his meds at home, saying that he is "not crazy." He was given an injection of Haloperidol 2 mg IM in the emergency department 2 hours ago. Currently he is thrashing in his bed yelling that he is "jumping out of his skin."

Nursing Diagnosis: Risk for Injury R/T Drug Side Effects

COLLECT DATA

Subjective	Objective
_____	_____
_____	_____
_____	_____
_____	_____
_____	_____
_____	_____

Would you report this data? Yes/No

If yes, to: _____

Nursing Care

_____
_____
_____
_____
_____
_____
_____
_____
_____
_____

How would you document this? _____
_____
_____
_____

Data Collected (use those that apply)

- BP 148/70, P 110, R 24
- Weight 188 lbs
- Client states, "I can't hold still!"
- Muscles of legs and arms are stiff
- Client's father states, "He is always difficult to get along with."
- Client is allergic to pollen
- Refused dinner this evening
- Client appears to be in distress
- Complains of jaw stiffness and discomfort
- When client protrudes his tongue, it quivers

Nursing Interventions (use those that apply; list in priority order)

- Call the physician and ask for an order for a sedative.
- Encourage the client to eat some soft foods for dinner.
- Assess VS q1h.
- Provide a low stimulation environment.
- Call the physician immediately to report extrapyramidal symptoms.
- Expect to give an anticholinergic medication.
- Tell the client that he is having a medication side effect called EPS that can be treated.
- Tell the client that nothing is wrong and he will be fine.
- Teach the client about all his medications now.
- Tell the client that he is allergic to haloperidol.
- Call for the resuscitation team.

NCLEX-PN® Exam Preparation

1 The chart indicates that a client is experiencing the negative symptoms of schizophrenia. What would the nurse expect to see?

A. hallucinations and delusional thinking
B. bizarre behavior
C. flat affect and little speech
D. difficulty with mental concentration

2 A client appears to be afraid. He is yelling about aliens and swinging his arms like he is trying to stop something from hitting him in the head. He also yells, "Stop them, stop them." What is the best way to document this situation? "The client is:

A. acting inappropriately and yelling."
B. a danger to others."
C. experiencing a frightening hallucination, apparently about aliens attacking him."
D. yelling, screaming, hitting, and disrupting all the other clients on the unit."

3 When a client is experiencing a frightening hallucination about aliens, what is the best first response by the nurse?

A. Reassure the client that he is safe in the hospital and there are no aliens.
B. Give the client more medication.
C. Tell the client that the aliens are friendly and not to worry.
D. Move the client to a private room where he will not disturb others.

4 What would you expect to find on a psychiatric unit that uses milieu therapy?

A. structured daily activities
B. a television on a news channel all day for orientation
C. plenty of stimulation: loud music and lots of people
D. strict rules to control client behavior

5 Which of the following clients is at greatest risk for violent behavior? A client who:

A. is experiencing catatonic symptoms.
B. has been following the nurse around all day.
C. refuses to eat or participate in her care.
D. is pacing the halls, clenching his fists, and talking angrily to unseen voices.

6 A client states that she is the Queen of England and has magical powers. What is this type of thinking called?

A. hallucinatory
B. manipulative
C. delusional
D. schizophrenic

7 What is the nurse's best response when a client newly diagnosed with schizophrenia asks, "What is wrong with me?"

A. "You are experiencing excessive neurotransmitter amines in your brain synapses."
B. "You have schizophrenia, which is a brain disorder that affects your thinking."
C. "You should ask your doctor."
D. "Nobody really understands schizophrenia."

8 Which of the following symptoms could indicate neuroleptic malignant syndrome in a client taking an antipsychotic medication?

A. dry mouth, orthostatic hypotension
B. high fever, muscle pain, unstable BP
C. urinary retention, dizziness, dry skin
D. photosensitivity, abnormal body movements, increased heart rate

9 A client with schizophrenia is hearing voices that no one else can hear. What is this symptom called? _____

10 A client with schizophrenia is experiencing all of the following symptoms. Choose all that are anticholinergic side effects of his psychotropic medications.

A. orthostatic hypotension
B. dry mouth
C. abnormal body movements
D. increased heart rate

Answers for Review Questions, as well as discussion of Care Plan and Critical Thinking Care Map questions, appear in Appendix V.

Chapter 49

Caring for Clients with Mood Disorders

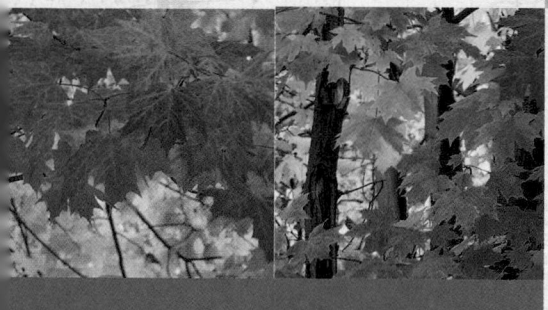

BRIEF Outline

Major Depressive Disorder
Bipolar Disorder

LEARNING Outcomes

After completing this chapter, you will be able to:

- Explain the pathophysiology of mood disorders in relation to brain neurotransmitters.
- Identify subjective and objective data to collect related to a client's mood.
- Assess clients for suicidal thinking.
- Safely and effectively administer antidepressant and mood stabilizing medications.
- Apply the nursing process to clients with mood disorders.

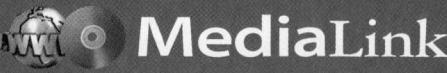

MediaLink

www.prenhall.com/burke
Use the address above to access the free, interactive Companion Website created for this textbook. Get hints, instant feedback, and textbook references to chapter-related NCLEX-style questions. Link to other interesting sites.

Audio Glossary:
Use the Companion Website, or the CD-ROM disk enclosed with your textbook, to hear the pronunciation of key terms in this chapter.

Everyone has had good and bad moods. We can all relate to a range of emotions that people normally experience in the course of their lives. When mood goes beyond the normal range of intensity, when elation or tragedy are persistent, are not a response to life experiences, and interfere with daily functioning, a disorder of mood exists.

Mood is a pervasive and sustained emotion that influences how a person perceives the world. Mood is like the overall climate: In Los Angeles, the climate is warm. A person with depression is usually sad. **Affect** (a'fekt) refers to the emotions a person is currently expressing. It is more changeable than mood. Affect is like the weather today: No matter what it is like usually, today it is snowing. Mood can be **elevated,** an exaggerated sense of energy or well-being; **euthymic,** in the normal range; **dysphoric,** sad or unpleasant; or **irritable,** easily annoyed, upset, or provoked to anger (American Psychiatric Association [APA], 2000).

There are several disorders of mood. In this chapter we will use Major Depressive Disorder and Bipolar I Disorder as our prototypes for the nursing management of mood disorders. Figure 49-1 ■ shows the characteristics of a major depressive episode.

Major Depressive Disorder

DEPRESSION

Because the symptoms of depression are similar to sadness, people often mistake depression (which is a mental disorder) with sadness (which is a normal response to a life experience). Depression takes sadness and lack of energy and motivation to another level that is not in the usual experience of unaffected people.

The American Psychiatric Association sets the standard for the definition of depression in the DSM-IV TR (2000).

Major Depressive Disorder is a disease that consists of one or more major depressive episodes. The diagnostic criteria for a major depressive episode include that the client must have five of the following symptoms during a 2-week period. At least one of the symptoms must be depressed mood or loss of interest or pleasure. The symptoms cause significant distress or impairment in social, occupational, or other important areas of functioning.

1. *Depressed mood* most of the day, nearly every day, as indicated by either subjective report (for example "I feel sad, or empty") or observation made by others (such as appears tearful). In children or adolescents, mood can be *irritable* instead of sad.
2. *Very diminished interest or pleasure* in all, or almost all, activities most of the day nearly every day (either by client report or report of others).
3. *Significant weight loss* while not dieting or *weight gain* (change of more than 5% of body weight in a month), or an increase or decrease of appetite nearly every day. *Note:* Children may fail to make expected weight gains.
4. *Insomnia* or *hypersomnia* (sleeping too much) nearly every day.
5. *Psychomotor agitation (increased activity)* or *psychomotor retardation (decreased purposeful activity)* nearly every day (observed by others, not just feeling restless or slow).
6. *Fatigue or loss of energy* nearly every day.
7. Feelings of *worthlessness or inappropriate or excessive guilt* nearly every day
8. *Diminished ability to think or concentrate,* or indecisiveness, nearly every day
9. *Recurrent thoughts of death* (not just fear of dying), recurrent suicidal thinking, a plan for committing suicide, or a suicide attempt.

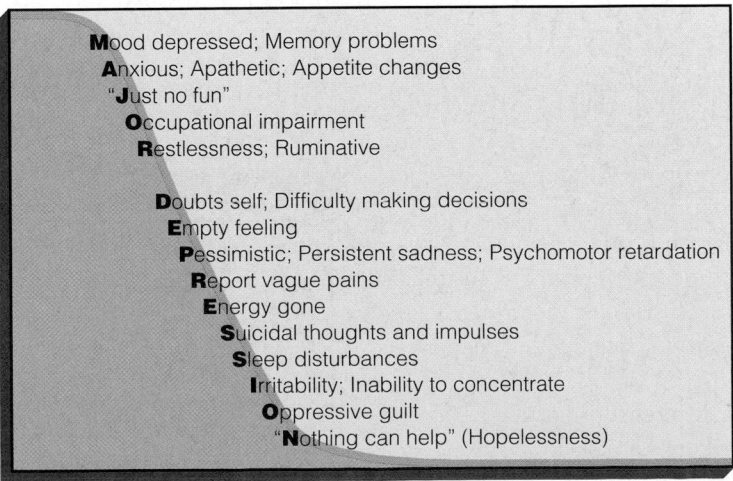

Mood depressed; Memory problems
Anxious; Apathetic; Appetite changes
"Just no fun"
Occupational impairment
Restlessness; Ruminative

Doubts self; Difficulty making decisions
Empty feeling
Pessimistic; Persistent sadness; Psychomotor retardation
Report vague pains
Energy gone
Suicidal thoughts and impulses
Sleep disturbances
Irritability; Inability to concentrate
Oppressive guilt
"Nothing can help" (Hopelessness)

Figure 49-1. ■ Characteristics of a major depressive episode.

Depression is not diagnosed if the symptoms are associated with general medical conditions, side effects of substances, or bereavement. Depressive episodes can range from mild to severe, with a range of functional impairment as well.

PATHOPHYSIOLOGY

Depression is a multifactorial disorder (that is, it can have a variety of causes). Major Depressive Disorder has a genetic component, a brain physiology component, and a psychosocial component. Each contributes, but none explains the disorder alone. Because multiple factors cause and affect the disorder, effective treatments must include psychosocial (teaching and counseling) and physiologic (usually medication) approaches.

Major depressive disorder is 1.5 to 3 times more common among first-degree biologic relatives of affected people than among the general population (APA, 2000). Researchers have found that people who have a variant of the gene that codes for a transporter of serotonin are more likely to develop depression after experiencing stress (Caspi et al., 2003). People inherit the tendency to respond to life stressors with the development of depression.

Recent advances in brain imaging have been used to assess brain function of people with depression. Positron emission tomography (PET) shows abnormal function in the prefrontal cortex of the cerebrum and in the limbic system during depressive episodes.

There is also a lot of evidence that an abnormality in brain neurotransmitter physiology causes depression. Brain neurotransmitters such as serotonin, norepinephrine, dopamine, acetylcholine, and gamma-aminobutyric acid (GABA) are likely involved. In schizophrenia, brain neurotransmitters are overactive. In depression, the opposite is true: The neurotransmitters have reduced function. The fact that antidepressant medications (which increase neurotransmitter function) are so effective is evidence that neurotransmitter function affects mood.

The endocrine system is also involved. The hypothalamus, pituitary, and adrenal glands, together called the *HPA axis,* control the physiologic responses to stress. These glands may be hyperactive in people with depression. The HPA axis also affects the 24-hour day–night cycle of body rhythms (circadian rhythms). In both depression and mania, the normal circadian rhythms are disrupted. Circadian rhythms affect many physiologic functions, including sleep and wakefulness, hormone secretion, mental alertness, and body temperature.

Children show no gender difference in risk, but after puberty females are twice as likely as males to be affected. A significant proportion of affected women report a worsening of depressive symptoms in the few days before menstruation. The lifetime risk of having a major depressive episode is 10% to 25% for women and 5% to 12% for men. At any given time, 3% to 5% of people in the United States are experiencing a major depressive episode. Most of these are not diagnosed or treated. The disorder affects people of all ethnicities and socioeconomic groups equally (APA, 2000).

It is common for people with depression to have other disorders simultaneously. The disorders that frequently occur with depression include schizophrenia, substance abuse, eating disorders, anxiety disorders, general medical conditions such as diabetes, cerebrovascular accident (CVA or stroke), and other chronic conditions.

Depressive symptoms may be caused by certain medications. Some antibiotics, antifungal, anti-inflammatory, antineoplastic, cardiovascular, and gastrointestinal drugs have been shown to cause depressive symptoms in some people.

Course of the Disease

The disorder may begin at any age. The average age of onset is in the mid-20s. A major life stressor precedes the first major depressive episode for many people (APA, 2000). However, it is not the stressor alone that causes depression. The person who becomes depressed is probably susceptible to depression after a stressful event. Box 49-1 ■ lists risk factors for the development of depression.

Some people experience only a single episode of depression. Most people continue to have episodes throughout their lives, with a course of exacerbations and remissions similar to other chronic disorders. Yet others experience almost a steady state of depressed mood. An untreated episode of depression can last for years.

Some clients experience psychotic symptoms associated with severe depression, such as hallucinations or delusional thinking. This psychotic depression is more disabling and often requires more intensive treatment than a depressive episode without psychotic features.

BOX 49-1

RISK FACTORS FOR DEPRESSION
- Previous depressive episode
- Female gender
- Family history of depression
- Stressful life events
- Substance abuse or dependency
- Postpartum period
- History of suicide attempt
- Chronic general medical condition

Postpartum Depression

Depression after childbirth can range from the "postpartum blues" to psychotic depression. It is very common for women to experience tearfulness, anxiety, impaired concentration, and lack of energy immediately after delivery. This normal case of "the blues" usually starts within 3 to 4 days after delivery and lasts no longer than 2 weeks. It usually resolves without medical treatment. The client may benefit from reassurance by the nurse that the condition is common and will resolve with time, rest, and family support. The client and her family should be encouraged to notify the care provider if the depressive symptoms do not resolve after 2 weeks.

Postpartum psychosis usually develops within 3 weeks after delivery. It is characterized by depressed mood, lack of concentration, guilt, lack of interest in the baby, rejection of the baby, or unreasonable fear that something bad will happen to the baby. The client may have an abnormal attitude toward bodily functions. The risk of suicide and infanticide should be assessed. Affected women usually improve within 2 to 3 months of treatment. Treatment depends on the individual client's symptoms. Women with a history of psychiatric disorders are more likely to develop postpartum psychosis.

Seasonal Affective Disorder

Seasonal affective disorder (SAD) is depression that is associated with shortened exposure to daylight. It happens in the fall and winter when the days become shorter, and resolves in the spring and summer. The symptoms are sleepiness, fatigue, lethargy, irritability, and increased appetite. It is thought to be a result of abnormal melatonin metabolism. The treatment is light therapy (*phototherapy*). In light therapy the client is exposed to bright light each morning and for a prescribed number of hours each day. Light therapy has been effective for clients with mild to moderate seasonal, nonpsychotic depression (Depression Guideline Panel, 1993).

MANIFESTATIONS

Major Depressive Disorder is a disabling disease that affects occupational and personal functioning. An affected person will have a depressed or low mood every day. Other symptoms include **anhedonia** (inability to feel pleasure); weight changes; difficulty sleeping; **psychomotor retardation;** feelings of worthlessness and guilt; constant fatigue or lack of energy; and recurrent thoughts of death or suicide. Children and adolescents may present with **psychomotor agitation** and irritability. A list of symptoms can never fully describe the human consequences of a disease. See Box 49-2 ■ for statements by people with depression describing their feelings.

BOX 49-2

CLIENTS SPEAK THEIR MINDS ON DEPRESSION

"I feel like I'm in a deep dark hole and can't even try to get out."

"Everything worth living for goes out of focus."

"I've been too tired to chew."

"People can be overstimulating, especially when they are cheerful."

"People want me to do things that I should really want to do. I just can't get the motivation for it, and it makes me feel guilty."

"My soul left and was replaced with lead."

"When I didn't answer your questions, it was because I didn't have the energy to talk."

"In 1980 I heard a bird call in my front yard. I didn't go outside until later, and saw a cat eating a bird. I could have saved that poor bird. When I am depressed, I think about it and feel so guilty."

Depression causes misery and disability (loss of function) for the people who have the disorder. It also causes difficulty in the relationships they have with other people. Depression causes people to lose the ability to enjoy the things in life that used to make them happy. It affects their ability to relate to other people. Depressed people miss work, lose their jobs, or have reduced effectiveness and productivity at work. Affected people often cannot continue their family and work responsibilities. They may not be able to do their activities of daily living. Most of the people who kill themselves are depressed at the time.

Depression has a high cost in human suffering as well as a financial cost to businesses that lose productivity. When a person has depression along with a general medical condition (such as diabetes or a stroke), the medical condition is likely to be worse than it would be if the depression were not present (Depression Guideline Panel, 1993). Depression is associated with increased disability and even reduced life expectancy in hospitalized clients with serious medical conditions (Roach, et al, 1998).

Stigma

Because of the stigma associated with mental illness, people are reluctant to seek help when they have the symptoms of depression. People with depression are less likely to accept treatment, to comply with treatment recommendations, and to continue treatment than are people with general medical conditions without depression.

Evidence of the stigma against people with mental illness includes the following (Depression Guideline Panel, 1993):

■ People are required in some states to report their mental illnesses when they apply for driver's licenses, jobs, security clearances, and other routine purposes, while those with other medical diseases are not (some of this has decreased since passage of the Americans with Disabilities Act).

- Insurance companies reimburse for mental illness treatment at a reduced rate compared with general medical illnesses.
- Physicians sometimes avoid entering the diagnosis of depression into medical records because they want to protect their clients from the stigma.
- At least 80% of all depression treatment takes place outside the mental health setting.
- Only 12% of people are willing to take medication for depression, while 70% would take medication for a headache.

People with depression may fear being stigmatized or discriminated against in hiring, promotion, and other societal opportunities. Until mental illness is seen on an equal plane with general medical disorders attitudinally, economically, socially, and politically, it will be underreported, underdiagnosed, and undertreated (Depression Guideline Panel, 1993).

Because the stigma against mental illness does exist, public education becomes even more important. Nurses and others must educate clients, their families, and communities about the disorder, its outcomes, and treatments. Knowledge can help people comply with treatment, be free from unnecessary guilt, and maintain hope (Depression Guideline Panel, 1993).

Suicide

In 1996 the World Health Organization urged member nations to create suicide prevention strategies. The U.S. surgeon general published a call to action in 1999, which included the risks for suicide (Box 49-3 ■) and the protective factors for suicide (Box 49-4 ■).

More Americans die each year from suicide than from homicide. An average of 85 Americans die from suicide each day. Suicide rates are highest among older adults. There is no recent change in the rates for this population. Most elderly suicide victims are seen by their primary care provider within a few weeks of their suicide and are experiencing a first episode of mild to moderate depression. This demonstrates a lost opportunity for identifying suicide risk and preventing suicide (U.S. Public Health Service, 1999). Clients often benefit from the opportunity to discuss feelings about suicide (see Box 49-5 ■).

The suicide rate in the United States has remained relatively stable during the last three decades. However, the rates for certain groups have increased significantly. The suicide rate among adolescents and young adults has nearly tripled. Among all persons ages 15 to 19, suicides increased 14% from 1980 to 1996. Among African American males

in the same age group, the rate increased 105%. Firearms-related suicides account for almost 100% of this increase in adolescent suicide. In the general population, firearms constitute the most common means of suicide in the United States (59%).

INTERDISCIPLINARY CARE

Effective treatment for depression is available. Once it is accurately identified, depression can almost always be treated successfully with medications, psychotherapy, or a

---

BOX 49-3

RISK FACTORS FOR SUICIDE

- Previous suicide attempt
- Mental disorders, especially mood disorders such as depression and bipolar disorder
- Co-occurring mental and alcohol or substance abuse disorders
- Family history of suicide
- Hopelessness
- Impulsive and/or aggressive tendencies
- Barriers to accessing mental health treatment
- Relationship, social, work, or financial losses
- General medical illness
- Easy access to lethal suicide methods, especially guns
- Unwillingness to seek help because of the stigma attached to mental and substance abuse disorders, and/or suicidal thoughts
- Influence of significant people—family members, celebrities, peers who have died by suicide—both through direct personal contact or inappropriate media representations
- Cultural or religious beliefs—for example, the belief that suicide is a noble resolution of a personal dilemma
- Local epidemics of suicide that have a contagious influence
- Isolation, a feeling of being cut off from other people

Source: U.S. Public Health Service. (1999). *The surgeon general's call to action to prevent suicide.* Washington, DC: Author.

BOX 49-4

PROTECTIVE FACTORS FOR SUICIDE

- Effective and appropriate clinical care for mental, physical, and substance abuse disorders
- Easy access to a variety of clinical interventions and support
- Restricted access to highly lethal methods of suicide
- Family and community support
- Support from ongoing medical and mental health care relationships
- Learned skills in problem solving, conflict resolution, and nonviolent handling of disputes
- Cultural and religious beliefs that discourage suicide and support self-preservation instincts

Source: U.S. Public Health Service. (1999). *The surgeon general's call to action to prevent suicide.* Washington, DC: Author.

TALKING ABOUT SUICIDE

A dangerous myth about suicide is that discussing it with someone who is not contemplating suicide may suggest the idea. In fact, most people with depression, whether they are contemplating suicide or not, benefit from talking about their feelings, especially the frightening ones. For people who are contemplating suicide, discussion of their feelings may be the only opportunity for prevention. Depression makes it hard for people to identify and explain their own feelings. Talking about and clarifying these feelings can help a depressed person gain perspective, interrupt negative thinking, or work on problem solving. Active listening is a powerful tool for nurses to use. Clients often express gratitude for the opportunity to express their feelings about suicide (Rives, 1999).

combination of the two (Depression Guideline Panel, 1993). Clients are individuals and respond to treatment differently, but when a client does not respond to one therapy, there are others to try. The goals of medical treatment for depression are:

- To decrease the depressive symptoms (depressed mood, decreased interest in daily activities, inability to experience pleasure, worthlessness, sleep disturbances, lack of motivation, inability to concentrate)
- To improve client's functional level
- To prevent recurrence.

There are four medical treatments for depression:

1. Medication
2. Psychotherapy
3. Electroconvulsive therapy (ECT)
4. Light therapy (discussed earlier under Seasonal Affective Disorder).

Clients experience the best treatment outcomes when their depression is treated with a combination of medications, cognitive-behavioral or other therapy, client and family education, and a treatment plan that includes significant others in the client's life. Electroconvulsive therapy (ECT) can also be an effective treatment for depression that does not respond to medications.

Medications

Medications have been shown to be effective for all types of depression. However, there is no single medication that works for everyone. There is also no single medication that is better or more effective than the others.

ANTIDEPRESSANT AGENTS. Although antidepressant medications have proven to be very effective, they do have limitations. People with depressive symptoms often wait until

their symptoms are almost intolerable before they seek help. Antidepressants require 2 to 6 weeks to achieve full effect; often several drugs are tried in an attempt to find effective treatment. Some people experience no improvement with antidepressant medications, others experience intolerable side effects. In other cases, side effects may be useful. For example, a client with depression who has trouble sleeping may be given an antidepressant with sedating effects at bedtime.

Depression appears to involve reduced neurotransmitter function in brain synapses and changes in receptors on brain neurons. See Chapter 47 for more information about brain neurotransmitter physiology. Figure 49-2 ■ diagrams brain neurotransmitters and illustrates the action of antidepressant drugs.

Antidepressants are given orally. Most act on two major brain neurotransmitters, serotonin (5HT) and norepinephrine (NE), which regulate mood. New antidepressants act on dopamine also.

The antidepressants may be organized into four groups:

1. Tricyclic antidepressants (TCAs) and related cyclic agents
2. Selective serotonin reuptake inhibitors (SSRIs)
3. Other, *novel* antidepressants
4. Monoamine oxidase inhibitors (MAOIs).

See Table 49-1 ■ for the nursing implications of antidepressant drugs.

The tricyclic antidepressants were the first choice of treatment for depression from the 1950s until the 1990s, when newer drugs with fewer side effects were introduced. TCAs block the reuptake of serotonin and norepinephrine, increasing the amount of these monoamine neurotransmitters in brain synapses (see Figure 49-2). A period of 2 to 4 weeks is required before TCAs cause a significant relief of depression symptoms. As a group,

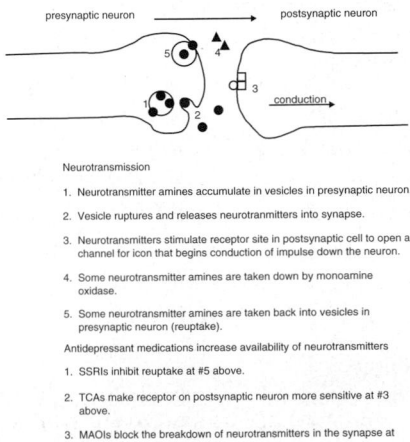

Figure 49-2. ■ Neurotransmission and antidepressant drug action.

TABLE 49-1

Nursing Implications for Pharmacology: Antidepressants

AGENTS/DRUGS	ACTION IN BRAIN SYNAPSES AND PURPOSE	NURSING RESPONSIBILITIES	CLIENT TEACHING
Tricyclic and related agents (TCAs) ■ Amitriptyline (Elavil) ■ Amoxapine (Ascendin) ■ Clomipramine (Anafranil) ■ Desipramine (Norpramin) ■ Doxepin (Sinequan) ■ Imipramine (Tofranil) ■ Maprotiline (Ludiomil) ■ Nortriptyline (Pamelor) ■ Protriptyline (Vivactil) ■ Trimipramine (Surmontil)	Block reuptake of serotonin and norepinephrine. Used to treat depression and as an adjunctive treatment for chronic pain.	Assess for side effects (S/Es): sedation, orthostatic hypotension, weight gain, anticholinergic effects, tachycardia or cardiac dysrhythmias. Assess VS, mental status. Notify physician if client has glaucoma. Assess for suicidal thinking; TCAs can be fatal in overdose. Older adults require lower doses. Use with caution in the elderly, who are more likely to have S/Es.	Efficacy takes 2–4 weeks. Make position changes slowly; sit before standing. Do not drink alcohol (causes potentially fatal CNS depression).
Selective serotonin reuptake inhibitors (SSRIs) ■ Citalopram (Celexa) ■ Escitalopram (Lexapro) ■ Fluoxetine (Prozac) ■ Fluvoxamine (Luvox) ■ Paroxetine (Paxil) ■ Sertraline (Zoloft)	Inhibit reuptake of serotonin. Used to treat depression; panic disorder (paroxetine); obsessive compulsive disorder (fluvoxamine, fluoxetine); premenstrual dysphoric disorder, bulimia nervosa (fluoxetine); anxiety (paroxetine); PTSD (sertraline).	Assess for S/Es: nausea, loose stools, sexual side effects (decreased libido), headache, anxiety or sedation, insomnia, slight anticholinergic symptoms, orthostatic hypotension. Assess VS, mental status. Low potential for harm in overdose. Decrease dose in elderly.	Efficacy takes 2–3 weeks, may take 5 weeks to reach peak effect. Avoid alcohol. Notify physician if taking herbal medicines (especially St. John's wort or tryptophan).
Novel antidepressants ■ Bupropion (Wellbutrin) ■ Duloxetine (Cymbalta) ■ Mirtazapine (Remeron) ■ Nefazodone (Serzone) ■ Reboxetine (Edronax, Vestra) ■ Trazodone (Desyrel) ■ Venlafaxine (Effexor)	Inhibit reuptake of norepinephrine, dopamine, and/or serotonin. Used to treat depression, aid to stop smoking (bupropion), insomnia (trazodone), anxiety disorder (reboxetine).	Assess for S/Es: anxiety, nausea, agitation or sedation, insomnia, weight loss, increased BP (venlafaxine), seizures (bupropion), liver failure (nefazodone), priapism (trazodone). Notify physician of seizure history. Assess VS, mental status.	Same as SSRIs.
Monoamine oxidase inhibitors (MAOIs) ■ Isocarboxazid (Marplan) ■ Phenelzine (Nardil) ■ Tranylcypromine (Parnate)	Block the enzyme monoamine oxidase that breaks down neurotransmitters. Used to treat depression that is not responsive to other agents.	Can cause hypertensive crisis when client eats foods high in tyramine or as a drug interaction with other antidepressants, meperidine, general anesthetics, sympathomimetics, bronchodilators, and methylphenidate. Assess VS, mental status. Can be fatal in overdose.	Takes 2–4 weeks for antidepressant effect. Client must carefully comply with diet restrictions. Call physician for throbbing headache, pounding heart, or stiff neck.
MAO-A inhibitor ■ Moclobemide (Manerix)	Reversible selective inhibitor of MAO-A. Used to treat depression.	Does not have the hypertensive side effect of MAOIs. Do not give with MAOIs or narcotics.	No diet restrictions.

BOX 49-6

ANTICHOLINERGIC SIDE EFFECTS

- Dry mouth
- Orthostatic hypotension
- Increased heart rate
- Constipation
- Urinary hesitancy or retention
- Pupil dilation (mydriasis)
- Blurred near vision
- Dry eyes
- Photophobia

BOX 49-7   FOCUS ON OLDER ADULTS

Antidepressants and the Older Adult

Older adults with depression tend to respond well to antidepressant drugs. There are some special considerations for this group, however:

- The elderly require *lower doses* due to decreased metabolic efficiency.
- Elders are at increased risk for *orthostatic hypotension*, which increases their risks for falls and injury.
- If older adults are *dehydrated*, they are at increased risk for medication side effects.

the tricyclics tend to cause sedation, orthostatic hypotension, weight gain, and anticholinergic side effects (Box 49-6 ■).

clinical ALERT

Clients with narrow-angle glaucoma may develop increased eye pressure due to pupil dilation when they take medications with anticholinergic side effects. The nurse should notify the physician if the client has a history of glaucoma.

Older adults may experience more severe anticholinergic effects, such as agitation, mental confusion, and paralytic ileus, and are at greater risk for developing orthostatic hypotension when taking TCAs. Older adults respond to lower doses than younger adults, due to slower and less efficient metabolism with aging. See Box 49-7 ■ for more information about elderly clients taking antidepressants.

clinical ALERT

The tricyclic antidepressants can be fatal in overdose. Because suicide is a risk of depression, the health care team must consider the possibility of the use of antidepressants by a client as a method of suicide.

If a client has significant suicidal thinking, a history of suicide attempts, or impulse control problems, another class of antidepressant is usually prescribed. The SSRIs are usually the first-choice drugs for the treatment of depression because they have fewer side effects than the other types of antidepressants, and they are just as effective. SSRIs take approximately 2 to 3 weeks to reduce depression symptoms effectively, and up to 5 weeks to reach peak effect.

The SSRIs have less severe anticholinergic, cardiovascular, and sedating side effects than the TCA or MAOI

antidepressants. They do, however, have a higher incidence of GI effects and sexual side effects (decreased libido, ejaculatory and orgasmic dysfunction) than the TCAs. Dosages of SSRIs should be decreased in the elderly.

When SSRIs are combined with antipsychotics, extrapyramidal symptoms are increased. Serotonin syndrome, a potentially fatal result of excess serotonin activity, can result from combining SSRIs with MAOIs, St. John's wort (herbal antidepressant), or tryptophan (an amino acid that is a serotonin precursor). The manifestations of serotonin syndrome include changes in mental status, agitation or restlessness, muscle spasms, hyperreflexia, diaphoresis, shivering, tremor, diarrhea, abdominal cramps, nausea, lack of coordination, and headache (Keltner et al., 2003).

clinical ALERT

A two-week "wash-out" period should occur between the use of SSRIs or TCAs and MAOIs. If the nurse suspects serotonin syndrome, hold the SSRI, and notify the physician immediately.

As their name implies, the group of novel antidepressants is composed of several unique individual drugs that act in a variety of ways to increase the amount of neurotransmitter available at the synapse. Bupropion (Wellbutrin, Zyban) inhibits dopamine and norepinephrine reuptake, and is more likely to cause anxiety, agitation, insomnia, nausea, and weight loss. It also increases the risk of seizures, especially at high doses. This drug is primarily used to help clients stop smoking.

Venlafaxine (Effexor) increases the availability of both serotonin and norepinephrine. It can cause nausea, decreased appetite, and insomnia. It may increase blood pressure, especially at high doses.

Mirtazapine (Remeron) increases norepinephrine and serotonin at the synapse. It causes sedation in approximately 20% of clients. Trazodone (Desyrel) and nefazodone (Serzone) block serotonin reuptake. Trazodone is primarily used to treat insomnia. Nefazodone has a lower risk of anxiety, sexual dysfunction, and insomnia. Rarely, nefazodone has been known to cause life-threatening liver failure (Keltner et al., 2003).

Reboxetine (Vestra) increases norepinephrine availability, and may help clients with severe depression. Its most common side effects are the anticholinergic effects (Keltner et al., 2003).

The **monoamine oxidase inhibitors (MAOIs)** block the enzyme monoamine oxidase that breaks down neurotransmitters in brain synapses, increasing available serotonin and norepinephrine (see Figure 49-2). They take approximately 2 to 4 weeks to have an antidepressant effect. MAOIs are effective antidepressant agents, but they are seldom prescribed because of their serious adverse effects. The MAOIs can cause:

- Hypertensive crisis when combined with foods containing the amino acid tyramine (see Box 49-8 ■)
- Potentially fatal drug interactions with SSRIs, other MAOIs, TCAs, meperidine (Demerol), CNS depressants including general anesthetics, sympathomimetics (such as over-the-counter cold, allergy, and weight loss remedies), methylphenidate (Ritalin), bronchodilators, and some antihypertensives
- Death in overdose.

clinical ALERT

MAOI drugs can cause hypertensive crisis when combined with other drugs, and foods containing tyramine. Symptoms are a throbbing headache, sense of speeding or pounding heart, and stiff neck. If you suspect hypertensive crisis, hold the MAOI, take vital signs, and notify the physician.

A relatively new MAOI, moclobemide (Manerix) is shorter acting and lacks the serious hypertensive side effects of the older MAOIs. It does not require a low tyramine diet, but should not be given with the older MAOIs or with narcotics (Keltner et al., 2003).

Psychotherapy

Psychotherapy is usually used in addition to medication therapy for major depression. Clients tend to have better outcomes when they are treated with a combination of medications and psychotherapy. Some of the psychosocial problems associated with depression (ability to relate to

---

BOX 49-8

FOODS TO AVOID WHEN TAKING MAOIs

The following foods are high in tyramine, and should be avoided by people taking MAOIs:

- Aged cheeses (all cheese is considered aged except cottage, cream, ricotta, and processed cheese slices)
- Foods containing aged cheeses, such as pizza, blue cheese dressing, etc.
- Preserved meats, such as pepperoni, sausage, salami, lunch meats, canned ham, pickled herring, dried fish
- Liver, other organ meats
- Broad fava beans, sauerkraut, and banana peel
- Draft beer (even alcohol-free), red wine
- Soy sauce, yeast or protein extract (concentrated) products
- While caffeine does not contain tyramine, large amounts of caffeine can cause a sympathomimetic effect. Coffee, cola, and tea should be used in moderation.

others, motivation) can be resolved by medications. Psychotherapy may be used in addition to medications to help the client learn to live with a chronic depressive disorder, to manage the specific symptoms, to promote effective coping skills, or for psychosocial rehabilitation. Clients experiencing a mild to moderate depressive episode without psychotic symptoms may benefit from psychotherapy alone.

COGNITIVE THERAPY. Cognitive therapy is the most effective psychotherapeutic approach for depression (Depression Guideline Panel, 1993). For depression, the objective of cognitive therapy is to reduce symptoms by identifying and correcting the client's distorted, negatively biased thinking (Beck & Rush, 1995). According to cognitive theory, depressed people have automatic negative thoughts even in the midst of positive life events. They have negative expectations of their environment, negative perceptions and expectations of self, and negative expectations for the future. Cognitive therapy approaches include identifying the client's erroneous negative thinking, developing new thinking patterns, and trying new behavior.

BEHAVIOR THERAPY. Behavior therapy is often used along with cognitive therapy. The behavioral approach to therapy is based on learning theory. The therapist and client work together to determine what behaviors to change. The client practices new ways to behave that are positive, replacing the old dysfunctional behavior. The principle in behavior therapy is that clients' thinking and feelings will follow their behavior. When people learn to act in a positive, self-confident way, they will feel positive and self-confident. Reinforcement of the client's successes will promote the persistence of positive effective behavior for coping.

INTERPERSONAL PSYCHOTHERAPY. The interpersonal psychotherapy approach involves identifying and resolving the client's interpersonal difficulties. Interpersonal problems are viewed as causal or aggravating factors of depression. According to the interpersonal theorists, the difficulties that lead to depression may be social isolation, prolonged grief, or early development of dysfunctional social behavior. The treatment focus is interpersonal relationships and social functioning.

Exercise

Moderate physical exercise has been shown to relieve mild to moderate depressive symptoms. The effects of exercise on depression may be due to the release of endorphins, which cause a sense of well-being. Even modest exercise has beneficial effects. The difficulty with exercise as a treatment for depression is that depressed people do not feel like exercising. Lack of energy and motivation are part of the disease. Regular exercise is also a very good preventive strategy for depression.

Electroconvulsive Therapy

Electroconvulsive therapy (ECT) is the application of electrical current to the brain, which induces a generalized seizure. The procedure is done while the client is under general anesthesia with muscle relaxation. A series of treatments is usually prescribed. The exact mechanism of action is not known, but ECT does increase circulating levels of brain neurotransmitters, which may be the way it relieves depression.

ECT is used for clients who have intense, prolonged symptoms with marked disability, especially if the client has not responded to adequate trials with medications or if psychotic features are present. ECT has been successful in inducing remission in people with severe psychomotor retardation. It may also be used for clients who cannot take medications, or those at imminent risk of suicide or having dangerous delusions. Clients tend to respond more quickly to ECT than they do to medication therapy (Depression Guideline Panel, 1993; Mendelowitz et al., 2000).

The most common side effects of ECT are transient memory loss and mental confusion. Some clients have had more severe memory loss. Rare mortality associated with the procedure was due to myocardial infarction, stroke, or cardiac rhythm abnormalities. Clients with cardiovascular disease should be treated and carefully assessed for the appropriateness of ECT. Because of the history of misuse of ECT, there is a stigma associated with its use.

Bipolar Disorder

Bipolar Disorder is our other prototype mood disorder. Bipolar refers to the experience of both poles of mood: mania and depression (Figure 49-3 ■). People with Bipolar Disorder, also called *manic-depressive disorder,* have experienced at least one manic episode or one mixed mood episode (with rapid cycling of depression and mania in the same day). Usually these individuals have also experienced one or more major depressive episodes.

The depressive episodes experienced by people with Bipolar Disorder are the same as those described in the preceding section on depression. The American Psychiatric Association (2000) defines manic episodes as follows: A manic

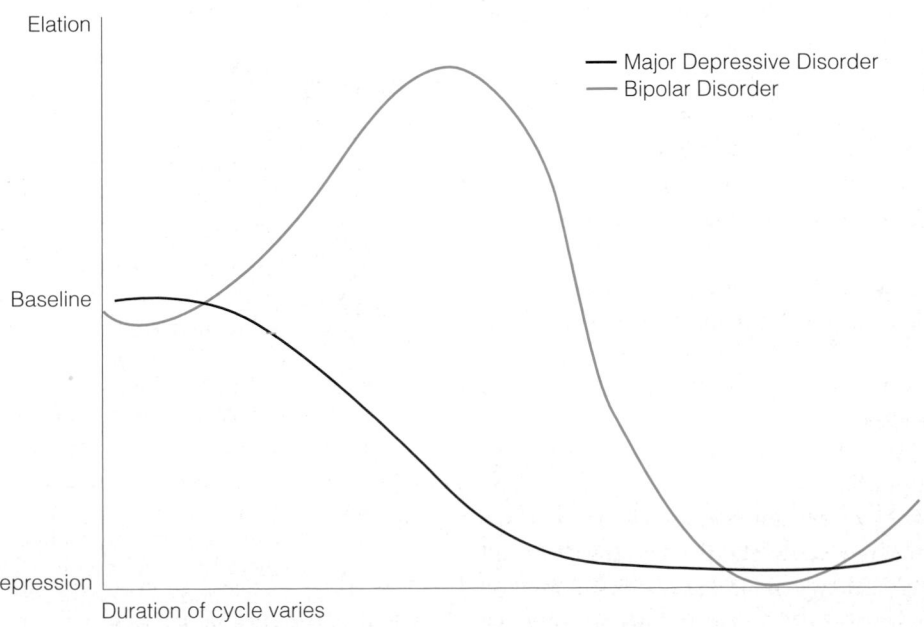

Figure 49-3. ■ Comparison of mood disorders.

episode is a distinct period of abnormal and persistently elevated, expansive, or irritable mood, lasting at least 1 week. The mood disturbance is sufficiently severe to cause marked impairment in occupational functioning or relationships with others, or to necessitate hospitalization to prevent harm to self or others. During the period of mood disturbance, three or more of the following symptoms have persisted to a significant degree (four if the mood is irritable, not elevated):

- Inflated self-esteem or grandiosity
- Decreased need for sleep
- More talkative than usual or pressure to keep talking
- Flight of ideas or subjective feeling that thoughts are racing
- Distractibility
- Increase in goal-oriented activity (either at work, at school, socially, or sexually) or psychomotor agitation
- Excessive involvement in pleasurable activities that have a high potential for painful consequences (engaging in unrestrained buying sprees, sexual indiscretions, or foolish business investments).

PATHOPHYSIOLOGY

Like Major Depressive Disorder, Bipolar I Disorder has a tendency to recur in families. There is evidence of a genetic etiology, but not of a single gene inheritance. First-degree biologic relatives of a person with bipolar disorder have a 4% to 24% chance of having the disease, the same recurrence rate as depression. Any given manic episode is likely to follow a stressor. Disordered sleep (such as experienced when traveling across time zones or working the night shift) may be a trigger (APA, 2000).

The brain neurotransmitters norepinephrine and dopamine are implicated in the cause of manic episodes. The same monoamine neurotransmitters whose decreased activity is implicated in depression are increased in mania. Hormones also interact with neurotransmitters in mood disorders. Hypothyroidism is correlated with depression and with rapid cycling of mood between depression and mania.

Mania is a biologic condition. Psychosocial factors are more important in the timing of manic episodes than in their cause.

MANIFESTATIONS

The mood a client feels while in a manic episode may be described as elated, euphoric, high, or unusually good. The mood is characterized by constant and indiscriminate energy and enthusiasm. Frequently the person alternates between elation and irritability. An affected person may play basketball enthusiastically for 24 hours, becoming angry when someone tries to take the ball. Clients may go on an extended shopping spree, buying gifts for everyone on credit, write an entire book, or gamble away an entire paycheck. The flurry of activity seems productive to the client, but can be really disorganized and unproductive.

Grandiose delusions are common. The client may believe that he is a famous musician or a successful novelist, without having any skill at music or writing. The client may feel qualified to give advice on any subject, such as how to conduct brain surgery or send a rocket to Mars. Clients may believe that they are superheroes.

People in mania have a decreased need for sleep. They may awaken several hours earlier than usual, feeling alert and energetic. When mania is severe, the affected person may go for days with no sleep and not feel tired. They may hold several conversations at the same time, or start many projects without finishing any (APA, 2000).

Manic speech is rapid and **pressured speech,** which means that it is so fast and determined that it is difficult to interrupt. The person's expressions may be dramatic, or may be related to sounds more than words, such as in clang association. The following is an example of *clang association:* "I went to the store, tell me more, open the door, I like to eat cake, may I have a rake?" If irritability is present, the person may make long speeches about angry subjects, such as why anyone would ever want to do nursing care plans. Rapid speech reflects rapid thinking. The person's thinking may be going so fast that the thoughts are disorganized and incoherent. Box 49-9 ■ describes Bipolar Disorder in the words of people who experience it.

The affected person is likely to be easily distractible. **Distractibility** is evidenced by an inability to screen out excess or irrelevant sensory stimuli. The person may not be able to distinguish which thoughts are pertinent to the

---

BOX 49-9

CLIENTS SPEAK THEIR MINDS ON BIPOLAR DISORDER

"Believe me, I have tried every drug I can find. Nothing feels so good as the natural high I get. I am smarter, stronger, quicker, happier, more alive, everything. When I get depressed, I think nothing can feel as bad as that. It is not like being alive. My life is a roller coaster, only more so."

"When Mom first starts to cycle up, she is great. She is so lively and excited, but it scares me. Once she took us to Disneyland, but she fought with some people there and didn't have enough money to get us home. It was so scary."

"Yes, I am feeling better. I am the CEO of Sears. Did you know that I put grocery departments in Sears? You and your family can join all the patients here for free groceries. I will also have free medications for everybody who needs them. Just go to any Sears and mention my name. They'll give you some new clothes for work."

situation and which are not. Manic clients may be distracted from a conversation by someone's clothing, colors, sounds, or even furnishings in the room (APA, 2000).

Unwarranted optimism, grandiosity, and poor judgment characterize their behaviors. Clients may spend an entire paycheck on lottery tickets, gamble, drive recklessly, and engage in unsafe sexual behavior, ignoring possible painful consequences. Affected people may spend money they do not have, do illegal things that have serious penalties, or hurt themselves or others in the moment without foreseeing future consequences (APA, 2000).

What may look like an exciting experience at the beginning can be devastating to affected people and their families. Manic episodes impair affected individuals' ability to function and may threaten their lives. Excess energy expenditure without adequate rest can lead to exhaustion. Often during a manic episode, people will be too busy to eat, thus decreasing their energy supply even more. Figure 49-4 ■ shows the characteristics of a manic episode.

People in a manic episode frequently lack insight about their illness and its effects on themselves and others. They often resist treatment. Sometimes involuntary hospitalization is necessary to protect clients from their own behavior. Involuntary hospitalization is indicated when a person is dangerous to self or others.

Course of the Disorder

The average age of onset of a first manic episode is in the early 20s. It affects women and men equally. More than 90% of all individuals who have one manic episode will go on to have more. The exact pattern of recurrence is individual, but without treatment the average rate of manic episodes is four in 10 years. A few individuals have more rapid cycling (four or more episodes per year).

Some children show a history of behavior problems before their first actual manic episode. Like depressive episodes, manic episodes tend to occur following psychosocial stressors. The episodes usually begin suddenly and last from a few weeks to several months. Manic episodes are briefer and end more abruptly than depressive episodes. Fifty to 70% of the time, a major depressive episode will come immediately before or after a manic episode. When a manic episode is accompanied by psychosis (hallucinations and delusions) it is more serious and more likely to lead to aggression or suicide (APA, 2000).

Concurrent Disorders

Disorders of substance use occur commonly with bipolar disorder. People who have substance use disorders in addition to bipolar disorder tend to experience more rapid cycling between mania and depression and have more *dysphoric* (unpleasant, unhappy) feelings in the manic phase (Sonne & Brady, 1999).

INTERDISCIPLINARY CARE

In the acute phase of a manic episode, the treatment priorities are ensuring client safety and treating the mood disorder. Medication continues to be the mainstay of treatment for Bipolar Disorder.

The desired treatment outcomes for clients with Bipolar Disorder are to:

- Eliminate the symptoms of the mood episode (either depression or mania)
- Stabilize the mood to prevent cycling between depression and mania
- Improve the client's self-care ability, function, and quality of life.

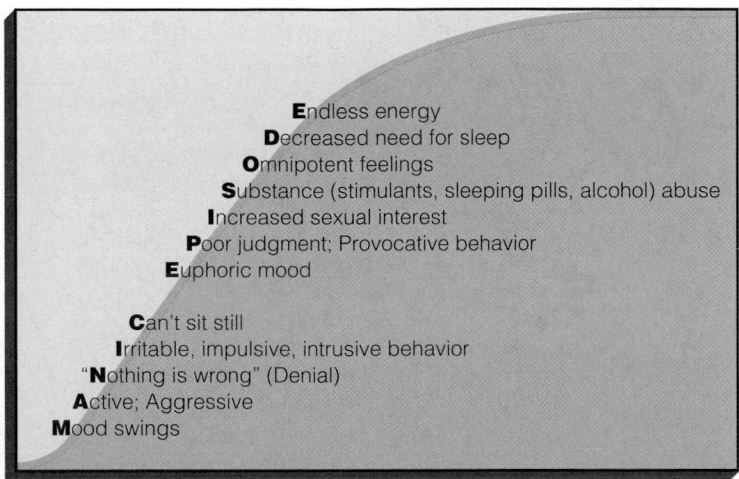

Figure 49-4. ■ Characteristics of a manic episode.

Medications

The symptoms of bipolar depression are the same as those in clients who have depression alone (unipolar depression). The depression associated with Bipolar Disorder does not respond well to antidepressant medications alone. Antidepressants given with either lithium or divalproex (an anticonvulsant) have been found to be effective in stabilizing mood (Bowden, 2003).

The classes of drugs used to treat manic episodes are mood stabilizers (antimanic agents), anticonvulsants (that act as mood stabilizers), benzodiazepines (to decrease anxiety and agitation while the other drugs are starting to work), and antipsychotics (if the client has psychotic symptoms). This chapter focuses on the mood-stabilizing, or antimanic, agents. In addition to the mood stabilizer, an antidepressant is often prescribed, often in lower doses than for people who have depression alone. The dose is kept low because antidepressant medications can trigger a manic episode in a person with bipolar disorder.

LITHIUM. Lithium, a naturally occurring element, was the first mood-stabilizing drug. It is a first-line treatment for acute mania due to bipolar disorder and for long-term prevention of recurrent episodes (Table 49-2 ■). Target symptoms of mania include irritability, euphoria, pressured speech, flight of ideas, motor hyperactivity, aggressive behavior, grandiosity, delusions, impulsiveness, and hallucinations.

Lithium's mechanism of action is not fully understood. It is thought to affect many neurotransmitter functions. It probably corrects an ion exchange abnormality in the neuron and normalizes neurotransmitter functions.

Before a client starts on lithium therapy, a full history and physical exam should be done, including a pregnancy

---

TABLE 49-2

Nursing Implications for Pharmacology: Mood Stabilizers

AGENTS/DRUGS	PURPOSE	NURSING RESPONSIBILITIES	CLIENT TEACHING
Lithium ■ Lithium carbonate ■ Eskalith ■ Eskalith CR ■ Lithonate ■ Lithotabs	To stabilize mood in Bipolar Disorder; to prevent and treat manic episodes.	Use with caution in elderly, thyroid disease, diabetes. Assess for toxicity. Therapeutic range is 0.5–1.5 mEq/L. Draw levels before A.M. dose. Check lithium (Li) levels weekly initially, then q2 mo. Monitor weight, stable Na intake, fluid and electrolyte balance, mental status. Pregnancy category D.	Dehydration, NSAIDs increase risk of toxicity. High Na intake increases Li excretion; maintain stable (not reduced) Na intake, replace losses due to sweating. Blood tests for Li levels necessary throughout treatment. Know symptoms of toxicity. Contraceptive teaching.
Anticonvulsant mood stabilizers: ■ Valproic acid (Depakene) ■ Sodium valproate (Depakon) ■ Divalproex sodium (Depakote) ■ Carbamazepine (Tegretol) ■ Lamotrigine (Lamictal)	To prevent and treat manic episodes. Carbamazepine and lamotrigine are used when valproate is not effective.	Assess for side effects (S/Es): weight gain, tremors, GI upset, transient hair loss, and thrombocytopenia (loss of blood clotting cells). Monitor liver function tests, mental status. Valproate: Mix liquid form with juice to reduce mouth irritation; carbonated beverages increase irritation. Carbamazepine: bone marrow suppression. Lamotrigine: Stevens–Johnson syndrome, d/c if rash develops, esp. in children. Pregnancy category: valproate D, others C.	Avoid alcohol and other CNS depressants. Regular blood tests are necessary to monitor blood cells and liver function. Contraceptive teaching.

test. Lithium is excreted by the kidneys and can have toxic effects on renal function. It inhibits several steps in thyroid hormone synthesis and metabolism, so thyroid function should be assessed. Lithium has a narrow therapeutic index, and toxicity is close to therapeutic blood levels.

In acute mania, lithium is effective in 1 to 2 weeks. It may take up to 4 weeks or longer for the symptoms to be fully relieved. A benzodiazepine or other agent may be needed to help the client during acute mania before the lithium is fully effective.

When the client is on a maintenance dose of lithium, the frequency and severity of both manic and depressive episodes are decreased. For some people lithium offers full symptom relief. For many it is only partially effective. The combination of lithium and one of the anticonvulsants may improve mood stability. Some people are not able to tolerate the side effects of lithium, which can be significant. See Box 49-10 ■ for a list of lithium side effects and toxic effects.

Lithium is a salt. Because of this, the sodium and fluid balances of the body affect lithium levels. The relationship between sodium and lithium is *inverse*. (As the client's serum sodium decreases, lithium level increases. When the sodium increases, lithium levels decrease.) Regular serum lithium levels are required to monitor each individual's status.

Client Teaching. Part of client education about lithium therapy is how to maintain consistent lithium and sodium levels. For example, if a person taking lithium played basketball for hours, losing sodium through perspiration, he would be at risk for lithium toxicity unless he replaced the lost sodium, maybe with a sports drink or a salty snack. He would also need to replace the water lost during exercise by drinking at intervals during the basketball game. The management of lithium therapy is difficult and can be a challenge for clients.

Treatment Compliance. Compliance with lithium therapy is an important issue. Clients sometimes find the side effects of the drug to be intolerable. There is a relatively high dropout rate for people on lithium therapy. Tolerability of treatment is especially important in Bipolar Disorder because people with Bipolar Disorder expect to live full occupational and social lives.

Trials of several drug combinations may be required before the most effective and agreeable treatment plan for an individual is found. It is no longer necessary for the treatment team to encourage a client to endure intolerable discomfort in exchange for prevention of mania (Bowden, 2003).

For the client to have the best possible outcomes, the nurse must ensure that the client understands and participates in the treatment plan. Lifestyle changes are necessary to maintain lithium/fluid and electrolyte balance and to prevent toxicity. People taking lithium require ongoing psychotherapeutic support.

ANTICONVULSANT MOOD STABILIZERS. Some anticonvulsants have proven to be clinically effective both in treating the symptoms of mania and in preventing recurrence of episodes. The anticonvulsant valproate is endorsed as a first-line drug for mood stabilizing in Bipolar Disorder (Mellman et al., 2001).

The antimanic effect of valproate is probably due to the following actions: decreased nerve cell irritability (less likely to conduct impulses), increase in GABA, increase in postsynaptic membrane response to GABA, and reduced calcium influx into nerve cells (Keltner et al., 2003).

The valproate agents valproic acid (Depakene), sodium valproate (Depakon), and divalproex sodium (Depakote) are especially effective for clients with rapidly cycling Bipolar Disorder, and for mania caused by a general medical condition. They act quickly and tend to be well tolerated without effects on cognition. Their side effects include transient hair loss, weight gain, tremors, GI upset, and thrombocytopenia (loss of blood clotting cells) with high doses (Keltner et al., 2003).

BOX 49-10

LITHIUM SIDE EFFECTS AND TOXICITY

Common Side Effects

- Fine hand tremors
- Polyuria
- Weight gain
- GI discomfort, mild nausea
- Subjective feeling of mental dullness
- Thyroid dysfunction

Early Toxicity (lithium level is > 2.0 mEq/L)

- Nausea/vomiting
- Diarrhea
- Coarse hand tremor
- Slurred speech
- Muscle weakness

Severe Toxicity (lithium level is > 2.5 mEq/L)

- Mental confusion
- Muscle irritability and decreased coordination
- Fever
- Seizures
- Decreased urine output
- Cardiac dysrhythmias (irregular pulse)
- Severe hypotension
- Coma
- Death

Carbamazepine (Tegretol) is another anticonvulsant proven effective for the treatment of Bipolar Disorder. Carbamazepine is used for clients who do not respond to lithium or valproate. It is thought to stabilize mood by inhibiting the **kindling process.** (Kindling is the process of small seizure activity that builds up into a major seizure or manic episode, like small pieces of wood kindle a larger fire.) Like the valproates, carbamazepine increases the amount of stimulus needed to cause seizures or mania. Carbamazepine can cause bone marrow suppression with decrease in red and white blood cell formation. Clients need to have regular blood cell counts taken while taking this drug.

Lamotrigine (Lamictal) is also used as a mood stabilizer. It acts by stabilizing nerve cell membranes and inhibiting neurotransmitter release. Lamotrigine can cause serious skin reactions, especially in children less than 16 years of age.

Psychotherapy

While bipolar disorder has a largely physiologic etiology, psychosocial therapy is still valuable. Living with bipolar disorder is challenging. At some point in a manic episode, the client may be feeling so wonderful that taking medications to stop this seems absurd. They may lack the insight to connect untreated mania with its many negative outcomes. Compliance with medication therapy is challenging, and often a problem for these clients.

Psychotherapy, in any of the same styles described under depression, can be a valuable tool to help clients with Bipolar Disorder to discuss and organize their feelings about having a chronic mental illness, consider the dilemmas of treatment, and work on development of insight into the real consequences of untreated Bipolar Disorder.

Group Therapy

When the acute phase of mania or depression has passed, client outcomes shift to coping with the disorder over the long term. Group therapy can be very valuable toward the goal of living with a chronic mental illness (or any chronic illness). The therapy or support group is composed of people who experience the same chronic mental illness. There may or may not be a mental health professional group facilitator. Local affiliates of the National Alliance for the Mentally Ill have support groups for clients and their families.

NURSING CARE

ASSESSING

Mood is reflected in the client's behavior and speech. When a client has a mood disorder, a mental status assessment on admission provides baseline information. (See Chapter 47 ⊙⊙ for more information on mental status assessment.) Over time, briefer assessments can be made of pertinent parts of mental status, and compared to the original assessment to document client progress.

Most cases of depression are not diagnosed or treated. Nurses in every area of specialty practice work with depressed people. It makes sense for nurses to routinely do screening assessments for depression. The Geriatric Depression Scale (Box 49-11 ■) is used for the elderly. The Beck Depression Inventory, short form (Box 49-12 ■) can be used to identify adults who are likely to be depressed. When the

BOX 49-11	ASSESSMENT

Geriatric Depression Scale (Short Form)

1. Are you basically satisfied with your life?	Yes/**No**
2. Have you dropped many of your activities and interests?	**Yes**/No
3. Do you feel that your life is empty?	**Yes**/No
4. Do you often get bored?	**Yes**/No
5. Are you in good spirits most of the time?	Yes/**No**
6. Are you afraid that something bad is going to happen to you?	**Yes**/No
7. Do you feel happy most of the time?	Yes/**No**
8. Do you often feel helpless?	**Yes**/No
9. Do you prefer to stay at home, rather than going out and doing new things?	**Yes**/No
10. Do you feel you have more problems with memory than most?	**Yes**/No
11. Do you think it is wonderful to be alive?	Yes/**No**
12. Do you feel pretty worthless the way you are now?	**Yes**/No
13. Do you feel full of energy?	Yes/**No**
14. Do you feel that your situation is hopeless?	**Yes**/No
15. Do you feel that most people are better off than you are?	**Yes**/No

Scoring: Bold responses indicate depression. A score of 5 or more indicates depression.

Source: Sheikh, J. I., & Yesavage, J. A. (1986). Geriatric depression scale: Recent evidence and development of a shorter form. *Clinical Gerontologist, 5,* 165–172.

BOX 49-12 | **ASSESSMENT**

Beck Depression Inventory, Short Form

Instructions: This is a questionnaire. On the questionnaire are groups of statements. Please read the entire group of statements in each category. Then pick out one statement in that group that best describes the way you feel today, that is, *right now*! Circle the number beside the statement you have chosen. If several statements in the group seem to apply equally well, circle each one.

Be sure to read all the statements in each group before making your choice.

A. (Sadness)
3 I am so sad or unhappy that I can't stand it.
2 I am blue or sad all the time and I can't snap out of it.
1 I feel sad or blue.
0 I do not feel sad.

B. (Pessimism)
3 I feel that the future is hopeless and that things cannot improve.
2 I feel I have nothing to look forward to.
1 I feel discouraged about the future.
0 I am not particularly pessimistic or discouraged about the future.

C. (Sense of failure)
3 I feel I am a complete failure as a person (parent, husband, wife).
2 As I look back on my life, all I can see is a lot of failures.
1 I feel I have failed more than the average person.
0 I do not feel like a failure.

D. (Dissatisfaction)
3 I am dissatisfied with everything.
2 I do not get satisfaction out of anything anymore.
1 I do not enjoy things the way I used to.
0 I am not particularly dissatisfied.

E. (Guilt)
3 I feel as though I am very bad or worthless.
2 I feel quite guilty.
1 I feel bad or unworthy a good part of the time.
0 I don't feel disappointed in myself.

F. (Self-dislike)
3 I hate myself.
2 I am disgusted with myself.
1 I am disappointed in myself.
0 I don't feel disappointed in myself.

G. (Self-harm)
3 I would kill myself if I had the chance.
2 I have definite plans about committing suicide.
1 I feel I would be better off dead.
0 I don't have any thought of harming myself.

H. (Social Withdrawal)
3 I have lost all of my interest in other people and don't care about them at all.
2 I have lost most of my interest in other people and have little feeling for them.
1 I am less interested in other people than I used to be.
0 I have not lost interest in other people.

I. (Indecisiveness)
3 I can't make any decisions at all anymore.
2 I have great difficulty in making decisions.
1 I try to put off making decisions.
0 I make decisions about as well as ever.

J. (Self-image change)
3 I feel that I am ugly or repulsive-looking.
2 I feel that there are permanent changes in my appearance and they make me look unattractive.
1 I am worried that I am looking old or unattractive.
0 I do not feel that I look any worse than I used to.

K. (Work difficulty)
3 I can't do any work at all.
2 I have to push myself very hard to do anything.
1 It takes extra effort to get started at doing something.
0 I can work about as well as before.

L. (Fatigability)
3 I get too tired to do anything.
2 I get tired from doing anything.
1 I get tired more easily than I used to.
0 I don't get any more tired than usual.

M. (Anorexia)
3 I have no appetite at all anymore.
2 My appetite is much worse now.
1 My appetite is not as good as it used to be.
0 My appetite is no worse than usual.

Scoring: 0–4 = None or mild depression.   8–15 = Moderate depression.
            5–7 = Mild depression.   16+ Severe depression.

Source: From Beck, A.T., Ward, C.H., Mendelson, M. et al. (1961). An inventory for measuring depression. *Arch Gen Psychiatr, 4,* 561–571. Copyright 1961. American Medical Association.

BOX 49-13

IS DEPRESSION THE SAME EVERYWHERE?
The answer to the question "Is depression the same everywhere?" is yes and no. People from all over the world suffer from depression. According to the World Health Organization, there is a worldwide epidemic of it. However, the signs and symptoms of depression vary from one culture and even subculture to another. Nurses must be aware of this in order to make accurate assessments and interpretations of client symptoms. African-Americans, Asian-Americans, and Latinos tend to experience more physical symptoms, such as headache, abdominal pain, and body aches than European-American clients do. When clients from these cultures have symptoms that are not explained by medical tests, depression should be considered. European-Americans are more likely to describe psychological symptoms, such as sadness and guilt feelings.

nurse identifies that a client is at risk for depression, the physician is notified. The client's cultural background is another important aspect of assessment. See Box 49-13 ■ for the relationship between culture and symptoms of depression.

Suicide Risk

Only when the nurse is aware of a client's suicidal thinking, or **suicidal ideation,** can the nurse intervene to help the client. The nurse can assess the dangerousness of the client's suicidal thoughts. Fleeting thoughts such as "I feel so bad, I wish I were dead" are not as dangerous as "I have a gun at home, and as soon as I am discharged I plan to shoot myself."

Imagine yourself asking a client: "Do you ever think about hurting yourself or other people?" This is a hard question. It is socially inappropriate. It is just not polite to talk about suicide, or to suggest that a person may be thinking about it. However, the nurse–client relationship is not social. In this professional relationship it is the nurse's goal to assess the client's safety, and to intervene to protect the client or others as necessary. It is difficult to ask people if they feel like hurting themselves or others, but if nurses do not ask, how will they provide appropriate care for the client?

In the general medical setting, every elderly client with a chronic illness, and every client who has the risk factors for suicide listed in Box 49-3 should be asked: "Do you feel like hurting yourself?" Add ". . . or other people" if there is a question of delusional or psychotic thinking.

The nurse can assess suicidal ideation (thinking) as follows:

1. Start with an assessment of whether the person has suicidal ideation: "Are you thinking about hurting yourself?" or "Do you think about killing yourself?"
2. If clients have suicidal ideation, determine if they have organized their thoughts about it enough to have a plan: "Do you have a plan?"

3. Assess lethality of the plan: "What is your plan?" or "How would you do it?" (more serious if planned means is firearm or hanging)
4. Assess if the client has access to the planned means of suicide: "Do you have access to a gun? . . . drugs? (the means in the client's plan)
5. **Inform the treatment team.** Failure to report suicidal ideation constitutes breach of the nurse's legal duty to protect the client.

Mental Status

Mood. One way to monitor a client's mood over time is to use a mood scale. Ask the client, "Please rate your mood on a scale of one to ten, where one is the lowest and ten is the best possible mood." Although the numbers themselves do not have real measurement value, the client's perception of how she or he feels may be quantified in this way. The nurse can compare the numbers over time to see if the client is feeling better or worse. The mood assessment is done at least once per shift and documented in the nurses' notes.

Appearance and Affect. Other aspects of mental status that are pertinent to a person with a mood disorder are appearance, *affect* (nonverbal expression of mood), behavior, motor activity, and thought processes. The appearance of a person with depression may be disheveled, if the client does not have the energy to bathe and change clothes. Mania may be expressed with flashy, bright clothing and outrageous makeup and jewelry.

Normal affect is called "broad," meaning that the client can express a broad range of emotions from happiness to sadness. A person with depression cannot usually express the full range of emotions. Depression limits emotions (affect) to sadness. This finding is expressed as "blunted affect." Emotions in mania may be restricted to excitement, elation, rage, or irritability.

Psychomotor Activity. Psychomotor activity would be slow (psychomotor retardation) in depression and agitated in mania. The depressed client may lie in bed all day or sit moving very little. Manic clients may be so active that they are in danger of exhaustion.

Thought Processes. Clients' thought processes also demonstrate how they are affected by mood disorders, and how they are responding to treatment. Everyone has occasional thought blocking, in which it is difficult to think of a word that you intended to say. However, thought blocking is very common and more severe in . . . uh . . . wait a minute . . . uh . . . umm . . . depression.

Flight of ideas, in which thoughts are moving so fast that the client's speech jumps from one subject to another frequently, is common in mania. Grandiosity is also common in mania. "I am the world's most famous author, and I will be glad to write my next book about you, if you will give me a candy bar" is a grandiose statement that would more likely be used by a person in mania than one in depression.

Thought processes might include psychotic features in either severe depression or severe mania. The content in depressive delusions or hallucinations would likely be frightening, persecutory, or very negative ("My boss hates me and wants to kill me"). In mania, delusions or hallucinations would be expansive and fantastic, such as "I will fly on over to my department store to pick up a new TV. No need for a plane."

DIAGNOSING, PLANNING, AND IMPLEMENTING

Priorities in Nursing Care. Common nursing diagnoses for clients with either depressive disorder or bipolar disorder include *Risk for Violence:* To self with Major Depressive Disorder, to self or others with Bipolar Disorder, *Impaired Social Interaction, Imbalanced Nutrition.* Hopelessness, Powerlessness, Chronic Low Self-Esteem, and Self-Care Deficit are common among people with depression. Disturbed Thought Processes is a common nursing diagnosis for clients with Bipolar Disorder. The same interventions listed in Chapter 48 ⬭ for the client experiencing Disturbed Thought Processes R/T psychosis would apply.

The desired outcomes for clients with psychiatric disorders fall into four categories: thinking (cognition), feeling (mood), physiology, and behavior (acting, or coping) (Figure 49-5 ■). Nursing care must be personalized for each individual client. The suggested interventions in this chapter are based on common concerns for clients with mood disorders. If a client has different concerns, creativity will be needed. Creativity is one of the cornerstones of nursing.

Risk for Violence (Self-Directed)

- Assess mental status, including suicidal ideation. *Mental status assessment includes information about client's mood and whether client has psychosis. (Psychosis increases suicide risk due to abnormal reality testing.)*
- If client does have suicidal ideation, assess for plan and whether client has the means to complete the plan. *It is more dangerous if client has a specific lethal plan and the means to complete it.*
- Share information about suicidal thinking with the treatment team. *Team must be involved to ensure client safety.*
- Remove potentially dangerous items from client's area (knives, lighters, razors, belts, glass, etc.). *Removing*

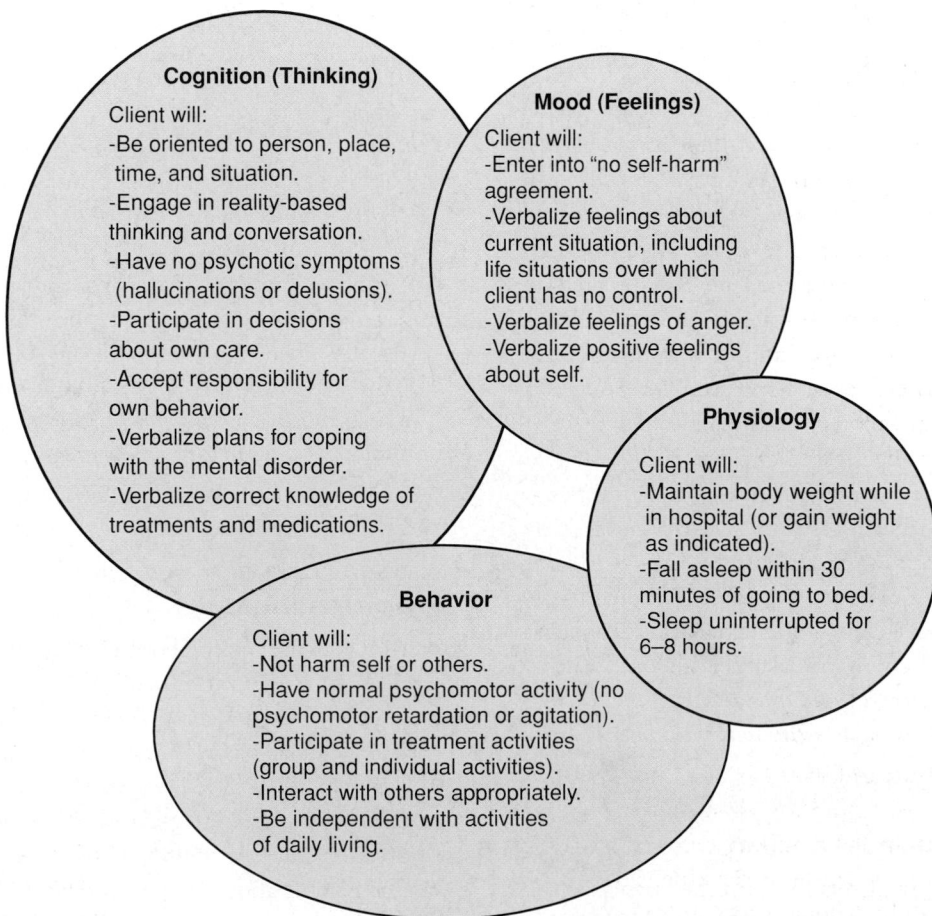

Figure 49-5. ■ Desired outcomes for clients with mood disorders.

dangerous items promotes safety by decreasing client's opportunity for impulsive self-harm. People experiencing mania are not likely to harm themselves intentionally, but have impaired judgment, so the nurse must anticipate the risks and must control the environment to promote safety.

- Assess client safety frequently during the night. *Client may feel unsupervised at night.*

- Remain with a client who is having feelings about harming self. *The nurse's presence shows regard for the client's safety and worth. The nurse can prevent harmful behavior. A client at high risk for suicidal behavior requires close observation.*

- Create a "no self-harm" contract with the client. *Although an agreement by the client not to harm self is not really binding, it suggests that the client is in control and responsible for her or his behavior. The contract emphasizes the worth of the client and the concern by the staff for her or his safety.*

Risk for Violence (Directed at Others)

- Remain calm. *Emotions are contagious. If the nurse is calm, it is easier for clients to remain in control of their behavior.*

- Provide low stimulation environment for a manic client. *People experiencing mania have a reduced ability to filter and process stimuli. The more sensory stimuli, the more difficult it is for the client to determine what is real, and to maintain control over behavior.*

- Make expectations for client behavior clear to client as soon as possible. Staff must be consistent in expectations of client. *Having clear, structured expectations can make it easier for client to comply with behavior expectations. Consistency among staff is important to avoid confusion and client manipulation of staff to change expectations.*

- Observe client closely and respond quickly to increasing agitation. Start with least restrictive approach: redirection, prn medication, isolation, and finally restraint as a last resort. *Early intervention may prevent violent behavior and injury to client and others.*

- Minimize group activities for client in mania. *Client in mania becomes easily overstimulated. May have difficulty responding appropriately with multiple people. One-to-one interactions are less stimulating and easier for client to manage.*

- Provide appropriate opportunities for physical activity. Walking is the ideal activity. Client may prefer another activity, such as ping-pong or basketball. *Client may feel compelled to be physically active and would thus find confinement very stressful. Walking is active without being exhausting if prolonged.*

Impaired Social Interaction

- Establish a trusting relationship with the client. *The nurse–client relationship is the foundation for nursing care and*

for understanding the client's needs. When the client trusts the nurse, she or he has an opportunity to have a sense of emotional security. A client who feels secure will be more likely to interact positively with others. The nurse provides a role model for how to communicate and behave in an individual relationship.

- Spend some time each shift interacting with the client individually. *The client may not be able to initiate interactions. The nurse is a role model for appropriate behavior. The nurse's choice to visit with the client is validating to the client. Long interactions may be stressful.*

- Provide structured activities to allow the client with depression to interact with others. Encourage client to participate (arts and crafts groups, listening to music in a group, walking or exercising in a group, discussing medications, reminiscing groups, etc.). *The depressed client is more likely to be able to interact with others if the situation is structured, because the demands on the individual are less. Positive interactions with others reinforce socializing.*

Imbalanced Nutrition

- If client is lethargic and overweight, offer lighter foods, snacks, and liquids. Discuss the value of regular exercise in improving one's spirits. Encourage the client to set a plan of regular, light exercise. *Client may be unable to focus on weight loss until depression is resolved, and may be too depressed to think of exercising. It is better to have a regular time for exercise than to try to get up and exercise when the depression is at its worst. Light, brief efforts are more possible to achieve and thus can improve self-esteem.*

- The client may feel too depressed to eat. *Offer fluids frequently and small amounts of nutritious foods as the client can tolerate them.*

- If client is highly active, pacing, or too busy to eat, provide nutritious "finger foods" (sandwiches, fruit, etc.) that client can eat while walking. Offer food and fluids frequently. *Client has high energy needs while in a manic phase, and may not be able to meet nutritional needs. Client may be able to eat foods that can be held in the hands when she or he is unable to sit down for a meal. Client is also at risk for dehydration from excessive activity, especially in hot weather.*

Hopelessness

- Allow client to talk about feelings and life events. Use therapeutic communication techniques to help client see that she or he has survived difficulties in the past and that she or he has strengths. *The knowledge that one has overcome obstacles before suggests that it is possible to do so again. When client recognizes own strengths, it provides a foundation for hope that the current trouble can be overcome.*

- Teach client about the disorder and medications and that the treatment team will not give up hope until the

BOX 49-14	NURSING CARE CHECKLIST

Talking with a Client Who Feels Hopeless

☑ Use open-ended questions, or broad opening statements when asking the client to express feelings.

Nurse: "Tell me about how you are feeling."

Client: "I feel bad."

☑ Clarify the client's message.

Nurse: "Can you give me some examples of how you feel bad?"

Client: "I am a failure, I lost my job, I hate myself, and I am so tired of it all."

Nurse: "Do you mean that you are tired of living?"

Client: "Yes."

☑ Make the implied message explicit. This is very important to do, even if it feels awkward.

Nurse: "Charlie, do you mean that you are thinking about killing yourself?"

Client: "Well, yes. I think about it a lot."

☑ Clarify and gather data for assessment.

Nurse: "You have a plan?"

Client: "I have a gun at home"

☑ Validate the importance of the client's feelings, give information about next steps, and assess the client's current safety.

Nurse: "Charlie, this is important. I will be talking with Dr. Rodgers and the other team members about your thoughts. We will work on a plan to help you. Are you thinking about hurting yourself here in the hospital?"

Client: "No."

☑ Obtain a "no self-harm" contract (an agreement with the client to disclose suicidal feelings before taking action to hurt self).

Nurse: "We want you to be safe. Will you promise me that if you do think you want to hurt yourself while you are here, you will not hurt yourself, but tell me or anyone on the staff, so we can help you?"

Client: "OK, I promise. I wish I wanted to live."

☑ Validate the client's importance, reassure the client that treatment can help, offer hope)

Nurse: "You are in the hospital so we can help you through times like this. There are effective treatments for depression, and we will not give up until you feel better. OK?"

Client: "OK."

client feels better. *Knowledge that the client is likely to have a positive response to treatment is hopeful. It may be beneficial to point out that depression has episodes and that this one will eventually resolve. Many clients worry that the staff will abandon them if they do not respond to treatment.*

- See Box 49-14 ■ for ideas about using therapeutic communication as an intervention for a client who feels hopeless.

EVALUATING

In the evaluation phase, the nurse looks back at the desired outcomes to decide if they were achieved. When clients have mood disorders, the nurse evaluates their cognition, mood, behavior, and physical findings related to these disorders (see Figure 49-5).

Documenting. Document changes in clients' mental status. These changes will form a record of clients' response to treatment.

CONTINUING CARE

Clients with mood disorders face many challenges related to their disorder and its treatment. Education is an important role for the nurse. The nurse should reinforce client teaching about medications, side effects, and the interaction between medication and diet or activities. Most clients will need ongoing psychotherapeutic support. Information about support groups, as well as emergency numbers, should be provided. The National Alliance for the Mentally Ill has support groups in many localities.

NURSING PROCESS CARE PLAN
Client with Depression

Ms. G. is a 70-year-old African American widowed woman who is a resident in a long-term care facility. She had a stroke a year ago, and has hemiplegia on her right side. She is right handed. She has a daughter who lives in another state, and a married son with one teenage granddaughter living nearby.

Assessment. The nurse is Craig C., LPN. He assessed that Ms. G. does not feed herself and has little appetite. She is alert and oriented to person and place. She cooperates with having her activities of daily living done for her, but she does not try to help. When she talks, it is only one or two words at a time. Her face always seems to look sad. Craig has worked with Ms. G. for the 3 months since she has been in this facility. He thinks Ms. G. is depressed. On the Geriatric Depression Scale she scored 12. In the conversation they had about the depression scale, Ms. G. said that she missed her family.

Diagnosis. Three priority nursing diagnoses were identified for this client:

- *Powerlessness* R/T disability and impaired communication
- *Self-Care Deficit,* bathing/hygiene, dressing/grooming, feeding, and toileting R/T hemiplegia and lack of motivation
- *Impaired Social Interaction* R/T lack of motivation and lack of opportunity to socialize with family and peers

Expected Outcomes. The expected outcomes for the plan of care are:

- Client will identify two areas in which she feels some control.
- Client will assist with all ADLs, feeding herself independently within 2 weeks.
- Client will interact with the staff, her peers, and her family.

Planning and Implementation. The charge nurse consulted with Ms. G.'s physician about the findings on the Geriatric Depression Scale. The physician agreed that Ms. G. is depressed. She prescribed fluoxetine 20 mg PO each morning. The following interventions were planned and implemented:

- *Offer simple choices first.* Ms. G. is given a choice of clothes to wear each day. She is asked if she wants to take her shower before or after breakfast, and where she wants to eat lunch (there are three dining rooms in this facility). She is asked which radio station she wants to listen to.

- *Encourage self-care.* The aides who supervised meals were asked to help her use her left hand to feed herself.
- *Encourage social contact.* The nurse called Ms. G.'s son and encouraged him to visit and to bring his family. He also arranged to visit with Ms. G. for a few minutes each day that he worked. (We know the nurse would have liked to have more time to talk with her, but this is a real story.) He had Ms. G. put on the list of residents who attend the news group (where the activity aide reads parts of the newspaper each morning).

Evaluation. Two weeks after the plan was started, Craig evaluated its effectiveness. With encouragement, Ms. G. had started to make choices about her clothes, radio stations, social activities, and visitors. She assisted in washing herself during her shower. She tried feebly, but was not much help with dressing. She was able to feed herself about 50% of her meals, and was able to call for help to get to the bathroom about 75% of the time.

Within 10 days after starting her new medication, she was smiling, more interested in her surroundings, had more appetite, and was more active. She is more talkative and enjoys visits from her family.

Critical Thinking in the Nursing Process

1. Why was it important for this client to make choices?
2. How successful was outcome 2 of Ms. G.'s plan? How might it be adapted after evaluation?
3. How does the range of social interactions that were set up for Ms. G. increase the likelihood that she will meet outcome 3?

Note: The bibliography listings for this and all chapters have been compiled at the back of the book.

Chapter Review

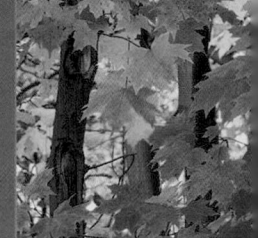

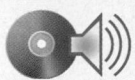 **KEY TERMS** by Topics

Use the audio glossary feature of either the CD-ROM or the Companion Website to hear the correct pronunciation of the following key terms.

Mood disorders
mood (elevated, euthymic, dysphoric, irritable), affect

Major Depressive Disorder
Major Depressive Disorder, anhedonia, psychomotor retardation, psychomotor agitation, monoamine oxidase inhibitors (MAOIs), electroconvulsive therapy (ECT)

Bipolar Disorder
distractibility, kindling process, suicidal ideation, pressured speech

KEY Points

- Mood disorders are caused by an interaction of genetic predisposition, brain function abnormalities, and environmental stressors (biologic and psychosocial factors).
- Depression is the most common mental disorder in the world.
- Nurses in every specialty area work with people who have mood disorders, especially depression.
- Most people who kill themselves were depressed.
- The suicide rate is highest in the elderly.
- Mood disorders are treatable and most people respond positively to medications.
- There is a stigma against people with mental disorders.
- Desired outcomes for people with mood disorders are in the areas of cognition, mood, behavior, and physiology.
- People with depression may experience anhedonia, lack of energy, lack of motivation, difficulty relating to other people, and psychomotor retardation, as well as sadness.
- Serious possible side effects are associated with the MAOI antidepressants, including hypertensive crisis when clients combine foods containing tyramine with these drugs.
- Serotonin syndrome can occur when MAOIs are combined with SSRIs or St. John's wort. Symptoms include agitation, muscle spasms, tremor, nausea, abdominal cramps, and headache.
- People with Bipolar Disorder in the manic phase have several challenges including lack of insight, poor judgment, and impulsive behavior.
- Lithium and valproate are both first-line drugs for bipolar disorder.

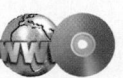 **EXPLORE MediaLink**

Additional interactive resources for this chapter can be found on the Companion Website at www.prenhall.com/burke. Click on Chapter 49 and "Begin" to select the activities for this chapter.

For chapter-related NCLEX-style review questions and an audio glossary, access the accompanying CD-ROM in this book.

☟ FOR FURTHER Study

For more information on psychopharmacology and mental status assessment, see Chapter 47.

See Chapter 48 for interventions for the client experiencing Disturbed Thought Processes.

Critical Thinking Care Map

Caring for a Client with Bipolar Disorder
NCLEX-PN® Focus Area: Physiologic Integrity

Case Study: David Clay is a 36-year-old European American male client with a diagnosis of Bipolar Disorder. He is hospitalized for a surgical repair of an ankle injury he experienced while he was playing basketball. Mr. Clay is a certified public accountant. He is having a manic episode that is less severe than his untreated episodes were, but he has been sleepless for three nights and he stayed home from work yesterday to play basketball all day. He did not eat or drink all day when he was playing basketball. He takes lithium carbonate extended release (Eskalith CR) 450 mg b.i.d. at home, and this is also ordered in the hospital. The morning dose is due now.

Nursing Diagnosis: Risk for Injury R/T lithium toxicity

COLLECT DATA

Subjective	Objective
_____	_____
_____	_____
_____	_____
_____	_____
_____	_____
_____	_____

Would you report this data? Yes/No

If yes, to: _____

Nursing Care

_____
_____
_____
_____
_____
_____
_____
_____
_____
_____

How would you document this? _____
_____
_____
_____

Data Collected
(use those that apply)

- Weight 185 lbs
- BP 130/80
- Pulse 108, irregular
- Client states, "My hands won't stop shaking."
- Slept 6 hours last night
- Skin is warm and dry
- Client's mother had bipolar disorder
- Client states, "Would you please read the menu to me, I can't see very well."
- When the physical therapist was teaching him to use crutches, the client was too weak to bear his own body weight on his unaffected leg
- Client is allergic to tree pollen
- Refused dinner last evening and breakfast today
- Client's wife states, "He has been under a lot of pressure at work lately."

Nursing Interventions
(use those that apply; list in priority order)

- Look in the client's chart to find his baseline vital signs.
- Call the physician to request an order for a sleeping pill, to help the client sleep to regain his strength.
- Teach client to drink 3 gallons of water daily.
- Hold the lithium dose that is due now.
- Call the physician to report the presence of symptoms of lithium toxicity.
- Teach the client and his wife that his strenuous exercise (playing basketball all day) is a good way to improve his cardiovascular fitness.

NCLEX-PN® Exam Preparation

1 What is the best way for the nurse to assess and document how a client's mood is subjectively responding to treatment over time?

A. Ask the client to draw a chart of his mood.
B. Measure the mood with the mental status assessment.
C. Ask the client to rate his mood on a 1–10 scale and document his report regularly.
D. Assess the client's response to medications, and if the client responds well to a low dose of medication, his mood is not as depressed as someone who requires a higher dose.

2 A newly married woman confides to the nurse that she tried to commit suicide during high school. She says she is afraid to become pregnant for fear that having a new baby might bring on those feelings again. Select the best information about postpartum depression for this client.

A. She is no more likely than any other young woman to experience postpartum depression.
B. She was probably just seeking attention in high school and has no risk of future depressive episodes.
C. She is at increased risk for another depressive episode considering her past experience.
D. She is worrying needlessly and should be encouraged to consider pregnancy.

3 A client complains that every winter she experiences feelings of extreme fatigue and irritability. She has been diagnosed with seasonal affective disorder. The nurse will teach her that the most effective treatment for this type of depression is:

A. light, or photo, therapy.
B. melatonin supplement.
C. psychoanalysis.
D. electroconvulsive treatment.

4 The nurse reads in the chart that a client is experiencing anhedonia. What symptom would the nurse expect to find? The client is:

A. hallucinating.
B. incapable of forming personal relationships.
C. overeating.
D. incapable of feeling pleasure.

5 People suffering from depression are often undiagnosed. The most likely reason for this is that:

A. physicians do not recognize the condition.
B. general practitioners feel underqualified to treat a mental disorder.
C. clients underreport their feelings, for fear of the stigma of being "mentally ill."
D. physicians do not value the depth of the psychologic feelings a client reports.

6 A client has just been started on an antidepressant medication. The client asked when the medication will work. The best response by the nurse is:

A. "You should feel over the depression immediately."
B. "It will take two to six weeks for the medication to reach its full effect."
C. "The medication usually takes one week to reach its potential."
D. "It may be six months before you feel the full effects of the medication."

7 What form of behavior would the nurse expect from a client who is having a manic episode with racing thoughts?

A. psychomotor agitation
B. hallucinations
C. powerlessness
D. thought blocking

8 A client with bipolar disorder is pacing constantly today while other clients are having a birthday party. There is music, noise, and food. Jim walks over to the table and starts grabbing handfuls of cake to eat as he paces up and down the halls. The nurse's best response to this behavior would be to:

A. let him continue to pace and eat.
B. medicate him with a prn antianxiety drug.
C. restrain him in his room.
D. ask him to go outside and take a walk with the nurse.

9 What side effect would the nurse expect if a client taking an MAOI eats pepperoni pizza?

10 What should the nurse do if a client scores high on the Geriatric Depression Scale?

Answers for Review Questions, as well as discussion of Care Plan and Critical Thinking Care Map questions, appear in Appendix V.

Chapter 50

Caring for Clients with Anxiety Disorders

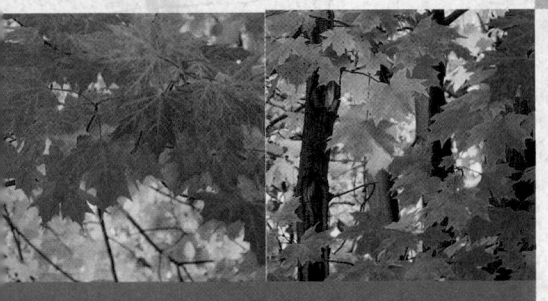

BRIEF Outline

Generalized Anxiety Disorder
Panic Disorder
Agoraphobia
Obsessive-Compulsive Disorder
Posttraumatic Stress Disorder
Social Phobia
Specific Phobias

LEARNING Outcomes

After completing this chapter, you will be able to:

- Collect subjective and objective data about clients' anxiety.
- Apply the nursing process to the care of clients with anxiety disorders.
- Explain the role of coping mechanisms in the management of anxiety.
- Plan nonpharmacologic nursing interventions to treat or prevent client anxiety.
- Safely administer antianxiety and sedative hypnotic agents.

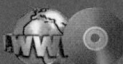

MediaLink

www.prenhall.com/burke
Use the address above to access the free, interactive Companion Website created for this textbook. Get hints, instant feedback, and textbook references to chapter-related NCLEX-style questions. Link to other interesting sites.

Audio Glossary:
Use the Companion Website, or the CD-ROM disk enclosed with your textbook, to hear the pronunciation of key terms in this chapter.

Anxiety is a normal response to stress. Everyone has experienced it. **Anxiety** is a feeling of uneasiness and activation of the autonomic nervous system in response to a vague, nonspecific threat (Carpenito, 2000). When anxiety becomes overwhelming, when it impairs a person's ability to function at home, school, or work, and affects relationships with other people, then it is a disorder. Anxiety disorders are serious medical illnesses that can grow worse if not treated.

PATHOPHYSIOLOGY

The experience of anxiety appears to originate in the subcortical or primitive brain, specifically in the limbic system (Rauch et al., 1995). During anxiety there is an increase in blood flow to the limbic system and the cerebral cortex. Figure 50-1 ■ shows the structures of the limbic system, and Table 50-1 ■ describes the functions of these structures and what happens when they function abnormally. The limbic system conducts stimuli to the sympathetic part of the autonomic nervous system. Sympathetic stimulation causes the symptoms we recognize as anxiety. From the limbic system, neural messages are also conducted to the cerebral cortex. In the association areas of the cerebral cortex, the individual experiences thoughts about anxiety. Thus, feelings, physiologic responses, and thoughts are all part of the anxiety experience.

Studies of twins and families suggest that there is a genetic influence on the development of anxiety disorders. As with other mental disorders, genetics is not the sole etiology of anxiety disorders. Life experiences also play an important part. Researchers are looking at how genetics and experience interact in anxiety disorders.

TABLE 50-1	
Functions of the Limbic System	
LIMBIC STRUCTURE	FUNCTIONS AND DYSFUNCTIONS
Thalamus	Relays sensory input from spinal cord. Regulates emotional aspects of sensory experiences. Dysfunction is involved in OCD, mood disorders, schizophrenia.
Amygdala	Coordinates actions of autonomic nervous system and endocrine system. Involved in control of emotions, nurturing behavior, fear conditioning. Controls memory of fear experiences. Dysfunction contributes to inappropriate fear and rage, anxiety, PTSD.
Hippocampus	Processes information between parts of the brain that receive sensory input and those that translate the input into action. Regulates immune system and memory storage. Dysfunction results in memory and learning impairments.
Hypothalamus	Composed of neurons that produce hormones. Integration center. Concentrates dopamine. Converts thinking and feelings into hormones that cause changes throughout the body through the autonomic nervous system. Dysfunction can cause excessive thirst and hunger. May be involved in eating disorders and schizophrenia. Implicated in side effects of psychotropic drugs.

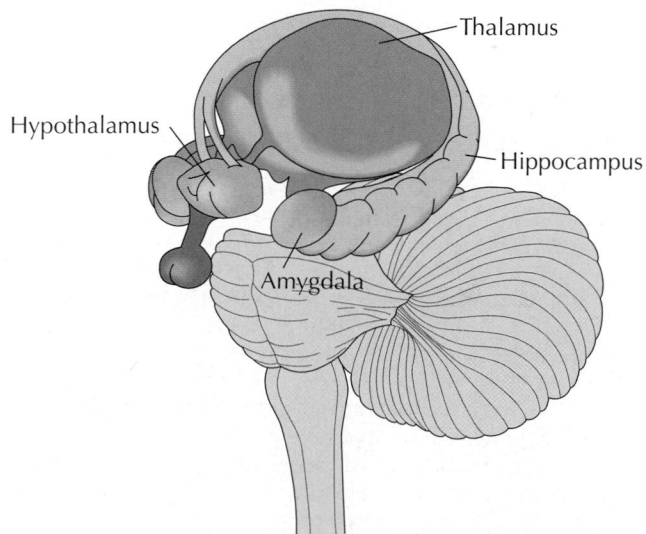

Figure 50-1. ■ The limbic system is surrounded by the cerebral cortex. It plays a role in motivation, emotion, and memory. It is composed of the thalamus, amygdala, hippocampus, and hypothalamus. (*Source:* Fontaine & Fletcher. (2003). *Mental health nursing* (5th ed.). Upper Saddle River, NJ: Pearson, Figure 7.4, page 161.)

From a behavioral point of view, experience can teach people different ways to respond to stressful events. An individual's experiences, both in childhood and adulthood, influence which situations cause anxiety, and the severity of the client's response.

Cognitive function can affect how a person perceives anxiety-producing stimuli. If a person focuses her or his thoughts on stressful events, this individual will be more prone to anxiety. Intelligence and the personality trait of introspection may put people at a higher risk for anxiety.

The sympathetic nervous system responds to the stress of fear or anxiety in the same way. Fear has survival value. When a person sees an alligator, fear motivates the person to run away. Anxiety is not as focused and often has no realistic source. Even when the individual experiencing anxiety knows the reason for it, the feeling of **dysphoria** (uncomfortable and distressed) is often out of proportion to the real danger. Low levels of anxiety can arouse the individual's

MANIFESTATIONS OF SYMPATHETIC STIMULATION

- Increased heart rate
- Increased blood pressure
- Dilated pupils
- Cool skin
- Piloerection (hair "standing on end")
- Decreased GI motility

attention and alertness, and even make it easier to learn new things, but as anxiety becomes more severe, it causes impairment of function. Anxiety and fear cause the same physiologic responses, which are the result of sympathetic nervous system stimulation (Box 50-1 ■).

MANIFESTATIONS

Levels of Anxiety

There are four degrees of anxiety (Peplau, 1989). Table 50-2 ■ shows the four levels and the behaviors the nurse might observe in a client at each level.

The *Diagnostic and Statistical Manual of Mental Disorders* (American Psychiatric Association [APA], 2000) lists several anxiety-related disorders, including Generalized Anxiety Disorder, Panic Disorder with or without Agoraphobia, Agoraphobia without Panic Disorder, and Obsessive-Compulsive Disorder (OCD) among others. They have many different manifestations. The feature they all have in common is anxiety.

Generalized Anxiety Disorder

Generalized Anxiety Disorder is characterized by excessive anxiety and worry occurring on most days for at least 6 months. The anxiety is about a number of different events or activities, and the individual finds it difficult to control. The affected person also has at least three of the following (APA, 2000):

- Restlessness
- Fatigue
- Difficulty concentrating
- Irritability
- Muscle tension
- Disturbed sleep.

The diagnosis of Generalized Anxiety Disorder in children requires only one of the above symptoms in addition to the persistent anxiety.

Affected people will report that they feel significant stress, have difficulty controlling the worry, or have related impairment in social or occupational functioning. In this disorder, the intensity, frequency, and duration of the anxiety are far out of proportion to the realistic likelihood or impact of the feared event. Thoughts of the feared event intrude on the individual's thinking, distracting her or him from other tasks. The focus of worry may shift from one concern to another. A few potential examples of concerns for these individuals are being late, personal performance, illness, family, job.

People with Generalized Anxiety Disorder usually realize that their anxiety is more intense than makes sense in

TABLE 50-2

Four Degrees of Anxiety

DEGREE OF ANXIETY	SUBJECTIVE EFFECTS	OBSERVABLE BEHAVIOR
Mild	Perceptual field widens slightly. Increased ability to see relationships among data.	Alert, more perceptive, able to recognize anxiety. Promotes motivation and growth.
Moderate	Perceptual field narrows slightly. Concentrates on the immediate focus, ignoring peripheral stimuli. Can change attention if directed.	Able to sustain attention on a focal point. Inattentive to stimuli outside this focus. May talk faster. VS begin to increase (except temperature). Able to recognize and express anxiety.
Severe	Perceptual field is greatly reduced. Does not notice external events. Unable to redirect focus even with outside direction.	Attention is focused on a small part of a specific area. Assumptions made may be erroneous due to incomplete perception. May be unaware of anxiety. VS increasing. Coping/relief measures used.
Panic	Perception is reduced to a detail. Perception is distorted. May jump from one detail to another, as in flight of ideas. Experienced as a threat to survival. Affected person feels dread, terror.	Feelings of unreality, confusion, terror, self-absorption. May be expressed with violence toward self or others. Loss of control. May include pacing or running. Automatic coping/relief behaviors used. Can result in exhaustion if prolonged.

the situation, but they still cannot control their worries. Their anxiety is accompanied by physical symptoms, especially fatigue, headaches, muscle tension, muscle pain, irritability, sweating, nausea, difficulty swallowing, trembling, and hot flashes. Relaxation seems impossible (NIMH, 2001).

Unlike people with other anxiety disorders, people with this disorder do not usually avoid anxiety-producing situations as a result of their disorder. When the disorder is mild, affected people can function, but at its worst it is very debilitating.

Generalized Anxiety Disorder affects about twice as many women as men in the general population. In treatment settings, the nurse can expect to see about equal numbers of women and men seeking treatment. In any given year, approximately 3% of the population will have this disorder. Over a lifetime, any individual has about a 5% chance of having it. This disorder is commonly associated with Major Depressive Disorder (APA, 2000).

Panic Disorder

People with Panic Disorder have recurrent, unexpected panic attacks followed by at least 1 month of persistent concern about having another one. They may worry about the possible complications of the attacks, or have a significant behavioral change associated with the attacks (APA, 2000).

A panic attack is characterized by an episode of intense fear or discomfort. During this episode four or more of the following are present (APA, 2000):

- Palpitations, pounding heart, or increased heart rate
- Sweating
- Trembling or shaking
- Sensations of shortness of breath or smothering
- Feeling of choking
- Chest pain or discomfort
- Nausea or abdominal distress
- Feeling dizzy, unsteady, light-headed, or faint
- Derealization (feeling of unreality) or depersonalization (being detached from oneself)
- Fear of losing control or going crazy
- Fear of dying
- Paresthesias (numbness or tingling)
- Chills or hot flushes.

People with Panic Disorder have panic attacks without warning. Sometimes the attacks are associated with a stressor, sometimes they are not. There is no way to predict when an attack will occur, so people often spend much time worrying about when the next one will strike. Panic attacks can occur at any time, even during sleep. An attack usually peaks in severity within 10 minutes, but some symptoms last much longer. Untreated, the disorder can be very disabling. Affected people often fear returning to the site or

situation of a previous attack, which can severely limit an individual's ability to function. For example, if a person experienced an anxiety attack at a grocery store and another attack on a bus, this individual may not be able to shop for groceries or go to work.

Not everyone who has a panic attack will go on to have Panic Disorder. Some people have one attack, with no recurrence.

clinical ALERT

People experiencing Panic Disorder often visit the hospital emergency department several times before they are accurately diagnosed. They may go for years before they find out that they have a real, treatable illness (NIMH, 2001). It is critical for emergency department nurses and physicians to be aware of Panic Disorder.

Imagine a person who comes to the hospital for help with a really terrifying panic episode, believing that she is dying. A physical assessment and EKG are done and show no abnormalities. The episode is resolving by the time the tests are done. The client is told that there is nothing wrong. The client may even be told that she has misused the emergency department. This client is suffering not only the effects of the panic attack, but also the devastation of not being taken seriously. Many people with treatable mental illnesses avoid treatment because they fear not being believed by health professionals.

Panic Disorder is often associated with other serious disorders such as depression, substance abuse, or alcoholism. The incidence of suicide is increased in people affected by this disorder. The disorder affects three times as many women as men, and affects 1% to 2% of the general population. The onset is usually between late adolescence and the mid-thirties, although it can begin at any age (APA, 2000).

Agoraphobia

Agoraphobia is characterized by anxiety about being in places or situations where escape may be difficult (or embarrassing), or when help might not be available in the case of a panic attack. Agoraphobic fears typically include situations that involve being alone away from home in a crowd or standing in line; on a bridge; or traveling in a plane, train, bus, or automobile. The fear-producing situations are avoided, endured with much anxiety and distress, or require the presence of a companion (APA, 2000).

Agoraphobia is commonly associated with Panic Disorder. People who seek treatment for the disorder almost always also have Panic Disorder. It is more likely to occur in females than in males. It can result in severe impairment in social and occupational functioning when the individual avoids multiple anxiety-producing situations (APA, 2000).

Not everyone who stays in the home has Agoraphobia, however. Agoraphobia causes people to confine themselves within their homes to avoid overwhelming anxiety. In some cultures women are expected to remain at home, and their public activities are greatly limited. If a woman from such a culture stays at home, she is acting in accordance with cultural expectations and does not have a diagnosis of Agoraphobia.

Obsessive-Compulsive Disorder

Obsessions are recurrent and intrusive thoughts that caused marked distress. The affected person recognizes that these thoughts are from her or his own mind, and tries to ignore or suppress the obsessive thoughts. **Compulsions** are repetitive behaviors or mental acts that the affected person feels driven to perform in response to obsessive thoughts. The objective of these behaviors is to reduce stress or to prevent some dreaded event. The compulsive behaviors are not realistically connected with the situations they are supposed to neutralize, or they are clearly excessive (APA, 2000).

Obsessive-Compulsive Disorder (OCD) is characterized by compulsions or obsessions, which the affected person recognizes are excessive or unreasonable. The obsessions or compulsions cause marked distress and take more than 1 hour each day, or significantly interfere with the affected person's daily occupational, academic, or personal functioning (APA, 2000).

Common obsessive thoughts involve dirt and germs, numbers or counting, symmetry and order, ideas that are against the individual's religious beliefs, or sexual thoughts that are disgusting to the affected individual. Some examples of compulsive rituals performed to control the obsessive thoughts are cleaning, hand washing, counting, touching or doing things in a certain order, or praying. There is no pleasure for the affected individual in performing the compulsive rituals, only temporary relief from the anxiety caused by not doing these things (NIMH, 2001).

Many people without OCD can identify with some compulsive behavior, such as checking several times that the stove is really off before leaving home. This behavior does not become OCD until it becomes distressing, consumes over an hour a day, or interferes with the individual's daily life.

OCD usually begins in adolescence or early adulthood. It can begin in childhood. It tends to affect males at an earlier age than females. Affected children often do not realize that the behavior is unreasonable. The majority of affected people experience OCD with a waxing and waning course. The disorder becomes more severe in the presence of stress. OCD occurs more often in first-degree relatives of people

with OCD and Tourette's Disorder than in the general population. OCD occurs in many cultures around the world. It affects approximately 1% to 2% of people at some time in their lives (APA, 2000).

Some people with OCD also have depression or other anxiety disorders. Some have eating disorders as well as OCD. The disorder can involve people so severely that their development or ability to function in their daily lives is affected.

Posttraumatic Stress Disorder

Posttraumatic Stress Disorder (PTSD) was first recognized in war veterans. It is a debilitating condition that follows an extreme traumatic stressor. The traumatic stressor can involve an event that threatens the individual's life, serious injury, or personal integrity; or witnessing an event including death or serious injury of another; or learning about the unexpected or violent death or serious harm to a significant other. The person's response to the event must involve intense fear, helplessness, or horror. Children respond with agitated or disorganized behavior. The characteristic symptoms of PTSD include the following, which are present for more than 1 month (APA, 2000):

- Persistent reexperiencing of the traumatic event
- Avoidance of stimuli associated with the trauma
- Numbing of general responsiveness (also called *psychic numbing* or *emotional anesthesia*)
- Increased arousal (difficulty sleeping, nightmares, exaggerated startle response, and hypervigilance or alertness for danger).

Traumatic events that might result in PTSD include, but are not limited to, violent personal assault (sexual assault, physical attack, robbery), military combat, being taken hostage, terrorist attack, torture, imprisonment as a prisoner of war or in a concentration camp, disasters, transportation crashes, or diagnosis of life-threatening illness. Children may develop PTSD as a result of sexual abuse even if there is no actual or threatened injury. The disorder is more likely to occur and to be more long lasting when the stressor is of intentional human action, such as rape or torture (APA, 2000).

People with PTSD can reexperience the traumatic event in various ways. Commonly, the person has repeated intrusive memories or dreams of the event. Some people experience flashbacks in which they relive the event, believing that it is actually happening. A flashback may include sights, sounds, smells, or feelings from the traumatic event.

Affected people feel distressed by situations that remind them of the event, and avoid these situations. For example, a person who was raped in an elevator may avoid all elevators. A person who was held in a prison camp with military guards may avoid anyone in uniform. Ordinary events can trigger memories and a flashback in susceptible individuals.

People with PTSD may have difficulty with interpersonal relationships. They may have difficulty trusting or being affectionate. Things they formerly enjoyed may not provide pleasure for them anymore. Irritability, aggression, even violence may be expressed when these would be out of character for the person before the incident. Depression sometimes occurs in people with PTSD. As with people affected by other anxiety disorders, people with PTSD may use alcohol and other substances to medicate their anxiety symptoms.

After extreme trauma, people often have some of the same symptoms as PTSD. The disorder is only diagnosed if symptoms persist for longer than a month. If a person is going to develop PTSD, it will usually occur within 3 months of the traumatic experience.

PTSD can occur at any age. Approximately half of people experience complete resolution of symptoms within 3 months. The most important factors affecting the likelihood of developing this disorder are severity of the traumatic event, duration of the trauma, and proximity of the individual's exposure. Approximately 8% of people in the United States will be affected at some time in their lives. The highest rates of occurrence of PTSD are in people who have survived rape, military combat and captivity, and ethnically or politically motivated imprisonment and genocide (APA, 2000).

Social Phobia

Social Phobia, also called Social Anxiety Disorder, is characterized by a marked and persistent fear of social or performance situations in which embarrassment may occur. A **phobia** is a persistent and irrational fear. Exposure to the social or performance situation (such as public speaking or speaking to a supervisor) almost always results in an immediate anxiety reaction. Adults and adolescents with Social Phobia recognize that their fear is excessive; affected children may not. People usually avoid the risky situations, but may endure them with dread. Social Phobia only exists if the fear, avoidance, or anxiety about encountering the social situation interferes significantly with the affected individual's daily routine, social, academic, or occupational life, or if the person is markedly distressed by the disorder. Anticipatory anxiety may begin weeks before an anticipated social event (APA, 2000).

In people less than age 18, the symptoms must have lasted for more than 6 months to make the diagnosis of Social Phobia. Temporary social anxiety in childhood or adolescence is quite common and does not constitute Social Phobia. Neither does fear of speaking in situations where fear may be justified, such as when the teacher calls on a student who did not do the homework.

Physical symptoms often accompany the anxiety in Social Phobia. These include blushing, excessive sweating, nausea, GI distress, tremors, and difficulty talking. Although they realize that their fears are irrational, people with this disorder are unable to control it. Even after they have done the dreaded deed, affected people continue to feel anxious about how they were perceived and judged by others. Making or keeping friends may be difficult. People with Social Phobia may medicate their symptoms with alcohol or drugs to make it possible for them to endure social situations.

Specific Phobias

A specific phobia is an excessive fear of a specific object or situation. It might be triggered by the presence of the feared object, or even the anticipation of it. Affected people have an immediate anxiety reaction in response to the feared situation, which may take the form of a panic attack. Some examples of specific phobias are animals, flying, heights or needles. See Table 50-3 ■ for examples of specific phobias and their clinical names. Adults with phobias recognize

TABLE 50-3	
Specific Phobias	
CLINICAL NAME	**FEARED OBJECT OR SITUATION**
Acrophobia	Heights
Agoraphobia	Open spaces
Apiphobia	Bees
Astraphobia	Lightning
Aviophobia	Flying
Claustrophobia	Closed spaces
Entomophobia	Insects
Gephyrophobia	Bridge crossing
Hematophobia	Blood
Hydrophobia	Water
Iatrophobia	Doctors
Microphobia	Germs
Monophobia (or Autophobia)	Being alone
Mysophobia	Dirt
Nyctophobia	Darkness, night
Pyrophobia	Fire
Xenophobia	Strangers

that their fears are unreasonable. People usually avoid the phobic stimulus, but may endure it with intense anxiety or dread. A person with a phobia will avoid the phobic stimulus or worry about it to the extent that the person's daily routine, occupational or academic functioning, social life, or quality of life are affected. People with phobias experience marked distress (APA, 2000).

Children often have fears of things that seem irrational to adults. A child with a fear is not diagnosed with a specific phobia unless the fear is specific, extreme, causes great distress, and has affected school or daily functioning for at least 6 months. Children with phobias may not realize that their fears are irrational. Anxiety in children may be expressed by crying, clinging, the inability to move or "freezing with fear," or tantrums.

People with phobias involving situations or objects that are easy to avoid may not feel the need to seek treatment. Phobias involving everyday experiences can be disabling. Fears of specific objects or situations are very common. Specific Phobia is not diagnosed unless the phobia significantly interferes with the individual's functioning or causes severe distress. Specific phobias often occur in people who also have other anxiety disorders, mood disorders, and substance-related disorders.

People who have a blood-injection-injury phobia have a history of fainting from a vasovagal response in about 75% of cases (APA, 2000). Nurses should be aware of the possibility of clients fainting during injections or, more frequently, blood draws. The potential for fainting is one of the reasons that clients should be in a sitting or recumbent position for injections or venipuncture.

clinical ALERT

The extreme fear in the phobia of blood or needles may result in the *vasovagal response* occurring. The client's heart and respiratory rates initially increase due to sympathetic stimulation. When the vagus nerve is stimulated, the heart rate and blood pressure fall, potentially resulting in a loss of consciousness.

The first symptoms of specific phobias usually occur in childhood, but can be in adulthood. Factors that predispose people to develop specific phobias include (APA, 2000):

- Traumatic events such as being trapped in a closet or attacked by an animal
- Unexpected panic attacks in the feared situation
- Observing others in the feared situation (seeing someone fall from a height)
- Seeing others demonstrate fear in the situation (mother is afraid of going to the dentist)
- Informational transmission (media coverage of bombing, natural disasters, plane crashes, or repeated parental warnings about dangers of some situation).

The subjects of specific phobias differ from one culture to another. Women are more frequently affected by phobias than men are, at a rate of 2:1. The prevalence of phobias decreases in the elderly. Some phobias tend to run in families, especially the fears of blood and injury (APA, 2000).

INTERDISCIPLINARY CARE

Coping with Anxiety

People use **coping behaviors** to adapt to or manage stress or change. To control anxiety, people develop patterns of coping behavior. Coping behaviors can be **adaptive** (healthy or likely to lead to positive resolution) or **maladaptive** (unhealthy). Coping behaviors are the conscious ways in which people deal with stress.

A person who uses active problem solving, while considering the rights of others, is using coping behavior adaptively. An example of using adaptive coping behavior is a nurse asking another nurse to help determine why a client's condition is changing. Maladaptive behavior might be expressed by negative or aggressive behavior toward others. An example of maladaptive active coping behavior is a nurse shouting at a nursing assistant who made a mistake.

UNCONSCIOUS DEFENSE MECHANISMS. Some methods of coping are part of our conscious thoughts, while others are unconscious. People use both conscious coping behaviors and unconscious defense mechanisms. These defense mechanisms may also be adaptive or maladaptive. See Table 50-4 ■ for specific examples of defense mechanisms.

Because the symptom of anxiety is associated with so many different physiologic and psychosocial problems, an accurate diagnosis must be made before treatment begins. It could be dangerous to treat the anxiety caused by hypoxia with an antianxiety agent. Some general medical disorders that frequently present with anxiety are listed in Box 50-2 ■.

BOX 50-2

GENERAL MEDICAL CONDITIONS ASSOCIATED WITH ANXIETY
- Hypoglycemia
- Hyperthyroidism
- Asthma
- Pneumonia
- Chronic obstructive pulmonary disease
- Pulmonary embolism
- Encephalitis
- Cardiac dysrhythmias
- Vitamin B_{12} deficiency
- Pheochromocytoma (adrenal tumor)
- Vestibular dysfunction
- Hyperthyroidism
- Neoplasms

TABLE 50-4

Defense Mechanisms

DEFENSE MECHANISM	DEFINITION	EXAMPLE
Acting Out	Using actions instead of thoughts or feelings to respond to stress or emotional distress.	A child who is afraid of being hospitalized kicks the nurse and knocks supplies off the hospital shelf.
Altruism	Dealing with emotional conflict by meeting the needs of others, receiving gratification either vicariously or from the reactions of others.	A young man's fiancée leaves him, and he joins the Peace Corps.
Anticipation	Experiencing emotional reactions in advance of a stressful event.	When first diagnosed with diabetes, a man begins to experience anticipatory grief for his eventual loss of function and health.
Compensation	Attempt (conscious or unconscious) to overcome perceived inadequacies.	A girl who is disappointed to have little athletic skill works hard to excel in academics.
Denial	Refusal to acknowledge a painful reality.	A person with alcoholism says: "I don't have a drinking problem, I can quit whenever I want."
Displacement	Transferring a feeling about one person or object to another, usually safer, one.	A patient is very angry with his doctor but yells at the nurse.
Dissociation	A breakdown in the usually integrated functions of consciousness, memory, or perception. Detachment from emotional significance.	A woman calmly describes her severe sexual abuse in childhood as though she were outside herself watching it happen.
Humor	Amusing or ironic aspects of a stressful experience are emphasized.	After making a mistake in front of the class, the teacher makes a joke about it.
Intellectualization	Excessive use of abstract thinking or using generalizations to control disturbing feelings.	A man analyzes and explains to a friend the interpersonal dynamics that led to his divorce.
Projection	Attributing one's own unacceptable feelings or thoughts to another.	A person who does not like children says: "Children just don't like me."
Rationalization	Concealing the true motivations (even to ourselves) behind our actions with incorrect but acceptable motivations.	Instead of admitting that he went to this college to be with his girlfriend, the student says that it is the best college in the state.
Reaction Formation	Substituting behavior or feelings that are the opposite of what one actually feels.	A woman does not like her supervisor at work, yet she gives the supervisor gifts and compliments.
Regression	Return to an earlier, less stressful level of adjustment.	A child returns to bedwetting after being hospitalized.
Repression	Removing unacceptable thoughts or wishes from consciousness.	A woman has no memory of being raped but may feel anxious when she goes near the area where it happened.
Sublimation	Unacceptable feelings are diverted into socially acceptable behavior.	A person is very angry and runs for hours on the track.
Suppression	Intentionally avoiding thinking about unacceptable or stressful feelings.	A woman does not have enough money to pay her bills and keeps herself busy with housework to avoid thinking about money.

There are effective treatments for anxiety disorders. Each disorder is treated specifically, but generally the most effective treatments are cognitive-behavioral therapy and medications.

Cognitive-Behavioral Therapy

A major goal of cognitive-behavioral therapy (CBT) is to reduce anxiety by eliminating beliefs or behaviors that help to maintain the anxiety disorder. CBT is effective for most anxiety disorders. It has two parts. In the cognitive therapy part, clients are helped to change thinking patterns that contribute to their anxieties. Cognitive therapy includes education about the physiology behind anxiety reactions (as presented earlier in this chapter). Avoidance of a feared object or situation prevents the person from learning that it is harmless. Cognitive therapy is based on the idea that thinking errors by the client produce mistaken negative beliefs that continue despite evidence to the contrary.

Cognitive restructuring is a therapeutic technique in which the client works to change patterns of negative thoughts that occur automatically. The client is helped to see the process of automatic negative anxiety-producing thoughts and negative self-talk. When clients see the basis for the erroneous negative thinking, they can see the situation realistically, and can then be helped to replace the negative self-talk with more supportive and self-calming thinking.

For example, a woman with Panic Disorder may think that her panic attacks are heart attacks. People with anxiety disorders tend to put the worst possible interpretation on physical symptoms. She can be helped to see that they are panic attacks, and are not life threatening. She can learn to replace the thought "I am dying!" with "I'm OK. This is a panic attack." She can discuss her experiences, looking for symptoms and events that come before the panic attacks, to help identify triggers. Finally, she can be helped to find new ways to think about the triggers that start panic attacks. In a similar way, a person with Social Phobia can be helped to see that other people are not really judging him to be incompetent when he walks into class.

The goal of the behavioral therapy part of CBT is to change the client's behavioral reaction to anxiety-provoking situations. One behavioral approach is to teach the client deep-breathing or relaxation techniques. People can use these techniques to cope with anxiety by deliberately relaxing or deep breathing in situations they expect to provoke anxiety, thus interrupting the automatic anxiety responses.

Exposure is an important aspect of behavioral therapy for anxiety disorders. In this therapy, clients confront the thing they fear. There are several approaches to the use of exposure in behavioral therapy. One approach, called *exposure and response prevention,* is often used in OCD. If clients fear dirt and germs, the therapist may encourage them to dirty their hands and then wait a certain amount of time before washing. The therapist helps the client to cope with the anxiety that results, and the client experiences a coping success. The compulsive rituals in OCD give the person some relief from anxiety, but the rituals also prevent the person from testing rational thoughts about danger. With repetition of this technique, the client will experience a series of successful situations in which he or she survives being dirty, and the anxiety will decrease over time (NIMH, 2001).

In another type of exposure exercise, a person with Social Phobia may be encouraged to spend a certain amount of time in a feared social situation, while fighting the desire to run away. The client may be asked to try making a small social error to see how others will respond. The therapist then discusses the reaction of others and helps the client see that the fear of judgment by others is not as brutal as the client feared. Repeated practice and discussion of feelings and coping techniques with the therapist can help reduce Social Phobia.

Behavioral therapy alone has long been used effectively to treat specific phobias. The person is gradually exposed to the feared object or situation. Initially the exposure may only be to pictures of the feared object. Later, when clients feel ready, they confront the actual feared situation in a safe setting. The therapist usually goes with the client to provide support and guidance (NIMH, 2001).

CBT or behavioral therapy usually takes about 12 weeks and can be done individually or in groups. As with all psychotherapy, CBT must be directed at the client's specific concerns. An effective approach for a person who has OCD and intrusive sexual thoughts will not be effective for a person who fears doctors.

Promoting Resilience

Resilience is the quality of being hardy or "stress resistant." Resilient people are "survivors" who are able to cope adaptively, and seem to flourish despite stress that other people cannot tolerate. Hardy, Concato, and Gill (2004) studied older people in the community and discovered several factors that are associated with resilience in the elder population. The resilience factors are:

- Self-efficacy (the belief that individuals have control over events in their own lives)
- High functional ability
- Independence with activities of daily living
- Good self-rated health
- Positive outlook on life.

Health care professionals may be able to promote resilience in clients by supporting their functional abilities and general health. This is also evidence of the importance of treating depression in the elderly.

MEDICATION

Medications from several classifications treat anxiety effectively. There is some controversy about the use of antianxiety medications, however. As a general rule, people are better off if they can develop the tools to solve their own problems without using drugs to solve problems. This is especially true for people who have transient or low-level anxiety or poor coping skills. The best approach to anxiety treatment for these clients is to promote adaptive coping skills. Medications should not be used when more adaptive approaches could realistically solve the problem.

Despite the potential hazards of antianxiety drugs for a few clients, there are many situations in which they are indicated. Some forms of anxiety, such as specific phobias, respond best to behavioral therapy alone. But most anxiety disorders require a combination of medication and psychotherapy for effective treatment. People with Panic Disorder may require the long-term prescription of antianxiety drugs if they are not able to function without them.

Nurses should be aware that many people with mental disorders require medications in order to function. People with depression require antidepressants; those with psychosis require antipsychotics, just as those with anxiety disorders often require antianxiety medications in order to function. Although the antianxiety medications are contraindicated as a problem-solving approach for the otherwise normal client, they are required for the well-being of many people with severe anxiety disorders. Nurses must be supportive of these individuals who need medications, because there is a loud message in our culture that says "Just Say No to Drugs" in any situation. The message from mental health care providers is "Take medications if you need them to treat mental disorders."

Nurses should educate clients that if one treatment is not effective, it is worth trying other treatment modalities. A combination of psychotherapy and medications proves to be the most effective for the most people. If one medication is not effective, another one is likely to work. People often must try several drugs before they find the one that works best for them.

Antianxiety and Sedative-Hypnotic Agents

Benzodiazepines (BZs) are the most widely prescribed drugs in the world today. They are used for anxiety, insomnia, alcohol withdrawal, skeletal muscle relaxation, acute management of seizures, severe agitation, Social Phobia, Generalized Anxiety Disorder, and Panic Disorder. The benzodiazepines continue to be the mainstay of anxiety management due to their efficacy, rapid onset, and generally favorable side effect profile (Stevens & Pollack, 2005). See Table 50-5 ■ for information about the BZ drugs.

The target symptoms for the antianxiety drugs are nervousness, sweating, increased heart rate, sense of dread, fearfulness, phobias, compulsiveness, nausea, vomiting, diarrhea,

---

TABLE 50-5

Benzodiazepine Antianxiety and Sedative-Hypnotic Agents

DRUG	DURATION OF ACTION	AVAILABLE IN INJECTABLE (IM & IV) FORM?
Antianxiety Agents		
Alprazolam (Xanax)	Intermediate acting	No
Chlordiazepoxide (Librium)	Long acting	Yes
Clonazepam (Klonopin)	Long acting	No
Clorazepate (Tranxene)	Long acting	No
Diazepam (Valium)	Long acting	Yes
Halazepam (Paxipam)	Intermediate acting	No
Lorazepam (Ativan)	Intermediate acting	Yes
Oxazepam (Serax)	Intermediate acting	No
Prazepam (Centrax)	Long acting	No
Sedative-Hypnotic Agents		
Estazolam (ProSom)	Intermediate acting	No
Flurazepam (Dalmane)	Long acting	No
Temazepam (Restoril)	Intermediate acting	No
Triazolam (Halcion)	Short acting	No
Quazepam (Doral)	Long acting	No

dizziness, irritability, headache, and dry mouth. The target symptoms for sedative-hypnotics are insomnia and sleep disorders. **Insomnia** includes difficulty falling asleep, staying asleep, or awakening too early and not being able to go back to sleep. The provider can choose the specific BZ based on which sleep problem the client has (a short-acting agent would be best for someone who has difficulty falling asleep). When the client is experiencing anxiety that is a symptom of another disorder, such as depression, the anxiety will probably resolve with treatment of the primary problem.

MECHANISM OF ACTION. Benzodiazepines are CNS depressants. They enhance the effects of gamma-aminobutyric acid (GABA), which is an inhibitory neurotransmitter. GABA makes the neuron less responsive to excitatory neurotransmitters such as norepinephrine, serotonin, and dopamine. The overall effect is to slow neuronal firing, which results in the CNS depressant properties of the BZs (Keltner et al., 2003).

SIDE EFFECTS. The benzodiazepines are CNS depressants and have some common side effects. The common side effects include sedation, drowsiness, dizziness, and decreased coordination. Older adults may have difficulty metabolizing the long-acting BZs and may have increasing blood levels. The shorter acting agents are a better choice for older adults. They are also more likely to suffer cognitive or memory side effects to long-term BZ therapy than are younger adults.

Occasionally clients will have a **paradoxical** (contradictory, opposite) **response** to the BZs. Instead of relaxation, they experience agitation or unstable emotions. The elderly, children, and people with brain damage are at increased risk. When a client has a paradoxical reaction, the BZ should be discontinued.

Other important concerns with the benzodiazepines are physical dependence and tolerance:

- Prolonged use of BZs causes a decrease in GABA receptors. Remember that GABA is an inhibiting transmitter. With a reduced capacity for inhibition, CNS stimulation results. When the BZ is discontinued abruptly, the CNS is stimulated, and unable to inhibit or regulate itself. The client experiences all the symptoms of CNS stimulation, including anxiety, agitation, increased blood pressure and pulse, and even possibly seizures. These CNS stimulation symptoms constitute BZ withdrawal. Withdrawal can be prevented by slowly decreasing (tapering) doses, instead of suddenly discontinuing a BZ in a client who has taken it regularly for an extended period (longer than 2 weeks). The presence of withdrawal does not constitute addiction (addiction is a psychologic process). These are safe drugs that must be prescribed with care and knowledge of their effects. Psychologic dependence occurs when clients believe that they cannot live or function without the drug to treat their anxiety.

- Prolonged regular use also causes tolerance (less response to the same dose, requiring increased doses to give the same effect). Clients become tolerant to the sedative effects relatively quickly. It takes longer to develop tolerance to the antianxiety effect.

DRUG INTERACTIONS. Overdoses of benzodiazepines alone are not commonly fatal. Fatalities involving the combination of BZs and alcohol are relatively common. An additive CNS depressant effect occurs when BZs are taken with CNS depressants such as alcohol, tricyclic antidepressants, MAOIs, anticonvulsants, antihistamines, or antipsychotics.

Non-Benzodiazepine Antianxiety Agents

Buspirone (BuSpar) is an effective non-benzodiazepine antianxiety agent. It differs from benzodiazepines in several ways. It does not bind to the same brain sites. It probably acts as a serotonin agonist. Buspirone is not effective against seizures, muscle spasm, or alcohol withdrawal, nor does it treat Panic Disorder effectively. Buspirone is not sedating, does not cause euphoria, and has no cross-tolerance with sedatives or alcohol. An example of cross-tolerance is seen in clients who are tolerant to large amounts of alcohol. They will also be tolerant to benzodiazepines, even if they have never taken them before. Buspirone does not cause dependence or withdrawal. It has virtually no abuse potential and is not a controlled substance. It begins to have antianxiety effects within 7 to 10 days, but may take up to 6 weeks to achieve full effect.

Propranolol is a blocker of beta-adrenergic receptors (beta blocker). Rather than acting directly on anxiety, it decreases some anxiety symptoms, such as increased heart rate. It is used in the treatment of Social Phobia, for such problems as performance anxiety. See Box 50-3 for a list of the non-benzodiazepine antianxiety agents.

BOX 50-3

NON-BENZODIAZEPINE ANTIANXIETY AND SEDATIVE-HYPNOTIC AGENTS

Antianxiety Agents
Classification: Azaspirone
  Generic name: Buspirone
  Trade name: (BuSpar)
Beta-Adrenergic Blockers
  Propranolol (Inderal)

Sedative-Hypnotic Agents
Imidazopyridine
  Zolpidem (Ambien)
Pyrazolopyrimidine
  Zaleplon (Sonata)
Antihistamines
  Diphenhydramine (Benadryl)

Non-Benzodiazepine Sedative-Hypnotic Agents

Zaleplon (Sonata) is a non-BZ sedative-hypnotic for the short-term treatment of insomnia. It binds to the benzodiazepine receptor and has a very rapid onset and duration of action. It is most effective for clients who have difficulty falling asleep. Clients who only have 4 hours before they have to get up can take it. It has some effects similar to the BZs: sedation and antianxiety, muscle relaxant, and anticonvulsant properties. It has no morning "hangover" effect.

Zolpidem (Ambien) is also used for short-term insomnia treatment. It is similar to Zaleplon in that it binds to BZ receptors and has fewer side effects than the BZs. This drug has a slightly longer half-life (2.5 vs. 1 hour for Zaleplon). It does not have antianxiety, anticonvulsant, or muscle-relaxant effects. It can cause daytime drowsiness, dizziness, and diarrhea.

Antihistamines, such as diphenhydramine (Benadryl), can be used for their sedating effects. Their advantage is that they do not cause dependence, although they are not as effective as the BZs. With prolonged use, clients become tolerant to the sedating side effect of antihistamines.

Barbiturates

The barbiturates, such as secobarbital and pentobarbital, are rarely used. The other sedative-hypnotic agents described earlier are more effective and safer. The barbiturates cause dependence and tolerance, they have a dangerous withdrawal syndrome, they are dangerous in overdose, and can cause fatalities due to interactions with alcohol and other CNS depressants. (For information about substance abuse and dependency, see Chapter 52. ⟳)

NURSING CARE

ASSESSING

During the nursing history, the nurse may identify that the client has a general medical condition that commonly has anxiety as a symptom. See Box 50-2 for a list of some of these disorders. In these clients, treating the general medical disorder treats anxiety symptoms. For example, if a client has anxiety symptoms due to hypoxia from an asthma attack, the treatment is her inhaler for bronchodilation, not an antianxiety medication.

The physical symptoms of anxiety usually begin with increased heart rate, blood pressure, and respiratory rate. Hildegard Peplau (1989) described four degrees or levels of anxiety, and a syndrome of symptoms that change as anxiety increases. Her idea is adapted in Table 50-2. See this table for a summary of the subjective effects and observable behavior of a person experiencing anxiety. The

---

BOX 50-4

NARRATIVE DOCUMENTATION EXAMPLE ON CLIENT WITH ANXIETY

The client is an 82-year-old woman who has been a resident of a long-term care facility for 1 year, since she had a CVA. She is unable to ambulate due to hemiplegia. She also has a diagnosis of Generalized Anxiety Disorder.

Nurse documentation on narrative notes: *Vital signs increased (HR 105, R 24, BP 154/96). Ct. was restless, unable to focus on one activity, moving items around on her bedside table repeatedly. Ct. states: "I am so nervous! I don't know what to do!" Ct. refused a back rub or music to decrease anxiety. PRN dose of Valium 2.5 mg. given 30 min. ago with good results. Ct. is working on a puzzle and states that she feels better.------------Ima Nurse, LPN*

---

nurse assesses not only whether the client has anxiety, but also the level of anxiety. (For information about assessment of mental status, see Chapter 47. ⟳)

Important assessments by nurses always include how clients respond to their illnesses and how they respond to their treatments. Nurses must document their objective findings, such as the client's vital signs and observed behaviors, as well as subjective symptoms such as the clients' statements on how they are feeling. Documentation should also include what factors cause or worsen anxiety if these are observed. In the intervention phase of the nursing process, the nurse will help the client recognize these factors that increase and decrease anxiety as a way of improving the client's insight.

Licensed nurses who are responsible for the care of clients who receive medications must know the desired effects and potential side effects of those medications. The nurse assesses the client's response to medications. See Box 50-4 ■ for an example of a narrative charting entry on a client with anxiety by a nurse that included objective and subjective assessment information and how the client responded to treatment. Note that the nurse tried nonpharmacologic interventions before medicating this client with her prn dose of diazepam.

If a client is experiencing an episode of anxiety, the client's perception of the threat represented by the situation is an important assessment. The nurse should also assess the client's use of alcohol or drugs as self-medication for anxiety at home. A history of insomnia or the regular use of medications for sleep may indicate chronic anxiety as well. Information about the client's usual coping methods can be helpful in planning care for the anxious client. See Box 50-5 ■ for some questions that might obtain information about the client's usual coping methods.

The nurse's own anxiety level is another important assessment. When the nurse is anxious, it is much easier for the client to feel anxious. Anxiety is "contagious" in this

Questions to Assess Coping Methods

"When you have a lot of stress, what do you do?"

"What do you usually do in situations like this?"

"What usually helps you when this happens?"

"Who can help you at a time like this?"

"Do you ever drink alcohol to help you through stressful times?"

"Where could you go for help?"

"What helps you get through a really bad day?"

way. Nurses need insight and enough self-understanding to know when they are anxious and what situations promote anxiety for them. Then nurses can use their own adaptive coping methods to reduce the anxiety enough to allow for a calm demeanor with the client. A calm nurse makes it easier for the client to remain calm.

DIAGNOSING, PLANNING, AND IMPLEMENTING

Anxiety is a nursing diagnosis. Nurses can diagnose and treat the symptom of anxiety independently. When a person has disabling anxiety such as in an anxiety disorder, a physician makes the diagnosis and care is collaborative. Some common nursing diagnoses for clients experiencing anxiety are *Anxiety, Ineffective Coping,* and *Post-Trauma Syndrome.*

The desired outcomes for people with anxiety are generally on three levels. First during the *acute phase* of anxiety, the desired outcomes are that the client will be free from self-inflicted harm, and will experience decreased anxiety symptoms. Second, during the *stabilization phase* of therapy, the client will begin to learn to verbalize own feelings, understand own stress response, and try new methods for anxiety reduction. Finally, *in the community* the client will develop adaptive methods for coping with stress, use support systems, and demonstrate adequate social and occupational function (Schultz & Videbeck, 2002).

Anxiety

- Assess for risk of self-harm. *People with some anxiety disorders (especially Panic Disorder and PTSD) are at risk for suicide.*
- Observe closely and provide safe environment. *People at risk for suicide require close observation, support, and no access to means of self-harm.*
- Have a calm, nonthreatening attitude while caring for client. *Anxiety is easily transmitted from one person to another. Client feels more secure when nurse is confident, calm, and nonthreatening.*

- Assure client that he or she is safe. Do not leave acutely anxious person alone. *People with high anxiety may fear for their lives. The presence of the nurse can convey a sense of protection and safety.*
- Maintain a low-stimulation environment (avoid loud noise, bright light). *Environmental stimuli can worsen anxiety because high anxiety reduces the client's ability to filter stimuli.*
- Keep communication simple and direct. *High levels of anxiety make it impossible for client to focus on anything more than brief concrete messages.*

Ineffective Coping

- Encourage client to express feelings. Therapeutic use of self by nurse. Provide time for 1:1 interaction. *Therapeutic use of self by nurse helps establish trust and the foundation for a therapeutic relationship, and 1:1 interaction provides client time to express feelings in a nonthreatening place.*
- Use therapeutic communication techniques. *Therapeutic communication techniques help client analyze own feelings and actions.*
- Help client to explore factors that lead to anxiety. *Understanding what comes before anxiety can begin the process of disarming these precipitating factors and learning to respond to them adaptively without anxiety.*
- Explore options for responding adaptively to stressors, and practice them if possible. *New coping skills can be discussed and planned first, but will be best incorporated into the client's life if an opportunity can be made to practice them.*
- Teach client to recognize anxiety as it develops and to take control of stopping the anxiety from escalating (relaxation or breathing techniques, exercise, meditation). *If clients can recognize anxiety early while they can still focus on problem solving, they can employ various techniques to reduce anxiety responses. Client preference indicates which intervention to use. Help clients recognize their own anxiety by describing client behavior and connecting it to anxious feelings. For example, the nurse could say, "I saw you pacing up and down the hall, or wringing your hands, or shaking, etc. Were you feeling nervous or anxious then?"*
- Teach the client to use progressive relaxation as a coping strategy. *Progressive relaxation is an effective technique for stress reduction. The directions for assisting the client through a progressive relaxation exercise are given in Box 50-6 ■. Note that in the directions the nurse tells the client to first tighten then relax each muscle group. The tightening serves to show the contrast between tension and relaxation. The nurse guides the client through the exercise the first time, then the client practices it alone. Finally, the client learns to use the relaxation technique when a stressful situation arises to stop the progression of anxiety.*

BOX 50-6	CLIENT TEACHING

Progressive Relaxation Exercise

Teach the client to use progressive relaxation as a way to cope with stress. Explain that progressive relaxation is an exercise involving first tightening then relaxing the major muscle groups from one end of the body to the other. This exercise can be done with the client sitting or lying down. Dim the lights. The exercise is best done with the eyes closed to enable the client to concentrate on relaxation.

The nurse reads the following:

- Take a deep breath in and hold it. Hold it in until it collects all the tension in your body, and then slowly let it out. The tension is leaving with the air. Take another slow, deep, relaxing breath. Let out the tension as you let out the air. Now breathe normally.
- Now tighten the muscles in your feet. Your toes are all tightened up. Now let them go. Wiggle the toes and let them relax. Now your calves and ankles. Point your feet up toward your head and hold them tight. Then point them to the floor and hold tight. Now wiggle your feet and relax them. They are free now. Tighten your thighs. Press them down and feel the tension. OK, shake your legs and loosen them up.
- Contract your abdomen. Hold the muscles down flat. Hold it tight. Now release. Hold your arms close to your body. Closer, tighter. Then release. Shake your arms to loosen them up. Now your hands. Tighten them into fists. Make them tight. Now let them go. Wiggle your fingers. Let them dance as they relax. Last, your mouth. Clench your teeth. Press your tongue to the roof of your mouth. Now let your tongue rest. Open your mouth and take a deep breath.
- Your whole body is relaxed now. Hold the breath in, then let it out, and with it goes that last bit of tension. You are relaxed. You can open your eyes.

Post-Trauma Syndrome

- Assess degree of anxiety or fear, and the degree of threat perceived by the client. *Understanding the client's perception is necessary for providing appropriate assistance to overcome the fear.*
- Be calm. Stay with client. *A calm demeanor on the part of the nurse will help the client feel calm. The client's feelings of danger and being threatened may be relieved by the presence of the nurse.*
- Keep communication simple. *A high level of anxiety will make it impossible for the client to process complicated information.*
- Assist client to correct any distortions of thinking. *Reality-based interactions will reinforce the safety of the hospital situation. The nurse can be the client's source of reality orientation.*

- Help client identify coping behaviors that have been useful in the past. *Client may benefit from using strategies previously found to be successful.*
- Identify supportive people in client's life. *Supportive people can help client cope with current situation and move on to live life fully after the traumatic event.*

EVALUATING

It is not the goal of the nurse to relieve all anxiety. Some anxiety is a necessary protective mechanism that allows people to be alert. Nurses try to help clients understand themselves, so they can learn new coping skills and keep anxiety at a manageable level.

Documenting. Evaluate effectiveness of nursing interventions by collecting data about and documenting the following: anxiety symptoms, client safety from self-harm, ability to demonstrate or report the use of new methods for coping with stress, ability to state plans for new adaptive coping methods, ability to state reasons for and side effects of medications for anxiety management, and client report that anxiety is reduced.

NURSING PROCESS CARE PLAN
Client with Generalized Anxiety Disorder

Mrs. Miedo is a 72-year-old Latina woman who has lived in a long-term care facility since she had a CVA 10 months ago. She was transferred to the skilled unit when she returned from the hospital to recover from surgery to repair a fractured hip. She was diagnosed with Generalized Anxiety Disorder as a young woman. She has not had severe anxiety symptoms for several years, until after the hip surgery. The nurse in the skilled unit is Eucharia.

Assessment. Mrs. Miedo's heart rate is 110, her respiratory rate is 26, and her BP is 158/98. She is oriented to person and place and is very alert, carefully watching anyone who enters her room. Her skin is pale and cool. She is having surgical pain. She is not sleeping well. When the nurse tried to teach Mrs. Miedo about her medications, she was not able to pay attention. She is restless. Her hands are always busy pulling and twisting the covers on her bed. She stated: "I don't know what to do. I am so nervous. Don't leave me." For Mrs. Miedo's anxiety, the physician ordered diazepam 5 mg PO t.i.d., and an additional 2.5 mg prn, also t.i.d.

Diagnosis. The following nursing diagnoses are established for Mrs. Miedo:

- *Pain* related to injury and surgery on hip

- *Anxiety* related to unfamiliar situation
- *Ineffective Coping* related to inadequate coping skills in new situation

Expected Outcomes. The expected outcomes for the plan care are that Mrs. Miedo will:

- Experience a manageable level of surgical pain throughout her stay in the skilled unit.
- Have reduced anxiety symptoms (VS will be within normal limits, she will state that she feels less nervous or anxious, and she will sleep at least 7 hours per night) within 2 days.
- Be able to express her feelings to the nurse and use strategies to relax herself within 1 week.

Planning and Implementation. The nurse will implement the following interventions:

- Introduce herself and asked if Mrs. Miedo has any questions about her care in the Skilled Unit.
- Give Mrs. Miedo the pain medication that the physician ordered q4h prn on a regular schedule every 4 hours instead of waiting for her to ask for it.
- Plan Mrs. Miedo's ambulation schedule so she will ambulate when the pain medication is at its peak (about 1 hour after the oral dose).
- Keep environmental stimuli to a minimum. This may include turning off the TV, turning on the radio so Mrs. Miedo can listen to music, and closing the drapes to keep out the bright light.
- Maintain a calm and confident manner with Mrs. Miedo. Keep questions short and communication concrete and simple.

- Check on Mrs. Miedo as often as possible, and assign the same nursing assistant to work with her every day.
- Assist the client with a progressive relaxation exercise.

Evaluation. When Mrs. M. took the pain medication on a regular schedule, her pain came under control very quickly. She needed less medication as time went on.

She came to trust the staff in the Skilled Unit. She was able to call the nurse when she started to feel anxious. Sometimes she needed prn diazepam, other times she responded to reassurance. She slept 8 hours each night after her pain was under control and she started taking the antianxiety medication. After 3 days she no longer needed the additional prn doses of diazepam. Her behavior indicated that she was feeling more relaxed. She smiled more, and the restlessness resolved. Her vital signs were within normal limits. Her anxiety was under control with the combination of the regular dose of diazepam and the nonpharmacologic nursing interventions. However, she was not able to do the relaxation technique independently.

Critical Thinking in the Nursing Process

1. Explain why the regular dosage of pain medication was better than the prn dosage for Mrs. Miedo in controlling both her pain and her anxiety.
2. What is the purpose of keeping the same nursing assistant on assignment to Mrs. Miedo every day?
3. What factor(s) might prevent Mrs. Miedo from doing self-relaxation exercises independently? Was this outcome realistic for Mrs. Miedo?

Note: The bibliography listings for this and all chapters have been compiled at the back of the book.

Chapter Review

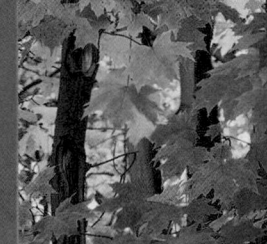

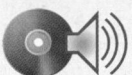 **KEY TERMS** by Topics

Use the audio glossary feature of either the CD-ROM or the Companion Website to hear the correct pronunciation of the following key terms.

Anxiety disorders
anxiety, dysphoria

Panic Disorder
obsession, compulsion

Social Phobia
phobia

Specific phobias
coping behavior, adaptive behavior, maladaptive behavior, resilience, insomnia, paradoxical response

KEY Points

- Anxiety is a universal human experience. It makes people alert to danger and more open to new learning. When it becomes so severe that it affects activities of daily living, occupational functioning, or quality of life, an anxiety disorder is present.

- Anxiety disorders are the most common psychiatric disorders in the United States, affecting 25% of the population each year.

- Many people with anxiety disorders do not seek help because they do not realize that they have a psychiatric problem, or they fear the stigma of mental illness.

- Effective medications and therapies are available to treat anxiety disorders.

- Client responses to anxiety include physiologic, behavioral, and cognitive changes.

- A calm and confident nurse is most therapeutic with anxious clients.

- Some client behaviors result in frustration, anger, and anxiety in nurses. Nurses can prevent these reactions by developing insight about how they react to client behavior.

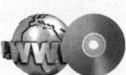 **EXPLORE MediaLink**

Additional interactive resources for this chapter can be found on the Companion Website at www.prenhall.com/burke. Click on Chapter 50 and "Begin" to select the activities for this chapter.

For chapter-related NCLEX-style review questions and an audio glossary, access the accompanying CD-ROM in this book.

FOR FURTHER Study

See Chapter 47 for more information about assessment of mental status.

See Chapter 52 to learn more about substance dependency and abuse.

Critical Thinking Care Map

Caring for a Client with Anxiety
NCLEX-PN® Focus Area: Psychosocial Integrity

Case Study: Kayla is a 22-year-old European American female client admitted to the surgical unit of a general hospital with abdominal pain. She had a cholecystectomy yesterday. She told the night nurse that she thinks she might die. She is scheduled for discharge tomorrow.

Nursing Diagnosis: Anxiety, Severe

COLLECT DATA

Subjective	Objective
_____	_____
_____	_____
_____	_____
_____	_____
_____	_____
_____	_____

Would you report this data? Yes/No

If yes, to: _____

Nursing Care

_____
_____
_____
_____
_____
_____
_____
_____
_____

How would you document this?_____
_____
_____

Data Collected
(use those that apply)

- VS: T 99°F, P 110, R 20, BP 130/86
- Client is married
- Has 1 child, age 10 months
- Client states, "Am I going to die from this?"
- Weight 152 lbs
- Skin is cool, diaphoretic
- States, "I think my incision is going to tear open."
- Client's hands are constantly moving, picking at the sheets
- Nurse stated in report: client slept approximately 3 hours last night
- Abdominal incision is well approximated, without exudate
- Nurse assesses that client has dry mouth
- Eyes are glancing around the room, darting from one thing to another
- Complains of feeling dizzy

Nursing Interventions
(use those that apply; list in priority order)

- Encourage the client to talk about her feelings.
- Accept the client as she is.
- Tell the client that she is fine, and that she should quit worrying so much.
- Acknowledge that client is anxious.
- Answer any questions the client has about her surgical incision.
- Assign a nursing assistant to sit with the client 24 hours per day.
- Keep communication simple and concrete.
- Explain the pathophysiology of cholecystitis, the procedure of cholecystectomy, and analgesic therapy in detail.
- Provide comfort measures.
- Be calm and confident with the client.
- Discuss healthy ways to talk about and relieve anxiety.
- Assess coping skills the client has used successfully in the past.
- Assess client's resources for support.
- Use progressive relaxation to help client relax.
- Give the client her prn pain medication to treat the anxiety.
- Give the client a book to read to distract her from her problems.

NCLEX-PN® Exam Preparation

1 A 30-year-old female client in the hospital emergency department is experiencing a panic attack. Select all the appropriate nursing actions for this client.

A. Restrain the client to keep her safe.
B. Assess for the risk of self-harm.
C. Have a calm approach to the client.
D. Keep communication simple.

2 A client started taking lorazepam (Ativan) for anxiety yesterday. Select all the likely side effects that the nurse will be assessing for.

A. agitation
B. sedation
C. insomnia
D. decreased muscle coordination

3 A client expresses nervousness about the MRI he will have in the morning. He is fidgeting with his sheets. The nurse's best first response to the client is to:

A. bring him his prn alprazolam (Xanax).
B. validate that you can see that he is anxious, and ask him what he thinks is the source of his "nervousness."
C. reassure him that MRIs are safe procedures and nothing to worry about.
D. turn on his television to divert his attention to something else.

4 Which of the following is a true statement about anxiety disorders?

A. People with Generalized Anxiety Disorder realize that the level of their anxiety is out of proportion to the stimulus, but they cannot control it.
B. Genetics alone is the source of anxiety disorders.
C. Antianxiety medications cause addiction and should not be used.
D. People with a higher level of intelligence are less likely to suffer from anxiety disorders than others.

5 A client diagnosed with agoraphobia has an abnormal fear of:

A. flying.
B. open spaces.
C. heights.
D. water.

6 When a nursing student starts to enter her client's room, she bursts into uncontrollable sobbing. She says that her mother died suddenly in that same room 2 months ago. This student is probably experiencing:

A. posttraumatic stress.
B. panic attack.
C. phobic attack.
D. acute stress disorder.

7 A client is being treated with cognitive-behavioral therapy for an anxiety disorder. The cognitive restructuring assists the client to:

A. avoid the situation or object that produces anxiety.
B. discuss his negative thoughts about certain anxiety-producing situations and objects.
C. replace negative self-talk with more supportive and positive self-talk.
D. accept his negative thoughts about certain situations and objects as being part of his normal life responses.

8 Select the best nursing intervention to assist the anxious client to adopt effective coping strategies.

A. Teach the client relaxation and/or deep-breathing techniques.
B. Leave the client alone to develop her own plan.
C. Provide reading material on coping strategies.
D. Tell the client what you would do in similar circumstances.

9 Which question would give the nurse the best information about the client's usual coping methods?

A. "Why did you let yourself get so sick?"
B. "What are your usual coping behaviors?"
C. "What usually helps you when things like this happen?"
D. "What do you think you should do about this?"

10 A nursing student is taking a test. He is having difficulty remembering the things he studied during the night. He is not aware of being anxious, but he is missing many questions because he is only able to focus on tiny details. His BP, pulse, and respirations are elevated. At what level is this student's anxiety?

A. mild
B. moderate
C. severe
D. panic

Answers for Review Questions, as well as discussion of Care Plan and Critical Thinking Care Map questions, appear in Appendix V.

Chapter 51

Caring for Clients with Personality Disorders

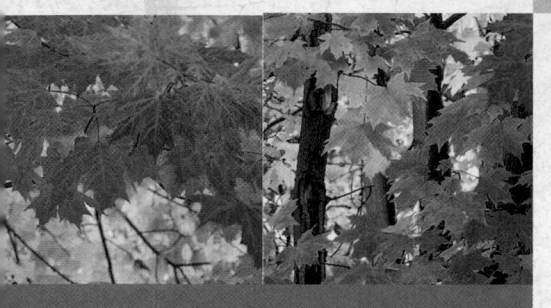

BRIEF Outline

Cluster A Personality Disorders: Odd/Eccentric
Paranoid Personality Disorder
Schizoid Personality Disorder
Schizotypal Personality Disorder

Cluster B Personality Disorders: Dramatic/Emotional/Erratic
Antisocial Personality Disorder
Borderline Personality Disorder
Histrionic Personality Disorder
Narcissistic Personality Disorder

Cluster C Personality Disorders: Anxious/Fearful
Avoidant Personality Disorder
Dependent Personality Disorder
Obsessive-Compulsive Personality Disorder

LEARNING Outcomes

After completing this chapter, you will be able to:
- Identify the major features of personality disorders.
- Perform basic client teaching about personality disorders.
- Adapt the nurse–client relationship to the special concerns of the client who has a personality disorder.
- Recognize client behaviors that are personality related.
- Apply the nursing process to clients with personality disorders.

MediaLink

www.prenhall.com/burke
Use the address above to access the free, interactive Companion Website created for this textbook. Get hints, instant feedback, and textbook references to chapter-related NCLEX-style questions. Link to other interesting sites.

Audio Glossary:
Use the Companion Website, or the CD-ROM disk enclosed with your textbook, to hear the pronunciation of key terms in this chapter.

Personality is the relatively stable way in which a person thinks, feels, and behaves. Personality includes the psychosocial traits and characteristics that make a person an individual.

Personality begins to form in early childhood and continues to develop through young adulthood. The overall pattern of personality is unique to each individual, but there are enough similarities observed in people that generalizations are possible. Personality is affected by genetic predispositions and by life experiences. It affects the defense mechanisms that each individual uses to respond to stress throughout life.

Naturally, people have a variety of different personality traits. People think, feel, and behave in various ways also. One of the strengths of the human race is our diversity.

Personality Disorders

While the normal range of human behavior, feelings, and thought is broad, it is possible for personality to be outside the normal range. A personality disorder is an enduring pattern of inner experience and behavior that has the following characteristics (American Psychiatric Association [APA], 2000):

- It deviates markedly from the expectations of the individual's culture.
- It is pervasive and inflexible.
- It begins in adolescence or young adulthood.
- It is stable over time.
- It leads to distress for the individual or impairment of functioning.

A person's personality significantly affects how this person responds to life events, including illnesses. A client's culture also affects the client's behavior and personality. Box 51-1 ■ shows the importance of considering a client's cultural background when interpreting behavior.

BOX 51-1

PERSONALITY AND CULTURE

Any judgment about a client's personality must take into account that person's ethnic, cultural, and social background. People who are immigrants from other cultures are especially at risk of being diagnosed with disorders of mental function and personality when they are acting or thinking in a way that is accepted in their culture of origin but not in their new home. For example, a Cuban immigrant stated to the nurse that her dead father talked to her and told her to be careful when talking to strangers. In the Cuban culture, "talking" with deceased people may mean the same as "This is what my father would have wanted me to do" in the Euro-American culture. The nurse can improve the cultural sensitivity of this client's care by talking with other Cuban people or learning more about the client's culture.

PATHOPHYSIOLOGY

Personality disorders are not the same as mental disorders or diseases, although people with mental disorders such as schizophrenia, Bipolar Disorder, or depression may have personality disorders as well. While there is a genetic physiologic influence on personality, such as a tendency toward anxiety or depression, these disorders are not considered physiologic.

Diagnosing personality disorders requires an evaluation of the person's long-term patterns of functioning. Personality patterns must be persistent to be significant. For a personality disorder to be present, the individual's symptoms cannot be caused by a general medical disorder or by substance abuse. The personality characteristics used for diagnosis must have persisted since the individual was an adolescent or young adult. Finally, they must be consistent over different situations (APA, 2000).

The American Psychiatric Association (2000) describes 10 specific types of personality disorders (see Table 51-1 ■). These disorders are grouped into three clusters by their similarities. The clusters are based on similar observed behaviors:

Cluster A. Odd and eccentric
Cluster B. Dramatic and emotional
Cluster C. Anxiety- and fear-based personality disorders.

MANIFESTATIONS

Impaired self-identity is a central problem in disorders of personality. Self-identity is a part of normal personality development. It includes an integration of social and occupational roles, chosen values and behaviors, gender roles, beliefs about sexuality and intimacy, goals, and political and religious beliefs. An adequately formed identity is necessary for goal-directed behavior and for satisfying interpersonal relationships. Self-identity is often minimal

---

TABLE 51-1

Personality Disorders by Cluster

CLUSTER	PERSONALITY DISORDER
A: Odd/eccentric	Paranoid Personality Disorder Schizoid Personality Disorder Schizotypal Personality Disorder
B: Dramatic/emotional	Antisocial Personality Disorder Borderline Personality Disorder Histrionic Personality Disorder Narcissistic Personality Disorder
C: Anxious/fearful	Avoidant Personality Disorder Dependent Personality Disorder Obsessive-Compulsive Personality Disorder

Source: From American Psychiatric Association. (2000). *Diagnostic and Statistical Manual of Mental Disorders* (4th ed., text revision). Washington, DC: Author.

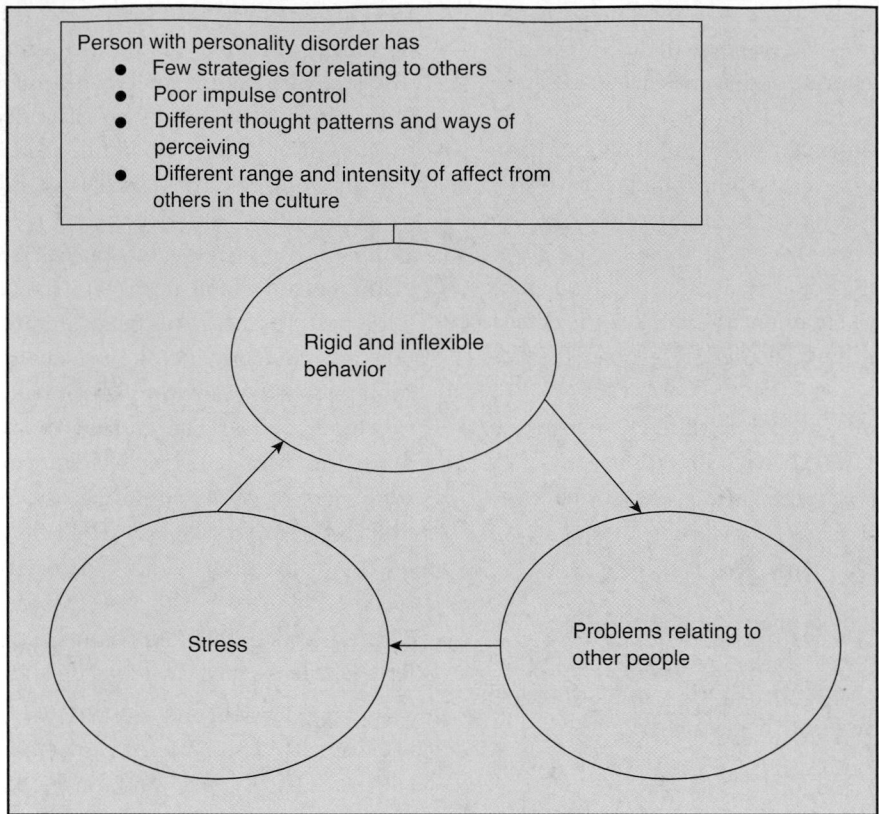

Figure 51-1. ■ Vicious cycle of personality disorders.

or absent in personality disorders (Limandri & Boyd, 2002).

Thinking patterns are distorted in personality disorders. The individual's ability to decode stimuli and to interpret environmental events is impaired. Maladaptive thinking patterns cause individuals to misinterpret the actions of others. The misinterpretations result in maladaptive responses by the affected person.

Emotions, in their intensity and quality, appear to be affected by disorders of personality. People affected by personality disorders have blunted or distorted emotional experiences. They tend to have more negative emotional experiences. Their ability to function in daily life and even to learn new things is affected.

Behavior is also affected by personality disorders. First, personality disorders cause *impulsive behavior*. These disorders appear to make it more difficult for people to foresee the consequences of their actions, or to control their impulses despite probable negative consequences.

Second, these disorders cause *inflexibility of behavior*. Affected people tend to be rigid. They are unable to change their usual behavior when circumstances suggest that a change is indicated. Normally, people learn to change their behavior when they try new behaviors and receive positive reinforcement from the new approach. The inflexibility in personality disorders makes it difficult for people to learn new ways to behave or cope.

This inflexibility traps the client in vicious cycles of behavior that are self-defeating. They become rigid and inflexible in role functions and personal interactions. The inflexibility provokes predicaments and problems. They continue to be inflexible, which creates more problems. The more inflexible they are, the more problems they have. The more problems they have, the more inflexible they are. This self-perpetuating circle reduces learning opportunities and alienates other people (Millon & Davis, 1999). See Figure 51-1 ■ for a diagram of this vicious cycle.

INTERDISCIPLINARY CARE

Personality disorders are difficult to treat, because personality is resistant to change. There are no medications that affect personality directly. Cognitive-behavioral therapy helps many people, but it takes time, commitment, and insight on the part of the client. Many people with personality disorders lack the insight to realize that they have a problem. Personality traits of "agreeableness" and "conscientiousness" tend to make people more responsive to therapy for disorders of personality. People usually do not seek treatment for personality disorders. These clients are seen in a variety of settings being treated for other things.

Medications

Pharmacologic treatment of personality disorders is based on treating specific target symptoms rather than the disorder itself. Antidepressants and mood stabilizing drugs are often used to treat symptoms of depression of mood lability. Antipsychotic drugs may be useful if a client experiences psychosis, which is occasionally a symptom in severe situations.

NURSING CARE

Often nurses find it frustrating to work with clients who have disorders of personality. These clients can be manipulative, socially inappropriate, and difficult. Over time these people have developed maladaptive methods of coping with life. Clients can control their behavior, but it is not within the ability of these clients to change their personalities completely. For these reasons, such clients need all the patience and skill nurses have to offer. Remember that the goal of the nurse is to provide professional care, not to be the friend of the client.

To work effectively with clients with personality disorders, nurses must understand themselves first. Nurses must have the insight to know what type of behavior causes them stress, so they can manage their own stress without giving it back to the client. Direct communication with clear expectations for client behavior, and clear and consistent limits, is important for these clients. Maladaptive behavior by these clients is a symptom of their disorders. Objective understanding of personality disorders will help nurses take an objective approach to client care.

Cluster A Personality Disorders: Odd/Eccentric

PARANOID PERSONALITY DISORDER

Paranoid Personality Disorder is a pattern of distrust and suspiciousness that other people are acting maliciously toward the affected individual. On the basis of imagined evidence, they may think that people are plotting against them or may attack them without reason. They may fight back when their victim never attacked in the first place. People with Paranoid Personality Disorder often imagine hidden threatening or demeaning messages in innocent remarks or actions. They find it difficult to forgive, and they hold grudges (APA, 2000).

Difficulty with interpersonal relationships is a hallmark of this disorder. Affected people tend to be so vigilant to the malicious intentions of others that they cannot form mutually satisfying relationships. They may form relationships in which they are in power or control. Paranoid Personality Disorder causes people to interpret the actions of others as deception and betrayal. They especially distrust the faithfulness or trustworthiness of a partner or friend (Millon & Davis, 1999).

This disorder causes a hostile and defensive nature. When the client's hostility arouses a hostile response in others, the suspicion that others are against the affected person is confirmed (APA, 2000).

Although people with paranoia may appear to be aggressive, their inner feelings are often fear and insecurity. These feelings often respond to reassurance about the person's safety. These clients are very aware of power relationships. They may respond better to information directly from the physician or charge nurse rather than from the staff nurse.

SCHIZOID PERSONALITY DISORDER

The most important features of Schizoid Personality Disorder are a pervasive pattern of detachment from social relationships and a restricted range of emotional expression (affect). People with this disorder of personality appear to receive little satisfaction from being part of a family or group. They prefer to be alone, and even choose hobbies that can be done in isolation from other people. They have little interest in sexual or other intimate relationships. They lack friends, and they appear indifferent to the opinions of others. People with Schizoid Personality Disorder rarely experience strong emotions such as anger or joy. They may only confide in their parents or sisters and brothers (APA, 2000).

Schizoid Personality Disorder may cause impairment in occupational as well as social functioning, unless the affected individual can find a suitable job working alone. Affected people find pleasure in few if any activities.

SCHIZOTYPAL PERSONALITY DISORDER

People with Schizotypal Personality Disorder have a consistent pattern of interpersonal deficits. They have discomfort in and reduced capacity for close relationships. They also have cognitive (thinking) or perceptual distortions, and eccentric behavior. The cognitive deficit may be **ideas of reference**, in which clients misinterpret everyday events as having a personal meaning for them. For example, the client may believe that her thoughts about the plants being dry caused it to rain, or that the arrival of the bus at exactly this moment is because she thought about it coming (APA, 2000).

People with Schizotypal Personality Disorder may be superstitious or preoccupied with paranormal activity that is outside the realm of belief of their culture, such as clairvoyance, telepathy, or mind reading. Their thinking and speech are likely to be odd. They may have suspicious or paranoid thoughts. Affect is likely to be restricted or inappropriate. **Inappropriate affect** occurs when the client has an emotional response that is not culturally appropriate for the situation, such as laughing when someone's pet dies. The behavior and appearance of affected people are also likely to be eccentric or peculiar. These clients will probably not have friends. They have excessive social anxiety that does not resolve as people become more familiar. Their social anxiety is more likely to be due to paranoid fears than to negative ideas about themselves (APA, 2000).

INTERDISCIPLINARY CARE

Because personality is such an integral part of the individual's identity, health care providers cannot simply identify a problem, plan an intervention, and make personality changes. Realistic short-term outcomes should be identified. For people affected by the odd/eccentric personality disorders, these outcomes will be related to small changes in thinking patterns and behavior, such as realistic interpretation of events, taking medications, eating meals, and cooperating with treatment. The long-term treatment goals for these clients are improved social skills, reality-based thinking, increased flexibility, and trust.

Social skills training can help these clients behave in more socially appropriate ways, thus making it easier for them to interact in the community. Often these clients do not enjoy being with other people. Still they require enough interpersonal contact to keep them oriented to reality, but not so much that they cannot cope.

NURSING CARE

ASSESSING

Priorities in Nursing Care. Collect subjective and objective data about the client's mental status (see Chapter 47). ⚭ Observe and describe the client's verbal and nonverbal behavior objectively in the chart. Pay particular attention to the client's anxiety level and ability to cooperate with others. Ask about medications the client takes at home.

DIAGNOSING, PLANNING, AND IMPLEMENTING

Table 51-2 ■ provides common nursing diagnoses for people with specific personality disorders, divided by cluster.

Disturbed Thought Processes

- Do not ignore the client's suspicions, but do not overemphasize the fears of the client either. If the client is re-

---

TABLE 51-2

Common Nursing Diagnoses for People with Personality Disorders

CLUSTER A: ODD/ECCENTRIC DISORDERS	CLUSTER B: DRAMATIC/EMOTIONAL DISORDERS	CLUSTER C: ANXIOUS/FEARFUL DISORDERS
Paranoid Personality Disorder ■ Defensive Coping ■ Disturbed Thought Processes ■ Impaired Social Interaction	**Antisocial Personality Disorder** ■ Risk for Other-Directed Violence ■ Ineffective Coping ■ Noncompliance (specify) ■ Impaired Social Interaction	**Avoidant Personality Disorder** ■ Chronic Low Self-Esteem ■ Social Isolation ■ Ineffective Coping
Schizoid and Schizotypal Personality Disorders ■ Impaired Social Interaction ■ Chronic Low Self-Esteem ■ Disturbed Thought Processes	**Borderline Personality Disorder** ■ Risk for Self-Mutilation ■ Risk for Other-Directed Violence ■ Ineffective Coping ■ Noncompliance (specify) ■ Chronic Low Self-Esteem ■ Risk for Suicide ■ Social Isolation	**Dependent Personality Disorder** ■ Ineffective Coping ■ Chronic Low Self-Esteem ■ Impaired Social Interaction ■ Social Isolation ■ Powerlessness
	Histrionic Personality Disorder ■ Ineffective Coping ■ Chronic Low Self-Esteem ■ Impaired Social Interaction	**Obsessive-Compulsive Personality Disorder** ■ Anxiety ■ Impaired Social Interaction ■ Ineffective Coping
	Narcissistic Personality Disorder ■ Impaired Social Interaction ■ Ineffective coping	

questing complicated confirmation that the medications are his, the nurse should respectfully and briefly reassure him that they are the correct medications, but not engage in any elaborate unnecessary plans. *Suspiciousness about medications or food being poisoned is common in these types of disorders. It may be enough to tell the client confidently that the nurse checked these medications personally, and they are accurate. The nurse could bring the medications still wrapped in their individual dose wrappers to reassure the client that they are the correct medications. When the reason for a client's suspiciousness is paranoia, excessive and elaborate proof (bringing in the client's chart with every medication, calling the pharmacist, etc.) does not really help.*

- Approach this client with a matter-of-fact, professional attitude. *Suspicious/paranoid clients will not respond to a friendly approach by the nurse, and may misinterpret friendliness as weakness or deceit.*

- Reassure clients that they are safe and that the staff is making every effort to provide accurate, quality care for them. *The nurse's confidence may be reassuring to the client. People with paranoia seem to be aggressive, but their feelings are often based on fear and insecurity.*

- Adhere strictly to the rules of the organization (such as visiting hours, medication times). *Any exceptions may appear to the client to have a devious intent. Strict adherence may be reassuring that there are limits in which the client is safe.*

- Try some corrective statements. Box 51-2 ■ gives examples of how to adjust unfounded observations toward more realistic thinking.

Impaired Social Interaction

- Make interpersonal interactions with the client brief and nonthreatening. *Clients who feel suspicious usually feel uncomfortable around other people. They need to interact with others to maintain mental health. Brief interactions may be easier to tolerate.*

- Assign consistent staff to work with this client. *Consistent one-to-one relationships promote the client's ability to form trust.*

- Provide low-stress opportunities for clients to be with other people, such as eating at a table with others at mealtime. *The client may not really want to socialize with other people, but the nurse knows that some contact with other people is important for mental health.*

- Provide some social skills training, such as redirecting behavior that is socially inappropriate. *If the client dresses or behaves in ways that the other clients accept, she or he may be more accepted.*

EVALUATING

Collect the following data to determine whether the client is achieving nursing care outcomes: how the client interacts with others, verbal and nonverbal behavior, and anxiety level.

BOX 51-2

CORRECTIVE STATEMENTS FOR DISTORTED THOUGHTS

Thought Distortion: "This is the worst thing that has ever happened."
Corrective Statement: "True, this is a bad thing, but it is not the worst thing that ever happened." (*Giving perspective allows client to see the real placement of this stressful event as it relates to life priorities.*)

Thought Distortion: "I could NEVER do anything so difficult."
Corrective Statement: "You have already done challenging things like this before, such as..." (*Giving examples makes the implied generalization specific.*)

Thought Distortion: "If only I hadn't made him mad, he wouldn't have beat me up."
Corrective Statement: "He is an adult and responsible for his own behavior. You are responsible for your own behavior, not his. (*Stating the mature reality of the situation helps the client see it from another point of view.*)

Thought Distortion: "My boyfriend left me. This will kill me. I can't go on."
Corrective Statement: "You have survived disappointments before. You are strong enough to handle this. Let's talk about how you feel." (*Allowing client to discuss and examine feelings increases insight and promotes the ability to learn from past experiences and to apply current learning to future situations.*)

Thought Distortion: "Nobody understands me."
Corrective Statement: "Let's talk about how you feel, so I can understand." (*Suggesting a problem-solving approach promotes adaptive coping.*)

Documenting. Document statements that indicate the client's thought processes, such as "Leave the light on. I want to see if anyone is coming to get me" or "There is too much going on here. Get me out."

Cluster B Personality Disorders: Dramatic/Emotional/Erratic

ANTISOCIAL PERSONALITY DISORDER

The essential characteristic of **Antisocial Personality Disorder** is a pervasive pattern of disregarding and violating the rights of others. To receive this diagnosis, clients must be at least 18 years old. They must have had Conduct Disorder in childhood by the age of 15. Conduct Disorder includes cruelty to people or animals, deceitfulness or theft, destruction of property, and serious violations of rules (APA, 2000).

People with Antisocial Personality Disorder tend to disregard societal expectations by breaking the law. For example, they may destroy the property of others, harass others, steal, or engage in illegal occupations (drug dealing, dog fighting, selling stolen property). People with this disorder manipulate others for their personal gain or pleasure (for money, sex, and power). They disregard the rights, feelings, and safety of others (APA, 2000).

Impulsiveness is a major feature of Antisocial Personality Disorder. People with this disorder make decisions suddenly, without planning ahead or considering the possible consequences. This leads to frequent change of jobs, residences, and relationships. People with this disorder tend to be aggressive and irritable. They may fight repeatedly or assault others frequently, including partners and children. Affected people may be friendly and likable until they are frustrated. This disorder results in disregard for the safety of self or others. Fast, reckless driving, substance use, or irresponsible sexual behavior may illustrate this aspect of the disorder (APA, 2000).

Affected people are irresponsible in all aspects of their lives: family, employment, interpersonal relationships, and finances. They live in the moment, not concerned with the past or the future. Rules are made for other people, not for them.

People with Antisocial Personality Disorder show little remorse for the negative consequences of their behavior. They may believe that they should do anything necessary to ensure that others will not control them. These clients often blame their victims for weakness or foolishness, without any guilt or sorrow over their suffering or loss (APA, 2000).

Approximately 1% of females are affected with Antisocial Personality Disorder, whereas 3% of males have the disorder. Nurses will encounter clients with this disorder much more often in substance abuse treatment or in *forensic* (legal) settings, such as prison (APA, 2000).

BORDERLINE PERSONALITY DISORDER

A psychoanalyst named Stern first used the term *borderline personality* in 1938. He was describing clients who seem to be on the border between anxiety and psychosis.

Marsha Linehan is a leading contemporary theorist on Borderline Personality Disorder. She and her colleagues believe that the disorder is caused by an interaction between biologic and social learning influences (nature and nurture). Their research focuses on the behavior patterns in the disorder, which include the following (Linehan, 1993; Koerner & Linehan, 2000):

- *Emotional vulnerability:* a pattern of difficulty managing negative emotions; high sensitivity to negative emotional stimuli; and slower than normal return to baseline emotional level than the average person
- *Self-invalidation:* failure to recognize own emotions, thoughts, behaviors; setting unrealistically high expectations for self; makes it impossible for self to be successful; intense shame and self-directed anger; and blames others for unrealistic expectations because client has no insight

- *Unrelenting crises:* experiences frequent, stressful negative events, some caused by self, others not
- *Inhibited grieving:* tries to over-control negative feelings, especially those associated with grieving such as guilt, sadness, shame, and anxiety
- *Active passivity:* affected person fails to work actively on solving own life problems; actively seeks help from others for problem solving, resulting in learned helplessness and hopelessness
- *Apparent competence:* tends to appear to be more competent than he or she really is; may be unable to apply what is learned in one situation to other situations; may fail to display nonverbal cues of early emotional distress.

The biosocial theorists propose that Borderline Personality Disorder occurs when a vulnerable individual interacts with an invalidating environment. An invalidating environment is one in which the individual's feelings and emotions are negated, disrespected, or punished. The invalidating environment is often abusive. The ultimate invalidation is sexual abuse, which is a common experience of people with the disorder (Linehan, 1993; Zanarini, 2000).

Manifestations

Borderline Personality Disorder includes a pattern of impulsiveness and instability in interpersonal relationships, self-image, and emotions. These symptoms begin by early adulthood and are present in a variety of contexts. Affected people have intense fear of abandonment. They make frantic efforts to avoid real or imagined abandonment by others. Being left by others may suggest to people with Borderline Personality Disorder that they are bad. They experience intense fears and inappropriate anger even when faced with expected separations (such as when a friend goes on vacation, someone is late for an appointment, or a favorite nurse has a day off work). Clients may even injure themselves in an effort to prevent abandonment (APA, 2000).

Affected people have a pattern of intense and unstable relationships. They may begin by idealizing a potential friend or partner, spending extensive amounts of time with them, and confiding their innermost thoughts early in the relationship. Then they might unexpectedly change to devaluing the person, saying that the formerly "perfect" friend or mate does not care enough. People with this disorder are able to cultivate relationships with others. However, they expect that the others will provide nurturance and be there to meet their considerable needs, on demand, at any moment (APA, 2000).

Borderline Personality Disorder is also characterized by an unstable self-image or sense of self. Life goals, plans, values, sexual identity, and friends may change abruptly and impulsively. The self-image of affected people is based on the feeling that they are bad. They may also have the sense

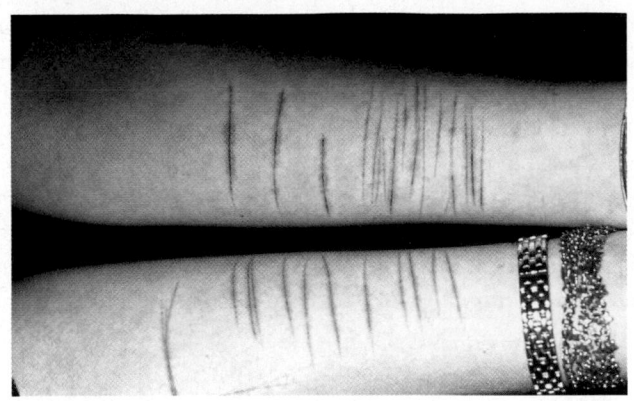

Figure 51-2. ■ Self-injury is sometimes used as a coping mechanism by clients with Borderline Personality Disorder.

that they do not exist at all, or that they have no feelings. This is most likely to occur when they are feeling a lack of support. People with this disorder respond best to a predictable, structured environment (APA, 2000).

Impulsivity is another hallmark of Borderline Personality Disorder. The diagnosis requires impulsivity in at least two areas that are potentially self-damaging (such as gambling, spending money irresponsibly, binge eating, unsafe sex, abusing substances, or self-injuring behavior) (APA, 2000).

Self-harm occurs in the majority of people with Borderline Personality Disorder. Completed suicide occurs in 8% to 10% of affected people. Self-injury without suicide intent, such as cutting, scratching, or burning self, occurs much more frequently (Figure 51-2 ■). Behavior aimed at harming but not killing oneself is called **parasuicidal behavior** (Linehan, 1993). While health professionals see parasuicidal behavior as a problem, clients with Borderline Personality Disorder tend to see it as a solution. While these clients do not enjoy hurting themselves, the pain becomes a mechanism for coping (Warner, 2004).

People with Borderline Personality Disorder also experience unstable emotions. Their baseline low mood is often interrupted with episodes of anger, panic, or despair. They rarely have periods of well-being or satisfaction. These clients often express intense or inappropriate anger, or have difficulty controlling their anger. They may have sarcastic or bitter outbursts. Inappropriate angry outbursts are often followed by shame and guilt, and contribute to the affected person's feeling of being bad or evil (APA, 2000).

Borderline Personality Disorder is much more common in women than in men, with women making up 75% of cases. It is estimated that 2% of the general population is affected, and 20% of psychiatric inpatients. Borderline Personality Disorder is five times more common among first-degree relatives of affected people than it is in the general population. There is also an increase in substance-related

disorders, Antisocial Personality Disorder, and mood disorders among family members (APA, 2000).

HISTRIONIC PERSONALITY DISORDER

The most important features of Histrionic Personality Disorder are excessive emotionality and attention-seeking behavior. People with Histrionic Personality Disorder need to be the center of attention. When they are not, they are uncomfortable or unhappy. They will often create a scene to bring attention to themselves (APA, 2000).

The appearance of affected individuals is often inappropriately sexually provocative. Affected people often behave seductively in social, work, and other settings. Their seductive behavior is beyond what is socially appropriate for the setting. Their emotional expression may be shallow and changeable. Affected people use physical appearance to draw attention to themselves. They spend inordinate time, energy, and money on clothes, jewelry, and grooming. Unflattering comments easily upset these people (APA, 2000).

Their speech is lacking in detail and excessively *impressionistic* (gives a general impression without evidence). An example of impressionistic speech is "He is the greatest man in the world" with no reason given for the greatness. Affected people have strong opinions and express them dramatically, yet there is rarely any foundation for the opinion. Their emotions are exaggerated theatrically. They may embarrass friends and acquaintances by being too intimate, sobbing uncontrollably over minor sentiments, or having temper tantrums. The emotions, though dramatic, are turned on and off quickly and may seem insincere (APA, 2000).

People with Histrionic Personality Disorder are very suggestible and easily influenced by others. They may be overly trusting, especially of authority figures. They often consider relationships to be more intimate than they really are. They have difficulty achieving close relationships. They may act dependent, while trying to control their partners with emotional manipulation. Affected people often alienate friends with their demands for attention. They may crave novelty and excitement. They have little tolerance for frustration or delayed gratification (APA, 2000).

Gender role stereotypes can affect the way people express this disorder. For example, a man with Histrionic Personality Disorder may spend lots of time bodybuilding, buy a sports car that he cannot afford, and exaggerate his sexual exploits. An affected woman may dress in seductive clothes, demand that her friends admire her new outfits, and exaggerate what a "dear friend" some important person is.

NARCISSISTIC PERSONALITY DISORDER

Narcissistic Personality Disorder is characterized by a pervasive pattern of grandiosity, need for admiration, and lack of empathy for others. Affected people have an inflated sense of self-importance. They routinely overestimate their abilities and inflate their accomplishments. They expect that others will have the same high opinion of them. They may be surprised if they do not receive the fame and fortune they think they deserve. While these clients inflate their own abilities, they tend to underestimate the abilities of others (APA, 2000).

People with Narcissistic Personality Disorder often have fantasies of unlimited success, power, beauty, or ideal love, and compare themselves with famous people. Affected people see themselves as superior to others and expect to be so recognized. They prefer to associate with other "special" people like themselves, and may ask to see the head surgeon, head nurse, or head hairdresser. Only the best is good enough. People with this disorder require excessive admiration and have a sense of entitlement. They feel entitled to especially favorable treatment and automatic compliance with their wishes (APA, 2000).

Affected people tend to exploit others, and have little empathy for others' feelings. They present an emotional coldness and lack of reciprocal interest. Narcissistic Personality Disorder causes people to have arrogant, conceited behavior and attitudes. These people are often envious of others, or believe that others are envious of them. They are quick to criticize, yet hate to be criticized. Their interpersonal relationships are usually impaired due to their insensitivity to others' feelings, their need for constant admiration, and the problems with entitlement. Many people with this disorder also have depression, eating disorders, and substance-related disorders.

INTERDISCIPLINARY CARE

The priority short-term goal for clients with Antisocial Personality Disorder is no harm to others. This client may be manipulative and physically violent, so these issues should be managed first. Other issues include anger management, coping skills, increasing self-awareness (insight) and learning to see an event from another person's point of view. The best personal approach to a client with this disorder is the most direct one. Nurses should tell the truth, clearly and concisely. The nurse should share perceptions about the emotional consequences of the client's behavior for others. Group therapy may help clients understand others' feelings. The staff must cooperate to consistently apply the treatment plan and facility policies.

The treatment priority for clients with Borderline Personality Disorder is no self-harm. Other treatment issues are dysfunctional mood and impulsive behavior. Treatment of this disorder is long term. It involves a treatment team of professionals (nurses, psychiatrist, social worker, psychologist, therapists) and the client working together.

Dialectical behavior therapy (DBT) (Linehan, 1993) is an approach to treating Borderline Personality Disorder that combines cognitive and behavioral therapies. In DBT treatment techniques include psychologic education, problem solving, monitoring moods, meditation, and social skills training. Clients actively practice new behaviors for coping and social skills.

Clients who use self-harming behavior for coping may benefit from alternative choices of behaviors to cope with their stress. The following are some suggestions for "things to try instead of hurting yourself" (Warner, 2004):

- Talk to someone.
- Delay your decision for 5 minutes.
- Hold an ice cube in each hand for 10 minutes.
- Put your hands in a bucket of ice water for 5 minutes.
- Take a hot or cold shower.
- Call a crisis line.
- Mark your arm with red lipstick.
- Yell, scream, or cry.
- Sing very loudly.
- Find a playground and swing as high as you can.
- Count things (ceiling tiles, colors, etc.).
- Masturbate.
- Pound on your bed until you are exhausted.

People with Histrionic Personality Disorder may seek out others to complete their lives and to take care of them. The treatment goal is for clients to begin to focus on themselves for problem solving, rather than expecting others to fulfill all their needs (Limandri & Boyd, 2002).

Clients with Narcissistic Personality Disorder are arrogant and have poor social skills. Treatment goals for them include developing coping skills that involve independent problem solving without exploitation of others.

NURSING CARE

ASSESSING

This group of personality disorders puts clients at risk for violence to themselves (Borderline Personality) and violence toward others (Antisocial Personality). Collect data about these clients' mental status and behavior. Document client behavior specifically and objectively. For example, "Client is difficult and inappropriate" is subjective and unspecific. A better note would be, "Client states 'I can't possibly take this medication unless the chief of surgery brings it to me.'"

DIAGNOSING, PLANNING, AND IMPLEMENTING

Sometimes clients with personality disorders in this group can disrupt an entire nursing unit with their behavior. See Box 51-3 ■ for strategies for preventing these clients from upsetting the unit.

BOX 51-3	NURSING CARE CHECKLIST

Preventing Personality Disordered Clients from Upsetting the Unit

☑ Make the unit rules clear. *People with some personality disorders (such as Antisocial, Borderline, Histrionic, and Narcissistic) may not have adaptive social and coping skills. They may be practiced in manipulating people in charge to give them exceptions to the rules. They may not believe that the rules are for them.*

Example: Unit policy is that televisions are turned off at 10 P.M. A client wants to watch TV until 3 A.M. "just this once."

☑ Stick to the rules consistently. This means everybody. *When staff responds to the manipulative client inconsistently, there is opportunity for the client to pit the staff against each other.*

Example: A client asked a nurse if he could have his pain medication a little bit early. The nurse gave it 30 minutes before it was scheduled. He asked the next nurse to do the same thing. She refused. The client told the first nurse that she is his favorite and that he only wants her to care for him, not the mean nurse who won't help him with his pain. Now the client wants the nurse to give him "just a little extra medicine, just this once, I really need it." Some of the nurses sympathize with the client's apparent pain, others think he is manipulative, and the entire unit is upset.

☑ When a client is causing staff to be upset, have a conference. *In the above situation, some nurses think one thing, others think another, and still others are unaware that there is a controversy. The client is treated differently each shift. The client is focusing on manipulating the staff, and the staff is focusing on controlling the client's behavior. When everyone works together and receives the same information (including the client), the client is best served.*

Example: A systematic approach to the situation would include an assessment of the client's problem (pain) with an appropriate prescription by the physician; an around-the-clock dosing schedule instead of prn doses so the client does not need to ask for the medication, it will automatically be given; adherence to the schedule by all nurses in the same way; feedback from the client about how pain is managed.

☑ Include the client in problem solving. *When a client's behavior is problematic, the client has an opportunity to learn how to change to more adaptive behavior only if the client is included in discussions of problem-solving strategies. Clients with personality disorders can benefit from discussions of how their behavior affects others because they often do not understand others' perspectives.*

Example: A client asks every staff member to give him coffee. He is drinking 20 cups of coffee a day. His nurse realizes this and tells the rest of the staff to limit the coffee. The client continues to ask and sometimes he receives coffee, other times he doesn't. He asks for coffee 50 times a day. When the client is included in the discussion and is told that he will be given three cups of regular coffee and three cups of decaffeinated coffee each day, and that he can choose when he drinks them, he limits his requests to the designated times.

☑ Remember who is the client and who is the professional. *It is easy to react emotionally when clients act inappropriately or make personal comments. When clients flatter or insult nurses, it is challenging not to respond personally, but it is critical for nurses to respond to clients professionally. The goal is not a friendship with the client, but professional client care. Maladaptive behavior by the client is a learning opportunity.*

Example: A client stated: "I don't want that fat one to be my nurse. I want my favorite nurse." A good response by the nurse is: "Your nurse is Jack. When you talk like that, it hurts people's feelings. How could you ask for what you want in a nicer way?"

Risk for Self-Directed Violence

- Help the client identify early internal cues of distress (such as pounding heart, sense of uneasiness, nervousness, etc.). *Identifying the symptoms of distress early can allow the client time to respond in an adaptive way.*
- Write the cues of distress listed by the client on a card and give it to the client (or the client can write the list on a card herself). *The client can refer to the card later in a time of distress.*
- Teach the client skills for tolerating a stressful event. The mnemonic "Wise mind ACCEPTS" can help the client remember new coping behaviors:
  - **A**ctivities to distract from stress
  - **C**ontributing to others such as volunteering or visiting a sick neighbor

- **C**omparing yourself to people less fortunate than you
- **E**motions that are opposite of what you are experiencing
- **P**ushing away from the situation for a while
- **T**houghts other than you are currently thinking
- **S**ensations that are intense, such as holding ice in your hand.

During a stressful situation, the client is not likely to be able to try new coping behaviors unless there has been advance planning.

- Use the five senses exercise to help people who have used self-harm for coping to find more enduring and adaptive ways to comfort themselves (Linehan, 1993). The five senses exercise follows:

  1. *Vision* (for example, go outside and look at the stars or flowers or autumn leaves)

2. *Hearing* (for example, listen to beautiful or invigorating music or the sounds of nature or the city)
3. *Smell* (for example, light a scented candle, boil a cinnamon stick in water)
4. *Taste* (for example, drink a soothing, warm nonalcoholic drink)
5. *Touch* (for example, take a hot bubble bath, pet your dog or cat, get a massage).

■ Tell all clients who have thoughts about self-harm or suicide to notify the staff if they feel like hurting themselves. An agreement to notify staff of thoughts of self-harm is called a "no self-harm" contract. Some nurses write out a statement for the client to sign that says, "I promise that if I feel like hurting myself I will tell the staff before I do it." *The idea is that clients are stating that they are in control of their own behavior. When the client tells the nurse of these feelings, the nurse will begin by encouraging the client to talk about and examine the feelings that led to the self-harm thinking. Alternatives to self-harm are then discussed. The nurse documents the conversation and reports it to the treatment team.*

Risk for Other-Directed Violence

■ Observe the client for increasing agitation or frustration. *These are the usual precursors to acting out violently (either physically or emotionally).*

■ If clients become agitated, direct them away from others into their rooms. *The reduction in sensory stimulation or removal from a frustrating stimulus may help the client regain control. This action may help the client learn the coping mechanism of seeking a quiet place.*

■ Do not tolerate verbal abuse. Calmly redirect the client, or state that the behavior is not acceptable. *Verbal abuse may precede violent acting out. Illness is not an excuse for abusing others verbally or otherwise. Clients benefit from the reminder of what appropriate behavior is and from the expectation that they can control themselves.*

■ Apply the rules consistently. *When clients use manipulation to get staff to change the rules for them, other staff members who uphold the rules are at risk of disapproval or targeting by antisocial clients.*

■ When a client is violent, get help. *When all talk-related and prn medication interventions have been tried, if a client is acting out the nurse should obtain help from the emergency response team, hospital security personnel, or the police.*

Cluster C Personality Disorders: Anxious/Fearful

AVOIDANT PERSONALITY DISORDER

People with Avoidant Personality Disorder have a pervasive pattern of social shyness, feelings of inadequacy, and hypersensitivity to negative evaluation. Because they fear disapproval or rejection, they avoid work or school activities that involve significant contact with other people. They assume other people to be critical and disapproving. Affected people would like to have social relationships, but they hesitate to join in social activities. They are preoccupied with thoughts of being criticized or rejected. They view themselves as socially inept, unappealing, or inferior. Their self-esteem is very low. They limit themselves in intimate relationships due to the fear of shame or ridicule. They are unusually reluctant to engage in new activities because of the chance of embarrassment. They may have a fearful and tense manner (APA, 2000).

In contrast to other personality disorders in which affected people have no desire to socialize with others, people with Avoidant Personality Disorder want to have contact with other people but find themselves unable to take the risk of rejection.

DEPENDENT PERSONALITY DISORDER

A need to be taken care of characterizes Dependent Personality Disorder. People with this disorder have submissive and clinging behavior; they fear separation and abandonment. They have difficulty making everyday decisions without excessive help and advice from others. They are passive and allow others to take responsibility for major areas of their lives. They have difficulty expressing disagreement due to fear of loss of support or approval. Doing things independently is difficult for these people because they have so little self-confidence. Dependent Personality Disorder is one of the most common disorders seen in mental health clinics (APA, 2000).

Affected people may fear abandonment so much that they will act as though they are incompetent and in need of help just to maintain the support of others. They submit to the will of others, even if the demands are unreasonable. They make great self-sacrifices and submit to abuse, even though other choices are available. When they are alone, affected individuals feel fearful and helpless because they feel unable to take care of themselves (APA, 2000).

People with Dependent Personality Disorder are preoccupied with the fear of being forced to take care of themselves. Even when there are no grounds to justify these fears, they have excessive and unrealistic fears of abandonment. These individuals have a pessimistic outlook and tend to minimize their own abilities and strengths. Their social relationships are limited to the few people on whom the individual is dependent (APA, 2000).

Like the other personality disorders, Dependent Personality Disorder is difficult to diagnose across cultures. The degree of dependent behavior that is considered normal varies across ages and cultures. So, the cultural expectations of the client must be considered when interpreting the client's behavior. An individual must have dependency behavior clearly in excess of what is expected by her or his culture to be diagnosed with this disorder (APA, 2000).

OBSESSIVE-COMPULSIVE PERSONALITY DISORDER

Obsessive-Compulsive Personality Disorder is characterized by a preoccupation with orderliness, perfectionism, and mental and personal control. Affected individuals prioritize orderliness and control so much that they cannot be flexible, open, or efficient. People with this disorder try to maintain a sense of control through painstaking attention to rules, trivial details, lists, and schedules, until the main point of the project is lost. Extraordinary attention is paid to detail and to checking repeatedly for possible mistakes. Affected people are oblivious to the fact that other people find the delays caused by their behavior to be aggravating. They expect themselves to be perfect. When this is not possible, it causes significant stress. They may be so involved in making every detail of a job perfect, that they can never finish it. They are excessively devoted to work to the exclusion of other activities such as family, friends, and fun (APA, 2000).

They are overly conscientious and inflexible about matters of morality. They adhere to very strict rules of performance, and may force others to do so as well. People with this disorder defer to authority, and insist on following rules without exception for any reason. They may criticize themselves without mercy for their own mistakes (APA, 2000).

People with Obsessive-Compulsive Personality Disorder may be unable to throw away things that are worn out or worthless, even when they have no sentimental value. They are reluctant to delegate tasks to others. They insist that everything be done their way, because only they can do things right. Affected people may hoard their resources out of an attitude that spending must be limited to provide for future emergencies. They are known for being rigid, indecisive, and stubborn. They plan ahead in meticulous detail and will not consider changes to their plans. It is difficult for people with this disorder to consider the perspectives of others. Their expression of emotion is tightly controlled, and they are often uncomfortable around people who are emotionally expressive (APA, 2000).

Obsessive-Compulsive Personality Disorder is not the same as Obsessive-Compulsive Disorder (OCD). OCD is characterized by true *obsessions* (uncontrollable desire to continue thinking about an idea or feeling) and *compulsions* (repetitive stereotyped acts done to relieve anxiety that are a response to obsessive thoughts). See Chapter 50 ⊕ for more information on OCD.

INTERDISCIPLINARY CARE

Long-term therapy is the only effective treatment for personality disorders. Treatment goals for clients with Avoidant Personality Disorder include improving self-esteem, developing a trusting relationship, developing adaptive coping skills, and improving social skills. Symptoms in some people with Avoidant Personality Disorder are reduced when they take antianxiety and antidepressant medications. Dependent Personality Disorder is seen in various practice settings. These clients expect caregivers to make their decisions for them. The challenge is to support these clients to make their own decisions without giving advice on how to act.

Clients with Obsessive-Compulsive Personality Disorder may seek medical help for anxiety or related symptoms. Antianxiety medications may be prescribed. Treatment will focus on how the client is affected by the disorder in such areas as coping, sleeping, nutrition, and interpersonal relationships.

NURSING CARE

ASSESSING

Priorities in Nursing Care. The physician or psychiatrist will make the medical diagnosis of a personality disorder. The role of the nurse is to help clients deal with the effects of the disorder. Collect information about the client's functional ability, mental status, and interpersonal relationships. Clients with personality disorders will often not understand how they are affected. Teaching usually does not help, because the problem is lack of insight, not lack of information. Family members may be a source of information about the client's functional ability at home.

DIAGNOSING, PLANNING, AND IMPLEMENTING

Anxiety

- Help clients identify the situations associated with their anxiety. *Early recognition of anxiety-producing situations will give the client a chance to take adaptive action.*
- Help anxious or dependent clients practice asking for what they need; give positive reinforcement when they identify their needs. *When clients have a thought distortion about being unworthy of care, they may benefit from a*

discussion of their perception. Practicing new behavior (asking for help and getting it) can encourage the client to continue this behavior.

- Give clients choices about their care whenever possible. *Choices, such as those relating to daily activities (when to bathe, meal choices, when to ambulate, where to put items at the bedside, etc.), can help the client have a sense of control. A sense of control can decrease anxiety.*

- Encourage clients to express their true feelings. *When clients believe that they are expected to always be compliant and agreeable, regardless of their own feelings, anxiety is worsened. Recognition and expression of feelings is therapeutic.*

- Reduce environmental stimuli. *Anxiety makes clients more sensitive to noises in the environment. The client is likely to feel calmer in a calm environment.*

- Maintain a calm approach to the anxious client. *The nurse's attitude can be "contagious" in that either calmness or anxiety can be transmitted to the client.*

- Promote a trusting relationship with the client. *A trusting nurse–client relationship can improve the client's self-esteem and reduce anxiety.*

EVALUATING

The desired outcomes for clients with personality disorders relate to resolving the effects these disorders have on clients. Nurses will intervene based on the individual client's needs, and evaluate whether the client achieves the following desired outcomes:

- Effective, adaptive coping behavior
- No harm to self or others
- Adequate sleep to feel rested during the day
- Appropriate interactions with other people
- Making positive statements about self
- Taking initiative to solve problems
- Following unit rules
- Asking for help directly and appropriately
- Reality-based thinking.

Documenting. Documentation focuses on clients' behavior, safety, mental status, and interpersonal interactions. Describe client behavior and statements that reflect mental status or clients' response to interventions. For example, you might document that a client sat in bed with her arms around her bent legs and stated, "I can't stay here. I am so scared." Chart your interventions, possibly a brief orientation to the unit and how to call the nurse, and reassurance of the client's safety. Include the client's response, "The client is visibly relaxed, and stated, 'Thanks, I feel better now.'"

Note: The bibliography listings for this and all chapters have been compiled at the back of the book.

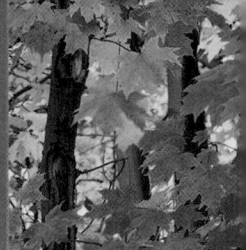

Chapter Review

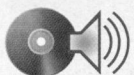 **KEY TERMS** by Topics

Use the audio glossary feature of either the CD-ROM or the Companion Website to hear the correct pronunciation of the following key terms.
Personality disorders
personality

Cluster A personality disorders: odd/eccentric
ideas of reference, inappropriate affect

Cluster B personality disorders: dramatic/emotional/erratic
parasuicidal behavior

KEY Points

- Personality disorders cause people to have abnormalities in perception or cognition, emotions, interpersonal functioning, and impulse control.

- Nurses often see people with personality disorders when they are hospitalized for reasons other than their personality disorder.

- Personality develops over years starting in childhood, and is very resistant to change.

- There is no medication to treat disorders of personality. Some people respond to long-term psychotherapy for changing the pervasive patterns of personality.

- Most people with personality disorders do not know that they are affected.

- Nurses can help people with personality disorders achieve personal growth.

- It can be very challenging to care for people with personality disorders. Nurses who work with them must understand themselves and their professional responsibilities to be most effective.

- The most successful nursing interventions will be based on realistic, practical, attainable goals.

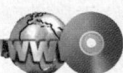 **EXPLORE MediaLink**

Additional interactive resources for this chapter can be found on the Companion Website at www.prenhall.com/burke. Click on Chapter 51 and "Begin" to select the activities for this chapter.

For chapter-related NCLEX-style review questions and an audio glossary, access the accompanying CD-ROM in this book.

FOR FURTHER Study

See Chapter 47 for information on mental status assessment.
See Chapter 50 for more information on anxiety disorders.

Critical Thinking Care Map

Caring for a Client with Ineffective Coping
NCLEX-PN® Focus Area: Psychosocial Integrity

Case Study: Ann Lee is a 68-year-old European American female client. She had acute diverticulitis and was admitted to the general hospital for a partial bowel resection yesterday. Ms. Lee also has Dependent Personality Disorder. She is recovering from her surgery. She is very compliant with requests made by the staff. She has never asked the staff for anything. The physician wrote an order for prn medication for incisional pain.

Nursing Diagnosis: Ineffective Coping

COLLECT DATA

Subjective	Objective
_____	_____
_____	_____
_____	_____
_____	_____
_____	_____
_____	_____
_____	_____

Would you report this data? Yes/No

If yes, to: _____

Nursing Care

_____
_____
_____
_____
_____
_____
_____
_____

How would you document this? _____
_____
_____

Data Collected (use those that apply)

- Client is married
- BP 158/90, P 110, R 24
- T 99.0
- Client states, "Yes, whatever you say."
- When asked if she needs pain medication, she states, "No, I don't want to bother you."
- When asked if she needs anything she states, "I don't know."
- Weighs 168 lbs
- Awake on all q2h checks during the night
- Bowel sounds hypoactive
- Ate 100% of clear liquid breakfast tray
- Ambulates when asked
- Abdominal surgical incision is dry and intact, without exudate; incision is well approximated
- Grimaces and sweats when ambulating or moving in bed
- States, "What do you think I should do?"

Nursing Interventions (use those that apply; list in priority order)

- Teach the client now about dressing changes at home.
- Call the physician immediately about the VS.
- Ask the client, "Are you in pain?"
- Say to the client, "Most people have a lot of pain after surgery. You have signs of pain; does your incision hurt?"
- Tell the client, "It is no trouble to give you some pain medication. I will be glad to get some if you need it."
- Say to the client, "Sometimes people don't like to ask for help. While you are in the hospital, we want to help you, so please tell us what you need."
- Tell the client, "Since you don't seem to want any help, I will leave you alone."
- Help the client practice identifying her needs.
- Document that the client is passive, inappropriate, and dishonest.
- Include offering pain med regularly in the plan of care.
- Visit the client regularly to determine whether she needs help.
- Discuss outpatient referral for therapy with treatment team.

NCLEX-PN® Exam Preparation

TEST-TAKING TIP Clarify what the question is asking. This sounds obvious, but sometimes the wrong answers are correct things to do, but they do not answer the question. Before you read the answers, you need to know if the question asks about a drug effect, a client behavior, or a nursing action. If it seems like more than one option is correct, go back and read the question again to clarify what it is asking.

1 The client with a Paranoid Personality Disorder responds best to a nurse who uses which of the following approaches?
A. friendly, outgoing
B. self-confident, matter-of-fact
C. shy, hesitant
D. quiet, uses brief encounters

2 A client in a long-term care facility who has cancer also has Schizoid Personality Disorder. You notice that the client says little to staff members and has no expression in his voice when he speaks. He has no visitors and receives no phone calls. As a nurse, you would conclude that:
A. this is the client's usual behavior.
B. the client is ashamed of his condition.
C. the client is depressed about his diagnosis.
D. the client is lonely.

3 As a new resident of an assisted living facility, a client refuses to ever eat in the optional dining room with other residents. She does not attend social functions, preferring to stay in her room. You know that she has a diagnosis of Schizotypal Personality Disorder. Your best approach to this client would be to:
A. insist she attend all social functions.
B. encourage other residents to visit her daily.
C. invite her to eat at least one meal a day in the dining room.
D. leave her alone.

4 A client with Antisocial Personality Disorder yells at the staff frequently. He is very demanding and expects to be exempt from the usual hospital rules. What is the best nursing approach to this client?
A. Allow him to break the rules to keep him happy.
B. Tell him that the rules apply to everyone, including him.
C. Ask the physician for an order for an anxiolytic medication.
D. Reassure him that he is safe in the hospital.

5 The treatment priority for a client with Borderline Personality Disorder is:
A. teaching appropriate social skills.
B. preventing self-injury.
C. teaching problem-solving techniques.
D. medicating for sleep disturbances.

6 A client on the psychiatric unit is continually disruptive in any group session by directing all attention to herself. She is constantly asking the other members of the group to help her solve her life problems. She refers to everyone in the group as her "dearest friends. "This client's behavior is consistent with which personality disorder?
A. Borderline
B. Avoidant
C. Schizotypal
D. Histrionic

7 A client is on a medical–surgical unit after gallbladder surgery. He is constantly belittling the nurses taking care of him and wants the surgeon called in the middle of the night to complain about his care. You suspect that he has a Narcissistic Personality Disorder. As his night primary nurse, your best approach would be to:
A. tell him you are sorry he is unhappy with his care. However, you will not call his surgeon, because that is not appropriate. His surgeon will visit in the morning, and he is welcome to voice his complaints at that time.
B. tell him you will call his surgeon and then do not call. If he asks, tell him no one answered.
C. tell him he is not the only client you have to take care of and you do not have time to cater to his every demand.
D. ask him how you can make him happier with his care. Make an extra effort to meet all his demands.

8 A client with Dependent Personality Disorder is very anxious. Which of the following nursing interventions are likely to relieve this client's anxiety? Select all that apply.
A. Establish a trusting nurse–client relationship.
B. Teach the client that she does not have to be anxious.
C. Maintain a calm approach to the client.
D. Encourage the client to express her feelings.

9 A hospitalized client has Antisocial Personality Disorder. Put the following nursing interventions in order of priority for this client.
A. Apply hospital rules consistently.
B. Encourage the client to participate in outpatient counseling.
C. Prevent emotional or physical harm to staff.
D. Encourage the client to express his needs in socially appropriate ways.

10 Which of the following medications is most likely to be prescribed for someone with Obsessive-Compulsive Personality Disorder who is in the hospital?
A. anxiolytic
B. antidepressant
C. antipsychotic
D. hypnotic

Answers for Review Questions, as well as discussion of Critical Thinking Care Map questions, appear in Appendix V.

Chapter 52

Caring for Clients with Substance Abuse or Dependency

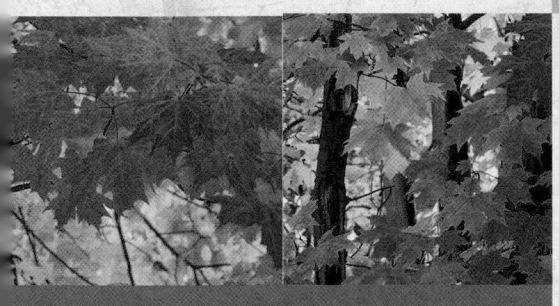

BRIEF Outline

Problem of Substance Abuse
Commonly Abused Substances
  Alcohol
  Other CNS Depressants
  CNS Stimulants

LEARNING Outcomes

After completing this chapter, you will be able to:

- Explain substance abuse, substance dependency, tolerance, and withdrawal.
- Collect information from clients who are using commonly abused drugs.
- Identify adverse effects caused by interactions between commonly abused substances and medications used in surgery or emergency care.
- Provide appropriate nursing interventions for a client in drug or alcohol withdrawal.
- Apply the nursing process to clients experiencing substance abuse or dependency.

MediaLink

www.prenhall.com/burke
Use the address above to access the free, interactive Companion Website created for this textbook. Get hints, instant feedback, and textbook references to chapter-related NCLEX-style questions. Link to other interesting sites.

Audio Glossary:
Use the Companion Website, or the CD-ROM disk enclosed with your textbook, to hear the pronunciation of key terms in this chapter.

Problem of Substance Abuse

Throughout human history, people have used substances to alter their perceptions; to elevate mood; to relieve pain, fear, anxiety or boredom; and to aid in religious ceremonies. Alcohol, the most commonly used psychoactive substance, can be used responsibly and enjoyably. Substance use becomes a problem when:

- It interferes with an individual's ability to function at work, home, or school
- It causes legal problems
- It puts anyone in danger
- It continues despite negative consequences.

Substance abuse is one of the most important health problems in the 21st century. As many as 20% of the adult population of the United States may meet the diagnostic criteria for an alcohol- or substance-related disorder (American Psychiatric Association [APA], 2000). Add to this number the family members, employers, employees, coworkers, people injured or killed by substance abusers, and babies born to women who abuse alcohol and other substances, and you can see how many people are affected. The annual financial cost to society is in the hundreds of billions of dollars. The toll in human morbidity and mortality is staggering. See Figure 52-1 ■ to learn about how often alcohol is a factor in fatal events.

The exact number of people with substance abuse and dependency is not known. The reason for this lack of infor-mation is that **denial** (refusal to acknowledge the existence of a real situation or feelings) is a common coping mechanism for people with these disorders and for the health professionals who work with them.

People with substance-related disorders usually do not receive treatment. Health professionals often do not ask the questions that could determine who is affected by substance use. Sometimes health professionals are not aware of how they can help. This chapter helps the nurse to identify clients with substance-related disorders and provides tools for intervening to help them.

The Diagnostic and Statistical Manual of Mental Disorders, Fourth Edition, Text Revision (DSM-IV-TR, APA, 2000) is the standard for the diagnosis and terminology of mental disorders, including substance-related disorders. The definitions from the DSM-IV-TR are relevant to all substances of abuse and dependence.

TYPES OF SUBSTANCE USE PROBLEMS

Substance Abuse

The DSM-IV-TR describes **substance abuse** as a maladaptive pattern of substance use despite adverse outcomes. It results in significant impairment or distress manifested by one or more of the following (APA, 2000):

1. Inability to fulfill major role obligations at work, school, or home (poor work performance or attendance, expulsions from school, neglect of children)

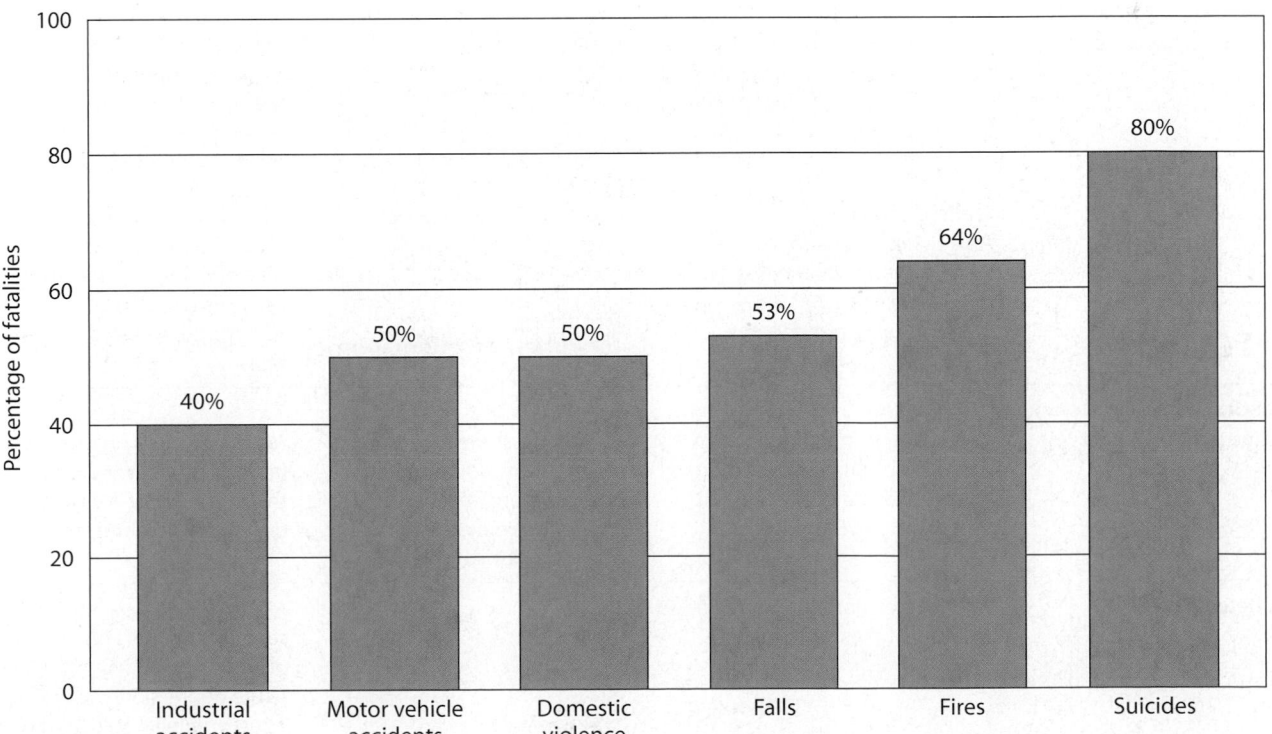

Figure 52-1. ■ Fatal events in which alcohol is a factor.

2. Recurrent substance use in physically hazardous situations (driving a car, operating a machine)
3. Recurrent legal or interpersonal problems
4. Continued use despite persistent social and interpersonal problems caused by use of the substance, such as fights or arguments with partner about intoxication.

Substance Dependency

Substance dependency is more severe than substance abuse. It is a maladaptive pattern of substance use leading to significant impairment or distress, manifested by three or more of the following (APA, 2000):

- Tolerance to the substance
- Withdrawal syndrome

- Substance either taken in higher amounts or for longer periods than intended
- Unsuccessful or persistent desire to decrease or control use
- A great deal of time spent in obtaining, using, and recovering from effects of the substance
- Reduction of important social, occupational, or recreational activities due to substance use
- Continued substance use despite knowledge of a persistent physical or psychologic problem that is likely caused by the substance.

Compulsive Substance Use

Compulsive substance use is repetitive substance use behavior for the purpose of reducing distress. Compulsive use is

---

TABLE 52-1

Comparison of Commonly Abused CNS Depressants and Stimulants

DRUG	EFFECTS OF USE	OVERDOSE SYMPTOMS	WITHDRAWAL SYMPTOMS AND THEIR ONSET (AFTER LAST DOSE)
CNS Depressants **Alcohol (beer, wine, liquor)**	Euphoria, loss of inhibition, ataxia, lack of coordination, reduced cognition, impaired judgment, nausea Tolerance with prolonged use	Respiratory depression, mental confusion, unconsciousness, death	6–8 hours CNS irritability, anxiety, increased vital signs, tremors, ataxia, diaphoresis, slurred speech, GI disturbance, disorientation, hallucinations, seizures, death
Opioids/narcotics (e.g., morphine, meperidine, methadone, oxycodone, heroin)	Analgesia, cough suppression, euphoria, loss of inhibition, lack of coordination, reduced cognition, impaired judgment, apathy, nausea constipation, constricted pupils Tolerance with prolonged use	Sedation, respiratory depression, mental confusion, unconsciousness, death	12–72 hours Watering eyes, CNS irritability, increased vital signs, tremors, diaphoresis, similar to alcohol but less likely to cause death
Sedatives, hypnotics, anxiolytics	Sedation, muscle relaxation, apathy, reduced cognition Anxiolytics cause reduced anxiety, muscle relaxation, and less sedation in low doses Tolerance with prolonged use.	Muscle weakness, respiratory depression, mental confusion, unconsciousness, death	Onset depends on type of sedative (short or long acting). CNS irritability, increased vital signs, tremors, slurred speech, diaphoresis, seizures Barbiturate withdrawal can be fatal
CNS Stimulants **Cocaine**	Local vasoconstriction, sudden rush of euphoria, elation, energy, talkativeness, anorexia, weight loss, elevated VS, grandiosity	Chest pain, slurred speech, mental confusion, vomiting, hallucinations, myocardial infarction, severe elevation of BP and P, shock, death	Acute depression, craving drug, fatigue, irritability, suicidal thoughts, loss of pleasure (anhedonia), not life threatening
Amphetamines	Euphoria, elation, energy, talkativeness, anorexia, weight loss, elevated VS, grandiosity	Same as cocaine	As with cocaine, withdrawal severity depends on amount of drug use Acute depression, craving drug, fatigue, irritability, suicidal thoughts, loss of pleasure (anhedonia)

often unwanted and time consuming (APA, 2000). Compulsive substance use represents ineffective coping behavior. Addiction is a commonly used, but not medically diagnostic, term that refers to psychologic and physiologic dependence and drug-seeking behavior.

Commonly Abused Substances

Substances that rapidly alter the mental state, by either stimulating or depressing the central nervous system, are the most commonly abused. The DSM-IV-TR lists 11 substances of abuse:

- Alcohol
- Opioids
- Sedatives, hypnotics, and anxiolytics
- Cocaine
- Amphetamines and similar drugs
- Hallucinogens

- Phencyclidine (PCP) and similar drugs
- Inhalants
- Cannabis
- Caffeine
- Nicotine.

Tables 52-1 ■ and 52-2 ■ provide summaries of the effects of these substances.

ALCOHOL

Ethyl alcohol (ethanol, beverage alcohol) is the most commonly abused substance. It is a central nervous system (CNS) depressant that is quickly absorbed into the blood after drinking. Initial symptoms of alcohol **intoxication** (a reversible set of physical, psychologic, and behavioral symptoms caused by use of the substance) are relaxation, loss of inhibition, **euphoria** (an exaggerated feeling of well-being), and decreased mental concentration. With increased use, symptoms progress to slurred speech, **ataxia**

TABLE 52-2

Comparison of Hallucinogens, Inhalants, Cannabis, Caffeine, and Nicotine

SUBSTANCE	EFFECTS OF USE	OVERDOSE SYMPTOMS	WITHDRAWAL SYMPTOMS
Hallucinogens LSD, DMT, mescaline, MDMA (Ecstasy)	Hallucinations and distorted perceptions, distortions of time and space, illusions, emotional lability, tremor, nausea and vomiting	Panic (may be drug reaction, not OD), seizures (rare)	No withdrawal; may experience flashbacks for several months after last dose
Phencyclidine (PCP)	Bizarre perceptions, disorientation, hallucinations, agitation, grandiosity, withdrawn or agitated or both, paranoid, dilated pupils, dry red skin	Seizures, coma, death	No withdrawal
Inhalants and Cannabis Inhalants *Hydrocarbons:* glue, gasoline, aerosol spray, solvents *Nitrites:* amyl nitrite, nitrous oxide	*Hydrocarbons:* euphoria, impaired judgment, nystagmus, ataxia, slurred speech, perceptual changes, sense of invulnerability *Nitrites:* prolonged erection or enhanced intercourse	*Hydrocarbons:* stupor, coma, cardiac depression and dysrhythmias, respiratory arrest, renal complications *Nitrites:* panic, hypotension, headache *Both:* brain damage	Similar to alcohol
Cannabis, marijuana, hashish	Mild euphoria, pleasure, confidence, grandiosity, relaxation, red eyes, dry mouth, increased appetite	None	No physical withdrawal May have craving
Caffeine and Nicotine Caffeine	Increased alertness, prolongs ability to work, elevates mood	Anxiety, cardiac dysrhythmias	Headache, fatigue
Nicotine	Pleasure, alertness, increased BP and P, decreased blood flow to heart muscle	None	Anxiety, depressed mood, anger, craving, increased appetite

---

BOX 52-1

MANIFESTATIONS OF ALCOHOL INTOXICATION BY BLOOD ALCOHOL CONCENTRATION

Blood Alcohol Concentration (g/dL)	Manifestations
0.05–0.10 (0.08–0.10 is legal level of intoxication in most states)	Relaxation, euphoria, decreased inhibitions, impaired judgment, changeable mood, decreased mental concentration, decreased fine motor coordination
0.15–0.25	Slurred speech, decreased motor function, ataxia, mood outbursts, aggressive behavior
0.3	Incoherent speech, mental confusion, stupor, vomiting, labored breathing
0.4	Unconsciousness, coma
0.5	Respiratory depression, death

(staggering gait), **labile** (changeable) mood, aggressive behavior, incoherent speech, vomiting, coma, respiratory depression, and death. See Box 52-1 ■ for manifestations of alcohol intoxication by blood alcohol concentrations.

Tolerance and Withdrawal

With continued use, the user develops **tolerance** to alcohol. This means that increasing amounts of alcohol are needed to achieve the same effect, or the same amount of alcohol causes less effect. If an individual drinks large amounts of alcohol regularly, the CNS experiences depression. Through its mechanism for maintaining homeostasis, the depressed CNS increases its own stimulation. The individual then requires more alcohol to achieve intoxication of the stimulated CNS. The process of increasing tolerance develops over years of alcohol dependency, until the individual must drink almost constantly to avoid the distressing symptoms of CNS stimulation.

When the alcohol-dependent individual stops drinking, the CNS is still stimulated. The homeostatic mechanism that balanced the depressant effects of the alcohol takes time to return to normal. Meanwhile, the individual suffers **withdrawal** symptoms. The alcohol withdrawal syndrome includes elevated vital signs, anxiety, tremors, diaphoresis, slurred speech, GI disturbances (vomiting, cramping, diarrhea), ataxia, nystagmus, disorientation, and, at its most severe, hallucinations, seizures, and death.

Alcohol withdrawal delirium (delirium tremens or DTs) is diagnosed when withdrawal is associated with severe cognitive symptoms such as confusion, delusions, and terrifying hallucinations. This delirium happens to people with a long (5- to 15-year) history of alcoholism. It is a medical emergency.

Note that the symptoms of alcohol withdrawal are generally the opposite of those of alcohol intoxication. The individual takes the CNS depressant substance; the CNS stimulates itself to maintain homeostasis. When the substance is withdrawn, the CNS is still stimulated, and the individual has CNS stimulation symptoms until the CNS eventually regains homeostasis without alcohol, and the symptoms subside. Alcohol withdrawal syndrome usually lasts about 4 days. See Table 52-1 for withdrawal symptoms.

The alcohol-dependent individual (**alcoholic**) may experience many episodes of withdrawal symptoms that he or she treats with alcohol. The statement "I feel bad (nervous, tired, angry, lonely, etc.); I need a drink" may be evidence of withdrawal symptoms. Nurses should be aware that substance withdrawal symptoms are often behind a client's desire to leave the hospital against medical advice.

Pattern of Use

The pattern of use of alcohol varies from one individual to another. Some people start drinking alcohol in childhood or adolescence, some in old age. Some drink daily, starting with "one or two drinks with dinner" and progressing to greater amounts and frequency. Some drink heavily on weekends or may abstain for long periods and then have a drinking binge.

For most people, drinking alcohol begins with a social motivation. For most people, drinking continues to be a social event. Some people begin to use alcohol as a coping mechanism, to relieve the everyday stress of life. In the early stage of alcoholism, the affected individual is likely to deny that alcohol is a problem, despite evidence otherwise and despite tolerance.

Alcohol dependency progresses to include memory blackouts during episodes of intoxication. At this stage, the alcohol is no longer a source of pleasure or relief, but a drug that is required by the individual. Commonly people in this phase begin to drink alone or drink secretly. They experience withdrawal symptoms. They wake up in the morning and need a drink to control tremors (an "eye-opener"). Denial is still the defense mechanism.

As the disease progresses, the individual completely loses control over the ability to choose whether or not to drink. Experiences include isolation from others, anger, aggression, loss of interest in any activity that previously brought pleasure, and malnutrition. The individual is willing to give up everything to maintain the addiction. It is common for people in this phase to have lost their jobs, families, friends, and self-respect.

The end stage of alcohol dependency is characterized by emotional and physical disintegration. The individual may experience psychosis. Every body system is affected by life-threatening complications. Abstention from alcohol results

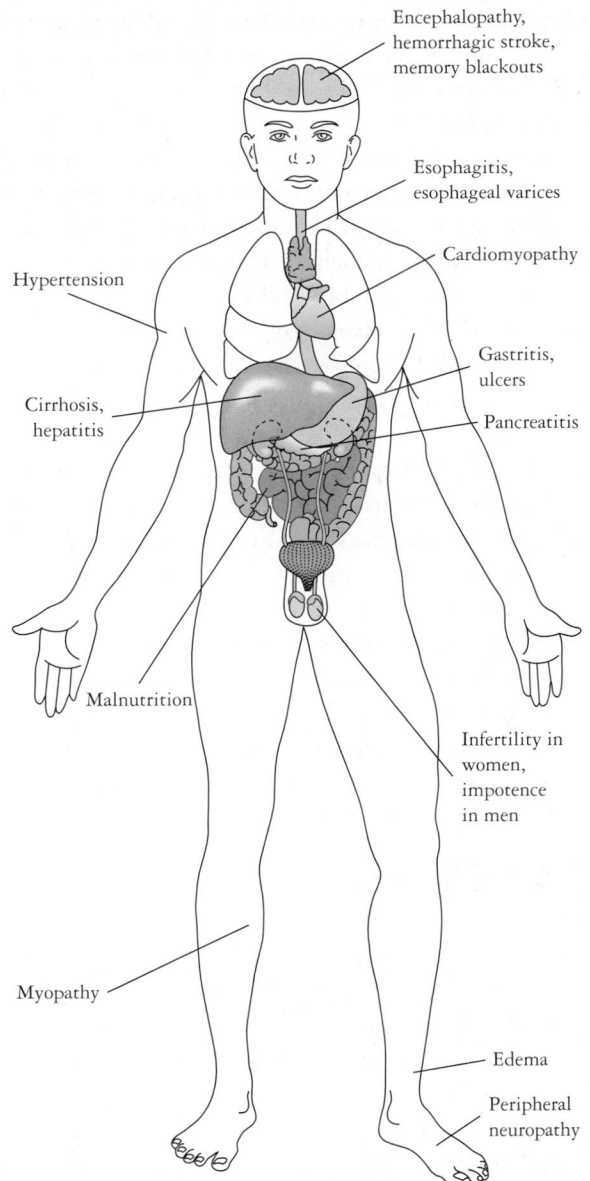

Figure 52-2. ■ Physiologic effects of alcoholism.

in life-threatening withdrawal. Thoughts of suicide are common.

Long-Term Physical Effects

Chronic use of alcohol takes a toll on the body. All body systems are affected over a period of years. Figure 52-2 ■ illustrates the physiologic effects. The gastrointestinal system is one of the first to show the effects of chronic alcoholism. Alcohol causes *gastritis* by inflaming the stomach lining. The protective mucous lining of the stomach is damaged by alcohol, allowing hydrochloric acid to erode the stomach wall. If the vascular structure in the stomach wall is involved, bleeding can occur. Ulcers may form in the stomach. Symptoms include gastric distress, nausea, vomiting, black stools, and abdominal distention. Esophagitis is caused by the irritant effect of alcohol on the esophagus, and by frequent vomiting. The primary symptom is esophageal pain.

Pancreatitis, either acute or chronic, may also be caused by chronic alcohol use. Chronic pancreatitis leads to pancreatic insufficiency, which causes malnutrition, weight loss, and diabetes mellitus. Acute pancreatitis happens 1 or 2 days after a binge of drinking alcohol. The symptoms include severe, constant epigastric pain, nausea, vomiting, and abdominal distention.

Alcoholic hepatitis affects an already damaged liver, usually after a prolonged binge of excessive alcohol consumption. The client has right upper quadrant abdominal pain, jaundice, an enlarged liver and spleen, vomiting, weakness, profound fatigue, and possibly ascites. *Cirrhosis* of the liver is the worst alcohol-related liver disorder. It is the end stage of chronic alcoholic liver disease. Liver cells are severely damaged and destroyed. They are replaced by scar tissue, which makes this disease irreversible. Cirrhosis causes portal hypertension, ascites, *esophageal varices* (varicose veins in the esophagus that can rupture and hemorrhage), and hepatic encephalopathy. Hepatic encephalopathy is caused by accumulation of ammonia. It results in impaired mental function and progresses to death.

Cardiomyopathy (muscle abnormality and weakening causing enlargement of the heart), heart failure, and cardiac dysrhythmias may occur. The risk of hemorrhagic stroke is increased. Other cardiovascular manifestations include hypertension (especially diastolic elevation), tachycardia, and edema.

Blackouts are an early sign of alcoholism, and reflect neurologic involvement. The affected individual remains conscious and appears to be functioning normally, but is completely unable to remember anything that occurs while intoxicated. After many years of alcohol abuse, a person may develop Korsakoff's syndrome and Wernicke's syndrome, which affect the entire neurologic system. These syndromes usually occur together, and are often called Wernicke-Korsakoff's syndrome.

Korsakoff's syndrome is a group of symptoms caused by a deficiency in the B vitamins, including thiamine, riboflavin, and folic acid. Amnesia, disorientation to time and place, **confabulation** (falsification of memory to fill in the gaps caused by cognitive deficits), and severe peripheral neuropathy characterize it. Symptoms of the neuropathy include tingling; muscle weakness; sore, burning muscles; abnormal sensation; and pain with movement. The extremities are affected, especially the legs. Because of their extreme pain, care must be taken when moving these clients.

Wernicke's syndrome (alcoholic encephalopathy) is characterized by ataxia, paralysis of eye muscles, nystagmus, and mental confusion. It is the result of severe vitamin B_1 deficiency from lack of adequate nutritional intake.

BOX 52-2

MANIFESTATIONS OF FETAL ALCOHOL SYNDROME

- Low birth weight
- Microcephaly (small head circumference, small brain)
- Facial anomalies
  - Flat mid-face
  - Flat nasal bridge
  - Small eyes
  - Short palpebral fissures (narrow eye openings)
  - Short nose
  - Flat philtrum (indistinct infranasal depression)
  - Thin upper lip
- Neurodevelopmental disorders
  - Developmental delay
  - Learning disabilities
  - Poor coordination
  - Distractibility/impulsivity

Early in the disorder, it may respond well to large doses of parenteral thiamine. If not treated early, it progresses to an irreversible, fatal condition that requires custodial care.

The reproductive system is affected as well. Men may become *impotent*. Women may stop menstruating and become infertile. Further, the unborn child of a pregnant woman may be seriously affected. Box 52-2 ■ describes effects of fetal alcohol syndrome.

When the musculoskeletal system is affected, osteoporosis can develop. Also, acute or chronic **myopathy** may occur, characterized by muscle cramps of sudden onset and later development of pain, tenderness, and edema of the skeletal muscles, especially of the legs. In chronic myopathy there is wasting and weakness of the skeletal muscles.

OTHER CNS DEPRESSANTS

Other depressants of the central nervous system are similar to alcohol in their effects on the CNS, intoxication symptoms, tolerance effects, and withdrawal symptoms. Table 52-1 provides a profile of the CNS depressants.

The Opiates

Opiates are naturally occurring substances derived from opium (such as morphine), semisynthetics (such as heroin), and drugs that resemble them (such as methadone, meperidine, oxycodone, or codeine). Opiates are narcotic drugs prescribed to relieve pain or diarrhea or to reduce cough. These drugs have alleviated immeasurable human pain, but when abused they have caused immense suffering as well.

EFFECTS OF OPIATES. Opiate drugs can cause physical dependence (tolerance and withdrawal); see Table 52-1. The opiate drugs decrease GI peristalsis, so they can be used therapeutically to treat severe diarrhea. When opiates are abused,

constipation can be severe, including fecal impaction. The nausea and vomiting that are commonly caused by opiates are due to stimulation of the medulla of the brain.

In therapeutic doses, opiates have little effect on the heart. Morphine is often used to treat cardiac clients for pain or to divert blood flow to the peripheral circulation, decreasing the work of the heart. In high doses, they cause hypotension by affecting the heart or reducing vascular resistance.

Nurses especially need to know about the respiratory effects of opioids. These drugs, which are used therapeutically to suppress cough, depress the respiratory center in the medulla of the brain. Respiratory depression is not likely to happen in therapeutic doses unless the client is narcotic naïve (has not been exposed to opiates recently). With high doses, though, respiratory depression may be life threatening. Chronic respiratory depression predisposes the client to pneumonia and other respiratory infections.

Opiate overdose is a medical emergency. Death can result from respiratory arrest and hypoxia. Opiate overdose is treated with a narcotic antagonist drug, such as naloxone hydrochloride (Narcan). This drug competes for opiate receptors and blocks or reverses the action of narcotic analgesics (opiates).

clinical ALERT

The nurse must be aware that naloxone has a shorter duration of action than narcotics. It may be necessary to give additional doses of naloxone if the client still has high levels of narcotics in the blood.

PATTERNS OF USE. While alcohol is legal and readily available, the opiates are either available only by prescription (narcotic analgesics) or are illegal under all circumstances (heroin). Opiate dependence is typically associated with a history of crimes committed to obtain drugs or the money to buy them. Health care professionals who are opiate dependent may steal medications from clients or their employers, write prescriptions for themselves, or manipulate physicians to write prescriptions for them.

Opioid dependence may begin at any age, but problems are most commonly observed in the late teens or early 20s (APA, 2000). Dependence develops over a period of many years, with periods of **abstinence** (complete lack of drug use). **Relapse** (returning to drug use after abstinence) is very common. Men are more commonly affected than women. Opiate-dependent individuals also experience other risks, such as developing hepatitis B or C, HIV infection, or other bloodborne diseases from needle use. Mortality in opiate-dependent people may be 2% per year. Death often results from overdose, accidents, or injuries (APA, 2000).

Sedative, Hypnotic, or Anxiolytic-Related Disorders

Sedatives, hypnotics, and anxiolytics include the benzodiazepines, the barbiturates, and similar drugs. Prescription sleeping medications and almost all of the anxiolytic (antianxiety) drugs are included. Like alcohol and the opiates, these substances depress the CNS. (For information about anxiety disorders, see Chapter 50. ∞)

OVERDOSE. CNS depressant drugs have additive effects when taken together. For example, when people use alcohol and a sedative drug at the same time, the CNS depressant effect is beyond what either substance would cause alone. Although the amount of sedative may be usual and the amount of alcohol may be what the person usually drinks, the two together could cause fatal respiratory depression. It is not uncommon for people to die as a result of this additive effect.

clinical ALERT

Nurses who work in emergency or trauma care must assess every client for substance use. Prescribed narcotics, sedatives, or anesthetics given to clients still under the influence of alcohol or other CNS depressant drugs cause additive CNS depression, which can be fatal.

Prescribed narcotic for pain + street drugs or alcohol = respiratory depression.

It is common for the substance-dependent individual to have a drug of choice, but to use a variety of other substances, including alcohol. This combination of abused substances is called **polysubstance abuse.** Benzodiazepines alone in overdose are rarely fatal, but barbiturates in overdose are often fatal, due to cardiac or respiratory arrest.

A relatively new, quick-acting sedative drug is flunitrazepam (Rohypnol). It is called the "date rape drug," because it can rapidly incapacitate a rape victim. One or two tablets dissolved in alcohol can render a person unconscious within minutes. The affected individual then has amnesia for several hours.

CNS STIMULANTS

Cocaine and Amphetamines

The clinical usefulness of this group of drugs is limited to the treatment of attention deficit hyperactivity disorder. Cocaine especially is a popular drug of abuse because of the immediate euphoria it induces. See Table 52-1 for intoxication and withdrawal symptoms.

Hallucinogens

Hallucinogens distort the user's perception of reality. The most common hallucinogens are LSD, mescaline, and PCP (phencyclidine). The CNS effects are unpredictable and may be influenced by the expectations of the user. Some individuals have frightening psychotic experiences. Hallucinations can lead to violent or self-injurious behavior. See Table 52-2 for a comparison of the hallucinogens with other drugs of abuse.

Synthetic or "designer" drugs are becoming increasingly popular. MDMA or Ecstasy is derived from amphetamine and methamphetamine, so it acts as both a stimulant and a hallucinogen.

Inhalants

Two kinds of inhalants (hydrocarbons and nitrites) are commonly abused. See Table 52-2 for their effects. The hydrocarbons can induce cardiac depression, renal injury, respiratory depression, and death from cardiac dysrhythmias or accidents while intoxicated (Keltner et al., 2003).

Cannabis

Delta-9-tetrahydrocannabinol (THC) is thought to be the chemical responsible for the psychoactive effects of marijuana and hashish. See Table 52-2 for its effects. Cannabis is the most widely used illegal substance in the United States. It has been therapeutically used to treat the anorexia, nausea, and vomiting associated with AIDS and cancer.

Caffeine and Nicotine

It may be surprising to find caffeine and nicotine on the list of substances of abuse. Still, these substances fit the model of dependence defined in the DSM-IV-TR. Both substances cause tolerance and withdrawal.

Caffeine is the most commonly used stimulant drug. The physiologic effects of caffeine explain why it is so popular as a performance enhancer. It prolongs the time the user can continue to work, improves mental alertness, and elevates mood (Table 52-2). The dose and frequency of use determine the effects and whether the user develops tolerance.

The average coffee drinker consumes 360 to 450 mg of caffeine per day. Intake of more than 600 mg of caffeine per day is considered excessive (Kneisl et al., 2004). See Figure 52-3 ■ for dosage information about common sources of caffeine.

Nicotine dependence is the most common substance dependence in the United States (American Society of Addiction Medicine, 1997). Smoking is especially common in the population of people who use alcohol and other substances. The consequences of smoking are also related to other substances present in tobacco. The incidence of cancer of the lungs, oral cavity, esophagus, pancreas, and prostate is increased significantly in tobacco users. The risk

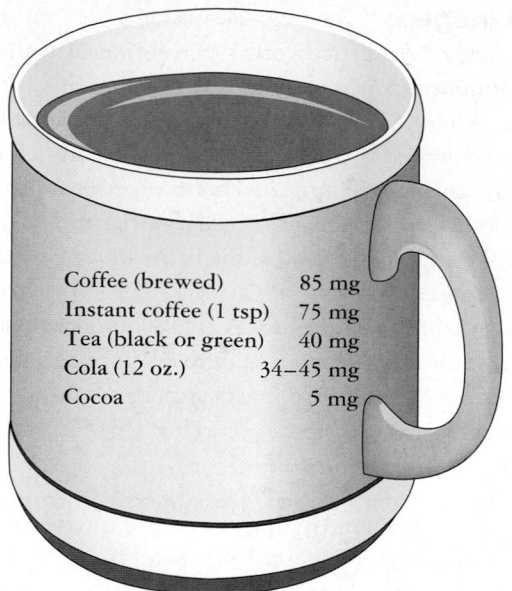

Coffee (brewed)	85 mg
Instant coffee (1 tsp)	75 mg
Tea (black or green)	40 mg
Cola (12 oz.)	34–45 mg
Cocoa	5 mg

Figure 52-3. ■ Common sources of caffeine, with doses per serving.

of cardiovascular disease, including stroke, myocardial infarction, and peripheral arterial disease, is increased by tobacco use as well. Accidents related to fire are also a concern (smoking in bed while drinking alcohol can be deadly).

Due to the widespread use of caffeine and nicotine, hospitalized clients are likely to experience caffeine or nicotine withdrawal. The headache that clients have after surgery may be better treated with a cup of coffee than medication. Some clients may consider leaving the hospital against medical advice so they can smoke cigarettes. These situations require the nurse's problem-solving skills.

Nurses should acknowledge that physiologic dependence as well as the psychologic habit of smoking make it difficult to quit. Smoking is not a character flaw; it is a significant health issue. Nurses should use the "five As" for every client who smokes, and the "five Rs" to help smokers who are not currently willing to quit (Gordon, Williams, & Lapin, 2001):

- **Ask** the client about tobacco use.
- **Advise** the client to quit.
- **Assess** the client's willingness to make an attempt to quit
- **Assist** the client to make an attempt to quit
- **Arrange** for follow-up contacts to prevent relapse.

The "five Rs" for smokers who are currently unwilling to quit:

- Provide motivational information that is personally **relevant** to the client.
- Discuss the **risks** associated with smoking and the **rewards** of quitting, such as improvements in functioning and self-efficacy.

- Ask the client about **roadblocks** or barriers to quitting.
- **Repeat** motivational strategies at every clinic visit because most smokers need to make repeated attempts to quit to be successful.

Steroid Abuse

Among the newer drugs of abuse are the anabolic-androgenic steroids. These are man-made substances related to male sex hormones. *Anabolic* refers to muscle building, and *androgenic* refers to increased masculine characteristics. These drugs are available only by prescription to treat clients with abnormally low testosterone, or to treat body wasting in clients with AIDS and other diseases that result in loss of lean muscle mass. Abuse of anabolic steroids can lead to serious health problems, some of which are irreversible.

Anabolic steroids are abused to enhance physical performance and to improve physical appearance. They are taken orally or injected, typically in cycles of weeks or months rather than continuously. Users may combine different types of steroids in an attempt to minimize negative effects.

The major side effects of abusing anabolic steroids include liver tumors, liver cancer, jaundice, edema, hypertension, increased LDL, and decreased HDL. Other side effects include severe acne, tremors, and aggression. Some users have psychiatric symptoms such as mood swings, paranoia, irritability, delusions, and impaired judgment. There are also gender-specific side effects (National Institute on Drug Abuse [NIDA], 2005):

- *For men:* shrinking of the testicles, reduced sperm count, infertility, baldness, breast development, increased risk of prostate cancer
- *For women:* growth of facial hair, male pattern baldness, changes in or cessation of the menstrual cycle, enlargement of the clitoris, deepened voice.

Steroid abuse among adolescents has increased since the early 1990s. While adolescent boys are more likely to abuse steroids, adolescent girls are using steroids in increasing numbers for the purpose of becoming leaner and more muscular. The anabolic steroids cause premature skeletal maturation and accelerated puberty changes. Adolescents who take steroids before their growth spurt is complete may remain short for the rest of their lives. Some people experience depression when they stop taking steroids, which may contribute to dependence on the drugs (NIDA, 2005).

INTERDISCIPLINARY CARE

Medical treatment of the client in the acute phase of alcohol or sedative withdrawal focuses on physiologic safety issues: symptom management, seizure prevention, stabilizing vital signs, and minimizing the effects of CNS stimulation. Management of the client in the rehabilitation phase is supportive. Nurses take a cooperative role with physicians, therapists, social workers, and others on the health care team.

Medications

Medical management includes prescription of medications and therefore must include consideration of drug interactions and cross-tolerance. Clients who use drugs or alcohol regularly are at risk for withdrawal, and those who have used drugs or alcohol recently are at risk for additive effects with prescribed drugs.

Nurses and physicians in emergency departments need to know that any client who is under the influence of drugs or alcohol on arrival is at risk for an overdose of CNS depressants. Clients who are taking narcotics, other CNS depressants (alcohol, barbiturates, sedatives, prescription sleep aids), or illegal drugs that depress the CNS (heroin, "downers") are at high risk of additive CNS depression. Commonly prescribed medications that cause additive CNS depression are the narcotic analgesics, sedatives, benzodiazepines, sleep agents, and anesthetic agents.

A person who is dependent on heroin or alcohol will be tolerant not only to these, but to other CNS depressants as well. This phenomenon is called **cross-tolerance.** Cross-tolerance is important to the anesthesiologist, who may find that the client needs more than the usual anesthetic to put him to sleep. It is also important to physicians and nurses, because clients who are tolerant to CNS depressants may need a higher than usual analgesic dose to relieve pain.

Treatment

There are several theories about chemical dependency and its causes. Current treatment methods are based on the concept that substance dependency is a chronic, progressive medical illness that is characterized by remissions and relapses, and that is eventually fatal if untreated. The etiology of substance abuse is a combination of genetic factors and cultural influences (nature and nurture). People who are dependent on substances have learned to use them to cope with their problems. These clients must have new skills to replace the functions substances play in their lives. A promise of abstinence alone is not a long-term solution. The ultimate goals of substance dependency treatment are (1) abstinence from substance use and (2) development of effective coping mechanisms to replace the need for substances as solutions to problems.

ACUTE PHASE OF TREATMENT. Substance dependency treatment has two major phases: acute and rehabilitation. In the *acute phase,* the person may be in a hospital or another inpatient or outpatient setting. The client often enters treatment while intoxicated. **Detoxification,** or removal of the substance from the body, begins the acute phase. The withdrawal syndrome also occurs acutely. Medical and nursing support are often needed during withdrawal.

Medications are used in the acute phase of treatment to provide safe withdrawal. For clients whose primary substance of abuse is alcohol, vitamin B_1 is given to prevent Wernicke-Korsakoff's syndrome.

Alcohol withdrawal is usually managed with a benzodiazepine anxiolytic agent, which is given in a decreasing dose over several days to treat and prevent withdrawal. Some health care workers have the attitude that if clients are allowed to suffer agonizing withdrawal, they will "learn a lesson" about why they should stop using drugs. On the contrary, withdrawal causes preoccupation and craving for the substance. There is no ethical justification for allowing clients to suffer needlessly. Alcohol and barbiturate withdrawals can be life threatening.

REHABILITATION PHASE. The second phase of substance dependency treatment is **rehabilitation.** This phase continues indefinitely. When clients have detoxified and are abstaining from substance use, rehabilitation begins.

Medications used in the rehabilitation phase of treatment are for the purpose of preventing relapse. Disulfiram (Antabuse) may be prescribed to deter clients from drinking alcohol. It causes a severe, uncomfortable reaction when the client drinks (flushing, throbbing headache, nausea, and vomiting).

Methadone, a synthetic opiate, is used as a replacement for heroin. A regular dose is prescribed, and the client basically trades one dependency for another. The goal is to prevent the risks of intravenous drug use (methadone is given orally) and the socially inappropriate behaviors associated with obtaining heroin (prostitution, burglary, robbery, etc.). Many people who use methadone lead productive lives.

Naltrexone (ReVia) is an opioid antagonist used to treat opiate overdose. It blocks the effects of any opioids used by the client. It has been found to reduce the cravings for alcohol in abstinent clients (Freed & York, 1997).

Clonidine (Catapres) is an antihypertensive drug. It is given to clients with opiate dependence to prevent some of the symptoms of withdrawal. Nurses should take the client's blood pressure before each dose, and hold the drug if the person is hypotensive.

The tasks of rehabilitation are to:

- Maintain sobriety (abstinence)
- Develop new coping skills
- Make a plan for relapse prevention
- Live life with all its responsibilities, joys, and frustrations.

Relapse is common. The best response to relapse is for the person to learn from the experience and to begin again on rehabilitation.

BOX 52-3

TWELVE STEPS OF ALCOHOLICS ANONYMOUS

We

1. Admitted that we were powerless over alcohol, that our lives had become unmanageable.
2. Came to believe that a Power greater than ourselves could restore us to sanity.
3. Made a decision to turn our wills and lives over to the care of God as we understood Him.
4. Made a searching and fearless moral inventory of ourselves.
5. Admitted to God, to ourselves, and to another human being the exact nature of our wrongs.
6. Were entirely ready to have God remove all these defects of character.
7. Humbly asked Him to remove our shortcomings.
8. Made a list of all persons we had harmed, and became willing to make amends to them all.
9. Made direct amends to such people whenever possible, except when to do so would injure them or others.
10. Continued to take personal inventory and when we were wrong promptly admitted it.
11. Sought through prayer and meditation to improve our conscious contact with God as we understood Him, praying only for knowledge of His will for us and the power to carry that out.
12. Having had a spiritual awakening as a result of these steps, we tried to carry this message to alcoholics and to practice these principles in all our affairs.

Source: Alcoholics Anonymous World Services, 1952. The Twelve Steps are reprinted with permission of Alcoholics Anonymous World Services, Inc. (A.A.W.S.). Permission to reprint the Twelve Steps does not mean that A.A.W.S. has reviewed or approved the contents of this publication, or that A.A.W.S. necessarily agrees with the views expressed herein. A.A. is a program of recovery from alcoholism *only*—use of the Twelve Steps in connection with programs and activities which are patterned after A.A., but which address other problems, or in any other non-A.A. context, does not imply otherwise.

Many people with substance abuse and dependency respond well to treatment. The most popular treatment program is Alcoholics Anonymous. This is a self-help group for alcoholics that is based on 12 steps, thus the name "Twelve-Step Program." Box 52-3 ■ lists the Twelve Steps of Alcoholics Anonymous. AA itself is for alcoholics only. Other 12-step programs are based on their principles. In all of these anonymous groups, people with similar problems share experience, strength, and hope. The groups offer a sense of community and unconditional support.

There are thousands of AA groups. Refer clients to their local telephone book or directory assistance for the closest meeting. There are also AA meetings for special interest groups, such as nonsmokers, women, lesbians, teachers, people who want to focus on religious aspects of

recovery, and so forth. Other 12-step programs include Overeaters Anonymous, Narcotics Anonymous, and Cocaine Anonymous.

Substance dependency is certainly a family illness. Al-Anon is a group for family members, especially spouses, of alcoholics. Ala-Teen is a similar group for teenage children of alcoholics. ACOA, or Adult Children of Alcoholics, serves people who grew up in alcoholic families. Partners of alcoholics often are **codependents**—they facilitate the alcoholic's problem by allowing for avoidance of the consequences for behavior related to drinking. For example, the codependent may provide excuses for the alcoholic at work or with family.

Dual Diagnosis

The term **dual diagnosis** refers to clients who have both a substance use disorder and a serious mental illness. El-Mallakh (1998) reports that up to 51% of people with severe mental illnesses also have substance use disorders. These individuals have two separate chronic illnesses, and they have a higher level of functional impairment than the general population of people with substance dependency. Many people self-medicate their psychiatric symptoms with alcohol or drugs. Both the mental disorder and the substance use must be treated together.

Substance Dependency among Nurses

It may seem unlikely for nurses to have problems with substance use, because they should know better. In fact, many nurses do use substances. Some reasons our profession is at especially high risk for substance use disorders are that:

- Nurses see medications as a solution to problems.
- Nurses have access to drugs at work and to physicians who prescribe them.
- Nurses often believe that they should work even when they are tired or sick, so they may use drugs to increase their ability to continue working.
- Nurses experience stress, emotional pain, anger, and frustration, which are symptoms that respond to drugs in the short term.
- Nurses think that if they know about drugs and drug abuse, addiction will not happen to them.

If nurses had adequate understanding of addiction and its early signs, we could identify it earlier in our coworkers and ourselves. Signs of an **impaired nurse** (one who is working under the influence of substances) include changes in the nurse's *behavior* (mood changes, irritability, forgetfulness, isolation from coworkers, inappropriate behavior). *Work performance* may be affected (multiple medication errors, missed deadlines, sloppy charting, inattention to detail, absenteeism, poor judgment, volunteering to give other nurses' narcotics, excessive wasting of narcotics, client complaints that pain medications are not effective, tampering with drug packaging, going to bathroom after administering narcotics). The nurse may also have *signs of drug use or withdrawal* (alcohol on breath, heavy use of breath mints and perfume, red eyes, ataxia, restlessness, anxiety, slurred speech, hyperactivity, family problems that interfere with work, tremors, runny nose).

Substance dependency is a chronic physiologic illness that requires treatment. Affected nurses deserve to be diagnosed and treated before they hurt their clients or themselves. If you suspect that a peer is impaired, notify a manager or hospital supervisor. The nurse is unlikely to be able to manage the problem alone. Check to see if your state board of nursing has a nurse monitoring or treatment program that can help affected nurses recover and return to the profession.

In the acute situation, your duty as a nurse is to protect your clients from an impaired nurse. In the big picture of caring for colleagues in your profession, your duty is to help your peers get treatment. The intervention to reach each of these outcomes is the same: Tell a supervisor (not just the unit charge nurse for the day), so clients will be safe and the nurse will be treated. This is no time to engage in denial.

NURSING CARE

ASSESSING

Assess the substance use history of every client. Notify the physician of recent use or regular use so appropriate measures can be taken to adjust doses of prescribed medications. Nursing assessment questions are listed in Box 52-4 ■. Note that the substance use assessment does not ask "Do you drink?" Because alcohol and drug use are associated with strong negative attitudes by society and with guilt by users, the client is most likely to believe that the right answer is "no." People use denial to cope with their substance abuse problems, and they often lie about or underestimate their use. The nurse must present a nonjudgmental attitude and be accepting of clients as people, whether they use drugs or not. (For more information about mental status assessment, see Chapter 47. 🔗)

Notice the assessment question that asks the client what purpose the substance serves. This promotes the nurse's ability to help the client find other choices for coping or entertainment.

A general screening tool for whether a client has problems with alcohol is the CAGE questionnaire (Ewing, 1984). Further inquiry is indicated if the client answers "yes" to any one of the following questions:

■ Have you ever felt you ought to **C**ut down on your drinking?

<table>
<tr><td>**BOX 52-4**</td><td>**ASSESSMENT**</td></tr>
</table>

Assessing for Substance Use

Note: This is a screening assessment. A more thorough assessment would be indicated in a substance abuse treatment setting.

■ How many cigarettes a day do you smoke?

■ How often do you drink alcohol?

■ About how much do you drink?

■ What kind of drugs do you use that are not prescribed?

■ What is your method of use (oral, smoking, inhaling, injecting)?

■ What purpose do these substances serve for you (relaxation, fun, to help you get through the day)?

■ Have you had any problems because of drinking or drug use (social, job, or legal)?

■ When was the last time you used alcohol or any drug, what was it, and how much?

■ Have people **A**nnoyed you by criticizing your drinking?

■ Have you ever felt bad or **G**uilty about your drinking?

■ Have you ever had a drink first thing in the morning to steady your nerves or get rid of a hangover (**E**ye-opener)?

DIAGNOSING, PLANNING, AND IMPLEMENTING

Risk for Injury R/T Alcohol Withdrawal

■ Take vital signs frequently. If they are elevated (T, P, R, and BP may be involved), medicate with benzodiazepines according to physician's orders. *Benzodiazepines either treat or prevent symptoms of alcohol withdrawal by balancing the CNS stimulation with a depressant effect until the client's CNS can return to homeostasis without alcohol.*

■ Assess for other withdrawal symptoms (anxiety, agitation, sweating, nausea, vomiting, tremors, and ataxia). *Treat with prn benzodiazepines as above. If withdrawal is so severe that the client has hallucinations or seizures, call the physician immediately. These may be symptoms of life-threatening withdrawal.*

■ If the client is nauseated, do not push fluids. Offer small amounts of fluids frequently. Offer high-calorie feedings. *Assess for dehydration. Clients in withdrawal are at risk for fluid and electrolyte disturbances. They are also at risk for inadequate nutrition. It is easier for the nauseated client to take foods and fluids in small amounts than in big meals.*

■ Maintain a low-stimulation environment for the client. *Clients in withdrawal are experiencing CNS stimulation. They will be more comfortable and less likely to have a seizure if they are in a quiet room with dim lights.*

■ Encourage expression of feelings about drinking or about what the client is experiencing. *People with alcohol dependency often have difficulty understanding their own feelings. Expressing them can begin the process of behavior change.*

Deficient Knowledge (Substance Abuse and its Consequences)

■ Assess what clients know and what they need to learn. Teach them about the process of drug abuse and dependency, and how people use drugs for coping, recreation, and company. Review the consequences to the client of substance use. *Because so many people deny the severity of the problem, nurses must be honest about what the consequences are (job loss, divorce, family estrangement, disease of every body system, etc.) When people know what the problem is physiologically and realistically, they can begin to do something about it.*

Ineffective Coping

■ Help plan for new healthy coping strategies to replace substance use. *The client may need to meet new people to make new friends if all of his old friends only get together to drink or use drugs. People need alternatives to substance use when they become too **H**ungry, **A**ngry, **L**onely, or **T**ired. (HALT is an acronym for feelings that lead to relapse into drug use.)*

■ Help make a list of fun, recreational activities. *Clients may not even know what to do for fun. Be sure the list is realistic and includes the client's preferences (taking a walk, basketball, calling a friend on the phone, listening to music, hiking, bike riding, outdoor work, reading, community service, spiritual activities, dancing, carpentry, painting, and appreciating nature are some ideas).*

■ Help clients identify their resources for various needs and stressful situations (e.g., a ride to the grocery store or the doctor's office, help caring for the cat if the client is in the hospital). His sponsor from Alcoholics Anonymous may be the one to call if he feels like drinking again, or if he wants to talk about how hard life is. *A practical list like this may be the thing the client turns to instead of drinking when he has a problem and cannot think of what to do.*

Other nursing diagnoses that commonly apply to people with substance use disorders are:

■ Compromised or Disabled Family Coping
■ Chronic Low Self-Esteem
■ Powerlessness
■ Fear
■ Ineffective Denial
■ Imbalanced Nutrition, Less than Body Requirements
■ Disturbed Sleep Pattern
■ Social Isolation
■ Spiritual Distress
■ Disturbed Sensory Perception
■ Risk for Violence

EVALUATING

To evaluate whether nursing interventions for clients with substance-use disorders are effective, look at the outcomes. Desired outcomes include:

■ Client will have a plan for healthy alternatives to substance use for coping.
■ Client will identify resources for obtaining help when needed (family, friends, Alcoholics Anonymous, social service agencies).
■ Client will identify risk factors for relapse and plan for relapse prevention.
■ Client will identify and verbalize feelings.
■ Client will assume responsibility for own behavior.
■ Client will use peer support to maintain sobriety.

Documenting. Documentation should include client's stated history of substance use, time and description of last drug use, symptoms of intoxication on admission (including smell of alcohol on breath), withdrawal symptoms and their treatment, and the client's response to medications given. Document any discussions the nurse has with the client about substance use and its significance to the client. Most people with substance abuse issues are hospitalized without any mention of substance use at all. Document the topics you have taught the client and client's response.

CONTINUING CARE

When people with substance use disorders are discharged from the hospital, there must be follow-up of their substance use issues. Clients may benefit from a written list of telephone numbers for counseling resources, drug abuse treatment, or Alcoholics Anonymous. When a person is not expected to abstain from substance use, the physician must consider this when prescribing medications for use at home. If a client is going to be discharged with sedatives or other medications that could interact with drugs of abuse, discuss the potential risks with the physician.

Nurses should remind clients that they are in control of their own behavior. Clients should be given resources for outpatient support. A promise "never to use again" will not make the person successful. People with substance dependency should always be referred to social services for assistance with discharge planning. See the following list of resources for clients and families.

Resources for Nurses, Clients, and Families

Alcoholics Anonymous World Services
475 Riverside
New York, NY 10115
www.aa.org; www.recovery.org/aa

Al-Anon Family Group Headquarters

1600 Corporate Landing Parkway

Virginia Beach, VA

1-888-4ALANON

www.Alanon.org

American Society of Addiction Medicine

www.asam.org

National Clearinghouse for Alcohol and Drug Information (NCADI)

Prevline: Prevention Online (This is the website for the Center for Substance Abuse Prevention, Substance Abuse and Mental Health Services Administration, and Center for Substance Abuse Treatment.)

www.health.org

National Institute on Drug Abuse (NIDA)

American Self Help Clearing House

www.nida.nih.gov

NURSING PROCESS CARE PLAN
Client with Ineffective Coping

A 30-year-old woman was hospitalized for hematemesis (vomiting blood) and abdominal pain 3 days ago. The medical diagnosis is acute gastritis due to chronic alcohol use. Her husband is a truck driver and is away from home most of the time.

Assessment. The nurse did a substance-use assessment and found that the woman uses alcohol most days. She drinks a bottle of wine at night after her children go to bed. After they go to school, she sometimes has a few drinks in the morning. She drinks because the only time she feels good is when she is drinking. Her parents were both alcoholics. She has no hobbies and states that her only reason for living is her children. The client states, "I don't even know what I like to do. The only time I feel good is when I'm drunk." Vital signs are T 99.2°F, P 90, R 18, BP 118/80.

Diagnosis. The nursing diagnosis is Ineffective Coping, related to inadequate role modeling and ineffective skills.

Expected Outcomes. The client will:

- Relate her feelings about alcohol dependency.
- List three resources for help when she needs it.
- Plan for four possible alternatives to drinking alcohol when she is under stress.

- Contact Alcoholics Anonymous while in the hospital, and plan to attend a meeting on the day she is discharged.
- List at least three things that she enjoys doing.

Planning and Implementation. The nurse will implement the following interventions:

- Spend time talking with the client each shift.
- Help the client make a list of people who can help her in various everyday situations (caring for the children, driving her to an AA meeting, being available to talk on the phone if she is lonely).
- Help the client make a list of alternatives to drinking. These items will be things that the client agrees that she would actually do. They may include going for a walk, writing a letter, working outdoors, taking the children to the park or the library, playing a game, listening to music, dancing, exercise, journaling, or volunteering.
- Show the client how to find the telephone number of the local Alcoholics Anonymous group in the phone book, and encourage the client to contact them.
- Assist the client to make a list of things she would enjoy doing. The nurse may make suggestions, but the client should choose the enjoyable things. These also become alternatives to drinking.

Evaluation. The client was discharged after 6 days in the hospital. She started attending Alcoholics Anonymous, but quit because she did not feel comfortable in the group meetings. Her sponsor convinced her to try an AA group for women only, which she likes and continues to attend. She and her husband are in couples counseling. He is scheduling his work so he can be at home more often. She has not had any alcohol since she left the hospital 4 weeks ago.

Critical Thinking in the Nursing Process

1. What are the situations that would put this client at greatest risk for relapse into drinking again?
2. What role did alcohol play in this woman's life?
3. If the client called the hospital unit and told the nurse that she feels like drinking and doesn't know what to do, what should the nurse say?

Note: The bibliography listings for this and all chapters have been compiled at the back of the book.

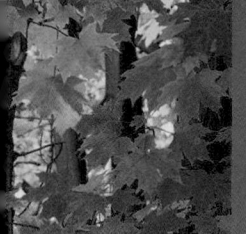

Chapter Review

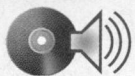 **KEY TERMS** by Topics

Use the audio glossary feature of either the CD-ROM or the Companion Website to hear the correct pronunciation of the following key terms.

Problems of substance abuse
denial, substance abuse, substance dependency

Commonly abused substances
intoxication, euphoria, ataxia, labile, tolerance, withdrawal, alcoholic, Korsakoff's syndrome, confabulation, Wernicke's syndrome, myopathy, abstinence, relapse, polysubstance abuse, cross-tolerance, codependent,

detoxification, rehabilitation, dual diagnosis, impaired nurse

KEY Points

- Substance abuse is a maladaptive pattern of substance use despite adverse outcomes. Substance dependency involves continuing to use the substance despite significant substance-related problems, including tolerance, withdrawal, and compulsive use.

- The DSM-IV-TR lists 11 substances of abuse: alcohol; opioids; sedatives, hypnotics, and anxiolytics; cocaine; amphetamines and similar drugs; hallucinogens; phencyclidine (PCP) and similar drugs; inhalants; cannabis; caffeine; and nicotine.

- The CNS depressant effects of prescribed drugs in the hospital, combined with the effects of drugs or alcohol the client used before admission, may cause severe respiratory depression.

- People who are tolerant to alcohol or narcotics need more analgesics than normal to obtain pain relief.

- Nurses should assess the substance use history of each client on admission.

- Understanding the personal consequences of drug and alcohol use is necessary for client rehabilitation.

- When substance abuse and dependency occur among nurses and other health care professionals, the first responsibility of the nurse is client safety and the second is to seek help for your colleague.

- The goal of substance use treatment is abstinence from substance use and development of skills to replace drug use for coping, enjoyment, or companionship.

- Clients with substance dependency need referral to social services for assistance and follow-up after discharge.

- Many people respond well to treatment for substance-related disorders: Keep hope alive.

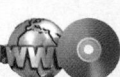 **EXPLORE Media**Link

Additional interactive resources for this chapter can be found on the Companion Website at www.prenhall.com/burke. Click on Chapter 52 and "Begin" to select the activities for this chapter.

For chapter-related NCLEX-style review questions and an audio glossary, access the accompanying CD-ROM in this book.

FOR FURTHER Study

See Chapter 47 for more information about mental status assessment.

Some substance use is self-medication for anxiety. See Chapter 50 for information about anxiety disorders.

Critical Thinking Care Map

Caring for a Client with Substance Dependency
NCLEX-PN® Focus Area: Psychosocial Integrity: Coping and Adaptation

Case Study: A 24-year-old male client is admitted to the medical–surgical unit with multiple trauma suffered in an automobile accident that happened while he was drinking. He has been on the unit for 4 days. His vital signs are stable now, although he has experienced alcohol withdrawal syndrome during the past several days. The substance-use history reveals that he drinks beer every day, usually "about two six-packs or so." The client states, "I don't have a drinking problem. I can quit whenever I want!"

Nursing Diagnosis: Ineffective Denial

COLLECT DATA

Subjective	Objective
_____	_____
_____	_____
_____	_____
_____	_____
_____	_____
_____	_____

Would you report this data? Yes/No

If yes, to: _____

Nursing Care

_____
_____
_____
_____
_____
_____
_____

How would you document this? _____
_____
_____
_____

Data Collected
(use those that apply)

- Client states, "I don't have a drinking problem. I can quit whenever I want!"
- Vital signs stable
- Blood alcohol content on admission 0.24 mg/dL
- Weight 165 lbs
- Skin warm, dry
- Requests pain medication (ordered q4h prn) approximately q1h
- States "I feel nervous."
- Has insomnia (sleeps less than 4 hours per night)
- Had seizures as a child
- Poor appetite: eats less than 50% of meals
- Client states, "If you don't let me out of here tomorrow, I'm leaving anyway."

Nursing Interventions
(use those that apply; list in priority order)

- Assess client's knowledge about alcoholism.
- Teach client about the disease of substance dependency.
- Weigh the client daily.
- Provide effective pain management.
- Minimize the amount of narcotics given to this client because he is an addict.
- Offer frequent feedings of high-protein foods.
- Confront the client with the reality of the consequences of alcoholism.
- Encourage the client to express his feelings about drinking and alcoholism.
- Ask the client why he wants to leave the hospital. If he doesn't say so, ask if he wants to drink alcohol.
- Ask the physician for an order for a sleeping medication for the client to take now and when he goes home.

NCLEX-PN® Exam Preparation

1   A client discovers he needs more than his usual pint of liquor to achieve the same effect. This phenomenon is called:

   A. tolerance.

   B. intoxication.

   C. addiction.

   D. abuse.

2   A client is admitted with a diagnosis of alcohol withdrawal. The nurse expects to find which of the following on assessment?

   A. B/P 110/70, P 72, R 20

   B. cooperative behavior

   C. anxiety, tremors

   D. warm, dry skin

3   A client is admitted with alcoholic encephalopathy (Wernicke's syndrome). The nurse expects to administer which of the following medications?

   A. Demerol (meperidine)

   B. Valium (diazepam)

   C. thiamine (vitamin B_1)

   D. Dilantin (phenytoin)

4   The physical assessment of a client admitted to the emergency department reveals pinpoint pupils, depressed respirations, and confusion. The physician diagnoses morphine overdose. Treatment includes:

   A. thiamine (vitamin B_1).

   B. Narcan (Naloxone HCl).

   C. Librium (chlordiazepoxide).

   D. $D_{50}W$.

5   A client is prescribed Xanax (alprazalom) for treatment of anxiety. Which of the following must the LPN/LVN include in the teaching plan?

   A. Take the drug every 4 hours.

   B. Avoid alcohol while taking the drug.

   C. The drug can cause drowsiness.

   D. Avoid driving until effects are known.

6   An LVN suspects her coworker is diverting narcotics on the nursing unit. What action by the nurse would be most effective?

   A. Confront the nurse with her suspicions.

   B. Notify the physician.

   C. Notify the charge nurse.

   D. Notify the nursing supervisor.

7   The nurse establishes a nursing diagnosis of *Deficient Knowledge* for a client with a history of substance abuse. The LPN/LVN reinforces a teaching plan to include:

   A. signs and symptoms of withdrawal.

   B. consequences to client of continued substance abuse.

   C. safe levels of drug use.

   D. antidotes to opiates.

8   A 28-year-old woman presented to the emergency department for treatment of cocaine addiction. The nurse expects her to exhibit which of the following behaviors during withdrawal from cocaine?

   A. anxiety

   B. hypertension

   C. depression

   D. seizures

9   Select all of the correct nursing interventions for a client experiencing alcohol withdrawal.

   A. Take vital signs frequently.

   B. Provide a low-stimulation environment.

   C. Withhold any medications that act on the CNS.

   D. Tell the client that this illness is his punishment for drinking.

10   A client on the medical–surgical unit had abdominal surgery this morning and now has a headache. She has been NPO since midnight last night. She might be experiencing withdrawal from what substance? _____

Answers for Review Questions, as well as discussion of Care Plan and Critical Thinking Care Map questions, appear in Appendix V.

Thinking Strategically About...

Juanita Santos, a 62-year-old woman, was admitted through the ER following an episode of hyperglycemia related to her adult-onset insulin-dependent diabetes mellitus (IDDM). She has poor short-term memory, but has good recall of events of her childhood. Her son states that she has had this memory problem for some time, but lately it has become a concern. Juanita loves to baby sit the grandchildren, but her daughter-in-law is reluctant to leave them with her. This is becoming a source of stress for the family. Juanita tells the ER nurse, "My family thinks I am useless now; they should just put me in a home."

NURSING ASSESSMENT

To further assess the client's mental status, what should the nurse do?

COMMUNICATION

Mrs. Santos is of Hispanic origin. Culturally Hispanics have a strong family connection. Her family is very concerned for her welfare as well as the children's safety. How could you as the nurse facilitate communication in order to relieve the family stress?

INTERDISCIPLINARY CARE

The family feels strongly that they want to care for Mrs. Santos at home. A discharge planning conference is being convened. Your RN team leader has asked you to attend, because you have a good relationship with the family and client. Also participating will be the RN, the diabetic educator, the psychiatric social worker, the home care nurse, and the physician. The son and daughter-in-law will also attend. As the LPN/LVN, what input could you give that would help with the transition from hospital to home?

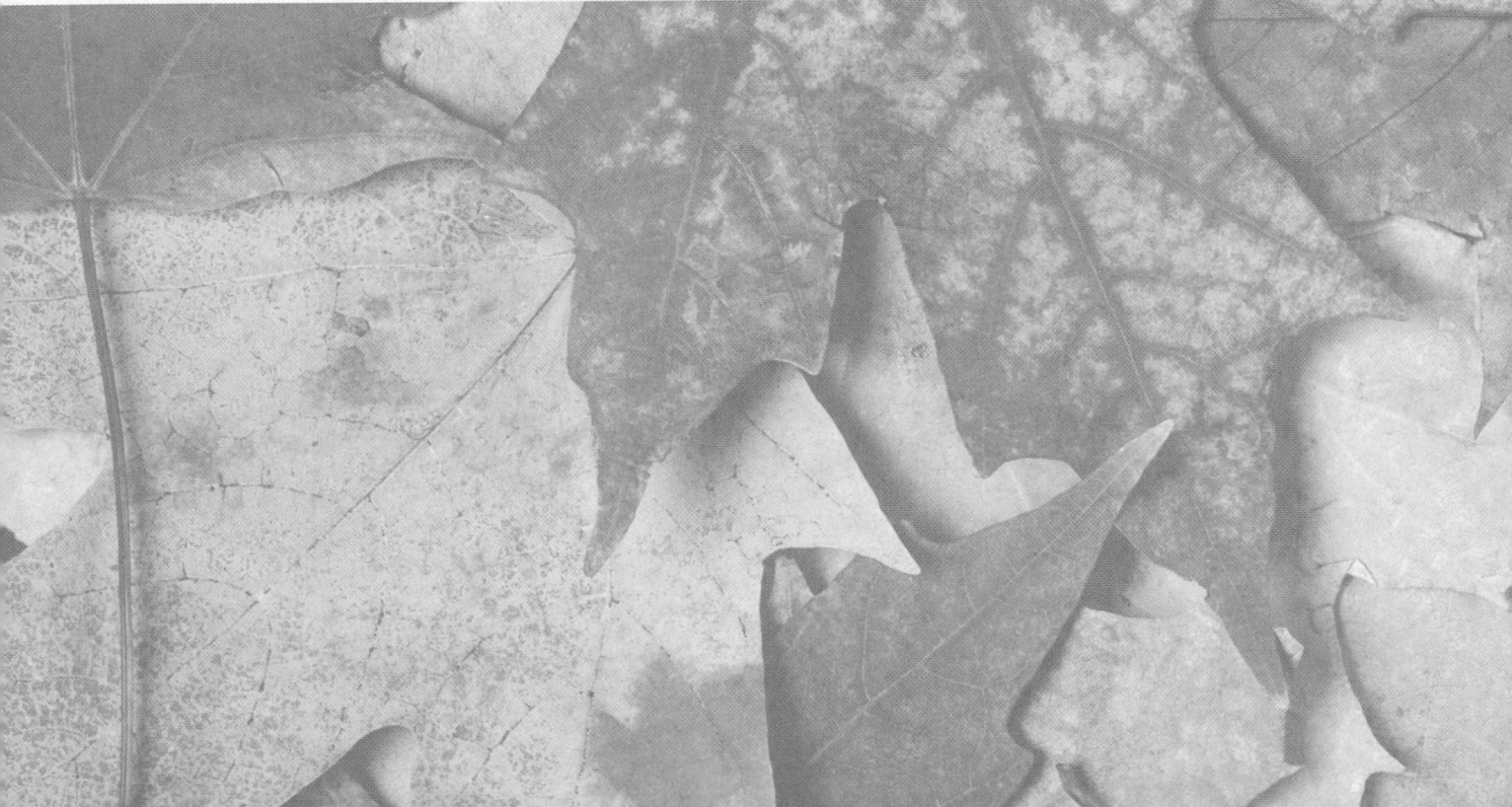

Appendix I

Standard Precautions

Standard precautions are designed to reduce the risk of transmission of microorganisms from both recognized and unrecognized sources of infection. They are the primary strategy for preventing nosocomial infections within institutions, and are important to protect healthcare workers as well. Standard precautions apply to (1) blood; (2) all body fluids, secretions, and excretions except sweat, regardless of whether or not they contain visible blood; (3) nonintact skin; and (4) mucous membranes. Standard precautions are applied to all clients receiving care in hospitals, regardless of their diagnosis or presumed infection status. These precautions are specifically designed for hospitals; however, they also may be implemented in extended and long-term care facilities, and to a more limited extent in providing home care or in other community-based care settings.

HANDWASHING

- Wash your hands (a) immediately after removing gloves, even if gloves appear to be intact; (b) between contacts with clients; and (c) after contacting blood, body fluids, secretions, excretions, and equipment or articles contaminated by them. You may need to wash your hands between tasks and procedures on the same client to prevent cross-contaminating different body sites.
- Use soap and warm water for handwashing when hands are visibly dirty or contaminated with blood or other body fluids. Use an antimicrobial agent for specific circumstances; e.g., to control an outbreak.
- If hands are not visibly soiled, an alcohol-based hand rub may be used for routinely decontaminating hands in all other situations.

GLOVES

- Wear clean, nonsterile gloves when touching blood, body fluids, secretions, excretions, and contaminated items.
- Put on clean gloves just before touching mucous membranes and nonintact skin.
- Change your gloves between tasks and procedures on the same client after contacting material that may contain a high concentration of microorganisms.
- Remove gloves promptly after use, before touching noncontaminated items and surfaces, and before going to another client; wash hands immediately after removing gloves.

MASK, EYE PROTECTION, FACE SHIELD

Wear a mask and eye protection or a face shield to protect mucous membranes of your eyes, nose, and mouth during procedures and client-care activities that are likely to generate splashes or sprays of blood, body fluids, secretions, or excretions.

GOWN

Wear a clean, nonsterile gown to protect your skin and prevent soiling of clothing during procedures and client-care activities that are likely to generate splashes or sprays of blood, body fluids, secretions, or excretions. Remove soiled gowns promptly, washing your hands immediately after gown removal.

EQUIPMENT

Handle used client-care equipment that is soiled with blood, body fluids, secretions, and excretions in a way that prevents exposing your skin and mucous membranes, contaminating your clothing, and transferring microorganisms to other clients or environments. Ensure that reusable equipment is cleaned and appropriately reprocessed before using for the care of another client. Ensure proper disposal of single-use items.

ENVIRONMENTAL CONTROL

Follow hospital procedures for routine care, cleaning, and disinfecting environmental surfaces, beds, bed rails, bedside equipment, and other frequently touched surfaces.

LINEN

Handle and transport linens soiled with blood, body fluids, secretions, and excretions in a manner that prevents exposing your skin and mucous membranes, contaminating your clothing, and transferring microorganisms to other clients and environments. Place soiled linen in leakage-resistant bags at the location where it is used.

OCCUPATIONAL HEALTH AND BLOODBORNE PATHOGENS

- Take care to prevent injuries when using needles, scalpels, and other sharps; when handling sharp instruments after procedures; when cleaning used instruments; and when disposing of used needles.
- Never recap used needles, manipulate them using both hands, or handle them in a manner that directs the point

of a needle toward any part of your body. If it is necessary to protect the needle prior to disposal, use a one-handed "scoop" technique or mechanical device to hold the needle sheath.

- Do not remove used needles from disposable syringes by hand; do not bend, break, or otherwise manipulate used needles by hand.
- Place used disposable syringes and needles, scalpel blades, and other sharp items in appropriate puncture-resistant containers located as close as practical to the area in which the items were used.
- Place reusable syringes and needles in a puncture-resistant container for transport to the reprocessing area.
- Use mouthpieces, resuscitation bags, or other ventilation devices as an alternative to mouth-to-mouth resuscitation methods whenever possible.

CLIENT PLACEMENT
Place clients who contaminate the environment or who do not (or are not expected to) assist in maintaining appropriate hygiene or environmental control, for example, an ambulatory, confused client with fecal incontinence, in a private room.

Source: Standard precautions. *(2005). U.S. Department of Health and Human Services, Centers for Disease Control and Prevention. Available: www.cdc.gov/ncidod/ dhqptgl_isolation_standard.html*

Appendix II

2005–2006 NANDA-Approved Nursing Diagnoses

Activity Intolerance
Activity Intolerance, Risk for
Adaptive Capacity: Intracranial, Decreased
Adjustment, Impaired
Airway Clearance, Ineffective
Anxiety
Anxiety, Death
Aspiration, Risk for
Attachment, Parent/Infant/Child, Risk for Impaired
Body Image, Disturbed
Body Temperature: Imbalanced, Risk for
Bowel Incontinence
Breastfeeding, Effective
Breastfeeding, Ineffective
Breastfeeding, Interrupted
Breathing Pattern, Ineffective
Cardiac Output, Decreased
Caregiver Role Strain
Caregiver Role Strain, Risk for
Communication, Readiness for Enhanced
Communication: Verbal, Impaired
Confusion, Acute
Confusion, Chronic
Constipation
Constipation, Perceived
Constipation, Risk for
Coping: Community, Ineffective
Coping: Community, Readiness for Enhanced
Coping, Defensive
Coping: Family, Compromised
Coping: Family, Disabled
Coping: Family, Readiness for Enhanced
Coping (Individual), Readiness for Enhanced
Coping, Ineffective
Decisional Conflict (Specify)
Denial, Ineffective
Dentition, Impaired
Development: Delayed, Risk for
Diarrhea
Disuse Syndrome, Risk for
Diversional Activity, Deficient
Dysreflexia, Autonomic
Dysreflexia, Autonomic, Risk for
Energy Field Disturbance
Environmental Interpretation Syndrome, Impaired
Failure to Thrive, Adult
Falls, Risk for
Family Processes, Dysfunctional: Alcoholism

Family Processes, Interrupted
Family Processes, Readiness for Enhanced
Fatigue
Fear
Fluid Balance, Readiness for Enhanced
Fluid Volume, Deficient
Fluid Volume, Deficient, Risk for
Fluid Volume, Excess
Fluid Volume, Imbalanced, Risk for
Gas Exchange, Impaired
Grieving, Anticipatory
Grieving, Dysfunctional
Grieving, Risk for Dysfunctional
Growth, Disproportionate, Risk for
Growth and Development, Delayed
Health Maintenance, Ineffective
Health Seeking Behaviors (Specify)
Home Maintenance, Impaired
Hopelessness
Hyperthermia
Hypothermia
Identity: Personal, Disturbed
Infant Behavior, Disorganized
Infant Behavior: Disorganized, Risk for
Infant Behavior: Organized, Readiness for Enhanced
Infant Feeding Pattern, Ineffective
Infection, Risk for
Injury, Risk for
Knowledge, Deficient (Specify)
Knowledge (Specify), Readiness for Enhanced
Latex Allergy Response
Latex Allergy Response, Risk for
Lifestyle, Sedentary
Loneliness, Risk for
Memory, Impaired
Mobility: Bed, Impaired
Mobility: Physical, Impaired
Mobility: Wheelchair, Impaired
Nausea
Neurovascular Dysfunction: Peripheral, Risk for
Noncompliance (Specify)
Nutrition, Imbalanced: Less than Body Requirements
Nutrition, Imbalanced: More than Body Requirements
Nutrition, Imbalanced: More than Body Requirements,
  Risk for
Nutrition, Readiness for Enhanced
Oral Mucous Membrane, Impaired
Pain, Acute

Pain, Chronic
Parenting, Impaired
Parenting, Readiness for Enhanced
Parenting, Risk for Impaired
Perioperative Positioning Injury, Risk for
Poisoning, Risk for
Post-Trauma Syndrome
Post-Trauma Syndrome, Risk for
Powerlessness
Powerlessness, Risk for
Protection, Ineffective
Rape-Trauma Syndrome
Rape-Trauma Syndrome: Compound Reaction
Rape-Trauma Syndrome: Silent Reaction
Religiosity, Impaired
Religiosity, Readiness for Enhanced
Religiosity, Risk for Impaired
Relocation Stress Syndrome
Relocation Stress Syndrome, Risk for
Role Conflict, Parental
Role Performance, Ineffective
Self-Care Deficit: Bathing/Hygiene
Self-Care Deficit: Dressing/Grooming
Self-Care Deficit: Feeding
Self-Care Deficit: Toileting
Self-Concept, Readiness for Enhanced
Self-Esteem, Chronic Low
Self-Esteem, Situational Low
Self-Esteem, Risk for Situational Low
Self-Mutilation
Self-Mutilation, Risk for
Sensory Perception, Disturbed (Specify: Visual, Auditory,
   Kinesthetic, Gustatory, Tactile, Olfactory)
Sexual Dysfunction
Sexuality Patterns, Ineffective
Skin Integrity, Impaired
Skin Integrity, Risk for Impaired
Sleep Deprivation
Sleep Pattern Disturbed
Sleep, Readiness for Enhanced
Social Interaction, Impaired
Social Isolation

Sorrow, Chronic
Spiritual Distress
Spiritual Distress, Risk for
Spiritual Well-Being, Readiness for Enhanced
Spontaneous Ventilation, Impaired
Sudden Infant Death Syndrome, Risk for
Suffocation, Risk for
Suicide, Risk for
Surgical Recovery, Delayed
Swallowing, Impaired
Therapeutic Regimen Management: Community,
   Ineffective
Therapeutic Regimen Management, Effective
Therapeutic Regimen Management: Family, Ineffective
Therapeutic Regimen Management, Ineffective
Therapeutic Regimen Management, Readiness
   for Enhanced
Thermoregulation, Ineffective
Thought Processes, Disturbed
Tissue Integrity, Impaired
Tissue Perfusion, Ineffective (Specify: Renal, Cerebral,
   Cardiopulmonary, Gastrointestinal, Peripheral)
Tissue Perfusion, Ineffective (Peripheral)
Transfer Ability, Impaired
Trauma, Risk for
Unilateral Neglect
Urinary Elimination, Impaired
Urinary Elimination, Readiness for Enhanced
Urinary Incontinence, Functional
Urinary Incontinence, Reflex
Urinary Incontinence, Stress
Urinary Incontinence, Total
Urinary Incontinence, Urge
Urinary Incontinence, Risk for Urge
Urinary Retention
Ventilation, Impaired Spontaneous
Ventilatory Weaning Response, Dysfunctional
Violence: Other-Directed, Risk for
Violence: Self-Directed, Risk for
Walking, Impaired
Wandering

Source: NANDA Nursing Diagnoses: Definitions and Classification, 2005–2006. Philadelphia: North American Nursing Diagnosis Association. Used with permission.

Appendix III

Common Laboratory Values

BLOOD	
Hematocrit	Male: 40–54% Female: 37–47%
Hemoglobin	Male: 13.5–18 g/dL Female: 12–16 g/dL
Red blood cells	Male: 4.6–6.0 mil/μL Female: 3.6–5.0 mil/μL
MCV	80–98 μm^3
MCH	26–34 pg
MCHC	32–36%
White blood cells	4,500–10,000/mm^3
Neutrophils	50–70% of total WBCs
Eosinophils	1–3%
Basophils	0.5–1%
Lymphocytes	25–35%
Monocytes	2–6%
Platelets	150,000–350,000 μL
ELECTROLYTES	
Sodium (Na$^+$)	135–145 mEq/L
Potassium (K$^+$)	3.5–5.0 mEq/L
Calcium (Ca^{2+})	8.5–10 mg/dL
Magnesium (Mg^{2+})	1.3–2.1 mEq/L or 1.6–2.6 mg/dL
Chloride (Cl$^-$)	98–106 mEq/L
Bicarbonate (HCO$_3{}^-$)	22–26 mEq/L
Phosphate/phosphorus (PO$_4{}^{2-}$)	2.5–4.5 mg/dL

BLOOD	
Serum osmolality	275–295 mOsm/kg
Carbon dioxide	24–30 mEq/L
pH	7.35–7.45
Blood urea nitrogen (BUN)	8–25 mg/dL
Creatinine	0.6–1.2 mg/dL
Bilirubin (Total)	0.3–1.2 mg/dL
Direct bilirubin	0–0.2 mg/dL
Indirect bilirubin	< 1.1 mg/dL
Glucose	70–110 mg/dL
Protein	6.0–8.0 g/dL
Albumin	3.5–5.0 g/dL
Low density lipoproteins (LDLs)	60–160 mg/dL
Low risk for CHD	< 130 mg/dL
High density lipoproteins (HDLs)	30–80 mg/dL
Low risk for CHD	46–59 mg/dL
Cholesterol	120–220 mg/dL
Desirable level	< 200 mg/dL
Prothrombin time (PT)	11–14 sec
Thyroxine (T$_4$)	4–12 μg/dL
T$_3$ resin uptake	25–35 relative % uptake
URINALYSIS	
Color	Yellow, clear
Specific gravity	1.010–1.035
pH	4.5–7.8
Protein	Negative
Glucosae	Negative
Ketones	Negative

Appendix IV

GLOSSARY

(Note: Glossary terms may appear in several chapters. The number(s) in parentheses in boldface after the glossary term show the primary chapter in which the term is defined. Other words or terms that may require definitions are italicized in the text and are defined there.)

A

Abscesses: pockets of accumulated pus (10)

Abstinence: voluntarily refraining from use of a drug that has been abused or from an activity such as sexual intercourse (36, 51, 52)

Acidosis: increased hydrogen ion concentration; a pH of less than 7.35 (5)

Acne: disorder of the sebaceous glands (45)

Acquired immunodeficiency syndrome (AIDS): last stage of HIV infection (11)

Active immunity: immunity acquired by having the disease or by artificial immunization for long-term immunity (11)

Active transport: process by which molecules are moved against a concentration gradient across cell membranes (5)

Acute illness: illness that occurs rapidly, lasts for a relatively short period of time, and is self-limiting (2)

Acute myocardial infarction (AMI or MI): myocardial cell necrosis (death) due to lack of blood and oxygen (26)

Acute pain: temporary pain that has a sudden onset and is localized (8)

Acute pulmonary edema: Accumulation of fluid in the interstitial spaces and alveoli of the lungs; may be classified as either cardiogenic (due to acute heart failure) or noncardiogenic (27)

Acute respiratory distress syndrome (ARDS): a severe form of respiratory failure due to acute damage to the alveoli (13, 24)

Adaptive behavior: positive, health-promoting coping behavior (50)

Addiction: condition of seeking drugs habitually (other than for a medical purpose) and of not being able to give them up without adverse psychologic and physiologic effects (8, 52)

Addisonian crisis: acute deficiency of cortisol that causes a life-threatening condition (16)

Addison's disease: autoimmune destruction of adrenal glands that causes deficient production of corticosteroids and mineral corticoid hormones (16)

Additive: the sum of the effects when two drugs with similar actions are taken (6)

Advance directives: legal documents that allow a person to plan for health care and financial affairs in the event of incapacity (14)

Adventitious: abnormal (e.g., abnormal breath sounds) (22)

Advocate: one who speaks for another (1)

Affect: the outward expression of emotion, more transient than mood (48, 49)

Ageism: a form of prejudice that stereotypes older adults (3)

Agonist: a drug that initiates an action (6)

Agranulocytosis: decrease in granulocytes; neutropenia (30)

Akathisia: restlessness; intense need to move (48)

Alcoholic: alcohol-dependent individual (52)

Alkalosis: decreased hydrogen ion concentration; a pH greater than 7.45 (5)

Allergen: substance such as dog hair or pollen that causes an allergic reaction (11)

Allodynia: pain resulting from a stimulus that normally would not cause pain, such as light touch (8)

Alopecia: hair loss (44)

Alterations in health: change in normal health state (2)

Alzheimer's disease: progressive deterioration of brain function resulting in dementia (39)

Ambulatory surgery: a surgical procedure performed on a nonhospitalized client under local or general anesthesia (9)

Amenorrhea: absence of menstruation (35)

Amputation: partial or total removal of a body part (42)

Amyotrophic lateral sclerosis (ALS): fatal neurologic disease causing loss of motor neuron function in the spinal cord and brainstem (39)

Anabolism: process by which tissues are built up (10)

Analgesics: pharmacologic agents used to relieve or reduce pain (8)

Anaphylactic shock: shock caused by a severe allergic reaction (13)

Anaphylaxis: an acute, immediate allergic reaction (11, 13)

Anastomosis: surgical connection of two tubular structures (19)

Androgens: male sex hormones (33)

Anemia: condition in which the hemoglobin concentration or the number of circulating RBCs is decreased (30)

Anergy: no response to common antigens given to test for immunocompetence (11)

Anesthesia: use of chemical substances to produce loss of sensation, reflex loss, or muscle relaxation during a surgical procedure, with or without the loss of consciousness (9)

Aneurysm: localized dilation of a blood vessel (28, 38)

Angina pectoris: chest pain that occurs when there is a temporary imbalance between myocardial blood supply and demand (26)

Anhedonia: inability to feel pleasure (48, 49)

Anorexia nervosa: an eating disorder marked by a disturbed body image, fear of gaining weight, and weight less than 85% of that expected for age and height (19)

Anorexia–cachexia syndrome: effect of cancer cells on metabolism; cancer cells divert nutrition to own use and inhibit food intake; they also break down body tissue and muscle proteins to support their growth (12)

Anoxia: lack of oxygen to body tissues (38)

Antagonist: prevents drug action (6)

Antibiotics: medications used to treat bacterial infections (10)

Antibody: an immunoglobulin that binds to and inactivates a specific antigen (11)

Antigen: substance that stimulates an immune response (11)

Anuria: absence of urine output (32)

Anxiety: feeling of uneasiness and activation of the autonomic nervous system in response to a nonspecific threat (50)

Aphasia: inability to speak or understand the spoken word (38)

Appendicitis: inflammation of the appendix (20)

Arteriosclerosis: disorder characterized by thickening, loss of elasticity, and calcification of arterial walls (28)

Arthralgia: joint pain (43)

Arthritis: inflammation of a joint (43)

Arthroplasty: reconstruction or replacement of a joint (43)

Arthroscopy: use of a flexible fiberoptic endoscope to view and/or repair joint structures and tissues (41)

Ascites: accumulation of serous fluid in the peritoneal cavity (21)

Assessment: collection of data about the client's individualized health and health care needs; first step of the nursing process (1, 5)

Asthma: a chronic inflammatory airway disorder with recurrent episodes of wheezing, breathlessness, chest tightness, and coughing (25)

Ataxia: staggering or unsteady gait (52)

Atelectasis: an area or areas of alveolar collapse and airlessness (25)

Atherosclerosis: disease in which the lining of medium and large arteries is affected by lesions called atheromas or plaque (26)

Aura: warning sign of a seizure or migraine headache; it may be a bright light, an unusual sound, or an abnormal taste or odor (38)

Auscultation: method of assessment that uses a stethoscope to listen for body sounds (5)

Autoantibodies: antibodies made against self-antigens (11)

Autograft: graft transplanted from one part of the body to another (11)

Autoimmune disorders: disorders in which the body reacts against itself (11)

Autologous: self (11)

Automatism: repetitive, nonpurposeful actions such as lip smacking or aimless walking (38)

Autonomic dysreflexia: an exaggerated sympathetic response associated with high spinal cord injuries (39)

Autotransfusion: process in which a client's own blood is collected and reinfused (13)

Azotemia: increased blood levels of nitrogenous wastes, including urea and creatinine (32)

B

Bactericidal: ability of an antibiotic to kill microorganisms (10)

Bacteriostatic: ability of an antibiotic to inhibit growth of microorganisms (10)

Barrel chest: a greater anterior–posterior (AP) chest diameter than lateral chest diameter (24)

Basal cell carcinoma: cancer that begins in the basal cell layer of the epidermis, usually on sun-exposed areas of the body (45)

B-cell lymphocytes (B cells): white blood cells responsible for humoral immunity that produce antibodies (11)

Bell's palsy: neurologic disorder resulting from inflammation of the facial nerve (39)

Benign prostatic hyperplasia (BPH): enlargement of the prostate gland (34)

Biliary colic: right upper quadrant pain associated with bile duct obstruction (21)

Biotransformation: process by which the body changes a drug from its original chemical structure into a form that can be eliminated by the body (6)

Block nursing: care, based on need, provided by the nurse to people who live on the same block as the nurse (4)

Blood pressure: force exerted by blood against the walls of the arteries (25)

Bone marrow transplant (BMT): transplantation of bone marrow from one person to another, or the harvest, preservation, and reinfusion of the client's own bone marrow (autologous BMT) (30)

Borborygmi: loud, hyperactive bowel sounds (19)

Bradykinesia: slowed voluntary movements and speech (39)

Brain abscess: collection of purulent material within the brain (38)

Brain death criteria: clinical criteria for determining when a client is dead (13)

Brain tumors: abnormal growths within the cranium (38)

Broad-spectrum antibiotics: antibiotics that act against a wide variety of pathogens (10)

Bronchitis: inflammation of the bronchi (24)

Bruit: harsh or musical sound (murmur) heard on auscultation of a blood vessel (28)

Buffer: substance that prevents major changes in pH by either removing or releasing hydrogen ions from a solution (5)

Bulimia nervosa: episodic binge eating and self-induced vomiting, laxative or diuretic use, or excessive exercise (19)

Burn: injury of tissue loss, damage, or irreversible destruction from exposure to a thermal, chemical, electrical, or radiation heat source (46)

Burn shock: type of hypovolemic shock resulting from the shift of a massive amount of fluid into the extravascular space (46)

C

Cancer: disease that results when normal cells mutate into abnormal ones and continue to reproduce within the body (12)

Candidiasis: infections caused by *Candida albicans,* a yeastlike fungus (45)

Carcinogens: cancer-causing agents (12)

Cardiac arrest: cessation of effective heart contractions and blood circulation; usually caused by ventricular fibrillation (26)

Cardiac dysrhythmia: disturbance or irregularity in the electrical system of the heart (26)

Cardiac output (CO): amount of blood pumped from the ventricles in 1 minute (25)

Cardiac reserve: ability of the heart to increase the cardiac output in response to metabolic demand (27)

Cardiac tamponade: compression of the heart by blood or fluid in the pericardial sac (27)

Cardiogenic shock: impaired tissue perfusion caused by pumping failure of the heart (13, 26)

Cardiomyopathy: disorder that affects the structure and function of the heart (27)

Cardioversion: restoration of a normal heart rhythm (normal sinus rhythm) using either electric shock or medications (26)

Caregivers: people who provide personal, individual assistance (1)

Carotid endarterectomy: surgical procedure to remove plaque from the carotid artery (38)

Carrier: person who transmits an infectious disease but does not show any clinical manifestations (10)

Catabolism: process by which body tissues are broken down (10, 19)

Cataract: clouding of the lens of the eye (40)

Ceiling effect: the limit of some drugs to produce a specific effect (6)

Cell-mediated immunity: immune response provided by direct action of the T cells (11)

Cellulitis: localized infection of the dermis and subcutaneous tissue (10, 45)

Cerebrovascular accident (CVA): sudden loss of neurologic function due to a blood clot or rupture of a cerebral artery; brain attack or stroke (38)

Cerumen: earwax (37)

Chain of infection: set of factors that must exist in order for an infection to develop (10)

Chancre: painless ulcer characteristic of primary syphilis (36)

Cheyne-stokes: periods of apnea for 10 to 60 seconds followed by gradual increased rate and depth of breathing (37)

Cholecystitis: inflammation of the gallbladder (21)

Cholelithiasis: formation of gallstones (21)

Chorea: constant, jerky, uncontrolled movements of the body (39)

Chronic illness: any impairment or deviation from normal functioning that affects more than one body system and that is permanent, leaves permanent disability, is irreversible, requires special teaching for rehabilitation, or requires a long period of care (2)

Chronic obstructive pulmonary disease (COPD): chronic and progressive air flow obstruction caused by chronic bronchitis and emphysema (24)

Chronic pain: pain that lasts longer than 6 months, may not be totally eliminated, or may end only with death; may be malignant (related to cancer) or nonmalignant (8)

Chyme: mixture of partly digested food and digestive juices (18)

Cirrhosis: chronic liver disease that destroys the structure and function of liver lobules (21)

Clonic contractions: alternate contraction and relaxation of muscles, causing jerky movements (38)

Clubbing: occurs when angle of nail base is greater than 180 degrees (44)

Codependent: a person who enables a person with substance dependency to avoid the consequences of substance use (often by making excuses or taking on their responsibilities) (52)

Cognition: the ability to perceive and understand one's world (3)

Cognitive: thinking and memory (48)

Colectomy: surgical removal of the colon (20)

Collateral circulation: Circulation developed to maintain blood flow to a tissue when the primary vessel is obstructed (28)

Colonization: the growth of bacteria on or in a body part (10)

Colostomy: opening of the colon through the abdominal wall to the skin surface (20)

Comfort measures only: order indicating that no further life-sustaining interventions are necessary and that the goal of care is a comfortable, dignified death (14)

Community-based nursing: care focused on individual and family health care needs, providing direct services to individuals to manage acute or chronic health problems and to promote self-care (4)

Compartment syndrome: constriction of blood vessels and nerves within a compartment by excess pressure in the compartment (42)

Compliance: distensibility (stretch) of the lungs (22)

Compulsion: repetitive behaviors or mental acts that the affected person feels driven to perform in response to obsessive thoughts (50)

Concrete thinking: literal thinking, without creativity (47)

Concussion: brain injury resulting from violent shaking or impact with an object (38)

Confabulation: falsification of memory to fill in the gaps caused by cognitive deficits (52)

Conjunctivitis: inflammation of the conjunctiva of the eye (40)

Conscious sedation: type of anesthesia that provides analgesia and amnesia but allows the client to remain conscious (9)

Constipation: infrequent or difficult passage of stools (20)

Contractility: the natural ability of cardiac muscle fibers to shorten during systole (25)

Contracture: abnormal flexion and fixation of a joint caused by muscle atrophy and shortening (42, 46)

Contralateral: opposite side (38)

Contusion: bleeding into soft tissue resulting from a blunt force (38, 42)

Convulsion: involuntary muscle contraction and relaxation (38)

Coping behavior: behaviors that help a person manage stress (50)

Corneal ulcers: superficial or deep ulceration of the cornea caused by infection, trauma, or contact lens overuse (40)

Coryza: profuse nasal discharge (23)

Crepitus: a grating sound or sensation (41)

Creutzfeldt-Jakob disease (CJD): rare, progressive neurologic disease causing brain degeneration (39)

Critical thinking: self-directed thinking that is focused on what to believe or do in a specific situation (1)

Crohn's disease: regional enteritis; a chronic, relapsing inflammatory disorder of the gastrointestinal tract (20)

Cross-tolerance: tolerance to other, similar types of substances (e.g., alcohol and heroin); for example, a client who is dependent on any CNS depressant will also be tolerant to other CNS depressants (52)

Cryptococcosis: an opportunistic infection by *Cryptococcus neoformans* that develops in the lungs and then travels to the brain or meninges (11)

Cryptorchidism: failure of one or both testes to descend through the inguinal ring into the scrotum (34)

Culture: attitudes, beliefs, customs, and behaviors that are passed from one generation to the next (47)

Cushing's syndrome: results from excessive production of corticosteroids from the adrenal glands (16)

Cyanosis: bluish, grayish, or dark purple skin tone caused by reduced oxygen content of the blood (24, 44)

Cystectomy: surgical removal of the urinary bladder (32)

Cystitis: inflammation of the urinary bladder (32)

Cystocele: herniation of the bladder into the vagina (35)

Cytomegalovirus (CMV): a viral infection with the cytomegalovirus that can affect the retina, gastrointestinal tract, or lungs (11)

Cytotoxic T cells: subset of T cells that attack viruses, fungi, and cancer cells (11)

D

Dawn phenomenon: rise in blood glucose levels between 5 and 8 A.M. (17)

Death: irreversible cessation of circulatory and respiratory functions or irreversible cessation of all functions of the entire brain, including the brainstem (14)

Debride: remove foreign material and dead or damaged tissue (43)

Debridement: process of removing dead tissue from a wound (46)

Debulking: surgery to remove a large part of a tumor when complete removal is impossible (38)

Deep venous thrombosis: a blood clot in one or more of the deep veins of the legs, pelvis, arms, or other areas of the body (28)

Dehiscence: separation in the layers of an incisional wound (9)

Delusion: false belief that is not accepted by one's culture and persists despite evidence that it is false. For example, saying "I am Spiderman." (48)

Dementia: different kinds of organic disorders that progressively affect mental function (3)

Demyelination: Destruction and degeneration of the myelin sheath covering nerve axons (39)

Denial: refusal to acknowledge the existence of a real situation or feelings as a mechanism for coping with stress (52)

Dermatitis: inflammation of the skin characterized by erythema and pain or pruritus (45)

Dermatome: area of skin supplied by a single sensory nerve (37)

Dermatophyte: tinea (fungal) infections of the skin (45)

Dermis: second, deeper layer of skin (44)

Desensitization: treatment of an allergy by giving several dilute injections that contain the allergen (11)

Detoxification: removal of a toxic substance from the body (52)

Diabetes insipidus: excessive urination caused by a lack of ADH (16)

Diabetes mellitus: chronic disorder of carbohydrate metabolism (17)

Diabetic ketoacidosis: life-threatening illness occurring in type 1 diabetics, characterized by hyperglycemia, metabolic acidosis, and coma (17)

Diabetic nephropathy: kidney disease caused by diabetes mellitus (17)

Diabetic neuropathy: disease of the peripheral and autonomic nerves caused by diabetes mellitus (17)

Diabetic retinopathy: disease of the retina caused by diabetes mellitus (17)

Diagnosis-related groups (DRGs): categories for reimbursement of inpatient services; the system pays a predetermined amount of money for the care of different persons with the same medical diagnosis (4)

Dialysis: diffusion of solutes from higher to lower concentration across a semipermeable membrane (32)

Diapedesis: movement of white blood cells from the circulation to the injury site (10)

Diarrhea: increase in the frequency, volume, and water content of stool (20)

Diastole: period of ventricular relaxation and filling (25)

Diffusion: process in which molecules move from an area of high concentration to an area of low concentration to become evenly distributed (5)

Dilemma: choice between two unpleasant alternatives (1)

Diplopia: double vision (40)

Disability: degree of observable and measurable impairment (4)

Disease: medical term describing alterations in structure and function of the body or mind (2)

Dislocation: separation of contact between two bones of a joint (42)

Disseminated intravascular coagulation (DIC): condition characterized by abnormal clotting and bleeding (13)

Distal paresthesia: subjective feeling of numbness or tingling in the toes and fingers (17)

Distractibility: an inability to screen out excess or irrelevant sensory stimuli, causing difficulty with focusing attention (49)

Diverticulitis: inflammation and perforation of a diverticulum, usually in the sigmoid colon (20)

Do-not-resuscitate (DNR): "no-code"; order written by the physician for a client near death, usually based on the wishes of the client and family that no cardiopulmonary resuscitation be performed for respiratory or cardiac arrest (14)

Dopamine: neurotransmitter (39)

Drug tolerance: process by which the body requires a progressively greater amount of a drug to achieve the same results (8)

Dual diagnosis: concurrent diagnoses of both a substance use disorder and a mental illness (51)

Durable power of attorney for health care: health care proxy; a legal document written by a competent, mentally healthy adult that gives another competent adult the right to make health care decisions on his or her behalf if he or she cannot (14)

Dysfunctional uterine bleeding (DUB): vaginal bleeding that is abnormal in amount, duration, or time of occurrence (35)

Dyskinesia: abnormal movement such as shuffling gait, tremor, slow movement, lack of facial expression (48)

Dysmenorrhea: pain associated with menstruation (35)

Dyspareunia: pain during sexual intercourse (35)

Dysphagia: difficult or painful swallowing (19, 23, 37)

Dysphoria: low, uncomfortable mood, but not as low as depression (50)

Dysphoric: sad or unpleasant (49)

Dyspnea: difficult or labored breathing (24)

Dystonia: muscle rigidity (48)

Dysuria: difficult or painful urination (31)

E

Ectopic: occurring in an abnormal location (35)

Edema: excess fluid in body tissues (5, 44)

Ejaculation: expulsion of seminal fluid from the male urethra (33)

Electrocardiogram (ECG): graphic record of the heart's electrical activity (25)

Electrolytes: substances that dissociate in solution to form charged particles, or ions (5)

Elevated mood: an exaggerated sense of energy or well-being (49)

Emancipated minors: individuals under age 18 who are responsible for their own welfare and live independently of their parents (9)

Embolus: blood clot or foreign matter that moves within the vascular system (28)

Emotional lability: extreme emotion and mood swings from crying to laughing (38)

Encephalitis: an acute inflammation of the white and gray matter of the brain and spinal cord (38)

Endocarditis: inflammation of the endocardium (27)

Endogenous pyrogens: chemicals, bacterial toxins, prostaglandins, and interleukin-1 that act on the hypothalamus to raise body temperature (10)

Endorphins: body's naturally produced morphines (painkillers) (8)

Endotoxins: harmful substances released from gram-negative bacteria (10)

Enteral: within or into the GI tract (19)

Epidermis: outermost part of the skin (44)

Epilepsy: chronic pattern of seizure activity; seizure disorder (38)

Epileptogenic focus: group of neurons that fire abnormally, causing a seizure (38)

Epistaxis: nosebleed (23)

Equianalgesic dose: having the same analgesic effect when administered to the same individual; drug dosages are equianalgesic if they have the same effect as morphine sulfate 10 mg IM (8)

Erectile dysfunction: impotence; inability to achieve and maintain an erection (34)

Erythema: reddening of the skin (44)

Erythrocyte: red blood cell (29)

Eschar: hard crust that forms over a burn wound (46)

Esophageal varices: enlarged, overdistended veins in the distal esophagus (21)

Estrogens: steroid hormones essential to developing and maintaining female secondary sex characteristics (33)

Ethics: principles of conduct concerned with moral duty, values, obligations, and the distinction between right and wrong (1)

Euphoria: an exaggerated feeling of well-being (52)

Euthanasia: (from the Greek for painless, easy, gentle, or good death) term commonly used to signify killing prompted by a humanitarian motive (14)

Euthymic: mood in the normal range (49)

Evaluation: the final step of the nursing process, which allows the nurse to determine whether the plan was effective and to continue, revise, or terminate the plan (1)

Evisceration: protrusion of body organs from a wound dehiscence (9)

Exacerbation: time period in some chronic illnesses when symptoms reappear following a remission (2)

Exophthalmos: forward protrusion of the eyeballs (15)

Exotoxins: harmful substances released from staphylococci, streptococci, and tetanus bacteria (10)

External otitis (swimmer's ear): inflammation of the ear canal (40)

Extracellular fluid (ECF): body fluid located outside of cells (5)

F

Family: a group of people who live together or in close contact and who take care of each other and provide assistance for their dependent members (2, 47)

Fasciculations: involuntary contractions of the voluntary muscles (39)

Filtration: process by which water and solutes move across capillary membranes, driven by fluid pressure (5)

Fistula: abnormal tubelike passage from one body cavity to another (10)

Flaccidity: decreased muscle tone (37)

Folliculitis: infection that begins at the hair follicle opening and extends down into the follicle (45)

Fracture: break in the continuity of a bone (42)

Full-thickness burn: burn (third-degree) that involves all layers of the skin and may extend into subcutaneous fat, connective tissue, muscle, and bone (46)

Furuncle: "boil"; infection of the hair follicle (45)

G

Gangrene: tissue death from reduced or absent blood supply (17, 42)

Gastrectomy: partial or total removal or resection of the stomach (19)

Gastritis: inflammation of the stomach lining (19)

Gastroenteritis: inflammation of the stomach and intestines (19)

Gastroesophageal reflux (GER): backward movement of gastric contents into the esophagus (19)

Gerontologic nursing: care of the older adult (3)

Glaucoma: disorder of increased intraocular pressure and gradual loss of peripheral vision (40)

Glomerular filtration rate (GFR): amount of fluid filtered from the blood into the glomerular capsule per minute (31)

Glomeruli: small clusters of capillaries in the kidney (31)

Glomerulonephritis: inflammation of the glomeruli (32)

Glomerulosclerosis: fibrosis of the glomerular capillaries in the kidneys (17)

Gluconeogenesis: process to make glucose in the liver (15)

Glycogenolysis: conversion of glycogen into glucose in the liver and muscles (15)

Glycosuria: presence of glucose in the urine (17)

Goiter: enlargement of the thyroid gland (16)

Gout: a disorder of purine metabolism characterized by the accumulation of urate crystals in joints and surrounding tissues (43)

Grief: emotional response to loss and its changes (14)

Guillain-Barré syndrome (GBS): acute progressive inflammation of the peripheral nervous system (39)

Gynecomastia: breast enlargement (34)

H

Half-life: the amount of time needed for elimination processes to decrease the original blood concentration by 50% (6)

Hallucination: sensory perception that seems real but occurs without external stimuli. Most common is hearing voices. (48)

Handicap: the total adjustment to disability that limits functioning at a normal level (4)

Health: state of complete physical, mental, and social well-being, not merely the absence of disease or infirmity (2)

Health–illness continuum: representation of health as a dynamic process, with high-level wellness at one extreme of the continuum and death at the opposite extreme (2)

Heart failure: inability of the heart to function as a pump to meet the needs of the body (27)

Heat stroke: life-threatening condition in which the body cannot cool itself (13)

Helper T cells: cells that turn on the immune system (11)

Hematemesis: vomiting blood (19)

Hematochezia: bright red blood in the stool (19)

Hematoma: collection of blood within a tissue, organ, or space caused by a break in a blood vessel (38, 42)

Hematuria: blood in the urine (may be microscopic or visible) (31)

Hemiplegia: paralysis on one side of the body (38)

Hemoglobin: oxygen-carrying protein in red blood cells (29)

Hemolysis: destruction of red blood cells (24, 29)

Hemophilia: hereditary clotting factor deficiencies (30)

Hemoptysis: bloody sputum (24)

Hemorrhage: excessive loss of blood (9)

Hemorrhoid: weakening and dilation of a vein of the anus or anal canal (20)

Hemostasis: blood clotting (29)

Hemothorax: blood in the pleural space (24)

Hepatic encephalopathy: brain dysfunction related to accumulation of substances normally detoxified by the liver (21)

Hepatitis: inflammation of the liver (21)

Hepatocytes: liver cells (18)

Herniated intervertebral disk: injury to the disk between two vertebrae that compresses the nearby spinal nerve root, resulting in motor and sensory changes and pain (39)

Herpes simplex: "fever blisters"; "cold sore" infections caused by herpesvirus I or II (45)

Herpes simplex 1 and 2: a herpes virus that causes skin eruptions of the oral, genital, or anal regions of the body (11)

Herpes zoster: "shingles"; viral infection of a dermatome section of the skin caused by varicella zoster, the herpes virus that causes chickenpox (45)

High-level wellness: way of functioning to reach one's maximum potential at a particular point in time (2)

Hirsutism: excessive hair growth or hair growth in unusual places, such as facial hair on women (16)

Histocompatibility: tissues compatible for transplantation to another person (11)

Home health care: health and social services provided in the home to people who are chronically ill, disabled, or recovering from an illness (4)

Homeostasis: body's tendency to maintain a state of physiologic balance in the presence of constantly changing conditions (5)

Homonymous hemianopia: loss of vision in half of the visual field (38)

Hormones: chemical messengers of the body (15)

Hospice: model (not a place) of care for clients and families, when client is faced with a limited life expectancy; it emphasizes quality rather than quantity of life (14)

Human immunodeficiency virus (HIV): retrovirus that causes HIV disease and AIDS (11)

Human papillomavirus: virus causing genital warts, a sexually transmitted disease (11)

Humoral immunity: immune response provided by antibodies (11)

Huntington's disease: progressive disease of the CNS system affecting personality, intellectual function, and movement (39)

Hydronephrosis: abnormal dilation of the renal pelvis and calyces (32)

Hyperglycemia: high blood glucose level (15)

Hyperkalemia: serum potassium level greater than 5.0 mEq/L (5)

Hyperosmolar hyperglycemic state (HHS): life-threatening illness occurring in type 2 diabetics, characterized by hyperglycemia, severe dehydration, and coma (17)

Hyperpituitarism: disease condition in which there is excessive function of the pituitary gland (16)

Hypersensitivity: altered immune response to an antigen that causes harm to the body (11)

Hypertension: blood pressure higher than 140 mm Hg systolic or 90 mm Hg diastolic on three separate readings several weeks apart (28)

Hypertrophic scar: overgrowth of dermal tissue that remains within the boundaries of the wound (46)

Hypervolemia: excess intravascular fluid (5)

Hypoglycemia: low blood glucose level (15, 17)

Hypokalemia: serum potassium level less than 3.5 mEq/L (5)

Hypopituitarism: disease condition in which there is deficient function of the pituitary gland (16)

Hypothyroidism: condition resulting from inadequate amounts of thyroid hormone (16)

Hypovolemic shock: shock caused by a decrease in intravascular volume (13)

Hypoxemia: low oxygen levels in the blood (PaO_2 < 80 mm Hg) (7, 25)

Hysterectomy: removal of the uterus (35)

I

Icterus: jaundice (21)

ICU psychosis: acute confusion after 2 to 3 days in the intensive care unit (13)

Ideas of reference: a cognitive deficit in which a person misinterprets everyday events as having a personal meaning; for example, a person may believe that her thoughts about the plants being dry caused it to rain (51)

Ileostomy: opening of the ileum through the abdominal wall to the skin surface (20)

Illness: response a person has to a disease (2)

Immunizations: vaccines that create immunity against a specific disease (11)

Immunocompetent: ability of the body's immune system to ward off pathogenic organisms (11)

Immunoglobulins: antibodies produced by B cells (11)

Immunosuppression: inability of the immune system to provide adequate immunity (10)

Impaired nurse: nurse with substance abuse problems, who may exhibit mood changes, irritability, forgetfulness, self-isolation, and inappropriate behavior (52)

Impairment: disturbance in structure or function resulting from physiologic or psychologic abnormalities (4)

Implementation: the fourth step in the nursing process—the "doing" phase—during which the nurse carries out planned interventions (1)

Impotence: erectile dysfunction; inability to achieve and maintain an erection (34)

Inappropriate affect: an emotional response that is not culturally appropriate for the situation, such as laughing when someone's pet dies (51)

Incision and drainage: procedure for draining pus from a wound (10)

Infection: condition in which pathogenic organisms trigger the inflammatory process (10)

Infectious disease: disease that is caused by a microorganism and can be transmitted to another person (10)

Infertility: inability to conceive during a year or more of unprotected intercourse (34)

Inflammation: nonspecific response that occurs when the body experiences any type of injury (10)

Influenza: flu; highly contagious viral upper respiratory disease (23)

Informed consent: a legal document required for certain diagnostic procedures or therapeutic measures, including surgery (9)

Inotropic: strengthening the contraction of the heart (27)

Inpatient surgery: surgery requiring admission to a hospital before and after the procedure (9)

Insight: self-understanding (47, 48)

Insomnia: difficulty falling asleep, staying asleep, or awakening too early (50)

Inspection: method of assessing by observing the client through the senses of seeing, smelling, and hearing (5)

Intermittent claudication: cramping or aching sensation in the calves, thighs, and buttocks that occurs with activity and is relieved by rest (28)

Interventions: purposeful actions performed by the nurse in implementing client care (1)

Intoxication: reversible set of physical, psychologic, and behavioral symptoms caused by use of a substance (52)

Intracellular fluid (ICF): body fluid contained within the cells (5)

Intracranial pressure (ICP): pressure exerted within the cranium by the brain, blood, and cerebrospinal fluid (38)

Intraocular lens: artificial lens inserted when a diseased lens is removed (40)

Intraoperative surgical phase: begins with entry into the operating room and ends with admittance to the postanesthesia care unit (PACU), or recovery room (9)

Invasiveness: organism's ability to invade the body and cause disease (10)

Irritable: easily annoyed, upset, or provoked to anger (49)

Ischemia: decreased blood flow to body tissue or organ (13)

Ischemic: inadequate blood and oxygen to meet the tissue's metabolic needs (26)

Isograft: transplant between identical twins (11)

J

Jacksonian march: seizure activity that may spread from one part of the body to another (38)

Jaundice: yellowness of the skin, sclera of the eyes, mucous membranes, and body fluids due to deposited bile pigment resulting from excess bilirubin in the blood (21, 44)

K

Keloid: scar that extends beyond the boundaries of the original wound (46)

Keratitis: inflammation of the cornea (40)

Ketonuria: presence of ketones in the urine (17)

Ketosis: build-up of ketones in the body (17)

Korsakoff's syndrome: group of symptoms caused by a deficiency in B vitamins, including thiamine, riboflavin, and folic acid (52)

Kyphosis: exaggeration of the normal posterior curve of the thoracic spine (43)

L

Labile: changeable (52)

Laparoscopy: exploration of the abdomen using an endoscope (20)

Laparotomy: surgical opening of the abdomen (20)

Laryngectomy: removal of the larynx (voice box) (23)

Laryngitis: inflammation of the larynx (23)

Laryngospasm: spasm of the muscles of the larynx (23)

Leukemia: malignant proliferation of WBCs (30)

Leukocyte: white blood cell (11, 29)

Leukocytosis: white blood cell count greater than normal (10)

Leukopenia: decreased white cell count below normal (10)

Libido: sexual desire (33)

Living will: legal document that formally expresses a person's wishes regarding life-sustaining treatment in the event of terminal illness or permanent unconsciousness (14)

Loading dose: an initial higher than normal dose of a drug (6)

Lobules: basic functional units of the liver (18)

Long-term care: care for persons with disabilities of all ages that lasts from a few days to several years; it includes skilled care, intermediate and long-term care, transitional care, nursing homes, retirement centers, and residential institutions (4)

Loss: occurs when a valued object, person, body part, or situation is lost or irreversibly changed (14)

Lower body obesity: peripheral obesity, characterized by a waist/hip ratio of <0.8 (19)

Lymphadenitis: enlarged, tender lymph nodes (10)

Lymphadenopathy: swelling and enlargement of the lymph nodes (30)

Lymphatic system: the lymphoid organs, including lymph vessels, lymph nodes, spleen, and thymus (29)

M

Macrophages: mature, large white blood cells that develop from monocytes (10)

Macular degeneration: loss of neurons in the area of central vision of the eye (40)

Malabsorption: condition of ineffective intestinal absorption of nutrients (20)

Maladaptive behavior: unhealthy coping behavior that does not promote integrity of the individual (50)

Malignant lymphomas: cancerous tumors of lymphoid tissue (30)

Malnutrition: long-term nutrient and calorie deficiencies resulting in health problems (19)

Mammography: x-ray imaging of breast tissue to detect breast cancer (33)

Manifestations: objective and subjective data (signs and symptoms) associated with a specific illness (2, 5)

Marfan syndrome: hereditary disorder affecting connective tissue, bones, muscles, and ligaments (28)

Mastectomy: removal of the breast (35)

Medical–surgical nursing: the health care and illness care of adults (1)

Melanoma: cutaneous or malignant melanoma; skin cancer that arises from melanocytes, the cells that produce skin pigment (45)

Melena: black, tarry stool that contains blood (19)

Memory cells: cells that provide immunity when reexposed to a past antigen (11)

Meninges: protective membranes covering the brain and spinal cord (37)

Meningitis: inflammation of the meninges of the brain and spinal cord (38)

Menopause: period during which menstrual activity permanently ceases (35)

Metabolic acidosis: increased hydrogen ion concentration and a pH of less than 7.35 due to inadequate bicarbonate in relation to the amount of acid in the body (7)

Metabolic alkalosis: Decreased hydrogen ion concentration and a pH greater than 7.45 due to an excess of bicarbonate (7)

Metabolism: biochemical reactions that occur in the body's cells (18)

Metastasis: process by which malignant neoplasms spread to distant sites; a secondary tumor formed by this process (12)

Metrorrhagia: bleeding between menstrual periods (35)

Microalbuminuria: presence of small amounts of albumin in the urine (17)

Milieu: therapeutic environment, or using the environment as part of therapy (48)

Mood: pervasive and sustained emotion that influences how a person perceives the world (49)

Multiple myeloma: malignancy in which plasma cells multiply uncontrollably and infiltrate bone marrow, lymph nodes, and other tissues (30)

Multiple organ dysfunction syndrome (MODS): irreversible complication of shock in which the body's systems fail (13)

Multiple sclerosis (MS): chronic, degenerative disease that damages the myelin sheath surrounding the axons of the CNS (39)

Muscular dystrophy: a group of inherited diseases that cause progressive muscle degeneration and wasting (43)

Mutation: change in an organism from its original form into a different form (10)

Myasthenia gravis: chronic autoimmune disorder that is characterized by muscle fatigue (39)

Myelin sheath: white fatty substance that insulates and protects some axons (37)

Myocardial infarction (MI): myocardial cell necrosis (death) due to lack of blood and oxygen (22)

Myocarditis: inflammation of the heart muscle (27)

Myopathy: condition characterized by muscle cramps of sudden onset, plus pain, tenderness, and edema of skeletal muscles (52)

Myxedema coma: life-threatening form of hypothyroidism (16)

N

Narrow-spectrum antibiotics: antibiotics that act against a few pathogens (10)

Natural immunity: person's natural resistance to foreign antigens (11)

Natural killer (NK) cells: white blood cells that can attack viruses and cancer cells (11)

Neoplasm: tumor; mass of abnormal cells that grows independently of its surrounding structures and has no physiologic purpose (12)

Nephron: functional unit of the kidney (31)

Nephrotoxins: agents that damage kidney tissue (32)

Neurogenic shock: shock caused by an interruption to the sympathetic nervous system (13)

Neuron: basic cell of the nervous system (37, 47)

Neuropathic pain: pain caused by damage to the CNS or peripheral nerves (8)

Neurotransmitter: chemical released during the transmission of an electrical impulse that assists or inhibits the impulse in crossing the synapse (37, 47)

Nevi: moles (45)

Nociceptors: nerve endings in the body that respond to noxious stimuli (8)

Nocturia: urinating more than one time at night (31)

Nonopioids: drugs such as acetaminophen and non-steroidal anti-inflammatory drugs (NSAIDs) that are used to treat mild to moderate pain (8)

Nosocomial infections: infections acquired in a health care setting (10)

Nursing diagnosis: the second step in the nursing process; a clinical judgment about individual, family, or community responses to actual or potential health problems/life processes (1)

Nursing process: series of activities nurses perform as they provide care to clients (1)

Nutrients: substances in food used for growth, maintenance, and repair of the body (18)

Nutrition: process of ingesting, absorbing, using, and eliminating food (18)

Nystagmus: involuntary eye movements (37)

O

Obesity: body weight more than 20% above ideal for gender, height, and age (19)

Objective data: observable or measurable pieces of data that can be seen, heard, touched, or smelled (also called *signs*) (5)

Obsession: recurrent and intrusive thoughts that cause marked distress (50)

Oncogenes: genes capable of triggering cancer (12)

Oncology: study of cancer; oncologists are physicians who specialize in cancer care (12)

Oophorectomy: removal of the ovary (35)

Opioid tolerance: process by which the body requires a progressively greater amount of an opioid drug to achieve the same results (8)

Opioids: drugs derived from opium (e.g., morphine) used to treat moderate to severe pain (8)

Orchiectomy: surgical removal of the testes (34)

Orthopnea: difficulty breathing while lying down (27)

Orthostatic hypotension: drop of greater than 10 mm Hg in blood pressure occurring with position change (7)

Osmolarity: concentration of particles in the blood (16)

Osmosis: transport process by which water moves across a semipermeable membrane from an area of lower solute concentration to an area of higher solute concentration (5)

Osmotic diuretic: A substance that pulls fluid from extracellular space (e.g., a drug, excess glucose in the blood) (17)

Osteoarthritis (OA): degenerative joint disease with progressive loss of joint cartilage in synovial joints (43)

Osteomyelitis: infection of the bone (43)

Osteoporosis: bone disorder characterized by loss of bone mass (43)

Ostomy: a surgically created opening from an organ to the surface of the body (20)

Otitis media: inflammation or infection of the middle ear (40)

Otorrhea: leakage of fluid from the external ear (38)

Outcomes: time-specific, achievable goals (1)

P

Pain: unpleasant sensory and emotional experience associated with actual or potential tissue damage (8)

Pain threshold: point at which each person recognizes pain (8)

Pain tolerance: amount and duration of pain a person can stand before seeking relief (8)

Palliative care: service provided to individuals who have an incurable illness; focused on promoting comfort by alleviating symptoms such as pain, nausea, dyspnea, and anxiety (14)

Pallor: paleness of skin (44)

Palpation: method of assessing by using the hands to touch and feel (5)

Pancreatitis: inflammation of the pancreas (21)

Paracentesis: removal of fluid from the peritoneal cavity (21)

Paradoxical response: contradictory, opposite from expected effect (50)

Paralytic ileus: slowing or stopping of peristalsis (20)

Paraplegia: paralysis of the lower half of the body (39)

Parasuicidal behavior: behavior aimed at harming but not killing oneself (51)

Parenchyma: essential, functional parts of an organ (21)

Parish nursing: nursing care provided in coordination with the pastor and staff of a faith community, to promote health and healing through counseling, referrals, teaching, and assessment of health care needs; a parish nurse may be employed by a hospital or a church (4)

Parkinson's disease (PD): chronic, progressive, degenerative neurologic disease that alters motor coordination (39)

Paroxysmal nocturnal dyspnea (PND): attacks of shortness of breath that occur at night, awakening the client (27)

Partial-thickness burn: burn (second-degree) that involves the entire dermis and may also involve the hair follicles (46)

Passive immunity: injection of preformed antibodies into an unprotected person for short-term immunity (11)

Pathogens: microorganisms that are capable of producing disease (10)

Pathologic fracture: fracture of a diseased or weakened bone that occurs with minimal force or trauma (43)

Patient-controlled analgesia (PCA): self-administration of opioid medications by a programmed infusion pump (8)

Pediculosis: infestation with lice (45)

Pelvic inflammatory disease: infection of the pelvic organs; often associated with sexually transmitted infections (35)

Peptic ulcer: break in the mucous lining of the gastrointestinal tract where it comes in contact with gastric juice (19)

Percussion: method of assessing by tapping the body to produce sound waves that provide information about underlying body structures or organs (5)

Pericardial friction rub: leathery, grating sound produced by the inflamed pericardial layers rubbing against the chest wall or pleura (27)

Pericarditis: inflammation of the pericardium (27)

Perimenopause: the period of several years around menopause during which estrogen levels decline (35)

Peripheral vascular resistance (PVR): force that opposes blood flow (25)

Peripheral vascular system: network of blood vessels that carry blood to peripheral tissues and then return it to the heart (25)

Peristalsis: alternating waves of contraction and relaxation of involuntary muscle (18)

Peritonitis: inflammation of the peritoneum, a double-layered membrane that lines the walls and organs of the abdominal cavity (20)

Personality: relatively stable way in which a person thinks, feels, and behaves (51)

Pertussis: an upper respiratory infection also known as *whooping cough* (23)

Petechiae: small, flat, purple or red spots on the skin or mucous membranes (30)

pH: measure of hydrogen ion concentration in a solution; as H^+ concentration increases, the solution becomes more acid and the pH falls; as H^+ concentration decreases, the solution becomes more alkaline and the pH rises (5)

Phagocytosis: process by which phagocytes ingest harmful bacteria and dead tissue cells (10)

Phantom pain: pain in a missing extremity resulting from nerve trauma during surgery (42)

Pharmacodynamics: the study of how drugs produce their effects in the body to result in a pharmacologic response (6)

Pharmacokinetics: the study of how drugs are processed by the body (6)

Pharmacology: the study of drugs and their uses in the body (6)

Pharyngitis: acute inflammation of the pharynx; sore throat (23)

Pheochromocytoma: tumor of the adrenal medulla that causes an increased release of catecholamines (16)

Phobia: persistent and irrational fear (50)

Photophobia: extreme sensitivity to light (40)

Physical dependence: adaptation of the body to chemical substances over an extended period of time; stopping the substance abruptly causes physical withdrawal symptoms (8)

Planning: the third step in the nursing process, in which the nurse develops a list of nursing interventions (1)

Plasma: the liquid part of the blood (29)

Plasmapheresis: procedure that removes plasma from the blood to take out immune substances that cause inflammation (39)

Platelets: small fragments of cytoplasm without nuclei; an essential component of the body's clotting mechanism (29)

Pleural effusion: collection of fluid in the pleural space (24)

Pneumatic antishock garment (PASG): inflatable garment applied to trauma victims in the prehospital setting to raise blood pressure (13)

***Pneumocystis carinii* pneumonia:** a fungus-like organism that causes pneumonia in clients with compromised immunity (11)

Pneumonia: inflammation of the respiratory bronchioles and alveoli (24)

Pneumothorax: accumulation of air in the pleural space (24)

Polycythemia: erythrocytosis; abnormally high red blood cell count and high hematocrit (30)

Polydipsia: excessive thirst (17)

Polyphagia: excessive hunger (17)

Polysubstance abuse: use of a variety of substances to induce an altered physical, mental, or emotional state (52)

Polyuria: excessive urine output (17)

Portal hypertension: elevated blood pressure in the portal vein (21)

Positive inotropic drugs: group of drugs used to increase cardiac output (13)

Postoperative surgical phase: begins with admission to the postanesthesia recovery area and ends with complete recovery from the surgical intervention (9)

Potentiation: when the action of one drug increases the effect of the second drug (6)

Premenstrual syndrome (PMS): complex of symptoms including irritability, depression, edema, and breast tenderness preceding the monthly menses (35)

Preoperative surgical phase: begins when the decision for surgery is made and ends when the client is transferred to the operating room (9)

Presbycusis: progressive hearing loss associated with aging (40)

Presbyopia: condition in which the lens of the eye becomes less elastic in older adults causing decreased near-sighted vision (37)

Pressure ulcers: bedsores; decubitus ulcers; ischemic lesions of the skin and underlying tissue caused by external pressure that impairs the flow of blood and lymph (45)

Pressured speech: rapid, persistent speech associated with mania, difficult to interrupt (49)

Primary hypertension: hypertension with no identified cause (28)

Primary intention: healing that takes place when a wound is uncomplicated and clean and has little tissue loss (9)

Prodromal phase: in schizophrenia, a period of time in which clients have symptoms, before they have a full psychotic episode (48)

Prophylactic: strategy to prevent an infection (10)

Prostatectomy: surgical removal of the prostate gland (34)

Proteinuria: protein in the urine (32)

Pruritus: subjective itching sensation producing an urge to scratch (45)

Psoriasis: chronic, noninfectious skin disorder characterized by raised, reddened, round circumscribed plaques of varied size, covered by silvery white scales (45)

Psychogenic pain: pain that results from emotional rather than physical causes (8)

Psychomotor agitation: increased activity (49)

Psychomotor retardation: decreased purposeful activity (49)

Psychosis: a disorder of thought that causes delusions, hallucinations, disorganized speech, or disorganized behavior (48)

Psychosocial: psychologic or social factors (47)

Psychosocial changes: life changes affecting relationships, income, or relocation (3)

Ptosis: drooping eyelid (37)

Pulmonary embolism: sudden blockage of a pulmonary artery that disrupts blood flow to the lungs (24)

Pulmonary hypertension: abnormal elevation of the pulmonary arterial pressure (24)

Pyelonephritis: inflammatory disorder affecting the renal pelvis and parenchyma (32)

Pyuria: cloudy, foul-smelling urine that contains pus (31)

Q

Quality assurance: includes the quality-control activities of evaluating, monitoring, or regulating the standard of services provided to the consumer (1)

R

Rabies: viral infection of the CNS caused by an animal bite (39)

Rectocele: herniation of the rectum into the vagina (35)

Red reflex: reddish-orange glow seen in the pupil when a beam of light is directed into it (40)

Reduction: restoration of normal alignment of a bone or joint (42)

Referred pain: pain that begins in one area of the body but is felt in another part (8)

Reflex: involuntary motor response to a stimulus (37)

Reflex arc: the neural pathway between the stimulus and the response organ (37)

Refraction: bending of light rays to focus on the retina (37)

Regurgitation: failure of a valve to close properly, allowing blood to flow back through it (27)

Rehabilitation: process of learning to live to one's maximum potential with a chronic impairment, disability, or substance dependency (4, 52)

Relapse: return to drug use after abstinence, or of an illness after a period of freedom from symptoms (52)

Relative hypovolemia: hypovolemia resulting from shift of fluids from the intravascular space to the interstitial space (13)

Reminiscence: recalling and telling stories of past life (3)

Remission: time period in a chronic illness when the disease is present, but there are no symptoms (2)

Renal colic: acute, severe, intermittent flank pain usually associated with renal calculi (32)

Renal failure: condition in which the kidneys are unable to remove accumulated waste products from the blood (32)

Renin–angiotensin system: blood pressure regulation system activated when there is reduced blood flow to the kidneys (13)

Resilience: flexibility in a stressful situation and the ability to return to normal afterward (50)

Respiration: exchange of gases between the person and the environment (22)

Respiratory acidosis: increased hydrogen ion concentration and a pH of less than 7.35 due to carbon dioxide retention (7)

Respiratory alkalosis: decreased hydrogen ion concentration and a pH of greater than 7.45 due to loss of carbon dioxide from the body (hyperventilation) (7)

Respiratory failure: inability of the lungs to oxygenate the blood and remove carbon dioxide well enough to meet the body's needs, even at rest (24)

Retinal detachment: separation of the retina from the vascular choroid layer of the eye (40)

Retroperitoneal: behind the peritoneum and outside the peritoneal cavity (18)

Reverse transcriptase: enzyme produced by HIV virus that converts RNA to DNA (11)

Rheumatic fever: a systemic inflammatory disease caused by an abnormal immune response to infection with group A beta-hemolytic streptococci (27)

Rheumatoid arthritis (RA): chronic, systemic inflammatory disorder resulting in persistent inflammation of the synovial tissue that lines joints (43)

Rhinitis: inflammation of the nasal cavities (23)

Rhinoplasty: surgical reconstruction of the nose (23)

Rhinorrhea: discharge of fluid from the nose (38)

Rhizotomy: surgical procedure that severs a nerve root to control pain (39)

Rule of nines: rapid method of estimating the extent of a burn by assigning percentages to parts of the body (46)

S

Salpingo-oophorectomy: removal of the fallopian tubes and ovaries (35)

Scabies: infestation caused by a mite (45)

Sciatica: pain that occurs along the sciatic nerve (39)

Scoliosis: lateral curvature of the spine (43)

Secondary hypertension: hypertension that results from a known cause (28)

Secondary intention: healing that occurs when a wound is large, gaping, and irregular (9)

Seizure: brief episode of abnormal electrical activity in nerve cells of the brain (38)

Senescence: the process of aging (3)

Septic shock: shock caused by overwhelming infection (13)

Septicemia: presence of bacteria in the blood (13)

Seroconversion: the presence of a disease's antibody in the blood (11)

Sexually transmitted infection (STI): any infection acquired as a result of sexual intercourse or intimate contact with an infected individual (36)

Shock: life-threatening condition characterized by inadequate blood flow to organs, tissues, and cells (9,13)

Shunt: movement of fluids from one area to another (13)

Sinusitis: inflammation of the mucous membranes of the sinuses (23)

Sleep apnea: temporary absence of breathing during sleep (23)

Somogyi effect: early morning hyperglycemia following an episode of hypoglycemia at night (17)

Spasticity: increased muscle tone (37)

Spinal cord tumors: benign or malignant tumors that develop within or outside of the spinal cord (39)

Spinal shock: temporary loss of reflex activity below the level of the spinal cord injury (39)

Sprain: injury to a ligament caused by a twisting motion (42)

Squamous cell carcinoma: malignant tumor of the squamous epithelium of the skin or mucous membranes (45)

Staging: system of classifying cancer by tumor size, lymph node involvement, and metastasis to distant sites (35)

Standard: statement or criterion that can be used by a profession and by the general public to measure quality of practice (1)

Standard Precautions: guidelines to protect the health care worker and prevent transmission of infectious organisms to other clients (10)

Status epilepticus: period of continuous tonic–clonic seizures (38)

Stem cell transplant: transplantation of stem cells from one person to another (30)

Stenosis: narrowing of a valve opening, which obstructs forward blood flow (27)

Stigma: negative attitude marking people as less valuable (47)

Stomatitis: inflammation of the oral mucosa (19)

Strain: microscopic muscle tear that causes bleeding into the tissues (42)

Stridor: high-pitched, harsh sound heard during inspiration, usually caused by partial airway obstruction (23)

Stroke volume (SV): amount of blood ejected from the heart with each contraction (13, 25)

Subarachnoid hemorrhage: bleeding into the subarachnoid space in the brain (38)

Subjective data: experiences (data) that only the client can describe, such as pain; also called symptoms (5)

Substance abuse: maladaptive pattern of substance use leading to significant impairment or distress (52)

Substance dependency: maladaptive pattern of substance use manifested by tolerance, withdrawal syndrome, increased use, ineffective attempts to stop use, increasing amounts of time devoted to obtaining substance, and social isolation (52)

Suicidal ideation: thinking about suicide (49)

Sundowning syndrome: behavior characterized by time disorientation and wandering in the evening (3, 39)

Superficial burn: first-degree burn that involves only the epidermal layer of skin (46)

Superinfection: overgrowth of bacteria that occurs when antibiotics eliminate the body's normal flora (10)

Suppressor T cells: cells that turn off the immune system, limiting the immune response (11)

Synapse: space between two neurons across which an electrical impulse passes (37, 47)

Synergism: when two drugs given together cause a greater response than each drug given separately (6)

Synovial joint: a joint in which synovial fluid separates the surfaces of the adjoining bones (41)

Systemic lupus erythematosus (SLE): chronic inflammatory connective tissue disease that affects multiple body systems (43)

Systole: ventricular contraction (25)

T

Tardive dyskinesia: late onset of movement disorder, irreversible side effect of antipsychotic medications (48)

T-cell lymphocytes (T cells): white blood cells responsible for cell-mediated immunity (11)

Tertiary intention: healing that occurs when substantial time passes before a wound is closed (9)

Tetanus: life-threatening disorder of the nervous system caused by an aerobic bacillus, *Clostridium tetani* (39)

Tetany: continuous spasm of the muscles; symptom complex of increased neuromuscular excitability associated with decreased ionized calcium levels (5, 16)

Tetraplegia: paralysis of the arms, legs, and trunk (39)

Thrombocytopenia: platelet count of less than 100,000 platelets per milliliter of blood (30)

Thrombus: blood clot (28)

Thymectomy: surgical removal of the thymus gland (39)

Thyroidectomy, subtotal: partial removal of the thyroid gland (16)

Thyroidectomy, total: complete removal of the thyroid gland (16)

Thyrotoxic crisis (thyroid storm): extreme state of hyperthyroidism (16)

Thyrotoxicosis: condition resulting from hypersecretion of the thyroid gland; also called hyperthyroidism (16)

Tinnitus: ringing in the ear (40)

Tolerance: need for more of a substance to achieve the same effect; diminished effect from continued use of the same amount of a substance (8, 52)

Tonic contractions: contraction in which the body becomes rigid with the arms and legs extended (38)

Tonsillectomy: surgical removal of the tonsils (23)

Tonsillitis: acute inflammation of the tonsils (23)

Total parenteral nutrition (TPN): the administration of an intravenous solution that meets all nutritional requirements except for fiber (19)

Toxic shock syndrome (TSS): form of septic shock caused by *Staphylococcus aureus* (13)

Toxoid: injection containing a weakened toxin, for example, tetanus toxoid (11)

Toxoplasmosis: an opportunistic infection with *Toxoplasma gondii* that can cause neurologic manifestations (11)

Tracheostomy: surgical opening into the trachea (23)

Traction: use of a pulling force to reduce a fracture or maintain alignment (42)

Transient ischemic attack (TIA): brief episode of reversible neurologic deficits (38)

Transmission-based Precautions: precautions against spread of infection through the air, by droplet, and through contact (10)

Transsphenoidal hypophysectomy: surgical procedure used to remove the pituitary gland (16)

Trauma: injury caused by applying more force to tissue than it is able to absorb (42)

Triage: system to identify who will receive medical attention first (13)

Trigeminal neuralgia: disease of the trigeminal nerve resulting in periodic, severe, one-sided facial pain (39)

Trismus: difficulty opening the jaw as seen in tetanus (39)

Tuberculosis: a chronic infectious disease caused by *Mycobacterium tuberculosis* (24)

Tympanic membrane: eardrum (37)

Type and cross-match: test to determine donor and recipient ABO types and Rh groups and their compatibility with one another (13)

U

Ulcerative colitis: chronic inflammatory bowel disorder of the mucosa and submucosa of the colon and rectum (20)

Upper body obesity: central obesity, characterized by a waist/hip ratio of >1 in men and >0.8 in women (19)

Uremia: a symptom complex caused by excess metabolic waste products in the blood (32)

Urinary incontinence: involuntary urination (32)

Urolithiasis: development of stones within the urinary tract (32)

Uterine prolapse: descent of the uterus into the vagina (35)

V

Vaccines: suspensions of live, attenuated, or killed microorganisms that promote active immunity against a specific organism (11)

Vaginitis: inflammation or infection of the vagina (35)

Valvular heart disease: deformity of one or more of the heart valves affecting blood flow through the chambers of the heart and/or to the pulmonary or systemic circulation (27)

Varicose veins: irregular, tortuous veins with incompetent valves (28)

Vasectomy: sterilization procedure in which a portion of the spermatic cord is removed (34)

Vasopressor drugs: drugs used to increase the blood pressure (13)

Venous insufficiency: stasis of venous blood flow in the lower extremities (28)

Venous thrombosis: formation of a blood clot (thrombus) on the wall of a vein, which obstructs the flow of blood back to the heart (28)

Ventilation: air movement into and out of the lungs (22)

Vertigo: sensation of whirling or rotation (40)

Virulence: power of a microorganism to cause an infection (10)

W

Warts: verrucae; lesions caused by the human papillomavirus (45)

Wernicke's syndrome: alcoholic encephalopathy; characterized by ataxia, paralysis of eye muscles, nystagmus, and mental confusion (52)

Widowhood: loss of a spouse from death (3)

Withdrawal: set of symptoms resulting from discontinuation or reduction of a substance after heavy or prolonged use (52)

X

Xenograft: transplant from animal to human (11)

CHAPTER 1

NCLEX-PN® ANSWERS (1) C—The nurse independently plans and implements client care based on nursing knowledge and skills. (2) B—The nurse as client advocate actively promotes the client's rights to autonomy and free choice. The nurse may speak for the client, mediate between the client and other persons, and protect the client's right to self-determination. (3) A—The nurse is responsible for the quality of client care through a process called quality assurance. Quality control activities include evaluating, monitoring, or regulating the standard of services provided to the client. (4) D—Nurses assess clients in two ways: an initial assessment, and ongoing, focused assessments. (5) A—Making a diagnosis is a complex process and always involves uncertainty. Critical thinking and reasoning are used to choose nursing diagnoses that best define the individual client's health problems. (6) B—Nursing interventions must be specific and individualized. The nurse identifies client problems and needed interventions, then works with the client to determine those that are needed and preferred by the individual client. (7) A—Implementation is the action or "doing" phase of the nursing process, when nurses carry out planned activities. (8) C—Documenting interventions is the final component of implementation, and it is a legal requirement. "If it isn't documented, it isn't done." (9) D—Nursing practice is structured by standards and codes of ethics that guide nursing practice and protect the public. (10) B—According to the ANA, the nurse has a moral obligation to provide care for the client with AIDS unless the risk exceeds the responsibility.

CHAPTER 2

NCLEX-PN® ANSWERS (1) A—Accidents are the leading cause of injury and death in people between ages 15 and 24. Unprotected sex with a variety of people and substance abuse are also major causes of concern for this age group. (2) A—Middle adults often have problems maintaining a healthy weight because they consume the same number of calories as when they were young, while decreasing physical activity. (3) B—Women should have an annual mammogram, beginning at age 40. Men should continue to do testicular self-examination. Vison examinations should be done each year. Regular amounts of exercise are recommended for this age group. (4) D—Although not always meeting traditional definitions, people (or even pets) who are significant to the client are the client's family. They should be an integral component of care

in all health care settings. (5) B—Wellness is an integrated method of functioning, oriented toward maximizing the individual's potential. Good health can exist as a relatively passive state of freedom from illness. (6) B—Cognitive development affects whether people view themselves as healthy or ill and may affect health practices. Educational level affects the ability to understand and follow guidelines for health. (7) C—The nurse promotes health by teaching activities that maintain wellness, providing information about diseases, and following healthy practices that serve as a model. (8) A—Illness is the highly individualized response a person has to disease. (9) D—An acute illness occurs rapidly, lasts for a relatively short period of time, and is self-limiting. It usually responds to self-treatment or to medical-surgical intervention. (10) A—Almost all people with a chronic illness need to live as normally as possible, despite their symptoms and treatment. Chronic illness can make a person feel alienated, lonely, and different from others.

CARE MAP ANSWERS (CLIENT WITH EARLY-ONSET DIABETES)

Correct Data *Subjective:* States "I'm not a good mother anymore"; states "I think I will just stop taking my insulin." *Objective:* Fasting blood glucose 180 (increased).

Correct Interventions Listen carefully to concerns; state "Tell me more about how you think diabetes controls you"; suggest joining a diabetes support group; ask her to keep a daily diary of self-management activities.

Report Yes, to her primary health care provider at the clinic.

Documentation 7/7/06. 1030. Blood glucose 180, makes statements that she is not a good mother, thinks she can't control her diabetes so might just as well stop taking insulin. Data reported to G. Walker, RN, NP, C. J. Tolch, LPN

CHAPTER 3

NCLEX-PN® ANSWERS (1) C—The rapid increase projected in the aging population by 2030s is largely the result of the "baby boom," which refers to the increased number of people born in the post–World War II period from 1946 to 1964. (2) A—Immunity theories are based on the knowledge that the immune system is affected by aging, with decreased defenses against foreign organisms and an increase in chronic illness. (3) B—Ageism is a form of prejudice in which older adults are stereotyped by characteristics of only a small number of their age group; a common myth is that older adults cannot learn new knowledge and skills. (4) D—Cognition means the ability to perceive and understand one's world; cognitive function does not normally change with aging. (5) B—Older adults like to tell stories about their past during reminiscence, allowing them to relive and restructure life experiences and facilitate achieving ego integrity. (6) A—When faced with widowhood, the remaining spouse is faced with not only adjusting to the loss of the loved person, but also to living alone. (7) D—The ability to function safely and independently at home alone depends on a variety of factors, but many older adults can continue living at home with the assistance of home health services, home-delivered meals, and senior transportation. (8) C—The leading causes of death in older adults are cardiovascular disease, cancer, and stroke. (9) B—Although medications do make life more comfortable for older adults, they carry a risk of adverse drug reactions and interactions that can cause adverse effects such as dizziness and numbness. These effects in turn may increase the risk for falling. (10) D—Nursing care to promote cognition in older adults includes ensuring that eyeglasses and hearing devices are used and that they have clean lenses and good batteries, respectively.

CHAPTER 4

NCLEX-PN® ANSWERS (1) C—Community-based nursing focuses on individual and family health care needs where they live, work, play, worship, and go to school. Community health nursing focuses on the health of a community. (2) B—Some of the most common community-based health care services include community centers, clinics, day care centers, block nursing, and parish nursing. (3) A—If a conflict arises, the nurses must remain the primary client's advocate, regardless of any negative response from the family. (4) B, D, and E—Specific criteria that the client must meet in order to secure Medicare reimbursement are to have a need for skilled care, be essentially homebound, and have a plan of care. (5) A—With shorter hospital stays, all clients should be evaluated for their ability to manage at home. The nurse should make a referral to a home health agency if the client has need for follow-up beyond the present clinical setting. (6) C—Nurses cannot close their eyes to an unsafe environment. Safety assessment in the home is both a nursing responsibility and a legal requirement. (7) D—The nurse cannot go into homes and change the family's living space and lifestyle. However, the nurse must alert the family to unsafe and hazardous conditions, suggest remedies, and document the family's response in the record. (8) B—Rehabilitation is the process of learning to live to one's maximum potential with a chronic impairment and of enabling a person to live with dignity, self-worth, and independence. (9) A—Rehabilitation promotes reintegration into the client's family and community through an interdisciplinary approach that includes in the plan of care physical function, mental health, interpersonal relationships, social interactions, and vocational status. It requires the expertise of a team of health care providers. (10) B—The plan of care developed for each client is individualized, based on the priority of needs from the client's and family's perspective.

CARE MAP ANSWERS (CLIENT WITH A HANDICAP)

Correct Data *Subjective:* States "I can't keep my present job"; states "I don't know where to go for help." *Objective:* Unable to bend left leg more than 15 degrees.

Correct Interventions Suggest career counseling; ask Kim if she has ever considered other types of employment; refer Kim to vocational rehabilitation services.

Report No, although it would be shared with other team members.

Documentation 8/5/06. 1300. Requesting information about other types of employment. Referred for career counseling and to vocational rehabilitation services. Jim Manning, LVN

CHAPTER 5

NCLEX-PN® ANSWERS (1) B—Objective data are observable or measurable pieces of information (such as the color of urine). Objective data can be seen, heard, touched, or smelled. (2) C—A focused assessment addresses a specific client problem. Assessing a client with abdominal pain includes assessing bowel movements, temperature, trauma, location, duration, and type of pain. (3) B—If the client is very young, very ill, unconscious, or confused, data may be collected from secondary sources, such as family or friends. (4) D—Open-ended questions give the client the chance to provide more information than do closed-ended questions. "Why" questions often make the client feel threatened or foolish. (5) C—Palpation is use of the hands to touch and feel. Light palpation is used for determining pulses, tenderness, skin texture, skin temperature, and skin moisture. (6) A—The nurse should wash his or her hands before and after the assessment, even if gloves need to be worn. (7) The pulse deficit is 15 (100 − 85). (8) B—Bowel sounds are auscultated by gently placing the stethoscope on the abdomen and listening in all four quadrants. Bowel sounds are clicks or gurgles made as intestinal contents move through the bowel; they should always be present. (9) C—Jaundice is a yellow color of the skin and mucous membranes. It is caused by liver or gallbladder disease, or by an excessive breakdown of red blood cells. Jaundice is usually first seen in the eyes and then in the skin and mucous membranes. (10) C—When recording blood pressure, the nurse should write "BP 120/70," not give a detailed description of the assessment method. Data should be organized in a logical way, and inferences or judgments should be avoided. The word *normal* should not be used; instead, write the specific assessment finding.

CARE MAP ANSWERS (CLIENT WITH RISK FOR EXCESS FLUID VOLUME)

Correct Data *Subjective:* States she had not taken her medications for more than a week and she does not follow her prescribed low-sodium diet. *Objective:* BP 180/96; R 30 with crackles and wheezes; AP 108, irregular; 4+ edema from toes to knees in both legs.

Correct Interventions Ask Cath if she would consider being seen by a social worker; monitor vital signs on a regular basis; monitor breath sounds, apical pulse, and peripheral pulses; measure circumference of lower legs.

Report Yes, to the home health manager or the primary health care provider.

Documentation 9/30/06. 0930. States she has not taken her medications for over a week. BP 180/96; R 30 with crackles and wheezes; AP 108 and irregular; 4+ edema in both lower legs. Data reported to R. Brunde, RN. L. Wilson, LPN

CHAPTER 6

NCLEX-PN® ANSWERS (1) C—Decreased serum albumin levels in older adults affect drug distribution. There is no effect on absorption, metabolism, or excretion. (2) A—This order is missing the number of milligrams. The nurse must call the physician for a complete order. Because the nurse is unsure when the physician will return to the health care facility, the nurse must call the physician. (3) B—Synergism is giving two drugs to cause a greater effect than each drug given separately. Aspirin and an anticoagulant potentiate each other, causing increased risk for bleeding. Nicotine increases the metabolism of anticonvulsants. Alcohol and a sedative drug have an additive effect, increasing sedative effects. (4) D—The nurse should question when multiple tablets are prescribed for a single dose. Illegible handwriting should be clarified with the physician who wrote the order. Atypical drug names should always be investigated further. Never use a medication dropper from one medication for another medication. (5) C—Because drugs are excreted by the kidneys, anyone with kidney disease is at an increased risk for adverse drug reactions. The other ages and conditions do not increase the risk for ADRs like liver or kidney disease. (6) 4, 5, 6, 1, 2, and 3—The IV route has the fastest absorption followed by sublingual, IM, subcutaneous, oral, and transdermal. (7) C—Vicodin is a Schedule III controlled substance. (8) A—Pediatric medication doses are calculated according to the child's body weight. Age, ethnicity, and sex do not affect dose calculation. (9) D—A loading dose (giving a larger than normal dose) is administered in clinical situations when it is necessary to reach therapeutic drug levels rapidly. (10) B—Teratogenic drugs must be avoided in women who are pregnant because they may cause harm to the fetus.

UNIT I WRAP-UP ANSWERS

TIME MANAGEMENT

After report, the nurse should first visit each client's room to introduce himself or herself and make a quick assessment of each client. The LPN can assess vital signs and surgical sites at this time (or delegate vital signs to UAP). It is important to check the MAR, Kardex, or chart for any new orders. Because Mr. Drew and Mr. Melezack are quiet at the moment, it will be a priority to deal with Mr. Ramos's agitation. Check to see if he can be medicated for anxiety. Make sure his catheter irrigation is running, and determine if the irrigation needs to be increased to flush out clots, which may be causing him discomfort. Bring in someone to sit with Mr. Ramos until he is calm again, and administer medication. Then inform his doctor of the agitation; discuss the need for physical restraints if he cannot be controlled by other means. At this point, if you are informed of Mr. Melezack's nausea and vomiting and pain, this will become your priority. While documenting, review lab work. When you find that Mr. Drew has not had an MI, you will need to schedule time to begin his discharge teaching. This is of lower priority, and may be accomplished at the end of visiting hours while you are providing HS care.

CLIENT TEACHING

Teach Mr. Drew some of the things that can be done to decrease recurrent angina: avoid overexertion; decrease anxiety and stress (causes blood vessels to constrict); avoid overeating (increases workload of the heart); avoid cold weather (constricts blood vessels to conserve heat); avoid hot, humid conditions (increase workload of the heart); avoid walking uphill and/or against the wind (increases workload of the heart). Also teach ways to control risk factors: stop smoking; decrease intake of fat content foods/cholesterol; decrease weight; increase exercise (gradually if not used to exercise); decrease hypertension by above activities; decrease stressors (some stress is normal) especially if they precipitate chest discomfort; take medication as prescribed by physician.

CRITICAL THINKING

Although the first concern is for the physiologic status of Mr. Ramos, the nurse must also be concerned with the stress the roommate is experiencing because of his behavior. While you are assessing your client, the nurse assigned to the roommate should (if possible) remove him from the area. He could be taken to the solarium in a wheelchair, if necessary, while arrangements are made to move him to a different room. It will be necessary to obtain an interpreter in order to assess Mr. Ramos's pain and anxiety level properly. It will be important to take the client's vital signs and observe the catheter bags for the condition of the drainage. It will be necessary to have a Spanish-speaking sitter stay with the client until he can be calmed down, because climbing out of bed could result in a fall and injury, and he could dislodge his IV or catheter if he climbs out of bed. Client safety is a priority; it will be necessary to medicate or temporarily restrain the client to prevent injury.

DOCUMENTING AND REPORTING

Date: 8/31/07. Time: 1630. Focus: NG tube. D: NGT clamped since 12 noon, clear liquid lunch; 50% consumed and tolerated. C/o stabbing abdominal pain 8/10. Vomited 500 mL drk. brown emesis. A: NGT unclamped; irrigated with 100 mL of NSS, connected to low intermittent wall suction. Medicated for pain Meperidine 75mg with Vistaril 25mg IM. Dr. Sample notified, order to continue suction. R: Client resting comfortably; pain 2/10. No c/o nausea. NGT drain moderate amt of drk. brown emesis. L. Fellows, LPN. Report client's condition to the charge nurse or RN team leader. Because NG tube cannot be removed, MD should be notified. Discuss client's needs with the care assistant and give instructions to provide mouth care, ice chips, partial bath, and gown and bed change as necessary.

CHAPTER 7

NCLEX-PN® ANSWERS (1) B—Females, in general, have more body fat and less body water than males. There is less water available in clients with a higher percentage of body fat. Individuals over the age of 65 also have decreased body water due to higher body fat content. (2) B—ADH regulates water excretion in the kidneys. The kidneys are less permeable to water. Copious amounts of dilute urine are produced. Serum osmolality decreases, blood pressure falls slightly, and the thirst mechanism in the brain is activated. (3) A—These signs and symptoms indicate a decrease in fluid volume, such as dehydration. Although the client is at risk for the other problems listed here, the assessment data directly relates to fluid volume status. (4) D—Decreased calcium level is manifested by increased muscle excitability. The parathyroid glands, involved in regulation of calcium in the body, may be inadvertently removed or damaged during a thyroidectomy. (5) C—Chronic alcoholism is a principal cause of hypomagnesemia. Excessive antacid use, in contrast, may cause hypermagnesemia. (6) A—The normal pH is 7.35 to 7.45. Respiratory alkalosis (pH > 7.45) occurs during hyperventilation. Other values listed are within the normal ranges. (7) A—The pancreas secretes bicarbonate into the small intestine. Vomiting, suctioning, and diarrhea contribute to the loss of bicarbonate. Overuse of baking soda increases the bicarbonate levels. (8) B—The client with a potassium imbalance is at risk for cardiac dysrhythmias. (9) A—Lasix is a loop diuretic that promotes water loss. Daily weights should be obtained; they are the most accurate measurement for water loss. Intake and output are also measured and compared. (10) B—As the acidosis is corrected, potassium tends to shift from extracellular fluid into the cells. As a result, hypokalemia may develop.

CARE PLAN HINTS

Fluid Volume Excess (1) Think how the heart adapts to increased blood volume to handle this increased workload. If necessary, you may wish to review Chapter 25. (2) Think about the effect of elevating the head of the bed on blood flow to the upper portion of the body, on the diaphragm, and on chest wall expansion. (3) Review Table 7-4. Be sure to adapt your teaching to Ms. Rainwater's specific needs. (4) As you formulate your response, think about going for 4, 8, 12, or more hours without drinking any fluids. Also review Ms. Rainwater's prescribed medications.

Hypokalemia (1) Review Ms. Ortiz's medications and her nursing assessment. (2) Think about the effect of hydrochlorothiazide on potassium excretion and balance; then consider the effect of hypokalemia on the effects of digitalis. Review Chapter 27 as necessary. (3) Review Box 7-12, and think about the components of a nutritionally balanced diet as you develop your response. Review Chapter 19 as needed.

CARE MAP ANSWERS (ACUTE RESPIRATORY ACIDOSIS)

Correct Data *Objective:* T 98.2, P 102, R 36 and shallow, BP 146/92; restless; oxygen at 4 L/min per nasal cannula; responds slowly to questions; ABGs: pH 7.38 (normal 7.35 to 7.45), $PaCO_2$ 48 mm Hg (normal 35 to 45 mm Hg), PaO_2 92 mm Hg (normal 80 to 100 mm Hg), HCO_3 24 mEq/dL (normal 22 to 26 mEq/L)

Report Yes, to charge nurse and/or physician.

Correct Interventions Monitor respiratory status and vital signs every 15 minutes for the first hour, then hourly; keep side rails in place, and call bell within reach; assess mental status, LOC, and color of skin, nail beds, and oral mucous membranes hourly; monitor ABGs, to be redrawn in 2 hours.

CHAPTER 8

NCLEX-PN® ANSWERS (1) B—Chronic pain is prolonged pain that lasts more than 6 months. It is usually nonresponsive to treatment. Acute pain is sudden, temporary, has an identified cause, and lasts less than 6 months. (2) C—Referred pain starts in one site but is perceived in another part of the body. It frequently occurs with visceral pain (pain from body organs lined with viscera), because the pain impulses travel along the same nerve paths. (3) D—Progression of cancer frequently produces pain that requires multiple therapies and is often unresponsive to treatment. Pain is caused by pressure on body organs, nerves, and metastasis to bone. (4) C—Phantom limb pain occurs in some individuals following the removal of an extremity. The client is aware that the part is missing, but the pain can be intense and difficult to treat. Medication should be administered to attempt relief. Nonpharmacologic approaches are ineffective. (5) A—Ibuprofen is an irritant to the gastric mucosa. Clients with gastric ulcer disease should use alternate medications for pain relief. (6) D—Allowing the client to describe his pain based on a pain scale provides an objective, individualized description of the pain. The nurse can make decisions for intervention based on this assessment. (7) B—This drug has a short half-life and will not accumulate and cause toxicity. Elderly patients may have impairment of liver and renal function that leads to increased risk for toxicity. Drugs such as meperidine and propoxyphene cause sedation and respiratory depression. Long-term use of acetaminophen may lead to liver damage. (8) C—Naloxone blocks the effects of opioid drugs and reverses sedation and respiratory depression that may result from excessive dosages. (9) C—Osteoarthritis requires long-term therapy with NSAIDs. A common side effect is gastric bleeding. Taking the drug with foods helps to reduce this risk. The physician should be consulted before medication is discontinued. Alcohol and aspirin should be avoided because they increase the risk of gastric irritation and bleeding. (10) A—Decreased peristalsis and constipation are common side effects of codeine. Assessment of bowel sounds is essential, especially in the elderly. Fluids should be increased to at least 3,000 mL/day if not contraindicated.

CARE PLAN HINTS

Pain (1) You would tell Ms. Akers to take pain medication on a regular basis; review the nursing diagnosis Acute Pain in the Nursing Process section of the chapter. (2) Review the Assessment section under Nursing Process and the pain rating scales. (3) Include in your discharge teaching the effects of opioids on the GI tract and methods to avoid constipation.

CARE MAP ANSWERS (ACUTE PAIN)

Correct Data *Subjective:* Says she feels tired and hopes she can sleep; dull pain in lower abdomen: "It hurts right here." *Objective:* P 100; BP 150/92; lying on her side with eyes closed.

Correct Interventions Offer a back massage at HS; give morphine sulfate 8 mg IM q4h PRN; listen attentively to Mrs. Bruski; teach Mrs. Bruski a relaxation technique.

CHAPTER 9

NCLEX-PN® ANSWERS (1) C—A and D are postoperative nursing diagnoses. B is an intraoperative nursing diagnoses. (2) B—Potassium level of 2.8 is below normal and places the client at risk for cardiac arrhythmias. (3) A—Discussion of risk factors is included in informed consent. Informed consent is the responsibility of the physician. (4) B, A, E, C, D—Assessment is needed before nursing intervention can be determined. Nursing measures to promote urination are appropriate before notifying the physician or preparing for straight catheterization. (5) C—The client should be in semi-Fowler's or Fowler's position for effective coughing and deep-breathing exercises. (6) A—Primary intention is normal wound healing. The wound edges are approximated and closed by staples or sutures. (7) B—The client is a married minor and can sign her own consent. (8) C—Assessment suggests impending shock. The client should be placed in the shock position to facilitate blood supply to vital organs. (9) D—A positive Homans' sign is suggestive of thrombophlebitis. Further assessment of the leg is indicated to support this finding. (10) D—The nurse must clarify this action with the physician. Alteration of physician orders is not an independent nursing action.

CARE PLAN HINTS

Inpatient Surgery (1) Review the section on Physical and Psychological Preparation. Also review preoperative teaching in this chapter, including postoperative breathing exercises, turning, coughing, deep breathing, and leg exercises. Discuss nutrition and pain management. (2) Think about the limitations Mrs. Overbeck will experience. What areas of follow-up exist in the postoperative period? What rehabilitation must occur? (3) Review the Preoperative section of this chapter, and see the nursing diagnoses there. What questions would you have if you were scheduled for this surgery?

CARE MAP ANSWERS (CLIENT AFTER SURGERY)

Correct Data *Subjective:* Incisional pain; complains of feeling warm and has chills; states she is "drinking lots of fluids." *Objective:* T 101.8°F, P 100; WBC 13,000 mm; light brown drainage on dressing; incision red, edematous, 2-cm opening; Cipro 250 mg q8h.

Report Yes, to charge nurse and/or physician.

Correct Interventions Empty Jackson Pratt drain q4h; monitor vital signs, especially temperature and pulse, q4h; report temperature above 100° to charge nurse; assess pedal pulses q8h; provide extra blankets for warmth; change dressing, using aseptic technique bid; assess wound status with each dressing change; Tylenol gr X PO q4h for temperature above 100°F; cleanse wound with normal saline qd, per physician's order; monitor urinary output; maintain fluid intake at least 2,000 mL/day; administer pain medications as needed; administer antibiotics as ordered; collect sample of wound drainage, send to lab for culture and sensitivity.

Documentation *Sample:* 1/04/06, 1600. T 102°F, P 102, R 36, BP 126/70. C/O chills. Two blankets removed, sheet provided for cover. Tylenol gr X given PO for fever. Dressing to right leg changed using aseptic technique. Incision red, edematous with small amount of light brown drainage. Steristrips intact. Opening in center of incision about 2 cm in length. Sterile gauze dressing reapplied. D. Moore, LPN

1645. T. 100.6°F, P 90. States she does not have chills at this time. Dressing dry and intact. D. Moore, LPN

CHAPTER 10

NCLEX-PN® ANSWERS (1) A—Urinary tract infections are the leading cause of nosocomial infections. The client has a Foley catheter that was inserted 4 days ago. The 1-week use of the antibiotic is significant but not as important as the invasive insertion of the Foley catheter. Peripheral vascular disease increases the susceptibility for a nosocomial infection, but is not a major factor in the hospital stay. (2) C—The normal WBC count is 4,500 to 10,000. An increased level indicates acute infection. (3) D—Allergy histories must always be discussed before giving any medication. The age and mental status are important factors. Old medications should be destroyed. Clients should be taught not to mix any drugs with alcohol. (4) B—The infection is an overgrowth of bacteria due to the side effects of the antibiotic. Nurses cannot diagnose medical conditions. You should address the problem and reassure the client. Never tell the client not to worry. "D" is incorrect, because it acknowledges the complaint but doesn't adequately address the client's concern. (5) D—Handwashing is extremely important in preventing infection. Antibiotic treatments should be completed as prescribed. Any fever should be reported because it may indicate an infection. Water intake should be at least 2 1/2 quarts per day to maintain body temperature and metabolism. (6) A—Although there is an increase in the growth of vancomycin-resistant organisms, vancomycin is still the drug of choice. (7) A—Cellulitis is a subcutaneous/connective tissue infection. Antibiotics must be given at the appropriate times to decrease the potential damage to the eye. Bed rest is unlikely order for this client. Morphine in frequent doses is contraindicated in older clients and may lead to respiratory depression. Lab values are important but may be checked at a later time. (8) B—Systemic infection produces the enlargement of lymph nodes throughout the body. Cellulitis, fistulas, and abscesses are all manifestations of local infection. (9) B—The *Pneumocystis carinii* organism is a fungus. It is considered to be an opportunistic disease in clients who are immunocompromised. (10) C—The chickenpox virus is spread through the air. Examples of droplet transmission include pneumonia and meningitis. Clients with acute diarrhea are placed on contact precautions. Standard precautions (universal precautions) include the use of gloves and handwashing.

CARE PLAN HINTS

MRSA Infection (1) Review the section on Infection Prevention and Control Techniques. (2) See the Nosocomial Infection section of this chapter. (3) Think about the chain of infection and about potential carriers of MRSA infection.

CARE MAP ANSWERS (CLIENT EXPOSED TO STAPHYLOCOCCUS AUREUS)

Correct Data *Subjective:* History of Type 2 diabetes. *Objective:* Roommate with *S. aureus* pneumonia; weight 140 lbs.; T 99°F; pressure ulcer on right great toe.

Correct Interventions Provide a diet high in protein; monitor vital signs every 4 hours; monitor skin for further breakdown; increase fluid intake as tolerated.

Report Yes, to physician.

Documentation 02/14/06, 0830. T 99°F. Has open wound on right great toe draining yellowish fluid. Foley draining dark yellow urine of 200 mL. Mark Belaqua, LVN

CHAPTER 11

NCLEX-PN® ANSWERS (1) C—Local injections may cause discomfort at the site. A heating pad will soothe the soreness. Redness at the injection site is common and does not indicate a severe reaction. Clients should remain in the clinic for at least 30 minutes after receiving an immunization to monitor for adverse reactions. (2) D—Cross-sensitivity may occur between certain foods and latex allergies. The nurse's main priority is to protect the nursing assistant from contact with latex. It is unprofessional to discuss personal medical problems with co-workers. This reaction is a Type I reaction but this knowledge serves no purpose at this time. The assistant is already aware that an allergic reaction is possible if pineapple is ingested. (3) A—Swelling of the lips may lead to edema in the throat. Breathing difficulties should be assessed immediately. Medication may be administered to counteract the inflammatory process. A medical history is important, as well as client teaching, after the initial assessment is completed. (4) B—Immunosuppressive agents decrease the ability of the immune system to fight infection. Emphasize the need to avoid large crowds and report signs of infection. Abnormal bleeding, decreased urine production, and jaundice should be reported immediately to the physician. (5) A—HIV is not transmitted by insects, sneezing, coughing, handshaking, sharing eating utensils, or linens. Answers B and C are not therapeutic communication techniques. These responses cast blame and discouragement. (6) C—A primary infection with HIV may produce few symptoms. Many clients manifest with flulike symptoms. Diarrhea, opportunistic infections, and night sweats develop later in the disease process. (7) D—Condoms must be used one time. Oil-based lubricants adversely affect the condom's ability to provide protection. Oral contraceptives may provide pregnancy protection but have no effect on viral transmission. Anal sex should be avoided. (8) B—Tuberculosis is a common manifestation in clients diagnosed with HIV. The Mantoux is the diagnostic test. MAC is caused by a bacteria found in the soil and also affects the respiratory system. Candidiasis is caused by a fungus. A protozoon is the causative agent for cryptosporidiosis; it produces watery diarrhea. (9) D—HIV encephalopathy is a progressive disorder that leads to mental confusion, motor deficits, and forgetfulness. All of these nursing interventions would be noted on the care plan. With dementia, safety is the primary consideration. (10) A—The first priority would be to remove the food from the client's room. Discuss medications for nausea and appetite enhancement before the next meal. Fluids should be limited with meals to encourage increased solid food consumption.

CARE PLAN HINTS

HIV Infection (1) Review the Interdisciplinary Care section for HIV in this chapter. (2) Note the recent medical events in Ms. Lu's record to determine the likely source of her infection. Recall the period of time in which the HIV would be "invisible" from that source. (3) Review with Ms. Lu the ways that HIV can be transmitted. Refer her and her fiancé for counseling regarding adoption or foster parenting.

CARE MAP ANSWERS (PNEUMOCYSTIS CARINII PNEUMONIA)

Correct Data *Subjective:* States "Short of breath when I walk"; easily fatigued. *Objective:* Crackless in the posterior bases; T 100.8°F; dry cough; RR 28, shallow; pulse oximetry 88%.

Report Yes, to physician.

Correct Interventions Instruct in use of incentive spirometer; monitor oxygen levels with pulse oximetry; encourage coughing and deep breathing; increase fluid intake as tolerated; place in semi-Fowler's position; give nasal oxygen at 3 L/min.

Documentation 3/15/06. 0915. Dry cough with crackles in the posterior bases. Respiratory rate 28 and shallow. Able to cough and deep breathe and use incentive spirometer every hour. Nasal oxygen in place at 3 L/min. Pulse oximetry 90%. E. Petro, LVN

CHAPTER 12

NCLEX-PN® ANSWERS (1) B—The liver is a common site of metastasis from lung tumors; the client is demonstrating manifestations of liver dysfunction. (2) C—A diet rich in whole grains, fruits, and vegetables with minimal red and processed meat is associated with a lower risk for colorectal cancer. While there appears to be a genetic link for many cancers, environmental factors also play a role in development of the disease. Screening is important for early detection of colon cancer, but annual exams are unnecessary due to the slow progression of tumors. (3) A—Expressing his feelings allows the client and nurse to identify possible sources of inability to sleep.

Assessment is needed before intervention. (4) A—Family members can provide needed care while the client adjusts to his diagnosis. The nurse should include the client in care as much as he will allow. (5) D—Choosing a head cover prior to losing her hair allows the client to prepare for the loss and make decisions in a less stressful environment. (6) C, E—Small frequent meals are more palatable when a patient is anorexic. Supplements such as Ensure or powdered drink mixes (e.g., Instant Breakfast) mixed with milk and ice cream provide needed calories for the anorexic client. Soft, cool foods are usually tolerated better than hot foods. (7) B—Placing the implant in a lead container prevents radiation exposure. Long-handled forceps reduce the nurse's risk by increasing the distance from the implant. Radioactive materials should not be disposed of in the trash or sewer system because of risk of contamination to individuals and the environment. (8) C—Rubbing or scratching increases irritation to the site and increases risk of infection. Skin should be cleansed with clear water; no ointments should be applied unless directed by the physician. Clients receiving external radiation are not radioactive, and therefore are not a risk to others. (9) A—Providing antiemetic medication prior to the treatment reduces the risk of nausea and vomiting. Nutritional needs should be met throughout the course of chemotherapy. (10) C—Decreased WBC increases the client's risk of infection. Temperature elevation is a systemic symptom of infection. Alopecia and nausea and vomiting are not complications of bone marrow depression. The platelet count is usually decreased with bone marrow depression. A platelet count of 200,000 is within normal limits.

CARE PLAN HINTS

Cancer (1) Review Nursing Care in this chapter, especially the assessment section and the nursing diagnoses *Imbalanced Nutrition: Less than Body Requirements* and *Risk for Infection*. (2) Review the nursing diagnosis *Pain* in the Nursing Care section of the chapter. (3) Use your knowledge of effective communication strategies to make the plan. Also remember any referrals that could be of value to Mr. Casey's daughter.

CARE MAP ANSWERS (CLIENT WITH ANOREXIA RELATED TO CANCER TREATMENT)

Correct Data *Subjective:* States she can't eat, that her mouth is sore, and it hurts to swallow; has lost weight. *Objective:* Height and weight; pale skin with poor turgor; red, swollen oral mucous membranes; dry, brittle hair; concentrated urine.

Correct Interventions Assess hemoglobin and hematocrit; encourage fluid intake; administer antiemetics; suggest eating soft, bland foods at room temperature; offer high-protein drinks; instruct on using soft toothbrush or toothette for oral hygiene.

Report Yes, to the physician or advanced practice nurse administering the chemotherapy.

Documentation Oral mucous membranes red and swollen, poor skin turgor. Weight 102. States that she has lost weight, can't eat, and that it hurts her to swallow. Data reported to H. Shaw, RN. R. Jones, LPN

CHAPTER 13

NCLEX-PN® ANSWERS (1) 4, 2, 3, 1, and 5—The nurse should stop the blood immediately and notify the charge nurse. Then start a normal saline infusion with intravenous tubing. Vital signs are then taken. Based on institutional policy, save the blood bag and return it to the lab. (2) D—Adult urine output should be no less than 30 mL/hr. The urine output is well below the norm and indicates a problem that should be corrected immediately. First, check the Foley for patency and palpate the bladder for distention. Notify the charge nurse immediately. The dark color of the urine indicates dehydration due to the client's blood loss. (3) B—The diagnosis of Anxiety is the most appropriate because there is no evidence of severe blood loss that could account for the restless state. The vital signs are stable and the dressing is dry. Infection does not develop until 72 hours postoperative. Knowledge Deficit relating to the prognosis of her surgery will be important once the anxiety is managed. (4) C—The appropriate response is to acknowledge the client's concern and to make an attempt to ascertain the waiting time. Ignoring the client will only increase his anxiety and frustration. The client may not care that other people need attention, or may not understand the levels of triage. Do not agree nor disagree with the long waiting times. (5) Progressive stage based on the absence of bowel sounds, thready pulse, rapid heart rate, and decreased level of consciousness. (6) A—Cirrhosis of the liver results in the fluid shifting into the interstitial spaces (ascites). This decreases the amount of fluid circulating in the bloodstream, resulting in hypovolemic shock. Anaphylactic shock occurs from a severe allergic reaction. Vital signs indicate that the heart is pumping effectively, so cardiogenic shock is not evident. Septic shock is caused by pathogenic toxins in the blood and results in high fevers. (7) C—Clients should be taught that many reactions are significantly more severe when exposed to the antigen the second time. Precautions should be initiated. Medic-Alert bracelets let medical personnel know that the client is allergic to bee venom. The pharmacist can teach about the antivenom drugs. The client's immediate family should learn appropriate interventions for handling an anaphylactic reaction. (8) D—Heat stroke is characterized by an extremely high temperature (as high as 106°F). Cool skin, profuse sweating, and nausea and vomiting are seen in heat exhaustion. (9) B—Diuretics increase the excretion of urine through the kidneys. Blood pressure drops slightly. Heart rhythm is regulated by antiarrhythmic drugs. LOC may or may not improve and is based on the overall effects of all the nursing and medical management.

(10) D—Safety issues within the client's home should be thoroughly discussed. Handrails in the bathroom, the removal of all loose rugs from the floors, and night-lights in the rooms are a few items that need to be addressed. The client should be able to maneuver with his walker prior to discharge. Food preparation and transportation are important once the safety issues are discussed.

CARE PLAN HINTS

Client with Septic Shock (1) Review Box 13-5 to differentiate between early and late septic shock manifestations. (2) Lactated Ringer's solution is used to increase volume, which will increase Ms. Huang's blood pressure. She also needs fluids to decrease her dehydration caused by the fever and indicated by her poor skin turgor. (3) She had surgery 4 days ago and is underweight. Surgery alters the body's protective mechanisms. Being underweight will reduce the healing ability of the skin.

CARE MAP ANSWERS (CLIENT AT ACCIDENT SCENE)

Correct Data *Subjective:* Allergic to penicillin; does not drink alcohol; complains of being thirsty; complains of left leg pain. *Objective:* Awake; scalp is bleeding; skin slightly pale and dry; left leg is twisted at an odd angle; shallow, slow respirations; denies and difficulty breathing; rapid radial pulse rate.

Correct Interventions Look for hazards in the area; call for help; keep head and neck in neutral position; cover client with a blanket; cover scalp wound with clean cloth.

CHAPTER 14

NCLEX-PN® ANSWERS (1) B—The grief process is highly individual in quality and duration depending on what the loss means to the person experiencing it. (2) B—In the anger stage, the person resists the loss, often directing his or her anger toward family and health care providers. (3) A—The age of the person experiencing the loss influences his or her understanding of and reaction to loss. An individual's reaction to loss is also affected by perception of a support system. (4) D—A do-not-resuscitate order is written by the physician for a client who is near death. The order is usually written based on the wishes of the client and family. (5) B—Nurses care for the dying client in intensive care units, emergency rooms, long-term care facilities, and the home. Regardless of the setting, the client's wishes about death should be respected. (6) A—Hospice is a model of care (rather than a place of care) for clients and their families, emphasizing quality rather than quantity of life for clients as they near the end of life. (7) D—Providing comfort and care to the dying is an active, desirable, and important component of nursing care. Using data from assessment to plan and provide symptom management is necessary for nurses to provide high-quality end-of-life care. (8) B—Near death, the client may have periods of apnea and/or

Cheyne–Stokes respirations. An accumulation of fluids in the lungs and oropharynx may lead to what is sometimes referred to as the "death rattle." These respiratory changes are normal at this time. (9) D—Anticipatory grieving is a combination of intellectual and emotional responses and behaviors by which people work through the grief process based on the perception of a potential loss. (10) C—Spending time listening to clients conveys acceptance of their emotional response to loss. The most appropriate interventions are to listen to how they are feeling and to be present.

CARE PLAN HINTS

Client Experiencing Loss (1) What are the benefits of scheduling a time for a meeting of the staff involved in Mrs. Rogers's care with Mrs. Rogers's daughter? Think about and practice statements to Mrs. Rogers's daughter that are nonthreatening and accepting. Consider why the use of questions like "Why don't you do more for your mother?" are not appropriate. (2) Consider the losses Mrs. Rogers has had. Review the material in the chapter on responses to loss. Think about the reasons the nurse would not say, "Oh, for gosh sakes. Why would you want to do that?" Compose two or three statements that would help you collect more information from Mrs. Rogers. (3) As defined by NANDA, social isolation is the aloneness experienced by the individual and perceived as imposed by others and as a negative or threatening state. Review the care plan and identify characteristics that provide clues to making this diagnosis.

CARE MAP ANSWERS (DYSFUNCTIONAL GRIEVING)

Correct Data *Subjective:* States, "I can't stand being alone"; difficulty sleeping; unable to continue normal routines. *Objective:* Weight loss of 25 pounds.

Correct Interventions Discuss time needed to resolve a loss; explain grief reactions; encourage expression of feelings; state, "This must have been very difficult for you."

Report Yes, to the nurse manager or physician.

Documentation 6/14/07. Has lost 25 pounds in past year. Makes statements that indicate she is still grieving the loss of her husband. J. Pequea, LPN

UNIT II WRAP-UP ANSWERS

CRITICAL THINKING

1. Signs included a low palpable systolic blood pressure of 80, tachycardia at 120 bpm, tachypnea at a rate of 36, and her skin was pale, cool, and diaphoretic. These are all signs of a possible fluid loss and a reduction in circulating volume.

2. Anytime a client is displaying signs of a reduction in circulating volume, a fluid volume deficit and a decrease in cardiac output can be expected. As this can lead to shock,

kidney failure, cardiac arrest with secondary anoxia, and death, fluid replacement is a must.

3. Blood type O-negative has neither A nor B antigens. It could be given immediately without waiting for the client's blood to be typed and crossmatched and would provide a lesser chance of a blood reaction. O-negative blood would be given to a woman of childbearing age because it does not have the Rh antigen attached (O-positive blood would be given to males and postmenopausal women in the same situation).

4. She had no obvious external bleeding and was displaying the symptoms of fluid loss: low blood pressure, elevated heart rate, rapid respiratory rate, cool, pale, diaphoretic skin.

PRIORITIES OF NURSING CARE

1. Knowing that oxygen is the most basic of needs, Ms. Sousa's respiratory status was first addressed by intubation and 100% oxygen. Blood was then administered through a second intravenous line, thereby addressing her fluid volume deficit.

COMMUNICATION

1. Provide the family with any information available about Ms. Sousa's situation, provide a comfortable waiting area for them while she is in surgery, assign a staff member to keep in contact with them so that they feel included and to let them know they have not been forgotten, and answer any questions they may have.

CHAPTER 15

NCLEX-PN® ANSWERS (1) A—ADH promotes water retention by the kidneys. ACTH controls cortisol secretion from adrenal cortex; epinephrine is released during stress; and aldosterone regulates blood volume. (2) C—Radioactive I-125 is harmless. The client is not required to fast before the test. Contrast dye is not injected nor are blood samples drawn. (3) D—Trousseau's is a sign of hypocalcemia and may indicate hypoparathyroidism. Kernig's sign is present with meningitis. Turner's sign is a blue discoloration around the flank and exists with hemorrhagic pancreatitis. Cushing's sign is not a sign of any disorder. (4) B—Glycosylated hemoglobin (Hb A1c) identifies glucose control during the past 3 months and is useful in diagnosing new-onset diabetes mellitus. The water deprivation test diagnoses posterior pituitary function and the secretion of ADH. 17-Ketosteroids and serum cortisol tests evaluate adrenal cortex function. (5) D—The hypothalamus is responsible for regulating temperature. The posterior pituitary gland regulates water balance and uterine contractions. The pancreas releases insulin and glucagon, which are necessary for blood glucose control. The adrenal medulla secretes epinephrine and norepinephrine for the body's stress response.

CHAPTER 16

NCLEX-PN® ANSWERS (1) Abnormal hypersecretion of growth hormone in adulthood results in acromegaly, which causes the manifestations listed. (2) A—Hemorrhage is life threatening. Be sure to assess the dressing behind the neck. Observe for edema and increased swallowing. Tetany usually occurs 1 to 7 days postop if the parathyroid glands were damaged, which decreases serum calcium levels. Dehydration does not occur during the immediate postop period and usually is not life threatening. The laryngeal nerve may be damaged during surgery but this is not life threatening. (3) A—Iodine is needed for the production of thyroid hormone. A decrease in this hormone causes the thyroid to enlarge, goiter, in order to increase the hormone production. Hyperthyroidism increases metabolism but does not cause a goiter. Hyper and hypo states of parathyroidism result in calcium imbalances. (4) D—Clients with hyperparathyroidism must increase activity to prevent calcium from leaving the bones and adding to already increased calcium levels. The client needs a well-balanced diet but there is no reason to increase calories. Room temperature is raised for clients with hypothyroidism. Reorientation is unnecessary because the client does not develop confusion. (5) C—Increased cortisol production by the adrenal cortex causes numerous physical and psychologic changes. The buffalo hump, moon face, edema, and purple striae on the abdomen add to the depression that is typically seen in patients with Cushing's syndrome. These clients have fluid volume excess not deficiency. While they are at risk for falls, they do not experience activity intolerance. Also, they do not develop constipation. (6) D—Hypoparathyroidism can cause respiratory distress. It is most important to ensure a patent airway first. All other interventions are important but not the highest priority for this client. (7) 2, 5, and 6—Clients allergic to shellfish, which contain iodine, cannot take potassium iodine (SSKI). SSKI should be mixed in milk or fruit juice and clients should be monitored for bradycardia. Antacids do not interfere with its absorption. SSKI does not cause rash or itching nor worsen asthma. (8) A—Clients with SIADH have a decreased urine output. Urine production must be monitored along with fluid restriction. A high-protein diet is not needed for this client. SIADH does not alter heart rate so checking the pulse is not required. The SIADH client has no increased risk of infection from crowds. (9) C—Synthroid is given for hypothyroidism, which causes bradycardia. By taking a thyroid drug, heart rate should return to normal. Decreased appetite and constipation are signs of hypothyroidism. Excessive weight loss could indicate side effects of hyperthyroidism. (10) B—With a lack of the mineralocorticoid aldosterone, blood volume and blood pressure are lower, which causes postural hypotension. Multiple bruises are noted with Cushing's syndrome. Peripheral edema and SOB are found in many disorders but not Addison's disease.

CARE PLAN HINTS

Graves' Disease (1) Review the pathophysiology of hyperthyroidism and the illustration of the multisystem effects of hyperthyroidism. (2) See the section on Graves' disease. Note the characteristic eye changes that occur with this disorder. (3) See the discussion of Interdisciplinary Care for Graves' disease. Review especially the pharmacology section. Consider what support Ms. Manuel might need in coping with her disorder.

CARE MAP ANSWERS (HYPOTHYROIDISM)

Correct Data *Subjective:* Rarely hungry, eats less than normal; weight gain of 10 lbs. in past 6 months. *Objective:* Yellowish, dry skin; edema in lower legs; puffy face; slurred speech.

Correct Interventions Provide information that helps Mrs. Lee understand why body changes occur from hypothyroidism; teach Mrs. Lee about reversible body changes.

Report Yes, to the physician.

Documentation 4/5/06. 1700. Complains of poor appetite but states has gained 10 lbs. in past 6 months. Skin is yellowish-colored and dry, with edema noted in lower legs. Face is puffy. Speech is slurred. J. Bergstrom, LPN

CHAPTER 17

NCLEX-PN® ANSWERS (1) B—The sliding scale permits periodic monitoring of blood glucose levels to provide better control. Fast-acting insulin (regular insulin) is used with the sliding scale to best mimic the natural action of the pancreas. (2) A—Clients experiencing Somogyi effect should be taught the symptoms of nighttime hypoglycemia, including tremors, night sweats, and restlessness. A bedtime snack or decreasing the evening dose of intermediate insulin may reduce the risk of developing the effect. (3) C—During periods of illness, blood glucose levels increase in response to physiologic stress and the body's need for glucose. It is important to continue taking insulin in order to prevent DKA or HHS. (4) D—Diabetes mellitus does not increase the client's risk of lung disease. The major concern is vasoconstriction, particularly of peripheral vessels, caused by nicotine in tobacco. Diabetic clients are at risk for circulatory alterations leading to pain, infection, gangrene, and eventual amputation of lower extremities. High blood pressure and the risk for MI and stroke may also develop. (5) A—Type 1 diabetes is caused by lack of insulin production. These individuals are insulin dependent and cannot be managed with oral antidiabetic medications. (6) D—The most likely time for a client to experience hypoglycemia as a result of receiving

NPH insulin is 6 to 12 hours following administration. (7) B—Diabetic ketoacidosis is characterized by hyperglycemia and spillage of ketones in the urine, which causes the classic acetone breath. The skin is very warm and dry as a result of dehydration. Slurred speech occurs with hypoglycemia. The pulse is usually rapid and weak. (8) Correct sequence is 5, 4, 2, 1, 3—Inspect regular insulin for clarity first. Next, NPH insulin is rolled between the palms to mix. Then clean the tops of both vials with alcohol. Inject air into NPH insulin and then the regular insulin. The regular insulin is withdrawn first to avoid mixing of the NPH in the regular insulin vial. (9) D—Regular soda, a rapid-acting glucose source, is given immediately to a conscious client with hypoglycemia. Giving insulin would decrease glucose levels further. Glucagon is only used with an unconscious client. Crackers and cheese are given after glucose levels have returned to normal because they take longer to act. (10) Correct teaching points are 1, 4, and 6—Toenails should be cut straight across to avoid development of ingrown toenails that can lead to infection. Diabetic clients should avoid open-toed shoes and heating pads to prevent injury. Lotion between the toes results in a warm, moist environment, which promotes bacterial and fungal growth. Shoes are best bought in the afternoon when feet are the largest. Clients must be taught to use a mirror daily to inspect all sides of the feet.

CARE PLAN HINTS

Insulin-Dependent Diabetes Mellitus (1) Name the factors in Mr. Meligrito's schedule that contributed to his condition. Review the appropriate medication dosages. (2) Review the section on treatment of diabetic ketoacidosis. Note whether this condition is more likely in Type 1 or Type 2 diabetics. Note the order and purpose of different intravenous solutions. (3) Recall the pathophysiology of these two types of diabetes. Review controllable factors, and see Box 17-4.

CARE MAP ANSWERS (DIABETES MELLITUS)

Correct Data *Subjective:* Does not complain of any discomfort in her feet; says she uses a hot water bottle on her feet at night. *Objective:* Red spots on top of the toes on her right foot; blister on the left heel.

Report Yes, to physician.

Correct Interventions Discuss the importance of not smoking; teach her to wear new shoes for short periods of time each day; instruct client in proper foot care; teach her to monitor red areas for signs of skin breakdown.

Documentation 08/13/06. Reviewed symptoms that would indicate skin breakdown. Discussed the importance of proper foot care, not smoking, and not using hot water bottles or heating pads on her feet. Repeated instructions correctly and says she will "take better care of her feet." Barbara Boucher, LPN

UNIT III WRAP-UP ANSWERS

CRITICAL THINKING

Jake has several acute problems that must be addressed. These include out-of-control blood glucose, renal disease, and a gangrenous infected foot. Following the report from the lab, the first intervention that the nurse would perform would be administration of insulin according to the sliding scale. After that, client teaching would be needed about the importance of fluid restriction, and a review of the prescribed diet should be done. If dialysis is to be performed on this day, the nurse should assist the client with his ADLs and perform any ordered wound care prior to the dialysis, since the treatment will take several hours. It is important to be sure that lab results and other documentation are on the chart so that the dialysis nurse has access to all pertinent information.

COLLABORATIVE CARE

These are expected results for a client with renal disease. Given the client's circumstances, it is not necessary to call the physician as long as the dialysis routine is being followed. As the LPN/LVN, you would want to consult with the dialysis nurse prior to administering insulin by the sliding scale.

COMMUNICATION

Teaching on the following topics will need to be addressed:

- **Diabetes care and control.** Although Jake has Type 2 (non-insulin-dependent) diabetes mellitus, he needs insulin to control his blood glucose while in the hospital. He will need to be taught how to monitor his blood sugar and how to self-administer insulin. Diet will also be important. The nurse should reinforce the teaching done by the dietitian. If Jake will be preparing his own meals, he will need to know what foods he can have and also learn about portion control. Foot care for both the infected and noninfected foot will be necessary. If the infection is not resolved, it may be necessary to amputate the gangrenous portion. The nurse needs to address prevention of additional infections, teach the proper way to cut toenails, and talk about wearing clean cotton socks each day. The client must be reminded to wear socks and shoes that fit properly. Teach client to get immediate attention for any cuts, blisters, or other injuries on the feet. The nurse can best evaluate the client's understanding of the teaching by asking him to provide a return demonstration for any procedures. Have him repeat any instructions that have been given. Carefully listen to his explanations and any questions that he asks in order to identify any misunderstanding of instructions.
- **Dialysis treatments.** Be sure that information concerning follow-up appointments and future dialysis treatments is included in discharge instructions. Transportation may be necessary, so be sure the client has the resources needed to get to appointments. If fluid restriction will be continued,

make sure the client understands that water as well as beverages at meals are included in the restriction.

CHAPTER 18

NCLEX-PN® ANSWERS
(1) B—Saliva contains amylase and lysozyme, enzymes that start the digestion of starch. (2) A—The cardiac, or lower esophageal sphincter, opens to allow food into the stomach, and normally is closed at other times. Stenosis, or tightening of this sphincter, will affect the movement of food from the esophagus into the stomach. (3) D—Dullness to percussion generally indicates solid tissue or a mass. The sigmoid colon is found in the left lower quadrant; the liver in the right upper quadrant. A dull percussion tone due to a full bladder is usually noted at midline. (4) C—In a colonoscopy, a flexible fiber-optic scope is inserted into the large intestine through the anus to visualize the mucous membranes and any abnormalities of the bowel. (5) A—Most food and nutrients are absorbed in the small intestine through the villi and microvilli.

CHAPTER 19

NCLEX-PN® ANSWERS
(1) C—Central or upper body obesity is identified by a waist-to-hip ratio of 1 or higher. Upper body obesity generally is associated with hyperlipidemia. While the client may have obese parents (parenteral obesity is a strong risk factor for obesity), that finding does not define upper body obesity. (2) A—A weight gain of 1 to 2 lbs per week is appropriate. A 1,500-kcal diet does not provide adequate kilocalories to support weight gain; an additional 3,500 kcal above metabolic needs is necessary to gain 1 lb. Excessive exercise increases kcal needs and will not promote weight gain. Unsaturated fats and whole-grain carbohydrates add calories to the diet. (3) B—Viscous lidocaine may be used to numb the mucous membranes in the mouth. Never use a strong mouthwash, because many of these contain alcohol that may cause severe burning of the mouth. The gag reflex may be assessed if viscous lidocaine has been swallowed. Raw fruits and vegetables can irritate inflamed mucous membranes, and should be limited or avoided. (4) A—Early symptoms of oral cancer are painless ulcers. Documenting the lesion and notifying the physician are your next priority. It is not an emergency, nor will you prepare the patient for a biopsy until the diagnosis is made by the physician. It is important for the client to report any changes in the ulceration. (5) 1, 4—Remaining upright after eating and raising the head of the bed on blocks reduces regurgitation of gastric contents into the lower esophagus. Continuing prescribed drugs for the full course of treatment is important to heal inflamed tissue of the esophagus. Cigarette smoke, alcohol, peppermint, and chocolate aggravate reflux and symptoms of GERD. (6) B—Cancers that erode through the esophageal wall may cause severe hemorrhage. Difficulty swallowing is an early sign of esophageal cancer, which may be followed by choking and weight loss. (7) B—During insertion of the NG tube, the gag reflex may be initiated. Briefly pause, allow the client a short rest, have her sip a small amount of water to help with the insertion, and resume the procedure. Do not initially remove the tube completely; this may increase anxiety and nasal trauma. Placement checks are done after the tube is inserted completely. (8) 4 hours. Divide 60 mL into 240 mL to calculate the number of hours that it will take for the feeding to run. (9) B—*Helicobacter pylori* bacteria has been found to increase the incidence of peptic ulcers. It will not affect the acid nor the mucus. Antibiotics are not usually given to prevent the appearance of this organism. (10) D—Dumping syndrome is characterized by stomach contents that rapidly flood the small intestine after a meal. Large amounts of water are pulled into the intestines, creating a volume deficit in the blood circulation. Proteins and fats are absorbed at a slower rate than sugars. Resting after a meal slows down the digestive process. Smaller, more frequent meals are generally more tolerated than three large meals.

CARE PLAN HINTS

Peptic Ulcer Disease (1) Review the pathophysiology of peptic ulcer disease and then note the conditions that made a relapse likely for Mr. O'Donnell. Recall the organism that is often a factor in PUD. (2) Remember the gastric side effects of NSAIDs and aspirin. See the Pharmacology section under this disorder. (3) Look at Mr. O'Donnell's lifestyle and occupation for clues. How does stress create an environment for PUD?

CARE MAP ANSWERS (OBESITY)

Correct Data *Subjective:* Exercise limited to "puttering around" and walking length of driveway; typically daily food intake: juice, oatmeal, muffin, coffee, cream; snack donuts and coffee; etc.; reports easily fatigued, SOB with activity. *Objective:* 30-lb. weight gain over 2 years; 5'10" tall, weight 201 lbs.; serum cholesterol 240 mg/dL (normal 150 to 200 mg/dL); HDL 37 mg/dL (normal > 45 mg/dL); LDL 180 mg/dL (normal < 130 mg/dL); 32% body fat.

Correct Interventions Assess weight weekly; discuss eating habits and strategies to reduce fat and calorie intake; identify eating cues and find strategies to reduce or eliminate eating cues; teach how to keep and use a food diary; discuss role of regular exercise in weight loss and control; discuss lifestyle and behavior-modification strategies to promote weight loss and control.

Documentation 8/14/06. Weight 198 lbs. Reports that he has started using low-fat creamer in his coffee and has given up his morning muffin and donut, having an English muffin with jam as a morning snack instead. He also reports that he is having raw vegetables and water with lunch, instead of chips and a soft drink. Before dinner he has a handful of pretzels with his wine. He and his wife started walking in the afternoon; he is now able to walk for 45 minutes "without becoming winded." Pleased with his progress; states his wife is a "great support—she went out and bought four new low-fat cookbooks!" Marie Langlios, LVN

CHAPTER 20

NCLEX-PN® ANSWERS (1) B—Severe diarrhea can lead to fluid volume deficit and hypovolemia. The first priority for the nurse is to assess fluid volume status (vital signs, orthostatic vitals, skin turgor, moisture of mucous membranes) because maintaining vascular volume is critical to maintain circulation and kidney function. (2) D—Older adults often have a bowel movement every two or three days. This pattern may be normal for the client; the nurse assesses for other indications of constipation, such as stool that is very hard or difficult to expel. (3) A—Rebound tenderness, characteristic of appendicitis, is characterized by relief of pain with pressure, followed by increased pain when pressure is relieved. (4) C—When using therapeutic communication, the nurse focuses on the client's concerns and feelings. Although stress does not cause irritable bowel syndrome, it often precipitates its manifestations. Discussing the client's feelings also helps establish the pattern of the disorder. (5) A—Antidiarrheal medications are not to be used until the cause of diarrhea has been determined because they could worsen or prolong the disease, or lead to complications. (6) B, C—Sulfasalazine increases photosensitivity (the risk for sunburn), and can decrease the effectiveness of oral contraceptives. Taking it with a full glass of water and avoiding use of aspirin and vitamin C while on the drug are important. Rash is an adverse effect that should be reported promptly to the physician. (7) C—Not allowed on this diet are fresh vegetables, rich desserts, raw or fresh fruits, or tough meats. (8) D—Increased pain with a rigid, boardlike abdomen may indicate perforation of the bowel and possible peritonitis, a potentially critical complication of bowel obstruction. (9) A—The passage of flatus and resumption of bowel sounds indicate the return of peristalsis, necessary for safe food introduction. Pain needs to be managed throughout recovery to promote mobility. Promoting mobility, such as in ambulation, will encourage return of normal peristalsis, but is not a requirement prior to introducing food. IV fluids provide fluid and electrolytes, but do not provide adequate calories unless total parenteral nutrition is used. (10) A—Because colorectal cancer is often a silent disease and treatment at an early stage has a high cure rate, the American Cancer Society recommends routine screening procedures for early detection. This includes annual digital rectal examination for all people over age 50, annual fecal occult blood test for people over age 50, and flexible sigmoidoscopy or colonoscopy at age 50 and every 5 to 10 years thereafter. Screening exams should be early and frequent for clients with inflammatory bowel disease, a history of

polyps, or a strong family history of colorectal cancer. Bowel cancer usually grows slowly. There may be 5 to 15 years of growth before symptoms occur. Manifestations depend on tumor location, type and extent, and complications. Bleeding is often what prompts clients to seek medical care.

CARE PLAN HINTS

Inflammatory Bowel Disease (1) Review the function of the colon, and the differences between the consistency and content of material entering the colon from the small intestine and feces that is expelled through the anus. Then review the manifestations of fluid volume deficit in Chapter 7. (2) Review the pathophysiology and manifestations of inflammatory bowel disease, and the effect of those manifestations on other body systems. (3) Think about placement of the stoma on the abdomen as you discuss possible clothing style options to suggest.

CARE MAP ANSWERS (COLORECTAL CANCER)

Correct Data *Subjective:* States "I really don't want a colostomy, but if that is what it takes to keep me well, I'm ready to get it over with." *Objective:* Intermittent constipation.

Correct Interventions Frequently assess stoma and peristomal skin condition; teach colostomy care; refer to the local United Ostomy Association; provide a list of local resources for ostomy supplies.

CHAPTER 21

NCLEX-PN® ANSWERS (1) B—Narcotic analgesics often are required for acute pain relief in cholelithiasis. (2) B—Nausea and vomiting after eating may indicate the T-tube is not functioning and/or blockage of the bile ducts. (3) D—Low-fat diets decrease stimulation of the gallbladder to release bile, thereby decreasing pain. (4) A—Hepatitis A is transmitted by the oral–fecal route and by consumption of contaminated food or water. (5) C—Hepatitis B is transmitted through blood and body fluid exposure, including contaminated needles, blood transfusions, and unprotected sexual relations. (6) D—Alcohol is hepatotoxic and use should be eliminated. (7) A, B—Decreased weight and abdominal girth may indicate a decrease in ascites. (8) B—Ammonia levels are elevated because of inability of the liver to metabolize protein products. Lactulose decreases the absorption of ammonia from the bowel. (9) B, A, C, D, E—Narcotic analgesics work quickly to relieve pain. Inserting the nasogastric tube removes gastric secretions that stimulate pancreatic enzyme release. The side-lying position with the head elevated reduces stress on abdominal muscles and tissues. Although these measures are important to promote comfort, they are of lower priority than the first three measures. (10) B—Fluid loss associated with vomiting, diaphoresis, third-space shifts, and nasogastric suction is common. Fluid initially is lost from vascular space, potentially impairing cardiac output and tissue perfusion.

CARE PLAN HINTS

Cholelithiasis (1) Review the pathophysiology of cholelithiasis and cholecystitis. Research cultural influences (Native American) on diet, and develop a diet plan that considers these influences. (2) Think about the location of the gallbladder and direction of bile drainage, as well as the effect of position on respiratory status. (3) Review Box 21-4, Nursing Care Checklist for clients having a laparoscopic cholecystectomy.

Cirrhosis (1) Review the effects of increased ammonia levels on mental function. Blood is a protein; think about what happens to it in the gut. (2) Review the pathophysiology of cirrhosis and its complications. (3) Check Chapter 7 for low-sodium foods, and review Chapter 32 for protein restriction guidelines.

CARE MAP ANSWERS (PANCREATITIS)

Correct Data *Subjective:* Thin, appears anxious and tired; states she lost 30 lbs. (13.6 kg) in the hospital; states main problems are lack of energy and lack of appetite. *Objective:* Weight 102 lbs. (46 kg), height 66 inches (168 cm); skin cool and dry, poor turgor; blood glucose 80 mg/dL.

Correct Interventions Plan daily rest periods, especially before meals; discuss dietary restrictions and how to adapt to usual diet; assist family to plan six small meals a day.

UNIT IV WRAP-UP ANSWERS

CRITICAL THINKING

1. Normal WBC is 5,000 to 10,000/mm^3.
2. WBCs or leukocytes are components of the blood that help defend the body against foreign invaders and infection. An elevated count usually indicates an infection or inflammation.
3. Wound care and clean dressing change; activity limitations such as avoidance of heavy lifting; observation and reporting to physician any elevation in temperature or change in appearance of incision, such as warmth, redness, or drainage; continue prescribed antibiotic therapy until complete; pain management, and the importance of follow-up care with the physician.

MANAGEMENT OF NURSING CARE

1. Usually no analgesics are administered until after a diagnosis is made; NPO status in case of surgery; heat is never used as the increase in circulation could cause appendix to rupture; laxatives and enemas are avoided as increased peristalsis could also cause the appendix to rupture.
2. Assess pain every two hours and provide analgesics as indicated; assess the incision twice each shift and change

dressing as needed, using aseptic technique, monitor the incision for signs of infection, such as drainage, redness, swelling, or heat; observe client for fever; encourage ambulation to stimulate peristalsis and to prevent respiratory complications.

CHAPTER 22

NCLEX-PN® ANSWERS (1) A, B, E—Intact airways, an intact thorax able to expand and contract during breathing, and an intact cardiovascular system are vital for the process of respiration, which includes air movement into and out of the lungs, the exchange of gases between the alveoli and blood, and transport of oxygen and carbon dioxide to and from the cells of the body. (2) B—The cough reflex is ineffective in clients who are comatose or unconscious. (3) D—The amount of radioactive ion used is small and rapidly excreted; no special precautions to avoid exposure of others to radioactivity are necessary. (4) C—Alpha$_1$-antitrypsin is a protein that is necessary to maintain lung structure. Low levels of this protein lead to emphysema. (5) B—Bronchodilators, smoking, and caffeine can interfere with PFT results and should be avoided the morning of the test. Fasting is not necessary, and the test is not painful.

CHAPTER 23

NCLEX-PN® ANSWERS (1) C—Antihistamines have many side effects, including drowsiness and a dry mouth. Some patients may have an allergic reaction with chest tightness or wheezing. Alcohol is contraindicated with most antihistamines, including Chlor-Trimeton. (2) D—Moist air helps to loosen secretions and provide comfort for the postoperative tonsillectomy client. Ice collars are used to decrease the potential for hemorrhage. The head of the bed should be elevated, with the patient's head turned to the side. The airway device must remain in place until the gag reflex returns. (3) B—Clients with pertussis are placed in respiratory isolation until about 5 days of antibiotic therapy have been completed. A physician's order is required before administering a narcotic cough suppressant. The disease is diagnosed by nasopharyngeal swab. Contacts of the client are treated with prophylactic antibiotic therapy. (4) A—Although the medical history and physical assessment are important aspects of nursing care, patient allergies to egg products must be ascertained. The influenza vaccine is produced in eggs. (5) B—Most viral URIs are self-limiting. Patient teaching that includes self-care should be stressed. Throat cultures are not always required. Antibiotics are not useful in the treatment of viral infections. Monitoring temperature may be done if the patient is febrile. (6) A—Impaired verbal communication is a primary nursing diagnosis for a patient with laryngitis. Talking will increase the inflammation of the larynx. There is no need for cough medications or effective coughing techniques with laryngitis. An increase in fluids will not influence the outcome of the condition to a great extent. (7) C, B, A, D, E—All of the answers are important, but controlling the bleeding and airway have the highest priority. (8) B—Obesity is a major factor for developing sleep apnea. Weight loss should be considered. Alcohol and hypnotics are contraindicated for patients with this condition. During sleep, the tongue relaxes and obstructs the airway. Obstructive sleep apnea is the most common form. (9) D—Persistent hoarseness, often without other symptoms, is an early sign of laryngeal cancer. The client should see his physician promptly, because early tumors often can be removed and the voice preserved. (10) C—In a total laryngectomy, the trachea and esophagus are separated and a tracheostomy is formed. There is no risk of choking during eating or drinking.

CARE PLAN HINTS

Upper Respiratory Infection (1) Review Table 23-1 for common manifestations. Review the Complementary Therapies and Continuing Care for measures to promote comfort during URI. (2) Review both the Pharmacology section under Interdisciplinary Care and Table 23-2. (3) Review the common manifestations and duration of uncomplicated URI and use this in teaching. Look at the manifestations of complications of URI such as pneumonia and sinusitis. Do these complications usually require emergency treatment? What symptoms should the client seek immediate care for? (*Hint:* Think ABCs.) Why is it usually more appropriate for a client to seek treatment by his or her primary care provider than in an ED? Look at continuity of care, cost, and utilization issues.

CARE MAP ANSWERS (TOTAL LARYNGECTOMY)

Correct Data *Subjective:* Complains that head "feels heavy." *Objective:* Tracheostomy tube present; O_2 per tracheostomy collar; oxygen saturation 94%; moderate edema noted right side of face and neck.

Correct Interventions Assess respiratory rate, lung sounds, and cough effectiveness every 2 hours; encourage to use deep breathing and coughing exercises hourly.

CHAPTER 24

NCLEX-PN® ANSWERS (1) B—Cigarette smoking is strongly associated with chronic bronchitis. The environment such as working in mines, silicone factories, or cotton mills may contribute to this disease. (2) B—A positive test indicates presence of antibodies to TB but does not necessarily indicate active disease and the ability to spread the organism. The husband should be tested because there is a risk of infection with people living in the same household, but there is no evidence that he is positive. (3) C—Manifestations of acute asthma attack include

chest tightness, wheezing, shortness of breath, and anxiety. Asthma can lead to respiratory distress if not managed properly. The medication effectiveness is also reported. (4) D—Rinsing the mouth after using the inhaler reduces systemic drug absorption and reduces the risk of thrush associated with some anti-inflammatory drugs used to treat asthma and COPD. Bronchodilators are used to treat acute attacks of asthma and before using anti-inflammatory drugs by MDI. (5) D—COPD clients have increased carbon dioxide in their blood, suppressing it as an effective stimulus for respirations; instead, a drop in blood oxygen levels stimulates the drive to breathe. Low doses of O_2 are useful for the COPD patient, particularly at night. High doses of O_2 suppress the drive to breathe and may result in respiratory failure. (6) A—Atelectasis is commonly seen with nonambulatory clients after surgery. Pain medication decreases respirations, which could lead to atelectasis. (7) B—A thoracentesis is performed by inserting a needle into the pleural space that surrounds the lungs in order to remove fluid or air. The mediastinum contains the heart and great vessels. The thoracic cavity refers to the chest. (8) B—The wound is covered with an occlusive dressing to prevent air from entering the pleural space, then the physician is notified. Reinsertion of the tube introduces bacteria and other possible contaminants into the pleural space. (9) B, D, E—These measures, along with wearing seat belts with shoulder harnesses in cars, are important measures to prevent lung and chest trauma. Pneumococcal vaccine is not recommended for young, healthy adults. Exercise, while beneficial, also is not a specific measure to prevent chest and lung trauma. (10) A—Restlessness and tachypnea (rapid respiratory rate) are early signs of hypoxia, a component of respiratory failure. Deep coma is a very late sign. Hypotension, tachycardia, and decreased urine output are indicative of decreased cardiac output, a later effect of respiratory failure.

CARE PLAN HINTS

COPD (1) Research the effects of secondhand smoke to respond to this question. (2) Review the control and function of the respiratory center in the central nervous system. Also review acid–base balance in Chapter 7. (3) Read the section on Respiratory Failure later in this chapter to identify its manifestations. Think about why the client with COPD would be vulnerable to developing respiratory failure.

CARE MAP ANSWERS (TUBERCULOSIS)

Correct Data *Subjective:* Homeless for past 10 years; uses shelters only during very cold or wet weather; complains of chronic cough that now is productive of pink sputum; often wakes up drenched with sweat in the middle of the night; complains of increasing fatigue. *Objective:* Vital signs: BP 152/86; P 92; R 20; and T 100.2°F (37.8°C); clean; answers questions appropriately and intelligently; very thin, almost emaciated; sputum Gram stain positive for acid-fast bacillus.

Correct Interventions Provide verbal and written information about tuberculosis; teach about prescribed medications, possible adverse effects, and importance of completing the entire prescribed regimen; emphasize importance of continued follow-up; refer to local incentive shelter program for directly observed medical therapy and meals.

Documentation Be sure to relate your documentation to the established goal, not to the care or interventions you provided.

UNIT V WRAP-UP ANSWERS

COORDINATION OF INTERDISCIPLINARY CARE

1. Quality, rather than quantity of life; palliative, rather than curative measures, emotional support for patient and family; and death with dignity.
2. Skilled nursing to help manage symptoms of his disease, home health aide to assist with hygiene cares, social worker to assist with grief counseling, chaplain services to assist with spiritual care, and volunteers to provide time-out for family caregivers.

CRITICAL THINKING

1. Chemotherapy drugs destroy cells that have a rapid rate of proliferation, such as bone marrow, neutrophils, hair follicles, cells lining the GI tract, and gonad cells; chemotherapy drugs do not distinguish between cancer cells and normal cells; signs and symptoms of toxic side effects occur when normal cells are destroyed; this creates common chemotherapy side effects, such as bone marrow suppression, neutropenia, hair loss, nausea and vomiting; and sterility.
2. The nurse must be an advocate for the client and provide support for whatever decision is made; the nurse can request interdisciplinary support and education for the client and family through consultation with the physician and social worker; the nurse can provide information regarding end-of-life care and client rights, the nurse can assist with providing answers to client/family questions.

CHAPTER 25

NCLEX-PN® ANSWERS (1) D—The pericardium is the outermost layer of the heart. The innermost layer is the endocardium, and the middle (muscle) layer is the myocardium. (2) B—The mitral valve separates the left atrium from the left ventricle. The atrioventricular valve on the right side of the heart is the tricuspid valve; the pulmonic and aortic valves lead from the ventricles to the pulmonary artery and aorta, respectively. (3) B—The QRS complex corresponds with ventricular systole (contraction). The P wave corresponds with atrial contraction, and the T wave with repolarization of the ventricles. The ST segment is the period between ventricular polarization as indicated by the QRS complex, and repolariza-

tion, as indicated by the T wave. (4) B, C, E—Blood vessel length and diameter and the viscosity of the blood affect peripheral vascular resistance, with vessel diameter being the primary factor in determining total peripheral resistance. (5) A—The echocardiogram is an imaging study that helps determine the size and movement of the heart, as well as some structural abnormalities.

CHAPTER 26

NCLEX-PN® ANSWERS (1) A—Many of the statin drugs, including atorvastatin, can impair liver function. Yellowing of the skin and sclera must be promptly reported to the physician to ensure that irreversible liver damage does not occur. (2) C—Anginal chest pain usually is relieved by rest and sublingual nitroglycerin (or other rapid-acting nitroglycerin preparations), whereas the chest pain associated with an acute myocardial infarction usually continues despite rest or administration of sublingual nitroglycerin. (3) D—Disruption of the integrity of the femoral artery by insertion of the catheter and sheath can result in either arterial bleeding or formation of a clot that impairs distal circulation to the affected extremity. (4) B—Hypotension (low blood pressure) and a urine output of less than 30 mL/hr are indicative of a fall in cardiac output and may indicate inadequate tissue perfusion. (5) A—Creatine kinase (CK) is an enzyme released from necrotic cardiac muscle cells. The blood level of CK rises within hours after an acute myocardial infarction and remains elevated for up to 48 hours. The hematocrit, and BUN should remain within normal limits following an MI. Blood glucose levels may increase slightly due to the stress response. (6) D—Lifestyle modifications, including dietary changes, can reduce the risk for myocardial infarction in the future. (7) C—The normal adult heart rate is 60 to 100 bpm. A rate lower than 60 is bradycardia, a rate greater than 100 is tachycardia. Sinus arrhythmia is an irregular heart rate characterized by increased heart rate on inspiration and decreased heart rate with expiration. (8) C—Assessment of the client is vital to determine whether the apparent heart rhythm is due to a mechanical problem (e.g., a loose monitor lead or wire) and/or is affecting cardiac output. (9) B—Immediate and effective CPR can be lifesaving for the client who experiences cardiac arrest and sudden cardiac death. (10) A, B, D—Correct electrode placement, client education, and ensuring safe, working equipment are important for effective cardiac monitoring.

CARE PLAN HINTS

Acute Myocardial Infarction (1) Review Box 26-9. Using your nursing diagnosis handbook, identify appropriate nursing diagnoses for the post-acute period of hospitalization. Also review the cardiac rehabilitation section (under Interdisciplinary Care for myocardial infarction) for the nursing care focus. (2) Review the scope of practice for an LPN/LVN in your state. Can you intervene independently or do you need to report this to the charge nurse? (3) Think about strategies to decrease Mrs. Williams's denial of the negative effects of smoking.

CARE MAP ANSWERS (AFTER CORONARY ARTERY BYPASS SURGERY)

Correct Data *Subjective:* History of progressive angina for 4 years; anterior wall myocardial infarction 2 years ago; treated with immediate thrombolytic therapy and percutaneous balloon angioplasty; strong family history of CHD (father died at age 51, brother died at age 48 of myocardial infarctions); does not smoke, uses alcohol occasionally; enjoys "good Southern-style cooking" and watching TV; rarely exercises other than dancing with wife and friends about once a month; usually works 50 to 60 hours per week at own contracting business; states "I have got to get back to work! You just can't sit around in my business—you have to make sure that the work is getting done on time." *Objective:* BP 138/72, P 86, regular, R 24, T 99.1°F PO; faint crackles left lung base; incision clean and dry, healing well; color good; O_2 sats 95% on 4 L O_2 per cannula; bowel sounds active; taking regular diet in small amounts.

Correct Interventions Teach about the heart and coronary heart disease, exercise and activities, lifestyle modifications, including diet and stress management; discuss emotional reactions to CHD and sexual activity after discharge, provide information about community resources for emotional support; help identify coping strategies for concerns about role in business.

CHAPTER 27

NCLEX-PN® ANSWERS (1) A—Left-sided heart failure affects cardiac output and the availability of blood and oxygen to meet the body's metabolic needs. As a result, fatigue and activity intolerance are common, early manifestations of heart failure. Heart failure is not painful, nor does it usually affect airway clearance. Fluid volume often increases in heart failure due to compensatory mechanisms. (2) B—The backward effects of right-sided heart failure affect the venous system and peripheral tissues. Increased pressure in the venous system causes peripheral edema. The heart rate increases, and urinary output may decrease. Pulmonary edema develops with left-sided failure. (3) C—A slow pulse may indicate digitalis toxicity. The physician should be notified as diagnostic tests may be necessary to determine the cause of the low pulse rate. (4) B—Cheese is high is sodium, as are smoked foods, indicating a need for further instruction about appropriate dietary selections. (5) C—Activity limitations are necessary to reduce the risk of heart damage associated with the acute carditis of rheumatic fever. Visits from family and friends should be encouraged as long as adequate rest is ensured. (6) D—Bacterial endocarditis occurs most frequently in clients who have had previous heart or valve damage that affects the flow of blood through the heart. The innermost layer of the heart is affected, and treatment is necessary to reduce the risk of permanent heart valve damage. (7) D—A pericardial friction rub is a manifestation of pericarditis, and therefore an expected assessment finding. Peripheral edema and respiratory wheezes are not expected findings, and should be reported to the physician. Pericarditis typically causes chest pain that increases with movement and breathing. (8) C—A collection of fluid or blood in the pericardial sac can obscure or muffle the heart sounds and affect cardiac filling and output. Filling is impaired to a greater extent during inspiration, leading to an ausculatory gap in the blood pressure as output falls. (9) A—The client needs information about possible complications to be reported to the physician. (10) B—Mechanical valve replacements necessitate anticoagulant therapy to prevent formation of clots on the valve. Until well regulated, this increases the client's risk for bleeding.

CARE PLAN HINTS

Heart Failure (1) Review Boxes 27-3, 27-5, and 27-6 for assessment data and guidelines for exercise in clients with heart failure as you design your plan. (2) Consider the underlying message and therapeutic communication strategies as you formulate your response. (3) Review the section of Chapter 7 on hypokalemia for the factors that can lead to this electrolyte imbalance. Think about the questions you might ask Mr. and Mrs. Jackson to help identify possible causes of his hypokalemia.

CARE MAP ANSWERS (MITRAL STENOSIS)

Correct Data *Subjective:* History of rheumatic fever; heart murmur; teeth cleaned two months ago; shortness of breath with walking short distance; weight loss and loss of appetite. *Objective:* Vital signs; presence of murmur; petechiae; poor color, O_2 sats 91%; apparent lack of understanding/concern by wife.

Report Yes.

Correct Interventions (Risk for Injury) Schedule appointments for IV antibiotic infusions, discuss prescribed outpatient intravenous antibiotic therapy, teach intravenous catheter care; discuss symptoms to report to physician; encourage rest before and after activity; discuss use of prophylactic antibiotic therapy.

CHAPTER 28

NCLEX-PN® ANSWERS (1) D—When an arterial thrombus develops, blood flow through the artery is occluded. Pain is the primary manifestation of arterial occlusion (tissue ischemia), and the affected extremity is cold and pale due to lack of circulation. (2) A—Instruct the client to keep the extremity in a dependent position; gravity helps to maintain blood flow to the distal tissues. (3) A—Heparin interferes with the normal clotting mechanism, preventing the formation of new clots and the extension of existing clots. (4) C—Stress management is particularly important for clients with Raynaud's disease. The client is encouraged to use relaxation techniques, massage therapy, hobbies, aromatherapy, and counseling to reduce and cope with stress. (5) C—Raynaud's is characterized by spasms of the small arteries and arterioles of the extremities. The arterial spasms limit blood flow to the fingers and, on occasion, the toes, ears, or nose. (6) B—People with stage 1 or stage 2 hypertension commonly have no symptoms other than an increased blood pressure. Hypertension is usually advanced when manifestations are seen. (7) A—Based on the lack of symptoms, clients often have difficulty understanding the importance of medication schedules. (8) D—Coumadin interferes with liver synthesis of clotting factors, preventing the clot formation. The client's symptoms and history are consistent with an intracranial bleed and clot formation. (9) C—Nicotine constricts blood vessels. The smaller the diameter of a vessel, the greater the friction against the walls of vessel and, thus, the greater impedance to blood flow. (10) A—Sudden, excruciating pain is a symptom of a dissecting aneurysm of the ascending aorta.

CARE PLAN HINTS

Hypertension (1) Review Box 28-2 as you read Mrs. Spezia's history and physicial assessment data. (2) Review the pathophysiology of and risk factors for hypertension. Think about how diet contributes to this disorder. (3) Review the timing and potential adverse effects of the prescribed medications. Think about hints and techniques clients can use to improve medication compliance.

CARE MAP ANSWERS (BUERGER'S DISEASE)

Correct Data *Subjective:* Has smoked over two packs of cigarettes a day for 20 years; calf pain with activity progressing over past 2 months; must rest frequently when walking; relates numbness and tingling of toes of left foot. *Objective:* Weak peripheral pulses in right leg; absent pedal and posterior tibial pulses in left foot; third, fourth, and fifth toes of left foot pale; right foot pink and warm; left foot cool to touch; skin on left leg shiny and thin; hairless below knee; moderate amount evenly distributed hair right leg.

Correct Interventions Assess pain at rest and during activity using a scale of 0 to 10; teach Buerger–Allen exercises; instruct to perform exercises three times per day; teach the importance of smoking cessation; teach foot care measures; encourage questions about the disease and its management.

UNIT VI WRAP-UP ANSWERS

CRITICAL THINKING

1. Mrs. Hipps' pastimes of reading and watching television contributed to a sedentary lifestyle. Frequent use of the leg muscles assists in venous return and helps prevent venous stasis, which is one of the main causes of clot formation.
2. Heat increases circulation to an inflamed area and subsequently assists in removal of debris and general clean up of the thrombosed area; heat also assists in pain reduction.

PRIORITIES OF NURSING CARE

1. Your first response should be to Mrs. Hipps. The most serious complication of a DVT is a pulmonary embolism, which is life threatening. Oxygen is the most basic of needs and Mrs. Hipps' change in color as reported by the CNA is probably due to lack of oxygen, rather than cold. Ask another coworker to assess Mr. Siron's pain and give an analgesic if appropriate. Direct the CNA to assist Mrs. Bigalow until you are able to assess her.

MANAGEMENT OF CARE

1. Monitor lab values related to the heparin and the warfarin, partial thromboplastin time and prothrombin time; observe for signs of bleeding, such as bleeding gums, tarry stools, bruising, or nose bleeds.
2. Measure the client prior to ordering the stockings to ensure proper fit; be aware that the stockings can act as tourniquets if allowed to roll down at the top; remove every shift, provide skin care, and inspect the skin for breakdown.
3. Ambulate at least every hour while reading or watching television, provide Chester with more frequent walks, do foot circles and stretch/flex of the feet every half-hour while sitting.

CHAPTER 29

NCLEX-PN® ANSWERS (1) B—Hemoglobin is the molecule in red blood cells that transports oxygen to the tissues. These levels are significantly lower than normal. (2) A, C—Erythropoietin is a hormone produced by the kidneys that stimulates the production of RBCs in the bone marrow. Clients with renal failure often have low RBC counts and hematocrits. (3) D—Neutrophils are the most plentiful WBC in circulating blood, accounting for 60% to 70% of circulating WBCs. While monocytes are plentiful in the body, many are found in body tissues, not circulating in the blood. (4) A—Thrombocytes (platelets) are an important part of the coagulation system, necessary to form stable blood clots. (5) C—The client is at risk for bleeding following bone marrow aspiration, particularly when the iliac crest is used.

CHAPTER 30

NCLEX-PN® ANSWERS (1) A—Clients with sickle cell crisis are in severe pain. Narcotic analgesics should be administered as soon as possible. (2) C—Lack of oxygen to the cells results in hypoxia and fatigue. Clients with anemia require frequent rest periods until correction of process can be accomplished. (3) B—Thrombocytopenia (low platelet count) places the client at risk for bleeding. The client should be protected from injury that could cause bleeding. (4) B—Contact sports place the client with hemophilia at risk for injury and bleeding. Golf is least likely to result in physical injury. (5) A, B, D, E—Acid pH of citrus juices increases pain and may injure open lesions on mucous membranes. (6) A—Coagulation in small blood vessels results in occlusion of small blood vessels and ischemia. Pillows under the knees further occlude vessels and promote ischemia. (7) A—Clients with multiple myeloma are at risk for pathologic fractures and experience severe pain. Nursing care should focus on prevention of fractures and controlling pain. (8) B—Elevation of extremities promotes lymphatic drainage and decreases edema. (9) A—Enlarged, painless, movable lymph nodes in the cervical area are a symptom of Hodgkin's disease. (10) D—Maintaining isolation precautions as prescribed at all times helps protect a client with an impaired immune system from infection.

CARE PLAN HINTS

Hodgkin's Disease (1) Review radiation and chemotherapy in Chapter 12. (2) Review measures to prevent infection in the Nursing Care and Continuing Care sections under Leukemia. (3) Think about issues such as insurance, savings, and job and economic status, as well as family responsibilities.

CARE MAP ANSWERS (ACUTE MYELOCYTIC LEUKEMIA)

Correct Data *Subjective:* States "I'm so tired, and I have these bruises all over me. I'm so afraid of the results of the bone marrow test. I don't know what we will do if I have cancer"; night sweats and intermittent fever for past 2 months; relates menstrual periods heavier than normal. *Objective:* 5′4″ (156 cm) tall, weighs 106 lbs. (48.1 kg); vital signs T 100°F; P 102; R 22; BP 130/82; numerous petechiae scattered over trunk and arms; ecchymoses on lower right arm and right calf; oral mucosa red, with several small ulcerations in buccal areas; low RBC count; low hemoglobin and hematocrit; low platelets; high WBC count; myeloblasts present.

Correct Interventions Place in a private room; limit visitors to husband and daughter; verbally and in writing remind staff, family, and client to practice good handwashing. Post a sign in the room as a reminder, and discuss the importance of handwashing with Mrs. Cole and her family; take and record vital signs every 4 hours.

UNIT VII WRAP-UP ANSWERS

CRITICAL THINKING

1. The object is to increase her folic acid level as quickly as possible; folic acid is water soluble and therefore not stored in the body; any excess is excreted rapidly in the urine so there is no danger of overdose.

2. Diet is deficient in foods that contain folic acid, and alcohol consumption increases folic acid requirements.

3. Folic acid is necessary for formation of red blood cells; a lack of this nutrient causes anemia, which in turn is manifested by weakness and fatigue.

4. Physiologic age changes include a decreased ability to absorb nutrients through the gastrointestinal tract, reduced saliva production, atrophy of oral mucosal epithelial cells, lack of teeth or poorly fitting dentures, and increased taste threshold; economic factors include living on a reduced, fixed income that precludes buying fresh fruits and vegetables, social factors include preparing meals for one person and eating most meals alone.

5. Oxidation of alcohol occurs in the liver; with high alcohol intake, necrosis of liver cells occurs with replacement by scar tissue; this cell damage is reflected by elevation of AST (SGOT), ALT (SGPT), and GGT.

COORDINATION OF INTERDISCIPLINARY CARE

1. Meals-on-wheels will usually deliver meals that can be consumed immediately or frozen to be reheated and eaten later; most senior centers provide a hot meal at midday for free or minimal charge; if finances preclude the purchase of nutritious food, a referral for a social work consultation may be of benefit.

MANAGEMENT OF CARE

1. Refer to a home health agency that provides physical therapy for strengthening exercises; assist her to develop a schedule of activities to do at home that will increase energy, such as short walks in her neighborhood or light housework.

2. Foods high in folic acid include leafy, green vegetables, liver, citrus fruits, yeast, dried beans, nuts, and grains.

3. Dysfunctional Grieving: Identify and express feelings about spouse's death freely, verbalize a sense of progress toward resolution of grief, identify positive coping mechanisms. Imbalanced Nutrition: Grain at least one pound per week, identify and eat a balanced diet that includes foods high in folic acid.

CHAPTER 31

NCLEX-PN® ANSWERS (1) A—The kidney is in the flank region. The spleen and pancreas are in the left upper quadrant of the abdomen; stomach in the epigastric region, and the bladder and uterus in the mid lower abdominal or suprapubic region. (2) C—The tubule (proximal convoluted, descending, ascending, and distal convoluted) is part of the nephron, the unit of the kidney responsible for urine formation. (3) D—Renal function declines with aging as nephron units are lost. This affects drug excretion, increasing the risk of toxicity. Doses of drugs such as digoxin often need to be lower for older adults. (4) C, D, E—The client voids at the start of the 24-hour period and discards this urine, saving all voided urine for the duration of the test. Toilet paper and feces in the saved urine can interfere with test results. (5) C—No more than a trace of protein should be present in the urine; this result should be reported to the physician.

CHAPTER 32

NCLEX-PN® ANSWERS (1) C—Assessment to determine if the bladder is distended is needed before further action is taken. (2) A—Lack of estrogen following a total hysterectomy results in decreased urethral resistance, placing the client at risk for stress incontinence. (3) B—Residual urine of 50 mL or less is within normal limits. (4) C—Kegel exercises help the client locate and tighten muscles of the pelvic floor. (5) B, D, E—Increasing fluid intake, wearing cotton briefs, and voiding before and following sexual intercourse reduce the risk of colonization of perineal tissues and the lower urethra with bacteria. (6) A—Recent infection with group A beta-hemolytic *Streptococcus* is a risk factor for acute glomerulonephritis. (7) C—All urine of clients with urinary calculi should be strained for presence of stones. Stones should be sent to the lab for analysis. (8) C—Client is at risk for urinary tract infection. Signs and symptoms should be reported to the physician promptly. (9) B—Protein is decreased to prevent azotemia. A high carbohydrate intake increases calories and spares protein breakdown. (10) A—The right arm should be used for blood pressure measurement to avoid injury to the AV fistula on the left arm.

CARE PLAN HINTS

Acute Glomerulonephritis (1) Review the principles of antibiotic therapy and the consequences of inadequate treatment in Chapter 10 and your pharmacology text. (2) Note Mr. Chang's age and living circumstances. How might these contribute to his risk for glomerulonephritis? (3) Think about the causes and pathophysiology of glomerulonephritis as you develop your teaching plan.

Bladder Cancer (1) Review the pathophysiology and risk factors for bladder cancer. (2) Review the procedures for changing an ostomy appliance in this chapter as well as in Chapter 20. (3) Consider the feelings behind Mr. Hussain's statement as you form your response.

CARE MAP ANSWERS (URINARY INCONTINENCE)

Correct Data *Subjective:* Relates urine leakage when laughing, coughing, and on hearing the sound of running water; often unable to reach bathroom in time at night; hysterectomy at age 52; estrogen replacement therapy for approximately 10 years after hysterectomy; urine leakage usually occurs in late afternoon and at night. *Objective:* Takes digoxin 0.125 mg qd, furosemide 40 mg bid, and KCI 20 mEq tid; moderate

cystourethrocele; atrophy of vaginal tissues; pelvic floor strength weak; urinalysis within normal limits; postvoiding residual urine 5 mL; average of nine daytime voidings and four at night.

Correct Interventions Teach how to identify pelvic floor muscles and perform Kegel exercises; encourage minimizing fluid intake after evening meal; change afternoon dose of furosemide from 9:00 P.M. to 4:00 P.M.; suggest commercial products for protecting clothing and furniture; schedule follow-up visits and evaluations to reinforce teaching.

UNIT VIII WRAP-UP ANSWERS

CRITICAL THINKING

1. Diabetes mellitus causes damage to capillary membranes; this impaired capillary function has a devastating effect on the microcirculation of the kidneys; the kidney's filtration mechanism is stressed, allowing blood proteins to leak into the urine; pressure in the blood vessels of the kidney increases and nephropathy results.
2. Greater mobility; not obligated to travel to dialysis center 3 to 5 times a week for treatment, the system is portable, fewer dietary restrictions than hemodialysis.
3. Risk of peritonitis; risk of exit-site infection; self-image problems associated with catheter placement.
4. Pruritus results from deposits on the skin of calcium, phosphate, and urea; the itching may be so severe that scratching can cause bleeding or secondary infections.
5. History of multiple abdominal surgical procedures; recurrent abdominal wall or inguinal hernias; excessive fat deposits in the abdomen; severe COPD; chronic back problems.

MANAGEMENT OF CARE

1. Never take a blood pressure on the affected arm; assess the fistula for patency by feeling for a thrill, which means palpating over the area for vibration, and listening for a bruit, which means auscultating over the area with a stethoscope for a whooshing sound.
2. Monitor the client for signs/symptoms of exit site infection, such as redness, tenderness, and drainage; monitor for signs/symptoms of peritonitis, such as cloudy dialysis solution return, abdominal pain, diarrhea, vomiting, abdominal distention, and fever.

CHAPTER 33

NCLEX-PN® ANSWERS (1) B—The fallopian tubes contain smooth muscle and are lined with cilia, which facilitate the movement of the ovum to the uterus. (2) B (testes), D (epididymis), A (vas deferens), E (seminal vesicle), C (urethra). (3) A—The hormone levels seen are typical of those following menopause, when estrogen levels fall, and FSH levels significantly increase. (4) C—The client will have some abdominal discomfort, and may experience shoulder pain or release of gas through the vagina following a laparoscopy, but severe pain is unusual and should be reported because it may signal a complication. (5) D—The PSA is performed fasting, and its results are affected by manipulation of the prostate gland, so it should be drawn either before or at least 2 weeks after a DRE.

CHAPTER 34

NCLEX-PN® ANSWERS (1) D—Discharge of seminal fluid into the bladder instead of through the urethra (retrograde ejaculation) is common following TURP. Nocturia is voiding more than one time at night. The subjective information presented is not indicative of impotence or decreased libido. (2) B—Blood clots promote bladder spasms and may obstruct urine flow. Continuous bladder irrigation is titrated to keep the output light pink or clear. When CBI is not used, irrigation may be done as needed to clear blood clots. Irrigation generally does not reduce the urge to void, unless the catheter is obstructed. Large amounts of irrigating fluid can cause hyponatremia, not prevent it. (3) A—Aspirin would promote excessive bleeding. Tub baths are avoided until the catheter is out, but showers are permitted. Sex should be delayed until healing is complete to avoid excessive bleeding. Extra fluid consumption keeps the bladder clear of blood, clots, and bacteria, thereby preventing painful bladder spasms and infection. (4) D, C, A, B, E. Chest pain and difficulty breathing could indicate an embolism or acute cardiac problem and need to be addressed immediately. Blood clots may obstruct the catheter or indicate hemorrhage, requiring attention; restoring urinary flow may relieve the bladder pain and catheter leakage. At this time, the client's poor appetite is of lowest priority. (5) B—Frequent ejaculation is thought to relieve congestion in the prostate. Fluids should be increased. This is not an infectious disorder. (6) C—PSA levels increase in prostate cancer, benign prostatic hypertrophy, and with aging, although the increase is greatest in prostate cancer. When combined with digital rectal examination, the PSA is used to screen for prostate cancer and monitor the response to treatment. (7) A—Orchiectomy removes the major source of testosterone, which feeds testicular tumor growth. Prostate cancer rarely metastasizes to the testes. (8) C—Patients should be advised to report an erection that lasts more than 4 hours. This drug is contraindicated with nitroglycerin and other nitrate drugs, and is used with caution in men with cardiovascular disease. It should not be taken more than once per day. (9) D—Acute scrotal pain may indicate testicular torsion, a medical emergency requiring immediate treatment to restore blood flow to the testicle. (10) C—All young men should be taught to do monthly testicular self-exam (TSE). This cancer does not usually present with pain, tenderness, blood in the urine, or other symptoms, so TSE is especially important.

CARE PLAN HINTS

Erectile Dysfunction (1) Review the long-term effects of diabetes presented in Chapter 17. (2) Review the explanation of the nocturnal penile tumescence and rigidity test presented earlier in Chapter 34, as well as your anatomy and physiology textbook on normal erectile function. Note that erections normally occur during REM sleep. (3) Think about Mr. and Mrs. Lawton's age group and possible cultural mores affecting the ability to openly discuss sexual concerns.

CARE MAP ANSWERS (PROSTATE CANCER)

Correct Data *Subjective:* Relates difficulty getting out of house to buy groceries due to embarrassment of being seen with drainage bag; reports inability to change from large drainage bag to leg bag due to arthritis. *Objective:* Fully dressed, carrying large night urinary drainage bag.

Correct Interventions Discuss the possibility of stress incontinence after the catheter is removed; reinforce the need for perineal muscle exercises while the catheter is still in place; explore available support systems to identify people to assist with catheter care; provide teaching for Mr. Turner and care assistants as appropriate.

CHAPTER 35

NCLEX-PN® ANSWERS (1) B, C—HRT relieves menopausal symptoms such as night sweats and hot flashes, and reduces the risk of fractures due to osteoporosis. It is associated with a higher risk for breast cancer and may actually increase the risk for coronary heart disease. The decision to begin HRT is an individual one. (2) B, C, D, E—Nonproliferative fibrocystic breast changes do not increase the risk for cancer. B, C, and E are measures to relieve discomfort. D has not been proven, but is reported by some to relieve symptoms. (3) A—Risk factors for cervical cancer include multiple sex partners, early sexual activity, and sexually transmitted infections. Pelvic examinations and Pap smears are important for early detection of cervical cancer, but do not reduce the risk. Tamoxifen is used to reduce the risk of breast cancer in women with high-risk factors. (4) B—Tamoxifen increases the risk for deep venous thrombosis and pulmonary embolism, particularly in women who smoke. (5) A—The upper outer quadrant, called the tail of Spence, is the most frequent location of breast cancers. When teaching breast self-exam, it is important to teach women to examine the breast tissue all the way to the axillary region. (6) B—She will need to know how to care for her drainage system. Permanent prostheses are not recommended until the scar is healed, no longer swollen, and not as painful. The arm should not be abducted to the level of the elbow above the shoulder until the drain comes out. She will be encouraged to flex and extend the elbow and do simple ADLs within 24 hours after surgery.

(7) D—The pill is often prescribed to help alleviate symptoms of primary dysmenorrhea. Locally applied heat relieves discomfort. NSAIDs are prostaglandin inhibitors, and therefore block one of the main causes of cramping. Orgasm also relieves symptoms in some women. (8) B—Bleeding in a postmenopausal women not on hormone replacement is never normal and is the most common symptom of endometrial cancer. (9) D—Menorrhagia is the appropriate term to describe menstrual bleeding that is excessive in amount or is prolonged. Amenorrhea is the absence of menstruation. Metrorrhagia is bleeding between menstrual periods, whereas Mittleschmerz is midcycle spotting associated with ovulation. (10) C—PID can cause tubal scarring and blockage, putting her at increased risk for infertility and tubal pregnancy. PID is usually caused by *Neisseria gonorrhoeae* and/or *Chlamydia trachomatis,* whereas cervical cancer is associated with HPV (genital warts). PID is caused by infectious organisms spread during unprotected sex, not by heredity. Toxic shock is caused by *Staphylococcus aureus;* it is related to poor hygiene during menstruation and use of super-absorbent tampons and diaphragms.

CARE PLAN HINTS

Cervical Cancer (1) Review the risk factors for cervical cancer. As you develop your outline, consider how you would modify what and how you present this information for different age or cultural groups. (2) Consider the risk for cervical cancer associated with HPV and how that affects your recommendations for follow-up Pap smears and exams. (3) Review the pathophysiology of cancer in Chapter 12.

CARE MAP ANSWERS (EXPERIENCING MENOPAUSE)

Correct Data *Subjective:* Hates thought of growing older; thinks her husband is losing interest in sex; wonders about decision not to have children.

Correct Interventions Refer to midlife women's support group at the local community center; arrange sexual counseling for Mr. and Mrs. Villagrana regarding techniques, positions, and modifications to accommodate midlife changes.

Documentation 12/20/06. Presents for annual gynecological exam. Relates problems with palpitations, hot flashes, night sweats, anxiety, and insomnia over past 15 months. Menstrual periods irregular, lasting only 1 to 3 days. LMP around 9/15/06. Wt. 152 lbs.; BP 140/70, P 74, R 18, T 98.2°F. Smokes 1 pack/day; relates high-fat, high-CHO, low-protein, low-fiber diet. Discussed risks and benefits of HRT; provided additional written information. Referred to midlife women's support group and to counselor for marital/sexual counseling. J. Voss, LPN.

CHAPTER 36

NCLEX-PN® ANSWERS (1) D—Untreated chlamydia ascends into the upper reproductive tract, and is a major cause of PID. Chlamydia is often asymptomatic in women. (2) B—Zithromax can be given in a single oral dose. Other antibiotics used for STIs may require multiple daily doses for 7 to 10 days. (3) A—Addresses the feelings in the client statement. B and C give unsolicited advice, which would block communication. She will receive prescriptions, but to follow her comments with D before recognizing her feelings changes the topic, also blocking communication. (4) D—Pap smears are important for this client because certain subtypes of HPV increase the risk for cervical cancer. HPV infection is painless. Warts are removed with topical treatments, not acyclovir. (5) C—Clients with gonorrhea often have another STI such as HIV, syphilis, or chlamydia. (6) A—Preventing spread of the infection to others is the most important reason for treatment of STIs. Although effective treatment will prevent tertiary syphilis, this is a less important goal than protection of the public health. (7) A—Penicillin G IM is the usual treatment for syphilis. If the client is allergic to penicillin, oral doxycycline (a tetracycline) can be used. (8) B—Condoms should be used during all sexual relations to prevent spread of the disease to the partner. Mutual monogamy does not prevent spreading the disease to the sexual partner, nor does oral sexual relations. (9) B—Sexually transmitted diseases can be spread by anal, oral, and vaginal intercourse. Some young clients do not consider oral contact to be intercourse, and since it avoids pregnancy, it is seen as a risk-free activity. (10) A, C, D, E—These STIs are reportable by law in all 50 states. The other measures, with the exception of cesarean delivery, are important to prevent spread of the disease to sexual partners and/or reinfection of the client following effective treatment. Cesarean delivery is not necessary following effective treatment and cure of the infection.

CARE PLAN HINTS

Gonorrhea (1) Review the manifestations of gonorrhea in men. (2) Review the pathophysiology and complications of gonorrhea in women. (3) Use some creative thinking to answer this question—think about how you might handle this situation.

CARE MAP ANSWERS (SYPHILIS)

Correct Data *Subjective:* Having unprotected sex with Ms. Jones and Ms. Simpson; syphilitic chancre on the shaft of the penis; believes that Ms. Jones is not having sex with anyone else, but is not sure; ELISA results negative for HIV; dark-field analysis of chancre exudate confirms syphilis.

Correct Interventions Administer and document IM injection of benzathine penicillin G as ordered; teach the importance of treatment to the health of their infant; discuss importance of abstaining from sexual activity until client and partners are cured and using condoms to prevent reinfection; explain the need for follow-up testing in 3 months and 6 months; notify Ms. Jones and Ms. Simpson of need for testing; send reminders for follow-up at 3- and 6-month intervals; provide a copy of STD prevention checklist.

UNIT IX WRAP-UP ANSWERS

CRITICAL THINKING

1. Side effects of chemotherapy; postoperative home care needs; prosthetic options for postmastectomy, both temporary and surgical reconstruction; community support groups for clients with breast cancer; and information about the availability of genetic counseling.
2. Nausea and vomiting are decreased by administration of ondansetron (Zofran), metoclopramide (Reglan), or a combination of phenothiazines, sedatives, steroids, and histamines. Bone marrow depression may be reversed by agents called colony-stimulating factors and erythropoietin.

MANAGEMENT OF CARE

1. Most chemotherapeutic agents cause myelosuppression (depression of bone marrow function). This means the client has decreased WBC (leukopenia), decreased RBC (anemia), and decreased platelets (thrombocytopenia). Monitor blood counts frequently. Protect the client from infection by limiting the type (no children) and number of visitors; no visitors with infection or recent vaccination; may need reverse isolation; careful hand washing before client contact, aseptic technique; avoid fresh fruits, raw meat, fish, and vegetable if WBC is less than 1000/mm^3.
2. Watch for and report any of the following: petechiae, bruising, prolonged bleeding from minor cuts/scratches, or blood in stool, urine, sputum, emesis; use soft toothbrush or toothettes, use electric razor, avoid activities that could result in trauma; avoid any medications that interfere with clotting such as aspirin.

COORDINATION OF INTERDISCIPLINARY CARE

1. Genetic counseling to assist in understanding the daughters' risk of breast cancer; breast cancer support group meetings, oncology nurses for further teaching about chemotherapy management, social services for consultation about employment changes.

CHAPTER 37

NCLEX-PN® ANSWERS (1) B—Older adults report reduced ability to discriminate between blue and green colors. They experience less tear secretion, reduced vision at night, and difficulty focusing on near objects. (2) D—Paste is used to attach electrodes to the scalp and should be washed out to increase client comfort. An EEG is noninvasive so there is no insertion site nor does it cause nausea and vomiting. Increasing fluids is unnecessary. (3) A, D, and E—These are actions of the sympathetic nervous system. Slowing of the heart rate and dilation of skin blood vessels are actions of the parasympathetic nervous system. (4) C—Cranial nerve VIII (vestibulocochlear) is responsible for hearing and equilibrium. Cranial nerve III (oculomotor) controls pupil constriction and eye movement; V (trigeminal) controls chewing and scalp sensations; and XI (accessory) controls neck and shoulder movement. (5) A—The nurse should ask if the client was wearing a helmet in order to assess the extent of injury. Difficulty sleeping does not relate to this case. It is important to know if the client has diabetes but not the most important for this client. Taking herbal preparations is not relevant for this client's situation.

CHAPTER 38

NCLEX-PN® ANSWERS (1) A—Blunt trauma may cause a contusion of the brain. If the skull is fractured, there may be leakage of cerebrospinal fluid into the ears or nose. Infection is a serious complication of brain injury. Headaches and dizziness are commonly seen after a blow to the head. Hematomas develop due to blood leaking underneath the skin. (2) B, C, and E—Use of birth control pills, atherosclerosis, and obesity increase stroke risk. Persons older than 65, those with excessive alcohol intake, and African Americans also have higher risk for CVA. (3) B—It is most important to monitor for CSF leak and hematoma formation. Client is kept flat afterward for 4 to 24 hours but can move legs. Fluids are increased not limited. Client should empty bladder before the procedure; not necessary afterward. (4) D—Dilantin causes gingival hyperplasia, which can be prevented by daily oral hygiene. It should be taken with meals. Dilantin does not cause fatigue, weakness, or brownish urine. (5) C—The earliest sign of increased intracranial pressure is level of consciousness. Irritability, personality changes, restlessness, and disorientation are early manifestations of ICP. Decreased heart rate, slow pupil responses, and projectile vomiting are seen during later stages. (6) A—The occipital lobe controls vision so a tumor is this area will cause visual deficits. Psychomotor seizures are common with temporal lobe tumors. Frontal lobe tumors cause motor deficits and expressive aphasia. (7) C—Status epilepticus is a life-threatening emergency, leading to physical exhaustion and respiratory distress. The first priority would be to maintain the airway. Anxiety and risk for injury also need to be addressed in the nursing care plan. There is no risk for cerebral perfusion alterations. (8) D—Patient education is a priority because most headaches are treatable at home. Helping a client understand what causes the migraines may help reduce the number of attacks. Diaries, comfort measures during an attack, and stress reduction classes are also important. (9) C—Meningitis is an inflammation of the spinal cord and meninges. It is usually secondary to an upper respiratory infection. Encephalitis is caused by a virus, in most cases. Brain abscesses occur from middle ear infection. A subdural hematoma is a collection of blood underneath the dura mater. (10) 2, 3, 6, 1, 5, 4—Loosen the gown and turn client on his side. If on floor, place pillow under head and clear area of objects that could cause injury. Provide supplemental oxygen. Pad the side rails as soon as possible.

CARE PLAN HINTS

Increased Intracranial Pressure and Altered Level of Consciousness (1) In a setting such as an accident, think of the ABCs of nursing assessment. Consider the effect on the body of a trauma like Mr. Straton experienced. (2) Consider the calming effect of family or significant others and how you can use them to assist in calming the client. (3) Review the Nursing Care section, especially the interventions under Imbalanced Nutrition: Less Then Body Requirements. Think how the family can participate in creating a plan of care.

CARE MAP ANSWERS (CEREBROVASCULAR ACCIDENT)

Correct Data *Subjective:* Eyes look pleading. *Objective:* Lack of eye contact; nods off while people speak to him; nods head to answer questions; makes a clenched fist of right hand when trying to speak.

Report Yes, to physician.

Correct Interventions Provide a large marker and tablet; use short, simple sentences when talking to Mr. Boren; contact speech therapy for consult; explain all health care procedures; maintain a calm, unhurried manner.

Documentation 09/21/06. Answers simple questions by nodding head to indicate "Yes." Tries to write with right hand by using marker and tablet. Contacted speech therapy for follow-up consult. R. Kitwell, LVN

CHAPTER 39

NCLEX-PN® ANSWERS (1) A—These are some of the manifestations of stage 1 Alzheimer's disease. (2) D—Pro-Banthine is used to control urinary frequency. Symmetrel controls fatigue, Decadron reduces inflammation, and Dantrium decreases muscle spasm. (3) A, B, and F—These are important points to teach the client taking Sinemet. It should be taken with food. Sinemet does not change urine color, or cause a rash or blurred vision. (4) A—Autonomic dysreflexia is an exaggerated sympathetic response in clients with a spinal cord injury above the T_6 level. Stimuli such as bladder or fecal impaction trigger a hypertensive crisis. (5) D—Guillain–Barré syndrome causes ascending paralysis that starts in the lower extremities. All other manifestations occur later. (6) C—C_5 spinal cord injuries can expect to operate an

electric wheelchair. C_1–C_3 injuries can operate a voice or sip-n-puff wheelchair only. C_6 and lower can learn self-transfer, whereas C_7 and lower can operate a manual wheelchair. (7) B—Elevate the client's head and place a small pillow under the knees for a herniated lumbar disk. (8) B—Clients with dysphasia may not be able to swallow the medication unless it is taken exactly on time. Doses taken too late may cause myasthenic crisis. (9) D—Clients must understand that stimulating trigger points can initiate an attack. They are taught to chew on the unaffected side. Unless they cannot eat, then a high-calorie, high-protein diet is needed. Fluids do not need to be increased. (10) C—The client should have a fluid intake of 2,400 to 3,000 mL in 24 hours to reduce the possibility of headache.

CARE PLAN HINTS

Alzheimer's Disease (1) Review the Continuing Care section. (2) Think about the ways that Alzheimer's disease alters thought processes. Reread the interventions under Disturbed Thought Processes in the chapter. (3) See the discussion of nursing interventions for self-care deficit. Think how you would present food to a person who becomes upset easily and who cannot focus. Think what types of foods would be appealing and easy to eat.

CARE MAP ANSWERS (HERNIATED INTERVERTEBRAL DISK)

Correct Data *Subjective:* Concerned about returning to work; complains of muscle weakness in left arm; unable to ride her bicycle. *Objective:* Decreased ability to use left hand; pain in the neck and shoulders; decreased reflexes in left arm.

Report Yes, to physician.

Correct Interventions Consult with physical therapist for mobility plan; instruct her to keep the cervical collar on at all times; give analgesics around the clock; teach her to not lift objects or twist neck.

Documentation 10/14/06. 1800. Contacted PT for follow-up consult. Instructed in how to apply cervical collar and in activities that should be avoided. Medicated with Vicodin 1 tablet for sharp shooting pain in the back of her neck. L. Johnson, LPN

CHAPTER 40

NCLEX-PN® ANSWERS (1) D—A fluorescein stain is placed in the eye and a slit lamp is used to diagnose a corneal abrasion. (2) A—Myopia, a common vision problem of the elderly, allows the client to see objects distinctly only when they are very close to the eye. (3) F, A, E, C, B, D—First warm the drops, tilt the head toward the unaffected side, then partially fill the ear dropper with medication. With the nondominant hand, pull the auricle up and backward, instill the drops, and place a loose cotton ball in the ear for 15 to 10 minutes. (4) C—Because the client's hearing is impaired, it is most important to reduce environmental noise before speaking with the client. Speaking in a higher pitch does not help the client hear. Use written messages when the client cannot hear. Most older clients are unwilling to learn sign language. (5) D—Increased sweating, wheezing, and breathing difficulty should be reported immediately to a health care provider. Stinging and bitter taste in the mouth are common with Dorzolamide (Trusopt). Darkening of the iris develops with latanoprost (Xalatan). (6) B—When irrigating the client's eye with solution, it is important to direct the flow of solution from the inner to the outer canthus, because the inner aspect of the eye is considered cleaner than the outer aspect. (7) A—Acute angle-closure glaucoma is an emergency condition that must be treated immediately. Darkness and emotional stress cause pupil dilation, which can trigger the condition. Medications and sunlight that cause pupil constriction do not affect this condition. Lying down will not help, it could only make the condition worse. (8) D—After surgery, place in semi-Fowler's position to decrease intraocular pressure in the affected eye. (9) B—Symptoms of open-angle glaucoma may include blurred vision, difficulty focusing on near objects, and halos around lights. (10) A—Because Ménière's disease causes a sensation of fullness or pressure in the ears that may be related to edema of the membranous labyrinth, a diet low in sodium is recommended.

CARE PLAN HINTS

Glaucoma and Cataracts (1) Pressing over the bridge of the nose occludes drainage of tears through the lacrimal duct, preventing systemic absorption of eyedrops. (2) Look up the systemic effects of beta blockers, focusing on their effects on the heart and lungs. (3) Think about local churches, home health providers, senior centers, advocates and agencies for older adults. Look at what is available in your own community.

CARE MAP ANSWERS (AGE-RELATED HEARING LOSS)

Correct Data *Objective:* Frequently asks nurse to repeat questions; ear canals clean, no redness, small amount of dark earwax noted; answers not always appropriate to the question; mental status exam is normal; ignores conversation at his table during meals; audiometric testing reveals significant hearing loss consistent with presbycusis.

Correct Interventions Use effective communication techniques; face Mr. Aaron when speaking with him; speak distinctly in a low voice; supplement verbal with nonverbal communication strategies; use a pocket talker as needed until hearing aids are available; ask Mr. Aaron's family to obtain headphones for radio and television use; teach Mr. Aaron how to use and care for hearing aids.

Documentation 10/27/06. 85 y.o. male with severe osteoarthritis of hands and hips. Alert and oriented. Significant hearing loss noted on audiometric testing. Referred for further testing and hearing aid fitting. Pocket talker provided for temporary use. J. Lemon, LVN

UNIT X WRAP-UP ANSWERS

CRITICAL THINKING

1. Manifestations of intracranial hematomas depend on the source of the bleed, venous being slower to develop than arterial; subdural hematomas are usually venous in nature and therefore slower to develop into a size large enough to cause manifestations; an acute hematoma is usually arterial, and manifestations are usually immediate.
2. Chronic alcoholism affects the liver's ability to manufacture the components necessary for blood coagulation; he is taking an anticoagulant, which slows clotting.
3. Worsening headache, decrease in level of consciousness, vomiting without nausea, elevated BP with wide pulse pressure, bradycardia.
4. Thrombi may form in the atria as a result of blood pooling due to ineffective atrial contraction; these clots may be ejected into circulation and pass to the brain, causing a stroke; therefore, long-term anticoagulant therapy is indicated.
5. Atrial fibrillation is associated with alcoholism.

PRIORITIES OF NURSING CARE

1. The first priority should be to assess Mr. Lee as straining to produce a stool can dangerously increase ICP; if a licensed coworker is not available to assess and treat Mrs. Smith's back pain, make this your second priority; have a coworker (the CNA could do this) obtain a set of vital signs on Mr. Hines and convey them to the physician, who is waiting for them; lastly, visit with Mr. Mullins, acknowledge his concerns, and notify the appropriate person to address them.

MANAGEMENT OF CARE

1. Restraints are contraindicated because the agitation of pulling against them will increase ICP; provide comfort measures since any pain or agitation will increase ICP; give sedatives as ordered; sedatives are ordered carefully on an individual basis as they can depress respirations and LOC; make sure Foley catheter is draining well; keep head of bed elevated 30 to 45 degrees to help decrease cerebral edema; limit activities that increase ICP such as suctioning, neck flexion, straining, coughing, sneezing; keep external stimuli to a minimum; administer bowel care as ordered to prevent straining.

COMMUNICATION

1. Provide them with any information available about Mr. Lee's condition; explain why a quiet environment, free of external stimuli, is important for prevention of increased ICP; explain the need for limited visitors; stay in contact with them, answering any questions they have; allow them to feel included in Mr. Lee's care.

CHAPTER 41

NCLEX-PN® ANSWERS (1) C—The epiphysis is the broad end of the bone; distal indicates the end further away from the trunk of the body. (2) D—Abduction is to move the extremity away from the midline of the body. (3) A, C, D—Flexion and extension of the wrist are used to assess wrist and forearm muscle strength. (4) A—Crepitus is a grating sensation or sound. (5) B—Drinking a large quantity of water following injection of the radioisotope promotes its distribution; the client can eat and drink before and during the procedure. No special radiation precautions are necessary because the amount of radioactivity is small. This in an invasive procedure that requires informed consent.

CHAPTER 42

NCLEX-PN® ANSWERS (1) C, D, E—Elevating the extremity facilitates venous return and helps prevent edema. Until the cast is completely dry, use only the palms of the hands. Handling with the fingers can leave dents that may cause pressure sores. Rough areas on the edges of the cast should be padded and taped to reduce skin irritation. (2) A—The prone position helps to prevent hip contracture. Place the client in a prone position every 4 hours. (3) D—It is important to keep the client in a position of abduction because adduction may dislocate the hip. Excessive hip flexion should also be avoided. (4) C—The client has manifestations of compartment syndrome including pain unrelieved by narcotics and paresthesias. Prompt intervention is required to preserve function of the extremity. (5) B—Teaching the client the RICE acronym (rest, ice, compression, elevation) will help her to remember how to care for the injury. (6) D—Fracture of a long bone is the principal risk for fat emboli. The manifestations may include confusion, petechiae, pulmonary edema, and acute respiratory distress syndrome. (7) D—Peripheral vascular disease is the major cause of amputation of the lower extremities. (8) A, B—When caring for a client in traction, maintain the pulling force and traction by maintaining the body alignment with the direction of the pull. Pin sites have a risk for infection and are cleansed regularly. Weights are not released on the client with skeletal traction, nor is the client allowed up to the bedside. Sliding when repositioning increases the risk of skin trauma and excoriation. (9) B—Use of ice constricts the vessels and helps to prevent or reduce edema. (10) A—Balanced suspension traction increases the client's mobility while maintaining appropriate bone position.

CARE PLAN HINTS

Hip Fracture (1) Review Chapter 9 to develop your response. (2) Review the section on traction that precedes hip fracture. (3) Think about all the health care professionals that will be involved, and don't forget other departments that are integral to client care, such as dietary, housekeeping, and the business office!

CARE MAP ANSWERS (BELOW-KNEE AMPUTATION)

Correct Data *Subjective:* Complaining of severe pain. *Objective:* Vital signs stable; stump splinted, covered by soft dressing; wound healing without signs of infection; refuses ROM exercises and turning; tolerating 1,800-cal ADA diet; yells, "Get out! I don't want anyone to see me like this" when anyone enters room.

Correct Interventions Encourage verbalization of feelings; contact the physician for a referral to a psychologist or social worker.

CHAPTER 43

NCLEX-PN® ANSWERS (1) B—Osteomyelitis may develop in the patient with open fractures or open wounds near a bone. The nurse should assess for other signs and symptoms of infection including chills, fever, and elevated WBC. Dressings should be changed as ordered. Evaluation of the drainage on the bandage is critical. The dressing should be dry and intact. Capillary refill should be within normal limits. A decreased capillary refill may indicate occlusion. Pain medications should be administered as necessary. (2) A, B, D, E, C—Safety, comfort, and promoting healing are the most important issues for discharge instruction. The walker and elevated toilet seat reduce the risk of falling and dislocation or damage of the hip. Effective pain management promotes activity and healing. Smoking constricts blood vessels and reduces oxygen delivery to tissues, slowing healing. Gradually increasing activities promotes the client's level of wellness. Calcium supplements may be ordered for the patient, because increased calcium may help prevent further bone loss and promote healing. (3) C— The tick should be removed with tweezers without jerking or twisting. It should not be crushed, and should be saved in alcohol. (4) D—Osteoarthritis affects the entire joint, causing deep, aching pain, stiffness following immobility, limited ROM, and crepitus with movement. (5) C—The SLE patient is sensitive to UV light and should avoid skin exposure, especially when rays are intense. No special diet is prescribed, and joint inflammation is treated as necessary. SLE is a chronic inflammatory disease that affects all body systems. (6) C— Sulfinpyrazone may cause peptic ulcers in some clients. They should report any symptoms of GI distress to their physician.

Water should be increased to at least 3 liters per day. Probenecid, sulfinpyrazone, and allopurinol are taken with food to prevent gastric upset. (7) B—Patients with chronic low back pain need to focus on rehabilitation and prevention of further injury. Appropriate body mechanics, back exercises, and environmental modifications need to be discussed. (8) C, D—Celecoxib is an NSAID that is taken on a regular basis to reduce inflammation and pain. It can be taken without regard to meals, but may increase the risk for GI bleeding. Abdominal pain, tarry stools, and other manifestations of GI bleed should be promptly reported to the physician. This and other NSAIDs may increase the risk for heart attack and stroke when taken in prescription strength for long periods. (9) A—This statement indicates the nurse's understanding and willingness to discuss the client's fears about the meaning of the mass. The other statements indicate inappropriate assumptions about the mass by the nurse. (10) A—Scoliosis is usually discovered during adolescence. It is found primarily in girls. Kyphosis is known as "hunchback." Paget's disease and osteomalacia are associated with inadequate mineralization of the bone.

CARE PLAN HINTS

Rheumatoid Arthritis (1) Review the normal inflammatory process in Chapter 10 and the pathophysiology of rheumatoid arthritis. (2) Review the long-term effects of excess corticosteroids (Chapter 16) to prepare your response to this question. (3) See Chapter 11 and 12 to review the short- and long-term adverse effects of methotrexate (a drug used for chemotherapy and as an immunosuppressant).

CARE MAP ANSWERS (OSTEOARTHRITIS AND TOTAL HIP REPLACEMENT)

Correct Data *Subjective:* Takes carbidopa/levodopa (Sinemet 25–100) 4 times a day for Parkinson's disease; no other chronic medical conditions; no known medication allergies; does not smoke; consumes only small amounts of alcohol. *Objective:* alert and oriented; speech is soft but clear; vital signs: BP 116/64; P 68 regular; R 18; T 97.4°F (36.3°C) PO; color good, skin warm and moist; peripheral pulses strong and equal in upper extremities; slightly weaker but equal in lower extremities; feet cool to touch, good capillary refill; walks with a limp, favoring right hip; shuffling gait noted.

Correct Interventions Help change position at least every 2 hours; encourage use of overhead trapeze to shift positions frequently; maintain sequential compression device and antiembolic stocking as ordered; remove for 1 hour daily; remind to use incentive spirometer hourly for first 24 hours, then at least every 2 hours while awake; assist out of bed three times a day after the first 24 hours; encourage frequent quadriceps-setting exercises and plantar and dorsiflexion of feet.

Documentation 1/8/07. Vital signs stable. Respirations 14, unlabored. Lung sounds clear throughout. Skin intact, wound healing well. Ambulating well accompanied by physical therapy. Taking oral analgesic bid with good pain relief. S. Campbell, LPN.

UNIT XI WRAP-UP ANSWERS

CRITICAL THINKING

1. The disease process of osteoporosis; lifestyle choices that have an impact on bone density; dietary requirements for her gender and age.
2. Bone is continually being formed by osteoblasts and resorbed by osteoclasts; usually these are equal so that bone mass is constant; in osteoporosis, the resorption is greater than the deposits and a gradual collapse of vertebra is seen.
3. Optimal exercises are weightbearing, forcing the individual to work against gravity; these include walking, hiking, stair climbing, and dancing. Low-impact exercises such as walking are preferred to high-impact exercises such as running due to the danger of fracture of osteoporotic bones.
4. Risk factors for osteoporosis include a diet low in calcium, excessive alcohol consumption, cigarette smoking, and an inactive lifestyle. These are all factors that Mrs. Bauer could change that could decrease loss of bone mass.
5. Yes, the risk factors for osteoporosis include female gender; thin, small framed; family history of osteoporosis; Caucasian or Asian-American; excessive use of alcohol; cigarette smoking; sedentary lifestyle; postmenopausal.

MANAGEMENT OF CARE

1. Three servings per day of dairy products with vitamin D, broccoli, spinach, canned salmon with bones; 20 to 30 minutes of weight bearing exercise three times per week or more is recommended.

COORDINATION OF INTERDISCIPLINARY CARE

1. Referral to a dietitian for dietary education about a high-calcium diet; physical therapy for education regarding appropriate exercise to decrease bone loss and prevent fractures.

CHAPTER 44

NCLEX-PN® ANSWERS (1) B, C, and F—These are common findings in the older adult. Blood supply and temperature regulation decrease rather than increase. Petechiae are an abnormal finding in all adults. (2) A—Tenting is seen in the elderly and in dehydration. The nurse assesses for it by pinching the skin over the collarbone. Edema is assessed by depressing the skin over the ankle. Palpating for moisture and looking for lesions in a group do not relate to tenting. (3) D—Exposure to radiation increases the risk for skin cancer. Other factors include men over 50, light-colored hair and eyes, living in high altitudes. (4) C—Vesicles are fluid-filled, palpable masses with thin translucent walls and defined borders. A macule is a flat, small area of skin color change. An elevated, reddish area with an irregular border is a wheal. A pustule is an elevated and pus-filled lesion. (5) B—Skin scraping is done to identify a fungal infection. Biopsy is used to rule out malignancy. Allergy testing is done with patch testing. Wood's light differentiates areas of pigmented from hypopigmented skin such as in vitiligo.

CHAPTER 45

NCLEX-PN® ANSWERS (1) A—The temperature should be decreased to provide comfort for skin lesions, but only after the bath is given. Cornstarch or baking soda baths help to relieve itching. Medication for itching such as Benadryl may be given, but pain medication generally is not needed for psoriasis. Rubbing the lesions may increase the chance for developing infection. (2) B, C, and E are all risk factors for herpes zoster. Cervical cancer and measles are important to note in the history but do not cause herpes zoster. Menstruation may trigger an outbreak of herpes simplex. (3) B—Antibiotics may result in superinfections such as mouth fungi, candidiasis. Furuncles are boils, tinea pedis is athlete's foot, and folliculitis is an infection of hair follicles. (4) D—Herpes is a sexually transmitted disease. Abstinence is recommended during an outbreak of the virus. Gloves should be worn to prevent the spread of the infection. The medication should be used daily. The type of bathing does not affect treatment of genital herpes. (5) D—Body lice are transmitted from contact with infested clothing or bed linens. Washing the items decrease the chance of reinfestation. Body lice may affect other family members or pets and can cause itching, especially at night. The best answer reflects the transmission of the lice. The lice must be eradicated from the household objects. (6) A—Most nonmelanoma skin cancers are directly related to exposure to sunlight. Fair-skinned people are at higher risk for skin cancer. Estrogen levels are not directly related. Liver spots are the result of hyperpigmentation of aging skin. (7) C—This client does not believe life will get better after the surgery. Anxiety, Fear, and Impaired Skin Integrity are all appropriate diagnoses for some cancer patients. Based on this statement, the client should be given more information regarding the success rate for cryosurgery and the treatment of basal cell carcinomas. (8) A—Patients should be able to identify changes in their own skin. Treatment and the prognosis for skin cancers need to be discussed at the appropriate time. Risk factors should be taught after the skin examination. (9) C—Redness over bony prominences suggests the beginning of skin breakdown. A decreased appetite could lead to a lack of protein and vitamins,

which are needed for intact skin. Contractures may also lead to loss of skin integrity due to immobility. Lack of mobility increases the mucous buildup in the lungs, causing a decrease in lung expansion. (10) D—High-protein and high-calorie diets decrease the likelihood that decubiti will develop. Massaging the skin may cause damage to the tissues. Clients should be turned and repositioned every 2 hours. Hot water may burn the skin.

CARE MAP ANSWERS (HERPES ZOSTER)

Correct Data *Subjective*: Reports chills and fever. *Objective*: T 99°F, open blisters on thorax.

Correct Interventions Teach how to apply topical medications; stress importance of avoiding intimate contact with family members; discuss need for careful handwashing; teach effects of pain medications.

Report Yes, to the primary health care provider at the clinic.

Documentation 04/29/06. Reports malaise, chills, and fever for past week. T 99°F. Has oozing fluid-filled blisters in a line over left thorax. Reports these are painful. Reports having chickenpox as a child. Is a migrant worker and is afraid lesions are the result of exposure to pesticides. E. Sanchez, LPN

CHAPTER 46

NCLEX-PN® ANSWERS (1) D—Electricity follows the path of least resistance. Lightning travels along bones, blood vessels, and nerve fibers. Although lightning may cause abnormal cardiac rhythms, the symptoms exhibited are directly related to the brain and central nervous system. There is a potential for loss of both urinary and pulmonary function, depending on the severity of the electrical discharge. (2) A—Full-thickness burns are also called third-degree burns. The skin appears dry, leathery, and firm to the touch. The pain receptors are destroyed. Second-degree burns are also known as partial thickness and include both deep and superficial partial-thickness injuries. Pain is present in various degrees, and the wound has blister formations. (3) B—The emergent or resuscitative stage consists of estimating the extent of burn damage, initiating first aid, and assessing for shock and respiratory distress. Carbon monoxide and other noxious fumes are prevalent in house fires, leading to pulmonary distress. Pain and urinary assessments are conducted in the acute stage. Mobility problems are addressed after the life-threatening problems are under control. (4) D—During reversal of burn shock, fluids shift from the extracellular spaces to the circulatory system. Older clients may develop excess fluid volume, which is manifested by pulmonary edema, distended neck veins, and cardiac arrhythmias. Heart failure signs and symptoms are dependent on which side of the heart is affected. Portal hypertension may occur with liver diseases. (5) A—The anterior trunk equals 18%, and the anterior and posterior aspect of the left arm equals 9%. (6) C—The intravenous route is the best route for managing pain. Most clients will initially be NPO. Intramuscular and rectal routes have slower absorption times. The skin may not accommodate injections due to the burn damage. (7) C—Curling's ulcer is common in clients with extensive burns. Enteral feedings are contraindicated with these clients. Peripheral IV therapy is usually not a viable option due to skin damage. A central venous line is inserted via the subclavian or jugular vein for administration of total parental nutrition. (8) A, C, D, and E—All burn clients should have aseptic wound care and daily weights. Burns to the extremities are at risk for compartment syndrome due to eschar, which can drastically reduce blood flow. It is essential to monitor peripheral pulses for signs of reduced blood flow. Injuries to extremities may also cause contractures so it is important to perform ROM exercises. VS should be checked at least every 4 hours. Aloe is only applied to minor burns. (9) B—Infection is a constant threat due to the decreased immune system in clients with major burns. Frequent vital signs are imperative. Touching the skin is inappropriate for determining body temperature. A set of vital signs should always be obtained prior to calling the physician. Dressings should be removed during wound care or on specific orders from the doctor. (10) D—Leukopenia may develop during the first 2 to 3 days of treatment. The nurse must monitor the client's WBC. Pain occurs more often with mafenide acetate (Sulfamylon). Dehydration and bleeding do not develop with this drug.

CARE PLAN HINTS

Major Burn (1) Review the content in the chapter about the pathophysiology of a major burn specific to the renal system and gastrointestinal system. Consider the need to measure urine hourly and the dangers of vomiting. (2) Review the discussion of narcotic analgesics in Chapter 8. Consider why this would be more necessary in a partial-thickness burn than in a full-thickness burn.

CARE MAP ANSWERS (CLIENT WITH MAJOR BURNS)

Correct Data *Objective:* Age; extent of burn; BP, P, R; urine output; confusion.

Correct Interventions Report and continue to monitor vital signs; report and continue to monitor urine output; report and continue to monitor confusion; determine body weight; monitor IV flow rate.

Report Yes, to the nurse manager of the ED or to the physician.

Documentation 2/23/07. 1300. 78-year-old woman with 40% TBSA burn. Confused. BP 92/62, P 110 and weak, R 36 and shallow. Urine output per Foley less than 20 mL per hour for past 2 hours. IV fluids infusing as ordered. A. Fu, LPN

UNIT XII WRAP-UP ANSWERS

CRITICAL THINKING

1. Asymmetry (Mr. Sanders's nevus has an uneven shape), Border irregularity (Mr. Sanders's lesion has irregular borders), Color not uniform (Mr. Sanders's nevus has various shades of brown), Diameter is greater than 6 mm (Mr. Sanders's mole is 3 cm in diameter). According to this rule, Mr. Sanders's lesion is definitely suspect.
2. Impaired skin integrity related to excision of melanoma from the left leg; risk for infection related to surgical incision on left leg; anxiety related to diagnosis of cancer.
3. Etiology is unknown, but ultraviolet rays are a common suspected factor due to increased incidence of melanoma in populations living near the equator and those using tanning beds on a regular basis.
4. Skin lesions or changes in lesions are usually thought of as minor and not life threatening; lack of insurance coverage prompts people to avoid seeking health care; lack of knowledge about malignant melanoma. Include a thorough skin assessment for all clients; routinely educate all clients about the dangers of sun exposure and use of tanning beds, prevention of sun exposure, how to assess their own skin using the ABCD rule, and the importance of seeing their physician immediately if suspect lesions are found.

COMMUNICATION

1. Avoid overexposure to the sun; wear wide-brimmed hats and long sleeves; apply broad spectrum sunscreens with SPF of 15 or greater approximately 20 minutes prior to sun exposure; avoid sun exposure between the hours of 10 A.M. and 4 P.M.; do not use indoor sunlamps or tanning beds; take special care to protect children from sunburns.

CHAPTER 47

NCLEX-PN® ANSWERS (1) B—This answer involves assessing the client's need before taking action. The client may speak English well enough to socialize without understanding medical terminology. The client should decide, not the interpreter. (2) C—Mental disorders are caused by too little or too much neurotransmitter activity. The brain continues to function, but the symptoms of mental illness occur (which symptoms is dependent on which neurotransmitter is involved). (3) B, E—The clients coping skills, self-concept, social support, and family roles are components of a psychosocial assessment. (4) A—The client's answer will be what he or she does to cope. Using medical terminology is often confusing for clients. (5) D—The nurse cannot tell if a client is suicidal by assessing behavior or unrelated verbalizations. This question must be asked.

CHAPTER 48

NCLEX-PN® ANSWERS (1) C—Flat affect and little speech are negative symptoms, which represent findings that are "less than" normal behavior. (2) C—"The client is experiencing a frightening hallucination, apparently about aliens attacking him" is the most objective, descriptive charting. (3) A—Reassure the client that he is safe in the hospital and there are no aliens. The nurse should reinforce reality. (4) A—Structured daily activities are a part of milieu therapy, in which the environment is therapeutic. (5) D—A client who is pacing the halls, clenching his fists, and talking angrily to unseen voices is probably hallucinating and most likely to be violent. (6) C—Delusional thinking (false belief). (7) B—"You have schizophrenia, which is a brain disorder that affects your thinking." This correctly answers the client's question in layperson's terms. Answer A is too technical. (8) B—High fever, muscle pain, and unstable BP are symptoms of NMS. (9) Hallucination, or auditory hallucinations. (10) A, B, D—These are all anticholinergic side effects. C is an extrapyramidal side effect.

CARE MAP ANSWERS (CLIENT WITH SCHIZOPHRENIA)

Correct Data Client states, "I can't hold still!"; muscles of legs and arms are stiff; client appears to be in distress; client complains of jaw tightness and discomfort; when client protrudes his tongue, it quivers.

Correct Interventions Provide a low stimulation environment; call the physician immediately to report extrapyramidal symptoms; expect to give an anticholinergic medication; tell the client that he is having medication side effects that can be treated.

CHAPTER 49

NCLEX-PN® ANSWERS (1) C—The best way to document if the client is feeling better is to use the 1–10 mood scale. (2) C—The client has a combination of factors that put her at risk for another episode of depression. She has had a previous depressive episode, is female, and has a history of a suicide attempt. With a new baby, she would be experiencing another stressful episode in her life and would be susceptible to postpartum depression. (3) A—Light therapy is the treatment of choice for SAD. It is the loss of light that seems to precipitate the symptoms. (4) D—Anhedonia is the medical term for the inability to experience pleasure and is a common symptom of depression. (5) C—Clients tend to be quiet about their feelings of depression, so that the physician is not aware of their psychologic state. The most common reason for this is the stigma society has placed on mental illness. It is often seen as a weakness on the part of the depressed person. (6) B—It will take 2 to 6 weeks for the maximum effect of the medication to be reached. (7) A—Racing thoughts are moving very fast and

are likely to result in fast-moving behavior (psychomotor agitation). (8) D—People in the manic state do not respond well to excessive environmental stimuli. Removing the client from the stimulation by taking him outside is the first line of intervention you should try. Walking with him allows him to continue his movement. Talk calmly and softly to help him de-escalate the agitation. 9. Hypertensive crisis. 10. Notify the physician or nurse practitioner.

CARE PLAN HINTS

1. Choices put her in charge. She's saying "yes" to life.
2. Outcome 2 was partially met. It might have been too high an expectation. She could be given more time to achieve this outcome.
3. Having some of the nurse's time, some of other residents' time, and some of family's time means Ms. G. is getting more types of contact and runs less risk of being disappointed if one is not available. She is participating in both individual and group interactions.

CARE MAP ANSWERS (CLIENT WITH BIPOLAR DISORDER)

Correct Data *Subjective:* States, "My hands won't stop shaking"; states, "Would you please read the menu to me, I can't see very well." *Objective:* Pulse 108, irregular; when the physical therapist was teaching him to use crutches, the client was too weak to bear his own body weight on his unaffected leg; refused dinner last evening and breakfast today.

Correct Interventions Look in the client's chart to find his baseline vital signs; hold the lithium dose that is due now; call the physician to report the presence of symptoms of lithium toxicity.

Report Yes, to physician.

Documentation 10/24/06. 0900. AP 108, irregular, ct. has hand tremors, anorexia (refused dinner and breakfast), blurred vision, and weakness (unable to bear his own weight on unaffected left leg). Dr. J. Joy called re: symptoms of lithium toxicity. Orders received to hold lithium, offer p.o. fluids, draw serum Li level STAT. L. Sheih, LPN

CHAPTER 50

NCLEX-PN® ANSWERS (1) B, C, D—Restraint is not indicated. A calm, reassuring approach by the nurse, keeping stimulation to a minimum, is correct. (2) B, D—The benzodiazepines cause sedation, drowsiness, dizziness, and decreased coordination. (3) B—This is a response to a specific situation and may not be an anxiety disorder. Validate his feelings, then assess for the source of his anxiety. Does he need more information about the process? Does he fear the results? Is he concerned about being in a small, closed space? (4) A—People with Generalized Anxiety Disorder are aware that they are not responding to situations appropriately, but they are unable to control those feelings without assistance. (5) B—This phobia concerns open spaces and is often associated with obsessive-compulsive disorder. (6) A—The nursing student is reliving the trauma of seeing her mother die suddenly in this room. Entering the room triggered the memory of this event. It is common for such episodes to occur within 3 months of the traumatic event. (7) C—The goal of CBT is for the client to view the situation realistically and replace inappropriate negative self-talk with positive thoughts that are supportive and calming. (8) A—Relaxation and deep-breathing responses are effective for many different anxiety-producing events. (9) C—See Box 50-5 for more help with assessing coping skills. (10) D—The student is having severe anxiety. See Table 50-2 for more information.

CARE PLAN HINTS

1. A steady dosage schedule ensures that Mrs. Miedo will experience some steady analgesic effect. Her pain will not be allowed to rise to an intolerable and anxiety-producing level. Regular checking in about her pain level reassures her that the nurses care and that they are monitoring her condition.

2. The stress of being in hospital and in pain has aggravated Mrs. Miedo's anxiety. Providing staff that are consistent and increasingly familiar is a simple way to create a safer feeling environment.

3. Mrs. Miedo may have cognitive impairment after the CVA that made it impossible for her to learn to do the self-relaxation exercises independently. This outcome was partially met. It was not completely realistic for Mrs. Miedo.

CARE MAP ANSWERS (CLIENT WITH ANXIETY)

Correct Data *Subjective:* VS: T 99°F, P 108, R 20, BP 130/86; client states, "Am I going to die from this?"; states, "I think my incision is going to tear open"; complains of feeling dizzy. *Objective:* Skin is cool, diaphoretic; client's hands are constantly moving, picking at the sheets; nurse stated in report: client slept approximately 3 hours last night; nurse assesses that client has dry mouth; eyes are glancing around the room, darting from one thing to another.

Correct Interventions Encourage the client to talk about her feelings; accept the client as she is; acknowledge that client is anxious; answer any questions the client has about her surgical incision; keep communication simple and concrete; provide comfort measures; be calm and confident with the client; discuss healthy ways to talk about and relieve anxiety; assess coping skills the client has used successfully in the past; assess client's resources for support; use progressive relaxation to help client relax.

Report Yes, to charge nurse or physician.

Documentation Client is very anxious: asks if she is dying; skin cool, diaphoretic, dry mouth, P, R, BP elevated, complains

of dizziness. Provided comfort measures, talked with client about her feelings. She participated in progressive relaxation exercise. Reported severe anxiety to charge nurse. Wendu Charles, LPN

CHAPTER 51

NCLEX-PN® ANSWERS (1) B—Clients with Paranoid Personality Disorder are suspicious of others. They have more confidence in a nurse who shows self-confidence and treats the client in a direct, matter-of-fact way. (2) A—The client with a Schizoid Personality Disorder typically avoids relationships even with caregivers. Not having visitors or receiving phone calls would validate the lack of social relationships. A flat affect is common. (3) C—As a client with Schizotypal Personality Disorder, this client would prefer to be alone because of severe social anxiety. The stress of being forced to interact with other residents could precipitate delusional thinking or perceptual alterations. Inviting her to one meal a day should be less threatening. Allow her to move at her own pace, and praise her when she is able to comply. (4) B—The client with an Antisocial Personality Disorder is often a very manipulative person to care for. Staff members need to all be consistent in care and in following all unit rules. (5) B—Although some of the other choices might be appropriate, your first priority would be to prevent self-injury. A common means of responding to stress for clients with Borderline Personality Disorder is to cut or burn themselves. (6) D—These behaviors are consistent with the self-centeredness of Histrionic Personality Disorder. (7) A—This client is demonstrating the symptoms of the Narcissistic Personality Disorder. You may briefly empathize with his stress, but you must consistently lay down the limits with what is appropriate and what is not. You must maintain a professional, no-nonsense approach. (8) A, C, D—Clients with anxiety respond well in a trusting relationship, when the nurse is calm, and when they understand their own feelings. (9) 3, 1, 4, 2—Safety is always a high priority. Consistency is critical for this client. Learning to express his feelings will be an ongoing effort, and finally his outpatient care is important but lowest of these priorities at this time. (10) A—The obsessive-compulsive behavior in persons with this personality disorder is worsened by anxiety. Hospitalization is likely to be stressful.

CARE MAP ANSWERS (CLIENT WITH INEFFECTIVE COPING)

Correct Data *Subjective:* Client states: "Yes, whatever you say"; when asked if she needs pain medication, she states, "No, I don't want to bother you"; when asked if she needs anything she states, "I don't know"; states, "What do you think I should do?" *Objective:* BP 158/90, P110, R24; grimaces and sweats when ambulating or moving in bed; awake on all q2h checks during the night.

Correct Interventions Ask the client, "Are you in pain?"; say to the client, "Most people have a lot of pain after surgery. You have signs of pain, does your incision hurt?"; tell the client, "It is no trouble to give you some pain medication. I will be glad to get some if you need it"; say to the client, "Sometimes people don't like to ask for help. While you are in the hospital, we want to help you, so please tell us what you need"; help the client practice identifying her needs; encourage the client to take the ordered pain med; include offering pain med regularly in the plan of care; visit the client regularly to determine whether she needs help; discuss outpatient referral for therapy with treatment team.

Report Yes, to charge nurse.

Documentation Ct. has signs of pain (elevated BP, P, R, sweating and grimacing with movement, sleeplessness) but is not asking for medication. Will encourage client to take ordered med and will continue to monitor for other needs. Zack Lee, LPN

CHAPTER 52

NCLEX-PN® ANSWERS (1) A—The body adjusts to constant use of a drug. As consumption continues, larger amounts are needed to give the desired effect. Once tolerance develops, many clients begin use of different, more potent substances. (2) C—When alcohol is withdrawn, the central nervous system is still stimulated. The client exhibits signs of stimulation including elevated vital signs, anxiety, tremors, and seizures. (3) C—Alcoholic encephalopathy is caused by vitamin B_1 deficiency related to inadequate nutritional intake. (4) B—Opiate overdose results in depressed central nervous system including marked respiratory depression. Narcan (naloxone HCl) reverses the sedative effects. (5) B—Clients must be cautioned to avoid combining alcohol and antianxiety drugs. These combinations can result in cardiac arrhythmias including cardiac arrest. (6) D—The nursing supervisor usually holds accountability and administrative authority for the unit and is aware of policy related to follow-up of situations in which narcotics are diverted. (7) B—Teaching the consequences of continued substance abuse gives the client information to make choices related to his or her behavior. (8) C—Opiates are central nervous system stimulants. When the drugs are withdrawn, the CNS is depressed. (9) A, B—Clients in alcohol withdrawal are experiencing CNS stimulation. Vital signs help assess the extent of this. (10) Caffeine. Caffeine withdrawal causes headache.

CARE PLAN HINTS

Ineffective Coping (1) Until very recently, this client had no other way to respond to the stressors in her life except to drink. She is at high risk for relapse. Any stressful event that she cannot manage with her new skills will put her in a position where she thinks about drinking because it is what she has always done. Health professionals can only give her alternatives.

Remember, we do not control her behavior. She must choose whether or not she will drink. Even if she has a relapse, there is still a good chance that she can recover from alcoholism in the long run. (2) Alcohol played the role of coping mechanism for her to make her feel better temporarily if she was upset or tired. Other people have many more tools for managing stressful situations. It will take time for her to develop new skills. (3) This person is no longer a client of the hospital nurses. The nurse's best response would be to refer the client back to her AA sponsor or other outpatient resource, saying kindly that the client is capable of managing the situation.

CARE MAP ANSWERS (CLIENT WITH SUBSTANCE DEPENDENCY)

Correct Data *Subjective:* States "I don't have a drinking problem. I can quit whenever I want"; states "I feel nervous"; had seizures as a child; states "If you don't let me out of here tomorrow, I'm leaving anyway." *Objective:* Vital signs stable; blood alcohol content: 0.24 mg/dL on admission; request pain meds q1h; insomnia; poor appetite.

Correct Interventions Assess his knowledge about alcoholism; teach client about disease process of alcoholism; provide effective pain management; offer frequent feeding; confront the client with the reality of the consequences of alcoholism; encourage the client to express his feelings about drinking and alcoholism; ask the client if he wants to leave the hospital to drink alcohol.

UNIT XIII WRAP-UP ANSWERS

NURSING ASSESSMENT

To further assess the client's mental status, the nurse should perform a Mini-Mental Status Exam.

COMMUNICATION

To facilitate communication, discuss with the family that Mrs. Santos feels like she is no longer an important part of the family since she is not able to provide child care. Provide the son and daughter-in-law an opportunity to talk about their feelings and to plan for her discharge. Explain the importance of involving the client in the planning to the extent that she is able.

INTERDISCIPLINARY CARE

Working closely with both the client and her family gives you the opportunity to observe them separately and as they interact. Many times a nurse can learn as much form what a client or family member does *not* say as from what they do say. If interactions are strained, it might not be best for the client to be discharged home without home care services. Family stress can be a catalyst for elder abuse. These observations can be important to the care conference. The nurse who has been providing direct care to the client will be able to provide the care conference with information about the client's mental status and self-care abilities. The nurse may also have suggestions about what the client needs to have a safe environment.

Bibliography

CHAPTER 1

Alfaro, R. (2005). *Applying nursing diagnoses and nursing process: A step-by-step guide* (6th ed.). Philadelphia: Lippincott.

American Hospital Association. (2004). *The patient care partnership: Understanding expectations, rights and responsibilities.* Available at www.hospitalconnect.com/aha/ptcommunication/partnership/index.html

American Nurses Association. (1980). *Nursing: A social policy statement.* Kansas City, MO: Author.

American Nurses Association. (1995). *Nursing's social policy statement.* Washington, DC: Author.

American Nurses Association. (1996). *Position statement on cultural diversity in nursing practice.* Washington, DC: Author.

American Nurses Association. (2001). *Code of ethics for nurses.* Washington, DC: Author.

American Nurses Association. (2004). *Nursing: Scope and standards of practice.* Washington DC: Author.

Davidhizar, R., & Shearer, R. (2003). The nurse manager in transition. *Journal of Practical Nursing, 53*(3), 18–19, 24.

Ellis, J., & Hartley, C. (2004). *Managing and coordinating care* (4th ed.). Philadelphia: Lippincott.

Gordon, M. (1994). *Nursing diagnosis: Process and application* (3rd ed.). New York: McGraw-Hill.

Green, C. (2000). *Critical thinking in nursing: Case studies across the curriculum.* Upper Saddle River, NJ: Prentice Hall.

International Council of Nurses. (2002). *The definition of nursing.* Geneva: Imprimeries Populaires.

Ketefian, S. (1987). Moral behavior in nursing. *Advances in Nursing Science, 9*(1), 10–19.

National Association for Practical Nurse Education and Service, Inc. (1997). *Licensed practical nursing: The work of the care-giver.* Silver Springs, MD: Author.

———. (2004). *NAPNES Standards of practice for licensed practical/vocational nurses.* Silver Springs, MD: Author.

North American Nursing Diagnosis Association. (2003). *NANDA nursing diagnoses: Definitions & classification 2003–2004.* Philadelphia: Author.

Spector, R. (2004). *Cultural diversity in health and illness* (6th ed.). Norwalk, CT: Appleton & Lange.

Stein, P. (2004). Pushing through barriers to advocate for a patient. *AORN Journal, 80*(3), 553, 555–556, 558.

Wilkinson, J. (2000). *Nursing process in action: A critical thinking approach* (7th ed.). Upper Saddle River, NJ: Prentice Hall Health.

Wilson, R. (2004). "I am JUST an LPN." *Nursing, 54*(2), 9.

CHAPTER 2

American Cancer Society. (2004). *Cancer prevention & early detection facts & figures.* Atlanta, GA: Author.

American Cancer Society. (2004). *ACS cancer detection guidelines.* Available at www.cancer.org/docroot/PE_2_3X_ACS_Cancer_Detection_Guidelines_36...

American Diabetic Association. (2001). *Vital statistics.* Alexandria, VA: Author.

Bradley, P. (2003). Family caregiver assessment: Essential for effective home health care. *Journal of Gerontological Nursing, 29*(2), 29–36.

Centers for Disease Control and Prevention. (2000a, December). CDC surveillance summaries, Dec. 2000, Tuberculosis morbidity in the United States: Final data, 2000. *Morbidity and Mortality Weekly Report, 40*(SS3), 23–28.

Centers for Disease Control and Prevention. (2000b, December). *Diabetes surveillance report, 2000:* Atlanta, GA: U.S. Department of Health and Human Services.

Centers for Disease Control and Prevention. (2000C, December). *HIV/AIDS surveillance report: U.S. HIV and AIDS cases reported through December 2000, 9*(2).

Centers for Disease Control and Prevention. (2003). *Preliminary data for 2003.* Washington, DC: U.S. Department of Health and Human Services.

Clemen-Stone, S., McGuire, S., & Eigsti, D. (2002). *Comprehensive community health nursing* (6th ed.). St. Louis, MD: Mosby.

D'Cruz, P. (2003). Family-focused interventions in health and illness. *Journal of Health Management, 5*(1), 37–56.

Dunn, H. (1959). High level wellness for man and society. *American Journal of Public Health, 49,* 786–972.

Duvall, E. (1977). *Marriage and family development* (5th ed.). Philadelphia, PA: Lippincott.

Edelman, C., & Mandle, C. (2002). *Health promotion throughout the life-span* (5th ed.). St. Louis, MO: Mosby.

Freiberg, K. L. (1992). *Human development: A lifespan approach* (4th ed.). Boston: Jones & Bartlett.

Giger, J., & Davidhizar, R. (2004). *Transcultural nursing: Assessment and intervention* (4th ed.). St. Louis, MO: Mosby.

Havighurst, R. J. (1972). *Human development and education* (3rd ed.). New York: Longman.

Joint National Committee. (1997). *The report of the Joint National Committee on detection, evaluation and treatment of high blood pressure.* Washington, DC: National Institutes of Health, National Heart, Lung, and Blood Institute.

Lubkin, I., & Larsen, P. (2002). *Chronic illness: Impact and interventions* (5th ed.). Boston: Jones & Bartlett.

NANDA International. (2005). *Nursing diagnosis: Definitions & classification 2005–2006.* Philadelphia: Author.

National Center for Health Statistics. (2001). *Health, United States, 2001* (DHHS Publication No. PHS 91-1232). Hyattsville, MD: Public Health Service.

Pender, N., Parsons, M., & Murdaugh, C. (2002). *Health promotion in nursing practice* (4th ed.). Upper Saddle River, NJ: Prentice Hall.

Suchman, E. (1972). Stages of illness and medical care. In E. Jaco (Ed.), *Patients, physicians and illness.* New York: Free Press.

U.S. Department of Health and Human Services. (2005). *Dietary guidelines for Americans 2005. Executive summary.* Available at www.health.gov/dietaryguidelines/dga2005/document/html/executivesummary.htm

World Health Organization (WHO). (1974). *Constitution of the World Health Organization.* Geneva: Author.

Zhou, H. H., Koshakji, R. J. P., Silberstein, D. J., Wilkinson, G. R., & Wood, A. J. J. (1989). Racial differences in drug response: Altered sensitivity to and clearance of propranolol in men of Chinese descent as compared with American whites. *New England Journal of Medicine, 320,* 565–570.

CHAPTER 3

Agency on Aging. (2001). Achieving cultural competence. *A guidebook for providers of services to older Americans and their families.* Available at www.aoa.gov/prof/adddiv/adddiv/asp

Aird, T., & McIntosh, M. (2003). Nursing tools and strategies to assess cognition and confusion. *British Journal of Nursing, 13*(10), 621–625.

Alzheimer's Disease Education & Referral Center. (2004). *Alzheimer's disease fact sheet.* Available at www.alzheimers.org/pubs/adfact/html

Centers for Disease Control and Prevention and Merck Institute of Aging & Health. (2004). *The state of aging and health in America 2004.* Available at www.cdc.gov/aging

Centers for Disease Control and Prevention. (2005). *Chronic disease-at-a-glance-healthy aging. The health and economic effects of an aging society.* Available at www.cdd.gov/nccdphp/aag/aag_aging.htm

Department of Health & Human Services, Administration on Aging. (2003). *Statistics—A profile of older Americans 2003.* Available at www.aoa.dhhs.gov/prof/Statistics/profile/2003/2.asp

Dunn, D. (2004). Preventing perioperative complications in an older adult. *Nursing, 34*(11), 36–41.

Eliopoulos, C. (2005). *Gerontological nursing* (6th ed.). Philadelphia: Lippincott Willams & Wilkins.

Erikson, E. (1963). *Childhood and society* (2nd ed.). New York: Norton.

Fulmer, T. (2004). Try this: Best practices in nursing care to older adults from the Hartford Institute for Geriatric Nursing. Elder abuse and neglect assessment. *AAACN Viewpoint, 26*(2), 3–4.

Havighurst, R. J. (1972). *Developmental tasks and education.* New York: David McKay.

Hoare, K. (2004). Care home placement: Can admission direct from acute hospital be justified? *Nursing Older People, 16*(6), 14–17.

Kohlberg, L. (1969). Stage and sequence: The cognitive-developmental approach to socialization. In D. Gaslin (Ed.), *Handbook of socialization: Theory and research* (pp. 347–380). Chicago: Rand-McNally.

Medical News Today. (2005). *Life expectancy in USA increases to 77.6 years; deaths from heart disease, cancer decline, report finds.* Available at www.medicalnewstoday.com/medicalnews.php?newsid=20557

Miller, C. (2003). Safe medication practices: Nursing assessment of medications in older adults. *Geriatric Nursing, 24*(5), 314–315, 317.

Miller, C. A. (2004). *Nursing for wellness in older adults. Theory and practice* (4th ed.). Philadelphia: Lippincott Williams & Wilkins.

National Institute of Neurological Disorders and Stroke. (2005). *NINDS Alzheimer's disease information page.* Available at www.ninds.nih.gov/disorders/alzheimersdisease/alzheimersdisease.htm

Naylor, M., Stephens, C., Bowles, K., & Bixby, M. (2005). Cognitively impaired older adults: From hospital to home. *American Journal of Nursing, 105*(2), 52–62.

Porth, C. M. (2005). *Pathophysiology: Concepts of altered health states* (7th ed). Philadelphia: Lippincott Williams & Wilkins.

Reed, P. (1996). Transcendence: Formulating nursing perspectives. *Nursing Science Quarterly, 9*(1), 2–4.

Roach, S. (2003). Sexual behavior of nursing home residents: Staff perceptions and responses. *Journal of Advanced Nursing, 48*(4), 371–379.

Senior Site. (2004). Learning to cope with chronic illness. Available at http://seniors-site.com/coping/chronic.html

Thompson, D. (2004). Geriatric incontinence. The long-term care challenge. *Urologic Nursing, 24*(4), 305–314, 356.

U.S. Census Bureau. (2001). *Baby boom brought biggest increases among people 45- to 54-years-old.* Available at www.census.gov/Press-Release/www/2001/cb01cn184.html

CHAPTER 4

Administration on Aging, U.S. Department of Health and Human Services. (2003). *Hospice care.* Available at www.aoa.gov

Administration on Aging, U.S. Department of Health and Human Services. (2003). *National family caregiver support program.* Available at www.aoa.gov/prof/aoaprog

American Nurses Association. (1998). *Scope and standards of parish nursing practice.* Washington, DC: Author.

American Nurses Association. (1999). *Scope and standards of home health nursing practice.* Washington, DC: Author.

Argyle, M., & Dean, J. (1965). Eye contact, distance and affiliation. *Sociometry, 28,* 285–304.

Center for Medicare & Medicaid Services. (2004). OASIS overview. Available at www.cms.hhs.gov/oasis/hhoview.asp

Clark, J. (2004). An aging population with chronic disease compels new delivery systems focused on new structures and practices. *Nursing Administration Quarterly, 28*(2), 105–115.

Clemen-Stone, S., McGuire, S., & Eigsti, D. (2002). *Comprehensive community health nursing: Family, aggregate and community practice* (6th ed.). St. Louis, MO: Mosby.

Giger, J., & Davidhizar, R. (2004). *Transcultural nursing: Assessment and intervention* (4th ed.). St. Louis, MO: Mosby Year Book.

Grindel-Waggoner, M. (1999). Home care: A history of caring, a future of challenges. *MEDSURG Nursing, 8*(2), 118–120.

Health Care Financing Administration. (2003). *Managed care in Medicare and Medicaid. Fact sheet.* Washington, DC: U.S. Department of Health and Human Services.

Health Care Financing Administration. (2004). *Medicare and home health care.* Washington, DC: U.S. Department of Health and Human Services.

Health Care Financing Administration. (2005). *Medicare & You 2004.* Washington, DC: U.S. Department of Health and Human Services.

Henderson, G., & Primeaux, M. (1981). *Transcultural health care.* Menlo Park, CA: Addison-Wesley.

Ketafian, S. (1987). Moral behavior in nursing. *Advances in Nursing Science, 9*(1), 10–19.

Leff, E., Blanchard, A., & Lemmah, M. (2004). Going home with hospice care. *Nursing, 34*(9), (Hospital Nursing), 32hn 6, 8,10.

Leininger, M. (1991). Transcultural care principles, human rights, and ethical considerations. *Journal of Transcultural Nursing, 3*(1), 21–23.

NANDA International. (2005). *Nursing diagnoses: Definitions & classification 2005–2006.* Philadelphia: Author.

National Association for Home Care. (2004). *Basic statistics about home care.* Washington, DC: Author.

National Association for Home Care. (2004). *How to choose a home care provider. What are my rights as a patient?* Available at www.nahc.org

Spector, R. (2004). *Cultural diversity in health and illness* (6th ed.). Upper Saddle River, NJ: Prentice Hall.

Stanhope, M., & Lancaster, J. (2004). *Community and public health nursing* (6th ed.). St. Louis, MO: Mosby.

Sue, D., & Sue, D. (1990). *Counseling the culturally different: Theory and practice* (2nd ed.). New York: John Wiley & Sons.

Volpato, M., & Cruz, D. (2003). Nursing diagnosis in medical-surgical patients. *International Journal of Nursing Terminologies and Classifications, 14*(4), Supplement 57.

Wilkinson, J. (2005). *Prentice Hall nursing diagnosis handbook with NIC interventions and NOC outcomes.* Upper Saddle River, NJ: Prentice Hall.

CHAPTER 5

Amella, E. (2004). Presentation of illness in older adults: If you think you know what you're looking for, think again. *American Journal of Nursing, 104*(10), 40–51.

Are you missing serious illness in older adults? Improve assessment of geriatric patients. *Hospital Home Health, 21*(9), 105–106.

Argyle, M., & Dean, J. (1965). Eye contact, distance and affiliation. *Sociometry, 28,* 285–304.

Dulak, S. (2004). Hands-on help: Assessing heart sounds. *RN, 67*(8) (Acute Care Focus), 24 ac 2k-4.

Dulak, S. (2004). A practical guide to a thorough history. *RN, Travel Nursing Today,* pp. 14–21.

Giger, J., & Davidhizar, R. (2004). *Transcultural nursing: Assessment and intervention* (4th ed.). St. Louis: Mosby.

Henderson, G., & Primeaux. (1981). *Transcultural health care.* Menlo Park, CA: Addison-Wesley.

Incredibly easy! Interpreting abnormal abdominal sounds. (2000). *Nursing, 30*(6), 28.

Jarvis, C. (2004). *Physical examination & health assessment.* St. Louis, MO: Mosby.

Narayan, M. (2003). Cultural assessment & care planning. *Home Healthcare Nurse, 21*(9), 611–620.

Stein, A. (2003). Aging is more than skin deep. Learn about the systemic effects and signs that may indicate abnormalities. *Nursing (Hospital Nursing), 33*(2), 32hn, 7–8.

Sue, D., & Sue, D. (2003). *Counseling the culturally different: Theory and practice* (4th ed.). New York: John Wiley & Sons.

Trim, J. (2004). Performing a comprehensive physiological assessment. *Nursing Times, 100*(50), 38–42.

Weber, J., & Kelley, J. (2002). *Health assessment in nursing* (2nd ed.). Philadelphia: Lippincott.

Woodrow, P. (2003). Assessing pulse in older people. *Nursing Older People, 15*(6), 38–40.

Wright, K. (2003). Conscientious record keeping: Its role in effective care. *Nursing & Residential Care, 5*(8), 376–379.

CHAPTER 6

Abrams, A. C. (2004). *Clinical drug therapy* (7th ed.). Philadelphia: Lippincott Williams & Wilkins.

Amella, E. J. (2004). Presentation of illness in older adults. *American Journal of Nursing, 104*(10), 40–51.

Brager, R. (2004). Is polypharmacy hazardous to your older patient's health? *Nursing2004, 34*(4), 32hn1–32hn4.

Holland, L. N., & Adams, M. P. (2003). *Core concepts in pharmacology.* Upper Saddle River, NJ: Prentice Hall.

Lehne, R. A. (2004). *Pharmacology for nursing care* (5th ed.). St. Louis, MO: Saunders.

Leibovitch, E. R., Deamer, R. L., & Sanderson, L. A. (2004). Food–drug interactions: Careful drug selection and patient counseling can reduce the risks in older patients. *Geriatrics, 59*(3), 19–22, 32–33.

Pagana, K. D., & Pagana, T. J. (2003). *Mosby's diagnostic and laboratory test reference* (6th ed.). St. Louis, MO: Mosby.

Smith, S. F., Duell, D. J., & Martin, B. C. (2004). *Clinical nursing skills.* Upper Saddle River, NJ: Prentice Hall.

CHAPTER 7

Astle, S. M. (2005). Restoring electrolyte balance. *RN, 68*(5), 34–40.

Burger, C. M. (2004). Hyperkalemia. *American Journal of Nursing, 104*(10), 66–70.

Burger, C. M. (2004). Hypokalemia. *American Journal of Nursing, 104*(11), 61–65.

Copstead, L. C., & Banasik, J. L. (2005). *Pathophysiology* (3rd ed.). St. Louis, MO: Elsevier/Saunders.

Edwards, S. L. (2005). Maintaining calcium balance: Physiology and implications. *Nursing Times, 101*(19), 58–61.

Elgart, H. N. (2004). Assessment of fluids and electrolytes. *AACN Clinical Issues: Advanced Practice in Acute and Critical Care, 15*(4), 607–621.

Fischbach, F. (2002). *Nurses' quick reference to common laboratory and diagnostic tests* (3rd ed.). Philadelphia: Lippincott.

Hayes, D. D. (2004). Calcium in the balance. *Nursing Made Incredibly Easy! 2*(2), 46–53.

Holland, N., & Adams, M. P. (2003). *Core concepts in pharmacology.* Upper Saddle River, NJ: Prentice Hall.

Holman, C., Roberts, S., & Nicol, M. (2005). Promoting adequate hydration in older people. *Nursing Older People, 17*(4), 31–32.

Metheny, N. M. (2000). *Fluid and electrolyte balance: Nursing considerations* (4th ed.). Philadelphia: Lippincott.

Mitchell, D. (2004). Consult stat. Here's an easy way to make sense of IV fluid therapy. *RN, 67*(10), 65–67, 39.

O'Keeffe, S. (2005). Clinician's guide to interpreting arterial blood gases (ABG's). *Clinical Times, 2*(3), 3.

Porth, C. M. (2005). *Pathophysiology: Concepts of altered health states* (7th ed.). Philadelphia: Lippincott.

Pruitt, W. C., & Jacobs, M. (2004). Interpreting arterial blood gases: Easy as ABC. *Nursing, 34*(8), 50–53.

Reid, J., Robb, E., Stone, D., Bowen, P., Baker, R., Irving, S., & Waller, M. (2004). Clinical. Improving the monitoring and assessment of fluid balance. *Nursing Times, 100*(20), 36–39.

Suhayda, R., & Walton, J. C. (2002). Preventing and managing dehydration. *Medsurg Nursing, 11*(6), 267–278.

Sweeney, J. (2005). Clinical queries. What causes sudden hypokalemia? *Nursing, 35*(4), 12.

Sweeney, J. (2005). Clinical queries. What causes hyponatremia? *Nursing, 35*(6), 18.

Tierney, L. M. Jr., McPhee, S. J., & Papadakis, M. A. (Eds.). (2005). *Current medical diagnosis & treatment* (44th ed.). New York: McGraw Hill.

Von Wissen, K., & Breton, C. (2004). Perioperative influences on fluid distribution. *Medsurg Nursing, 13*(5), 304–311.

Wilkinson, J. M. (2005). *Nursing diagnosis handbook* (8th ed.). Upper Saddle River, NJ: Prentice Hall.

Woodrow, P. (2003). Assessing fluid balance in older people: Fluid replacement. *Nursing Older People, 14*(10), 29–30.

Zembrzuski, C. (2004). Try this: Best practices in nursing care to older adults. Nutrition and hydration. *Medsurg Nursing, 13*(1), 60–61.

CHAPTER 8

Abrams, A. C. (2004). *Clinical drug therapy* (7th ed.). Philadelphia: Lippincott Williams & Wilkins.

Acello, B. (2003). Following the guideline for pain control in the elderly. *Nursing2003, 33*(10), 17.

Davidhizar, R., Shearer, R., & Giger, J. (1997, Nov./Dec.) Pain and the culturally diverse client. *Today's Surgical Nurse,* 35–38.

Durrance, S. A. (2003). Older adults and NSAIDs: Avoiding adverse reactions. *Geriatric Nursing, 24*(6), 349–352.

Giger, J., & Davidhizar, R. (2004). *Transcultural nursing: Assessment and intervention* (4th ed.). St. Louis, MO: Mosby Year Book.

Lafleur, K. (2004). Taking the fifth (vital sign). *RN, 67*(7), 30–37.

Lehne, R. A. (2004). *Pharmacology for nursing care* (5th ed.). St. Louis, MO: Saunders.

Levy, R. (1993). *Ethnic and racial differences in responses to medicines.* Reston, VA: National Pharmaceutical Council.

Lipton, J., & Marbach, J. (1984). Ethnicity and the pain experience. *Social Science Medicine, 17,* 1279–1298.

McCaffery, M., & Pasero, C. (1999). *Pain: Clinical manual* (2nd ed.). St. Louis, MO: Mosby.

McCaffery, M., & Thorpe, D. (1988). Differences in perception of pain and the development of adversarial relationships among health care providers. *Advances in Pain Research and Therapy, 11,* 113–122.

Melzack, R., & Wall, P. (1965). Pain mechanisms: A new theory. *Science, 150,* 971–979.

Panke, J. T. (2002). Difficulting in managing pain at the end of life. *AJN, 102*(7), 26–34.

Porth, C. M. (2005). *Pathophysiology: Concepts of altered health states* (7th ed.). Philadelphia: Lippincott Williams & Wilkins.

Prebe, L., Guveyan, J., & Sinatra, R. (1992). Client characteristics influencing postoperative pain management. St. Louis, MO: Mosby Year Book, 140–150.

Salerno, E. (1995). Race, culture, and medications. *Journal of Emergency Nurses, 21,* 560–562.

Schaffer, S. D., & Yucha, C. B. (2004). Relaxation and pain management. *AJN, 104*(8), 75–82.

Siedlecki, S. L. (2004). Assessing chronic pain. *Nursing2004, 34*(5), 17.

Watson, A. C., & Coyne, P. J. (2003). Recognizing the faces of cancer pain. *Nursing2003, 33*(4), 32hn1–32hn8.

Yezierski, R. P., Radson, E., & Vanderah, T. W. (2004). Understanding chronic pain. *Nursing2004, 34*(4), 22–23.

CHAPTER 9

Association of periOperative Registered Nurses. (2005). AORN guidance statement: Preoperative patient care in the ambulatory surgery setting. *AORN Journal, 81*(4), 871–872, 874, 874–878.

Association of periOperative Registered Nurses. (2005). AORN guidance statement: Postoperative patient care in the ambulatory surgery setting. *AORN Journal, 81*(4), 881–884, 886–888.

Beyea, S. C. (2004). Evidence-based practice in perioperative nursing. *American Journal of Infection Control, 32*(2), 97–100.

Boyle, H. J. (2005). Patient advocacy in the perioperative setting. *AORN Journal, 82*(2), 250–252, 254–262.

Crenshaw, J. T., & Winslow, E. H. (2002). Preoperative fasting: Old habits die hard. *American Journal of Nursing, 102*(5), 36–44.

Dunn, D. (2004). Preventing perioperative complications in an older adult. *Nursing, 34*(11), 36–42.

Fessey, E. (2005) Implementing nurse-led discharge from day surgery. *Nursing Times, 101*(16), 32–34.

Garza, S. F. (2004). Periop care for the morbidly obese. *RN, 67*(3), 26ac1–6.

Joint Commission on Accreditation of Healthcare Organizations (JCAHO). (2003). *Universal Protocol for Preventing Wrong Site, Wrong Procedure, Wrong Person Surgery™.* Available: www.jcaho.org/accredited+organizations/patient+safety/universal+protocol

Joint Commission on Accreditation of Healthcare Organizations (JCAHO). (2003). *Implementation expectations for the Universal Protocol for Preventing Wrong Site, Wrong Procedure and Wrong Person Surgery™.* Available: www.jcaho.org/accredited+organizations/patient+safety/universal+protocol

Lehne, R. A. (2004). *Pharmacology for Nursing Care* (5th ed.). Philadelphia: Saunders.

NANDA International. (2005). *Nursing Diagnoses: Definitions and classification 2005–2006.* Philadelphia: Author.

Perry, J., & Jagger, J. (2005). Exposure safety. Pass with care in the OR. *Nursing, 35*(2), 70.

Porth, C. M. (2005). *Pathophysiology: Concepts of altered health states* (7th ed.). Philadelphia: Lippincott.

Roark, J. (n.d.) *Current surgical skin prep standards due for review.* Available: www.infectioncontroltoday.com/articles

Rothrock, J. C. (2003). *Alexander's care of the patient in surgery* (12th ed.). St. Louis, MO: Mosby.

Way, L. W., & Doherty, G. M. (2003). *Current surgical diagnosis & treatment* (11th ed.). New York: McGraw Hill.

Wilkinson, J. M. (2005). *Nursing diagnosis handbook* (8th ed.). Upper Saddle River, NJ: Prentice Hall.

Winslow, E. H., Crenshaw, J. T., & Warner, M. A. (2002). Counterpoint. Best practices shouldn't be optional. *American Journal of Nursing, 102*(6), 59, 63.

CHAPTER 10

Abrams, A. C. (2004). *Clinical drug therapy* (7th ed.). Philadelphia: Lippincott Williams & Wilkins.

Capriotti, T. (2003). Preventing nosocomial spread of MRSA is in your hands. *MedSurg Nursing, 12*(3), 193–196.

Centers for Disease Control and Prevention. (2003). *Community-acquired MRSA Frequently asked questions.* Available at www.cdc.gov/ncidod/hip/ARESIST/mrsa_comm_faq_print.htm

Centers for Disease Control and Prevention. (2004). *Anthrax Q&A: Preventive therapy.* Available at www.bt.cdc.gov/agent/anthrax/faq/preventive.asp

Centers for Disease Control and Prevention. (2004). *MRSA—Methicillin-resistant* Staphylococcus aureus *information for healthcare personnel.* Available at www.cdc.gov/ncidod/hip/ARESIST/mrsahcw.htm

Centers for Disease Control and Prevention. (2004). *Standard Precautions.* (developed 1996). Available at www.cdc.gov/ncidod/hip/ISOLAT/std_prec_excerpt.htm

Centers for Disease Control and Prevention. (2004). *What you should know about a smallpox outbreak.* Available at www.cdc.gov/smallpox

Giger, J., & Davidhizar, R. (2004). *Transcultural nursing: Assessment and intervention* (4th ed.). St. Louis, MO: Mosby Year Book.

Karber, S., & Fasano, N. (2003). What you need to know about the smallpox vaccine. *Nursing2003, 33*(6), 36–43.

Kluckhohn, A., & Strodtbeck, F. (1961). *Variations in value orientations.* New York: Row, Peterson.

Kozier, B., Erb, G., Berman, A., & Snyder, S. (2004). *Fundamentals of nursing* (7th ed.). Upper Saddle River, NJ: Prentice Hall.

Lehne, R. A. (2004). *Pharmacology for nursing care* (5th ed.). St. Louis, MO: Saunders.

Pagana, K. D., & Pagana, T. J. (2003). *Mosby's diagnostic and laboratory test reference* (6th ed.). St. Louis, MO: Mosby.

Porth, C. M. (2005). *Pathophysiology: Concepts of altered health states* (7th ed.). Philadelphia: Lippincott Williams & Wilkins.

Rotter, J. (1966). Generalized expectancies for internal versus external locus of reinforcement. *Psychological Monographs, 80*(1), 1–28.

Sheff, B. (2003). Multidrug-resistant microorganisms still making waves. *Nursing2003 33*(11), 59–63.

Wilson, B. A., Shannon, M. T., & Stang, C. L. (2004). *Nurses's drug guide 2004.* Upper Saddle River, NJ: Prentice Hall.

Wooten, J. M., & Salkind, A. R. (2003). Superbugs—Unmasking the threat. *RN, 66*(3), 37–44.

CHAPTER 11

Abrams, A. C. (2004). *Clinical drug therapy* (7th ed.). Philadelphia: Lippincott Williams & Wilkins.

Gardner, P., & Pabbatireddy, S. (2004). Vaccines for women age 50 and older. *Emerging Infectious Diseases, 10*(11), 1990–1994.

Gerberding, J. L. (2004). Women and infectious diseases. *Emerging Infectious Diseases, 10*(11), 1965–1967.

Godwin, C. (2004). What's new in the fight against AIDS. *RN, 67*(4), 46–53.

Hinkle, J. L. (2004). The new adult immunization schedule. *Journal of Neuroscience Nursing, 36*(3), 167–172.

Kenny, P. E. (2004). The changing face of AIDS. *Nursing 2004, 34*(9), 56–63.

Lehne, R. A. (2004). *Pharmacology for nursing care* (5th ed.). St. Louis, MO: Saunders.

The Medical Letter. (2003). *Rapid tests for HIV infection.* New Rochelle, NY: The Medical Letter, Inc.

The Medical Letter. (2003). *Enfuvirtide (Fuzeon) for HIV infection.* New Rochelle, NY: The Medical Letter, Inc.

National Institute of Allergy and Infectious Diseases. (2003). *Understanding the immune system.* Washington, DC: National Institute of Allergy and Infectious Diseases.

National Institute of Allergy and Infectious Diseases. (2003). *Understanding vaccines.* Washington, DC: National Institute of Allergy and Infectious Diseases.

National Institute of Allergy and Infectious Diseases. (2004). *HIV/AIDS Statistics.* Available at www.aiaid.gov/factsheets/aidsstat.htm

Pagana, K. D., & Pagana, T. J. (2003). *Mosby's diagnostic and laboratory test reference* (6th ed.). St. Louis, MO: Mosby.

Parini, S. (2003). Vaccination do's and don'ts. *Nursing 2003, 33*(12), 58–63.

Porth, C. M. (2005). *Pathophysiology: Concepts of altered health states* (7th ed.). Philadelphia: Lippincott Williams & Wilkins.

CHAPTER 12

American Cancer Society. (2005a). *Cancer facts and figures—2005.* Atlanta, GA: Author.

American Cancer Society. (2005b). *Cancer facts and figure for African Americans—2005–2006.* Atlanta, GA: Author.

Aziz, N. M., & Rowland, J. H. (2002). Cancer survivorship research among ethnic minority and medically underserved groups. *Oncology Nursing Forum, 29*(5), 789–816.

Beriwal, S., Singh, S., & Garcia-Young, J. A. (2002). Tumor lysis syndrome in extensive-stage small-cell lung cancer. *American Journal of Clinical Oncology, 25*(5), 474–475.

Cairo, M. S., & Bishop, M. (2004). Tumour lysis syndrome: New therapeutic strategies and classification. *British Journal of Haematology, 127*(1), 3–11.

Cantril, C. A., & Haylock, P. J. (2004). Emergency. Tumor lysis syndrome. *American Journal of Nursing, 104*(4), 49–52.

Copstead, L. C., & Banasik, J. L. (2005). *Pathophysiology* (3rd ed.). St. Louis, MO: Elsevier/Saunders.

Dowd, S., Poole, V., Davidhizar, R., & Giger, J. (1998). Death, dying, and grief in a transcultural context: Application of the Giger and Davidhizar Assessment Model. *The Hospice Journal, 13*(4), 33–55.

Facione, N. C., Giancarlo, C., & Chan, L. (2000). Perceived risk and help-seeking behavior for breast cancer: A Chinese-American perspective. *Cancer Nursing, 23*(4), 258–267.

Fu, M. R. (2004). Post-breast cancer lymphedema and management. *Recent Advances: Research Updates, 5*(1), 125–138.

Fu, M. R., Anderson, C. M., McDaniel, R., & Armer, J. (2002). Patients' perception of fatigue in response to biochemotherapy as a treatment for metastatic melanoma. *Oncology Nursing Forum, 29*(6), 961–966.

Habib, G. S., & Saliba, W. R. (2002). Tumor lysis syndrome after hydrocortisone treatment in metastatic melanoma: A case report and review of the literature. *American Journal of the Medical Sciences, 323*(3), 155–157.

Haynes, M. A., & Smedley, B. D. (Eds.). (1999). *The unequal burden of cancer: An assessment of NIH research and programs for ethnic minorities and the medically underserved.* Washington, DC: National Academy Press.

Holdsworth, M. T., Nguyen, P. (2003). Role of I.V. allopurinol and rasburicase in tumor lysis syndrome. *American Journal of Health-System Pharmacy, 60*(21), 2213–2222.

Kasper, D. L., Braunwald, E., Fauci, A. S., Hauser, S. L., Longo, D. L., & Jameson, J. L. (Eds.). (2005). *Harrison's principles of internal medicine* (16th ed.). New York: McGraw-Hill.

Legha, S., Ring, S., Eton, O., Bedikian, A., Buzaid, A. C., Plager, C., & Papadopoulos, N. (1998). Development of a biochemotherapy regiment with concurrent administration of cisplatin, vinblastine, dacarbazine, interferon alfa, and interleukin-2 for patients with metastatic melanoma. *Journal of Clinical Oncology, 16*(5), 1752–1759.

Perry, H. (1993). *Mourning and funeral customs of African Americans. Ethnic variations in dying, death, and grief* (pp. 51–67). Washington, DC: Taylor & Francis.

Porth, C. M. (2005). *Pathophysiology: Concepts of altered health states* (7th ed.). Philadelphia: Lippincott.

Rosenblatt, P., Walsh, R., & Jackson, D. (1976). *Grief and mourning in cultural perspective.* New Haven, CT: HRAF Press.

Some, M. (1993). *Ritual: Power, healing, and community.* Newberg, OR: Swan Raven and Company.

Talamanes, M., Lawler, W., & Espino, D. (1995). Hispanic American elders: Caregiving norms surrounding dying and the use of hospice services. *The Hospice Journal, 10*(2), 35–49.

Wu, T. Y., & Yu, M.Y. (2003). Reliability and validity of the mammography screening beliefs questionnaire among Chinese American women. *Cancer Nursing, 26*(2), 131–142.

CHAPTER 13

Blank-Reid, C. (2004). Abdominal trauma. *Nursing 2004, 34*(9), 36–41.

Broderick, M. (2004). Pediatric poisoning. *RN, 67*(9), 37–43.

Diehl-Oplinger, L., & Kaminski, M. F. (2004). Choosing the right fluid to counter hypovolemic shock. *Nursing 2004, 34*(3), 52–54.

Landry, D. W., & Oliver, J. A. (2004, February). Insights into shock. *Scientific American,* pp. 37–41.

Lehne, R. A. (2004). *Pharmacology for nursing care* (5th ed.). St. Louis, MO: Saunders.

Mower-Wade, D., & Kang, T. M. (2004). Sepsis: When defense turns deadly. *Nursing 2004, 34*(7), 32cc1–32cc4.

National Center for Injury Prevention and Control. (2004). *Injuries among children and adolescents.* Available at www.cdc.gov/ncipc/factsheets/children.htm

National Center for Injury Prevention and Control. (2004). *Injuries among older adults.* Available at www.cdc.gov/ncipc/lderadults.htm

Porth, C. M. (2005). *Pathophysiology: Concepts of altered health states* (7th ed.). Philadelphia: Lippincott Williams & Wilkins.

Steffen, K. A. (2003). When your trauma patient is over 65. *Nursing 2003, 33*(4), 53–56.

CHAPTER 14

American Association of Colleges of Nursing. (1999a). *Peaceful death: Recommended competencies and curricular guidelines for end-of-life nursing care*. Washington, DC: Author.

American Association of Colleges of Nursing. (1999b). *Position statement: Moral distress*. Available from info@aacn.org

American Association of Colleges of Nursing. (2004). *About ELNEC*. Available at www.aacn/nche.edu/elnec/about.htm

American Association of Retired Persons. (2003). *End of life: Talking about your final wishes*. Available at www.aarp.org/life/endoflife/Articles/a2003-12-02-endoflife-finalwishes.html

American Geriatrics Society. (2002). *Position statement: The care of dying patients*. Available at http://americangeriatrics.org/products/positionpapers/careofd.html

American Nurses Association. (1992). *Position statement on nursing and the Patient Self-Determination Act*. Kansas City: Author.

American Nurses Association. (1992). *Report from the task force on the nurse's role in end of life decisions*. Kansas City: Author.

American Nurses Association. (2003). *Position statements: Pain management and control of distressing symptoms in dying patients*. Available at www.nursingworld.org/readroom/position/ethics/etpain.htm

Bialk, J. (2004). Ethical guidelines for assisting patients with end-of-life decision making. *Medsurg Nursing, 13*(2), 87–90.

Collins, F. (2004). An evaluation of palliative care services in the community. *Nursing Times, 100*(33), 34–37.

Dochterman, J., & Bulechek, G. (2004). *Nursing interventions classification (NIC)* (4th ed.). St. Louis, MO: Mosby.

Dunne, K. (2004). Grief and its manifestations. *Nursing Standard, 18*(45), 45–53.

Florida Department of Elder Affairs and the Florida Partnership for End-of-life Care. (2004). *Making choices: Beginning to plan for end-of-life care*. Available at http://elderaffairs.state.fl.us

Henneman, E., & Karras, G. (2004). Determining brain death in adults: A guideline for use in critical care. *Critical Care Nurse, 24*, 50–56. Available at http://ccn.aacnjournals.org/cgi/contents/full/24/5/50

International Council of Nurses. (1997). *Basic principles of nursing care*. Washington, DC: American Nurses Publishing.

Kruse, B. (2004). The meaning of letting go: The lived experience for caregivers of persons at end of life. *Journal of Hospice and Palliative Nursing, 6*(4), 215–222.

Kübler-Ross, E. (1969). *On death and dying*. New York: Macmillan.

Kübler-Ross, E. (1978). *To live until we say goodbye*. Englewood Cliffs, NJ: Prentice Hall.

Kübler-Ross, E. (1997). *On death and dying: What the dying have to teach doctors, nurses, clergy, and their own families*. New York: Simon & Schuster.

Lewis, I., & McBride, M. (2004). Anticipatory grief and chronicity: Elders and families in racial/ethnic minority groups. *Geriatric Nursing, 25*(1), 44–47.

Lipson, J. G., Dibble, S. L., & Minarik, P. A. (Eds.). (1996). *Culture & nursing care: A pocket guide*. San Francisco: UCSF Nursing Press.

Poor, B., & Poirrier, G. (2001). *End of life nursing care*. Boston: Jones & Bartlett.

Rancour, P. (2002). Catapulting through life stages: When younger adults are diagnosed with life-threatening illnesses. *Journal of Psychosocial Nursing and Mental Health Services, 40*(2), 32–37, 52–53.

Reed, P. G. (1996). Transcendence: Formulating nursing perspectives. *Nursing Science Quarterly, 9*(1), 2–4.

Spector, R. (2004). *Cultural diversity in health and illness* (6th ed.). Upper Saddle River, NJ: Prentice Hall.

Teasdale, K. (2004). Care of the bereaved when postmortems are required. *Nursing Times, 100*(36), 32–33.

Tierney, L. M., McPhee, S. J., & Papadakis, M. A. (2004). *Current medical diagnosis & treatment* (43rd ed.). New York: McGraw Hill.

Tuttas, C. (2002). The facts of end-of-life care. *Journal of Nursing Care Quality, 16*(2), 10–16.

Wiese, K. (2003). Grief, loss and bereavement. *Prairie Rose, 72*(4), 20–27.

Yetman, L. (2004). Helping patients make their wishes known. *Home Healthcare Nurse, 22*(8), 576.

CHAPTER 15

Danter, J. H. (2003). Geriatric assessment. *Nursing2003, 33*(12), 52.

Pagana, K. D., & Pagana, T. J. (2003). *Mosby's diagnostic and laboratory test reference* (6th ed.). St. Louis, MO: Mosby.

Porth, C. M. (2005). *Pathophysiology: Concepts of altered health states* (7th ed.). Philadelphia: Lippincott Williams & Wilkins.

CHAPTER 16

Abrams, A. C. (2004). *Clinical drug therapy* (7th ed.). Philadelphia: Lippincott Williams & Wilkins.

Holcomb, S. S. (2003). Detecting thyroid disease, part 1. *Nursing 2003, 33*(8), 32cc1–32cc4.

Holcomb, S. S. (2003). Detecting thyroid disease, part 2. *Nursing 2003, 33*(9), 32cc1–32cc4.

Kumrow, D., & Dahlen, R. (2002). Thyroidectomy: Understanding the potential complications. *MEDSURG Nursing, 11*(5), 228–235.

Lehne, R. A. (2004). *Pharmacology for nursing care* (5th ed.). St. Louis, MO: Saunders.

National Cancer Institute. (2004). *Thyroid cancer: Treatment*. Available at www.nci.nih.gov/cancertopics/pdq/treatment/thyroid/HealthProfessional

National Institute of Diabetes and Digestive and Kidney Diseases. (2004). *Addison's disease: Adrenal insufficiency*. Bethesda, MD: Author.

National Institute of Diabetes and Digestive and Kidney Diseases. (2004). *Cushing's fact sheet*. Bethesda, MD: Author.

Porth, C. M. (2005). *Pathophysiology: Concepts of altered health states* (7th ed.). Philadelphia: Lippincott Williams & Wilkins.

Schori-Ahmed, D. (2003). Thyroid disease. *RN, 66*(6), 38–43.

CHAPTER 17

Abrams, A. C. (2004). *Clinical drug therapy* (7th ed.). Philadelphia: Lippincott Williams & Wilkins.

American Diabetes Association. (2004). Diagnosis and classification of diabetes mellitus. *Diabetes Care, 27*(Supplement 1), S5–S10.

American Diabetes Association. (2004). Insulin administration. *Diabetes Care, 27*(Supplement 1), S106–S107.

American Diabetes Association. (2004). Nutrition principles and recommendations in diabetes. *Diabetes Care, 27*(Supplement 1), S36–S46.

American Diabetes Association. (2004). Physical activity/exercise and diabetes. *Diabetes Care, 27*(Supplement 1), S5–S10.

Fain, J. A. (2004). Blood glucose meters: Different strokes for different folks. *Nursing2004, 34*(11), 48–51.

Jack, L., Boseman, L., & Vinicor, F. (2004). Aging Americans and diabetes. A public health and clinical response. *Geriatrics, 59*(4), 14–16.

Lehne, R. A. (2004). *Pharmacology for nursing care* (5th ed.). St. Louis, MO: Saunders.

National Diabetes Information Clearinghouse. (2004). *Complementary and alternative medical therapies for diabetes*. Bethesda, MD: Author.

National Diabetes Information Clearinghouse. (2004). *Pancreatic islet transplantation.* Bethesda, MD: Author.

Olohan, K., & Zappitelli, D. (2003). The insulin pump. *American Journal of Nursing, 103*(4), 48–57.

Porth, C. M. (2005). *Pathophysiology: Concepts of altered health states* (7th ed.). Philadelphia: Lippincott Williams & Wilkins.

CHAPTER 18

Assessment made incredibly easy! (2004). Philadelphia: Springhouse.

Balance your nutrition: Update on recommended daily intakes-1. (2004). Available: http://www.balanceyournutrition.com/BYN_updateRDA.htm

Gallo, J. J., Fulmer, T., Paveza, G. J., & Reichel, W. (2000). *Handbook of geriatric assessment* (3rd ed.). Gaithersburg, MD: Aspen.

Fischbach, F. T., & Dunning, M. B. (2005). *Nurses' quick reference to common laboratory and diagnostic tests* (4th ed.). Philadelphia: Lippincott.

Jarvis, C. (2004). *Physical examination & health assessment.* St. Louis, MO: Mosby.

Kee, J. (2005). *Prentice Hall handbook of laboratory & diagnostic tests with nursing implications.* Upper Saddle River, NJ: Prentice Hall.

Mehta, M. (2003). Assessing the abdomen: Use sight, sound and touch to screen for abnormalities. *Nursing, 33*(5), 54–55.

United States Department of Health. (2005). *Dietary guidelines for Americans 2005. Key recommendations for the general population.* Available: http://www.health.gov/dietaryguidelines/dga2005/recommendations.htm

CHAPTER 19

Barry, D. (2004). An emerging model of behavior change in women maintaining weight loss. *Nursing Science Quarterly, 17*(3), 242–252.

Carlson, D. S., & Pfadt, E. (2004). Perforated peptic ulcer. *Nursing, 34*(12), 88.

Copstead, L. C., & Banasik, J. L. (2005). *Pathophysiology* (3rd ed.). St. Louis, MO: Elsevier Saunders.

Davidhizar, R., & Brownson, K. (2000). Literacy, cultural diversity, and client education. *Home HealthCare Management Practitioner, 12*(2), 38–44.

DiMaria-Ghalili, R. A., & Amella, E. (2005). Nutrition in older adults. *American Journal of Nursing, 105*(3), 40–50.

Doak, D., Doak, L., & Root, J. (1996). *Teaching patients with low literacy skills* (2nd ed.). Philadelphia: Lippincott.

Fontaine, K. L. (2005). *Healing practices: Alternative therapies for nursing* (2nd ed.). Upper Saddle River, NJ: Prentice Hall Health.

Gunter, D. A. (2004). A nursing guide to the assessment of GERD in long term care. *Director, 12*(4), 221,223–227.

Kasper, D. L., Braunwald, E., Fauci, A. S., Hauser, S. L., Longo, D. L., & Jameson, J. L. (Eds.). (2005). *Harrison's Principles of internal medicine* (16th ed.). New York: McGraw-Hill.

Metheny, N. A., & Titler, M. G. (2001). Assessing placement of feeding tubes. *American Journal of Nursing, 101*(5), 36–45.

National Institutes of Health (NIH). (2004). *Statistics related to overweight and obesity.* Available: www.niddk.nih.gov/win

Padula, C. A., Kenny, A., Planchon, C., & Lamoureax, C. (2004). Enteral feedings: What the evidence says. *American Journal of Nursing, 104*(7), 62–69.

Porth, C. M. (2005). *Pathophysiology: Concepts of altered health states* (6th ed.). Philadelphia: Lippincott.

Reid, M. B., & Allard-Gould, P. (2004). Malnutrition and the critically ill elderly patient. *Critical Care Nursing Clinics of North America, 16*(4), 531–536.

Reising, D. L., & Neal, R. S. (2005). Enteral tube flushing. *American Journal of Nursing, 105*(3), 58–63.

Rothrock, J. C. (2003). *Alexander's care of the patient in surgery* (12th ed.). St Louis, MO: Mosby.

Smith, G. D. (2004). The management of acute upper gastrointestinal bleeding. *Nursing Times, 100*(26), 40–43.

U. S. Preventive Services Task Force. (2003). Behavioral counseling in primary care to promote a healthy diet: Recommendations and rationale. *American Journal of Nursing, 103*(8), 81–82, 85–86, 89–90.

U. S. Preventive Services Task Force. (2004). Screening for obesity in adults: Recommendations and rationale. *American Journal of Nursing, 104*(5), 94, 97–98, 100.

CHAPTER 20

American Cancer Society. (2005). *Cancer facts and figures 2005.* Atlanta: Author.

Ayers, D. M. M. (2003). Using a colonoscopy to survey intestinal health. *Nursing, 33*(3), 65

Banks, N., & Razor, B. (2003). Preopertive stomal site assessment and marking. *American Journal of Nursing, 103*(3), 64A–64C, 64E.

Beitz, J. M. (2004). Diverticulosis and diverticulitis: Spectrum of a modern malady. *Journal of the WOCN, 31*(2), 75–84.

Bohrn, M., & Siewert, B. (2004). Acute abdominal pain: What not to miss. *Patient Care for the Nurse Practitioner, 2004* (Mar), 8p.

Bristow, N. (2004). Clinical. Treatment and management of acute appendicitis. *Nursing Times, 100*(43), 34–36.

Brooks, D. (2004). Understanding colon cancer screening tests. *Clinical Advisor, 7*(4), 23–24, 27–30, 31.

Copstead, L. C., & Banasik, J. L. (2005). *Pathophysiology* (3rd ed.). St. Louis, MO: Elsevier/Saunders.

Fletcher, K. (2005). Elimination: Geriatric self-learning module. *MEDSURG Nursing, 14*(2), 127–131.

Fontaine, K. L. (2005). *Healing practices: Alternative therapies for nursing* (2nd ed.). Upper Saddle River, NJ: Prentice Hall Health.

Hughes, E. (2005). Caring for the patient with an intestinal obstruction. *Nursing Standard, 19*(47), 56–64, 66, 68.

Jagot, C. (2004). Clinical. The importance of improving awareness of colorectal cancer. *Nursing Times, 100*(14), 30–31.

Kasper, D. L., Braunwald, E., Fauci, A. S., Hauser, S. L., Longo, D. L., & Jameson, J. L. (Eds.). (2005). *Harrison's Principles of internal medicine* (16th ed.). New York: McGraw-Hill.

Lalchan, E. (2005). Improving care of patients with inflammatory bowel disease. *Nursing Times, 101*(1), 46.

Mauk, K. L. (2005). Healthier aging. Preventing constipation in older adults. *Nursing, 35*(6), 22–23.

NANDA International. (2005). *Nursing Diagnoses: Definitions and Classification 2005–2006.* Philadelphia: Author.

Nightingale, A. (2004). An overview of the diagnosis and management of Crohn's disease. *Gastrointestinal Nursing, 2*(4), 31–39.

Pearson, C. (2004), Clinical. Inflammatory bowel disease. *Nursing Times, 100*(9), 86–90.

Porth, C. M. (2005). *Pathophysiology: Concepts of altered health states* (7th ed.). Philadelphia: Lippincott.

Rayhorn, N. (2003). Inflammatory bowel disease (IBD). *Nursing, 33*(11 Part 1), 54–55.

Rigby, D., & Powel, M. (2005). Causes of constipation and treatment options. *Primary Health Care, 15*(2), 41–50.

Roush, K. (2005). Fecal incontinence: What to know about this often-hidden problem. *American Journal of Nursing, 105*(6), 62–63.

Sargent, C., & Murphy, D. (2003). What you need to know about colorectal cancer. *Nursing, 33*(2), 37–41.

Sidebotham, J. (2003). Managing the complications of diverticular disease. *Nursing Times, 99*(12), 28–29.

Tierney, L. M. Jr., McPhee, S. J., & Papadakis, M. A. (Eds.). (2005). *Current medical diagnosis & treatment* (44th ed.). New York: McGraw Hill.

Trouble down below: Understanding small-bowel obstruction. (2005). *Nursing, 35*(7), Critical Care 32cc4, 32cc6–32cc7.

Veronesi, J. (2004). Inflammatory bowel disease. *Nursing Times, 100*(43), 34–36.

What you need to know about. . . peritonitis. (2003). *Nursing Times, 99*(31), 26.

Wilkes, G. M. (2005). Therapeutic options in the management of colon cancer: 2005 update. *Clinical Journal of Oncology Nursing, 9*(1), 31–44, 61–63.

Wilkinson, J. M. (2005). *Nursing diagnosis handbook* (8th ed.). Upper Saddle River, NJ: Prentice Hall.

Wondergem, F. (2005). Relieving constipation. *Journal of Community Nursing, 19*(5), 16.

Woodward, S. (2005). Complementary therapies in bowel care. *Gastrointestinal Nursing, 3*(3), 31–34.

CHAPTER 21

Alexander, D., Schaffer, S., & Zeilman, C. (2003). Noninfectious liver disorders: Assessment and diagnosis. *Nurse Practitioner: American Journal of Primary Health Care, 28*(12), 12–17, 21–24, 26–27.

Alper, B. S. (2004). Evidence-based medicine. Enteral feeding preferred for acute pancreatitis. *Clinical Advisor, 7*(9), 112.

American Cancer Society. (2005). *Cancer facts and figures 2005*. Atlanta: Author.

Brettler, S. J. (2003). Primary biliary cirrhosis: Defenses gone awry. *RN, 66*(9), 38–44.

Burruss, N., & Holz, S. (2005). Understanding acute pancreatitis. *Nursing, 35*(3), 32hn1–32hn2, 32hn4.

Christensen, T. (2004). The treatment of oesophageal varices using a Sengstaken-Blakemore tube: Considerations for nursing practice. *Nursing in Critical Care, 9*(2), 58–63.

Copley, L. (2005). Hepatitis C: The silent killer. *Practice Nurse, 29*(3), 41–42, 44.

Copstead, L. C., & Banasik, J. L. (2005). *Pathophysiology* (3rd ed.). St. Louis, MO: Elsevier/Saunders.

Durston, S. (2004). Cirrhosis: Scarred for life. *Nursing Made Incredibly Easy! 2*(6), 14–15, 17–25, 35.

Durston, S. (2005). What you need to know about viral hepatitis. *Nursing, 35*(8), 36–42.

Fontaine, K. L. (2005). *Healing practices: Alternative therapies for nursing* (2nd ed.). Upper Saddle River, NJ: Prentice Hall Health.

Gungabissoon, U. (2003). The epidemiology and control of hepatitis C infection. *Nursing Times, 99*(31), 24–25.

Harkness, G. A. (2003). Emerging infections. Hepatitis C: The 'silent stalker.' *American Journal of Nursing, 103*(9), 24–25.

Hepatitis A vaccination. (2005). *Nursing Times, 101*(23), 27.

Hepatitis B vaccine. (2005). *Nursing Times, 101*(21), 29.

Holland, N., & Adams, M. P. (2003). *Core concepts in pharmacology.* Upper Saddle River, NJ: Prentice Hall.

Hughes, E. (2004). Continuing professional development. Understanding the care of patients with acute pancreatitis. *Nursing Standard, 18*(18), 45–52, 54–55.

Kaplan, M. M., & Keeffe, E. B. (2003). What do abnormal liver function test results really mean? *Patient Care for the Nurse Practitioner.* 2003 May.

Kasper, D. L., Braunwald, E., Fauci, A. S., Hauser, S. L., Longo, D. L., & Jameson, J. L. (Eds.). (2005). *Harrison's Principles of internal medicine* (16th ed.). New York: McGraw-Hill.

Knight, J. A. (2005). Liver function tests: Their role in the diagnosis of hepatobiliary diseases. *Journal of Infusion Nursing, 28*(2). 108–117.

NANDA International. (2005). *Nursing Diagnoses: Definitions and Classification 2005–2006.* Philadelphia: Author.

National Center for Complementary and Alternative Medicine. (2004). *Research report. Hepatitis C and complementary and alternative medicine: 2003 update.* National Institutes of Health: NCCAM Publication No. D004. Available: http://nccam.nih.gov/health/hepatitisc/

Parker, M. (2004). Acute pancreatitis. *Emergency Nurse, 11*(10), 28–35.

Porth, C. M. (2005). *Pathophysiology: Concepts of altered health states* (7th ed.). Philadelphia: Lippincott.

Rothrock, J. C. (2003). *Alexander's care of the patient in surgery* (12th ed.). St. Louis, MO: Mosby.

Tierney, L. M. Jr., McPhee, S. J., & Papadakis, M. A. (Eds.). (2005). *Current medical diagnosis & treatment* (44th ed.). New York: McGraw Hill.

Wilkinson, J. M. (2005). *Nursing diagnosis handbook* (8th ed.). Upper Saddle River, NJ: Prentice Hall.

Wilson, T. R. (2005). The ABCs of hepatitis. *Nurse Practitioner: American Journal of Primary Health Care, 30*(6), 12–15, 18, 20–23.

CHAPTER 22

Assessment made incredibly easy! (2004). Philadelphia: Springhouse.

Benham, L., Benbow, H., & Hansen, C. (2003). Respiratory care. The development of a respiratory assessment tool. *Nursing Times, 99*(23) 52–53, 55.

Gallo, J. J., Fulmer, T., Paveza, G. J., & Reichel, W. (2000). *Handbook of geriatric assessment* (3rd ed.). Gaithersburg, MD: Aspen.

Fischbach, F. T., & Dunning, M. B. (2005). *Nurses' quick reference to common laboratory and diagnostic tests* (4th ed.). Philadelphia: Lippincott.

Jarvis, C. (2004). *Physical examination & health assessment.* St. Louis, MO: Mosby.

Kee, J. (2005). *Prentice Hall handbook of laboratory & diagnostic tests with nursing implications.* Upper Saddle River, NJ: Prentice Hall.

Mehta, M. (2003). Peak technique. Respiratory assessment: How to make sense of what your senses tell you. *Nursing Made Incredibly Easy! 1*(2), 56–59.

CHAPTER 23

American Cancer Society. (2005). *Cancer facts and figures 2005*. Atlanta: Author.

American Cancer Society. (2005). *Laryngeal and hypopharyngeal cancer.* Available: www.cancer.org

Centers for Disease Control and Prevention. (2005). *CDC guidelines and recommendations. Updated infection control measures for the prevention and control of influenza in health-care facilities.* Author.

Copstead, L. C., & Banasik, J. L. (2005). *Pathophysiology* (3rd ed.). St. Louis, MO: Elsevier/Saunders.

Davey, M. J. (2003). Understanding obstructive sleep apnoea. *Nursing Times, 99*(22), 26–27.

deCastro, A. B. (2005). Health and safety. Preventing exposure to influenza: Steps health care workers can take. *American Journal of Nursing, 105*(1), 112.

Fontaine, K. L. (2005). *Healing practices: Alternative therapies for nursing* (2nd ed.). Upper Saddle River, NJ: Prentice Hall Health.

Goldrick, B. A. (2004). Emerging infections. Influenza 2004–2005: What's new with the flu. *American Journal of Nursing, 104*(10), 34–36.

Jull, A. (2003). Review: Specific signs and symptoms can help practitioners to diagnose acute purulent sinusitis in general practice. *Evidence-Based Nursing, 6*(1), 24.

Kasper, D. L., Braunwald, E., Fauci, A. S., Hauser, S. L., Longo, D. L., & Jameson, J. L. (Eds.). (2005). *Harrison's Principles of internal medicine* (16th ed.). New York: McGraw-Hill.

Malcolm, A. (2005). The nurse role in managing and treating sleep disorders. *Nursing Times, 101*(23), 34–37.

McCance, K. L., & Huether, S. E. (2002). *Pathophysiology: The biologic basis for disease in adults & children* (4th ed.). St. Louis, MO: Mosby.

McErlane, K., & Pence, C. (2004). Action stat. Epistaxis. *Nursing, 34*(8), 88.

Merritt, S. L., & Johnson, J. (2004). Beats & breath. Obstructive sleep apnea-hypopnea syndrome: Nurses may detect a problem often overlooked by other providers. *American Journal of Nursing, 104*(7), 49–52.

NANDA International. (2005). *Nursing Diagnoses: Definitions and Classification 2005–2006.* Philadelphia: Author.

Nosing into flu season: Learn how to administer influenza vaccine intranasally in a few steps. (2004). *Nursing, 34*(9), 49.

Porth, C. M. (2005). *Pathophysiology: Concepts of altered health states* (7th ed.). Philadelphia: Lippincott.

Rothrock, J. C. (2003). *Alexander's care of the patient in surgery* (12th ed.). St. Louis, MO: Mosby.

St. John, R. E. (2004). Contemporary issues in adult tracheostomy management. *Critical Care Nursing Clinics of North America, 16*(3), 413–430.

Schweon, S., & Mangan, D. (2003). Don't underestimate group A strep. *RN, 66*(8), 28–33.

Tierney, L. M., McPhee, S. J., & Papadakis, M. A. (2005). *Current medical diagnosis & treatment* (44th ed.). New York: Lange Medical Books/McGraw-Hill.

The Voice Center. (2002). *Speech after a total laryngectomy.* Available: www.voicecenter.com/alaryngeal_speech.htm

Wilkinson, J. M. (2005). *Nursing diagnosis handbook with NIC interventions and NOC outcomes* (8th ed.). Upper Saddle River, NJ: Prentice Hall Health.

Willard, R. M., & Dreher, H. M. (2005). Wake-up call for sleep. *Nursing, 35*(3), 46–49.

Wilson, T., & Olson-Burgess, C. (2004). Are you up to date on immunizations? *The Nurse Practitioner, 29*(9), 33–34, 36, 38, 43.

CHAPTER 24

American Lung Association. (2005). *Asthma in adults fact sheet.* Available: www.lungusa.org

American Thoracic Society, CDC, & Infectious Diseases Society of America. (2003). Treatment of tuberculosis. *MMWR Recommendations and Reports, 55*(RR11), 1–77. Available: http://cdc.gov/mmwr/preview/mmwrhtml/rr5211al.htm

Aronson, B. S., & Marquis, M. (2004). Care of the adult patient with cystic fibrosis. *Medsurg Nursing, 13*(3), 143–154.

Barry, R. M. (2004). Penetrating chest wounds. *RN, 67*(5), 36, 42.

Bauer, J. (2004). RN news watch: Clinical highlights. Rapid treatment can be a lifesaver in elderly pneumonia patients. *RN, 67*(5), 20, 47, 70–71.

Bell, C. (2004). The treatment of patients with TB and the role of the nurse. *Nursing Times, 100*(36), 48–50.

Bialous, S. A., & Sarna, L. (2004). Sparing a few minutes for tobacco cessation. *American Journal of Nursing, 104*(12), 54–62.

Boyle, A. H., & Locke, D. L. (2004). Update on chronic obstructive pulmonary disease. *Medsurg Nursing, 13*(1), 42–48.

Capriotti, T. (2005). Changes in inhaler devices for asthma and COPD. *Medsurg Nursing, 14*(3), 185–194.

Cardin, T., & Marinelli, A. (2004). Pulmonary embolism. *Critical Care Nursing Quarterly, 27*(4), 310–324.

Charlebois, D. (2005). Early recognition of pulmonary embolism: The key to lowering mortality. *Journal of Cardiovascular Nursing, 20*(4), 254–259.

Cheever, K. H. (2005). An overview of pulmonary arterial hypertension: Risks, pathogenesis, clinical manifestations, and management. *Journal of Cardiovascular Nursing, 20*(2), 108–118.

Clinical rounds: Bioterrorism. How to identify inhalation anthrax. (2004). *Nursing, 34*(10), 34–35.

Coleman, P. R. (2004). Pneumonia in the long-term care setting: Etiology, management and prevention. *Journal of Gerontological Nursing, 30*(4), 14–23, 54–55.

Copstead, L. C., & Banasik, J. L. (2005). *Pathophysiology* (3rd ed.). St. Louis, MO: Elsevier/Saunders.

Covey, M. K., & Larson, J. L. (2004). Beats & breaths. Exercise and COPD. *American Journal of Nursing, 104*(5), 40–43.

Darlison, L. (2005). Respiratory care. Lung cancer: An update on current diagnostic techniques and treatment. *Nursing Times, 101*(14), 42–44, 46.

de Castro, A. B. (2004). Health & safety. Respiratory protection: Preventing exposure to communicable agents. *American Journal of Nursing, 104*(12), 88.

Dent, M. (2004). Hospital-acquired pneumonia: The "gift" that keeps on taking. *Nursing 34*(2), 48–51.

Dreher, H. M., Dean, J. L., Moriarty, D. M., Kaiser, R., Willard, R., O'Donnell, S., Virella, J., O'Brien, C., Marcolongo, C., Regn, K., Constans, C., Sowden, R., & Phung, L. (2004). What you need to know about SARS now. *Nursing, 34*(1), 58–63.

Fontaine, K. L. (2005). *Healing practices: Alternative therapies for nursing* (2nd ed.). Upper Saddle River, NJ: Prentice Hall Health.

Hilton, P. (2004). Clinical. Evaluating the treatment options for spontaneous pneumothorax. *Nursing Times, 100*(28), 32–33.

Jacobs, M. (2005). Ease the stress of managing ARDS. *Nursing Made Incredibly Easy! 3*(1), 6–15, 17–18.

Kane, C., & Galanes, S. (2004). Adult respiratory distress syndrome. *Critical Care Nursing Quarterly, 27*(4), 325–335.

Kasper, D. L., Braunwald, E., Fauci, A. S., Hauser, S. L., Longo, D. L., & Jameson, J. L. (Eds.). (2005). *Harrison's Principles of internal medicine* (16th ed.). New York: McGraw-Hill.

Kleinpell, R. M., & Elpern, E. H. (2004). Community-acquired pneumonia: Updates in assessment and management. *Critical Care Nursing Quarterly, 27*(3), 231–240.

Koschel, M. J. (2004). Emergency. Pulmonary embolism. *American Journal of Nursing, 104*(6), 46–50.

Lenaghan, N. A. (2000). The nurse's role in smoking cessation. *Medsurg Nursing, 9*(6), 298–302.

Lindgren, V. A., & Ames, N. J. (2005). Caring for patients on mechanical ventilation: What research indicates is best practice. *American Journal of Nursing, 105*(5), 50–61.

Markou, N. K., Myrianthefs, P. M., & Baltopoulos, G. J. (2004). Respiratory failure: An overview. *Critical Care Nursing Quarterly, 27*(4), 353–379.

Merrel, P., & Mayo, D. (2004). Inhalation injury in the burn patient. *Critical Care Nursing Clinics of North America, 16*(1), 27–38.

NANDA International. (2005). *Nursing Diagnoses: Definitions and Classification 2005–2006.* Philadelphia: Author.

National Heart, Lung, and Blood Institute. (2003). *Expert panel report: Guidelines for the diagnosis and management of asthma. Update on selected topics 2002.* Bethesda, MD: Author. NIH Publication No. 02-5074.

National Heart, Lung, and Blood Institute. (2004). *Morbidity & mortality: 2004 chart book of cardiovascular, lung, and blood diseases.* Bethesda, MD: Author.

National Heart, Lung, and Blood Institute, & World Health Organization. (2005). *Global initiative for chronic obstructive lung disease. Pocket guide to COPD diagnoses, management, and prevention.* Bethesda, MD: Author.

O'Neill, P. (2004). Hospital nursing. Nutrition series: Nutrition for a patient with COPD can be complicated. *Nursing, 34*(12), 32hn6, 32hn8.

Petty, M. (2003). Lung and heart-lung transplnatation: Implications for nursing care when hospitalized outside the transplant center. *Medsurg Nursing, 12*(4), 250–259.

Porth, C. M. (2005). *Pathophysiology: Concepts of altered health states* (7th ed.). Philadelphia: Lippincott.

Roman, M. (2005). Clinical 'how to.' Tracheostomy tubes. *Medsurg Nursing, 14*(2), 143–144.

Rothrock, J. C. (2003). *Alexander's care of the patient in surgery* (12th ed.). St. Louis, MO: Mosby.

Schleder, B. J. (2004). Taking charge of hospital-acquired pneumonia. *The Nurse Practitioner, 29*(3), 50–53.

Simmons, P., & Simmons, M. (2004). Informed nursing practice: The administration of oxygen to patients with COPD. *Medsurg Nursing, 13*(2), 82–85.

Smyth, M. (2005). Acute respiratory failure, part 1. Failure in oxygenation. *American Journal of Nursing, 105*(5), Critical Care Extra, 72GG–72JJ, 72MM, 7200.

Smyth, M. (2005). Acute respiratory failure, part 2. Failure of ventilation: Exploring the other cause of acute respiratory failure. *American Journal of Nursing, 105*(6), Critical Care Extra 72AA–72DD.

Sniffing out pneumonia: The nose knows. (2004). *Nursing, 34*(7), 35.

Steinbis, S. (2004). What you should know about pulmonary hypertension. *The Nurse Practitioner, 29*(4), 8–10, 13–15, 19.

Tierney, L. M. Jr., McPhee, S. J., & Papadakis, M. A. (Eds.). (2005). *Current medical diagnosis & treatment* (44th ed.). New York: McGraw Hill.

Understanding pleural effusion. (2004). *Nursing, 34*(8), 64.

U. S. Centers for Disease Control and Prevention. (2005). New draft guidelines from CDC for preventing tuberculosis transmission in healthcare. *Home Healthcare Nurse, 23*(4), 240.

Veronesi, J. F. (2004). Blunt chest injuries. *RN, 67*(3), 48, 55.

Way, L. W., & Doherty, G. M. (2003). *Current surgical diagnosis & treatment* (11th ed.). New York: McGraw Hill.

What you need to know about . . . Lung cancer. (2004). *Nursing Times, 100*(13), 31.

Wilkinson, J. M. (2005). *Nursing diagnosis handbook* (8th ed.). Upper Saddle River, NJ: Prentice Hall.

Wing, S. (2004). Pleural effusion: Nursing care challenge in the elderly. *Geriatric Nursing, 25*(6), 348–354.

Woods, A., & Hathaway, L. (2004). Treating community-acquired pneumonia. *Nurse Practitioner, 29*(6), 11.

CHAPTER 25

Coviello, J. (2004). Cardiac assessment 101: A new look at the guidelines for cardiac homecare patients. *Home Healthcare Nurse, 22*(2), 116–123.

Dulak, S. (2004). Hands-on help assessing heart sounds. *RN, 67*(8) Acute Care Focus, 24acl–4.

Eliopoulos, E. (2005). *Gerontological nursing* (6th ed.). Philadelphia: Lippincott Williams & Wilkins.

Jarvis, C. (2004). *Physical examination & health assessment.* St. Louis, MO: Mosby.

Kee, J. (2005). *Prentice Hall handbook of laboratory & diagnostic tests with nursing implications.* Upper Saddle River, NJ: Prentice Hall.

Weber, J., & Kelley, J. (2002). *Health assessment in nursing* (2nd ed.). Philadelphia: Lippincott.

CHAPTER 26

American Heart Association. (2005). *Heart disease and stroke statistics— 2005 update.* Dallas, TX: American Heart Association.

Blumenthal, R. S., & Margolis, S. (2005). *The Johns Hopkins white papers. Heart attack prevention.* Redding, CT: Medletter Associates, Inc.

Copstead, L. C., and Banasik, J. L. (2005). *Pathophysiology* (3rd ed.). St. Louis, MO: Saunders.

DeVon, H. A., & Zerwic, J. J. (2004). Differences in the symptoms associated with unstable angina and myocardial infarction. *Progress in Cardiovascular Nursing, 19*(1) 6–11.

Foley, S. (2005). Update on risk factors for atherosclerosis: The role of inflammation and apolipoprotein E. *Medsurg Nursing, 14*(1), 43–50.

Granger, B. B., & Miller, C. M. (2001). Acute coronary syndrome. *Nursing, 31*(11), 36–43.

Granot, M., Goldstein-Ferber, S., & Azzam, A. S. (2004). Gender differences in the perception of chest pain. *Journal of Pain and Symptom Management, 27*(2), 149–155.

Hummard, J. (2004). Management of atrial fibrillation. *Nursing Times, 100*(6), 42–44.

Kasper, D. L., Braunwald, E., Fauci, A. S., Hauser, S. L., Longo, D. L., & Jameson, J. L. (2005). *Harrison's Principles of internal medicine* (16th ed.). New York: McGraw-Hill.

McSweeney, J. C., & Coon, S. (2004). Women's inhibitors and facilitators associated with making behavioral changes after myocardial infarction. *Medsurg Nursing, 13*(1), 49–56.

National Cholesterol Education Program. (2002). *Third report of the National Cholesterol Education Program (NCEP) Expert Panel on detection, evaluation, and treatment of high blood cholesterol in adults (Adult Treatment Panel III). Final report.* Bethesda, MD: National Heart, Lung, and Blood Institute, National Institutes of Health.

National Heart, Lung, and Blood Institute (NHLBI). (2004). *Morbidity & mortality: 2004 chart book of cardiovascular, lung, and blood diseases.* Bethesda, MD: National Institutes of Health.

NHLBI. (2005). Statement from Elizabeth G. Nabel, M.D., Director of the National Heart, Lung, and Blood Institute of the National Institutes of Health on the Findings of the Women's Health Study. *NIH News,* March 7. Available: www.nhlbi.hih.gov

NANDA International. (2005). *NANDA's Nursing Diagnoses: Definitions & Classification 2005–2006.* Philadelphia: Author.

Pelter, M. M., & Adams, M. G. (2004). Premature beats. *American Journal of Critical Care, 13*(6), 519–520.

Porth, C. M. (2005). *Pathophysiology: Concepts of altered health states* (7th ed.). Philadelphia: Lippincott.

Quigley, M. P. (2004). Promoting cardiac rehabilitation. *Nursing, 34*(8), 24.

Rosenfeld, A. G. (2004). Treatment-seeking delay among women with acute myocardial infraction: Decision trajectories and their predictors. *Nursing Research, 53*(4), 225–236.

Ryan, C. J., DeVon, H. A., & Zerwic, J. J. (2005). Typical and atypical symptoms: Diagnosing acute coronary syndromes accurately. *American Journal of Nursing, 105*(2), 34–36.

Shaffer, R. S. (2002). ICD therapy: The patient's perspective. *American Journal of Nursing, 102*(2), 46–49.

Tierney, L. M., McPhee, S. J., & Papadakis, M. A. (2005). *Current medical diagnosis & treatment* (44th ed.). New York: McGraw-Hill.

U. S. Department of Health & Human Services. (2005). *Dietary guidelines for Americans 2005.* U. S. Department of Agriculture. Available: www.healthierus.gov/dietaryguidelines

U. S. Preventive Services Task Force. (2002). Aspirin for the primary prevention of cardiovascular events: Recommendations and rationale. *American Journal of Nursing, 102*(3), 67, 69–70.

U. S. Preventive Services Task Force. (2002). Screening for lipid disorders in adults: Recommendations and rationale. *American Journal of Nursing, 102*(6), 91, 93, 95.

Wilkinson, J. M. (2005). *Nursing diagnosis handbook with NIC interventions and NOC outcomes* (8th ed.). Upper Saddle River, NJ: Prentice Hall Health.

Woods, S. L., Froelicher, E. S., Motzer, S. A., & Bridges, E. (2004). *Cardiac nursing* (5th ed.). Philadelphia: Lippincott.

Zerwic, J. J., & Ryan, C. J. (2004). Delays in seeking MI treatment. *American Journal of Nursing, 104*(1), 81–83.

CHAPTER 27

American Heart Association. (2005). *Heart Disease and Stroke Statistics—2005 Update.* Dallas, Texas: American Heart Association.

Ammon, S. (2001). Managing patients with heart failure. *American Journal of Nursing, 101*(12), 34–40.

Artinian, N. T. (2003). The psychosocial aspects of heart failure. *American Journal of Nursing, 103*(12), 32–42.

Bither, C. J., & Apple, S. (2001). Home management of the failing heart. *American Journal of Nursing, 101*(12), 41–45.

Bolton, M. M., & Wilson, B. A. (2005). The influence of race on heart failure in African-American women. *Medsurg Nursing, 14*(1), 8–15.

Bond, A. E., Nelson, K., Germany, C. L., & Smart, A. N. (2003). The left ventricular assist device. *American Journal of Nursing, 103*(1), 32–40.

Capriotti, T. (2002). Current concepts and pharmacologic treatment of heart failure. *Medsurg Nursing, 11*(2), 71–83.

Copstead, L. C., & Banasik, J. L. (2005). *Pathophysiology* (3rd ed.). St. Louis, MO: Elsevier/Saunders.

Deaton, C., Bennett, J. A., & Riegel, B. (2004). State of the science for care of older adults with heart disease. *Nursing Clinics of North America, 39*(3), 495–528.

Fischbach, F. (2005). *Nurses' quick reference to common laboratory and diagnostic tests* (4th ed.). Philadelphia: Lippincott.

Fontaine, K. L. (2005). *Healing practices: Alternative therapies for nursing* (2nd ed.). Upper Saddle River, NJ: Prentice Hall Health.

Goldrick, B. A. (2003). Emerging infections. Endocarditis associated with body piercing. *American Journal of Nursing, 103*(1), 26–27.

Hunt, S. A., Baker, D. W., Chin, M. H., Ciquegrani, M. P., Feldman, A. M., Francis, G. S., Ganiats, T. G., Goldstein, S., Gregoratos, G., Jessup, M. L., Noble, R. J., Packer, M., Silver, M. A., and Stevenson, L. W. (2001) ACC/AHA guidelines for the evaluation and management of chronic heart failure in the adult: Executive summary: A report of the American College of Cardiology/American Heart Association Task Force on Practice Guidelines (Committee to Revise the 1995 Guidelines for the Evaluation and Management of Heart Failure). *Circulation, 104,* 2996–3007.

Kasper, D. L., Braunwald, E., Fauci, A. S., Hauser, S. L., Longo, D. L., & Jameson, J. L. (Eds.). (2005). *Harrison's Principles of internal medicine* (16th ed.). New York: McGraw-Hill.

King, J. E. (2004). How to classify heart failure. *Nursing, 34*(5), 15.

Luggen, A. S., & Parton, A. (2004). Gerontologic nurse practitioner care guidelines: Early management of heart failure. *Geriatric Nursing, 25*(4), 251–253.

Miracle, V. A. (2001). Put the brakes on pericarditis. *Nursing, 31*(4), 44–45.

Munson, B. L. (2005). Myths and facts . . . About infective endocarditis. *Nursing, 35*(2), 71.

NANDA International. (2005). *Nursing Diagnoses: Definitions and Classification 2005–2006.* Philadelphia: Author.

National Heart, Lung, and Blood Institute, National Institutes of Health. (2004). *Morbidity & mortality: 2004 chart book of cardiovascular, lung, and blood diseases.* Bethesda, MD: Author.

Piña, I. L., Apstein, C. S., Balady, G. J., Belardinelli, R., Chaitman, B. R., Duscha, B. D., Fletcher, B. J., Fleg, J. L., Myers, J. N., & Sullivan, M. J. (2003). *AHA Scientific Statement. Exercise and heart failure.* American Heart Association. Available: http://www.circulationaha.org

Porth, C. M. (2005). *Pathophysiology: Concepts of altered health states* (7th ed.). Philadelphia: Lippincott.

Pugh, L. C., Havens, D. S., Xie, S., Robinson, J. M., & Blaha, C. (2001). Case management for elderly persons with heart failure: The quality of life and cost outcomes. *Medsurg Nursing, 10*(2), 71–75.

Steinbis, S. (2003). Hypertophic obstructive cardiomyopathy and septal ablation. *Critical Care Nurse, 23*(3), 47–50.

Tierney, L. M. Jr., McPhee, S. J., & Papadakis, M. A. (Eds.). (2005). *Current medical diagnosis & treatment* (44th ed.). New York: McGraw Hill.

Way, L. W., & Doherty, G. M. (2003). *Current surgical diagnosis & treatment* (11th ed.). New York: Lange Medical/McGraw-Hill.

Wilkinson, J. M. (2005). *Nursing diagnosis handbook* (8th ed.). Upper Saddle River, NJ: Prentice Hall.

Woods, S. L., Froelicher, E. S., Motzer, S. A., & Bridges, E. (2004). *Cardiac nursing* (5th ed.). Philadelphia: Lippincott.

Yee, C. A. (2005). Endocarditis: The infected heart. *Nursing Management, 36*(2), 25–30.

CHAPTER 28

American Heart Association. (2005). *Heart disease and stroke statistics—2005 update.* Dallas, TX: Author.

Aortic aneurysms: Synthetic graft prevents ruptures. (2005). *Nursing, 35*(6), 34.

Applying antiembolism stockings isn't just pulling on socks. (2004). *Nursing, 34*(8), 48–49.

Beese-Bjurstrom, S. (2004). Hidden danger: Aortic aneurysms & dissections. *Nursing, 34*(2), 36–42.

Bonner, L. (2004). Clinical. The prevention and treatment of deep vein thrombosis. *Nursing Times, 100*(29), 38–42.

Chant, T. (2004). Clinical update: Peripheral vascular disease. *Primary Health Care, 14*(8), 29–34.

Copstead, L. C., & Banasik, J. L. (2005). *Pathophysiology* (3rd ed.). St. Louis, MO: Elsevier/Saunders.

Dee, R. (2003). Issues in geriatrics. Getting a leg up on varicose veins. *Clinical Advisor, 6*(1), 65–67.

Fontaine, K. L. (2005). *Healing practices: Alternative therapies for nursing* (2nd ed.). Upper Saddle River, NJ: Prentice Hall Health.

Kasper, D. L., Braunwald, E., Fauci, A. S., Hauser, S. L., Longo, D. L., & Jameson, J. L. (Eds.). (2005). *Harrison's Principles of internal medicine* (16th ed.). New York: McGraw-Hill.

Moll, S., & Severson, M. A. (2004). Deep vein thrombosis: The hidden threat. *CareManagement, Supplement,* 5–47.

Nadeau, C., & Varrone, J. (2003). Treat DVT with low molecular weight heparin. *Nurse Practitioner: American Journal of Primary Health Care, 28*(10), 22–23, 26, 29–31.

National Heart, Lung, and Blood Institute. (2003). *Facts about the DASH eating plan.* NIH Publication No. 03-4082. Available: http://nhlbi.hih.gov

National Heart, Lung, and Blood Institute: National High Blood Pressure Education Program. (2004a). *The seventh report of the Joint National Committee on prevention, detection, evaluation, and treatment of high blood pressure.* Bethesda, MD: National Institutes of Health.

National Heart, Lung, and Blood Institute. (2004b). *Morbidity & mortality: 2004 chart book of cardiovascular, lung, and blood diseases.* Bethesda, MD: National Institutes of Health.

North American Nursing Diagnosis Association. (2005). *NANDA nursing diagnoses: Definitions & classification 2005–2006.* Philadelphia: NANDA.

Porth, C. M. (2005). *Pathophysiology: Concepts of altered health states* (7th ed.). Philadelphia: Lippincott.

Rice, K. L. (2005). How to measure ankle/brachial index. *Nursing, 35*(1), 56–57.

Ruff, D. (2005). Conservative management of varicose veins. *Nursing Times, 101*(4), 51–52, 54.

Then, K. L., & Ranking, J. A. (2004). Hypertension: A review for clinicians. *Nursing Clinics of North America, 39*(4) 793–814.

Tierney, L. M., McPhee, S. J., & Papadakis, M. A. (2005). *Current medical diagnosis & treatment* (44th ed.). New York: McGraw-Hill.

U. S. Preventive Services Task Force. (2004). Screening for high blood pressure: Recommendations and rationale. *American Journal of Nursing, 104*(11), 82–85, 87.

U. S. Preventive Services Task Force. (2005). Screening for abdominal aortic aneurysm: Recommendation statement. *The American Journal for Nurse Practitioners, 9*(5), 55–60.

Way, L. W., & Doherty, G. M. (2003). *Current surgical diagnosis & treatment* (11th ed.). New York: McGraw-Hill

Wipke-Tevis, D. D., Stotts, N. A., Williams, D. A., Froelicher, E. S., & Hunt, T. K. (2001). Tissue oxygenation, perfusion, and position in patients with venous leg ulcers. *Nursing Research, 50*(1), 24–32.

Wilkinson, J. M. (2005). *Nursing diagnosis handbook* (8th ed.). Upper Saddle River, NJ: Prentice Hall.

Woods, A. (2004). Loosening the grip of hypertension. *Nursing, 34*(12), 36–45.

CHAPTER 29

Board, J., & Harlow, W. (2002). Lymphoedema 1: Components and function of the lymphatic system. *British Journal of Nursing, 11*(5), 304–309.

Eliopoulos, E. (2005). *Gerontological nursing* (6th ed.). Philadelphia: Lippincott Williams & Wilkins.

Fischbach, F. (2005). *Nurses' quick reference to common laboratory and diagnostic tests* (4th ed.). Philadelphia: Lippincott.

Jarvis, C. (2004). *Physical examination & health assessment.* St. Louis, MO: Mosby.

Kee, J. (2005). *Prentice Hall handbook of laboratory & diagnostic tests with nursing implications.* Upper Saddle River, NJ: Prentice Hall.

Navuluri, R. (2001). Understanding hemostasis. *American Journal of Nursing, 101*(9), Hospital extra: 24B, 24C.

Rempher K. J., & Little, J. (2004). Assessment of red blood cell and coagulation laboratory data. *AACN Clinical Issues, 15*(4), 622–637.

Weber, J., & Kelley, J. (2002). *Health assessment in nursing* (2nd ed.). Philadelphia: Lippincott.

Woodrow, P. (2003). Assessing blood results in older people: Hematology and liver function tests. *Nursing Older People, 15*(3), 29–31.

CHAPTER 30

American Cancer Society. (2005). *Cancer facts and figures 2005.* Atlanta: Author.

Bennett, L. (2005). Understanding sickle cell disorders. *Nursing Standard, 19*(32), 52–61.

Blackhouse, R. (2004). Understanding disseminated intravascular coagulation. *Nursing Times, 100*(36), 38–42.

Breed, C. D. (2003). Diagnosis, treatment, and nursing care of patients with chronic leukemia. *Seminars in Oncology Nursing, 19*(2), 109–117.

Campbell, K. (2005). Laboratory diagnosis and investigation of anaemia. *Nursing Times, 101*(22), 36–39.

Cantril, C. A., & Haylock, P. J. (2004). Tumor lysis syndrome. *American Journal of Nursing, 104*(4), 49–52.

Cashion, A. (2002) Genetics in transplantation. *Medsurg Nursing 11*(2), 91–94.

Coleman, E. A., Hutchins, L., & Goodwin, J. (2004). An overview of cancer in the older adult. *Medsurg Nursing, 13*(2), 75–80, 109.

Cope, D. (2004). Tumor lysis syndrome. *Clinical Journal of Oncology Nursing, 8*(4), 415–416.

Copstead, L. C., & Banasik, J. L. (2005). *Pathophysiology* (3rd ed.). St. Louis, MO: Elsevier/Saunders.

Dowsett, C. (2005). Managing leg ulceration in patients with sickle cell disorder. *Nursing Times, 101*(16), 48–49.

Dressler, D. K. (2004). DIC: Coping with a coagulation crisis. *Nursing, 34*(5), 58–62.

Fischbach, F. (2005). *Nurses' quick reference to common laboratory and diagnostic tests* (4th ed.). Philadelphia: Lippincott.

Fontaine, K. L. (2005). *Healing practices: Alternative therapies for nursing* (2nd ed.). Upper Saddle River, NJ: Prentice Hall Health.

Francis, J. L., & Drexler, A. J. (2005). Striking back at heparin-induced thrombocytopenia. *Nursing, 35*(9), 48–51.

Holcomb, S. S. (2005). Patient education series. Anemia. *Nursing, 35*(3), 53.

Johnson, L. (2005). Managing acute and chronic pain in sickle cell disease. *Nursing Times, 101*(8), 40–43.

Kasper, D. L., Braunwald, E., Fauci, A. S., Hauser, S. L., Longo, D. L., & Jameson, J. L. (Eds.). (2005). *Harrison's Principles of internal medicine* (16th ed.). New York: McGraw-Hill.

King, M. (2005). Helping to understand the pathophysiology of anaemia. *Nursing Times, 101*(9), 42.

Krimmel, T. (2003). Disseminated intravascular coagulation. *Clinical Journal of Oncology Nursing, 7*(4),479–481.

Maningo, J. (2002). Peripheral blood stem cell transplant: Easier than getting blood from a bone. *Nursing, 32*(12), 52–55.

Munson, B. L. (2005). Myths & facts . . . about polycythemia vera. *Nursing, 35*(5), 28.

NANDA International. (2005). *Nursing Diagnoses: Definitions and Classification 2005–2006.* Philadelphia: Author.

National Heart, Lung, and Blood Institute, National Institutes of Health. (2002). *Morbidity & mortality: 2002 chart book of cardiovascular, lung, and blood diseases.* Bethesda, MD: Author.

Porth, C. M. (2005). *Pathophysiology: Concepts of altered health states* (7th ed.). Philadelphia: Lippincott.

Rogers, B. (2005). Looking at lymphoma and leukemia. *Nursing, 35*(7), 56–63.

Sadler, G. R., Wasserman, L., Fullerton, J. T., & Romero, M. (2004). Supporting patients through genetic screening for cancer risk. *Medsurg Nursing, 13*(4), 233–246.

Simmons, P. (2003). A primer for nurses who administer blood products. *Medsurg Nursing, 12*(3), 184–190.

Tierney, L. M. Jr., McPhee, S. J., & Papadakis, M. A. (Eds.). (2005). *Current medical diagnosis & treatment* (44th ed.). New York: McGraw Hill.

Treating the older patient with leukemia, lymphoma, and myeloma. (2004). *ONS News, 19*(9 Suppl), 77–78.

Viele, C. S. (2003). Diagnosis, treatment and nursing care of acute leukemia. *Seminars in Oncology Nursing, 19*(2), 109–117.

Waldman, A. R. (2003). Understanding non-Hodgkin's lymphomas. *Clinical Journal of Oncology Nursing, 7*(1), 93–96.

Wilkinson, J. M. (2005). *Nursing diagnosis handbook* (8th ed.). Upper Saddle River, NJ: Prentice Hall.

CHAPTER 31

Eliopoulos, C. (2005). *Gerontological nursing* (6th ed.). Philadelphia: Lippincott Williams & Wilkins.

Fischbach, F. (2005). *Nurses' quick reference to common laboratory and diagnostic tests* (4th ed.). Philadelphia: Lippincott.

Jarvis, C. (2004). *Physical examination & health assessment.* St. Louis, MO: Mosby.

Kee, J. (2005). *Prentice Hall handbook of laboratory & diagnostic tests with nursing implications.* Upper Saddle River, NJ: Prentice Hall.

Mehta, M. (2003). Assessing the abdomen: Use sight, sound and touch to screen for abnormalities. *Nursing, 33*(5), 54–55.

Palmer, M. (2004). Physiologic and psychologic age-related changes that affect urologic clients. *Urologic Nursing, 24*(4), 247–252, 257.

Uphold, C. R., & Graham, M. V. (2003). *Clinical guidelines in adult health* (3rd ed.). Gainsville, FL: Barmarrae Books.

Weber, J., & Kelley, J. (2002). *Health assessment in nursing* (2nd ed.). Philadelphia: Lippincott.

CHAPTER 32

American Cancer Society. (2005). *Cancer facts and figures 2005.* Atlanta: Author.

Barone, C. P., Martin-Watson, A. L., & Barone, G. W. (2004). The postoperative care of the adult renal transplant recipient. *Medsurg Nursing, 13*(5), 296–302.

Bissett, L. (2004). The control of urinary tract infection in hospitalised older people. *Nursing Times, 100*(8), 54–56.

Blais, D. (2004). Urinary tract infections among the institutionalized older adult. *Perspectives, 28*(2), 23–27, 29–34.

Boyd, L. A. (2003). Intravesical Bacillus Calmette-Guerin for treating bladder cancer. *Urology Nursing, 23*(3), 189–191, 199.

Buccalo, S. (1997). Window on another world: An "English" nurse looks at the Amish culture and their health care beliefs. *Journal of Multicultural Nursing and Health, 3*(2), 53–58.

Burrows-Hudson, S. (2005). Chronic kidney disease: An overview. *American Journal of Nursing, 105*(2), 40–49.

Campoy, S., & Elwell, R. (2005). Pharmacology & CKD: How chronic kidney disease and its complications alter drug response. *American Journal of Nursing, 105*(9), 60–72.

Cannon, J. D. (2004). Recognizing chronic renal failure ... the sooner, the better. *Nursing, 34*(1), 50–53.

Copstead, L. C., & Banasik, J. L. (2005). *Pathophysiology* (3rd ed.). St. Louis, MO: Elsevier/Saunders.

Davidhizar, R., Bechtel, G., & Giger, J. (1999, April). The influence of time and culture on health patterns. *Competency Matters, 2*(1), 13–15.

Fontaine, K. L. (2005). *Complementary & alternative therapies for nursing practice* (2nd ed.). Upper Saddle River, NJ: Prentice Hall.

Frerick, J. (2004). Gerontologic nurse practitioner care guidelines: Urinary tract infection. *Geriatric Nursing, 24*(3), 185–187.

Giger, J., & Davidhizar, R. (2004). *Transcultural nursing: Assessment and intervention* (4th ed.). St. Louis, MO: Mosby Year Book.

Holcomb, S. S. (2005). Evaluating chronic kidney disease risk. *Nurse Practitioner: American Journal of Primary Health Care, 30*(4), 12–14, 17–18, 23–27.

Kaplow, R., & Barry, R. (2002). Continuous renal replacement therapies. *American Journal of Nursing, 102*(11), 26–33.

Kasper, D. L., Braunwald, E., Fauci, A. S., Hauser, S. L., Longo, D. L., & Jameson, J. L. (Eds.). (2005). *Harrison's Principles of internal medicine* (16th ed.). New York: McGraw Hill.

Kelley, K. T. (2004). How peritoneal dialysis works. *Nephrology Nursing Journal, 31*(5), 481–482, 488–491.

Legg, V. (2005). Complications of chronic kidney disease. *American Journal of Nursing, 105*(6), 40–49.

McCance, K. L., & Huether, S. E. (2006). *Pathophysiology: The biologic basis for disease in adults & children* (5th ed.). St. Louis, MO: Mosby.

McCarley, P. B., & Salai, P. B. (2005). Cardiovascular disease in chronic kidney disease. *American Journal of Nursing, 105*(4), 40–52.

McLoughlin, C. (2004). Antimuscarinic drugs. *Professional Nurse, 20*(1), 50–51.

Naish, W. (2003). Intermittent self-catheterisation for managing urinary problems. *Professional Nurse, 18*(10), 585–587.

National Kidney and Urologic Diseases Information Clearinghouse. (2004). *Kidney and urologic disease statistics for the United States.* NIH Publication No. 04-3895. Available: www.niddk.nih.gov/kudiseases/kidney/pubs/kustats

Palmer, M. H., & Newman, D. K. (2004). Bladder matters: Urinary incontinence in nursing homes. *American Journal of Nursing, 104*(11), 57–59.

Paton, M. (2003). Continuous renal replacement therapy: Slow but steady. *Nursing, 33*(6), 48–50.

Porth, C. M. (2005). *Pathophysiology: Concepts of altered health states* (7th ed.). Philadelphia: Lippincott.

Rothrock, J. C. (2003). *Alexander's care of the patient in surgery* (12th ed.). St. Louis, MO: Mosby.

Simmons, R. (2005). Conservative and surgical approaches to the treatment of overactive bladder. *Professional Nurse, 20*(6), 31–33.

Small, K. R., & McMullen, M. (2005). When clear becomes cloudy: A review of acute tubular necrosis, a form of renal failure. *American Journal of Nursing, 105*(1), Critical Care Extra: 72AA–BB, 72EE, 72GG.

Sofer, D. (2003). Chronic kidney disease: The emerging epidemic. *American Journal of Nursing, 103*(12), 23.

Tierney, L. M. Jr., McPhee, S. J., & Papadakis, M. A. (Eds.). (2005). *Current medical diagnosis & treatment* (44th ed.). New York: McGraw Hill.

Uphold, C. R., & Graham, M. V. (2003). *Clinical guidelines in adult health* (3rd ed.). Gainsville, FL: Barmarrae Books.

U. S. Renal Data System (USRDS). (2005). *2005 Annual data report: Atlas of end-stage renal disease in the United States.* Bethesda, MD: National Institutes of Health, National Institute of Diabetes and Digestive and Kidney Diseases.

Wareing, M. (2003). Urinary retention: Issues of management and care. *Emergency Nursing, 11*(8), 24–27.

Way, L. W., & Doherty, G. M. (2003). *Current surgical diagnosis & treatment* (11th ed.). New York: McGraw Hill.

Wilkinson, J. M. (2005). *Nursing diagnosis handbook* (8th ed.). Upper Saddle River, NJ: Prentice Hall.

Woods, A. (2005). Managing UTIs in older adults. *Nursing, 35*(3), 12.

Zabat, E. (2003). When your patient needs peritoneal dialysis. Brush up on this necessary but infrequently used skill that you may need if your patient has chronic renal failure. *Nursing, 33*(8), 52–54.

CHAPTER 33

Eliopoulos, C. (2005). *Gerontological Nursing* (6th ed.). Philadelphia: Lippincott Williams & Wilkins.

Fischbach, F. (2005). *Nurses' quick reference to common laboratory and diagnostic tests* (4th ed.). Philadelphia: Lippincott.

Jarvis, C. (2004). *Physical examination & health assessment.* St. Louis, MO: Mosby.

Kee, J. (2005). *Prentice Hall handbook of laboratory & diagnostic tests with nursing implications.* Upper Saddle River, NJ: Prentice Hall.

Uphold, C. R., & Graham, M. V. (2003). *Clinical guidelines in adult health* (3rd ed.). Gainsville, FL: Barmarrae Books.

Weber, J., & Kelley, J. (2002). *Health assessment in nursing* (2nd ed.). Philadelphia: Lippincott.

CHAPTER 34

American Cancer Society. (2005). *Cancer facts and figures 2005.* Atlanta: Author.

Burt, J., Caelli, K., Moore, K., & Anderson, M. (2005). Radical prostatectomy: Men's experiences and postoperative needs. *Journal of Clinical Nursing, 14*(7), 883–890.

Calabrese, D. A. (2004). Prostate cancer in older men. *Urologic Nursing, 24*(4), 258–264, 268–269.

Carlson, S. L. (2004). Prostate disease. *RN, 67*(9), 54–60.

Clinical. Erectile dysfunction. (2005). *Nursing Times, 101*(4), 28.

Copstead, L. C., & Banasik, J. L. (2005). *Pathophysiology* (3rd ed.). St. Louis, MO: Elsevier/Saunders.

Crouch, D. (2004). Sex, drugs and cardiac care. *Nursing Times, 100*(46), 26–27.

Diabetes and erectile dysfunction. (2004). *Practice Nurse, 2004*(Supplement), 1–4, 5–8.

Fischbach, F. (2005). *Nurses' quick reference to common laboratory and diagnostic tests* (4th ed.). Philadelphia: Lippincott.

Fontaine, K. L. (2005). *Healing practices: Alternative therapies for nursing* (2nd ed.). Upper Saddle River, NJ: Prentice Hall Health.

Hallam-Jones, R. (2004). Assessing and treating erectile dysfunction. *Practice Nursing, 15*(12), 615–616, 618, 620.

Jack, G. S., & Zeitlin, S. I. (2005). Treatment strategies for the patient with chronic prostatitis. *Patient Care for the Nurse Practitioner, 2005*(Aug), 6 p.

Johnson, B. K. (2004). Prostate cancer and sexuality: Implications for nursing. *Geriatric Nursing, 25*(6), 341–347.

Kasper, D. L., Braunwald, E., Fauci, A. S., Hauser, S. L., Longo, D. L., & Jameson, J. L. (Eds.). (2005). *Harrison's Principles of internal medicine* (16th ed.). New York: McGraw Hill.

Kellogg-Spadt, S. (2005). Sex Rx. Erectile dysfunction: What your patients should know. *The American Journal for Nurse Practitioners, 9*(9), 62–63.

Kelly, D. (2004). Male sexuality in theory and practice. *Nursing Clinics of North America, 39*(2), 341–356.

Kirby, R. S. (2004). Men's health. Selecting long-term medical therapy for BPH. *Patient Care for the Nurse Practitioner, 2004*(Aug), 10 p.

Lewis, J. H., Rosen, R., & Goldstein, I. (2005). Erectile dysfunction. *Nursing, 35*(2), 64.

Lewis, J. H., Rosen, R., & Goldstein, I. (2004). Erectile dysfunction in primary care. *Nurse Practitioner: American Journal of Primary Health Care, 29*(12), 42–46, 48–50, 55–57.

Mason, T. M. (2005). Information needs of wives of men following prostatectomy. *Oncology Nursing Forum, 32*(3), 557–563.

McCance, K. L., & Huether, S. E. (2006). *Pathophysiology: The biologic basis for disease in adults & children* (5th ed.). St. Louis, MO: Mosby.

McCullagh, J., & Lewis, G. (2005). Testicular cancer: Epidemiology, assessment and management. *Nursing Standard, 19*(25), 45–53, 55.

McCullagh, J., Lewis, G., & Warlow, C. (2005). Promoting awareness and practice of testicular self-examination. *Nursing Standard, 19*(51), 41–49.

McGlynn, B., Al-Saffar, N., Begg, H., Gurun, M., Hollins, G., McPhee, S., Meddings, R., & Tindall, M. (2004). Management of urinary incontinence following radical prostatectomy. *Urologic Nursing, 24*(6), 475–482, 515.

NANDA International. (2005). *Nursing Diagnoses: Definitions and Classification 2005–2006.* Philadelphia: Author.

Patterson, A. (2004). Improving information for men with postoperative urinary incontinence. *Nursing Times, 100*(48), 52–53.

Porth, C. M. (2005). *Pathophysiology: Concepts of altered health states* (7th ed.). Philadelphia: Lippincott.

Rothrock, J. C. (2003). *Alexander's care of the patient in surgery* (12th ed.). St. Louis, MO: Mosby.

Stevenson, T. D., & McNeill, J. A. (2004). Surgical management of testicular cancer. *Clinical Journal of Oncology Nursing, 8*(4), 355–360.

Stotts, R. C. (2004). Cancers of the prostate, penis, and testicles: Epidemiology, prevention, and treatment. *Nursing Clinics of North America, 39*(2), 327–340.

Tierney, L. M. Jr., McPhee, S. J., & Papadakis, M. A. (Eds.). (2005). *Current medical diagnosis & treatment* (44th ed.). New York: McGraw Hill.

Weeks, B., & Ficorelli, C. T. (2005). Health matters: Promoting health and wellness. The ABCs of BPH. *Nursing, 35*(10), 68–69.

Wilkinson, J. M. (2005). *Nursing diagnosis handbook* (8th ed.). Upper Saddle River, NJ: Prentice Hall.

Wooten, J. (2004). Men's health: Erectile dysfunction. *RN, 67*(10), 40–46.

CHAPTER 35

Abernethy, K. (2005). Guiding women through menopause—the role of the nurse. *Nurse 2 Nurse, 4*(11), 36–38, 40.

American Cancer Society. (2005). *Cancer facts and figures 2005.* Atlanta: Author.

Barber, D. (2004). Endometriosis: Diagnosis and management of symptoms. *Community Practitioner, 77*(6), 227–228.

Breedlove, G., & Busenhart, C. (2005). Clinical rounds. Screening and detection of ovarian cancer. *Journal of Midwifery & Women's Health, 50*(1), 51–54.

Copstead, L. C., & Banasik, J. L. (2005). *Pathophysiology* (3rd ed.). St. Louis, MO: Elsevier/Saunders.

De Gaetano, C., & Lichtman, S. M. (2004). Care of elderly women with ovarian cancer. *Geriatric Nursing, 25*(6), 329–335.

Dell, D. D. (2005). Spread the word about breast cancer. *Nursing, 35*(10), 56–64.

Dunleavey, R. (2004). Clinical. Incidence, pathophysiology and treatment of cervical cancer. *Nursing Times, 100*(44), 38–41.

Durain, D. (2004). Primary dysmenorrhea: Assessment and management update. *Journal of Midwifery & Women's Health, 49*(6), 520–528, 555–556.

Dyer, K. (2005). Myths & facts . . . about endometriosis. *Nursing, 35*(4), 68.

Elsley, K., Chan, L. C., & Waldrop, J. B. (2004). Advisor forum. Fighting vaginal infections. *Clinical Advisor, 7*(3), 80, 85.

Falsetti, D. (2005). HPV infection and cervical cancer risk. *The American Journal for Nurse Practitioners, 9*(7/8), 21–23, 25–27.

Fischbach, F. (2005). *Nurses' quick reference to common laboratory and diagnostic tests* (4th ed.). Philadelphia: Lippincott.

Fontaine, K. L. (2005). *Healing practices: Alternative therapies for nursing* (2nd ed.). Upper Saddle River, NJ: Prentice Hall Health.

Gross, B., & MacDonald, C. E. (2004). Advisor forum. Pap smears and the elderly. *Clinical Advisor, 7*(7), 68–69.

Iannacchione, M. A. (2004). The vagina dialogues: Do you douche? *American Journal of Nursing, 104*(1), 40–42, 44–45.

Israel, R. (2004). Uterine tumors: A new look at an old problem. *Clinical Advisor, 7*(8), 34, 37–38, 41.

Jones, A. E. (2004). Managing the pain of primary and secondary dysmenorrhoea. *Nursing Times, 100*(10), 40–43.

Kasper, D. L., Braunwald, E., Fauci, A. S., Hauser, S. L., Longo, D. L., & Jameson, J. L. (Eds.). (2005). *Harrison's Principles of internal medicine* (16th ed.). New York: McGraw Hill.

Kirshbaum, M. (2005). Promoting physical exercise in breast cancer care. *Nursing Standard, 19*(41), 41–48.

Martin, V. R. (2005). Straight talk about ovarian cancer. *Nursing, 35*(4), 36–42.

McCance, K. L., & Huether, S. E. (2006). *Pathophysiology: The biologic basis for disease in adults & children* (5th ed.). St. Louis, MO: Mosby.

McCready, C., & Waldrop, J. B. (2005). Advisor forum. Preventing toxic shock syndrome. *Clinical Advisor, 8*(9), 50.

NANDA International. (2005). *Nursing Diagnoses: Definitions and Classification 2005–2006.* Philadelphia: Author.

Newton, S. E., Robinson, J., & Kozac, J. (2004). Balanced analgesia after hysterectomy: The effect on outcomes. *Medsurg Nursing, 13*(3), 176–180, 199.

Parkman, C. A. (2005). CAM trends. Current studies on alternative therapies for menopause. *Case Manager, 16*(4), 26–28.

Porth, C. M. (2005). *Pathophysiology: Concepts of altered health states* (7th ed.). Philadelphia: Lippincott.

Rothrock, J. C. (2003). *Alexander's care of the patient in surgery* (12th ed.). St. Louis, MO: Mosby.

Shinn, S. E. (2004). Taking a stand against cervical cancer. *Nursing, 34*(5), 36–42.

Smith, P. E. (2005). Menopause: Assessment, treatment, and patient education. *Nurse Practitioner: American Journal of Primary Health Care, 30*(2), 32–33, 36–38, 39–40+.

Sontheimer, D., & Alper, B. S. (2005). Stat consult. Pelvic inflammatory disease. *Clinical Advisor, 8*(6), 78, 80–81.

Tierney, L. M. Jr., McPhee, S. J., & Papadakis, M. A. (Eds.). (2005). *Current medical diagnosis & treatment* (44th ed.). New York: McGraw Hill.

Varma, R., & Gupta, J. (2004). Endometriosis—A persisting medical and nursing challenge. *Nurse 2 Nurse, 3*(12), 13–16.

Vickers, M. (2005). HRT and breast cancer: Is there an association? *Practice Nursing, 16*(3), 130–132, 138.

Wilkinson, J. M. (2005). *Nursing diagnosis handbook* (8th ed.). Upper Saddle River, NJ: Prentice Hall.

CHAPTER 36

Adderley-Kelly, B., & Stephens, E. M. (2005). Chlamydia: A major health threat to adolescents and young adults. *ABNF Journal, 16*(3), 52–55.

Bechtel, G., & Davidhizar, R. (1998). Culture, personal space, and health. *Competence Matters, 1*(2), 20. Birmingham, AL: University of Alabama at Birmingham.

Blair, M. (2004). Sexually transmitted diseases: An update. *Urologic Nursing, 24*(6), 467–474.

Blenkinsopp, A., Paxton, P., Blenkinsopp, J., & Reid, S. (2004). Nurse prescribers. Sexual health—*Chlamydia* and trichomonas infections. *Primary Health Care, 14*(10), 33–34.

Bonsu, I. K. (2005). Clinical knowledge: How contraception nurses can improve teenage sexual health. *Nursing Times, 101*(7), 34–36.

Chamberlain-Webber, J. (2005). Tackling the sexual health crisis head on. *Professional Nurse, 20*(7), 10–15.

Clavon, A. M., & Waldrop, J. B. (2005). Advisor forum. Testing for multiple STDs. *Clinical Advisor, 8*(6), 53.

Copstead, L. C., & Banasik, J. L. (2005). *Pathophysiology* (3rd ed.). St. Louis, MO: Elsevier/Saunders.

Dunleavey, R. (2004). Clinical. Incidence, pathophysiology and treatment of cervical cancer. *Nursing Times, 100*(44), 38–44.

Fey, M. C., & Beal, M. W. (2004). Role of human papilloma virus testing in cervical cancer prevention. *Journal of Midwifery & Women's Health, 49*(1), 4–13.

Fischbach, F. (2005). *Nurses' quick reference to common laboratory and diagnostic tests* (4th ed.). Philadelphia: Lippincott.

Fontaine, K. L. (2005). *Healing practices: Alternative therapies for nursing* (2nd ed.). Upper Saddle River, NJ: Prentice Hall Health.

Giger, J., & Davidhizar, R. (2004). *Transcultural nursing: Assessment and intervention* (4th ed.). St. Louis, MO: Mosby Year Book.

Gonorrhoea. (2005). *Nursing Times, 101*(13), 27.

Gorman, E. R., & Harris, A. L. (2004). Trichomoniasis: Current knowledge and case studies. *Clinical Excellence for Nurse Practitioners, 8*(3), 117–120.

Kasper, D. L., Braunwald, E., Fauci, A. S., Hauser, S. L., Longo, D. L., & Jameson, J. L. (Eds.). (2005). *Harrison's Principles of internal medicine* (16th ed.). New York: McGraw Hill.

McCance, K. L., & Huether, S. E. (2006). *Pathophysiology: The biologic basis for disease in adults & children* (5th ed.). St. Louis, MO: Mosby.

Meleis, A. (1996). Arab Americans. In J. Lipson, S. Dibble, & P. Minarik (Eds.), *Culture and nursing care.* San Francisco: UCSF Nursing Press.

Mixed picture on STDs. (2005). *Clinical Advisor, 8*(1), 21.

NANDA International. (2005). *Nursing Diagnoses: Definitions and Classification 2005–2006.* Philadelphia: Author.

Owens, J. A., & Leslie, N. S. (2005). The worry that goes with warts. *Clinical Excellence for Nurse Practitioners, 9*(3), 137–140.

Phillips, K. D., Dudgeon, W. D., Becker, J., & Bopp, C. M. (2004). Sexually transmitted diseases in men. *Nursing Clinics of North America, 39*(2), 357–377.

Porth, C. M. (2005). *Pathophysiology: Concepts of altered health states* (7th ed.). Philadelphia: Lippincott.

Stamm, C. A., Kabir, K., & McGregor, J. A. (2004). Women's health. Treatable and preventable: STIs in young women. *Patient Care for the Nurse Practitioner, 2004*(May), 15 p.

'STIs happen to other people.' (2005). *Community Practitioner, 78*(7), 231.

Tierney, L. M. Jr., McPhee, S. J., & Papadakis, M. A. (Eds.). (2005). *Current medical diagnosis & treatment* (44th ed.). New York: McGraw Hill.

Uphold, C. R., & Graham, M. V. (2003). *Clinical guidelines in adult health* (3rd ed.). Gainesville, FL: Barmarrae Books.

Wilkinson, J. M. (2005). *Nursing diagnosis handbook* (8th ed.). Upper Saddle River, NJ: Prentice Hall.

Young, F. (2005). Genital chlamydia: Practical management in primary care: a steep rise in chlamydia means that community health professionals must be more aware of transmission, diagnosis and treatment. *The Journal of Family Health Care, 15*(1), 19–21.

CHAPTER 37

Amella, E. J. (2004). Presentation of illness in older adults. *American Journal of Nursing, 104*(10), 40–51.

Crimlisk, J. T., & Grande, M. M. (2004). Neurologic assessment skills for the acute medical surgical nurse. *Orthopaedic Nursing, 23*(1), 3–9.

Pagana, K. D., & Pagana, T. J. (2003). *Mosby's diagnostic and laboratory test reference* (6th ed.). St. Louis, MO: Mosby.

Porth, C. M. (2005). *Pathophysiology: Concepts of altered health states* (7th ed.). Philadelphia: Lippincott Williams & Wilkins.

CHAPTER 38

Bettler, S. J. (2004). Traumatic brain injury. *RN, 67*(4), 32–37.

Gambrell, M., & Flynn, N. (2004). Seizures 101. *Nursing2004, 34*(8), 36–41.

Lehne, R. A. (2004). *Pharmacology for nursing care* (5th ed.). St. Louis, MO: Saunders.

McCance, K. L., & Huether, S. E. (2002). *Pathophysiology: The biologic basis for disease in adults and children* (4th ed.). St. Louis, MO: Mosby.

National Center for Injury Prevention and Control. (2004). *Traumatic brain injury in the United States.* Available at www.cdc.gov/ncipc/pub-res/TBI_in_US_04/TBI_ED.htm

National Institute of Neurological Disorders and Stroke. (2005). *Migraine information page.* Available at www.ninds.nih.gov/disorders/migraine.htm

National Institute of Neurological Disorders and Stroke. (2005). *Stroke: Hope through research.* Available at www.ninds.nih.gov/disorders/stroke/detail_stroke_pr.htm

National Institute of Neurological Disorders and Stroke. (2005). *Traumatic brain injury: Hope through research.* Available at www.ninds.nih.gov/disorders/tbi/detail_tbi_pr.htm

Pagana, K. D., & Pagana, T. J. (2003). *Mosby's diagnostic and laboratory test reference* (6th ed.). St. Louis, MO: Mosby.

Porth, C. M. (2005). *Pathophysiology: Concepts of altered health states* (7th ed.). Philadelphia: Lippincott Williams & Wilkins.

Sole, M. L., Klein, D. G., & Moseley, M. J. (2005). *Introduction to critical care nursing* (4th ed.). St. Louis, MO: Elsevier.

Wilson, B. A., Shannon, M. T., & Stang, C. L. (2004). *Nurses's drug guide 2004.* Upper Saddle River, NJ: Prentice Hall.

CHAPTER 39

Brandabur, M. M. (2005). *Complementary and alternative medicine and Parkinson disease.* Available at www.parkinson.org

Courts, N. F., Buchanan, E. M., & Werstlein, P. O. (2004). Focus groups: The lived experience of participants with multiple sclerosis. *Journal of Neuroscience Nursing, 36*(1), 42–47.

Lehne, R. A. (2004). *Pharmacology for nursing care* (5th ed.). St. Louis, MO: Saunders.

National Institute of Neurological Disorders and Stroke. (2005). *Multiple sclerosis: Hope through research.* Available at www.ninds.nih.gov/disorders/multiple_sclerosis/detail.htm

National Institute of Neurological Disorders and Stroke. (2005). *NINDS deep brain stimulation for Parkinson's disease.* Available at www.ninds.nih.gov/disorders/deep_brain_stimulation/pr.htm

National Institute of Neurological Disorders and Stroke. (2005). *Spinal cord injury: Hope through research.* Available at www.ninds.nih.gov/disorders/sci/detail_sci_pr.htm

National Spinal Cord Injury Statistical Center. (2004). *Spinal cord injury facts and figures at a glance.* Available at www.spinalcord.uab.edu

Pagana, K. D., & Pagana, T. J. (2003). *Mosby's diagnostic and laboratory test reference* (6th ed.). St. Louis, MO: Mosby.

Porth, C. M. (2005). *Pathophysiology: Concepts of altered health states* (7th ed.). Philadelphia: Lippincott Williams & Wilkins.

Skidmore-Roth, L. (2004). *Mosby's handbook of herbs & natural supplements* (2nd ed.). St. Louis, MO: Mosby.

Sole, M. L., Klein, D. G., & Moseley, M. J. (2005). *Introduction to critical care nursing* (4th ed.). St. Louis, MO: Elsevier.

CHAPTER 40

Glaucoma Research Foundation. (2005). *Alternative medicine.* Available at www.glaucoma.org/treating/treatme_meds.html

Kerns, B. L., & Mason, J. D. (2004). Red eye: A guide through the differential diagnosis. *Emergency Medicine, 36*(9), 31–40.

Lehne, R. A. (2004). *Pharmacology for nursing care* (5th ed.). St. Louis, MO: Saunders.

Pagana, K. D., & Pagana, T. J. (2003). *Mosby's diagnostic and laboratory test reference* (6th ed.). St. Louis, MO: Mosby.

Porth, C. M. (2005). *Pathophysiology: Concepts of altered health states* (7th ed.). Philadelphia: Lippincott Williams & Wilkins.

Wilson, B. A., Shannon, M. T., & Stang, C. L. (2004). *Nurses's drug guide 2004.* Upper Saddle River, NJ: Prentice Hall.

CHAPTER 41

Eliopoulos, C. (2005). *Gerontological Nursing* (6th ed.). Philadelphia: Lippincott Williams & Wilkins.

Fischbach, F. (2005). *Nurses' quick reference to common laboratory and diagnostic tests* (4th ed.). Philadelphia: Lippincott Williams & Wilkins.

Hathaway, L. (2004). Peak technique. Pump up your musculoskeletal assessment. *Nursing Made Incredibly Easy! 2*(3), 46–47, 49–50.

Jarvis, C. (2004). *Physical examination & health assessment.* St. Louis, MO: Mosby.

Kee, J. (2005). *Prentice Hall handbook of laboratory & diagnostic tests with nursing implications.* Upper Saddle River, NJ: Prentice Hall.

Uphold, C. R., & Graham, M. V. (2003). *Clinical guidelines in adult health* (3rd ed.). Gainsville, FL: Barmarrae Books.

Weber, J., & Kelley, J. (2002). *Health assessment in nursing* (2nd ed.). Philadelphia: Lippincott.

CHAPTER 42

Altizer, L. (2003). Hand and wrist fractures . . . first part of a 2-part series. *Orthopaedic Nursing, 22*(2), 131–138.

Altizer, L. (2003). Hand and wrist fractures. *Orthopaedic Nursing, 22*(3), 232–239.

Altizer, L. (2004). Compartment syndrome. *Orthopaedic Nursing, 23*(6), 391–396.

Altizer, L. (2005). Hip fractures. *Orthopaedic Nursing, 24*(4), 283–294.

Bailey, J. (2003). Getting a fix on orthopedic care. *Nursing, 33*(6), 58–64.

Bechtel, G., & Davidhizar, R. (1998). Culture, personal space, and health. *Competence Matters, 1*(2), 20. Birmingham, AL: University of Alabama at Birmingham.

Brasier, K., & Parker, A. (2004). Digital replantation following amputation due to trauma. *Nursing Times, 100*(41), 40–42.

Childs, S. G. (2004). Cervical whiplash syndrome: Hyperextension-hyperflexion injury. *Orthopaedic Nursing, 23*(2), 106–112.

Clontz, A. S., Annonio, D., & Walker, L. (2004). Trauma nursing: Amputation. *RN, 67*(7), 38–44.

Copstead, L. C., & Banasik, J. L. (2005). *Pathophysiology* (3rd ed.). St. Louis, MO: Elsevier/Saunders.

Davis, P. (2003). Wound care. Skeletal pin traction: Guidelines on postoperative care and support. *Nursing Times, 99*(21), 46–48.

DiNucci, E. M. (2005). Energy healing: A complementary treatment for orthopaedic and other conditions. *Orthopaedic Nursing, 24*(4), 259–269.

Folate pills cut risk of high BP, hip fracture. (2005). *Clinical Advisor, 8*(4), 12.

Fontaine, K. L. (2005). *Healing practices: Alternative therapies for nursing* (2nd ed.). Upper Saddle River, NJ: Prentice Hall Health.

Frakes, M. A., & Evans, T. (2004). Major pelvic fractures. *Critical Care Nurse, 24*(2), 18–24, 26–32.

Giger, J., & Davidhizar, R. (2004). *Transcultural nursing: Assessment and intervention* (4th ed.). St. Louis, MO: Mosby Year Book.

Hall, E. (1966). *Hidden dimension.* New York: Doubleday.

Managing pelvic fractures. (2003). *Nursing, 33*(12), 43.

McCance, K. L., & Huether, S. E. (2006). *Pathophysiology: The biologic basis for disease in adults & children* (5th ed.). St. Louis, MO: Mosby.

NANDA International. (2005). *Nursing Diagnoses: Definitions and Classification 2005–2006.* Philadelphia: Author.

Porth, C. M. (2005). *Pathophysiology: Concepts of altered health states* (7th ed.). Philadelphia: Lippincott.

Predicting hip fracture risk. (2004). *Nursing, 34*(4), 35.

Rothrock, J. C. (2003). *Alexander's care of the patient in surgery* (12th ed.). St. Louis, MO: Mosby.

Ryan, J., & Phelan, M. (2004). Fracture risk: The bare bones. *Nursing in the Community, 5*(2), 25–26, 28.

Siddle, L. (2004). The challenge and management of phantom limb pain after amputation. *British Journal of Nursing, 13*(11), 664–667.

Smith, B. L. (2005). How to manage that pelvic fracture. *RN, 68*(8), 30–35.

Smith, G. R. (2004). Trauma library in review. Rib fracture pain and disability: Can we do better? *Journal of Trauma Nursing, 11*(1), 40.

Sprauve, D. (2003). Action stat. Hip fracture. *Nursing, 33*(11 Part 1), 88.

Think 'osteoporosis' if older woman has fracture history. (2005). *Practice Nurse, 29*(6), 8.

Uphold, C. R., & Graham, M. V. (2003). *Clinical guidelines in adult health* (3rd ed.). Gainesville, FL: Barmarrae Books.

Wilkinson, J. M. (2005). *Nursing diagnosis handbook* (8th ed.). Upper Saddle River, NJ: Prentice Hall.

Young, T. (2004). The healing of amputation wounds. *Nursing Standard, 18*(45), 74, 76, 78.

Zemke, L. (2005). They cut off your what? Strategies for managing amputation clients. *CareManagement, 11*(1), 24–26.

CHAPTER 43

Acupuncture, magnets relieve knee pain. (2005). *Clinical Advisor, 8*(3), 10.

Alper, B. S. (2005). Evidence-based medicine. Exercising reduces pain and disability from knee osteoarthritis. *Clinical Advisor, 8*(8), 108–109.

Bauer, J., & Roman, L. (Eds.) (2005). Clinical highlights. Adding acupuncture helps patients with arthritic knees. *RN, 68*(3), 27.

Becker, M. (2004). Osteoporosis: Essentials for diagnosis and management. *The American Journal for Nurse Practitioners, 8*(2), 49–57.

Brown, S. (2003). Clinical. Systemic lupus erythematosus. *Nursing Times, 99*(40), 30–32.

Brown, S. (2005). Managing systemic lupus erythematosus. *Nurse 2 Nurse, 4*(11), 28–30.

Bruce, M. L., & Peck, B. (2005). New rheumatoid arthritis treatments. *Holistic Nursing Practice, 19*(5), 197–206.

Burks, K. (2005). Osteoarthritis in older adults: Current treatments. *Journal of Gerontological Nursing, 31*(5), 11–19, 59–60.

Chatterjee, M. (2004). Nurses improve arthritis care. *Nursing Times, 100*(24), 6.

Copstead, L. C., & Banasik, J. L. (2005). *Pathophysiology* (3rd ed.). St. Louis, MO: Elsevier/Saunders.

D'Arcy, Y. (2005). Controlling pain. Following new guidelines to treat fibromyalgia pain. *Nursing, 35*(10), 17–18.

Edmonds, A. R., & Holm, G. B. (2004). Managing pain in osteoarthritis and rheumatoid arthritis. *CE-Today for Nurse Practitioners, 3*(7), 19–27.

Fontaine, K. L. (2005). *Healing practices: Alternative therapies for nursing* (2nd ed.). Upper Saddle River, NJ: Prentice Hall Health.

Holcomb, S. S. (2005). Boning up on osteoporosis. *Nursing Made Incredibly Easy! 3*(2), 6–7, 9–12, 14–15+.

Kamienski, M. (2003). Gout: Not just for the rich and famous! Everyman's disease. *Orthopaedic Nursing, 22*(1), 16–22.

Kasper, D. L., Braunwald, E., Fauci, A. S., Hauser, S. L., Longo, D. L., & Jameson, J. L. (Eds.). (2005). *Harrison's Principles of internal medicine* (16th ed.). New York: McGraw Hill.

Knisley, J., & Johnson, M. (2004). Lyme disease: Knowledge is the best prevention. *Nurse Practitioner: American Journal of Primary Health Care, 29*(8), 34–37, 39–40, 43–45.

Lucas, B. (2004). Nursing management issues in hip and knee replacement surgery. *British Journal of Nursing, 13*(13), 782–787.

McCance, K. L., & Huether, S. E. (2006). *Pathophysiology: The biologic basis for disease in adults & children* (5th ed.). St. Louis, MO: Mosby.

McClintock, R. (2004). What can you say about systemic lupus erythematosus? *Nursing, 34*(8), Hospital Nursing 32hn1–32hn2, 32hn4.

NANDA International. (2005). *Nursing Diagnoses: Definitions and Classification 2005–2006.* Philadelphia: Author.

Oliver, S., & Hill, J. (2005). Continuing professional development. Arthritis in the older person: Part 1. *Nursing Older People, 17*(4), 25–29.

Oliver, S., & Ryan, S. (2004). Effective pain management for patients with arthritis. *Nursing Standard, 18*(50), 43–52, 54.

Ostrov, B. E., & Kase, E. M. (2004). Intricacies in the diagnosis and treatment of gout. *Patient Care for the Nurse Practitioner, 2004* (Oct. 1), 2 p.

Overstreet, M. L. (2005). Lyme disease: The dangerous hitchhiker. *Nursing Made Incredibly Easy! 3*(3), 38–39, 41–44.

Peterson, J. (2005). Understanding fibromyalgia and its treatment options. *Nurse Practitioner: American Journal of Primary Health Care, 30*(1), 48–57.

Porth, C. M. (2005). *Pathophysiology: Concepts of altered health states* (7th ed.). Philadelphia: Lippincott.

Pullen, R. L., Cannon, J. D., & Rushing, J. D. (2003). Managing organ-threatening systemic lupus erythematosus. *Medsurg Nursing, 12*(16), 368–379.

Rooney, J. (2004). Don't get out of joint: Understanding the differences between osteoarthritis and rheumatoid arthritis. *Nursing Made Incredibly Easy! 2*(2), 26–31, 33–35.

Rooney, J. (2004). Oh, those aching joints: What you need to know about arthritis. *Nursing, 34*(11), 58–64.

Rothrock, J. C. (2003). *Alexander's care of the patient in surgery* (12th ed.). St. Louis, MO: Mosby.

Schettler, A. E., & Gustafson, E. M. (2004). Osteoporosis prevention starts in adolescence. *Journal of the American Academy of Nurse Practitioners, 16*(7), 274–282.

Schultz, M. A., Hernández, N. E., & Hernández, J. (2004). Help patients cope with fibromyalgia. *RN, 67*(9), 45, 46–50, 74–75.

Shaver, J. L. (2004). Fibromyalgia syndrome in women. *Nursing Clinics of North America, 39*(1), 195–204.

Sheff, E. K. (2005). Solving the mystery of osteomyelitis. *Nursing, 35*(7), Hospital Nursing 32hn1–32hn3.

Taylor, A. C., & de Beer, J. (2004). What to do when the complaint is a worn-out knee. *Patient Care for the Nurse Practitioner, 2004*(Aug.), 7 p.

Think 'osteoporosis' if older woman has fracture history. (2005). *Practice Nurse, 29*(6), 8.

Tierney, L. M. Jr., McPhee, S. J., & Papadakis, M. A. (Eds.). (2005). *Current medical diagnosis & treatment* (44th ed.). New York: McGraw Hill.

Waxman, J. (2005). The best approach to relieving fibromyalgia. *Clinical Advisor, 8*(8), 22, 25–27.

Wilkinson, J. M. (2005). *Nursing diagnosis handbook* (8th ed.). Upper Saddle River, NJ: Prentice Hall.

CHAPTER 44

Pagana, K. D., & Pagana, T. J. (2003). *Mosby's diagnostic and laboratory test reference* (6th ed.). St. Louis, MO: Mosby.

Porth, C. M. (2005). *Pathophysiology: Concepts of altered health states* (7th ed.). Philadelphia: Lippincott Williams & Wilkins.

CHAPTER 45

Abrams, A. C. (2004). *Clinical drug therapy* (7th ed.). Philadelphia: Lippincott Williams & Wilkins.

Agency for Health Care Policy and Research. (1992). *Pressure ulcers in adults: Prediction and prevention.* Rockville, MO: U.S. Department of Health and Human Services.

American Academy of Dermatologists. (2004). *What is eczema?* Available at www.skincarephysicians.com/eczemanet

Lehne, R. A. (2004). *Pharmacology for nursing care* (5th ed.). St. Louis, MO: Saunders.

Mayo Clinic. (2004). *Boils and carbuncles.* Available at www.mayoclinic.com

National Cancer Institute. (2005). *What you need to know about melanoma.* Available at www.cancer.gov/cancertopics/wynto/melanoma/allpages

Porth, C. M. (2005). *Pathophysiology: Concepts of altered health states* (7th ed.). Philadelphia: Lippincott Williams & Wilkins.

Quillen, T. F. (2004). Easing the heartbreak of prosiasis. *Nursing2004, 34*(11), 18–19.

U.S. Preventive Services Task Force (2004). Counseling to prevent skin cancer: Recommendations and rationale. *American Journal of Nursing, 104*(4), 87–91.

CHAPTER 46

Abrams, A. C. (2004). *Clinical drug therapy* (7th ed.). Philadelphia: Lippincott Williams & Wilkins.

Friedman, M. (1986). *Family nursing: Theory and assessment.* East Norwalk, CT: Appleton-Century-Crofts.

Giger, J., & Davidhizar, R. (2004). *Transcultural nursing: Assessment and intervention* (4th ed.). St. Louis, MO: Mosby Year Book.

Lehne, R. A. (2004). *Pharmacology for nursing care* (5th ed.). St. Louis, MO: Saunders.

Murray, R., Meili, P., & Zentner, J. (1993). The family—the basic unit for the developing person. In Murray, R., & Zentner, J. (Eds.), *Nursing concepts for health promotion* (5th ed.). Englewood Cliffs, NJ: Prentice Hall.

National Institutes of Health. (2005). *Trauma, burn, shock, and injury: Facts and figures.* Available at www.nigms.nih.gov/news/facts/traumaburnfactsfigures.html

Osborn, K. (2003). Nursing burn injuries. *Nursing Management, 34*(5), 49–56.

Porth, C. M. (2005). *Pathophysiology: Concepts of altered health states* (7th ed.). Philadelphia: Lippincott Williams & Wilkins.

Regojo, P. S. (2003). Burn care basics. *Nursing2003, 33*(3), 50–53.

Sole, M. L., Klein, D. G., & Moseley, M. J. (2005). *Introduction to critical care nursing* (4th ed.). St. Louis, MO: Elsevier.

Wilson, B. A., Shannon, M. T., & Stang, C. L. (2004). *Nurses's drug guide 2004.* Upper Saddle River, NJ: Prentice Hall.

CHAPTER 47

American Psychiatric Association. (2000). *Diagnostic and statistical manual of mental disorders* (4th ed., text revision). Washington, DC: Author.

Hockenberry, M. J. (2005). *Wong's essentials of pediatric nursing* (7th ed.) St. Louis, MO: Mosby.

Murray, C., & Lopez, A. (1996). *The global burden of disease: A comprehensive assessment of mortality and disability from disease, injuries, and risk factors in 1990 and projected to 2020.* Cambridge, MA: Harvard University Press.

National Institute of Mental Health. (2001). *The numbers count: Mental disorders in America.* (NIMH Publication No. 01-4584). Retrieved June 15, 2005, from www.nimh.nih.gov/publicat/numbers/cfm

Patterson, J. (1995). Promoting resilience in families experiencing stress. *Pediatric Clinics of North America, 42,* 1, 47–63.

Torrey, E. F. (2001). *Surviving schizophrenia: A manual for families, consumers, and providers* (4th ed.). New York: Quill, HarperCollins.

CHAPTER 48

Amador, X. (2001). *I am not sick, I don't need help! Helping the seriously mentally ill accept treatment.* Peconic, NY: Vida Press.

American Psychiatric Association. (2000). *Diagnostic and statistical manual of mental disorders* (4th ed., text revision). Washington, DC: Author.

Anders, R. L. (2000). Assessment of inpatient treatment of persons with schizophrenia: Implications for practice. *Archives of Psychiatric Nursing, 14*(5), 213–221.

Battle, Y., et al. (1999). Seasonality and infectious diseases in schizophrenia: The birth hypothesis revisited. *Journal of Psychiatric Research, 33,* 501.

Dixon, L., & Rebori, T. A. (1995). Psychosocial treatment of substance abuse in schizophrenic patients. In T. A. Kerr (Ed.), *Contemporary issues in treatment of schizophrenia.* Washington, DC: American Psychiatric Press.

Frederick, J., & Cotanch, P. (1995). Self help techniques for auditory hallucinations. *Issues in Mental Health Nursing, 16,* 213.

Goff, D. C., & Coyle, J. T. (2001). The emerging role of glutamate in the pathophysiology and treatment of schizophrenia. *American Journal of Psychiatry, 158*(9), 1367–1376.

Harrison, P. J., & Owen, M. J. (2003). Genes for schizophrenia? Recent findings and their pathophysiological implications. *Lancet, 361,* 417–419.

Keltner, N. L., Schwecke, L. H., & Bostrom, C. E. (2003). *Psychiatric nursing* (4th ed.). St. Louis, MO: Mosby.

Kennedy, M. G., Schepp, K. G., & O'Connor, F. W. (2000). Symptom self-management and relapse in schizophrenia. *Archives of Psychiatric Nursing, 14*(6), 266–275.

Mills, J. (2000). Dealing with voices and strange thoughts. In C. Gamble & G. Brennan (Eds.), *Working with serious mental illness: A manual for clinical practice.* London: Bailliere Tindall.

Rankin, E. A. (2000). *Quick reference for psychopharmacology.* Albany, NY: Delmar.

Schultz, J. M., & Videbeck, S. L. (2002). *Lippincott's manual of psychiatric nursing care plans* (6th ed.). Philadelphia: Lippincott.

Stuart, G. W., & Laraia, M. T. (2001). *Principles and practice of psychiatric nursing* (7th ed.). St. Louis, MO: Mosby.

Torrey, E. F. (1997). *Out of the shadows: Confronting America's mental illness crisis.* New York: John Wiley.

Torrey, E. F. (2001). *Surviving schizophrenia: A manual for families, consumers, and providers* (4th ed.). New York: Harper Collins.

Videbeck, S. L. (2004). *Psychiatric mental health nursing.* Philadelphia: Lippincott.

CHAPTER 49

American Psychiatric Association. (2000). *Diagnostic and statistical manual of mental disorders* (4th ed., text revision). Washington, DC: Author.

Beck, A. T., & Rush, A. J. (1995). Cognitive therapy. In H. I. Kaplan & B. J. Sadock (Eds.), *Comprehensive textbook of psychiatry IV* (Vol. 2). Baltimore: Williams & Wilkins.

Bowden, C. L. (2003). Improving bipolar outcomes across the life cycle. In *American Psychiatric Association 156th Annual Meeting, Bipolar CME.* Retrieved July 31, 2003, from www.medscape.com/viewprogram/2469_pnt

Caspi, A., Sugden, K., Moffitt, T., Taylor, A., Craig, I., Harrington, H., McClay, J., Mill, J., Martin, J., Braithwaite, A., & Poulton, R. (2003). Influence of life stress on depression: Moderation by a polymorphism in the 5-HTT gene. *Science, 301,* 386.

Depression Guideline Panel. (1993). *Depression in primary care: Volume 2. Treatment of major depression. Clinical practice guideline, Number 5* (AHCPR Pub. No. 93-0551). Rockville, MD: U.S. Department of Health and Human Services, Public Health Service, Agency for Health Care Policy and Research.

Keltner, N. L., Schwecke, L. H., & Bostrom, C. E. (2003). *Psychiatric nursing* (4th ed.). St. Louis, MO: Mosby.

Mellman, T. A., Miller, A. L., Weissman, E. M., Crimson, M. L., Essock, S. M., & Marder, S. R. (2001). Evidence-based pharmacologic treatment for people with severe mental illness: A focus on guidelines and algorithms. *Psychiatric Services, 52*(5), 619–625.

Mendelowitz, A. J., Dawkins, K., & Lieberman, J. A. (2000). Antidepressants. In J. A. Lieberman & A. Tasman (Eds.), *Psychiatric drugs.* Philadelphia: W. B. Saunders.

Post, R. M. (1992). Transduction of psychosocial stress in the neurobiology of affective disorders. *American Journal of Psychiatry, 149,* 999.

Rives, W. (1999). Emergency department assessment of suicidal patients. *Psychiatric Clinics of North America, 22*(4), 779–787.

Roach, M. J., et al. (1998). Depressed mood and survival in seriously ill hospitalized adults, *Archives of Internal Medicine, 158,* 397.

Roy, A. (1999). Psychiatric emergencies: Suicide. In H. I. Kaplan & B. J. Sadock (Eds.), *Comprehensive textbook of psychiatry* (7th ed., Vol. 2). Philadelphia: Lippincott.

Sheikh, J. I., & Yesavage, J. A. (1986). Geriatric depression scale: Recent evidence and development of a shorter form. *Clinical Gerontologist, 5,* 165–172.

Sonne, S. C., & Brady, K. T. (1999). Substance abuse and bipolar comorbidity. *Psychiatric Clinics of North America, 22*(3), 609–628.

Thase, M. E. (1999). Mood disorders: Neurobiology. In H. I. Kaplan & B. J. Sadock (Eds.), *Comprehensive textbook of psychiatry* (7th ed. Vol. 1). Philadelphia: Lippincott.

U.S. Public Health Service. (1999) *The surgeon general's call to action to prevent suicide.* Washington, DC: Author.

CHAPTER 50

American Psychiatric Association (2000). *Diagnostic and statistical manual of mental disorders* (4th ed., text revision). Washington, DC: Author.

Carpenito, L. (2000). *Handbook of Nursing Diagnosis* (8th ed.). Philadelphia: Lippincott Williams & Wilkins.

Fontaine, K. L. (2003). *Mental health nursing* (5th ed.). Upper Saddle River, NJ: Pearson.

Goodwin, D. W. (1986). *Anxiety.* New York: Oxford University Press.

Hardy, S. E., Concato, J., & Gill, T. M. (2004). Resilience of community-dwelling older persons. *Journal of the American Gerontological Society, 52*(2), 257–263.

Hendrix, M. L., & Dickey, M. (2004). *Anxiety disorder* (NIH Publication No. 00-3879). Retrieved May 7, 2005, from www.nimh.nih.gov/anxiety/

Keltner, N. L., Schwecke, L. H., & Bostrom, C. E. (2003). *Psychiatric nursing* (4th ed.). St. Louis, MO: Mosby.

Kushner, M. G., Sher, K. J., & Beltman, B. D. (1990). The relation between alcohol problems and the anxiety disorders. *American Journal of Psychiatry, 147*(6), 685–695.

National Institute of Mental Health (2001). *Anxiety disorder* (NIH Publication No. 00-3879). Retrieved August 25, 2002 from http://www.nimh.nih.gov/anxiety/anxiety.cfm

Peplau, H. (1989). Theoretical constructs: Anxiety, self, and hallucinations. In A. O'Toole & S. Welt (Eds.), *Interpersonal theory in nursing practice. Selected works of Hildegard E. Peplau.* New York: Springer.

Rankin, E. A. (2000). *Quick reference for psychopharmacology.* Albany, NY: Delmar.

Rauch, S. L., Baer, L., Breiten, H. C., Fischman, A. J., Manzo, P. A., Moretti, C., & Jenike, M. A. (1995). A positron emission tomographic study of simple phobic symptom provocation. *Archives of General Psychiatry, 52,* 20–28.

Schultz, J. M., & Videbeck, S. L. (2002). *Psychiatric nursing care plans.* Philadelphia: Lippincott.

Spear, H. L. (1996). Anxiety: When to worry, what to do. *RN, 59*(7), 40–45.

Stevens, J. C., & Pollack, M. H. (2005). Benzodiazepines in clinical practice: Consideration of their long term use and alternative agents. *Journal of Clinical Psychiatry, 66*(Suppl 2), 21–27.

Stuart, G. W. (2001). Anxiety responses and anxiety disorders. In G. W. Stuart & M. T. Laraia (Eds.), *Principles and practice of psychiatric nursing* (7th ed.). St. Louis, MO: Mosby.

CHAPTER 51

American Psychiatric Association. (2000). *Diagnostic and statistical manual of mental disorders* (4th ed., text revision). Washington, DC: Author.

Gallop, R., Lancee, W., & Shugar, G. (1993). Residents' and nurses' perceptions of difficult to treat short-stay patients. *Hospital and Community Psychiatry, 44,* 352–357.

Koerner, K., & Linehan, M. (2000). Research on dialectical behavior therapy for patients with borderline personality disorder. *Psychiatric Clinics of North America, 23*(1), 151–167.

Limandri, B., & Boyd, M. A. (2002). Personality and impulse control disorders. In M. A. Boyd (Ed.), *Psychiatric nursing: Contemporary practice.* Philadelphia: Lippincott.

Linehan, M. (1993). *Cognitive-behavioral treatment of borderline personality disorder.* New York: The Guilford Press.

Mayo Clinic Staff. (2004). *Personality disorders.* Retrieved June 15, 2005, from www.mayoclinic.com/invoke.cfm?id=DS00562

Millon, T., & Davis, R. (1999). *Personality disorders in modern life.* New York: John Wiley & Sons.

National Institute of Mental Health. (2001). *Borderline personality disorder* (NIH Publication No. 01-4928). Retrieved June 13, 2005, from www.mental-health-matters.com/articles/nimh001.php?artID=227

Stern, A. (1938). Psychoanalytic investigation of and therapy in the borderline group of neuroses. *Psychoanalytic Quarterly, 7,* 467–489.

Warner, C. E. (2004). *Borderline personality disorder: Struggling, understanding, succeeding.* Eau Claire, WI: PESI HealthCare.

Wood, D. (2003). *What is paranoid personality disorder? A mental health matters article.* Retrieved June 13, 2005, from www.mental-health-matters.com/articles/dw001.php?artID=66

Zanarini, M. C. (2000). Childhood experiences associated with the development of borderline personality disorder. *Psychiatric Clinics of North America, 23*(1), 89–101.

CHAPTER 52

American Psychiatric Association. (2000). *Diagnostic and statistical manual of mental disorders* (4th ed., text revision). Washington, DC: Author.

American Society of Addiction Medicine. (1997). Public policy statement on nicotine dependence and tobacco. *Journal of Addiction Disorders 16,* 99.

El-Mallakh, P. (1998). Treatment models for clients with co-occurring addictive and mental disorders. *Archives of Psychiatric Nursing, 12*(2), 71.

Ewing, J. A. (1984). Detecting alcoholism: The CAGE questionnaire. *Journal of the American Medical Association, 252,* 1902–1907.

Freed, P. E., & York, L. N. (1997). Naltrexone: A controversial therapy for alcohol dependence. *Journal of Psychosocial Nursing, 35*(7), 24–28.

Gordon, C., Williams, B., & Lapin, P. (2001). New program to help seniors quit smoking. *Nursing Spectrum, 2*(10), 18–19.

Keltner, N. L., Schwecke, L. H., & Bostrom, C. E. (2003). *Psychiatric nursing* (4th ed.). St. Louis, MO: Mosby.

Kneisl, C. R., Wilson, H. S., & Trigoboff, E. (2004). *Contemporary psychiatric-mental health nursing.* Upper Saddle River, NJ: Pearson Education.

Lehman, A. (1987). Assessment and classification of clients with psychiatric and substance abuse problems. *Hospital and Community Psychiatry, 40*(10), 1019.

McCloskey, J. C., & Bulechek, G. M. (Eds.). (2000). *Nursing intervention classification (NIC)* (4th ed.). St. Louis, MO: Mosby.

Mynatt, S. (1996). A model of contributing risk factors to chemical dependency in nurses. *Journal of Psychosocial Nursing, 34,* 13.

Naegle, M. A., & D'Avanzo, C. E. (2001). *Addictions and substance abuse strategies for advanced practice nursing.* Upper Saddle River, NJ: Prentice Hall Health.

National Institute on Drug Abuse, National Institutes of Health. (2005). *NIDA InfoFacts: Steroids (anabolic-androgenic).* Retrieved May 29, 2005, from www.drugabuse.gov/infofacts/Steroids.html

Index

Note: Figures and tables, denoted by *f* and *t*, are generally cited only when they appear outside the text discussion.

A

A-delta fibers, 138, 139*f*, 140, 140*f*
AACN (American Association of Colleges of Nursing), 310
Abacavir, 242*t*
ABCD rule, 1103
Abdomen
    acute abdomen, 445
    muscles, 1008*f*
    in older adult, 62
    palpation, 391
    physical assessment, 64*t*, 68–69, 68*f*
    preparation for surgery, 176*f*
    quadrants and associated organs, 68, 68*f*, 392*f*
Abdominal aortic aneurysm, 677, 677*t*
Abdominal breathing, 558, 559
Abdominal procedures
    abdominoperineal resection, 456
    laparoscopy, 813
        appendectomy, 444
        female reproductive system, 812, 812*f*
    ultrasound, 812*t*
    x-ray, 394*t*
        bowel obstruction, 461
        cardiovascular, 602*t*
Abducens nerve, 900*t*
Ablation
    in cardiac dysrhythmia, 634
    endometrial, 844
Abrasion, 297*f*
    corneal, 342, 976
    dermabrasion for acne, 1094
Abscess, 194
    anorectal, 466
    brain. *See* Brain abscess
    incision and drainage, 194
    lung, 550
    pancreatic, 490
    in peritonitis, 445
    peritonsillar, 515
Absence seizure, 932
Absorbents, for diarrhea, 433–434, 435*t*
Absorption of drugs
    in older adult, 79
    process and rate, 77, 77*f*
    routes, 77, 78*t*
Abstinence
    from drug use, 1228
    from sexual activity, 881
Abuse, spiral fracture in, 1029. *See also* Alcohol use and abuse; Substance use and abuse
Acarbose, for diabetes mellitus, 366*t*
Acceptance, in death and dying, 307–308
Accessory nerve, 900*t*
Accidents. *See* Burn injury; Injury; Trauma
Accommodation (visual), 65, 902
ACE inhibitors. *See* Angiotensin-converting enzyme (ACE) inhibitors

Acebutolol, for cardiac dysrhythmia, 632*t*
Acetaminophen, 143, 144*t*
    for cerebral aneurysm, 932
    for headaches, 940
    for increased intracranial pressure, 916
    for osteoarthritis, 1057
    for otitis media, 991
Acetazolamide
    for glaucoma, 983*t*
    for heart failure, 645*t*–646*t*
Acetylcholine
    mental disorders and, 1138*t*
    in Parkinson's disease, 952–953
Acetylsalicylic acid. *See* Aspirin
Acid-base balance
    assessment, 126, 126*t*
    regulation, 123–124, 124*f*
Acid-base disorders, 123–135. *See also specific disorder*
    acidosis *vs.* alkalosis, 124–125
    assessment, 125–126, 126*t*
    metabolic acidosis, 125*f*, 126–129
    metabolic alkalosis, 125*f*, 129–130
    respiratory acidosis, 125*f*, 130–132, 135
    respiratory alkalosis, 125*f*, 132–133
Acid-fast bacilli smear, 547
Acid-fast stain, 506, 508*t*
Acid therapy for warts, 1100
Acidosis, 124–125, 124*f*. *See also specific condition*
    etiology and manifestations, 128*t*
    metabolic, 125*f*, 126–129
    respiratory, 125*f*, 130–132
Acne, 1092–1096
    client education/continuing care, 1096
        medications, 1094*t*
        therapeutic baths, 1093
    interdisciplinary care, 1092–1094
        complementary therapy, 1094
        diagnostic tests, 1093
        medications, 1094, 1094*t*
        surgery, 1094
        therapeutic baths, 1093
    nursing care
        assessing, 1094–1095
        body image, 1095
        deficient knowledge, 1096
        diagnosing, planning, and implementing, 1095–1096
        evaluating, 1096
        skin integrity, 1095
    pathophysiology and manifestations, 1092, 1092*f*
Acne rosacea, 1092
Acne vulgaris, 1092
Acoustic neuroma, 921*t*
Acquired hemolytic anemia, 716
Acquired hernia, 462
Acquired immunodeficiency syndrome. *See* HIV/AIDS
Acromegaly, 336
Acrophobia, 1193*t*
ACTH (adrenocorticotropic hormone), 326*t*, 327*f*
Acting out, 1195*t*
Action potential, 595
Activated partial thromboplastin time (APTT), 687, 706*t*

Active immunity, 226
Active transport, 94–95, 95*f*
Activity. *See* Exercise
Activity intolerance, nursing care
    in Addison's disease, 353
    in anemia, 719
    in heart failure, 648–649
    in hepatitis, 479
    in hypothyroidism, 345
    in lung cancer, 566–567
    in pneumonia, 543
    in rheumatic fever/heart disease, 652
    in valvular heart disease, 662
Acupuncture, 148
Acute, 22*t*
Acute abdomen, 445
Acute asthma, 551, 551*f*
Acute bacterial pneumonia, 539
Acute bronchitis
    interdisciplinary care, 538
    nursing care, 538
    pathophysiology and manifestations, 538
Acute cholecystitis, 472
Acute coronary syndromes, 609
Acute endocarditis, 653
Acute epiglottitis, 516
Acute gastritis. *See* Gastritis
Acute glomerulonephritis, 767–768
Acute gouty arthritis, 1068
Acute heart failure, 644
Acute illness, 23
Acute inflammation
    pain in, 198
    pathophysiology and manifestations, 193–194, 195*f*
Acute lymphoblastic leukemia, 721, 721*t*
Acute mastoiditis, 990
Acute myelocytic leukemia, 721, 721*t*
    critical thinking care map, 740
Acute myocardial infarction (AMI), 618–625
    client education/continuing care, 624
    interdisciplinary care
        cardiac rehabilitation, 622
        diagnostic tests, 620, 620*f*
        invasive devices, 622, 622*f*
        laboratory tests, 620, 620*t*
        medical management, 620–621
        medication, 621
        revascularization, 621–622
    nursing care
        assessing, 622, 623
        coping, 623–624
        diagnosing, planning, and implementing, 622–624
        evaluating, 624
        fear, 624
        pain, 622–623
        tissue perfusion, 623
        nursing process care plan, 624–625
    pathophysiology and manifestations, 618–620
        cocaine-induced AMI, 619
        complications, 619–620
        in women and older adults, 619
Acute otitis media, 990, 990*f*

Group A beta-hemolytic streptococcus, 515, 651
Group therapy, for bipolar disorder, 1178
Growth hormone (GH)
    function, 326t, 327f
    normal values, 330t
Guaifenesin, for pneumonia, 540
Guanabenz, for hypertension, 672t
Guanfacine, for hypertension, 672t
Guided imagery for pain management, 148
Guillain-Barré syndrome
    interdisciplinary care, 958
    nursing care, 958
    pathophysiology and manifestations, 958
Guillotine amputation, 1038
Gynecologic surgery site preparation, 176f
Gynecomastia, 329, 822

H

H₂ receptor antagonists, preoperative
        administration, 168t
HAART (highly active antiretroviral therapy),
        237–238, 241
Haemophilus ducreyi, 878t
Haemophilus influenzae meningitis, 936t
Hair
    health history, 1083
    in middle adult years, 17t
    in older adult, 35t, 62, 1087
    physical examination, 62, 63t, 65, 1085
    preoperative removal of, 168, 176–177, 176f
    structure and function, 1082t, 1083, 1083f
    in young adult, 16t
Halazepam, for anxiety, 1197t
Half-life of drugs, 79
Hallucination, 1147t
    client experiencing, nursing care checklist, 1158
    in schizophrenia, 1149
        auditory, client education/continuing care, 1159
Hallucinogens, 1225t, 1229
Hallux valgus
    client education/continuing care, 1056
    nursing care
        infection risk, 1056
        pain, 1056
    pathophysiology and manifestations, 1055, 1055f
Halo vest
    nursing care checklist, 965
    for spinal cord injury, 964, 964f
Haloperidol
    for Huntington's disease, 957
    Parkinson's disease and, 952
    for schizophrenia, 1156
HALT, substance abuse and, 1234
Hammertoe
    client education/continuing care, 1056
    nursing care
        infection risk, 1056
        pain, 1056
    pathophysiology and manifestations, 1055, 1055f
Hand
    fracture, 1029t
    preparation for surgery, 176f
Hand washing, 208
Handicap, 52
Handicapped client, critical thinking care map, 55
Handouts, literacy levels and, 431

Hashimoto's thyroiditis, 344
Hashish. *See* Cannabis
Hawthorn, for heart failure, 646
HCO₃, in arterial blood gases, 126, 126t
HDL. *See* High-density lipoprotein
Head
    imaging, in respiratory dysfunction, 509t
    physical examination, 63t, 65–66, 65f, 66f
    preparation for surgery, 176f
    tissue perfusion in inhalation injury, nursing
        care, 578
Head injury, 912–920
    client education/continuing care, 919–920
    complications
        cerebral edema, 914–915, 915t
        increased intracranial pressure, 912–914
    interdisciplinary care
        diagnostic tests, 915–916
        ICP monitoring, 916–917
        medications, 916
        surgery, 917, 917f
    nursing care
        assessing, 917, 918
        breathing pattern, 918
        diagnosing, planning, and implementing, 917–919
        evaluating, 919–920
        infection risk, 919
        mobility, 919
        nutrition, 918–919
        skin integrity, 919
        tissue perfusion, 917–918
    nursing process care plan, increased intracranial
        pressure and altered level of consciousness, 920
    pathophysiology and manifestations, 912, 913t
Headaches, 939–941
    client education/continuing care, 941
    increased intracranial pressure and, 914
    interdisciplinary care
        complementary therapy, 940
        medications, 940
    nursing care
        assessing, 941
        pain, 940–941
    pathophysiology and manifestations, 939t
        cluster headache, 940
        migraine, 940
        tension headache, 940
    risk factors, 939t
Healing
    of fracture, 1021, 1022f–1023f
    in inflammatory response, 193
    of wounds. *See* Wound healing
Health, 20–21, 20f. *See also* Health maintenance
Health care clinics, 44
Health care proxy, 310
Health care settings, 44–45
    infection in. *See* Nosocomial infections
    latex allergy sources in, 229
Health care surrogate, 310
Health history, 59–60, 59t
    cardiovascular, 598
    endocrine, 328–329
    gastrointestinal, 389, 391
    hematologic/lymphatic, 706
    information included in, 59t
    integumentary, 1083–1084

musculoskeletal, 1010
neurologic, 903–904
reproductive, 807–808
urinary, 748–749
Health-illness continuum, 20, 20f
Health maintenance
    healthy behaviors
        mental disorders and, 1159
        in middle adult, 18
        in older adult, 38
        in young adult, 17
    ineffective, nursing care
        in glaucoma, 984
        in hypertension, 674
        in low back pain, 1072–1073
        in sexually transmitted infections, 879–880, 882
    in older adult, 39–40, 39t–40t, 40f
    promoting, 21, 21t
Healthy Eating Pyramid, 400f, 401
Hearing. *See also* Ear
    assessment, 904
        in older adult, 62, 905
    at end-of-life, 312
    process of, 903
Hearing aids, 995, 997f
Hearing loss, 995–998
    age-related, critical thinking care map, 1000
    client education/continuing care, 998
    interdisciplinary care
        amplification, 995, 997f
        diagnostic tests, 995
        surgery, 995–996
    nursing care
        assessing, 996
        diagnosing, planning, and implementing,
            996–997
        evaluating, 998
        sensory perception, 996–997
        social isolation, 997–998
        verbal communication, 997
    in otosclerosis, 992–993
    pathophysiology and manifestations
        conductive hearing loss, 995
        presbycusis, 995
        sensorineural hearing loss, 995
Heart. *See also* Cardiovascular system
    antipsychotics and, 1155
    assessment, 63t–64t, 67, 67f, 69f
    cardiac cycle, 596, 596f
    cardiac output, 596
    conduction system, 595–596, 595f
    coronary circulation, 595
    in older adult, 642
    primary dysfunction. *See* Cardiac disorders
    secondary conditions affecting
        alcoholism, 1227, 1227f
        hypertension, 670t
    size and location, 594, 594f
    structure, 594–595, 594f, 595f
    transplantation, 647, 647f
Heart block, 626
Heart disease. *See* Coronary heart disease; Rheumatic
        fever and rheumatic heart disease; Valvular
        heart disease
Heart failure, 642–650
    acute *vs.* chronic, 644

Iron preparations
 for anemia, 717, 717t
 for dysfunctional uterine bleeding, 844
 in renal failure, 787
 Z-track administration checklist, 718
Iron tests, 707, 708t
Irreducible hernia, 463
Irregular bones, 1006, 1007f
Irrelevant data, 10
Irreversible stage of shock, 285, 287
Irreversible sterility, 263
Irrigation
 closed *vs.* intermittent open system of gastric
  lavage, 415
 of colostomy, checklist, 460
 of ear, 990
 of eye, 977
 of infected sinus, 518
Irritable bowel syndrome (IBS)
 interdisciplinary care
  diagnostic tests, 441
  treatment, 441
 nursing care, 441
 pathophysiology and manifestations, 440
Irritable mood
 in depression, 1165
 in menopause, 841
Irritant laxatives, 439t
IRV (inspiratory reserve volume), 509, 510f
Ischemia
 in renal failure, 784
 during shock, 286
Ischemic, 609
Islets of Langerhans, 328
Isocarboxazid, for depression, 1170t
Isoelectric line, 600
Isoetharine, for asthma, 552t
Isograft, 232
Isolated systolic hypertension, 669
Isolation
 medical
  precautions, 208, 211
  Standard Precautions, 211
 social, nursing care
  in hearing loss, 997–998
  in urinary incontinence, 761
Isoniazid
 inactivation, biologic variability in, 28, 890
 for tuberculosis, 548t
Isoproterenol, for asthma, 552t
Isosorbide dinitrate, for angina pectoris, 613t
Isosorbide mononitrate, for angina pectoris, 613t
Isotonic solutions, 94, 94f
Isotretinoin, for acne, 1094, 1094t
Isradipine
 for angina pectoris, 613t
 for hypertension, 673t
Isthmus, 327
Itch-scratch-itch cycle, 1091
IV therapy, 98–102
 absorption rate, 77, 78t
 analgesic, 145, 146f
 common fluids in, 100t
 IV set, 100f
 nitroglycerin, for myocardial infarction, 621
 over-the-needle catheter, 102f

 procedure checklists, 99
  changing bag, tubing, and dressing site, 101
  initiating infusion, 103
 in shock, 293
 sites, 102f
IVP (intravenous pyelography), 751
 nursing care checklist, 752

J

Jackknife surgical position, 178t
Jacksonian march, 932
Jaundice, 62
 assessment, 1083
 in hepatitis, 477
Jejunum, 387
Joint and connective tissue disorders. *See also*
  specific disorder
 ankylosing spondylitis, 1071
 fibromyalgia, 1071–1072
 gout, 1068–1070
 low back pain, 1072–1073
 Lyme disease, 1070–1071
 muscular dystrophy, 1073
 osteoarthritis, 1056–1060
 rheumatoid arthritis, 1060–1065
 systemic lupus erythematous, 231, 1065–1068
Joint dislocation and subluxation
 interdisciplinary care, 1035
 nursing care, 1035
 pathophysiology and manifestations, 1035
Joint replacement. *See also* Hip
 nursing care checklist, 1058
 in osteoporosis, 1057–1058, 1058f
Joints
 dislocation and subluxation, 1035
 disorders. *See* Joint and connective tissue disorders
 motion, 1007t
 in older adult, 1007
 repetitive use injury, 1035–1037
 ROM assessment, 1010, 1011t
 types of, 1006–1007
Junctional dysrhythmias, 630
Juvenile-onset diabetes mellitus, 358. *See also*
  Diabetes mellitus
Juxtaglomerular apparatus, 748

K

Kanamycin, 209t
Kaolin and pectin, 435t
Kaposi's sarcoma, 240, 243t
Kcal (kilocalories), 389
Kegel exercises
 in fecal incontinence, 442
 in pelvic organ prolapse, 861
 in urinary incontinence, 761
Keloids, 1085t, 1122
Keratin, 1082
Keratitis, 974
Keratotomy, 978
Ketoacidosis, 367–368
Ketoconazole, 211t
 for skin infections, 1099, 1099t
Ketone bodies, 359
Ketones, 748t
 in diabetes mellitus, 360–361
 in endocrine disorders, 331t

Ketonuria, 367
Ketoprofen
 for inflammation, 197t
 for rheumatoid arthritis, 1062t
Ketorolac, 144t
 for inflammation, 197t
Ketosis, in diabetes mellitus, 359
Kidney(s). *See also* Renal system
 primary dysfunction. *See* Renal and urinary tract
  disorders
 secondary conditions affecting
  hypertension, 670t
  shock, 286f, 287
 structure and function, 746–747, 746f, 747f
  age-related functional change, 748, 749t
  blood pressure regulation, 598
  body fluid regulation, 95
  endocrine function, 748
  internal anatomy, 747f
  urine formation, 747–748
 trauma to, 777
 tumors. *See* Renal cancer
Kidney function tests, 105
Kidney stones. *See* Urinary calculi
Kidney transplant, 790–791, 791f
 nursing care checklist, 791
Kilocalories (kcal), 389
Kindling process, 1178
Kinetic continuous rotation bed, 299f
Knee
 above-knee amputation
  bandage technique, 1038, 1038f
  critical thinking care map, 1042
 ROM assessment, 1011t
 total knee replacement, 1057–1058, 1058f
Knowledge deficit. *See* Deficient knowledge, nursing care
Kock's ileostomy/pouch
 in bladder cancer, 778, 778t, 779f
 in inflammatory bowel disease, 451f
Korsakoff's syndrome, 1227
KUB (kidney, ureter, bladder) x-ray, 651
Kübler-Ross, Elisabeth, 307
Kupffer cells, 286, 388, 388f
Kwell, 1100
Kyphosis, 1046–1047
 client education/continuing care, 1047
 interdisciplinary care, 1046–1047
 nursing care, injury risk, 1047
 in osteoporosis, 1047, 1048f
 pathophysiology and manifestations, 1046, 1046f

L

Labetalol, for hypertension, 672t
Labia, 806–807, 806f
Labile mood, in intoxication, 1226
Laboratory tests. *See specific test, disorder, or condition*
Labyrinthitis
 client education/continuing care, 994
 interdisciplinary care, 993
 nursing care
  assessing, 993–994
  diagnosing, planning, and implementing, 994
  evaluating, 994
  sleep pattern, 994
  trauma risk, 994
 pathophysiology and manifestations, 993

Parenchymal cells, liver cancer and, 489
Parenteral drug administration, 77, 78*t*
Parenteral feedings, 405–406
Paresthesias, 714
Parietal cells, 386
Parietal lobe, 897*f*
Parietal lobe tumors, 921
Parietal pericardium, 594
Parietal pleura, 503, 503*f*
Parish nursing, 45
Parkinson's disease, 952–956
   client education/continuing care, 954*t*, 955–956
   etiology, 952
   interdisciplinary care
      complementary therapy, 953
      electrical stimulation, 953
      medications, 953, 954*t*
      surgery, 953
   nursing care
      assessing, 954, 955
      diagnosing, planning, and implementing,
         954–955
      evaluating, 955–956
      mobility, 955
      nutrition, 955
      verbal communication, 955
   pathophysiology and manifestations, 952–953, 953*f*
Paroxetine
   for depression, 1170*t*
   for premenstrual syndrome, 842
Paroxysm, 538
Paroxysmal nocturnal dyspnea (PND), 644
Partial assessment, 58
Partial gastrectomy, 425, 425*f*
Partial laryngectomy, 529
Partial seizures, 932
Partial-thickness burn, 1115*t*, 1116, 1116*f*
Partial thromboplastin time (PTT), 166, 167*t*, 706*t*
PASG (pneumatic antishock garment), 290, 290*f*
Passive immunity, 226
Passivity, in personality disorder, 1212
Patch (lesion), 1084*t*
Patch test, 230, 1086*t*
Pathogens, 200. *See also* Infection; Infection control;
      Microorganisms; Nosocomial infections
Pathologic fracture, 1021
   in multiple myeloma, 727
   in osteoporosis, 1047
Patient-controlled analgesia (PCA), 145, 146*f*
   in bone fracture, 1028
Patient Self-Determination Act, 310
PCA (patient-controlled analgesia), 145, 146*f*, 1208
PCM (protein-calorie malnutrition), 403
PCOS (polycystic ovary syndrome), 848
PCP. *See Pneumocystis carinii* pneumonia
PCR. *See* Percutaneous coronary revascularization
PDR (Physicians' Desk Reference), 77
Peak action, 79
Peak and trough levels, antibiotic, 206–207
Peak expiratory flow rate (PEFR), 551, 555
Peau d'orange skin, 864, 864*f*
Pediculosis
   client education/continuing care, 1101–1102
   interdisciplinary care, 1099
      diagnostic tests, 1099
      medications, 1100

nursing care
   acute pain, 1100
   assessing, 1100
   diagnosing, planning, and implementing,
      1100–1101
   evaluating, 1101–1102
   infection risk, 1101
   sleep pattern, 1100
pathophysiology and manifestations, 1098–1099
Pediculosis capitis, 1098
Pediculosis corporis, 1098
Pediculosis pubis, 1098–1099
PEEP (positive end-expiratory pressure), 581, 581*t*
PEFR (peak expiratory flow rate), 551, 555
Pelvic examination nursing care checklist, 809
Pelvic exenteration, in cervical cancer, 854
Pelvic floor exercises. *See* Kegel exercises
Pelvic fracture, 1030*t*
Pelvic inflammatory disease (PID), 851–853
   client education/continuing care, 852–853
   complications, 878*t*
   HIV/AIDS-related, 240
   interdisciplinary care
      diagnostic tests, 851
      medications, 851
      surgery, 852
   nursing care
      assessing, 852
      deficient knowledge, 852
      diagnosing, planning, and implementing, 852
      evaluating, 852–853
      injury risk, 852
   pathophysiology and manifestations, 851, 878*t*
Pelvic organ prolapse
   interdisciplinary care, 861
   nursing care, 861–862
   pathophysiology and manifestations, 861, 861*f*
Pelvic surgery risks, 845
Pelvic ultrasound, 812*t*
Penbutolol, for hypertension, 672*t*
Penectomy, 830
Penetrating trauma, 296
Penicillamine, for rheumatoid arthritis, 1062
Penicillin(s), 209*t*
   for meningitis, 937
   resistance to, 203*t*, 204
   for skin infections, 1099
   for STIs, 879*t*, 886
Penicillin-resistant *Streptococcus pneumoniae,* 203*t*, 204
Penicillinase-resistant agents, 209*t*
Penis
   assessment, 750, 750*f*
   cancer, 830
   client education/continuing care, 830
   ejaculatory dysfunction, 833–834
   erectile dysfunction, 830–833
   genital herpes on, 882*f*
   genital warts on, 883*f*
   nursing care, 830
   phimosis, 829
   priapism, 829–830
   structure and function, 804, 804*f*
Penrose drain, 181
Pentazocine, equianalgesic dosage chart, 145*t*
Pentoxifylline, for peripheral atherosclerosis, 681
Peptic ulcer, 420

Peptic ulcer disease (PUD), 420–425
   client education/continuing care, 418*t*–419*t*,
      423–424
   interdisciplinary care
      of complications, 421
      diagnostic tests, 421
      diet, 421
      medications, 418*t*–419*t*, 421
      surgery, 422
   manifestations and complications, 420–421
   nursing care
      assessing, 422
      cardiac output, 423
      diagnosing, planning, and implementing,
         422–423
      evaluating, 423–424
      nutrition, 423
      pain, 422–423
   nursing process care plan, 424–425
   pathophysiology, 420, 420*f*, 421*f*
Perception of pain. *See* Sensory perception
Percussion
   guidelines and methods, 61, 61*f*
   of kidney, 750, 750*f*
   in pneumonia, 541–542, 541*f*
Percutaneous balloon valvuloplasty, 661, 661*f*
Percutaneous cholecystostomy, 473
Percutaneous coronary revascularization (PCR)
   in angina pectoris, 614
   complications and nursing care, 615
   in myocardial infarction, 621–622
Percutaneous lithotripsy, 774, 774*f*
Percutaneous transluminal coronary angioplasty (PTCA)
   in angina pectoris, 614, 614*f*
   nursing care checklist, 612
Perforation
   of appendix, 443
   of colon, 449
   of eye, 976–977
   in peptic ulcer disease, 421
Pergolide, for Parkinson's disease, 954*t*
Perianal surgery nursing care checklist, 466
Pericardial effusion, 277, 656
Pericardial frictional rub, 656
Pericardiocentesis, 656, 656*f*
   nursing care checklist, 657
Pericarditis, 655–658
   client education/continuing care, 657–658
   interdisciplinary care, 656
      pericardiocentesis, 656, 656*f*, 657
   myocardial infarction and, 619
   nursing care
      breathing pattern, 657
      cardiac output, 657
      pain, 656–657
   pathophysiology and manifestations, 656
Pericardium, 594
Perimenopause, 839. *See also* Menopause
Perimetrium, 805*f*, 806
Perineal prostatectomy, 823*t*
Periodontal disease, 387–388
Periorbital ecchymosis, 912, 977
Periorbital edema, 65
Periosteum, 1006
Peripheral atherosclerosis, 680–683
   client education/continuing care, 682–683

SINGLE PC LICENSE AGREEMENT AND LIMITED WARRANTY

READ THIS LICENSE CAREFULLY BEFORE OPENING THIS PACKAGE. BY OPENING THIS PACKAGE, YOU ARE AGREEING TO THE TERMS AND CONDITIONS OF THIS LICENSE. IF YOU DO NOT AGREE, DO NOT OPEN THE PACKAGE. PROMPTLY RETURN THE UNOPENED PACKAGE AND ALL ACCOMPANYING ITEMS TO THE PLACE YOU OBTAINED THEM. *THESE TERMS APPLY TO ALL LICENSED SOFTWARE ON THE DISK EXCEPT THAT THE TERMS FOR USE OF ANY SHAREWARE OR FREEWARE ON THE DISKETTES ARE AS SET FORTH IN THE ELECTRONIC LICENSE LOCATED ON THE DISK:*

1. GRANT OF LICENSE and OWNERSHIP: The enclosed computer programs and data ("Software") are licensed, not sold, to you by Pearson Education, Inc. ("We" or the "Company") and in consideration of your purchase or adoption of the accompanying Company textbooks and/or other materials, and your agreement to these terms. We reserve any rights not granted to you. You own only the disk(s) but we and/or our licensors own the Software itself. This license allows you to use and display your copy of the Software on a single computer (i.e., with a single CPU) at a single location for <u>academic</u> use only, so long as you comply with the terms of this Agreement. You may make one copy for back up, or transfer your copy to another CPU, provided that the Software is usable on only one computer

2. RESTRICTIONS: You may <u>not</u> transfer or distribute the Software or documentation to anyone else. Except for backup, you may <u>not</u> copy the documentation or the Software. You may <u>not</u> network the Software or otherwise use it on more than one computer or computer terminal at the same time. You may <u>not</u> reverse engineer, disassemble, decompile, modify, adapt, translate, or create derivative works based on the Software or the Documentation. You may be held legally responsible for any copying or copyright infringement which is caused by your failure to abide by the terms of these restrictions.

3. TERMINATION: This license is effective until terminated. This license will terminate automatically without notice from the Company if you fail to comply with any provisions or limitations of this license. Upon termination, you shall destroy the Documentation and all copies of the Software. All provisions of this Agreement as to limitation and disclaimer of warranties, limitation of liability, remedies or damages, and our ownership rights shall survive termination.

4. LIMITED WARRANTY AND DISCLAIMER OF WARRANTY: Company warrants that for a period of 60 days from the date you purchase this SOFTWARE (or purchase or adopt the accompanying textbook), the Software, when properly installed and used in accordance with the Documentation, will operate in substantial conformity with the description of the Software set forth in the Documentation, and that for a period of 30 days the disk(s) on which the Software is delivered shall be free from defects in materials and workmanship under normal use. The Company does not warrant that the Software will meet your requirements or that the operation of the Software will be uninterrupted or error-free. Your only remedy and the Company's only obligation under these limited warranties is, at the Company's option, return of the disk for a refund of any amounts paid for it by you or replacement of the disk. THIS LIMITED WARRANTY IS THE ONLY WARRANTY PROVIDED BY THE COMPANY AND ITS LICENSORS, AND THE COMPANY AND ITS LICENSORS DISCLAIM ALL OTHER WARRANTIES, EXPRESS OR IMPLIED, INCLUDING WITHOUT LIMITATION, THE IMPLIED WARRANTIES OF MERCHANTABILITY AND FITNESS FOR A PARTICULAR PURPOSE. THE COMPANY DOES NOT WARRANT, GUARANTEE OR MAKE ANY REPRESENTATION REGARDING THE ACCURACY, RELIABILITY, CURRENTNESS, USE, OR RESULTS OF USE, OF THE SOFTWARE.

5. LIMITATION OF REMEDIES AND DAMAGES: IN NO EVENT, SHALL THE COMPANY OR ITS EMPLOYEES, AGENTS, LICENSORS, OR CONTRACTORS BE LIABLE FOR ANY INCIDENTAL, INDIRECT, SPECIAL, OR CONSEQUENTIAL DAMAGES ARISING OUT OF OR IN CONNECTION WITH THIS LICENSE OR THE SOFTWARE, INCLUDING FOR LOSS OF USE, LOSS OF DATA, LOSS OF INCOME OR PROFIT, OR OTHER LOSSES, SUSTAINED AS A RESULT OF INJURY TO ANY PERSON, OR LOSS OF OR DAMAGE TO PROPERTY, OR CLAIMS OF THIRD PARTIES, EVEN IF THE COMPANY OR AN AUTHORIZED REPRESENTATIVE OF THE COMPANY HAS BEEN ADVISED OF THE POSSIBILITY OF SUCH DAMAGES. IN NO EVENT SHALL THE LIABILITY OF THE COMPANY FOR DAMAGES WITH RESPECT TO THE SOFTWARE EXCEED THE AMOUNTS ACTUALLY PAID BY YOU, IF ANY, FOR THE SOFTWARE OR THE ACCOMPANYING TEXTBOOK. BECAUSE SOME JURISDICTIONS DO NOT ALLOW THE LIMITATION OF LIABILITY IN CERTAIN CIRCUMSTANCES, THE ABOVE LIMITATIONS MAY NOT ALWAYS APPLY TO YOU.

6. GENERAL: THIS AGREEMENT SHALL BE CONSTRUED IN ACCORDANCE WITH THE LAWS OF THE UNITED STATES OF AMERICA AND THE STATE OF NEW YORK, APPLICABLE TO CONTRACTS MADE IN NEW YORK, AND SHALL BENEFIT THE COMPANY, ITS AFFILIATES AND ASSIGNEES. HIS AGREEMENT IS THE COMPLETE AND EXCLUSIVE STATEMENT OF THE AGREEMENT BETWEEN YOU AND THE COMPANY AND SUPERSEDES ALL PROPOSALS OR PRIOR AGREEMENTS, ORAL, OR WRITTEN, AND ANY OTHER COMMUNICATIONS BETWEEN YOU AND THE COMPANY OR ANY REPRESENTATIVE OF THE COMPANY RELATING TO THE SUBJECT MATTER OF THIS AGREEMENT. If you are a U.S. Government user, this Software is licensed with "restricted rights" as set forth in subparagraphs (a)-(d) of the Commercial Computer-Restricted Rights clause at FAR 52.227-19 or in subparagraphs (c)(1)(ii) of the Rights in Technical Data and Computer Software clause at DFARS 252.227-7013, and similar clauses, as applicable.

Should you have any questions concerning this agreement or if you wish to contact the Company for any reason, please contact in writing: Prentice-Hall, New Media Department, One Lake Street, Upper Saddle River, NJ 07458.